```
FRRLS-PT ADULT
31022006528290
616 FERRI'S
Ferri's clinical advisor
:
```

Y0-BNB-614

PEACHTREE CITY LIBRARY
201 WILLOWBEND ROAD
PEACHTREE CITY, GA 30269-1623

Ferri's
CLINICAL ADVISOR

Instant Diagnosis and Treatment

Ferri's CLINICAL ADVISOR

Instant Diagnosis and Treatment

FRED F. FERRI, M.D., F.A.C.P.
Clinical Associate Professor
Brown University School of Medicine
Chief, Division of Internal Medicine
St. Joseph's Health Services and Fatima Hospital
Providence, Rhode Island

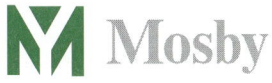 Mosby

St. Louis Baltimore Boston Carlsbad Chicago Minneapolis New York Philadelphia Portland
London Milan Sydney Tokyo Toronto

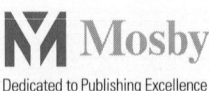

A Times Mirror
Company

Publisher: Susie H. Baxter
Senior Developmental Editor: Laura C. Berendson
Project Manager: Patricia Tannian
Production Editor: Heidi Fite-Crowley
Book Design Manager: Gail Morey Hudson
Manufacturing Manager: Dave Graybill
Cover Design: Teresa Breckwoldt

Copyright © 1999 by Mosby–Year Book, Inc.

All rights reserved. No part of this publication may be reproduced, stored in a retrieval system, or transmitted, in any form or by any means, electronic, mechanical, photocopying, recording, or otherwise, without written permission of the publisher.

Permission to photocopy or reproduce solely for internal or personal use is permitted for libraries or other users registered with the Copyright Clearance Center, provided that the base fee of $4.00 per chapter plus $.10 per page is paid directly to the Copyright Clearance Center, 222 Rosewood Drive, Danvers, MA 01923. This consent does not extend to other kinds of copying, such as copying for general distribution, for advertising or promotional purposes, for creating new collected works, or for resale.

Printed in the United States of America
Composition by The Clarinda Company
Printing/binding by Von Hoffmann Press, Inc.

Mosby–Year Book, Inc.
11830 Westline Industrial Drive
St. Louis, Missouri 63146

Library of Congress Cataloging in Publication Data

Ferri's clinical advisor: instant diagnosis and treatment/ [edited by] Fred F. Ferri. -- 1st ed.
    p. cm.
    Includes bibliographical references and index.
    ISBN 0-8151-0317-4
    1. Clinical medicine—Handbooks, manuals, etc. 2. Primary care (Medicine)—Handbooks, manuals, etc. I. Ferri, Fred F.
    DNLM: 1. Primary Health Care handbooks. 2. Diagnosis handbooks.
3. Therapeutics handbooks. WB 39 M8935 1998]
RC55.M67   1998
616—dc21
DNLM/DLC
for Library of Congress   98-3837
                                                                                 CIP

98 99 00 01 02 / 9 8 7 6 5 4 3 2 1

Section Editors

GEORGE T. DANAKAS, M.D., F.A.C.O.G.
Clinical Assistant Professor
Department of Obstetrics and Gynecology
State University of New York at Buffalo
Buffalo, New York
Section I

FRED F. FERRI, M.D., F.A.C.P.
Clinical Associate Professor
Brown University School of Medicine
Chief, Division of Internal Medicine
St. Joseph's Health Services and Fatima Hospital
Providence, Rhode Island
Sections I-VII, Appendix

JOSEPH R. MASCI, M.D.
Associate Director of Medicine
Elmhurst Hospital Center
Elmhurst, New York
Associate Professor of Medicine
Mount Sinai School of Medicine
New York, New York
Section I

LONNIE R. MERCIER, M.D.
Clinical Instructor
Department of Orthopedic Surgery
Creighton University School of Medicine
Omaha, Nebraska
Section I

WILLIAM H. OLSON, M.D.
Professor, Department of Neurology
University of Louisville School of Medicine
Louisville, Kentucky
Section I

Contributors

PHILIP J. ALIOTTA, M.D., M.S.H.A., F.A.C.S.
Clinical Instructor, Department of Urology
School of Medicine and Biomedical Sciences
State University of New York at Buffalo
Buffalo, New York
Adjunct Clinical Professor
New York College of Osteopathic Medicine
New York City, New York
Section I

GEORGE O. ALONSO, M.D.
Attending Physician, Division of Infectious Diseases
Elmhurst Hospital Center
Elmhurst, New York
Instructor in Medicine, Mount Sinai School of Medicine
New York, New York
Section I

HARINDER BRAR, M.D.
Clinical Instructor
Departments of Internal Medicine and Pediatrics
State University of New York at Buffalo
Buffalo, New York
Section I

MANDEEP K. BRAR, M.D.
Clinical Assistant Professor
Department of Obstetrics and Gynecology
State University of New York at Buffalo
Buffalo, New York
Section I

Contributors

JEFFREY CONSTANTINE, M.D.
Clinical Instructor
Department of Obstetrics and Gynecology
Sisters Hospital
Buffalo, New York
Section I

MARIA A. CORIGLIANO, M.D., F.A.C.O.G.
Clinical Assistant Professor
Department of Obstetrics and Gynecology
State University of New York at Buffalo
Buffalo, New York
Section I

CLAUDIA L. DADE, M.D.
Attending Physician, Division of Infectious Diseases
Elmhurst Hospital Center
Elmhurst, New York
Instructor in Medicine, Mount Sinai School of Medicine
New York, New York
Section I

JANE V. EASON, M.D.
Attending Physician, Division of Infectious Diseases
Elmhurst Hospital Center
Elmhurst, New York
Instructor in Medicine, Mount Sinai School of Medicine
New York, New York
Section I

RIFAAT S. EL-MALLAKH, M.D.
Assistant Professor
Department of Psychiatry and Behavioral Sciences
University of Louisville School of Medicine
Louisville, Kentucky
Section I

CANDICE C. GREEN, M.D.
Clinical Instructor
Department of Obstetrics and Gynecology
State University of New York at Buffalo
Buffalo, New York
Section I

MICHAEL GRUENTHAL, M.D., Ph.D.
Assistant Professor, Department of Neurology
University of Louisville School of Medicine
Louisville, Kentucky
Section I

MICHELE HALPERN, M.D.
Attending Physician
Division of Infectious Diseases
New Rochelle Hospital
New Rochelle, New York
Section I

KAREN HOUCK, M.D.
Clinical Instructor
Department of Obstetrics and Gynecology
State University of New York at Buffalo
Buffalo, New York
Section I

WAN J. KIM, M.D.
Clinical Instructor
Department of Obstetrics and Gynecology
State University of New York at Buffalo
Buffalo, New York
Section I

MELVYN KOBY, M.D.
Associate Clinical Professor of Ophthalmology
University of Louisville School of Medicine
Louisville, Kentucky
Section I

WON S. LEE, M.D.
Clinical Instructor
Department of Obstetrics and Gynecology
State University of New York at Buffalo
Buffalo, New York
Section I

JOSEPH J. LIEBER, M.D.
Chief, Medical Consultation Service
Elmhurst Hospital Center
Elmhurst, New York
Clinical Associate Professor of Medicine
Mount Sinai School of Medicine
New York, New York
Section I

EUGENE J. LOUIE-NG, M.D.
Clinical Instructor
Department of Obstetrics and Gynecology
State University of New York at Buffalo
Buffalo, New York
Section I

DENNIS J. MIKOLICH, M.D.
Chief, Division of Infectious Disease
VA Medical Center
Clinical Associate Professor of Medicine
Brown University School of Medicine
Providence, Rhode Island
Section I

TAKUMA NEMOTO, M.D.
Research Associate Professor of Surgery
State University of New York at Buffalo
Buffalo, New York
Section I

Contributors

PETER NICHOLAS, M.D.
Chief, Division of Infectious Diseases
Elmhurst Hospital Center
Elmhurst, New York
Associate Professor of Medicine
Mount Sinai School of Medicine
New York, New York
Section I

PETER PETROPOULOS, M.D.
Ambulatory Care Department, VA Medical Center
Clinical Instructor of Medicine
Brown University School of Medicine
Providence, Rhode Island
Section I

MAURICE POLICAR, M.D.
Attending Physician, Division of Infectious Diseases
Elmhurst Hospital Center
Elmhurst, New York
Assistant Professor of Medicine
Mount Sinai School of Medicine
New York, New York
Section I

LUTHER K. ROBINSON, M.D.
Associate Professor of Pediatrics
Director, Dysmorphology and Clinical Genetics
State University of New York at Buffalo
Buffalo, New York
Section I

HARVEY M. SHANIES, M.D., Ph.D.
Chief, Pulmonary Division, Elmhurst Hospital Center
Elmhurst, New York
Clinical Associate Professor of Medicine
Mount Sinai School of Medicine
New York, New York
Section I

DEBORAH L. SHAPIRO, M.D.
Chief, Division of Rheumatology
Elmhurst Hospital Center
Elmhurst, New York
Clinical Assistant Professor of Medicine
Mount Sinai School of Medicine
New York, New York
Section I

MARIA ELENA SOLER, M.D.
Clinical Instructor
Department of Obstetrics and Gynecology
State University of New York at Buffalo
Buffalo, New York
Section I

YUKIO SONODA, M.D.
Clinical Instructor
Department of Obstetrics and Gynecology
State University of New York at Buffalo
Buffalo, New York
Section I

DENNIS M. WEPPNER, M.D., F.A.C.O.G., F.A.C.S.
Associate Professor of Clinical Gynecology/Obstetrics
State University of New York at Buffalo
Clinical Chief, Department of Gynecology/Obstetrics
Buffalo General Hospital
Buffalo, New York
Section I

LAUREL M. WHITE, M.D.
Clinical Assistant Professor
Department of Obstetrics and Gynecology
Division of Maternal Fetal Medicine
State University of New York at Buffalo
Buffalo, New York
Section I

JOHN M. WIECKOWSKI, M.D., Ph.D., F.A.C.O.G.
Director, Reproductive Medicine/IVF
Williamsville, New York
Section I

MATTHEW L. WITHIAM-LEITCH, M.D., Ph.D.
Clinical Instructor
Department of Obstetrics and Gynecology
State University of New York at Buffalo
Buffalo, New York
Section I

BETH J. WUTZ, M.D.
Clinical Assistant Professor of Medicine
Division of Internal Medicine/Pediatrics
Buffalo General Hospital
State University of New York at Buffalo
Buffalo, New York
Section I

SCOTT J. ZUCCALA, D.O.
Clinical Assistant Professor
Department of Obstetrics and Gynecology
State University of New York at Buffalo
Buffalo, New York
Section I

To my family
Their constant support and encouragement made this book a reality

Preface

This book is intended to be a clear and concise reference for the primary care physician. It is available in clinical text and CD-ROM format. Its user-friendly format was designed to provide a fast and efficient way to identify important clinical information and to provide practical guidance in patient management. The book is divided into seven unique sections, which make this book one of the most valuable medical information references to primary care physicians.

Section I covers 450 medical disorders of crucial importance to primary care physicians. Medical topics in this section are arranged alphabetically, and the material in each topic is presented in outline format for ease of retrieval. Key, quick-access information is consistently highlighted in color, and clinical photographs in full color are used to further illustrate selected medical conditions. ICD-9-CM codes are included to help expedite claims submission and reimbursement. References focus on current, peer-reviewed journal articles rather than outdated textbooks and old review articles. All topics in this section use the following structured approach:
1. Basic Information (Definition, Synonyms, ICD-9-CM Codes, Epidemiology and Demographics, Physical Findings, Etiology)
2. Diagnosis (Differential Diagnosis, Workup, Laboratory Tests, Imaging Studies)
3. Treatment (Nonpharmacologic Therapy, Acute General Rx, Chronic Rx, Disposition, Referral)
4. Miscellaneous (Comments, References)

Section II consists of the differential diagnosis, etiology, and classification of nearly 200 signs and symptoms. This is a practical section that allows the user investigating a physical complaint or abnormal laboratory value to follow a "workup" leading to a diagnosis. The physician then can easily look up the presumptive diagnosis in Section I for the information specific to that illness.

Section III provides over 90 clinical algorithms to guide and expedite the patient's workup and therapy. This section is particularly valuable in today's managed care environment.

Section IV includes normal laboratory values and interpretation of results of 170 tests. Laboratory tests are part of most patient encounters. By providing interpretation of abnormal results, this section facilitates the diagnosis of medical disorders and further adds to the comprehensive, "one stop" nature of our text.

Section V focuses on preventive medicine and offers essential guidelines from the U.S. Preventive Services Task Force. Information in this section on clinical preventive services includes recommendations for the periodic health examination, screening for major diseases and disorders, patient counseling, and immunizations and chemoprophylaxis recommendations.

Section VI includes a review of the medical literature. Clinically relevant articles from over 1000 journals published worldwide are reviewed annually, and abstracts of key articles are reported along with commentaries on these articles placing them in perspective.

Section VII consists of medication comparison tables covering hundreds of commonly prescribed medications. This section facilitates the use of cost-effective medications by comparing the cost of similar medications and illustrating significant differences among medications in the same therapeutic class.

The appendix of our book emphasizes the practical features of patient management by providing extensive sections on disease prevention, patient evaluation, nutrition, growth and development, and emergency medicine. Medical tables, graphs, and formulas are used extensively to simplify difficult topics and enhance recollection of principal points.

Preface

As practicing physicians we all realize the importance of patient education and the need for clear communication with our patients. Toward that end, we have included on a companion CD-ROM easy-to-use, practical patient instruction sheets, organized alphabetically and covering the majority of the topics in this book.* They are a valuable addition to patient care and useful to improve physician-patient communication, patient satisfaction, and quality of care. For ease of identification, each clinical topic in Section I of the book with a corresponding patient teaching guide on the CD is marked with *"(PTG)"* after the topic name, at the top of the page in the book. Additionally the cross references to the CD are included in the table of contents.

In conclusion, I strongly believe that we have produced a state of the art information system with significant differences from existing texts. I hope that its user-friendly approach, its numerous unique features, and yearly updates will make our book and CD-ROM valuable medical references not only to primary care physicians, but also to physicians in other specialties, medical students, and allied health professionals.

Fred F. Ferri, M.D.

---

*If you have not ordered *Ferri's Clinical Advisor: Instant Diagnosis and Treatment* on CD-ROM, call 1-800-633-6699 for more information.

Contents

Section I	Clinical Topics, 1-533
Section II	Differential Diagnosis, Etiology, and Classification of Common Signs and Symptoms, 535-667
Section III	Clinical Algorithms, 669-778
Section IV	Laboratory Tests and Interpretation of Results, 779-839
Section V	Clinical Preventive Services, 841-895
Section VI	Review of Medical Literature, 897-964
Section VII	Medications: Comparison Tables, 965-1001
Appendix	Essential Facts and Formulas, 1003-1071

Detailed Contents

SECTION I   CLINICAL TOPICS (Color plates following p. 6)

Abruptio placentae, 3
Abscess, pelvic, 4
Abuse, child *(PTG)*, 5
Abuse, drug *(PTG)*, 7
Abuse, geriatric *(PTG)* (see Abuse, elderly), 9
Acetaminophen poisoning, 10
Achilles tendon rupture *(PTG)*, 11
Acne vulgaris *(PTG)*, 12
Acquired immunodeficiency syndrome *(PTG)*, 13
Acromegaly *(PTG)*, 14
Addison's disease *(PTG)*, 15
Agoraphobia and panic *(PTG)*, 16
Alcoholism *(PTG)*, 18
Aldosteronism, primary *(PTG)*, 19
Alzheimer's disease *(PTG)*, 20
Amaurosis fugax *(PTG)*, 21
Amblyopia, 22
Amebiasis *(PTG)*, 23
Amyloidosis, 24
Amyotrophic lateral sclerosis, 25
Anaerobic infections, 26
Anal fissure, 28
Anaphylaxis, 29
Anemia, aplastic *(PTG)*, 30
Anemia, autoimmune hemolytic, 31
Anemia, iron deficiency *(PTG)*, 32
Anemia, pernicious *(PTG)*, 33
Anemia, sickle cell *(PTG)*, 34
Aneurysm, abdominal aorta, 36
Angina pectoris *(PTG)*, 37
Ankle fracture *(PTG)*, 39
Ankle sprain *(PTG)*, 40
Ankylosing spondylitis *(PTG)*, 41
Anorectal fistula, 42
Anorexia nervosa *(PTG)*, 43
Anxiety (generalized anxiety disorder) *(PTG)*, 45

Aortic regurgitation *(PTG)*, 46
Aortic stenosis *(PTG)*, 47
Appendicitis, acute, 48
Arthritis, granulomatous, 49
Arthritis, infectious (bacterial) *(PTG)*, 50
Arthritis, juvenile rheumatoid *(PTG)*, 51
Arthritis, psoriatic *(PTG)*, 52
Arthritis, rheumatoid *(PTG)*, 53
Asbestosis *(PTG)*, 54
Ascariasis *(PTG)*, 55
Asthma *(PTG)*, 56
Atelectasis *(PTG)*, 58
Atrial fibrillation *(PTG)*, 59
Atrial flutter *(PTG)*, 60
Atrial septal defect *(PTG)*, 61
Attention deficit hyperactivity disorder *(PTG)* (see ADHD), 62
Autistic disorder *(PTG)* (see Autism), 63
Babesiosis, 64
Balanitis *(PTG)*, 66
Basal cell carcinoma *(PTG)*, 67
Bell's palsy *(PTG)*, 68
Bipolar disorder *(PTG)*, 69
Bite wounds *(PTG)* (see Bites, animal; bites, insect; bites, marine envenomations; bites, snakes; bites, spider), 70
Bladder cancer *(PTG)*, 71
Blepharitis, 73
Bone tumor, primary malignant, 74
Botulism, 75
Brain neoplasm, 76
Breast abscess, 77
Breast cancer *(PTG)*, 78
Breech birth, 80
Bronchiectasis *(PTG)*, 81

Bronchitis, acute *(PTG)*, 82
Brucellosis, 83
Bulimia nervosa *(PTG)*, 84
Bursitis *(PTG)*, 85
Candidiasis, 86
Carcinoid syndrome, 87
Cardiac tamponade, 88
Cardiomyopathy, dilated *(PTG)*, 89
Cardiomyopathy, hypertrophic *(PTG)*, 90
Cardiomyopathy, restrictive *(PTG)*, 91
Carotid sinus syndrome *(PTG)*, 92
Carpal tunnel syndrome *(PTG)*, 93
Cataracts *(PTG)*, 94
Cat-scratch disease *(PTG)*, 95
Cavernous sinus thrombosis, 97
Celiac disease *(PTG)*, 98
Cellulitis *(PTG)*, 99
Cerebral palsy, 100
Cerebrovascular accident *(PTG)*, 101
Cervical cancer *(PTG)*, 102
Cervical disc syndromes *(PTG)* (see Cervical disc disease), 103
Cervical dysplasia *(PTG)*, 104
Cervical polyps *(PTG)*, 106
Cervicitis *(PTG)*, 107
Chagas' disease, 108
Chancroid *(PTG)*, 110
Charcot's joint *(PTG)*, 111
Charcot-Marie-Tooth disease, 112
Chickenpox *(PTG)*, 113
Chlamydia genital infections *(PTG)* (see Chlamydia infection), 114
Cholangitis, 115

Detailed Contents

Cholecystitis, 116
Cholelithiasis *(PTG)*, 117
Cholera, 118
Chronic fatigue syndrome, 119
Chronic obstructive pulmonary disease *(PTG)*, 120
Cirrhosis *(PTG)*, 121
Claudication, 123
Coccidioidomycosis, 124
Colorectal cancer *(PTG) (see Colon cancer)*, 127
Condyloma acuminatum *(PTG)*, 129
Congestive heart failure *(PTG)*, 130
Conjunctivitis *(PTG)*, 132
Contraception *(PTG)*, 133
Conversion disorder, 135
Corneal abrasion, 136
Corneal ulceration, 137
Costochondritis *(PTG)*, 138
Creutzfeldt-Jakob disease, 139
Crohn's disease *(PTG)*, 140
Cryptococcosis *(PTG)*, 141
Cushing's disease and syndrome *(PTG)*, 142
Cystic fibrosis *(PTG)*, 143
Delirium tremens, 144
Depression, major *(PTG)*, 145
Dermatitis, atopic *(PTG)*, 146
Dermatitis, contact *(PTG)*, 147
Diabetes insipidus *(PTG)*, 148
Diabetes mellitus *(PTG)*, 149
Diabetic ketoacidosis, 151
Diffuse interstitial lung disease *(PTG) (see Diffuse interstitial pulmonary disease)*, 153
Diphtheria, 154
Disseminated intravascular coagulation *(PTG)*, 155
Diverticular disease *(PTG)*, 156
Down syndrome *(PTG)*, 157
Dupuytren's contracture, 158
Dysfunctional uterine bleeding *(PTG)*, 159
Dysmenorrhea *(PTG)*, 161
Echinococcosis, 162
Eclampsia, 163
Ectopic pregnancy, 164
Ejaculation, premature, 165
Encephalitis, acute viral, 166
Encopresis *(PTG)*, 167
Endocarditis, infective *(PTG)*, 168
Endometrial cancer *(PTG)*, 169
Endometriosis *(PTG)*, 170
Endometritis, 172
Enuresis *(PTG)*, 173
Epicondylitis, 174
Epididymitis *(PTG)*, 175
Epiglottitis *(PTG)*, 176
Episcleritis, 177
Epstein-Barr virus infections, 178
Erectile dysfunction *(PTG)*, 179
Erythema multiforme *(PTG)*, 180
Fatty liver of pregnancy, acute, 181
Femoral neck fracture *(PTG)*, 182
Fibrocystic breast disease *(PTG)*, 183
Fibromyalgia *(PTG)*, 184
Filariasis, 185
Folliculitis *(PTG)*, 187
Food poisoning, bacterial *(PTG)*, 188
Friedreich's ataxia, 190
Frozen shoulder *(PTG)*, 191
Gastric cancer, 192
Gastritis *(PTG)*, 193
Gastroesophageal reflux disease *(PTG)*, 194
Giardiasis *(PTG)*, 195
Gilbert's disease *(PTG)*, 196
Gingivitis *(PTG)*, 197
Glaucoma, chronic open-angle (chronic simple glaucoma), 198
Glaucoma, primary closed-angle (narrow-angle glaucoma) *(PTG) (see Glaucoma, primary angle closure)*, 199
Glomerulonephritis, acute *(PTG)*, 200
Glossitis *(PTG)*, 202
Gonorrhea *(PTG)*, 203
Goodpasture's syndrome, 204
Gout *(PTG)*, 205
Granuloma inguinale *(PTG)*, 206
Graves' disease *(PTG)*, 207
Guillain-Barré syndrome, 208
Headache, cluster *(PTG)*, 209
Headache, migraine *(PTG)*, 210
Headache, tension-type *(PTG)*, 211
Heart block, complete, 212
Heart block, second-degree *(PTG)*, 213
Heat exhaustion and heat stroke *(PTG)*, 214
Hemochromatosis *(PTG)*, 215
Hemophilia *(PTG)*, 216
Hemorrhoids, 217
Hepatic encephalopathy, 218
Hepatitis A *(PTG)*, 219
Hepatitis B *(PTG)*, 220
Hepatitis C *(PTG)*, 222
Hepatorenal syndrome, 223
Herpangina *(PTG)*, 224
Herpes simplex *(PTG)*, 225
Herpes simplex, genital *(PTG)*, 227
Herpes zoster *(PTG)*, 228
Histoplasmosis, 229
HIV infection *(PTG)*, 232
Hodgkin's disease *(PTG)*, 233
Hookworm *(PTG)*, 235
Hordeolum (stye), 236
Human granulocytic ehrlichiosis, 237
Huntington's chorea, 238
Hydrocephalus, normal pressure, 239
Hypercholesterolemia *(PTG)*, 240
Hyperemesis gravidarum, 241
Hyperlipoproteinemia, primary *(PTG)*, 242
Hyperosmolar coma, 243
Hyperparathyroidism *(PTG)*, 244
Hypertension, 245
Hyperthyroidism, 247
Hypoaldosteronism, 249
Hypothermia *(PTG)*, 250
Hypothyroidism *(PTG)*, 251
Idiopathic thrombocytopenic purpura *(PTG)*, 252
Impetigo *(PTG)*, 253
Inappropriate secretion of antidiuretic hormone *(PTG) (see Syndrome of inappropriate antidiuretic hormone secretion)*, 254
Incontinence *(PTG) (see Urinary incontinence)*, 255
Influenza *(PTG)*, 257
Insomnia *(PTG)*, 258
Irritable bowel syndrome *(PTG)*, 259
Kaposi's sarcoma *(PTG)*, 260
Klinefelter's syndrome *(PTG)*, 261
Korsakoff's psychosis, 262
Labyrinthitis *(PTG)*, 263
Lactose intolerance *(PTG)*, 264
Lambert-Eaton myasthenic syndrome, 265

Detailed Contents xv

Laryngitis *(PTG)*, 266
Lead poisoning *(PTG)*, 267
Legg-Calvé-Perthes disease *(PTG)*, 268
Leptospirosis, 269
Leukemia, acute lymphoblastic, 270
Leukemia, acute myelogenous, 271
Leukemia, chronic lymphocytic *(PTG)*, 272
Leukemia, chronic myelogenous *(PTG)*, 273
Leukemia, hairy cell *(PTG)*, 274
Listeriosis, 275
Lumbar disc syndromes *(PTG)*, 276
Lung neoplasm, primary *(PTG)*, 277
Lyme disease *(PTG)*, 279
Lymphangitis *(PTG)*, 280
Lymphedema, 281
Lymphogranuloma venereum *(PTG)*, 283
Lymphoma, non-Hodgkin's *(PTG)*, 284
Macular degeneration, 285
Malaria *(PTG)*, 286
Mastoiditis *(PTG)*, 289
Meigs' syndrome, 290
Melanoma *(PTG)*, 291
Meniere's disease *(PTG)*, 292
Meningioma *(PTG)*, 293
Meningitis, bacterial, 294
Meningitis, viral, 295
Meningomyelocele, 296
Menopause *(PTG)*, 297
Metatarsalgia *(PTG)*, 299
Mitral regurgitation *(PTG)*, 300
Mitral stenosis *(PTG)*, 301
Mitral valve prolapse *(PTG)*, 302
Mixed connective tissue disease, 303
Mononucleosis *(PTG)*, 304
Motion sickness *(PTG)*, 305
Multiple myeloma *(PTG)*, 306
Multiple sclerosis *(PTG)*, 307
Mumps *(PTG)*, 308
Munchausen's syndrome, 310
Muscular dystrophy, 311
Myasthenia gravis *(PTG)*, 312
Myelodysplastic syndromes *(PTG)*, 313
Myocardial infarction, 314
Myocarditis *(PTG)*, 316

Myxedema coma, 317
Narcolepsy *(PTG)*, 318
Nephrotic syndrome *(PTG)*, 319
Neuroblastoma, 320
Neuroleptic malignant syndrome, 321
Nosocomial infections, 322
Obsessive-compulsive disorder *(PTG)*, 325
Ocular foreign body, 326
Optic atrophy, 327
Optic neuritis, 328
Osgood-Schlatter disease *(PTG)*, 329
Osteoarthritis *(PTG)*, 330
Osteochondritis dissecans *(PTG)*, 331
Osteomyelitis *(PTG)*, 332
Osteoporosis *(PTG)*, 333
Otitis externa *(PTG)*, 335
Otitis media *(PTG)*, 337
Otosclerosis (otospongiosis), 339
Ovarian cancer *(PTG)*, 340
Ovarian tumor, benign, 341
Paget's disease of the bone *(PTG)*, 342
Paget's disease of the breast *(PTG)*, 343
Pancreatitis, acute, 344
Pancreatitis, chronic *(PTG)*, 346
Parkinson's disease *(PTG)*, 347
Paroxysmal atrial tachycardia *(PTG)*, 349
Pediculosis *(PTG)*, 350
Pedophilia, 351
Pelvic inflammatory disease *(PTG)*, 352
Peptic ulcer disease *(PTG)*, 354
Pericarditis *(PTG)*, 356
Peripheral nerve dysfunction, 358
Peritonitis, secondary, 359
Peritonitis, spontaneous bacterial, 360
Pertussis *(PTG)*, 361
Pharyngitis/tonsillitis *(PTG)*, 362
Pheochromocytoma *(PTG)*, 363
Phobias *(PTG)*, 364
Pilonidal disease, 365
Pituitary adenoma, 366
Pityriasis rosea *(PTG)*, 368
Pneumonia, aspiration, 369
Pneumonia, bacterial *(PTG)*, 370
Pneumonia, *Mycoplasma* *(PTG)*, 372

Pneumonia, *Pneumocystis carinii* *(PTG)*, 374
Pneumonia, viral *(PTG)*, 375
Poliomyelitis, 378
Polyarteritis nodosa, 379
Polycythemia vera *(PTG)*, 380
Polymyalgia rheumatica *(PTG)*, 381
Posttraumatic stress disorder *(PTG)*, 382
Precocious puberty, 383
Preeclampsia, 384
Premenstrual syndrome *(PTG)*, 386
Prolactinoma *(PTG)*, 388
Prostate cancer *(PTG)*, 389
Prostatic hyperplasia, benign, 390
Pruritus ani *(PTG)*, 392
Pruritus vulvae, 393
Pseudogout *(PTG)*, 394
Pseudomembranous colitis *(PTG)*, 395
Psittacosis, 396
Psoriasis *(PTG)*, 397
Pulmonary edema, 398
Pulmonary embolism, 399
Pyelonephritis *(PTG)*, 401
Rabies, 402
Ramsay Hunt syndrome, 403
Raynaud's phenomenon *(PTG)*, 404
Reiter's syndrome *(PTG)*, 406
Renal failure, acute *(PTG)*, 407
Renal failure, chronic *(PTG)*, 408
Renal tubular acidosis, 409
Respiratory distress syndrome, acute, 410
Retinal detachment, 412
Retinal hemorrhage, 413
Retinitis pigmentosa, 414
Retinoblastoma, 415
Retinopathy, diabetic, 416
Rh incompatibility, 417
Rhabdomyolysis *(PTG)*, 418
Rheumatic fever *(PTG)*, 419
Rhinitis, allergic *(PTG)*, 420
Rickets, 421
Rosacea *(PTG)*, 422
Rotator cuff syndrome *(PTG) (see Rotator cuff tendinitis/tear)*, 423
Salmonellosis *(PTG)*, 424
Sarcoidosis *(PTG)*, 426
Scabies *(PTG)*, 427
Schizophrenia *(PTG)*, 428

Scleritis, 430
Scoliosis (PTG), 431
Seizure disorder, absence (PTG) (see Seizure disorder, petit mal), 432
Seizure disorder, generalized tonic-clonic (PTG) (see Seizure disorder, grand mal), 433
Seizure disorder, partial (PTG) (see Seizure disorder, Jacksonian), 434
Seizures, febrile (PTG), 435
Septicemia, 436
Sheehan's syndrome, 437
Shigellosis (PTG), 438
Sialadenitis (PTG), 439
Sinusitis (PTG), 440
Sjögren's syndrome (PTG), 442
Sleep apnea, obstructive (PTG), 443
Somatization disorder, 444
Spinal cord compression, 445
Spontaneous miscarriage, 446
Sporotrichosis, 448
Squamous cell carcinoma, 450
Status epilepticus, 451
Stevens-Johnson syndrome (PTG), 452
Strabismus, 453
Subarachnoid hemorrhage, 454
Suicide (PTG), 455
Syncope (PTG), 456
Syphilis (PTG), 458
Syringomyelia, 459
Systematic lupus erythematosus (PTG), 460
Tabes dorsalis, 462
Tapeworm infestation (PTG), 463
Tarsal tunnel syndrome (PTG), 464
Temporal arteritis, 465
Tetanus, 466
Therapeutic insemination (frozen donor semen), 467
Therapeutic insemination (husband/partner), 468
Thoracic outlet syndrome, 470
Thromboangiitis obliterans (Buerger's disease), 471
Thrombophlebitis, superficial, 472
Thrombosis, deep vein, 473
Thrombotic thrombocytopenic purpura, 474
Thyroid carcinoma (PTG) (see Thyroid neoplasms), 475
Thyroid nodule (PTG), 476
Thyroiditis (PTG), 477
Thyrotoxic storm, 478
Tinea corporis (PTG), 479
Tinea cruris (PTG), 480
Tinea versicolor (PTG), 481
Torticollis, 482
Tourette's syndrome (PTG), 483
Toxic shock syndrome (PTG), 484
Toxoplasmosis (PTG), 486
Tracheitis (PTG), 488
Transfusion reaction, hemolytic, 489
Transient ischemic attack (PTG), 490
Trichinosis (PTG), 491
Trichomoniasis (PTG) (see Vaginitis, trichomonas), 492
Trigeminal neuralgia (PTG), 493
Tropical sprue, 494
Tuberculosis, miliary, 495
Tuberculosis, pulmonary (PTG), 497
Tularemia, 500
Turner's syndrome, 502
Typhoid fever, 504
Ulcerative colitis (PTG), 505
Urethritis, gonococcal (PTG) (see Urethritis), 506
Urethritis, nongonococcal (PTG) (see Urethritis), 507
Urinary tract infection (PTG), 508
Urolithiasis (PTG) (see Renal calculi), 510
Urticaria, 512
Uterine malignancy (PTG), 513
Uterine myomas (PTG), 514
Uterine prolapse (PTG) (see Pelvic organ prolapse), 515
Uveitis, 516
Vaginal bleeding during pregnancy, 517
Vaginal malignancy, 518
Vaginismus, 519
Vaginosis, bacterial (PTG), 520
Varicose veins, 521
von Willebrand's disease (PTG), 522
Vulvar cancer, 523
Vulvovaginitis, bacterial, 524
Vulvovaginitis, estrogen deficient, 525
Vulvovaginitis, fungal (PTG) (see Vaginitis, Candida), 526
Vulvovaginitis, prepubescent, 527
Vulvovaginitis, trichomonas (PTG), 528
Warts (PTG), 529
Wegener's granulomatosis (PTG), 531
Wernicke's encephalopathy, 532
Yellow fever, 533

SECTION II DIFFERENTIAL DIAGNOSIS, ETIOLOGY, AND CLASSIFICATION OF COMMON SIGNS AND SYMPTOMS

Abdominal distention, 537
Abdominal pain, by location, 537
Abdominal pain, poorly localized, 538
Abdominal pain, by age groups, 539
Abdominal pain, in pregnancy, 539
Abortion, recurrent, 540
Acidosis, anion gap, 540
Acidosis, lactic, 541
Acidosis, metabolic, 541
Acidosis, respiratory, 542
Adrenal masses, 542
Alkalosis, metabolic, 542
Alkalosis, respiratory, 543
Alopecias, 543
Amenorrhea, 544
Amnesia, 545
Androgen resistance syndromes, 546
Anemia, iron deficiency, 547
Anemia, megaloblastic, 547
Anergy, cutaneous, 548
Anisocoria, 549
Arthritis, axial skeleton, 549
Arthritis, crystal-induced, 550
Arthritis, monoarticular and oligoarticular, 550

Detailed Contents xvii

Arthritis, polyarticular, 551
Ascites, 552
Ataxia, 552
Back pain, 553
Bleeding disorders, 555
Bleeding, gastrointestinal: by location, 555
Bleeding, gastrointestinal: diagnostic considerations by age, 556
Breast mass, 556
Bullous diseases, 557
Cardiac murmurs, 558
Cerebrospinal fluid abnormalities, 559
Cestode tissue infections, 559
Chest pain in children, 560
Chest pain, nonpleuritic, 560
Chest pain, pleuritic, 560
Clubbing, 561
Coagulopathy, congenital, 561
Coma, 562
Constipation, 563
Cough, 563
Cutaneous signs of internal malignancy, 564
Cutaneous eruptions, drug-induced, 565
Cyanosis, 566
Delirium, 566
Dementia, 567
Dermatitis, 568
Diarrhea, drug-induced, 568
Diarrhea in patients with AIDS, 569
Dizziness, 569
Dysphagia, 570
Dyspnea, 570
Dysuria, 571
Edema, generalized, 571
Edema of lower extremities, 571
Elevated hemidiaphragm, 572
Epilepsy, 572
Epistaxis, 573
Eosinophilia, 573
Exanthems, 574
Eye pain, 576
Facial pain, 576
Facial paralysis, 576
Fever and rash, 577
Fever of unknown origin, 580
Flushing, 580
Fungal infections in the central nervous nystem, 581
Galactorrhea, 582

Gay bowel syndrome, 582
Genital lesions, 583
Goiter, 584
Granulomatous disorders, 584
Granulomatous lung disease, 585
Groin pain in active people, 587
Gynecomastia, 587
Halitosis, 588
Headache, 588
Headache and facial pain, 589
Hearing loss, acute, 590
Hematuria, 590
Hemiparesis/Hemiplegia, 590
Hemoptysis, 591
Hepatomegaly, 591
Hip pain in children and adults, 592
Hirsutism and hypertrichosis, 592
Hoarseness, 593
Hypercalcemia, laboratory differential diagnosis, 593
Hypercapnia, 594
Hypercoagulable states, 594
Hyperinsulinism, 595
Hyperkalemia, 595
Hyperkinetic movement disorders, 596
Hypermagnesemia, 598
Hyperventilation, 598
Hypocalcemia, laboratory differential diagnosis, 599
Hypoglycemia syndromes, test results, 600
Hypogonadism, 601
Hypokalemia, 602
Hypomagnesemia, 603
Impotence, 603
Infectious diseases in compromised host, 604
Infectious diseases in travelers, 605
Insomnia in the elderly, 606
Intestinal helminths, 607
Intestinal pseudo-obstruction, 608
Jaundice, 609
Jugular venous distention, 609
Knee pain, 610
Leg cramps, nocturnal, 614
Leg pain with exercise, 615
Leg ulcers, 616
Liver disease in pregnancy, 617
Liver function tests in liver disease, 618

Lymphadenopathy, 619
Lymphocyte abnormalities in peripheral blood, 620
Malabsorptive disorders, 621
Mediastinal masses or widening on chest x-ray, 622
Metastatic neoplasms, 622
Micropenis, 622
Miosis, 623
Muscle weakness, 623
Mydriasis, 624
Myelopathy and myelitis, 624
Nail disorders, 625
Nausea and vomiting, 625
Neck mass, 626
Nematode tissue infections, 629
Neurologic deficit, focal, 630
Neurologic deficit, multifocal, 630
Neuropathies, 631
Nystagmus, 631
Pancytopenia, 632
Papilledema, 632
Paraplegia, 632
Paresthesias, 633
Pelvic mass, 633
Pelvic pain, 633
Photosensitivity, 634
Pleural effusions, 634
Pleural effusions, drug-induced, 635
Polycythemias, 635
Polyneuropathy, drug-induced, 635
Polyneuropathy, symmetric, 636
Polyuria, 636
Popliteal swelling, 636
Proteinuria, 637
Pruritus, 637
Puberty, delayed, 638
Puberty, precocious, 638
Pulmonary function abnormalities, 639
Pulmonary lesions, 639
Pulmonary nodule, solitary, 639
Purpura, 640
Rectal pain, 640
Red eye, 640
Renal cystic diseases, 641
Renal failure, serum and radiographic abnormalities, 641
Renal failure, urinary abnormalities, 642
Respiratory failure, hypoventilatory, 642

Detailed Contents

Rhinitis, chronic, 643
Short stature, 647
Shoulder pain, 648
Skin lesions, primary, 649
Skin lesions, secondary, 651
Skin lesions, special, 653
Spherocytosis, 654
Splenomegaly, 654
Spondyloarthropathies, 655
Spondyloarthropathies, seronegative, 656
ST segment elevation, 657
Swollen limb, 657
Synovial fluid abnormalities, 658
Tall stature, 658
Testicular size variations, 659
Thrombocytopenia, 659
Thyroid nodule, cold, 659
Trematode tissue infections, 660
Tremor, 660
Uropathy, obstructive, 661
Urticaria, 661
Vaginal bleeding abnormalities, 662
Vaginal bleeding, pregnancy, 662
Vaginitis, 663
Vasculitic syndromes, 663
Ventricular failure, 664
Vertigo, 664
Visual field defects, 665
Visual loss, 666
Vomiting, 666
Weight gain, 666
Weight loss, 667
Wheezing, 667

SECTION III CLINICAL ALGORITHMS

Abdominal pain, 671
Adrenal mass, 672
Amenorrhea, 673
Anemia, 674
Anorexia, 675
Antinuclear antibody abnormality, 676
Arthralgia limited to one or few joints, 677
Ascites, 678
Asystole, 679
Back pain, 680
Bleeding, early pregnancy, 687
Bleeding, gastrointestinal, 688
Bleeding, vaginal, 689
Bleeding disorder, congenital, 692
Breast, nipple discharge evaluation, 693
Breast, radiologic evaluation, 695
Breast, routine screen or palpable mass evaluation, 697
Code status determination before cardiac arrest, 699
Contraceptive use, oral, 700
Cough, chronic, 702
Creatine kinase elevation, 703
Dementia, 704
Developmental delay, 706
Diarrhea, acute, 707
Diarrhea, chronic, 708
Diarrhea, chronic, in patients with HIV infection, 709
Edema, generalized, 710
Edema, regional, 711
Fecal occult blood evaluation, 712
Genital ulcer disease, 713
Glomerular disease, 714
Head injury, 715
Hearing loss, 716
Heartburn, 718
Hematuria, 719
Herpetic and postherpetic neuralgia, 720
Hirsutism, 721
Hypercalcemia, 722
Hypernatremia, 723
Hypocalcemia, 724
Hypoglycemia, fasting, 725
Hypokalemia, 726
Hyponatremia, 727
Hypophosphatemia, 728
Infertility, 729
Jaundice and hepatobiliary disease, 731
Leg ulcer, 732
Liver function test abnormalities, 733
Lymphadenopathy, generalized, 734
Lymphadenopathy, localized, 735
Macrocytosis, 736
Malabsorption, 737
Muscle cramps and aches, 738
Neck pain, 739
Nephrolithiasis, 740
Neutropenia, 741
Neutrophilia, 742
Pain management, cancer patient, 743
Pap smear abnormality, 744
Pelvic mass, 745
Pelvic pain, reproductive-age woman, 746
Polycythemia, 747
Pruritus, generalized, 748
Puberty, delayed, 749
Puberty, precocious, 750
Pulmonary nodule, 751
Pulseless electrical activity (PEA), 752
Purpura, palpable, 753
Rhinorrhea, 754
Scrotal mass, 755
Sexual dysfunction, 756
Sleep disorders, 757
Spinal injury, cervical, 760
Splenomegaly, 761
Tachycardia, narrow complex, 762
Tachycardia, wide complex, 763
Thrombocytopenia, 764
Thrombolytic therapy in acute MI, 765
Thyroid disease, nodular, 766
Thyroid tests, diagnostic approach, 767
Tinnitus, 768
Trauma, abdomen, 769
Trauma, chest, 770
Trauma, kidneys, 772
Unconscious patient, 773
Urticaria, chronic, 774
Vaginal discharge, 775
Ventricular fibrillation or pulseless ventricular tachycardia, 776
Ventricular tachycardia, 777

SECTION IV LABORATORY TESTS AND INTERPRETATION OF RESULTS

Acetone (serum or plasma), 781
Acid-base reference values, 781
Acid phosphatase (serum), 782
Alanine aminotransferase (ALT, SGPT), 782
Albumin (serum), 782
Aldolase (serum), 782
Alkaline phosphatase (serum), 782
Ammonia (serum), 783
Amylase (serum), 783
Angiotensin-converting enzyme (ACE level), 784
Anion gap, 784
Anti-DNA, 784
Antimitochondrial antibody, 784
Antineutrophil cytoplasmic antibody (ANCA), 784
Antinuclear antibody (ANA), 784
Anti-streptolysin O titer (Streptozyme, ASLO titer), 786
Antithrombin III, 786
Aspartate aminotransferase (AST, SGOT), 786
Basophil count, 786
Bilirubin, direct (conjugated bilirubin), 787
Bilirubin, indirect (unconjugated bilirubin), 787
Bilirubin, total, 787
Bleeding time (modified Ivy method), 787
Calcitonin (serum), 788
Calcium (serum), 788
Cancer antigen 125, 789
Carboxyhemoglobin, 789
Carcinoembryonic antigen (CEA), 790
Carotene (serum), 790
Cerebrospinal fluid (CSF), 790
Ceruloplasmin (serum), 790
Chloride (serum), 791
Cholesterol, total, 791
Chromosomal abnormalities in malignancy, 792
Circulating anticoagulant (lupus anticoagulant), 792
Coagulation factors, 792
Cold agglutinins titer, 793
Complement, 793
Complete blood count (CBC), 795
Coombs, direct, 795
Coombs, indirect, 796
Copper (serum), 796
Cortisol (plasma), 797
C-peptide, 797
C-reactive protein, 797
Creatine kinase (CK, CPK), 797
Creatine kinase isoenzymes, 797
Creatinine (serum), 798
Creatinine clearance, 798
Cryoglobulins (serum), 798
Drug monitoring, 798
Eosinophil count, 798
Epstein-Barr viral (EBV) infection, 800
Erythrocyte sedimentation rate (ESR; Westergren), 800
Extractable nuclear antigen (ENAcomplex, anti-RNP antibody, anti-Sm, anti-Smith), 801
Fecal fat, quantitative (72-hr collection), 801
Ferritin (serum), 801
α-1 Fetoprotein, 801
Fibrin degradation product (FDP), 801
Fibrinogen, 801
Folate (folic acid), 802
Free thyroxine index, 802
Gastrin (serum), 802
Glomerular basement membrane antibody, 803
Glucose, fasting, 803
Glucose, postprandial, 803
Glucose tolerance test, 803
Glucose-6-phosphate dehydrogenase screen (blood), 803
γ-Glutamyl transferase (GGT), 803
Glycated (glycosylated) hemoglobin (HbA$_{1c}$), 804
Ham test (acid serum test), 804
Haptoglobin (serum), 804
Hematocrit, 805
Hemoglobin, 805
Hemoglobin electrophoresis, 805
Hepatitis A antibody, 806
Hepatitis A viral infection, 806
Hepatitis B surface antigen, 806
Hepatitis B viral infection, 806
Hepatitis C viral infection, 806
Hepatitis D viral infection, 806
Heterophil antibody, 813
High-density lipoprotein (HDL) cholesterol, 813
HLA antigens, 813
Human immunodeficiency virus antibody, type 1 (HIV-1), 813
Immune complex assay, 815
Immunoglobulins, 815
International normalized ratio (INR), 815
Iron-binding capacity (TIBC), 815
Lactate dehydrogenase (LDH), 816
Lactate dehydrogenase isoenzymes, 816
Legionella titer, 816
Leukocyte alkaline phosphatase (LAP), 817
Lipase, 817
Low-density lipoprotein (LDL) cholesterol, 817
Lymphocytes, 817
Magnesium (serum), 817
Mean corpuscular volume (MCV), 817
Monocyte count, 817
Neutrophil count, 819
5′ Nucleotidase, 819
Oncogenes, 819
Osmolality, serum, 819
Partial thromboplastin time (PTT), 819
Phosphate (serum), 821
Platelet count, 821
Potassium (serum), 822
Prolactin, 822
Prostatic specific antigen (PSA), 822
Protein (serum), 822
Protein electrophoresis (serum), 823
Prothrombin time (PT), 823
Protoporphyrin (free erythrocyte), 823
Red blood cell (RBC) count, 823
Red blood cell distribution width (RDW), 824
Red blood cell mass (volume), 825
Red blood cell morphology, 825

xx Detailed Contents

Renin (serum), 825
Reticulocyte count, 826
Rheumatoid factor, 826
Schilling test, 826
Smooth muscle antibody, 826
Sodium (serum), 828
Sucrose hemolysis test (sugar water test), 829
T_3 (triiodothyronine), 829
T_4 free (free thyroxine), 829
Testosterone, 829
Thrombin time (TT), 829
Thyroid-stimulating hormone (TSH), 829
Thyroxine (T_4), 829
Transferrin, 830
Triglycerides, 830
Tuberculin test (PPD), 831
Tumor markers, 831
Urea nitrogen (BUN), 831
Uric acid (serum), 831
Urinalysis, 833
Urine amylase, 833
Urine bile, 833
Urine calcium, 833
Urine cAMP, 833
Urine catecholamines, 834
Urine chloride, 834
Urine copper, 834
Urine cortisol, free, 834
Urine creatinine (24 hr), 834
Urine eosinophils, 834
Urine glucose (qualitative), 834
Urine hemoglobin, free, 834
Urine hemosiderin, 834
Urine 5-hydroxyindole-acetic acid (urine 5-HIAA), 834
Urine indican, 835
Urine ketones (semiquantitative), 835
Urine metanephrines, 835
Urine myoglobin, 835
Urine nitrite, 835
Urine occult blood, 835
Urine osmolality, 835
Urine pH, 835
Urine phosphate, 836
Urine potassium, 836
Urine protein (quantitative), 836
Urine sediment, 836
Urine sodium (quantitative), 836
Urine specific gravity, 836
Urine vanillylmandelic acid (VMA), 836
VDRL, 837
Viscosity (serum), 837
Vitamin B_{12}, 838
Wet-mount microscopic procedures, 839
D-Xylose absorption, 839

SECTION V CLINICAL PREVENTIVE SERVICES

PART A
The Periodic Health Examination

Age-Specific Charts, 843
Table 5-1 Birth to 10 years, 843
Table 5-2 Ages 11-24 years, 845
Table 5-3 Ages 25-64 years, 847
Table 5-4 Age 65 and older, 849
Table 5-5 Pregnant women, 851

PART B
Screening

Cardiovascular Diseases, 853

1 Screening for Asymptomatic Coronary Artery Disease, 853
2 Screening for High Blood Cholesterol and Other Lipid Abnormalities, 853
3 Screening for Hypertension, 854
4 Screening for Asymptomatic Carotid Artery Stenosis, 855
5 Screening for Peripheral Arterial Disease, 855
6 Screening for Abdominal Aortic Aneurysm, 855

Neoplastic Diseases, 856

7 Screening for Breast Cancer, 856
8 Screening for Colorectal Cancer, 856
9 Screening for Cervical Cancer, 857
10 Screening for Prostate Cancer, 858
11 Screening for Lung Cancer, 858
12 Screening for Skin Cancer—*Including Counseling to Prevent Skin Cancer*, 858
13 Screening for Testicular Cancer, 859
14 Screening for Ovarian Cancer, 859
15 Screening for Pancreatic Cancer, 859
16 Screening for Oral Cancer, 859
17 Screening for Bladder Cancer, 860
18 Screening for Thyroid Cancer, 860

Metabolic, Nutritional, and Environmental Disorders, 860

19 Screening for Diabetes Mellitus, 860
20 Screening for Thyroid Disease, 860
21 Screening for Obesity, 861
22 Screening for Iron Deficiency Anemia—*Including Iron Prophylaxis*, 861
23 Screening for Elevated Lead Levels in Childhood and Pregnancy, 862

Infectious Diseases, 863

24 Screening for Hepatitis B Virus Infection, 863
25 Screening for Tuberculous Infection—*Including Bacille Calmette-Guérin Immunization*, 863
26 Screening for Syphilis, 864
27 Screening for Gonorrhea—*Including Ocular Prophylaxis in Newborns*, 864
28 Screening for Human Immunodeficiency Virus Infection, 865
29 Screening for Chlamydial Infection—*Including Ocular Prophylaxis in Newborns*, 866
30 Screening for Genital Herpes Simplex, 867
31 Screening for Asymptomatic Bacteriuria, 868
32 Screening for Rubella—*Including Immunization of Adolescents and Adults*, 868

Vision and Hearing Disorders, 869
33 Screening for Visual Impairment, 869
34 Screening for Glaucoma, 869
35 Screening for Hearing Impairment, 869

Prenatal Disorders, 870
36 Screening Ultrasonography in Pregnancy, 870
37 Screening for Preeclampsia, 870
38 Screening for D (Rh) Incompatibility, 871
39 Intrapartum Electronic Fetal Monitoring, 871
40 Home Uterine Activity Monitoring, 871

Congenital Disorders, 872
41 Screening for Down Syndrome, 872
42 Screening for Neural Tube Defects—*Including Folic Acid/Folate Prophylaxis*, 872
43 Screening for Hemoglobinopathies, 873
44 Screening for Phenylketonuria, 874
45 Screening for Congenital Hypothyroidism, 874

Musculoskeletal Disorders, 874
46 Screening for Postmenopausal Osteoporosis, 874
47 Screening for Adolescent Idiopathic Scoliosis, 875

Mental Disorders and Substance Abuse, 875
48 Screening for Dementia, 875
49 Screening for Depression, 875
50 Screening for Suicide Risk, 876
51 Screening for Family Violence, 876
52 Screening for Problem Drinking, 876
53 Screening for Drug Abuse, 878

PART C
Counseling
54 Counseling to Prevent Tobacco Use, 880
55 Counseling to Promote Physical Activity, 881
56 Counseling to Promote a Healthy Diet, 881
57 Counseling to Prevent Motor Vehicle Injuries, 882
58 Counseling to Prevent Household and Recreational Injuries, 883
59 Counseling to Prevent Youth Violence, 884
60 Counseling to Prevent Low Back Pain, 885
61 Counseling to Prevent Dental and Periodontal Disease, 885
62 Counseling to Prevent HIV Infection and Other Sexually Transmitted Diseases, 886
63 Counseling to Prevent Unintended Pregnancy, 887
64 Counseling to Prevent Gynecologic Cancers, 887

PART D
Immunizations and Chemoprophylaxis
65 Childhood Immunizations, 889
66 Adult Immunizations—*Including Chemoprophylaxis against Influenza A*, 891
67 Postexposure Prophylaxis for Selected Infectious Diseases, 893
68 Postmenopausal Hormone Prophylaxis, 894
69 Aspirin Prophylaxis for the Primary Prevention of Myocardial Infarction, 895
70 Aspirin Prophylaxis in Pregnancy, 895

SECTION VI REVIEW OF MEDICAL LITERATURE

Year Book of Cardiology, 901

Edited by: Schlant RC, Collins JJ, Gersh BJ, Graham T, Kaplan NM, Waldo AL

Borghi C et al: Factors Associated with the Development of Stable Hypertension in Young Borderline Hypertensives, 901

Gill JB et al: Prognostic Importance of Myocardial Ischemia Detected by Ambulatory Monitoring Early after Acute Myocardial Infarction, 901

Grossman E et al: Should a Moratorium Be Placed on Sublingual Nifedipine Capsules Given for Hypertensive Emergencies and Pseudoemergencies?, 903

Howard G: Insulin Sensitivity and Atherosclerosis, 903

Williams PT: High-Density Lipoprotein Cholesterol and Other Risk Factors for Coronary Heart Disease in Female Runners, 904

Year Book of Family Practice, 905

Edited by: Berg AO, Bowman MA, Davidson RC, Dexter WW, Scherger JE

Abrams SA et al: Absorption by 1-Year-Old Children of an Iron Supplement Given with Cow's Milk or Juice, 905

Ettinger B et al: Reduced Mortality Associated with Long-Term Postmenopausal Estrogen Therapy, 905

Hahn SR et al: The Difficult Patient: Prevalence, Psychopathology, and Functional Impairment, 906

Hemminki E and Meriläinen J: Long-Term Effects of Cesarean Sections: Ectopic Pregnancies and Placental Problems, 907

Hyams JS et al: Abdominal Pain and Irritable Bowel Syndrome in Adolescents: A Community-Based Study, 907

Jamieson DJ and Steege JF: The Prevalence of Dysmenorrhea, Dyspareunia, Pelvic Pain, and Irritable Bowel Syndrome in Primary Care Practices, 908

Joorabchi B and Devries JM: Evaluation of Clinical Competence: The Gap between Expectation and Performance, 909

Kristiansson P et al: Back Pain during Pregnancy: A Prospective Study, 910

Liberthson RR: Sudden Death from Cardiac Causes in Children and Young Adults, 911

Muller JE: Triggering Myocardial Infarction by Sexual Activity: Low Absolute Risk and Prevention by Regular Physical Exertion, 911

Saigal S et al: Self-Perceived Health Status and Health-Related Quality of Life of Extremely Low-Birth-Weight Infants at Adolescence, 913

Sharpe M et al: Cognitive Behavior Therapy for the Chronic Fatigue Syndrome: A Randomized Controlled Trial, 913

Werler MM et al: Pre-Pregnant Weight in Relation to Risk of Neural Tube Defects, 914

Ytterstad B: The Harstad Injury Prevention Study: The Epidemiology of Sports Injuries. An 8-Year Study, 915

Year Book of Geriatrics and Gerontology, 915

Edited by: Burton JR, Beck JC, Otswald SK, Rabins PV, Reuben DB, Roth J, Shapiro JR, Whitehouse PJ

Bergstrom N et al: Multi-Site Study of Incidence of Pressure Ulcers and the Relationship between Risk Level, Demographic Characteristics, Diagnoses, and Prescription of Preventive Interventions, 915

Graafmans WC et al: Falls in the Elderly: A Prospective Study of Risk Factors and Risk Profiles, 917

Jonker C et al: Memory Complaints and Memory Impairment in Older Individuals, 918

Moore AA and Siu AL: Screening for Common Problems in Ambulatory Elderly: Clinical Confirmation of a Screening Instrument, 919

Nichol KL et al: Immunizations in Long-Term Care Facilities: Policies and Practice, 921

Strawbridge WJ et al: Successful Aging: Predictors and Associated Activities, 922

Tamblyn RM et al: Do Too Many Cooks Spoil the Broth? Multiple Physician Involvement in Medical Management of Elderly Patients and Potentially Inappropriate Drug Combinations, 923

Year Book of Medicine, 924

Edited by: Klahr S, Cline MJ, Petty TL, Frishman WH, Greenberger NJ, Malawista SE, Mandell GL, O'Rourke RA

Becker U et al: Prediction of Risk of Liver Disease by Alcohol Intake, Sex, and Age: A Prospective Population Study, 924

Bhatia S et al: Malignant Neoplasms following Bone Marrow Transplantation, 926

Brivet FG et al: Acute Renal Failure in Intensive Care Units—Causes, Outcome, and Prognostic Factors of Hospital Mortality: A Prospective, Multicenter Study, 927

Cavill I: Guidelines for the Prevention and Treatment of Infection in Patients with an Absent or Dysfunctional Spleen, 928

Diabetes Control and Complications Trial Research Group: Effects of Intensive Diabetes Therapy on Neuropsychological Function in Adults in the Diabetes Control and Complications Trial, 929

Fort JM et al: Bowel Habit after Cholecystectomy: Physiological Changes and Clinical Implications, 930

Fries JF et al: Reduction in Long-Term Disability in Patients with Rheumatoid Arthritis by Disease-Modifying Antirheumatic Drug-Based Treatment Strategies, 931

Gabbay FH et al: Triggers of Myocardial Ischemia during Daily Life in Patients with Coronary Artery Disease: Physical and Mental Activities, Anger and Smoking, 932

Gray-Donald K et al: Nutritional Status and Mortality in Chronic Obstructive Pulmonary Disease, 933

Grodstein F et al: Postmenopausal Estrogen and Progestin Use and the Risk of Cardiovascular Disease, 934

Halm EA: Echocardiography for Assessing Cardiac Risk in Patients Having Non-Cardiac Surgery, 935

Harding SM et al: Asthma and Gastroesophageal Reflux: Acid Suppressive Therapy Improves Asthma Outcome, 936

Hatala R et al: Once-Daily Aminoglycoside Dosing in Immunocompetent Adults: A Meta-Analysis, 937

Hylek EM et al: An Analysis of the Lowest Effective Intensity of Prophylactic Anticoagulation for Patients with Non-Rheumatic Atrial Fibrillation, 937

Jaakkola MS et al: Effect of Passive Smoking on the Development of Respiratory Symptoms in Young Adults: An 8-Year Longitudinal Study, 938

Jones DC and Hayslett JP: Outcome of Pregnancy in Women with Moderate or Severe Renal Insufficiency, 939

Klag MJ et al: Blood Pressure and End-Stage Renal Disease in Men, 939

Leibowitz G et al: Pre-Clinical Cushing's Syndrome: An Unexpected Frequent Cause of Poor Glycemic Control in Obese Diabetic Patients, 940

Niskanen LK et al: Evolution, Risk Factors, and Prognostic Implications of Albuminuria in NIDDM, 941

Papazian L et al: Effect of Ventilator-Associated Pneumonia on Mortality and Morbidity, 942

Peters RK et al: Long-Term Diabetogenic Effect of Single Pregnancy in Women with Previous Gestational Diabetes Mellitus, 943

Smith JA et al: Pregnancy in Sickle Cell Disease: Experience of the Cooperative Study of Sickle Cell Disease, 944

Stefanski A et al: Early Increase in Blood Pressure and Diastolic Left Ventricular Malfunction in Patients with Glomerulonephritis, 944

Thompson WH et al: Controlled Trial of Oral Prednisone in Outpatients with Acute COPD Exacerbation, 945

Tynell E et al: Acyclovir and Prednisolone Treatment of Acute Infectious Mononucleosis: A Multicenter, Double-Blind, Placebo-Controlled Study, 946

van Boven AJ: Reduction of Transient Myocardial Ischemia with Pravastatin in Addition to the Conventional Treatment in Patients with Angina Pectoris, 947

Year Book of Neurology and Neurosurgery, 947

Edited by: Bradley WG, Wilkins RH

Evans SC et al: MRI of "Idiopathic" Juvenile Scoliosis: A Prospective Study, 947

Knudsen FU et al: Long Term Outcome of Prophylaxis for Febrile Convulsions, 948

Year Book of Obstetrics, Gynecology, and Women's Health, 948

Edited by: Mishell DR, Herbst AL, Kirschbaum TH

Baird DD et al: Vaginal Douching and Reduced Fertility, 948

Bucher HC et al: Effect of Calcium Supplementation on Pregnancy-Induced Hypertension and Preeclampsia: A Meta-Analysis of Randomized Controlled Trials, 949

Creinin MD et al: Methotrexate and Misoprostol for Early Abortion: A Multicenter Trial. I. Safety and Efficacy, 950

Newell M-L et al: Detection of Virus in Vertically Exposed HIV-Antibody-Negative Children, 952

Nygaard IE et al: Efficacy of Pelvic Floor Muscle Exercises in Women with Stress, Urge, and Mixed Urinary Incontinence, 952

Petitti DB et al: Stroke in Users of Low-Dose Oral Contraceptives, 954

Rossing MA et al: Oral Contraceptive Use and Risk of Breast Cancer in Middle-Aged Women, 955

Scott LL et al: Acyclovir Suppression to Prevent Cesarean Delivery after First-Episode Genital Herpes, 956

van der Schouw YT et al: Age at Menopause as a Risk Factor for Cardiovascular Mortality, 956

Year Book of Pulmonary Disease, 958

Edited by: Petty TL

Bonnefoi H and Smith IE: How Should Cancer Presenting as a Malignant Pleural Effusion Be Managed?, 958

Leatherman JW et al: Muscle Weakness in Mechanically Ventilated Patients with Severe Asthma, 959

Mooe T et al: Sleep-Disordered Breathing in Men with Coronary Artery Disease, 960

Pépin J-L et al: Long-Term Oxygen Therapy at Home: Compliance with Medical Prescription and Effective Use of Therapy, 961

Prandoni P et al: The Long-Term Clinical Course of Acute Deep Venous Thrombosis, 962

Renkema TEJ et al: Effects of Long-Term Treatment with Corticosteroids in COPD, 963

SECTION VII MEDICATIONS: COMPARISON TABLES

ACE inhibitors, 967
Acid secretion inhibitors, 968
Adrenergic antagonists, 969
Antiarrhythmic agents, 969
Antibiotic dosage, 970
Anticonvulsants, 972
Antidepressants, 973
Antidiabetic agents, 974
Antiemetics, 975
Antihistamines, 976
Antipsychotics, 977
Antiretroviral agents, 978
Antiseptic solutions, 979
Benzodiazepines, 980
β-Adrenergic blocking agents, 981
Calcium channel blockers, 982

Cephalosporins, 983
Chemotherapeutic agents, 984
Contraceptives, oral, 986
Corticosteroids, 987
Diuretics, 988
Fluoroquinolones, 989
Insulin preparations, 990
Laxatives, 991
Lipid-lowering agents, 993
Macrolide antibiotics, 994
Narcotic analgesics, 995
Nitrates, 996
Nonsteroidal antiinflammatory drugs (NSAIDs), 997
Topical steroid preparations, 999
Ventricular arrhythmia therapeutic agents, 1000

APPENDIX ESSENTIAL FACTS AND FORMULAS

Disease Prevention, 1005

Childhood immunization schedule, 1005
Immunizations for adults, 1006
Immunizations during pregnancy, 1012
Administration of vaccines and immune globulins, 1017
Vaccinations for international travel, 1019
Hepatitis B prophylaxis, 1020
HIV chemoprophylaxis after occupational exposure, 1021
Endocarditis prophylaxis, 1022

Patient Evaluation, 1025

Mini-mental state examination, 1025
Orthopedic maneuvers, 1026
Office hearing tests, 1027
Screening of geriatric patients for hearing handicaps, 1027

International prostate symptom score (I-PSS), 1028
Katz index of activities of daily living, 1029
Evaluation for alcohol abuse, 1030
Hamilton anxiety scale, 1032
Zung depression scale, 1033
Geriatric depression scale, 1034
Evaluation for sports participation, 1034

Growth and Development, 1038

Developmental milestones, 1038
Physical growth curves, 1040
Sexual maturation stages, 1041

Medical Tables, Graphs, and Formulas, 1042

Commonly used formulas, 1042
Acid-base map, 1043
Nomogram for calculation of body surface area, 1043

Events of the cardiac cycle, 1044
Spinal dermatomes, 1044

Nutrition, 1045

Food guide pyramid, 1045
Nomogram for body mass index, 1045
Nutritional assessment, 1046
Recommended daily dietary allowances, 1047
Height-weight correlations for adults, 1048
Commercial formulas for nutritional support, 1049

Oncology, 1050

Breast self-examination, 1050
Cancer risk factor screening for women, 1051
Possible strategies for follow-up of selected cancers, 1052

Emergency Medicine, 1053

Toxicology treatment protocols, 1053
Treatment guidelines for STDs following sexual assault, 1056
Bite wounds guidelines, 1057
Thrombolytic therapy in AMI, 1058
Burn area estimation, 1059

Community Resources, 1060

Treatment of Bacterial Endocarditis, 1061

Medical Record Abbreviations, 1063

Ferri's
CLINICAL ADVISOR

Instant Diagnosis and Treatment

SECTION I

Clinical Topics

Abruptio placentae

BASIC INFORMATION

DEFINITION
Abruptio placentae is the separation of placenta from the uterine wall before delivery of the fetus. There are three classes of abruption based on maternal and fetal status, including an assessment of uterine contractions, quantity of bleeding, fetal heart rate monitoring, and abnormal coagulation studies (fibrinogen, PT, PTT).
- Grade I: mild vaginal bleeding, uterine irritability, stable vital signs, reassuring fetal heart rate, normal coagulation profile (fibrinogen: 450 mg %)
- Grade II: moderate vaginal bleeding, hypertonic uterine contractions, orthostatic blood pressure measurements, unfavorable fetal status, fibrinogen 150 mg % to 250 mg %
- Grade III: severe bleeding (may be concealed), hypertonic uterine contractions, overt signs of hypovolemic shock, fetal death, thrombocytopenia, fibrinogen <150 mg %

ICD-9-CM CODES
641.2 Premature separation of placenta

EPIDEMIOLOGY AND DEMOGRAPHICS
INCIDENCE (IN U.S.): 1/86-206 births; incidence by grade: I = 40%, II = 45%, III = 15%; 80% occur before the onset of labor.
RISK FACTORS: Hypertension (greatest association), trauma, polyhydramnios, multifetal gestation, smoking, use of crack-cocaine, chorioamnionitis, preterm premature rupture of membranes
RECURRENCE RATE: 5% to 17%; with 2 prior episodes, 25%

PHYSICAL FINDINGS
- Triad of uterine bleeding (concealed or per vagina), hypertonic uterine contractions or signs of preterm labor, and evidence of fetal compromise
- More than 80% of cases have external bleeding; 20% of cases have no bleeding but have indirect evidence of abruption, such as failed tocolysis for preterm labor.
- Tetanic uterine contractions are found in only 17% of cases, unless grade II or III abruption.

ETIOLOGY
- Primary etiology is unknown.
- Hypertension: found in 40% to 50% of grade III abruptions
- Rapid decompress of uterine cavity, such as is found with polyhydramnios or multifetal gestation
- Blunt external trauma (motor vehicle accident, spousal abuse)

DIAGNOSIS

DIFFERENTIAL DIAGNOSIS
Placenta previa, cervical or vaginal trauma, labor, cervical cancer, rupture of membranes. The differential diagnosis of vaginal bleeding in pregnancy is described in Box 2-120.

WORKUP
- Initial assessment should evaluate for the source of bleeding, ruling out placenta previa and associated conditions that contraindicate any type of vaginal examination, i.e., pelvic speculum examination.
- Continuous fetal heart monitoring is indicated for all viable gestations (60% incidence of fetal distress in labor); may show early signs of maternal hypovolemia (late decelerations or fetal tachycardia) before overt maternal vital sign changes.
- Actual amount of blood loss is often greater than initially perceived because of the possibility of concealed retroplacental bleeding and the apparent "normal" vital signs. The relative hypervolemia of pregnancy initially protects the gravida until late in the course of bleeding, when abrupt and sudden cardiovascular collapse can occur without warning.

LABORATORY TESTS
- Baseline Hgb and Hct help quantify blood loss and, even more important, with every four to six determinations can demonstrate significant trends during expectant management.
- Coagulation profile: platelets, fibrinogen, prothrombin and partial prothrombin time. DIC can develop with severe abruption. If fibrinogen is <150 mg %, estimated blood loss equals 2000 ml, and if fibrinogen is <100 mg %, consider FFP to prevent further bleeding.
- Type and antibody screen is important to identify Rh-negative patients that may need Rh immune globulin.

IMAGING STUDIES
Ultrasound should include fetal presentation and status, amniotic fluid volume, placental location, as well as any evidence of hematoma (retroplacental, subchorionic, or preplacental).

TREATMENT

Treatment is dependent on gestational age of the fetus, severity of the abruption, and maternal status. Stabilization of the mother is the first priority.

ACUTE GENERAL Rx
- Initial assessment for signs of maternal hemodynamic compromise or hemorrhagic shock; large bore intravenous access, with crystalloid fluid resuscitation using a replacement of 3 ml LR solution for every 1 ml estimated blood loss.
- Indwelling Foley catheter to monitor urine output and maternal volume status, with a goal of 30 ml/hr urine output.
- Assess fetal status and gestational age, using sonogram and continuous fetal heart rate monitoring.
- Because of the unpredictable nature of abruptions, cross-matched blood should be made available during the initial resuscitation period.

CHRONIC Rx
- In the term fetus or where lung maturity has been documented, delivery is indicated.
- In the preterm fetus or with an immature lung profile, consideration should be given for betamethasone 12.5 mg IM q24h for two doses and then delivery, depending on the severity of the abruption and the likelihood of fetal complications from preterm birth.
- C-section should be reserved for cases of fetal distress or for standard obstetric indications.
- In very select cases, such as severe prematurity with a stable mother and mild contractions, magnesium sulfate can be used for tocolysis, 6 g IV loading dose then 3 g/hr maintenance, to allow for course of steroids.

DISPOSITION
Because of the unpredictable nature of abruptions expectant management should occur only under very controlled circumstances.

REFERRAL
Abruptio placentae places mother and fetus in a high-risk situation and should be managed by a qualified obstetrician in a facility with capability for neonatal and maternal resuscitation and ability to perform emergency C-sections.

MISCELLANEOUS

REFERENCES
Gabbe S, Niebyl JR, Simpson JL: *Obstetrics: normal and problem pregnancies*, ed 3, New York, 1996, Churchill Livingstone.
Hurd W et al: Selective management of abruptio placentae: a prospective study, *Obstet Gynecol* 61:467, 1983.

Author: **Scott J. Zuccala, D.O.**

Abscess, pelvic

BASIC INFORMATION

DEFINITION
Pelvic abscess in an acute or chronic infection, most commonly involving the pelvic viscera, initially localized and thus creating its own unique environment, so that treatment and possible cure require specific therapy.
There are four categories based on etiologic factors:
- Ascending infection, spreading from cervix through endometrial cavity to adenexa, forming a tubo-ovarian complex
- Infection occurring in the pueperium, which spreads to the adenexa from the endometrium or myometrium via hematogenous or lymphatic route
- Abscess complicating pelvic surgery
- Involvement of the pelvic viscera secondary to spread from contiguous organs, such as appendicitis or diverticulitis

SYNONYMS
Tubo-ovarian abscess (TOA)
Vaginal cuff abscess

ICD-9-CM CODES
614.2 Salpingitis and oophoritis not specified as acute, subacute, or chronic

EPIDEMIOLOGY AND DEMOGRAPHICS
INCIDENCE:
- 34% of hospitalized patients with PID
- 1% to 2% of patients undergoing hysterectomy, majority with vaginal approach
- Peak incidence third to fourth decade
- 25% to 50% are nulliparous

RISK FACTORS: Same risk factors as for PID, although in 30% to 50% of patients there is no prior history of salpingitis before abscess forms.

PHYSICAL FINDINGS
- Abdominal or pelvic pain (90%)
- Fever or chills (50%)
- Abnormal bleeding (21%)
- Vaginal discharge (28%)
- Nausea (26%)
- Up to 60% to 80% present in the absence of fever or leukocytosis; lack of these findings should not rule out diagnosis

ETIOLOGY
- Mixed flora of anaerobes, aerobes, and facultative anaerobes, such as *E. coli, B. fragilis, Prevotella* species, aerobic streptococci, *Peptococcus,* and *Peptostreptococcus*
- *N. gonorrhea* and *Chlamydia* are the major etiologic factors in cervicitis and salpingitis but are rarely found in abscess cavity cultures.

DIAGNOSIS

DIFFERENTIAL DIAGNOSIS
- Pelvic neoplasms, such as ovarian tumors and leiomyomas
- Inflammatory masses involving adjacent bowel or omentum, such as ruptured appendicitis or diverticulitis
- Pelvic hematomas, as may occur after C-section or hysterectomy
- Fig. 3-64 describes the diagnostic approach to patients with a pelvic mass; the differential diagnosis of pelvic mass is described in Box 2-92.
- The differential diagnosis of pelvic pain is described in Box 2-93.
- Physical examination
- Sonogram or CT scan: commonly employed because owing to associated pain and guarding, a suboptimal abdominal or pelvic examination is the rule rather than the exception
- Most common cause of preventable death: physician delay in diagnosis

LABORATORY TESTS
- CBC including WBC with differential, Hgb, and Hct
- Aerobic as well as anaerobic cultures of cervix, blood, urine, sputum, peritoneal cavity (if entered) and abscess cavity before starting antibiotics
- Pregnancy test in patients of reproductive age if the possibility of pregnancy exists

IMAGING STUDIES
- Sonogram: noninvasive, inexpensive study to confirm diagnosis, estimate size of abscess, and monitor response to therapy; sensitivity >90%
- CT scan: used for both diagnosis and therapy (CT-guided drainage)
  1. Primary focus where sonogram provided insufficient information, as with intraabdominal vs. pelvic abscesses
  2. Success rate with CT-guided abscess drainage: unilocular, 90%; and multilocular, 40%

TREATMENT

Major concerns:
1. Desire for future fertility
2. Likelihood of rupture of abscess cavity, with resulting peritonitis, septic shock, and morbid sequelae

ACUTE GENERAL Rx
- Decision as to whether patient requires immediate surgery (uncertain diagnosis or suspicion of rupture) or management with IV antibiotics, reserving surgery for those with inadequate clinical response (i.e., 48 to 72 hr of therapy, with persistent fever or leukocytosis, increasing size of mass, or suspicion of rupture)
- Poor response to medical therapy in those with adnexal masses >8 cm, bilateral disease, or immunocompromise
- Antibiotic combinations:
  1. Clindamycin 900 mg IV q8h or metronidazole 500 mg IV q6-8h plus gentamicin either 5 to 7 mg/kg q24h or 1.5 mg/kg q8h
  2. Alternatives: ampicillin sulbactam 3 g IV q6h or cefoxitin 2 g IV q6h or cefotetan 2 g IV q12h plus doxycyline 100 mg IV q12h
- During medical management, high index of suspicion for acute rupture, such as acute worsening of abdominal pain or new-onset tachycardia and hypotension, mandating immediate surgical intervention after patient stabilization
- Surgical options:
  1. Laparoscopy with drainage and irrigation
  2. Transvaginal colpotomy (abscess must be midline, dissect rectovaginal septum, and be adherent to vaginal fornix)
  3. Laparotomy, including total abdominal hysterectomy with bilateral salpingo-oophorectomy or unilateral salpingo-oophorectomy

DISPOSITION
- Of patients treated with medical therapy, response in 75%, with a 50% pregnancy rate
- No response in 30% to 40%; can be treated with either CT-guided drainage or surgical intervention, keeping in mind that unilateral adenexectomy may give equal chance of cure vs. hysterectomy, yet preserve reproductive potential

REFERRAL
If patient has a TOA, refer to gynecologist.

MISCELLANEOUS

COMMENTS
If *Actinomycoses* species is isolated from culture, treatment with penicillin is required for an extended period of time (6 wk to 3 mo).

REFERENCES
American College of Obstetrics and Gynecology: *Antimicrobial therapy for gynecologic infections,* Technical bulletin No 153, March, 1991.
Sweet RL, Gibbs RS: *Infectious diseases of the female genital tract,* ed 3, Baltimore, 1995, Williams & Wilkins.

Author: **Scott J. Zuccala, D.O.**

Abuse, child (PTG)

BASIC INFORMATION

DEFINITION
Child abuse refers to the intentional maltreatment by a caregiver of any child under the age of 18 yr. Four categories generally defined:
1. Neglect: failure to provide basic needs such as food, shelter, supervision
2. Physical abuse: infliction of bodily injury or harm
3. Sexual abuse: passive or active use or exposure of children to sexual acts
4. Emotional abuse: humiliating, coercive behavior that retards a child's psychologic development

SYNONYMS
Child maltreatment
Child neglect
Sexual abuse
"Shaken baby syndrome"
"Battered-child syndrome"

ICD-9-CM CODES
995.5 Child maltreatment syndrome

EPIDEMIOLOGY AND DEMOGRAPHICS
INCIDENCE (IN U.S.):
- 1.2 cases/100,000 persons/yr (70% physical abuse, 25% sexual abuse, 5% neglect)
- Death rate 1000 to 4000 children/yr
- 10% of emergency injuries for children <5 yr of age

PREVALENCE (IN U.S.): Over 5% of children <18 yr of age
PREDOMINANT SEX: Females may be at a slightly greater risk.
PREDOMINANT AGE:
- Incidence of all forms of abuse increases with age; teenagers are at twice the risk as infants.
- Risk of death is much higher in children <5 yr.
- Of the 1000 to 4000 annual deaths attributable to abuse, 80% are in children <5 yr, and 40% are in children <1 yr of age. For children <6 mo of age, abuse is the second cause of death (sudden infant death is first).

PEAK INCIDENCE:
- Approximately one third before the age of 1 yr, one third between 1 yr and 6 yr, and one third above age 6 yr
- Handicapped children at a much greater risk throughout childhood

GENETICS:
- No genetic factors are known.
- Sexual abuse is equally distributed throughout all socioeconomic groups, but physical abuse and neglect are more prevalent in lower socioeconomic groups, since abuse increases with severe stress, family violence, and substance abuse.
- Approximately 30% of abused children will abuse their children.

PHYSICAL FINDINGS
- Presence of multiple injuries of various ages, particularly in the setting of a discrepancy in the history and severity of injury
- Injuries of childhood usually on bony prominences; soft tissue injuries more frequently inflicted by others
- Burns in 10% of abused children; usually result from cigarettes or immersion of buttock or extremities in scalding hot water
- Retinal hemorrhage diagnostic for "shaken baby syndrome," since it occurs with head injury or sudden compression of the chest (Purtscher's retinopathy)
- Subdural bleeding exceedingly rare in children unless child has suffered shaking or significant head trauma
- Presence of sperm or acid phosphatase in the vaginal vault diagnostic of intercourse within 72 hr and indicates sexual abuse of female child
- Sexually transmitted diseases in a child highly suggestive of sexual abuse
- Disruption of normal genital anatomy frequently associated with recurrent sexual abuse (e.g., a lax anal sphincter, thickening or darkening of labial skin, significantly enlarged hymen opening)

ETIOLOGY
- Sexual abuse of girls: passive mother and domineering father (or stepfather)
- Physical abuse: severe psychosocial stressors such as poverty, unemployment, drug abuse, or marital discord
- History of abuse in the parent or the presence of violence in the family of origin: may predispose to child abuse
- Neglect associated with similar factors, particularly if child's birth was unplanned

DIAGNOSIS

DIFFERENTIAL DIAGNOSIS
Distinction from accidental injuries is crucial.

Abuse, child (PTG)

WORKUP
- History from the child, caregivers, and other individuals living in the home to reconstruct events and determine any inconsistency or implausibility in the story (Caution is required not to taint the history with the way in which it is obtained or the interviewer's own bias.)
- Physical examination to determine developmental parameters (height, weight) and to document extent and age of bruises
- Examinations for sexual abuse performed within the first 72 hr to be conducted by a rape-crisis team

LABORATORY TESTS
- Examine fluids in the vaginal vault for sperm and acid phosphatase if intercourse was believed to have occurred within 72 hr.
- Culture oral, vaginal, and anal orifices for sexually transmitted diseases.
- Do bleeding studies if bruising is thought to be secondary to clotting abnormality.
- Examine nutritional, hematopoietic, and endocrine parameters for patients with neglect or failure to thrive.

IMAGING STUDIES
- For children ages 2 to 5 yr: obtain a bone survey (skull, thorax, pelvis, spine, arms, and legs).
- In children older than 5 yr: obtain more focused x-rays.
- Do brain imaging if head trauma or shaking is suspected.
- Take color photographs of skin lesions if legal action is anticipated. (NOTE: Parental consent is not required for photos documenting suspected child abuse.)

TREATMENT

NONPHARMACOLOGIC THERAPY
- Gear initial interventions toward stabilizing the injuries and preventing further abuse.
- Contact Child Protective Services. (NOTE: Physicians are mandated to report suspected abuse.)
- Where hospitalization is not required, arrange for emergency foster care if possible.
- If a child is returned to abusive environment, 5% mortality rate and 35% severe injury rate is to be expected.

ACUTE GENERAL Rx
Pharmacologic intervention is limited to that required to stabilize the injuries.

CHRONIC Rx
- Treatment in abusive families is generally poor. A review of several studies including some 3000 families found that a third of abusive parents will continue abuse while in treatment and half may revert to abuse at end of treatment.
- Separation of child via foster care may be traumatic to the child.
- Preventative programs for young single mothers at high risk are thought to be more effective than other interventions.
- Treatment of sexual abusers is marred by a high recurrence rate.
- In <5% of cases the abuse is related to a psychotic illness that can be treated directly.

DISPOSITION
- Victims of abuse and neglect may die or suffer lifelong emotional or physical disability.
- Abused children are more aggressive and have greater interpersonal difficulties. As adults they suffer from depression, anxiety, and substance abuse at twice the rate in the general population, and some 30% are likely to abuse their children.
- Victims of sexual abuse will experience problems with sexual identity and function. Of women with borderline personality disorder, 60% have suffered physical or sexual abuse.

REFERRAL
- The physician is mandated to report suspected abuse to Child Protective Services.
- Rape crisis teams exist in most urban areas and usually are better prepared to deal with issues of sexual abuse.
- Individuals at high risk may benefit from prophylactic counseling.
- Most abused children need some therapy to cope with abuse and resulting separation from the family of origin.
- U.S. Preventive Services Task Force Recommendations regarding counseling to prevent youth violence are described in Section V, Chapter 59; recommendations regarding screening for family violence are described in Section V, Chapter 51.

MISCELLANEOUS

REFERENCES
Brodsky BS, Cloitre M, Dulit RA: Relationship of dissociation to self-mutilation and childhood abuse in borderline personality disorder, *Am J Psychiatry* 152:1788, 1995.

Wissow LS: Child abuse and neglect, *N Engl J Med* 332:1425, 1995.

Author: **Rif S. El-Mallakh, M.D.**

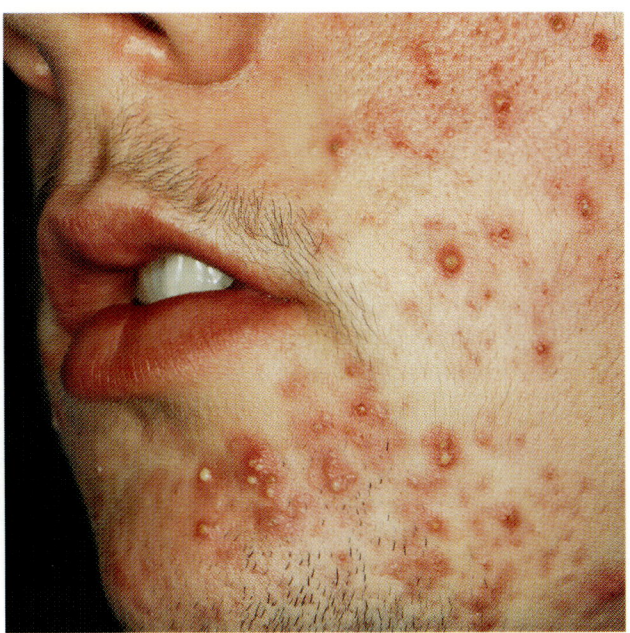

Plate 1 Acne vulgaris. Papular and pustular acne (moderate). Many pustules are present, and several have become confluent on the chin area. (From Habif TB: *Clinical dermatology: a color guide to diagnosis and therapy*, ed 3, St Louis, 1996, Mosby.)

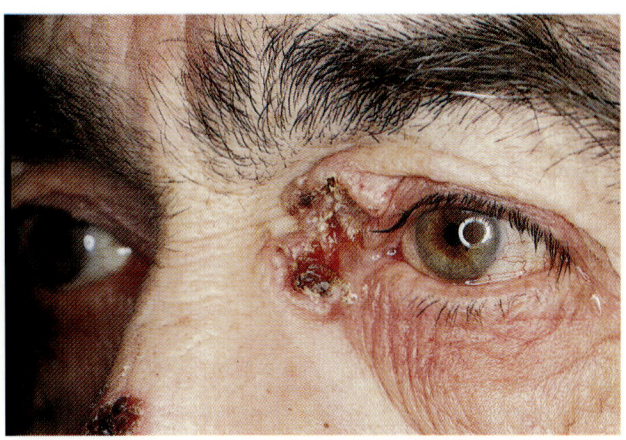

Plate 2 Basal cell carcinoma. Note rolled translucent border and central ulceration in typical facial location. (From Noble J et al: *Textbook of primary care medicine*, ed 2, St Louis, 1995, Mosby.)

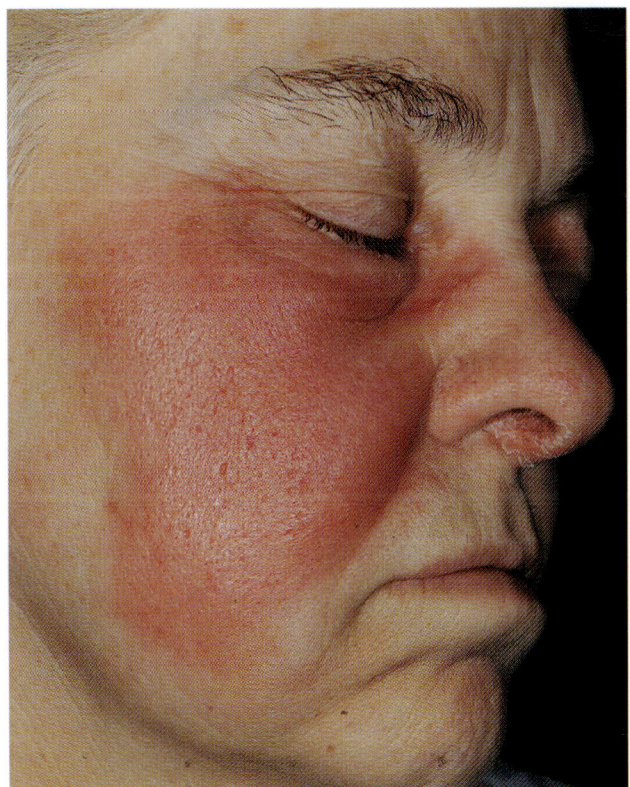

Plate 3 Erysipelas. Streptococcal cellulitis. The acute phase with intense erythema. (From Habif TB: *Clinical dermatology: a color guide to diagnosis and therapy*, ed 3, St Louis, 1996, Mosby.)

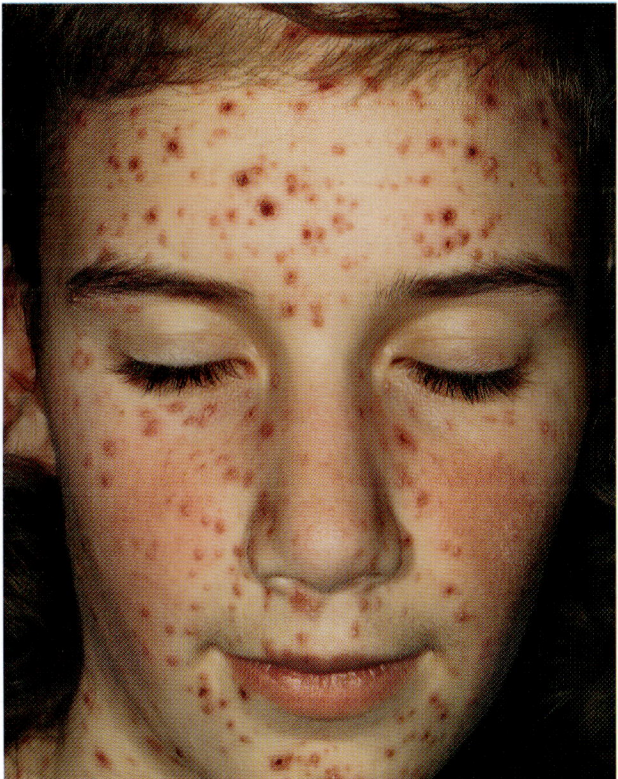

Plate 4 Chicken pox. Lesions present in all stages of development. (From Habif TB: *Clinical dermatology: a color guide to diagnosis and therapy*, ed 3, St Louis, 1996, Mosby.)

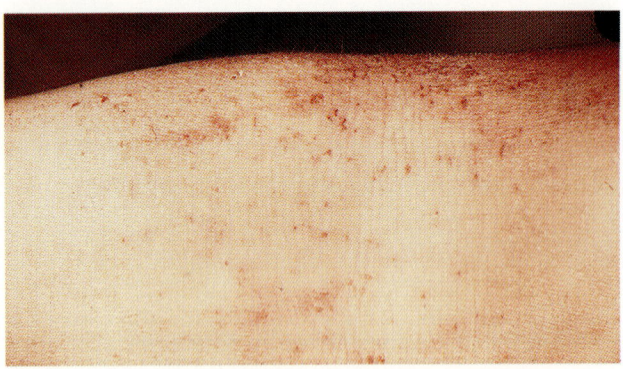

Plate 5 Lichenification (atopic dermatitis). Note erythema and pinpoint excoriations in antecubital fossa (typical location for atopic dermatitis—flexural). (From Noble J et al: *Textbook of primary care medicine,* ed 2, St Louis, 1995, Mosby.)

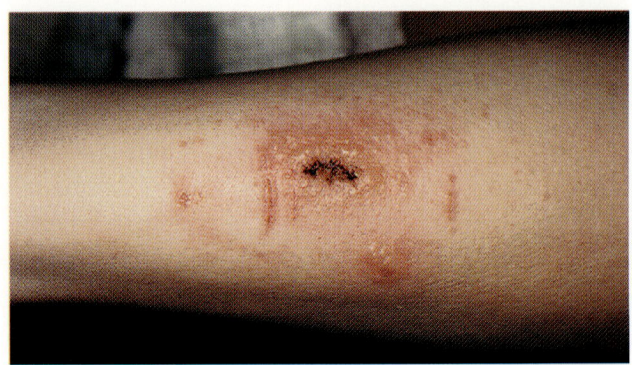

Plate 6 Allergic contact dermatitis (poison oak, acute vesicular reaction, and linear features). Dark central pigmentation is oxidized oleoresin. (From Noble J et al: *Textbook of primary care medicine,* ed 2, St Louis, 1995, Mosby.)

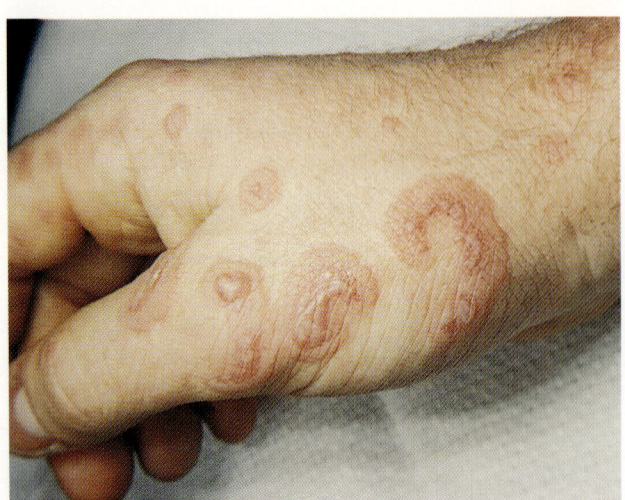

Plate 7 Iris and arcuate lesions of erythema multiforme. Note erythematous lesions with multiform configurations—target, arcuate, and vesicles (From Noble J et al: *Textbook of primary care medicine,* ed 2, St Louis, 1995, Mosby.)

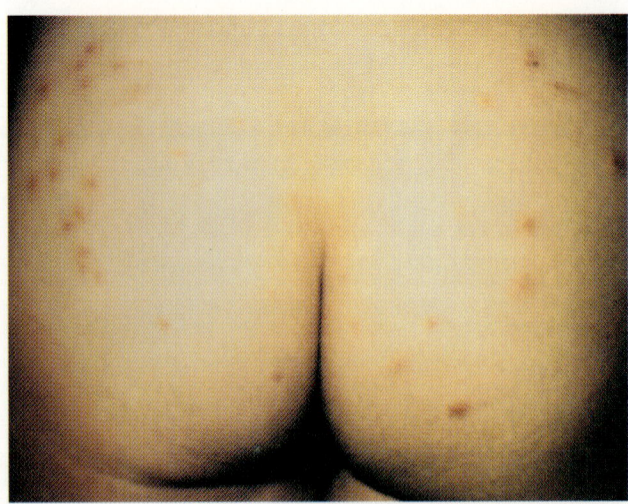

Plate 8 Hot tub folliculitis. (From Stein JH: *Internal medicine,* ed 5, St Louis, 1998, Mosby.)

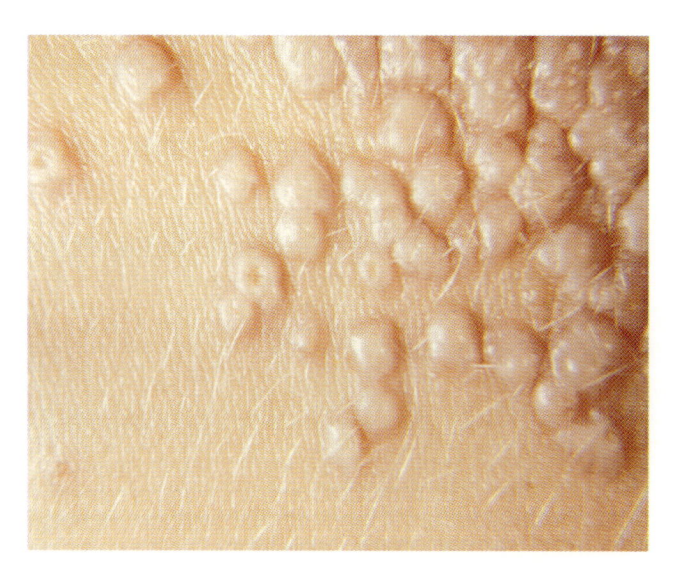

Plate 9 Vesicles (herpes simplex). Note umbilication characteristic of viral infection and herpetiform grouping. (From Noble J et al: *Textbook of primary care medicine,* ed 2, St Louis, 1995, Mosby.)

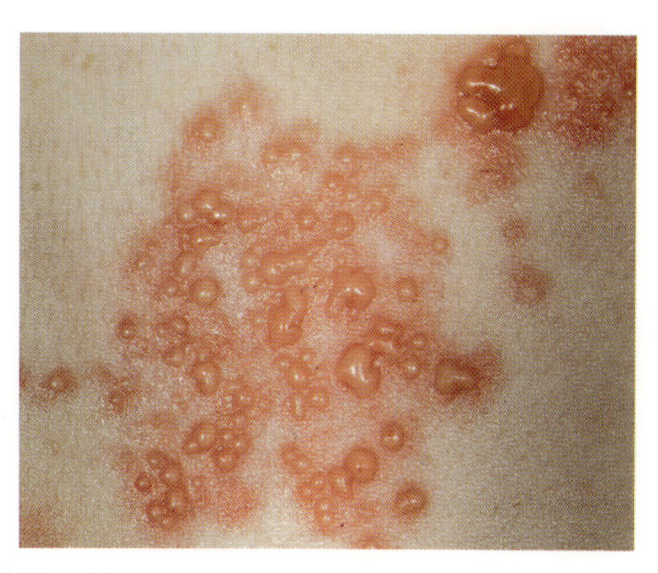

Plate 10 Herpes zoster. A group of vesicles that vary in size. Vesicles of herpes simplex are of uniform size (see Plate 9). (From Habif TB: *Clinical dermatology: a color guide to diagnosis and therapy,* ed 3, St Louis, 1996, Mosby.)

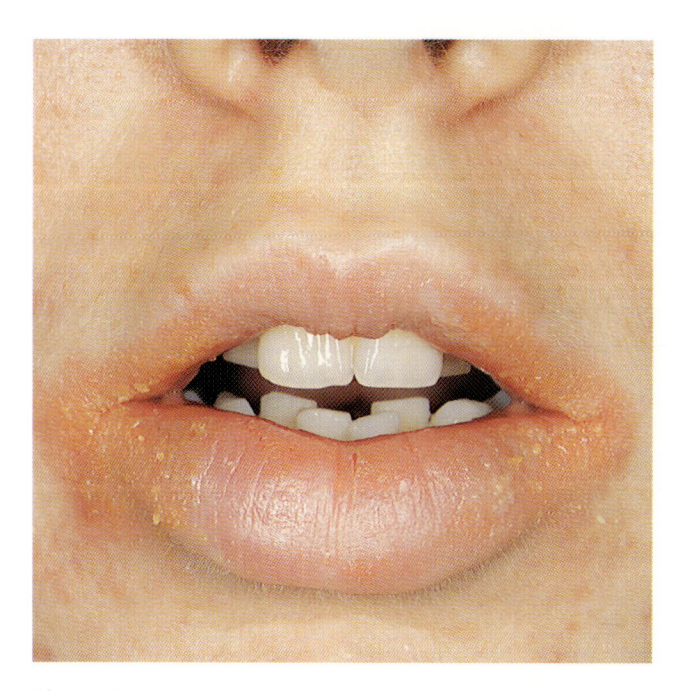

Plate 11 Impetigo. Serum and crust at the angle of the mouth is a common presentation for impetigo. (From Habif TB: *Clinical dermatology: a color guide to diagnosis and therapy,* ed 3, St Louis, 1996, Mosby.)

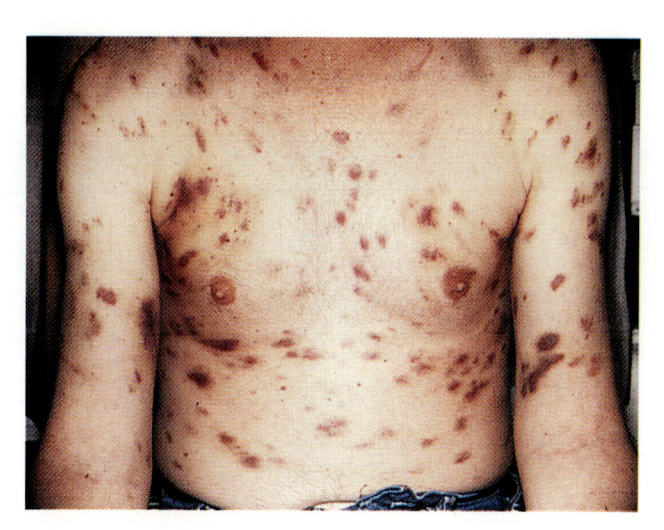

Plate 12 Kaposi's sarcoma. More advanced lesions. Note widespread hemorrhagic plaques and nodules. (From Noble J et al: *Textbook of primary care medicine,* ed 2, St Louis, 1995, Mosby.)

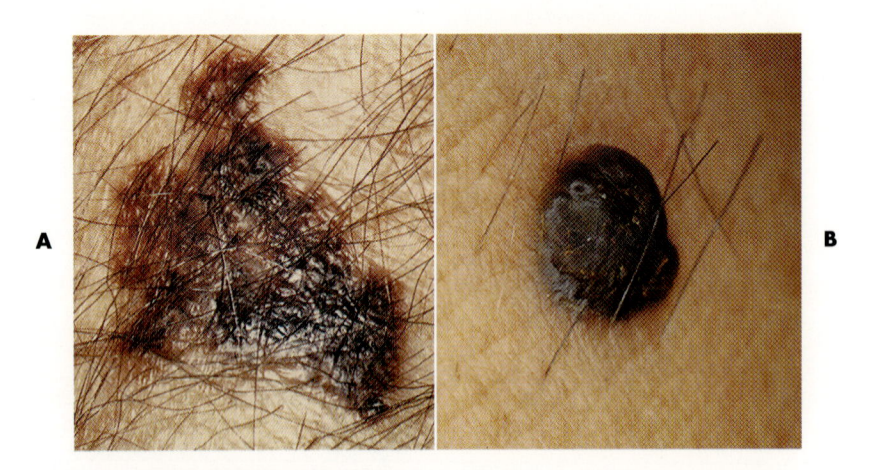

Plate 13 Malignant melanoma. **A**, Superficial spreading melanoma. **B**, Nodular melanoma. (From Stein JH: *Internal medicine,* ed 4, St Louis, 1998, Mosby.)

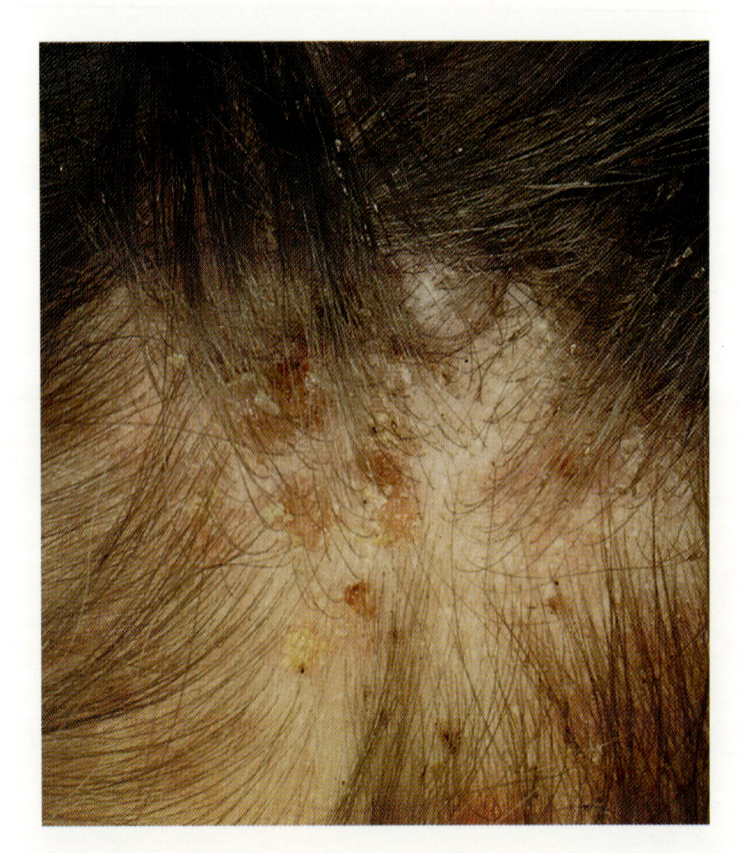

Plate 14 Pediculosis capitis. A heavy infestation with secondary pyoderma. (From Habif TB: *Clinical dermatology: a color guide to diagnosis and therapy,* ed 3, St Louis, 1996, Mosby.)

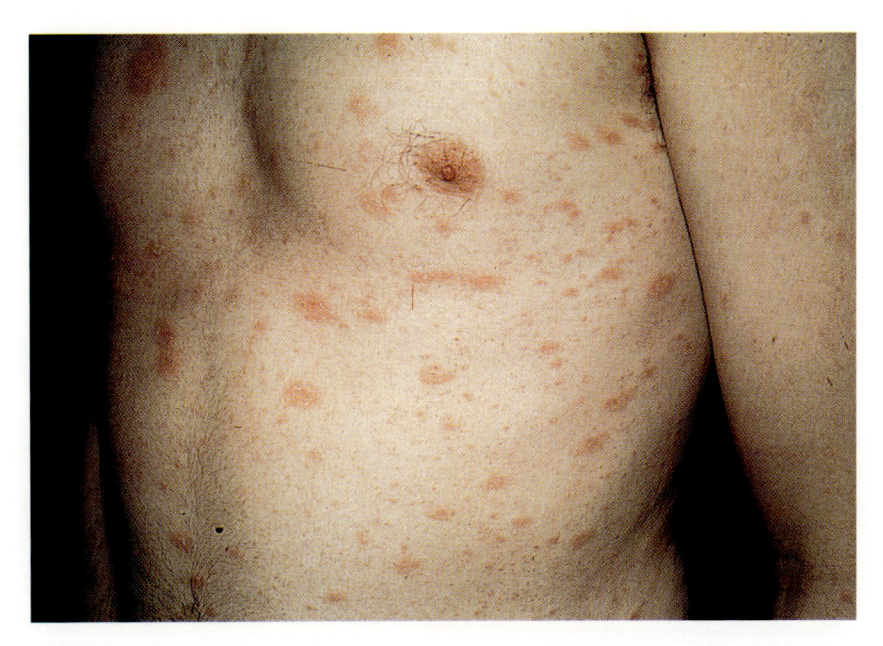

Plate 15 Scale (pityriasis rosea). Shows example of how unique scaling (collarette of fine scale within several lesions), distribution and shape of lesions (oval lesions with long axis paralleling natural skin cleavage lines); and color (salmon-pink) help in diagnosing skin disease. (From Noble J et al: *Textbook of primary care medicine,* ed 2, St Louis, 1995, Mosby.)

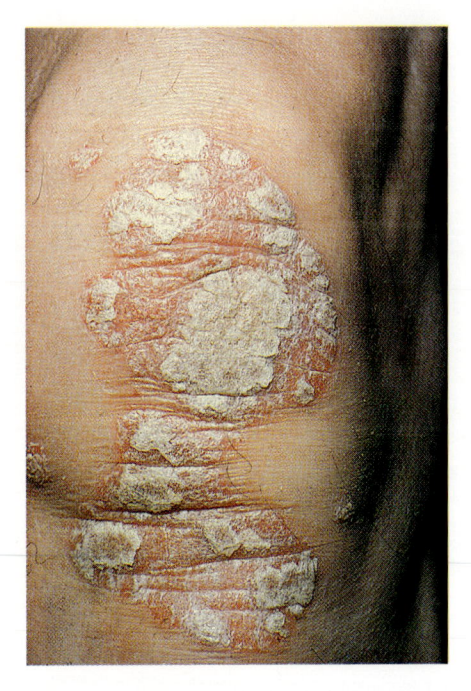

Plate 16 Plaques (psoriasis). Note special physical characteristic of scale (silvery, micaceous). Typical location: extensor surfaces (knee). (From Noble J et al: *Textbook of primary care medicine,* ed 2, St Louis, 1995, Mosby.)

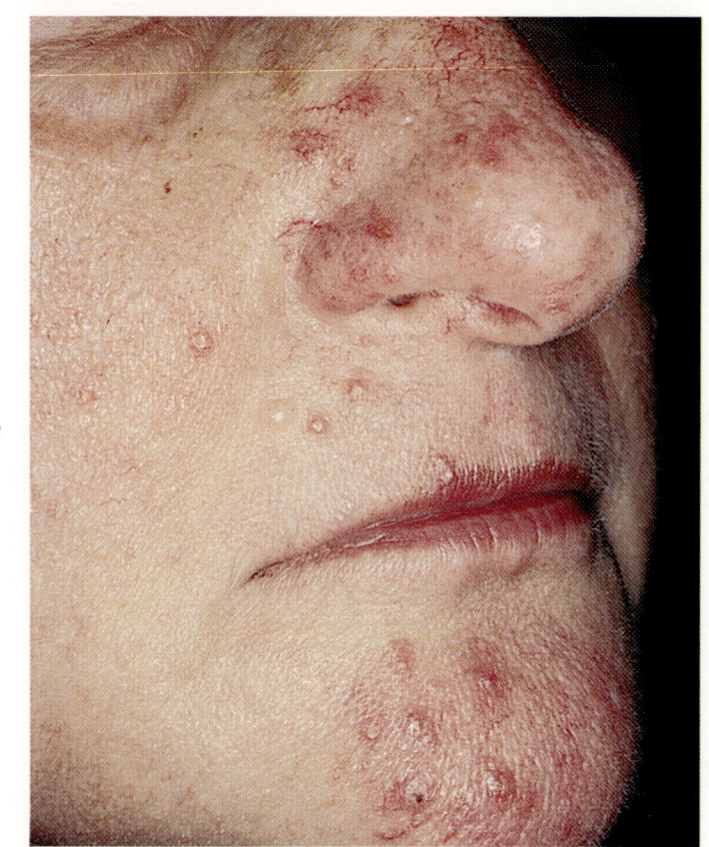

Plate 17 Pustules (rosacea). Note also the presence of telangiectasia. (From Noble J et al: *Textbook of primary care medicine,* ed 2, St Louis, 1995, Mosby.)

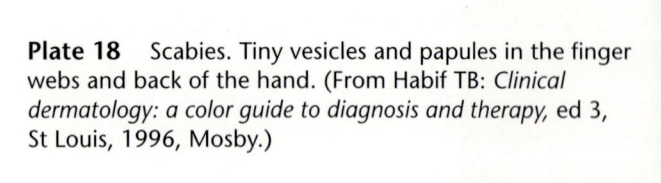

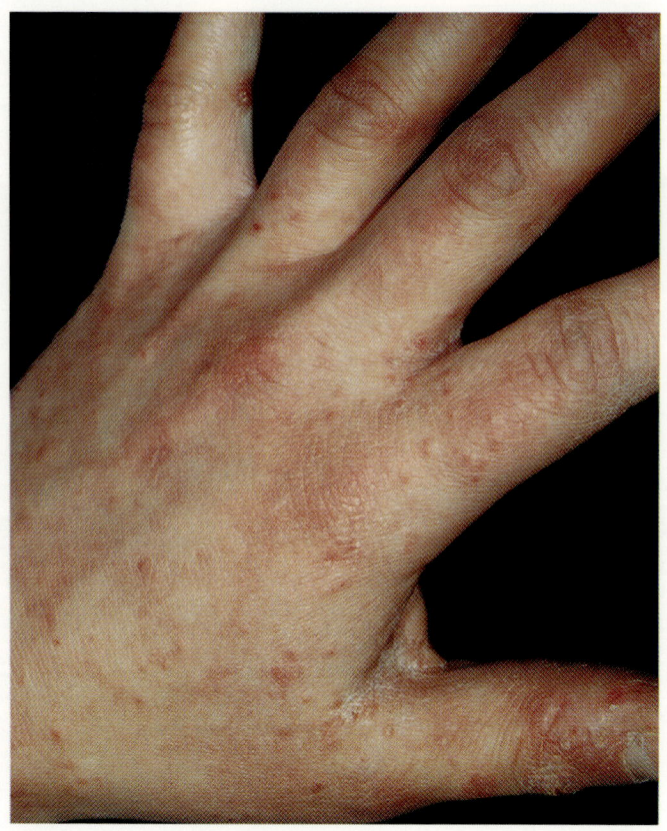

Plate 18 Scabies. Tiny vesicles and papules in the finger webs and back of the hand. (From Habif TB: *Clinical dermatology: a color guide to diagnosis and therapy,* ed 3, St Louis, 1996, Mosby.)

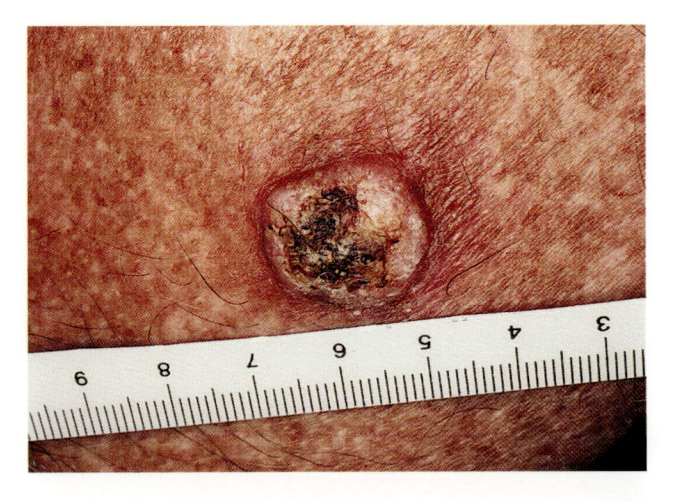

Plate 19 Squamous cell carcinoma. Nodular hyperkeratotic lesion with central erosion. (From Noble J et al: *Textbook of primary care medicine,* ed 2, St Louis, 1995, Mosby.)

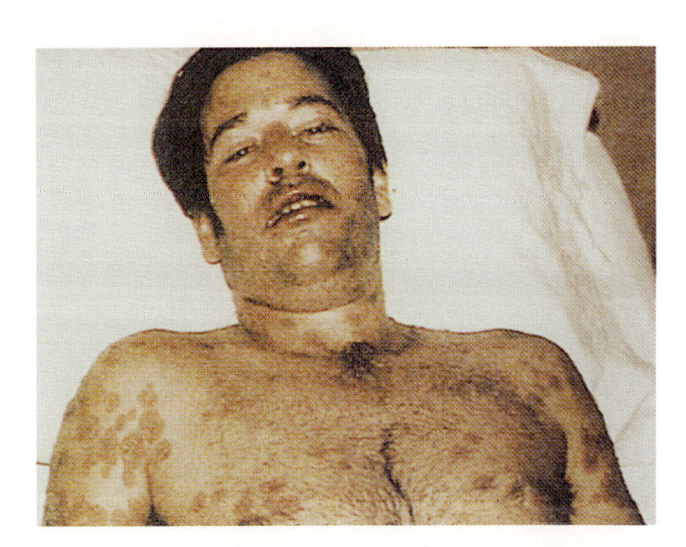

Plate 20 Stevens-Johnson syndrome. (From Stein JH: *Internal medicine,* ed 5, St Louis, 1998, Mosby.)

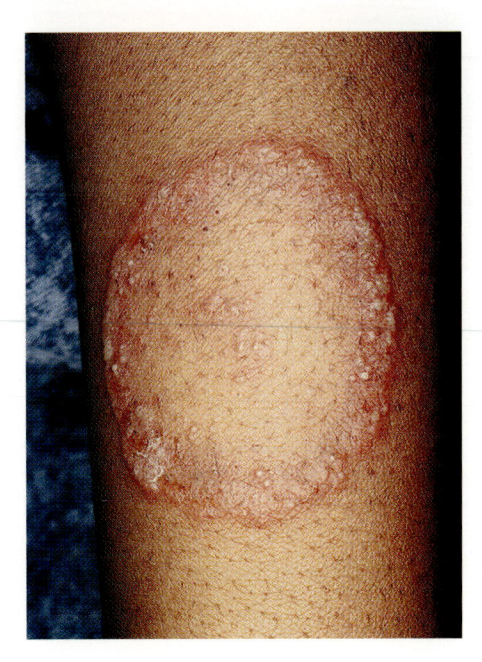

Plate 21 Annular lesion (tinea corporis). Note raised erythematous scaling border and central clearing. (From Noble J et al: *Textbook of primary care medicine,* ed 2, St Louis, 1995, Mosby.)

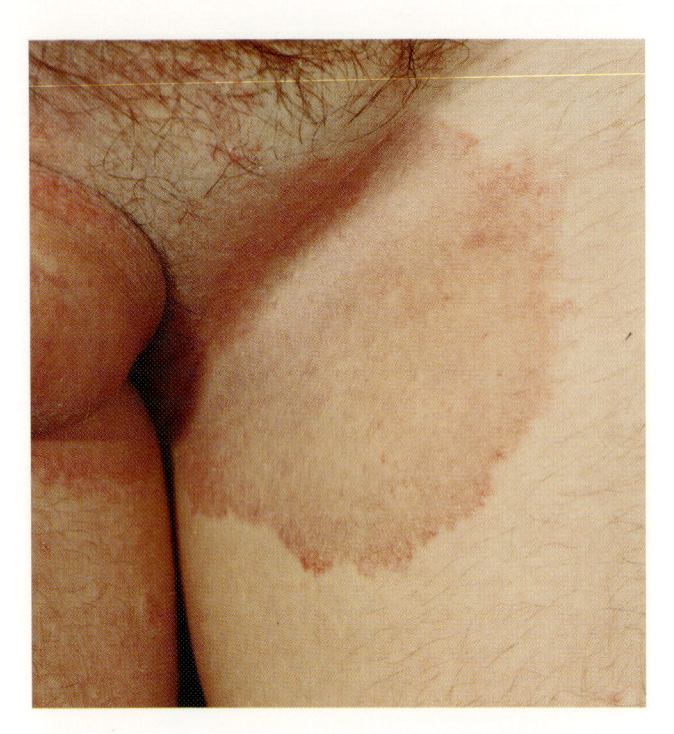

Plate 22 Tinea cruris. A half moon–shaped plaque has a well-defined, scaling border. (From Habif TB: *Clinical dermatology: a color guide to diagnosis and therapy,* ed 3, St Louis, 1996, Mosby.)

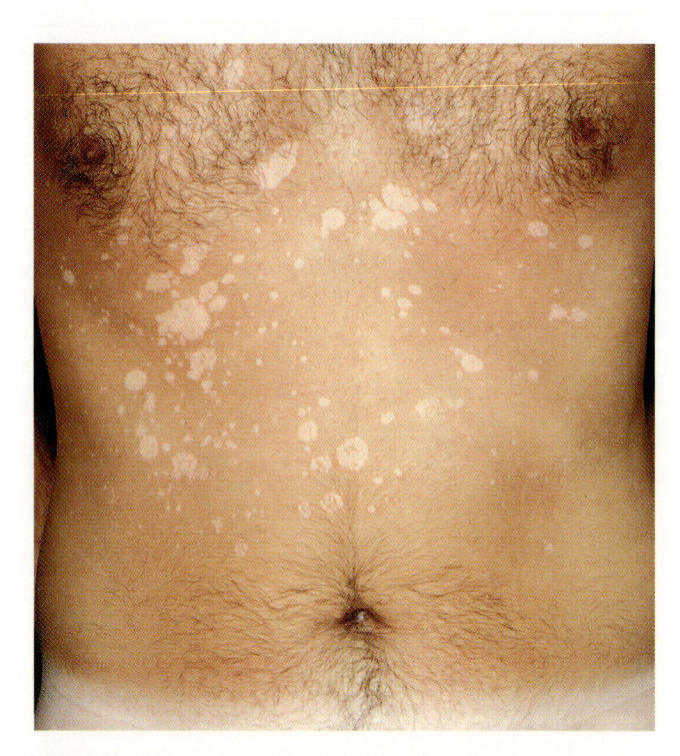

Plate 23 The classic presentation of tinea versicolor with white, oval or circular patches on tan skin. (From Habif TB: *Clinical dermatology: a color guide to diagnosis and therapy,* ed 3, St Louis, 1996, Mosby.)

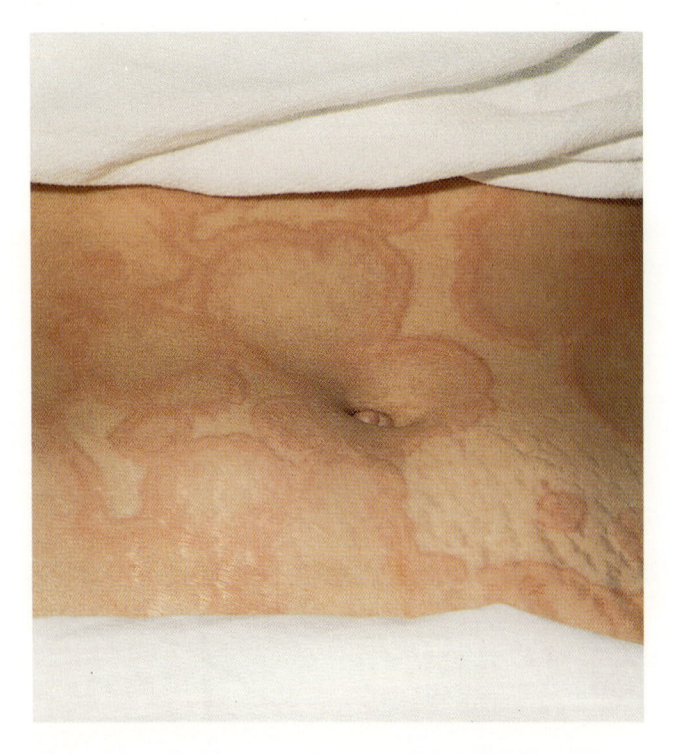

Plate 24 Wheal (urticaria). Note central clearing, giving annular configuration. (From Noble J et al: *Textbook of primary care medicine,* ed 2, St Louis, 1995, Mosby.)

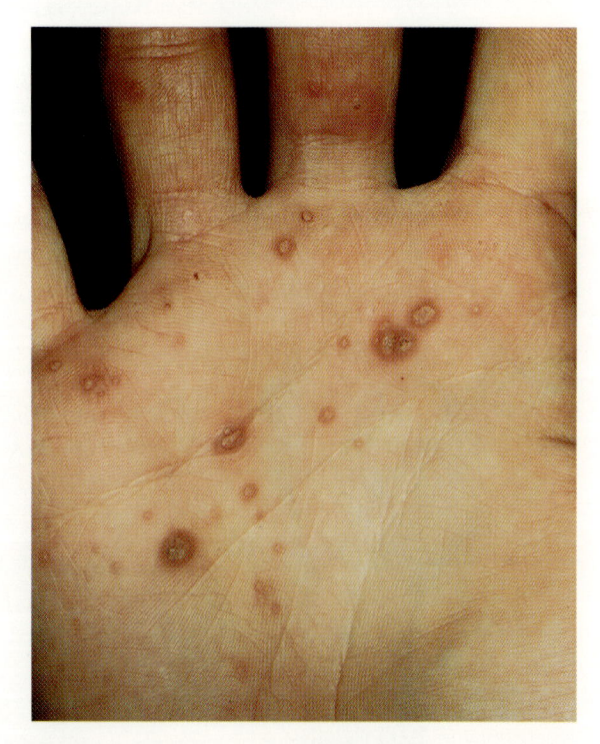

Plate 25 Common warts with thrombosed vessels (black dots) on the surface. (From Habif TB: *Clinical dermatology: a color guide to diagnosis and therapy,* ed 3, St Louis, 1996, Mosby.)

Abuse, drug (PTG)

CLINICAL TOPICS

BASIC INFORMATION

DEFINITION
Drug abuse is a recurring pattern of harmful use of a substance despite adverse consequences of the substance in work, school, relationships, the legal system, or personal health. This may occur concurrently with or independently from *substance dependence*, in which there is the presence of physiologic tolerance, discontinuation-induced withdrawal, or inability to willfully control rate or discontinue substance.

SYNONYMS
Substance abuse
Addiction

ICD-10-CM CODES
Defined by specific substance F10-F19 (DSM-IV code is also defined by specific substance 291-292, 303-305).

EPIDEMIOLOGY AND DEMOGRAPHICS
INCIDENCE (IN U.S.): For alcohol the incidence is 7%/yr.
PREVALENCE (IN U.S.):
- For alcohol: lifetime
- For cocaine abuse: lifetime prevalence is 0.2%
- For marijuana abuse: lifetime prevalence is 4%
- For amphetamine abuse: lifetime prevalence is 2%
- For hallucinogens: rate is 0.3%
- For opiates: rate is 0.7%
- For nicotine: lifetime prevalence of dependence is 20%.

PREDOMINANT SEX:
- Males abuse substances more frequently than females.
- The rates of male:female substance abusers are as follows:
  Alcohol 5:1
  Opiates 3-4:1
  Amphetamines 3-4:1
  Hallucinogens 2:1
  Marijuana 1-2:1
  Cocaine 1:1

PREDOMINANT AGE:
- Problematic use of substances may begin in early life (8 to 10 yr).
- The near age of onset of problem drinking is about 25 for men and 30 for women.

PEAK INCIDENCE:
- For most substances: 18 to 30 yr of age
- Men: average >20 yr of heavy drinking
- Women: average 15 yr of heavy drinking

GENETICS:
- There is evidence of a nonspecific genetic factor.
- Vulnerability to alcohol abuse is increased in Asians with the alcohol dehydrogenase type 2 isozyme and the aldehyde dehydrogenase type 2 isozyme.

PHYSICAL FINDINGS
- Abuse of several substances generally occurs together; e.g., alcohol abuse is often found in association with abuse or dependence of nicotine.
- Symptoms of anxiety, depression, insomnia, cognitive and memory dysfunction, and emotional/behavioral dyscontrol are frequent.
- Alcohol and cocaine abuse are specifically associated with violence and accidents; e.g., more than half of all murderers *and* their victims are intoxicated at the time of the crime.

ETIOLOGY
Two models of addiction: (1) Conditioning—substance use paired with enforcing and triggering stimuli, and (2) Homeostatic—either preexisting abnormalities or drug-induced abnormalities lead to initial or continued use of the drug.

DIAGNOSIS

DIFFERENTIAL DIAGNOSIS
- Psychiatric disorders such as depression, mania, social phobia, or other anxiety disorders that coexist or occur as a consequence of substance abuse
- Cannot diagnose these disorders accurately in the setting of active substance abuse

WORKUP
- The history is crucial for diagnosis of any substance abuse disorder; because of frequent denial and poor insight into problem substance abuse, collateral information from family, friends, and coworkers is often helpful.
- Observation of problematic behavior during intoxication or withdrawal is diagnostic.

Abuse, drug (PTG)

- Physical examination findings are limited and not diagnostic (e.g., needle scars from repeated intravenous injections, rhinorrhea secondary to intranasal cocaine).

LABORATORY TESTS
Most helpful tests: toxicology screen or blood alcohol level

IMAGING STUDIES
- Not helpful in routine diagnosis and management of substance abuse, but possibly useful in the management of sequelae of substance abuse; e.g., head CT scan to evaluate the alcohol abuse-associated increased risk of subdural hematomas or increased evidence of cerebral atrophy
- Liver ultrasound to evaluate for alcohol-related fatty changes
- Two-dimensional echo for intravenous drug use-associated valvular vitiations

TREATMENT

NONPHARMACOLOGIC THERAPY
- Relapse prevention by avoidance of trigger stimuli or by uncoupling trigger stimuli from substance ingestion
- Self-help groups such as Alcoholics Anonymous, Narcotics Anonymous, and Al-Anon

ACUTE GENERAL Rx
- Acute interventions are usually confined to safe withdrawal in the setting of dependence.
- Benzodiazepines are safe and effective in acute alcohol withdrawal.
- Anticonvulsants, particularly carbamazepine, are used effectively in Europe.
- β-Blockers and clonidine should be avoided in alcohol withdrawal, since they mask markers of the severity of the withdrawal (blood pressure and pulse rate).
- Clonidine alleviates the discomfort of opiate and nicotine withdrawal.
- Nicotine patches and gum reduce withdrawal symptoms.

CHRONIC Rx
- Few agents are useful in prevention of substance abuse relapse.
- Disulfram (Antabuse) workup and metronidazole (Flagyl): possible interaction with alcohol causes physical discomfort.
- Naltrexone helps reduce craving for alcohol.
- Adjunctive use of antidepressants or lithium is helpful when substance use is associated with anxiety and mood symptoms.
- Methadone replacement is used in opiate abuse/dependence (controversial).

DISPOSITION
- Substance abuse is a chronic relapsing illness.
- The goal of treatment is always abstinence, but success of treatment is measured by return of function and increasing duration between relapses.
- When substance abuse is complicated by another psychiatric illness, prognosis for both conditions is quite poor.

REFERRAL
- Always refer to self-help groups (AA, NA) for patient, Al-Anon for significant others.
- Intensive substance abuse treatment is nearly always indicated in substance-dependent individuals.
- Individuals with a coexisting primary psychiatric illness and substance abuse nearly always require the care of a psychiatrist.

MISCELLANEOUS

COMMENTS
U.S. Preventive Services Task Force Recommendations regarding screening for drug abuse are described in Section V, Chapter 53.

REFERENCES
Meyer RE: The disease called addiction: emerging evidence in a 200-year debate, *Lancet* 347:162, 1996.

Widiger TA, Smith GT: Substance use disorder: abuse, dependence, and dyscontrol, *Addiction* 89:267, 1994.

Author: **Rif S. El-Mallakh, M.D.**

CLINICAL TOPICS — Abuse, geriatric (PTG)

BASIC INFORMATION

DEFINITION
Geriatric abuse is the willful infliction of physical pain or injury; emotional pain, injury, humiliation, or intimidation; exploitation or misappropriation of money or property; or neglect by the designated caregiver of nutritional, hygiene, or medical needs.

SYNONYMS
Elder abuse
Battered elder syndrome

ICD-9-CM CODES
995.81 Adult maltreatment syndrome

EPIDEMIOLOGY AND DEMOGRAPHICS
INCIDENCE (IN U.S.): Unknown
PREVALENCE (IN U.S.):
- 3.2% in a large study in Boston
- Estimated up to 10% of individuals >65 yr of age
- Only 15% of elder abuse comes to the attention of authorities.
- Most (>60%) abuse is committed by one spouse against another.
- Approximately 25% of abuse is committed by an adult child of the victim who is living in the same home and is usually financially dependent on the victim.

PREDOMINANT SEX:
- No data available
- Women thought to be at greater risk

PREDOMINANT AGE: Risk increases as level of disability, not age, increases
PEAK INCIDENCE: >80 yr old

PHYSICAL FINDINGS
- Physical abuse with multiple injuries at various stages with implausible or inconsistent descriptions of their origins
- Extreme fear, hypervigilance, or withdrawal
- Torn or blood-stained underwear or new onset of a sexually transmitted disease signaling sexual abuse
- Toxicologic evidence of unprescribed medications

ETIOLOGY
- Relatives with mental illness or substance abuse
- Excessive dependence on the elderly individual for financial, housing, and other necessities
- A history of violence, particularly within the family

DIAGNOSIS

DIFFERENTIAL DIAGNOSIS
Risk increases as the elder's level of disability increases. Consequently, poor hygiene, poor nutrition, confusion, psychosis in the setting of dementia, and poor compliance with prescribed treatments may all occur without ongoing abuse.

WORKUP
- Interview patient separately from the suspected abuser.
- Build trust; patients may be reticent.
- Ask direct questions.
- Be aware that physical findings are usually unexplained injuries or burns.

LABORATORY TESTS
- Toxicology screens or therapeutic drug monitoring
- If sexual abuse suspected, screening for sexually transmitted diseases

IMAGING STUDIES
X-rays as indicated

TREATMENT

NONPHARMACOLOGIC THERAPY
- Reporting abuse to Adult Protective Services is mandatory in most states. This also provides the physician access to specialized personnel who can aid in evaluation and disposition.
- Separate patient and abuser.
- If the burden of care underlies the abuse, refer to respite services.

ACUTE GENERAL Rx
As indicated for injury or pain relief

CHRONIC Rx
If the patient's level of disability does not allow for independent living, institutionalization may be required.

REFERRAL
Referral to Adult Protective Services is mandatory in 42 states.

MISCELLANEOUS

COMMENTS
U.S. Preventive Services Task Force Recommendations for screening for family violence are described in Section V, Chapter 51.

REFERENCES
Lachs MS, Pillemer K: Abuse and neglect of elderly persons, *N Engl J Med* 332:437, 1995.

Author: **Rif S. El-Mallakh, M.D.**

Acetaminophen poisoning

BASIC INFORMATION

DEFINITION
Acetaminophen poisoning is a disorder manifested by hepatic necrosis, jaundice, somnolence, and eventual death if not treated appropriately. Pathologically there is hepatic necrosis.

SYNONYMS
Paracetamol poisoning

ICD-9-CM CODES
965.4 Acetaminophen poisoning

EPIDEMIOLOGY AND DEMOGRAPHICS
- Potentially toxic ingestions of acetaminophen-containing medications exceed 100,000 cases annually.
- Death rate is approximately 1/1000 persons. Nearly 50% of exposures occur in children <6 yr.
- Hepatic nephrosis is most likely to occur in individuals who are chronically malnourished, who regularly abuse alcohol, and who are using other potentially hepatotoxic medications.

PHYSICAL FINDINGS
- The physical examination may vary depending on the number of hours lapsed from the ingestion of acetaminophen.
- Initially, symptoms may be mild or absent and may consist of diaphoresis, malaise, nausea, and vomiting.
- After the initial 12 to 24 hr, patient may complain of RUQ pain with associated vomiting, diaphoresis, and subsequent somnolence.
- In massive overdoses, jaundice may occur within the initial 72 hr.
- Subsequent coma, somnolence, and confusion follow and can ultimately lead to death if not treated appropriately.

ETIOLOGY
The amount of acetaminophen necessary for hepatic toxicity varies with the patient's body size and hepatic function. Using standardized nomograms[1], calculating the acetaminophen plasma level and the number of hours after ingestion, the clinician can determine potential hepatic toxicity.

---

[1] Rumack BH, Matthew H: Acetaminophen poisoning and toxicity, *Pediatrics* 55:871, 1975.

DIAGNOSIS

DIFFERENTIAL DIAGNOSIS
- Liver disease from alcohol abuse or hepatitis
- Ingestion of other hepatotoxic substances

WORKUP
Initial workup is aimed at confirming acetaminophen overdose with plasma acetaminophen level and assessment of hepatic damage and the potential damage to other organ systems, such as kidneys, pancreas, and heart (see "Laboratory Tests").

LABORATORY TESTS
- Initial laboratory evaluation consists of plasma acetaminophen level with a second level drawn approximately 4 to 6 hr after the initial level. Subsequent levels can be obtained q2-4h until the levels stabilize or decline. These levels can be plotted using the Rumack-Matthew nomogram to calculate potential hepatic toxicity.
- Transaminases (AST, ALT), bilirubin level, prothrombin time, BUN, creatinine should be initially obtained on all patients.
- Serum and urine toxicology screen for other potential toxic substances is also recommended on admission.

TREATMENT

NONPHARMACOLOGIC THERAPY
Consultation with Poison Control Center for management recommendations is recommended in patients with large ingestions of acetaminophen and/or ingestion of other toxic substances.

ACUTE GENERAL Rx
- Perform gastric lavage and administer activated charcoal if the patient is seen within 1 hr of ingestion or the clinician suspects polydrug ingestion.
- Determine blood levels 4 hr after ingestion; if in the toxic range, start *N*-acetylcysteine (Mucomyst), 140 mg/kg PO as a loading dose, followed by 70 mg/kg PO q4h for 48 hr. (*N*-acetylcysteine therapy should be started within 24 hr of acetaminophen overdose.) If charcoal therapy was initially instituted, lavage the stomach and recover as much charcoal as possible; then instill *N*-acetylcysteine, increasing the loading dose by 40%.
- Monitor acetaminophen level; use graph to plot possible hepatic toxicity.
- Provide adequate IV hydration (e.g., $D_5\frac{1}{2}NS$ at 150 ml/hr).
- If acetaminophen level is nontoxic, acetylcysteine therapy may be discontinued.

DISPOSITION
Most patients will recover fully without persisting hepatic abnormalities. Hepatic failure is particularly unusual in children <6 yr.

REFERRAL
Psychiatric referral is recommended following intentional ingestions.

MISCELLANEOUS

COMMENTS
- Patient education regarding child safety issues is recommended in all cases of childhood acetaminophen poisoning.
- Instructions on avoidance of alcohol use and proper nutrition is also advisable in patients with acetaminophen poisoning and coexisting alcohol abuse or poor nutritional status.

REFERENCES
Kulig K: Initial management of ingestion of toxic substances, *N Engl J Med* 326:1679, 1992.

Livitz TL et al: 1994 annual report of the American Association of Poison Control Centers Toxic Exposure Surveillance System, *Am J Emerg Med* 13:551, 1995.

Vale JA, Proud AT: Paracetamol poisoning, *Lancet* 346:547, 1995.

Weinstock MS: General management of poisoning and drug overdose. In Ferri FF: *Practical guide to acute medical patient*, ed 4, St Louis, 1998, Mosby.

Author: **Fred F. Ferri, M.D.**

Achilles tendon rupture (PTG)

BASIC INFORMATION

DEFINITION
Achilles tendon rupture refers to the loss of continuity of the tendo Achilles, usually from attrition.

ICD-9-CM CODES
845.09 Achilles tendon rupture

EPIDEMIOLOGY AND DEMOGRAPHICS
PREDOMINANT AGE: 30 to 55 yr

PHYSICAL FINDINGS
Injury frequently occurs during an activity that puts great stress on the tendon. Sudden "pop" is often felt followed by weakness and swelling.
- Patient walks flat-footed and is unable to stand on the ball of the foot.
- Tenderness and hemorrhage are present at the site of injury and a sulcus is usually palpable but may be obscured by an organizing clot if the examination is delayed.
- Although active plantar flexion is usually lost, some plantar flexion occasionally remains because of the activity of the other posterior compartment muscles.
- Thompson's test is usually positive. Test measures plantar flexion of the foot when the calf is squeezed with the patient kneeling on a chair; normal foot plantarflexes with calf compression but movement is absent when tendo Achilles is ruptured.
- Excessive passive dorsiflexion of the foot is also present on the injured side.

ETIOLOGY
- Relative hypovascularity predisposing to tendon rupture in several tendons (Achilles, biceps, and supraspinatus)
- With advancing age, vascular supply to the tendon further compromised
- Repetitive trauma leading to degeneration of this critical area and weakness
- Rupture of tendo Achilles usually 2.5 to 5 cm from the insertion of the tendon into the os calcis
- Most common causative event leading to rupture: sudden dorsiflexion of the plantar flexed foot (landing from a height) or sudden pushing off with the weight on the forefoot

DIAGNOSIS

DIFFERENTIAL DIAGNOSIS
- Incomplete (partial) tendo Achilles rupture
- Partial rupture of gastrocnemius muscle, often medial head (previously thought to be "plantaris tendon rupture")

WORKUP
- Clinical diagnosis of tendo Achilles rupture is usually obvious.
- If bony injury is suspected, plain roentgenograms are indicated.
- Other studies are usually unnecessary.

TREATMENT
- Early referral is necessary for surgical repair.
- If surgery is contraindicated, a short leg cast applied with the foot in equinus will allow healing.
- In cases of neglected rupture, reconstruction is usually indicated.

DISPOSITION
- Prognosis for recovery after surgical repair of the acute rupture is good, but recurrence is not uncommon regardless of treatment.
- Tendo Achilles must be protected from excessive activity for up to 1 year.
- Results of reconstruction for neglected cases are worse than with primary repair.

MISCELLANEOUS

REFERENCES
Lea RB, Smith L: Nonsurgical treatment of tendo Achilles rupture, *J Bone Joint Surg (Am)* 54:1398, 1972.

Phillips, BB: Tendo calcaneus injuries. In Chrenshaw AH (ed): *Campbell's operative orthopedics*, ed 8, St Louis, 1992, Mosby.

Author: **Lonnie R. Mercier, M.D.**

Acne vulgaris (PTG)

BASIC INFORMATION

DEFINITION
Acne vulgaris is a chronic disorder of the pilosebaceous apparatus resulting in inflammation and subsequent formation of papules, pustules, nodules, comedones, and scarring.

SYNONYMS
Acne

ICD-9-CM CODES
706.1 Acne vulgaris

EPIDEMIOLOGY AND DEMOGRAPHICS
- Acne is the most common skin disease in the U.S.
- It is most common in teenagers (highest incidence between ages of 16 and 18 yr).

PHYSICAL FINDINGS
- Open comedones (blackheads), closed comedones (whiteheads)
- Greasiness (oily skin)
- Presence of scars from prior acne cysts
- Various stages of development and severity may be present concomitantly
- Common distribution of acne: face, back, and upper chest
- Inflammatory papules, pustules, and ectatic pores (see color plate 1)

ETIOLOGY
- Overactivity of the sebaceous glands and blockage in the ducts
- Exacerbated by environmental factors (hot, humid, tropical climate), medications (e.g., iodine in cough mixtures, hair greases), industrial exposure to halogenated hydrocarbons

DIAGNOSIS

DIFFERENTIAL DIAGNOSIS
- Gram-negative folliculitis
- Staphylococcal pyoderma
- Acne rosacea
- Drug eruption
- Sebaceous hyperplasia
- Angiofibromas, basal cell carcinomas, osteoma cutis
- Occupational exposures to oils or grease
- Steroid acne

WORKUP
History and physical examination:
- Inquire about previous treatment
- Careful drug history
- Family history, history of cyclic menstrual flares
- History of use of cosmetics and cleansers
- Oral contraceptive use

LABORATORY TESTS
- Laboratory evaluation is generally not helpful.
- Patients who are candidates for therapy with isotretinoin (Accutane) should have baseline liver enzymes, cholesterol, and triglycerides checked, since this medication may result in elevation of lipids and liver enzymes.
- A negative serum pregnancy test should also be obtained in females 1 wk prior to initiation of isotretinoin; it is also imperative to maintain effective contraception during and 1 mo after therapy with Isotretinoin ends because of its teratogenic effects.

TREATMENT

NONPHARMACOLOGIC THERAPY
- Contrary to popular belief, diet has little or no bearing on acne. Greasy foods do not cause acne. If the patient, however, feels that a particular food is exacerbating the acne, it should be avoided.
- Acne is not caused by dirt; therefore, excessive washing is unnecessary.
- Long-term exposure to coal tar, machine oil, lubricating oils, and greases should be avoided; use of hair pomades containing oils should also be avoided; topical exposure to cocoa butter can also exacerbate acne and should be avoided.

ACUTE GENERAL Rx
Treatment generally varies with the severity of acne.
- Comedones can be treated with tretinoin (Retin-A); it is applied generally once qhs; large open comedones (blackheads) should be expressed.
- Patients should be reevaluated after 4 to 6 wk. Benzoyl peroxide gel (2.5% or 5%) may be added if the comedones become inflamed or form pustules. Topical antibiotics (erythromycin, clindamycin lotions or pads) can also be used in patients with significant inflammation.
- Pustular acne can be treated with tretinoin and benzoyl peroxide gel applied on alternate evenings; drying agents (sulfacetamide-sulfa lotions [Novacet, Sulfacet]) are also effective when used in combination with benzoyl peroxide; oral antibiotics (tetracycline 500 mg to 2 g qd or erythromycin 1 g qd given in two to three divided doses) are effective in patients with moderate to severe pustular acne; patients not responding well to these antibiotics can be switched over the minocycline 50 to 100 mg bid; however, this medication is more expensive.
- Patients with nodular cystic acne can be treated with periodic intralesional (triamcinolone) Kenalog injections by dermatologist.
- Isotretinoin is indicated for acne resistant to antibiotic therapy and severe acne; dosage is 0.5 to 1 mg/kg/day in two divided doses (maximum of 2 mg/kg/day); duration of therapy is generally 20 wk for a cumulative dose ≥120 mg/kg for severe cystic acne; before using this medication patients should undergo baseline laboratory evaluation (see above). This drug is absolutely contraindicated during pregnancy because of its teratogenicity.

REFERRAL
Referral for intralesional injection and dermabrasion should be considered in patients with severe acne unresponsive to conventional therapy.

MISCELLANEOUS

COMMENTS
Indications for systemic therapy of acne are:
- Painful deep papules or nodules
- Extensive lesions
- Active acne with severe scarring or hyperpigmentation
- Patient's morale

Patients should be educated that in most cases acne can be controlled but not cured and that at least 4 to 6 wk of initial therapy should be required before significant improvement is noted.

REFERENCES
Goulden D et al: Current indications for isotretinoin as a treatment for acne vulgaris, *Dermatology* 190:284, 1995.
Habif TP: *Clinical dermatology*, ed 3, St Louis, 1996, Mosby.
Lucky AW: Hormonal correlates of acne and hirsutism, *Am J Med* 98:89S, 1995.
Sykes NL, Webster GF: Acne, a review of optimum treatment, *Drugs* 48:59, 1994.

Author: **Fred F. Ferri, M.D.**

Acquired immunodeficiency syndrome (PTG)

BASIC INFORMATION

DEFINITION
Acquired immunodeficiency syndrome (AIDS) is a disorder caused by infection with the human immunodeficiency virus, type 1 (HIV-1) and marked by progressive deterioration of the cellular immune system leading to secondary infections or malignancies.

SYNONYMS
AIDS

ICD-9-CM CODES
042.9 AIDS, unspecified

EPIDEMIOLOGY AND DEMOGRAPHICS
INCIDENCE (IN U.S.):
- 27.1 cases/100,000 persons
- Varies widely by location
- 85% of cases in large cities

PREVALENCE (IN U.S.): 62 cases/100,000 persons
PREDOMINANT SEX: Males 87%, females 13% (through 1994)
PREDOMINANT AGE: 80% between ages 20 and 40 yr
PEAK INCIDENCE: See above
GENETICS:
- Familial disposition: no clear genetic predisposition
- Congenital infection:
  1. Transmittable from an infected mother to the fetus in utero in as many as 30% of pregnancies.
  2. No specific congenital malformations associated with infection; low birth weight and spontaneous abortion is possible.
- Neonatal infection: transmission possible to the neonate intrapartum or postpartum through breast-feeding

PHYSICAL FINDINGS
- Nonspecific findings: fever, weight loss, anorexia
- Specific syndromes:
  1. Seen in association with opportunistic infection and malignancies, so-called indicator diseases
  2. Most common:
     Respiratory infections (*Pneumocystis carinii* pneumonia, TB, bacterial pneumonia, fungal infection)
     CNS infections (toxoplasmosis, cryptococcal meningitis, TB)
     GI (cryptosporidiosis, isosporiasis, cytomegalovirus); Box 2-33 describes organisms associated with diarrhea in patients with AIDS
     Eye infections (cytomegalovirus, toxoplasmosis)
     Kaposi's sarcoma (cutaneous or visceral) or lymphoma (nodal or extranodal)
- Possibly asymptomatic
- Diagnosis of AIDS if T-lymphocyte subset analysis demonstrating CD4 cell count <200 or <14% of total lymphocyte in the presence of proven HIV infection even in the absence of other infections

ETIOLOGY
- Caused by infection with human immunodeficiency virus, type 1 (HIV-1, HIV)
- Transmitted by heterosexual or male homosexual contact, needle-sharing (during IV drug use), transfusion of contaminated blood or blood products, and from infected mother to fetus or neonate as described above

DIAGNOSIS

DIFFERENTIAL DIAGNOSIS
- Other wasting illnesses mimicking the nonspecific features of AIDS:
  1. TB
  2. Neoplasms
  3. Disseminated fungal infection
  4. Malabsorption syndromes
  5. Depression
- Other disorders associated with dementia or demyelination producing encephalopathy, myelopathy, or neuropathy

WORKUP
- Prompt evaluation of respiratory, CNS, GI complaints
- U.S. Preventive Services Task Force Recommendations regarding screening for HIV infection are described in Section V, Chapter 28.

LABORATORY TESTS
- HIV antibody testing
- T-lymphocyte subset analysis: performed to determine the degree of immunodeficiency
- Viral load assay: to plan long-term antiviral therapy
- CSF examination: for meningitis
- Serologic tests for syphilis, hepatitis B, hepatitis C, and toxoplasmosis

IMAGING STUDIES
- Cerebral CT for encephalopathy or focal CNS complications (e.g., toxoplasmosis, lymphoma)
- Pulmonary gallium scanning to aid in the diagnosis of a *Pneumocystis carinii* pneumonia

TREATMENT

NONPHARMACOLOGIC THERAPY
- Maintain adequate caloric intake
- Encourage good oral hygiene, regular dental care

ACUTE GENERAL Rx
Acute management of opportunistic infections and malignancies are reviewed elsewhere in this text under specific AIDS-related disorders.

CHRONIC Rx
For all HIV-infected patients, particularly those meeting the case definition of AIDS:
- Preventive therapy for *Pneumocystis carinii* pneumonia and TB (see specific chapters elsewhere in this text)
- Antiretroviral therapy employing combinations of nucleoside derivative agents: zidovudine (AZT), didanosine (DDI), zalcitabine (DDC), lamivudine (3TC), stavudine (D4T) with or without the addition of protease inhibitors (saquinavir, ritonavir, indinavir) according to current recommendations based on clinical stage and viral load studies; Table 7-12 compares currently available antiviral agents.
- An approach to evaluating chronic diarrhea in patients with HIV infection is described in Fig. 3-29; Table 3-4 describes common GI pathogens associated with HIV infection.

DISPOSITION
AIDS is a chronic disease whose course is often marked by increasingly severe complications and worsening disability.

REFERRAL
All patients with AIDS: to a physician knowledgeable and experienced in the management of the disease and its complications

MISCELLANEOUS

COMMENTS
- Multidisciplinary involvement by nursing, social service, and medical personnel is required for care of patients with AIDS.
- Investigational treatment protocols are available at many large medical centers and through community consortia in high-prevalence areas.
- U.S. Preventive Services Task Force Recommendations on counseling to prevent HIV infection and other STDs are described in Section V, Chapter 62.

REFERENCES
Carpenter CCJ et al: Antiretroviral therapy for HIV infection in 1996: recommendations of an international panel, *JAMA* 276(2):146, 1996.

Masci JR: *Outpatient management of HIV infection*, St Louis, 1996, Mosby.

Author: **Joseph R. Masci, M.D.**

Acromegaly (PTG)

BASIC INFORMATION

DEFINITION
Acromegaly is a chronic debilitating disease with an insidious onset, resulting from the effects of either hypersecretion of growth hormone (GH) or increased amounts of a insulin-like growth factor I (IGF-I).

SYNONYMS
Marie's disease

ICD-9-CM CODES
253.0 Acromegaly

EPIDEMIOLOGY AND DEMOGRAPHICS
INCIDENCE: 3 to 4 new cases/1,000,000 persons
PREVALENCE: 50 to 60 cases/1,000,000 persons, with some estimates as high as 90 cases/1,000,000 persons
PREDOMINANT SEX: No sexual predominance
MEAN AGE AT DIAGNOSIS: Males: 40 yr; females: 45 yr
RISK FACTORS:
- Increased mortality, primarily from cardiovascular and respiratory causes
- Death in 50% of untreated patients by age 50 (twice the rate of the general population)
- Increased prevalence of colon carcinoma as well as other malignancies

PHYSICAL FINDINGS
- Coarse features resulting from growth of soft tissue
- Coarse, oily skin
- Hands and feet that are spade-like, fleshy, and moist
- Prognathism, which can give an underbite
- Carpal tunnel syndrome
- Excessive sweating
- Arthralgias and severe osteoarthritis
- History of increased hat, glove, and/or shoe size
- Hypertension
- Skin tags
- Muscle weakness and decreased exercise capacity
- Headache, often severe
- Diabetes mellitus
- Visual field defects

ETIOLOGY
Cause is usually a pituitary adenoma, affecting the anterior lobe.

DIAGNOSIS

DIFFERENTIAL DIAGNOSIS
Ectopic production of growth hormone-releasing hormone (GHRH) from a carcinoid or other neuroendocrine tumor

WORKUP
1. First screening test: Measure serum IGF-I level.
   a. Direct measurement of the GH level is not as useful, since it is secreted in a pulsatile fashion and a random level may be falsely normal.
   b. Upper limits of a normal IGF-I level, depending on the assay: >380 ng/mL or 2.5 U/mL.
2. Failure to suppress serum GH to less than 2 ng/mL after 100 g oral glucose is considered conclusive.
   a. Patients may show suppression of GH or a paradoxical response.
   b. Patients will not suppress GH to 2 ng/mL or less (the normal response).
   c. GHRH level >300 ng/mL is indicative of an ectopic source of GH.

LABORATORY TESTS
- Elevated serum phosphate
- Elevated urine calcium

IMAGING STUDIES
- Imaging studies of choice: MRI of the pituitary and hypothalamus
- CT of the pituitary and hypothalamus used initially

TREATMENT

SURGERY
Treatment of choice: transsphenoidal microsurgical adenomectomy
- Surgical failure rate: about 13.3% for microadenomas (tumors <10 mm) and 11.1% for macroadenomas (tumors >10 mm confined to the sella)
- Preoperative IGF-I level: indicator of surgical outcome with higher levels in the surgical failure group

RADIOTHERAPY
- Irradiation to reduce further growth of the tumor in most patients
- Major complication: hypopituitarism, which may occur in up to 50% of patients; this complication is more likely in patients who had surgery irradiation

MEDICAL Rx
- Indicated when patients have failed surgical therapy, when surgery is contraindicated, and in patients waiting for the effects of radiotherapy to begin
- Octreotide
  1. A somatostatin analogue given tid at a dose of 100 μg subcutaneously
  2. Important side effects: biliary sludge and gallstones; nausea, cramps, and steatorrhea; suppression of GH levels to about 5 μg/L in 52% of patients, IGF-I levels normalized to about 53%
  3. Important in the preoperative shrinkage of pituitary tumors and softening of adenomatous tissue
- Bromocriptine
  1. A dopamine analogue given at a dosage of 10 to 60 mg orally tid to qid
  2. Less effective than octreotide
  3. Important advantages: less expensive than octreotide and taken orally
  4. Important side effects: orthostatic hypotension, lightheadedness, nausea, constipation, and nasal stuffiness
  5. Suppresses GH levels to <5 μg/L in about 20% of patients; normalizes GH levels in approximately 10%, and shrinks pituitary adenomas in 10% to 20%; IGF-I levels normalized to about 10%

CHRONIC Rx
Combination of bromocriptine and octreotide may be synergistic, allowing a lower combination dosage than alone.

DISPOSITION
- Patients receiving radiotherapy need long-term follow-up to monitor the potential development of hypopituitarism.
- Continuation of medical therapy should be based on the normalization of IGF-I levels.

MISCELLANEOUS

REFERENCES
Jaffe CA, Barkan AL: Acromegaly: recognition and treatment, *Drugs* 47(3):425, 1994.

Krishna AY, Phillips LS: Management of acromegaly: a review, *Am J Med Sci* 308(6):370, 1994.

Author: **Candace C. Green, M.D.**

Addison's disease (PTG)

BASIC INFORMATION

DEFINITION
Addison's disease is characterized by inadequate secretion of corticosteroids resulting from partial or complete destruction of the adrenal glands.

SYNONYMS
Primary adrenocortical insufficiency

ICD-9-CM CODES
255.4 Addison's disease

EPIDEMIOLOGY AND DEMOGRAPHICS
PREVALENCE: 5 cases/100,000 persons
PREDOMINANT SEX: Female:male ratio of 2:1

PHYSICAL FINDINGS
- Hyperpigmentation: more prominent in palmar creases, buccal mucosa, pressure points (elbows, knees, knuckles), perianal mucosa, and around areolas of nipples
- Hypotension
- Generalized weakness
- Amenorrhea and loss of axillary hair in females

ETIOLOGY
- Autoimmune destruction of the adrenal glands (80% of cases)
- Tuberculosis (15% of cases)
- Carcinomatous destruction of the adrenal glands
- Adrenal hemorrhage (anticoagulants, trauma, coagulopathies, pregnancy, sepsis)
- Adrenal infarction (arteritis, thrombosis)
- Other: sarcoidosis, amyloidosis, postoperative, fungal infections, AIDS

DIAGNOSIS

DIFFERENTIAL DIAGNOSIS
Sepsis, hypovolemic shock, acute abdomen, apathetic hyperthyroidism in the elderly, myopathies, GI malignancy, major depression, anorexia nervosa, hemochromatosis, salt-losing nephritis, chronic infection

WORKUP
- If the clinical picture is highly suggestive of adrenocortical insufficiency, the diagnosis can be made with the rapid ACTH (Cortrosyn) test:
  1. Give 250 μg ACTH by IV push and measure cortisol levels at 0 and 30 min.
  2. Cortisol level <20 μg/dl at 30 or 60 min is suggestive of adrenal insufficiency.
  3. Measure plasma ACTH. A high ACTH level confirms primary adrenal insufficiency.
- Secondary adrenocortical insufficiency (caused by pituitary dysfunction) can be distinguished from primary adrenal insufficiency by the following:
  1. Normal or low plasma ACTH level following rapid ACTH (Cortrosyn) test
  2. Absence of hyperpigmentation
  3. No significant impairment of aldosterone secretion (because aldosterone secretion is under control of the renin-angiotensin system)
  4. Additional evidence of hypopituitarism (e.g., hypogonadism, hypothyroidism)

LABORATORY TESTS
- Increased potassium, decreased sodium and chloride
- Decreased glucose
- Increased BUN/creatinine ratio (prerenal azotemia)
- Mild normocytic, normochromic anemia, neutropenia, lymphocytosis, eosinophilia (significant dehydration may mask hyponatremia and anemia)
- PPD and antiadrenal antibodies

IMAGING STUDIES
- Chest x-ray examination may reveal a small-sized heart.
- Abdominal x-ray film: adrenal calcifications may be noted if the adrenocortical insufficiency is secondary to TB or fungus.
- Abdominal CT scan: small adrenal glands generally indicate either idiopathic atrophy or long-standing TB, whereas enlarged glands are suggestive of early TB or potentially treatable diseases.

TREATMENT

NONPHARMACOLOGIC THERAPY
- Perform periodic monitoring of serum electrolytes, vital signs, and body weight; liberal sodium intake is suggested.
- Periodic measurement of bone density may be helpful in identifying patients at risk for the development of osteoporosis.

Patients should carry a Medic Alert bracelet and an emergency pack containing hydrocortisone 100 mg ampule, syringe, and needle. Patients and partners should be educated on how to give IM injection in case of vomiting or coma.

ACUTE GENERAL Rx
Addisonian crisis is an acute complication of adrenal insufficiency characterized by circulatory collapse, dehydration, nausea, vomiting, hypoglycemia, and hyperkalemia.
1. Draw plasma cortisol level; do not delay therapy while waiting for confirming laboratory results.
2. Administer dexamethasone sodium phosphate 4 mg q12h or hydrocortisone 100 mg IV q6h for 24 hr; if patient shows good clinical response, gradually taper dosage and change to oral maintenance dose (usually prednisone 7.5 mg/day).
3. Provide adequate volume replacement with D_5NS solution until hypotension, dehydration, and hypoglycemia are completely corrected. Large volumes (2 to 3 L) may be necessary in the first 2 to 3 hr to correct the volume deficit and hypoglycemia and to avoid further hyponatremia.

Identify and correct any precipitating factor (e.g., sepsis, hemorrhage).

CHRONIC Rx
- Give hydrocortisone 15 to 20 mg PO every morning and 5 to 10 mg in late afternoon or prednisone 5 mg in morning and 2.5 mg hs.
- Give fludroxycortisone acetate 0.1 mg/day: this mineralocorticoid is necessary if the patient has primary adrenocortical insufficiency.
- Instruct patients to increase glucocorticoid replacement in times of stress and to receive parenteral glucocorticoids if diarrhea or vomiting occurs.

DISPOSITION
- Lifelong medical supervision is necessary to monitor adequacy of therapy and prevent complications.
- Adrenal function is rarely recovered.
- Life expectancy is in the normal range if adequately treated.

REFERRAL
Hospital admission and endocrinology consult for Addisonian crisis

MISCELLANEOUS

COMMENTS
Patient education material may be obtained from the National Addison's Disease Foundation, 505 Northern Blvd., Suite 200, Great Neck, NY 11021, phone: (516) 487-4992.

REFERENCES
Oelkers W: Adrenal Insufficiency, *N Engl J Med* 335:1206, 1996.

Author: **Fred F. Ferri, M.D.**

Agoraphobia and panic (PTG)

BASIC INFORMATION

DEFINITION
In the U.S., agoraphobia is considered part of the continuum of panic attacks and panic disorder. In Europe, agoraphobia is conceptualized as a phobic condition independent of panic. A *panic attack* is a relatively brief, sudden episode of intense fear or apprehension, often associated with a sense of impending doom and various uncomfortable and disquieting physical symptoms. *Panic disorder* is diagnosed if at least one panic attack is followed by a significant degree of concern about future attacks or a major change in behavior related to these attacks. Agoraphobia is anxiety about, or avoidance of, places or situations in which the ability to leave suddenly is limited or impossible in the event of having a panic attack.

SYNONYMS
Anxiety attacks
Fear attacks

ICD-10-CM CODES
F 41.0 Panic disorder without agoraphobia (DSM-IV: 300.01)
F 40.01 Panic disorder with agoraphobia (DSM-IV: 300.01)

EPIDEMIOLOGY AND DEMOGRAPHICS
INCIDENCE (IN U.S.): 1% 1-mo incidence of panic attacks
PREVALENCE (IN U.S.):
- 15% lifetime prevalence of panic attacks
- Panic disorder much more uncommon, with a lifetime prevalence of 1.5% to 3.5%; chronicity of condition reflected by a similar 1-yr prevalence rate of 1% to 2%
- Agoraphobia relatively rare; 0.3% to 1% lifetime prevalence

PREDOMINANT SEX:
- Women more commonly affected (>85% of clinical population)
- Panic disorder twice as common in women
- Panic disorder with agoraphobia three times as common in women

PREDOMINANT AGE:
- Age of onset earlier in males (24 yr) than females (28 yr)
- Onset after age 45 yr rare

PEAK INCIDENCE:
- Chronic condition with a waxing and waning course
- Bimodal incidence peaks noted, with the first peak between ages 15 and 24 yr and second peak between 35 and 44 yr

GENETICS:
- Risk of developing panic disorder in first-degree relatives of individuals with panic disorder four to seven times that of general population
- Findings in twin studies: about 60% of contributing factors to panic are genetic

PHYSICAL FINDINGS
- Panic disorder
  1. Present either with a panic attack or with fear and anxiety related to anticipation of a future panic attack
  2. Typical presentation: unexpected, untriggered periods of intense anxiety and fear with associated physiologic changes (e.g., palpitations, sweating, tremulousness, shortness of breath, chest pain, GI distress, faintness, derealization, paresthesia)
  3. Emergency or physician visits frequently occasioned by physical symptoms

- Agoraphobia
  1. Rare complaints to physician
  2. Activities usually self-limited by avoiding public situations where the patient might experience a panic attack and would be unable to exit readily, such as the following:
     Crowded public areas (stores, public transportation, church)
     Individual interactions (hairdresser, neighborhood meetings)
  3. On exposure to or anticipation of exposure to such situations, significant anxiety occurs

ETIOLOGY
Hypotheses (NOTE: There is sufficient data to support each model.)
1. Central dyscontrol of autonomic arousal (typically localized to the locus ceruleus)
2. Cognitive overreaction to relatively mild physiologic cues
3. Dysfunction of a central suffocation alarm mechanism

DIAGNOSIS

DIFFERENTIAL DIAGNOSIS
- Medical conditions
  1. Arrhythmias
  2. Hyperthyroidism
  3. Hyperparathyroidism
  4. Seizure disorders
  5. Respiratory diseases
  6. Pheochromocytoma
- Therapeutic (theophylline, steroids) and recreational (cocaine, amphetamine, caffeine) drugs and drug withdrawal (alcohol, barbiturates, benzodiazepines)

- Phobias (e.g., specific phobia or social phobia)
- Obsessive-compulsive disorder (cued by exposure to the object of the obsession)
- Posttraumatic stress disorder (cued by recall of a stressor)

WORKUP
- Emergency presentation: cardiac, respiratory, or neurologic symptoms
- History and physical examination to rule out a concomitant medical condition

NOTE: Panic disorder and agoraphobia are not diagnoses of exclusion, but exclusion of other conditions is usually required.

LABORATORY TESTS
- Thyroid profile
- Electrolyte measures, including calcium
- Toxicology screen
- ECG
- Acute cases: possible monitoring and cardiac enzymes to rule out arrhythmia or ischemia

IMAGING STUDIES
- For temporal lobe dysfunction (e.g., temporal lesions or as ictal or interictal manifestation of temporal lobe seizures): brain CT scan or MRI and/or an EEG in some patients
- Holter monitor to rule out occult or episodic arrhythmias
- Chest x-ray examination, ABG, or pulmonary function tests if respiratory compromise suspected

TREATMENT

NONPHARMACOLOGIC THERAPY
- Psychotherapy: generally very effective; long-term follow-up studies of panic patients suggest that therapy is possibly superior to pharmacologic interventions
- Interpersonal and cognitive-behavioral therapy modalities: most extensively studied

ACUTE GENERAL Rx
- Benzodiazepines, particularly alprazolam: very effective in acute setting
- Low-dose alprazolam for patients with rare panic attacks and asymptomatic interattack periods (0.25 to 0.5 mg orally or sublingually on a PRN basis)

CHRONIC Rx
- Because panic disorder patients, as a group, have a low likelihood of abusing benzodiazepines, uncomplicated cases managed with low-dose benzodiazepines on a scheduled or PRN basis
- Preferred pharmacologic agents: antidepressants with a significant serotonin reuptake inhibitory action
- Imipramine quite effective in both panic disorder and agoraphobia
- Newer antidepressants (paroxetine, sertraline, and fluoxetine) quite effective in preventing panic attacks and ameliorating agoraphobia

DISPOSITION
- Typical course chronic but with significant waxing and waning (common to have long periods of remission)
- Presence of agoraphobia associated with a more chronic course
- Findings with long-term follow-up studies: 6 to 10 yr posttreatment, some 30% in remission, 40% to 50% improved with residual symptoms, and the remainder either unchanged or worse

REFERRAL
Referral needed if:
- Patients do not respond to a serotonin reuptake inhibitor
- Therapy is the preferred treatment

MISCELLANEOUS

REFERENCES
Eaton WW et al: Panic and panic disorder in the United States, *Am J Psychiatry* 151:413, 1994.

Roth M: The panic-agoraphobic syndrome: a paradigm of the anxiety group of disorders and its implications for psychiatric practice and theory, *Am J Psychiatry* 153:111, 1996.

Sheehan DV, Harnett-Sheehan K: The role of SSRIs in panic disorder, *J Clin Psychiatry* 57(suppl 10):51, 1996.

Author: **Rif S. El-Mallakh, M.D.**

Alcoholism (PTG)

BASIC INFORMATION

DEFINITION
Although it is impossible to define alcoholism precisely, among the commonly used screening instruments for this disorder are the CAGE questionnaire (Box A-8), short Michigan Alcoholism Screening Test (SMAST) (Box A-7), National Council on Alcoholism criteria, and DSM-III-A criteria.

SYNONYMS
Alcohol abuse
Substance abuse

ICD-9-CM CODES
303.9 Alcoholism

EPIDEMIOLOGY AND DEMOGRAPHICS
INCIDENCE (IN U.S.):
- See "Prevalence."
- 20% achieve abstinence without help, 70% achieve sobriety for 1 yr.

PREVALENCE (IN U.S.): 7% of population 18 yr or older

PREDOMINANT SEX:
- Lifetime risk for males 8% to 10%
- Lifetime risk for females 3% to 5%

PEAK INCIDENCE: 20 to 40 yr

GENETICS: More common with a family history of alcoholism and in patients of Irish, Scandinavian, and Native American descent

PHYSICAL FINDINGS
- Recurring minor trauma
- GI bleeding
- Pancreatitis
- Liver disease
- Odor of alcohol on breath
- Tremulousness
- Tachycardia
- Peripheral neuropathy
- Recent memory loss
- Box A-9 describes the CIWA-Ar scale for assessing severity of alcohol withdrawal syndrome.

ETIOLOGY
- Social and genetic factors important
- Risk factors:
  1. Broken homes
  2. Unemployment
  3. Divorce
  4. Recurrent depression
  5. Addiction to another substance, including tobacco

DIAGNOSIS

WORKUP
- Screening tests (CAGE or SMAST; see Boxes A-7 and A-8)
- Blood studies
- Stool for occult blood

LABORATORY TESTS
- γ-Glutamyltransferase (GGT)
- Aspartate aminotransferase (SGOT, AST)
- Mean corpuscular volume (MCV)

IMAGING STUDIES
Indicated only if there is a history of trauma

TREATMENT

NONPHARMACOLOGIC THERAPY
Abstinence

ACUTE GENERAL Rx
- Observe for delirium tremens (DTs): if sympathetic symptoms occur, administer diazepam or other benzodiazepines (see Table 7-14).
- IM thiamine is mandatory in DTs and in acute extraocular disorders.

CHRONIC Rx
See "Referral."

DISPOSITION
See "Referral."

REFERRAL
- To Alcoholics Anonymous or Adult Children of Alcoholics
- Family members to Al-Anon or Al-A-Teen

MISCELLANEOUS

COMMENTS
- Frequently underdiagnosed by the primary care physician
- U.S. Preventive Services Task Force Recommendations for screening for problem drinking are described in Section V, Chapter 52.

REFERENCES
Magruder-Habib K, Durand AM, Frey KA: Alcohol abuse and alcoholism in primary health care settings, *J Fam Pract* 32:406, 1991.

Meyer RE: Toward a comprehensive theory of alcoholism, *Ann NY Acad Sci* 708:238, 1994.

Olson WH et al: Alcoholism. In: *Symptom oriented neurology*, Chicago, 1989, Year Book.

Schuckit MA, Irwin M: Diagnosis of alcoholism, *Med Clin North Am* 72:1133, 1988.

Author: **William H. Olson, M.D.**

Aldosteronism, primary (PTG)

BASIC INFORMATION

DEFINITION
Primary aldosteronism is a clinical syndrome characterized by hypokalemia, hypertension, low plasma renin activity (PRA), and excessive aldosterone secretion.

SYNONYMS
Conn's syndrome
Hyperaldosteronism

ICD-9-CM CODES
255.1 Primary aldosteronism

EPIDEMIOLOGY AND DEMOGRAPHICS
INCIDENCE/PREVALENCE: 1% to 2% of patients with hypertension; more common in females

PHYSICAL FINDINGS
- Generally asymptomatic
- If significant hypokalemia is present, possible muscle cramping, weakness, paresthesias
- Hypertension
- Polyuria, polydipsia

ETIOLOGY
- Aldosterone-producing adenoma (>60%)
- Idiopathic hyperaldosteronism (>30%)
- Glucocorticoid-suppressible hyperaldosteronism (<1%)
- Aldosterone-producing carcinoma (<1%)

DIAGNOSIS

DIFFERENTIAL DIAGNOSIS
- Diuretic use
- Hypokalemia from vomiting, diarrhea
- Renovascular hypertension
- Other endocrine neoplasm (pheochromocytoma, deoxycorticosterone-producing tumor, renin-secreting tumor)

WORKUP
In patients with hypokalemia and a low PRA (1), confirming tests for primary hyperaldosteronism include the following:
- 24-hr urine test for aldosterone and potassium levels (potassium >40 mEq and aldosterone >15 µg).
- Captopril test: administer 25 to 50 mg of captopril (ACE inhibitor) and measure plasma renin and aldosterone levels 1 to 2 hr later. A plasma aldosterone level >15 ng/dl confirms the diagnosis of primary aldosteronism. This test is more expensive and is best reserved for situations in which the 24-hr urine for aldosterone is ambiguous.
- 24-hr urinary tetrahydroaldosterone (<65 µg/24 hr) and saline infusion test (plasma aldosterone >10 ng/dl), can also be used in ambiguous cases.
- The renin-aldosterone stimulation test (posture test) is helpful in differentiating IHA from aldosterone-producing adenoma (APA). Patients with APA have a decrease in aldosterone levels at 4 hr, whereas patients with IHA have an increase in their aldosterone levels.
- Bilateral adrenal venous sampling may be done to localize APA when adrenal CT scan is equivocal. In APA, ipsilateral/contralateral aldosterone level is >10:1, and ipsilateral venous aldosterone concentration is very high (>1000 ng/dl).

LABORATORY TESTS
- Hypokalemia
- Low ambulatory PRA (≤1)
- Possible alkalosis and hypernatremia

IMAGING STUDIES
- Adrenal CT scan (with 3-mm cuts) to localize neoplasm
- Adrenal scanning with iodocholesterol (NP-59) to localize APA

TREATMENT

NONPHARMACOLOGIC THERAPY
- Regular monitoring and control of blood pressure
- Low-sodium diet, tobacco avoidance, maintenance of ideal body weight, and regular exercise program

ACUTE GENERAL Rx
- Control of blood pressure and hypokalemia with spironolactone, amiloride, or ACE inhibitors
- Surgery (unilateral adrenalectomy) for APA

CHRONIC Rx
Chronic medical therapy with spironolactone, amiloride, or ACE inhibitors to control blood pressure and hypokalemia is necessary in all patients with bilateral idiopathic hyperaldosteronism.

DISPOSITION
Unilateral adrenalectomy normalizes hypertension and hypokalemia in 70% of patients with APA after 1 yr. After 5 yr, 50% of patients remain normotensive.

REFERRAL
Surgical referral for unilateral adrenalectomy following confirmation of unilateral APA or carcinoma

MISCELLANEOUS

COMMENTS
- Frequent monitoring of blood pressure and electrolytes postoperatively is necessary, since normotension after unilateral adrenalectomy may take up to 4 mo.
- Fig. 3-2 describes a diagnostic approach to patients with adrenal mass.

REFERENCES
Blumenfeld JD et al: Diagnosis and treatment of primary hyperaldosteronism, *Ann Intern Med* 121:877, 1994.
Litchfield WR, Druhy RG: Primary aldosteronism, *Metab Clin North Am* 24: 593, 1995.
Noble J (ed): *Textbook of primary care medicine*, ed 2, St Louis, 1996, Mosby.
Author: **Fred F. Ferri, M.D.**

Alzheimer's disease (PTG)

BASIC INFORMATION

DEFINITION
DSM-IV defines Alzheimer's as follows:
A. The development of multiple cognitive deficits manifested by both:
  1. Memory impairment (impaired ability to learn new information and to recall previously learned information)
  2. One (or more) of the following cognitive disturbances:
     a. Aphasia (language disturbance)
     b. Apraxia (impaired ability to carry out motor activities despite intact motor function)
     c. Agnosia (failure to recognize or identify objects despite intact sensory function)
     d. Disturbance in executive functioning (i.e., planning, organizing, sequencing, abstracting)
B. The cognitive deficits in criteria A1 and A2 each cause significant impairment in social or occupational functioning and represent a significant decline from a previous level of functioning.
C. The course is characterized by gradual onset and continuing cognitive decline.
D. The cognitive deficits in criteria A1 and A2 are not a result of any of the following:
  1. Other central nervous system conditions that cause progressive deficits in memory and cognition (e.g., cerebrovascular disease, Parkinson's disease, Huntington's disease, subdural hematoma, normal-pressure hydrocephalus, brain tumor)
  2. Systemic conditions that are known to cause dementia (e.g., hypothyroidism, vitamin B_{12} or folic acid deficiency, niacin deficiency, hypercalcemia, neurosyphilis, HIV infection)
  3. Substance-induced conditions
E. The deficits do not occur exclusively during the course of a delirium.
F. The disturbance is not better accounted for by another Axis I disorder (e.g., major depressive disorder, schizophrenia).

ICD-9-CM CODES
331.0 Alzheimer's disease

EPIDEMIOLOGY AND DEMOGRAPHICS
INCIDENCE (IN U.S.): 3.5% of Americans ages 65 to 74 yr
PREDOMINANT SEX: Female
PREDOMINANT AGE: 85+ yr
PEAK INCIDENCE: 65 to 74 yr
GENETICS:
- Patients with trisomy 21 (Down syndrome) develop Alzheimer's in middle age.

PHYSICAL FINDINGS
Families often bring patient to medical attention because of memory problems (e.g., repetitive questions, misplacement of items, missed appointments, getting lost away from home), hallucinations, disruptive behavior, insomnia, and anxiety/depression disorders. Initial screen of cognitive function: diagnosis requires a documentation of a decline in cognition from a previous level. Perform Folstein Mini-Mental State Examination (see Fig. A-1).
- Orientation to time and space: based on intact registration and recall (short-term memory); orientation to space is preserved longer than orientation to time.
- Registration: depends on hearing and paying attention, if patient unable to complete task, consider the diagnosis of delirium (see above).
- Attention and calculation: to avoid educational bias, use simple tasks such as saying the days of the week forward and backward or counting backward from 20 to 0; since this function is preserved very late in Alzheimer's disease, if patient unable to complete task, consider a frontal lobe dementia such as Pick's disease or delirium.
- Recall: patients with early stages of dementia will make first errors in this function, often with no other errors in the examination. Errors in orientation follow next.
- Language: patients with early stages of Alzheimer's disease will have specific difficulty drawing a clock showing a given time. This is a measure of the characteristic visual-spatial impairment.
- Consider comprehensive neuropsychologic testing by a qualified neuropsychologist to confirm screening mental status testing. This testing can help differentiate parietal-temporal dementias (AD or PD) from frontal-temporal dementias, such as Pick's, or focal dementias, such as vascular dementias.

DIAGNOSIS

WORKUP
- U.S. Preventive Services Task Force Recommendations for screening for dementia are described in Section V, Chapter 48.
- Screening tests for dementia are described in Table 3-3.
- Lumbar puncture if infection suspected

LABORATORY TESTS
- CBC
- Serum electrolytes
- Glucose
- BUN/creatinine
- Liver and thyroid function tests
- Serum B_{12}
- Syphilis serology
- HIV, sedimentation rate, urinalysis

IMAGING STUDIES
- CT scan or MRI to rule out hydrocephalus, mass lesions

TREATMENT

NONPHARMACOLOGIC THERAPY
Patients must have a caregiver; enrollment in adult day care centers is helpful.

ACUTE GENERAL Rx
None

CHRONIC Rx
- Estrogen replacement may reduce incidence in women.
- Tacrine (Cognex) may be helpful in early Alzheimer's disease. Frequent monitoring of liver enzymes is necessary.
- Donepezil (Aricept) 5 mg PO at hs initially may be used in mild to moderate dementia.

MISCELLANEOUS

COMMENTS
The physician must make a thorough search for the treatable causes of dementia.

REFERENCES
DSM-IV: Diagnostic and Statistical Manual of Mental Disorders, ed 4; Washington DC, 1994, American Psychiatric Association.

Fretwell MD: Cognitive Dysfunction. In Ferri FF, Fretwell MD, Wachtel (eds): *Practical Guide to the Care of the Geriatric Patient,* ed 2, St Louis, 1997, Mosby. Ferri, Fretwell, Wachtel eds.

Golden R: Dementia and Alzheimer's disease: indications, diagnosis, and treatment, *Minn Med* 78:25, 1995.

Sandson TA, Sperling RA, Price BH: Alzheimer's disease: an update, *Compr Ther* 21:480, 1995.

Author: **William H. Olson, M.D.**

Amaurosis fugax (PTG)

BASIC INFORMATION

DEFINITION
Amaurosis fugax is a temporary loss of vision in one eye caused by transient interference with its blood supply.

ICD-9-CM CODES
362.34 Amaurosis fugax

EPIDEMIOLOGY AND DEMOGRAPHICS
INCIDENCE (IN U.S.): An uncommon presentation of carotid artery disease
PEAK INCIDENCE: 55 yr and older

PHYSICAL FINDINGS
- There are usually no physical findings.
- Acute stage: cholesterol emboli are possible in retinal artery (Hollenhorst plaque): carotid bruits or other evidence of generalized atherosclerosis.
- If embolus is cardiac in origin, atrial fibrillation is often present.

ETIOLOGY
Usually embolic

DIAGNOSIS

DIFFERENTIAL DIAGNOSIS
- Embolic from carotid artery, aorta and great vessels, heart
- Ocular causes: glaucoma, central retinal vein or artery occlusion
- Neurologic causes: optic neuritis, multiple sclerosis, optic nerve compression
- Systemic disorders: migraine, giant cell arteritis, blood dyscrasia

WORKUP
- Careful examination of retina
- Auscultation of arteries for bruits
- Examination of all pulses

LABORATORY TESTS
- CBC with sedimentation rate
- PT and PTT
- Serum chemistries, including lipid profile
- Anticardiolipin antibody, Protein C and Protein S should be considered in younger patients with a personal or family history of coagulopathy or strokes at a young age.
- VDRL and toxicology screen are discretionary tests based on patient's age and history.

IMAGING STUDIES
- Carotid Dopplers followed by MRA or four-vessel angiography as indicated
- Transthoracic echocardiography (TTE) is indicated to screen for embolization in patients with evidence of heart disease and in patients without an evident source for their transient neurologic deficit. Transesophageal echocardiography (TEE) is more sensitive for detecting cardiac sources of embolization (ventricular mural thrombus, patent foramen ovale, aortic arch, mitral valve disorders), however it is more uncomfortable and expensive and is best reserved for patients with an unknown source of TIA or when cardiac embolization cannot be completely ruled out on TTE.

TREATMENT

NONPHARMACOLOGIC THERAPY
- Diet
- Exercise
- Cessation of tobacco use if thought to be atherosclerotic in origin

ACUTE GENERAL Rx
- Treat as an emergency.
- Give aspirin, heparin if there is no intracranial hemorrhage.

CHRONIC Rx
Reduce risks by carotid endarterectomy if stenosis >80%. Control hypertension and manage risk factors for increased cholesterol levels.

DISPOSITION
If significant stenosis not found and emboli are from carotid, consider other causes in differential diagnosis.

REFERRAL
Vascular surgeon or neurosurgeon if significant stenosis found
- Carotid endarterectomy is indicated in the following settings:
  1. High-grade (≥ 70%) isolateral stenosis and surgery can be done early and at low risk
  2. Greater than 50% stenosis associated with a large carotid artery ulcer
  3. Multiple TIAs despite medical therapy, in the setting of high-grade or ulcerative ipsilateral disease, and surgery can be done at low to medium risk
  4. Crescendo attacks in the setting of high-grade or ulcerative ipsilateral disease and surgery can be done at low to medium risk.
- Patient preference and the experience of the surgical team should be considered whenever surgery is contemplated.

MISCELLANEOUS

COMMENTS
Although amaurosis fugax is relatively rare, this classic presentation of carotid artery disease is often accompanied by a transient contralateral hemiparesis.

REFERENCES
Amaurosis Fugax Study Group: Current management of amaurosis fugax, *Stroke* 21:201, 1990.
Burdo RM: Amaurosis fugax: an overview, *J Clin Neuro-Ophthalmol* 9:195, 1989.
Feinberg AW: The evaluation of amaurosis fugax, *Hosp Pract* 27:47, 1992.
Feinberg AW: Recognition and significance of amaurosis fugax, *Heart Disease and Stroke* 2:392, 1993.

Author: **William H. Olson, M.D.**

Amblyopia

BASIC INFORMATION

DEFINITION
Amblyopia refers to a decrease in vision in one or both eyes in the presence of an otherwise normal ophthalmologic examination.

SYNONYMS
- Deprivation amblyopia
- Occlusion amblyopia
- Strabismus amblyopia
- Refractive amblyopia
- Organic or toxic amblyopias
- Lazy eye

ICD-9-CM CODES
368.00 Amblyopia

EPIDEMIOLOGY AND DEMOGRAPHICS
INCIDENCE (IN U.S.): 1% to 4% of the general population
PREVALENCE (IN U.S.): High incidence in premature infants with drug-dependent mothers and in neurologically impaired children
PREDOMINANT SEX: None
PREDOMINANT AGE: Childhood
PEAK INCIDENCE: Childhood

PHYSICAL FINDINGS
Decreased vision using best refraction in the presence of normal corneal, lens, retinal, and optic nerve appearance

ETIOLOGY
- Visual deprivation
- Strabismus
- Occlusion with patching
- Refractive error organic lesions in the nervous system
- Toxins

DIAGNOSIS

DIFFERENTIAL DIAGNOSIS
- Central nervous system (CNS) disease
- Optic nerve disorders
- Corneal or other eye diseases

WORKUP
- Complete eye examination
- Motility evaluation
- U.S. Preventive Services Task Force Recommendations for screening for visual impairment are described in Section V, Chapter 33.

LABORATORY TESTS
Usually none

IMAGING STUDIES
Usually not necessary unless CNS lesion suspected

TREATMENT

NONPHARMACOLOGIC THERAPY
- Glasses
- Patches
- Removal of the cause of the amblyopia if possible
- Surgery to align the eyes

CHRONIC Rx
Patching or optics, including prisms

DISPOSITION
Immediate patching, alternating eyes daily

REFERRAL
To ophthalmologist if vision is compromised

MISCELLANEOUS

COMMENTS
The earlier the referral, the better the outcome.

REFERENCES
Rubin SE, Nelson LB: Amblyopia: diagnosis and management, *Pediatr Clin North Am* 40:727, 1993.

Author: **Melvyn Koby, M.D.**

Amebiasis (PTG)

BASIC INFORMATION

DEFINITION
Amebiasis is an infection caused by the protozoal parasite *Entameba histolytica*. Although primarily an infection of the colon, amebiasis may cause extraintestinal disease, particularly liver abscess.

SYNONYMS
Amebic dysentery (when severe intestinal infection)

ICD-9-CM CODES
006.9 Amebiasis

EPIDEMIOLOGY AND DEMOGRAPHICS
INCIDENCE (IN U.S.): Highest in institutionalized patients, sexually active homosexual men
PREVALENCE (IN U.S.): 4% (80% of infections asymptomatic)
PREDOMINANT SEX:
- Equal sex distribution in general
- Striking male predominance of liver abscess

PREDOMINANT AGE: Second through sixth decades
PEAK INCIDENCE: Peaks at age 2 to 3 yr and >40 yr
GENETICS: Infection more likely to be fulminant in young infants

PHYSICAL FINDINGS
- Often nonspecific
- Approximately 20% of cases symptomatic
  1. Diarrhea, which may be bloody
  2. Abdominal and back pain
- Abdominal tenderness in 83% of severe cases
- Fever in 38% of severe cases
- Hepatomegaly, RUQ tenderness, and fever in almost all patients with liver abscess (may be absent in fulminant cases)

ETIOLOGY
- Caused by the protozoal parasite *E. histolytica*
- Transmission by the fecal-oral route
- Infection usually localized to the large bowel, particularly the cecum where a localized mass lesion (ameboma) may form
- Extraintestinal infection when the organism invades the bowel mucosa and gains access to the portal circulation

DIAGNOSIS

DIFFERENTIAL DIAGNOSIS
- Severe intestinal infection possibly confused with ulcerative colitis or other infectious enterocolitis syndromes, such as those caused by *Shigella, Salmonella, Campylobacter*, or invasive *Escherichia coli*
- In elderly patients: ischemic bowel possibly producing a similar picture

WORKUP
- Three stool specimens over a period of 7 to 10 days to exclude the diagnosis (sensitivity 50% to 80%)
- Concentration and staining the specimen with Lugol's iodine or methylene blue to increase the diagnostic yield
- Available culture (rarely necessary in routine cases)

LABORATORY TESTS
- Stool examination is generally reliable.
- Mucosal biopsy is occasionally necessary.
- Serum antibody may be detected and is particularly sensitive and specific for extraintestinal infection or severe intestinal disease.
- Aspiration of abscess fluid is used to distinguish amebic from bacterial abscesses.

IMAGING STUDIES
Abdominal imaging studies (sonography or CT scan) to diagnose liver abscess

TREATMENT

ACUTE GENERAL Rx
- Metronidazole (750 mg PO tid for 10 days) is used in the treatment of mild to severe intestinal infection and amebic liver abscess, it may be administered intravenously when necessary.
- Follow with iodoquinol (650 mg PO tid for 20 days) to eradicate persistent cysts.
- For asymptomatic patients with amebic cysts on stool examination, use iodoquinol or paromomycin (500 mg PO tid for 7 days).
- Avoid antiperistaltic agents in severe intestinal infections to avoid risk of toxic megacolon.
- Liver abscess is generally responsive to medical management but surgical intervention indicated for extension of liver abscess into pericardium or, occasionally, for toxic megacolon.

DISPOSITION
Host immunity incomplete and reinfection rate high for patients remaining at risk

REFERRAL
- For consultation with infectious diseases specialist for extraintestinal infection or persistent or relapsing intestinal infection
- For surgical consultation:
  1. For toxic megacolon
  2. For impending rupture of or extension of liver abscess into adjacent structures

MISCELLANEOUS

COMMENTS
- Infection with other intestinal parasites, particularly *Giardia lamblia*, may coexist with amebiasis.
- Clinical algorithms for evaluation of patients with diarrhea are described in Fig. 3-28.

REFERENCES
Reed SL: New concepts regarding the pathogenesis of amebiasis, *Clin Infect Dis* 21(suppl 2):S182, 1995.

Author: Joseph R. Masci, M.D.

Amyloidosis

BASIC INFORMATION

DEFINITION
Amyloidosis is a generic term describing the deposition of amyloid fibrils in body tissues. *Amyloid* is an amorphous, eosinophilic material, it is birefringent and usually extracellular. Electron microscopy reveals nonbranching fibrils that are soluble and relatively resistant to proteolytic digestion.

ICD-9-CM CODES
277.3 Amyloidosis

EPIDEMIOLOGY AND DEMOGRAPHICS
Amyloidosis affects primarily males between the ages of 60 and 70 yr.

PHYSICAL FINDINGS
- Findings are variable with organ system involvement. Symmetric polyarthritis, peripheral neuropathy, and carpal tunnel syndrome may be present with joint involvement.
- Signs and symptoms of nephrotic syndrome may be present with renal involvement.
- Fatigue and dyspnea may occur with pulmonary involvement.
- Diarrhea, macroglossia, malabsorption, and weight loss may occur with GI involvement.

ETIOLOGY
There are several chemically documented amyloidoses that can be principally subdivided into:
1. Acquired systemic amyloidosis (immunoglobulin light chain, multiple myeloma, hemodialysis amyloidosis)
2. Heredofamilial systemic (polyneuropathy, familial Mediterranean fever)
3. Organ-limited (Alzheimer's disease)
4. Localized endocrine (pancreatic islet, medullary thyroid carcinoma)

DIAGNOSIS

DIFFERENTIAL DIAGNOSIS
Variable, depending on the organ involvement:
- Renal involvement (toxin or drug-induced necrosis, glomerulonephritis, renal vein thrombosis)
- Interstitial lung disease (sarcoidosis, connective tissue disease, infectious etiologies)
- Restrictive cardiac (endomyocardial fibrosis, viral myocarditis)
- Carpal tunnel (rheumatoid arthritis, hypothyroidism, overuse)
- Mental status changes (multiinfarct dementia)
- Peripheral neuropathy (alcohol abuse, vitamin deficiencies, diabetes mellitus)

WORKUP
Diagnostic approach is aimed at demonstration of amyloid deposits in tissues. This may be accomplished with rectal biopsy (positive in >60% of cases). Renal, myocardial, and bone marrow biopsy are other potential options. Abdominal fat pad biopsy can also be diagnostic.

LABORATORY TESTS
- Initial laboratory evaluation should include CBC, TSH, renal functions studies, urinalysis, and serum and urine protein electrophoresis.
- Various laboratory abnormalities include proteinuria (found in >70% of cases), anemia, renal insufficiency, hypothyroidism, and elevated monoclonal proteins.

IMAGING STUDIES
- Chest x-ray may reveal hilar adenopathy and mediastinal adenopathy.
- Echocardiography is indicated if cardiac involvement is suspected.

TREATMENT

NONPHARMACOLOGIC THERAPY
Life-style changes with low-salt diet in patients with CHF; protein and sodium restrictions in patients with renal failure

ACUTE GENERAL Rx
Therapy is variable, depending on the type of amyloidosis. Amyloidosis associated with plasma cell disorders may be treated with melphalan and prednisone, along with colchicine. Colchicine may also be effective in renal amyloidosis.

CHRONIC Rx
Renal transplantation is needed in patients with renal amyloidosis. Peritoneal dialysis in place of hemodialysis in patients with renal failure may improve hemodialysis amyloidosis by clearing β-2 microglobulin.

DISPOSITION
Prognosis varies with the form of amyloidosis:
- In reactive amyloidosis, eradication of the predisposing disease slows and can occasionally reverse the progression of amyloid disease. Survival of 5 to 10 yr after diagnosis is not uncommon.
- Patients with familial amyloidotic polyneuropathy generally have a prolonged course lasting 10 to 15 yr.
- Amyloidosis associated with immunocytic processes carries the worst prognosis (life expectancy <yr).
- The progression of amyloidosis associated with renal hemodialysis can be improved with newer dialysis membranes that can pass β-2 microglobulin.

REFERRAL
Surgical referral for biopsy of subcutaneous abdominal fat, skin, gingival, or rectal tissue

MISCELLANEOUS

COMMENTS
Additional information on amyloidosis can be obtained from the National Organization for Rare Disorders (NORD), Box 8923, New Fairfield, CT 06812.

REFERENCES
Gertz MA et al: Dialysis support of patients with primary systemic amyloidosis, *Arch Intern Med* 152:2245, 1992.

Glenner GG: The amyloidoses. In Stein JH (ed): *Internal medicine*, ed 4, St Louis, 1994, Mosby.

Vogelgesang SA, Klirple GL: The many guises of amyloidosis: clinical presentations and disease associations, *Postgrad Med* 96:126, 1994.

Author: Fred F. Ferri, M.D.

Amyotrophic lateral sclerosis

BASIC INFORMATION

DEFINITION
Amyotrophic lateral sclerosis (ALS) is a disease affecting upper and lower motor neurons, characterized pathologically by degeneration of motor neurons in the brain stem and spinal cord and by degeneration of neurons in the motor cortex and corticospinal tracts.

SYNONYMS
ALS
Lou Gehrig's disease

ICD-9-CM CODES
335.20 Amyotrophic lateral sclerosis

EPIDEMIOLOGY AND DEMOGRAPHICS
INCIDENCE: 0.5 to 2 cases/100,000 persons
PREVALENCE: 5 in 100,000 persons
GENETICS: 5% of cases are familial in an autosomal dominant pattern; some but not all families map to the gene for superoxide dismutase on chromosome 21.

PHYSICAL FINDINGS
- Lower motor neuron signs (weakness, wasting, fasciculations)
- Upper motor neuron signs (Babinski's sign, clonus)
- Unexplained weight loss, slurring of speech
- Difficulty walking and swallowing

ETIOLOGY
- The cause of ALS is unknown.
- A familial form is transmitted in an autosomal dominant pattern.
- Ingestion of the cycad nut may be associated with ALS-Parkinson-dementia complex of Guam.

DIAGNOSIS

DIFFERENTIAL DIAGNOSIS
- Cervical spondylotic myelopathy
- Spinal stenosis with compression of lumbosacral nerve roots
- Lead axonal neuropathy
- Multifocal motor neuropathy with conduction block
- Syphilitic myelitis with amyotrophy
- Delayed effects of electrical injury to spinal cord
- Late-onset hexosaminidase deficiency
- Polyglucosan body disease
- Syringomyelia
- Spinal AV malformations

WORKUP
- EMG and nerve conduction studies
- Lumbar puncture and CSF analysis
- Bone marrow examination to exclude myeloma, Waldenstrom disease, or other lymphoproliferative disease if CSF protein content exceeds 75 mg/dl

LABORATORY TESTS
- Serum protein immunofixation electrophoresis on warm blood (allowed to clot at 37° C to avoid loss of the monoclonal proteins as a cryoglobulin)
- Quantitative immunoglobulin analysis
- Antibodies to GM1 and myelin-associated glycoprotein
- Heavy metal testing: generally not indicated

IMAGING STUDIES
Chest x-ray examination
MRI in selected cases to exclude disorders listed in differential diagnosis

TREATMENT

NONPHARMACOLOGIC THERAPY
- Family planning for chronic illness (discussion of living will, financial matters, and DNR orders)
- Emotional support for patient and family members
- Prosthetic devices (e.g., wheelchair)
- Discussion regarding preparation for tracheostomy

ACUTE GENERAL Rx
Riluzole (Rilutek) is the only medication approved to extend survival in patients with ALS. Dosage is 50 mg q12h, at least 1 hr before or 2 hr after meals. Benefits are marginal and the medication is very expensive.

CHRONIC Rx
Supportive care to prevent complications (aspiration, decubitus ulcerations, malnutrition)

DISPOSITION
- Mean duration of symptoms is 2 to 4 yr.
- About 20% of patients survive >5 yr.
- There have been reports of spontaneous arrest of the disease.

REFERRAL
- Referral to a neurologist is recommended to confirm diagnosis.
- Surgical referral for tracheostomy may be needed to prevent aspiration as the disease progresses.
- Psychiatric referral for counseling on associated anxiety and depression may be necessary in selected cases.
- Nursing home placement and/or hospice may be necessary in advanced stages of the disease.

MISCELLANEOUS

COMMENTS
Patient education material may be obtained through the ALS Association, 21021 Ventura Boulevard, Suite 321, Woodland Hills, CA 91364, phone: (800)782-4727; or the Muscular Dystrophy Association, 3561 East Sunrise Drive, Tucson, AZ 85718-3204; phone: (602) 529-2000.

REFERENCES
Hewer RL: The management of motor neuron disease. In Leigh PN, Swash M (eds): *Motor neuron disease: biology and management,* London, 1995, Springer-Verlag.
Rowland LP et al: Amyotrophic lateral sclerosis. In Johnson RT, Griffin JW (eds): *Current therapy in neurologic disease,* ed 5, St Louis, 1996, Mosby.

Author: **Fred F. Ferri, M.D.**

Anaerobic infections

BASIC INFORMATION

DEFINITION
An anaerobic infection is caused by one of a group of bacteria that require a reduced oxygen tension for growth.

ICD-9-CM CODES
See specific condition.

EPIDEMIOLOGY AND DEMOGRAPHICS
INCIDENCE (IN U.S.): Statistics incomplete for various reasons: unavailable specimens, fastidious organisms, inadequate culture techniques

PHYSICAL FINDINGS
- May occur at any site, but most are anatomically related to mucosal surfaces
- Should be suspected when there is foul-smelling tissue, soft-tissue gas, necrotic tissue, or abscesses
- Head and neck
  1. Odontogenic infections from dental or soft tissue possibly progressing to periapical abscesses, at times extending to bone
  2. Both anaerobic and aerobic pathogens in chronic sinusitis, chronic mastoiditis, and chronic otitis media
  3. Peritonsillar abscess possible
  4. Complications: deep neck space infections, brain abscesses, mediastinitis
- Pleuropulmonary
  1. May involve anaerobes present in the oropharynx
  2. Aspiration more common in persons with altered mental status or seizures
  3. Anaerobic bacteria more likely in those with gingivitis or periodontitis
  4. Manifestations: necrotizing pneumonia, empyema, lung abscess
- Intraabdominal
  1. Disruption of intestinal integrity leading to infection involving anaerobic bacteria
  2. Bacteria from colonic neoplasm, perforated appendicitis, diverticulitis, or bowel surgery, causing bacteremia, peritonitis, at times intraabdominal abscesses
  3. Resulting infections usually mixed, containing both anaerobes and aerobes
- Female genital tract
  1. Anaerobes in bacterial vaginosis, salpingitis, endometritis, pelvic abscesses, septic abortion; infections tend to be mixed
  2. Possible pelvic thrombophlebitis when resolving pelvic infection is accompanied by new or persistent fever
- Other anaerobic infections
  1. Skin and soft-tissue infection at any site
  2. More commonly associated infections: synergistic gangrene, bite wound infections, infected decubitus ulcers
  3. Clinical significance of anaerobes in diabetic foot infections unclear
  4. Anaerobic bacteremia uncommon with source usually intraabdominal, followed by female genital tract, pleuropulmonary, and head and neck infections
  5. Osteomyelitis especially when associated with decubitus ulcers or vascular insufficiency
  6. Facial bone osteomyelitis from adjacent infections of the teeth or sinuses

ETIOLOGY
- Most commonly endogenous, arising from bacteria that normally line mucosal surfaces
- Disruption of mucosal barriers resulting from various conditions (trauma, ischemia, surgery, perforation), with infection occurring when organisms gain access to normally sterile sites, causing tissue destruction and abscess formation
- Synergy between different anaerobes or between anaerobes and aerobes important
- Most commonly involved: gram-negative anaerobic bacilli
  1. *Bacteroides*
     a. Many organisms, including those in the *B. fragilis* group, which can be found in most intraabdominal infections
     b. May also play a part in infections of the female genital tract, only occasionally causing infections above the diaphragm
  2. *Prevotella:* may be involved in oral and pleuropulmonary infections, as well as infections of the female genital tract
  3. *Porphyromonas:* important in dental infections
  4. *Fusobacterium:* may be involved in infections related to oral flora (pleuropulmonary, otitis, sinusitis, brain abscess)
- Gram-positive anaerobic cocci
  1. *Peptostreptococcus* and anaerobic *Streptococcus*
  2. More commonly associated with head and neck infections, female genital tract infections, and, at times, skin and soft-tissue infections
- Anaerobic gram-positive bacilli
  1. Less common
  2. Include *Clostridium difficile*-associated diarrhea and *C. perfringens* wound infections

3. Bacteremia with *C. septicum*, *C. perfringens*, or *C. tertium* possibly associated with colonic malignancy
4. Potent toxins produced by *C. botulinum* and *C. tetani* potential cause of severe disease

DIAGNOSIS

DIFFERENTIAL DIAGNOSIS
- Clinically similar to focal infections caused by other organisms, but have an increased propensity toward tissue destruction and abscess formation
- Aerobic gram-negative organisms involved in gas formation, although more commonly associated with anaerobes
- Abscesses differentiated from other space-occupying lesions
- Diarrhea associated with *C. difficile* a mimic of other causes of infectious diarrhea

WORKUP
- Specimens submitted for culture processed within 30 min
- Large volume of material more likely to have significant growth; swabs less efficient for transporting infected material

LABORATORY TESTS
- Elevated WBC count, with extremely high WBC counts sometimes seen with pseudomembranous colitis
- Positive stool *C. difficile* toxin assay
- Increased lactate levels in ischemia or perforation
- Possible positive blood or wound cultures, but failure to grow anaerobes in culture may be common, attributed to inadequate culturing techniques and/or fastidious organisms

IMAGING STUDIES
- Plain film of an affected area to show gas in tissues, free air resulting from a perforated viscus, or an air/fluid level inside an abscess
- Ultrasound, CT scan, or MRI to reveal abscesses or tissue destruction

TREATMENT

NONPHARMACOLOGIC THERAPY
- Removal of necrotic tissue
- Drainage of abscesses (accomplished by CT scan-guided percutaneous drainage)

ACUTE GENERAL Rx
Oral antibiotics with anaerobic activity: clindamycin, metronidazole, and chloramphenicol
- Broader spectrum of activity with amoxicillin/clavulanate
- Penicillin VK in odontogenic infections
- Oral metronidazole for *C. difficile*-associated diarrhea, with oral vancomycin reserved for recurrent or recalcitrant infections

Parenteral antibiotics for more serious illness
- IV Clindamycin, metronidazole, and chloramphenicol
- Cephalosporins (anaerobic or mixed infections): cefoxitin and cefotetan
- Extended-spectrum penicillins (i.e., piperacillin) and combination β-lactamase plus β-lactamase inhibitor drugs
  1. Significant anaerobic activity, plus various degrees of broad-spectrum coverage
  2. Include ampicillin/sulbactam, ticarcillin/clavulanate, and piperacillin/tazobactam
- Imipenem: a broad-spectrum agent with extensive anaerobic activity
- SMX/TMP and fluoroquinolones: ineffective

CHRONIC Rx
Some infections (lung abscess, osteomyelitis, and empyema) require weeks to months of therapy.

DISPOSITION
- Most infections are curable if adequate surgical and medical therapy is provided.
- Those involving sites with compromised vasculature are more likely to require surgical manipulation, including amputation.

REFERRAL
If other than mild disease

MISCELLANEOUS

COMMENTS
- Chloramphenicol is associated with aplastic anemia, although this is an extremely rare complication.
- Imipenem is a possible cause of thrombocytopenia and may lower the seizure threshold, especially in elderly patients with renal insufficiency.

REFERENCES
Finegold SM: Overview of clinically important anaerobes, *Clin Infect Dis* 20(suppl 2):S205, 1995.

Author: **Maurice Policar, M.D.**

Anal fissure

BASIC INFORMATION

DEFINITION
A fissure is a tear in the epithelial lining of the anal canal (i.e., from the dentate line to the anal verge).

SYNONYMS
Anorectal fissure
Anal ulcer

ICD-9-CM CODES
565.0 Anal fissure

EPIDEMIOLOGY AND DEMOGRAPHICS
- Can occur at any age
- Most common in young and middle-aged adults
- Occurs in men > women
- Women more likely to have anterior fissure than men (10% vs. 1%, respectively)
- Most common cause of rectal bleeding in infants
- Common in women before and after childbirth

PHYSICAL FINDINGS
With separation of the buttock will see a tear in the posterior midline or, less frequently, in the anterior midline
- Acute anal fissure:
  1. Sharp burning or tearing pain exacerbated by bowel movements
  2. Bright-red blood on toilet paper, a streak of blood on the stool or in the water
- Chronic anal fissure:
  1. Pruritus ani
  2. Pain seldom present
  3. Intermittent bleeding
  4. Sentinel tag at the caudal aspect of the fissure, hypertrophied anal papilla at the proximal end
- Underlying disease possible if the fissure:
  1. Is ectopically located
  2. Extends proximal to the dentate line
  3. Is broad-based or deep
  4. Is especially purulent

ETIOLOGY
- Most initiated after passage of a large, hard stool
- May result from frequent defecation and diarrhea
- Bacterial infections: TB, syphilis, gonorrhea, chancroid, lymphogranuloma venereum
- Viral infections: herpes simplex virus, cytomegalovirus, human immunodeficiency virus
- Inflammatory bowel disease (IBD): Crohn's disease, ulcerative colitis
- Trauma: surgery (hemorrhoidectomy), foreign bodies, anal intercourse
- Malignancy: carcinoma, lymphoma, Kaposi's sarcoma

DIAGNOSIS

DIFFERENTIAL DIAGNOSIS
- Proctalgia fugax
- Thrombosed hemorrhoid

WORKUP
- Digital rectal examination after lubricating the entire anus with anesthetic jelly (i.e., 2% lidocaine) and waiting 5 to 10 min
- Anoscopy
- Proctosigmoidoscopy to exclude inflammatory or neoplastic disease
- Biopsy if doubt exists about the etiology of the condition
- All studies done under adequate anesthesia

IMAGING STUDIES
- Colonoscopy or barium enema: if diagnosis of IBD or malignancy is suspected
- Small bowel series: occasionally obtained for similar reasons
- Biopsy to reveal caseating granuloma if TB is suspected
- Wet prep with darkfield examination to demonstrate treponemes if syphilis is suspected

TREATMENT

NONPHARMACOLOGIC THERAPY
- Sitz baths
- High-fiber diet
- Increased oral fluid intake

ACUTE GENERAL Rx
- Bulk producing agent (i.e., Metamucil)/stool softener
- Local anesthetic jelly (may exacerbate pruritus ani)
- Suppositories *not* recommended
- Surgery

CHRONIC Rx
Surgery: lateral internal anal sphincterotomy

DISPOSITION
Outpatient surgery

REFERRAL
- If fissure does not resolve with conservative therapy in 4 to 6 wk
- If patient prefers surgery for acute fissure
- If patient has chronic fissure

MISCELLANEOUS

COMMENTS
HIV-positive patients should be referred to clinicians who are well versed in the myriad infectious and neoplastic conditions that masquerade as anal ulcers in these patients.

REFERENCES
Barnett JL, Raper SE: Anorectal diseases. In Yamada T, Alpers DH, Owyang C: *Textbook of gastroenterology,* ed 2, Philadelphia, 1995, Lippincott.

Beart R: Chapter 97. In Sciarra JJ: *Gynecology and obstetrics,* Philadelphia, 1997, Lippincott.

Author: **Maria Elena Soler, M.D.**

Anaphylaxis

BASIC INFORMATION

DEFINITION
Anaphylaxis is a sudden-onset, life-threatening event characterized by a constellation of signs and symptoms involving one or more organs or tissues. Its clinical presentation may include respiratory, cardiovascular, cutaneous or gastrointestinal manifestations.

SYNONYMS
Anaphylactoid reaction

ICD-9-CM CODES
995.0 Anaphylactic shock
995.60 Anaphylaxis due to food
999.4 Anaphylaxis due to immunization
977.9 Anaphylaxis due to drugs
989.5 Anaphylaxis following stings

EPIDEMIOLOGY AND DEMOGRAPHICS
INCIDENCE: 20,000 to 50,000 persons/yr in the U.S.

PHYSICAL FINDINGS
- Urticaria, pruritus, skin flushing, angioedema
- Dyspnea, cough, malaise, difficulty swallowing
- Wheezing, tachycardia, diarrhea

ETIOLOGY
Virtually any substance may induce anaphylaxis in a given individual.
- Commonly implicated medications are antibiotics, insulin, allergen extracts, opiates, vaccines, NSAIDs, contrast media, streptokinase
- Foods and food additives, nuts, egg whites, shellfish, fish, milk, fruits and berries
- Blood products, plasma, immunoglobulin, cryoprecipitate, whole blood
- Venoms such as snake venom, fire ant venom, bee sting
- Latex

DIAGNOSIS

DIFFERENTIAL DIAGNOSIS
- Endocrine disorders (carcinoid, pheochromocytoma)
- Globus hystericus, anxiety disorder
- Systemic mastocytosis
- Pulmonary embolism, serum sickness, vasovagal reactions

WORKUP
Workup is aimed mainly at eliminating other conditions that may mimic anaphylaxis. (e.g., vasovagal syncope may be differentiated by the presence of bradycardia as opposed to the tachycardia seen in anaphylaxis; the absence of hypoxemia in ABG analysis may be useful to exclude pulmonary embolism or foreign body aspiration)

LABORATORY TESTS
- Laboratory evaluation is generally not helpful, since the diagnosis of anaphylaxis is a clinical one.
- ABG analysis may be useful to exclude pulmonary embolism, status asthmaticus, and foreign body aspiration.
- Elevated serum and urine histamine levels can be useful for diagnosis of anaphylaxis, but these tests are not commonly available.

IMAGING STUDIES
Generally not helpful.
- Chest x-ray is indicated in patients presenting with acute respiratory compromise.
- Radiologic evaluation for epiglottitis is useful in patients with acute respiratory compromise.
- ECG should be considered in all patients with sudden loss of consciousness or complaints of chest pains or dyspnea and in any elderly patient.

TREATMENT

NONPHARMACOLOGIC THERAPY
- IV access should be rapidly established, and intravenous fluids (i.e., saline) should be administered.
- Supplemental oxygen and cardiac monitoring are also recommended.

ACUTE GENERAL Rx
- Epinephrine should be rapidly administered as a SC or IM injection at a dose of 0.01 ml/kg of aqueous epinephrine 1:1000 (maximum adult dose 0.3 to 0.5 ml). The dose may be repeated approximately q5-10min if there is persistence or recurrence of symptoms. Endotracheal epinephrine should be considered if IV access is not possible during life-threatening reactions.
- Administration of H_1- and H_2-receptor antagonists is also recommended in the initial treatment of anaphylaxis.
  1. Administer diphenhydramine 25 to 50 mg IV or IM.
  2. Cimetidine 300 mg IV over 3 to 5 min, or ranitidine 50 mg IV, should be given initially; subsequent doses of H_1- and H_2-blockers can be given orally q6h for 48 hr.
- Corticosteroids are not useful in the acute episode because of their slow onset of action; however, they should be administered in most cases to prevent prolonged or recurrent anaphylaxis. Commonly used agents are hydrocortisone sodium succinate 250 to 500 mg IV q4-6h in adults (4 to 8 mg/kg for children) or methylprednisolone 60 to 125 mg IV in adults (1 to 2 mg/kg in children).
- Aerosolized β-agonists (i.e., albuterol, 2.5 mg, repeat PRN 20 min) are useful to control bronchospasm.
- Additional useful agents in specific circumstances: atropine for refractory bradycardia, dopamine for refractory hypotension (despite volume expansion), and glucagon in patients on β-blocking drugs.

DISPOSITION
Prognosis is generally good if treated immediately.

MISCELLANEOUS

COMMENTS
- Patient education regarding the nature of the illness and preventive measures is recommended.
- Prescription for prefilled epinephrine syringe (EpiPen) should be given and the patient should be instructed on the use of this emergency epinephrine kit in case of recurrent anaphylactic episodes.
- Patients should also be advised to carry or wear Medic Alert ID describing substances that have caused anaphylaxis.
- Avoidance of radiologic contrast is also recommended.

REFERENCES
Sandler SG et al: IgA anaphylactic transfusion reactions, *Transfus Med Rev* 9(1):1, 1995.
Sloop GD, Friedberg RC: Complications of blood transfusions: how to recognize or respond to noninfectious reactions, *Postgrad Med* 98(1):159, 1995.
Wittbrod ET, Spinler SA: Prevention of anaphylactoid reactions in high-risk patients receiving radiographic contrast media, *Ann Pharmacother* 28(2):236, 1994.

Author: **Fred F. Ferri, M.D.**

Anemia, aplastic (PTG)

BASIC INFORMATION

DEFINITION
Aplastic anemia is a bone marrow failure resulting from a variety of causes and characterized by stem cell destruction or suppression leading to pancytopenia.

SYNONYMS
Refractory anemia
Hypoplastic anemia

ICD-9-CM CODES
284.9 Aplastic anemia
284.8 Acquired aplastic anemia
284.0 Congenital aplastic anemia

EPIDEMIOLOGY AND DEMOGRAPHICS
- There is no predominant age or sex for the acquired form.
- The annual incidence of aplastic anemia in the U.S. is 3 to 9 cases/1,000,000 persons.

PHYSICAL FINDINGS
- Skin pallor, ecchymosis, petechiae, retinal hemorrhage
- Possible fever, mouth and tongue ulceration, pharyngitis
- Possible short stature or skeletal and nail anomalies in the congenital form
- Possible audible systolic ejection murmur with profound anemia

ETIOLOGY
- In most patients with acquired aplastic anemia, bone marrow failure results from immunologically mediated, tissue-specific organ destruction.
- Common etiologic factors in aplastic anemia:
  Toxins (e.g., benzine, insecticides)
  Drugs (e.g., Felbatol, cimetidine, busulfan and other myelosuppressive drugs, gold salts, chloramphenicol, sulfonamides, trimethadione, quinacrine, phenylbutazone)
  Ionizing irradiation
  Infections (e.g., hepatitis C, HIV)
  Idiopathic
  Inherited (Fanconi's anemia)
  Other: immunologic, pregnancy

DIAGNOSIS

DIFFERENTIAL DIAGNOSIS
- Bone marrow infiltration from lymphoma, carcinoma, myelofibrosis
- Severe infection
- Hypoplastic acute lymphoblastic leukemia in children
- Hypoplastic myelodysplastic syndrome or hypoplastic acute myeloid leukemia in adults
- Hypersplenism
- Hairy cell leukemia

WORKUP
- Diagnostic workup consists primarily of bone marrow aspiration and biopsy and laboratory evaluation (CBC and examination of blood film).
- Bone marrow examination generally reveals paucity or absence of erythropoietic and myelopoietic precursor cells; patients with pure red cell aplasia demonstrate only absence of RBC precursors in the marrow.
- A clinical algorithm for the diagnosis of anemia is described in Fig. 3-5.

LABORATORY TESTS
- CBC reveals pancytopenia. Macrocytosis and toxic granulation of neutrophils may also be present. Isolated cytopenias may occur in the early stages.
- Reticulocyte count reveals reticulocytopenia.
- Additional initial laboratory evaluation should include Ham test to exclude paroxysmal nocturnal hemoglobinuria (PNH) and testing for hepatitis C.

IMAGING STUDIES
- Chest x-ray examination
- Abdominal sonogram or CT scan to evaluate for splenomegaly
- Radiography of hand and forearm in patients with constitutional anemia
- CT scan of thymus region if thymoma-associated RBC aplasia is suspected

TREATMENT

NONPHARMACOLOGIC THERAPY
- Discontinuation of any offending drugs or agents
- Evaluation for bone marrow transplantation

ACUTE GENERAL Rx
- Aggressive treatment for prevention of infections
- Platelet and RBC transfusions PRN; however, avoidance of transfusions in patients who are candidates for bone marrow transplantation
- Immunosuppressive therapy with antithymocyte globulin (ATG) and/or cyclosporine (CSP); ATG in combination with prednisone (1 to 2 mg/kg/day initially) to avoid complications of serum sickness
- Transplantation of allogeneic marrow as treatment of choice in patients with severe aplastic anemia who have HLA-matched donors

CHRONIC Rx
Long-term patient monitoring with physical examination and routine laboratory evaluation to screen for relapse

DISPOSITION
- Patients with severe aplastic anemia who have marrow transplants before the onset of transfusion-induced sensitization have an excellent probability of long-term survival and normal life; age is a significant factor; the incidence of graft vs. host disease increases with age and is >90% in patients >30 yr of age.
- Following bone marrow transplantation from an HLA-identical sibling, >70% of patients are long-term survivors and can be considered cured.

REFERRAL
Hematology referral is indicated in all patients with aplastic anemia.

MISCELLANEOUS

COMMENTS
Additional patient information on aplastic anemia can be obtained from Aplastic Anemia Foundation of America, PO Box 22689, Baltimore, MD 21203; phone number: (410) 955-2803.

REFERENCES
Paquette RL et al: Long-term outcome of aplastic anemia in adults treated with antithymocyte globulin: comparison with bone marrow transplantation, *Blood* 85:283, 1995.
Soutar RL, King BJ: Bone marrow transplantation, *Br Med J* 310:31, 1995.
Young NS, Barrett AJ: The treatment of severe acquired aplastic anemia, *Blood* 85:3367, 1995.
Young NS, Maciejewski J: The pathophysiology of acquired aplastic anemia, *N Engl J Med* 336:1365, 1997.

Author: **Fred F. Ferri, M.D.**

Anemia, autoimmune hemolytic

BASIC INFORMATION

DEFINITION
Autoimmune hemolytic anemia is anemia secondary to premature destruction of red blood cells caused by the binding of autoantibodies and/or complement to red blood cells.

ICD-9-CM CODES
283.0 Autoimmune hemolytic anemia

EPIDEMIOLOGY AND DEMOGRAPHICS
Autoimmune hemolytic anemia is most common in women <50 yr.

PHYSICAL FINDINGS
- Pallor
- Tachycardia
- Hepatomegaly, splenomegaly

ETIOLOGY
- Warm antibody mediated: IgG (often idiopathic or associated with leukemia, lymphoma, thymoma, myeloma, viral infections, and collagen-vascular disease)
- Cold antibody mediated: IgM and complement in majority of cases (often idiopathic, at times associated with infections, lymphoma, or cold agglutinin disease)
- Drug induced: three major mechanisms:
  1. Antibody directed against Rh complex (e.g., methyldopa)
  2. Antibody directed against RBC-drug complex (hapten-induced, e.g., penicillin)
  3. Antibody directed against complex formed by drug and plasma proteins; the drug-plasma protein-antibody complex causes destruction of RBC (innocent bystander, e.g., quinidine).

DIAGNOSIS

DIFFERENTIAL DIAGNOSIS
- Hemolytic anemia caused by membrane defects (paroxysmal nocturnal hemoglobinuria, spur-cell anemia, Wilson's disease)
- Nonimmune mediated (microangiopathic hemolytic anemia, hypersplenism, cardiac valve prosthesis, giant cavernous hemangiomas, march hemoglobinuria, physical agents, infections, heavy metals, certain drugs [nitrofurantoin, sulfonamides])

WORKUP
- Evaluation consists primarily of laboratory evaluation to confirm hemolysis and to exclude other causes of the anemia.
- A clinical algorithm for evaluation of anemia is described in Fig. 3-5.
- Box 2-13 describes the differential diagnosis of megaloblastic anemia.

LABORATORY TESTS
- Initial labs: CBC (anemia), reticulocyte count (elevated), liver function studies (elevated indirect bilirubin, LDH), evaluation of peripheral smear, Coombs' test (positive direct Coombs' test indicates presence of antibodies or complement on the surface of RBC, positive indirect Coombs' test implies presence of anti-RBC antibodies freely circulating in the patient's serum), haptoglobin level (decreased).
- IgG antibody and IgM antibody
- Hepatitis serology, ANA

IMAGING STUDIES
Chest x-ray
CT scan of chest and abdomen to rule out lymphoma should also be considered

TREATMENT

NONPHARMACOLOGIC THERAPY
- Discontinuation of any potentially offensive drugs
- Plasmapheresis-exchange transfusion for severe life-threatening cases only
- Avoid cold exposure in patients with cold antibody

ACUTE GENERAL Rx
- Prednisone 1 to 2 mg/kg qd in divided doses initially
- Splenectomy in patients responding inadequately to corticosteroids when RBC sequestration studies indicate splenic sequestration
- Immunosuppressive drugs and/or immunoglobulins only after both corticosteroids and splenectomy (unless surgery is contraindicated) have failed to produce an adequate remission
- Danazol, usually used in conjunction with corticosteroids (may be useful in warm antibody autoimmune hemolytic anemia)

DISPOSITION
Prognosis is generally good unless anemia is associated with underlying disorder with a poor prognosis (e.g., leukemia, myeloma).

REFERRAL
Surgical referral for splenectomy in refractory cases

MISCELLANEOUS

COMMENTS
Monitor for potential complications such as thromboembolism or severe anemia with shock.

REFERENCES
Jefferies LC: Transfusion therapy in autoimmune hemolytic anemia, *Hematol Oncol Clin North Am* 8:1087, 1994.
Schreiber AD: Acquired hemolytic disorders. In Bennett JC, Plum S (eds): *Cecil's textbook of medicine,* ed 20, Philadelphia, 1996, WB Saunders.

Author: **Fred F. Ferri, M.D.**

Anemia, iron deficiency (PTG)

BASIC INFORMATION

DEFINITION
Iron deficiency anemia is anemia secondary to inadequate iron supplementation or excessive blood loss.

ICD-9-CM CODES
280.9 Iron deficiency anemia
648.2 Iron deficiency anemia complicating pregnancy

EPIDEMIOLOGY AND DEMOGRAPHICS
Dietary iron deficiency occurs frequently in infants as a result of unsupplemented milk diets. It is also frequently seen in women during their reproductive years, as a result of heavy menstrual periods, and during pregnancy (increased demand).

PHYSICAL FINDINGS
- Most patients have a normal examination.
- Skin pallor and conjunctival pallor may be present.

ETIOLOGY
- Blood loss from GI or menstrual bleeding (GU blood loss less frequently the cause)
- Dietary iron deficiency (rare in adults)
- Poor iron absorption in patients with gastric or small bowel surgery
- Repeated phlebotomy
- Increased requirements (e.g., during pregnancy)
- Other: traumatic hemolysis (abnormally functioning cardiac valves), idiopathic pulmonary hemosiderosis (iron sequestration in pulmonary macrophages), paroxysmal nocturnal hemoglobinuria (intravascular hemolysis)

DIAGNOSIS

DIFFERENTIAL DIAGNOSIS
- Anemia of chronic disease
- Sideroblastic anemia
- Thalassemia trait
- The differential diagnosis of iron deficiency is described in Table 2-5.

WORKUP
- Diagnostic workup consists primarily of laboratory evaluation. Most patients with iron deficiency anemia are asymptomatic in the early stages. With progressive anemia, the major complaints are fatigue, dizziness, exertional dyspnea, pagophagia (ice eating), pica. Patient's history may also suggest GI blood loss (melena, hematochezia, hemoptysis).
- A clinical algorithm for the evaluation of anemia is described in Fig. 3-5.

LABORATORY TESTS
- Laboratory results vary with the stage of deficiency.
- Absent iron marrow stores and decreased serum ferritin are the initial abnormalities.
- Decreased serum iron and increased TIBC are the next abnormalities.
- Hypochromic microcytic anemia is present with significant iron deficiency.
- Peripheral smear in patients with iron deficiency generally reveals microcytic hypochromic RBCs with a wide area of central pallor, anisocytosis, and poikilocytosis when severe.
- Laboratory abnormalities consistent with iron deficiency are low serum ferritin level, elevated RBC distribution width (RDW) with values generally >15, low MCV, elevated TIBC, and low serum iron.

TREATMENT

NONPHARMACOLOGIC THERAPY
Patients should be instructed to consume foods containing large amounts of iron, such as liver, red meat, and legumes.

ACUTE GENERAL Rx
- Treatment consists of ferrous sulfate 325 mg PO qd-tid for at least 6 mo. Calcium supplements can decrease iron absorption; therefore, these two medications should be staggered.
- Parenteral iron therapy is reserved for patients with poor tolerance, noncompliance with oral preparations, or malabsorption.
- Transfusion of packed RBCs is indicated in patients with severe symptomatic anemia (e.g., angina) or life-threatening anemia.

CHRONIC Rx
Patients should be instructed to continue their iron supplements for at least 6 mo or longer to correct depleted body iron stores.

DISPOSITION
Most patients respond rapidly to iron supplementation with improvement in CBC and general well-being. GI side effects from oral iron therapy are frequent and may require decreased dose to once daily.

REFERRAL
GI referral for evaluation of GI malignancy is recommended in all patients with iron deficiency and suspected GI blood loss.

MISCELLANEOUS

COMMENTS
- If the diagnosis of iron deficiency anemia is made, it is mandatory to try to locate the suspected site of iron loss.
- U.S. Preventive Services Task Force Recommendations for screening for iron deficiency anemia are described in Section V, Chapter 22.

REFERENCES
Massey, AC: Microcytic anemia: differential diagnosis and management of iron deficiency anemia, *Med Clin North Am* 76(3):549, 1992.
Newton W: Laboratory diagnosis of iron-deficiency anemia, *J Fam Pract* 41:404, 1995.
Rochey DC, Cello JP: Evaluation of the GI tract in patients with iron deficiency, *New Engl J Med* 329: 1691, 1993.

Author: **Fred F. Ferri, M.D.**

CLINICAL TOPICS   Anemia, pernicious (PTG)   33

BASIC INFORMATION

DEFINITION
Pernicious anemia is an autoimmune disease resulting from antibodies against intrinsic factor and gastric parietal cells.

SYNONYMS
Megaloblastic anemia resulting from vitamin B_{12} deficiency

ICD-9-CM CODES
281.0 Pernicious anemia

EPIDEMIOLOGY AND DEMOGRAPHICS
- Increased incidence in females and older adults (diagnosis is unusual before age 35)
- The overall prevalence of undiagnosed PA over age 60 yr is 1.9%
- Prevalence is highest in women (2.7%), particularly in black women (4.3%)

PHYSICAL FINDINGS
- Mucosal pallor, glossitis
- Peripheral sensory neuropathy with paresthesias initially and absent reflexes in advanced cases
- Loss of joint position sense, pyramidal or long track signs
- Possible splenomegaly and mild hepatomegaly
- Generalized weakness and delirium/dementia

ETIOLOGY
- Antigastric parietal cell antibodies in >70% of patients, antiintrinsic factor antibodies in >50% of patients
- Atrophic gastric mucosa

DIAGNOSIS

DIFFERENTIAL DIAGNOSIS
- Nutritional vitamin B_{12} deficiency
- Malabsorption
- Chronic alcoholism (multifactorial)
- Chronic gastritis related to *Helicobacter pylori* infection
- Folic acid deficiency
- Myelodysplasia
- The differential diagnosis of megaloblastic anemia is described in Box 2-13. A clinical algorithm for evaluation of anemia is described in Fig. 3-5.

WORKUP
- The clinical presentation of pernicious anemia varies with the stage. Initially, patient may be asymptomatic. In advanced stages, patients may present with impaired memory, depression, gait disturbances, paresthesias, and complaints of generalized weakness.
- Investigation consists primarily of laboratory evaluation.
- Endoscopy and biopsy for atrophic gastritis may be performed in selected cases.
- Diagnosis is crucial because failure to treat may result in irreversible neurologic deficits.

LABORATORY TESTS
- CBC generally reveals macrocytic anemia and leukopenia with hypersegmented neutrophils.
- MCV is generally significantly elevated in the advanced stages.
- Reticulocyte count is low/normal.
- Falsely low serum cobalamin levels can occur in patients with severe folate deficiency, in patients using high doses of ascorbic acid, and when cobalamin levels are measured following nuclear medicine studies (radioactivity interferes with cobalamin RIA measurement).
- Falsely high normal levels in patients with cobalamin deficiency can occur in severe liver disease or chronic granulocytic leukemia.
- The absence of anemia or macrocytosis does not exclude the diagnosis of cobalamin deficiency. Anemia is absent in 20% of patients with cobalamin deficiency, and macrocytosis is absent in >30% of patients at the time of diagnosis. It can be blocked by concurrent iron deficiency or anemia of chronic disease and may be masked by thalassemia trait.
- Schilling test is abnormal in part I (refer to Section IV), part II corrects to normal after administration of intrinsic factor.
- Laboratory tests used for detecting cobalamin deficiency in patients with normal vitamin B_{12} levels include serum and urinary methylmalonic acid level (elevated), total homocysteine level (elevated), intrinsic factor antibody (positive).
- Additional laboratory abnormalities can include elevated LDH, direct hyperbilirubinemia, and decreased haptoglobin.

TREATMENT

NONPHARMACOLOGIC THERAPY
Avoid folic acid supplementation without proper vitamin B_{12} supplementation.

ACUTE GENERAL Rx
Traditional therapy of a cobalamin deficiency consists of IM injections of vitamin B_{12} 1000 μg/wk for the initial 4 to 6 wk followed by 1000 μg/mo IM indefinitely. When hematological parameters have returned to normal range, intranasal cyanocobalamin may be used in place of cyanocobalamin. The initial dose of intranasal cyanocobalamin (Nascobal) is one spray (500 μg) in one nostril once per week. Monitor response and increase dose if serum B_{12} levels decline. Consider return to intramuscular vitamin B_{12} supplementation if decline persists.

CHRONIC Rx
Parenteral vitamin B_{12} 1000 μg/mo or intranasal cyanocobalamin 500 μg/wk (see above) for the remainder of life

DISPOSITION
Anemia generally resolves with appropriate treatment. Neurologic deficits, if present at diagnosis, may be permanent.

REFERRAL
GI referral for endoscopy upon diagnosis of pernicious anemia and surveillance endoscopy every 5 yr to rule out gastric carcinoma

MISCELLANEOUS

COMMENTS
- Patients must understand that therapy is lifelong.
- Self-injection of vitamin B_{12} may be taught in selected patients.

REFERENCES
Carmel R: Prevalence of undiagnosed pernicious anemia in the elderly, *Arch Intern Med* 156:1097, 1996.

Pruth RK, Tefferi A: Pernicious anemia revisited, *Mayo Clin Proc* 69:144, 1994.

Sumner AE et al: Elevated methylmalonic acid and total homocysteine levels show high prevalence of vitamin B_{12} deficiency after gastric surgery, *Ann Intern Med* 124:469, 1996.

Author: **Fred F. Ferri, M.D.**

Anemia, sickle cell (PTG)

BASIC INFORMATION

DEFINITION
Sickle cell anemia is a hemoglobinopathy characterized by the production of hemoglobin S caused by substitution of the amino acid valine for glutamic acid in the sixth position of the γ-globin chain. When exposed to lower oxygen tension, RBCs assume a sickle shape resulting in stasis of RBCs in capillaries. Painful crises are caused by ischemic tissue injury resulting from obstruction of blood flow produced by sickled erythrocytes.

SYNONYMS
Sickle cell disease
Hemoglobin S disease

ICD-9-CM CODES
286.60 Sickle cell anemia

EPIDEMIOLOGY AND DEMOGRAPHICS
- Sickle cell hemoglobin S is transmitted by an autosomal recessive gene. It is found mostly in blacks (1 in 400 black Americans).
- Sickle cell trait occurs in nearly 10% of black Americans.
- There is no predominant sex.

PHYSICAL FINDINGS
- Physical examination is variable depending on the degree of anemia and presence of acute vasoocclusive syndromes or neurologic, cardiovascular, GU, and musculoskeletal complications.
- There is no clinical laboratory finding that is pathognomonic of painful crisis of sickle cell disease. The diagnosis of a painful episode is made solely on the basis of the medical history and physical examination.
- Bones are the most common site of pain. Dactylitis, or hand-foot syndrome (acute, painful swelling of the hands and feet), is the first manifestation of sickle cell disease in many infants. Irritability and refusal to walk are other common symptoms. After infancy, musculoskeletal pain can be symmetric, asymmetric, or migratory, and it may or may not be associated with swelling, low-grade fever, redness, or warmth.
- In both children and adults, sickle vasoocclusive episodes are difficult to distinguish from osteomyelitis, septic arthritis, synovitis, rheumatic fever, or gout.
- When abdominal or visceral pain is present, care should be taken to exclude sequestration syndromes (spleen, liver) or the possibility of an acute condition such as appendicitis, pancreatitis, cholecystitis, urinary tract infection, PID, or malignancy.
- Pneumonia ("chest syndrome") develops during the course of 20% of painful events and can present as chest and abdominal pain. In adults, chest pain may be a result of vasoocclusion in the ribs and often precedes a pulmonary event. The lower back is also a frequent site of painful crisis in adults.
- Musculoskeletal and skin abnormalities seen in sickle cell anemia include leg ulcers (particularly on the malleoli) and limb girdle deformities caused by avascular necrosis of the femoral and humeral heads.
- Endocrine abnormalities include delayed sexual maturation and late physical maturation, especially evident in boys.
- Neurologic abnormalities on examination may include seizures and altered mental status.
- Infections, particularly involving *Salmonella*, *Mycoplasma*, and *Streptococcus*, are relatively common.
- Severe splenomegaly secondary to sequestration often occurs in children prior to splenic atrophy.

DIAGNOSIS

DIFFERENTIAL DIAGNOSIS
- Thalassemia
- Iron deficiency anemia, leukemia
- The differential diagnosis of patients presenting with a painful crisis is discussed in "Physical findings" (see above).

WORKUP
- Screening of all newborns regardless of racial background is recommended. Screening can be performed with sodium metabisulfite reduction test (Sickledex test).
- Hemoglobin electrophoresis will also confirm the diagnosis and is useful to identify hemoglobin variants such as fetal hemoglobin and hemoglobin A2.

LABORATORY TESTS
- Anemia (resulting from chronic hemolysis), reticulocytosis, leukocytosis, and thrombocytosis are common.
- Elevations of bilirubin and LDH are also common.
- Peripheral blood smear may reveal sickle cells, target cells, poikilocytosis and hypochromia.
- Elevated BUN and creatinine may be present in patients with progressive renal insufficiency.
- Urinalysis may reveal hematuria and proteinuria.

IMAGING STUDIES
- Chest x-ray examination is useful in patients presenting with "chest syndrome." Cardiomegaly may be present on chest x-ray examination.
- Bone scan is useful to rule out osteomyelitis (usually secondary to salmonella). MRI scan is also effective in diagnosing osteomyelitis.
- CT scan or MRI of brain is often needed in patients presenting with neurologic complications such as TIA, CVA, seizures, or altered mental status.

Anemia, sickle cell (PTG)

TREATMENT

NONPHARMACOLOGIC THERAPY
- Patients should be instructed to avoid conditions that may precipitate sickling crisis, such as hypoxia, infections, acidosis, and dehydration.
- Maintain adequate hydration (PO or IV).
- Correct hypoxia.

ACUTE GENERAL Rx
- Aggressively diagnose and treat suspected infections (salmonella osteomyelitis and pneumococcal infections occur more frequently in patients with sickle cell anemia because of splenic infarcts and atrophy).
- Provide pain relief during the vaso-oclusive crisis. Medications should be administered on a fixed time schedule with a dosing interval that does not extend beyond the duration of the desired pharmacologic effect.
  1. Meperidine is contraindicated in patients with renal dysfunction or CNS disease because its metabolite, normeperidine (which is excreted by the kidneys) can cause seizures.
  2. Narcotics should be given on a fixed schedule (not PRN for pain), with rescue dosing for breakthrough pain as needed.
  3. Except when contraindications exist, concomitant use of NSAIDs should be standard treatment.
  4. Nurses should be instructed not to give narcotics if the patient is heavily sedated or respirations are depressed.
  5. When the patient shows signs of improvement, narcotic drugs should be tapered gradually to prevent withdrawal syndrome. It is advisable to observe the patient on oral pain relief medications for 12 to 24 hr before discharge from the hospital.
- Aggressively diagnose and treat any potential complications (e.g., septic necrosis of the femoral head, priapism, bony infarcts, and acute "chest syndrome").
- Avoid "routine" transfusions. Indications for transfusion: aplastic crises, severe hemolytic crises (particularly during third trimester of pregnancy).
- Hydroxyurea (500 to 750 mg/day) increases hemoglobin F levels and reduces the frequency of painful crises.

CHRONIC Rx
- Guidelines for prompt management of fever, infections, pain, and specific complications should be reviewed.
- Genetic counseling is recommended in all cases.
- Avoid unnecessary transfusions. Exchange transfusions may be necessary for patients with acute neurologic signs, aplastic crisis, or undergoing surgery.
- Allogeneic stem cell transplantation can be curative in young patients with symptomatic sickle cell disease; however, the death rate from the procedure is nearly 10%, the marrow recipients are likely to be infertile, and there is an undefined risk of chemotherapy-induced malignancy.

REFERRAL
- Hospitalization is generally recommended for most crises and complications.
- Psychosocial counseling and support structures should be developed.

MISCELLANEOUS

COMMENTS
- Patients and their families should receive genetic counseling and should be made aware of the difference between sickle cell trait and sickle cell disease.
- Regular immunizations and pneumococcal vaccination are recommended.
- Patients should be instructed on a well-balanced diet and appropriate folic acid supplementation.

REFERENCES
US Department of Health and Human Services: *Management of painful crises in sickle cell disease,* NIH Pub No 96-2117, 1995.

Walters MC et al: Bone marrow transplantation for sickle cell disease, *N Engl J Med* 335:369, 1996.

Ware RE et al: Hydroxyurea: an alternative to transfusion therapy for stroke in sickle cell anemia, *Am J Hematol* 50:140, 1995.

Author: **Fred F. Ferri, M.D.**

Aneurysm, abdominal aorta

BASIC INFORMATION

DEFINITION
An abdominal aortic aneurysm is a permanent localized dilatation of the abdominal aortic artery to at least 50% when compared with the normal diameter. The normal diameter in men is 2.3 cm, and in women it is 1.9 cm.

SYNONYMS
AAA

ICD-9-CM CODES
441.4 Aneurysm abdominal (aorta)
441.3 Ruptured abdominal aortic aneurysm

EPIDEMIOLOGY AND DEMOGRAPHICS
- The incidence of abdominal aortic aneurysms has been rising from 12.2 cases/100,000 persons to 36.2 cases/100,000 persons from 1951 to 1980.
- The prevalence ranges from 2% to 5% in men >60 yr.
- AAA is predominantly a disease of the elderly, affecting men > women (4:1).
- Rupture of an abdominal aortic aneurysm is the tenth leading cause of death in men >55 yr (15,000 deaths/yr in the U.S.).
- The risk of rupture is 2% in 5 yr in aneurysms <4 cm and 25% to 40% in aneurysms >5 cm.
- Mortality after rupture is >90%. Of those patients who reach the hospital, it is estimated 50% will survive.

PHYSICAL FINDINGS
- Pulsatile epigastric mass that may or may not be tender.
- Discoloration and pain of the feet if the thrombus within the aneurysm embolizes.
- Shock, hypoperfusion, abdominal distention if rupture occurs.
- Rare presentations include hematemesis or melena with abdominal and back pain in patients with aortoenteric fistulas. Aortocaval fistula produces loud abdominal bruits.

ETIOLOGY
Multifactorial
- Atherosclerotic (degenerative or nonspecific)
- Genetic, e.g., Ehlers-Danlos syndrome
- Trauma
- Cystic medial necrosis (Marfan's syndrome)
- Arteritis, inflammatory
- Mycotic, infected (syphilis)

DIAGNOSIS

DIFFERENTIAL DIAGNOSIS
Almost 75% of abdominal aneurysms are asymptomatic and are discovered on routine examination or serendipitously when ordering studies for other complaints. This must be considered in the differential of anyone presenting with abdominal pain or back pain.

IMAGING STUDIES
- Abdominal ultrasound is nearly 100% accurate in identifying an aneurysm and estimating the size to within 0.3 to 0.4 cm. It is not very good in estimating the proximal extension to the renal arteries or involvement of the iliac arteries.
- CT scan is recommended for preoperative aneurysm imaging and estimating the size to within 0.3 mm. There are no false-negatives, and the CT scan can localize the proximal extent, detect the integrity of the wall, and rule out rupture.
- Angiography gives detailed arterial anatomy, localizing the aneurysm relative to the renal and visceral arteries. This is the definitive preoperative study for surgeons.
- MRI can also be used, but it is more expensive and not as readily available.

TREATMENT

NONPHARMACOLOGIC THERAPY
- Treat atherosclerotic risk factors (diet and exercise for blood pressure, cholesterol, and diabetes, and abstinence from tobacco).
- Definitive treatment depends on the size of the aneurysm (see "Chronic Rx").

ACUTE GENERAL Rx
- Abdominal aortic rupture is an emergency. Surgery is the only chance for survival.
- Surgical mortality rates for ruptured aneurysms average 50% compared with 4% for elective repair of the nonruptured aorta.

CHRONIC Rx
Diagnosing, sizing, and repairing the asymptomatic patient is crucial.
- For aneurysms 5 cm or greater, prosthetic graft replacement is recommended, providing there is no contraindication (e.g., MI within 6 mo, refractory CHF, life expectancy <2 yr, severe residual from CVA).
- For aneurysms between 4 and 5 cm, there is still controversy. Some recommend surgery and others recommend follow-up every 6 mo with ultrasound to look for expansion. If there is >0.5 cm expansion in this group, most would proceed with surgery.
- For aneurysms <4 cm, most would follow-up with ultrasounds every 6 mo to 1 yr.

DISPOSITION
For aneurysms <5 cm, the course is variable but estimates of expansion rates average 0.4 cm/yr, with larger aneurysms expanding more rapidly.

REFERRAL
Vascular surgical referral should be made in asymptomatic patients with aneurysms 4 cm or greater or in rapidly expanding aneurysms of .5 cm, especially if symptoms are present.

MISCELLANEOUS

COMMENTS
- The majority of abdominal aortic aneurysms are infrarenal. Surgical risk is increased in patients with co-existing coronary artery disease, pulmonary disease (Pao_2 <50 mm Hg, FEV_1 <1L), liver cirrhosis, and chronic renal failure (Cr >3 mg/dl). Detailed cardiac workup with radionuclide perfusion studies for ischemia and aggressive perioperative hemodynamic monitoring help identify high-risk patients and decrease postoperative complications.
- U.S. Preventive Services Task Force Recommendations regarding screening for abdominal aortic aneurysm are described in Section V, Chapter 6.

REFERENCES
Ernst CB: Abdominal aortic aneurysm, *N Engl J Med* 328:1167,1993.
Mitchell MB, Rutherford RB, Krupski WC: *Infrarenal aortic aneurysms, vascular surgery,* ed 4, Philadelphia, 1995, WB Saunders.

Author: **Peter Petropoulos, M.D.**

CLINICAL TOPICS   **Angina pectoris (PTG)**   37

BASIC INFORMATION

DEFINITION
Angina pectoris is characterized by discomfort that occurs when myocardial oxygen demand exceeds the supply. Myocardial ischemia can be asymptomatic (silent ischemia), particularly in diabetics. Angina is classified as follows:

1. **CHRONIC (STABLE):**
   - Usually follows a precipitating event, e.g., climbing stairs, sexual intercourse, a heavy meal, emotional stress, cold weather
   - Generally same severity as previous attacks; relieved by the customary dose of nitroglycerin
   - Caused by a fixed coronary artery obstruction secondary to atherosclerosis
2. **UNSTABLE (REST OR CRESCENDO):**
   - Recent onset
   - Increasing severity, duration, or frequency of chronic angina
   - Occurs at rest or with minimal exertion
3. **PRINZMETAL'S VARIANT:**
   - Occurs at rest
   - Manifests electrocardiographically as episodic ST-segment elevations
   - Caused by coronary artery spasms with or without superimposed coronary artery disease
   - Patients also more likely to develop ventricular arrhythmias
4. **MICROVASCULAR ANGINA (SYNDROME X):**
   - Refers to patients with normal coronary angiograms and no coronary spasm but chest pain resembling angina and positive exercise test
   - Defective endothelium-dependent dilation in the coronary microcirculation contributing to the altered regulation of myocardial perfusion and the ischemic manifestations in these patients
   - Excellent prognosis
5. **ANGINA CAUSED BY AORTIC STENOSIS AND IDIOPATHIC HYPERTROPHIC SUBAORTIC STENOSIS (IHSS)**
6. **COCAINE-INDUCED CORONARY VASOCONSTRICTION**

ICD-9-CM CODES
411.1 Angina, stable
413 Angina pectoris
413.1 Prinzmetal's angina
413.9 Angina, unspecified

EPIDEMIOLOGY AND DEMOGRAPHICS
- Angina is most common in middle-aged and elderly males.
- Females are usually affected after menopause.
- Prevalence of angina pectoris in people older than 30 yr is >3%.
- Within 12 mo of initial diagnosis, 10% to 20% of patients with diagnosis of stable angina progress to MI or unstable angina.

PHYSICAL FINDINGS
- Although there is significant individual variation, most patients usually complain of substernal chest pain (pressure, tightness, heaviness, sharp pain, sensation similar to intestinal gas or dysphagia).
- The pain is of short duration (30 sec to 30 min), nonpleuritic, and often accompanied by shortness of breath, nausea, diaphoresis, and numbness or pain in the left arm, jaw, or shoulder.

ETIOLOGY
UNCONTROLLABLE RISK FACTORS FOR ANGINA:
- Advanced age
- Male sex
- Genetic predisposition

MODIFIABLE RISK FACTORS FOR ANGINA:
- Smoking (risk is almost double)
- Hypertension (risk is double if systolic blood pressure is >180 mm Hg)
- Hyperlipidemia
- Glucose intolerance or diabetes mellitus
- Obesity (weight >30% over ideal)
- Hypothyroidism
- Left ventricular hypertrophy (LVH)
- Sedentary life-style
- Oral contraceptive use
- Cocaine use (Cocaine is used by >5,000,000 Americans regularly and is responsible for >64,000 ER evaluations yearly to rule out myocardial ischemia.)
- Low serum folate levels (Folate is required for conversion of homocysteine to methionine.) Hyperhomocystinemia has a toxic effect on vascular endothelium and interferes with proliferation of arterial wall smooth muscle cells. Folate deficiencies are associated with an increased risk of fatal coronary heart disease.)

DIAGNOSIS

DIFFERENTIAL DIAGNOSIS
Noncardiac pain mimicking angina may be caused by:
- Pulmonary diseases (pulmonary hypertension, pulmonary embolism, pleurisy, pneumothorax, pneumonia)
- GI disorders (peptic ulcer disease, pancreatitis, esophageal spasm, esophageal reflux, cholecystitis, cholelithiasis)
- Musculoskeletal conditions (costochondritis, chest wall trauma, cervical arthritis with radiculopathy, muscle strain, myositis)
- Acute aortic dissection
- Herpes zoster

WORKUP
- The most important diagnostic factor is the history.
- The physical examination is of little diagnostic help and may be totally normal in many patients.
- An ECG taken during the acute episode may show transient T-wave inversion or ST-segment depression or elevation, but some patients may have a normal tracing. (Table 2-62, Section II describes the differential diagnosis of ST-segment elevation.)
- Perform exercise tolerance test.

LABORATORY TESTS
- Cardiac isoenzymes (CK-MB q8h × 2) should be obtained to rule out MI.
- Cardiac troponin I is also a specific marker of myocardial necrosis and is useful in evaluating patients with unstable angina (a cardiac troponin I level > 0.4 ng/ml may be indicative of non–Q wave infarction).

IMAGING STUDIES
- Chest x-ray may show cardiomegaly or pulmonary vascular congestion.
- Echocardiography is indicated only in patients with suspected valvular abnormalities; it is also useful to evaluate LV function.
- Ambulatory (Holter) electrocardiographic monitoring can detect silent ischemia (ischemic ECG changes without accompanying symptoms), which occur in >50% of patients with unstable angina despite intensive medical therapy, and it can identify a subset of patients at risk for early unfavorable outcomes.
- Coronary angiography is performed to define the location and extent of coronary disease; this is indicated in selected patients who are candidates for CABG surgery or angioplasty.

TREATMENT

NONPHARMACOLOGIC THERAPY
- Aggressive modification of preventable risk factors (weight reduction in obese patients, regular aerobic exercise program, correction of folate deficiency, estrogen replacement in postmenopausal women, low-cholesterol and low-sodium diet, cessation of cigarette smoking)
- Correction of possible aggravating factors (e.g., anemia, thyrotoxicosis, hypertension, hypercholesterolemia)

Angina pectoris (PTG)

ACUTE GENERAL Rx
The major classes of antiischemic agents are nitrates, β-adrenergic blockers, calcium channel blockers, aspirin and heparin; they can be used alone or in combination.
- Nitrates cause venodilation and relaxation of vascular smooth muscle; the decreased venous return from venodilation decreases diastolic ventricular wall tension (preload) and thereby reduces mechanical activity (and myocardial oxygen consumption) during systole. Relaxation of vascular smooth muscle increases coronary blood flow and reduces systemic pressure. Tolerance to nitrates can be minimized by avoiding sustained blood levels with a daily nitrate-free period (e.g., omission of bedtime dose of oral isosorbide dinitrate or 12 hr on/12 hr off transdermal nitroglycerin therapy).
- β-Adrenergic blockers achieve their major antianginal effect by reducing heart rate and systolic blood pressure.
- Calcium channel blockers play a major role in preventing and terminating myocardial ischemia induced by coronary artery spasm. They are particularly effective in treating microvascular angina. Short-acting calcium channel blockers should be avoided. Calcium channel blockers should generally also be avoided after complicated MI (CHF) and in patients with CHF secondary to systolic dysfunction (unless necessary to control heart rate).
- Aspirin has been proven effective for prevention of MI and coronary death in males >50 yr old. Dosage varies from 81 mg to 325 mg qd or 325 mg qod.
- IV heparin is useful in patients with unstable angina and reduces the frequency of MI and refractory angina. Patients with unstable angina treated with aspirin plus heparin have a 32% reduction in the risk of MI and death compared with those treated with aspirin alone; therefore, unless heparin is contraindicated, most hospitalized patients with unstable angina should be treated with both aspirin and heparin.

The pharmacologic treatment of ischemic chest pain resulting from the use of cocaine differs from that of patients with the usual type of myocardial ischemia:
- These patients should be initially treated with oxygen, benzodiazepines, aspirin, and nitroglycerin.
- Calcium antagonists (e.g., verapamil) or phentolamine should be considered as second line therapy.
- β-Blockers should be avoided because they enhance cocaine-induced coronary vasoconstriction, increase blood, and increase likelihood of seizures.

CHRONIC Rx
Use of lipid-lowering drugs (e.g., statins) is cost effective in patients with coronary heart disease and hyperlipidemia refractory to diet and exercise.

DISPOSITION
- The Framingham study showed that the overall mortality for angina in medically treated patients is 4%.
- Mortality drops to 1.5% if angina is based on one- or two-vessel disease and rises to 9% if the patient has three-vessel disease and poor exercise tolerance.

REFERRAL
- CABG surgery is recommended for patients with left main coronary disease or symptomatic three-vessel disease, since the survival rate is significantly improved in these patients. When CABG is done for relief of severe angina, it brings complete relief of angina in approximately 70% of patients, partial relief in another 20%.
- Minimally invasive direct coronary artery bypass (MIDCAB) is a recent variation of CABG for patients in whom sternotomy and cardiopulmonary bypass is either contraindicated or unnecessary. In this procedure, the left internal mammary is anastomosed to the LAD through a thoracic incision without cardiopulmonary bypass.
- Percutaneous transluminal coronary angioplasty (PTCA) should be considered for patients with one- or two-vessel disease. Patients selected for PTCA must also be candidates for CABG. The types of lesions best suited for angioplasty are proximal lesions, noncalcified, concentric, and preferably shorter than 5 mm. Approximately 80% of patients show immediate benefit after PTCA. Restenosis with recurrence of angina occurs in approximately 30% of patients, usually within the first few months after PTCA. In these patients, PTCA can be repeated.
- The development of coronary stents has broadened the number of patients that can be treated in the cardiac laboratory. These mesh props provide a safety net during PTCA and reduce restenosis rates afterwards in about 30% of patients. The major limitations of stenting are the 4% risk of MI after this procedure, bleeding complications when anticoagulants are used after stenting, and the higher cost associated with the use of stents.

MISCELLANEOUS

REFERENCES
Antman EM et al: Cardiac specific troponin I levels to predict the risk of mortality in patients with acute coronary syndromes, *N Engl J Med* 335:1342, 1996.

Butler RR, Habelson W: Radionuclide imaging in the evaluation of heart disease, *Am Fam Physician* 55:221, 1997.

Hollander JE: The management of cocaine-associated myocardial ischemia, *N Engl J Med* 333:1267, 1995.

Johannenson M et al: Cost effectiveness of simvastatin treatment to lower cholesterol levels in patients with coronary heart disease, *N Engl J Med* 336:332, 1997.

Versaci F et al: A comparison of coronary artery stenting with angioplasty for isolated stenosis of the proximal left anterior descending artery, *N Engl J Med* 336:817, 1997.

Author: **Fred F. Ferri, M.D.**

CLINICAL TOPICS

Ankle fracture (PTG)

BASIC INFORMATION

DEFINITION
Ankle fractures involve the lateral, medial, or posterior malleolus of the ankle and may occur either alone or in some combination. Associated ligamentous injuries are included.

ICD-9-CM CODES
824.8 Ankle fracture (malleolus) (closed)
824.2 Lateral malleolus fracture (fibular)
824.0 Medial malleolus fracture (tibial)

PHYSICAL FINDINGS
- Deformity usually dependent on extent of displacement
- Pain, tenderness, and hemorrhage at the site of injury
- Gentle palpation of ligamentous structures (especially deltoid ligament) to determine the extent of soft tissue injury
- Evaluation of distal neurovascular status; results recorded

ETIOLOGY
- The ankle depends on its ligamentous and bony support for stability. The joint, or *mortise*, is an inverted U with the dome of the talus fitting into the medial and lateral malleoli. The posterior margin of the tibia is often called the *third* or *posterior malleolus*.
- Most common ankle fractures are the result of eversion or lateral rotation forces on the talus (in contrast to common sprains, which are caused usually by inversion).

DIAGNOSIS

IMAGING STUDIES
Standard AP and lateral views accompanied by an AP taken 15° internally rotated. The last view is taken to properly visualize the mortise.

TREATMENT

All fractures: elevation and ice to control swelling for 48 to 72 hr.

ACUTE GENERAL Rx
- Clinical and roentgenographic assessment of the status of the ankle mortise and stability of the injury is mandatory to determine treatment.
- There is potential for displacement if both sides of the joint are significantly injured (e.g., fracture of the lateral malleolus with deltoid ligament injury).
- Deviation of the position of the talus in the mortise could lead to traumatic arthritis.
- If there is no widening of the ankle mortise, many injuries can be safely treated with simple casting without reduction or surgical intervention:
  1. Undisplaced or avulsion fractures of either malleolus below the ankle joint line:
     a. Stability of the joint is not compromised and a short leg walking cast or ankle support is sufficient.
     b. Weight bearing is allowed as tolerated.
     c. In 4 to 6 wk, protection may be discontinued.
  2. Isolated undisplaced fractures of either the medial, lateral, or posterior malleolus:
     a. Usually stable and require only the application of a short leg walking cast with the ankle in the neutral position.
     b. Immobilization should be continued for 8 wk.
     c. Fracture line of lateral malleolus may persist roentgenographically for several months but immobilization beyond 8 wk is usually unnecessary.
     d. Undisplaced bimalleolar fractures are treated with a long leg cast flexed 30° at the knee to prevent motion and displacement of the fracture fragments.
     e. In 4 wk, a short leg walking cast may be applied for an additional 4 wk.
  3. Isolated fractures of the lateral malleolus that are slightly displaced:
     a. May be treated with casting if no medial injury is present.
     b. A below-knee walking cast is applied with ankle in the neutral position and weight bearing is allowed as tolerated.
     c. Six weeks of immobilization is sufficient.
     d. If medial tenderness is present, suggesting deltoid ligament rupture, a carefully molded cast may suffice if weight bearing is not allowed and the patient is followed closely for signs of instability, especially after swelling recedes. If significant widening of the medial ankle mortise (increase in the "medial clear space") develops as a result of lateral displacement of the talus, referral for possible reduction is indicated.
     e. If signs of instability are already present at initial examination (widening of the medial clear space with medial tenderness), referral is indicated.
  4. Undisplaced fracture of the distal fibular epiphysis:
     a. Diagnosed clinically.
     b. There is tenderness over the epiphyseal plate.
     c. Roentgenographic findings are often negative.
     d. A short leg walking cast is applied for 4 wk.
     e. Growth disturbance is rare.
  5. Isolated posterior malleolar fractures involving less than 25% of the joint surface on the lateral roentgenogram:
     a. Safely treated by applying a short leg walking cast.
     b. Fractures involving >25% of the weight bearing surface should be referred because of the potential for instability and subsequent traumatic arthritis.

CHRONIC Rx
- Early motion is encouraged through a home exercise program.
- Protection from reinjury is appropriate for 4 to 6 wk following cast removal.
- Temporary increase in lower extremity swelling that frequently occurs after short leg cast removal may benefit from the use of support hose.

DISPOSITION
Significant factors involved in the development of traumatic arthritis:
- Amount of joint trauma at the time of injury
- Eventual position of the talus in the mortise

Fracture nonunion is uncommon unless displacement is significant.

REFERRAL
Orthopedic consultation for:
- Unstable ankle joint
- Widened ankle mortise
- Posterior malleolar fracture over 25% of joint with incongruity
- Marked displacement of fracture fragment

MISCELLANEOUS

REFERENCES
Michelson JD: Current concepts review: fractures about the ankle, *J Bone Joint Surg* 77(A):142, 1995.
Stiehl JB: Complex ankle fracture dislocations with syndesmotic diastasis, *Orthop Rev* 19:499, 1990.

Author: **Lonnie R. Mercier, M.D.**

Ankle sprain (PTG)

BASIC INFORMATION

DEFINITION
An ankle sprain is an injury to the ligamentous support of the ankle. Most (85%) involve the lateral ligament complex. The anterior inferior tibiofibular (AITF) ligament, deltoid ligament, and interosseous membrane may also be injured. Damage to the tibiofibular syndesmosis is sometimes called a *high sprain* because of pain above the ankle.

ICD-9-CM CODES
845.00 Sprain, ankle or foot

EPIDEMIOLOGY AND DEMOGRAPHICS
PREVALENCE: 1 case/10,000 people each day
PREDOMINANT SEX: Varies according to age and level of physical activity

PHYSICAL FINDINGS
- Often a history of a "pop"
- Variable amounts of tenderness and hemorrhage
- Possible abnormal anterior drawer test (pulling the plantar flexed foot forward to determine if there is any abnormal increase in forward movement of the talus in the ankle mortise)
- Inversion sprains: tender laterally; syndesmotic injuries: area of tenderness is more anterior and proximal
- Evaluation of motor function

ETIOLOGY
- Lateral injuries usually result from inversion and plantar flexion injuries.
- Eversion and rotational forces may injure the deltoid or AITF ligament or the interosseous membrane.

DIAGNOSIS

DIFFERENTIAL DIAGNOSIS
Fracture of the ankle or foot, particularly involving the distal fibular growth plate in the immature patient

WORKUP
- History and clinical examination are usually sufficient to establish the diagnosis.
- Plain radiographs are always needed.

IMAGING STUDIES
Roentgenographic evaluation
1. Usually normal but always performed
2. Should include the fifth metatarsal base
3. All minor avulsion fractures noted
Varying opinions on the usefulness of arthrograms, tenograms, and stress films

TREATMENT

ACUTE GENERAL Rx
Ankle sprains are often graded I, II, or III, according to severity, with Grade III injury implying complete rupture.
- Rest
- Ice
- Compression
- Elevation
- Varying opinions regarding the initial use of NSAIDs
- In 48 to 72 hr, active range of motion and weight bearing as tolerated
- In 4 to 5 days, exercise against resistance added
- Possible cast immobilization for some patients who require early independent walking, short leg orthoses also available for the same purpose
- Surgery is rarely recommended, even for Grade III sprains, reports of equally satisfactory outcomes with nonsurgical treatment

CHRONIC Rx
- Lateral heel and sole wedge to prevent inversion
- Protective taping or bracing during vigorous activities
- Strengthening exercises

DISPOSITION
- Lateral sprains of any severity may cause lingering symptoms for weeks and months.
  1. Some syndesmotic sprains take even longer to heal.
  2. Heterotopic ossification may even develop in the interosseous membrane, but long-term results do not seem to be affected by such ossification.
- Continuing lateral symptoms may require surgical reconstruction, although late traumatic arthritis or chronic instability are rare regardless of treatment.

REFERRAL
For orthopedic consultation for cases that fail to respond to conservative treatment

MISCELLANEOUS

COMMENTS
If healing seems delayed, the following conditions should be considered:
1. Talar dome fracture
2. Reflex sympathetic dystrophy
3. Chronic tendinitis
4. Peroneal tendon subluxation
5. Other occult fracture
6. Peroneal weakness

Repeat plain roentgenograms, bone scan, or MRI may be indicated.

REFERENCES
Cox JS: Surgical and nonsurgical treatment of acute ankle sprains, *Clin Orthop Relat Res* 198:118, 1985.
Kannus P, Renstrom, P: Current concepts review: treatment for acute tears of the lateral ligaments of the ankle, *J Bone Joint Surg* 73:305, 1991.

Author: **Lonnie R. Mercier, M.D.**

Ankylosing spondylitis (PTG)

BASIC INFORMATION

DEFINITION
Ankylosing spondylitis is a chronic inflammatory condition involving the sacroiliac joints and axial skeleton. It is one of a group of several overlapping syndromes, including spondylitis, associated with Reiter's syndrome, psoriasis, and IBD. Patients are typically seronegative for the rheumatoid factor, and these disorders are now commonly called *rheumatoid variants* or *seronegative spondyloarthropathies*.

SYNONYMS
Marie-Strumpell disease

ICD-9-CM CODES
720.0 Ankylosing spondylitis

EPIDEMIOLOGY AND DEMOGRAPHICS
PREVALENCE: 0.15% of male population (rare in blacks)
PREDOMINANT AGE AT ONSET: 15 to 35 yr
PREDOMINANT SEX: male:female ratio of 10:1

PHYSICAL FINDINGS
- Morning stiffness
- Fatigue, weight loss, anorexia, and other systemic complaints in more severe forms
- Bilateral sacroiliac tenderness (sacroilitis)
- Limited lumbar spine motion
- Loss of chest expansion measured at the nipple line <2.5 cm, reflecting rib cage involvement
- Occasionally, peripheral joint involvement (large joints are more commonly affected)
- Possible extraskeletal manifestations affecting the cardiovascular system (aortic insufficiency, heart block, cardiomegaly), lungs (pulmonary fibrosis), and eye (uveitis)

ETIOLOGY
Unknown

DIAGNOSIS

DIFFERENTIAL DIAGNOSIS
- Other spondyloarthropathies (see Table 2-61 and Box 2-112)
- A clinical algorithm for the evaluation of back pain is described in Fig. 3-11.

WORKUP
The modified New York criteria are often used for diagnosis:
- Low back pain of at least 3 mo duration improved by exercise and not relieved by rest
- Limitation of lumbar spine movement in sagittal and frontal planes
- Decreased chest expansion below normal values for age and sex
- Bilateral sacroiliitis of minimal grade or greater
- Unilateral sacroiliitis of moderate grade or greater

LABORATORY TESTS
- Elevated sedimentation rate
- Absence of rheumatoid factor and ANA
- Possible mild hyperchromic anemia
- Presence of HLA/B27 antigen in >90% of patients

IMAGING STUDIES
- Early roentgenographic features are those of bilateral sacroiliitis on plain films.
- Vertebral bodies may become demineralized and a typical "squaring off" occurs.
- With progression, calcification of the annulus fibrosis and paravertebral ligaments develop giving rise to the so-called bamboo spine appearance.
- End result may be a forward protruding cervical spine and fixed dorsal kyphosis.

TREATMENT

NONPHARMACOLOGIC THERAPY
- Exercises primarily to maintain flexibility; general aerobic activity also important
- Postural training
  1. Patients must be instructed to sit in the erect position and to avoid stooping; otherwise, a flexion contracture of the spine may develop.
  2. Sleeping should be in the supine position on a firm mattress; pillows should not be placed under the head or knees.

CHRONIC Rx
NSAIDs: indomethacin is often successful in relieving symptoms; newer nonsteroidal agents may be tried as well.

DISPOSITION
- Most patients have a normal life span.
- The usual course of the disease is not life-threatening, but death may occur as a result of aortic insufficiency or secondary amyloidosis with renal disease.

REFERRAL
- Orthopedic consultation for pain or deformity
- Ophthalmologic consultation for occular complications
- Rheumatology consultation for uncontrolled symptoms

MISCELLANEOUS

COMMENTS
Years may pass between the onset of symptoms and the ultimate diagnosis because of the frequency of nonspecific low back pain from other disorders.

REFERENCES
Amor B, Dougades M: Management of refractory ankylosing spondylitis and related spondyloarthropathies, *Rheum Dis Clin North Am* 21(1):117, 1995.

Ball, GV: Ankylosing spondylitis. In McCarty DJ (ed) *Arthritis and allied conditions*, ed 11, Philadelphia, 1989, Lea and Febiger.

Author: **Lonnie R. Mercier, M.D.**

Anorectal fistula

BASIC INFORMATION

DEFINITION
A fistula is an inflammatory track with a secondary (external) opening in the perianal skin and a primary (internal) opening in the anal canal at the dentate line. It originates in an abscess in the intersphincteric space of the anal canal. Fistulas can be classified as follows:
1. Intersphincteric: fistula track passes within the intersphincteric plane to the perianal skin; most common
2. Transsphincteric: fistula track passes from the internal opening, through the internal and external sphincter, and into the ischiorectal fossa to the perianal skin; frequent
3. Suprasphincteric: After passing through the internal sphincter, fistula tract passes above the puborectalis and then tracts downward, lateral to the external sphincter, into the ischiorectal space to the perianal skin; uncommon; if abscess cavity extends cephalad, a supralevator abscess possibly palpable on rectal examination
4. Extrasphincteric: fistula tract passes from the rectum, above the levators, through the levator muscles to the ischiorectal space and perianal skin; rare.

With a horseshoe fistula, the track passes from one ischiorectal fossa to the other behind the rectum.

SYNONYMS
Fistula-in-ano

ICD-9-CM CODES
565.1 Anal fistula

EPIDEMIOLOGY AND DEMOGRAPHICS
- Common in all ages
- Occurs equally in men and women
- Associated with constipation
- Pediatric age group: more common in infants; boys > girls

PHYSICAL FINDINGS
- Acute stage: perianal swelling, pain, and fever
- Chronic stage: history of rectal drainage or bleeding; previous abscess with drainage
- Tender external fistulous opening, within 2 to 3 cm of the anal verge, with purulent or serosanguineous drainage on compression; greater the distance from the anal margin, greater the probability of a complicated upward extension
- Goodsall's rule:
  1. Location of the internal opening related to the location of the external opening.
  2. With external opening anterior to an imaginary line drawn horizontally across the midpoint of the anus: fistulous tract runs radially into the anal canal.
  3. With opening posterior to the transanal line: track is usually curvilinear, entering the anal canal in the posterior midline.
  4. Exception to this rule: an external, anterior opening that is >3 cm from the anus. In this case the tract may curve posteriorly and end in the posterior midline.
- If perianal abscess recurs, presence of a fistula is suggested.

ETIOLOGY
- Most common: nonspecific cryptoglandular infection (skin or intestinal flora)
- Fistulas more common when intestinal microorganisms are cultured from the anorectal abscess
- Tuberculosis
- Lymphogranuloma venereum
- Actinomycosis
- Inflammatory bowel disease (IBD): Crohn's disease, ulcerative colitis
- Trauma: surgery (episiotomy, prostatectomy), foreign bodies, anal intercourse
- Malignancy: carcinoma, leukemia, lymphoma
- Treatment of malignancy: surgery, radiation

DIAGNOSIS

DIFFERENTIAL DIAGNOSIS
- Hidradenitis suppurativa
- Pilonidal sinus
- Bartholin's gland abscess or sinus
- Infected perianal sebaceous cysts

WORKUP
- Digital rectal examination:
  1. Assess sphincter tone and voluntary squeeze pressure
  2. Determine the presence of an extraluminal mass
  3. Indentify an indurated track
  4. Palpate an internal opening or pit
- Gentle probing of external orifice to avoid creating a false tract; 50% do not have clinically detectable opening
- Anoscopy
- Proctosigmoidoscopy to exclude inflammatory or neoplastic disease
- All studies done under adequate anesthesia

LABORATORY TESTS
- CBC
- Rectal biopsy if diagnosis of IBD or malignancy suspected; biopsy of external orifice is useless

IMAGING STUDIES
- Colonoscopy or barium enema if:
  1. Diagnosis of IBD or malignancy is suspected
  2. History of recurrent or multiple fistulas
  3. Patient < 25 yr old
- Small bowel series: occasionally obtained for reasons similar to above
- Fistulography: unreliable; but may be helpful in complicated fistulas

TREATMENT

NONPHARMACOLOGIC THERAPY
Sitz baths

ACUTE GENERAL Rx
- Treatment of choice: surgery
- Broad-spectrum antibiotic given if:
  1. Cellulitis present
  2. Patient is immunocompromised
  3. Valvular heart disease present
  4. Prosthetic devices present
- Stool softener/laxative

CHRONIC Rx
- Surgery
- Surgical goals are as follows:
  1. Cure the fistula.
  2. Prevent recurrence.
  3. Preserve sphincter function.
  4. Minimize healing time.
- Methods for the management of anal fistulas: fistulotomy, setons, rectal advancement flaps, colostomy

DISPOSITION
Outpatient surgery

REFERRAL
Refer to a surgeon with expertise in this area.

MISCELLANEOUS

COMMENTS
- HIV-positive and diabetic patients with perirectal abscesses/fistula are true surgical emergencies.
- Risk of septicemia, Fournier's gangrene, and other septic complications make immediate drainage imperative.

REFERENCES
Barnett JL, Raper SE: Anorectal diseases. In Yamada T, Alpers DH, Owyang C: *Textbook of gastroenterology,* ed 2, Philadelphia, 1995, Lippincott.

Beart R: Chapter 97. In Sciarra JJ: *Gynecology and obstetrics,* Philadelphia, 1997, Lippincott.

Author: **Maria Elena Soler, M.D.**

Anorexia nervosa (PTG)

BASIC INFORMATION

DEFINITION
Anorexia nervosa is a prolonged illness characterized by severe self-induced weight loss and a specific psychopathology (see "Workup").

ICD-9-CM CODES
307.1 Anorexia nervosa

EPIDEMIOLOGY AND DEMOGRAPHICS
INCIDENCE/PREVALENCE (IN U.S.): Anorexia nervosa occurs in 0.2% to 1.3% of the general population, with an annual incidence of 5 to 10 cases/100,000 persons.
PREDOMINANT SEX: Female:male ratio is 9:1. Approximately 0.5% to 1% of women between the ages of 15 and 30 yr have anorexia nervosa.
PREDOMINANT AGE: Adolescence to young adulthood is the predominant age. Mean age of onset is 17 yr.

PHYSICAL FINDINGS
- Patient is emaciated and bundled in clothing.
- Skin is dry and has excessive growth of lanugo. Skin may also be yellow-tinged from carotenodermia.
- Brittle nails, thinning scalp hair are present.
- Bradycardia, hypotension, hypothermia, and bradypnea are common.
- Female fat distribution pattern is no longer evident.
- Axillary and pubic hair is preserved.
- Peripheral edema may be present.

ETIOLOGY
- Etiology is unknown, but likely multifactorial (sociocultural, psychologic, familial, and genetic factors).
- A history of sexual abuse has been reported in as many as 50% of patients with anorexia nervosa.

DIAGNOSIS

DIFFERENTIAL DIAGNOSIS
- Depression with loss of appetite
- Schizophrenia
- Conversion disorder
- Occult carcinoma, lymphoma
- Endocrine disorders: Addison's disease, diabetes mellitus, hypo- or hyperthyroidism, panhypopituitarism
- GI disorders: celiac disease, Crohn's disease, intestinal parasitosis
- Infectious disorders: AIDS, TB
- A clinical algorithm for the evaluation of anorexia is described in Fig. 3-6.

WORKUP
A diagnosis can be made using the following DSM-IV diagnostic criteria for anorexia nervosa:
1. Refusal to maintain body weight (BW) at or above a minimally normal weight for age and height (e.g., weight loss leading to maintenance of BW <85% of that expected or failure to make expected weight gain during a period of growth, leading to BW <85% of that expected)
2. Intense fear of gaining weight or becoming fat, even though underweight
3. Disturbance in the way in which BW or shape is experienced, undue influence of BW or shape on self-evaluation, or denial of the seriousness of the current low BW
4. In postmenarchal females, amenorrhea, i.e., the absence of at least three consecutive menstrual cycles (A woman is considered to have amenorrhea if her periods occur only following hormone, e.g., estrogen, administration.)

Anorexia nervosa (PTG)

Specify type:
   Restricting type: During the current episode of anorexia nervosa, the person has not regularly engaged in binge-eating or purging behavior (i.e., self-induced vomiting or the misuse of laxatives, diuretics, or enemas).
   Binge-eating/purging type: During the current episode of anorexia nervosa, the person has regularly engaged in binge-eating or purging behavior (i.e., self-induced vomiting or the misuse of laxatives, diuretics, or enemas).

Baseline ECG should be performed on all patients with anorexia nervosa. Routine monitoring of patients with prolonged QT interval is necessary; sudden death in these patients is often caused by ventricular arrhythmias related to QT interval prolongation.

LABORATORY TESTS
- Endocrine abnormalities:
  1. Decreased FSH, LH, T_4, T_3, estrogens, urinary 17-OH steroids, estrone, and estradiol
  2. Normal free T_4, TSH
  3. Increased cortisol, GH, rT_3, T_3RU
  4. Absence of cyclic surge of LH
- Leukopenia, thrombocytopenia, anemia, reduced ESR, reduced complement levels, reduced CD4 and CD8 cells may be present.
- Metabolic alkalosis, hypocalcemia, hypokalemia, hypomagnesemia, hypercholesterolemia, and hypophosphatemia may be present.
- Increased plasma β-carotene levels are useful to distinguish these patients from others on starvation diets.

TREATMENT

NONPHARMACOLOGIC THERAPY
- A multidisciplinary approach with psychologic, medical, and nutritional support is necessary.
- A goal weight should be set and the patient should be initially monitored at least once a week in the office setting. The target weight is 100% of ideal BW for teenagers and 90% to 100% for older patients.
- Weight gain should be gradual (1 to 3 lb/wk) to prevent gastric dilatation.
- Electrolyte levels should be strictly monitored.
- Mealtime should be a time for social interaction, not confrontation.
- Postprandially, sedentary activities are recommended. The patient's access to a bathroom should be monitored to prevent purging.

ACUTE GENERAL Rx
Pharmacologic treatment generally has no role in anorexia nervosa unless major depression or another psychiatric disorder is present. SSRIs can be used to alleviate the depressed mood and moderate obsessive-compulsive behavior in some individuals.

CHRONIC Rx
- Psychotherapy continued for years and focused specifically on self-image, family and peer interactions, and relapse prevention is an integral part of a successful recovery.
- Family therapy is also recommended, especially in younger patients.

DISPOSITION
- The long-term prognosis is generally poor and marked by recurrent exacerbations.
- Mortality rates vary from 5% to 20%. Frequent causes of death are electrolyte abnormalities, starvation, or suicide.

REFERRAL
Hospitalization should be considered in the following situations:
1. Severe dehydration or electrolyte imbalance
2. ECG abnormalities (prolonged QT interval, arrhythmias)
3. Significant physiologic instability (hypotension, orthostatic changes)
4. Intractable vomiting, purging, or bingeing
5. Patient having suicidal thoughts
6. Weight loss exceeds 30% of ideal BW and is unresponsive to outpatient treatment

MISCELLANEOUS

REFERENCES
American Psychiatric Association: *Diagnostic and statistical manual of mental disorders,* ed 4, Washington, DC, 1994, The Association.

Hobbs WL, Johnson CA: Anorexia nervosa: an overview, *Am Fam Physician* 54:1273, 1996.

Rome ES: Eating disorders in adolescents and young adults: what's a primary care clinician to do? *Cleveland Clin J Med* 63:387, 1996.

Author: **Fred F. Ferri, M.D.**

Anxiety (generalized anxiety disorder) (PTG)

BASIC INFORMATION

DEFINITION
Anxiety may present as a symptom in a wide range of psychiatric and medical conditions. Generalized anxiety disorder (GAD) is a condition in which the individual experiences excessive anxiety, fear, and worry for most of the time, continuously for at least 6 mo. The subjective anxiety must be accompanied by at least three somatic symptoms (e.g., restlessness, irritability, sleep disturbance, muscle tension, difficulty concentrating, or fatigability).

SYNONYMS
Anxiety neurosis
Chronic anxiety
GAD

ICD-9-CM CODES
F41.1 (DSM-IV Code 300.02)

EPIDEMIOLOGY AND DEMOGRAPHICS
INCIDENCE (IN U.S.): 31% in 1 yr
PREVALENCE (IN U.S.):
- In general population: 4.1% to 6.6% lifetime
- In primary care setting: 2.9% (It is the most common anxiety disorder in this setting.)

PREDOMINANT SEX: Females are more frequently affected (2:1 ratio), but they present for treatment less frequently (3:2 female:male).
PREDOMINANT AGE:
- 30% of patients report onset of symptoms prior to age 11 yr.
- 50% of patients have onset prior to age 18 yr.

PEAK INCIDENCE: Chronic condition with onset in early life
GENETICS: Concordance rates in dizygotic twins and monozygotic twins are not different (0% to 5%), but detailed analysis of 1033 female twin pairs finds that heredity contributes about 30% of the factors that may cause GAD.

PHYSICAL FINDINGS
- Report of being "anxious" all of their lives
- Excessive worry, usually regarding family, finances, work, or health
- Sleep disturbance, particularly early insomnia
- Muscle tension (typically in the muscles of neck and shoulders)
- Headaches (muscle tension)
- Difficulty concentrating
- Day form fatigue
- Gastrointestinal symptoms compatible with IBD (one third of patients)
- Physical consequences of anxiety are the driving force for patients seeking medical attention.
- Comorbid psychiatric illness (e.g., dysthymia or major depression) and substance abuse (e.g., alcohol abuse) are frequent.

ETIOLOGY
- There is no clear etiology.
- Several hypotheses centering on neurotransmitter (catecholamines, indolamines) and developmental psychology are used as framework for treatment recommendations.

DIAGNOSIS

DIFFERENTIAL DIAGNOSIS
- Wide range of psychiatric and medical conditions; however, for a diagnosis of GAD to be made a person must experience anxiety with coexisting physical symptoms the majority of the time continuously for at least 6 mo.
- Cardiovascular and pulmonary disease
- Hyperthyroidism
- Parkinson's disease
- Myasthenia gravis
- Consequence of recreational drug use (e.g., cocaine, amphetamine, and PCP) or withdrawal (e.g., alcohol or benzodiazepines)

WORKUP
- History: required for diagnosis
- Physical examination: confirm the patient's physical complaints
- Exclusion of organic basis for the complaints possibly requiring additional workup

TREATMENT

NONPHARMACOLOGIC THERAPY
- Cognitive-behavioral therapy
- Relaxation training
- Biofeedback
- Psychodynamic psychotherapy

NOTE: Studies directly comparing medications with psychotherapy are not available, but the general clinical impression is that the psychotherapies are probably superior to pharmacotherapies.

ACUTE GENERAL Rx
- Acute treatment is rarely indicated because GAD is a chronic condition.
- Occasionally patients are in acute distress, requiring physician to respond quickly; benzodiazepines given under these conditions as drug of choice for both daytime anxiety and initial insomnia.

CHRONIC Rx
- Benzodiazepines provide long-term symptom control with only occasional problems with tolerance or abuse; however, rate of relapse after discontinuation of benzodiazepines may be twice the rate after discontinuation of the available nonbenzodiazepine anxiolytic, buspirone.
- Buspirone is effective without any potential for tolerance or abuse.
- Tricyclic antidepressants are useful if an element of comorbid depression exists.
- Sedating antidepressants are also useful in ameliorating initial insomnia.
- Trazodone and Serzone possibly have unique benefits for these patients.

DISPOSITION
- This condition is chronic with periodic exacerbations.
- Treatment is given to provide a significant degree of improvement, but symptoms and dysfunction may persist.

REFERRAL
- If the symptoms are refractory to treatment
- If the case is complicated with a comorbid psychiatric condition
- If treatment response is suboptimal with residual dysfunction

MISCELLANEOUS

COMMENTS
The Hamilton Anxiety scale is described in Box A-10.

REFERENCES
Mancuso DM, Townsend MH, Mercante DE: Long-term follow-up of generalized anxiety disorder, *Comp Psychiatry* 34:441, 1993.

Sanderson WC, Barlow DH: A description of patients diagnosed with DSM-III-R generalized anxiety disorder, *J Nerv Ment Dis* 178:588, 1990.

Author: **Rif S. El-Mallakh, M.D.**

Aortic regurgitation (PTG)

BASIC INFORMATION

DEFINITION
Aortic regurgitation is retrograde blood flow into the left ventricle from the aorta secondary to incompetent aortic valve.

SYNONYMS
Aortic insufficiency
AI
AR

ICD-9-CM CODES
424.1 Aortic valve disorders

EPIDEMIOLOGY AND DEMOGRAPHICS
- The most common cause of isolated severe aortic regurgitation is aortic root dilatation.
- Infectious endocarditis is the most frequent cause of acute aortic regurgitation.

PHYSICAL FINDINGS
- Widened pulse pressure (markedly increased systolic blood pressure, decreased diastolic blood pressure) is present.
- Bounding pulses, head "bobbing" with each systole (de Musset's sign) are present; "water hammer" or collapsing pulse (Corrigan's pulse) can be palpated at the wrist or on the femoral arteries ("pistol shot" femorals) and is caused by rapid rise and sudden collapse of the arterial pressure during late systole; capillary pulsations (Quincke's pulse) may occur at the base of the nail beds.
- A to-and-fro "double Duroziez" murmur may be heard over femoral arteries with slight compression.
- Popliteal systolic pressure is increased over brachial systolic pressure ≥40 mm Hg (Hill's sign).
- Cardiac auscultation reveals:
  1. Displacement of cardiac impulse downward and to the patient's left
  2. S_3 heard over the apex
  3. Decrescendo, blowing diastolic murmur heard along left sternal border
  4. Low-pitched apical diastolic rumble (Austin-Flint murmur) caused by contact of the aortic regurgitant jet with the left ventricular wall
  5. Early systolic apical ejection murmur

ETIOLOGY
- Infective endocarditis
- Rheumatic fibrosis
- Trauma with valvular rupture
- Congenital bicuspid aortic valve
- Myxomatous degeneration
- Syphilitic aortitis
- Rheumatic spondylitis
- SLE
- Aortic dissection

DIAGNOSIS

DIFFERENTIAL DIAGNOSIS
- Patent ductus arteriosus, pulmonary regurgitation, and other valvular abnormalities
- The differential diagnosis of cardiac murmurs is described in Box 2-21 and Table 2-13.

WORKUP
- Echocardiogram, chest x-ray, ECG, and cardiac catheterization (selected patients)
- Medical history and physical examination focused on the following clinical manifestations:
  1. Dyspnea on exertion
  2. Syncope
  3. Chest pain
  4. CHF

IMAGING STUDIES
- Chest x-ray study
  1. Left ventricular hypertrophy (chronic aortic regurgitation)
  2. Aortic dilation
  3. Normal cardiac silhouette with pulmonary edema: possible in patients with acute aortic regurgitation
- ECG: left ventricular hypertrophy
- Echocardiography: coarse diastolic fluttering of the anterior mitral leaflet; LVH in patients with chronic aortic regurgitation
- Cardiac catheterization: assesses degree of left ventricular dysfunction, confirms the presence of a wide pulse pressure, assesses surgical risk, and determines if there is coexistent coronary artery disease

TREATMENT

NONPHARMACOLOGIC THERAPY
- Avoidance of competitive sports and strenuous activity
- Salt restriction

ACUTE GENERAL Rx
MEDICAL:
- Digitalis, diuretics, ACE inhibitors, and sodium restriction for CHF; nitroprusside in patients with acute aortic regurgitation
- Long-term vasodilator therapy with nifedipine for reducing or delaying the need for aortic valve replacement in asymptomatic patients with severe aortic regurgitation and normal left ventricular function
- Bacterial endocarditis prophylaxis for surgical and dental procedures (see Boxes A-1, A-2, and A-3 and Tables A-11 and A-12 in Appendix)

SURGICAL:
Reserved for:
- Symptomatic patients with chronic aortic regurgitation despite optimal medical therapy
- Patients with acute aortic regurgitation (i.e., infective endocarditis) producing left ventricular failure
- Evidence of systolic failure:
  1. Echocardiographic fractional shortening <25%
  2. Echocardiographic and diastolic dimension >55 mm
  3. Angiographic ejection fraction <50% or end-systolic volume index (ESVI) >60 ml/m^2
- Evidence of diastolic failure:
  1. Pulmonary pressure >45 mm Hg systolic
  2. Left ventricular end-diastolic pressure (LVEDP) >15 mm Hg at catheterization
  3. Pulmonary hypertension detected on examination
- In general, the "55 rule" has been used to determine the timing of surgery: surgery should be performed before EF <55% or end-systolic dimension >55 mm.

DISPOSITION
Variable depending on underlying condition and left ventricular function; aortic regurgitation (except when secondary to infective endocarditis) is generally well tolerated, and patients remain asymptomatic for years.

REFERRAL
Surgical referral (see "Acute General Rx" for indications)

MISCELLANEOUS

COMMENTS
The operative mortality rate for aortic regurgitation is 3% to 5%.

REFERENCES
Carabello BA, Crawford FA: Valvular heart disease, *N Engl J Med* 337:32, 1997.

Klodas E et al: Aortic regurgitation complicated by extreme left ventricular dilatation: long-term outcome after surgical correction, *J Am Coll Cardiol* 77:670, 1996.

Tornos NP et al: Clinical outcome of severe symptomatic chronic aortic regurgitation: a long-term prospective follow-up study, *Am Heart J* 130:333, 1995.

Author: **Fred F. Ferri, M.D.**

Aortic stenosis (PTG)

BASIC INFORMATION

DEFINITION
Aortic stenosis is obstruction to systolic left ventricular outflow across the aortic valve. Symptoms appear when the valve orifice decreases to <1 cm^2 (normal orifice is 3 cm^2). The stenosis is considered severe when the orifice is <0.5 cm^2/m^2 or the pressure gradient is 50 mm Hg or higher.

SYNONYMS
Aortic valvular stenosis
AS

ICD-9-CM CODES
424.1 Aortic valvular stenosis

EPIDEMIOLOGY AND DEMOGRAPHICS
- Aortic stenosis is the most common valve lesion in adults in Western countries.
- Calcific stenosis (most common cause in patients >60 yr old) occurs in 75% of patients.

PHYSICAL FINDINGS
- Rough, loud systolic diamond-shaped murmur, best heard at base of heart and transmitted into neck vessels; often associated with a thrill or ejection click; may also be heard well at the apex
- Absence or diminished intensity of sound of aortic valve closure (in severe aortic stenosis)
- Late, slow-rising carotid upstroke with decreased amplitude
- Strong apical pulse
- Narrowing of pulse pressure in later stages of aortic stenosis

ETIOLOGY
- Rheumatic inflammation of aortic valve
- Progressive stenosis of congenital bicuspid valve
- Idiopathic calcification of the aortic valve
- Congenital (major cause of aortic stenosis in patients <30 yr)

DIAGNOSIS

DIFFERENTIAL DIAGNOSIS
- Hypertrophic cardiomyopathy
- Mitral regurgitation
- Ventricular septal defect
- Aortic sclerosis
- The differential diagnosis of cardiac murmurs is described in Box 2-21 and Table 2-13.

WORKUP
- Echocardiography
- Chest x-ray examination, ECG
- Cardiac catheterization in selected patients (see below)
- Medical history focusing on symptoms and potential complications:
  1. Angina
  2. Syncope (particularly with exertion)
  3. CHF
  4. GI bleeding: in patients with associated hemorrhagic telangiectasia (AVM)

IMAGING STUDIES
- Chest x-ray examination
  1. Poststenotic dilation of the ascending aorta
  2. Calcification of aortic cusps
  3. Pulmonary congestion (in advanced stages of aortic stenosis)
- ECG:
  1. Left ventricular hypertrophy (found in >80% of patients)
  2. ST-T wave changes
  3. Atrial fibrillation: frequent
- Echocardiography: thickening of the left ventricular wall; if the patient has valvular calcifications, multiple echos may be seen from within the aortic root and there is poor separation of the aortic cusps during systole. Gradient across the valve can be estimated but is less precise than with cardiac catheterization.
- Cardiac catheterization: indicated in symptomatic patients; it confirms the diagnosis and estimates the severity of the disease by measuring the gradient across the valve, allowing calculation of the valve area. It also detects coexisting coronary artery stenosis that may need bypass at the same time as aortic valve replacement.

TREATMENT

NONPHARMACOLOGIC THERAPY
- Strenous activity should be avoided.
- Sodium restriction is needed if CHF is present.

ACUTE GENERAL Rx
MEDICAL:
- Diuretics and sodium restriction are needed if CHF is present; digoxin is used only to control rate of atrial fibrillation.
- ACE inhibitors are contraindicated.
- Calcium channel blocker verapamil may be useful only to control rate of atrial fibrillation.
- Antibiotic prophylaxis is necessary for surgical and dental procedures (see Boxes A-1, A-2, and A-3 and Tables A-11 and A-12 in Appendix).

SURGICAL:
- Valve replacement is the treatment of choice in symptomatic patients because the 5-yr mortality rate after onset of symptoms is extremely high, even with optimal medical therapy; valve replacement is indicated if cardiac catheterization establishes a pressure gradient >50 mm Hg and valve area <1 cm^2.
- Balloon aortic valvotomy for adult acquired aortic stenosis is useful only for palliation.

DISPOSITION
- 15% to 20% of patients with severe aortic stenosis die before age 20 yr.
- The 5-yr survival rate in adults is 40%.
- The average duration of symptoms before death is as follows: angina, 60 mo; syncope, 36 mo; CHF, 24 mo.
- About 75% of patients with symptomatic aortic stenosis will be dead 3 yr after onset of symptoms unless the aortic valve is replaced.

REFERRAL
- Surgical referral for valve replacement in symptomatic patients.
- Surgical mortality rate for valve replacement is 3% to 5%; however, it varies with patient's age (>8% in patients >75 yr old).

MISCELLANEOUS

COMMENTS
- Balloon valvuloplasty is useful in infants and children or poor surgical candidates who do not have calcified valve apparatus; it can be done as an intermediate procedure to stabilize high-risk patients before surgery.
- When performed in adults who have calcified valves, balloon valvuloplasty is useful only for short-term reduction in severity of aortic stenosis when surgery is contraindicated, since restenosis occurs rapidly.

REFERENCES
Carabello BA, Crawford FA: Valvular heart disease, *N Engl J Med* 337:32, 1997.

Kennedy KD et al: Natural history of moderate aortic stenosis, *J Am Coll Cardiol* 17:313, 1991.

Otto CM et al: Three-year outcome after balloon aortic valvuloplasty, *Circulation* 89:642, 1995.

Author: Fred F. Ferri, M.D.

Appendicitis, acute

BASIC INFORMATION

DEFINITION
Appendicitis is the acute inflammation of the appendix.

ICD-9-CM CODES
540.9 Appendicitis
540.0 Appendicitis with generalized peritonitis

EPIDEMIOLOGY AND DEMOGRAPHICS
- Appendicitis occurs in 10% of the population, most commonly between the ages of 10 and 30 yr.
- It is the most common abdominal surgical emergency.
- Incidence of appendicitis has declined over the past 30 yr.
- Male:female sex ratio is 3:2 until mid-20s; it equalizes after age 30 yr.

PHYSICAL FINDINGS
- Abdominal pain: initially the pain may be epigastric or periumbilical; it subsequently localizes to the RLQ within 12 to 18 hr. Pain can be found in back or right flank if appendix is retrocecal or in other abdominal locations if there is malrotation of the appendix.
- Pain with right thigh extension (psoas sign), low grade fever: temperature may be >38° C if there is appendiceal perforation.
- Pain with internal rotation of the flexed right thigh (obturator sign) is present.
- RLQ pain on palpation of the LLQ (Rovsing's sign): physical examination may reveal right-sided tenderness in patients with pelvic appendix.
- Point of maximum tenderness is in the RLQ (McBurney's point).
- Nausea, vomiting, tachycardia, cutaneous hyperesthesias at the level of T12 can be present.

ETIOLOGY
Obstruction of the appendiceal lumen with subsequent vascular congestion, inflammation, and edema; common causes of obstruction are:
- Fecaliths: 30% to 35% of cases (most common in adults)
- Foreign body: 4% (fruit seeds, pinworms, tapeworms, roundworms, calculi)
- Inflammation: 50% to 60% of cases (submucosal lymphoid hyperplasia [most common etiology in children, teens])
- Neoplasms: 1% (carcinoids, metastatic disease, carcinoma)

DIAGNOSIS

DIFFERENTIAL DIAGNOSIS
- Intestinal: regional enteritis, incarcerated hernia, fecal diverticulitis, intestinal obstruction, perforated ulcer, perforated cecum, Meckel's diverticulitis
- Reproductive: ectopic pregnancy, ovarian cyst, torsion of ovarian cyst, salpingitis, tubo-ovarian abscess, Mittelschmerz endometriosis, seminal vesiculitis
- Renal: renal and ureteral calculi, neoplasms, pyelonephritis
- Vascular: leaking aortic aneurysm
- Psoas abscess
- Trauma
- Cholecystitis

WORKUP
- Patients presenting with RLQ pain, nausea, vomiting, anorexia and RLQ rebound tenderness should undergo prompt clinical and laboratory evaluation. Imaging studies are generally not necessary in typical appendicitis. They are useful when the diagnosis is uncertain.
- A clinical algorithm for the evaluation of abdominal pain is described in Fig. 3-1.

LABORATORY TESTS
- CBC with differential reveals leukocytosis with a left shift in 90% of patients with appendicitis. Total WBC count is generally lower than 20,000/mm^3. Higher counts may be indicative of perforation. Less than 4% have a normal WBC and differential. A low Hgb and Hct in an older patient should raise suspicion for carcinoma of the cecum.
- Microscopic hematuria and pyuria may occur in <20% of patients.

IMAGING STUDIES
- Appendiceal CT scan as a noninvasive diagnostic aid has an accuracy of more than 90%. It improves patient care and reduces the use of hospital resources.
- Ultrasound is useful, especially in younger women when diagnosis is unclear. Normal ultrasonographic findings should not deter surgery if the history and physical examination are indicative of appendicitis.
- Laparoscopy may be useful as both a diagnostic and a therapeutic modality.

TREATMENT

NONPHARMACOLOGIC THERAPY
- NPO
- Do not administer analgesics or antibiotics until the diagnosis is made (may mask signs of peritonitis).

ACUTE GENERAL Rx
- Immediate appendectomy (laparoscopic or open), correction of fluid and electrolyte imbalance with vigorous IV hydration and electrolyte replacement
- IV antibiotic prophylaxis to cover gram-negative bacilli and anaerobes (cefotetan, clindamycin and gentamicin, or metronidazole with gentamicin)

DISPOSITION
In general, prognosis is excellent. Mortality is <1% in young adults without complications; however, it exceeds 10% in elderly patients with ruptured appendix.

REFERRAL
Surgical referral as soon as diagnosis is suspected

MISCELLANEOUS

COMMENTS
Perforation is common (20% in adult patients). Indicators of perforation are pain lasting >24 hr, leukocytosis >20,000/mm^3, temperature >102° F, palpable abdominal mass, and peritoneal findings.

REFERENCES
Rao P et al: Effect of computed tomography of the appendix on treatment of patients and the use of hospital resources, N Engl J Med 338:141, 1998.
Temple CL et al: The natural history of appendicitis in adults: a prospective study, Ann Surg 221:278, 1995.

Author: **Fred F. Ferri, M.D.**

CLINICAL TOPICS   Arthritis, granulomatous   49

BASIC INFORMATION

DEFINITION
The prototype of granulomatous arthritis is tuberculous arthritis. Atypical mycobacteria, sarcoidosis, and sporotrichosis can cause granulomatous involvement of the synovium, but these entities are much less common.

SYNONYMS
Tuberculous arthritis
Pott's disease

ICD-9-CM CODES
711.40 Arthropathy associated with other bacterial disease
730.88 Other infection involving bone

EPIDEMIOLOGY AND DEMOGRAPHICS
INCIDENCE (IN U.S.): Unknown
PREVALENCE (IN U.S.): Unknown
PREDOMINANT SEX: Male = female
PREDOMINANT AGE: Rare in childhood
PEAK INCIDENCE: No seasonal predilection

PHYSICAL FINDINGS
- Often no constitutional symptoms (fever and weight loss)
- Possibly no clinical or radiographic evidence of pulmonary TB
- Spinal infection most often in the thoracic or upper lumbar area, with back pain as the most common symptom
- Considerable local muscle spasm possible
- Kyphosis and neurologic symptoms resulting from spinal cord compression in advanced disease
- Chronic monoarticular arthritis in the peripheral joints
- Single joint involved in 85% of patients
- Pain, swelling, limitation of motion, and joint stiffness less dramatic than in acute bacterial arthritis; possibly present for months to years
- Seen more often in persons from developing countries, elderly patients, and hemodialysis patients

ETIOLOGY
- Hematogenous spread of organisms from a distant site of infection or by direct spread from bone
- Most commonly affected area: 50% of cases in the spine; next most commonly affected area: large joints (knee and hip)
- Primary infection beginning in the lungs and spreading to the highly vascular synovium
- Tuberculous osteomyelitis commonly involving an adjacent joint
- In peripheral joints, a granulomatous reaction in the synovium causing joint effusion and eventual destruction of underlying bone
- In the spine, infection of the intervertebral disc spreading to adjacent vertebrae
- Osteomyelitis of vertebrae causing collapse, kyphosis, or gibbous deformity, and possibly paraspinal "cold" abscess

DIAGNOSIS

DIFFERENTIAL DIAGNOSIS
- Sarcoidosis
- Fungal arthritis
- Metastatic cancer
- Primary or metastatic synovial tumors

WORKUP
- High index of suspicion needed
- Gold standard: synovial biopsy
- Joint aspiration and culture of the synovial fluid performed while awaiting biopsy
- Positive synovial fluid smear for acid-fast bacilli in 20% of cases; positive culture in 80%
- Elevated synovial fluid protein, low glucose
- Considerable variation in synovial fluid WBC count, but values of 10,000 to 20,000 cells/mm^3 typical; may be predominantly polymorphonuclear leukocytes
- Usually positive tuberculin skin test
- Anergy in elderly patients or in advanced disease
- In spinal infections, percutaneous or open biopsy to obtain accurate C&S data

LABORATORY TESTS
Peripheral WBC count and ESR are elevated but nonspecific.

IMAGING STUDIES
- Plain radiographs of the affected joint
  1. Typically demonstrate bony destruction with little new bone formation
  2. Osteopenia and soft tissue swelling in early infections
  3. Later, erosions at the joint margins
  4. In the spine, disc space narrowing with vertebral collapse (wedging) causing characteristic kyphosis
- CT scan: useful in early diagnosis of infections of the spine and to detect paraspinal abscess
- Technetium and gallium scintigraphic scans: may be positive, but do not permit differentiation from inflammation or osteoarthritis

TREATMENT

NONPHARMACOLOGIC THERAPY
Encourage range-of-motion exercises of the affected joint to prevent contractures.

ACUTE GENERAL Rx
- Combination chemotherapy
  1. If sensitive TB suspected, give isoniazid 5 mg/kg/day (maximum 300 mg/day) plus rifampin 10 mg/kg/day (maximum 600 mg/day) for at least 6 mo and pyrazinamide 15 to 30 mg/kg/day (maximum 2 g/day) for at least the first 2 mo plus ethambutol 15 to 25 mg/kg/day until sensitivity results are available.
  2. Most patients are treated successfully with chemotherapy alone.
  3. Urgent surgical intervention is necessary if spinal cord compression causes neurologic changes.
- Surgical debridement in cases of extensive bone involvement

CHRONIC Rx
In long-standing extensive disease, arthrodesis of weight-bearing joints

DISPOSITION
Loss of cartilage and destruction of underlying bone if treatment is not initiated promptly

REFERRAL
- To a physician experienced in the management of TB
- For consultation with an infectious diseases specialist if drug resistance is suspected or documented
- For neurosurgical and/or orthopedic consultation if neurologic impairment suspected

MISCELLANEOUS

COMMENTS
- As TB has become more prevalent in the U.S. in the last 10 to 20 yr, TB arthritis and osteomyelitis have also become more common.
- Early diagnosis is crucial for successful management.
- A clinical algorithm for the evaluation of arthralgia limited to one or few joints is described in Fig. 3-8.

REFERENCES
Furia JP, Box GG, Lintner DM: Tuberculous arthritis of the knee presenting as a meniscal tear, *Am J Orthop* 25(2):138, 1996.
Sternbach G: Percival Pott: tuberculous spondylitis, *J Emerg Med* 14(1):79, 1996.
Author: **Deborah L. Shapiro, M.D.**

Arthritis, infectious (bacterial) (PTG)

BASIC INFORMATION

DEFINITION
Bacterial arthritis is a highly destructive form of joint disease most often caused by hematogenous spread of organisms from a distant site of infection. Direct penetration of the joint as a result of trauma or surgery and spread from adjacent osteomyelitis may also cause bacterial arthritis. Any joint in the body may be affected. Gonococcal arthritis causes a distinct clinical syndrome and is often considered separately.

SYNONYMS
Septic arthritis
Pyogenic arthritis

ICD-9-CM CODES
711 Pyogenic arthritis, site unspecified

EPIDEMIOLOGY AND DEMOGRAPHICS
INCIDENCE (IN U.S.): Unknown
PREVALENCE (IN U.S.): Unknown
PREDOMINANT SEX: Gonococcal arthritis in males
PREDOMINANT AGE: Gonococcal arthritis in sexually active adults
PEAK INCIDENCE:
- Gonococcal arthritis: young adults
- Other bacterial causes: all ages

PHYSICAL FINDINGS
- Hallmark: acute onset of a swollen, painful joint
- Limited range of motion of the joint
- Effusion, with varying degrees of erythema and increased warmth around the joint
- Single joint affected in 80% to 90% of cases of nongonococcal arthritis
- Gonococcal dermatitis-arthritis syndrome
  1. Typical pattern is a migratory polyarthritis or tenosynovitis
  2. Small pustules on the trunk or extremities
- Febrile patient at presentation
- Most commonly affected joints in adult: knee and hip, but any joint may be involved; in children: hip

ETIOLOGY
- Bacteria spread from another locus of infection
  1. Highly vascular synovium is invaded by hematogenously spread bacteria.
  2. WBC enzymes cause necrosis of synovium, cartilage, and bone.
  3. Extensive joint destruction is rapid if infection is not treated with appropriate IV antibiotics and drainage of necrotic material.
- Predisposing factors: rheumatoid arthritis, prosthetic joints, advanced age, immunodeficiency
- The most common nongonococcal organisms are *Staphylococcus aureus*, β-hemolytic streptococci, and gram-negative bacilli.

DIAGNOSIS

DIFFERENTIAL DIAGNOSIS
- Gout
- Pseudogout
- Trauma
- Hemarthrosis
- Rheumatic fever
- Adult or juvenile rheumatoid arthritis
- Spondyloarthropathies such as Reiter's syndrome
- Osteomyelitis
- Viral arthritides
- Septic bursitis

WORKUP
- Joint aspiration, Gram stain, and culture of the synovial fluid
- Immediate arthrocentesis before other studies are undertaken or antibiotics instituted

LABORATORY TESTS
- Joint fluid analysis
  1. Synovial fluid leukocyte count is usually elevated >50,000 cells/mm^3 with a differential count of 80% or more polymorphonuclear cells.
  2. Counts are highly variable, with similar findings in gout, pseudogout, or rheumatoid arthritis.
  3. The differential diagnosis of synovial fluid abnormalities is described in Table 2-64.
- Blood cultures
- Culture of possible extraarticular sources of infection
- Elevated peripheral WBC count and ESR (nonspecific)

IMAGING STUDIES
- X-ray examination of the affected joint to rule out osteomyelitis
- CT scan for early diagnosis of infections of the spine, hips, and sternoclavicular and sacroiliac joints
- Technetium and gallium scintigraphic scans (positive, but do not permit differentiation of infection from inflammation)
- Indium-labeled WBC scans (less sensitive, but more specific)

TREATMENT

NONPHARMACOLOGIC THERAPY
- Affected joints aspirated daily to remove necrotic material and to follow serial WBC counts and cultures
- If no resolution with IV antibiotics and closed drainage: open debridement and lavage, particularly in nongonococcal infections
- Prevention of contractures:
  1. After acute stage of inflammation, range-of-motion exercises of the affected joint
  2. Physical therapy helpful

ACUTE GENERAL Rx
- IV antibiotics immediately after joint aspiration and Gram stain of the synovial fluid
- For infections caused by gram-positive cocci: penicillinase-resistant penicillin, such as nafcillin (2 g IV q4h), unless there is clinical suspicion of methicillin-resistant *Staphylococcus aureus*, in which case vancomycin (1 g IV q12h)
- Infections caused by gram-negative bacilli: treated with a third-generation cephalosporin or an antipseudomonal penicillin plus an aminoglycoside, pending C&S results
- For suspected gonococcal infection, including young adults when the synovial fluid Gram stain is nondiagnostic: ceftriaxone 1 g IV q24h

CHRONIC Rx
See indications for surgical drainage.

DISPOSITION
- With prompt treatment, complete resolution is expected.
- Delay in treatment may result in permanent destruction of cartilage and loss of function of the affected joint.

REFERRAL
To an orthopedist for open drainage if the infected joint fails to improve on appropriate antibiotics and closed aspiration

MISCELLANEOUS

COMMENTS
- Any patient with an acute monoarticular arthritis should undergo an urgent joint aspiration to rule out septic arthritis, even if there is a history of gout.
- A clinical algorithm for the evaluation of arthralgia limited to one or few joints is described in Fig. 3-8.

REFERENCES
Kaandorp CJ et al: Risk factors for septic arthritis in patients with joint disease: a prospective study, *Arth Rheum* 38(12):1819, 1995.

Author: **Deborah L. Shapiro, M.D.**

Arthritis, juvenile rheumatoid (PTG)

BASIC INFORMATION

DEFINITION
Juvenile rheumatoid arthritis is arthritis beginning before the age of 16 yr.

SYNONYMS
Still's disease
Juvenile chronic arthritis
Juvenile polyarthritis

ICD-9-CM CODES
714.3 Juvenile chronic polyarthritis

EPIDEMIOLOGY AND DEMOGRAPHICS
PREVALENCE (IN U.S.): 250,000 to 300,000 cases
PREVALENT SEX: female:male ratio of 2:1
PREVALENT AGE: Two peak incidences between ages of 1 and 3 yr and ages 8 and 12 yr.

PHYSICAL FINDINGS
Usually one of three types:

SYSTEMIC OR ACUTE FEBRILE JUVENILE RHEUMATOID ARTHRITIS (20% OF CASES):
- Characterized by extraarticular manifestations, especially spiking fevers and a typical rash that frequently appears in the evening and may be elicited by gently scratching the skin in susceptible areas (Koebner's phenomenon)
- Possible splenomegaly, generalized lymphadenopathy, pericarditis, and myocarditis
- Often, minimal articular findings overshadowed by systemic symptoms

PAUCIARTICULAR OR OLIGOARTICULAR FORM (50% OF CASES):
- Involves fewer than 5 joints
- Usually involves the larger joints, such as the knees, elbows, and ankles
- Systemic features often minimal, and only one to three joints usually involved
- Rarely causes impairment but chronic iridocyclitis develops in approximately 30% of cases with this form, and permanent loss of vision will develop in a high percentage of these patients
- Accelerated growth of the affected limb from chronic hyperemia possibly resulting in a temporary leg length discrepancy that is eventually equalized in most cases on control of the inflammation

POLYARTICULAR JUVENILE RHEUMATOID ARTHRITIS (30% OF CASES):
- Involves 5 or more joints
- Resembles the adult disease in its symmetric involvement of the small joints of the hands and feet
- Cervical spine involvement common and may produce marked loss of motion
- Early closure of the ossification centers of the mandible, often producing a markedly receding chin, a characteristic of this form
- Systemic manifestations similar to the febrile variety but not as dramatic

ETIOLOGY
Unknown

DIAGNOSIS

DIFFERENTIAL DIAGNOSIS
- Infectious causes of fever
- SLE
- Rheumatic fever
- Drug reaction
- Serum sickness
- "Viral arthritis"
- Lyme arthritis

WORKUP
Initial laboratory and imaging studies are often nonspecific in children with rheumatoid arthritis.

LABORATORY TESTS
- Increased ESR
- Low-grade anemia
- Very high peripheral WBC count
- Rheumatoid factor: rarely demonstrable in the serum of children
- Anti-nuclear antibodies: often found in children with ocular complications

IMAGING STUDIES
- Roentgenographic findings are similar to those in adult, with soft tissue swelling and osteoporosis early in the disease.
- Joint destruction is less frequent.
- Bony erosion and cyst formation may be present as a result of synovial hypertrophy.

TREATMENT

NONPHARMACOLOGIC THERAPY
Proper management requires close cooperation among primary physician, therapist, rheumatologist, and orthopedist.
- Rest
- Physical and occupational therapy
- Patient and family education
- Proper diet and weight-maintenance

ACUTE GENERAL Rx
- Aspirin (stopped during childhood viral illnesses to avoid Reye's syndrome)
- Other NSAIDs
- DMARDs
- Intraarticular steroids
- Systemic corticosteroids

DISPOSITION
- Complete remission occurs in the majority of patients and may occur at any age.
- 70% to 85% of children regain normal function.
- Mortality rate is 2%.
- Children with a protracted systemic phase of the disease are most at risk for developing serious intercurrent infection and potentially fatal amyloidosis.
- Myocarditis may develop in the systemic form.
- Blindness is the most serious complication of the pauciarticular form; joint deformity is the most serious problem of polyarticular disease.

REFERRAL
- For ophthalmology consultation when ocular involvement is suspected (Frequent eye examinations, especially in oligoarticular form)
- For orthopedic consultation for corrective surgery

MISCELLANEOUS

COMMENTS
Patient information on juvenile rheumatoid arthritis can be obtained from the National Arthritis Foundation, 1330 West Peachtree Street, Atlanta, GA 30309; phone: 1-800-283-7800.

REFERENCES
Ansell BM, Swann M: The management of chronic arthritis of children, *J Bone Joint Surg* 65(b)5:536, 1983.
Calabro JJ: Juvenile rheumatoid arthritis. In McCarty DJ (ed): *Arthritis and allied conditions,* ed 11, Philadelphia, 1989, Lea and Febiger.
Hackett J et al: Juvenile rheumatoid arthritis, *Hand Clin* 12(3):573, 1996.

Author: **Lonnie R. Mercier, M.D.**

Arthritis, psoriatic (PTG)

BASIC INFORMATION

DEFINITION
Psoriatic arthritis is an inflammatory spondyloarthritis occurring in patients with psoriasis who are usually seronegative for rheumatoid factor. It is often included in a class of disorders called *rheumatoid variants*.

ICD-9-CM CODES
696.0 Psoriatic arthritis

EPIDEMIOLOGY AND DEMOGRAPHICS
PREVALENCE: 5% to 10% of patients with psoriasis (psoriasis affects 1% to 1.5% of general population)
PREVALENT SEX: Males = females
PREVALENT AGE: 30 to 55 yr

PHYSICAL FINDINGS
- Usually gradual clinical onset
- Asymmetric involvement of scattered joints
- Selective involvement of the DIP joints (described in "classic" cases but only present in 5% of patients)
- Symmetric arthritis similar to RA in 15% of patients
- Possible development of predominant sacroiliitis in a small number of cases
- Advanced form of hand involvement (arthritis mutilans) in some patients
- Dystrophic changes in the nails (pitting, ridging) in many patients with DIP involvement

ETIOLOGY
Unknown

DIAGNOSIS

DIFFERENTIAL DIAGNOSIS
- Rheumatoid arthritis
- Erosive osteoarthritis
- Gouty arthritis
- Ankylosing spondylitis
- The differential diagnosis of spondyloarthropathies is described in Table 2-61 and Box 2-112.

WORKUP
- Early diagnosis may be difficult to establish because the arthritis may develop before skin lesions appear.
- Laboratory studies show no specific abnormalities in most cases.

LABORATORY TESTS
- Slight elevation of ESR
- Possible mild anemia
- Possible HLA-B27 antigen (especially in patients with sacroiliitis)

IMAGING STUDIES
- Peripheral joint findings similar to those in rheumatoid arthritis but erosive changes in the distal phalangeal tufts characteristic of psoriatic arthritis
- Bony osteolysis; periosteal new bony formation
- Changes in axial skeleton: sacroiliitis, development of vertebral syndesmophytes (osteophytes) that often bridge adjacent vertebral bodies
- Paravertebral ossification
- Spinal changes: do not have same appearance as ankylosing spondylolitis; however, spine abnormalities are less common than sacroiliitis

TREATMENT

NONPHARMACOLOGIC THERAPY
- Rest
- Splinting
- Joint protection
- PT

ACUTE GENERAL Rx
- NSAIDs
- Occasional intraarticular steroid injections
- DMARDs: rarely are required

DISPOSITION
- Different from rheumatoid arthritis in both prognosis and response to treatment
- Generally, mild joint symptoms in psoriatic arthritis
- Disease-free intervals lasting for several years in many patients

REFERRAL
Orthopedic consultation for painful joint deformity

MISCELLANEOUS

REFERENCES
Bennett RM: Psoriatic arthritis. In McCarty DJ (ed): *Arthritis and allied conditions,* ed 11, Philadelphia, 1989, Lea and Febiger.
Laurent MR: Psoriatic arthritis, *Clin Rheumatic Dis* 11:61, 1985.
Author: **Lonnie R. Mercier, M.D.**

Arthritis, rheumatoid (PTG)

BASIC INFORMATION

DEFINITION
Rheumatoid arthritis (RA) is a systemic disorder characterized by chronic joint inflammation that most commonly affects peripheral joints.

ICD-9-CM CODES
714.0 Rheumatoid arthritis

EPIDEMIOLOGY AND DEMOGRAPHICS
PREVALENCE: 5 cases/1000 adults
PREVALENT AGE: 35 to 45 yr
PREDOMINANT SEX:
- Female:male ratio of 3:1
- After age 50 yr, sex difference less marked

PHYSICAL FINDINGS
- Usually gradual onset; common prodromal symptoms of weakness, fatigue, and anorexia
- Initial presentation: multiple symmetric joint involvement, most often in the hands and feet
- Joint effusions, tenderness, and restricted motion usually present early in the disease
- Eventual characteristic deformities: subluxations, dislocations, and joint contractures
- Extraarticular findings:
  1. Tendon sheaths and bursae frequently affected by chronic inflammation
  2. Possible tendon rupture
  3. Rheumatoid nodules over bony prominences such as the elbow and shaft of the ulna
  4. Splenomegaly, pericarditis, and vasculitis

ETIOLOGY
Unknown

DIAGNOSIS

DIFFERENTIAL DIAGNOSIS
- SLE
- Seronegative spondyloarthropathies (see Table 2-61)
- Polymyalgia rheumatica

According to the American College of Rheumatology, RA exists when four of seven criteria are present, with criteria 1 to 4 being present for at least 6 wk.
1. Morning stiffness over 1 hr
2. Arthritis in three or more joints with swelling
3. Arthritis of hand joints with swelling
4. Symmetric arthritis
5. Rheumatoid nodules
6. Roentgenographic changes typical of RA
7. Positive serum rheumatoid factor

LABORATORY TESTS
- Increase in rheumatoid factor in 80% of cases (rheumatoid factor also present in the normal population)
- Possible mild anemia
- Usually, elevated acute phase reactants (ESR, C-reactive protein)
- Possible mild leukocytosis
- Usually, turbid joint fluid, which forms a poor mucin clot; elevated cell count, with an increase in polymorphonuclear leukocytes

IMAGING STUDIES
Plain radiography
- Usually reveals soft tissue swelling and osteoporosis early
- Eventually, joint space narrowing, erosion, and deformity visible as a result of continued inflammation and cartilage destruction

TREATMENT

NONPHARMACOLOGIC THERAPY
Proper management requires close cooperation among primary physician, therapist, rheumatologist, and orthopedist.
- Patient education is important.
- Rest with proper exercise and splinting can prevent or correct joint deformities.
- Maintain proper diet and control obesity.

CHRONIC Rx
- NSAIDs: commonly used as the initial treatment to relieve inflammation; (drug of choice for most patients: aspirin, but other NSAIDs also effective; see Table 7-29)
- Disease-modifying drugs (DMARDs): begun when NSAIDs are not effective; usually slow-acting drugs that require more than 8 wk to become effective
- Oral prednisone
- Intrasynovial steroid injections

DISPOSITION
- Remissions and exacerbations are common, but condition is chronically progressive in the majority of cases.
- Joint degeneration and deformity often lead to disability.
- Early diagnosis and treatment are important and can improve quality of life.

REFERRAL
Orthopedic consultation for corrective surgery

MISCELLANEOUS

COMMENTS
Patient information on rheumatoid arthritis can be obtained from the National Arthritis Foundation, 1330 West Peachtree Street, Atlanta, GA 30309; phone: 1-800-283-7800.

REFERENCES
Harris ED: Treatment of rheumatoid arthritis for now and the future. In Kelly WN et al (eds): *Textbook of rheumatology (update 18)*, New York, 1995, WB Saunders.

Author: **Lonnie R. Mercier, M.D.**

Asbestosis (PTG)

BASIC INFORMATION

DEFINITION
Asbestosis is a slowly progressive diffuse interstitial fibrosis resulting from dose-related inhalation exposure to fibers of asbestos.

ICD-9-CM CODES
501 Asbestosis

EPIDEMIOLOGY AND DEMOGRAPHICS
- In U.S.: 5 to 10 new cases/100,000 persons/yr
- Prolonged interval (20 to 30 yr) between exposures to inhaled fibers and clinical manifestations of disease
- Most common in workers involved in the primary extraction of asbestos from rock deposits and in those involved in the fabrication and installation of products containing asbestos (e.g., Naval shipyards in World War II, installation of floor tiles, ceiling tiles, acoustic ceiling coverings, wall insulation and pipe coverings in public buildings)

PHYSICAL FINDINGS
- Insidious onset of shortness of breath with exertion is usually the first sign of asbestosis.
- Dyspnea becomes more severe as the disease advances; with time, progressively less exertion is tolerated.
- Cough is frequent and usually paroxysmal, dry, and nonproductive.
- Scant mucoid sputum may accompany the cough in the later stages of the disease.
- Fine end respiratory crackles (rales, crepitations) are heard more predominately in the lung bases.
- Digital clubbing, edema, jugular venous distention are present.

ETIOLOGY
Inhalation of asbestos fibers

DIAGNOSIS

DIFFERENTIAL DIAGNOSIS
- Silicosis
- Siderosis, other pneumonoconioses
- Lung cancer
- Atelectasis

WORKUP
Documentation of exposure history, diagnostic imaging, pulmonary function testing

LABORATORY TESTS
- Generally not helpful
- Possible mild elevation of ESR, positive ANA and RF (These tests are nonspecific and do not correlate with disease severity or activity.)
- Pulmonary function testing: decreased vital capacity, decreased total lung capacity, decreased carbon monoxide gas transfer
- ABGs: hypoxemia, hypercarbia in advanced stages

IMAGING STUDIES
Chest x-ray examination:
- Small, irregular shadows in lower lung zones
- Thickened pleural, calcified plaques (present under diaphragms and lateral chest wall)

CT scan of chest confirms the diagnosis.

TREATMENT

NONPHARMACOLOGIC THERAPY
- Smoking cessation, proper nutrition, exercise program to maximize available lung function
- Home oxygen therapy PRN
- Removal of patient from further asbestos fiber exposure

ACUTE GENERAL Rx
- Prompt identification and treatment of respiratory infections
- Supplemental oxygen on a PRN basis
- Annual influenza vaccination, pneumococcal vaccination

CHRONIC Rx
See "Acute General Rx."

DISPOSITION
- There is no specific treatment for asbestosis.
- Death is usually secondary to respiratory failure from cor pulmonale.
- Patients with asbestosis have increased risk for mesotheliomas, lung cancer, and TB.
- Survival in patients following development of mesothelioma is 4 to 6 yr.

REFERRAL
To pulmonologist initially

MISCELLANEOUS

COMMENTS
Patient information on asbestosis can be obtained from the American Lung Association, 1740 Broadway, New York, NY 10019.

REFERENCES
Davis GS, Calhoun WJ: Occupational and environmental causes of interstitial lung disease. In Schwarz MI, King, TE (eds): *Interstitial lung disease*, ed 2, St Louis, 1993, Mosby.

Newman LS: Occupational illness, *N Engl J Med* 333:1128, 1995.

Author: **Fred F. Ferri, M.D.**

Ascariasis (PTG)

BASIC INFORMATION

DEFINITION
Ascariasis is a parasitic infection caused by the nematode *Ascaris lumbricoides*. The majority of those infected are asymptomatic; however, clinical disease may arise from pulmonary hypersensitivity, intestinal obstruction, and secondary complications.

ICD-9-CM CODES
127.0 Ascariasis

EPIDEMIOLOGY AND DEMOGRAPHICS
INCIDENCE (IN U.S.):
- Unknown
- Three times the infection rates found in blacks as in whites

PREVALENCE (IN U.S.): Estimated at 4,000,000, the majority of which live in the rural southeastern part of the country

PREDOMINANT SEX: Both sexes probably equally affected, with a possible slight female preponderance

PREDOMINANT AGE: Most common in children, with estimated mean age of approximately 5 yr based on surveys in highly endemic areas

PEAK INCIDENCE: Unknown

NEONATAL INFECTION: Probable transmission, though not specifically studied

PHYSICAL FINDINGS
- Occurs approximately 9 to 12 days after ingestion of eggs (corresponding to the larvae migration through the lungs)
- Nonproductive cough
- Substernal chest discomfort
- Fever
- In patients with large worm burdens, especially children, intestinal obstruction associated with perforation, volvulus, and intussception
- Migration of worms into the biliary tree giving clinical appearance of biliary colic and pancreatitis as well as acute appendicitis with movement into that appendage
- Rarely, infection with *A. lumbricoides* producing interstitial nephritis and acute renal failure
- In endemic areas in Asia and Africa, malabsorption of dietary proteins and vitamins as a consequence of chronic worm intestinal carriage

ETIOLOGY
- Transmission is usually hand to mouth, but eggs may be ingested via transported vegetables grown in contaminated soil.
- Eggs are hatched in the small intestine, with larvae penetrating intestinal mucosa and migrating via the circulation to the lungs.
- Larval forms proceed through the alveoli, ascend the bronchial tree, and return to the intestines after swallowing, where they mature into adult worms.
- Estimated time until the female adult worm to begin producing eggs is 2 to 3 mo.
- Eggs are passed out of the intestines with feces.
- Within human host, adult worm lifespan is 1 to 2 yr.

DIAGNOSIS

DIFFERENTIAL DIAGNOSIS
- Radiologic manifestations and eosinophilia to be distinguished from drug hypersensitivity and Löffler's syndrome
- The differential diagnosis of intestinal helminths is described in Table 2-38.

LABORATORY TESTS
- Examination of the stool for *Ascaris* ova
- Expectoration or fecal passage of adult worm
- Eosinophilia: most prominent early in the infection and subsides as the adult worm infestation established in the intestines

IMAGING STUDIES
- Chest x-ray examination to reveal bilateral oval or round infiltrates of varying size (Löffler's syndrome); NOTE: infiltrates are transient and eventually resolve.
- Plain films of the abdomen and contrast studies to reveal worm masses in loops of bowel
- Ultrasonography and endoscopic retrograde cholangiopancreatography (ERCP) to identify worms in the pancreaticobiliary tract

TREATMENT

NONPHARMACOLOGIC THERAPY
Aggressive IV hydration, especially in children with fever, severe vomiting, and resultant dehydration

ACUTE GENERAL Rx
- Mebendazole (Vermox)
  1. Drug of choice for intestinal infection with *A. lumbricoides*
  2. 100 mg PO tid given for 3 days
- Albendazole, given as a single 400-mg dose orally
- Both mebendazole and albendazole are contraindicated in pregnancy.
- Pyrantel pamoate (Antiminth)
  1. Given at a dose of 11 mg/kg PO (maximum dose of 1 g/day)
  2. Considered safe for use in pregnant women
- Piperazine citrate
  1. Recommended in cases of intestinal or biliary obstruction
  2. Administered as a syrup, given via nasogastric tube, a 150 mg/kg loading dose, followed by six doses of 65 mg/kg q12h
  3. Considered safe in pregnancy, but cannot be given concurrently with chlorpromazine
- Complete obstruction should be managed surgically.

DISPOSITION
Overall prognosis is good.

REFERRAL
To surgeon in cases of complete obstruction or suspected secondary complication (e.g., perforation or volvulus)

MISCELLANEOUS

Although not recommended as treatment, at least one case has been described of an adult worm having been excreted by an asymptomatic patient following whole body irradiation.

COMMENTS
Given the known transmission of the parasite, routine hand washing and proper disposal of human waste would significantly decrease the prevalence of this disease.

REFERENCES
Asrat T, Rogers N: Acute pancreatitis caused by biliary *Ascaris* in pregnancy, *J Perinatol* 15(4):330, 1995.

Villamizar E et al: *Ascaris lumbricoides* infestation as a cause of intestinal obstruction in children: experience with 87 cases, *J Pediatr Surg* 31(1):201, 1996.

Author: **George O. Alonso, M.D.**

Asthma (PTG)

BASIC INFORMATION

DEFINITION
The American Thoracic Society defines asthma as a "disease characterized by an increased responsiveness of the trachea and bronchi to various stimuli and manifested by a widespread narrowing of the airways that changes in severity either spontaneously or as a result of treatment." *Status asthmaticus* can be defined as a severe continuous bronchospasm.

SYNONYMS
Bronchospasm
Reactive airway disease
Bronchial asthma

ICD-9-CM CODES
493.9 Asthma, unspecified
493.1 Intrinsic asthma
493.0 Extrinsic asthma

EPIDEMIOLOGY AND DEMOGRAPHICS
- Asthma affects 5% of the population.
- It is more common in children (10% of children, 5% of adults).

PHYSICAL FINDINGS
Physical examination varies with the stage and severity of asthma and may reveal only increased inspiratory and expiratory phases of respiration. Physical examination during status asthmaticus may reveal:
- Tachycardia and tachypnea
- Use of accessory respiratory muscles
- Pulsus paradoxus (inspiratory decline in systolic blood pressure >10 mm Hg)
- Wheezing: absence of wheezing (silent chest) or decreased wheezing can indicate worsening obstruction
- Mental status changes: generally secondary to hypoxia and hypercapnia and constitute an indication for urgent intubation
- Paradoxic abdominal and diaphragmatic movement on inspiration (detected by palpation over the upper part of the abdomen in a semirecumbent position): important sign of impending respiratory crisis, indicates diaphragmatic fatigue
- The following abnormalities in vital signs are indicative of severe asthma:
  1. Pulsus paradoxus >18 mm Hg.
  2. Respiratory rate >30 breaths/min.
  3. Tachycardia with heart rate >120 beats/min.

ETIOLOGY
- Intrinsic asthma: occurs in patients who have no history of allergies; may be triggered by upper respiratory infections or psychologic stress
- Extrinsic asthma (allergic asthma): brought on by exposure to allergens (e.g., dust mites, cat allergen)
- Exercise-induced asthma: seen most frequently in adolescents; manifests with bronchospasm following initiation of exercise and improves with discontinuation of exercise
- Drug-induced asthma: often associated with use of NSAIDs, β-blockers, sulfites, certain foods and beverages

DIAGNOSIS

DIFFERENTIAL DIAGNOSIS
- CHF
- COPD
- Pulmonary embolism (in adult and elderly patients)
- Foreign body aspiration (most frequent in younger patients)
- Pneumonia and other upper respiratory infections
- Rhinitis with postnasal drip
- TB
- Hypersensitivity pneumonitis
- Anxiety disorder
- Wegener's granulomatosis
- Diffuse interstitial lung disease

WORKUP
Medical history, physical examination, pulmonary function studies and peak flow meter determination, blood gas analysis and oximetry (during acute bronchospasm), chest radiography if infection is suspected

LABORATORY TESTS
Laboratory tests can be normal if obtained during a stable period. The following laboratory abnormalities may be present during an acute bronchospasm:
- ABGs can be used in staging the severity of an asthmatic attack:
  Mild: decreased Pao_2 and $Paco_2$, increased pH.
  Moderate: decreased Pao_2, normal $Paco_2$, normal pH.
  Severe: marked decreased Pao_2, increased $Paco_2$, and decreased pH.
- CBC, leukocytosis with "left shift" may indicate the existence of bacterial infection.
- Sputum: eosinophils, Charcot-Leyden crystals; PMNs, and bacteria may be found on Gram stain in patients with pneumonia.
- Useful diagnostic tests for asthma:
  1. Pulmonary function studies: during acute severe bronchospasm, FEV_1 is <1 L and peak expiratory flow rate (PEFR) <80 L/min
  2. Methacholine challenge test
  3. Skin test: to assess the role of atopy (when suspected)

IMAGING STUDIES
- Chest x-ray film: usually normal, may show evidence of thoracic hyperinflation (e.g., flattening of the diaphragm, increased volume over the retrosternal air space).
- ECG: tachycardia, nonspecific ST-T wave changes; may also show cor pulmonale, right bundle-branch block, right axial deviation, counterclockwise rotation.

TREATMENT

NONPHARMACOLOGIC THERAPY
- Avoidance of triggering factors (e.g., salicylates, sulfites)
- Encouragement of regular exercise (e.g., swimming)
- Patient education regarding warning signs of an attack and proper use of medications (e.g., correct use of inhalers)

ACUTE GENERAL Rx
The Expert Panel of the National Asthma Education and Prevention Program (NAEPP) recommends the following stepwise approach in the pharmacologic management of asthma in adults and children older than 5 yr:
STEP 1 (MILD INTERMITTENT ASTHMA): No daily medications are needed.
- Short-acting inhaled β-2 agonists as needed (e.g., albuterol [Ventolin, Proventil], terbutaline [Brethaire], bitolterol [Tornalate], pirbuterol [Maxair]).

STEP 2 (MILD PERSISTENT ASTHMA): Daily treatment may be needed.
- Low-dose inhaled corticosteroid (e.g., beclomethasone [Beclovent, Vanceril], flunisolide [AeroBid], triamcinolone [Azmacort]) can be used.
- Cromolyn (Intal) or nedocromil (Tilade) can also be used.
- Sustained-release theophylline is an alternative; however, it is not preferred therapy; additional considerations for long-term control are the use of zafirlukast (Accolade) or zileuton (Zyflo).
- Quick relief of asthma can be achieved with short-acting inhaled β-2 agonists (see above).

STEP 3 (MODERATE PERSISTENT ASTHMA): Daily medication is recommended.
- Low-dose or medium-dose inhaled corticosteroids (see above) plus long-acting inhaled β-2 agonist (salmeterol [Serevent]), sustained-release theophylline, or long-acting oral β-2 agonists (e.g., albuterol, sustained-release tablets).

- Use short-acting inhaled β-agonists on a PRN basis for quick relief.

STEP 4 (SEVERE PERSISTENT ASTHMA):
- Daily treatment with high-dose inhaled corticosteroids plus long-acting inhaled β-agonists (e.g., sustained-release theophylline or long-acting oral β-2 agonist plus long-term systemic corticosteroids (e.g., methylprednisolone, prednisolone, prednisone)can be used.
- Short-acting β-2 agonists can be used on a PRN basis for quick relief.

Treatment of *status asthmaticus* is as follows:
- Oxygen generally started at 2 to 4 L/min via nasal cannula or Venti-Mask at 40% FiO_2; further adjustments are made according to the ABGs.
- Sympathomimetics: various agents and modalities are available.
  1. Epinephrine (1:1000 dilution)
     a. Dosage range is 0.3 to 0.5 ml SC; may repeat after 15 to 20 min.
     b. Onset of action is within 15 min.
     c. Duration is 1 to 4 hr.
     d. Use with caution in patients >40 yr or anyone with heart disease.
  2. Terbutaline (Brethine)
     a. May be given SC, 0.25 mg q6-8h.
     b. Clinically significant increase in FEV_1 occurs within 15 min and persists 90 min to 4 hr.
     c. Generally, has fewer cardiac stimulating effects than epinephrine; however, systemic vasodilation with compensatory tachycardia can occur.
  3. Metaproterenol (Alupent)
     a. May be administered via aerosol nebulizer, bulb nebulizer, or IPPB (e.g., 0.3 ml of metaproterenol in 3 ml of saline solution, given via nebulizer).
     b. Onset of action is within 5 min; duration is 3 to 4 hr.
  4. Isoetharine (Bronkosol): 0.25 to 0.5 ml in 3 ml of saline solution via nebulizer q4h is also effective; however, its duration is less than that of metaproterenol.
  5. Albuterol (Proventil, Ventolin): 0.5 to 1 ml (2.5 to 5 mg) in 3 ml of saline solution tid or qid via nebulizer.
- Corticosteroids
  1. Early administration is advised, particularly in patients using steroids at home.
  2. Patients may be started on hydrocortisone (Solu-Cortef) 2.5 to 4 mg/kg or methylprednisolone (Solu-Medrol) 0.5 to 1 mg/kg IV loading dose, then q6h PRN; higher doses may be necessary in selected patients (particularly those receiving steroids at home); steroids given by inhalation, (e.g., beclomethasone 2 inhalations qid; maximum 20 inhalations/day) are also useful for controlling bronchospasm and tapering oral steroids and should be used in all patients with severe asthma.
  3. Rapid but judicious tapering of corticosteroids will eliminate serious steroid toxicity; long-term low-dose methotrexate may be an effective means of reducing the systemic corticosteroids requirement in some patients with severe refractory asthma.
  4. The most common errors regarding steroid therapy in acute bronchospasms are the use of "too little, too late" and too rapid tapering with return of bronchospasm.
- Atropine analog (e.g., ipratropium bromide [Atrovent] 2 inhalations qid, maximum 12 inhalations in 24 hr) is useful in patients not responding well to β-agonists and whose bronchospasm is secondary to bronchitis; when ipratropium is used with a β-2 agonist there is additive effect.
- Theophylline or aminophylline
  1. Its role in acute exacerbation of asthma has been questioned; IV theophylline or aminophylline has been used in patients with asthma because of its primary bronchodilating effect and its antiinflammatory actions.
  2. Most authorities now believe that aminophylline should not be used routinely in the treatment of acute exacerbations of asthma. The addition of aminophylline may be justified for those patients who do not respond to β-agonists, corticosteroids, and anticholinergic medications. Aminophylline has potential toxic effects (e.g., cardiac arrhythmias, seizures).
  3. When used, frequent monitoring of blood levels is indicated to prevent toxicity, particularly in elderly patients.
- IV hydration: judicious use is necessary to avoid CHF.
- IV antibiotics are indicated when there is suspicion of bacterial infection (e.g., infiltrate on chest x-ray, fever, or leukocytosis).
- Intubation and mechanical ventilation are indicated when above measures fail to produce significant improvement.
- General anesthesia: halothane may reverse bronchospasm in a severe asthmatic who cannot be ventilated adequately by mechanical means.
- IV magnesium sulfate supplementation in children with low or borderline-low magnesium levels may improve acute bronchospasm. Several reports in recent literature point to the beneficial effect on bronchospasm with a 20-min infusion of 1.2 g of magnesium sulfate in patients with acute asthma attack.

DISPOSITION
Most children with asthma experience spontaneous remission during adulthood. The outlook is somewhat better in patients with extrinsic asthma.

REFERRAL
Hospital admission in patients with status asthmaticus

MISCELLANEOUS

COMMENTS
Additional patient information on asthma can be obtained from the Asthma and Allergy Foundation of American, Suite 305, Washington, DC 20036.

REFERENCES
Corbridge TC, Hall, JB: The assessment and management of adulthood status asthmaticus, *Am J Resp Crit Care Med* 151:1296, 1995.

National Asthma Education and Prevention Program: *Expert panel report 2: guidelines for diagnosis and management of asthma*, Bethesda, Md, 1997, National Institute of Health.

Shuttari MF: Asthma: diagnosis and management, *Am Fam Physician* 52:2225, 1996.

Weinberg M, Hendle L: Theophylline and asthma, *N Engl J Med* 334:1380, 1996.

Author: **Fred F. Ferri, M.D.**

Atelectasis (PTG)

BASIC INFORMATION

DEFINITION
Atelectasis is the collapse of lung volume.

ICD-9-CM CODES
518.0 Atelectasis

EPIDEMIOLOGY AND DEMOGRAPHICS
- Occurs frequently in patients receiving mechanical ventilation with higher Fio_2
- Dependent regions of the lung are more prone to atelectasis: they are partially compressed, not as well ventilated, and there is no spontaneous drainage of secretions with gravity

PHYSICAL FINDINGS
- Decreased or absent breath sounds
- Abnormal chest percussion
- Cough, dyspnea, decreased vocal fremitus and vocal resonance
- Diminished chest expansion, tachypnea, tachycardia

ETIOLOGY
- Mechanical ventilation with higher Fio_2
- Chronic bronchitis
- Cystic fibrosis
- Endobronchial neoplasms
- Foreign bodies
- Infections (e.g., TB, histoplasmosis)
- Extrinsic bronchial compression from neoplasms, aneurysms of ascending aorta, enlarged left atrium
- Sarcoidosis
- Silicosis
- Anterior chest wall injury, pneumothorax
- Alveolar injury (e.g., toxic fumes, aspiration of gastric contents)
- Pleural effusion, expanding bullae
- Chest wall deformity (e.g., scoliosis)
- Muscular weaknesses or abnormalities (e.g., neuromuscular disease)
- Mucus plugs from asthma, allergic bronchopulmonary aspergillosis, postoperative state

DIAGNOSIS

DIFFERENTIAL DIAGNOSIS
- Neoplasm
- Pneumonia
- Encapsulated pleural effusion
- Abnormalities of brachiocephalic vein and of the left pulmonary ligament

WORKUP
- Chest x-ray
- CT scan and fiberoptic bronchoscopy (selected patients)

IMAGING STUDIES
- Chest x-ray will confirm diagnosis.
- CT scan is useful in patients with suspected endobronchial neoplasm or extrinsic bronchial compression.
- Fiberoptic bronchoscopy (selected patients) is useful for removal of foreign body or evaluation of endobronchial and peribronchial lesions.

TREATMENT

NONPHARMACOLOGIC THERAPY
- Deep breathing, mobilization of the patient
- Incentive spirometry
- Tracheal suctioning
- Humidification
- Chest physiotherapy with percussion and postural drainage

ACUTE GENERAL Rx
- Positive pressure breathing (CPAP by face mask, positive end-expiratory pressure [PEEP] for patients on mechanical ventilation)
- Use of mucolytic agents (e.g., acetylcysteine [Mucomyst])
- Recombinant human DNase (Dornase alpha) in patients with cystic fibrosis
- Bronchodilator therapy in selected patients

CHRONIC Rx
Chest physiotherapy, humidification of inspired air, frequent nasotracheal suctioning

DISPOSITION
Prognosis varies with the underlying etiology.

REFERRAL
- Bronchoscopy for removal of foreign body or plugs unresponsive to conservative treatment
- Surgical referral for removal of obstructing neoplasms

MISCELLANEOUS

COMMENTS
Patients should be educated that frequent changes of position are helpful in clearing secretions. Sitting the patient upright in a chair is recommended to increase both volume and vital capacity relative to the supine position.

REFERENCES
Celli BR: Physiologic and mechanical aids to lung expansion, *Clin Chest Med* 14(2): 257, 1993.

Author: **Fred F. Ferri, M.D.**

BASIC INFORMATION

DEFINITION
Atrial fibrillation is totally chaotic atrial activity caused by simultaneous discharge of multiple atrial foci.

SYNONYMS
AF
A-fib

ICD-9-CM CODES
427.31 Atrial fibrillation

EPIDEMIOLOGY AND DEMOGRAPHICS
The prevalence of atrial fibrillation increases with age, from 2% in the general population to 5% in patients older than 60 yr.

PHYSICAL FINDINGS
Clinical presentation is variable:
- Most common complaint: palpitations
- Fatigue, dizziness, light-headedness in some patients
- A few completely asymptomatic patients
- Cardiac auscultation revealing irregularly irregular rhythm

ETIOLOGY
- Coronary artery disease
- MS, MR, AS, AR
- Thyrotoxicosis
- Pulmonary embolism, COPD
- Pericarditis
- Myocarditis, cardiomyopathy
- Tachycardia-bradycardia syndrome
- Alcohol abuse
- MI
- WPW syndrome
- Other causes: left atrial myxoma, atrial septal defect, carbon monoxide poisoning, pheochromocytoma, idiopathic

DIAGNOSIS

DIFFERENTIAL DIAGNOSIS
- Multifocal atrial tachycardia
- Atrial flutter
- Frequent atrial premature beats

WORKUP
New-onset atrial fibrillation: ECG, echocardiogram, Holter monitor, and laboratory evaluation

LABORATORY TESTS
- TSH, T_4
- Electrolytes

IMAGING STUDIES
- ECG
  1. Irregular, nonperiodic wave forms (best seen in V1) reflecting continuous atrial reentry
  2. Absence of P waves
  3. Conducted QRS complexes showing no periodicity
- Echocardiography to evaluate left atrial size and detect valvular disorders
- Holter monitor: useful to evaluate paroxysmal atrial fibrillation

TREATMENT

NONPHARMACOLOGIC THERAPY
- Avoidance of alcohol in patients with suspected excessive alcohol use
- Avoidance of caffeine and nicotine

ACUTE GENERAL Rx
- Use β-blockers, digoxin, verapamil, or diltiazem for acute rate control.
- Cardioversion is indicated if the ventricular rate is >140 bpm and the patient is symptomatic (particularly in acute MI, chest pain, dyspnea, CHF) or when there is no conversion to normal sinus rhythm after 3 days of therapy with digoxin and quinidine. The likelihood of cardioversion-related clinical thromboembolism is low in patients with atrial fibrillation lasting <48 hr.
- Anticoagulate with warfarin (unless patient has specific contraindications).
- Long-term anticoagulation with warfarin (adjusted to maintain an INR of 2 to 3) is indicated in all patients with atrial fibrillation and associated cardiovascular disease, including the following:
  1. Rheumatic valvular disease (MS, MR, AI)
  2. Aortic stenosis
  3. Prostatic mitral valve
  4. History of previous embolism
  5. Known cardiac thrombus
  6. CHF
  7. Cardiomyopathy with poor left ventricular function
  8. Nonrheumatic heart disease (e.g., hypertensive cardiovascular disease, coronary artery disease, AST)
9. Anticoagulation is generally not recommended in young patients with lone atrial fibrillation.

CHRONIC Rx
- Anticoagulation with warfarin (see "Acute General Rx")
- Rate control with digoxin

DISPOSITION
Factors associated with maintenance of sinus rhythm following cardioversion:
- Left atrium diameter <60 mm
- Absence of mitral valve disease
- Short duration of atrial fibrillation

REFERRAL
Surgical treatment of atrial fibrillation:
- The Maze procedure with its recent modifications creating electrical barriers to the macroreentrant circuits that are thought to underlie atrial fibrillation is being performed with good results in several medical centers (preservation of sinus rhythm in >95% of patients without the use of long-term antiarrhythmic medication). Clear indications for its use remain undefined. Generally surgery is reserved for patients with rapid heart rate refractory to pharmacologic therapy or who cannot tolerate pharmacologic therapy.
- Catheter-based radiofrequency ablation procedures designed to eliminate atrial fibrillation are being investigated.

MISCELLANEOUS

COMMENTS
Aspirin may be a suitable alternative to warfarin in men >70 yr with increased risk of bleeding.

REFERENCES
Aboaf AB, Wolff TS: Paroxysmal atrial fibrillation: a common but neglected entity, *Arch Intern Med* 156:362, 1996.

Blackshear JL et al: Management of atrial fibrillation in adults: prevention of thromboembolism and symptomatic treatment, *Mayo Clin Proc* 71:150, 1996.

Weegner MJ et al: Risk for clinical thromboembolism associated with cardioversion to sinus rhythm in patients with atrial fibrillation lasting less than 48 hours, *Ann Intern Med* 126:615, 1997.

Zarembski DJ et al: Treatment of resistant atrial fibrillation, *Arch Intern Med* 155:1885, 1995.

Author: **Fred F. Ferri, M.D.**

Atrial flutter (PTG)

BASIC INFORMATION

DEFINITION
Atrial flutter is a rapid atrial rate of 280 to 340 bpm with varying degrees of intraventricular block.

ICD-9-CM CODES
427.32 Atrial flutter

EPIDEMIOLOGY AND DEMOGRAPHICS
Atrial flutter is common during the first week after open heart surgery.

PHYSICAL FINDINGS
- Fast pulse rate (approximately 150 bpm)
- Symptoms of cardiac failure, lightheadedness, and angina pectoris

ETIOLOGY
- Atherosclerotic heart disease
- MI
- Thyrotoxicosis
- Pulmonary embolism
- Mitral valve disease
- Cardiac surgery
- COPD

DIAGNOSIS

DIFFERENTIAL DIAGNOSIS
- Atrial fibrillation
- Paroxysmal atrial tachycardia

WORKUP
- ECG
- Laboratory evaluation

LABORATORY TESTS
- Thyroid function studies
- Serum electrolytes

IMAGING STUDIES
ECG
- Regular, "sawtooth," or "F" wave pattern, best seen in II, III, and AVF and secondary to atrial depolarization
- AV conduction block (2:1, 3:1, or varying)

TREATMENT

NONPHARMACOLOGIC THERAPY
- Valsalva maneuver or carotid sinus massage usually slows the ventricular rate (increases grade of AV block) and may make flutter waves more evident.
- Electrical cardioversion is given at low energy levels (20 to 25 J).

ACUTE GENERAL Rx
- In absence of cardioversion, IV diltiazem or digitalization may be tried to slow the ventricular rate and convert flutter to fibrillation. Esmolol, verapamil, and adenosine may also be effective.
- Atrial pacing may also terminate atrial flutter.

CHRONIC Rx
- Chronic atrial flutter may respond to amiodarone.
- Radiofrequency ablation to interrupt the atrial flutter is also effective for patients with chronic or recurring atrial flutter.

DISPOSITION
Over 85% of patients convert to regular sinus rhythm following cardioversion with as little as 25 to 50 J.

REFERRAL
For radiofrequency ablation in patients with chronic or recurring atrial flutter

MISCELLANEOUS

COMMENTS
Patient education material can be obtained from American Heart Association, 7320 Greenville Avenue, Dallas, TX 75231.

REFERENCES
Kirkorian G et al: Radiofrequency ablation of atrial flutter: efficacy of anatomically guided approach, *Circulation* 90:2804, 1994.

Author: **Fred F. Ferri, M.D.**

BASIC INFORMATION

DEFINITION
Atrial septal defect (ASD) is an abnormal opening in the atrial septum that allows for blood flow between the atria. There are several forms:
- Ostium primum: defect low in the septum
- Ostium secundum: occurs mainly in the region of the fossa ovalis
- Sinus venous defect: less common form, involves the upper part of the septum

SYNONYMS
ASD

ICD-9-CM CODES
429.71 Atrial septal defect

EPIDEMIOLOGY AND DEMOGRAPHICS
- 80% of cases of ASD involve persistence of ostium secundum.
- Incidence is higher in females.
- ASD accounts for 8% to 10% of congenital heart abnormalities.

PHYSICAL FINDINGS
- Pansystolic murmur best heard at apex secondary to mitral regurgitation (ostium primum defect)
- Widely split S_2
- Visible and palpable pulmonary artery pulsations
- Ejection systolic flow murmur
- Prominent right ventricular impulse
- Cyanosis and clubbing (severe cases)
- Exertional dyspnea
- Patients with small defects: generally asymptomatic

ETIOLOGY
Unknown

DIAGNOSIS

DIFFERENTIAL DIAGNOSIS
- Primary pulmonary hypertension
- Pulmonary stenosis
- Rheumatic heart disease
- Mitral valve prolapse
- Cor pulmonale

WORKUP
- ECG
- Chest x-ray examination
- Echocardiography
- Cardiac catheterization

IMAGING STUDIES
- ECG
  1. Ostium primum defect: left axis deviation, RBBB, prolongation of PR interval
  2. Sinus venous defect: leftward deviation of P axis
  3. Ostium secundum defect: right axis deviation, right bundle-branch block
- Chest x-ray: cardiomegaly, enlargement of right atrium and ventricle, increased pulmonary vascularity, small aortic knob
- Echocardiography with saline bubble contrast and Doppler flow studies: may demonstrate the defect and the presence of shunting
- Cardiac catheterization: confirms the diagnosis in patients who are candidates for surgery

TREATMENT

NONPHARMACOLOGIC THERAPY
Avoidance of strenuous activity in symptomatic patients

ACUTE GENERAL Rx
- Children and infants: closure of ASD before age 10 yr is indicated if pulmonary:systemic flow ratio is >1.5:1.
- Adults: closure is indicated in symptomatic patients with shunts >2:1.
- Surgery should be avoided in patients with pulmonary hypertension with reversed shunting (Eisenmenger's syndrome) because of increased risk of right heart failure.
- Transcatheter closure is advocated in children when feasible.
- Surgical closure is indicated in all patients with ostium primum defect and significant shunting unless patient has significant pulmonary vascular disease.

CHRONIC Rx
See "Acute General Rx."

DISPOSITION
- Mortality is high in patients with significant ostium primum defect.
- Patients with small shunts have a normal life expectancy.
- Surgical mortality varies with the age of the patient and the presence of cardiac failure and systolic pulmonary artery hypertension; mortality ranges from <1% in young patients (<45 yr old) to >10% in elderly patients with presence of heart failure and systolic pulmonary hypertension.

REFERRAL
Surgical referral in patients with significant left:right shunts and elevated pulmonary:systemic flow ratios

MISCELLANEOUS

COMMENTS
Patient education materials can be obtained from American Heart Association, 7320 Greenville Avenue, Dallas, TX 75231.

REFERENCES
Konstantinides S et al: A comparison of surgical and medical therapy for atrial septal defect in adults, *New Engl J Med* 233:469, 1995.

Author: **Fred F. Ferri, M.D.**

Atrial deficit hyperactivity disorder (PTG)

BASIC INFORMATION

DEFINITION
Attention deficit hyperactivity disorder (ADHD) follows a persistent pattern (lasting at least 6 mo) of inattention or hyperactivity/impulsivity that is greater than expected for age and that begins before age 7 yr. The disorder is further defined by dysfunction in at least two settings (e.g., home, school, day care).

SYNONYMS
Hyperactivity
Attention deficit disorder (ADD)

ICD-9-CM CODES
F90.X (DMS-IV 314.XX)

EPIDEMIOLOGY AND DEMOGRAPHICS
PREVALENCE (IN U.S.): 35% of school-age children
PREDOMINANT SEX: MALES > FEMALES, WITH RATES RANGING FROM 4:1 TO 9:1
PREDOMINANT AGE:
- Onset must occur before age 7 yr.
- At least 20% experience spontaneous remissions by adolescence; however, the disorder may persist into adulthood.

PEAK INCIDENCE: Diagnosis is usually made after child begins school (ages 6 to 9 yr).
GENETICS:
- Familial pattern in many patients with ADHD
- Specific thyroid hormone abnormality in a very small fraction of familial ADHD

PHYSICAL FINDINGS
- Usually diagnosed in elementary school where achievement is compromised and behavioral dyscontrol is less tolerated
- Wide array of symptoms, including difficulty sustaining attention, frequent careless mistakes, failure to follow instructions, difficulty organizing activities, distractability, forgetfulness, fidgeting, inability to sit still or play quietly, excessive activity or speech, inability to await turn, or intrusiveness
- May exhibit bossiness, stubbornness, demoralization, mood lability, and poor self-esteem
- IQ scores slightly lower than the general population

ETIOLOGY
- Probability of multiple etiologies
- Associated and possibly etiologic factors: comorbid Tourette's, a history of abuse or neglect, lead poisoning, previous encephalitis, drug exposure in utero, low birth weight, and mental retardation
- Thyroid hormone metabolism abnormalities identified in a pedigree of familial ADHD

DIAGNOSIS

DIFFERENTIAL DIAGNOSIS
- In early childhood, may be difficult to distinguish from normal active children.
- ADHD may overlap symptoms in children with disruptive behavior such as conduct disorder or oppositional defiant disorders.
- School and behavioral problems are associated with a learning disability (these disorders often coexist).
- Bipolar disorder may be confused with ADHD, but it can be distinguished by the episodic nature of bipolar illness and the pervasive presence of ADHD.

WORKUP
- History with collateral information from parents and teachers is central to the diagnosis.
- Neurologic examination is used to uncover nonspecific, nonvocal, soft neurologic signs that frequently can be found in ADHD children.
- Questionnaires for parents and adolescents aid in the diagnosis.
- Psychologic testing is useful to diagnose a learning disability.

TREATMENT

NONPHARMACOLOGIC THERAPY
Children generally do better in special education settings with behavioral management of the disruptive behavior.

ACUTE GENERAL Rx
- Stimulants: mainstay of treating ADHD; include methylphenidate (Ritalin), dextroamphetamine (Dexedrine), and pemoline (Cylert)
- Adjuncts: antidepressants (rare cardiac deaths in children and adolescents warrant caution); serotonin reuptake inhibiting antidepressants (safer but efficacy not as well documented), clonidine, and neuroleptics

DISPOSITION
- Severity generally decreases with age.
- In late adolescence, the symptom severity is quite mild in many individuals.
- Full or partial aspects of the disorder are possibly persistent into mid-adulthood and require ongoing pharmacotherapy.

REFERRAL
- If diagnosis is complicated by coexisting conditions
- If treatment with stimulants is not adequately effective

MISCELLANEOUS

REFERENCES
Wender EH: Attention-deficit hyperactivity disorders in adolescence, *J Develop Behav Ped* 16:192, 1995.
Author: **Rif S. El-Mallakh, M.D.**

Autistic disorder (PTG)

BASIC INFORMATION

DEFINITION
The term *autistic disorder* refers to impairment in the development of language, communication, and reciprocal social interaction along with a restricted behavioral repertoire, with onset prior to age 3 yr.

SYNONYMS
Autism
Early infantile autism
Childhood autism
Kanner's autism

ICD-10-CM CODES
F84.0 Autistic disorder
(DSM-IV code 299.0 Autistic disorder)

EPIDEMIOLOGY AND DEMOGRAPHICS
PREVALENCE (IN U.S.): 2 to 5 cases/10,000 persons (10 to 15 cases/10,000 persons when broader definitions are used)
PREDOMINANT SEX: Male:female ration of 3-4:1
PREDOMINANT AGE: Lifelong illness
PEAK INCIDENCE: Before age 3 yr
GENETICS: Unknown genetic component; risk for sibling of affected individual: increases to 3%

PHYSICAL FINDINGS
- Marked impairment in the understanding and use of both verbal and nonverbal communication (probably underlies the profound impairment in social interactions)
- Stereotypic behavior or language

ETIOLOGY
- Majority of cases of autism are not associated with a medical condition.
- There is a significant increase in comorbid seizure disorder (25%) and mental retardation.
- Autism is sometimes associated with other neurologic conditions (e.g., encephalitis, phenylketonuria, Fragile X, and others), suggesting that it may result from nonspecific neuronal injury.
- Specific abnormality that produces autistic symptoms has not been identified.

DIAGNOSIS

DIFFERENTIAL DIAGNOSIS
- Other pervasive developmental disorders
- Rett's syndrome: occurs in females, exhibits head growth deceleration, loss of previously acquired motor skills, and incoordination
- Childhood disintegration disorder: development normal until age 2 yr, followed by regression
- Childhood-onset schizophrenia: follows period of normal development
- Asperger's syndrome: lacks the language developmental abnormalities of autism
- Isolated symptoms of autism: when occurring in isolation, defined as disorders, e.g., selective mutism, expressive language disorder, mixed receptive-expressive language disorder, or stereotypic movement disorder

WORKUP
A two-part process:
1. Establish the diagnosis.
2. Determine if there are any associated medical conditions.

LABORATORY TESTS
- PKU screen (usually done at birth in the U.S.)
- Chromosome analysis to rule out fragile-X in both boys and girls (Carrier girls may exhibit mild symptoms.)

IMAGING STUDIES
- EEG to rule out coexisting seizure disorder
- Head CT scan or MRI to rule out tuberous sclerosis
- Possible BAER to rule out hearing deficit
- IQ testing to help determine functional level of the child

TREATMENT

NONPHARMACOLOGIC THERAPY
- A behavioral training program that is consistent in both the home and school environments is important.
- Educational needs should focus on language and social development.
- Most children need a highly structured environment.
- Educating the parents and teachers is of great value.

ACUTE GENERAL Rx
- Haloperidol or other high-potency neuroleptics are helpful in reducing aggression and stereotypy.
- Serotonin reuptake inhibitor antidepressants (fluoxetine, clomipramine, sertraline, paroxetine) are possibly useful in children with coexisting depression or with marked obsessive or ritualistic behaviors.
- Naltrexone is useful for children with self-injurious behaviors.
- Valproic acid and carbamazepine are preferred to phenytoin or phenobarbital for seizure control.

CHRONIC Rx
- Extended use of all medications used for acute management
- Potential for tardive dyskinesia with chronic use of neuroleptics
- Large doses of vitamin B_6 and magnesium supplementation (mild ameliorating effect)

DISPOSITION
- Most children (70%) will require some degree of assistance as adults, will not be able to work, and will not achieve proper social adjustment.
- Some 10% (particularly if IQ is in the normal range and speech is achieved by age 5 yr) may have a reasonable outcome.
- Children with Asperger's syndrome may have a very good outcome despite ongoing symptoms.

REFERRAL
Assistance may be needed in diagnosis, management, parental teaching, or intervention with the school system.

MISCELLANEOUS

REFERENCES
Bauer S: Autism and the pervasive developmental disorders. Part I. *Ped in Rev* 16:130, 1995.
Bauer S: Autism and the pervasive developmental disorders. Part II. *Ped in Rev* 16:168, 1995.
Authors: **Rif S. El-Mallakh, M.D.** and **Peter E. Tanguay, M.D.**

Babesiosis (PTG)

BASIC INFORMATION

DEFINITION
Babesiosis is a tick-transmitted protozoan disease of animals, caused by intraerythrocytic parasites of the genus *Babesia*. Humans are incidentally infected, resulting in a nonspecific febrile illness.

ICD-9-CM CODES
088.82 Babesiosis

EPIDEMIOLOGY AND DEMOGRAPHICS
INCIDENCE (IN U.S.): Unknown
PREVALENCE (IN U.S.):
- In areas of high endemicity, seropositivity ranging from 9% (Rhode Island) to 21% (Connecticut)
- Highest number of reported cases in New York

PREDOMINANT SEX: Males (most likely through increased exposure to vectors during recreational or occupational activities)
PREDOMINANT AGE: Severity apparently increasing with age >40 yr
PEAK INCIDENCE: Spring and summer months, May through September
GENETICS: None known
CONGENITAL INFECTION: At least one case of probable vertical transmission
NEONATAL INFECTION: At least two cases of perinatal transmission

PHYSICAL FINDINGS
- Incubation period 1 to 4 wk, or 6 to 9 wk in transfusion-associated disease
- Gradual onset of irregular fever, chills, diaphoresis, headache, myalgia, arthralgia, fatigue, and dark urine
- On physical examination: petechiae, frank or mild hepatosplenomegaly, and jaundice
- Infection with *B. divergens* producing a more severe illness with a rapid onset of symptoms and increasing parasitemia progressing to massive intravascular hemolysis and renal failure

ETIOLOGY
- Vector: Deer tick, *Ixodes scapularis* (also known as *I. dammini*)
  1. Feeds on rodents during the spring and summer while in its larval and nymphal stages and on deer as an adult
  2. During the warmer months in endemic areas, humans are readily infected while engaging in outdoor activities
- *Babesia microti*, along with *B. divergens* and *B. bovis*, account for most human infections.
- In the U.S., cases caused by *B. microti* are acquired on offshore islands of the northeastern coast, including Nantucket Island, Cape Cod, and Martha's Vineyard in Massachusetts; Block Island in Rhode Island; and Long Island, Fire Island, and Shelter Island in New York; as well as the nearby mainland including Connecticut.
- Sporadic cases reported from California, Georgia, Maryland, Minnesota, Virginia, Wisconsin, and most recently the WA-1 strain from Washington State and the MO-1 strain from Missouri.
- *B. divergens* and *B. bovis* are implicated in human disease in Europe, where the disease remains rare and predominantly associated with asplenia.
- Majority of cases are asymptomatic.
- Believed to be transmissible by transfusion, through platelets and erythrocytes.
- Mixed infections (*B. microti* and *Borrelia burgdorferi*) are estimated to occur in 10% (Rhode Island and Connecticut) to 60% (New York) of cases.

DIAGNOSIS

DIFFERENTIAL DIAGNOSIS
- Amebiasis
- Ehrlichiosis
- Hepatic abscess
- Leptospirosis
- Malaria
- Salmonellosis, including typhoid fever
- Acute viral hepatitis
- Hemorrhagic fevers

WORKUP
Should be suspected in any febrile patient living or traveling in an endemic area, irrespective of exposure history to ticks or tick bites, especially if asplenic

CLINICAL TOPICS   Babesiosis (PTG)   65

LABORATORY TESTS
- CBC to reveal mild to moderate pancytopenia
- Abnormally elevated serum chemistries, including creatinine, liver function profile, lactate dehydrogenase, and direct and total bilirubin levels
- Urinalysis to reveal proteinuria and hemoglobinuria
- Examination of Giemsa- or Wright-stained thick and thin blood films for intraerythrocytic parasites
  1. In its classic, though infrequently seen, form a "tetrad" or "Maltese Cross" composed of four daughter cells attached by cytoplasmic strands is observed.
  2. More commonly, smaller forms composed of a single chromatin dot are eccentrically located within bluish cytoplasm.
  3. Parasitized erythrocytes may be multiply infected but not enlarged, or they may show evidence of pigment deposition, seen with *Plasmodium* species.
- Diagnosis achieved serologically by indirect immunofluorescence assay (IFA) is specific for *B. microti*.
  1. Titer of ≥1:64 is indicative of seropositivity, whereas one ≥1:256 is considered diagnostic of acute infection.
  2. Assay is hampered by the inability to distinguish between exposed patients and those who are actively infected.
  3. Immunoglobulin M indirect immunofluorescent-antibody test may be highly sensitive and specific for diagnosis.

TREATMENT

NONPHARMACOLOGIC THERAPY
Supportive care with adequate hydration

ACUTE GENERAL Rx
- In patients with intact spleens: predominantly asymptomatic or if symptomatic, generally self-limited
- Therapy reserved for the severely ill patient, especially if asplenic or immunosuppressed
- Combination of quinine sulfate 650 mg PO tid plus clindamycin 600 mg PO tid (1.2 g parenterally bid) taken for 7 to 10 days: effective but may not eliminate parasites
- Exchange transfusions in addition to therapy with quinine and clindamycin: successful treatment for severe infections in asplenic patients associated with high levels of *B. microti* or *B. divergens* parasitemia

DISPOSITION
Prognosis is usually good and fatal outcomes are rare.

REFERRAL
- For prompt consultation with an infectious disease specialist if the diagnosis is acutely suspected, especially in the asplenic, elderly, or immunocompromised patient
- For hospitalization for the severely ill patient who may require exchange transfusions in addition to antibiotic therapy

MISCELLANEOUS

COMMENTS
- Prevention of babesiosis in asplenic or immunocompromised hosts is best achieved by avoidance of areas where the vector is endemic, especially during the months of May through September.
- If residence or travel in endemic areas is unavoidable, advise patients to perform daily cutaneous self-examination, wear light-colored clothing (to facilitate removal of ticks), and apply tick repellent (diethyltoluamide and dimethylphthalate) to skin or clothing.
- Advise a daily inspection for ticks in family pets, e.g. cats and dogs.
- Infection with *B. divergens*, especially in the asplenic patient, is often fatal.

REFERENCES
Boustani MR, Gelfand JA: Babesiosis, *Clin Infect Dis* 22:611, 1996.
Herwaldt BL et al: A fatal case of babesiosis in Missouri: identification of another piroplasm that infects humans, *Ann Intern Med* 124:643, 1996.
Krause PJ et al: Concurrent Lyme disease and babesiosis: evidence for increased severity and duration of illness, *JAMA* 275(21):1657, 1996.
Krause PJ et al: Efficacy of immunoglobulin M serodiagnostic test for rapid diagnosis of acute babesiosis, *J Clin Microbiol* 34(8):2014, 1996.
Author: **George O. Alonso, M.D.**

Balanitis (PTG)

BASIC INFORMATION

DEFINITIONS
Balanitis is an inflammation of the superficial tissues of the penile head.

ICD-9-CM CODES
112.2 Balanitis

EPIDEMIOLOGY AND DEMOGRAPHICS
INCIDENCE (IN US): Unknown
PREVALENCE (IN US): Unknown
PREDOMINANT SEX: Exclusive to males
PEAK INCIDENCE: All ages, especially in sexually active men

PHYSICAL FINDINGS
- Itching and tenderness
- Pain, dysuria, and local edema
- Rarely, ulceration and lymph node enlargement
- Severe ulcerations leading to superimposed bacterial infections
- Inability to void: unusual, but a more distressing and serious complication

ETIOLOGY
- Poor hygiene causing erosion of tissue with erythema and promoting growth of *Candida albicans*
- Sexual contact, urinary catheters, and trauma
- Allergic reactions to condoms or medications

DIAGNOSIS

DIFFERENTIAL DIAGNOSIS
- Leukoplakia
- Reiter's syndrome
- Lichen planus
- Balanitis xerotica obliterans
- Psoriasis
- Carcinoma of the penis
- Erythroplasia of Queyrat

WORKUP
- Sexually active males: assessment for evidence of other sexually transmitted diseases
- Biopsy if lesions do not heal

LABORATORY TESTS
- VDRL
- Serum glucose
- Wet mount
- KOH prep
- Microculture

TREATMENT

NONPHARMACOLOGIC THERAPY
- Maintenance of meticulous hygiene
- Retraction and bathing of prepuce several times a day
- Warm sitz baths to ease edema and erythema
- Consideration of circumcision, especially when symptoms are severe or recurrent
- With Foley catheters, strict catheter care strongly advised

MEDICATIONS
- Analgesics, such as acetaminophen and/or codeine
- Clotrimazole 1% cream applied topically twice daily to affected areas
- Bacitracin or Neosporin ointment applied topically four times daily
- With more severe bacterial superinfection: cephalexin 500 mg orally qid
- Topical corticosteroids added four times daily if dermatitis severe
- Patients with suspected urinary tract infections: trimethoprim-sulfa DS twice daily or ciprofloxacin 500 mg PO bid after obtaining appropriate cultures

REFERRAL
- For surgical evaluation for circumcision if symptoms are recurrent, especially if phimosis or meatitis occur (NOTE: Severe phimosis with an inability to void may require prompt slit drainage.)
- For biopsy to rule out other diagnosis such as premalignant or malignant lesions if lesions are not healing

MISCELLANEOUS

REFERENCES
Gangai MP: Balanitis and posthitis. In Kaufman JJ (ed): *Current urologic therapy,* Philadelphia, 1986, WB Saunders.

Webster SB: Candidal vaginitis and balanitis. In Moschella S, Hurley H (eds): *Dermatology,* vol 1, Philadelphia, 1992, WB Saunders.

Author: **Joseph J. Lieber, M.D.**

Basal cell carcinoma (PTG)

BASIC INFORMATION

DEFINITION
Basal cell carcinoma is a malignant tumor of the skin arising from basal cells of the lower epidermis and adnexal structures. Histologically, there are five major types (nodular, superficial, micronodular, infiltrative, morpheaform). The most common type is nodular (21%); the least common is morpheaform (1%); a mixed pattern is present in approximately 40% of cases. Basal cell carcinoma advances by direct expansion and destroys normal tissue.

SYNONYMS
BCC

ICD-9-CM CODES
179.9 Basal cell carcinoma, site unspecified
173.3 Basal cell carcinoma, face
173.4 Basal cell carcinoma, neck, scalp
173.5 Basal cell carcinoma, trunk
173.6 Basal cell carcinoma of the limb
173.7 Basal cell carcinoma, lower limb

EPIDEMIOLOGY AND DEMOGRAPHICS
- Most common cutaneous neoplasm in humans (>400,000 cases/yr)
- 85% appear on the head and neck region
- Most common site: nose (30%)
- Increased incidence with age >40 yr
- Increased incidence in men
- Risk factors: fair skin, increased sun exposure, use of tanning salons with ultraviolet A or B radiation, history of irradiation (e.g., Hodgkin's disease), personal or family history of skin cancer, impaired immune system

PHYSICAL FINDINGS
Variable with the histologic type:
- Nodular: dome-shaped, painless lesion that may become multilobular and frequently ulcerates (rodent ulcer); prominent telangiectatic vessels are noted on the surface; border is translucent, elevated, pearly white (see color plate 2); some nodular basal cell carcinomas may contain pigmentation giving the appearance similar to a melanoma.
- Superficial: circumscribed scaling black appearance with a thin raised pearly white border; a crust and erosions may be present; occurs most frequently on the trunk and extremities.
- Morpheaform: flat or slightly raised yellowish or white appearance (similar to localized scleroderma); appearance similar to scars, surface has a waxy consistency.

ETIOLOGY
Sun exposure and use of tanning salons with equipment that emits ultraviolet A or B radiation

DIAGNOSIS

DIFFERENTIAL DIAGNOSIS
- Keratoacanthoma
- Melanoma (pigmented basal cell carcinoma)
- Xeroderma pigmentosa
- Basal cell nevus syndrome
- Molluscum contagiosum
- Sebaceous hyperplasia
- Psoriasis

WORKUP
Biopsy to confirm diagnosis

TREATMENT

NONPHARMACOLOGIC THERAPY
Avoidance of excessive tanning, use of sun screens to prevent damage from excessive sun exposure

ACUTE GENERAL Rx
Variable with tumor size, location, and cell type:
- Excision surgery: preferred method for large tumors with well-defined borders on the legs, cheeks, forehead, and trunk
- Mohs' micrographic surgery: preferred for lesions in high-risk areas (e.g., nose, eyelid), very large primary tumors, recurrent basal cell carcinomas, and tumors with poorly defined clinical margins
- Electrodesiccation and curettage: useful for small (<6 mm) nodular basal cell carcinomas
- Cryosurgery with liquid nitrogen: useful in basal cell carcinomas of the superficial and nodular types with clearly definable margins; no clear advantages over the other forms of therapy; generally reserved for uncomplicated tumors
- Radiation therapy: generally used for basal cell carcinomas in areas requiring preservation of normal surround tissues for cosmetic reasons (e.g., around lips); also useful in patients who cannot tolerate surgical procedures or for large lesions and surgical failures

CHRONIC Rx
Periodic evaluation for at least 5 yr because of increased risk of recurrence of another basal cell carcinoma (>40% risk within 5 yr of treatment)

DISPOSITION
- More than 90% of patients are cured.
- Nodular and superficial basal cell carcinomas are the least aggressive.
- Morpheaform lesions have the highest incidence of positive tumor margins (>30%) and the greatest recurrence rate.

REFERRAL
Surgical referral for biopsy and removal of the malignancy

MISCELLANEOUS

COMMENTS
U.S. Preventive Services Task Force Recommendations regarding screening for skin cancer are described in Section V, Chapter 12.

REFERENCES
Fleming ID et al: Principles of management of basal and squamous cell carcinoma of the skin, *Cancer* 75(2S):699, 1995.
Habif TP: *Clinical dermatology,* ed 3, St Louis, 1996, Mosby.
Marghoob AA: Basal and squamous cell carcinomas, *Postgrad Med* 102:139, 1997.

Author: **Fred F. Ferri, M.D.**

Bell's palsy (PTG)

BASIC INFORMATION

DEFINITION
Bell's palsy is facial weakness affecting the muscles supplied by the seventh cranial nerve (facial nerve).

SYNONYMS
Idiopathic facial paralysis

ICD-9-CM CODES
351.0 Bell's palsy

EPIDEMIOLOGY AND DEMOGRAPHICS
INCIDENCE: 25 cases/100,000 persons
GENETICS: A predisposition to cranial neuropathies, especially seventh and third nerve palsies, has been reported.
RISK FACTORS: Diabetes, pregnancy, age >30 yr

PHYSICAL FINDINGS
- Unilateral paralysis of the facial muscles (<1% of facial palsies are bilateral)
- Ipsilateral loss of taste
- Possible ipsilateral ear pain
- Increased or decreased unilateral eye tearing

ETIOLOGY
- The cause is most likely viral (herpes simplex).
- Herpes zoster can cause Bell's palsy in association with herpetic blisters affecting the outer ear canal or the area behind the ear.
- Bell's palsy can also be one of the manifestations of Lyme disease.

DIAGNOSIS

DIFFERENTIAL DIAGNOSIS
- Neoplasms affecting the base of the skull or the parotid gland
- Bacterial infectious process (meningitis, otitis media, osteomyelitis of the base of the skull)
- Brain stem stroke
- Multiple sclerosis
- Sarcoidosis
- Head trauma with fracture of temporal bone
- Other: Guillain-Barré, carcinomatous or leukemic meningitis, leprosy, Melkersson-Rosenthal syndrome

Box 2-44 describes the differential diagnosis of facial palsy.

WORKUP
Bell's palsy is a clinical diagnosis. A focused history and neurologic examination will confirm the diagnosis.

LABORATORY TESTS
- FBS to evaluate for diabetes
- VDRL in selected patients
- Lyme titer in endemic areas

IMAGING STUDIES
- Contrast-enhanced MRI to exclude neoplasms is indicated only in patients with atypical features or course.
- Chest x-ray examination may be useful to exclude sarcoidosis or to rule out TB in selected patients before treating with steroids.

TREATMENT

NONPHARMACOLOGIC THERAPY
- Reassure patient that the disease is most likely a result of a virus attacking the nerve, not a stroke. It is also important to inform the patient that the prognosis is good.
- Avoid corneal drying by applying skin tape to the upper lid to keep the palpebral fissure narrowed. Lacri-Lube ophthalmic ointment at night and artificial tears during the day are also useful to prevent excessive drying.
- The patient should use dark glasses when going outside to minimize sun exposure.

ACUTE GENERAL Rx
- Although the benefits of corticosteroid therapy remain unproven, most practitioners use a brief course of prednisone therapy.
- If used, prednisone therapy should be started within 4 days of onset of Bell's palsy.
- Optimal steroid dose is unknown. Prednisone can be given as one 50-mg tablet qd for 7 days without tapering or can be started at 80 mg and tapered by 5 mg/day until finished.

CHRONIC Rx
Patients should be monitored for evidence of corneal abrasion and ulceration or hemifacial spasm.

DISPOSITION
- Of affected individuals, 95% recover satisfactorily within few months.
- Recurrence is experienced in 5% of Bell's palsy cases.

REFERRAL
- Persistent redness or irritation of the eye requires referral to an ophthalmologist.
- Neurology referral is recommended if diagnosis is unclear or if the clinical course is atypical.

MISCELLANEOUS

COMMENTS
A patient brochure discussing facial nerve problems can be obtained from the American Academy of Otolaryngology—Head and Neck Surgery (AAO-HNS), phone: (703) 519-1528.

REFERENCES
Chang GY, Keane JR: Bell's palsy and herpes zoster oticus. In Johnson RT, Griffin JW (eds): *Current therapy in neurologic disease*, ed 5, St Louis, 1996, Mosby.

Author: **Fred F. Ferri, M.D.**

Bipolar disorder (PTG)

BASIC INFORMATION

DEFINITION
Bipolar disorder is an episodic, recurrent, and frequently progressive condition in which the afflicted individual suffers periods of mania and, possibly, depression. Depressive episodes are not essential for the diagnosis. However, the individual must experience at least one manic episode in which he/she experiences at least 1 wk of continuous symptoms of elevated, expansive, or irritable mood in association with three or four of the following:
- Decreased need for sleep
- Grandiosity
- Pressured speech
- Subjective or objective flight of ideas
- Distractibility
- Increased level of goal-directed activity
- Problematic behavior

SYNONYMS
Manic-depression
Cycloid psychosis

ICD-9-CM CODES
296.4-6 Circular manic, circular depressed, circular type mixed

EPIDEMIOLOGY AND DEMOGRAPHICS
INCIDENCE (IN U.S.): Approximately 1% of the population
PREVALENCE (IN U.S.): 0.4% to 1.6%
PREDOMINANT SEX: Equal distribution among male and female
PREDOMINANT AGE: Lifelong condition with age of onset 14 to 30 yr
PEAK INCIDENCE: Onset in 20s
GENETICS:
- Concordance rates for monozygotic twins: 0.7 to 0.9, for dizygotic twins: 0.2 to 0.4
- Risk of offspring with one affected parent: 0.2 to 0.4, with two affected parents: 0.4 to 0.7
- Displays the phenomenon of genetic anticipation (earlier onset with successive generations), which is a hallmark phenomenon of trinucleotide repeat diseases
- CAG trinucleotide repeats increased by approximately 30 repeats but location unknown
- Displays a parent of origin effect in which there is a higher frequency of the disease in maternal relatives
- Susceptibility locus mapped to chromosome 18p

PHYSICAL FINDINGS
- Mania associated with psychomotor activation that is usually goal-directed but not necessarily productive
- Elevated and frequently labile mood
- Flight of ideas with rapid, loud, pressured speech
- Psychosis with delusions, hallucinations, and formal thought disorder possible
- Depressive episodes resembling major depression (see "Major Depression"); however, retardation usually extreme
- Catatonia possible in severe cases

ETIOLOGY
- Unknown
- Hypotheses:
  1. Abnormalities of membrane function
  2. Second messenger abnormalities
  3. Noradrenergic excess

DIAGNOSIS

DIFFERENTIAL DIAGNOSIS
- Secondary manias caused by medical disorder (e.g., renal disease, AIDS, stroke, digoxin toxicity) are frequent.
- Onset of mania after age 40 yr is suggestive of secondary mania.
- Less severe, and probably distinct, conditions of bipolar type II and cyclothymia are possible.
- Cross-sectional examination of acutely manic patient can be confused with schizophreniform or a paranoid psychosis.

WORKUP
- History
- Physical examination
- Mental status examination

LABORATORY TESTS
- Because of high rate of secondary manias, initial presentation to confirm health of all major organ systems (routine chemistries, complete blood count, urinalysis, sedimentation rate)
- Low threshold for examination of CSF

IMAGING STUDIES
Imaging of anatomy (CT scan or MRI) as well as function (EEG) should be part of initial workup.

TREATMENT

NONPHARMACOLOGIC THERAPY
- Psychotherapy to help patients cope with consequences of the disease and improve compliance with medications
- Bright light therapy in the northern latitudes in individuals exhibiting a seasonal pattern of winter depression

ACUTE GENERAL Rx
- First-line agents for acute mania: lithium, valproate, and carbamazepine
- Useful adjuncts to acute treatment: antipsychotics and benzodiazepines
- Problematic because antidepressants can induce manic episodes

CHRONIC Rx
- Goal of long-term treatment: prevention
- Best agents for prophylaxis: lithium, valproate, and carbamazepine
- Useful second-line agents: antipsychotics (particularly the atypical agents such as clozapine)
- Long-term use of antidepressants: frequently destabilizes patient and leads to more frequent relapses

DISPOSITION
- Course is variable.
- Over 90% of people having a single manic episode are likely to experience others.
- Uncontrolled manic or depressive episodes can lead to additional episodes ("illness begets illness").
- Untreated suicide rate approaches 20%; drops to only 8% to 10% with treatment.
- Psychosocioeconomic consequences of both mania and depression can be severe and disabling.
- Cost of condition is about $48 billion annually (in 1991 dollars).

REFERRAL
- If use of antidepressant contemplated
- If patient is severely manic or suicidal

MISCELLANEOUS

REFERENCES
El-Mallakh RS: *Lithium: actions and mechanisms,* Washington, DC, 1996, American Psychiatric Press.

Goodwin F, Jamison KR: *Manic-depressive illness,* New York, 1991, Oxford University Press.

Author: **Rif S. El-Mallakh, M.D.**

Bite wounds (PTG)

BASIC INFORMATION

DEFINITION
A bite wound can be animal or human, accidental or intentional.

ICD-9-CM CODES
879.8 Bite wound, unspecified site

EPIDEMIOLOGY AND DEMOGRAPHICS
- Bite wounds account for 1% of emergency department visits.
- Over 1,000,000 bites occur in humans annually in the U.S.
- Dog bites account for 85% to 90% of all bites; cat bites, 10% to 20%. Typically the animal is owned by the victim.
- Infection rates are highest for cat bites (30% to 50%), followed by human bites (15% to 30%) and dog bites (5%).
- The extremities are involved in 75% of bites.
- The annual incidence of fatal dog bites in the U.S. is approximately 20 bites/yr.

PHYSICAL FINDINGS
- The appearance of the bite wound is variable (e.g., puncture wound, tear, avulsion).
- Cellulitis, lymphangitis, and focal adenopathy may be present in infected bite wounds.
- Patient may experience fever and chills.

ETIOLOGY
- Increased risk of infection: human and cat bites, closed fist injuries, wounds involving joints, puncture wounds, face and lip bites, bites with skull penetration, bites in immunocompromised hosts
- Most frequent infecting organisms:
  1. *Pasteurella multocida:* responsible for majority of infections within 24 hr of dog and cat bites
  2. *Capnocytophaga canimorsus* (formerly DF-2 bacillus): a gram-negative organism responsible for late infection, usually following dog bites
  3. Gram-negative organisms (*Pseudomonas, Hemophilus):* often found in human bites
- *Streptococcus* spp., *Staphylococcus aureus*
- *Eikenella corrodens* in human bites

DIAGNOSIS

DIFFERENTIAL DIAGNOSIS
- Bite from a rabid animal (often the attack is unprovoked)
- Factitious injury

WORKUP
- Determination of the time elapsed since the patient was bitten, status of rabies immunization of the animal, and underlying medical conditions that might predispose the patient to infection (e.g., DM, immunodeficiency)
- Documentation of bite site, notification of appropriate authorities (e.g., police department, animal officer)

LABORATORY TESTS
- Generally not necessary
- Hct if there has been significant blood loss
- Wound cultures (aerobic and anaerobic) if there is evidence of sepsis or victim is immunocompromised patient; cultures should be obtained before irrigation of the wound but after superficial cleaning

IMAGING STUDIES
X-rays are indicated when bony penetration is suspected or if there is suspicion of fracture or significant trauma; x-rays are also useful for detecting presence of foreign bodies (when suspected).

TREATMENT

NONPHARMACOLOGIC THERAPY
Local care with debridement, vigorous cleansing, and saline irrigation of the wound; debridement of devitalized tissue

ACUTE GENERAL Rx
- Avoid suturing of hand wounds and any wounds that appear infected.
- Puncture wounds should be left open.
- Give antirabies therapy and tetanus toxoid as needed (see Box A-14 in Appendix).
- Use empiric antibiotic therapy in high-risk wounds (e.g., cat bite, hand bites, face bites, genital area bites, bites with joint or bone penetration, human bites, immunocompromised host): Dicloxacillin 500 mg qid, for 5 to 7 days or amoxicillin-clavulanate (Augmentin) 500 to 875 mg bid for 7 days or cefuroxime (Ceftin) 250 to 500 mg bid for 7 days.
- In hospitalized patients, IV antibiotics of choice are cefoxitin 1 to 2 g q6h, ampicillin-sulbactam 1.5 to 3g q6h, ticarcillin-clavulanate 3 g q6h, or ceftriaxone 1 to 2 g q24h.

DISPOSITION
Prognosis is favorable with proper treatment.

REFERRAL
Hospitalization and IV antibiotic therapy for infected human bites, bites with injury to joints, nerves, tendons, or any animal bites unresponsive to oral therapy

MISCELLANEOUS

COMMENTS
All patients should be evaluated for tetanus and rabies (see Box A-14 in Appendix).

REFERENCES
Dumyati G et al: Animal and human bite wounds: immunization, prophylaxis, treatment, *Consultant* 37:1501, 1997.

Lewis KT, Stilles M: Management of cat and dog bites, *Am Fam Physician* 52:479, 1995.

Wiggins ME, Akelman E, Weiss A: Management of dog bites and dog bite infections of the hand, *Orthopedics* 17:617, 1994.

Author: **Fred F. Ferri, M.D.**

Bladder cancer (PTG)

BASIC INFORMATION

DEFINITION
Bladder cancer is a heterogeneous spectrum of neoplasms ranging from non–life-threatening, low-grade, superficial papillary lesions to high-grade invasive tumors, which often have metastasized at the time of presentation. It is a field change disease in which the entire urothelium from the renal pelvis to the urethra may be susceptible to malignant transformation.
Types: Transitional cell carcinoma (TCCa), squamous cell carcinoma, and adenocarcinoma.

ICD-9-CM CODES
Primary: 188.9
Secondary: 198.1
CIS: 233.7
Benign: 223.3
Uncertain Behavior: 236.7
Unspecified: 239.4

EPIDEMIOLOGY AND DEMOGRAPHICS
Each year approximately 49,000 new cases are diagnosed and over 10,000 deaths are attributed to bladder cancer.
PREDOMINANT SEX: In males, it is the fourth most common cancer; it accounts for 10% of all cancers. In females, it is the eighth most common cancer; it accounts for 4% of all cancers.
RISK: The lifetime risk of developing bladder cancer is 2.8% in white males, 0.9% in black males; 1% in white females, and 0.6% in black females.
PEAK INCIDENCE: Incidence increases with age, high >60 yr, uncommon <40 yr.
GENETICS: It is thought to be multifactorial in etiology involving both genetic and environmental interactions. Overall, it is estimated that approximately 20% to 25% of the male population in the U.S. with bladder cancer has the disease as a result of occupational exposure.
DISTRIBUTION: In North America, transitional cell carcinomas comprise 93%, squamous cell carcinomas comprise 6%, and adenocarcinomas account for 1% of bladder cancers.
PATHOGENESIS: Two pathways exist for bladder cancer (TCCa):
1. Papillary superficial disease occasionally leading to invasive cancer (75%)
2. Carcinoma-in-situ and solid invasive cancer with high risk of disease progression (25%)

At presentation, 72% of cancers are localized to the bladder, 20% of the cancers extend to the regional lymph nodes, and 3% present with distant metastases. 80% of superficial TCCa recur with up to 30% progressing to a higher stage or grade. Younger patients most commonly develop low grade papillary noninvasive TCCa and are less likely to have recurrences when compared with older patients with similar lesions. Involvement of the upper tracts with tumor occurs in 25 to 5% of the cases.

STAGING (BASED ON THE TNM SYSTEM):
T_0 No tumor in specimen
T_{is} CIS
T_a Papillary Tcc_a noninvasive
T_1 Papillary Tcc_a into lamina propria
T_2 Tcc_a invasive of superficial ms
T_{3a} Invasive of deep ms
T_{3b} Invasive of perivesical fat
T_{4a} Invasive of adjacent pelvic organ
T_{4b} Invasive of pelvic wall with fixation
Invasive of nodal status:
N_0 No nodal involvement
N_{1-3} Pelvic nodes
N_4 Nodes above bifurcation
N_x Unknown
Invasive of metastatic status:
M_0 No distant metastases
M_1 Distant metastases
M_x Unknown

MOLECULAR EPIDEMIOLOGY: TCCa is usually a field change disease with tumors arising at different times and sites in the urothelium suggesting a polyclonal etiology of bladder cancer. Bladder cancers have been associated with abnormalities on chromosomes 1,4,11,5,7,3,9,21,18,13,8; with alterations in suppressor genes P53, retinoblastoma gene, and P16; and alterations in oncogenes H-ras and epidermal growth factor receptor.

PHYSICAL FINDINGS
- Gross painless hematuria
- Microhematuria
- Frequency, urgency, occasional dysuria

With locally invasive to distant metastatic disease, the presentation can include:
- Abdominal pain
- Flank pain
- Lymphedema
- Renal failure
- Anorexia
- Bone pain

ETIOLOGY
Bladder cancer is a potentially preventable disease associated with specific etiologic factors:
- Cigarette smoking
- Occupational exposures: dye workers, textile workers, tire and rubber workers, petroleum workers
- Chemical exposures: O-toluidine, 2-naphthylamine, Benzidine, 4-aminobiphenyl, and nitrosamines
- Exposure to HPV type 16

Squamous carcinomas are associated with:
- Schistosomiasis
- Urinary calculi
- Indwelling catheters
- Bladder diverticula

Miscellaneous causes:
- Phenacetin abuse
- Cyclophosphamide
- Pelvic irradiation
- Tuberculosis

Adenocarcinomas are associated with:
- Exstrophy
- Endometriosis
- Neurogenic bladder
- Urachal abnormalities
- As a secondary site for distant metastases from other organs (i.e., colon cancer)

DIAGNOSIS

- History and physical examination
- Urinalysis
- Cystoscopy with bladder barbotage and biopsy
- Transurethral resection of bladder tumor(s)

DIFFERENTIAL DIAGNOSIS
- Urinary tract infection
- Frequency-urgency syndrome
- Interstitial cystitis
- Stone disease
- Endometriosis
- Neurogenic bladder

LABORATORY TESTS
BLADDER TUMOR MARKERS: BTA (BTA, BARD Diagnostic Sciences, Inc.), Nuclear Matrix Protein (NMP 22, Matritech), Autocrine Motility Factor Receptor (AMFR), Hyaluronidase, Immunocytology (Lewis X-Antigen), and Aura-Tek Fibrinogen Degradation Products

RADIOLOGIC TESTS:
- IVP, renal ultrasound, retrograde pyelography, CT scan, and MRI.

Bladder cancer (PTG)

- One or a combination of studies can be used. In the absence of skeletal symptoms, bone scan is not recommended.

TREATMENT

NONPHARMACOLOGIC THERAPY
- Initially, transurethral resection of bladder tumor (TURBT)
- Loop biopsy of the prostatic urethra if high grade TCCa is suspected
- If superficial disease, follow-up protocol with repeat TURBT and/or the use of intravesical agents is recommended
- For advanced bladder cancer, radical cystectomy with urethrectomy (unless orthotopic diversion is planned) and either ileal loop conduit or orthotopic diversion

BLADDER PRESERVATION APPROACHES: Following cystectomy for muscle invasive disease, 50% or more of the patients will develop metastases. Most patients develop metastases at distant sites, a third relapse locally. Bladder preservation management is offered in those individuals who refuse surgery or who might not be suitable radical cystectomy patients. Bladder-sparing protocols include extensive TURBT or partial cystectomy with external beam or interstitial radiotherapy and systemic chemotherapy. Radiotherapy as a single treatment modality is not effective. The best predictor of successful bladder preservation is a complete response following the combination of initial TURBT and two cycles of CMV (cisplatin, methotrexate, vinblastine) chemotherapy seen with stages T2-T3a.

INDICATIONS FOR PARTIAL CYSTECTOMY:
- Tumor within a bladder diverticula
- solitary, primary, and muscle-invasive or high-grade lesion of a region of the bladder that allows complete excision with adequate surgical margins
- Inability to adequately resect tumor by TURBT alone because of size or location
- Tumor overlying a ureteral orifice requiring ureteral reimplantation
- Biopsy of a radiation induced ulceration
- Palliation of severe local symptoms
- Patient refusal or urinary diversion
- Poor-risk patient who is not a diversion candidate

Contraindications:
- Multiple tumors
- CIS
- Cellular atypia on biopsy
- Prostatic invasion
- Invasion of the trigone
- Inability to achieve adequate surgical margins
- Prior radiotherapy
- Inability to maintain adequate bladder volume after resection
- Evidence of extravesical tumor extension
- Poor surgical risk

ACUTE GENERAL R_X
INDICATIONS FOR INTRAVESICAL CHEMOTHERAPY:
- High grade tumor
- Tumor size >5 cm
- Tumor multiplicity
- Presence of CIS
- Positive urinary cytologies following a resection
- Incomplete tumor resection. Intravesical agents: thiotepa, adriamycin, mitomycin C, AD-32, BCG, interferon, bropirimine, Epodyl, interleukin-2, and Keyhole-Limpet hemocyanin. Photodynamic therapy with hematoporphyrin derivatives have also been used.

INDICATIONS FOR CYSTECTOMY:
- Large tumors not amenable to complete TURBT
- High-grade tumor
- Multiple tumors with frequent recurrences
- Diffuse CIS not responsive to intravesical chemotherapy
- Prostatic urethra involvement
- Irritative bladder symptoms with upper tract deterioration
- Muscle-invasive disease
- Disease outside of the bladder

SYSTEMIC CHEMOTHERAPY: Used as neoadjuvant and adjuvant therapy for systemic disease. The most effective agents are cisplatin, methotrexate, vinblastine, adriamycin (MVAC). Other agents include: mitoxantrone, vincristine, etoposide (VP16), 5FU, ifosfamide, Taxol, Gemcitabine, Piritrexim, and gallium nitrate. Chemotherapy in combination can provide palliation and modest survival benefit.

RADIOTHERAPY: Conflicting reports suggest that superficial bladder cancer is more sensitive to radiotherapy. Squamous changes within the tumor and secretion of human chorionic gonadotropin by the lesion are associated with poor response to radiotherapy. Only 20% to 30% of patients with invasive bladder cancer can be cured by external beam radiation therapy alone. It is used in combination with surgery or with systemic agents to treat bladder cancer primarily in those patients who are not surgical candidates or who refuse surgery.

CHRONIC R_X
FOLLOW-UP RECOMMENDATIONS FOR SUPERFICIAL BLADDER CANCER:
- Cystoscopy, bladder barbotage, and bimanual examination every 3 mo for 2 yr, then every 6 mo for 2 yr, thereafter, annually.
- Upper tract studies are based on the risk of upper tract tumor development, generally every 2 to 5 yr.

FOLLOW-UP RECOMMENDATIONS FOR ADVANCED DISEASE:

Bladder Preservation:
- Cystoscopy, barbotage, bimanual examination, biopsy (when indicated), every 3 mo for 2 yr, then every 6 mo for 2 yr, yearly thereafter.
- CT scan of abdomen and pelvis every 6 mo for 2 yr in addition to chest x-ray examination, liver function testing, and serum creatinine.

Cystectomy with Ileal Loop/Orthotopic Bladder:
- Neobladder endoscopy and IVP yearly.
- CT scan of abdomen and pelvis every 6 mo for 2 yr in addition to chest x-ray examination, liver function tests, and serum creatinine.
- Loopogram every 6 mo for 2 yr, then yearly.

MISCELLANEOUS

COMMENTS
- The most useful prognostic parameters for bladder tumor recurrence and subsequent cancer progression are tumor grade, depth of tumor penetration, multifocal tumors, frequency of recurrence, tumor size, carcinoma-in-situ, lymphatic invasion, papillary or solid tumor configuration.
- U.S. Preventive Services Task Force Recommendations for screening for bladder cancer are described in Section V, Chapter 17.

REFERENCES
Catalona WJ: Urothelial tumors of the urinary tract. In Walsh PC et al (eds): *Campbell's urology*, Philadelphia, 1992, WB Saunders.

Korman HJ, Watson RB, and Soloway MS: Bladder cancer: clinical aspects and management. In Stamey T (ed): *Monographs in urology*, Montverde, Fla, 1966, Medical Directions Publishing.

Vogelzang NJ et al (eds): *Comprehensive textbook of genitourinary oncology*, Baltimore, Md, 1996, Williams & Wilkins.

Author: **Philip J. Aliotta, M.D., M.S.H.A.**

Blepharitis

BASIC INFORMATION

DEFINITION
Blepharitis is an acute or, most often, chronic inflammation of the eyelid margins.

ICD-9 CM CODES
373.0 Blepharitis

PHYSICAL FINDINGS
- Chronically infected lids are usually diffusely erythematous, with collarettes (fibrin exudate) at the base of the lashes.
- Lid margins thicken over time, with associated loss of eyelashes (madarosis), misdirected growth of lashes (trichiasis), and overflow or inspissation of the meibomian glands.
- Associated conjunctivitis with erythema and edema is frequent, but it is usually without discharge.
- Chalazia is possible.
- Superficial punctate erosions of the inferior cornea epithelium are common.
- More severe findings, such as corneal pannus, ulcerative keratitis, or lid ectropion, are less common.

ETIOLOGY
- Staphylococcal infection
- Seborrhea
- Rosacea
- Dry eye
- Meibomian gland abnormalities
- Two categories of blepharitis:
  1. Anterior blepharitis, most often associated with staphylococcal infection or seborrheic dermatitis
  2. Posterior blepharitis, associated with meibomian gland dysfunction

DIAGNOSIS

DIFFERENTIAL DIAGNOSIS
- Dry eye syndrome
- Eyelid malignancies
- Herpes simplex blepharitis
- Molluscum contagiosum
- Phthiriasis palpebrarum
- Phthirus pubis (pubic lice)
- Demodex folliculorum (transparent mites)
- Allergic blepharitis

WORKUP
- Scrapings of the eyelids to show polymorphonuclear leukocytes and gram-positive cocci
- Empirical treatment of patients based on the physical findings (cultures usually not obtained)

LABORATORY TESTS
Eyelid cultures and antibiotic sensitivity testing (usually not done unless patient fails to respond to initial treatment regimen)

TREATMENT

NONPHARMACOLOGIC THERAPY
- Once or twice daily regimen of massage, scrubs, application of antibiotic ointment, and possibly oral antibiotics
- Hot compress applied to closed lids for 5 to 10 min; heat loosens debris from the lid margins and increases meibomian gland fluidity
- Firm massage of the lid margins to enhance the flow of secretions from glands, followed by cleansing of the lids with cotton-tipped applicators dipped in a 50:50 mixture of baby shampoo and water
- Lashes and lid margins scrubbed vigorously while the eyelids are closed, followed by thorough rinsing

ACUTE GENERAL Rx
- Following local massage and cleansing, mainstay of treatment: application of topical antibiotic ointment to the eyelid margins
  1. Most effective topical antibiotics available are bacitracin and erythromycin ophthalmic ointments.
  2. Ointment is applied one to four times daily, depending on the severity of the inflammation, for 1 to 2 wk.
  3. Treatment is continued once daily, at bedtime, for another 4 to 8 wk.
  4. Treatment is continued for 1 mo after all signs of inflammation have disappeared.
- In patients with rosacea:
  1. Tetracycline 250 mg orally four times daily or doxycycline 100 mg orally twice daily along with local treatment
  2. Dosing reduced to once daily for several months, depending on the clinical situation
- Recalcitrant cases with antibiotic resistance:
  1. Vancomycin eyedrops 1%
  2. Ciprofloxacin and ofloxacin eyedrops (commercially available, but efficacy has not been not established)

CHRONIC Rx
- By definition, this is a chronic condition for which there is frequently no cure.
- Treatment is as described above.

DISPOSITION
Treatment failure is often a result of inadequate instruction of the patient and poor compliance.

REFERRAL
To an ophthalmologist if patient fails to respond to local therapy

MISCELLANEOUS

REFERENCES
Baum J: Infections of the eye, *Clin Infect Dis* 21:479, 1995.

Weinstock FJ, Weinstock MB: Common eye disorders: six patients to treat, pitfalls to avoid, *Postgrad Med* 99(4):119, 1996.

Author: Jane V. Eason, M.D.

Bone tumor, primary malignant

BASIC INFORMATION

DEFINITION
Primary malignant bone tumors are invasive, anaplastic, and have the ability to metastasize. Most arise from the marrow (myeloma), but tumors may develop from bone, cartilage, fat, and fibrous tissues.

FIBROSARCOMA AND LIPOSARCOMA: Extremely rare. They are similar to those tumors arising in soft tissue. Leukemia and lymphoma are excluded from this discussion.

OSTEOSARCOMA: A rare primary malignant tumor of bone characterized by malignant tumor cells that produce osteoid or bone. Several variants have been described: parosteal sarcoma, periosteal sarcoma, multicentric, and telangiectatic forms.

CHONDROSARCOMA: A malignant cartilage tumor that may develop primarily or secondarily from transformation of a benign osteocartilaginous exostosis or enchondroma.

EWING'S SARCOMA: A malignant tumor of unknown histogenesis.

MULTIPLE MYELOMA: A neoplastic proliferation of plasma cells.

SYNONYMS
Multiple myeloma:
1. Plasma cell myeloma
2. Plasmacytoma

ICD-9-CM CODES
203.0 Multiple myeloma
170.9 Neoplasma, bone (periosteum), primary, malignant
M9180/3 Osteosarcoma
N9220/3 Chondrosarcoma
M9260/3 Ewing's sarcoma

EPIDEMIOLOGY AND DEMOGRAPHIC
MULTIPLE MYELOMA:
- The most common tumor in bone
- Age at onset: usually >40
- Male:female ratio of 2:1

OSTEOGENIC SARCOMA:
- Average age at onset: 10 to 20 yr
- Males > females
- Parosteal sarcoma in older patients

CHONDROSARCOMA:
- Age at onset: 40 to 60 yr
- Male:female ratio of 2:1

EWING'S SARCOMA:
- Age at onset: 10 to 15 yr

PHYSICAL FINDINGS
MULTIPLE MYELOMA:
- May present as a systemic process or, less commonly, as a "solitary" lesion
- Early manifestations: anorexia, weight loss, and bone pain; majority of cases present initially with back pain that often leads to the detection of a destructive skeletal lesion
- Other organ systems eventually becoming involved, resulting in more bone pain, anemia, renal insufficiency, and/or bacterial infections, usually as a result of the dysproteinemia typical of this disorder
- Possible secondary amyloidosis, leading to cardiac failure or nephrotic syndrome

OSTEOSARCOMA:
- Most originating in the metaphysis
- 50% to 60% about the knee
- Possible pain and swelling, but otherwise healthy patient
- Osteosarcoma in conjunction with Paget's disease, manifested primarily as a sudden increase in bone pain

CHONDROSARCOMA:
- Tumor most commonly involving the pelvis, upper femur, and shoulder girdle
- Painful swelling

EWING'S SARCOMA:
- Painful soft tissue mass often present
- Possibly increased local heat
- Midshaft of a long bone usually affected (in contrast to other tumors)
- Weight loss, fever, and lethargy

DIAGNOSIS

DIFFERENTIAL DIAGNOSIS
- Osteomyelitis
- Metastatic bone disease

The age of the patient and the initial radiographic features often determine the next appropriate diagnostic steps.

LABORATORY TESTS
- Slightly elevated alkaline phosphatase in osteosarcoma
- In Ewing's sarcoma: reflective of systemic reaction; include anemia, an increase in WBC count, and an elevated sedimentation rate
- In multiple myeloma:
  1. Bence Jones protein in the urine
  2. Anemia and elevated sedimentation rate
  3. Characteristic dysproteinemia on serum protein electrophoresis
  4. Diagnostic feature: peak in the electrophoretic pattern suggestive of a monoclonal gammopathy
  5. Rouleaux formation in the peripheral blood smear
  6. Often, presence of hypercalcemia, but alkaline phosphatase levels usually normal

IMAGING STUDIES
- Classic osteogenic sarcoma penetrates the cortex early in many cases.
  1. A blastic (dense), lytic (lucent), or mixed response may be seen in the affected bone.
  2. An aggressive perpendicular sunburst pattern may be present as a result of periosteal reaction, and peripheral Codman's triangles are often noted.
  3. Margins of the tumor are poorly defined.
- Speckled calcifications in a destructive radiolucent lesion are usually suggestive of chondrosarcoma.
- Ewing's sarcoma is characterized radiographically by mottled, irregular destructive changes with periosteal new bone formation. The latter may be multilayered, producing the typical "onion skin" appearance.
- Typical roentgenographic finding in multiple myeloma is the "punched out" lesion with sharply demarcated edges.
  1. Multiple lesions are usual.
  2. Diffuse osteoporosis may be the only finding in many cases.
  3. Pathologic fractures are common.

TREATMENT

The evaluation and treatment of malignant bone tumors is complicated. Diagnostic studies and treatment should be supervised by an orthopedic cancer specialist and oncologist.

DISPOSITION
- In the past 20 yr, dramatic improvements have been made in the treatment protocols for osteosarcoma with the use of adjuvant multidrug regimens and limb-sparing surgery.
- 70% 5-yr survival rates have been obtained in some series.
- Prognosis of multiple myeloma remains poor despite new therapies.
  1. Complete remissions are uncommon.
  2. Survival with a solitary lesion may be long, but most patients succumb after a median of 3 yr.
- Prognosis for Ewing's sarcoma has improved with a combination of chemotherapy, local resection, and radiation therapy.
- Chondrosarcomas are not sensitive to chemotherapy or radiation, and prognosis will depend upon the grade of the tumor and the ability to obtain an adequate resection.

MISCELLANEOUS

REFERENCES
Dahlin DC, Unni KK: *Bone tumors: general aspects and data in 8542 cases,* Springfield, Ill, 1986, Charles C. Thomas.
Mercuri M et al: The management of malignant bone tumors in children and adolescents, *Clin Orthop* 264:156, 1991.

Author: **Lonnie R. Mercier, M.D.**

CLINICAL TOPICS   Botulism (PTG)   75

BASIC INFORMATION

DEFINITION
Botulism is an illness caused by a neurotoxin produced by *Clostridium botulinum.* Three types of disease can occur: food-borne botulism, wound botulism, and infant botulism.

ICD-9-CM CODES
005.1 Botulism

EPIDEMIOLOGY AND DEMOGRAPHICS
INCIDENCE (IN U.S.): Approximately 22 cases/yr

PHYSICAL FINDINGS
- Symptoms usually begin 12 to 36 hr following ingestion.
- Severity of illness is related to the quantity of toxin ingested.
- Significant findings:
  1. Cranial nerve palsies, with ocular and bulbar manifestations being most frequent (ptosis, ophthalmoplegia, dysphagia, and dysarthria)
  2. Usually bilateral nerve involvement that may progress to a descending flaccid paralysis
  3. Typically, absence of sensory findings; sensorium intact
  4. GI symptoms (nausea, vomiting, diarrhea, or cramps)
  5. Usually no fever
- Wound botulism
  1. Occurs mostly in injecting drug users (subcutaneous heroin injection—"skin popping") or with traumatic injury.
  2. Presentation is similar to that of food-borne disease, except for a longer incubation period and the absence of GI symptoms.
  3. Wound infection is not always apparent.

ETIOLOGY
- Cause is one of several types of neurotoxins (usually A, B, or E) produced by *C. botulinum,* an anaerobic, gram-positive bacillus.
- In food-borne variety, disease is caused by ingestion of preformed toxin.
- In wound botulism, toxin is elaborated by organisms that contaminate a wound.
- In infant botulism, toxin is produced by organisms in the GI tract.

DIAGNOSIS

DIFFERENTIAL DIAGNOSIS
- Myasthenia gravis
- Guillain-Barré syndrome
- Tick paralysis
- CVA

WORKUP
Search made for toxin and the organism (see "Laboratory Tests")

LABORATORY TESTS
- Samples of food and stool are cultured for the organism.
- Food, serum, and stool are sent for toxin assay.

TREATMENT

NONPHARMACOLOGIC THERAPY
- Supportive care with intubation if respiratory failure occurs
- Debridement of the wound in wound botulism

ACUTE GENERAL Rx
- Give trivalent equine botulinum antitoxin as early as possible.
  1. Give one vial by IM injection and one vial IV.
  2. The antitoxin is available from the Centers for Disease Control and Prevention [(404) 639-2206]; it is derived from horse serum, so there is a significant incidence of serum sickness.
  3. Skin testing, and possible desensitization, is recommended before treatment.
- Give wound botulism patients penicillin, 2 million U IV q4h.

CHRONIC Rx
- Supportive
- Rehabilitation/physical therapy

DISPOSITION
- Highest mortality in the first case in an outbreak, with subsequent cases receiving rapid treatment
- Complete recovery for most individuals

REFERRAL
Immediate for all cases to an ER and an infectious disease consultant

MISCELLANEOUS

COMMENTS
- Routine cooking inactivates the toxin, but spores are resistant to environmental factors. At room temperature, spores can germinate and produce toxin.
- Most outbreaks are associated with home-canned foods, especially vegetables.
- Patients must be closely monitored for progression to respiratory paralysis.
- Notify public health authorities.

REFERENCES
Gollober M et al: Wound botulism—California, 1995, *MMWR* 44:889, 1995.
Townes JM et al: An outbreak of type A botulism associated with a commercial cheese sauce, *Ann Intern Med* 125:558, 1996.

Author: **Maurice Policar, M.D.**

Brain neoplasm (PTG)

BASIC INFORMATION

DEFINITION
Brain neoplasms are primary (non-metastatic) tumors arising from one of many intracranial cellular substrates.

SYNONYMS
Brain tumors
Primary tumors of the central nervous system

ICD-9-CM CODES
225.0 Brain neoplasm (benign)
239.2 Brain neoplasm (unspecified)

EPIDEMIOLOGY AND DEMOGRAPHICS
INCIDENCE (IN U.S.): Male: 9.2 cases/100,000 persons/yr; female: 8.1 cases/100,000 persons/yr
PREVALENCE (IN U.S.): Not reported
PREDOMINANT SEX: Male > female
PREDOMINANT AGE: Male: 75+ yr; female: 65 to 74 yr
PEAK INCIDENCE: Over age 64 yr
GENETICS:
- Some tumor types are associated with specific chromosomal abnormalities.
- Incidence is increased in certain inherited diseases (e.g., neurofibromatosis, tuberous sclerosis).

PHYSICAL FINDINGS
- Varies with tumor location, size, and rate of growth
- Generally: progressive signs and symptoms
- Headache as presenting symptom is seen in 20% of patients and develops later in 60%
- Seizures in 33% of patients

ETIOLOGY
- Most cases are idiopathic.
- Specific chromosomal abnormalities and prior cranial radiation are sometimes implicated.

DIAGNOSIS

DIFFERENTIAL DIAGNOSIS
- Stroke
- Abscess
- Metastatic tumors

WORKUP
- Thorough history and physical examination to help resolve differential diagnosis
- Imaging studies and histologic confirmation if needed

LABORATORY TESTS
CSF cytology may yield histologic diagnosis.

IMAGING STUDIES
- MRI with contrast is highly sensitive.
- CT scan is useful if calcification or hemorrhage suspected.

TREATMENT

NONPHARMACOLOGIC THERAPY
- Surgical removal or debulking possibly required.
- Radiation is useful for certain types of tumors.

ACUTE GENERAL Rx
Steroids (e.g., dexamethasone 4 mg PO q6h) may be used as a temporizing measure to reduce edema.

CHRONIC Rx
Surgical removal, radiation, and/or chemotherapy, depending in tumor type and location

DISPOSITION
- Varies as a function of histologic type and age
- Overall relative survival rates: 25% in adults, 59% in children

REFERRAL
All cases warrant evaluation by an oncologist.

MISCELLANEOUS

REFERENCES
Jaeckle KA: Clinical presentation and therapy of nervous system tumors. In Bradley et al (eds): Neurology in clinical practice, Boston, 1996, Butterworth-Henneman.

Author: **Michael Gruenthal, M.D., Ph.D.**

Breast abscess

BASIC INFORMATION

DEFINITION
Breast abscess is an acute inflammatory process resulting in the formation of a collection of pus. Typically there is painful erythematous mass formation in the breast occasionally with draining through the overlying skin or nipple duct opening.

SYNONYMS
Subareolar abscess
Lactational or puerperal abscess

ICD-9-CM CODES
6.110 Abscess of the breast
675.0 Abscess of the nipple related to childbirth
675.1 Abscess of the breast related to childbirth

EPIDEMIOLOGY AND DEMOGRAPHICS
- 10% to 30% of all breast abscesses are lactational.
- Acute mastitis occurs in 2.5% of nursing mothers, with 1 in 15 of these women developing abscess.

PHYSICAL FINDINGS
Painful erythematous induration involving the part of the breast leading to fluctuant abscess

ETIOLOGY
- Lactational abscess: milk stasis and bacterial infection leading to mastitis, then to abscess, with *Staphylococcus aureus* the most common causative agent
- Subareolar abscess:
  1. Central ducts involved, with obstructive nipple duct changes leading to bacterial infection
  2. Cultured organisms mixed, including anaerobes, staphylococci, streptococci, and others

DIAGNOSIS

DIFFERENTIAL DIAGNOSIS
- Inflammatory carcinoma
- Advanced carcinoma with erythema, edema, and/or ulceration
- Rarely, tuberculous abscess
- Hydradenitis of breast skin
- Sebaceous cyst with infection

WORKUP
- Clinical examination sufficient
- If abscess suspected, referral to surgeon for incision, drainage, and biopsy
- If possible abscess or advanced carcinoma, referral for workup required

LABORATORY TESTS
- Perform C&S test of abscess contents.
- If mammogram or ultrasound prevented by discomfort, perform after resolution of abscess if required.

TREATMENT

NONPHARMACOLOGIC THERAPY
- Established abscess: incision and drainage, preferably with general anesthesia
- Biopsy of abscess cavity wall to exclude carcinoma

ACUTE GENERAL Rx
- Antibiotics: the pathogen is generally staphylococci in lactational abscess.
- If acute mastitis is treated early, resolution without drainage is possible.
- Subareolar abscess: broad-spectrum antibiotic treatment and drainage is needed to control acute phase.

CHRONIC Rx
Further surgical treatment for recurrences or fistula

DISPOSITION
- Lactational abscess: possible to continue breast-feeding without apparent risk of infection to the infant
- Subareolar abscess:
  1. Notorious for recurrence or complication of fistula formation
  2. Patient informed and referred for subsequent care

REFERRAL
- If abscess drainage required
- For surgical consultation if subareolar abscess involved

MISCELLANEOUS

REFERENCES
Harris J et al: *Breast diseases*, ed 2, Philadelphia, 1991, Lippincott.
Author: **Takuma Nemoto**, M.D.

Breast cancer (PTG)

BASIC INFORMATION

DEFINITION
The term *breast cancer* refers to invasive carcinoma of the breast, whether ductal or lobular.

SYNONYMS
Carcinoma of the breast

ICD-9-CM CODES
174.9 Malignant neoplasm female breast

EPIDEMIOLOGY AND DEMOGRAPHICS
- Nearly exclusively the disease of women, with only 1% of breast cancers in males
- Steady increase in its incidence in the U.S., with 180,000 new patients annually
- Annual mortality of 44,000
- Risk steadily increases with age
- Genetically defined group of women with BRCA-1 or BRCA-2 identified to carry lifetime risk as high as 85%

PHYSICAL FINDINGS
- Increasing number of small breast cancers found by mammograms
- Patients usually completely free of physical findings
- Palpable tumors possibly as small as 1 cm or even smaller
- Size of the mass and its location measured and documented
- Skin and/or nipple retraction and skin edema/erythema/ulcer/satellite nodule
- Nodal enlargement in axilla and supraclavicular areas
- Advanced disease: clinical signs of pleural effusion and/or hepatomegaly
- Rare instances: clear, serous, or bloody discharge only symptom
- Nipple evaluation (see "Paget's disease of the breast")

ETIOLOGY
- Precise mechanism of carcinogenesis not understood
- Possibly interaction of ovarian estrogen, nonovarian estrogen, estrogens of exogenous origin with breast tissue of varied carcinogenic susceptibility to develop cancer
- Other known or suspected variables: childbearing, breast-feeding practice, diet, physical activities, body mass, alcoholic intake
- Have identified families with known high risk
- Women with BRCA-1 and BRCA-2 associated with high risk

DIAGNOSIS

DIFFERENTIAL DIAGNOSIS
The following nonmalignant breast lesions can simulate breast cancer on both physical and mammogram examinations:
1. Fibrocystic changes
2. Fibroadenoma
3. Hamartoma

IMAGING STUDIES
- Mammograms: 30% to 50% of breast cancers detected by screening mammograms only as a spiculated mass, a mass with or without microcalcifications, or a cluster of microcalcifications

WORKUP
- Physical examination:
  1. Mass detected by patient or medical professional: workup required
  2. Negative mammogram: breast cancer not ruled out
  3. Sonogram: to demonstrate mass to be cyst, usually eliminating need for further workup
- To establish diagnosis:
  1. Positive aspiration cytology on a clinically and mammographically malignant mass—highly accurate but still requires open biopsy confirmation
  2. Stereotactic core needle biopsy diagnosis: reliable with invasive carcinoma identified, but negative or equivocal results require careful evaluation
  3. Atypical hyperplasia or in situ carcinoma found by core needle biopsy: open surgical biopsy confirmation still required
  4. Excisional or incisional biopsy: establishes diagnosis

NOTE: Do not rely on negative mammogram or negative aspiration cytology to exclude malignancy. Make appropriate referral. Obtain imaging studies such as bone scan, chest x-ray examination, CT scan of abdomen or CT scan of liver.

TREATMENT

NONPHARMACOLOGIC THERAPY
- Early breast cancer: primarily surgical or surgical and radiotherapeutic

- Choice in 60% to 70% of women between modified mastectomy and breast-conserving treatment, which consists of lumpectomy, axillary dissection, and breast irradiation

ACUTE GENERAL Rx
- May require adjuvant chemotherapy or endocrine therapy
- Evaluation and treatment by medical oncologist

DISPOSITION
- Prognosis after curative therapy: depends on size of tumor, extent of nodal metastasis, and pathologic grade of tumor
  1. Patient with 1 cm tumor with no axillary node metastasis: 10-yr disease-free survival rate of 90%
  2. Patient with 3 cm tumor with metastasis in four nodes: 10-yr disease-free survival rate of 15% if no systemic adjuvant therapy given
  3. Outlook for most patients is between these extremes
- Systemic adjuvant therapy: improves prognosis significantly

CHRONIC RX
- Follow-up required after proper treatment of primary breast cancer includes:
  1. Periodic clinical evaluations
  2. Annual mammograms
  3. Other tests as indicated
  4. Patient instruction in monthly breast self-examination technique

REFERRAL
Referral is necessary as soon as breast cancer is even remotely suspected.

MISCELLANEOUS

Breast cancer in pregnancy and lactation:
1. Frequency in women 40 yr old or younger reported to be 15%
2. May carry worse prognosis because disease discovery delayed by engorged and nodular breast changes and/or because disease progression more rapid in pregnancy
3. Survival rates similar to those for nonpregnant early-stage breast cancer patients in same age group
4. Mass usually found by patient or obstetrician
5. Expedient workup recommended, including mammography and sonography
6. Diagnosis to be made without delay
7. Choice of mastectomy or lumpectomy with axillary dissection for treatment
8. Adjuvant chemotherapy delayed until third trimester or after delivery
9. Irradiation to breast after lumpectomy delayed until after delivery

Duct carcinoma in situ (DCIS, intraductal carcinoma):
1. "New" disease mostly found by mammogram as cluster of microcalcification and/or density
2. Less often, presents as palpable mass or nipple discharge
3. Before mammogram screening, DCIS accounted for 1% of all breast cancers
4. Now, 15% to 20% or even higher proportion present with DCIS
5. Formerly treated with mastectomy, now lumpectomy
6. Cure rates 98% to 99%
7. No axillary dissection required
8. With radiation, breast recurrences reduced
9. Mastectomy possibly required with extensive and/or high-grade DCIS
10. Systemic adjuvant treatment is not indicated

Inflammatory carcinoma:
1. Rare but rapidly progressive and often lethal form of breast cancer
2. Presents as erythematous and edematous breast resembling mastitis
3. Biopsy required, including skin
4. Treatment with combination chemotherapy followed by surgery and radiation therapy
5. Prognosis once dismal, now 5-yr disease-free survival in 50% of patients

COMMENTS
- Patient education material can be obtained from the following:
  1. SHARE: Self-Help for Women with Breast Cancer, 19 W 44th Street, No 415, New York, NY 10036-5902.
  2. Y-ME National Organization of Breast Cancer Information and Support, 18220 Harwood Avenue, Homewood, IL 80430.
- Refer to Fig. A-12 for breast self-examination.
- Breast radiologic evaluation is described in algorithm 3-19; evaluation of nipple discharge is noted in Fig. 3-18, and evaluation of palpable mass is described in Fig. 3-20.

REFERENCES
Harris JR et al: *Disease of the breast*, Philadelphia, 1996, Lippincott-Raven.

Author: **Takuma Nemoto, M.D.**

Breech birth

BASIC INFORMATION

DEFINITION
Breech presentation exists when the fetal longitudinal axis is such that the cephalic pole occupies the uterine fundus. Three types exist, with respective percentages at term, frank (48% to 73%, flexed hips, extended thighs), complete (4.6% to 11.5%, flexed hips and knees), and footling (12% to 38%, hips extended).

ICD-9-CM CODES
652.2 Breech presentation without mention of version

EPIDEMIOLOGY AND DEMOGRAPHICS
INCIDENCE: Gestational age dependent: 3% to 4% overall, 14% at 29 to 32 wk, 33% at 21 to 24 wk
PERINATAL MORTALITY: 9% to 25%, or three to five times increase over vertex presentation at term. If one corrects for the associated increase in congenital anomalies and complications of prematurity, the morbidity and mortality approaches that of the vertex presentation at term regardless of route of delivery.

PHYSICAL FINDINGS
- Maintain a high index of suspicion
- Lack of presenting part on vaginal examination
- Fetal heart tones heard above the umbilicus
- Leopold maneuvers revealing mobile fetal part in the uterine fundus

ETIOLOGY
- Abnormal placentation (fundal), uterine anomalies (fibroids, septae), pelvic or adnexal masses, alterations in fetal muscular tone, or fetal malformations.
- Associated conditions: trisomy 13, 18, 21, Potter syndrome, myotonic dystrophy, prematurity

DIAGNOSIS

DIFFERENTIAL DIAGNOSIS
Vertex, oblique, or transverse lie

WORKUP
- If possible, determine reason for breech presentation, history of uterine anomalies, gestational age, or associated fetal congenital anomalies.
- Assess fetal status, either by continuous fetal heart rate monitoring or ultrasound.
- Assess pelvis to determine feasibility of vaginal delivery.
- Assess risk for safety of vaginal vs. abdominal delivery.

IMAGING STUDIES
Ultrasound to evaluate for:
- Fetal anomalies, such as hydrocephalous
- Placental location
- Position of fetal head relative to spine (check for hyperextension)
- Estimated fetal weight (2500 to 3800 g)
- Type of breech (frank, complete, footling)

CRITERIA FOR TRIAL OF LABOR
- Estimated fetal weight 2000 to 3800 g
- Frank breech
- Adequate pelvis
- Flexed fetal head
- Continuous fetal monitoring
- Normal progress of labor
- Bedside availability of anesthesia and capability for immediate C-section
- Informed consent
- Obstetrician trained in vaginal breech delivery

CRITERIA FOR C-SECTION
- Estimated fetal weight <1500 g or >4000 g
- Footling presentation (20% risk of cord prolapse, usually late in course of labor)
- Inadequate pelvis
- Hyperextended fetal head (21% risk of spinal cord injury)
- Nonreassuring fetal status
- Abnormal progress of labor
- Lack of trained obstetrician

TREATMENT

ACUTE GENERAL Rx
- Vaginal delivery in selected patient: allow maternal expulsive forces to deliver fetus until scapula visible (avoiding traction); with flexion and/or Piper forceps, deliver fetal head.
- Perform C-section for the above mentioned reasons.
- External cephalic version, success 60% to 75%, after 37 wk, contraindicated with placental abruption, low-lying placenta, maternal hypertension, previous uterine incision, multiple gestation, nonreasurring fetal status.

COMPLICATIONS
- Head entrapment: leading cause of death (with the exception of anomalous fetuses), 88 cases/1000 deliveries, avoid by maintaining flexion of fetal head, use of Piper forceps or Dührssen's incisions. Before 36 wk, HC > AC, thus fetal predisposition. Tentorial tears secondary to hyperextended head. Association with trisomy 21 in 3% to 5% of cases. Avoid hyperextension of head during delivery.
- Cord prolapse: usually occurs late in the course of labor. Incidence depends on type of breech—frank (0.5%), complete (4% to 5%), footling (10%).
- Nuchal arm: arm extended above fetal head, occurs when there is undue traction before delivery of fetal scapulas. Treatment depends on bringing trapped arm across infant's face.

DISPOSITION
If confounding variables are corrected for, such as prematurity and associated congenital anomalies (6.3% of breeches vs. 2.4% in general population), route of delivery plays a less important role in fetal outcome than previously thought.

REFERRAL
An obstetrician trained in delivery of the vaginal breech is a prerequisite for attempting vaginal route, although it must explained to the patient that with C-section certain risks (such as hyperextension of the fetal head with resultant spinal cord injury) may be minimized but not eliminated.

MISCELLANEOUS

COMMENTS
For breech presentation, in general, mortality is increased thirteenfold and morbidity sevenfold. The main reasons are an increase in congenital anomalies, perinatal hypoxia, birth injury, and prematurity.
There is no contraindication to induction of labor in the breech presentation, nor is labor prohibited in a primigravida.

REFERENCES
American College of Obstetricians and Gynecologists: *Technical bulletin No 95*, August 1986.
Flanagan TA et al: Management of term breech presentation, *Am J Obstet Gynecol* 156:1492, 1987.
Gabbe S, Niebyl J, Simpson JL: *Obstetrics: normal and problem pregnancies,* ed 3, New York, 1996, Churchill Livingstone.
Author: Scott J. Zuccala, D.O.

BASIC INFORMATION

DEFINITION
Bronchiectasis is the abnormal dilation and destruction of bronchial walls, which may be congenital or acquired.

ICD-9-CM CODES
494.0 Bronchiectasis

EPIDEMIOLOGY AND DEMOGRAPHICS
- Cystic fibrosis is responsible for nearly 50% of all cases of bronchiectasis.
- Acquired primary bronchiectasis is uncommon because of rapid diagnosis of pulmonary infections and frequent use of antibiotics.

PHYSICAL FINDINGS
- Moist crackles at lung bases
- Cough with expectoration of large amount of purulent sputum
- Fever, night sweats, generalized malaise, weight loss
- Hemoptysis
- Halitosis, skin pallor
- Clubbing (infrequent)

ETIOLOGY
- Cystic fibrosis
- Lung infections (pneumonia, lung abscess, TB, fungal infections, viral infections)
- Abnormal host defense (panhypogammaglobulinemia, Kartagener's syndrome, AIDS, chemotherapy)
- Localized airway obstruction (congenital structural defects, foreign bodies, neoplasms)
- Inflammation (inflammatory pneumonitis, granulomatous lung disease, allergic aspergillosis)

DIAGNOSIS

DIFFERENTIAL DIAGNOSIS
- TB
- Asthma
- Chronic bronchitis or chronic sinusitis
- Interstitial fibrosis
- Chronic lung abscess
- Foreign body aspiration
- Cystic fibrosis
- Lung carcinoma

WORKUP
Sputum for Gram stain and C&S, chest x-ray examination, bronchoscopy, spirometry

LABORATORY TESTS
- Sputum for Gram stain, C&S, and acid fast bacteria (AFB)
- CBC with differential (leukocytosis with left shift, anemia)
- Serum protein electrophoresis to evaluate for hypogammaglobulinemia
- Antibody test for aspergillosis
- Sweat test in patients with suspected cystic fibrosis

IMAGING STUDIES
- Chest x-ray examination: hyperinflation, crowded lung markings, small cystic spaces at the base of the lungs
- High resolution CT scan of the chest: to detect cystic lesions and exclude underlying obstruction from neoplasm
- Bronchography only when surgery is contemplated
- Pulmonary function tests: generally reveal obstructive or mixed ventilatory defect
- Bronchoscopy: helpful to evaluate hemoptysis, rule out obstructive lesions, and remove mucus plugs

TREATMENT

NONPHARMACOLOGIC THERAPY
- Postural drainage and chest percussion
- Adequate hydration
- Supplemental oxygen for hypoxemia

ACUTE GENERAL Rx
- Antibiotic therapy is based on the results of sputum, Gram stain, and C&S; in patients with inadequate or inconclusive results, empiric therapy with amoxicillin/clavulanate 500 mg to 875 mg q12h, TMP-SMX q12h, doxycycline 100 mg bid, or cefuroxime 250 mg bid for 10 to 14 days is recommended.
- Bronchodilators are useful in patients with demonstrable air flow obstruction.

CHRONIC Rx
- Avoidance of tobacco
- Maintenance of proper nutrition and hydration
- Prompt identification and treatment of infections
- Pneumococcal vaccination and annual influenza vaccination

DISPOSITION
Prognosis is variable with severity of the disease and underlying etiology of bronchiectasis.

REFERRAL
Surgical referral for partial lung resection in patients with localized severe disease unresponsive to medical therapy or in patients with massive hemoptysis

MISCELLANEOUS

COMMENTS
Patient education material on bronchiectasis can be obtained from the American Lung Association, 1740 Broadway, New York, NY 10019.

REFERENCES
Marwah OS: Bronchiectasis: hard to identify, treat, and prevent, *Postgrad Med* 97:149, 1995.

McGuiness G et al: Bronchiectasis: CT evaluation, *Am J of Roentgenol* 160:253, 1993.

Author: **Fred F. Ferri, M.D.**

Bronchitis, acute (PTG)

BASIC INFORMATION

DEFINITION
Acute bronchitis is the inflammation of trachea and bronchi.

ICD-9-CM CODES
466.0 Acute bronchitis

EPIDEMIOLOGY AND DEMOGRAPHICS
Highest incidence in smokers, older adults, young children, and in winter months

PHYSICAL FINDINGS
- Cough, usually worse in the morning, often productive
- Low-grade fever
- Substernal discomfort worsened by coughing
- Postnasal drip, pharyngeal injection
- Rhonchi that may clear after cough, occasional wheezing

ETIOLOGY
- Viral infection (rhinovirus, influenza virus, adenovirus, respiratory syncytial virus)
- Atypical organisms (*mycoplasma, Chlamydia pneumoniae*)
- Bacterial infections (*Hemophilus influenza, Moraxella, Streptococcus pneumoniae*).

DIAGNOSIS

DIFFERENTIAL DIAGNOSIS
- Pneumonia
- Asthma
- Sinusitis
- Bronchiolitis
- Aspiration
- Cystic fibrosis
- Pharyngitis
- Cough secondary to medications
- Neoplasm (elderly patients)
- Influenza

WORKUP
Seldom necessary (e.g., to rule out pneumonia, neoplasm)

LABORATORY TESTS
- Tests are generally not necessary.
- CBC may reveal mild leukocytosis.
- Sputum culture, Gram stain, and blood cultures are generally not indicated.

IMAGING STUDIES
Chest x-ray examination is usually reserved for patients with suspected pneumonia, influenza, or underlying COPD and no improvement with therapy.

TREATMENT

NONPHARMACOLOGIC THERAPY
- Avoidance of tobacco and other pulmonary irritants
- Increased fluid intake
- Use of vaporizer to increase room humidity

ACUTE GENERAL Rx
- Inhaled bronchodilators (e.g., albuterol, metaproterenol) PRN
- Cough suppression with guaifenesin; addition of codeine for cough suppression (e.g., Robitussin-AC) if cough is severe and is significantly interrupting patients sleep pattern
- Use of antibiotics (TMP-SMX, amoxicillin, doxycycline, cefuroxime) for acute bronchitis only in patients with concomitant COPD and purulent sputum or in patients unresponsive to conservative treatment

CHRONIC Rx
Avoidance of tobacco and other pulmonary irritants

DISPOSITION
Complete recovery within 7 to 10 days in most patients

REFERRAL
For pulmonary function testing only in patients with recurrent bronchitis and suspected underlying asthma

MISCELLANEOUS

COMMENTS
Patient education material may be obtained from the American Lung Association, 1740 Broadway, New York, NY 10019.

REFERENCES
Hueston W: A comparison of albuterol and erythromycin for the treatment of acute bronchitis, *J Fam Pract* 33(5):476, 1991.

Orr PH et al: Randomized placebo-controlled trials of antibiotics for acute bronchitis: a critical review of the literature, *J Fam Pract* 36(5):507, 1993.

Author: **Fred F. Ferri, M.D.**

Brucellosis

BASIC INFORMATION

DEFINITION
Brucellosis is a zoonotic infection caused by one of four species of *Brucella*. It commonly presents as a nondescript febrile illness.

SYNONYMS
Malta fever
Bang's disease

ICD-9-CM CODES
023.9 Brucellosis

EPIDEMIOLOGY AND DEMOGRAPHICS
INCIDENCE (IN U.S.): About 100 cases/yr (may be underreported)
PREDOMINANT SEX: Male
PREDOMINANT AGE: Adult
CONGENITAL INFECTION: Although infection can cause abortion in animals, there is no clear increase in the abortion rate in humans.
NEONATAL INFECTION: Can occur if mother is infected during pregnancy.

PHYSICAL FINDINGS
- Incubation period is 1 wk to 3 mo.
- Patients may be asymptomatic or have nonspecific symptoms such as fever, sweats, malaise, weight loss, and depression.
- Fever is the most common finding.
- Hepatomegaly, splenomegaly, or lymphadenopathy are possible.
- Localized disease:
  1. Related to a single organ
  2. Includes endocarditis, meningitis, and osteomyelitis (especially vertebral)

ETIOLOGY
- Caused by infection with *Brucella* species:
  1. Most commonly *melitensis*, but also *suis*, *abortus*, or *canis*
  2. A small, gram-negative coccobacillus
- Acquired through breaks in the skin or by inhalation or ingestion of organisms.
- Most cases occur after exposure to animals (sheep, goats, swine, cattle, or dogs), or animal products (i.e., milk, hides, tissue).
- Most cases (in U.S.) occur in men with occupational exposure to animals (farmers, ranchers, veterinarians, abattoir workers).
- Laboratory acquisition is possible.
- May occur in tourists to other countries who ingest goat milk or cheese.

DIAGNOSIS

DIFFERENTIAL DIAGNOSIS
Many febrile conditions without localizing manifestations (i.e., TB, endocarditis, typhoid fever, malaria, autoimmune diseases)

WORKUP
- Cultures of blood, bone marrow, or other tissue (lymph node, liver) should be sent and held for 4 wk, since *Brucella* grows slowly in vitro.
- Granulomas on biopsy are suggestive of diagnosis.

LABORATORY TESTS
- WBC count: normal or low
- Serology:
  1. Serum agglutination test (SAT) to detect antibodies to *B. abortus, melitensis,* and *suis*
  2. Specific antibody test to identify antibodies to *B. canis*
  3. False-negative SAT possibly resulting from a prozone effect

IMAGING STUDIES
- Radiographs to show splenic calcifications in chronic disease
- Bone scan and radiographs of the spine to suggest osteomyelitis
- Ultrasound or CT scan of the abdomen to show an enlarged liver or spleen
- Echocardiogram to reveal vegetations in endocarditis

TREATMENT

NONPHARMACOLOGIC THERAPY
- Drainage of abscesses
- Valve replacement for endocarditis

ACUTE GENERAL Rx
Combination antibiotics required:
- Doxycycline 100 mg PO bid plus streptomycin 15 mg/kg IM qd for 6 wk
- Less effective: doxycycline 100 mg PO bid plus rifampin 600 mg PO qd or sulfamethoxazole 800 mg/trimethoprim 160 mg one DS tablet PO qid

Courses <6 wk are associated with higher relapse rates; longer courses are recommended for complicated disease.

CHRONIC Rx
See "Acute General Rx."

DISPOSITION
Relapse is possible weeks to months after the completion of therapy, usually because of noncompliance with a prolonged medical regimen or a persistent focus of infection that requires surgical drainage.

REFERRAL
For all cases to an infectious disease specialist

MISCELLANEOUS

COMMENTS
- Alert the microbiology laboratory to the possibility of *Brucella*.
- Do not use doxycycline in children or pregnant women.
- Avoid aminoglycosides in pregnant women.

REFERENCES
Young, EJ: An overview of human brucellosis, *Clin Infect Dis* 21:283, 1995.
Author: **Maurice Policar, M.D.**

Bulimia nervosa (PTG)

BASIC INFORMATION

DEFINITION
Bulimia nervosa is a prolonged illness characterized by a specific psychopathology (see below).

ICD-9-CM CODES
783.6 Bulimia

EPIDEMIOLOGY AND DEMOGRAPHICS
INCIDENCE/PREVALENCE: Affects 1% to 4% of the general population, 17% of college students
PREDOMINANT SEX: Female:male ratio of 9:1
PREDOMINANT AGE: Adolescence to young adulthood; mean age of onset: 17 yr

PHYSICAL FINDINGS
- Parotid and salivary gland swelling
- Scars on the back of the hand and knuckles (Russell's sign) from rubbing against the upper incisors when inducing vomiting
- Eroded enamel, particularly on the lingual surface of the upper teeth; pyorrhea and other gum disorders possible
- Petechial hemorrhages of the cornea, soft palate, or face possibly noted after vomiting
- Loss of gag reflex, well-developed abdominal musculature
- Usually no emaciation; normal physical examination possible

ETIOLOGY
Etiology is unknown but likely multifactorial (sociocultural, psychologic, familial factors). Bulimia is much more common in Western societies where there is a strong cultural pressure to be slender.

DIAGNOSIS

DIFFERENTIAL DIAGNOSIS
- Schizophrenia
- GI disorders
- Neurologic disorders (seizures, Kleine-Levin syndrome, Klüver-Bucy syndrome)
- Brain neoplasms
- Psychogenic vomiting

WORKUP
- The following questions are useful to screen patients for bulimia:
  1. "Are you satisfied with your eating habits?"
  2. "Do you ever eat in secret?"
- Answering "no" to the first question and/or "yes" to the second question has 100% sensitivity and 90% specificity for bulimia.
- A diagnosis can also be made using the following DSM-IV diagnostic criteria for bulimia nervosa:
  1. Recurrent episodes of binge eating (rapid consumption of a large amount of food in a discrete period of time)
  2. A feeling of lack of control over eating behavior during the eating binges
  3. Self-induced vomiting, use of laxatives or diuretics, strict dieting or fasting, or rigorous exercise to prevent weight gain
  4. A minimum of two binge-eating episodes a week for at least 3 mo
  5. Persistent overconcern with body shape and weight

LABORATORY TESTS
- Electrolyte abnormalities secondary to vomiting (hypokalemia and metabolic alkalosis) or to diarrhea from laxative abuse (hypokalemia and hyperchloremic metabolic acidosis)
- Hyponatremia, hypocalcemia, hypomagnesemia (caused by laxative abuse)
- Elevated cortisol, decreased LH, decreased FSH

TREATMENT

NONPHARMACOLOGIC THERAPY
- Cognitive behavioral therapy to control abnormal behaviors
- Use of food diaries, nutritional counseling, and planning meals at least a day in advance is useful to counter abnormal eating behaviors
- Correction of electrolyte abnormalities

ACUTE GENERAL Rx
- Antidepressants (fluoxetine at higher doses [40 to 60 mg/day], or tricyclics [desipramine 100 to 250 mg/day] are useful in severely depressed patients and in those that fail to benefit from cognitive behavioral therapy.
- Prompt recognition and treatment of complications:
  1. Ipecac cardiotoxicity from laxative abuse
  2. Electrolyte abnormalities (see above)
  3. Esophagitis and Mallory-Weiss tears; esophageal rupture from repeated vomiting
  4. Aspiration pneumonia and pneumomediastinum
  5. Menstrual irregularities (including amenorrhea)
  6. GI abnormalities: acute gastric dilatation, pancreatitis, abdominal pain, constipation

CHRONIC Rx
- Psychotherapy continued for years and focused specifically on self-image and family and peer interactions is an integral part of successful recovery.
- Family therapy is also recommended, especially in younger patients.

DISPOSITION
Course is variable and marked by frequent recurrence of exacerbations.

REFERRAL
- In addition to the primary care physician, the multidisciplinary team should include a dietician, a psychiatrist, and a family therapist.
- Hospitalization should be considered for patients with severe electrolyte abnormalities or those with suicidal thoughts.

MISCELLANEOUS

COMMENTS
Bulimia has a close association with depression, bipolar disorder, obsessive-compulsive disorder, alcoholism, and substance abuse.

REFERENCES
American Psychiatric Association: *Diagnostic and statistical manual of mental disorders,* ed 4, Washington, DC, 1994, The Association.

Rome ES: Eating disorders in adolescents and young adults: what's a primary care clinician to do? *Cleveland Clin J Med* 63:387, 1996.

Author: **Fred F. Ferri, M.D.**

Bursitis (PTG)

BASIC INFORMATION

DEFINITION
Bursitis is an inflammation of a bursa and is usually aseptic. A *bursa* is a closed sac lined with a synovial-like membrane that sometimes contains fluid that is found or that develops in an area subject to pressure or friction.

SYNONYMS
Housemaid's knee (prepatellar bursitis)
Weaver's bottom (ischial gluteal bursitis)
Baker's cyst (gastrocnemius-semimembranosus bursa)

ICD-9-CM CODES
726.19 Subacromial bursitis
726.33 Olecranon bursitis
726.5 Ischiogluteal bursitis (hip)
726.5 Iliopsoas bursitis (hip)
726.61 Anserine bursitis
726.5 Trochanteric bursitis
726.65 Prepatellar bursitis
727.51 Baker's cyst
726.79 Retrocalcaneal bursitis

PHYSICAL FINDINGS
- Swelling, especially if bursa is superficial (olecranon, prepatellar)
- Local tenderness with pain on pressure against bursa
- Pain with joint movement
- Referred pain
- Palpable occasional fibrocartilaginous bodies (most common in olecranon and prepatellar bursae)

ETIOLOGY
- Acute trauma
- Repetitive trauma
- Sepsis

DIAGNOSIS

DIFFERENTIAL DIAGNOSIS
- Degenerative joint disease
- Tendinitis (sometimes occurs in conjunction with bursitis)
- Cellulitis (if bursitis is septic)
- Infectious arthritis

WORKUP
Aspiration with Gram stain and C & S

IMAGING STUDIES
- Plain radiography to rule out other potential or coexisting bone or joint problems
- MRI

TREATMENT

NONPHARMACOLOGIC THERAPY
- If chronic, elimination of cause of pressure or irritation
- Use of relief pads, avoidance of direct pressure
- Rest
- Elevation
- Ice for acute trauma

ACUTE GENERAL Rx
- Septic:
  1. Appropriate antibody coverage and drainage
  2. Aspiration of purulent fluid with a large-bore needle (if there is no rapid clinical response, incision and drainage are indicated)
- Nonseptic:
  1. Aspiration of blood from acute trauma
  2. Application of compression dressing

CHRONIC Rx
- Aspiration if excessive fluid volume present, followed by application of compression dressing to prevent fluid reaccumulation (repeat aspiration may be required)
- Steroid injection into bursa
- NSAIDs (see Table 7-29)

DISPOSITION
- Many bursal sacs "dry up" eventually.
- Nonsurgical treatment is effective in most cases.

REFERRAL
For orthopedic consultation to assist in treatment of sepsis or for excision of chronic enlarged bursa when indicated

MISCELLANEOUS

COMMENTS
- Injection of trochanteric bursa may require spinal needle in large patient.
- Sterile bursae should not be incised and drained because a chronic draining sinus tract may develop.
- Involvement of the iliopsoas bursa may cause groin pain, although the diagnosis is difficult to make because of the inaccessibility of the area to direct examination. (This also makes steroid injection impossible even if the diagnosis could be established.)

REFERENCES
Bluestein HG: In Stein J (ed): *Periarticular rheumatic complaints in internal medicine*, ed 4, St Louis, 1994, Mosby.
Smith DL et al: Septic and nonseptic olecranon bursitis, *Arch Intern Med* 149:1581, 1989.
Author: **Lonnie R. Mercier, M.D.**

Candidiasis (PTG)

BASIC INFORMATION

DEFINITION
Candidiasis is an inflammatory process involving the vulva and/or the vagina and is caused by superficial invasion of epithelial cells by *Candida* species.

SYNONYMS
Moniliasis
Thrush
Candidosis

ICD-9-CM CODES
112.1 Moniliasis
112.0 Thrush
112 Candidosis

EPIDEMIOLOGY AND DEMOGRAPHICS
- This is the second most common form of vaginitis in the U.S. It is estimated that up to 75% of women will have at least one episode of vulvovaginal candidiasis (VVC) during their childbearing years and about 45% will have a second attack. A small subpopulation of probably <5% of adult women has recurrent, often intractable episodes. *Candida* may be isolated in up to 20% of asymptomatic women of childbearing age.
- Factors that predispose to development of symptomatic VVC include pregnancy, antibiotic use, and diabetes. Antibiotic use disturbs normal vaginal flora and allows overgrowth of fungi; pregnancy and diabetes are associated with decrease in cell-mediated immunity.
- Factors associated with increased rates of asymptomatic vaginal colonization: pregnancy, high-estrogen oral contraceptives, uncontrolled diabetes mellitus, attendance at STD clinics.

PHYSICAL FINDINGS
Symptoms of VVC consist of:
- Vulvar pruritus with vaginal discharge that typically resembles cottage cheese
- Erythema and edema of labia and vulvar skin; possible discrete pustulopapular peripheral lesions (satellite lesions)
- Vagina may be erythematous with an adherent, whitish discharge
- Cervix may appear normal.
- Symptoms characteristically exacerbated in the week preceding menses with some relief after onset of menstrual flow.

ETIOLOGY
- *Candida* are dimorphic fungi (spores and mycelial forms).
- *C. albicans* is responsible for 85% to 90% of vaginal yeast infections.
- *C. glabrata*, *C. tropicalis* (nonalbicans species) also cause vaginitis and may be more resistant to conventional therapy.

DIAGNOSIS

DIFFERENTIAL DIAGNOSIS
- Bacterial vaginosis
- Trichomoniasis

WORKUP
- Discharge may vary from watery to homogeneously thick. May have complaints of vaginal soreness, dyspareunia, vulvar burning, and irritation. External dysuria may be present.
- Usually normal vaginal pH (<4.5).
- Budding yeast forms or mycelia will appear in as many as 80% of cases. Saline wet prep of vaginal secretions usually are normal; may be increased in inflammatory cells in severe cases.
- Whiff test negative (KOH).
- 10% KCL useful and more sensitive than wet mount for microscopic identification.
- Can make a presumptive diagnosis based on symptomatology in the absence of microscopy proven fungal elements if the pH and wet prep are normal. Fungal culture is recommended to confirm diagnosis.
- In chronic/recurrent, burning replaces itching as prominent symptom. Confirm diagnosis with direct microscopy and culture. Many may actually have chronic or atrophic dermatitis.

LABORATORY TESTS
If sending cultures, send on Nickerson's media or semiquantitative slide-stix cultures. There is no reliable serologic technique for diagnosis.

TREATMENT

ACUTE GENERAL Rx
TOPICAL BUTOCONAZOLE: 2% vaginal cream 5 g intravaginally for 3 days
TOPICAL CLOTRIMAZOLE:
  1% cream 5 g intravaginally for 7 to 14 days
  100-mg vaginal tablet for 7 days
  100-mg vaginal tablets, two tablets for 3 days
  500-mg vaginal tablet, single dose
TOPICAL MICONAZOLE:
  2% cream 5 g intravaginally for 7 days
  200-mg vaginal suppository for 3 days
  100-mg vaginal suppository for 7 days
TOPICAL TIOCONAZOLE: 6.5% ointment 5 g intravaginally, single dose
TOPICAL TERCONAZOLE:
  0.4% cream 5 g intravaginally for 7 days
  0.8% cream 5 g intravaginally for 3 days
  80-mg suppository for 3 days
ORAL FLUCONAZOLE: 150-mg single PO dose

CHRONIC Rx
Ketoconazole 400 mg PO qd or fluconazole 200 mg PO qd until symptoms resolve. Then maintenance on prophylactic doses of these agents for 6 mo. (ketoconazole 100 mg/day, fluconazole 150 mg weekly)

DISPOSITION
Usually relatively limited in duration and occurrence. If chronic or recurrent, may consider screening for diabetes, HIV or other immune deficiencies.

MISCELLANEOUS

COMMENTS
Azoles are more effective than nystatin. Symptoms usually take 2 to 3 days to resolve. Adjunctive treatment with weak topical steroid such as 1% hydrocortisone cream may help with relief of symptoms.

REFERENCES
Benenson AS (ed): *Control of communicable diseases in man*, ed 15, Washington, D.C., 1990, American Public Health Association.
Drugs for sexually transmitted diseases, *Med Lett Drugs Ther* 37(964): 117, 1995.
Reef et al: Treatment options for vulvovaginal candidiasis, *Clin Infect Dis* 20 (suppl 1):S80, 1995.
Woods GL: Update on laboratory diagnosis of sexually transmitted diseases, *Clin Lab Med* 15(3):665, 1995.
Author: **Eugene Louie-Ng, M.D.**

Carcinoid syndrome

BASIC INFORMATION

DEFINITION
Carcinoid syndrome is a symptom complex characterized by paroxysmal vasomotor disturbances, diarrhea, and bronchospasm. It is caused by the action of amines and peptides (serotonin, bradykinin, histamine) produced by tumors arising from enterochromaffin cells.

SYNONYMS
Flush syndrome
Argentaffinoma syndrome

ICD-9-CM CODES
259.2 Carcinoid syndrome

EPIDEMIOLOGY AND DEMOGRAPHICS
INCIDENCE: Carcinoid tumors are found incidentally in 0.5% to 0.75% of autopsies.

PHYSICAL FINDINGS
- Cutaneous flushing (75% to 90%)
    1. The patient usually has red-purple flushes starting in the face, then spreading to the neck and upper trunk.
    2. The flushing episodes last from a few minutes to hours (longer-lasting flushes may be associated with bronchial carcinoids).
    3. Flushing may be triggered by emotion, alcohol, or foods, or it may occur spontaneously.
    4. Dizziness, tachycardia, and hypotension may be associated with the cutaneous flushing.
- Diarrhea (>70%): often associated with abdominal bloating and audible peristaltic rushes
- Intermittent bronchospasm (25%): characterized by severe dyspnea and wheezing
- Facial telangiectasia

ETIOLOGY
- The carcinoid syndrome is caused by neoplasms originating in the endocrine argentaffin cells.
- Carcinoid tumors are principally found in the following organs: appendix (40%), small bowel (20%; 15% in the ileum), rectum (15%), bronchi (12%), esophagus, stomach, colon (10%), ovary, biliary tract, pancreas (3%).
- Carcinoid tumors do not usually produce the syndrome unless liver metastases are present or the primary tumor does not involve the GI tract.

DIAGNOSIS

DIFFERENTIAL DIAGNOSIS
The carcinoid syndrome must be distinguished from idiopathic flushing (IF); patients with IF more often are females, younger, and with a longer duration of symptoms; palpitations, syncope, and hypotension occur primarily in patients with IF.

LABORATORY TESTS
- The biochemical marker for carcinoid syndrome is increased 24-hr urinary 5-hydroxyindoleacetic acid (5-HIAA), a metabolite of serotonin (5-hydroxytryptamine).
- False elevations can be seen with ingestion of certain foods (bananas, pineapples, eggplant, avocados, walnuts) and certain medications (acetaminophen, caffeine, guaifenesin, reserpine); therefore patients should be on a restricted diet and should avoid these medications when the test is ordered.

IMAGING STUDIES
- Chest x-ray examination is useful to detect bronchial carcinoids.
- CT scan of abdomen or a liver and spleen radionuclide scan are useful to detect liver metastases (palpable in >50% of cases).
- Iodine-123 labeled somatostatin (123-ISS) can detect carcinoid endocrine tumors with somatostatin receptors.
- Scanning with radiolabeled vasoactive intestinal peptide (VIP) can visualize intestinal tumors and metastases that express receptors for VIP.

TREATMENT

NONPHARMACOLOGIC THERAPY
Avoidance of ethanol ingestion (may precipitate flushing)

ACUTE GENERAL Rx
- Surgical resection of the tumor can be curative if the tumor is localized or palliative and result in prolonged asymptomatic periods if metastases are present. Surgical manipulation of the tumor can, however, cause severe vasomotor abnormalities and bronchospasm (carcinoid crisis).
- Percutaneous embolization and ligation of the hepatic artery can decrease the bulk of the tumor in the liver and provide palliative treatment of tumors with hepatic metastases.
- Cytotoxic chemotherapy: combination chemotherapy with 5-fluorouracil and streptozotocin can be used in patients with unresectable or recurrent carcinoid tumors.
- Control of clinical manifestations:
    1. Diarrhea usually responds to diphenoxylate with atropine (Lomotil).
    2. Flushing can be controlled by the combination of H_1- and H_2-receptor antagonists (e.g., diphenhydramine 25 to 50 mg PO q6h and ranitidine 150 mg bid).
    3. Somatostatin analog (SMS 201-995) is effective for both flushing and diarrhea in most patients.
    4. Bronchospasm can be treated with aminophylline and/or albuterol.
- Nutritional support: supplemental niacin therapy may be useful to prevent pellagra, since the tumor uses dietary tryptophan for serotonin synthesis resulting in a nutritional deficiency in some patients.

CHRONIC Rx
- Subcutaneous somatostatin analog has been used successfully for long-term control of symptoms in patients with unresectable neoplasms.
- Echocardiography and monitoring for right-sided CHF is recommended for patients with unresectable disease because endocardial fibrosis, involving predominantly the endocardium, chordae, and valves of the right side of the heart, can occur and result in right-sided CHF.

DISPOSITION
- Prognosis varies with the stage and location of the tumor.
- Carcinoids of the appendix and rectum have a low malignancy potential and rarely produce the clinical syndrome; metastases are also uncommon if the size of the primary lesion is <2 cm in diameter.

MISCELLANEOUS

REFERENCES
Virgolini I et al: Vasoactive intestinal peptide-receptor imaging for the localization of intestinal adenocarcinomas and endocrine tumors, N Engl J Med 331:1116, 1994.
Author: **Fred F. Ferri, M.D.**

Cardiac tamponade

BASIC INFORMATION

DEFINITION
Cardiac tamponade is compression of the heart by fluid within the pericardial sac that impairs dilation and filling of the ventricles during diastole.

ICD-9-CM CODES
423.9 Unspecified diseases of the pericardium

PHYSICAL FINDINGS
Acute cardiac tamponade (e.g., penetrating wounds, iatrogenic, aortic dissection, etc.)
1. Beck's triad
   a. Decrease in systemic arterial pressure
   b. Elevated central venous pressure
   c. Small, quiet heart

Chronic accumulating pericardial effusion leading to tamponade
1. Pericardial friction rub may be present
2. Tachypnea and tachycardia
3. Raised jugular venous distention (prominent x descent with absent y descent)
4. Pulsus paradoxus (>10 mm Hg fall in systolic blood pressure during inspiration)
5. Soft heart sounds

ETIOLOGY
Acute
1. Penetrating trauma
2. Aortic dissection
3. Myocardial rupture after treatment of MI with thrombolytics and/or heparin
4. Iatrogenic (central line and pacemaker insertions, post-coronary bypass surgery)

Chronic accumulating pericardial effusion leading to tamponade
1. Malignancy (e.g., lung, breast, lymphoma)
2. Viral pericarditis (e.g., coxsackie, HIV)
3. Uremia
4. Bacterial, fungal, and tuberculosis
5. Myxedema (rare)
6. Collagen-vascular disease (e.g., SLE, RA, scleroderma)
7. Radiation

DIAGNOSIS

DIFFERENTIAL DIAGNOSIS
COPD, constrictive pericardial disease, restrictive cardiomyopathy, right ventricular infarction, and pulmonary embolism can all lead to elevated jugular venous pressure, decrease systemic pressure, and pulsus paradoxus.

WORKUP
Cardiac tamponade is a clinical diagnosis made at the bedside by noting the above mentioned physical findings. The echocardiogram will support the clinical diagnosis. Thereafter, one must pursue the etiology with specific laboratory work (see below).

LABORATORY TESTS
- Electrolytes, BUN, Cr, ESR, thyroid function tests, ANA, RF, PPD, blood cultures, viral titers, and pericardial fluid analysis and cultures will all help in identifying or excluding a possible etiology of the effusion leading to tamponade.
- 12-lead ECG findings are suggestive but not diagnostic.
  1. Low voltage (<5 mm QRS amplitude in the limb leads and <10 mm in the chest leads
  2. PR depression
  3. Electrical alternans (alternating amplitude of the QRS complex in any or all leads)

IMAGING STUDIES
- The chest x-ray examination is not very specific. The heart size can be normal in acute tamponade or massive (water bottle configuration) in slow-forming effusions.
- The echocardiogram can detect effusions as small as 20 ml and can strongly suggest tamponade physiology (collapse of the right atrium and right ventricle during diastole).
- Right-sided cardiac catheterization and intrapericardial pressure measurements confirm the diagnosis.
- Typical findings are diastolic equalization of pressures (pulmonary artery pressure = right ventricular diastolic pressure = right atrial pressure = intrapericardial pressure).

TREATMENT

NONPHARMACOLOGIC THERAPY
Cardiac tamponade should be treated urgently. Avoid drugs that will reduce preload and exacerbate tamponade (e.g., nitrates, diuretics).

ACUTE GENERAL Rx
- The acute forms of tamponade as mentioned earlier (see "Etiology") usually require emergency cardiothoracic surgery.
- Provide hemodynamic support with volume expansion and vasopressors along with emergency subxiphoid pericardiocentesis in the suspected tamponade code situation (e.g., electromechanical dissociation, patient in shock).

CHRONIC Rx
- Depends on etiology
- Semiacute treatment includes:
  1. Right-side heart catheter with echocardiographic guided pericardiocentesis (can be done by cardiology). The catheter can be left in place for 48 hr to allow for continued drainage until a more definitive procedure is performed or the etiology is resolved (e.g., dialysis for uremia, levothyroxine for myxedema).
- Other surgical drainage procedures include:
  1. Subxiphoid pericardial drainage
  2. Limited pericardiectomy draining the pericardial fluid into the left hemithorax
  3. Complete pericardiectomy

DISPOSITION
The prognosis of cardiac tamponade depends on the underlying cause.

REFERRAL
- Cardiology consultation is made if the clinical suspicion of tamponade exists.
- Cardiothoracic surgeon consultation is made when tamponade is confirmed.

MISCELLANEOUS

COMMENTS
As little as 200 ml of fluid can lead to acute cardiac tamponade, whereas in the chronic formation, the pericardial sac can hold up to 5 L of fluid before tamponade occurs.

REFERENCES
Ameli S: Cardiac tamponade pathophysiology, diagnosis, and management, *Cardiol Clin* 9(4):665, 1991.

Braunwald E: Heart disease: a textbook of cardiovascular medicine, ed 5, Philadelphia, 1997, WB Saunders.

Hancock EW: Cardiac tamponade, *Heart Dis Stroke* 155, 1994.

Author: **Peter Petropoulos, M.D.**

Cardiomyopathy, dilated (PTG)

BASIC INFORMATION

DEFINITION
Cardiomyopathies are a group of diseases primarily involving the myocardium and characterized by myocardial dysfunction that is not the result of hypertension, coronary atherosclerosis, valvular dysfunction, or pericardial abnormalities. In dilated cardiomyopathy, the heart is enlarged, and both ventricles are dilated.

SYNONYMS
Congestive cardiomyopathy

ICD-9-CM CODES
425.4 Other primary cardiomyopathies

EPIDEMIOLOGY AND DEMOGRAPHICS
- The prevalence of dilated cardiomyopathy in the general adult population is approximately 1%.
- Incidence increases with age and approaches 10% at age 80 yr.

PHYSICAL FINDINGS
- Increased jugular venous pressure
- Small pulse pressure
- Pulmonary rales, hepatomegaly, peripheral edema
- S_3, S_4
- Mitral regurgitation, tricuspid regurgitation (less common)

ETIOLOGY
- Idiopathic
- Alcoholism
- Collagen-vascular disease (SLE, RA, polyarteritis, dermatomyositis)
- Postmyocarditis
- Peripartum (last trimester of pregnancy or 6 mo postpartum)
- Heredofamilial neuromuscular disease
- Toxins (cobalt, lead, phosphorus, carbon monoxide, mercury, doxorubicin, daunorubicin)
- Nutritional (beri-beri, selenium deficiency, carnitine deficiency, thiamine deficiency)
- Cocaine, heroin, organic solvents ("glue sniffer's heart")
- Irradiation
- Acromegaly, osteogenesis imperfecta, myxedema, thyrotoxicosis, diabetes
- Hypocalcemia
- Antiretroviral agents (zidovudine, didanosine, zalcitabine)
- Phenothiazines
- Infections (viral, rickettsial, mycobacterial, toxoplasmosis, trichinosis, Chagas' disease)
- Hematologic (e.g., sickle cell anemia)

DIAGNOSIS

DIFFERENTIAL DIAGNOSIS
- Frank pulmonary disease
- Valvular dysfunction
- Pericardial abnormalities
- Coronary atherosclerosis
- Psychogenic dyspnea

WORKUP
- Chest x-ray examination, ECG, echocardiogram
- Medical history with emphasis on the following symptoms:
  1. Dyspnea on exertion, orthopnea, PND
  2. Palpitations
  3. Systemic and pulmonary embolism

IMAGING STUDIES
CHEST X-RAY EXAMINATION:
- Massive cardiac enlargement
- Interstitial pulmonary edema

ECG:
- Left ventricular hypertrophy with ST-T wave changes
- RBBB or LBBB
- Arrhythmias (atrial fibrillation, PVC, PAC, ventricular tachycardia)

ECHOCARDIOGRAM:
- Low ejection fraction with global akinesia

TREATMENT

NONPHARMACOLOGIC THERAPY
- Bed rest when CHF is present
- Treatment of underlying disease (SLE, alcoholism)

ACUTE GENERAL Rx
- Treat CHF (cause of death in 70% of patients) with sodium restriction, diuretics, ACE inhibitors and digitalis.
- Vasodilators (combined with nitrates and ACE inhibitors) are effective agents in dilated cardiomyopathy.
- Prevent thromboembolism with oral anticoagulants.
- Low-dose β-blockade with metoprolol may improve ventricular function by interrupting the cycle of reflex sympathetic activity and controlling tachycardia.
- Diltiazem has also been reported to have a long-term beneficial effect in idiopathic dilated cardiomyopathy.
- Preliminary studies have revealed that growth hormone administered for 3 mo to patients with idiopathic dilated cardiomyopathy increased myocardial mass and reduced the size of the left ventricular chamber, resulting in improvement in hemodynamics and clinical status.
- Use antiarrhythmic treatment as appropriate.

DISPOSITION
Annual mortality is 20% in patients with moderate heart failure, and it exceeds 50% in patients with severe heart failure.

REFERRAL
Consider heart transplant for young patients (<60 yr old) who are no longer responsive to medical therapy.

MISCELLANEOUS

COMMENTS
Patients should be encouraged to restrict alcohol and sodium intake.

REFERENCES
Dec WG, Fuster V: Idiopathic dilated cardiomyopathy, *New Engl J Med* 331:1564, 1994.

Fazio S et al: A preliminary study of growth hormone in the treatment of dilated cardiomyopathy, *New Engl J Med* 334:809, 1996.

Kasper EK et al: The causes of dilated cardiomyopathy: a clinical pathologic review of 673 cases, *J Am Coll Cardiol* 23:568, 1994.

Author: **Fred F. Ferri, M.D.**

Cardiomyopathy, hypertrophic (PTG)

BASIC INFORMATION

DEFINITION
Cardiomyopathies are a group of diseases primarily involving the myocardium and characterized by myocardial dysfunction that is not the result of hypertension, coronary atherosclerosis, valvular dysfunction, or pericardial abnormalities. In hypertrophic cardiomyopathy there is marked hypertrophy of the myocardium and disproportionally greater thickening of the intraventricular septum than that of the free wall of the left ventricle (asymmetric septal hypertrophy [ASH]).

SYNONYMS
Idiopathic hypertrophic subaortic stenosis (IHSS)
Hypertrophic obstructive cardiomyopathy (HOCM)
ASH

ICD-9-CM CODES
425.4 Cardiomyopathy, hypertrophic nonobstructive
425.1 Cardiomyopathy, hypertrophic obstructive
746.84 Cardiomyopathy, hypertrophic congenital

EPIDEMIOLOGY AND DEMOGRAPHICS
The disease occurs in two major forms:
1. A familial form, usually diagnosed in young patients and gene mapped to chromosome 14q
2. A sporadic form, usually found in elderly patients

PHYSICAL FINDINGS
- Harsh, systolic, diamond-shaped murmur at the left sternal border or apex that increases with Valsalva maneuver and decreases with squatting
- Paradoxic splitting of S_2 (if left ventricular obstruction is present)
- S_4
- Double or triple apical impulse
- Increased obstruction
  1. Drugs: digitalis, β-adrenergic stimulators (isoproterenol, dopamine, epinephrine), nitroglycerin, vasodilators, diuretics, alcohol
  2. Hypovolemia
  3. Tachycardia
  4. Valsalva maneuver
  5. Standing position
- Decreased obstruction
  1. Drugs: β-adrenergic blockers, calcium channel blockers, disopyramide, α-adrenergic stimulators
  2. Volume expansion
  3. Bradycardia
  4. Hand grip exercise
  5. Squatting position

ETIOLOGY
- Autosomal dominant trait with variable penetrance
- Sporadic occurrence

DIAGNOSIS

DIFFERENTIAL DIAGNOSIS
- Coronary atherosclerosis
- Valvular dysfunction
- Pericardial abnormalities
- Chronic pulmonary disease
- Psychogenic dyspnea

WORKUP
- Chest x-ray examination, ECG, echocardiography
- Medical history with emphasis in the following manifestations:
  1. Dyspnea
  2. Syncope (usually seen with exercise)
  3. Angina (decreased angina in recumbent position)
  4. Palpitations
- 24-hr Holter monitor to screen for potential lethal arrhythmias (principal cause of syncope or sudden death in obstructive cardiomyopathy)

IMAGING STUDIES
- Chest x-ray examination: normal or cardiomegaly
- ECG: left ventricular hypertrophy, abnormal Q waves in anterolateral and inferior leads
- Echocardiography: ventricular hypertrophy, ratio of septum thickness to left ventricular wall thickness >1.3:1, increased ejection fraction

TREATMENT

NONPHARMACOLOGIC THERAPY
Advise avoidance of alcohol; alcohol use (even in small amounts) results in increased obstruction of the left ventricular outflow tract.

ACUTE GENERAL Rx
- Propranolol 160 to 240 mg/day. The beneficial effects of β-blockers on symptoms (principally dyspnea and chest pain) and exercise tolerance appear to be largely a result of a decrease in the heart rate with consequent prolongation of diastole and increased passive ventricular filling. By reducing the inotropic response, β-blockers may also lessen myocardial oxygen demand and decrease the outflow gradient during exercise, when sympathetic tone is increased.
- Verapamil also decreases left ventricular outflow obstruction by improving filling and probably reducing myocardial ischemia.
- IV saline infusion in addition to propranolol or verapamil is indicated in patients with CHF.
- Disopyramide is a useful antiarrhythmic.
- Use antibiotic prophylaxis for surgical procedures (see Boxes A-1, A-2, and A-3 and Tables A-11 and A-12 in Appendix).
- Avoid use of digitalis, diuretics, nitrates, and vasodilators.
- Encouraging results have been reported on the use of pacing for hemodynamic and symptomatic benefit in patients with drug-resistant hypertrophic obstructive cardiomyopathy.
- Amiodarone is useful for the prevention of recurrences of atrial fibrillation.

DISPOSITION
Patients with hypertrophic cardiomyopathy are at increased risk of sudden death, especially if there is onset of symptoms during childhood. Adult patients can be considered low risk if they have no symptoms or mild symptoms and also if they have none of the following:
- A family history of premature death caused by hypertrophic cardiomyopathy
- Nonsustained ventricular tachycardia during Holter monitoring
- A marked outflow tract gradient
- Substantial hypertrophy (>20 mm)
- Marked left atrial enlargement
- Abnormal blood pressure response during exercise

REFERRAL
Surgical treatment (myotomy-myectomy) is reserved for patients who have both a large outflow gradient (≥50 mm Hg) and severe symptoms of heart failure that are unresponsive to medical therapy. The risk of sudden death from arrhythmias is not altered by surgery.

MISCELLANEOUS

COMMENTS
Screening of family members with echocardiography is indicated.

REFERENCES
Glickson M et al: Expanding indications for permanent pacemakers, *Ann Intern Med* 123:443, 1995.
Spirito P et al: The management of hypertrophic cardiomyopathy, *N Engl J Med* 336:775, 1997.

Author: **Fred F. Ferri, M.D.**

BASIC INFORMATION

DEFINITION
Cardiomyopathies are a group of diseases primarily involving the myocardium and characterized by myocardial dysfunction that is not the result of hypertension, coronary atherosclerosis, valvular dysfunction, or pericardial abnormalities. Restrictive cardiomyopathies are characterized by decreased ventricular compliance, usually secondary to infiltration of the myocardium.

ICD-9-CM CODES
425.4 Other primary cardiomyopathies

EPIDEMIOLOGY AND DEMOGRAPHICS
Relatively uncommon cardiomyopathy that is most frequently caused by amyloidosis, myocardial fibrosis (after open heart surgery), and radiation

PHYSICAL FINDINGS
- Edema, ascites, hepatomegaly, distended neck veins
- Fatigue, weakness (secondary to low output)
- Kussmaul's sign: may be present
- Regurgitant murmurs
- Possible prominent apical impulse

ETIOLOGY
- Infiltrative and storage disorders (glycogen storage disease, amyloidosis, sarcoidosis, hemochromatosis)
- Scleroderma
- Radiation
- Endocardial fibroelastosis
- Endomyocardial fibrosis
- Idiopathic
- Toxic effects of anthracycline
- Carcinoid heart disease, metastatic cancers
- Diabetic cardiomyopathy
- Eosinophilic cardiomyopathy (Löffler's endocarditis)

DIAGNOSIS

DIFFERENTIAL DIAGNOSIS
- Coronary atherosclerosis
- Valvular dysfunction
- Pericardial abnormalities
- Chronic lung disease
- Psychogenic dyspnea

WORKUP
- Chest x-ray examination, ECG, echocardiogram
- Cardiac catheterization, MRI (selected cases)

IMAGING STUDIES
- Chest x-ray examination:
  1. Moderate cardiomegaly
  2. Possible evidence of CHF (pulmonary vascular congestion, pleural effusion)
- ECG:
  1. Low voltage with ST-T wave changes
  2. Possible frequent arrhythmias, left axis deviation, and atrial fibrillation
- Echocardiogram: increased wall thickness and thickened cardiac valves (especially in patients with amyloidosis)
- Cardiac catheterization to distinguish restrictive cardiomyopathy from constrictive pericarditis
  1. Constrictive pericarditis: usually involves both ventricles and produces a plateau of elevated filling pressures
  2. Restrictive cardiomyopathy: impairs the left ventricle more than the right (PCWP > RAP, PASP > 50 mm Hg)
- MRI to distinguish restrictive cardiomyopathy from constrictive pericarditis (thickness of the pericardium >5 mm in the latter)

TREATMENT

NONPHARMACOLOGIC THERAPY
Control CHF by restricting salt.

ACUTE GENERAL Rx
- Cardiomyopathy caused by hemochromatosis may respond to repeated phlebotomies to decrease iron deposition in the heart.
- Sarcoidosis may respond to corticosteroid therapy.
- Corticosteroid and cytotoxic drugs may improve survival in patients with eosinophilic cardiomyopathy.
- There is no effective therapy for other causes of restrictive cardiomyopathy.

CHRONIC Rx
Death usually results from CHF or arrhythmias; therefore therapy should be aimed at controlling CHF by restricting salt, administering diuretics, and treating potentially fatal arrhythmias.

DISPOSITION
Prognosis varies with the etiology of the cardiomyopathy.

REFERRAL
Cardiac transplantation can be considered in patients with refractory symptoms and idiopathic or familial restrictive cardiomyopathies.

MISCELLANEOUS

REFERENCES
Katritisi SD et al: Primary restrictive cardiomyopathy: clinical and pathologic characteristics, *J Am Coll Cardiol* 18:123, 1991.

Author: **Fred F. Ferri, M.D.**

Carotid sinus syndrome (PTG)

BASIC INFORMATION

DEFINITION
Dizziness, presyncope, or syncope in a patient with carotid sinus hypersensitivity is defined as *carotid sinus syndrome*. Carotid sinus hypersensitivity is the exaggerated response to carotid stimulation resulting in bradycardia, hypotension, or both.

SYNONYMS
Carotid sinus syncope
CSS

ICD-9-CM CODES
337.0 Idiopathic peripheral autonomic neuropathy
Carotid sinus syncope or syndrome

EPIDEMIOLOGY AND DEMOGRAPHICS
- The incidence of carotid sinus hypersensitivity is 10% in the adult population.
- The incidence increases with age.
- Men are affected more often than women (2:1).
- Carotid sinus syndrome is rarely found before the age of 50 yr.

PHYSICAL FINDINGS
Properly performed carotid sinus massage at the bedside is diagnostic. This maneuver can elicit three types of responses in the appropriate patient (see "Diagnosis").
1. Carotid sinus massage (CSM) should be done in the supine position while monitoring the patient's blood pressure by cuff and heart rate by ECG.
2. CSM should not be performed on patients with carotid bruits or recent TIA/CVA.
3. CSM should only be performed on one artery at a time.
4. CSM should be applied for approximately 5 sec.

ETIOLOGY
- Idiopathic
- Head and neck tumors (e.g., thyroid)
- Significant lymphadenopathy
- Carotid body tumors
- Prior neck surgery

DIAGNOSIS

- The diagnosis of CSS is made when carotid sinus hypersensitivity is diagnosed by CSM and no other cause of syncope is identified.
- CSM can elicit three types of responses that are diagnostic of carotid sinus hypersensitivity:
  1. Cardioinhibitory type: CSM producing asystole for at least 3 sec
  2. Vasodepressor type: CSM producing a decrease in systolic blood pressure of 50 mm Hg or 30 mm Hg in the presence of neurologic symptoms
  3. Mixed type: CSM producing both types of responses
- It is not absolutely necessary to produce symptoms with CSM to diagnose CSS.

DIFFERENTIAL DIAGNOSIS
All causes of syncope, e.g., cardiac tachyarrhythmias and bradyarrhythmias, cardiac valvular disease and obstructive cardiomyopathy, cerebrovascular events, seizures, drug-induced, autonomic dysfunction, orthostasis/hypovolemia, cough, micturition, hypoxemia, and hypoglycemia

WORKUP
The workup must exclude other causes of syncope as guided by the history and the physical examination. Blood tests, cardiac noninvasive studies (Holter, echocardiograms, ECG, tilt test, treadmill testing), cardiac invasive testing (electrophysiologic studies), EEG, and CT scan should be ordered in the appropriate clinical setting.

TREATMENT

NONPHARMACOLOGIC THERAPY
Avoidance of triggering factors such as straining or applying neck pressure from tight collars, shaving, or rapid head turning.

ACUTE GENERAL Rx
Treatment will vary according to the type of carotid hypersensitivity response (e.g., cardioinhibitory, vasopressor or mixed) and symptoms present (see "Chronic Rx"). Acute treatment is usually not needed, since most patients at presentation will be hemodynamically stable but present with either a fall resulting in an injury (e.g., hip fracture, laceration) or a complaint of true syncope with no injury.

CHRONIC Rx
For asymptomatic carotid sinus hypersensitivity of either the cardioinhibitory or vasodepressor type, it is generally agreed that pacemaker implantation is not necessary.
For patients with CSS with a cardioinhibitory response to CSM:
- Dual-chamber permanent pacemaker is indicated.
- Controversy exists as to whether to implant the pacemaker after the first syncopal episode or after a recurrent episode.

For patients with CSS with a vasodepressor response to CSM:
- Measures to maintain systolic blood pressure are tried:
  1. Sympathomimetics (Ephedrine has been tried with success but has significant side effects, e.g., palpitations, tremors.)
  2. Fludrocortisone with its mineralocorticoid effect also has been tried with limited success.
  3. Dual-chamber pacemaker is *not* indicated in the patient with pure vasodepressor response.
  4. Elastic knee-high or thigh-high stockings help to maintain systolic blood pressure.
  5. Carotid sinus denervation is reserved for those patients refractory to the above mentioned treatment.

For patients with CSS with a mixed response to CSM:
- Dual-chamber permanent pacemaker and atropine can effectively treat the bradycardic response but have no major effect on the hypotensive response. The vasodepressor response should be treated as mentioned above.

DISPOSITION
CSS occurs in the elderly population and presents with falls or syncope often resulting in injury. Up to 50% of the patients who present with symptoms will have recurrent symptoms. This is reduced in the group of patients where pacemaker is indicated. There is no difference in survival in this group of patients when compared with the general population.

REFERRAL
Cardiology referral is indicated if a pacemaker is considered.

MISCELLANEOUS

COMMENTS
The most common type of response to CSM in this population is cardioinhibitory response followed by mixed and vasodepressor responses.

REFERENCES
Braunwald E: *Heart disease: a textbook of cardiovascular medicine*, ed 5, Philadelphia, 1997, WB Saunders.
McIntosh SJ: Clinical characteristics of vasodepressor, cardioinhibitory, and mixed carotid sinus syndrome in the elderly, *Am J Med* 95(2):203, 1993.
McIntosh SJ: Carotid sinus syndrome in the elderly, *J Royal Soc Med* Vol 87: 798, 1994.

Author: **Peter Petropoulos, M.D.**

Carpal tunnel syndrome (PTG)

BASIC INFORMATION

DEFINITION
Carpal tunnel syndrome is a common entrapment neuropathy involving the median nerve at the wrist.

ICD-9-CM CODES
354.0 Carpal tunnel syndrome

EPIDEMIOLOGY AND DEMOGRAPHICS
PREVALENT AGE: 30 to 60 yr (bilateral up to 50%)
PREVALENT SEX: Females are affected two to five times as often as males

PHYSICAL FINDINGS
- Nocturnal pain
- Occasional median nerve sensory impairment (often only index and long fingers)
- Positive Tinel's sign at wrist (tapping over the median nerve on the flexor surface of the wrist produces a tingling sensation radiating from the wrist to the hand)
- Positive Phalen's test (reproduction of symptoms after 1 min of gentle, unforced wrist flexion)
- Carpal compression test: Pressure with the examiner's thumb over the patient's carpal tunnel for 30 sec elicits symptoms
- Thenar atrophy in long-standing cases

ETIOLOGY
- Idiopathic in most cases
- Space-occupying lesions in carpal tunnel (tenosynovitis, ganglia, aberrant muscles)
- Often associated with hypothyroidism, hormonal changes of pregnancy
- Job-related mechanical overuse may be a risk factor
- Traumatic injuries to wrist

DIAGNOSIS

DIFFERENTIAL DIAGNOSIS
- Cervical radiculopathy
- Chronic tendinitis
- Vascular occlusion
- Reflex sympathetic dystrophy
- Osteoarthritis
- Other arthritides
- Other entrapment neuropathies

IMAGING STUDIES
Routine roentgenograms may be helpful in establishing cause or ruling out other conditions.

ELECTRODIAGNOSTIC STUDIES
Nerve conduction velocity tests and electromyography are useful in establishing the diagnosis and ruling out other syndromes.

TREATMENT

ACUTE GENERAL Rx
- Elimination of repetitive trauma
- Occupational splints or braces
- NSAIDs (see Table 7-29)
- Injection of carpal canal (avoiding median nerve)

DISPOSITION
Prognosis is variable. Some cases resolve spontaneously. Relief from local injection appears transient and symptoms recur in the majority of cases following injection.

REFERRAL
Surgical referral in cases of failed medical management

MISCELLANEOUS

REFERENCES
Kuschner et al: Tinel's sign and Phalen's test in carpal tunnel syndrome, *Orthopedics* 15:1297, 1992.
Slater RR, Bynum DK: Diagnosis and treatment of carpal tunnel syndrome, *Orthop Review* 22:1095, 1993.
Author: **Lonnie R. Mercier, M.D.**

Cataracts (PTG)

BASIC INFORMATION

DEFINITION
Cataracts are the clouding and opacification of the crystalline lens of the eye. The opacity may occur in the cortex, the nucleus of the lens, or the posterior ubscapular region, but it is usually in a combination of areas.

SYNONYMS
Congenital cataracts (e.g., from rubella)
Metabolic cataracts (e.g., caused by diabetes)
Collagen-vascular disease cataracts (caused by lupus)
Hereditary cataracts
Age-related senile cataracts
Traumatic cataracts
Toxic or drug-induced cataracts (e.g., caused by steroids)

ICD-9-CM CODES
366 Cataract

EPIDEMIOLOGY AND DEMOGRAPHICS
INCIDENCE (IN U.S.): Highest cause of treatable blindness; cataract removal most frequent surgical procedure in patients >>65 yr old (1,300,000 operations/yr, with an annual cost of approximately $3 billion).
PREDOMINANT AGE: Elderly; some stage of cataract development is present in >50% of persons 65 to 74 yr old and 65% of those >75 yr old.
PEAK INCIDENCE:
- In early life: congenital and hereditary causes predominant
- In older age group: senile cataracts (after 40 yr of age)

GENETICS: Hereditary with such syndromes as galactosemia, homocystinuria, diabetes

PHYSICAL FINDINGS
Cloudiness and opacification of the crystalline lens of the eye

ETIOLOGY
- Heredity
- Trauma
- Toxins
- Age-related
- Drug-related
- Congenital
- Inflammatory

DIAGNOSIS

DIFFERENTIAL DIAGNOSIS
- Corneal lesions
- Retinal lesions

WORKUP
Complete eye examination, including slit lamp examination, funduscopic examination, and brightness acuity testing

LABORATORY TESTS
- Rarely, urinary amino acid screening and CNS imaging studies
- Fasting glucose

TREATMENT

NONPHARMACOLOGIC THERAPY
- Wait until vision is severely compromised before doing surgery.
- Surgery is indicated when corrected visual acuity in the affected eye is >20/50 in the absence of other ocular disease; however, surgery may be justified when visual acuity is 20/40 or better in specific situations (especially disabling glare, monocular diplopia).

ACUTE GENERAL Rx
None necessary

CHRONIC Rx
- Change glasses as cataracts develop.
- Myopia is common, and glasses can be adjusted until surgery is contemplated.

DISPOSITION
Refer if sight compromised.

REFERRAL
Refer to ophthalmologist for extraction when vision is compromised (see "Nonpharmacologic Treatment").

MISCELLANEOUS

COMMENTS
Success rate with surgery is 95% to 98%.

REFERENCES
Hockwin O: Cataract classification, *Doc Ophthalmol* 88:263, 1995.
Paton D, Craig JA: Management of cataracts, *Clin Symp* 42:2, 1990.
Author: **Melvyn Koby, M.D.**

Cat-scratch disease (PTG)

BASIC INFORMATION

DEFINITION
Cat-scratch disease (CSD) is a syndrome consisting of gradually enlarging regional lymphadenopathy occurring after contact with a feline. Atypical presentations are characterized by a variety of neurologic manifestations as well as granulomatous involvement of the eye, liver, spleen, and bone. The disease is usually self-limiting, and recovery is complete; however, patients with atypical presentations, especially if immunocompromized, may suffer significant morbidity and mortality.

SYNONYMS
Cat-scratch fever
Benign inoculation lymphoreticulosis
Nonbacterial regional lymphadenitis

ICD-9-CM CODES
078.3 Cat-scratch disease

EPIDEMIOLOGY AND DEMOGRAPHICS
PREVALENCE: Unknown
INCIDENCE (IN U.S.):
- Unknown
- Majority of reported cases in children

PEAK INCIDENCE: August through January
GENETICS: Unknown

PHYSICAL FINDINGS
- Classic, most common finding: regional lymphadenopathy occurring within 2 wk of a scratch or contact with felines
- Tender, swollen lymph nodes most commonly found in the head and neck, followed by the axilla, the epitrochlear, inguinal, and femoral areas
- Erythematous overlying skin, showing signs of suppuration from involved lymph nodes
- On careful examination: evidence of cutaneous inoculation in the form of a nonpruritic, slightly tender, pustule or papule
- Fever in most patients
- Malaise and headache in fewer than a third of patients
- Atypical presentations in fewer than 15% of cases
  1. Usually in association with lymphadenopathy and low-grade or frank fever (>101° F, >38.3° C)
  2. Include granulomatous involvement of the conjunctiva (Parinaud's ocularglandular syndrome) and focal masses in the liver, spleen, and mesenteric nodes
- CNS involvement: encephalopathy, encephalitis, transverse myelitis, seizure activity, and coma
- Possible osteomyelitis in children

ETIOLOGY
- Major cause: *Bartonella (Rochalimaea) henselae;* another recently reclassified gram-negative bacteria, *Afipia felis,* also implicated
- Mode of transmission: presumably by direct inoculation through the scratch, bite, or lick of a cat, especially a kitten
- Limited evidence in support of an arthropod (flea) as an alternate vector of infection
- Rarely, associated with dogs, monkeys, and inanimate objects with which a feline has been in recent contact
- Approximately 2 wk after introduction of the bacteria into the host, regional lymphatic tissues displaying granulomatous infiltration associated with gradual hypertrophy
- Possible dissemination to distant sites (e.g., liver, spleen, and bone), usually characterized by focal masses or discrete parenchymal lesions

DIAGNOSIS

DIFFERENTIAL DIAGNOSIS
Granulomas of this syndrome must be differentiated from those associated with tularemia, tuberculosis, sarcoidosis, sporotrichosis, toxoplasmosis, lymphogranuloma venerum, fungal diseases, and benign and malignant tumors.

WORKUP
Diagnosis should be considered in patients who present with a predominant complaint of gradually enlarging regional (focal) lymphadenopathy, often with fever and a recent history of having contact with a cat.

LABORATORY TESTS
- Three of four of the following criteria are required:
  1. History of animal contact in the presence of a scratch, dermal, or eye lesion
  2. Culture of lymphatic aspirate that is negative for other causes
  3. Positive CSD skin test
  4. Biopsied lymph node histology consistent with CSD

Cat-scratch disease (PTG)

- Enhanced culture techniques and serologies will augment establishment of the diagnosis.
- Histopathologically, Warthin-Starry silver stain has been used to identify the bacillus.
- Routine laboratory findings:
  1. Mild leukocytosis or leucopenia
  2. Infrequent eosinophilia
  3. Elevated ESR
- Abnormalities of bilirubin excretion and elevated hepatic transaminases are usually secondary to hepatic obstruction by granuloma, mass, or lymph node
- In patients with neurologic manifestations, lumbar puncture usually reveals normal CSF, although there may be a mild pleocytosis and modest elevation in protein.

TREATMENT

NONPHARMALOGICAL THERAPY
- Warm compresses to the affected nodes
- In cases of encephalitis or coma: supportive care

ACUTE GENERAL Rx
- There is no consensus over therapy, especially as the disease is self-limited in a majority of cases.
- It would be prudent to treat severely ill patients, especially if immunocompromised, with antibiotic therapy, since these patients tend to suffer dissemination of infection and increased morbidity.
- *Bartonella* is usually sensitive to aminoglycosides, tetracycline, erythromycin, and the quinolones.
- When the isolate is proven by culture, the patient should receive antibiotic therapy as directed by the obtained sensitivities.
- Antipyretics and NSAIDs may also be used.

DISPOSITION
Overall prognosis is good.

REFERRAL
- To an appropriate subspecialist to evaluate specific lesions
- For diagnostic aspiration or excision in presence of regional lymphadenopathy, bone lesions, and mesenteric lymph nodes and organs
- To ophthalmologist for ocular granulomas
  1. Usually diagnosed clinically
  2. Rarely require excision

MISCELLANEOUS

COMMENTS
- A typical presentation of this syndrome may be as fever of unknown origin.
- Hepatic and splenic granulomas, coronary valve infections may offer few physical clues to diagnosis, emphasizing the need for a complete history.
- Feline to feline transmission of the bacteria is possible via an arthropod (flea) vector (demonstrated in limited experimental data).
- Further study is needed for complete elucidation of human acquisition of infection, by animal, arthropod or both.
- Chronically immunocompromised patients considering the acquisition of a young feline should be made aware of the possible risk of infection.
- No signs of illness may be apparent in bacteremic kittens.

REFERENCES
Case records of the Massachusetts General Hospital: weekly clinicopathological exercises, Case 2-1997, *New Engl J Med* 336(3):205, 1997.

Comer JA et al: Antibodies to *Bartonella* species in inner city intravenous drug users in Baltimore, Md, *Arch Intern Med* 156(21):2491, 1996.

Greene CE et al: *Bartonella henselae* infection in cats: evaluation during primary infection, treatment, and rechallenge infection, *J Clin Microbiol* 34(7):1682, 1996.

Liston TE, Koehler JE: Granulomatous hepatitis and necrotizing splenitis due to *Bartonella henselae* in a patient with cancer: case report and review of hepatosplenic manifestations of *Bartonella* infection, *Clin Infect Dis* 22:951, 1996.

Soheilian M et al: Intermediate uveitis and retinal vasculitis as manifestations of cat-scratch disease, *Am J Ophthalmol* 122(4):582, 1996. Tan TQ et al: *Bartonella (Rochalimaea) henselae* hepatosplenic infection occurring simultaneously in two siblings, *Clin Infect Dis* 22:721, 1996.

Zinzindohoue F et al: Portal triad involvement in cat-scratch disease, *Lancet* 348(9035):1178, 1996.

Author: **George O. Alonso, M.D.**

Cavernous sinus thrombosis

BASIC INFORMATION

DEFINITION
Cavernous sinus thrombosis is an uncommon diagnosis usually stemming from infections of the face or paranasal sinuses resulting in thrombosis of the cavernous sinus and inflammation of its surrounding anatomic structures, including cranial nerves III, IV, V (ophthalmic and maxillary branch), VI, and the internal carotid artery.

SYNONYMS
Intracranial venous sinus thrombosis or thrombophlebitis

ICD-9-CM CODES
325 Phlebitis and thrombophlebitis of intracranial venous sinus

EPIDEMIOLOGY AND DEMOGRAPHICS
- Cavernous sinus thrombosis is rare.
- Before antibiotics the mortality from cavernous sinus thrombosis was 80% to 100%.
- With antibiotics, the mortality rates range between 20% and 30%.
- Morbidity remains high (between 25% and 50%).

PHYSICAL FINDINGS
The classic findings include:
- Ptosis
- Proptosis
- Chemosis
- Cranial nerve palsies (III, IV, V, VI)
  1. Sixth nerve palsy is the most common.
  2. Sensory deficits of the ophthalmic and maxillary branch of the fifth nerve are common.

Other findings:
- Decrease visual acuity and blindness may occur.
- Venous engorgement and papilledema on funduscopic examination may be found.
- Fever, tachycardia, sepsis may be present.
- Headache with nuchal rigidity may occur.
- Pupil may be dilated and sluggishly reactive.

ETIOLOGY
- *Staphylococcus aureus* is the most common infectious microbe found in 50% to 60% of the cases.
- *Streptococci* is the second leading cause.
- Gram-negative rods and anaerobes may also lead to cavernous sinus thrombosis.
- The most common primary site of infection leading to cavernous sinus thrombosis is sphenoid sinusitis; however, other sites of infection, including the middle ear, orbit, eye, eyelid, and face, can result in the same sequelae.

DIAGNOSIS

- The diagnosis of cavernous sinus thrombosis is made clinically.
- Proptosis, ptosis, chemosis, and cranial nerve palsy beginning in one eye and progressing to the other eye establishes the diagnosis.

DIFFERENTIAL DIAGNOSIS
- Orbital cellulitis
- Internal carotid artery aneurysm
- CVA
- Migraine headache
- Allergic blepharitis
- Thyroid exophthalmus
- Brain tumor
- Meningitis
- Mucormycosis
- Trauma

WORKUP
Cavernous sinus thrombosis is a clinical diagnosis with laboratory tests and imaging studies confirming the clinical impression.

LABORATORY TESTS
- CBC, ESR, blood cultures, and sinus cultures help establish and identify an infectious primary source.
- Lumbar puncture is necessary to rule out meningitis.

IMAGING STUDIES
- Sinus films are helpful in the diagnosis of sphenoid sinusitis. Opacification, sclerosis, and air fluid levels are typical findings.
- CT scan is the best study to diagnose sphenoid sinusitis; however, CT scan is not very sensitive in diagnosing cavernous sinus thrombosis.
- MRI is the imaging study of choice to diagnose cavernous sinus thrombosis.
- Cerebral angiography can be performed, but it is invasive and not very sensitive.
- Orbital venography is difficult to perform, but it is excellent in diagnosing occlusion of the cavernous sinus.

TREATMENT

NONPHARMACOLOGIC THERAPY
Recognizing the primary source of infection (e.g., facial cellulitis, middle ear, and sinus infections) and treating the primary source expeditiously is the best way to prevent cavernous sinus thrombosis.

ACUTE GENERAL Rx
- Broad-spectrum intravenous antibiotics are used until a definite pathogen is found.
  1. Nafcillin 1.5 g IV q4h
  2. Cefotaxime 1.5 to 2 g IV q4h
  3. Metronidazole 15 mg/kg load followed by 7.5 mg/kg IV q6h
- Anticoagulation with heparin is controversial. Retrospective studies show conflicting data. This decision should be made with subspecialty consultation.
- Steroid therapy is also controversial.

CHRONIC Rx
Surgical drainage with sphenoidotomy is indicated if the primary site of infection is thought to be the sphenoid sinus.

DISPOSITION
Cavernous sinus thrombosis can be a life-threatening, rapidly progressive infectious disease with high morbidity and mortality rates despite antibiotic use.

REFERRAL
If the diagnosis is suspected, this should be considered a medical emergency. Depending on the primary site of infection, appropriate consultation should be made (e.g., ENT, ophthalmology, and infectious disease).

MISCELLANEOUS

COMMENTS
Realizing the cavernous sinus lies just above and lateral to the sphenoid sinus and drains the middle portion of the face via the superior and inferior ophthalmic veins and knowing that cranial nerves III, IV, V, and VI pass alongside or through the cavernous sinus make the clinical findings and diagnosis easier to understand.

REFERENCES
Kriss TC, Kriss VM, Warf BC: Cavernous sinus thrombophlebitis: case report, *Neurosurg* 39(2):385, 1996.

Author: **Peter Petropoulos, M.D**

Celiac disease (PTG)

BASIC INFORMATION

DEFINITION
Celiac disease is a chronic disease characterized by malabsorption and diarrhea precipitated by ingestion of food products containing gluten.

SYNONYMS
Gluten enteropathy
Celiac sprue

ICD-9-CM CODES
579.0 Celiac disease

EPIDEMIOLOGY AND DEMOGRAPHICS
- Estimates of the incidence and prevalence of celiac sprue in the U.S. range from 50 to 500 cases/100,000 persons; it is highest in whites of northern European ancestry.
- Incidence is highest during infancy and the initial 36 mo (secondary to the introduction of foods containing gluten), in the third decade (frequently associated with pregnancy and severe anemia during pregnancy), and in the seventh decade.
- There is a slight female predominance.

PHYSICAL FINDINGS
- Physical examination may be entirely within normal limits.
- Weight loss, short stature, and failure to thrive in children and infants.
- Weight loss, fatigue, and diarrhea are common in adults.
- Abdominal pain, nausea, and vomiting are unusual.
- Pallor as a result of iron deficiency anemia is common.
- Manifestations of calcium deficiency, such as tetany and seizures, are rare and can be exacerbated by coexistent magnesium deficiency.

ETIOLOGY
Sensitivity to gluten

DIAGNOSIS

DIFFERENTIAL DIAGNOSIS
- IBD
- Laxative abuse
- Intestinal parasitic infestations
- Other: irritable bowel syndrome, tropical sprue, chronic pancreatitis, Zollinger-Ellison syndrome, cystic fibrosis (children), lymphoma, eosinophilic gastroenteritis, short bowel syndrome, Whipple's disease

WORKUP
Initial evaluation consists of laboratory tests followed by radiographic studies and upper GI endoscopy with biopsy of duodenum or proximal jejunum.

LABORATORY TESTS
- Iron deficiency anemia
- Folic acid deficiency
- Vitamin B_{12} deficiency, hypomagnesemia, hypocalcemia
- Antigliadin IgA and IgG antibodies are elevated in >90% of patients; however, they are nonspecific. IgA reticulin antibodies and IgA endomysial antibodies are more specific for celiac sprue.
- Biopsy of the small bowel reveals absence or shortening of villi, intraepithelial lymphocytes, and crypt lengthening and hyperplasia. Several biopsy specimens should be obtained for proper diagnosis.
- Tests for malabsorption are abnormal: fecal fat estimation for 72 hr is elevated (>7 g/day), d-xylose testing reveals malabsorption of sugar.

IMAGING STUDIES
Small bowel follow-through reveals altered mucosal folds and luminal dilation.

TREATMENT

NONPHARMACOLOGIC THERAPY
Patients should be instructed on gluten-free diet (avoidance of wheat, rye, barley, and oats).

ACUTE GENERAL Rx
- Correct nutritional deficiencies with iron, folic acid, vitamin B_{12} as needed.
- Prednisone 20 to 60 mg qd gradually tapered is useful in refractory cases.

CHRONIC Rx
- Lifelong gluten-free diet is necessary.
- Repeat small bowel biopsy following treatment generally reveals significant improvement. It is also useful to evaluate for increased risk of small bowel T-cell lymphoma in these patients (10%), especially in untreated patients.

DISPOSITION
Prognosis is good with adherence to gluten-free diet. Rapid improvement is usually seen within a few days of treatment.

REFERRAL
GI referral for small bowel biopsy

MISCELLANEOUS

COMMENTS
- Patient education material can be obtained from the American Celiac Society, 45 Gifford Ave., Jersey City, NJ 07304.
- Celiac disease should be considered in patients with unexplained metabolic bone disease or hypocalcemia, especially because GI symptoms may be absent or mild.

REFERENCES
Ferguson A et al: Clinical and pathological spectrum of celiac disease: active, silent, latent, potential, *Gut* 34:150, 1993.
Shaker JL et al: Hypocalcemia and skeletal disease as presenting features of celiac disease, *Arch Intern Med* 157:1013, 1997.

Author: **Fred F. Ferri, M.D.**

BASIC INFORMATION

DEFINITION
Cellulitis is a superficial inflammatory condition of the skin. It is characterized by erythema, warmth, and tenderness of the area involved.

SYNONYMS
Erysipelas (cellulitis generally secondary to group A β-hemolytic streptococci)

ICD-9-CM CODES
682.9 Cellulitis

EPIDEMIOLOGY AND DEMOGRAPHICS
Cellulitis occurs most frequently in diabetics, immunocompromised hosts, and in patients with venous and lymphatic compromise.

PHYSICAL FINDINGS
Variable with the causative organism
- Erysipelas: superficial-spreading, warm, erythematous lesion distinguished by its indurated and elevated margin (see color plate 3); lymphatic involvement and vesicle formation are common.
- Staphylococcal cellulitis: area involved is erythematous, hot, and swollen; differentiated from erysipelas by nonelevated, poorly demarcated margin; local tenderness and regional adenopathy are common; up to 85% of cases occur on the legs and feet.
- *H. influenzae* cellulitis: area involved is a blue-red/purple-red color; occurs mainly in children; generally involves the face in children and the neck or upper chest in adults.
- *Vibrio vulnificus*: larger hemorrhagic bullae, cellulitis, lymphadenitis, myositis; often found in critically ill patients in septic shock.

ETIOLOGY
- Group A β-hemolytic streptococci (may follow a streptococcal infection of the upper respiratory tract)
- Staphylococcal cellulitis
- *H. influenza*
- *Vibrio vulnificus*: higher incidence in patients with liver disease (75%) and in immunocompromised hosts (corticosteroid use, diabetes mellitus, leukemia, renal failure)
- *Erysipelothrix rhusiopathiae*: common in people handling poultry, fish, or meat
- *Aeromonas hydrophila*: generally occurring in contaminated open wound in fresh water
- Fungi (cryptococcus, neoformans): immunocompromised granulopenic patients
- Gram-negative rods (*Serratia, Enterobacter, Proteus, Pseudomonas*): immunocompromised or granulopenic patients

DIAGNOSIS

DIFFERENTIAL DIAGNOSIS
- Necrotizing fasciitis
- DVT
- Peripheral vascular insufficiency
- Paget's disease of the breast
- Thrombophlebitis
- Acute gout
- Psoriasis
- Candida intertrigo
- Pseudogout
- Osteomyelitis

WORKUP
Physical examination and laboratory evaluation

LABORATORY TESTS
- Gram-stain and culture (aerobic and anaerobic)
  1. Aspirated material from:
     a. Advancing edge of cellulitis
     b. Any vesicles
  2. Swab of any drainage material
  3. Punch biopsy (in selected patients)
- Blood cultures
- ASLO titer (in suspected streptococcal disease)

Despite the above measures the cause of cellulitis remains unidentified in most patients.

IMAGING STUDIES
CT or MRI in patients with suspected necrotizing fasciitis (deep-seated infection of the subcutaneous tissue that results in the progressive destruction of fascia and fat): patients present with diffuse swelling of an arm or leg followed by the appearance of bullae filled with clear fluid or maroon, violaceous fluid.

TREATMENT

NONPHARMACOLOGIC THERAPY
Immobilization and elevation of the involved limb

ACUTE GENERAL Rx
Erysipelas
- PO: penicillin V 250 mg to 500 mg qid
- IM: penicillin G (procaine) 600,000 U bid
- IV: penicillin G (aqueous) 4 to 6 million U/day

NOTE: Use erythromycin, cephalosporins, clindamycin, or vancomycin in patients allergic to penicillin.

Staphylococcus cellulitis
- PO: dicloxacillin 250 to 500 mg qid
- IV: nafcillin, 1 to 2 g q4-6h
- Cephalosporins (cephalothin, cephalexin, cephradine) also provide adequate antistaphylococcal coverage except for MRSA.
- Use vancomycin in patients allergic to penicillin or cephalosporins and in patients with methicillin-resistant *S. aureus* (MRSA).

H. influenzae cellulitis
- PO: amoxicillin, cefaclor, cefixime, or cefuroxime
- IV: cefuroxime or ampicillin; TMP-SMZ in patients allergic to penicillin
- Amoxicillin is ineffective in ampicillin-resistant strains (approximately 30%), IV cefuroxime is indicated in severely ill patients.

Vibrio vulnificus
- Aminoglycoside plus tetracycline or chloramphenicol
- IV support and admission into ICU (mortality rate >50% in septic shock)

Erysipelothrix
- Penicillin

Aeromonas hydrophila
- Aminoglycosides
- Chloramphenicol

DISPOSITION
Prognosis is good with prompt treatment.

REFERRAL
For surgical debridement in addition to antibiotics in patients with suspected necrotizing fasciitis

MISCELLANEOUS

REFERENCES
Brook I, Frazier EH: Clinical features and aerobic and anaerobic microbiological characteristics of cellulitis, *Arch Surg* 130:786, 1995.

Habif TP: *Clinical dermatology*, ed 3, St Louis, 1996, Mosby.

Author: **Fred F. Ferri, M.D.**

Cerebral palsy

BASIC INFORMATION

DEFINITION
Cerebral palsy refers to a group of motor impairment syndromes secondary to lesions or anomalies of the brain that arise in the early stages of development.

SYNONYMS
Little's disease
Congenital static encephalopathy
Congenital spastic paralysis

ICD-9-CM CODES
343 Infantile cerebral palsy
343.9 Infantile cerebral palsy, unspecified

EPIDEMIOLOGY AND DEMOGRAPHICS
INCIDENCE (IN U.S.): 1.5 to 2.5 cases/1000 live births
PREVALENCE (IN U.S.): Close to incidence (0 nonprogressive disease)
PREDOMINANT SEX: Male = female
PREDOMINANT AGE: 3 to 5 yr
PEAK INCIDENCE: At birth

PHYSICAL FINDINGS
- Mental retardation (30%)
- Seizures (30%)
- Hemiplegia
- Diplegia
- Extrapyramidal findings
- Delay in motor milestones
- Hypotonia

ETIOLOGY
Multifactorial: low birth weight, congenital malformations, thyroid or estrogen therapy during pregnancy, low Apgar scores, difficult delivery, prematurity, hyperbilirubinemia

DIAGNOSIS

DIFFERENTIAL DIAGNOSIS
Spinal cord abnormalities

WORKUP
Follow motor milestones and primitive reflexes

LABORATORY TESTS
- Thyroid function
- Urine amino acid screen
- Chromosomal analysis

IMAGING STUDIES
CT scan, MRI, and ultrasonography may show periventricular leukomalacia and/or periventricular hemorrhage.

TREATMENT

NONPHARMACOLOGIC THERAPY
- Physical therapy
- Special education

ACUTE GENERAL Rx
Not applicable unless seizures are present.

CHRONIC Rx
- Physical therapy
- Special schooling
- Treatment of seizures, if present

DISPOSITION
Have child remain at home if at all possible.

REFERRAL
If the child is seriously handicapped, physical medicine and rehabilitation referrals are especially helpful.

MISCELLANEOUS

COMMENTS
- Prevention is the most rational approach and involves close monitoring of pregnancy, ultrasound, and the avoidance of all drugs and alcohol.
- Patient education information on cerebral palsy can be obtained from the United Cerebral Palsy Association, 7 Penn Plaza, Suite 804, New York, NY 10001; phone: 1-800-USA-1UCP.

REFERENCES
Eicher PS, Batshaw ML: Cerebral palsy, *Pediatr Clin North Am* 40:537, 1993.
Kuban KCK, Leviton A: Cerebral palsy, *New Engl J Med* 330:188, 1994.
Paneth N: The causes of cerebral palsy: recent evidence, *Clin Invest Med* 16:95, 1993.
Stanley FJ: The etiology of cerebral palsy, *Early Hum Dev* 36:81, 1994.
Taft LT: Cerebral palsy, *Pediatr Rev* 16:411, 1995.
Author: **William H. Olson, M.D.**

Cerebrovascular accident (PTG)

BASIC INFORMATION

DEFINITION
Cerebrovascular accident (CVA) describes acute brain injury caused by decreased blood supply.

SYNONYMS
Stroke
CVA

ICD-9-CM CODES
436 Acute, but ill-defined, cerebrovascular disease

EPIDEMIOLOGY AND DEMOGRAPHICS
INCIDENCE (IN U.S.):
- Occurs in 5 to 10/100,000 persons <40 yr of age
- Occurs in 10 to 20/100,000 persons >65 yr of age

PREVALENCE (IN U.S.): Estimated at 2,000,000 persons
PREDOMINANT SEX: Incidence is 30% higher in males
PREDOMINANT AGE: 60+ yr
PEAK INCIDENCE: 80 to 84 yr
GENETICS: Family history a risk factor, but no distinct genetic etiology has been identified.

PHYSICAL FINDINGS
Motor and/or sensory and/or cognitive deficits, depending on distribution and extent of involved vascular territory.

ETIOLOGY
- From 70% to 80% are caused by ischemic infarcts; 20% to 30% are hemorrhagic.
- 80% of ischemic infarcts are from occlusion of large vessels caused by atherosclerotic vascular disease, 15% are caused by cardiac embolism, 5% are from other causes, including hypercoagulable states and vasculitis.
- Small vessel occlusion is most often caused by lipohyalinosis along with chronic hypertension.

DIAGNOSIS

DIFFERENTIAL DIAGNOSIS
- TIA
- Migraine
- Seizure
- Mass lesion

WORKUP
- Thorough history and physical examination, including detailed neurologic and cardiovascular evaluation to identify vascular territory and likely etiology
- Mandatory ECG
- Possible echocardiography, Holter monitor, carotid Doppler, transcranial Doppler studies, or angiography to determine etiology

LABORATORY TESTS
- CBC
- Platelet count
- PT
- PTT
- ESR
- VDRL
- Glucose
- Electrolytes
- Urinalysis
- Additional tests, depending on suspected etiology

IMAGING STUDIES
- CT scan without contrast to identify hemorrhage
- Possibly MRI to identify abnormalities in the posterior fossa and some mass lesions
- Possibly MRI or x-ray angiography to identify aneurysms or other vascular malformations

TREATMENT

NONPHARMACOLOGIC THERAPY
- Antiembolism stockings in patients with decreased mobility
- Carotid endarterectomy in suitable patients with carotid territory stroke associated with 70% to 99% ipsilateral carotid stenosis, performed by an experienced surgeon with low morbidity and mortality
- Modification of risk factors

ACUTE GENERAL Rx
- Judicious control of blood pressure; patients with chronic hypertension may extend the area of infarction if the blood pressure is lowered into the "normal" range.
- If patient presents <3 hr after onset of a nonhemorrhagic stroke, thrombolytic therapy in a specialized stroke center may be beneficial.

CHRONIC Rx
- Antiplatelet therapy (aspirin or ticlopidine) reduces the risk of subsequent stroke.
- Anticoagulation may be indicated in patients with cardioembolic stroke.

DISPOSITION
One yr mortality: 28% to 40%

REFERRAL
- If uncertain about diagnosis, etiology, or management
- For intracerebral hemorrhage (possible neurosurgical intervention)

MISCELLANEOUS

REFERENCES
Nadeau SE: Stroke, *Geriatr Med* 73:1351, 1989.
Author: **Michael Gruenthal, M.D., Ph.D.**

Cervical cancer (PTG)

BASIC INFORMATION

DEFINITION
Cervical cancer is penetration of the basement membrane and infiltration of the stroma of the uterine cervix by malignant cells.

SYNONYMS
Cervical intraepithelial neoplasia

ICD-9-CM CODES
180 Malignant neoplasm of cervix uteri

EPIDEMIOLOGY AND DEMOGRAPHICS
INCIDENCE: There are approximately 15,000 new cases annually, with 4000 to 5000 associated deaths. The U.S. has an age-adjusted mortality of 2.6 cases/100,000 persons for cervical cancer.
PREDOMINANCE: Higher incidence rates occur in developing countries. Among the U.S. population, Hispanics have a higher incidence than African-Americans, who likewise have a higher incidence than whites.
RISK FACTORS: Smoking, early age at first intercourse, multiple sexual partners, nonbarrier methods of birth control, infection with high-risk HPV (types 16 and 18), multiparity.

PHYSICAL FINDINGS
- Unusual vaginal bleeding, particularly postcoital
- Vaginal discharge and/or odor
- Advanced cases may present with lower extremity edema or renal failure.
- In early stages there may be little or no obvious cervical lesion, more advanced cases may present with large, bulky, friable lesions encompassing the majority of the vagina.

ETIOLOGY
- Dysplastic cells progress to invasive carcinoma.
- Thought to be linked to the presence of HPV types 16, 18, 45, and 56 via interaction of E6 oncoproteins on p53 gene product.

DIAGNOSIS

DIFFERENTIAL DIAGNOSIS
- Cervical polyp or prolapsed uterine fibroid
- Preinvasive cervical lesions
- Neoplasia metastatic from a separate primary

WORKUP
- Thorough history and physical examination
- Pelvic examination with careful rectovaginal examination
- Colposcopy with directed biopsy and endocervical curettage

LABORATORY TESTS
- CBC, chemistry profile
- Squamous cell carcinoma (SCC) antigen in research setting

IMAGING STUDIES
- Chest x-ray examination
- IVP
- Depending on stage, may need cystoscopy, sigmoidoscopy or BE, CT scan or MRI, lymphangiography

TREATMENT

NONPHARMACOLOGIC THERAPY
- FIGO stage Ia: cone biopsy or simple hysterectomy
- FIGO stage Ib or IIa: type III radical hysterectomy and pelvic lymphadenectomy *or* pelvic radiation therapy
- Advanced or bulky disease: multimodality therapy (radiation, chemotherapy and/or surgery)

ACUTE GENERAL Rx
Cervical cancer may present with massive and acute vaginal bleeding requiring volume and blood replacement, vaginal packing or other hemostatic modalities, and/or high-dose local radiotherapy.

CHRONIC Rx
- Physical examination with Pap smear every 3 mo for 2 yr, every 6 mo during the third to fifth year, and annually thereafter
- Chest x-ray examination annually

DISPOSITION
Five-year survival varies by stage:
- Stage I 60% to 90%
- Stage II 40% to 80%
- Stage III <60%
- Stage IV <15%

Early detection by Pap smear imperative to long-term improvements in survival.

REFERRAL
Gynecologic oncologist for all invasive disease

MISCELLANEOUS

COMMENTS
U.S. Preventive Services Task Force Recommendations regarding screening for cervical cancer are described in Section V, Chapter 9. Counseling recommendations regarding prevention of gynecologic cancers are described in Section V, Chapter 64.

REFERENCES
Cannistra SA, Niloff JM: Cancer of the uterine cervix, *New Engl J Med* 334(15):1030, 1996.
Hatch K: Cervical cancer. In Berek JS, Hacker NF (eds): *Practical gynecologic oncology*, ed 2, Baltimore, Md, 1994, Williams & Wilkins.
Morris M. et al: Cervical intraepithelial neoplasia and cervical cancer, *Obstet Gynecol Clin North Am* 23(2):347, 1996.

Author: **Karen Houck, M.D.**

Cervical disc syndromes (PTG)

BASIC INFORMATION

DEFINITION
Cervical disc syndromes refer to diseases of the cervical spine resulting from disc disorder, either herniation or degenerative change (spondylosis). When posterior osteophytes compress the anterior spinal cord, lower extremity symptoms may result, a condition termed *cervical spondylotic myelopathy*.

ICD-9-CM CODES
722.4 Degenerative intervertebral cervical disc
722.71 Degenerative cervical disc with myelopathy

EPIDEMIOLOGY AND DEMOGRAPHICS
PREVALENCE: 10% of general adult population (symptoms in 50% of population at some time in their life)
PREDOMINANT SEX: Male = female
PREDOMINANT AGE: 30 to 60 yr

PHYSICAL FINDINGS
- Neck pain, radicular symptoms, or myelopathy, either alone or in combination
- Limited neck movement
- Pain with neck motion, especially extension
- Referred unilateral interscapular pain, resulting in a local trigger point
- Radicular arm pain (usually unilateral), numbness, and tingling possible, most commonly involving the C6 (C5-C6 disc) or C7 (C6-C7 disc) nerve root
- Weakness and reflex changes (C6-biceps, C7-triceps)
- Myelopathy possibly resulting in gait disturbance, weakness, and even spasticity
- Sensory examination usually not helpful

ETIOLOGY
Unknown

DIAGNOSIS

DIFFERENTIAL DIAGNOSIS
- Rotator cuff tendinitis
- Carpal tunnel syndrome
- Thoracic outlet syndrome
- Brachial neuritis

A clinical algorithm for evaluation of neck pain is described in Fig. 3-58.

WORKUP
In most cases, the diagnosis can be established on a clinical basis alone.

IMAGING STUDIES
- Plain roentgenograms within the first few weeks
  1. Usually normal in soft disc herniation
  2. With chronic degenerative disc disease, usually loss of height of the disc space, anterior and posterior osteophyte formation, and encroachment on the intervertebral foramen by osteophytes
- Myelography, CT scanning, and MRI indicated in patients whose symptoms do not resolve or when other spinal pathology suspected
- Electrodiagnostic studies to confirm the diagnosis or rule out peripheral nerve disorders

TREATMENT

NONPHARMACOLOGIC TREATMENT
- Rest and cervical collar if needed
- Local modalities such as heat
- Physical therapy

ACUTE GENERAL Rx
- NSAIDs
- "Muscle relaxants" for their sedative effect
- Analgesics as needed
- Epidural steroid injection for radicular pain

DISPOSITION
- Usually improve with time
- Surgical intervention in <5%

REFERRAL
Orthopedic or neurosurgical consultation for intractable pain or neurologic deficit

MISCELLANEOUS

COMMENTS
- Pain relief with physical therapy seems anecdotal and short-lived; any overall improvement usually parallels what would have probably occurred naturally.
- Sometimes carpal tunnel syndrome and cervical radiculopathy occur together; this is termed the *double-crush syndrome* and results from nerve compression at two separate levels. Proximal compression may decrease the ability of the nerve to tolerate a second, more distal compression.
- Surgical intervention is indicated primarily for relief of radicular pain caused by nerve root compression or for the treatment of myelopathy; it is generally not helpful when chief complaint is neck pain alone.

REFERENCES
Bernhardt M et al: Current concepts review: cervical spondylotic myelopathy, *J Bone Joint Surg* 75(A):119, 1993.
Levine MJ, Albert TJ, Smith MD: Cervical radiculopathy: diagnosis and nonoperative management, *J Am Acad Orthop Surg* 4:305, 1996.

Author: **Lonnie R. Mercier, M.D.**

Cervical dysplasia (PTG)

BASIC INFORMATION

DEFINITION
Cervical dysplasia refers to atypical development of immature squamous epithelium that does not penetrate the basement epithelial membrane. Characteristics include increased cellularity, nuclear abnormalities, and increased nuclear to cytoplasm ratio. A progressive polarized loss of squamous differentiation exists beginning adjacent to the basement membrane and progressing to the most advanced stage (severe dysplasia), which encompasses the complete squamous epithelial layer thickness.

Classification systems:
Modified Papanicolaou: Class I, II, III, IV, and V
Dysplasia: Normal, atypia-mild, moderate and severe, carcinoma in situ, and cancer
CIN: Normal, atypia-CIN I, II, or III, and cancer
Bethesda classification:
Normal/benign, AGCUS, ASCUS, LGSIL (including HPV), HGSIL, and cancer

SYNONYMS
Class III or class IV Pap smear
Cervical intraepithelial neoplasia (CIN)
Low-grade or high-grade squamous intraepithelial lesion (LGSIL or HGSIL)

ICD-9-CM CODES
622.1 Dysplasia of cervix (uteri)

EPIDEMIOLOGY AND DEMOGRAPHICS

PEAK INCIDENCE:
- Age 35 yr
- Abnormal Pap smear rate revealing dysplasia approximates 2% to 5%, depending on population risk factors and false-negative rate variance
- False-negative rate approaching 40%
- Average age adjusted incidence of severe dysplasia 35 cases/100,000 persons

PREVALENCE:
- Dysplasia: peak age, 26 yr (3600 cases/100,000 persons)
- CIS: peak age, 32 yr (1100 cases/100,000 persons)
- Invasive cancer: peak age, 77 yr (800 cases/100,000 persons)

PHYSICAL FINDINGS
- Cervical lesions associated with dysplasia usually are not visible to the naked eye; therefore physical findings are best viewed by colposcopy of a 3% acetic acid-prepared cervix.
- Patients evaluated by colposcopy are identified by abnormal cervical cytology screening from Pap smear screening
- Colposcopic findings:
  1. Leukoplakia (white lesion seen by the unaided eye that may represent condyloma, dysplasia, or cancer)
  2. Acetowhite epithelium with or without associated punctation, mosaicism, abnormal vessels
  3. Abnormal transformation zone (abnormal iodine uptake, "cuffed" gland openings)

ETIOLOGY
- Not clearly elucidated
- May be caused by abnormal reserve cell hyperplasia resulting in atypical metaplasia resulting in dysplastic epithelium
- Strongly associated and initiated by oncogenic HPV infection (high-risk HPV types 16, 18, 31, 33, 35, 45, 51, 52, 56, and 58; low-risk HPV types 6, 11, 42, 43, and 44)
- Risk factors:
  1. Any heterosexual coitus
  2. Coitus during puberty (T-zone metaplasia peak)
  3. DES exposure
  4. Multiple sexual partners
  5. Lack of prior Pap smear screening
  6. History of STD
  7. Other genital tract neoplasia
  8. HIV
  9. TB
  10. Substance abuse
  11. "High-risk" male partner (HPV)
  12. Low socioeconomic status
  13. Early first pregnancy
  14. Tobacco use
  15. HPV

DIAGNOSIS

DIFFERENTIAL DIAGNOSIS
- Metaplasia
- Hyperkeratosis
- Condyloma
- Microinvasive carcinoma
- Glandular epithelial abnormalities
- Adenocarcinoma in situ
- VIN
- VAIN
- Metastatic tumor involvement of the cervix

WORKUP
Periodic history and physical examination (including cytologic screening), depending on age, risk factors, and history of preinvasive cervical lesions
- Consider screening for sexually transmitted disease (Gc, chlamydia, VDRL, HIV)
- Abnormal cytology (HGSIL/LGSIL, initial ASCUS in high-risk patients, recurrent ASCUS in low-risk/postmenopausal patients) and grossly evident suspicious lesions; refer for colposcopy and possible directed biopsy/ECC (examination should include cervix, vagina, vulva, and anus)
- For glandular cell abnormalities (AGCUS): refer for colposcopy, possible directed biopsy/ECC, and consider endometrial sampling

- In pregnancy: abnormal cytology followed by colposcopy in the first trimester and at 28 to 32 wk; only high-grade lesions suspicious for cancer biopsied; ECC contraindicated

LABORATORY TESTS
- Gc, chlamydia to rule out STD
- Pap cytology screening (requires appropriate sampling, preparation, cytologist interpretation and reporting)
- Colposcopy and directed biopsy, ECC for indications (see "Workup")
- HPV-DNA typing considered

IMAGING STUDIES
- Cervicography
- Computer-enhanced Pap cytology screening (i.e., PAPNET)

TREATMENT

NONPHARMACOLOGIC TREATMENT
- Superficial ablative techniques (cryosurgery, CO_2 laser, and electrocoagulation diathermy) considered for colposcopy-identified dysplasia (moderate to severe dysplasia or CIS) and negative ECC; mild dysplasia followed conservatively in a compliant patient
- Cone biopsy (LEEP, CO_2 laser, "cold knife" cone biopsy) considered for colposcopy-identified dysplasia (moderate to severe dysplasia or CIS) and positive ECC or if there is a two grade or more discrepancy between the Pap smear, colposcopy, and biopsy or ECC findings
- Hysterectomy if patient has completed child bearing and has persistent or recurrent severe dysplasia or CIS
- In pregnancy: treatment for cervical dysplasia deferred until after delivery

ACUTE GENERAL Rx
Topical 5-fluorouracil (5-FU) is rarely used for recurrent cervicovaginal lesions.

CHRONIC Rx
- Because of the risk for persistent and recurrent dysplasia, long-term follow-up is individualized based on patient risk factors, Pap smear and colposcopy results, treatment history, and presence of high-risk HPV.(i.e., Pap smear q3-4mo/1 yr, then q6mo/1 yr, then annually [if all normal], or repeat colposcopy examination and treat as indicated).
- Mild dysplasia with negative ECC should be followed conservatively in a compliant patient as a majority of these lesions persist or regress.

DISPOSITION
- Because of the large numbers of women in high-risk groups, the prevalence of HPV, and the high false-negative Pap smear rate, routine Pap smear screening should be reinforced for all women, especially those with a history of cervical dysplasia.
- Success rates for treatment approach 80% to 90%.
- Detection of persistence or recurrence requires careful follow-up.
- Cervical treatment possibly results in infertility (cervical stenosis or incompetence), which requires careful consideration and discretion for use of LEEP and cone biopsy.
- Appropriate counseling and informed consent needed when considering any form of management of cervical dysplasia.
- There has been no case of cervical dysplasia progressing to invasive cancer with appropriate screening, diagnosis, treatment and follow-up.

REFERRAL
- Patients with abnormal Pap cytology should not be followed by repeat Pap smear screening.
- Patients with identified abnormal cytology should be evaluated by a skilled colposcopist (defined as documented didactic and Preceptorship training including 50 cases of identified pathology, ongoing colposcopy activity with a minimum of 2 cases/wk, Q.A. Log, and periodic CME).
- If treatment is required, patient should be referred to a gynecologist or gynecologic oncologist skilled in the diagnosis and treatment of preinvasive cervical disease.

MISCELLANEOUS

COMMENTS
- Patient education material available from American College of Obstetricians and Gynecologists.
- A clinical algorithm for workup of Pap smear abnormalities is described in Fig. 3-63.
- U.S. Preventive Services Task Force Recommendations regarding counseling to prevent gynecologic cancer are described in Section V, Chapter 64.

REFERENCES
Barek JS, Hacker NF: *Practical gynecologic oncology,* ed 2, Baltimore, 1994, Williams & Wilkins.
Disaia PJ, Creasman WT: *Clinical gynecologic oncology,* ed 3, St Louis, 1989, Mosby.
Jones HW, Wentz AC, Burnett CS: *Novaks textbook of gynecology,* ed 11, Baltimore, 1988, Williams & Wilkins.
Author: **Dennis M. Weppner, M.D.**

Cervical polyps (PTG)

BASIC INFORMATION

DEFINITION
A cervical polyp is a growth protruding from the cervix or endocervical canal. Polyps that arise from the endocervical canal are called endocervical polyps. If they arise from the ectocervix, they are called cervical polyps.

ICD-9-CM CODES
622.7 Mucous polyp of cervix

EPIDEMIOLOGY AND DEMOGRAPHICS
Cervical polyps are common. Found in approximately 4% of all gynecologic patients. Most commonly present in perimenopausal and multigravid women between the ages of 30 and 50 yr. Endocervical polyps are more common than cervical polyps and are almost always benign. Malignant degeneration is extremely rare.

PHYSICAL FINDINGS
Polyps may be single or multiple and vary in size from being extremely small (a few mm) to large (4 cm). They are soft, smooth, reddish-purple to cherry-red in color. They bleed easily when touched. Very large polyps can cause some cervical dilatation. There may be vaginal discharge associated with cervical polyps if the polyp has become infected.

ETIOLOGY
- Most unknown
- Inflammatory
- Traumatic
- Pregnancy

DIAGNOSIS

DIFFERENTIAL DIAGNOSIS
- Endometrial polyp
- Prolapsed myoma
- Retained products of conception
- Squamous papilloma
- Sarcoma
- Cervical malignancy

WORKUP
Polyps are most commonly asymptomatic and are usually found at the time of annual gynecologic pelvic examination. Polyps are also found in women who present for evaluation of intermenstrual or postcoital bleeding and for profuse vaginal discharge. Polyps are painless. Unless a patient has a bleeding abnormality that necessitates her being evaluated by a physician, polyps would go undiagnosed until her next Pap smear was obtained.

TREATMENT

NONPHARMACOLOGIC THERAPY
Simple surgical excision can be done in the office. The physician should be prepared for bleeding, which can easily be controlled with silver nitrate or Monsel's solution. Most commonly, a polyp is excised by grasping it at the stalk and twisting it off. Polyps can also be excised by electrocautery or, in the case of very large polyps, in an outpatient surgical suite. Sexual intercourse and tampon usage is to be avoided until the patient's follow-up visit. Also, douching is not to be performed.

ACUTE GENERAL Rx
Generally, no medication is needed.

CHRONIC Rx
Patient is followed up in 2 wk for recheck of the surgical excision site unless there is active bleeding, in which case she would be seen immediately. The cervix should be checked at the patient's routine gynecologic visits.

DISPOSITION
Since these are almost always benign, usually no further treatment is needed. Annual gynecologic examinations should be performed to check for any regrowths.

REFERRAL
To a gynecologist for removal of polyps

MISCELLANEOUS

COMMENTS
A Pap smear should be obtained prior to removing the polyp. If an abnormal Pap smear is obtained, more than likely the cause will be secondary to the polyp. If a colposcopic evaluation is needed, this should also be performed. During pregnancy, the cervix is highly vascularized. If the polyps are stable and benign-appearing, they should just be observed during the pregnancy and removed only if they are causing bleeding.

REFERENCES
Copeland L: *Textbook of gynecology*, Philadelphia, 1993, WB Saunders.
Herbst et al: *Comprehensive gynecology*, ed 2, St Louis, 1992, Mosby.

Author: **George T. Danakas, M.D.**

Cervicitis (PTG)

BASIC INFORMATION

DEFINITION
Cervicitis is an infection of the cervix. It may result from direct infection of the cervix, or it may be secondary to uterine or vaginal infection.

SYNONYMS
Endocervicitis
Ectocervicitis
Mucopurulent cervicitis

ICD-9-CM CODES
616.0 Cervicitis
098.15 Acute gonococcal cervicitis
079.8 Chlamydia infection

EPIDEMIOLOGY AND DEMOGRAPHICS
Cervicitis accounts for 20% to 25% of patients presenting with abnormal vaginal discharge, and this effects women only. It is most common in adolescents, but it can be found in any sexually active woman. Practicing unsafe sex with multiple sexual partners increases the risk of developing cervicitis as well as other sexually transmitted diseases.

PHYSICAL FINDINGS
Cervicitis is usually asymptomatic or associated with mild symptoms. Copious vaginal discharge, pelvic pain, and dyspareunia may be present if cervicitis is severe. The cervix can be erythematous and tender on palpation during bimanual examination. The cervix may also bleed easily when obtaining cultures or a Pap smear.

ETIOLOGY
- Chlamydia
- Trichomonas
- Neisseria gonorrhoeae
- Herpes simplex
- Trichomonas vaginalis
- Human papillomavirus

DIAGNOSIS

DIFFERENTIAL DIAGNOSIS
- Carcinoma of the cervix
- Cervical erosion
- Cervical metaplasia

WORKUP
The patient usually presents with a vaginal discharge or history of postcoital bleeding. Otherwise the patient is diagnosed asymptomatically during routine examination. On examination there is gross visualization of yellow, mucopurulent material on the cotton swab.

LABORATORY TESTS
On a smear there will be ten or more polymorphonuclear leukocytes per microscopic field. Positive Gram stain is found. Cultures should be obtained for Chlamydia and N. gonorrhoeae. Use a wet mount to look for trichomonads. Obtain a Pap smear.

TREATMENT

NONPHARMACOLOGIC THERAPY
Cervicitis is treated in an outpatient setting. Cryosurgery is an option for treatment of cervicitis with negative cultures and negative biopsies. Safe sex should be practiced with the use of condoms. Partners should be treated in all cases of infection proven by culture.

ACUTE GENERAL Rx
Since Chlamydia and N. gonorrhoeae make up >50% of the cause of infectious cervicitis, if it is suspected, treat without waiting for culture results. Administer ceftriaxone 125-mg IM single dose followed by doxycycline 100 mg PO bid for 7 days. If the patient is pregnant, treat with azithromycin (Zithromax) 1-g single dose instead of using doxycycline, which is contraindicated in pregnant or nursing mothers. If Trichomonas is the etiologic agent, treat with metronidazole 2-g single dose. For herpes, treat with acyclovir 200 mg PO five times qd for 7 days.

DISPOSITION
Cervicitis responds well to antibiotics. Possible complications to watch for are a subsequent PID and infertility (found in 5% to 10% of patients). Repeat cultures should be performed after treatment. Sexual relations can be resumed after negative cultures.

REFERRAL
If subsequent PID develops, consider hospital admission for IV antibiotics.

MISCELLANEOUS

COMMENTS
Patient educational material can be obtained from local health clinics and clinics for sexually transmitted diseases.

REFERENCES
Centers for Disease Control: Sexually transmitted disease treatment guideline, *MMWR* 47(RR-1), 1998.
Herbst et al: *Comprehensive gynecology*, ed 2, St Louis, 1992, Mosby.
Sweet RL, Gibbs RS: *Infections of the female genital tract*, Baltimore, Md, 1990, Williams & Wilkins.

Author: **George T. Danakas, M.D.**

Chagas' disease (PTG)

BASIC INFORMATION

DEFINITION
Chagas' disease is a infection caused by the protozoan parasite, *Trypanosoma cruzi*. The disease is characterized by an acute nonspecific febrile illness that may be followed, after a variable latency period, by chronic cardiac, GI, and neurologic sequelae.

SYNONYMS
American trypanosomiasis

ICD-9-CM CODES
086.2 Chagas' disease

EPIDEMIOLOGY AND DEMOGRAPHICS
INCIDENCE (IN U.S.):
- Four cases of autochthonous transmission in California and Texas
- In the last two decades, six cases of laboratory-acquired infection, three cases of transfusion-associated transmission, and nine cases of imported disease reported to the Centers for Disease Control (none of the imported cases involved returning tourists)

PREVALENCE (IN U.S.): At least 5 % of Salvadoran and Nicaraguan immigrants infected, according to the limited surveys

PREDOMINANT SEX: Male = female
PREDOMINANT AGE:
- In highly endemic areas, mean age of acute infection: approximately 4 yr old
- Variable age distribution for both types of chronic disease, depending on geography
- Mean age of onset: usually between 35 and 45 yr

PEAK INCIDENCE: Unknown
GENETICS:
Congenital Infection: Congenital transmission has been documented with attendant high fetal mortality and morbidity in surviving infants.
Neonatal Infection: In rural areas, within substandard housing, transmission is likely to occur.

PHYSICAL FINDINGS
- Inflammatory lesion that develops about 1 wk after contamination of a break in the skin with infected insect feces (chagoma)
  1. Area of induration and erythema
  2. Usually accompanied by local lymphadenopathy
- Presence of Romaña sign, which consists of unilateral painless palpebral and periocular edema, when conjunctiva is portal of entry
- Constitutional symptoms of fever, fatigue, and anorexia, along with edema of the face and lower extremities, generalized lymphadenopathy, and mild hepatosplenomegaly after the appearance of local signs of disease
- Myocarditis in a small proportion of patients, sometimes with resultant CHF
- Uncommonly, possible CNS disease, such as meningoencephalitis, which carries a poor prognosis
- Symptoms and signs of disease persisting for weeks to months, followed by spontaneous resolution of the acute illness; patient then in the indeterminate phase of the disease (asymptomatic with attendant subpatent parasitemia and reactive antibodies to *T. cruzi* antigens)
- Chronic disease may become manifest years to decades after the initial infection:
  1. Most common organ involved: heart, followed by GI tract, and to a much lesser extent the CNS
     a. Cardiac involvement takes the form of arrhythmias or cardiomyopathy, but rarely both.
     b. Cardiomyopathy is bilateral but predominantly affects the right ventricle and is often accompanied by apical aneurysms and mural thrombi.
     c. Arrhythmias are a consequence of involvement of the bundle of His and have been implicated as the leading cause of sudden death in adults in highly endemic areas.
     d. Right-sided heart failure, thromboembolization, and rhythm disturbances associated with symptoms of dizziness and syncope are characteristic.
  2. Patients with megaesophagus: dysphasia, odynophagia, chronic cough, and regurgitation, frequently resulting in aspiration pneumonitis
  3. Megacolon: abdominal pain and chronic constipation, which, when severe, may lead to obstruction and perforation
  4. CNS symptoms: most often secondary to embolization from the heart or varying degrees of peripheral neuropathy

ETIOLOGY
- *T. cruzi*
  1. Found only in the Americas, ranging from the southern half of the U.S. to southern Argentina
  2. Transmitted to humans by various species of blood sucking reduviid ("kissing") insects, primarily those of the genera *Triatoma, Panstrongylus,* and *Rhodnius*
  3. Usually found in burrows and trees where infected insects transmit the parasite to nonhuman mammals (e.g., opossums and armadillos), which constitute the natural reservoir
  4. Intrusion into enzootic areas for farmland, allowing insects to take up residence in rural dwellings, thus including humans and domestic animals in the cycle of transmission
  5. Initial infection of insects by ingesting blood from animals or humans that have circulating flagellated trypanosomes (trypomastigotes)
  6. Multiplication of ingested parasites in the insect midgut as epimastigotes, then differentiation into infective metacyclic trypomastigotes in the hindgut whereby the parasites are discharged with the feces during subsequent blood meals
  7. Transmission to the second mammalian host through contamination of mucous membranes, conjunctivas, or wounds with insect feces containing infected forms
- In the vertebrate host
  1. Movement of parasites into various cell types, intracellular transformation and multiplication in the cytoplasm as amastigotes, and thereafter differentiation into trypomastigotes
  2. Following rupture of the cell membrane, parasitic invasion of local tissues or hematogenous spread to distant sites, maintaining a parasitemia infective for vectors
- In addition to insect vectors, *T. cruzi* is transmitted through blood transfusions, transplacentally, and, occasionally, secondary to laboratory accidents.

DIAGNOSIS

DIFFERENTIAL DIAGNOSIS
Acute disease
- Early African trypanosomiasis
- New World cutaneous and mucocutaneous leishmaniasis

Chronic disease
- Idiopathic cardiomyopathy
- Idiopathic achalasia
- Congenital or acquired megacolon

WORKUP
Principal considerations in diagnosis:
- A history of residence where transmission is known to occur
- Recent receipt of a blood product while in an endemic area
- Occupational exposure in a laboratory

LABORATORY TESTS
For acute diagnosis:
- Demonstration of *T. cruzi* in wet preparations of blood, buffy coat, or Giemsa-stained smears
- Xenodiagnosis, a technique involving laboratory-reared insect vectors fed on subjects with suspected infection thereafter examined for parasites, and culture of body fluids in liquid media to establish diagnosis
  1. Hampered by the length of time required for completion
  2. Of limited use in clinical decision making with regard to drug therapy
  3. Although xenodiagnosis and broth culture are considered to be more sensitive than microscopic examination of body fluids, sensitivities may not exceed 50%.
- Recent advances in serologic testing, including immunoblot assay, in situ indirect fluorescent antibody, and PCR-based techniques
  1. Show increased sensitivity and specificity for *T. cruzi* in acute and chronic infections
  2. Not widely available, limiting their usefulness in the diagnosis of acute disease

For chronic *T. cruzi* infection:
- Traditional serologic tests including: complement fixation (CF), indirect immunofluorescence (IIF), indirect hemagglutination, enzyme-linked immunosorbent assay (ELISA), and radioimmune precipitation assay
- Persistent problem with these tests: in addition to sensitivity and specificity, false-positive results

TREATMENT

NONPHARMACOLOGIC THERAPY
- Chronic chagasic heart disease: mainly supportive
- Megaesophagus: symptoms usually amenable to dietary measures or pneumonic dilatation of the esophagogastric junction
- Chagasic megacolon: in its early stages responsive to a high-fiber diet, laxatives, and enemas

ACUTE GENERAL Rx
Nifurtimox (Lampit, Bayer 2502):
- Only drug available in the U.S. for the treatment of acute, congenital, or laboratory-acquired infection
- Recommended oral dosage for adults: 8 to 10 mg/kg/day given in four divided daily doses and continued for 90 to 120 days
- Parasitologic cure in approximately 50% of those treated; should be begun as early as possible

Benznidazole, a nitroimidazole derivative:
- Has demonstrated similar efficacy as nifurtimox in limited trials
- Recommended oral dosage: 5 mg/kg/day for 60 days

CHRONIC Rx
- In patients with indeterminate phase or chronic disease: no evidence of benefit with pharmacologic therapy
- In patients exhibiting bradyarrhythmias: pacemakers
- In individuals with congestive heart failure:
  1. Treat with modalities appropriate for dilated, especially right-sided, cardiomyopathic disease.
  2. Cardiac transplant is a controversial alternative for end-stage cardiomyopathy; however, reactivation rate found to be low and amenable to therapy without subsequent infection of the allograft in one study.
  3. Myotomies or esophageal resection is reserved for patients with advanced disease.
- In advanced chagasic megacolon associated with chronic fecal impaction, perforation, or, less commonly, volvulus: surgical resection

DISPOSITION
Based on few prospective studies, most patients infected with *T. cruzi* will not develop symptomatic Chagas' disease.

REFERRAL
- For consultation with an infectious disease specialist or communication with the Centers for Disease Control when the disease is acutely suspected
- To a cardiologist for pacemaker implantation for patients with bradyarrhythmias
- To a surgeon for symptomatic disease in individuals with chagasic megaesophagus or megacolon

MISCELLANEOUS

COMMENTS
- In recipients of solid organ or bone marrow transplants, patients with AIDS, or those receiving chemotherapy, there may be reactivation of indeterminate phase disease.
- Prognosis in patients with chagasic cardiomyopathy who develop CHF is poor, with death often ensuing in a matter of months.
- Patients with chagasic esophageal disease have an increased incidence of esophageal malignancy.

REFERENCES
Altclas J et al: Chagas' disease after bone marrow transplantation, *Bone Marrow Transplant* 18(2):447, 1996.

de Carvalho VB et al: Heart transplantation in Chagas' disease: 10 years after the initial experience, *Circulation* 94(8):1815, 1996.

Kirchhoff LV: American trypanosomiasis (Chagas' disease), *Gastroenterol Clin North Am* 25(3):517, 1996.

Levy AM et al: In situ indirect fluorescent antibody: a new specific test to detect ongoing chagasic infections, *J Clin Lab Anal* 10(2):98, 1996.

Sgambatti de Andrade ALS et al: Randomized trial of efficacy of benznidazole in treatment of early *Trypanosoma cruzi* infection, *Lancet* 348:1407, 1996.

Umezawa ES et al: Immunoblot assay using excreted-secreted antigens of *Trypanosoma cruzi* in serodiagnosis of congenital, acute and chronic Chagas' disease, *J Clin Microbiol* 34(9):2143, 1996.

Author: **George O. Alonso, M.D.**

Chancroid (PTG)

BASIC INFORMATION

DEFINITION
Chancroid is a sexually transmitted disease characterized by painful genital ulceration and inflammatory inguinal adenopathy.

SYNONYMS
Soft chancre
Ulcus molle

ICD-9-CM CODES
099.0 Chancroid

EPIDEMIOLOGY AND DEMOGRAPHICS
- Exact incidence is unknown.
- Occurs more frequently in men (male:female ratio of 10:1).
- Cases reported in 1987: 5047 and rising.
- Clinical infection is rare in women.
- There is a higher incidence in uncircumcised men and in tropical and subtropical regions.
- Incubation period is 4 to 7 days but may take up to 3 wk.

PHYSICAL FINDINGS
- One to three extremely painful ulcers, accompanied by tender inguinal lymphadenopathy (especially if fluctuant)
- May present with inguinal bubo and several ulcers
- In women: initial lesion in the fourchette, labia minora, urethra, cervix, or anus; inflammatory pustule or papule that ruptures leaving a shallow, nonindurated, shallow ulceration, usually 1- to 2-cm diameter with ragged, undermined edges
- Unilateral lymphadenopathy develops 1 wk later in 50% of patients

ETIOLOGY
Hemophilus ducreyi, a bacillus

DIAGNOSIS

DIFFERENTIAL DIAGNOSIS
- Other genitoulcerative diseases such as syphilis, herpes, LGV, granuloma inguinale
- A clinical algorithm for the initial management of genital ulcer disease is described in Fig. 3-33.

WORKUP
Diagnosis based on history and physical examination is often inadequate. Must rule out syphilis in women because of the consequences of inappropriate therapy in pregnant women. Base initial diagnosis and treatment recommendations on clinical impression of appearance of ulcer and most likely diagnosis for population. Definitive diagnosis is made by isolation of organism from ulcers by culture or Gram stain.

LABORATORY TESTS
Darkfield microscopy, RPR, HSV cultures, *H. ducreyi* culture, HIV testing recommended

TREATMENT

NONPHARMACOLOGIC THERAPY
Fluctuant nodes should be aspirated through healthy adjacent skin to prevent formation of draining sinus. I&D not recommended, delays healing. Use warm compresses to remove necrotic material.

ACUTE GENERAL Rx
- Erythromycin 500 mg PO qid for 7 days
- *or* Ceftriaxone 250 mg IM (single dose)
- *or* Azithromycin 1 g PO (single dose)
- *or* Ciprofloxacin 500 mg PO bid for 3 days

DISPOSITION
All sexual partners should be treated with a 10-day course of one of the above regimens.

MISCELLANEOUS

COMMENTS
- In the U.S. HSV-1 or syphilis are the most common causes of genital ulcers followed by chancroid, LGV, and granuloma inguinale.
- U.S. Preventive Services Task Force Recommendations regarding prevention of HIV and other STDs are described in Section V, Chapter 62.

REFERENCES
Benenson AS (ed): *Control of communicable diseases in man,* ed 15, Washington, DC, 1990, American Public Health Association.

Drugs for sexually transmitted diseases, *Med Lett Drugs Ther* 37(964): 117, 1995.

Schulte JM, Schmid GP: Recommendations for treatment of chancroid, *Clin Infect Dis* 20(suppl 1): S39, 1995.

Woods GL: Update on laboratory diagnosis of sexually transmitted diseases, *Clin Lab Med* 15(3):665, 1995.

Author: **Eugene J. Louie-Ng, M.D.**

Charcot's joint (PTG)

BASIC INFORMATION

DEFINITION
Charcot's joint is a chronic, progressive joint degeneration, often devastating, seen most commonly in peripheral weight bearing joints and vertebrae, which develops as a result of the loss of normal sensory innervation of the joint. It was described by Charcot as a result of tabes dorsalis.

SYNONYMS
Neuropathic arthropathy

ICD-9-CM CODES
094.0 Charcot's arthropathy

EPIDEMIOLOGY AND DEMOGRAPHICS
PREVALENCE:
- 1 case/750 patients with diabetes mellitus; 5 cases/100 of those with peripheral neuropathy (foot is most commonly involved)
- 20% to 40% of patients with syringomyelia (shoulder most commonly involved)
- 5% to 10% of patients with tabes dorsalis; usually >60 yr (spine, hip, and knee most commonly involved)

PHYSICAL FINDINGS
Neuropathic joint disease is relatively painless, often in spite of considerable destruction.
- Often, diffusely warm, swollen, and occasionally erythematous involved joint, the latter suggesting sepsis
- Possible progression of joint instability; Palpable osseous debris; crepitus common
- Often, frank dislocation, leading to bony deformity, especially in more superficial joints

ETIOLOGY
The most widely accepted theory is the "neurotraumatic" theory:
- Impairment and loss of joint sensitivity decreases the protective mechanism about the joint.
- Rapid destruction occurs.
- Chronic inflammation and repetitive effusions develop, eventually contributing to joint instability and incongruity.

DIAGNOSIS

DIFFERENTIAL DIAGNOSIS
- Osteomyelitis
- Infectious arthritis
- Osteoarthritis
- Rheumatoid and other inflammatory arthritides

WORKUP
- An underlying neurologic disorder must always be present.
- Diabetes mellitus with peripheral neuropathy is the most common cause.
- Syringomyelia, tabes dorsalis, Charcot-Marie-Tooth disease, congenital indifference to pain, alcoholism, and spinal dysraphism can all lead to the disorder.

LABORATORY TESTS
In questionable cases, aspiration, sometimes including biopsy, to rule out sepsis

IMAGING STUDIES
Plain roentgenography
- Sufficient to establish diagnosis in most cases, especially if etiology is known
- Findings: variable degrees of destruction and dislocation

TREATMENT

ACUTE GENERAL Rx
- Protection of effusions, sprains, and fractures until all hyperemic response has
- Braces, special shoes with molded inserts, and elevation of the extremity
- Patient education with avoidance of weight bearing when lower extremity joints are involved
- Surgery: only limited value

DISPOSITION
Once the full-blown neuropathic joint has developed, treatment is difficult.

MISCELLANEOUS

REFERENCES
Alpert SW, Koval KJ, Zuckerman JD: Neuropathic arthropathy: review of current knowledge, *J Am Acad Orthop Surg* 4:100, 1996.

Calabro JJ, Garg SL: Neuropathic joint disease, *Am Fam Physician* 7:90, 1973.

Author: **Lonnie R. Mercier, M.D.**

Charcot-Marie-Tooth disease

BASIC INFORMATION

DEFINITION
Charcot-Marie-Tooth disease is a heterogeneous group of noninflammatory inherited peripheral neuropathies.

SYNONYMS
Peroneal muscular atrophy
Hereditary motor and sensory neuropathy (HMSN)
Idiopathic dominantly inherited hypertrophic polyneuropathy

ICD-9-CM CODES
356.1 Charcot-Marie-Tooth disease, paralysis, or syndrome

EPIDEMIOLOGY AND DEMOGRAPHICS
PREDOMINANT AGE: Onset usually 10 to 20 yr but can be delayed to 50 to 60 yr
PREDOMINANT SEX: Male:female ratio of 3:1

PHYSICAL FINDINGS
- Variable presentation from family to family but affected individuals in a family tend to have similar symptomatology
- Usually, gradual onset, with slowly progressive disorder
- Foot deformity producing a high arch (cavus) and hammer toes
- Atrophy of the lower legs producing a stork-like appearance (muscle wasting does not involve the upper legs)
- Nerve enlargement
- Sensory loss or other neurologic signs, although the sensory involvement is usually mild
- Scoliosis
- Decreased proprioception that often interferes with balance and gait
- Painful paresthesias
- In late cases, possible involvment of hands
- Absence of DTRs in many cases
- Poorly healing foot ulcers in some patients

ETIOLOGY
Chronic segmental demyelination of peripheral nerves with hypertrophic changes caused by remyelination

DIAGNOSIS

DIFFERENTIAL DIAGNOSIS
- Other inherited neuropathies
- Toxic, metabolic, and nutritional polyneuropathies

WORKUP
- The Early onset, slow progression, and familial nature of the disorder is usually sufficient to establish diagnosis.
- Electrophysiologic studies are often diagnostic and may also be helpful in defining various subtypes of this group of neuropathies.
- Occasionally, muscle and nerve (sural) biopsy may be required.

TREATMENT

ACUTE GENERAL Rx
- Genetic counseling
- Supportive physical therapy and occupational therapy
- Prevention of injury to limbs with diminished sensibility
- Bracing

CHRONIC Rx
Occasionally, surgery to add stability and restore a plantigrade foot

DISPOSITION
- Disability is usually mild and compatible with a long life.
- 10% to 20% of patients are asymptomatic
- A small number of cases are nonambulators by the sixth or seventh decades.

REFERRAL
- For orthopedic consultation for bracing and treatment of deformity
- For genetic counseling

MISCELLANEOUS

COMMENTS
Patient information on Charcot-Marie-Tooth disease is available from the Muscular Dystrophy Association, 3300 East Sunrise Drive, Tucson, Arizona 85718; phone: 1-800-572-1717.

REFERENCES
Harding, AE: From the syndrome of Charcot, Marie, and Tooth to disorders of peripheral myelin proteins, *Brain* 118(3):809, 1995.
Ionasescu, VV: Charcot-Marie-Tooth neuropathies: from clinical description to molecular genetics, *Muscle Nerve*, 18(3):267, 1995.

Author: **Lonnie R. Mercier, M.D.**

Chickenpox (PTG)

BASIC INFORMATION

DEFINITION
Chickenpox is a common illness characterized by acute onset of diffuse papulovesicular rash.

SYNONYMS
Varicella

ICD-9-CM CODES
052.9 Varicella

EPIDEMIOLOGY AND DEMOGRAPHICS
- The incubation period of chickenpox ranges from 9 to 21 days.
- Peak incidence is in the springtime.
- The predominant age is 5 to 10 yr.
- Infectious period begins 2 days before onset of clinical symptoms and lasts until all lesions have crusted.
- Most patients will have lifelong immunity following an attack of chickenpox; protection from chickenpox following varicella vaccine is approximately six yr.

PHYSICAL FINDINGS
- Findings vary with the clinical course. Initial symptoms consist of fever, chills, backache, generalized malaise, and headache.
- Symptoms are generally more severe in adults.
- Initial lesions generally occur on the trunk (centripetal distribution); these lesions consist primarily of a 3- to 4-mm red papules with an irregular outline and a clear vesicle on the surface (dew drop on a rose petal appearance).
- Intense pruritus generally accompanies this stage.
- New lesion development generally ceases by the fourth day with subsequent crusting by the sixth day.
- Lesions generally spread to the face and the extremities (centrifugal spread).
- Patients generally present with lesions at different stages at the same time (see color plate 4).
- Crusts generally fall off within 5 to 14 days.
- Fever is usually highest during the eruption of the vesicles; temperature generally returns to normal following disappearance of vesicles.
- Signs of potential complications (e.g., bacterial skin infections, neurologic complications, pneumonia, hepatitis) may be present on physical examination.
- Mild constitutional symptoms (e.g., anorexia, myalgias, headaches, restlessness) may be present (most common in adults).
- Excoriations may be present if scratching is prominent.

ETIOLOGY
Varicella-zoster virus is a human herpesvirus III that can manifest with either varicella or herpes zoster (i.e., shingles, which is a reactivation of varicella).

DIAGNOSIS

DIFFERENTIAL DIAGNOSIS
- Other viral infection (see Section II, Table 2-21 for differential diagnosis of exanthems)
- Impetigo
- Scabies
- Drug rash
- Urticaria
- Dermatitis herpetiformis

WORKUP
Diagnosis is usually made based on patient's history and clinical presentation.

LABORATORY TESTS
- Laboratory evaluation is generally not necessary.
- CBC may reveal leukopenia and thrombocytopenia.
- Serum varicella titers (significant rise in serum varicella IgG antibody level), skin biopsy, or Tzanck smear are used only when diagnosis is in question.

TREATMENT

NONPHARMACOLOGIC THERAPY
- Use antipruritic lotions for symptomatic relief.
- Avoid scratching to prevent excoriations and superficial skin infections.
- Use a mild soap for bathing, hands should be washed often.

ACUTE GENERAL Rx
- Use acetaminophen for fever and myalgias; aspirin should be avoided because of the increased risk of Reye's syndrome.
- Oral acyclovir (20 mg/kg qid for 5 days) initiated at the earliest sign (within 24 hr of illness) is useful in healthy, nonpregnant individuals 13 yr of age or older to decrease the duration and severity of signs and symptoms. Immunocompromised hosts should be treated with IV acyclovir 500 mg/m^2 or 10 mg/kg q8h IV for 7 to 10 days.
- Varicella-zoster immunoglobulin (VZIG) is effective in preventing chickenpox in susceptible individuals. Dose is 12.5 U/kg IM (up to a maximum of 625 U). May repeat dose 3 wk later if the exposure persists; VZIG must be administered as early as possible after presumed exposure.
- Varicella vaccine is available for children and adults; protection lasts at least 6 yr. Patients with HIV or other immunocompromised patients should not receive the live attenuated vaccine.
- Pruritus from chickenpox can be controlled with antihistamines (e.g., hydroxyzine 25 mg q6h) and oral antipruritic lotions (e.g., calamine).
- Oral antibiotics are not routinely indicated and should be used only in patients with secondary infection and infected lesions (most common infective organisms are *Streptococcus* sp. and *Staphylococcus* sp.).

DISPOSITION
- The course is generally benign in immunocompetent adults and children.
- Infants who develop chickenpox are incapable of controlling the infection and should be given varicella-zoster immunoglobulin or γ-globulin if VZIG is not available.

REFERRAL
Hospitalization and IV acyclovir is recommended in immunocompromised patients with chickenpox and in patients who develop neurologic complications or pneumonia.

MISCELLANEOUS

COMMENTS
- VZIG can be obtained from the nearest regional Red Cross Blood Center or the Center for Disease Control and Prevention in Atlanta, Georgia.
- Varicella immunization (Varivax) is recommended for all who have not had chickenpox; dose for adults and adolescents (≥13 yr old) is two 0.5-ml doses 4 to 8 wk apart.

REFERENCES
Enders G et al: Consequences of varicella and herpes zoster in pregnancy: perspective study of 1709 cases, *Lancet* 343:1548, 1994.

Habif TP: *Clinical dermatology*, ed 3, St Louis, 1996, Mosby.

Author: **Fred F. Ferri, M.D.**

Chlamydia genital infections (PTG)

BASIC INFORMATION

DEFINITION
Genital infection with *Chlamydia trachomatis* may result in urethritis, epididymitis, cervicitis, and acute salpingitis, but often it is asymptomatic in women (see "Pelvic inflammatory disease").

ICD-9-CM CODES
597.80 Urethritis
604.0 Epididymitis
616.0 Cervicitis
381.51 Acute salpingitis

EPIDEMIOLOGY AND DEMOGRAPHICS
- *Chlamydia trachomatis* is the most common cause of sexually transmitted disease in the U.S. Over 4,000,000 infections occur annually, although the exact number is unknown because reporting is not required in all states. Occurrence is common worldwide, and recognition has been increasing steadily over the last two decades in the U.S., Canada, Australia, and Europe.
- Most women with endocervical or urethral infections are asymptomatic.
- Up to 45% of cases of gonococcal infection may have concomitant chlamydial infection.
- Infertility or ectopic pregnancy can result as a complication from symptomatic or asymptomatic chronic infections of the endometrium and fallopian tubes.
- Conjunctival and pneumonic infection of the newborn may result from infection in pregnancy.

PHYSICAL FINDINGS
Clinical manifestations may be similar to those of gonorrhea: mucopurulent endocervical discharge, with edema, erythema and easily induced endocervical bleeding caused by inflammation of endocervical columnar epithelium. Less frequent manifestations may include bartholinitis, urethral syndrome with dysuria and pyuria, perihepatitis (Fitz-Hugh-Curtis syndrome).

ETIOLOGY
- *Chlamydia trachomatis*, serotypes D through K
- Obligate, intracellular bacteria

DIAGNOSIS

DIFFERENTIAL DIAGNOSIS
Gonorrhea, nongonococcal urethritis (nonchlamydial etiologies)

WORKUP
Diagnosis based on laboratory demonstration of evidence of infection in intraurethral or endocervical swab by various tests. The intracellular organism is less readily recovered from the discharge.

LABORATORY TESTS
- Cell culture is the reference method for diagnosis (single culture sensitivity 80% to 90%), but it is labor intensive and takes 48 to 96 hr; it is not suited for large screening programs
- Nonculture methods:
  Direct fluorescent antibody (DFA) tests
  Enzyme immunoassay (EIA)
  DNA probes
  Polymerase chain reaction (PCR)
- With the exception of PCR, the other tests are probably less specific than cell culture and may yield false-positive results.
- Since this is an intracellular organism, purulent discharge is not an appropriate specimen. An adequate sample of infected cells must be obtained.

TREATMENT

Urethritis, cervicitis, conjunctivitis (except for LGV):
- Azithromycin 1 g oral × 1 *or*
- Doxycycline 100 mg PO bid for 7 days
- Alternatives:
  1. Ofloxacin 300 mg PO bid for 7 days
  2. Erythromycin 500 mg PO qid for 7 days

Infection in pregnancy:
- Erythromycin 500 mg PO qid for 7 days
- Alternatives:
  1. Amoxicillin 500 mg PO tid for 10 days
  2. Azithromycin 1 g oral x 1

DISPOSITION
See "Gonorrhea." In all patients being treated for chlamydia, presumptive treatment for concomitant infection with gonorrhea should be done. Also see "Treatment" in "Pelvic inflammatory disease."

MISCELLANEOUS

COMMENTS
U.S. Preventive Services Task Force Recommendations on counseling to prevent HIV infection and other STDs are described in Section V, Chapter 62.

REFERENCES
Benenson AS (ed): *Control of communicable diseases in man,* ed 15, Washington, DC, 1990, American Public Health Association.
Drugs for sexually transmitted diseases, *Med Lett Drugs Ther* 37(964): 117, 1995.
Weber, Johnson: New treatments for *Chlamydia trachomatis* genital infection, *Clin Infect Dis* 20(suppl 1):S66. 1995.
Woods GL: Update on laboratory diagnosis of sexually transmitted diseases, *Clin Lab Med* 15(3):665, 1995.

Author: **Eugene J. Louie-Ng, M.D.**

Cholangitis

BASIC INFORMATION

DEFINITION
Cholangitis refers to an inflammation and/or infection of the hepatic and common bile ducts associated with obstruction of the common bile duct.

SYNONYMS
Biliary sepsis
Ascending cholangitis
Suppurative cholangitis

ICD-9-CM CODES
576.1 Cholangitis

EPIDEMIOLOGY AND DEMOGRAPHICS
INCIDENCE (IN U.S.): Complicates approximately 1% of cases of cholelithiasis
PREVALENCE (IN U.S.): <2 cases/1000 hospital admissions
PREDOMINANT SEX:
- Females, for cholangitis secondary to gallstones
- Males, for cholangitis secondary to malignant obstruction and HIV infection

PREDOMINANT AGE: Seventh decade and older; unusual <50 yr of age
PEAK INCIDENCE: Seventh decade

PHYSICAL FINDINGS
- Usually acute onset of fever, chills, abdominal pain, jaundice, and tenderness over the RUQ of the abdomen
- All signs and symptoms in only 50% to 85% of patients
- Often, dark coloration of the urine resulting from bilirubinuria
- Complications:
  1. Bacteremia (50%) and septic shock
  2. Hepatic abscess and pancreatitis

ETIOLOGY
Obstruction of the common bile duct causing rapid proliferation of bacteria in the biliary tree
- Most common cause of common bile duct obstruction: stones, usually migrated from the gallbladder
- Other causes: prior biliary tract surgery with secondary stenosis, tumor (usually arising from the pancreas or biliary tree), and parasitic infections from *Ascaris lumbricoides* or *Fasciola hepatica*
- Iatrogenic after contamination of an obstructed biliary tree by endoscopic retrograde cholangiopancreatoscopy (ERCP) or percutaneous transhepatic cholangiography (PTC)
- Primary sclerosing cholangitis (PSC)
- HIV-associated sclerosing cholangitis: associated with infection by CMV, cryptosporidium, *Microsporida*, and *Mycobacterium avium* complex

DIAGNOSIS

DIFFERENTIAL DIAGNOSIS
- Biliary colic
- Acute cholecystitis
- Liver abscess
- PUD
- Pancreatitis
- Intestinal obstruction
- Right kidney stone
- Hepatitis
- Pyelonephritis

WORKUP
- Blood cultures
- CBC
- Liver function tests

LABORATORY TESTS
- Usually, elevated WBC count with a predominance of polynuclear forms
- Elevated alkaline phosphatase and bilirubin in chronic obstruction
- Elevated transaminases in acute obstruction
- Positive blood cultures in 50% of cases, typically with enteric gram-negative aerobes (e.g., *E. coli*, *Klebsiella pneumonia*), enterococci, or anaerobes

IMAGING STUDIES
- Ultrasound:
  1. Allows visualization of the gallbladder and bile ducts to differentiate extrahepatic obstruction from intrahepatic cholestasis
  2. Insensitive but specific for visualization of common duct stones
- CT scan:
  1. Less accurate for gallstones
  2. More sensitive than ultrasound for visualization of the distal common bile duct
  3. Also allows better definition of neoplasm
- ERCP:
  1. Confirms obstruction and its level
  2. Allows collection of specimens for culture and cytology
  3. Indicated for diagnosis if ultrasound and CT scan are inconclusive
  4. May be indicated in therapy (see "Treatment")

TREATMENT

NONPHARMACOLOGIC THERAPY
Biliary decompression
- May be urgent in severely ill patients or those unresponsive to medical therapy within 12 to 24 hr
- May also be performed semielectively in patients who respond

- Options:
  1. ERCP with or without sphincterotomy or placement of a draining stent
  2. Percutaneous transhepatic biliary drainage for the acutely ill patient who is a poor surgical candidate
  3. Surgical exploration of the common bile duct

ACUTE GENERAL Rx
- Nothing by mouth
- Intravenous hydration
- Broad-spectrum antibiotics directed at gram-negative enteric organisms, anaerobes, and enterococcus: if infection nosocomial or the patient in shock, strong consideration of broader coverage to include hospital organisms such as *Pseudomonas aeruginosa*, resistant *Staphylococcus aureus*, and others

CHRONIC Rx
Repeated decompression may be necessary, particularly when obstruction is related to neoplasm.

DISPOSITION
Excellent prognosis if obstruction amenable to definitive surgical therapy, otherwise relapses are common.

REFERRAL
- To biliary endoscopist if obstruction is from stones or a stent needs to be placed
- To interventional radiologist if external drainage is necessary
- To a general surgeon in all other cases
- To an infectious disease specialist if blood cultures are positive or the patient is in shock or otherwise severely ill

MISCELLANEOUS

REFERENCES
Levison ME, Bush LM: Peritonitis and other intraabdominal infections. In Mandell GL, Bennett JE, Dolin R (eds): *Mandell, Douglas, and Bennett's principles and practice of infectious diseases*, New York, 1995, Churchill Livingstone.

Nash JA, Cohen SA: The gallbladder and biliary tract in the acquired immunodeficiency syndrome, *Gastroenterol Clin North Am* 26 (2):323, 1997.

Reese RE, Hruska JF: Gastrointestinal and intraabdominal infections. In Reese RE, Betts RF (eds): *A practical approach to infectious diseases*, Boston, 1996, Little, Brown.

Author: **Michele Halpern, M.D.**

Cholecystitis

BASIC INFORMATION

DEFINITION
Cholecystitis is an acute or chronic inflammation of the gallbladder generally secondary to gallstones (>95% of cases)

SYNONYMS
Gallbladder attack

ICD-9-CM CODES
575.0 Acute cholecystitis
574.0 Calculus of the gallbladder with acute cholecystitis
575.1 Cholecystitis without mention of calculus

EPIDEMIOLOGY AND DEMOGRAPHICS
- Acute cholecystitis occurs most commonly in females during the fifth and sixth decades.
- The incidence of gallstones is 0.6% in the general population and much higher in certain ethnic groups (>75% of Native Americans by age 60 yr).

PHYSICAL FINDINGS
- Pain and tenderness in the right hypochondrium or epigastrium; pain possibly radiating to the infrascapular region
- Palpation of the RUQ eliciting marked tenderness and stoppage of inspired breath (Murphy's sign)
- Guarding
- Fever (33%) and vomiting
- Jaundice (25% to 50% of patients)
- Palpable gallbladder (20% of cases)
- Nausea and vomiting (>70% of patients)
- Fever and chills (>25% of patients)
- Medical history often revealing ingestion of large, fatty meals before onset of pain in the epigastrium and RUQ

ETIOLOGY
- Gallstones (>95% of cases)
- Ischemic damage to the gallbladder, critically ill patient (acalculous cholecystitis)
- Infectious agents, especially in patients with AIDS (CMV, cryptosporidium)
- Strictures of the bile duct
- Neoplasms, primary or metastatic

DIAGNOSIS

DIFFERENTIAL DIAGNOSIS
- Hepatic: hepatitis, abscess, hepatic congestion, neoplasm, trauma
- Biliary: neoplasm, stricture
- Gastric: PUD, pyloric stenosis, neoplasm, alcoholic gastritis, hiatal hernia
- Pancreatic: pancreatitis, neoplasm, stone in the pancreatic duct or ampulla
- Renal: calculi, infection, inflammation, neoplasm, ruptured kidney
- Pulmonary: pneumonia, pulmonary infarction, right-sided pleurisy
- Intestinal: retrocecal appendicitis, intestinal obstruction, high fecal impaction
- Cardiac: myocardial ischemia (particularly involving the inferior wall), pericarditis
- Cutaneous: herpes zoster
- Trauma
- Fitz-Hugh-Curtis syndrome (perihepatitis)
- Subphrenic abscess
- Dissecting aneurysm
- Nerve root irritation caused by osteoarthritis of the spine

WORKUP
Laboratory evaluation and imaging studies

LABORATORY TESTS
- Leukocytosis (12,000 to 20,000) is present in >70% of patients.
- Elevated alkaline phosphatase, ALT, AST, bilirubin; bilirubin elevation >4 mg/dl is unusual and suggests presence of choledocholithiasis.
- Elevated amylase may be present (consider pancreatitis if serum amylase elevation exceeds 500 U).

IMAGING STUDIES
- Nuclear imaging (HIDA scan): sensitivity and specificity exceed 90% for acute cholecystis. This test is only reliable when bilirubin is <5 mg/dl. A positive test will demonstrate obstruction of the cystic or common hepatic duct; the test will not demonstrate the presence of stones.
- Ultrasound of the gallbladder will demonstrate the presence of stones and also dilated gallbladder with thickened wall and surrounding edema in patients with acute cholecystitis.
- CT scan of abdomen is useful in cases of suspected abscess, neoplasm, or pancreatitis.
- Plain film of the abdomen generally is not useful, since <25% of stones are radiopaque.

TREATMENT

NONPHARMACOLOGIC THERAPY
Provide IV hydration, withhold oral feedings.

ACUTE GENERAL Rx
- Cholecystectomy (laparoscopic is preferred, open cholecystectomy is acceptable); conservative management with IV fluids and antibiotics may be justified in some high-risk patients in order to convert an emergency procedure into an elective one with a lower mortality.
- ERCP with sphincterectomy and stone extraction can be performed in conjunction with laparoscopic cholecystectomy for patients with choledochal lithiasis; approximately 7% to 15% of patients with cholelithiasis also have stones in the common bile duct.
- IV fluids, broad-spectrum antibiotics, pain management (meperidine PRN) should be used.

DISPOSITION
- Prognosis is good; elective laparoscopic cholecystectomy can be performed as outpatient procedure.
- Hospital stay (when necessary) varies from overnight with laparoscopic cholecystectomy to 4 to 7 days with open cholecystectomy.
- Complication rate is approximately 1% (hemorrhage and bile leak) for laparoscopic cholecystectomy and <0.5% (infection) with open cholecystectomy.

REFERRAL
Hospitalization and surgical referral in all patients with acute cholecystitis

MISCELLANEOUS

COMMENTS
Patients should be instructed that stones may recur in bile ducts.

REFERENCES
Barrie PS, Fischer E: Acute acalculous cholecystitis, *J Am Coll Surg* 180:232, 1995.
Gruber PJ et al: Presence of fever and leukocytosis in acute cholecystitis, *Ann Emerg Med* 28:273, 1996.
Hobbs KEF: Laparoscopic cholecystectomy, *Gut* 36:161, 1995.
Johnston DE, Kaplan MN: Pathogenesis and treatment of gallstones, *New Engl J Med* 238:412, 1993.

Author: **Fred F. Ferri, M.D.**

Cholelithiasis (PTG)

BASIC INFORMATION

DEFINITION
Cholelithiasis is the presence of stones in the gallbladder.

SYNONYMS
Gallstones

ICD-9-CM CODES
574.2 Calculus of the gallbladder without mention of cholecystitis
574.0 Calculus of the gallbladder with acute cholecystitis

EPIDEMIOLOGY AND DEMOGRAPHICS
- Gallstone disease can be found in 20,000,000 Americans. Of these, 2% to 3% (500,000 to 600,000) are treated with cholecystectomies each year.
- Annual medical expenditures for gallbladder surgeries in the U.S. exceed $5,000,000,000.
- Incidence of gallbladder disease increases with age. Highest incidence is in the fifth and sixth decades. Predisposing factors for gallstones are female sex, pregnancy, age >40 yr, family history of gallstones, obesity, ileal disease, oral contraceptives, diabetes mellitus, rapid weight loss, estrogen replacement therapy, ethnicity (e.g., Native American).
- Patients with gallstones have a 20% chance of developing biliary colic or its complications at the end of a 20-yr period.

PHYSICAL FINDINGS
- Physical examination is entirely normal unless patient is having a biliary colic; 80% of gallstones are asymptomatic.
- Typical symptoms of obstruction of the cystic duct include intermittent, severe, cramping pain affecting the RUQ.
- Pain occurs mostly at night and may radiate to the back or right shoulder. It can last from a few minutes to several hours.

ETIOLOGY
- 75% of gallstones contain cholesterol and are usually associated with obesity, female sex, diabetes mellitus; mixed stones are most common (80%), pure cholesterol stones account for only 10% of stones.
- 25% of gallstones are pigment stones (bilirubin, calcium, and variable organic material) associated with hemolysis and cirrhosis. These tend to be black pigment stones that are refractory to medical therapy.
- 50% of mixed-type stones are radiopaque.

DIAGNOSIS

DIFFERENTIAL DIAGNOSIS
- PUD
- GERD
- IBD
- Pancreatitis
- Neoplasms
- Nonulcer dyspepsia

LABORATORY TESTS
Generally normal unless patient has biliary obstruction (elevated alkaline phosphatase, bilirubin).

IMAGING STUDIES
- Ultrasound of the gallbladder will detect small stones and biliary sludge (sensitivity, 95%; specificity, 90%); the presence of dilated gallbladder with thickened wall is suggestive of acute cholecystitis.
- Nuclear imaging (HIDA scan) can confirm acute cholecystitis (>90% accuracy) if gallbladder does not visualize within 4 hr of injection and the radioisotope is excreted in the common bile duct.

TREATMENT

NONPHARMACOLOGIC THERAPY
Life-style changes (avoidance of diets high in polyunsaturated fats, weight loss—however, avoid rapid weight loss—in obese patients)

ACUTE GENERAL Rx
- The management of gallstones is affected by the clinical presentation.
- Asymptomatic patients do not require therapeutic intervention.
- Surgical intervention is generally the ideal approach for symptomatic patients. Laparoscopic cholecystectomy is generally preferred over open cholecystectomy because of the shorter recovery period.
- Patients who are not appropriate candidates for surgery because of co-existing illness or patients who refuse surgery can be treated with oral bile salts: ursodiol (Actigall) 8 to 10 mg/kg/day in two to three divided doses, for 16 to 20 mo or chenodiol (Chenix) 250 mg bid initially, increasing gradually to a dose of 60 mg/kg qd. Candidates for oral bile salts are patients with cholesterol stones (radiolucent, noncalcified stones), with a diameter of ≤ 15 mm and having three or fewer stones.
- Direct solvent dissolution with methyl *tert*- butyl ether (MTBE) can be used in patients with multiple stones with diameter ≥3 cm; this method should be used only by physicians experienced with contact dissolution. Administration of the solvent is either through percutaneous transhepatic placement of a catheter into the gallbladder or endoscopic retrograde catheter placement with subsequent continuous infusion and aspiration of the solvent either manually or by automatic pump system. MTBE is a powerful cholesterol solvent and can dissolve stones in a few hours (>90% dissolution over a 12-hr infusion).
- Extracorporeal shock wave lithotripsy (ESWL) is another form of medical therapy. It can be used in patients with stone diameter of ≤ 3 cm and having three or fewer stones.
- Candidates for medical therapy must have a functioning gallbladder and must have absence of calcifications on CT scans.

DISPOSITION
- Recurrence rate after bile acid treatment is approximately 50% in 5 yr. Periodic ultrasound is necessary to assess the effectiveness of treatment.
- Gallstones recur after dissolution therapy with MTBE in >40% of patients within 5 yr.
- Following extracorporeal shock wave lithotripsy, stones recur in approximately 20% of patients after 4 yr.

REFERRAL
Surgical referral for cholecystectomy in symptomatic patients who are surgical candidates

MISCELLANEOUS

REFERENCES
Johnston DE, Kaplan MM: Pathogenesis and treatment of gallstones, *New Engl J Med* 328:412, 1993.
Nunez G et al: Strategies for nonsurgical management of gallstone disease, *Contemp Intern Med* 9:21, 1997.
Tait N, Little JM: The treatment of gallstones, *Br Med J* 311:99, 1995.
Author: **Fred F. Ferri, M.D.**

Cholera

BASIC INFORMATION

DEFINITION
Cholera is an acute diarrheal illness caused by *Vibrio cholerae*.

ICD-9-CM CODES
001 Cholera

EPIDEMIOLOGY AND DEMOGRAPHICS
INCIDENCE (IN U.S.): Approximately 50 cases/yr, mostly in travelers returning from endemic areas
PREDOMINANT AGE:
- In nonendemic areas, attack rates equal in all age groups
- In epidemic areas, children >2 yr old most commonly infected

PEAK INCIDENCE:
- None in the U.S.
- Summer and fall in endemic areas

GENETICS:
Neonatal Infection: Illness uncommon before age 2 yr, probably because of passive immunity

PHYSICAL FINDINGS
- Asymptomatic illness or a mild diarrhea
- Classic illness: abrupt onset of voluminous watery diarrhea, which may lead to severe dehydration, acidosis, shock, and death
- Vomiting early in the illness, but usually absence of fever and abdominal pain
- Typical "rice water" stools, pale with flecks of mucus and no blood
- Possibly prominent muscle cramps attributable to loss of fluid and electrolytes
- Untreated illness: results in hypovolemic shock and death in hours to days
- With adequate fluid and electrolyte repletion, a self-limited illness that resolves in a few days
- Antimicrobials to shorten the course of illness

ETIOLOGY
Responsible organism is one of several strains of *V. cholerae*, with most infections from the 01 serotype, the *El Tor* biotype.
- In U.S., one outbreak occurred from the ingestion of illegally imported crab, and sporadic infection has been associated with the consumption of contaminated shellfish in Gulf Coast states.
- Most cases occur in returning travelers.
- Transmission during epidemics results from ingestion of contaminated water and, in some instances, contaminated food.

DIAGNOSIS

DIFFERENTIAL DIAGNOSIS
- Mild illness mimicking gastroenteritis from a variety of etiologies
- Sudden, voluminous diarrhea causing marked dehydration uncommon in other illnesses

A differential diagnosis of infectious diseases in travelers is described in Table 2-36.

WORKUP
- Send stool for culture and microscopy.
- NOTE: Treatment should not be delayed while awaiting culture results.

LABORATORY TESTS
- Possibly elevated WBC count; increased Hgb as a result of hemoconcentration
- Elevated BUN and creatinine suggesting prerenal azotemia
- Hypoglycemia
- Stool cultures on appropriate media to grow the organism
- Wet mount of stool under dark-field or phase contrast microscopy to show organisms with characteristic darting motility

TREATMENT

NONPHARMACOLOGIC THERAPY
Adequate fluid and electrolyte replacement:
- Usually achieved using oral rehydration solutions containing salts and glucose
- IV fluid and electrolyte replacement sometimes required

ACUTE GENERAL Rx
Antimicrobial therapy to decrease shedding of fluid and organisms and shorten the course of illness:
- Doxycycline 100 mg PO bid for 5 days *or*
- Septra one DS tablet PO bid for 5 days

CHRONIC Rx
It is likely that asymptomatic chronic carriers exist, but since they are difficult to identify and their role in transmission of disease appears limited, there is no recommendation for treatment of these individuals.

DISPOSITION
Mortality of adequately hydrated patients is <1%.

REFERRAL
If more than mild illness occurs

MISCELLANEOUS

COMMENTS
- Currently, there is no indication for vaccination of travelers to endemic areas: the risk of infection is small, protection from available vaccines is limited, and side effects are prominent and frequent.
- Doxycycline should not be used to treat children or pregnant women.

REFERENCES
Seas C et al: Practical guidelines for the treatment of cholera, *Drugs* 51:966, 1996.

Author: **Maurice Policar, M.D.**

CLINICAL TOPICS   Chronic fatigue syndrome   119

BASIC INFORMATION

DEFINITION
Chronic fatigue syndrome (CFS) is characterized by four or more of the following symptoms, present concurrently for at least 6 mo:
- Impaired memory or concentration
- Sore throat
- Tender cervical or axillary lymph nodes
- Muscle pain
- Multijoint pain
- New headaches
- Unrefreshing sleep
- Postexertion malaise

SYNONYMS
Yuppie flu
CFS
Chronic Epstein-Barr syndrome

ICD-9-CM CODES
780.7 Chronic fatigue syndrome
300.8 Neurasthenia

EPIDEMIOLOGY AND DEMOGRAPHICS
PREVALENCE IN USA: 100 to 300 cases/100,000 persons
PREDOMINANT AGE: Young adulthood and middle age
PREDOMINANT SEX: Female > male

PHYSICAL FINDINGS
- There are no physical findings specific for CFS.
- The physical examination may be useful to identify fibromyalgia and other rheumatologic conditions that may coexist with CFS.

ETIOLOGY
- The etiology of CFS is unknown.
- Many experts suspect that a viral illness may trigger certain immune responses leading to the various symptoms. Most patients often report the onset of their symptoms with a flulike illness.
- Initial reports indicated a possible role for Epstein-Barr virus, but subsequent studies disproved this theory.

DIAGNOSIS

DIFFERENTIAL DIAGNOSIS
- Psychosocial: depression, dysthymia, anxiety-related disorders, and other psychiatric diseases
- Infectious diseases (SBE, Lyme disease, fungal diseases, mononucleosis, HIV, chronic hepatitis B or C, TB, chronic parasitic infections
- Autoimmune diseases: SLE, myasthenia gravis, multiple sclerosis, thyroiditis, RA
- Endocrine abnormalities: hypothyroidism, hypopituitarism, adrenal insufficiency, Cushing's syndrome, diabetes mellitus, hyperparathyroidism, pregnancy, reactive hypoglycemia
- Occult malignant disease
- Substance abuse
- Systemic disorders: chronic renal failure, COPD, cardiovascular disease, anemia, electrolyte abnormalities, liver disease
- Other: inadequate rest, sleep apnea, narcolepsy, fibromyalgia, sarcoidosis, medications, toxic agent exposure, Wegener's granulomatosis

WORKUP
Because CFS is a clinical diagnosis and the symptoms are generally subjective, the history and physical examination are essential for excluding other causes of fatigue. A detailed mental status examination is necessary. Abnormalities should be further evaluated with appropriate psychiatric, psychologic, or neurologic examination.

LABORATORY TESTS
- No specific laboratory tests exist for diagnosing CFS. Initial laboratory tests are useful to exclude other conditions that may mimic or may be associated with CFS.
  1. Screening laboratory tests: CBC, ESR, ALT, total protein, albumin, globulin, alkaline phosphatase, calcium, phosphorus, glucose, BUN, creatinine, electrolytes, TSH, and urinalysis are useful.
  2. Serologic tests for Epstein-Barr virus, *Candida albicans*, human herpesvirus 6, and other studies for immune cellular abnormalities are not useful; these tests are expensive and generally not recommended.
- Other tests may be indicated depending on the history and physical examination (e.g., ANA, RF in patients presenting with joint complaints or abnormalities on physical examination).

IMAGING STUDIES
Generally not recommended unless history and physical examination indicate specific abnormalities (e.g., chest x-ray examination in any patient suspected of TB or sarcoidosis)

TREATMENT

NONPHARMACOLOGIC THERAPY
- Education and counseling help to develop realistic goals and expectations.
- Support groups (see below) are useful.
- Patients should be reassured that the illness is not fatal and that most patients improve over time.
- An initially supervised exercise program to preserve and increase strength is beneficial for most patients.

ACUTE GENERAL Rx
Therapy is generally palliative. The following medications may be helpful:
- Antidepressants: The choice of antidepressant varies with the desired side effects. Patients with difficulty sleeping or fibromyalgia-like symptoms may benefit from low-dose tricyclics (doxepin 10 mg hs or amitriptyline 25 mg qhs). When sedation is not desirable, low-dose SSRIs (sertraline 50 mg qd) often help alleviate fatigue and associated symptoms.
- NSAIDs can be used to relieve muscle and joint pain and headaches.
- Fludrocortisone is useful in the subset of CFS patients with associated neurally-mediated hypotension. "Alternative" medications (herbs, multivitamins, nutritional supplements) are very popular with many CFS patients but are generally not very helpful.

CHRONIC Rx
Psychiatric referral and treatment is helpful in coping with the disease in the majority of patients.

DISPOSITION
Moderate to complete recovery at 1 yr occurs in 22% to 60% of patients with CFS.

MISCELLANEOUS

COMMENTS
Patient support and literature can be obtained from the National CFS Association, 3521 Broadway, Kansas City, MO 64111 or the American Association for Chronic Fatigue Syndrome, Box 895, Olney, MD 20830.

REFERENCES
Buchwald D et al: Chronic fatigue and the chronic fatigue syndrome: prevalence in a Pacific Northwest health care system, *Ann Intern Med* 123:81, 1995.
Fukuda K et al: The chronic fatigue syndrome: a comprehensive approach to its definition and study, *Ann Intern Med* 121:953, 1994.
Author: **Fred F. Ferri, M.D.**

Chronic obstructive pulmonary disease (PTG)

BASIC INFORMATION

DEFINITION
Chronic obstructive pulmonary disease (COPD) is a disorder characterized by the presence of airway obstruction. Patients with COPD are classically subdivided in two major groups based on their appearance:
1. "Blue bloaters" are patients with chronic bronchitis; the name is derived from the bluish tinge of the skin (secondary to chronic hypoxemia and hypercapnia) and from the frequent presence of peripheral edema (secondary to cor pulmonale); chronic cough with production of large amounts of sputum is characteristic.
2. "Pink puffers" are patients with emphysema; they have a cachectic appearance but pink skin color (adequate oxygen saturation); shortness of breath is manifested by pursed-lip breathing and use of accessory muscles of respiration.

SYNONYMS
COPD
Emphysema
Chronic bronchitis

ICD-9-CM CODES
496 COPD
492.8 Emphysema

EPIDEMIOLOGY AND DEMOGRAPHICS
- COPD affects 15,000,000 Americans and is responsible for >80,000 deaths/yr.
- Highest incidence is in males >40 yr.

PHYSICAL FINDINGS
- Blue bloaters (chronic bronchitis): peripheral cyanosis, productive cough, tachypnea, tachycardia
- Pink puffers (emphysema): dyspnea, pursed-lip breathing with use of accessory muscles for respiration, decreased breath sounds
- Possible wheezing in both patients with chronic bronchitis and emphysema
- Features of both chronic bronchitis and emphysema in many patients with COPD

ETIOLOGY
- Tobacco abuse
- Occupational exposure to pulmonary toxins
- Atmospheric pollution
- α-1 antitrypsin deficiency (rare)

DIAGNOSIS

DIFFERENTIAL DIAGNOSIS
- CHF
- Asthma
- Respiratory infections
- Bronchiectasis
- Cystic fibrosis
- Neoplasm
- Pulmonary embolism
- Sleep apnea, obstructive
- Hypothyroidism

WORKUP
Chest x-ray examination, pulmonary function testing, blood gases (in patients with acute exacerbation)

LABORATORY TESTS
- CBC may reveal leukocytosis with "shift to the left" during acute exacerbation.
- Sputum may be purulent with bacterial respiratory tract infections.
- ABGs: normocapnia, mild to moderate hypoxemia may be present.
- α-1 antitrypsin level is low in patients with α-1 antitrypsin deficiency (do not order this test routinely).
- Pulmonary function testing: abnormal diffusing capacity, increased total lung capacity and/or residual volume, fixed reduction in FEV_1 are present with emphysema; normal diffusing capacity, reduced FEV_1 are present with chronic bronchitis.

IMAGING STUDIES
Chest x-ray examination:
- Hyperinflation with flattened diaphragm, tenting of the diaphragm at the rib, and increased retrosternal chest space
- Decreased vascular markings and bullae in patients with emphysema
- Thickened bronchial markings and enlarged right side of the heart in patients with chronic bronchitis

TREATMENT

NONPHARMACOLOGIC THERAPY
- Weight loss in patients with chronic bronchitis
- Avoidance of tobacco use and elimination of air pollutants
- Oxygen therapy on a PRN basis

ACUTE GENERAL Rx
- Acute exacerbation of COPD can be treated with:
  1. Aerosolized β-agonists (e.g., metaproterenol, isoetharine) or SC administration of epinephrine or terbutaline 0.1 to 0.5 ml
  2. Inhaled solution of ipratropium 0.5 mg q4-8h
  3. IV aminophylline
  4. IV methylprednisolone 50- to 100-mg bolus, then q6-8h; taper as soon as possible.
  5. Judicious oxygen administration (hypercapnia and further respiratory compromise may occur after high-flow oxygen therapy); use of a Venturi-type mask delivering an inspired oxygen fraction of 24% to 28% is preferred to nasal cannula.
  6. Noninvasive positive pressure ventilation delivered by a facial or nasal mask in the treatment of chronic restrictive thoracic disease may obviate the need for intratracheal intubation.
- Antibiotics are indicated in suspected respiratory infection.
  1. *Hemophilus influenzae, Streptococcus pneumoniae* are frequent causes of acute bronchitis.
  2. Oral antibiotics of choice are ampicillin, TMP-SMX, doxycycline, cefuroxime, or cefaclor.
  3. The use of antibiotics is beneficial in exacerbations of COPD presenting with increased dyspnea and sputum purulence (especially if the patient is febrile).
- Guaifenesin can improve cough symptoms and mucus clearance.
- Pulmonary toilet: careful nasotracheal suction is indicated in patients with excessive secretions and inability to expectorate.
- Intubation and mechanical ventilation may be necessary if above measures fail to provide improvement.

DISPOSITION
- Following the initial episode of respiratory failure, 5-yr survival is approximately 25%.
- Development of cor pulmonale or hypercapnia and persistent tachycardia are poor prognostic indicators.

MISCELLANEOUS

COMMENTS
- All patients with COPD should receive pneumococcal vaccine and yearly influenza vaccine.
- Patient education material on COPD can be obtained from the American Lung Association, 1740 Broadway, New York, NY 10019.

REFERENCES
American Thoracic Society: Standards for the diagnosis and cure of patients with chronic obstructive pulmonary disease, *Am J Resp Care Med* 152:S120, 1995.
Ball P: Epidemiology and treatment of chronic bronchitis and its exacerbations, *Chest* 108:43, 1995.

Author: **Fred F. Ferri, M.D.**

Cirrhosis (PTG)

BASIC INFORMATION

DEFINITION
Cirrhosis is defined histologically as the presence of fibrosis and regenerative nodules in the liver. It can be classified as micronodular, macronodular, and mixed; however, each form may be seen in the same patient at different stages of the disease. Cirrhosis manifests clinically with portal hypertension, hepatic encephalopathy, and variceal bleeding.

ICD-9-CM CODES
571.5 Cirrhosis of the liver
571.2 Cirrhosis of the liver secondary to alcohol

EPIDEMIOLOGY AND DEMOGRAPHICS
- Cirrhosis is the eleventh leading cause of death in the U.S. (death rate 9 deaths/100,000 persons/yr).
- Alcohol abuse and viral hepatitis are the major causes of cirrhosis in the U.S.

PHYSICAL FINDINGS
SKIN: Jaundice, palmar erythema (alcohol abuse), spider angiomata, ecchymosis (thrombocytopenia or coagulation factor deficiency), dilated superficial periumbilical vein (caput medusae), increased pigmentation (hemochromatosis), xanthomas (primary biliary cirrhosis), needle tracks (viral hepatitis)
EYES: Kayser-Fleischer rings (corneal copper deposition seen in Wilson's disease; best diagnosed with slit lamp examination), scleral icterus
BREATH: Fetor hepaticus (musty odor of breath and urine found in cirrhosis with hepatic failure)
CHEST: Possible gynecomastia in men
ABDOMEN: Tender hepatomegaly (congestive hepatomegaly), small, nodular liver (cirrhosis), palpable, nontender gallbladder (neoplastic extrahepatic biliary obstruction), palpable spleen (portal hypertension), venous hum auscultated over periumbilical veins (portal hypertension), ascites (portal hypertension, hypoalbuminemia)
RECTAL EXAMINATION: Hemorrhoids (portal hypertension), guaiac-positive stools (alcoholic gastritis, bleeding esophageal varices, PUD, bleeding hemorrhoids)
GENITALIA: Testicular atrophy in males (chronic liver disease, hemachromatosis)
EXTREMITIES: Pedal edema (hypoalbuminemia, failure of right side of the heart), arthropathy (hemachromatosis)
NEUROLOGIC: Flapping tremor, asterixis (hepatic encephalopathy), choreoathetosis, dysarthria (Wilson's disease)

ETIOLOGY
- Alcohol abuse
- Secondary biliary cirrhosis, obstruction of the common bile duct (stone, stricture, pancreatitis, neoplasm, sclerosing cholangitis)
- Drugs (e.g., acetaminophen, isoniazid, methotrexate, methyldopa)
- Hepatic congestion (e.g., CHF, constrictive pericarditis, tricuspid insufficiency, thrombosis of the hepatic vein, obstruction of the vena cava)
- Primary biliary cirrhosis
- Hemochromatosis
- Chronic active hepatitis caused by hepatitis B or C
- Wilson's disease
- α-1 antitrypsin deficiency
- Infiltrative diseases (amyloidosis, glycogen storage diseases, hemachromatosis)
- Nutritional: jejunoileal bypass
- Others: parasitic infections (schistosomiasis), idiopathic portal hypertension, congenital hepatic fibrosis, systemic mastocytosis, autoimmune hepatitis, hepatic steatosis, IBD

DIAGNOSIS

DIFFERENTIAL DIAGNOSIS
Refer to "Etiology."

WORKUP
Diagnostic workup is aimed at identifying the most likely cause of cirrhosis. The history is extremely important:
- Alcohol abuse: alcoholic liver disease
- History of hepatitis B (chronic active hepatitis, primary hepatic neoplasm, or hepatitis C)
- History of IBD (primary sclerosing cholangitis)
- History of pruritus, hyperlipoproteinemia, and xanthomas in a middle-aged or elderly female (primary biliary cirrhosis)
- Impotence, diabetes mellitus, hyperpigmentation, arthritis (hemachromatosis)
- Neurologic disturbances (Wilson's disease, hepatolenticular degeneration)
- Family history of "liver disease" (hemochromatosis [positive family history in 25% of patients], α-1 antitrypsin deficiency)
- History of recurrent episodes of RUQ pain (biliary tract disease)
- History of blood transfusions, IV drug abuse (hepatitis C)
- History of hepatotoxic drug exposure
- Coexistence of other diseases with immune or autoimmune features (ITP, myasthenia gravis, thyroiditis, autoimmune hepatitis)

LABORATORY TESTS
- Decreased Hgb and Hct, elevated MCV, increased BUN and creatinine (the BUN may also be "normal" or low if the patient has severely diminished liver function), decreased sodium (dilutional hyponatremia), decreased potassium (as a result of secondary aldosteronism or urinary losses)
- Decreased glucose in a patient with liver disease indicating severe liver damage
- Other laboratory abnormalities:
  1. Alcoholic hepatitis and cirrhosis: there may be mild elevation of ALT and AST, usually <500 IU; AST > ALT (ratio >2:3).
  2. Extrahepatic obstruction: there may be moderate elevations of ALT and AST to levels <500 IU.
  3. Viral, toxic, or ischemic hepatitis: there are extreme elevations (>500 IU) of ALT and AST.
  4. Transaminases may be normal despite significant liver disease in patients with jejunoileal bypass operations or hemachromatosis or after methotrexate administration.
  5. Alkaline phosphatase elevation can occur with extrahepatic obstruction, primary biliary cirrhosis, and primary sclerosing cholangitis.
  6. Serum LDH is significantly elevated in metastatic disease of the liver; lesser elevations are seen with hepatitis, cirrhosis, extrahepatic obstruction, and congestive hepatomegaly.
  7. Serum γ-glutamyl transpeptidase (GGTP) is elevated in alcoholic liver disease and may also be elevated with cholestatic disease (primary biliary cirrhosis, primary sclerosing cholangitis).

8. Serum bilirubin may be elevated; urinary bilirubin can be present in hepatitis, hepatocellular jaundice, and biliary obstruction.
9. Serum albumin: significant liver disease results in hypoalbuminemia.
10. Prothrombin time: an elevated PT in patients with liver disease indicates severe liver damage and poor prognosis.
11. Presence of hepatitis B surface antigen implies acute or chronic active hepatitis B.
12. Presence of antimitochondrial antibody suggests primary biliary cirrhosis, chronic active hepatitis.
13. Elevated serum copper, decreased serum ceruloplasmin, and elevated 24-hr urine may be diagnostic of Wilson's disease.
14. Protein immunoelectrophoresis may reveal decreased α-1 globulins (α-1 antitrypsin deficiency), increased IgA (alcoholic cirrhosis), increased IgM (primary biliary cirrhosis), increased IgG (chronic active hepatitis, cryptogenic cirrhosis).
15. An elevated serum ferritin and increased transferrin saturation are suggestive of hemachromatosis.
16. An elevated blood ammonia suggests hepatocellular dysfunction; serial values are not useful in following patients with hepatic encephalopathy because there is poor correlation between blood ammonia level and degree of hepatic encephalopathy.
17. Serum cholesterol is elevated in cholestatic disorders.
18. Antinuclear antibodies (ANA) may be found in autoimmune hepatitis.
19. Alpha fetoprotein: levels >1000 pg/ml are highly suggestive of primary liver cell carcinoma.
20. Anti–hepatitis C virus identifies patient with prior hepatitis C virus infection.
21. Elevated level of serum globulin (especially γ-globulins) may occur with autoimmune hepatitis.

IMAGING STUDIES

- Ultrasonography is the procedure of choice for detection of gallstones and dilatation of common bile ducts.
- CT scan is useful for detecting mass lesions in liver and pancreas, assessing hepatic fat content, identifying idiopathic hemochromatosis, early diagnosing of Budd-Chiari syndrome, dilatation of intrahepatic bile ducts, and detection of varices and splenomegaly.
- Technetium-99m sulfur colloid scanning is useful for diagnosing cirrhosis (there is a shift of colloid uptake to the spleen, bone marrow), identifying hepatic adenomas (cold defect is noted), diagnosing Budd-Chiari syndrome (there is increased uptake by the caudate lobe).
- ERCP is the procedure of choice for diagnosing periampullary carcinoma, common duct stones; it is also useful in diagnosing primary sclerosing cholangitis.
- Percutaneous transhepatic cholangiography (PTC) is useful when evaluating patients with cholestatic jaundice and dilated intrahepatic ducts by ultrasonography; presence of intrahepatic strictures and focal dilation are suggestive of PSC.
- Percutaneous liver biopsy is useful in evaluating hepatic filling defects, diagnosing hepatocellular disease or hepatomegaly, evaluating persistently abnormal liver function tests, and diagnosing hemachromatosis, primary biliary cirrhosis, Wilson's disease, glycogen storage diseases, chronic hepatitis, autoimmune hepatitis, infiltrative diseases, alcoholic liver disease, drug induced liver disease, and primary or secondary carcinoma.

TREATMENT

NONPHARMACOLOGIC THERAPY
Avoid any hepatotoxins (e.g., ethanol, acetaminophen); improve nutritional status.

ACUTE GENERAL Rx
- Correct any mechanical obstruction to bile flow (e.g., calculi, strictures).
- Provide therapy for underlying cardiovascular disorders in patients with cardiac cirrhosis.
- Remove excess body iron with phlebotomy and deferoxamine in patients with hemachromatosis.
- Remove copper deposits with D-penicillamine in patients with Wilson's disease.
- Long-term ursodiol therapy will slow the progression of primary biliary cirrhosis. It is, however, ineffective in primary sclerosing cholangitis.
- Glucocorticoids (prednisone 20 to 30 mg/day initially or combination therapy of prednisone and azathioprine) is useful in autoimmune hepatitis.
- Liver transplantation may be indicated in otherwise healthy patients (age <65 yr) with sclerosing cholangitis, chronic hepatitis cirrhosis, or primary biliary cirrhosis with prognostic information suggesting <20% chance of survival without transplantation; contraindications to liver transplantation are AIDS, most metastatic malignancies, active substance abuse, uncontrolled sepsis, uncontrolled cardiac or pulmonary disease.

CHRONIC Rx
Treatment of complications of portal hypertension (ascites, esophagogastric varices, hepatic encephalopathy, and hepatorenal syndrome)

DISPOSITION
Prognosis varies with the etiology of the patient's cirrhosis and whether there is ongoing hepatic injury. Mortality rate exceeds 80% in patients with hepatorenal syndrome.

REFERRAL
- Hospital admission for bleeding varices, hepatic encephalopathy, or onset of hepatorenal syndrome
- Liver transplantation in suitable candidates

MISCELLANEOUS

COMMENTS
Patient education material is available through the National Digestive Disease Information Clearinghouse, Box NDDIC, Bethesda, MD 20892.

REFERENCES
Roberts LR, Kamath PS: Pathophysiology and treatment of variceal hemorrhage, *Mayo Clin Proc* 71:973, 1996.
Roberts LR, Kamath PS: Ascites in hepatorenal syndrome: pathophysiology and management, *Mayo Clin Proc* 71:874, 1996.
Runyon BA: Care of patients with ascites, *New Engl J Med* 330:337, 1994.
Author: **Fred F. Ferri, M.D.**

Claudication

BASIC INFORMATION

DEFINITION
Claudication refers to leg pain brought on by exertion and relieved with rest.

SYNONYMS
Intermittent claudication

ICD-9-CM CODES
443.9 Peripheral vascular disease, unspecified
440.21 Intermittent claudication due to atherosclerosis

EPIDEMIOLOGY AND DEMOGRAPHICS
INCIDENCE: 3 to 8 cases/1000 persons
PREVALENCE: 2% to 4% in the general population
RISK: Major risk factors of tobacco, hypertension, diabetes, and hypercholesterolemia increase the chance of developing claudication. Cigarette smoking is the major determinant of disease progression.

PHYSICAL FINDINGS
- Diminished pulses
- Bruits over the distal aorta, iliac or femoral arteries heard
- Pallor of the distal extremities on elevation
- Rubor with prolonged capillary refill on dependency
- Cool skin temperature
- Trophic changes of hair loss and muscle atrophy noted
- Nonhealing ulcers, necrotic tissue, and gangrene possible

ETIOLOGY
Primary cause of claudication is atherosclerosis with subsequent stenosis of peripheral vessels and inability to supply blood to working muscle.

DIAGNOSIS

The history of buttock, thigh, or calf pain or fatigue brought on by exertion and relieved by rest along with the above mentioned physical findings makes the diagnosis of claudication fairly certain. Noninvasive studies help confirm the diagnosis.

DIFFERENTIAL DIAGNOSIS
Spinal stenosis, muscle cramps, degenerative osteoarthritic joint disease particularly of the lumbar spine and hips, compartment syndrome may all resemble claudication.

WORKUP
- Noninvasive vascular testing confirms the clinical impression of claudication and aids in locating the major occlusive site. Noninvasive testing uses continuous-wave Doppler to measure systolic arterial pressures and reports the ankle-brachial index (ABI) and segmental systolic pressures as well as Doppler waveforms.
- Ankle-brachial index (ABI): The ratio of ankle pressure to brachial pressure is usually about 1.
  1. In claudication the ABI ranges from 0.5 to 0.8.
  2. In patients with rest pain or impending limb loss, ABI $\leq$ 0.3.
- Segmental systolic pressures usually are measured from the high thigh, above the knee, below the knee, and the ankle. Normally there should not be >20 mm Hg difference in pressures between adjacent segments. If the gradient is >20 mm Hg, significant narrowing is suspected in the intervening segment.
- Both ABI and segmental pressures can be done before and after exercise.

IMAGING STUDIES
- Duplex ultrasound can be used to locate the occluded areas and assess the patency of the distal arterial system or prior vein grafts.
- MRA and spiral CT angiography are newer imaging techniques available.
- Angiography remains the gold standard for imaging peripheral arterial occlusions. Complications can occur, and the study should be done only if surgical reconstruction is being considered.

TREATMENT

NONPHARMACOLOGIC THERAPY
- Avoidance of tobacco is vital.
- Diet to control diabetes and blood pressure as well as to reduce cholesterol should be followed.
- Exercise must be emphasized. Exercise along with abstaining from tobacco is the best medical treatment available for the exertional claudication patient. Exercise will increase walking distances before symptoms occurs and provides an overall better functioning status. Walking 30 to 60 min/day for 5 days at about 2 mi/hr is recommended.

ACUTE GENERAL Rx
Most patients with claudication respond to conservative management mentioned above. If this fails, medicines can be tried (see "Chronic Rx"). Surgical reconstruction has its specific indications reserved for patients with impending limb loss (see "Chronic Rx").

CHRONIC Rx
- Pentoxifylline (Trental) has been approved for use in patients with intermittent claudication who have not responded well to conservative measures. Pentoxifylline 400 mg tid for 3 mo should be tried. If there is no improvement in symptoms, the medicine can be discontinued.
- Surgical reconstruction is indicated in patients with refractory rest pain, limb ischemia, nonhealing ulcers, or gangrene and in a select group of patients with functional disability. Common surgical procedures:
  1. Aortoiliofemoral reconstruction: perioperative mortality <3%.
  2. Infrainguinal bypass, e.g., femoropopliteal, femorotibial: perioperative mortality, 2% to 5%.
  3. Extraanatomic bypass, e.g., axillofemoral or femorofemoral bypass.
  4. Angioplasty is used on short, discrete stenotic lesions in the iliac or femoropopliteal artery.
  5. Atherectomy, stents, and lasers are newer techniques.

DISPOSITION
Intermittent claudication progressing to an ischemic leg or limb loss is an unusual course especially if maintaining to the conservative treatment of exercise and abstaining from tobacco.

REFERRAL
Consultation with the vascular surgeon is recommended in the patient with threatened limb loss, rest pain, nonhealing ulcers, functional disability from pain, and gangrene.

MISCELLANEOUS

COMMENTS
Claudication is a marker for generalized atherosclerosis. This group of patients have a higher risk of death from cardiovascular events than from limb loss. This should be kept in mind when deciding to proceed with surgical evaluation. Every effort should be made toward conservative measures.

REFERENCES
Cooke JP: Medical therapy of peripheral arterial occlusive disease, *Surg Clin North Am* 75(4):569, 1995.
Hiatt WR: Clinical trials for claudication, *Circulation* 92(3): 614, 1995.
McDermott M: Intermittent claudication: the natural history, *Surg Clin North Am* 75(4):581, 1995.
Santilli JD: Claudication: diagnosis and treatment, *Am Fam Physician* 53(4):1245, 1996.
Author: **Peter Petropoulos, M.D.**

124 Coccidioidomycosis

BASIC INFORMATION

DEFINITION
Coccidioidomycosis is an infectious disease caused by the fungus, *Coccidioides immitis*. It is usually asymptomatic and characterized by a primary pulmonary focus with infrequent progression to chronic pulmonary disease and dissemination to other organs.

SYNONYMS
San Joaquin Valley fever

ICD-9-CM CODES
114.0 Coccidioidax pneumonia
114.1 Cutaneous or extrapulmonary (primary) coccidioidomycosis
114.3 Disseminated or prostate coccidioidomycosis
114.5 Pulmonary coccidioidomycosis
114.2 Meninges coccidioidomycosis
114.4 Chronic coccidioidomycosis

EPIDEMIOLOGY AND DEMOGRAPHICS
PREVALENCE: Unknown
INCIDENCE (IN U.S.): Estimated annual infection rate 100,000 persons, predominantly in southwest U.S.
PREDOMINANT SEX: Males, between the ages of 25 to 55 yr
PEAK INCIDENCE: Unknown
GENETICS
Familial Disposition: Unknown
Congenital Infection: Documented, but considered to occur rarely
Neonatal Infection
- Occurs equally between the sexes
- Clinical disease more severe than in older children and adults

PHYSICAL FINDINGS
- Asymptomatic infections or illness consistent with a nonspecific upper respiratory tract infection in at least 60%
- Symptoms of primary infection—cough, malaise, fever, chills, night sweats, anorexia, weakness, and arthralgias (desert rheumatism)—in remaining 40% within 3 wk of exposure
- Skin rashes, such as erythema nodosum and erythema multiforme, usually with a significant female preponderance
- Scattered rales and areas that are dull on percussion with auscultation
- Spontaneous improvement within 2 wk of illness, with complete recovery usual
- Subsequent pulmonary residua in the form of pulmonary nodules and cavities in <10% of those patients with primary infection; half of these patients asymptomatic
- In a small portion of these patients: a progressive pneumonitis, often with a fatal outcome
- Some, especially if immunocompromised and/or diabetic, progressing to chronic pulmonary disease
- Over many years, granuloma rupture leading to the new cavity formation and continued fibrosis, often accompanied by hemoptysis
- Possible bronchiectasis with acute or chronic disease
- Disseminated or extrapulmonary disease in approximately 0.5% of acutely infected patients
  1. Early signs of probable dissemination: fever, malaise, hilar adenopathy, and elevated ESR persisting in the setting of primary infection
  2. Most organs are susceptible to dissemination, with heart and GI tract generally spared
- Musculoskeletal involvement
  1. Occurs one third of the time in disseminated disease
  2. Usually presents with local pain, swelling of a joint, bone, or muscle
  3. Majority of bone lesions unifocal and usually involve the skull, metacarpals, metatarsals, and tibia
  4. Vertebral column possibly affected with usually multiple lesions involving the arch and contiguous ribs and sparing the intravertebral disc
  5. Joint lesions predominantly unifocal, most commonly involving the ankle and knee, and often accompanying adjacent sites of osteomyelitis
- Meningeal involvement
  1. Occurs approximately one third of the time with dissemination
  2. Usually presents within 6 mo of primary infection or may appear concurrently
  3. Mass lesions rare, with approximately 40 cases reported this century
  4. Usually, absence of classic signs of meningeal irritation, but possible focal deficits, seizure activity, and stiff neck
  5. Most common complaint: headache
  6. Presenting symptoms: fever, weakness, confusion, lethargy, vomiting
- Cutaneous involvement, excluding rash
  1. Variable in appearance, taking the form of pustules, papules, plaques, nodules, ulcers, abscesses, or proliferative lesions
  2. Lesions most characteristically verrucous
  3. Dissemination and fatal outcomes most common in men, pregnant women, neonates, immunocompromised hosts, and individuals of dark-skinned races, especially those of African, Filipino, Mexican, and Native American ancestry

ETIOLOGY
- *Coccidioides immitis* is endemic to the American continent, including north, central (Middle), and southern parts.

- In U.S., most cases are acquired in Arizona, California, New Mexico, and Texas.
- Endemic areas coincide with the Lower Sonoran Life Zone, with semi-arid climate, sparse flora, and alkaline soil.
- Fungus exists in the mycelial phase in soil, having barrel-shaped hyphae (arthroconidia).
- Windswept spores from easily fragmented arthroconidia are dispersed to infect other soil (saprophytic cycle) or are inhaled by animals, including rodents and humans.
- Arthrospore deposits in the alveoli, then fungus converts to thick-walled spherule.
- Internal spherical spores (endospores) are released through spherule rupture and mature into new spherules (parasitic cycle).
- Fungus incites a granulomatous reaction in host tissue, usually with caseation necrosis.

DIAGNOSIS

DIFFERENTIAL DIAGNOSIS
- Acute pulmonary coccidioidomycoses:
  1. Community-acquired pneumonias caused by *Mycoplasma* and *Chlamydia*
  2. Granulomatous diseases, e.g., *Mycobacterium tuberculosis* and sarcoidosis
  3. Other fungal diseases, such as *Blastomyces dermatitidis* and *Histoplasma capsulatum*
- Coccidioidomas: true neoplasms

WORKUP
- Suspected in patients with a history of residence or travel in an endemic area, especially during periods favorable to spore dispersion (e.g., dust storms and drought followed by heavy rains)
- Suspected with a patient history of handling fomites from endemic areas (e.g., fruit and cotton), as in textile workers or fruit handlers

LABORATORY TESTS
- CBC to reveal eosinophilia, especially with erythema nodosum
- Routine chemistries: usually normal but may reveal hyponatremia
- Elevated serum levels of IgE; associated with progressive disease
- CSF cell counts and chemistry: pleocytosis with mononuclear cell predominance associated with hypoglycorrhachia and elevated protein level
- Definitive diagnosis based on demonstration of the organism by culture from body fluids or tissues
  1. Greatest yield with pus, sputum, synovial fluid, and soft tissue aspirations, varying with the degree of dissemination
  2. Possible positive cultures of blood, gastric aspirate, pleural effusion, peritoneal fluid, and CSF, but less frequently obtained
  3. In patients with AIDS: failure of sputum cultures to grow the fungus, so pulmonary biopsy is needed
- Serologic evaluations
  1. Latex agglutination and complement fixation
  2. Elevated serum complement-fixing antibody (CFA) titers ≥1:32 (Smith and Saito) strongly correlated with disseminated disease, except with meningitis where lower titers seen
  3. Variable discriminating titers depending on method, so must be based on reference ranges provided
  4. In meningeal disease: CFA detected in CSF except with high serum CFA titers secondary to concurrent extraneural disease
  5. Enzyme-linked immunosorbent assay (ELISA) against a 33-kDa spherule antigen to detect and monitor CNS disease
- Coccidioidin, the mycelial phase antigen, and spherulin, the parasitic phase antigen
  1. Positive (>5 mm) 1 mo following onset of symptomatic primary infection
  2. Useful in assessing prior infection
  3. Negative skin test with primary infection: latent or future dissemination

IMAGING STUDIES
Chest x-ray examination:
- Reveals unilateral infiltrates, hilar adenopathy, or pleural effusion in primary infection
- Shows areas of fibrosis containing usually solitary, thin-wall cavities that persist as residua of primary infection
- Possible coccidioidoma, a coin-like lesion representing a healed area of previous pneumonitis

TREATMENT

NONPHARMACOLOGIC THERAPY
- Supportive care in mild symptomatic disease
- In patients with extrapulmonary manifestations involving draining skin, joint and soft tissue infection: local wound care to avoid possible bacterial superinfection

ACUTE GENERAL Rx
- In general, drug therapy is not required for patients with asymptomatic pulmonary disease and most patients with mild symptomatic primary infection.
- Chemotherapy is indicated under the following circumstances:
  1. Severe symptomatic primary infection
  2. High serum CFA titers
  3. Persistent symptoms >6 wk

4. Prostration
  5. Progressive pulmonary involvement
  6. Pregnancy
  7. Infancy
  8. Debilitation
  9. Concurrent illness (e.g., diabetes, asthma, COPD, malignancy)
  10. Acquired or induced immunosuppression
  11. Racial group with known predisposition for disseminated disease
- Amphotericin B is the classic therapy for disseminated extraneural disease, dose 1 to 1.5 mg/kg/day, qd for the first week and qid thereafter, for a total dose of 1 to 2.5 g or until clinical and serologic remission is accomplished.
  1. Local instillation into body cavities such as sinuses, fistulae, and abscesses have been adjuncts to therapy.
  2. Liposomal Amphotericin B is probably equally effective, but further studies are needed.
  3. Duration of therapy for extraneural disease is undefined but probably about 1 yr.
- Fluconazole and itraconazole
  1. Oral therapy with 200 to 400 mg/day and itraconazole 200 mg bid (appear to be equally efficacious with respect to clinical cure and relapse rate)
  2. Continued for life, based on relapse rate after cessation
- Ketoconazole 200 to 400 mg/day may be used for extraneural disease, but it is associated with GI intolerance and may block steroid hormone synthesis at high doses.
- With meningeal disease:
  1. Intrathecal amphotericin B remains the traditional treatment modality, given alone or preceding the use of oral agents.
  2. Begin in doses of 0.01 to 0.025 mg/day, gradually increasing the dose as tolerated, to 0.5 mg/day with the patient in Trendelenburg position.
  3. If given via Ommaya reservoir, as in ventriculitis, dose may be increased to 1.5 mg/day if tolerated.
  4. Concomitant parenteral therapy with amphotericin B is used for simultaneous extraneural disease at standard doses and with purely meningeal disease in smaller doses, although not strictly indicated.
  5. Intrathecal therapy is usually given three times a week for at least 3 mo, then discontinued or gradually tapered until once every 6 wk through 1 yr of therapy.
  6. Patients need routine monitoring of CSF, CFA, cell count, and chemistries for at least 2 yr following cessation of therapy.
- For osteomyelitis, soft-tissue closed space infections, and pulmonary fibrocavitary disease: surgical debridement, drainage or resection, respectively, in addition to oral azole therapy or parenteral administration of amphotericin B

CHRONIC Rx
For chronically immunocompromised patients, lifelong therapy with oral azoles or amphotericin B

DISPOSITION
- Prognosis for primary symptomatic infection is good.
- Immunocompromised patients are most likely to have disseminated disease and higher morbidity and mortality.

REFERRAL
- To surgeon for the evaluation of chronic hemoptysis, enlarging cavitary lesions despite chemotherapy and intrapleural rupture, osteomyelitis, and other synovial or soft-tissue closed space infections
- For neurosurgical consultation in patients with meningeal disease to establish the delivery route of intrathecal drug therapy

MISCELLANEOUS

COMMENTS
- Infected body fluids contained within a closed moist environment (e.g., sputum in a specimen cup) provide the opportunity for the fungus to revert to its hyphal form whereby spores may be made airborne on opening of the container. Purulent drainage into a cast, allowing conversion of fungus to the saprophytic phase, has been responsible for acute disease when the cast was opened and the spores were unintentionally made airborne.
- Patients with a remote history of exposure, especially if immunosuppressed by medication or disease, may reactivate primary disease and suffer rapid dissemination.

REFERENCES
Banuelos AF et al: Central nervous system abscesses due to *Coccidioides* species, *Clin Infect Dis* 22:240, 1996.

Dewsnup DH et al: Is it ever safe to stop azole therapy for *Coccidioides immitis* meningitis? *Ann Intern Med* 124(3):305, 1996.

Galgiani JN et al: Cerebrospinal fluid antibodies detected by ELISA against a 33-kDa antigen from spherules of coccidioides immitis in patients with coccidioidal meningitis, *J Infect Dis* 173:499, 1996.

Low WS et al: *Coccidioides immitis* subperiosteal abscess of the temporal bone in a child, *Arch Otolaryngol Head Neck Surg* 122(2):189, 1996.

Wagner JA et al: Disseminated coccidioidomycosis diagnosed by culture of a central venous catheter tip, *Clin Infect Dis* 22:180, 1996.

Author: **George O. Alonso, M.D.**

Colorectal cancer (PTG)

BASIC INFORMATION

DEFINITION
Colorectal cancer is a neoplasm arising from the luminal surface of the large bowel: descending colon (40% to 42%), rectosigmoid and rectum (30% to 33%), cecum and ascending colon (25% to 30%), transverse colon (10% to 13%).

ICD-9-CM CODES
154.0 Colorectal cancer

EPIDEMIOLOGY AND DEMOGRAPHICS
- Colorectal cancer is the second leading cause of cancer deaths in the U.S.
- Peak incidence is in the seventh decade of life.
- 50% of rectal cancers are within reach of the examiner's finger, 50% of colon cancers are within reach of the flexible sigmoidoscope.
- Colorectal cancer accounts for 14% of all cases of cancer (excluding skin malignancies) and 14% of all yearly cancer deaths.
- Risk factors:
  1. Hereditary polyposis syndromes
     a. Familial polyposis (high risk)
     b. Gardner's syndrome (high risk)
     c. Turcot's syndrome (high risk)
     d. Peutz-Jeghers syndrome (low to moderate risk)
  2. IBD, both ulcerative colitis and Crohn's disease
  3. Family history of "cancer family syndrome"
  4. Heredofamilial breast cancer and colon carcinoma
  5. History of previous colorectal carcinoma
  6. Women undergoing irradiation for gynecologic cancer
  7. First-degree relatives with colorectal carcinoma
  8. Age >40 yr
  9. Possible dietary factors (diet high in fat or meat, beer drinking, reduced vegetable consumption)
  10. Hereditary nonpolyposis colon cancer (HNPCC): autosomal-dominant disorder characterized by early age on onset (mean age of 44 yr) and right-sided or proximal colon cancers, synchronous and metachronous colon cancers, mucinous and poorly differentiated colon cancers

PHYSICAL FINDINGS
- Physical examination may be completely unremarkable.
- Digital rectal examination can detect approximately 50% of rectal cancers.
- Palpable abdominal masses may indicate metastasis or complications of colorectal carcinoma (abscess, intussusception, volvulus).
- Abdominal distention and tenderness are suggestive of colonic obstruction.
- Hepatomegaly may be indicative of hepatic metastasis.

ETIOLOGY
See "Risk Factors."

DIAGNOSIS

DIFFERENTIAL DIAGNOSIS
- Diverticular disease
- Strictures
- IBD
- Infectious or inflammatory lesions
- Adhesions
- Arteriovenous malformations
- Metastatic carcinoma (prostate, sarcoma)
- Extrinsic masses (cysts, abscesses)

WORKUP
- The clinical presentation of colorectal malignancies is initially vague and nonspecific (weight loss, anorexia, malaise). It is useful to divide colon cancer symptoms into those usually associated with the right colon and those commonly associated with the left colon, since the clinical presentation varies with the location of the carcinoma.
  1. Right colon
     a. Anemia (iron deficiency secondary to chronic blood loss)
     b. Dull, vague, and uncharacteristic abdominal pain may be present or patient may be completely asymptomatic.
     c. Rectal bleeding is often missed because blood is mixed with feces.
     d. Obstruction and constipation are unusual because of large lumen and more liquid stools.
  2. Left colon
     a. Change in bowel habits (constipation, diarrhea, tenesmus, pencil-thin stools)
     b. Rectal bleeding (bright red blood coating the surface of the stool)
     c. Intestinal obstruction is frequent because of small lumen.
- Early diagnosis of patients with surgically curable disease (Duke's A, B) is necessary, since survival time is directly related to the stage of the carcinoma at the time of diagnosis. Appropriate screening recommendations are discussed in Section V.

128 Colorectal cancer (PTG)

- Duke's and UICC classification for colorectal cancer:
  - A Confined to the mucosa-submucosa (I)
  - B Invasion of muscularis propria (II)
  - C Local node involvement (III)
  - D Distant metastasis (IV)

LABORATORY TESTS
- Positive fecal occult blood test
- Microcytic anemia
- Elevated plasma carcinoembryonic antigen (CEA)
- Liver function tests

IMAGING STUDIES
- Air-contrast barium enema only in patients refusing colonoscopy or unable to tolerate colonoscopy
- CT scan of abdomen to assist in preoperative staging
- Chest x-ray examination to look for evidence of metastatic disease
- Colonoscopy with biopsy (primary assessment tool)

TREATMENT

NONPHARMACOLOGIC THERAPY
Decrease fat intake to 30% of total energy intake, increase fiber, fruit, and vegetable consumption.

ACUTE GENERAL Rx
- Surgical resection: 70% of colorectal cancers are resectable for cure at presentation; 45% of patients are cured by primary resection.
- Radiation therapy is a useful adjunct to fluorouracil and levamisole therapy for stage II or III rectal cancers.
- Adjuvant chemotherapy with combination of 5-fluorouracil (5-FU) and levamisole substantially increases cure rates for patients with stage III colon cancer and should be considered standard treatment for all such patients and selected patients with high-risk stage II colon cancer.
- Irinotecan (Camptosar) can be used for the treatment of metastatic colorectal cancer refractory to other drugs including 5-FU; it may offer a few months of palliation but is expensive and associated with significant toxicity.

CHRONIC Rx
Follow-up is indicated with:
- Fecal occult blood testing every 6 mo for 4 yr, then yearly
- Colonoscopy yearly for the initial 2 yr, then every 3 yr
- CEA level should be obtained baseline; if elevated, it can be used postoperatively as a measure of completeness of tumor resection or to monitor tumor recurrence; if used to monitor tumor recurrence, CEA should be obtained every 2 mo for 2 yr, then every 4 mo for 2 yr and then yearly. The role of CEA for monitoring patients with resected colon cancer has been questioned because of the small number of cures attributed to CEA monitoring despite the substantial cost in dollars and physical and emotional stress associated with monitoring.

DISPOSITION
The 5-yr survival varies with the stage of the carcinoma:
- Duke's A 5-yr survival, >80%
- Duke's B 5-yr survival, 60%
- Duke's C 5-yr survival, 20%
- Duke's D 5-yr survival, 3%

Overall 5-yr disease-free survival is approximately 50% for colon cancer.

REFERRAL
- Surgical referral for resection
- Oncology referral for adjuvant chemotherapy in selected patients
- Radiation oncology referral for patients with stage II or III rectal cancers

MISCELLANEOUS

COMMENTS
- Patient education material on colorectal cancer can be obtained from the National Cancer Institute, Department of Health and Human Services, Public Inquiries Section, Office of Cancer Communications, Building 31, Room 101-118, 9000 Rockville Pike, Bethesda, MD 20892.
- U.S. Preventive Services Task Force Recommendations regarding screening for colorectal cancer are described in Section V, Chapter 8. American Cancer Society guidelines for screening and surveillance for early detection of colorectal polyps and cancer are available from *CA Cancer J Clin* 47: 154, 1997.

REFERENCES
Burke W et al: Recommendations for follow-up care of individuals with uninherited predisposition to cancer, *JAMA* 277:918, 1997.

Moertl GC et al: Fluorouracil plus levamisole as effective adjuvant therapy after resection of stage III colon carcinoma: a final report, *Ann Intern Med* 122:321, 1995.

Shibata D et al: The DCC protein in prognosis of colorectal cancer, *New Engl J Med* 335:1727, 1996.

Toribara N, Sleisenger M: Screening for colorectal cancer, *New Engl J Med* 332:861, 1995.

Author: **Fred F. Ferri, M.D.**

Condyloma acuminatum (PTG)

BASIC INFORMATION

DEFINITION
Condyloma acuminatum is a sexually transmitted viral disease of the vulva, vagina, and cervix that is caused by the human papilloma virus (HPV).

SYNONYMS
Genital warts
Venereal warts
Anogenital warts

ICD-9-CM CODES
078.11 Condyloma acuminatum

EPIDEMIOLOGY AND DEMOGRAPHICS
- Seen mostly in young adults with a mean age of onset of 16 to 25 yr
- A sexually transmitted disease spread by skin-to-skin contact
- Highly contagious, with 25% to 65% of sexual partners developing it
- Virus shed from both macroscopic and microscopic lesions
- Average incubation time 2 mo (range: 1 to 8 mo)
- Predisposing conditions: diabetes, pregnancy, local trauma, and immunosuppression (e.g., transplant patients, those with HIV infection).

PHYSICAL FINDINGS
- Usually found in genital area, but can be present elsewhere
- Lesions usually in similar positions on both sides of perineum
- Initial lesions pedunculated, soft papules about 2 to 3 mm in diameter, 10 to 20 mm long; may occur as single papule or in clusters
- Size of lesions varies from pinhead to large cauliflower-like masses
- Usually asymptomatic, but if infected, can cause pain, odor, or bleeding
- Vulvar condyloma more common than vaginal and cervical

ETIOLOGY
- HPV DNA type 6 and 11 usually found in exophytic warts and have no malignant potential
- HPV type 16 and 18 usually found in flat warts and are associated with increased risk of malignancy
- Recurrence associated with persisting viral infection of adjacent normal skin in 25% to 50% of cases

DIAGNOSIS

DIFFERENTIAL DIAGNOSIS
- Abnormal anatomic variants or skin tags around labia minora and introitus
- Dysplastic warts

WORKUP
- Colposcopic examination of lower genital tract from cervix to perianal skin with 3% to 5% acetic acid
- Biopsy of vulvar lesions that lack the classic appearance of warts that become ulcerated or fail to respond to treatment
- Biopsy of flat white or ulcerated cervical lesions

LABORATORY TESTS
- Pap smear
- Cervical cultures for *N. gonorrhea* and *Chlamydia*
- Serologic test for syphilis
- HIV testing offered
- Wet mount for trichomoniasis, *Candida albicans,* and *Gardnerella vaginalis*
- Testing for diabetes (blood glucose)

TREATMENT

NONPHARMACOLOGIC THERAPY
- Keep genital area dry and clean.
- Keep diabetes, if present, well controlled.
- Advise use of condoms to prevent spread of infection to sexual partner.

ACUTE GENERAL Rx
Keratolytic agents:
- Podophyllin
  1. Acts by poisoning mitotic spindle and causing intense vasospasm
  2. Applied directly to lesion weekly and washed off in 6 hr
  3. Used in minimal vulvar or anal disease
  4. Applied cautiously to nonkeratinized epithelial surfaces
  5. Contraindicated in pregnancy
  6. Discontinued if lesions do not disappear in 6 wk; switch to other treatment
- Trichloroacetic acid (30% to 80% solution)
  1. Acts by precipitation of surface proteins
  2. Applied twice monthly to lesion
  3. Indicated for vulvar, anal, and vaginal lesions; can be used for cervical lesions
  4. Less painful and irritating to normal tissue than podophyllin
- Fluorouracil
  1. Causes necrosis and sloughing of growing tissue
  2. Can be used intravaginally or for vulvar, anal, or urethral lesions
  3. Better tolerated; 3 g (two thirds of vaginal applicator) applied weekly for 12 wk
  4. Possible vaginal ulceration and erythema
  5. Patient's vagina examined after four to six applications
  6. 80% cure rate

Physical agents:
- Cryotherapy
  1. Can be used weekly for 3 to 6 wk
  2. 62% to 79% success rate
  3. Not suitable for large warts
- Laser therapy
  1. Done by physician with necessary expertise and equipment
  2. Painful; requires anesthesia
- Electrocautery or excision
  1. For recurrent, very large lesions
  2. Local anesthesia needed

Immunotherapy:
- Interferon
  1. Injected intralesionally at a dose of 3 million U/m^2 three times weekly for 8 wk
  2. Side effects: fever, chills, malaise, headache
- Autologous vaccine
  1. Made from host's own condyloma acuminatum; not very effective

DISPOSITION
Follow closely with pelvic examinations and Pap smears every 3 mo for 6 mo, every 6 mo for 12 mo, and then yearly if no evidence of recurrence.

REFERRAL
Consult gynecologist in case of extensive lesions or lesion resistant to treatment with keratolytic agents (podophyllin and trichloroacetic acid).

MISCELLANEOUS

COMMENTS
- Obtain patient education material from the American College of Obstetricians and Gynecologists.
- A clinical algorithm for the evaluation of genital ulcer disease is described in Fig. 3-33.
- U.S. Preventive Services Task Force Recommendations for counseling to prevent HIV infection and other STDs are described in Section V, Chapter 62.

REFERENCES
American College of Obstetricians and Gynecologists: Genital human papillomavirus infections, *ACOG technical bulletin* No 105, June 1987.

Herbst AL et al: *Comprehensive gynecology,* ed 2, St Louis, 1992, Mosby.

Krebs H: Treatment of vaginal condylomata acuminata by weekly topical application of 5-fluorouracil, *Obstet Gynecol* 70:68, 1987.

Precis V: *Human papillomavirus infection,* Washington, DC, 1994, American College of Obstetricians and Gynecologists.

Author: **Mandeep K. Brar, M.D.**

Congestive heart failure (PTG)

BASIC INFORMATION

DEFINITION
Congestive heart failure is a pathophysiologic state characterized by congestion in the pulmonary or systemic circulation. It is caused by the heart's inability to pump sufficient oxygenated blood to meet the metabolic needs of the tissues.

SYNONYMS
CHF
Cardiac failure
Heart failure

ICD-9-CM CODES
428.0 Congestive heart failure

EPIDEMIOLOGY AND DEMOGRAPHICS
CHF is the most common admission diagnosis in elderly patients.

PHYSICAL FINDINGS
The findings on physical examination in patients with CHF vary depending on the severity and whether the failure is right-sided or left-sided.
- Common clinical manifestations are:
  1. Dyspnea on exertion initially, then with progressively less strenuous activity, and eventually manifesting when patient is at rest; caused by increasing pulmonary congestion
  2. Orthopnea caused by increased venous return in the recumbent position
  3. Paroxysmal nocturnal dyspnea (PND) resulting from multiple factors (increased venous return in the recumbent position, decreased PaO_2, decreased adrenergic stimulation of myocardial function)
  4. Nocturnal angina resulting from increased cardiac work (secondary to increased venous return)
  5. Cheyne-Stokes respiration: alternating phases of apnea and hyperventilation caused by prolonged circulation time from lungs to brain
  6. Fatigue, lethargy resulting from low cardiac output
- Patients with failure of the left side of the heart will have the following abnormalities on physical examination: pulmonary rales, tachypnea, S_3 gallop, cardiac murmurs (AS, AR, MR), paradoxical splitting of S_2.
- Patients with failure of right side of the heart manifest with jugular venous distention, peripheral edema, perioral and peripheral cyanosis, congestive hepatomegaly, ascites hepatojugular reflux.

ETIOLOGY
LEFT VENTRICULAR FAILURE:
- Systemic hypertension
- Valvular heart disease (AS, AR, MR)
- Cardiomyopathy, myocarditis
- Bacterial endocarditis
- Myocardial infarction
- IHSS

Left ventricular failure is further differentiated according to systolic dysfunction (low ejection fraction) and diastolic dysfunction (normal or high ejection fraction), or "stiff ventricle". It is important to make this distinction because treatment is significantly different (see "Treatment").
- Common causes of systolic dysfunction are post-MI, cardiomyopathy, myocarditis.
- Causes of diastolic dysfunction are hypertensive cardiovascular disease, valvular heart disease (AS, AR, MR, IHSS), restrictive cardiomyopathy.

RIGHT VENTRICULAR FAILURE:
- Valvular heart disease (mitral stenosis)
- Pulmonary hypertension
- Bacterial endocarditis (right-sided)
- Right ventricular infarction

BIVENTRICULAR FAILURE:
- Left ventricular failure
- Cardiomyopathy
- Myocarditis
- Arrhythmias
- Anemia
- Thyrotoxicosis
- AV fistula
- Paget's disease
- Beriberi

DIAGNOSIS

DIFFERENTIAL DIAGNOSIS
- Cirrhosis
- Nephrotic syndrome
- Venous occlusive disease
- COPD, asthma
- Pulmonary embolism
- ARDS
- Heroin overdose
- Pneumonia

WORKUP
Chest x-ray examination, echocardiography, cardiac catheterization (selected patients)

LABORATORY TESTS
CBC (to rule out anemia, infections), BUN, creatinine, liver enzymes, TSH

IMAGING STUDIES
- Chest x-ray examination:
  1. Pulmonary venous congestion
  2. Cardiomegaly with dilation of the involved heart chamber
  3. Pleural effusions
- Two-dimensional echocardiography is useful to assess global and regional left ventricular function and estimate ejection fraction.
- Cardiac catheterization remains the best method to evaluate ventricular diastolic properties; however, it is invasive.

TREATMENT

NONPHARMACOLOGIC THERAPY
- Determine if CHF is secondary to systolic or diastolic dysfunction and treat accordingly.
- Identify and correct precipitating factors (i.e., anemia, thyrotoxicosis, infections, increased sodium load, β-blockers, medical noncompliance).
- Decrease cardiac work load in patients with systolic dysfunction: restrict patients to bed rest with chair and commode privileges; the risk of thromboembolism during this period can be minimized by using heparin 5000 U SC q12h.
- Restrict sodium intake.

ACUTE GENERAL Rx
TREATMENT OF CHF SECONDARY TO SYSTOLIC DYSFUNCTION:
1. Diuretics: indicated in patients with systolic dysfunction and volume overload
   a. Furosemide: 20 to 80 mg/day produces prompt venodilation and diuresis. IV therapy may produce diuresis when oral therapy has failed; when changing from IV to oral furosemide, doubling the dose is usually necessary to achieve an equal effect.
   b. Thiazides are not as powerful as furosemide but are useful in mild to moderate CHF.
   c. The addition of metolazone to furosemide enhances diuresis.
   d. Frequent monitoring of renal function and electrolytes is recommended in all patients receiving diuretics.

2. ACE inhibitors:
   a. They cause dilation of the arteriolar resistance vessels and venous capacity vessels, thereby reducing both preload and afterload.
   b. They are associated with decreased mortality and improved clinical status when used in patients with CHF caused by systolic dysfunction. They are also indicated in patients with ejection fraction <40%.
   c. They can be used as first line therapy or they can be added to diuretics in patients with CHF poorly controlled with only diuretic therapy.
   d. Therapy with ACE inhibitors should be initiated at low dose (e.g., enalapril 2.5 mg qd or bid) to prevent hypotension.
3. Digitalis is useful because of its positive inotropic and vagotonic effects in patients with CHF secondary to systolic dysfunction; it is of limited value in patients with mild CHF and normal sinus rhythm. It is more beneficial in patients with rapid atrial fibrillation, severe CHF or ejection fraction of <30%; it can be added to diuretics and ACE inhibitors in patients with severe CHF. In patients with chronic heart failure and normal sinus rhythm, digoxin does not reduce mortality, but it does reduce the rate of hospitalization both overall and for worsening heart failure.
4. Direct vasodilating drugs (hydralazine, isosorbide) are useful in the therapy of systolic dysfunction with CHF because they can reduce the systemic vascular resistance and pulmonary venous pressure, especially when used in combination. They are less effective than ACE inhibitors, and tolerance develops for these agents. The combination of hydralazine and isosorbide is useful in patients who cannot tolerate ACE inhibitors and in patients remaining symptomatic even while taking an ACE inhibitor.
5. Inotropic agents (e.g., dobutamine, nitroprusside, milrinone, amrinone) are useful in treating severe heart failure in patients responding poorly to oral therapeutic medications, or in patients being maintained awaiting cardiac transplantation.
6. Anticoagulants:
   a. Anticoagulation is not recommended for patients in sinus rhythm and no prior history of stroke, left ventricular thrombi, or arteriolar emboli.
   b. Anticoagulation therapy is appropriate for patients with heart failure and atrial fibrillation or a history of embolism.
7. Surgical revascularization should be considered in patients with both heart failure and severe limiting angina.

TREATMENT OF CHF SECONDARY TO DIASTOLIC DYSFUNCTION: Therapeutic options are determined by the cause
1. Hypertension
   a. Calcium channel blockers (verapamil)
   b. ACE inhibitors
   c. β-Blockers or verapamil to control heart rate and prolong diastolic filling
   d. Diuretics: vigorous diuresis should be avoided, since a higher filling pressure may be needed to maintain cardiac output in patients with diastolic dysfunction
2. Aortic stenosis
   a. Diuretics
   b. Contraindicated medications: ACE inhibitors, nitrates, digitalis (except to control rate of atrial fibrillation)
   c. Aortic valve replacement in patients with critical stenosis
3. Aortic insufficiency and mitral regurgitation
   a. ACE inhibitors increase cardiac output and decrease pulmonary wedge pressure. They are agents of choice along with diuretics.
   b. Hydralazine combined with nitrates can be used if ACE inhibitors are not tolerated.
4. IHSS
   a. β-Blockers and/or verapamil
   b. Contraindicated medications (they increase outlet obstruction by decreasing the size of the left ventricle in end systole): diuretics, digitalis, ACE inhibitors, hydralazine
   c. Restoration of intravascular volume with IV saline solution if necessary in acute pulmonary edema
   d. Septal myotomy in selected patients

TREATMENT OF CHF SECONDARY TO MITRAL STENOSIS:
1. Diuretics
2. Control of the heart rate and atrial fibrillation with digitalis, verapamil, and/or β-blockers is critical to allow emptying of left atrium and relief of pulmonary congestion.
3. Repairing or replacing the mitral valve is indicated if CHF is not readily controlled by the above measures.
4. Balloon valvuloplasty is useful in selected patients.

DISPOSITION
- Annual mortality ranges from 10% in stable patients with mild symptoms to >50% in symptomatic patients with advanced disease.
- Sudden death secondary to ventricular arrhythmias occurs in >40% of patients with heart failure.
- Cardiac transplantation has a 5-yr survival rate of >70% in many centers and represents a viable option in selected patients.

REFERRAL
Hospital admission in patients inadequately controlled with oral medications.

MISCELLANEOUS

COMMENTS
Patient education information on congestive heart failure can be obtained from the American Heart Association, 7320 Green Mill Avenue, Dallas, TX 75231.

REFERENCES
Cohn JN: The management of chronic heart failure, *New Engl J Med* 335:490, 1996.
Constanzo MR et al: Selection and treatment of candidates for heart transplantation, *Circulation* 92:3593, 1995.
Karon BL: Diagnosis and outpatient management of congestive heart failure, *Mayo Clin Proc* 70:1080, 1995.
Senni M, Redfield M: Congestive heart failure in elderly patients, *Mayo Clin Proc* 72:453, 1997.
Author: **Fred F. Ferri, M.D.**

Conjunctivitis (PTG)

BASIC INFORMATION

DEFINITION
The term *conjunctivitis* refers to an inflammation of the conjunctiva resulting from a variety of causes, including allergies and bacterial, viral, and chlamydial infections.

SYNONYMS
"Red eye"
Acute conjunctivitis
Subacute conjunctivitis
Chronic conjunctivitis
Purulent conjunctivitis
Pseudomembranous conjunctivitis
Papillary conjunctivitis
Follicular conjunctivitis
Newborn conjunctivitis

ICD-9-CM CODES
372.30 Conjunctivitis, unspecified

EPIDEMIOLOGY AND DEMOGRAPHICS
INCIDENCE (IN U.S.): Newborn 1.6% to 12%
PREVALENCE (IN U.S.):
- Very common
- Often seasonal and can be extremely contagious

PREDOMINANT AGE: Occurs at any age
PEAK INCIDENCE: More common in the fall when viral infections and pollens increase

PHYSICAL FINDINGS
- Injection and chemosis of conjunctivae with discharge
- Cornea clear
- Vision usually normal

ETIOLOGY
- Bacterial
- Viral
- Chlamydial
- Allergic

DIAGNOSIS

DIFFERENTIAL DIAGNOSIS
- Acute glaucoma
- Corneal lesions
- Acute iritis
- Episcleritis
- Scleritis
- Uveitis
- Canalicular obstruction

WORKUP
- History and physical examination
- Reports of itching, pain, visual changes

LABORATORY TESTS
Cultures are useful if not successfully treated with antibiotic medications; initial culture is usually not necessary.

TREATMENT

NONPHARMACOLOGIC THERAPY
- Warm compresses if infective conjunctivitis
- Cold compresses in irritative or allergic conjunctivitis

ACUTE GENERAL Rx
- Antibiotic drops (gentamicin ophthalmic solution; one or two drops q2-4h)
- Caution: be careful with steroid treatment

CHRONIC Rx
- Depends on cause
- If allergic (most common) or viral (herpes): treat underlying allergy and manage eyes symptomatically

DISPOSITION
Follow carefully for the first 2 wk to make sure secondary complications do not occur.

REFERRAL
To ophthalmologist if symptoms refractory to initial treatment

MISCELLANEOUS

COMMENTS
Do not use steroids indiscriminately; use only when the diagnosis is certain.

REFERENCES
Gigliotti F: Acute conjunctivitis, *Pediatr Rev* 16:203, 1995.
Author: **Melvyn Koby, M.D.**

Contraception (PTG)

BASIC INFORMATION

DEFINITION
Contraception refers to the various options that a sexually active couple have to prevent pregnancy. These options can be either medical or non-medical and used by men or women or both. The options are as follows:
- No contraception: failure rate 85% both typical and perfect
- Abstinence
  1. 12.4% of unmarried men
  2. 13.2% of unmarried women
  3. More frequently practiced before age 17 yr
  4. No intercourse experienced by 13% of women ages 30 to 34 yr old
  5. Failure rate 0%
- Withdrawal
  1. Used in only 2% of sexually active women
  2. Failure rate with perfect use, 4%; with typical use, 19%
- Rhythm method (natural family planning)
  1. Failure rate with perfect use 1% to 9%; with typical use, 20%
  2. Symptothermal type: mucus method and ovulation pain combined with basal body temperature
  3. Ovulation (Billing's method): takes into account mucus quality
  4. Basal body temperature method: uses biphasic temperature chart
  5. Lactation amenorrhea method: effective in fully breast-feeding women, especially 70 to 100 days after delivery; depends on number of feedings per day
- Barriers
  1. Diaphragm and cervical cap: failure rate 5% to 9% in nulliparous women, 20% in multiparous women
  2. Female condom: failure rate with perfect use, 5.1%; with typical use, 12.4%; FDA labeling states 25% failure rate
  3. Male condom: failure rate with perfect use, 3%; with typical use, 12%
  4. Spermicides (aerosols, foam, jellies, creams, tabs): failure rate with perfect use, 3%; with typical use, 21%
- Oral contraceptives
  1. Failure rate with perfect use, <1%; with typical use, 3%
  2. Come in combinations of estrogen/progestin or progestin only
- Hormonal implants
  1. Norplant
     a. Most typically used in U.S.
     b. Failure rate in first 5 yr: 1%
     c. Failure rate after 6 yr: 2%
  2. Depo-Provera: failure rate 0.3% in first year of use
- Mini pill (progesterone only pill)
  1. Failure rate with typical use, 1.1% to 13.2%
  2. With perfect use, 5 pregnancies/1000 women
- Emergency postcoital contraception
  1. Decreases pregnancy rate by 75% with women treated immediately postcoitally
  2. Involves hormonal use or IUD insertion
- IUD
  1. Progestasert: failure rate with perfect use 2%; with typical use 3%
  2. Copper T (380-A): failure rate with perfect use 0.8%; with typical use 3%
- Female sterilization (tubal ligation): failure rate with perfect use 0.2%; with typical use 3%
- Male sterilization: failure rate of 0.1% in first year

SYNONYMS
Birth control
Family planning

ICD-9-CM CODES
V25.01 Oral contraceptives
V25.02 Other contraceptive measures
V25.09 Family planning
V25.1 IUD
V25.2 Sterilization

EPIDEMIOLOGY AND DEMOGRAPHICS
For women at risk for pregnancy, ranges for most commonly used birth control are dependent, as follows:
- Oral contraceptives: 3% (40 to 44 yr old) to 60% (20 to 24 yr old)
- Condoms: 9% (40 to 44 yr old) to 26% (15 to 19 yr old)
- Diaphragm: 0.8% (15 to 19 yr old) to 8% (30 to 34 yr old)
- Periodic abstinence: 0.7% (15 to 19 yr old) to 3% (35 to 39 yr old)
- Withdrawal: 1.1% (40 to 44 yr old) to 3% (20 to 30 yr old)
- IUD: 0% (15 to 19 yr old) to 3% (30 to 34 yr old)
- Spermicides: 0.8% (15 to 19 yr old) to 2.7% (35 to 39 yr old)
- No method: 6.3% (35 to 39 yr old) to 19.8% (15 to 19 yr old)
- Sterilization
  Female: 0.2% (15 to 19 yr old) to 47% (40 to 44 yr old)
  Male: 0.2% (15 to 19 yr old) to 21% (40 to 44 yr old)

Women are more likely to use contraception. The only two male forms available are condoms and vasectomy (sterilization).

DIAGNOSIS

WORKUP
- Thorough medical history
- Thorough surgical history
- Obstetric history (fertility desired?)
- Gynecologic history, including:
  1. History of previous sexually transmitted diseases
  2. Number of partners
  3. Previous difficulties with contraception
  4. Frequency of intercourse
- Family history

LABORATORY TESTS
- Pap smear
- Cultures, aerobic and *Chlamydia*
- Pregnancy test if suspected pregnancy
- Lipid profile if family history of premature vascular event

TREATMENT

NONPHARMACOLOGIC THERAPY
- Male condoms
  1. 95% latex (rubber), 5% skin or natural membrane
  2. Proper use: place on an erect penis and leave one-half inch empty space at the tip of the condom; use with non-oil-based lubricants.
  3. Effectiveness increased when used with spermicides
- Female condoms
  1. Composed of polyurethane, with one end open and one end closed
  2. Proper use: place closed end over cervix, open end hanging out of vagina to cover penis and scrotum.
  3. Highly effective against HIV

- Spermicides
  1. Types: nonoxynol, octoxynol
  2. Forms: jellies, creams, foams, suppositories, tablets, soluble films
  3. Proper use: put in immediately before intercourse; may be used with other barrier methods.
- Diaphragm and cervical cap
  1. Must be fitted by practitioner, used with contraceptive gels, and refitted with weight gain or loss
  2. Diaphragm sizes: 50 to 95 mm; cervical cap sizes: 22, 25, 28, and 31 mm
  3. Proper use of diaphragm: put in immediately before intercourse and keep in for 6 hr after intercourse; must not remain in the vagina for longer than 24 hr.
  4. Proper use of cervical cap: fit over the cervix exactly; must not remain in place for longer than 48 hr.
- Lactation amenorrhea method
  1. Depends on number of breast-feedings per day; effective as birth control for 6 mo if 15 or more feedings, lasting 10 minutes, are accomplished daily
  2. Not a common practice in the U.S.
- Withdrawal
  1. Withdrawal of the penis from the vagina before ejaculation
  2. Dependent on self-control
- Rhythm method
  1. Dependent on awareness of physiology of male and female reproductive tracts
  2. Sperm viable in vagina for 2 to 7 days
  3. Ovum life span 24 hr
- Sterilization
  1. Male:
     a. Vasectomy to interrupt vas deferentia and block passage of sperm to seminal ejaculate
     b. Scalpel and nonscalpel techniques available
     c. More easily performed procedure than female sterilization and does not require general anesthesia
  2. Female:
     a. Leading method of birth control in U.S. in women older than 30 yr
     b. Interrupts fallopian tubes, blocking passage of ovum proximally and sperm distally through tube
     c. Several types; modified Pomeroy done during cesarean section or laparoscopic done in nonpregnant females most common

ACUTE GENERAL Rx
- Combination oral contraceptives (see Table 7-19)
  1. Taken daily for 21 days, pill-free interval of 7 days
  2. Less than 50 µg ethynyl estradiol in most common combination oral contraceptives; progestins most commonly used in combination pills are norethindrone, levonorgestrel, norgestrel, norethindrone acetate, ethyodiol, diacetate, norgestimate, or desogestrel; triphasic combination oral contraceptives available (give varying doses of progestin and estrogens throughout cycle)
- Monophasic oral contraceptives
  1. Offer same dose of progestin and estrogen throughout cycle; taken daily at same time
  2. If taken with antibiotics, efficacy affected by inadequate gastrointestinal absorption in most cases; only rifampin truly reduces pill's effectiveness
- Mini pill
  1. Progestin only; taken without a break
  2. Causes much irregular bleeding because of the lack of estrogen effect on the lining of the uterus
- Norplant
  1. Progestin only; inserted under the skin
  2. Six levonorgestrel implants placed subcutaneously in upper inner arm effective for 5 yr
- Depo-Provera
  1. Medroxyprogesterone acetate given every 3 mo in IM injection form
  2. Major side effect: irregular bleeding
  3. Fertility return possibly delayed up to 18 mo after discontinuation
- Postcoital contraception
  1. Done on emergency basis, usually secondary to noncompliance with birth control or failure of birth control (e.g., condom breakage) at the time of ovulation
  2. Methods:
     a. IUD insertion within 7 days of coitus
     b. Hormonal methods (combination pills and danazol) given within 48 hr of coitus
- IUD
  1. Device inserted into uterus to prevent sperm and ovum from uniting in fallopian tube
  2. Types available in U.S.:
     a. Progestasert: a T-shaped device that is an ethylene vinyl acetate copolymer T; vertical stem contains 38 mg progesterone and must be changed yearly
     b. ParaGard (Copper T/380-A): a polyethylene T wrapped with a fine copper wire that is effective for 10 yr of use

CHRONIC Rx
- With all of the above types of birth control, patient is followed at least yearly, or as necessary, if problems arise.
- Full history, physical examination, and Pap smear, including cultures when needed, are performed yearly.
- Patients with medical problems are followed about every 6 mo when taking hormonal therapy.

DISPOSITION
- Follow yearly or more frequently according to patient's side effects.
- Tailor birth control to patient according to different needs or side effects present at different times in life.

REFERRAL
With hormonal contraception, if neurologic or cardiac symptoms arise, stop method immediately, evaluate, and refer to internist when appropriate.

MISCELLANEOUS

COMMENTS
- Patient education information available through American College of Obstetricians and Gynecologists (ACOG) at 1-800-673-8444 and through various drug companies representing and supplying the particular type of contraception.
- A clinical algorithm on the use of oral contraceptives is described in Fig. 3-22.
- U.S. Preventive Services Task Force Recommendations regarding counseling to prevent unintended pregnancy are described in Section V, Chapter 63.

REFERENCES
Corigliano MA, Danakas GT, Pietrantoni M: *Practical guide to the care of gynecologic/obstetric patient,* St Louis, 1997, Mosby.

Hatcher RA et al: *Contraceptive technology,* ed 16, New York, 1994, Irvington Publishers.

Author: **Maria A. Corigliano, M.D.**

CLINICAL TOPICS **Conversion disorder** 135

BASIC INFORMATION

DEFINITION
Conversion disorder is an alteration or loss of voluntary motor or sensory function suggestive of a physical disorder but without demonstrable physical cause and related to a psychologic stress or a conflict.

SYNONYMS
Hysteria
Hysterical conversion
Pseudoneurologic illness
Nondisease
Psychosomatic illness
Persistent somatization
Functional illness

ICD-9-CM CODES
300.11 Conversion disorder

EPIDEMIOLOGY AND DEMOGRAPHICS
INCIDENCE (IN U.S.): 22 cases/100,000 persons/yr (in Iceland, 11 cases/100,000 persons/yr)
PREVALENCE (IN U.S.): 11 to 300 cases/100,000 persons
PREDOMINANT SEX: More common in women (2-10:1)
PREDOMINANT AGE: Generally a disease of adults
PEAK INCIDENCE: Older than 10 yr and younger than 35 yr
GENETICS: Monozygotic twins have increased risk, but dizygotic twins do not.

PHYSICAL FINDINGS
- Dysfunction of voluntary activity or sensation
- Most common symptoms: amnesia, difficulty swallowing, speech dysfunction, deafness, visual problems, loss of sensation, fainting, pseudoseizures, gait abnormalities, paresis, and paralysis
- In women: left side of the body more commonly affected
- Other presentations, such as hyperemesis
- In children <10 yr old: gait difficulties or pseudoseizures
- Physical abnormalities (if present) insufficient to explain the presentation
- Proximal psychologic issue identifiable

ETIOLOGY
The term *conversion* was coined by Freud and Breuer, who proposed that psychic energy of a conflict is converted into physical symptoms; this remains one of the best theoretical formulations.

DIAGNOSIS

DIFFERENTIAL DIAGNOSIS
- Malingering: dysfunction is consciously created for the purpose of secondary gain or avoidance of noxious duties
- Factitious disorder (e.g., Munchausen's syndrome): dysfunction is consciously created for the purpose of assuming the patient role
- Somatization: a related disorder in which psychologic difficulties present with a wide range of somatic complaints that affect several organ systems

WORKUP
Physical examination and laboratory evaluation must be sufficient to rule out a physical cause for the dysfunction.

LABORATORY TESTS
- No specific laboratory tests
- Goal of tests: to exclude physical cause for the dysfunction

IMAGING STUDIES
Goal of tests: to exclude physical cause for the dysfunction

TREATMENT

NONPHARMACOLOGIC THERAPY
- Psychotherapy that attempts to address the underlying psychologic conflicts is generally recommended.
- Affected individuals generally are not ideal psychotherapy candidates; supportive psychotherapy is possibly the only reasonable intervention.
- Patients are frequently suggestible, so interventions such as suggestion and hypnosis may be useful.

ACUTE GENERAL Rx
Amobarbital (Sodium Amytal) interviews are sometimes used both diagnostically and therapeutically; conversion may disappear under the influence of Amytal.

CHRONIC Rx
Conversion has a high recurrence rate, so ongoing psychotherapy may be cost effective.

DISPOSITION
- Among hospitalized patients with conversion disorder, remission typically occurs within 2 wk. However, recurrence may occur in 20% to 25% of patients within 1 yr. Recurrences foretell future recurrences.
- Symptoms of pseudoseizures and tremor are less likely to remit than symptoms of paralysis, aphonia, or blindness.

REFERRAL
If supportive interventions are not helpful, disability is extreme, or there is no improvement in 2 wk

MISCELLANEOUS

COMMENTS
Many patients "elaborate" on symptoms to convince the physician they are ill; this may considerably complicate appropriate diagnosis and therapy.

REFERENCES
El-Mallakh RS, Liebowitz NR, Hale MS: Hyperemesis gravidarum as conversion disorder, *J Nerv Mental Dis* 178:655, 1990.
Silver FW: Management of conversion disorder, *Am J Phys Med Rehabil* 75:134, 1996.

Author: **Rif S. El-Mallakh, M.D.**

Corneal abrasion

BASIC INFORMATION

DEFINITION
A corneal abrasion is a loss of surface epithelial tissue of the cornea caused by trauma.

SYNONYMS
Corneal erosion
Corneal contusion

ICD-9-CM CODES
918.1 Corneal abrasion

EPIDEMIOLOGY AND DEMOGRAPHICS
INCIDENCE (IN U.S.): A universal problem
PREDOMINANT AGE: Any age
PEAK INCIDENCE: Childhood through active adulthood

PHYSICAL FINDINGS
- Haziness of the cornea
- Disruption of the corneal surface
- Redness and infection of the conjunctiva
- Pain
- Sensation of a foreign body

ETIOLOGY
Trauma (direct mechanical event)

DIAGNOSIS

DIFFERENTIAL DIAGNOSIS
- Acute angle glaucoma
- Herpes ulcers and other corneal ulcers
- Foreign body in the cornea (be certain it is not a keratitis)

WORKUP
- Fluorescein staining, slit lamp evaluation
- Assessment of visual acuity
- Intraocular pressure

TREATMENT

NONPHARMACOLOGIC THERAPY
- Warm compresses
- Pressure dressing
- Removal of any foreign particles if present

ACUTE GENERAL Rx
- Topical antibiotics
- Pressure patching of eye with eyelid closed
- Cycloplegics

CHRONIC Rx
Topical antibiotics to prevent secondary infection

DISPOSITION
Follow-up until abrasion has cleared and vision has returned to normal

REFERRAL
To ophthalmologist if patient experiences no relief within 24 hr

MISCELLANEOUS

COMMENTS
Never give patient topical anesthetic to use at home because these can cause decomposition of the cornea and permanent damage.

REFERENCES
Leone CR: Periorbital trauma, *Int Ophthalmol Clin* 35:1, 1995.
Lubeck D, Greene JS: Corneal injuries, *Emerg Med Clin North Am* 6:73, 1988.
Torok PG, Mader TH: Corneal abrasions: diagnosis and management, *Am Fam Physician* 53:2521, 1996.
Author: **Melvyn Koby, M.D.**

Corneal ulceration

BASIC INFORMATION

DEFINITION
Corneal ulceration refers to the disruption of the corneal surface and/or deeper layers caused by trauma or infection.

SYNONYMS
Infectious keratitis
Bacterial keratitis
Viral keratitis
Fungal keratitis

ICD-9-CM CODES
370.0 Corneal ulcer NOS

EPIDEMIOLOGY AND DEMOGRAPHICS
INCIDENCE (IN U.S.): 4-6 cases/mo seen by average general ophthalmologist
PREVALENCE (IN U.S.): Common
PREDOMINANT SEX: Either
PREDOMINANT AGE: All ages

PHYSICAL FINDINGS
- Localized, well-demarcated, infiltrative lesion with corresponding focal ulcer or oval, yellow-white stromal suppuration with thick mucopurulent exudate and edema
- Eye possibly painful, with conjunctival edema and infection

ETIOLOGY
- Complication of contact lens wear, trauma, or diseases such as herpes simplex keratitis, keratoconjunctivitis sicca
- Viral causes often contagious

DIAGNOSIS

DIFFERENTIAL DIAGNOSIS
- *Pseudomonas* and *pneumococcus* infection—virulent
- *Moraxella, staphylococci, alpha streptococcus* infection—less virulent
- Herpes simplex infection or disease caused by other viruses

WORKUP
- Fluorescein staining, slit lamp
- Appearance often typical

LABORATORY TESTS
Microscopic examination and culture of scrapings

TREATMENT

NONPHARMACOLOGIC THERAPY
- Warm compresses
- Remove eyelid crusting

ACUTE GENERAL Rx
- An ophthalmic emergency
- Bacterial infection: subconjunctival cefazolin or gentamicin
- Fungal infection: hospitalization and topical application of antifungal agents

DISPOSITION
Ideally treated by an ophthalmologist if the patient does not rapidly respond to antibiotics (within 24 hr).

MISCELLANEOUS

COMMENTS
Do not use topical steroids because herpes, fungal, or other ulcers may be aggravated, leading to perforation of the cornea.

REFERENCES
Scribbick AT, Scribbick FW: Clinical pearls: right-eye pain, corneal ulcer, *Acad Emerg Med* 1:412, 1994.
Shingleton BJ: Eye injuries, *N Engl J Med* 325:408, 1991.

Author: **Melvyn Koby, M.D.**

Costochondritis (PTG)

BASIC INFORMATION

DEFINITION
Costochondritis is a poorly defined chest wall pain of uncertain cause.

SYNONYMS
- Benign chest wall pain syndrome
- Costosternal syndrome
- Costosternal chondrodynia

ICD-9-CM CODES
733.6 Costochondritis

EPIDEMIOLOGY AND DEMOGRAPHICS
PREVALENCE: Unknown
PREVALENT SEX: Women > men
PREVALENT AGE: Over age 40 yr

PHYSICAL FINDINGS
- Tenderness of costochondral junctions (second through fifth) and/or sternum
- Pain with coughing and deep breathing
- Both sides of chest equal in frequency of involvement

ETIOLOGY
- Unknown
- May be a form of regional fibrositis
- May be referred pain from cervical or thoracic spine

DIAGNOSIS

DIFFERENTIAL DIAGNOSIS
- Tietze's syndrome
- Cardiovascular disease
- GI disease
- Pulmonary disease
- Osteoarthritis

WORKUP
There are no laboratory or radiographic abnormalities.

TREATMENT

ACUTE GENERAL Rx
- Explanation, reassurance
- Tricyclic antidepressants for sleep disturbance
- Aerobic exercise program

DISPOSITION
- The duration of the disorder is variable
- Spontaneous remission is the rule.

MISCELLANEOUS

COMMENTS
In spite of the name, no inflammation is present. After other more serious conditions are ruled out, the treatment is strictly symptomatic and supportive.

REFERENCES
Fam AG, Smythe HA: Musculoskeletal chest wall pain, *Can Med Assoc J* 133:379, 1985.
Kaye, BR: Chest pain: not always a cardiac problem, *J Musculoskeletal Med* 37, March 1993.

Author: **Lonnie R. Mercier, M.D.**

Creutzfeldt-Jakob disease

BASIC INFORMATION

DEFINITION
Creutzfeldt-Jakob disease is a progressive, dementing process caused by an infectious agent known as a *prion*.

SYNONYMS
Subacute spongiform encephalopathy
Gerstmann-Sträussler syndrome

ICD-9-CM CODES
046.1 Creutzfeldt-Jakob disease

EPIDEMIOLOGY AND DEMOGRAPHICS
INCIDENCE (IN U.S.): 1 case/1,000,000 persons/yr
PREVALENCE (IN U.S.): After diagnosis, death occurs in 6 mo to 1 yr
PREDOMINANT SEX: Men = women
PEAK INCIDENCE: Over 50 yr
PEAK AGE: 60 yr
GENETICS: 5% to 15% familial

PHYSICAL FINDINGS
Subacute dementia and myoclonus

ETIOLOGY
Infectious "slow virus" prion

DIAGNOSIS

DIFFERENTIAL DIAGNOSIS
- Alzheimer's disease
- Other dementias (vascular, endocrine, vitamin deficiency, infectious syphilis)

The U.S. Preventive Services Task Force Recommendations for screening for dementia are described in Section V, Chapter 48. A clinical algorithm for the evaluation of dementia is described in Fig. 3-25.

WORKUP
- Evaluate for curable causes of dementia.
- Brain biopsy can be diagnostic, but it is usually not performed.

LABORATORY TESTS
- EEG may show burst-suppression pattern.
- Rule out curable causes of dementia.

IMAGING STUDIES
CT scan to rule out NPH, space-occupying lesions

TREATMENT

NONPHARMACOLOGIC THERAPY
Constant caregiver usually necessary

ACUTE GENERAL Rx
No known therapy

CHRONIC Rx
No known therapy

DISPOSITION
Nursing home often required

REFERRAL
If NPH or brain tumor found

MISCELLANEOUS

COMMENTS
- Not known to be transmissible except through direct contact with brain
- Autopsy important to confirm diagnosis

REFERENCES
Will RG: Epidemiology of Creutzfeldt-Jakob disease, *Br Med Bull* 49:960, 1993.

Author: **William H. Olson, M.D.**

Crohn's disease (PTG)

BASIC INFORMATION

DEFINITION
Crohn's disease is an inflammatory disease of the bowel of unknown etiology, most commonly involving the terminal ileum and manifesting primarily with diarrhea, abdominal pain, fatigue, and weight loss.

SYNONYMS
Regional enteritis
Inflammatory bowel disease (IBD)

ICD-9-CM CODES
555.9 Crohn's disease, unspecified site
555.0 Crohn's disease, small intestine
555.1 Crohn's disease involving large intestine

EPIDEMIOLOGY AND DEMOGRAPHICS
PREVALENCE: 1 case/1000 persons; most common in Caucasians and Jews

PHYSICAL FINDINGS
- Abdominal tenderness, mass, or distention
- Hyperactive bowel sounds in patients with partial obstruction, bloody diarrhea
- Delayed growth and failure of normal development in children
- Perianal and rectal abscesses, mouth ulcers, and atrophic glossitis
- Extraintestinal manifestations: joint swelling and tenderness, hepatosplenomegaly, erythema nodosum, clubbing, tenderness to palpation of the sacroiliac joints

ETIOLOGY
Unknown

DIAGNOSIS

DIFFERENTIAL DIAGNOSIS
- Ulcerative colitis
- Infectious diseases (TB, Yersinia, salmonella, *Shigella*, *Campylobacter*)
- Parasitic infections (amebic infection)
- Pseudomembranous colitis
- Ischemic colitis in elderly patients
- Lymphoma
- Colon carcinoma
- Diverticulitis
- Radiation enteritis
- Collagenous colitis
- Fungal infections (*Histoplasma*, *Actinomyces*)
- Gay bowel syndrome (in homosexual patient)
- Carcinoid tumors
- Celiac sprue
- Mesenteric adenitis

LABORATORY TESTS
- Decreased Hgb and Hct from chronic blood loss
- Hypokalemia, hypomagnesemia, hypocalcemia, and low albumin from chronic diarrhea possible
- Vitamin B_{12} and folate deficiency
- Endoscopic features of Crohn's disease include asymmetric and discontinued disease, deep longitudinal fissures, cobblestone appearance, presence of strictures. Crypt distortion and inflammation are also present. Granulomas may be present.

IMAGING STUDIES
- Barium imaging studies reveal deep ulcerations (often longitudinal and transverse), segmental lesions (skip lesions, strictures, fistulas, cobblestone appearance of mucosa caused by submucosal inflammation); "thumbprinting" is common, "string sign" in terminal ileum may be noted.
- In 5% to 10% of patients with IBD, a clear distinction between ulcerative colitis and Crohn's disease cannot be made. Generally, Crohn's disease can be distinguished from ulcerative colitis by presence of transmural involvement and the frequent presence of noncaseating granulomas and lymphoid aggregates.

TREATMENT

NONPHARMACOLOGIC THERAPY
- Nutritional supplementation is needed in patients with advanced disease. TPN may be necessary in selected patients.
- Low-residue diet is necessary when obstructive symptoms are present.
- If diarrhea is prominent, increased dietary fiber and lowering of fat in the diet are sometimes helpful.
- Psychotherapy is useful for situational adjustment crises. A trusting and mutually understanding relationship and referral to self-help groups is very important because of the chronicity of the disease and the relatively young age of the patients.
- Avoid oral feedings during acute exacerbation to decrease colonic activity: a low-roughage diet may be helpful in early relapse.

ACUTE GENERAL Rx
- Sulfasalazine, 500 mg PO qid initially, increased qd or qod by 1 g until therapeutic dosages of 4 to 6 g/day are achieved. The oral salicylates, mesalamine (Asacol, Rowasa) are as effective as sulfasalazine but more expensive; they may be useful in patients allergic to the sulfa moiety of sulfasalazine molecule. Corticosteroids (prednisone) 40 to 60 mg/day is useful for acute exacerbation. Steroids are usually tapered over approximately 2 to 3 mo. Some patients require a low dose for prolonged period of maintenance.
- Immunosuppressive drugs, such as azathioprine (Imuran), 150 mg/day or methotrexate or cyclosporine can be used for severe, progressive disease.
- Metronidazole (Flagyl) 250 mg qid is useful for colonic fistulas.
- Hydrocortisone (Cortenema) enema bid or tid is useful for proctitis.
- Most patients who have anemia associated with Crohn's disease respond to intravenous iron alone. Erythropoietin is useful in patients with anemia refractory to treatment with iron and vitamins.

CHRONIC Rx
- Monitoring of disease activity with symptom review and laboratory evaluation (CBC and sedimentation rate)
- Liver tests and vitamin B_{12} levels monitored on a yearly basis

REFERRAL
- GI referral is needed for endoscopic procedures.
- Surgical referral is needed for complications such as abscess formation, obstruction, fistulas, toxic megacolon, refractory disease, or severe hemorrhage. A conservative surgical approach is necessary, since surgery is not curative. Multiple surgeries may also result in short bowel syndrome.

MISCELLANEOUS

COMMENTS
Patient education material on Crohn's disease may be obtained from the Crohn's and Colitis Foundation of America, 386 Park Avenue South, 17th Floor, New York, NY 10016.

REFERENCES
Egan LJ, Sandborn WJ: Methotrexate for inflammatory bowel disease: pharmacology and preliminary results, *Mayo Clin Proc* 71:69, 1996.

Schreiber S et al: Recombinant erythropoietin for the treatment of anemia in inflammatory bowel disease, *N Engl J Med* 334:619, 1996.

Author: **Fred F. Ferri, M.D.**

Cryptococcosis (PTG)

BASIC INFORMATION

DEFINITION
Cryptococcosis is an infection caused by the fungal organism *Cryptococcus neoformans*.

ICD-9-CM CODES
117.5 Cryptococcosis

EPIDEMIOLOGY AND DEMOGRAPHICS
INCIDENCE (IN U.S.)
- 1 to 2 cases/1,000,000 (non-HIV-infected) persons annually
- 6% to 7% in HIV-infected persons

PREDOMINANT SEX: Equal sex distribution when corrected for HIV status
PREDOMINANT AGE: Less than 2 yr of age; 20 to 40 yr of age
PEAK INCIDENCE: 20 to 40 yr (parallel to AIDS epidemic)
NEONATAL INFECTION: Very uncommon

PHYSICAL FINDINGS
- Over 90% present with meningitis; almost all have fever and headache.
- Meningismus, photophobia, mental status changes are seen in approximately 25%.
- Focal intracranial infection occurs in rare cases with focal deficit, increased intracranial pressure.
- Most common infections outside the CNS:
  1. In the lungs (fever, cough, dyspnea)
  2. In the skin (cellulitis, papular eruption)
  3. In the lymph nodes (lymphadenitis)
  4. Potential involvement of virtually any organ

ETIOLOGY
- Caused by the fungal organism *C. neoformans*
- Transmission by the respiratory route
- Disseminates to the CNS in most cases, usually without recognizable lung involvement
- Almost always in the setting of AIDS or other disorders of cellular immune function (hematologic malignancies, long-term corticosteroid therapy, immunosuppressive therapy following organ transplantation)

DIAGNOSIS

DIFFERENTIAL DIAGNOSIS
- Acute or subacute meningitis (caused by *Neisseria meningitidis*, *Streptococcus pneumoniae*, *Hemophilus influenzae*, *Listeria monocytogenes*, *Mycobacterium tuberculosis*, *Histoplasma capsulatum*, viruses)
- Intracranial mass lesion (neoplasms, toxoplasmosis, TB)
- Pulmonary involvement confused with *Pneumocystis carinii* pneumonia when diffuse or confused with TB or bacterial pneumonia when focal or involving the pleura
- Skin lesions confused with bacterial cellulitis or molluscum contagiosum

WORKUP
- Lumbar puncture to exclude cryptococcal meningitis; a differential diagnosis of common fungal infections in the CNS is described in Table 2-24.
- CT scan of the head when focal lesion or increased intracranial pressure are suspected
- Biopsy of enlarged lymph nodes and skin lesions if feasible

LABORATORY TESTS
- Culture and India ink stain (60% to 80% sensitive in culture-proven cases), examination of the CSF in all cases when CNS involvement is suspected
- Blood and serum cryptococcal antigen assay (>90% sensitivity and specificity)
- Culture and histologic examination of biopsy material

IMAGING STUDIES
- CT scan or MRI of the head if focal neurologic involvement is suspected
- Chest x-ray examination to exclude pulmonary involvement

TREATMENT

ACUTE GENERAL Rx
- Therapy is initiated with IV amphotericin B (0.5 mg/kg/qd).
- After stabilization (usually several weeks), consider fluconazole (200 to 400 mg qd PO) for additional 6 to 8 wk.
- Alternative: IV fluconazole for initial therapy in patients unable to tolerate amphotericin B.

CHRONIC Rx
Fluconazole (200 mg PO qd) is highly effective in preventing a relapse in HIV-infected patients.

DISPOSITION
Without maintenance therapy, relapse rate is >50% among AIDS patients.

REFERRAL
- For consultation with infectious diseases specialist in all cases
- For neurologic consultation if level of consciousness is depressed or focal lesion is present

MISCELLANEOUS

COMMENTS
Cryptococcosis is considered an AIDS-defining infection when it occurs in the absence of other known causes of immunodeficiency; thus all patients should be advised to be HIV tested and, if positive, referred for evaluation and follow-up by a physician experienced in the management of HIV infection.

REFERENCES
Kirchner JT: Opportunistic fungal infections in patients with HIV disease: combating cryptococcosis and histoplasmosis, *Postgrad Med* 99(6):209, 1996.

Author: **Joseph R. Masci, M.D.**

Cushing's disease and syndrome (PTG)

BASIC INFORMATION

DEFINITION
- Cushing's syndrome is the occurrence of clinical abnormalities associated with glucocorticoid excess secondary to exaggerated adrenal cortisol production or chronic glucocorticoid therapy.
- Cushing's disease is Cushing's syndrome caused by pituitary ACTH excess.

ICD-9-CM CODES
255.0 Cushing's disease or syndrome

PHYSICAL FINDINGS
- Hypertension
- Central obesity with rounding of the facies (moon facies); thin extremities
- Hirsutism, menstrual irregularities, hypogonadism
- Skin fragility, ecchymoses, red-purple abdominal striae, acne, poor wound healing, hair loss, facial plethora, hyperpigmentation (when there is ACTH excess)
- Psychosis, emotional lability, paranoia
- Muscle wasting with proximal myopathy

NOTE: The above characteristics are not commonly present in Cushing's syndrome secondary to ectopic ACTH production. Many of these tumors secrete a biologically inactive ACTH that does not activate adrenal steroid synthesis. These patients may have only weight loss and weakness.

ETIOLOGY
- Iatrogenic from chronic glucocorticoid therapy (common)
- Pituitary ACTH excess (Cushing's disease; 60%)
- Adrenal neoplasms (30%)
- Ectopic ACTH production (neoplasms of lung, pancreas, kidney, thyroid, thymus; 10%)

DIAGNOSIS

DIFFERENTIAL DIAGNOSIS
- Alcoholic pseudo-Cushing's syndrome (endogenous cortisol overproduction)
- Obesity associated with diabetes mellitus
- Adrenogenital syndrome

WORKUP
- In patients with a clinical diagnosis of Cushing's syndrome the initial screening test is the overnight dexamethasone suppression test:
  1. Dexamethasone 1 mg PO given at 11 PM
  2. Plasma cortisol level measured 9 hr later (8 AM)
  3. Plasma cortisol level <5 µg/100 ml excludes Cushing's syndrome
- Serial measurements (two or three consecutive measurements) of 24-hr urinary free cortisol and creatinine (to ensure adequacy of collection) are undertaken if overnight dexamethasone test is suggestive of Cushing's syndrome. Persistent elevated cortisol excretion indicates Cushing's syndrome.
- The low-dose (2 mg) dexamethasone suppression test is useful in order to exclude pseudo-Cushing's syndrome if the above results are equivocal. CRH stimulation after low-dose dexamethasone administration (dexamethasone-CRH test) is also used to distinguish patients with suspected Cushing's syndrome from those who have mildly elevated urinary free cortisol level and equivocal findings.
- The high-dose (8 mg) dexamethasone test and measurement of ACTH by RIA are useful to determine the etiology of Cushing's syndrome.
  1. ACTH undetectable or decreased and lack of suppression indicates adrenal etiology of Cushing's syndrome.
  2. ACTH normal or increased and lack of suppression indicates ectopic ACTH production.
  3. ACTH normal or increased and partial suppression suggest pituitary excess (Cushing's disease).

LABORATORY TESTS
- Hypokalemia, hypochloremia, metabolic alkalosis, hyperglycemia, hypercholesterolemia
- Increased 24-hr urinary free cortisol (>100 µg/24 hr)

IMAGING STUDIES
- CT scan of adrenal glands in suspected adrenal Cushing's syndrome
- MRI of pituitary gland with gadolinium in suspected pituitary Cushing's syndrome
- Additional imaging studies to localize neoplasms of the lung, pancreas, kidney, thyroid, or thymus in patients with ectopic ACTH production

TREATMENT

ACUTE GENERAL Rx
The treatment of Cushing's syndrome varies with its cause:
- Pituitary adenoma: transsphenoidal microadenomectomy is the therapy of choice in adults. Pituitary irradiation is reserved for patients not cured by transsphenoidal surgery. In children, pituitary irradiation may be considered as initial therapy, since 85% of children are cured by radiation. Stereotactic radiotherapy (photon knife or gamma knife) is effective and exposes the surrounding neuronal tissues to less irradiation than conventional radiotherapy. Total bilateral adrenalectomy is reserved for patients not cured by transsphenoidal surgery or pituitary irradiation.
- Adrenal neoplasm:
  1. Surgical resection of the affected adrenal
  2. Glucocorticoid replacement for approximately 9 to 12 mo after the surgery to allow time for the contralateral adrenal to recover from its prolonged suppression
- Bilateral micronodular or macronodular adrenal hyperplasia: bilateral total adrenalectomy
- Ectopic ACTH:
  1. Surgical resection of the ACTH-secreting neoplasm
  2. Control of cortisol excess with metyrapone, aminoglutethimide, mifepristone, or ketoconazole
  3. Control of the mineralocorticoid effects of cortisol and 11-deoxycorticosteroid with spironolactone
  4. Bilateral adrenalectomy: a rational approach to patients with indolent, unresectable tumors

CHRONIC Rx
Patient education regarding maintenance of proper weight and side effects of drug therapy

DISPOSITION
Prognosis is favorable in patients with surgically amenable disease.

REFERRAL
- Endocrinology referral for diagnostic testing when diagnosis is equivocal
- Surgical and/or radiotherapy referral for all patients with pituitary adenomas
- Surgical referral for adrenal neoplasms and for resectable ectopic ACTH-secreting neoplasms

MISCELLANEOUS

COMMENTS
Screening for MEN I should be considered in patients with Cushing's disease.

REFERENCES
Orth DN: Cushing's syndrome, *N Engl J Med* 332:791, 1995.

Author: **Fred F. Ferri, M.D.**

BASIC INFORMATION

DEFINITION
Cystic fibrosis is an autosomal recessive disorder characterized by dysfunction of exocrine glands.

ICD-9-CM CODES
277.0 Cystic fibrosis

EPIDEMIOLOGY AND DEMOGRAPHICS
- It is the most common fatal hereditary disorder of Caucasians in the U.S. (1 case/2500 Caucasians).
- Median survival is 30 yr.

PHYSICAL FINDINGS
- Failure to thrive in children
- Increased anterior/posterior chest diameter
- Basilar crackles and hyperresonance to percussion
- Digital clubbing
- Chronic cough
- Abdominal distention
- Greasy, smelly feces

ETIOLOGY
Chromosome 7 gene mutation (CFTR gene) resulting in abnormalities in chloride transport and water flux across the surface of epithelial cells; the abnormal secretions cause obstruction of glands and ducts in various organs and subsequent damage to exocrine tissue (recurrent pneumonia, atelectasis, bronchiectasis, diabetes mellitus, biliary cirrhosis, cholelithiasis, intestinal obstruction, increased risk of GI malignancies)

DIAGNOSIS

DIFFERENTIAL DIAGNOSIS
- Immunodeficiency states
- Celiac disease
- Asthma
- Recurrent pneumonia

WORKUP
Pilocarpine iontophoresis test, PFTs, chest x-ray examination, gene analysis

LABORATORY TESTS
- Pilocarpine iontophoresis ("sweat test"): diagnostic of cystic fibrosis in children if sweat chloride is >60 mmol/L (>80 mmol/L in adults) on two separate tests on consecutive days
- Sputum C&S and Gram stain (frequent bacterial infections with *Staphylococcus aureus, Pseudomonas, Hemophilus influenza*)
- Low albumin level, increased 72-hr fecal fat excretion
- ABGs: hypoxemia
- Pulmonary function studies: decreased TLC, forced vital capacity, pulmonary diffusing capacity

IMAGING STUDIES
- Chest x-ray examination: may reveal focal atelectasis, peribronchial cuffing, bronchiectasis, increased interstitial markings, hyperinflation
- High resolution chest CT scan: bronchial wall thickening, cystic lesions, ring shadows (bronchiectasis)

TREATMENT

NONPHARMACOLOGIC THERAPY
- Postural drainage and chest percussion
- Encouragement of regular exercise and proper nutrition
- Psychosocial evaluation and counseling of patient and family members

ACUTE GENERAL Rx
- Antibiotic therapy based on results of Gram stain and C&S of sputum (PO ciprofloxacin or floxacillin for *Pseudomonas*, cephalosporins for *S. aureus*, IV aminoglycosides plus ceftazidine for life-threatening *Pseudomonas* infections)
- Bronchodilators for patients with air flow obstruction
- Chronic pancreatic enzyme replacement
- Alternate-day prednisone (2 mg/kg) possibly beneficial in children with cystic fibrosis (decreased hospitalization rate, improved pulmonary function); routine use of corticosteroids not recommended in adults
- Proper nutrition and vitamin supplementation
- Recombinant human deoxyribonuclease (DNase, [Dornase alpha]) 2.5 mg qd or bid given by aerosol for patients with viscid sputum; useful but expensive (annual cost to the pharmacist is >$10,000); most beneficial in patients with FVC values >40% of predicted
- Treatment of glucose intolerance and diabetes mellitus

CHRONIC Rx
Pneumococcal vaccination, yearly influenza vaccination

DISPOSITION
- Over 50% of children with cystic fibrosis live beyond age 20 yr.
- Lung transplantation is the only definitive treatment; 3-yr survival following transplantation exceeds 50%.

REFERRAL
- To regional ambulatory care cystic fibrosis center
- For lung transplantation in selected patients
- For screening of family members with DNA analysis

MISCELLANEOUS

COMMENTS
Patient education material can be obtained from Cystic Fibrosis Foundation, 6931 Arlington Road, Suite 2000, Bethesda, MD 20814.

REFERENCES
Crystal RG: Cystic fibrosis: from the gene to the cure, *Am J Respir Crit Care Med* 151:S45, 1995.
Hodson ME: Aerosolized Dornase Alpha (RHDNase) for therapy of cystic fibrosis, *Am J Respir Crit Care Med* 151:S70, 1995.

Author: **Fred F. Ferri, M.D.**

Delirium tremens

BASIC INFORMATION

DEFINITION
Delirium tremens refers to overactivity of the central nervous system after cessation of alcohol intake. The time interval is variable; it usually occurs within 1 wk after reduction or cessation of heavy alcohol intake and persists for 1 to 3 days.

SYNONYMS
Alcohol withdrawal syndrome
DTs
Alcoholic delirium

ICD-9-CM CODES
291.00 Alcohol withdrawal delirium

EPIDEMIOLOGY AND DEMOGRAPHICS
INCIDENCE (IN U.S.): Up to 500,000 cases annually
PREDOMINANT SEX: Male
PEAK INCIDENCE: 30 yr and older
PEAK AGE: Teenage years and older
GENETICS: More common with patients who have relatives that are alcoholic

PHYSICAL FINDINGS
- Initially: anxiety, insomnia, tremulousness
- Early: tachycardia, sweating, anorexia, agitation, headache, GI distress
- Late: seizures, visual hallucinations, delirium

ETIOLOGY
Alcoholism

DIAGNOSIS

DIFFERENTIAL DIAGNOSIS
Be alert for coexisting illness, trauma, and drug usage.

WORKUP
- Frequent rating of symptoms (hallucinations, tremor, sweating, agitation, orientation)
- The CIWA-Ar Scale (see Box A-9) can be used to measure the severity of alcohol withdrawal.

LABORATORY TESTS
- Electrolytes
- Close monitoring of glucose levels
- Drug screen

IMAGING STUDIES
CT scan of head if there is a history of head trauma

TREATMENT

NONPHARMACOLOGIC THERAPY
Refer to drug rehabilitation program.

ACUTE GENERAL Rx
- Prescribe diazepam 150 to 200 mg/day or chlordiazepoxide 400 to 600 mg/day.
- For severe withdrawal, consider adrenergic blockers (0.1 to 0.3 tid of clonidine) and thiamine (100 mg IV qd initially).

CHRONIC Rx
Alcoholics Anonymous has a good record in breaking addiction.

DISPOSITION
Refer to drug rehabilitation program.

REFERRAL
If cardiac arrhythmias are prominent or respiratory distress develops

MISCELLANEOUS

COMMENTS
This is a potentially lethal disease if not carefully treated. Mortality is 15% in untreated patients.

REFERENCES
Griffin RE, Gross GA, Teitelbaum HS: Delirium tremens: a review, *JAMA* 93:924, 1993.
Lohr RH: Treatment of alcohol withdrawal in hospitalized patients, *Mayo Clin Proc* 70:777, 1995.
Yost DA: Alcohol withdrawal syndrome, *Am Fam Physician* 54:657, 1996.
Author: **William H. Olson, M.D.**

Depression, major (PTG)

BASIC INFORMATION

DEFINITION
Major depression is an episodic, frequently recurrent syndrome lasting at least 2 wk with five of the following symptoms: depressed mood; diminished interest, pleasure, energy, self-worth, ability to think and concentrate; altered sleep pattern, appetite, and level of psychomotor activity.

SYNONYMS
Unipolar depression
Depressive episode

ICD-9-CODES
296.2 Major depressive disorder, single episode

EPIDEMIOLOGY AND DEMOGRAPHICS
INCIDENCE (IN U.S.): 10% of men; 20% of women
PREVALENCE (IN U.S.): 2.5% of men; 8% of women
PREDOMINANT SEX: Female > male
PREDOMINANT AGE: 25 to 44 yr
PEAK INCIDENCE: 30 to 40 yr
GENETICS:
- Clear evidence of familial predominance
- No established pattern of inheritance

PHYSICAL FINDINGS
- Psychomotor retardation with slowed thinking, slowed responses, slowed physical movements, depressed affect and mood, sleep disturbance, appetite disturbance
- May be associated with mood-congruent delusional thinking (paranoid and melancholic themes)
- May be associated with active or passive suicidal ideation

ETIOLOGY
- Unknown
- Several factors possible: neuroendocrine response to unremitting stress, hormones, social/developmental factors

DIAGNOSIS

DIFFERENTIAL DIAGNOSIS
- Hypothyroidism
- Neurosyphilis
- Major organ system disease (e.g., cardiovascular, liver, renal, neuronal diseases, and others) with depressive symptoms
- Elderly patients: frequently coexists with dementia

WORKUP
- History
- Physical examination
- Mental status examination
- The Zung Depression Scale is described in Fig. A-3.
- Box A-11 describes the Geriatric Depression Scale.
- U.S. Preventive Services Task Force Recommendations regarding screening for depression are described in Section V, Chapter 49. Screening recommendations for suicide risk are described in Section V, Chapter 50.

LABORATORY TESTS
All done to rule out other major organ system disease:
- Routine chemistries
- CBC with differential
- Sedimentation rate
- Thyroid function studies

IMAGING STUDIES
With unusual presentations (e.g., associated with new-onset severe headache, focal neurologic signs, a cognitive or sensory disturbance), the following are performed:
- EEG (diffuse slowing indicates metabolic encephalopathy)
- Anatomic brain imaging (CT scan or MRI)

TREATMENT

NONPHARMACOLOGIC THERAPY
- Many forms of psychotherapy are helpful.
- Behavioral, cognitive, and interpersonal psychotherapies have efficacy rates of 40% to 50%.

ACUTE GENERAL Rx
- Many antidepressants are available (see Table 7-8), all with efficacy rates of 60% to 65%.
- Serotonin reuptake inhibitors generally are first-line agents.
- Therapy should be continued for 6 to 12 mo.
- Several treatment-refractory strategies are available.

CHRONIC Rx
The risk of recurrence exceeds 90% in individuals having experienced three or more depressive episodes; for these individuals continuous prophylactic therapy is recommended.

DISPOSITION
- Course is variable.
- Additional episodes are experienced by >60% of individuals having one depressive episode.
- There can be increasing or decreasing numbers of episodes into old age.
- Depression associated with physical disorders generally does not resolve until physical disorder improves.

REFERRAL
- If treatment refractory
- If patient imminently suicidal

MISCELLANEOUS

REFERENCES
El-Mallakh RS et al: Clues to depression in primary care practice, *Postgrad Med* 100:85, 1996.
Author: **Rif S. El-Mallakh, M.D.**

Dermatitis, atopic (PTG)

BASIC INFORMATION

DEFINITION
Atopic dermatitis is an eczematous eruption that is pruritic, symmetric, and associated with personal family history of allergic manifestations (atopy).

SYNONYMS
Eczema
Atopic neurodermatitis
Atopic eczema

ICD-9-CM CODES
691.8 Atopic dermatitis

EPIDEMIOLOGY AND DEMOGRAPHICS
- Incidence is between 5 and 25 cases/1000 persons.
- Highest incidence is among children (5%).
- Onset of disease before age 5 yr in 85% of patients.
- Over 50% of children with generalized atopic dermatitis develop asthma and allergic rhinitis by age 13 yr.

PHYSICAL FINDINGS
- There are no specific cutaneous signs for atopic dermatitis.
- The primary lesions are a result of itching caused by severe and chronic pruritus. The repeated scratching modifies the skin surface producing lichenification, dry and scaly skin, and redness.
- The lesions are typically on the neck, face, upper trunk, and bends of elbows and knees (see color plate 5).
- There is dryness, thickening of the involved areas, discoloration, blistering, and oozing.
- Papular lesions are frequently found in the antecubital and popliteal fossae.
- In children, red scaling plaques are often confined to the cheeks and the perioral and perinasal areas.
- Inflammation in the flexural areas and lichenified skin is a very common presentation children.
- Constant scratching may result in areas of hypopigmentation or hyperpigmentation (more common in blacks).
- In adults, redness and scaling in the dorsal aspect of the hands or about the fingers is the most common expression of atopic dermatitis; oozing and crusting may be present.
- Secondary skin infections may be present (*Staphylococcus aureus*, dermatophytosis, herpes simplex).

ETIOLOGY
Unknown; elevated T-lymphocyte activation, defective cell immunity, and B cell IgE overproduction may play a significant role.

DIAGNOSIS

DIFFERENTIAL DIAGNOSIS
- Scabies
- Psoriasis
- Dermatitis herpetiform
- Contact dermatitis
- Photosensitivity
- Seborrheic dermatitis
- Candidiasis
- Lichen simplex chronicus
- Other: Wiskott-Aldrich syndrome, PKU, mycosis fungoides, ichthyosis, HIV dermatitis, nonnummular eczema, histiocytosis X

A comparison of the various types of dermatitis is described in Section II, Table 2-19.

WORKUP
Diagnosis is based on the presence of three of the following major features and three minor features.

MAJOR FEATURES:
- Pruritus
- Personal or family history of atopy-asthma, allergic rhinitis, atopic dermatitis
- Facial and extensor involvement in infants and children
- Flexural lichenification in adults

MINOR FEATURES:
- Elevated IgE
- Eczema-perifollicular accentuation
- Recurrent conjunctivitis
- Ichthyosis
- Nipple dermatitis
- Wool intolerance
- Cutaneous *S. aureus* infections or herpes simplex infections
- Food intolerance
- Hand dermatitis (nonallergic irritant)
- Facial pallor, facial erythema
- Cheilitis
- White dermographism

LABORATORY TESTS
- Tests are generally not helpful.
- Elevated IgE levels are found in 80% to 90% of atopic dermatitis.
- Blood eosinophilia correlates with disease severity.

TREATMENT

NONPHARMACOLOGIC THERAPY
Avoidance of triggering factors:
- Sudden temperature changes, sweating, low humidity in the winter
- Contact with irritating substances (e.g., wool, cosmetics, some soaps and detergents, tobacco)
- Foods that provoke exacerbations (e.g., eggs, peanuts, fish, soy, wheat, milk)
- Stressful situations
- Allergens and dust
- Excessive hand washing

ACUTE GENERAL Rx
- Emollients can be used to prevent dryness.
- Topical corticosteroids (e.g., 1% to 2.5% hydrocortisone) may be helpful. Consider intermediate-potency steroids (e.g., triamcinolone, fluocinolone) for more severe cases and limit potent corticosteroids (e.g., betamethasone, desoximetasone, clobetasol) for severe cases.
- Topical steroids should be applied qd to bid to affected areas.
- Oral antihistamines (e.g., hydroxyzine, diphenhydramine) are effective in controlling pruritus and inducing sedation, restful sleep, and prevention of scratching during sleep.
- Oral prednisone, IM triamcinolone, Goeckerman regimen, PUVA are generally reserved for severe cases.

DISPOSITION
- Resolution occurs in approximately 40% of patients by adulthood.
- Most patients have a course characterized by remissions and intermittent flares.

REFERRAL
Dermatology referral in patients refractory to conservative therapy (see "Acute General Rx.")

MISCELLANEOUS

COMMENTS
Patients should be reassured that atypic dermatitis is not an emotional disorder and that prognosis is generally benign.

REFERENCES
Cooper KD: Atopic dermatitis: recent trends in pathogenic therapy, *Investigational Dermatology* 102:128, 1994.
Habif TP: *Clinical dermatology*, ed 3, St Louis, 1996, Mosby.

Author: **Fred F. Ferri, M.D.**

BASIC INFORMATION

DEFINITION
Contact dermatitis is an eczematous dermatitis resulting from exposure to substances in the environment. It can be subdivided into "irritant" contact dermatitis (nonimmunologic physical and chemical alteration of the epidermis) and "allergic" contact dermatitis (delayed hypersensitivity reaction).

SYNONYMS
Irritant contact dermatitis
Allergic contact dermatitis

ICD-9-CM CODES
692 Contact dermatitis and other eczema

EPIDEMIOLOGY AND DEMOGRAPHICS
- 20% of all cases of dermatitis in children are caused by allergic contact dermatitis.
- Rhus dermatitis (poison ivy, poison oak, and poison sumac) are responsible for most cases of contact dermatitis.
- Frequent causes of irritant contact dermatitis are soaps, detergents, and organic solvents.

PHYSICAL FINDINGS
IRRITANT CONTACT DERMATITIS:
- Mild exposure may result in dryness, erythema, and fissuring of the affected area (e.g., hand involvement in irritant dermatitis caused by exposure to soap, genital area involvement in irritant dermatitis caused by prolonged exposure to wet diapers).
- Eczematous inflammation may result from chronic exposure.

ALLERGIC CONTACT DERMATITIS:
- Poison ivy dermatitis can present with vesicles and blisters; linear lesions (as a result of dragging of the resins over the surface of the skin by scratching) are a classic presentation (see color plate 6).
- The pattern of lesions is asymmetric; itching, burning, and stinging may be present.
- The involved areas are erythematous, warm to touch, swollen, and may be confused with cellulitis.

ETIOLOGY
- Irritant contact dermatitis: cement (construction workers), rubber, ragweed, malathion (farmers), orange and lemon peels (chefs, bartenders), hair tints, shampoos (beauticians), rubber gloves (medical, surgical personnel)
- Allergic contact dermatitis: poison ivy, poison oak, poison sumac, rubber (shoe dermatitis), nickel (jewelry), balsa of Peru (hand and face dermatitis), neomycin, formaldehyde (cosmetics)

DIAGNOSIS

DIFFERENTIAL DIAGNOSIS
- Impetigo
- Lichen simplex chronicus
- Atopic dermatitis
- Nummular eczema
- Seborrheic dermatitis
- Psoriasis
- Scabies

WORKUP
- Medical history: gradual onset vs. rapid onset, number of exposures, clinical presentation, occupational history
- Physical examination: contact dermatitis in the neck may be caused by necklaces, perfumes, after shave lotion; involvement of the axillae is often secondary to deodorants, clothing; face involvement can occur with the cosmetics, airborne allergens, after shave lotion

LABORATORY TESTS
- Patch testing is useful to confirm the diagnosis of contact dermatitis; it is indicated particularly when inflammation persists despite appropriate topical therapy and avoidance of suspected causative agent; patch testing should not be used for irritant contact dermatitis since this is a nonimmunologic-mediated inflammatory reaction.
- Gram stain and cultures are indicated only in cases of suspected secondary infection or impetigo.

TREATMENT

NONPHARMACOLOGIC THERAPY
Avoidance of suspected allergens

ACUTE GENERAL Rx
- Removal of the irritant substance by washing the skin with plain water or mild soap within 15 min of exposure is helpful in patients with poison ivy, poison oak, or poison sumac dermatitis.
- Cold or cool water compresses for 20 to 30 min five to six times a day for the initial 72 hr are effective during the acute blistering stage.
- Oral corticosteroids (e.g., prednisone 20 mg bid for 6 to 10 days) are generally reserved for severe, widespread dermatitis.
- IM steroids (e.g., Kenalog) are used for severe reactions and in patients requiring oral corticosteroids but unable to tolerate PO
- Oral antihistamines (e.g., hydroxyzine 25 mg q6h) will control pruritus, especially at nighttime; calamine lotion is also useful for pruritus; however, it can lead to excessive drying.
- Colloidal oatmeal (Aveeno) baths can also provide symptomatic relief.
- Patients with mild to moderate erythema may respond to topical steroid gels or creams.
- Patients with shoe allergy should change their socks at least once a day; use of aluminum chloride hexahydrate in a 20% solution (Drysol) qhs will also help control perspiration.
- Use hypoallergenic surgical gloves in patients with rubber and surgical glove allergy.

DISPOSITION
Allergic contact dermatitis generally resolves within 2 to 4 wk if reexposure to allergen is prevented.

REFERRAL
For patch testing in selected patients (see "Laboratory Tests")

MISCELLANEOUS

COMMENTS
Commercially available corticosteroid dose packs should be avoided, since they generally provide an inadequate amount of medication.

REFERENCES
Habif, TP: *Clinical dermatology,* ed 3, St Louis, 1996, Mosby.
Klaus MV, Wieselphier JS: Contact dermatitis, *Am Fam Physician* 48:629, 1993.
Lepoittevin J et al: Studies in patients with corticosteroid contact allergy: understanding cross reactivity among different steroids, *Arch Dermatol* 131:31, 1995.
Patil S, Maibach HI: Effect of age and sex on the elicitation of irritant contact dermatitis, *Contact Dermatitis* 30(5):257, 1994.

Author: **Fred F. Ferri, M.D.**

Diabetes insipidus (PTG)

BASIC INFORMATION

DEFINITION
Diabetes insipidus is a polyuric disorder resulting from insufficient production of antidiuretic hormone (ADH) (pituitary [neurogenic] diabetes insipidus) or unresponsiveness of the renal tubules to ADH (nephrogenic diabetes insipidus).

ICD-9-CM CODES
253.5 Diabetes insipidus

EPIDEMIOLOGY AND DEMOGRAPHICS
GENETICS:
- Nephrogenic diabetes insipidus can be inherited as sex-linked recessive.
- There is also a rare autosomal dominant form of neurogenic diabetes insipidus.

PHYSICAL FINDINGS
- Polyuria: urinary volumes ranging from 2.5 to 6 L/day
- Polydipsia (predilection for cold or iced drinks)
- Neurologic manifestations (seizures, headaches, visual field defects)
- Evidence of volume contractions

NOTE: The above physical findings and clinical manifestations are generally not evident until vasopressin secretory capacity is reduced <20% of normal.

ETIOLOGY
NEUROGENIC DIABETES INSIPIDUS:
- Idiopathic
- Neoplasms of brain or pituitary fossa (craniopharyngiomas, metastatic neoplasms from breast or lung)
- Posttherapeutic neurosurgical procedures (e.g., hypophysectomy)
- Head trauma (e.g., basal skull fracture)
- Granulomatous disorders (sarcoidosis or TB)
- Histiocytosis (Hand-Schuller-Christian disease, eosinophilic granuloma)
- Familial (autosomal dominant)
- Other: interventricular hemorrhage, aneurysms, meningitis, postencephalitis, multiple sclerosis

NEPHROGENIC DIABETES INSIPIDUS:
- Drugs: lithium, amphotericin B, demeclocycline, methoxyflurane anesthesia
- Familial: X-linked
- Metabolic: hypercalcemia or hypokalemia
- Other: sarcoidosis, amyloidosis, pyelonephritis, polycystic disease, sickle cell disease, postobstructive

DIAGNOSIS

DIFFERENTIAL DIAGNOSIS
- Diabetes mellitus
- Primary polydipsia
- Osmotic diuresis (glucose, mannitol, urea)
- Box 2-98 describes the differential diagnosis of polyuria.

WORKUP
The diagnostic workup is aimed at showing that the polyuria is caused by the inability to concentrate urine and determining whether the problem is secondary to decreased ADH or insensitivity to ADH. This is done with the water deprivation test:
1. Following baseline measurement of weight, ADH, plasma sodium, and urine and plasma osmolarity, the patient is deprived of fluids under strict medical supervision.
2. Frequent (q2h) monitoring of plasma and urine osmolarity follows.
3. The test is generally terminated when plasma osmolarity is >295 or the patient loses ≥3.5% of initial body weight.
4. Diabetes insipidus is confirmed if the plasma osmolarity is >295 and the urine osmolarity is <500.
5. To distinguish nephrogenic from neurogenic diabetes insipidus, the patient is given 5 U of vasopressin (ADH) and the change in urine osmolarity is measured. A significant increase (>50%) in urine osmolarity following administration of ADH is indicative of neurogenic diabetes insipidus.

LABORATORY TESTS
- Decreased urinary specific gravity (≤1.005)
- Decreased urinary osmolarity (usually <200 mOsm/kg)
- Hypernatremia, increased plasma osmolarity, hypercalcemia, hypokalemia

IMAGING STUDIES
MRI of the brain if neurogenic diabetes insipidus is confirmed

TREATMENT

NONPHARMACOLOGIC THERAPY
- Patient education regarding control of fluid balance and prevention of dehydration with adequate fluid intake
- Daily weight

ACUTE GENERAL Rx
Therapy varies with the degree and type of diabetes insipidus:

NEUROGENIC DIABETES INSIPIDUS:
1. Desmopressin acetate (DDAVP) 10 to 40 μg qd intranasally in one to three divided doses or in tablet form 0.05 mg bid. Usual oral dose is 0.1 to 1.2 mg/day in two to three divided doses. Desmopressin is also available in injectable form given as 2 to 4 μg/day SC or IV in two divided doses.
2. Vasopressin tannate in oil: 2.5 to 5 U IM q24-72h; useful for long-term management because of its long life.
3. In mild cases of neurogenic diabetes insipidus, the polyuria may be controlled with HCTZ 50 mg qd or chlorpropamide (Diabinese) 250 mg qd.

NEPHROGENIC DIABETES INSIPIDUS:
1. Adequate hydration
2. Low-sodium diet and chlorothiazide to induce mild sodium depletion
3. Polyuria of diabetes insipidus secondary to lithium can be ameliorated by using amiloride (5 mg PO bid initially, increased to 10 mg bid after 2 wk)

CHRONIC Rx
Patients should be aware of the danger of dehydration and the need for liberal water intake.

DISPOSITION
Prognosis varies with the etiology of the diabetes insipidus.

REFERRAL
Endocrinology evaluation for diagnostic testing

MISCELLANEOUS

COMMENTS
Patients should be instructed to wear a medical identification tag or bracelet identifying their medical illness.

REFERENCES
Blevins LS Jr, Wand GS: Diabetes insipidus, *Crit Care Med* 20:69, 1992.
Noble J (ed): *Primary care medicine*, ed 2, St Louis, 1996, Mosby.

Author: **Fred F. Ferri, M.D.**

Diabetes mellitus (PTG)

BASIC INFORMATION

DEFINITION
Diabetes mellitus (DM) refers to a syndrome of hyperglycemia resulting from many different causes (see "Etiology"). It can be classified into type 1 insulin-dependent (formerly IDDM) and type 2 non-insulin-dependent (formerly NIDDM) DM. Because "insulin-dependent" and "non-insulin-dependent" refer to stage at diagnosis, when a type 2 diabetic needs insulin, he remains classified as type 2 and does not revert to type 1. The World Health Organization (WHO) diagnostic criteria for DM include a fasting blood sugar (FBS) ≥140 mg/dl and a glucose level ≥200 mg/dl 2 hr after 75 g glucose load (Glucola).
Recent criteria (1997) from the American Diabetes Association (ADA) define DM as (1) a fasting plasma glucose ≥ 126 mg/dl or (2) a nonfasting plasma glucose ≥ 200 mg/dl or (3) an oral glucose tolerance test (OGTT) ≥ 200 mg/dl in the 2-hr sample. Furthermore, the ADA also defines a value of 110 mg/dl on fasting blood sugar as the upper limit of normal for glucose. A fasting glucose between 110 mg/dl and 126 mg/dl is classified as "Impaired Fasting Glucose" (IFG). When results of the oral glucose test are between 110 mg/dl and 200 mg/dl, the patient is also classified as having IFG.

SYNONYMS
IDDM (insulin-dependent diabetes mellitus)
NIDDM (non-insulin-dependent diabetes mellitus)
Type 1 diabetes mellitus (insulin-dependent diabetes mellitus)
Type 2 diabetes mellitus (non-insulin-dependent diabetes mellitus)

ICD-9-CM CODES
250.0 Diabetes mellitus (NIDDM)
250.1 Insulin-dependent diabetes mellitus without complication (IDDM)

EPIDEMIOLOGY AND DEMOGRAPHICS
- DM affects 5% to 7% of the U.S. population. Prevalence in Pima Indians is 35%.
- Incidence increases with age, with 2% in persons ages 20 to 44 yr to 18% in persons 65 to 74 yr of age.
- Diabetes accounts for 8% of all legal blindness and is the leading cause of end-stage renal disease in the U.S.
- Patients with diabetes are twice as likely as nondiabetic patients to develop cardiovascular disease.

PHYSICAL FINDINGS
1. Physical examination varies with the presence of complications and may be normal in early stages.
2. Diabetic retinopathy:
    a. Nonproliferative (background diabetic retinopathy):
        (1) Initially: microaneurysms, capillary dilation, waxy or hard exudates, dot and flame hemorrhages, AV shunts
        (2) Advanced stage: microinfarcts with cotton wool exudates, macular edema
    b. Proliferative retinopathy: characterized by formation of new vessels, vitreal hemorrhages, fibrous scarring, and retinal detachment
3. Cataracts and glaucoma occur with increased frequency in diabetics.
4. Peripheral neuropathy: patients often complain of paresthesias of extremities (feet more than hands); the symptoms are symmetric, bilateral, and associated with intense burning pain (particularly during the night).
    a. Mononeuropathies involving cranial nerves III, IV, and VI, intercostal nerves, and femoral nerves are also common.
    b. Physical examination may reveal:
        (1) Decreased pinprick sensation, sensation to light touch, and pain sensation
        (2) Decreased vibration sense
        (3) Loss of proprioception (leading to ataxia)
        (4) Motor disturbances (decreased DTR, weakness and atrophy of interossei muscles); when the hands are affected, the patient has trouble picking up small objects, dressing, and turning pages in a book.
        (5) Diplopia, abnormalities of visual fields
5. Autonomic neuropathy:
    a. GI disturbances: esophageal motility abnormalities, gastroparesis, diarrhea (usually nocturnal)
    b. GU disturbances: neurogenic bladder (hesitancy, weak stream, and dribbling), impotence
    c. Orthostatic hypotension: postural syncope, dizziness, lightheadedness
6. Nephropathy: Pedal edema, pallor, weakness, uremic appearance
7. Foot ulcers: occur frequently and are usually secondary to peripheral vascular insufficiency, repeated trauma, (unrecognized because of sensory loss), and superimposed infections
8. Neuropathic arthropathy (Charcot joints): bone or joint deformities from repeated trauma (secondary to peripheral neuropathy
9. Necrobiosis lipoidica diabeticorum: plaquelike reddened areas with a central area that fades to white-yellow found on the anterior surfaces of the legs; in these areas the skin becomes very thin and can ulcerate readily.

ETIOLOGY
IDIOPATHIC DIABETES:
Type 1 (IDDM)
- Hereditary factors:
    1. Islet cell antibodies (found in 90% of patients within the first year of diagnosis)
    2. Higher incidence of HLA types DR3, DR4
    3. 50% concordance in identical twins
- Environmental factors: viral infection (possibly coxsackie virus, mumps virus)
Type 2 (NIDDM)
- Hereditary factors: 90% concordance in identical twins
- Environmental factor: obesity

DIABETES SECONDARY TO OTHER FACTORS:
- Hormonal excess: Cushing's syndrome, acromegaly, glucagonoma, pheochromocytoma
- Drugs: glucocorticoids, diuretics, oral contraceptives
- Insulin receptor unavailability (with or without circulating antibodies)
- Pancreatic disease: pancreatitis, pancreatectomy, hemochromatosis
- Genetic syndromes: hyperlipidemias, myotonic dystrophy, lipoatrophy
- Gestational diabetes

DIAGNOSIS

Diagnosis is made on the basis of:
- Fasting glucose ≥140 mg/dl (WHO criteria) or ≥ 126 mg/dl (ADA criteria)
- Glucose level 2 hr after 75 g glucose load (Glucola) ≥200 mg/dl
- Elevated glycosylated hemoglobin (Hb A1c) level (this test is not recommended for diagnosis at this time by the ADA)
- U.S. Preventive Services Task Force Recommendations on screening for diabetes mellitus are described in Section V, Chapter 19.

DIFFERENTIAL DIAGNOSIS
- Diabetes insipidus
- Stress hyperglycemia
- Diabetes secondary to hormonal excess, drugs, pancreatic disease

Diabetes mellitus (PTG)

TREATMENT

NONPHARMACOLOGIC THERAPY
1. Diet
   a. Calories
      (1) The diabetic patient can be started on 15 calories/lb of ideal body weight; this number can be increased to 20 calories/lb for an active person and 25 calories/lb if the patient does heavy physical labor.
      (2) The calories should be distributed as 55% to 60% carbohydrates, 25% to 35% fat, and 15% to 20% protein.
      (3) The emphasis should be on complex carbohydrates rather than simple and refined starches and on polyunsaturated instead of saturated fats in a ratio of 2:1.
   b. Seven food groups
      (1) The exchange diet of the ADA includes protein, bread, fruit, milk, and low- and intermediate-carbohydrate vegetables.
      (2) The name of each exchange is meant to be all inclusive (e.g., cereal, muffins, spaghetti, potatoes, rice are in the bread group; meats, fish, eggs, cheese, peanut butter are in the protein group).
      (3) The *glycemic index* compares the rise in blood sugar after the ingestion of simple sugars and complex carbohydrates with the rise that occurs after the absorption of glucose; equal amounts of starches do not give the same rise in plasma glucose (pasta equal in calories to a baked potato causes less of a rise than the potato): thus it is helpful to know the glycemic index of a particular food product.
      (4) Fiber: insoluble fiber (bran, celery) and soluble globular fiber (pectin in fruit) delay glucose absorption and attenuate the postprandial serum glucose peak; they also appear to lower the elevated triglyceride level often present in uncontrolled diabetics.
2. Exercise increases the cellular glucose uptake by increasing the number of cell receptors. The following points must be considered:
   a. Exercise program must be individualized and built up slowly.
   b. Insulin is more rapidly absorbed when injected into a limb that is then exercised, and this can result in hypoglycemia.
3. Weight loss: to ideal body weight if the patient is overweight

ACUTE GENERAL Rx
- When the above measures fail to normalize the serum glucose, metformin or a sulfonylurea should be added to the regimen.
- Because metformin does not produce hypoglycemia when used as a monotherapy, it is preferred for most patients. It is contraindicated in patients with renal insufficiency.
- Sulfonylureas work best when given before meals because they increase the postprandial output of insulin from the pancreas. All sulfonylureas are contraindicated in patients allergic to sulfa.
- Acarbose works by competitively inhibiting pancreatic amylase and small intestinal glucosidases, thereby reducing alimentary hyperglycemia. Its major side effects are flatulence, diarrhea, and abdominal cramps.
- Troglitazone reduces insulin resistance and is useful in addition to insulin in type 2 diabetics whose hyperglycemia is inadequately controlled despite insulin therapy.
- Table 7-8 in Section VII compares the various oral antidiabetic agents.
- Insulin is indicated for the treatment of all type 1 DM and type 2 DM patients who cannot be adequately controlled with diet and oral agents.
- Table 7-23 in Section VII compares the various insulin preparations.

DISPOSITION
The Diabetes Control and Complications Trial (DCCT) proved that intensive treatment decreases the development and progression of complications of DM. Each patient should be made aware of these findings.
- Retinopathy occurs in approximately 15% of diabetic patients after 15 yr and increases 1%/yr after diagnosis.
- The frequency of neuropathy in type II diabetics approaches 70% to 80%.
- Nephropathy occurs in 35% to 45% of patients with type 1 DM and in 20% of type 2 DM.
- Infections are generally more common in diabetics because of multiple factors, such as impaired leukocyte function, decreased tissue perfusion secondary to vascular disease, repeated trauma because of loss of sensation, and urinary retention secondary to neuropathy.
- Diabetic ketoacidosis and hyperosmolar coma are described in detail in Section I.

MISCELLANEOUS

COMMENTS
- Since normalization of serum glucose level is the ultimate goal, every patient should measure his blood glucose unless contraindicated by senility or blindness.
- For blood glucose monitoring, glucose oxidase strips are used in conjunction with a meter to give a digital reading. The testing can be done once day, but the time should be varied each day so that over a period of time the serum glucose level before meals and at bedtime can be assessed frequently without pricking the patient's fingers four times daily.
- Glycosylated hemoglobin should be measured at least twice yearly; measurement of microalbumin in the urine on a yearly basis is also recommended.

REFERENCES
DCCT Research Group: The effect of intensive treatment of diabetes on the development and progression of long-term complications in insulin-dependent diabetes mellitus, *New Engl J Med* 329:977, 1993.

Hanley CH: Diabetes mellitus. In Ferri FF: *Practical guide to the care of the medical patient,* ed 4, St Louis, 1998, Mosby.

Author: **Fred F. Ferri, M.D.**

CLINICAL TOPICS   Diabetic ketoacidosis   151

BASIC INFORMATION

DEFINITION
Diabetic ketoacidosis (DKA) is a life-threatening complication of diabetes mellitus resulting from severe insulin deficiency and manifested clinically by severe dehydration and alterations in the sensorium.

SYNONYMS
DKA

ICD-9-CM CODES
250.1 Diabetic ketoacidosis

EPIDEMIOLOGY AND DEMOGRAPHICS
INCIDENCE/PREVALENCE: 46 episodes/10,000 diabetics; cause of 14% of all hospital admissions of diabetic patients
PREDOMINANT AGE: 1 to 25 yr

PHYSICAL FINDINGS
- Evidence of dehydration (tachycardia, hypotension, dry mucous membranes, sunken eyeballs, poor skin turgor)
- Clouding of mental status
- Tachypnea with air hunger (Kussmaul's respiration)
- Fruity breath odor (caused by acetone)
- Lipemia retinalis in some patients
- Possible evidence of precipitating factors (infected wound, pneumonia)
- Abdominal or CVA tenderness in some patients

ETIOLOGY
Metabolic decompensation in diabetics usually precipitated by an infectious process (up to 40% of cases). Poor compliance with insulin therapy and severe medical illness (e.g., CVA, MI) are other common causes.

DIAGNOSIS

DIFFERENTIAL DIAGNOSIS
- Hyperosmolar nonketotic state
- Alcoholic ketoacidosis
- Uremic acidosis
- Metabolic acidosis secondary to methyl alcohol, ethylene glycol
- Salicylate poisoning

WORKUP
- Laboratory evaluation (see below) to confirm diagnosis and evaluate precipitating factors
- Admission ECG to evaluate electrolyte abnormalities and rule out myocardial ischemia/infarction as a contributing factor

LABORATORY TESTS
- Glucose level reveals severe hyperglycemia (serum glucose generally >300 mg/dl).
- ABGs reveal acidosis: arterial pH usually <7.3 with P_{CO_2} <40 mm Hg.
- Serum electrolytes:
  1. Serum bicarbonate is usually <15 mEq/L.
  2. Serum potassium may be low, normal, or high. There is always significant total body potassium depletion regardless of the initial potassium level.
  3. Serum sodium is usually decreased as a result of hyperglycemia, dehydration, and lipemia. Assume 1.6 mEq/L decrease in extracellular sodium for each 100 mg/dl increase in glucose concentration.
  4. Calculate the anion gap (AG):

  $$AG = Na^+ - (Cl^- + HCO_3^-)$$

  In DKA the anion gap is increased; hyperchloremic metabolic acidosis may be present in unusual circumstances when both the glomerular filtration rate and the plasma volume are well maintained.
- CBC with differential, urinalysis, urine and blood cultures to rule out infectious precipitating factor.
- Serum calcium, magnesium, and phosphorus; the plasma phosphate and magnesium levels may be significantly depressed and should be rechecked within 24 hr because they may decrease further with correction of DKA.
- BUN and creatinine generally reveal significant dehydration.
- Amylase, liver enzymes should be checked in patients with abdominal pain.

IMAGING STUDIES
Chest x-ray examination is helpful to rule out infectious process. The initial chest x-ray may be negative if the patient has significant dehydration. Repeat chest x-ray examination after 24 hr if pulmonary infection is strongly suspected.

TREATMENT

NONPHARMACOLOGIC THERAPY
- Monitor mental status, vital signs, and urine output qh until improved, then monitor q2-4h.
- Monitor electrolytes, renal function, and glucose level (see below).

ACUTE GENERAL Rx
FLUID REPLACEMENT (THE USUAL DEFICIT IS 6 TO 8 L):
1. Do not delay fluid replacement until laboratory results have been received.
2. The initial fluid replacement should be with 0.9%NS. Careful monitoring for fluid overload is necessary in elderly patients and those with a history of CHF.

Diabetic ketoacidosis (PTG)

3. The rate of fluid replacement varies with the age of the patient and the presence of significant cardiac or renal disease.
- The usual rate of infusion is 500 ml to 1 L over the first hour; 300 to 500 ml/hr for the next 12 hr.
- Continue the infusion at a rate of 200 to 300 ml/hr, using 0.45%NS until the serum glucose level is <300 ml/dl, then change the hydrating solution to D_5W to prevent hypoglycemia, replenish free water, and introduce additional glucose substrate (necessary to suppress lipolysis and ketogenesis).

INSULIN ADMINISTRATION:
1. The patient should be given an initial loading IV bolus of 0.15 to 0.2 U/kg of regular insulin followed by a constant infusion at a rate of 0.1 U/kg/hr (e.g., 25 U of regular insulin in 250 ml of 0.9% saline solution at 70 ml/hr equals 7 U/hr for a 70 kg patient).
2. Monitor serum glucose qh for the first 2 hr, then monitor q2-4h.
3. The goal is to decrease serum glucose level by 80 mg/dl/hr (following an initial drop because of rehydration); if the serum glucose level is not decreasing at the expected rate, double the rate of insulin infusion.
4. When the serum glucose level approaches 250 mg/dl, decrease the rate of insulin infusion to 2 to 3 U/hr and continue this rate until the patient has received adequate fluid replacement, HCO_3^- is close to normal, and ketones have cleared.
5. Approximately 30 to 60 min before stopping the IV insulin infusion, administer a SC dose of regular insulin (dose varies with the patient's demonstrated insulin sensitivity); this SC dose of regular insulin is necessary because of the extremely short life of the insulin in the IV infusion.
6. When the patient is able to eat, regular insulin is administered before each meal and at hs. It is best to use sliding scale doses of regular insulin until maintenance doses are established. In newly diagnosed diabetics, the total daily dose to maintain metabolic control ranges from 0.5 to 0.8 U/kg/day. Split dose therapy with regular and NPH insulin may be given, with two thirds of the total daily dose administered in the morning and one third in the evening.

ELECTROLYTE REPLACEMENT:
Potassium Replacement: The average total potassium loss in DKA is 300 to 500 mEq.
- The rate of replacement varies with the patient's serum potassium level, degree of acidosis (decreased pH, increased potassium level), and renal function (potassium replacement should be used with caution in patient with renal failure).
- As a rule of thumb, potassium replacement may be started when there is no ECG evidence of hyperkalemia (tall, narrow, or tent-shaped T waves, decreased or absent P waves, short QT intervals, widening of QRS complex).
- In patients with normal renal function, potassium replacement can be started by adding 20 to 40 mEq KCl/L of IV hydrating solution if serum potassium is 4 to 5 mEq/L, more if serum potassium level is lower than 4 mEq/L.
- Monitor serum potassium level qh for the first 2 hr, then monitor q2-4h.

Phosphate Replacement: If the serum PO_4 is <1.5 mEq/L, give 2.5 mg/kg IV over 6 hr of elemental phosphate. Routine replacement of phosphate (in absence of laboratory evidence of significant hypophosphatemia) is not indicated. Rapid IV phosphate administration can cause hypocalcemia.

Magnesium Replacement: Replacement indicated only in the presence of significant hypomagnesemia or refractory hypokalemia.

BICARBONATE THERAPY: Routine use of bicarbonate in DKA is contraindicated, since it can worsen hypokalemia and intracellular acidosis and cause cerebral edema. Bicarbonate therapy should be used only if the arterial pH is <7. In these patients 44 to 88 mEq of sodium bicarbonate can be added to a liter of 0.45% NS q2-4h until pH increases >7.

DISPOSITION
- Average mortality in DKA is 5% to 10%.
- In children <10 yr of age, DKA causes 70% of diabetes-related deaths.

REFERRAL
Patients with DKA should be admitted to the ICU.

MISCELLANEOUS

COMMENTS
Potential complications of DKA therapy include hypoglycemia, cerebral edema, cardiac arrhythmias, shock, MI, and acute pancreatitis.

REFERENCES
DeFronzo RA, Matsuda M, Barrett EJ: Diabetic ketoacidosis: a combined metabolic-nephrologic approach to therapy, *Diabetic Rev* 2 (2):209, 1994.

Kitabchi AE, Wall BM: Diabetic Ketoacidosis, *Med Clin North Am* 79:9, 1995.

Author: **Fred F. Ferri, M.D.**

Diffuse interstitial lung disease (PTG)

BASIC INFORMATION

DEFINITION
Diffuse interstitial pulmonary disease is a group of blood disorders involving the lung interstitium and characterized by inflammation of the alveolar structures and progressive parenchymal fibrosis.

SYNONYMS
Interstitial lung disease
ILD

ICD-9-CM CODES
136.3 Acute interstitial lung disease
515 Chronic interstitial lung disease

EPIDEMIOLOGY AND DEMOGRAPHICS
- The incidence of interstitial lung disease is 5 cases/100,000 persons
- There are >100 known disorders that can cause interstitial lung disease (see "Etiology").

PHYSICAL FINDINGS
- The patient generally presents with progressive dyspnea and nonproductive cough; other clinical manifestations vary with the underlying disease process.
- Physical examination typically shows end respiratory dry rales (Velcro rales), cyanosis, clubbing, and right-sided heart failure.

ETIOLOGY
- Occupational and environmental exposure: pneumoconiosis, asbestosis, organic dust, gases, fumes, berylliosis, silicosis
- Granulomatous lung disease: sarcoidosis, infections (e.g., fungal, mycobacterial)
- Drug-induced: bleomycin, busulfan, methotrexate, chlorambucil, cyclophosphamide, BCNU (carmustine), gold salts, tetrazolium chloride, amiodarone, tocainide, penicillin, zidovudine, sulfonamide
- Radiation pneumonitis
- Connective tissue diseases: SLE, rheumatoid arthritis, dermatomyositis
- Idiopathic pulmonary fibrosis: bronchiolitis obliterans, interstitial pneumonitis, DIP
- Infections: viral pneumonia, *Pneumocystis* pneumonia
- Others: Wegener's granulomatosis, Goodpasture's syndrome, eosinophilic granuloma, lymphangitic carcinomatosis, chronic uremia, chronic gastric aspiration, hypersensitivity pneumonitis, lipoid pneumonia, lymphoma, lymphoid granulomatosis

DIAGNOSIS

DIFFERENTIAL DIAGNOSIS
- CHF
- Chronic renal failure
- Lymphangitic carcinomatosis
- Sarcoidosis
- Allergic alveolitis

The differential diagnosis of granulomatous lung disease is described in Table 2-28.

WORKUP
Chest x-ray examination, ABGs, PFTs, bronchoscopy with bronchioloalveolar lavage, biopsy, laboratory evaluation

LABORATORY TESTS
- ABGs provide only limited information; initially ABGs may be normal but with progression of the disease, hypoxemia may be present.
- Antineutrophil cytoplasmic antibody (c-ANCA) is frequently positive in Wegener's granulomatosis.
- Antiglomerular basement membrane (anti-GBM) and anti-pulmonary basement membrane antibody are often present in Goodpasture's syndrome.

IMAGING STUDIES
Chest x-ray examination may be normal in 10% of patients.
- Ground-glass appearance is often an early finding.
- A coarse reticular pattern is usually a late finding.
- CHF causing interstitial changes on chest x-ray film must always be ruled out.
- Differential diagnosis of interstitial patterns include the following: pulmonary fibrosis, pulmonary edema, PCP, TB, sarcoidosis, eosinophilic granuloma, pneumoconiosis, and lymphangitic spread of carcinoma.
- Pulmonary function testing: findings are generally consistent with restrictive disease (decreased VC, TLC, and diffusing capacity).
- Bronchoscopy with bronchioloalveolar lavage is useful to characterize the pulmonary inflammatory response; the effector cell population in patients with interstitial lung disease consists of two major cell types:
  1. Lymphocytes (e.g., sarcoidosis, berylliosis, silicosis, hypersensitive pneumonitis)
  2. Neutrophils (e.g., asbestosis, collagen-vascular disease, idiopathic pulmonary fibrosis)
- Open lung biopsy or transbronchial biopsy is useful to identify the underlying disease process and exclude neoplastic involvement; transbronchial biopsy is less invasive but provides less tissue for analysis (this factor may be important in patients with irregular pulmonary involvement).
- Gallium-67 scanning plays a limited role in the evaluation of interstitial lung disease because it is not specific and a negative result does not exclude the disease (e.g., patients with end-stage fibrosis may have a negative scan).

TREATMENT

NONPHARMACOLOGIC THERAPY
Avoidance of tobacco (may adversely effect pulmonary function)

ACUTE GENERAL Rx
- Removal of offending agent (e.g., environmental exposure)
- Treatment of infectious process with appropriate antibiotic therapy
- Supplemental oxygen in patients with significant hypoxemia
- Corticosteroids in symptomatic patients with sarcoidosis
- Immunosuppressive therapy in selected cases (e.g., cyclophosphamide in patients with Wegener's granulomatosis)
- Treatment of any complications (e.g., pneumothorax, pulmonary embolism)

DISPOSITION
Overall mortality is 50% within 5 yr of diagnosis.

REFERRAL
- Surgical referral for biopsy
- Pulmonary referral for bronchoscopy and bronchoalveolar lavage (selected patients)
- Lung transplantation (selected patients)

MISCELLANEOUS

COMMENTS
Although open lung biopsy is the gold standard for diagnosis, it may be inappropriate in elderly patients; therefore individual consideration is advisable.

REFERENCES
Raghu G: Interstitial lung disease: a diagnostic approach. Are CT scans, lung biopsy indicated in every patient? *Am J Respir Crit Care Med* 151:909, 1995.

Schwartz DA et al: Determinants of survival in idiopathic pulmonary fibrosis, *Am J Respir Crit Care Med* 149:450, 1994.

Author: **Fred F. Ferri, M.D.**

Diphtheria (PTG)

BASIC INFORMATION

DEFINITION
Diphtheria is an infection of the mucous membranes or skin caused by *Corynebacterium diphtheriae*.

ICD-9-CM CODES
032.9 Diphtheria

EPIDEMIOLOGY AND DEMOGRAPHICS
INCIDENCE (IN U.S.):
- Fewer than 5 cases/yr since 1980 (<0.002 cases/100,000 persons)
- Last culture-confirmed indigenous case in 1988

PREDOMINANT AGE: Adult years

PHYSICAL FINDINGS
RESPIRATORY DIPHTHERIA:
- Commonly presenting as pharyngitis, but any part of the respiratory tract may be involved, including the nasopharynx, larynx, trachea, or bronchi
- Areas of gray or white exudate coalescing to form a "pseudomembrane" that bleeds when removed
- Possible fever and dysphagia
- Complications: respiratory tract obstruction and pneumonia
- Systemic effects of the toxin: myocarditis and polyneuritis (frequently involving a bulbar distribution)
- Occurs mostly in nonimmune individuals; usually milder and less likely to be complicated in those adequately immunized

CUTANEOUS DIPHTHERIA:
- Usually complicates existing skin lesion (i.e., impetigo or scabies)
- Resembles the underlying condition

ETIOLOGY
- Caused by *C. diphtheriae*, an aerobic, gram-positive rod
- Transmitted by close contact through droplets of nasopharyngeal secretions
- Symptomatic disease of the respiratory system caused by toxin-producing strains (tox$^+$)
- Systemic effects of toxin: ranging from nausea and vomiting to polyneuropathy, myocarditis, and vascular collapse
- Presence of strains not producing toxin (tox$^-$) in the respiratory tract of asymptomatic carriers and in skin lesions of cutaneous diphtheria

DIAGNOSIS

DIFFERENTIAL DIAGNOSIS
- Streptococcus pharyngitis
- Viral pharyngitis
- Mononucleosis

WORKUP
- Presence of a pseudomembrane in the oropharynx suggestive of diagnosis (not always present)
- Gram stains of secretions to show club-shaped organisms, which appear as "Chinese letters"
- Nasolaryngoscopy to identify lesions in the nares, nasopharynx, larynx, or tracheobronchial tree
- Electrocardiogram
- Possible ICU monitoring

LABORATORY TESTS
- Cultures of mucosal lesions or of nasal discharge
  1. Positive culture for *C. diphtheriae* confirms the diagnosis.
  2. Laboratory is notified of the suspected diagnosis so that appropriate culture medium (Tinsdale agar) is used.
- Testing of all isolated organisms for toxin production

IMAGING STUDIES
Chest x-ray examination to rule out pneumonia

TREATMENT

NONPHARMACOLOGIC THERAPY
- Intubation or tracheostomy if signs of respiratory distress occur
- Nasogastric or parenteral nutrition in those with bulbar signs
- ICU monitoring for patients with signs of systemic toxicity
- Cardiac pacing in patients with heart block
- Respiratory isolation

ACUTE GENERAL Rx
- Administration of diphtheria antitoxin once a clinical diagnosis is made
- If tests for hypersensitivity to horse serum are negative: 50,000 U given for mild to moderate disease or 60,000 to 120,000 U for critically ill patients
- IV infusion of antitoxin over 60 min
- Serum sickness in 10% of treated individuals; those with hypersensitivity to horse serum should be desensitized before administration of antitoxin
- Antibiotics to eradicate the organism in carriers or patients
- For respiratory diphtheria:
  1. Erythromycin 500 mg qid PO or IV or IM penicillin 600,000 U bid for 14 days
  2. Carriers or patients with cutaneous disease: erythromycin 500 mg PO qid or rifampin 600 mg PO qd for 7 days

CHRONIC Rx
Antibiotics to limit toxin production and eradicate carrier state, thereby preventing transmission

DISPOSITION
Complete recovery with adequate supportive measures and antitoxin

REFERRAL
- Hospitalization and referral to an infectious disease specialist for all suspected patients
- To an otolaryngologist for evaluation in cases of respiratory diphtheria
- All cases reported to the Public Health Authorities

MISCELLANEOUS

COMMENTS
- Most cases are imported by travelers to epidemic areas, so recent epidemics in Europe are a cause for concern.
- Vaccination with diphtheria toxoid (attenuated toxin) is safe and effective in the form of DPT or Td; Td boosters should be given to adults every 10 yr.
- According to serologic studies, 20% to 60% of U.S. adults >20 yr of age are susceptible to diphtheria.

REFERENCES
Vuopio-Varkila J et al: Diphtheria acquired by U.S. citizens in the Russian Federation and Ukraine—1994, *MMWR* 44:243, 1995.

Author: **Maurice Policar, M.D.**

BASIC INFORMATION

DEFINITION
Disseminated intravascular coagulation (DIC) is an acquired thromboembolic disorder characterized by generalized activation of the clotting mechanism.

SYNONYMS
Consumptive coagulopathy
DIC

ICD-9-CM CODES
286.6   Disseminated intravascular coagulation

EPIDEMIOLOGY AND DEMOGRAPHICS
Greater than 50% of cases are associated with gram-negative sepsis or other septicemic infections.

PHYSICAL FINDINGS
- Wound site bleeding, epistaxis, gingival bleeding, hemorrhagic bullae
- Petechiae, ecchymosis, purpura
- Dyspnea, localized rales, delirium
- Oliguria, anuria, GI bleeding, metrorrhagia

ETIOLOGY
- Infections (e.g., gram-negative sepsis, viral or fungal infection)
- Obstetric complications (e.g., dead fetus, amniotic fluid embolism, abruptio placentae, septic abortion, eclampsia)
- Tissue trauma (e.g., burns, hypothermia-rewarming)
- Neoplasms (e.g., adenocarcinomas [GI, prostate, lung, breast], acute promyelocytic leukemia)
- Quinine, cocaine-induced rhabdomyolysis
- Other: SLE, vasculitis, aneurysms, polyarteritis, cavernous hemangiomas

DIAGNOSIS

DIFFERENTIAL DIAGNOSIS
- Hepatic necrosis: normal or elevated Factor VIII concentrations
- Vitamin K deficiency: normal platelet count
- Hemolytic uremic syndrome
- Thrombocytopenic purpura
- Renal failure, SLE, sickle cell crisis, dysfibrinogenemias

WORKUP
Diagnostic workup includes laboratory screening to confirm the diagnosis and exclude conditions noted in the differential diagnosis.

LABORATORY TESTS
- Peripheral blood smear generally shows RBC fragments and low platelet count.
- Diagnostic characteristics of DIC are increased PT, PTT, TT, fibrin split products, D-Dimer; decreased fibrinogen level, thrombocytopenia.
- Coagulopathy secondary to DIC must be differentiated from that secondary to liver disease or vitamin K deficiency.
  1. Vitamin K deficiency manifests with prolonged PT and normal PTT, TT, platelet, and fibrinogen level; PTT may be elevated in severe cases.
  2. Patients with liver disease have abnormal PT and PTT; TT and fibrinogen are usually normal unless severe disease is present; platelets are usually normal unless splenomegaly is present.
  3. Factors V and VIII are low in DIC, but they are normal in liver disease with coagulopathy.

IMAGING STUDIES
Imaging studies are generally not useful. Chest x-ray examination may be helpful to exclude infectious processes in patients presenting with pulmonary symptoms such as dyspnea, cough, or hemoptysis.

TREATMENT

NONPHARMACOLOGIC THERAPY
No specific precautions regarding activity level are necessary unless thrombocytopenia is severe.

ACUTE GENERAL Rx
- Correct underlying cause (e.g., antimicrobial therapy for infection).
- Give replacement therapy with FFP and platelets in patients with significant hemorrhage:
  1. FFP 10 to 15 ml/kg can be given with a goal of achieving a PT within 2 to 3 sec of control.
  2. Platelet transfusions are given when platelet count is <10,000 (or higher if major bleeding is present).
  3. Cryoprecipitate 1 U/5 kg is reserved for hypofibrinogen states.
- Heparin therapy at a dose lower than that used in venous thrombosis may be useful in selected cases to increase neutralization of thrombin (e.g., DIC associated with acute promyelocytic leukemia).

CHRONIC Rx
Follow-up management includes coagulation screening to assess factor replacement therapy. Laboratory abnormalities generally correct with treatment of the underlying disorder. Chronic laboratory monitoring is not required.

DISPOSITION
Mortality in severe DIC exceeds 75%. Death generally results from progression of the underlying disease and complications such as acute renal failure, intracerebral hematoma, shock, or cardiac tamponade.

REFERRAL
Hematology consultation is recommended in all cases of DIC.

MISCELLANEOUS

COMMENTS
The treatment of chronic DIC is controversial. Low-dose SC heparin and/or combination antiplatelet agents such as aspirin and dipyridamole may be useful.

REFERENCES
Bick RL: Disseminated intravascular coagulation: objective criteria for diagnosis and management, *Med Clin North Am* 78: 511, 1994.
Gilbert JA, Scalzi RP: Disseminated intravascular coagulation, *Emerg Med Clin North Am* 11(2):465, 1993.
Levi M et al: Pathogenesis of disseminated intravascular coagulation in sepsis, *JAMA* 270:975, 1993.
Author: **Fred F. Ferri, M.D.**

Diverticular disease (PTG)

BASIC INFORMATION

DEFINITION
- Colonic diverticula are herniations of mucosa and submucosa through the muscularis. They are generally found along the colon's mesenteric border at the site where the vasa recta penetrates the muscle wall (anatomical weak point).
- *Diverticulosis* is the asymptomatic presence of multiple colonic diverticula.
- *Diverticulitis* is an inflammatory process or localized perforation of diverticulum.

ICD-9-CM CODES
562.10 Diverticulosis of colon
562.11 Diverticulitis of colon

EPIDEMIOLOGY AND DEMOGRAPHICS
- Incidence of diverticulosis in the general population is 35% to 50%.
- Diverticulosis is more common in western countries, affecting >30% of people >40 yr and >50% of people >70 yr.

PHYSICAL FINDINGS
- Physical examination in patients with diverticulosis is generally normal.
- Painful diverticular disease can present with LLQ pain, often relieved by defecation; location of pain may be anywhere in the lower abdomen because of the redundancy of the sigmoid colon.
- Diverticulitis can cause muscle spasm, guarding, and rebound tenderness predominantly affecting the LLQ.

ETIOLOGY
Diverticular disease is believed to be secondary to low intake of dietary fiber.

DIAGNOSIS

DIFFERENTIAL DIAGNOSIS
- Irritable bowel syndrome
- IBD
- Carcinoma of colon
- Endometriosis
- Ischemic colitis
- Infections (pseudomembranous colitis, appendicitis, pyelonephritis, PID)
- Lactose intolerance

LABORATORY TESTS
- WBC count in diverticulitis reveals leukocytosis with left shift.
- Microcytic anemia can be present in patients with chronic bleeding from diverticular disease. MCV may be elevated in acute bleeding secondary to reticulocytosis.

IMAGING STUDIES
- Barium enema will demonstrate multiple diverticula and muscle spasm ("sawtooth" appearance of the lumen) in patients with painful diverticular disease. Barium enema can be hazardous and should not be performed in the acute stage of diverticulitis because it may produce free perforation.
- A CT scan of the abdomen can be used to diagnose acute diverticulitis; typical findings are thickening of the bowel wall, fistulas, or abscess formation.
- Evaluation of suspected diverticular bleeding:
  1. Arteriography if the bleeding is faster than 1 ml/min (advantage: the possible infusion of vasopressin directly into the arteries supplying the bleeding as well as selective arterial embolization; disadvantages: its cost and invasive nature)
  2. Technetium-99m sulfa colloid
  3. Technetium-99m labeled RBC (can detect bleeding rates as low as 0.12 to 5 ml/min)

TREATMENT

NONPHARMACOLOGIC THERAPY
- Increase in dietary fiber intake and regular exercise to improve bowel function
- NPO and IV hydration in severe diverticulitis; NG suction if ileus or small bowel obstruction is present

ACUTE GENERAL Rx
TREATMENT OF DIVERTICULITIS:
- IV antibiotics (PO in mild cases):
  1. Ampicillin (to treat enterococcus) in mild diverticulitis
  2. Aggressive treatment of gram-negative aerobes and *Bacteroides fragilis* in moderate to severe diverticulitis (possible antibiotic choices: cefotetan, cefoxitin, or an aminoglycoside plus clindamycin or metronidazole)
- Surgical treatment consisting of resection of involved areas and reanastomosis (if feasible); otherwise a diverting colostomy with reanastomosis performed when infection has been controlled; surgery should be considered in patients with:
  1. Repeated episodes of diverticulitis (two or more)
  2. Poor response to appropriate medical therapy (failure of conservative management
  3. Abscess or fistula formation
  4. Obstruction
  5. Peritonitis
  6. Immunocompromised patients, first episode in young patient (<40 yr old)
  7. Inability to exclude carcinoma (10% to 20% of patients diagnosed with diverticulosis on clinical grounds are subsequently found to have carcinoma of the colon)

DIVERTICULAR HEMORRHAGE: 70% of diverticular bleeding occurs in the right colon.
  1. Bleeding is painless and stops spontaneously in the majority of patients (60%); it is usually caused by erosion of a blood vessel by a fecalith present within the diverticular sac.
  2. Medical therapy consists of blood replacement and correction of volume and any clotting abnormalities.
  3. Surgical resection is necessary if bleeding does not stop spontaneously after administration of 4 to 5 U of PRBCs or recurs with severity within a few days; if attempts at localization are unsuccessful, total abdominal colectomy with ileoproctostomy may be indicated (high incidence of rebleeding if segmental resection is performed without adequate localization).

CHRONIC Rx
Asymptomatic patients with diverticulosis can be treated with a high-fiber diet or fiber supplements.

DISPOSITION
- Most patients with diverticulitis respond well to antibiotic management and bowel rest. Up to 30% of patients with diverticulitis will eventually require surgical management.
- Diverticular bleeding can recur in 15% to 20% of patients within 5 yr.

REFERRAL
Surgical referral when considering resection (see "Acute General Rx")

MISCELLANEOUS

REFERENCES
Jones DJ: Diverticular disease, *Br Med J* 304:1435, 1992.
Schoep ZD Jr: Uncomplicated diverticulitis: indications for surgery and surgical management, *Surg Clin North Am* 73:965, 1993.
Author: **Fred F. Ferri, M.D.**

Down syndrome (PTG)

BASIC INFORMATION

DEFINITION
Down syndrome is a chromosomal abnormality causing mental retardation and multiple organ defects.

SYNONYMS
Trisomy 21

ICD-9-CM CODES
758.0 Down syndrome

EPIDEMIOLOGY AND DEMOGRAPHICS
INCIDENCE (IN U.S.): 1 in 700 births
PREVALENCE (IN U.S.): 300,000 persons
PREDOMINANT SEX: Male:female ratio of 1:3 to 1:0
PREDOMINANT AGE: Newborn to early adulthood
PEAK INCIDENCE: Newborn
GENETICS:
- Nondisjunction causing trisomy 21
- Increases with increasing maternal age

PHYSICAL FINDINGS
- Microcephaly
- Flattening of occiput and face
- Upward slant to eyes with epicanthal folds
- Brushfield spots in iris
- Broad stocky neck
- Small feet, hands, and digits
- Palmar crease
- Associated with congenital heart disease, malformations of the GI tract, cataracts, hypothyroidism, hip dysplasia

ETIOLOGY
Nondisjunction of chromosome 21

DIAGNOSIS

DIFFERENTIAL DIAGNOSIS WORKUP
- Prenatal diagnosis is possible with ultrasound and amniocentesis.
- Anticipate associated congenital abnormalities.

LABORATORY TESTS
- CBC (transient leukemoid reaction)
- Chromosomal karyotype
- Thyroid screen
- Auditory brain stem responses

IMAGING STUDIES
Echocardiogram

TREATMENT

NONPHARMACOLOGIC THERAPY
Usual outcome is that the patient remains at home until young adulthood, when they often enter a small group home.

CHRONIC Rx
- See "Nonpharmacologic Therapy."
- Frequent visits to pediatrician or special clinic are necessary.

DISPOSITION
Down syndrome clinics use a preventative checklist to anticipate many clinical challenges.

REFERRAL
Refer if not experienced in following children with Down syndrome.

MISCELLANEOUS

COMMENTS
- All patients develop early Alzheimer's disease.
- This disease accounts for approximately one third of moderate to severe cases of mental retardation and presents many medical and ethical challenges.
- The U.S. Preventive Services Task Force Recommendations for screening for Down Syndrome are described in Section V, Chapter 41.

REFERENCES
Hayes A, Batshaw M: Down syndrome, *Pediatr Clin North Am* 40:523, 1993.
Author: **William H. Olson, M.D.**

Dupuytren's contracture (PTG)

BASIC INFORMATION

DEFINITION
Dupuytren's contracture is a disease of the palmar fascia characterized by nodular fibroblastic proliferation that often results in progressive contractures of the fascia and flexion deformity of the fingers.

ICD-9-CM CODES
728.6 Dupuytren's contracture

EPIDEMIOLOGY AND DEMOGRAPHICS
PREVALENCE: Varies depending on nationality
PREVALENT AGE: 40 to 60 yr
PREVALENT SEX: male:female ratio of 10:1

PHYSICAL FINDINGS
- Usually asymptomatic
- Most common complaints: deformity and interference with the use of the hand by the flexed, contracted fingers
- Process usually begins in the ulnar side of the hand, often starting at the ring finger
- Isolated painless nodules that eventually harden and mature into a longitudinal cord that extends into the finger
- Lesion often begins in the distal palmar crease
- Overlying skin adherent to the fascia
- Later stages: fibrous cord begins to contract and pull the finger into flexion
- Possible involvment of other fingers, particularly small finger

ETIOLOGY
Unknown

DIAGNOSIS

DIFFERENTIAL DIAGNOSIS
Soft tissue tumor

TREATMENT

NONPHARMACOLOGIC THERAPY
- Stretching exercises
- Local heat

DISPOSITION
Rate of development is variable.

REFERRAL
- If joint contracture begins to develop
- For excision of rare nodule that is painful (at any stage)

MISCELLANEOUS

COMMENTS
- Dupuytren's contracture develops earlier and more often in certain families.
- The disorder is more common in Scandinavians, and some Northern Europeans have a 25% prevalence over age 60 yr.
- About 5% of patients develop a similar condition elsewhere, such as Peyronie's disease or Ledderhose disease (involvement of the plantar fascia).
- Soft tissue "pads" in the knuckles may also be present.
- Individuals with these additional findings are considered to have Dupuytren's diathesis, and their disease is generally more severe and recurrent.

REFERENCES
Boswick JA Jr et al: Symposium: Dupuytren's contracture, *Contemp Orthop* 16:71, 1988.
Hill NA: Current concepts review: Dupuytren's contracture, *J Bone Joint Surg* 67(A):1439, 1985.
Author: **Lonnie R. Mercier, M.D.**

Dysfunctional uterine bleeding (PTG)

BASIC INFORMATION

DEFINITION
Dysfunctional uterine bleeding (DUB) describes abnormal uterine bleeding in the absence of disease in the pelvis, pregnancy, or medical illness. Specific types of abnormal bleeding include the following:
- Hypermenorrhea: excessive bleeding in amount during normal duration of regular menstrual cycles.
- Hypomenorrhea: decreased bleeding in amount in regular menstrual cycles.
- Menorrhagia: regular normal intervals, excessive flow and duration.
- Metrorrhagia: irregular intervals, excessive flow and duration.
- Menometrorrhagia: irregular or excessive bleeding during menstruation and between periods.
- Oligomenorrhea: intervals greater than 35 days.
- Polymenorrhea: intervals less than 21 days.

SYNONYMS
DUB

ICD-9-CM CODES
626 Disorders of menstruation and other abnormal bleeding from female genital tract
626.2 Hypermenorrhea
626.1 Hypomenorrhea
626.2 Menorrhagia
626.6 Metrorrhagia
626.2 Menometrorrhagia
626.1 Oligomenorrhea
626.2 Polymenorrhea

EPIDEMIOLOGY AND DEMOGRAPHICS
- Most cases of DUB occur in postmenarcheal and perimenopausal age groups.
- During reproductive age, <20% of abnormal bleeding results from anovulatory DUB.

PHYSICAL FINDINGS
- A clinical diagnosis of exclusion
- Thorough physical and pelvic examination to exclude the other causes of abnormal bleeding
  1. Includes thyroid, breasts, liver, presence or absence of ecchymotic lesions
  2. Patient possibly obese and hirsute (polycystic ovarian disease)
  3. No evidence of any vulvar, vaginal, cervical lesions, uterine (fibroid) or ovarian tumor, urethral caruncle, urethral diverticula, hemorrhoids, anal fissure, colorectal lesions
  4. Bimanual pelvic examination: Normal-sized or slightly enlarged uterus

ETIOLOGY AND PATHOGENESIS
- 90% is caused by anovulation.
- 10% is ovulatory in origin; can be caused by dysfunction of corpus luteum or mid-cycle bleeding.

DIAGNOSIS

DIFFERENTIAL DIAGNOSIS
- Pregnancy-related cause
- Anatomic uterine causes:
  1. Leiomyomas
  2. Adenomyosis
  3. Polyps
  4. Endometrial hyperplasia
  5. Cancer
  6. Sexually transmitted diseases
  7. Intrauterine contraceptive devices
- Anatomic nonuterine causes:
  1. Cervical neoplasia, cervicitis
  2. Vaginal neoplasia, adhesions, trauma, foreign body, atrophic vaginitis, infections, condyloma
  3. Vulvar trauma, infections, neoplasia, condyloma, dystrophy, varices
  4. Urinary tract: urethral caruncle, diverticulum, hematuria
  5. GI tract: hemorrhoids, anal fissure, colorectal lesions
- Systemic diseases:
  1. Exogenous hormone intake
  2. Coagulopathies: Von Willebrand's disease, thrombocytopenia, hepatic failure
  3. Endocrinopathies: thyroid disorder, hypo- and hyperthyroidism, diabetes mellitus
  4. Renal diseases
- Table 2-66 describes a differential diagnosis of vaginal bleeding abnormalities.

WORKUP
- A detailed history and thorough physical examination, including a pelvic examination to exclude above causes.
- Figs. 3-14, 3-15, and 3-16 describe clinical algorithms for the evaluation of vaginal bleeding.

LABORATORY TESTS
- CBC with platelets; Possible iron deficiency anemia or thrombocytopenia
- Prothrombin (PT); partial thromboplastin and bleeding time if coagulopathy is suspected
- Serum human chorionic gonadotropin (hCG)
- Chemistry profile, including liver function tests
- Thyroid profile

Dysfunctional uterine bleeding (PTG)

- Stool testing for occult blood
- Urinalysis for hematuria
- Pap smear
- Cultures for gonorrhea and chlamydia
- Serum gonadotropins and prolactin
- Serum androgens
- Endometrial biopsy in women >30 yr old and barely >20 yr old
- Hysterogram and hysteroscopy

IMAGING STUDIES
Pelvic ultrasound, including measurement of endometrial thickness

TREATMENT

NONPHARMACOLOGIC THERAPY
Increase iron intake in the form of pills and in a diet rich in iron.

ACUTE GENERAL Rx
- Progestational agents:
  1. Progesterone in oil, 100 to 200 mg
  2. Medroxyprogesterone acetate, 20 to 40 mg qd for 15 days
  3. Megestrol acetate, 40 to 120 mg qd
  4. Oral contraceptives: any oral contraceptive pill, one tablet qid for 5 to 7 days, followed by one tablet low-dose estrogen qd for 21 days; causes one heavy withdrawal bleeding, should then be on cyclical Provera or continue on oral contraceptives
- Estrogens:
  1. Conjugated estrogen (Premarin) 25 mg IV q4h until bleeding is under control (in cases of severe or life-threatening bleeding); maximum three doses
  2. For prolonged bleeding that is not life-threatening: Premarin 1.25 mg (Estrace 2.0 mg) q4h for 24 hr, followed by Provera to bring on withdrawal bleeding; then sequential regimen of estrogen and progestin (Premarin 1.25 mg qd for 24 days; Provera 10 mg for 10 days) or oral contraceptives
- Surgical treatment:
  1. Dilatation and curettage
  2. Hysterectomy

CHRONIC Rx
- Progestational agents:
  1. Medroxyprogesterone acetate 10 mg qd for 12 days, then cyclically to induce monthly withdrawal bleeding
  2. Norethindrone 1 mg qd for 12 days
  3. Depo-Provera 150 mg IM and then 150 mg every 3 mo
  4. Oral contraceptives one tablet qd
- Clomiphene citrate: patients with anovulatory bleeding who want to become pregnant
- Others:
  1. Antiprostaglandins
  2. Danazol
  3. Gonadotropic-releasing hormone analogs (GNRH)
  4. Human menopausal gonadotropin (HMG)
- Surgical treatment:
  1. Dilatation and curettage
  2. Endometrial ablation
  3. Hysterectomy

DISPOSITION
Cyclical treatment on birth control pills or Provera for several cycles, then discontinue pill and watch patient for onset of regular menses

REFERRAL
To gynecologist in case of failure of treatment

MISCELLANEOUS

COMMENTS
Patient education material may be obtained from the American College of Obstetricians and Gynecologists, 409 12th Street SW, Washington, DC 20024-2188; phone: (202)638-5577.

REFERENCES
American College of Obstetricians and Gynecologists: Dysfunctional uterine bleeding, *ACOG Technical Bulletin,* No 134, Washington, DC, 1989.

Kim M: Dysfunctional uterine bleeding. In Copeland LJ: *Textbook of gynecology,* Philadelphia, 1993, WB Saunders.

Speroff L: Dysfunctional uterine bleeding in clinical gynecologic endocrinology and infertility, ed 5, Baltimore, 1994, Williams & Wilkins.

Author: **Mandeep K. Brar, M.D.**

BASIC INFORMATION

DEFINITION
Dysmenorrhea is pain with menstruation, usually as cramping and usually centered in the lower abdomen. It is defined as *primary dysmenorrhea* when there is no associated organic pathology and *secondary dysmenorrhea* when there is demonstrable organic pathology.

SYNONYMS
Menstrual cramps
Painful periods

ICD-9-CM CODES
625.3 Dysmenorrhea

EPIDEMIOLOGY AND DEMOGRAPHICS
Approximately 50% of menstruating women are affected by dysmenorrhea, with approximately 10% of them having severe dysmenorrhea with incapacitation for 1 to 3 days/mo. Dysmenorrhea is most common in the age group from 20 to 24 yr, and primary dysmenorrhea usually appears within 6 to 12 mo after menarche.

PHYSICAL FINDINGS
- Sharp, crampy, midline, lower abdomen pain without a lower quadrant or adnexal component but possible radiation to the lower back and upper thighs
- Unremarkable pelvic examination in nonmenstruating patient
- Accompanying symptoms: nausea, vomiting, headaches, anxiety fatigue, diarrhea, fainting, and abdominal bloating
- Cramps usually lasting <24 hr and seldom lasting >2 to 3 days
- Secondary dysmenorrhea: dyspareunia is a common complaint and bimanual pelvic-abdominal examination may demonstrate uterine or adnexal tenderness, fixed uterine retroflexion, uterosacral nodularity, a pelvic mass, or an enlarged, irregular uterus.

ETIOLOGY
Prostaglandin $F_{2\alpha}$ (PG $F_{2\alpha}$) is the agent responsible for dysmenorrhea. It stimulates uterine contractions, cervical stenosis or narrowing, and increased vasopressin release. Behavior and psychologic factors have also been implicated in the etiology of primary dysmenorrhea. Primary dysmenorrhea only occurs in ovulatory cycles. Secondary dysmenorrhea is usually caused by endometriosis, adenomyosis, leiomyomas and, less commonly, chronic salpingitis, IUD use, or congenital or acquired outflow tract obstruction, including cervical stenosis.

DIAGNOSIS

DIFFERENTIAL DIAGNOSIS
- Adenomyosis
- Adhesions
- Allen-Masters syndrome
- Cervical structures or stenosis
- Congenital malformation of Mullerian system
- Ectopic pregnancy
- Endometriosis, endometritis
- Imperforate hymen
- IUD use
- Leiomyomas
- Ovarian cysts
- Pelvic congestion syndrome, pelvic inflammatory disease
- Polyps
- Transverse vaginal septum

WORKUP
- Primary dysmenorrhea: characteristic history, physical examination normal with the absence of an identifiable cause of pelvic pain
- Secondary dysmenorrhea: history of onset generally >2 yr after menarche, physical examination may reveal uterine irregularity, cul-de-sac tenderness, or nodularity or pelvic masses

LABORATORY TESTS
- No specific tests diagnostic for dysmenorrhea
- Elevated WBC count in the presence of infection
- HCG to rule out ectopic pregnancy

IMAGING STUDIES
- Ultrasound scan of the pelvic to evaluate the presence of leiomyomas, ovarian cysts, or ectopic pregnancy
- Hysterosalpingogram to assess the uterine cavity to rule out endometrial polyps, submucosal or intraluminal leiomyomas

TREATMENT

NONPHARMACOLOGIC THERAPY
- Applying heat to the lower abdomen with hot compresses, heating pads, or hot water bottles seems to offer some relief.
- Offer reassurance that this is a treatable condition.

ACUTE GENERAL Rx
- Nonsteroidal antiinflammatory drugs such as ibuprofen 400 to 600 mg q4-6h or naproxen sodium 550 mg q12h, mefenamic acid 500 mg initial dose followed by 250 mg q6h PRN, aspirin 650 mg q 4-6h, or oral contraceptives
- Nifedipine 30 mg qd in difficult cases of dysmenorrhea
- Secondary dysmenorrhea: treatment directed to the specific underlying condition; surgery plays a greater role
- Endometriosis: use of nonsurgical approaches, such as using danazol, gonadotropin-releasing hormone, agonists, and oral contraceptives

CHRONIC Rx
Acupuncture and transcutaneous electrical nerve stimulation (TENS) may be tried. In cases where medical therapy has not worked, laparoscopy should be considered, as well as other surgical treatments depending on the secondary cause of the dysmenorrhea.

DISPOSITION
The majority of patients are satisfactorily treated with good outcomes. It is thought that primary dysmenorrhea generally improves with age and parity and that secondary dysmenorrhea usually has good results with adequate treatment. Possible chronic complications with primary dysmenorrhea that hasn't been adequately treated can lead to anxiety and depression. With certain causes of secondary dysmenorrhea infertility can become a problem.

REFERRAL
If a secondary cause of dysmenorrhea is revealed, refer to the appropriate specialist for further medical or surgical treatment (gynecologist, pain management center).

MISCELLANEOUS

COMMENTS
Patient education materials can be obtained through various pharmaceutical companies (e.g., booklet on "Painful Periods" from Warner Lambert, Inc.)

REFERENCES
Dawood MY: Dysmenorrhea, *Clin Obstet Gynecol* 33(1):168, 1990.
Speroff L: *Clinical gynecologic endocrinology and infertility,* ed 5, Baltimore, Md, 1994, Williams & Wilkins.
Author: **George T. Danakas, M.D.**

Echinococcosis

BASIC INFORMATION

DEFINITION
Echinococcosis is a chronic infection caused by the larval stage of several animal cestodes (flat worms) of the genus *Echinococcus*.

SYNONYMS
Hydatid disease

ICD-9-CM CODES
122.9 Echinococcus infection

EPIDEMIOLOGY AND DEMOGRAPHICS
INCIDENCE (IN U.S.): Seen primarily in immigrants; varies widely depending on areas of origin.
PREVALENCE (IN U.S.): See "Incidence."
PREDOMINANT SEX: Male = female
PREDOMINANT AGE: 20 to 50 yr of age
PEAK INCIDENCE: Presumed to be acquired in childhood or early adulthood in most cases.

PHYSICAL FINDINGS
- Signs of an enlarging mass lesion in a visceral site such as the liver, lungs, kidneys, bone, or CNS
- Occasional cyst rupture causing allergic manifestations such as urticaria, angioedema, or anaphylaxis that bring the patient to medical attention
- Incidental discovery of cysts by abdominal or thoracic imaging studies performed for other reasons

ETIOLOGY
- Four species of *Echinococcus*: *E. granulosus*, *E. multilocularis*, *E. oligarthrus* and *E. vogeli*.
  1. *E. granulosus* is the cause of cystic hydatid disease.
  2. *E. multilocularis* and *E. vogeli* are the causes of alveolar and polycystic disease.
- The disease is transmitted to humans by infected canines (domestic or wild dogs, wolves, foxes) and seen most commonly in livestock-producing areas of the Middle East, Africa, Australia, New Zealand, Europe, and the Americas, including the southwestern U.S.
- Eggs are present in the feces of infected canines; human infection occurs by ingestion of viable eggs in contaminated food.
- It is common in many areas of the world, especially the Middle East.

DIAGNOSIS

DIFFERENTIAL DIAGNOSIS
- Cystic neoplasms
- Abscess (amebic or bacterial)
- Congenital polycystic disease
- Table 2-15 describes the differential diagnosis of cestode tissue infections.

WORKUP
- Antibody assay
- Imaging study (CT scan, ultrasonography)
- Histologic examination of cyst or contents obtained by aspiration or resection (if possible) to confirm diagnosis

LABORATORY TESTS
Antibody assays (ELISA and Western blot): >90% sensitive and specific for liver cysts, but less accurate for cysts in other sites

IMAGING STUDIES
Ultrasonography and/or CT scan:
- Both are extremely sensitive for the detection of cysts, especially in the liver.
- Both lack specificity and are inadequate to establish the diagnosis of echinococcosis with certainty.

TREATMENT

NONPHARMACOLOGIC THERAPY
- Treatment of choice for echinococcal cysts is surgical resection, when feasible.
- If resection is not feasible, perform percutaneous drainage with instillation of 95% ethanol to prevent dissemination of viable larvae.
- Surgical therapy is followed by medical therapy with albendazole (see "Acute General Rx").

ACUTE GENERAL Rx
For echinococcosis confined to the liver:
- Albendazole (400 mg twice daily for 28 days followed by 14 days of rest for at least three cycles)
- Mebendazole (50 to 70 mg/kg qd) if albendazole not available

CHRONIC Rx
See "Acute General Rx."

DISPOSITION
- Long-term follow-up is necessary following surgical or medical therapy because of the high incidence of late relapse.
- Antibody assays and imaging studies are repeated every 6 to 12 mo for several years following successful surgical or medical therapy.

REFERRAL
- All patients for evaluation for possible surgical resection of cysts
- For consultation with a physician experienced in the medical and surgical management of echinococcosis

MISCELLANEOUS

COMMENTS
Surgical resection, if indicated, should be performed by surgeons experienced in the management of echinococcal cysts.

REFERENCES
Donovan SM et al: Imported echinococcosis in southern California, *Am J Trop Med Hyg* 53(6):668, 1995.

Author: **Joseph R. Masci, M.D.**

Eclampsia

BASIC INFORMATION

DEFINITION
Eclampsia is the occurrence of seizures or coma in a woman with preeclampsia, occurring at >20 wk gestation, or <48 hr postpartum. Atypical eclampsia occurs at <20 wk gestation or as much as 14 days postpartum.

SYNONYMS
Toxemia
Seizures of pregnancy

ICD-9-CM CODES
642.6 Eclampsia

EPIDEMIOLOGY AND DEMOGRAPHICS
INCIDENCE: 1 case/150 to 3000 pregnancies; 2% to 4% of those with preeclampsia
RISK FACTORS: Multifetal gestation (3.6% in twin gestation), molar pregnancy, nonimmune hydrops fetalis, uncontrolled hypertension, preexisting hypertension or renal disease
GENETICS: Increased incidence with first-degree relatives (sister or mother) having had eclampsia

PHYSICAL FINDINGS
- Seizure begins as facial twitching then spreads to generalized clonic-tonic state, with cessation of respiration, followed by a postictal period of amnesia, agitation, and confusion.
- 40% have severe hypertension, 40% have mild to moderate hypertension, and 20% are normotensive.
- Generalized edema with rapid weight gain (>2 lb/wk) may be one of the earliest signs of eclampsia.
- Persistent occipital headache and hyperreflexia with clonus occur in 80% of patients with eclampsia; epigastric pain exists in 20% of these patients.

ETIOLOGY
Although the exact etiology is unknown, the common pathway relates to abnormalities in autoregulation of cerebral blood flow. This may involve transient vasospasm, ischemia, cerebral hemorrhage, and edema, occurring by a mechanism involving hypertensive encephalopathy, decreased colloid osmotic pressure, and prostaglandin imbalance.

DIAGNOSIS

DIFFERENTIAL DIAGNOSIS
- Preexisting seizure disorder
- Metabolic abnormalities (hypoglycemia, hyponatremia, hypocalcemia)
- Substance abuse
- Head trauma, infection (meningitis, encephalitis)
- Intracerebral bleeding or thrombosis
- Amniotic fluid embolism
- Space-occupying brain lesions or neoplasms
- Pseudoseizure

WORKUP
- Rule out other causes of seizures during pregnancy.
- Atypical presentations such as prolonged postictal state, status epilepticus, gestational age <20 wk or >48 hr postpartum, or signs of meningitis, substance abuse, or severe uncontrolled hypertension should prompt a search for other seizure etiologies.

LABORATORY TESTS
- Proteinuria: Severe (49%), mild to moderate (29%), absent (22%)
- Hct: elevated secondary to hemoconcentration
- Platelet count: decreased; LFTs elevated in HELLP syndrome
- BUN and creatinine: elevated with renal involvement
- Serum electrolytes, glucose, calcium, toxicology profile: to rule out other causes of seizures
- Hyperuricemia: >6.9 mg/dl found in 70% of eclamptics
- ABG: maternal acidemia and hypoxia

IMAGING STUDIES
- CT scan or MRI indicated in atypical presentation, suspected intracerebral bleeding, focal neurologic deficit.
- There are abnormal findings, including cerebral edema, hemorrhage, and infarction, in 50% of patients.

TREATMENT

NONPHARMACOLOGIC THERAPY
- Airway protection (risk of aspiration)
- Supportive care during acute event

ACUTE GENERAL Rx
- Maintain airway, adequate oxygenation, and IV access.
- Fetal resuscitation, involving maternal oxygenation, left lateral positioning, and continuous fetal heart rate monitoring is needed.
- Give magnesium sulfate 6 g IV load over 20 min, then 3 g/hr maintenance, for recurrent seizure prophylaxis. If repeated convulsion, may give an additional 2 g IV over 3 to 5 min. About 10% to 15% of patients will have a second seizure after initial loading dose. Check magnesium level 1 hr after loading dose, then q6h (therapeutic range 4 to 6 mg/dl). Antidote for toxicity is calcium gluconate 10 ml of 10% solution. Phenytoin has been used as an alternative in patients in whom magnesium sulfate is contraindicated (renal insufficiency, heart block, myasthenia gravis, hypoparathyroidism).
- Give sodium amobarbital 250 mg IV over 3 min for persistent seizures.
- Treat blood pressure if >160 mm Hg/110 mm Hg, with either labetalol 20- to 40-mg IV bolus, hydralazine 10 mg IV or nifedipine 10 to 20 mg sublingual q20min.
- Evaluate patient for delivery.

CHRONIC Rx
- The first priority is stabilization of the mother in terms of adequate oxygenation, hemodynamics, and laboratory abnormalities, such as associated coagulopathies.
- Cervical status and gestational age should be assessed. If unfavorable cervix and <30 wk consider C-section, otherwise consider induction.
- Controlled epidural is the anesthesia of choice for labor or C-section.
- Avoid general anesthesia in uncontrolled hypertension to minimize risk of catastrophic cerebral events.

DISPOSITION
The maternal mortality rate for eclampsia averages 5% to 6%. Morbidity is 25%, including placental abruption (10%), maternal apnea with fetal asphyxia, aspiration pneumonia, pulmonary edema (4%), renal failure, cardiopulmonary arrest, and coma.

REFERRAL
Because of the potential for serious permanent maternal and fetal sequelae, all cases should be managed by a team approach of obstetrician, neonatologist, and intensivist.

MISCELLANEOUS

COMMENTS
- Eclampsia antepartum, 50%; intrapartum, 20%; and postpartum, 30%
- Postseizure there is an associated period of fetal bradycardia from 1 to 9 min; if there is evidence of fetal compromise beyond that time, consider alternative etiologies such as placental abruption (23% incidence).

REFERENCES
Repke JT: Eclampsia: a challenging obstetric emergency, *Female Patient* 21:75, 1996.
Usta IH, Sibai BM: Emergent management of puerperal eclampsia, *Obstet Gynecol Clin North Am* 22:315, 1995.
Author: Scott J. Zuccala, D.O.

Ectopic pregnancy

BASIC INFORMATION

DEFINITION
An ectopic pregnancy (EP) is one in which a fertilized ovum implants outside the endometrial lining of the uterus.

SYNONYMS
Abdominal pregnancy (1% to 2%)
Cervical pregnancy (0.5%)
Interstitial pregnancy (2% to 3%)
Ovarian pregnancy (1%)
Tubal pregnancy (97%)

ICD-9-CM CODES
633 Ectopic pregnancy

EPIDEMIOLOGY AND DEMOGRAPHICS
- 1% to 2% of pregnancies
- 13% of maternal deaths

PREVALENCE (IN U.S.): Increasing number of EP; 17,800 reported cases in 1970 and 108,000 reported cases in 1992.

RISK FACTORS: Previous salpingitis, previous EP, previous tubal ligation, previous tuboplasty, IUD use, progestin-only pill, and assisted reproductive techniques

PHYSICAL FINDINGS
- Abdominal tenderness: 95%
- Adnexal tenderness: 87% to 99%
- Peritoneal signs: 71% to 76%
- Adnexal mass: 33% to 53%
- Enlarged uterus: 6% to 30%
- Shock: 2% to 17%
- Amenorrhea or abnormal vaginal bleeding: 75%
- Shoulder pain: 10%
- Tissue passage: 6% to 7%

ETIOLOGY
- Anatomic obstruction to zygote passage
- Abnormalities in tubal motility
- Transperitoneal migration of the zygote

DIAGNOSIS

DIFFERENTIAL DIAGNOSIS
- Corpus luteum cyst
- Rupture or torsion of ovarian cyst
- Threatened or incomplete abortion
- PID
- Appendicitis
- Gastroenteritis
- Dysfunctional uterine bleeding
- Degenerating uterine fibroids
- Endometriosis

WORKUP
1. The classic presentation of EP includes the triad of abnormal vaginal bleeding, pelvic pain, and an adnexal mass. Consider in all women with abdominal-pelvic pain and a positive pregnancy test.
2. Culdocentesis is clinically useful when other diagnostic modalities are not readily available.
   - Positive tap means nonclotting blood with Hct >12%.
   - Negative tap means clear or blood-tinged fluid.
   - Nondiagnostic tap means clotted blood or no fluid.
3. Laparoscopy

LABORATORY TESTS
- hCG: if normal IUP, 85% have doubling time of 2 days. If abnormal gestation, will show <66% increase of QhCG within 2 days. However, 13% of ectopic pregnancies have a normal doubling time.
- Progesterone: decreased production in EP, <5 ng/ml strongly predictive of abnormal pregnancy. If >25 ng/ml, strongly predictive of normal IUP.
- Dropping Hct associated with tubal rupture.
- Leukocytosis

IMAGING STUDIES
- Ultrasound: presence of an IUP rules out EP.
- If QhCG >6000 mIU/ml, should see IUP on abdominal scan, and QhCG >1500 mIU/ml for transvaginal scan.
- Findings on ultrasound in EP include:
  1. Empty uterus
  2. Adnexal mass
  3. Cul-de-sac fluid
  4. Fetal sac in tube
  5. Fetal cardiac activity in adnexa

TREATMENT

NONPHARMACOLOGIC THERAPY
Surgery: can be performed by laparoscopy if patient is stable or by laparotomy if patient is unstable. Salpingiosis: direct injection of chemotherapy into ectopic via laparoscopy, transvaginal ultrasound, or hysteroscopy.
- Conservative surgery-salpingostomy or segmental resection depends on tubal location and size of ectopic.
- Salpingectomy should be considered in the following circumstances:
  1. Ruptured tube
  2. Future fertility not desired
  3. Recurrent ectopic in the same tube
  4. Uncontrolled hemorrhage

ACUTE GENERAL Rx
- If the patient is stable and compliant may consider medical management with methotrexate. Patient should not have contraindications to methotrexate such as: hepatic or renal disease, thrombocytopenia, leukopenia, or significant anemia. There should be no evidence of hemoperitoneum on transvaginal ultrasound. Ectopic should be <4 cm mass with QhCG <30,000 mIU/ml.
- Most common regimen is methotrexate 50 mg/m^2 body surface area. May require second dose or surgical intervention if QhCG increases or plateaus after 7 days.

CHRONIC Rx
Persistent EP results from residual trophoblastic tissue or secondary implantation after conservative surgery. There is a 5% incidence of persistent ectopic with conservative treatment.

DISPOSITION
If diagnosed and treated early (before rupture) prognosis is excellent for good recovery. Follow QhCG weekly until negative. Use reliable contraception until hCG negative. With subsequent pregnancies, follow QhCG and perform early ultrasound to confirm IUP. There is a 12% recurrence rate for EP.

REFERRAL
Should obtain gynecologic consultation if EP is suspected.

MISCELLANEOUS

COMMENTS
Patient information can be obtained though American College of Obstetricians and Gynecologists, 409 12th St SW, Washington, DC 20024-2188.

REFERENCES
Leach RE, Ory SJ: Modern management of ectopic pregnancy, *J Reprod Med* 34:324, 1989.
Ory SJ: Surgery for ectopic pregnancy. In Gershenson et al: *Operative gynecology*, Philadelphia, 1993, WB Saunders.
Sklar A: Evaluation of lower abdominal and pelvic pain. In Danakas GT, Pietrantoni M: *Practical guide to the care of the gynecologic/obstetric patient*, St Louis, 1997, Mosby.

Author: **George T. Danakas, M.D.**

Ejaculation, premature

BASIC INFORMATION

DEFINITION
Premature ejaculation is a persistent and recurrent problem in which a male experiences orgasm or ejaculation in the early phases of sexual contact and before he wishes it. Other definitions have emphasized elapsed time after intromission (with durations of 30 sec to several min), number of thrusts, or rate of partner satisfaction.

SYNONYMS
Rapid ejaculation
Early ejaculation
Inadequate ejaculatory control

ICD-10-CODES
F52.4 Premature ejaculation (DSM-IV Code 302.75)

EPIDEMIOLOGY AND DEMOGRAPHICS
INCIDENCE (IN U.S.): Reported as 21% in 1988; 46% in 1970
PREVALENCE (IN U.S.): 7% to 38%
PREDOMINANT SEX: Only males affected
PREDOMINANT AGE: None defined
PEAK INCIDENCE: Adolescence and young adulthood
GENETICS: No identifiable genetic factors

PHYSICAL FINDINGS
- Complaint of ejaculation before, upon, or shortly after penetration
- Frequently associated anxiety either related to sexual activity or more generalized anxiety disorder
- Premature ejaculation secondary to a medical condition frequently associated with low anxiety, low desire, and/or erectile insufficiency

ETIOLOGY
- Unclear etiology; different theoretical frameworks emphasizing anxiety related to performance or personal interactions, behavioral concepts of learned expectations related to early experience, or heightened penile sensitivity
- Organic factors in a small fraction of individuals (e.g., abdominal or pelvic trauma or surgery, neuropathies, or urologic pathology such as prostatic urethritis)

DIAGNOSIS

DIFFERENTIAL DIAGNOSIS
- In as many as 25% of men with complaints of premature ejaculation, partner is anorgasmic.
- In young adolescents, premature ejaculation is normally experienced as a consequence of heightened excitation.

WORKUP
- History with a specific emphasis on sexual activities, beliefs, orientation, and gender identity
- History of relationships
- Collateral information from sexual partner when possible
- Additional history regarding surgery, trauma, and myologic symptoms
- History of prescribed and recreational drugs revealing contributory factors (e.g., tricyclic antidepressants, alcohol, opiates)

LABORATORY TESTS
Urinalysis and urine culture after prostatic massage may uncover a urinary or prostatic infection.

IMAGING STUDIES
None indicated

TREATMENT

NONPHARMACOLOGIC THERAPY
- Behavioral and psychotherapeutic interventions: strongly guided by a specific theoretical framework; often inadequate data to suggest the superiority of any particular approach
- Use of condoms frequently recommended to reduce penile sensitivity
- Use of pause-squeeze technique, in which 4 sec of moderate pressure is applied to the frenulum to reduce ejaculatory urge

ACUTE GENERAL Rx
- Topical anesthetics (benzodiazepines) increase ejaculatory latency.
- Anxiolytics may be useful in individuals with anxiety.
- Serotonin reuptake inhibiting antidepressants, which frequently delay orgasm in both men and women, are a common intervention but have not been extensively studied.

DISPOSITION
- Premature ejaculation is frequently a chronic, lifelong problem.
- There is gradual improvement with age but few spontaneous remissions.
- Impact of successful therapy may be prolonged.

REFERRAL
If behavioral sex therapy or psychotherapy is indicated or if significant urologic abnormalities are discovered

MISCELLANEOUS

REFERENCES
Grenier G, Byers ES: Rapid ejaculation: a review of conceptual, etiological, and treatment issues, *Arch Sex Behav* 24:447, 1995.
St Lawrence JS, Madakasira S: Evaluation and treatment of premature ejaculation: a critical review, *Int J Psychiatry Med* 22:77, 1992.

Author: **Rif S. El-Mallakh, M.D.**

Encephalitis, acute viral

BASIC INFORMATION

DEFINITION
Acute viral encephalitis is an acute febrile syndrome with evidence of meningeal involvement and of derangement of the function of the cerebrum, cerebellum, or brain stem.

SYNONYMS
Arboviral encephalitis
Brain stem encephalitis
Acute necrotizing encephalitis
Rasmussen encephalitis
Encephalitis lethargica

ICD-9-CM CODES
049.9 Viral encephalitis NOS

EPIDEMIOLOGY AND DEMOGRAPHICS
INCIDENCE (IN U.S.): About 20,000 cases/yr are reported to the CDC.
PREVALANCE (IN U.S.): Unknown
PREDOMINANT SEX: Male = female
PREDOMINANT AGE: Any age.
PEAK INCIDENCE: Any age.
GENETICS: No specific genetic or congenital predisposition

ETIOLOGY
- Can be caused by a host of viruses, with herpes simplex the most common virus identified
- Arboviruses: agents causing Eastern equine encephalitis, Western equine encephalitis, St. Louis encephalitis, Venezualian equine encephalitis, California virus encephalitis, Japanese B encephalitis, Murray Valley encephalitis, Russian spring-summer encephalitis, as well as other less known agents
- Also implicated: rabies-causing agents, CMV, Ebstein-Barr, varicella-zoster, echo virus, mumps, adenovirus, coxsackie, rubeola, and herpes viruses
- Meningoencephalitis: acute retroviral infection

PHYSICAL FINDINGS
- Initially, fever and evidence of meningeal irritation
- Headache and stiff neck
- Later, development of signs of cortical dysfunction: lethargy, coma, stupor, weakness, seizures, facial weakness, as well as brain stem findings
- Cerebellar findings: ataxia, nystagmus, hypotonia; myoclonus, cranial nerve palsies, and abnormal tendon reflexes
- Patients with rabies: hydrophobia, anxiety, facial numbness, psychosis, coma, or dysarthria
- Rarely, movement disorders, such as chorea, hemiballismus, or dystonia
- Recall of a prodromal viral-like illness (this finding is not at all uniform)

DIAGNOSIS

DIFFERENTIAL DIAGNOSIS
- Bacterial infections: brain abscess, toxic encephalopathies, TB
- Protozoal infections
- Behçet's disease
- Lupus encephalitis
- Sjögren's syndrome
- Multiple sclerosis
- Syphilis
- Cryptococcus
- Toxoplasmosis
- Brucellosis
- Leukemic or lymphomatous meningitis
- Other metastatic tumors
- Lyme disease
- Cat-scratch disease
- Vogt-Koyangai-Harada syndrome
- Mollaret's meningitis

WORKUP
- Lumbar puncture to reveal pleocytosis, usually lymphocytic although neutrophils may be seen early on
- Usually, elevated CSF protein
- Normal or low CSF glucose
- In herpes simplex encephalitis: RBCs and xanthochromia
- EEG changes showing periodic high-voltage sharp waves in the temporal regions and slow wave complexes suggestive of herpes encephalitis
- CT scan and MRI to reveal edema and hemorrhage in the frontal and temporal lobes
- Arbovial infections suspected during outbreaks in specific areas
- Rising titers of neutralizing antibodies from the acute to the convalescent stage demonstrated but often not helpful in the acutely ill patient
- Polymerase chain reaction that amplifies DNA from the CSF for herpes simplex encephalitis
- Rarely, brain biopsy to assist in the diagnosis; viral culture of cerebral tissue obtained if biopsy done
- Classic herpetic skin lesions suggestive of herpes encephalitis
- In diagnosing arboviral encephalitis:
  1. Presence of antiviral IgM within the first few days of symptomatic disease; detected and quantified by ELISA
  2. Unusual to recover an arbovirus from the blood or CSF

LABORATORY TESTS
- Aside from the lumbar puncture, most other laboratory studies are nonspecific.
- Skin lesions and urine may be cultured for herpes simplex and CMV.

TREATMENT

ACUTE GENERAL Rx
- Supportive care, frequent evaluation, and neurologic examination
- Ventilatory assistance for patients who are moribund or at risk for aspiration
- Avoidance of infusion of hypotonic fluids to minimize the risk of hyponatremia
- For patients who develop seizures: anticonvulsant therapy and follow-up in a critical care setting
- For comatose patients:
  1. Aggressive care to avoid decubiti, contractures, and DVT
  2. Close attention to weights, input/output, and serum electrolytes
- Acyclovir 30 mg/kg/day IV for 14 days for herpes simplex encephalitis
- Short courses of corticosteroids to control brain edema and prevent herniation
- In patients with suspected rabies:
  1. Human rabies immune globulin (HRIG) should be given at a dose of 20 U/kg.
  2. Active immunization may be stimulated by recently developed rabies vaccine, which is grown on a human diploid cell line (HDCV) and has reduced the number of doses needed to five.
  3. If suspect animal can be found, observe closely for 10 days to detect rabid behavior.
  4. If signs are seen, animal should be sacrificed and it's brain examined for signs of rabies.
- No specific pharmacologic therapy for most other viral pathogens

CHRONIC Rx
Some patients may develop permanent neurologic sequela; these patients will gain benefit from intensive rehabilitation programs, including physical, occupational, and speech therapy.

REFERRAL
- For infectious disease and/or neurologic consultation when diagnosis is unclear, especially in patients with severe neurologic syndromes
- To neurologic intensive care for severely ill patients if quickly available

MISCELLANEOUS

REFERENCES
Griffin DE: Encephalitis, myelitis, and neuritis. In *Mandell, Douglas, and Bennett's principles and practices of infectious diseases,* ed 4, New York, 1995. Churchill Livingstone.

Author: **Joseph J. Lieber, M.D.**

Encopresis (PTG)

BASIC INFORMATION

DEFINITION
Encopresis is the voluntary or involuntary passage of stool into inappropriate places, in children over the developmental age of 4 yr, with the absence of direct physiologic causes.

SYNONYMS
Functional incontinence of stool

ICD-9-CM CODES
787.6 Incontinence of feces
307.7 Encopresis

EPIDEMIOLOGY AND DEMOGRAPHICS
INCIDENCE (IN U.S.): 1% of 5 yr olds
PREVALENCE (IN U.S.): 3% of the pediatric population
PREDOMINANT SEX: Male > female
PREDOMINANT AGE: 4 to 9 yr of age
PEAK INCIDENCE: 4 to 5 yr of age
GENETICS: Factors that contribute to slow gut motility may predispose to encopresis

PHYSICAL FINDINGS
- When constipation and overflow incontinence is causative, defecation is usually uncomfortable or painful, so patient avoids defecation with consequent stool retention.
- Stool is usually poorly formed and leakage is continuous (occurring during sleep and wakefulness).
- Encopresis resolves when the constipation is resolved.
- When there is no constipation with overflow incontinence, stool is more likely to be normal in character.
- Soiling is intermittent and usually in a prominent location.
- Coexisting oppositional-defiant or conduct disorders are frequent.

ETIOLOGY
- Approximately 96% of children will have bowel movements between three times daily to once every other day. When bowel movements are less frequent, stool becomes drier and harder and much more uncomfortable to pass. Children may avoid the discomfort by avoiding elimination, but this only results in worsening constipation.
- Soiling results from more liquid stool that leaks around the main stool mass.
- Constipation may begin gradually as a result of a slow decrease in elimination frequency or more acutely after an illness, dehydration, or prolonged bed rest.
- In encopresis without constipation and overflow incontinence, soiling is usually intentional. This frequently occurs in the setting of comorbid oppositional-defiant disorder or conduct disorder.
- Incontinence can also result from anal masturbation.

DIAGNOSIS

DIFFERENTIAL DIAGNOSIS
- Hirschsprung's disease
- Cerebral palsy
- Myelomeningocele
- Pseudoobstruction
- Anorectal lesions
- Malformations
- Trauma
- Rectal prolapse
- Hypothyroidism
- Medications

WORKUP
- History: pay particular attention to frequency of elimination, character of the stool, associated pain, and presence of enuresis (with which it is frequently associated).
- Physical examination: pay particular attention to the abdomen, anus, rectum, and saddle sensation.

LABORATORY TESTS
- Thyroid profile
- Electrolytes (including calcium)
- Adrenal function
- Urinalysis and urine culture

IMAGING STUDIES
- Abdominal x-rays to determine extent of obstruction or megacolon
- Anorectal manometric studies to determine sphincter function if Hirschsprung's disease is suspected; if abnormal, followed up with a barium enema and rectal biopsy

TREATMENT

NONPHARMACOLOGIC THERAPY
- Psychotherapy or family therapy in chronic encopresis
- Biofeedback to improve sphincter function

ACUTE GENERAL Rx
- Disimpaction with hypertonic phosphate (30 ml/5 kg body weight) or isotonic saline enemas
- Resistant cases: repeated instillation of 200 to 600 ml of milk of magnesia enemas
- If child does not permit enemas: oral disimpaction with large doses of mineral oil or lactulose until stool mass is cleared (NOTE: this is frequently more painful and more uncomfortable than an enema)

CHRONIC Rx
- Prevention of recurrence of constipation by increased dietary fiber and the use of laxatives
- In immediate postdisimpaction period (3 mo following acute treatment) laxatives needed because bowel tone remains low
- Laxatives possibly required for several years or indefinitely

DISPOSITION
In most cases encopresis is self-limited and of relatively brief duration; it is rarely chronic.

REFERRAL
If patient is resistant to treatment, complicated family factors are involved, or encopresis is purposeful

MISCELLANEOUS

REFERENCES
Loening-Baucke V: Encopresis and soiling, *Pediatr Clin North Am* 43:279, 1996.

Author: **Rif S. El-Mallakh, M.D.**

Endocarditis, infective (PTG)

BASIC INFORMATION

DEFINITION
Infective endocarditis is an infection of the endocardial surface of the heart or mural endocardium.
ACUTE ENDOCARDITIS: Usually caused by *Staphylococcus aureus, Streptococcus pyogenes,* pneumococcus, and *Neisseria* organisms; classic clinical presentation of fever, positive blood cultures, vascular and immunologic phenomenon
SUBACUTE ENDOCARDITIS: Usually caused by viridans streptococci in the presence of valvular pathology; less toxic, often indolent presentation with lower fevers, night sweats, fatigue
INFECTIVE ENDOCARDITIS IN INJECTION DRUG USERS: Often involving *S. aureus* or *Pseudomonas aeruginosa* with variation that may be geographically influenced; tricuspid or multiple valvular involvement; high mortality rate of 50% to 60%
EARLY PROSTHETIC VALVE ENDOCARDITIS: Usually caused by *S. epidermidis* within 2 mo of valve replacement; other organisms include *S. aureus,* gram-negative bacilli, diphtheroids, *Candida* organisms
LATE PROSTHETIC VALVE ENDOCARDITIS: Typically develops >60 days after valvular replacement; involved organisms similar to early prosthetic valve endocarditis, including viridans streptococci, enterococci, and group D streptococci
NOSOCOMIAL ENDOCARDITIS: Secondary to intravenous catheters, TPN lines, pacemakers; coagulase negative staphylococci, *S. aureus,* and streptococci most common

SYNONYMS
Bacterial endocarditis

ICD-9-CM CODES
421.0 Infective endocarditis
996.61 Prosthetic valve endocarditis

EPIDEMIOLOGY AND DEMOGRAPHICS
INCIDENCE (IN U.S.): 1.7 to 3.8 cases/100,000 persons/yr
NOSOCOMIAL ENDOCARDITIS: 14% to 28% of cases
PREVALENCE (IN U.S.): 0.3 to 3 cases/1000 hospital admissions
PREDOMINANT SEX:
Male > female
PREDOMINANT AGE: 45 to 65 yr
PEAK INCIDENCE: Females: often <35 yr old; males: 45 to 65 yr old

PHYSICAL FINDINGS
- Fever may be variable in presentation; may be high, hectic, or absent.
- Fever, chills, fatigue, and rigors occur in 25% to 80% of patients.
- Heart murmur may be absent in right-sided endocarditis.
- Embolic phenomenon with peripheral manifestations are found in 50% of patients.
- Skin manifestations include petechiae, Osler nodes, splinter hemorrhages, Janeway lesions.
- Splenomegaly is more common with subacute course.

ETIOLOGY
Streptococcal and staphylococcal infections are the most common causes of infective endocarditis. Variation in incidence may occur that is influenced by the patient's risk for developing infection.
ACUTE ENDOCARDITIS:
- *S. aureus*
- *Streptococcus pneumonia*
- Streptococcal species and groups A through G
- *Haemophilus influenza*

SUBACUTE ENDOCARDITIS:
- Viridans streptococci (α-hemolytic)
- *Str. bovis*
- Enterococci
- *S. aureus*

ENDOCARDITIS IN IV DRUG ADDICTS:
- *S. aureus*
- *P. aeruginosa*
- *Candida* species
- Enterococci

PROSTHETIC VALVE (EARLY):
- *S. epidermidis*
- *S. aureus*
- Gram-negative bacilli
- Group D streptococci

PROSTHETIC VALVE (LATE):
- *S. epidermidis*
- Viridans streptococci
- *S. aureus*
- Enterococci and Group D streptococci

NOSOCOMIAL ENDOCARDITIS:
- Coagulase negative staphylococcus
- *S. aureus*
- Streptococci: viridans, group B, enterococcus

DIAGNOSIS

DIFFERENTIAL DIAGNOSIS
- Brain abscess
- FUO
- Pericarditis
- Meningitis
- Rheumatic fever
- Osteomyelitis
- Salmonella
- TB
- Bacteremia
- Pericarditis
- Glomerulonephritis

WORKUP
Physical examination to evaluate for the above physical findings followed by laboratory testings (see below)

LABORATORY TESTS
- Blood cultures: three sets in first 24 hr
- More culturing if patient has received prior antibiotic
- CBC (anemia possibly present, subacute)
- WBC (leukocytosis is higher in acute endocarditis)
- ESR (elevated)
- Positive rheumatoid factor (subacute endocarditis)
- False-positive VDRL
- Proteinuria, hematuria, RBC casts

IMAGING STUDIES
- Echocardiogram: two-dimensional
- Transesophageal echocardiography: more sensitive in detecting vegetations if two-dimensional is negative, especially helpful with prosthetic valves or in detecting perivalvular disease

TREATMENT

Initial IV antibiotic therapy (before culture results) is aimed at the most likely organism:
- In patients with prosthetic valves or patients with native valves who are allergic to penicillin: vancomycin plus rifampin and gentamicin
- In IV drug users: nafcillin or oxacillin plus gentamicin
- In native valve endocarditis: combination of penicillin and gentamicin; a penicillase-resistant penicillin (oxacillin or nafcillin) can be used if acute bacterial endocarditis is present or if *S. aureus* is suspected as one of the possible causative organisms

Antibiotic therapy after identification of the organism should be guided by susceptibility testing (MIC, MBC).

MISCELLANEOUS

COMMENTS
For endocarditis prophylaxis, refer to Boxes A-1, A-2, A-3 and Tables A-11 and A-12 in Appendix.

REFERENCES
Wilson WR et al: Antibiotic treatment of adults with infective endocarditis due to streptococci, enterococci, staphylococci, and HACEK microorganisms, *JAMA* 274:1706, 1995.

Author: **Dennis J. Mikolich, M.D.**

BASIC INFORMATION

DEFINITION
Endometrial cancer is a malignant transformation of endometrial stroma and/or glands typified by irregular nuclear membranes, nuclear atypia, mitotic activity, loss of glandular pattern irregular cell size.

SYNONYMS
Uterine cancer (some forms)

ICD-9-CM CODES
182 Malignant neoplasm of body of uterus

EPIDEMIOLOGY AND DEMOGRAPHICS
INCIDENCE: 21.2 cases/100,000 persons; approximately 30,000 new cases annually
PREDOMINANCE: Median age at onset: 63 yr; only 5% occur in women <40 yr
RISK FACTORS: Obesity, diabetes, nulliparity, early menarche and late menopause, unopposed estrogen therapy, tamoxifen use, endometrial atypical hyperplasia

PHYSICAL FINDINGS
- Abnormal uterine bleeding or postmenopausal bleeding in 90%
- Pyometra or hematometra
- Abnormal Pap smear

ETIOLOGY
Endogenous or exogenous chronic unopposed estrogen stimulation of the endometrium

DIAGNOSIS

DIFFERENTIAL DIAGNOSIS
- Atypical hyperplasia
- Other genital tract malignancy
- Polyps
- Atrophic vaginitis

WORKUP
- Complete history and physical examination
- Endometrial biopsy or dilation and curettage
- Assessment of operative risk

LABORATORY TESTS
- CBC
- Chemistry profile including liver function tests
- Consider CA-125 level

IMAGING STUDIES
- Chest x-ray examination
- Possible CT scan, BE, and/or pelvic ultrasound

TREATMENT

NONPHARMACOLOGIC THERAPY
- Surgery is the mainstay of treatment, with or without radiation, depending on tumor stage and grade.
- Surgery consists of pelvic washings, total abdominal hysterectomy and bilateral salpingo-oophorectomy, omental biopsy, and selective pelvic and periaortic lymphadenectomy, depending on stage and grade.
- Brachytherapy and/or teletherapy are added in an advanced stage.
- Chemotherapy (cisplatin, adriamycin) or tamoxifen may also be used.

ACUTE GENERAL Rx
- A thorough workup should be completed before any therapy for endometrial cancer.
- Surgery is the treatment of choice.

CHRONIC Rx
- Physical and pelvic examination every 3 mo for 2 yr, then every 6 mo for 2 yr, annually thereafter
- Yearly Pap smear
- Hormone replacement (combination) a consideration in low risk patients

DISPOSITION
The majority of cases present early, where the 5-yr survival is generally good:
- Stage I   75% to 100%
- Stage II   60%
- Stage III   50%
- Stage IV   20%

Some histologic types (clear cell, serous papillary) have poorer survival rates.

REFERRAL
A gynecologist may manage early stage disease, otherwise refer to a gynecologic oncologist.

MISCELLANEOUS

COMMENTS
U.S. Preventive Services Task Force Recommendations regarding counseling to prevent gynecologic cancers are described in Section V, Chapter 64.

REFERENCES
Baker TR: Endometrial carcinoma. In Piver MS (ed): *Handbook of gynecologic oncology,* ed 2, Boston, 1996, Little, Brown.

Burke TW et al: Cervical intraepithelial neoplasia and cervical cancer, *Obstet Gynecol Clin North Am* 23(2):411-456, 1996.

Noumoff JS, Faruqi S: Endometrial adenocarcinoma, *Microsc Res Tech* 25(3): 246-54, 1993.

Author: **Karen Houck, M.D.**

Endometriosis (PTG)

BASIC INFORMATION

DEFINITION
Endometriosis is defined as the presence of functioning endometrial glands and stroma outside the uterine cavity.

ICD-9-CM CODES
617.9 Endometriosis

EPIDEMIOLOGY AND DEMOGRAPHICS
PREVALENCE:
- Women of reproductive age: 2% to 5%
- Infertile women: 20% to 40%

MOST COMMON AGE OF DIAGNOSIS: 25 to 29 yr

GENETICS:
- Multifactorial inheritance pattern
- 6.9% occurrence rate in first-degree female relatives

PHYSICAL FINDINGS
- Classic triad is dysmenorrhea, dyspareunia, and infertility.
- Presence of pelvic pain *not correlated* with the total area of endometriosis, type of lesion, or volume of disease, but it *is correlated* with the depth of infiltration.
- Most severe discomfort is associated with lesions >1 cm in depth.
- Bimanual examination may reveal tender uterosacral ligaments, cul-de-sac nodularity, induration of the rectovaginal septum, fixed retroversion of the uterus, adnexal mass, and generalized or localized tenderness.

ETIOLOGY
- Reflux and direct implantation theory: retrograde menstruation with implantation of viable endometrial cells to surrounding pelvic structures
- Coelomic metaplasia theory: transformation of multipotential cells of the coelomic epithelium into endometrium-like cells
- Vascular dissemination theory: transport of endometrial cells to distant sites via the uterine vascular and lymphatic systems
- Autoimmune disease theory: disorder of immune surveillance allows growth of endometrial implants

DIAGNOSIS

DIFFERENTIAL DIAGNOSIS
- Ectopic pregnancy
- Acute appendicitis
- Chronic appendicitis
- PID
- Pelvic adhesions
- Hemorrhagic cyst
- Hernia
- Psychologic disorder
- Irritable bowel syndrome
- Uterine leiomyomata
- Adenomyosis
- Nerve entrapment syndrome
- Scoliosis
- Muscular/skeletal strain
- Interstitial cystitis

WORKUP
- Thorough history and physical examination, including inquiry about physical and emotional abuse
- Colonoscopy if rectal bleeding present
- Laparoscopy for definitive diagnosis
- Revised American Fertility Society (RAFS) scale to classify endometriosis (since 1985):
  Stage I   minimal
  Stage II   mild
  Stage III moderate
  Stage IV   severe

LABORATORY TESTS
Cancer antigen 125 [CA125]
- Also elevated in ovarian epithelial neoplasm, myomas, adenomyosis, acute PID, ovarian cysts, pancreatitis, chronic liver disease, menstruation, and pregnancy
- CA125 value >35U/mL: positive predictive value of 0.58 and a negative predictive value of 0.96 for the presence of endometriosis

IMAGING STUDIES
- Ultrasound: for evaluating adnexal mass; cannot reliably distinguish endometriomas from other benign or malignant ovarian conditions
- MRI:
  1. Highly accurate in detecting endometriomas
  2. Limited sensitivity in detecting diffuse pelvic endometriosis

TREATMENT

NONPHARMACOLOGIC THERAPY
Expectant management (observation for 5 to 12 mo) for stage I or stage II endometriosis-associated infertility

ACUTE GENERAL Rx
NSAIDs (see Table 7-29) for symptomatic relief of dysmenorrhea

CHRONIC Rx
PHARMACOLOGIC MANAGEMENT:
Estrogen-progesterone:
- State of "pseudopregnancy" created by continuous use of combination oral contraceptives for 6 to 12 mo

- Effective in alleviating pain in 75% to 89% of patients
- Breakthrough bleeding treated by increasing the dose of these agents or by administering conjugated estrogens 1.25 mg/day for 2 wk

Danazol:
- Initial dose 200 mg PO bid
- If no improvement within 6 wk, dosage increased to 300 or 400 mg PO bid
- Treatment generally continued for 6 mo, after which up to 90% of patients with mild to moderate endometriosis experience alleviation of pelvic pain
- Treatment begun after menses to avoid fetal exposure

Progestins:
- Medroxyprogesterone acetate 10 to 30 mg PO qd and occasionally up to 100 mg PO qd
- Alternatively, 100 mg IM every 2 wk for four doses, followed by 200 mg IM monthly for 4 mo
- Breakthrough bleeding treated with ethynyl estradiol (20 µg/day) or conjugated estrogens (1.25 mg/day) for 1 to 2 wk
- Comparison with danazol: progestins cost less, have a more tolerable side-effect profile, and have comparable efficacy with regard to pain relief, so are often the first-line drug

Gonadotropin-releasing Hormone Analogues:
- Leuprolide acetate and goserelin SC; nafarelin acetate intranasally
- Use limited to 6 mo
- As effective as danazol for relief of pelvic pain

SURGICAL MANAGEMENT:
Conservative:
- Directed at enhancing fertility
- Removal or destruction of endometriotic implants by excision, electrocautery, or laser
- Yields cumulative pregnancy rate of approximately 52%
- No increase in fertility for patients with mild to moderate endometriosis but significant increase for those with severe endometriosis
- Also indicated for treatment of pain unresponsive to pharmacologic management

Definitive:
- Directed at relieving endometriosis-associated pain
- Total abdominal hysterectomy with bilateral salpingo-oophorectomy and complete excision or ablation of endometriosis
- Thorough abdominal exploration to ensure removal of all disease
- Must be prepared to manage possible GI and urinary tract endometriosis
- 90% effective in pain relief
- Estrogen replacement therapy (ERT) to be considered in all women undergoing definitive surgical management; after ERT, recurrence rate 0% to 5% in women with endometriosis confined to the pelvis but 18% in women with bowel involvement

MANAGEMENT OF ENDOMETRIOSIS-ASSOCIATED INFERTILITY:
Conservative surgery:
- Yields significantly increased pregnancy rate than does expectant management, in part because of correction of mechanical factors such as adhesions

Assisted reproductive technologies:
- Can be used to circumvent unknown mechanism of endometriosis-associated infertility
- Superovulation with clomiphene citrate or human menopausal gonadotropins; clomiphene citrate results in threefold pregnancy rate over either danazol or expectant management
- Further improvement with intrauterine insemination combined with superovulation
- In vitro fertilization if above unsuccessful

DISPOSITION
Tends to recur unless definitive surgery is performed

REFERRAL
To a reproductive endocrinologist for advanced surgical management or infertility management

MISCELLANEOUS

COMMENTS
Patient information can be obtained through the following organizations: Endometriosis Association, 8585 North 76th Place, Milwaukee, WI 53225, 414-355-2200 or 800-992-ENDO; Women's Reproductive Health Network, P.O. Box 30167, Portland, OR 97230-9067; phone: 503-667-7757.

REFERENCES
Hesla JS, JA Rock: Endometriosis. In Rock JA, Thompson JD: *Te Linde's operative gynecology*, ed 8, Philadelphia, 1997, Lippincott-Raven.
Johnson KM: Endometriosis: the immunoendocrine factor, *Female Patient* 21:15, 1996.
Lu PY, Ory SJ: Endometriosis: current management, *Mayo Clin Proc* 70:453, 1995.

Author: **Wan J. Kim, M.D.**

Endometritis

BASIC INFORMATION

DEFINITION
Endometritis is defined as a uterine infection following delivery or abortion.

SYNONYMS
Endomyometritis
Endoperimetritis
Metritis

ICD-9-CM CODES
615.9 Endometritis

EPIDEMIOLOGY AND DEMOGRAPHICS
- Overall rate of postpartum infection: estimated between 1% and 8%
- Most common genital tract infection following delivery
- Usually presents early in postpartum period; more commonly seen following C-section than vaginal delivery; also seen with an incomplete abortion (spontaneous abortion, legal abortion, or illegal abortion)
- Possible following any uterine manipulation in the presence of an undiagnosed cervicitis or vaginitis

PHYSICAL FINDINGS
- Postpartum oral temperature >37.8° C
- Localized uterine tenderness, purulent or foul lochia; physical examination revealing uterine or parametrial tenderness
- Nonspecific signs and symptoms such as malaise, abdominal pain, chills, and tachycardia.

ETIOLOGY
Endometritis is usually associated with multiple organisms: Group A or B streptococci, *Staphylococcus aureus* and *Bacteroides* species, *Neisseria gonorrhoeae, Chlamydia trachomatis,* enterococci, *Gardnerella vaginitis, E. coli,* and *Mycoplasmas*.

DIAGNOSIS

DIFFERENTIAL DIAGNOSIS
Causes of postoperative or postprocedural infections

WORKUP
Diagnosis based on symptoms of fever, malaise, abdominal pain, uterine tenderness, and purulent, foul vaginal discharge

LABORATORY TESTS
CBC, blood cultures, and uterine culture

IMAGING STUDIES
Ultrasound may be useful if retained products are considered a possible source of infection.

TREATMENT

ACUTE GENERAL Rx
- In treating endometritis after a vaginal delivery, ampicillin 2 g IV q6h plus gentamicin loading dose IV or IM (2 mg/kg of body weight), followed by a maintenance dose (1.5 mg/kg of body weight) q8h are used.
- Regimen should be continued for at least 48 hr after substantial clinical improvement. If response is not adequate, check cultures and treat with appropriate antibiotics.
- Endometritis following C-section should be treated with ampicillin 2 g IV q6h plus gentamicin loading dose IV or IM (2 mg/kg of body weight), followed by a maintenance dose (1.5 mg/kg of body weight) q8h and clindamycin 900 mg IV q8h. If *Chlamydia* is one of the etiologic agents, add doxycycline 100 mg PO bid for completion of a 14-day course of therapy.

CHRONIC Rx
Watch for recurrent infection.

DISPOSITION
With appropriate antibiotic therapy, 95% to 98% cure rate.

REFERRAL
For patients who do not respond within 48 to 72 hr of appropriate antibiotic therapy, obtain an infectious disease consult or gynecologic consultation.

MISCELLANEOUS

REFERENCES
Centers for Disease Control: Sexually transmitted disease treatment guideline, ed 2, *MMWR* 42:RR-15, 1993.
Suite RL, Gibbs RS: *Infections of the female genital tract,* Baltimore, Md, 1990, Williams & Wilkins.

Author: **George T. Danakas, M.D.**

Enuresis (PTG)

BASIC INFORMATION

DEFINITION
Enuresis refers to the voiding of urine into clothes or in bed that is usually involuntary but occasionally intentional in individuals who are expected to be continent (i.e., >5 yr of age). The diagnosis is made if voiding occurs at least twice a week for 3 mo.

SYNONYMS
Urinary incontinence
Bed-wetting
Self-wetting

ICD-9-CM CODES
F98.0
DMS-IV Code 307.6

EPIDEMIOLOGY AND DEMOGRAPHICS
PREVALENCE (IN U.S.):
- Age 5: 7% of males and 3% of females
- Age 10: 3% of males and 2% of females
- Age 18: 1% of males and even fewer females

PREDOMINANT SEX: Twice as many males as females

PREDOMINANT AGE: By definition, enuresis does not begin before age 5 yr, at which time the prevalence is highest and decreases steadily through life.

PEAK INCIDENCE: Early childhood, ages 5 to 10 yr

GENETICS:
- Approximately 75% of children with enuresis have a first-degree relative with enuresis.
- Concordance rate may be higher in monozygotic twins than dizygotic twins.

PHYSICAL FINDINGS
Three subtypes are defined:
- Nocturnal only: usually occurs in first third of sleep, frequently during REM sleep; child may recall a dream with voiding.
- Diurnal only: more frequent in girls and rarely after age 9 yr; voiding occurs in early afternoon on school days.
- Combined nocturnal and diurnal enuresis

ETIOLOGY
- No clear etiology
- Hypotheses: lax toilet training, stress, inability to concentrate urine, and altered smooth muscle physiology
- Diurnal enuresis associated with a higher rate of urinary tract infections

DIAGNOSIS

DIFFERENTIAL DIAGNOSIS
- May be associated with encopresis and sleep disorders such as sleep terrors
- Must rule out organic causes associated with polyuria or urgency but may coexist if enuresis was present before or after treatment of the associated medical condition

WORKUP
History and physical examination to rule out anatomic abnormalities
NOTE: Since children frequently experience shame, gentleness and care must be exercised when questioning or examining the child.

LABORATORY TESTS
- Urinalysis to determine specific gravity
- Urine culture to rule out urinary tract infection
- Serum studies to rule out diabetes and fluid balance abnormalities

IMAGING STUDIES
- In complicated cases: sleep studies possibly useful
- If an anatomic abnormality suspected: renal ultrasound or IVP possibly indicated

TREATMENT

NONPHARMACOLOGIC THERAPY
- Scheduled voiding to reduce the frequency of enuretic episodes
- Conditioning, psychotherapy, and bed alarms: all reported as useful but not found to be adequate by the children's caregivers

ACUTE GENERAL Rx
- Imipramine: used with mixed results; the use of tricyclic antidepressants in children is problematic because of the risk of sudden death.
- Serotonin reuptake inhibitors: lack of adequate trials is notable.

DISPOSITION
- After age 5 yr, the rate of spontaneous remissions is 5% to 10%/yr.
- Usually the disorder resolves by adolescence.
- Fewer than 1% will experience enuresis as adults.

REFERRAL
If coexisting psychiatric condition complicates the course of treatment

MISCELLANEOUS

REFERENCES
Muffatt MEK: Nocturnal enuresis: psychological implications of treatment and nontreatment, *J Pediatrics* 114:697, 1989.

Author: **Rif S. El-Mallakh, M.D.**

Epicondylitis

BASIC INFORMATION

DEFINITION
Epicondylitis is an inflammation of the musculotendinous origin of the common extensors at the lateral elbow or the flexor pronator group at the medial elbow.

SYNONYMS
Tennis elbow (lateral epicondylitis)
Golfer's elbow (medial epicondylitis)

ICD-9-CM CODES
726.31 Medial epicondylitis
726.32 Lateral epicondylitis

EPIDEMIOLOGY AND DEMOGRAPHICS
PREVALENCE: 10% to 15% of regular (2 hr/wk) tennis players
PREVALENT AGE: 20 to 40 yr

PHYSICAL FINDINGS
- Local tenderness over affected epicondyle
- Reproduction of pain by resistance against wrist extension (lateral) or flexion (medial)

ETIOLOGY
- Unknown
- Overuse probably causing minor tendinous tears resulting in inflammation

DIAGNOSIS

DIFFERENTIAL DIAGNOSIS
- Cervical radiculopathy
- Intraarticular elbow pathology (osteoarthritis, osteochondritis dissecans, loose body)
- Radial nerve compression
- Ulnar neuropathy
- Medial collateral ligament instability

IMAGING STUDIES
Traction spur or minor soft-tissue calcification may be present on plain radiography.

TREATMENT

- Rest, restricted activities
- Ice after exercise
- Stretching exercise program
- NSAIDs (see Table 7-29)
- Local steroid/lidocaine injection
- Counterforce brace
- Proper technique in sports activities

DISPOSITION
Disorder is self-limited in most cases. Resolution of symptoms may take months to years.

REFERRAL
- If symptoms fail to respond to medical management
- For surgical consideration

MISCELLANEOUS

REFERENCES
Jobe FW, Ciccott MG: Lateral and medial epicondylitis of the elbow, *J Am Acad Orthop Surg* 2:1, 1994.
Regan WD: Lateral elbow pain in the athlete: a clinical review, *Clin J Sport Med* 1:53, 1991.

Author: **Lonnie R. Mercier, M.D.**

Epididymitis (PTG)

BASIC INFORMATION

DEFINITION
Epididymitis is an inflammatory reaction of the epididymis caused by either an infectious agent or local trauma.

SYNONYMS
Nonspecific bacterial epididymitis
Sexually transmitted epididymitis

ICD-CM-9 CODES
604.90 Nonvenereal epididymitis
098.0 Gonococcal epididymitis

EPIDEMIOLOGY AND DEMOGRAPHICS
INCIDENCE (IN U.S.): Cause of >600,000 visits to physicians per year
PREDOMINANT SEX: Exclusive to males
PREDOMINANT AGE: All ages affected but usually in sexually active men or older males
PEAK INCIDENCE: Sexually active years
CONGENITAL: Congenital urologic structural disorders possibly predisposing to infections

PHYSICAL FINDINGS
- Tender swelling of the scrotum with erythema
- Dysuria and/or urethral discharge
- Fever and signs of systemic illness (less common)
- Pain and redness on scrotal examination
- Hydrocele or even epididymo-orchitis, especially late
- Chronic draining scrotal sinuses with a "beadlike" enlargement of the vas deferens in tuberculous disease

ETIOLOGY
- In young, sexually active men, the most common infectious agents isolated are *N. gonorrhoeae* and *Chlamydia trachomatis*.
- In men >35 yr or with underlying urologic disease:
  1. Gram-negative aerobic rods are predominant.
  2. Similar organisms are found in men following invasive urologic procedures.
  3. Gram-positive cocci are rarely seen in these groups.
  4. Mycobacteria is also a cause of epididymitis.
- Young, prepubertal boys may present with epididymitis caused by coliform bacteria; almost always a complication of underlying urologic disease such as reflux.

DIAGNOSIS

DIFFERENTIAL DIAGNOSIS
- Orchitis
- Testicular torsion, trauma, or tumor
- Epididymal cyst
- Hydrocele
- Varicocele
- Spermatocele

WORKUP
- Consideration of a full assessment of the urologic tract in patients with bacterial infection, especially if recurrent
- Imaging with sonogram or IVP (possibly procedures of choice)
- If discharge is present: cultures and Gram stain
- In sexually active men: gonococcal cultures of the throat and rectum possibly of value
- If testicular torsion a consideration: radionuclear imaging

LABORATORY TESTS
- Urinalysis and urine culture if dysuria is present or if urinary tract infection is suspected
- VDRL in sexually active men
- PPD placed and chest x-ray viewed if TB suspected
- Rarely, biopsy to assure the diagnosis of tuberculous epididymitis

TREATMENT

ACUTE GENERAL Rx
- Ice packs and scrotal elevation for relief of pain
- Analgesia with acetaminophen with or without codeine or NSAIDs (such as ibuprofen or Naprosyn)
- Antibiotics to cover suspected pathogens
- In sexually active men, doxycycline 100 mg PO bid or tetracycline 500 mg PO qid for 10 days to cover both *gonococci* and *chlamydiae*; ceftriaxone 1 g IV or IM may be adequate for *gonococci* alone
- Best treatment for older men with gram-negative bacteria and leukocyturia: trimethoprim-sulfa DS orally twice daily or ciprofloxacin 500 mg orally bid, both for 10 to 14 days
- *Pseudomonas* covered by ciprofloxacin or ceftazidime (1 g IV q6-8h)
- Gentamicin in toxic appearing patients (1 mg/kg IV q8h following a loading dose of 2 mg/kg): doses must be adjusted for renal function and these agents may be more toxic
- Vancomycin (1 g IV q12h) to cover suspected gram-positive infections
- Surgical aspiration of local abscesses or even open surgical drainage
- Diabetics: especially prone to develop more extensive scrotal infections, including Fournier's gangrene
- Reinforcement of compliance with antibiotics to avoid partial treatment

CHRONIC Rx
- Repair of underlying structural defects is considered especially if infections are severe or recur.
- Surgical repair of reflux in young boys should be undertaken promptly and at a young age when possible.

DISPOSITION
Usually self-limited

REFERRAL
- If abscess or chronic structural problems suspected
- If other diagnosis, such as testicular torsion, strongly considered

MISCELLANEOUS

REFERENCES
Krieger JN: Prostatitis, epididymitis, and orchitis. In Mandell G, Douglas RG, and Bennett J (eds): *Principles and practices of infectious diseases*, ed 4, New York., 1995, Churchill Livingstone.

Author: **Joseph J. Lieber, M.D.**

Epiglottitis (PTG)

BASIC INFORMATION

DEFINITION
Epiglottitis is a rapidly progressive cellulitis of the epiglottis and adjacent soft tissue structures with the potential to cause abrupt airway obstruction.

SYNONYMS
Supraglottitis
Cherry-red epiglottitis

ICD-9-CM CODES
464.30 Epiglottitis

EPIDEMIOLOGY
INCIDENCE (IN U.S.): Highest in young children, 2 to 4 yr old
INCIDENCE (IN U.S.): Unknown
PREDOMINANT SEX: Males
PEAK INCIDENCE: Peaks in young boys ages 2 to 4 yr, but it is reported in adults as well

PHYSICAL FINDINGS
- Irritability, fever, dysphonia, and dysphagia
- Respiratory distress, with child tending to lean up and forward
- Often, drooling or oral secretions
- Often, presence of tachycardia and tachypnea
- On visualization, edematous and cherry-red epiglottis
- Often, no classic barking cough as seen in croup
- Possibly fulminant course (especially in children), leading to complete airway obstruction

ETIOLOGY
- In children, *Haemophilus influenza* type b is usual.
- In adults, *H. influenza* can be isolated from blood and/or epiglottis (about 26% of cases).
- Pneumococci, streptococci, and staphylococci are also implicated.
- Role of viruses in epiglottitis unclear.

DIAGNOSIS

DIFFERENTIAL DIAGNOSIS
- Croup
- Angioedema
- Peritonsillar abscess
- Retropharyngeal abscess
- Diphtheria
- Foreign body aspiration
- Lingual tonsillitis

WORKUP
- Cultures of blood and urine
- Lateral neck radiograph to show an enlarged epiglottis, ballooning of the hypopharynx, and normal subglottic structures
  1. Radiographs are of only moderate sensitivity and specificity and take time to perform.
  2. Epiglottis should be visualized directly to secure diagnosis and only when prepared to urgently secure the airway.
  3. Visualization of the epiglottis may be safer in adults than in children.
- Cultures of the epiglottis

LABORATORY TESTS
- CBC: may reveal a leukocytosis with a shift to the left
- Chest x-ray examination: may reveal evidence of pneumonia in close to 25% of cases
- Cultures of blood, urine, and the epiglottis, as noted above

TREATMENT

ACUTE GENERAL Rx
- Maintenance of adequate airway is critical.
- Early placement of an endotracheal or nasotracheal tube in a child is advised.
- Closely follow adult patient and defer intubation, provided the airway reveals no signs of obstruction.
- In children, visualization and intubation are best done in the most controlled environment, such as an operating room; pay close attention to vital signs, oxygen saturation, respiratory rate, input, and output, since abrupt deterioration can occur.
- Use antibiotics such as ceftriaxone (80 to 100 mg/kg/day in two divided doses), cefotaxime (50 to 180 mg/kg/day in four divided doses), or ampicillin (200 mg/kg/day in four divided doses) with chloramphenicol (75 to 100 mg/kg/day in four divided doses).
- If possible, obtain cultures before initiating antibiotics, but do not delay antibiotic therapy if cultures cannot be obtained quickly.
- Treat adult patients with similar antibiotic regimens.
- Give close family contacts of the patient who are <4 yr old rifampin 20 mg/kg/day for 4 days (up to 600 mg/day) for prophylaxis.
- Role of epinephrine or corticosteroids in the management of epiglottitis is not firmly established.

REFERRAL
For effective management:
- Close cooperation between the pediatrician or internist, anesthesiologist, and otorhinolaryngologist, especially when epiglottis is visualized and when the patient requires endotracheal intubation
- Best managed in a critical care setting or ICU

MISCELLANEOUS

REFERENCES
Burns JE, Hendley JO: Epiglottitis. In Mandell G, Douglas RG, and Bennett J (eds): *Principles and practices of infectious diseases,* ed 4, New York, 1995, Churchill Livingstone.

Author: **Joseph J. Lieber, M.D.**

Episcleritis

BASIC INFORMATION

DEFINITION
Episcleritis is an inflammation of the episclera, or thin layer of vascular elastic tissue between the sclera and conjunctiva.

ICD-9-CM CODES
379.0 Scleritis and episcleritis

EPIDEMIOLOGY AND DEMOGRAPHICS
INCIDENCE (IN U.S.): Relatively rare in an ophthalmologic practice
PREDOMINANT SEX: None
PREDOMINANT AGE: 43 yr
PEAK INCIDENCE: Most common in middle and old age

PHYSICAL FINDINGS
- Red, vascular injection of conjunctiva with engorged and enlarged blood vessels beneath the conjunctions
- Pain in area of inflammation

ETIOLOGY
Associated with collagen-vascular diseases

DIAGNOSIS

DIFFERENTIAL DIAGNOSIS
- Acute glaucoma
- Conjunctivitis
- Scleritis
- Subconjunctival hemorrhage
- Congenital or lymphoid masses
- Table 2-53 describes the differential diagnosis of "Red Eye."

WORKUP
Eye examination

LABORATORY TESTS
Studies for collagen-vascular disease

TREATMENT

NONPHARMACOLOGIC THERAPY
Warm compresses

ACUTE GENERAL Rx
Topical steroids

CHRONIC Rx
Topical steroids and nonsteroidal anti-inflammatory drugs

DISPOSITION
Close follow-up needed

REFERRAL
To ophthalmologist if patient unresponsive to treatment after a few days

MISCELLANEOUS

COMMENTS
Usually related to systemic disease

REFERENCES
Sainz de la Maza M, Jabbur NS, Foster CS: Severity of scleritis and episcleritis, *Ophthalmology* 101:389, 1994.

Author: **Melvyn Koby, M.D.**

Epstein-Barr virus infections

BASIC INFORMATION

DEFINITION
Epstein-Barr virus infection refers to a disease caused by *Epstein-Barr virus* (EBV), a human herpesvirus.

SYNONYMS
Infectious mononucleosis

ICD-9-CM CODES
075 Mononucleosis

EPIDEMIOLOGY AND DEMOGRAPHICS
INCIDENCE (IN U.S.): 45 cases/100,000 persons/yr of infectious mononucleosis (IM)
PREDOMINANT SEX: Neither, although peak incidence occurs about 2 years earlier in women
PREDOMINANT AGE:
- Infectious mononucleosis: occurs most commonly between the ages of 15 and 24 yr.
- EBV infection: occurs earlier in life in lower socioeconomic groups.

PHYSICAL FINDINGS
- Most EBV infections either are asymptomatic or cause a nonspecific illness.
- Incubation period is 1 to 2 mo, possibly followed by a prodrome of anorexia, malaise, headache, and chills; after several days, clinical triad of pharyngitis, fever, and adenopathy may appear, accompanied by fatigue and malaise.
- Pharyngitis is usually the most severe symptom; exudates are common.
- Lymphadenopathy is most prominent in the cervical region but may be diffuse.
- Splenomegaly is possible, most commonly during the second week of illness.
- Rash is uncommon, but will occur in nearly all patients who receive ampicillin.
- Possible IM presentation: fever and adenopathy without pharyngitis.
- Although complications may be severe, they are also uncommon and tend to resolve completely.
- Involvement of the hematologic, pulmonary, cardiac, or nervous systems possible; splenic rupture is rare.
- IM is usually a self-limited illness, but symptoms of malaise and fatigue may last months before resolving.
- Besides IM, EBV is also related to lymphoproliferative syndromes in transplant recipients and in AIDS patients.
- Increasing evidence showing an association between EBV infection and both African Burkitt's lymphoma and nasopharyngeal carcinoma.

ETIOLOGY
- Ubiquitous virus
- Prevalence is higher in lower socioeconomic groups than in age-matched controls in more affluent groups.
- Infection during childhood is much less likely to cause significant illness.
- Frequency of IM in late adolescence is attributed to the onset of social contact between the sexes.
- Close personal contact is usually necessary for transmission, although EBV is occasionally transmitted by blood transfusion; transfer via saliva while kissing may be responsible for many cases.

DIAGNOSIS

DIFFERENTIAL DIAGNOSIS
- Heterophile-negative infectious mononucleosis caused by CMV
- Although clinical presentation similar, CMV more frequently follows transfusion
- Bacterial and viral causes of pharyngitis
- Toxoplasmosis
- Acute retroviral syndrome of HIV
- Lymphoma

WORKUP
Heterophile antibody and CBC

LABORATORY TESTS
- Increased WBC common, with a relative lymphocytosis and neutropenia
- Hallmark of IM: atypical lymphocytes (not pathognomonic)
- Mild thrombocytopenia
- Falling Hct signaling splenic rupture
- Elevated hepatocellular enzymes and cryoglobulins in most cases
- Heterophile antibody
  1. As measured by the Monospot test, may be positive at presentation or may appear later in the course of illness.
  2. Negative test is repeated if clinical suspicion is high.
- Virus-specific antibodies possibly responding to IM: determination of these EBV-specific antibodies is rarely necessary to diagnose IM

IMAGING STUDIES
Chest x-ray examination:
- May rarely show infiltrates
- Possible elevated left hemidiaphragm with splenic rupture

TREATMENT

NONPHARMACOLOGIC THERAPY
- Supportive
- Rest advocated by some; impact on outcome not clear
- Splenectomy if rupture occurs
- Transfusions for severe anemia or thrombocytopenia

ACUTE GENERAL Rx
- Pharmacologic therapy is not indicated in uncomplicated illness.
- Use of steroids:
  1. Suggested in patients who have severe thrombocytopenia or hemolytic anemia, or impending airway obstruction resulting from enlarged tonsils
  2. Prednisone 60 to 80 mg PO qd for 3 days, then tapered over 1 to 2 wk
- There is no role for antiviral agents such as acyclovir in the management of IM.

CHRONIC Rx
An extremely rare, chronic form of IM with persistent fevers and other objective findings has been described and should be differentiated from chronic fatigue syndrome, which is not related to EBV.

DISPOSITION
Eventual resolution of all symptoms

REFERRAL
If more than mild illness

MISCELLANEOUS

COMMENTS
Avoidance of contact sports during the first month of illness, since splenic rupture can occur even in the absence of clinically detectable splenomegaly.

Author: **Maurice Policar, M.D.**

Erectile dysfunction (PTG)

BASIC INFORMATION

DEFINITION
Erectile dysfunction is the inability to achieve or sustain an erection of adequate rigidity to make intercourse possible.

SYNONYMS
Impotence
Male erectile disorder
Sexual dysfunction (a nonspecific term)

ICD-9-CM CODES
F52.2 Male erectile disorder (DSM-IV Code: 302.72 Male erectile disorder)

EPIDEMIOLOGY AND DEMOGRAPHICS
INCIDENCE (IN U.S.): Unknown
PREVALENCE (IN U.S.):
- Increases with age
- Nearly 2% for men in their 40s, 25% for men in their 60s, 80% for men in their 80s

PREDOMINANT SEX: By definition, only in males
PREDOMINANT AGE: Increases with age
PEAK INCIDENCE: Over 70 yr old

PHYSICAL FINDINGS
- Psychogenic impotence: inability to obtain erection, inability to obtain or maintain an adequate erection, or the loss of erection before completion of sexual intercourse; nocturnal penile tumescence usually normal
- Organic impotence: inability to obtain an erection or inability to obtain an adequate erection; nocturnal penile tumescence usually abnormal

ETIOLOGY
- Psychogenic erectile dysfunction resulting from a wide range of experiential, historical, or even psychotic processes
- Organic impotence resulting from a wide variety of insults to neurologic, hormonal, or vascular structures
- Medications (antihypertensives, antidepressants, antipsychotics, histamine blockers, nicotine, alcohol, and others) commonly causative
- Endocrinopathies such as diabetes, hypogonadism, hypo- or hyperthyroidism, and hyperprolactinemia
- Neurogenic causes including spinal cord lesions, cortical lesions, and peripheral neuropathies

DIAGNOSIS

DIFFERENTIAL DIAGNOSIS
- Treatment dependent on the etiology
- Psychogenic dysfunction distinguished from organic
- Etiology of organic dysfunction to be determined
- Erectile dysfunction possible in the setting of another psychiatric condition (e.g., depression or obsessive-compulsive disorder)
- Box 2-69 describes the differential diagnosis of impotence.

WORKUP
- History (often including partner report) with a focus on risk factors (e.g., smoking, alcohol)
- Report of nocturnal erections
- Physical examination to rule out neuronal damage, direct penile damage (e.g., fibrosis), or testicular atrophy
- Fig. 3-75 describes a clinical algorithm for evaluation of sexual dysfunction.

LABORATORY TESTS
Screen for endocrinopathy with am testosterone levels, fasting glucose, and thyroid profile.

IMAGING STUDIES
- Nocturnal penile tumescence very specific for distinguishing psychogenic and organic causes
- Vascular etiologies screened by the penile-brachial pressure index (measures the loss of systolic blood pressure between the arm and penis) or with Doppler studies
- Neurogenic etiologies examined by the bulbocavernosus reflex or the pudendal-evoked response
- Intracorporeal injection of prostaglandin E_1 to distinguish vascular and nonvascular etiologies (erection is achieved in patients with nonvascular etiologies)

TREATMENT

NONPHARMACOLOGIC THERAPY
- Various psychotherapeutic approaches: cognitive behavioral therapy preferred because it is the most focused; success rates decrease with advancing age and duration of symptoms.
- Sex therapy and couples' therapy are used to address technical or social issues that contribute to the impotence.
- Vacuum devices (70% to 90% effective) work for many men, but they are difficult to use and cumbersome.

ACUTE GENERAL Rx
- Intracavernosal injections of vasodilators (e.g., papaverine or prostaglandin E_1 pellet)
- Oral medications such as pentoxifylline and yohimbine (limited success)

CHRONIC Rx
- Psychogenic impotence: open-ended, insight psychotherapies possibly curative but time-consuming and require extraordinary motivation
- Successful acute approaches maintained over time, but intracavernosal injections of papaverine associated with penile scarring
- For men failing other approaches: penile prosthesis (does not address issues of sexual drive or orgasm)
- Testosterone therapy in elderly hypogonadal males

DISPOSITION
- When erectile dysfunction is secondary to an organic cause, it does not remit unless the organic cause is corrected; therefore, it is usually a chronic condition.
- Psychogenic acquired erectile dysfunction will remit spontaneously in 15% to 30% of the cases.
- Lifelong erectile dysfunction is usually a chronic and unremitting condition.
- Situational erectile dysfunction may remit with changes in social environment, but it usually recurs.

REFERRAL
If psychotherapy, sex therapy, or invasive organic treatment required

MISCELLANEOUS

REFERENCES
Korenman SG: Advances in the understanding and management of erectile dysfunction, *J Clin Endocrinol Metab* 80:1985, 1995.

O'Keefe M, Hunt DK: Assessment and treatment of impotence, *Med Clin North Am* 79:415, 1995.

Wespes E, Schulman C: Venous impotence: pathophysiology, diagnosis and treatment, *J Urol* 149:1238, 1993.

Author: Rif S. El-Mallakh, M.D.

Erythema multiforme (PTG)

BASIC INFORMATION

DEFINITION
Erythema multiforme is an inflammatory disease believed to be secondary to immune complex formation and subsequent deposition in the skin and mucous membranes.

SYNONYMS
EM

ICD-9-CM CODES
695.1 Erythema multiforme

EPIDEMIOLOGY AND DEMOGRAPHICS
- Predominant age: 20 to 40 yr
- Often associated with herpes simplex and other infectious agents, drugs, and connective tissue diseases

PHYSICAL FINDINGS
- Symmetrical skin lesions with a classic "target" appearance (caused by the centrifugal spread of red maculopapules to circumference of 1 to 3 cm with a purpuric, cyanotic, or vesicular center) are present (see color plate 7).
- Lesions are most common in the back of the hands and feet and extensor aspect of the forearms and legs. Trunk involvement can occur in severe cases.
- Urticarial papules, vesicles, and bullae may also be present and generally indicate a more severe form of the disease.
- Individual lesions heal in 1 or 2 wk without scarring.
- Bullae and erosions may also be present in the oral cavity.

ETIOLOGY
- Immune complex formation and subsequent deposition in the cutaneous microvasculature may play a role in the pathogenesis of erythema multiforme.
- The majority of EM cases follow outbreaks of herpes simplex.
- In >50% of patients, no specific cause is identified.

DIAGNOSIS

DIFFERENTIAL DIAGNOSIS
- Chronic urticaria
- Secondary syphilis
- Pityriasis rosea
- Contact dermatitis
- Pemphigus vulgaris
- Lichen planus
- Serum sickness
- Drug eruption
- Granuloma annulare

WORKUP
- Medical history with emphasis on drug ingestion
- Laboratory evaluation in patients with suspected collagen-vascular diseases
- Skin biopsy when diagnosis is unclear

LABORATORY TESTS
- CBC with differential
- ANA
- Serology for *Mycoplasma pneumoniae*
- Urinalysis

TREATMENT

NONPHARMACOLOGIC THERAPY
- Mild cases generally do not require treatment; lesions resolve spontaneously within 1 mo.
- Potential drug precipitants should be removed.

ACUTE GENERAL Rx
- Treatment of associated diseases (e.g., acyclovir for herpes simplex, erythromycin for mycoplasma infection).
- Prednisone 40 to 80 mg/day for 1 to 3 wk may be tried in patients with many target lesions; however, the role of systemic steroids remains controversial.
- Levamisole, an immunomodulator, may be effective in treatment of patients with chronic or recurrent oral lesions (dose is 150 mg/day for 3 consecutive days used alone or in combination with prednisone).

DISPOSITION
The rash of EM generally evolves over a 2-wk period and resolves within 3 to 4 wk without scarring. A severe bullous form can occur (see "Stevens-Johnson syndrome").

REFERRAL
Hospital admission in patients with Stevens-Johnson syndrome

MISCELLANEOUS

COMMENTS
The risk of recurrence of erythema multiforme exceeds 30%.

REFERENCES
Cote B et al: Clinical pathological relation in erythema multiforme in Stevens-Johnson syndrome, *Arch Dermatol* 131:1268, 1995.
Habif TP: *Clinical dermatology*, ed 3, St Louis, 1996, Mosby.

Author: **Fred F. Ferri, M.D.**

Fatty liver of pregnancy, acute

BASIC INFORMATION

DEFINITION
Acute fatty liver of pregnancy (AFLP) is characterized histologically by microvesicular fatty cytoplasmic infiltration of hepatocytes with minimal hepatocellular necrosis.

SYNONYMS
Acute fatty metamorphosis
Acute yellow atrophy

ICD-9-CM CODES
646.7 Liver disorders in pregnancy

EPIDEMIOLOGY AND DEMOGRAPHICS
INCIDENCE:
- Approximately 1 in 10,000 pregnancies
- Equal frequencies in all races and at all maternal ages

AVERAGE GESTATIONAL AGE: 37 wk (range 28 to 42 wk)

RISK FACTORS:
- Primiparity
- Multiple gestation
- Male fetus

GENETICS: Some with a familial deficiency of long- chain 3-hydroxyacyl-CoA dehydrogenase (LCHAD)

PHYSICAL FINDINGS
- Initial manifestations:
  1. Nausea and vomiting (70%)
  2. Pain in RUQ or epigastrium (50% to 80%)
  3. Malaise and anorexia
- Jaundice often in 1 to 2 wk
- Late manifestations:
  1. Fulminant hepatic failure
  2. Encephalopathy
  3. Renal failure
  4. Pancreatitis
  5. GI and uterine bleeding
  6. Disseminated intravascular coagulation
  7. Seizures
  8. Coma
- Liver
  1. Usually small
  2. Normal or enlarged in preeclampsia, eclampsia, HELLP (hemolysis, elevated liver enzymes, and low platelets) syndrome, and acute hepatitis
  3. Coexistent preeclampsia in up to 46% of patients

ETIOLOGY
- Postulated that inhibition of mitochondrial oxidation of fatty acids may lead to microvesicular fatty infiltration of liver.
- Fatty metamorphosis of preeclamptic liver disease thought to be of different etiology.

DIAGNOSIS

DIFFERENTIAL DIAGNOSIS
- Acute gastroenteritis
- Preeclampsia or eclampsia with liver involvement
- HELLP syndrome
- Acute viral hepatitis
- Fulminant hepatitis
- Drug-induced hepatitis caused by halothane, phenytoin, methyldopa, isoniazid, hydrochlorothiazide, or tetracycline
- Intrahepatic cholestasis of pregnancy
- Gallbladder disease
- Reye's syndrome
- Hemolytic-uremic syndrome
- Budd-Chiari syndrome
- SLE
- Table 2-41 describes the differential diagnosis of liver disease in pregnancy.

WORKUP
- A clinical diagnosis is based predominantly on physical and laboratory findings.
- Most definitive diagnosis is through liver biopsy with oil red O staining and electron microscopy.
- Liver biopsy is reserved for atypical cases only and only after any existing coagulopathy corrected with FFP.

LABORATORY TESTS
Tests to determine the following:
- Hypoglycemia (often profound)
- Hyperammonemia
- Elevated aminotransferases (usually <500 U/mL)
- WBC count >15,000
- Hyperbilirubinemia (usually <10 mg/dl)
- Low albumin
- DIC (in 75%)

IMAGING STUDIES
- Ultrasound: best used to rule out other diseases in the differential diagnosis such as gallbladder disease
- CT scan: plays minimal role because of a high false- negative rate

TREATMENT

NONPHARMACOLOGIC THERAPY
- Patient is admitted to intensive care unit for stabilization.
- Fetus is delivered; spontaneous resolution usually follows delivery.
- Mode of delivery is based on obstetric indications and clinical assessment of disease severity.

ACUTE GENERAL Rx
- Decrease in endogenous ammonia through dietary protein restriction; neomycin 6 to 12 g/day PO to decrease presence of ammonia-producing bacteria; magnesium citrate 30 to 50 ml PO or enema to evacuate nitrogenous wastes from colon
- Administration of intravenous fluids with glucose to keep glucose levels >60 mg/dl
- Coagulopathy corrected with FFP
- Avoidance of drugs metabolized by liver
- Aggressive avoidance and treatment for nosocomial infections; consideration of prophylactic antibiotics

CHRONIC Rx
Orthotopic liver transplantation is the only treatment for irreversible liver failure.

DISPOSITION
- Before 1980, both maternal and fetal mortalities: approximately 85%
- After 1980, both maternal and fetal mortalities: below 20%
- Usually rapid return of liver function to normal after delivery
- Minimal risk of recurrence with future pregnancies

REFERRAL
To tertiary health care facility as soon as diagnosis is suspected

MISCELLANEOUS

REFERENCES
Cunningham FG et al: Gastrointestinal disorders. In Cunningham FG et al (eds): *Williams' obstetrics,* ed 20, Stamford, Conn, 1997, Appleton & Lange.
Davidson KM: Acute fatty liver of pregnancy, *Postgrad Obstet Gynecol* 15:1, 1995.
Knox TA, Olans LB: Liver disease in pregnancy, *New Engl J Med* 335:569, 1996.
Sawai SK: Acute fatty liver of pregnancy. In Foley MR, Strong TH, Jr: *Obstetric intensive care: a practical manual,* Philadelphia, 1997, WB Saunders.

Author: **Wan J. Kim, M.D.**

Femoral neck fracture (PTG)

BASIC INFORMATION

DEFINITION
A femoral neck fracture occurs within the capsule of the hip joint between the base of the head and the intertrochanteric line.

SYNONYMS
Intracapsular fracture

ICD-9-CM CODES
820.8 Femoral neck fracture

EPIDEMIOLOGY AND DEMOGRAPHICS
PREVALENCE: Lifetime risk in women approximately 16%
PREVALENT SEX: Females 3:1 male
PREVALENT AGE: 90% over age 60

PHYSICAL FINDINGS
- A hip or groin pain
- Affected limb usually shortened and externally rotated in displaced fractures
- Impacted fractures: possibly no deformity and only mild pain with hip motion
- Mild external bruising

ETIOLOGY
- Trauma
- Age-related bone weakness, usually caused by osteoporosis
- Increased risk fractures in elderly (decline in muscle function, use of psychotrophic medication, etc)

DIAGNOSIS

DIFFERENTIAL DIAGNOSIS
Pathologic fracture

WORKUP
Diagnosis usually obvious based on clinical and radiographic findings

IMAGING STUDIES
- Standard roentgenograms consisting of an AP of the pelvis and a cross-table lateral of the hip to confirm the diagnosis
- If initial roentgenograms negative and diagnosis of an occult femoral neck fracture suspected, hospital admission and further radiographic assessment with either bone scanning or MRI
- Bone scanning most sensitive at 48-72 hours.

TREATMENT

- Orthopedic consultation
- Surgery indicated in most cases

DISPOSITION
- Mortality rate within 1 yr in elderly patients is 25% to 30%.
- Dementia is a particularly poor prognostic sign.

MISCELLANEOUS

COMMENTS
- Complications: nonunion and avascular necrosis
- Intracapsular fractures:
  1. Occasionally occur in nonambulatory patients
  2. Usually treated nonsurgically, especially in the demented patient with limited pain perception
  3. Early bed-to-chair mobilization and vigilant nursing care to avoid skin breakdown
  4. Fracture usually pain free in a short time even if solid bony healing does not occur

REFERENCES
Cummings S, Black D, Rubin S: Lifetime risks of hip, colles, or vertebral fractures and coronary artery disease among white postmenopausal women, *Arch Intern Med* 149:2445, 1989.

Koval KS, Xuckerman JD: Hip fractures: I. Overview and evaluation and treatment of femoral neck fractures, *J Am Acad Orthop Surg* 2:141, 1994.

Swiontkowski MF: Current concepts review: intracapsular fractures of the hip, *J Bone Joint Surg* 76(A):129, 1994.

Author: **Lonnie R. Mercier, M.D.**

Fibrocystic breast disease (PTG)

BASIC INFORMATION

DEFINITION
Fibrocystic breast disease (FCD) is a "nondisease," in which are included nonmalignant breast lesions such as microcystic and macrocystic changes, fibrosis, ductal or lobular hyperplasia, adenosis, apocrine metaplasia, fibroadenoma, papilloma, papillomatosis, and other changes. Atypical ductal or lobular hyperplasia is associated with a moderate increase in breast cancer risk.

SYNONYMS
Cystic changes
Chronic cystic mastitis
Mammary dysplasia

ICD-9-CM CODES
610.0 Solitary cyst of the breast
610.1 Fibrocystic disease of the breast

EPIDEMIOLOGY AND DEMOGRAPHICS
- Ubiquitous in premenopausal women after 20 yr of age
- Palpable nodular changes in the breast termed *FCD* clinically; such changes observable in more than half of adult women 20 to 50 yr of age

PHYSICAL FINDINGS
- Tender breasts
- Nodular areas
- Dominant mass
- Thickening
- Nipple discharge
- Can vary with menstrual cycle

ETIOLOGY
- Although frequently seen and diagnosed, mechanism of development not understood.
- Because found in majority of healthy breasts, regarded as nonpathologic process.
- With hormone replacement therapy, may be carried into menopausal age.

DIAGNOSIS

DIFFERENTIAL DIAGNOSIS
- If presenting as dominant mass or masses: exclude possible carcinoma.
- Carcinoma: detection is difficult with FCD, particularly among premenopausal women.
- If presenting with nipple discharge: differentiate from discharge of possible malignant origin.

WORKUP
- Exclude breast carcinoma if breast mass, thickening, discharge, and pain present.
- Perform biopsy of suspected area for histologic confirmation.

IMAGING STUDIES
Mammography and ultrasound studies required:
- For mammographic changes (suspicious densities, microcalcifications, architectural distortion): careful evaluation, including possibly biopsy to exclude breast cancer
- Ultrasound study: to establish cystic nature of clinical or mammographic mass lesion

TREATMENT

NONPHARMACOLOGIC THERAPY
- Not considered a "disease" and does not require treatment
- Surgical intervention diagnostic to eliminate possibility of breast cancer
- Periodic physician examination to follow patients with FCD who have pronounced nodular features
- Aspiration for palpable cysts (NOTE: Cysts often recur; repeat aspiration is not always required unless pain is a problem.)

ACUTE GENERAL Rx
Majority of women require no treatment.

CHRONIC Rx
For breast pain:
- Danocrine (Danazol): limited success reported
- Bromocriptine or tamoxifen: used less frequently
- Limited caffeine intake: not as successful in controlling pain or nodularity as originally suggested

DISPOSITION
- Careful evaluation to exclude suspicious changes for breast cancer, then reassurance and periodic reevaluation as required
- Regular self-examination, annual physician examination, and annual mammograms for women with atypical ductal or lobular hyperplasia

REFERRAL
- For further evaluation and/or biopsy if there are suspicious changes that may be associated with FCD (including changing of dominant mass or thickening, persistent or spontaneous discharge, suspicious mammographic changes or lesions)
- To alleviate anxiety associated with breast symptoms or changes

MISCELLANEOUS

COMMENTS
Patient education material is available from American College of Obstetricians and Gynecologists, 408 12th Street SW, Washington, DC 20024-2188.

REFERENCES
Donegan WL, Spratt JA: *Cancer of the breast*, Philadelphia, 1995, WB Saunders.

Author: Takuma Nemoto, M.D.

Fibromyalgia (PTG)

BASIC INFORMATION

DEFINITION
Fibromyalgia is a poorly defined disorder characterized by multiple trigger points and referred pain.

SYNONYMS
Myofascial pain syndrome
Fibrositis
Psychogenic rheumatism
Nonarticular rheumatism

ICD-9-CM CODES
729.0 Rheumatism, unspecified and fibrositis
729.1 Myalgia and myositis, unspecified

EPIDEMIOLOGY AND DEMOGRAPHICS
PREVALENCE: 1% to 2% of the general population
PREVALENT SEX: Female:male ratio of 9:1
PREVALENT AGE: 30 to 50 yr

PHYSICAL FINDINGS
Tender "nodules" and tender points

ETIOLOGY
- Unknown
- Pain magnification may play a role

DIAGNOSIS

DIFFERENTIAL DIAGNOSIS
- Polymyalgia rheumatica
- Referred discogenic spine pain
- Rheumatoid arthritis
- Localized tendinitis
- Connective tissue disease
- Osteoarthritis
- Thyroid disease

WORKUP
- Subsets of this disorder are often described:
  1. If symptoms develop in conjunction with other conditions (rheumatoid disease or acute stress)
  2. If findings are more regionally distributed, such as those in the neck following motor vehicle accidents
- The primary condition is often suggested by the following criteria from the American College of Rheumatology:
  1. History of widespread pain
  2. Pain in eleven of eighteen selected tender spots on digital palpation (mainly in the spine, elbows, and knees)

LABORATORY TESTS
There are no abnormalities in fibromyalgia, but laboratory assessment may be required to rule out other conditions and may include:
- CBC, ESR, rheumatoid factor, ANA
- CPK, T_4

TREATMENT

ACUTE GENERAL Rx
- Self-management
- Explanation, reassurance
- Tricyclic antidepressants for sleep disturbance
- Aerobic and stretching exercise, particularly swimming
- Mild analgesics; avoidance of chronic narcotic use
- Trigger point injections
- Physical therapy

DISPOSITION
- Prognosis is uncertain.
- Symptoms come and go for years in spite of an aggressive multifaceted approach to treatment.

MISCELLANEOUS

COMMENTS
- Before making this diagnosis, all other more likely disorders should be ruled out.
- The term "fibrositis" is often used, but no inflammation has ever been found.
- The number of trigger points needed to establish the diagnosis is debated.

REFERENCES
Croft P, Schollum N, Silman A: Population study of tender point counts and pain as evidence of fibromyalgia, *Br Med J* 309:696, 1994.

Smythe HA: Nonarticular rheumatism and psychogenic musculoskeletal syndromes. In McCarty DJ (ed): *Arthritis and allied conditions,* ed 11, Philadelphia, 1989, Lea and Febiger.

Wolfe F et al: The American College of Rheumatology 1990 criteria for the classification of fibromyalgia: report of the multicenter criteria committee, *Arthritis Rheum* 33:160, 1990.

Author: **Lonnie R. Mercier, M.D.**

Filariasis

BASIC INFORMATION

DEFINITION
Filariasis is a general term for an infection caused by nematodes (roundworms) of the genera *Wuchereria* and *Brugia*, found in the tropical and subtropical regions of the world. The disease is variably characterized by acute lymphatic inflammation or chronic lymphatic obstruction associated with intermittent fevers or recurrent episodes of dyspnea and bronchospasm.

SYNONYMS
Lymphatic filariasis

ICD-9-CM CODES
125.0 Bancroftian
125.1 Brugian
125.9 Filariasis

EPIDEMIOLOGY AND DEMOGRAPHICS
INCIDENCE (IN U.S.): Unknown
PREDOMINANT SEX: Male
PREDOMINANT AGE: For both males and females, risk is greatest between the ages of 15 to 35 yr.
PEAK INCIDENCE: Unknown

PHYSICAL FINDINGS
- Clinical manifestations result from acute lymphatic inflammation or chronic lymphatic obstruction.
- Many patients are asymptomatic despite the presence of microfilaremia.
- Episodes of lymphangitis and lymphadenitis are associated with fever, headache, and back pain.
- Acute funiculitis and epididymitis or orchitis may also be present; all usually resolve within days to weeks but tend to recur.
- Chronic infections may be associated with lymphedema, most commonly manifested by hydrocele.
- It is a progressive disease, leading to nonpitting edema and brawny changes that may involve a whole limb.
- Elephantiasis occurs in about 10% of patients, with skin of the scrotum or leg becoming thickened and fissured; patient is thereafter plagued by recurrent ulceration and infection.
- Chyluria, a condition that develops when lymphatic vessels rupture into the urinary tract, may occur.

ETIOLOGY
Caused by one of three types of nematode parasites, all of which are transmitted to humans by mosquitoes.
- *W. bancrofti*: distributed in Africa, areas of central and South America, the Pacific Islands, and the Caribbean Basin
- *B. malayi*: restricted to southeast Asia
- *B. timori*: confined to the Indonesian archipelago

After bite of an infected mosquito:
- Filarial larvae move into lymphatic vessels and nodes, settling and maturing over 3 to 15 mo into adult male and female worms.
- After fertilization, the female nematode produces large numbers of larvae or microfilariae that enter into the blood stream via the lymphatics.
- Nocturnal periodicity, characteristic of B. malayi, is an increased presence of microfilariae in the circulation during the night.
- Microfilariae of *W. bancrofti* are maximal during late afternoon.
- Most microfilariae remain in the body as immature forms for 6 mo to 2 yr.
- Infected larvae are ingested by mosquitoes, then transmitted to humans where the microfilariae mature into new adult worms.

Acute and chronic inflammatory and granulomatous changes in the lymphatic channels:
- Result from complex interaction of adult worms and host's immune systems
- Eventually lead to fibrosis and obstruction
- Most likely to develop into obstructive lymphatic disease with recurrent exposure over many years

DIAGNOSIS

DIFFERENTIAL DIAGNOSIS
- Elephantiasis is distinguished from other causes of chronic lymphedema, including Milroy's disease, postoperative scarring, and lymphedema of malignancy.
- The differential diagnosis of nematode tissue infections is described in Table 2-47.

WORKUP
Diagnosis is suspected in individuals who have resided in endemic areas for at least 3 to 6 mo or more and complain of recurrent episodes of lymphangitis, lymphadenitis, scrotal edema, or thrombophlebitis, with or without fever.

LABORATORY TESTS
- Demonstration of microfilariae on a blood smear for definitive diagnosis
- For patients from southeastern Asia: blood sample drawn at night, especially between midnight and 2 AM
- Occasionally, microfilaremia in chylous urine or hydrocele fluid
- Prominent eosinophilia only during periods of acute lymphangitis or lymphadenitis
- Serologic tests for antibody, including enzyme-linked immunosorbent assay and indirect fluorescent antibody (often unable to distinguish among the various forms of filariasis or between acute and remote infection)
- Immunoassays (such as Circulating Filaria Antigen [CFA]): more successful in antigen detection in patients who are microfilaremic than in those who are amicrofilaremic

IMAGING STUDIES
- Chest x-ray examination: reticular nodular infiltrates (tropical pulmonary eosinophilia syndrome)
- In men proven to be microfilaremic, scrotal ultrasonography to aid in the detection of adult worms

TREATMENT

NONPHARMACOLOGIC THERAPY
- Standard of care for elephantiasis:
  1. Elevation of the affected limb
  2. Use of elastic stockings
  3. Local foot care
- General wound care for chronic ulcers and prevention of secondary infection

ACUTE GENERAL Rx
- Diethylcarbamazine citrate (DEC) to reduce microfilaremia by 90%
  1. Effect on adult worms, especially those of the *Wuchereria* species, less certain
  2. Given in an oral dose of 6 mg/kg qd for 12 to 14 days
- Ivermectin alone or in combination with diethylcarbamazine citrate to decrease microfilaremia
- Both drugs are similar in efficacy and tolerability; advantage of ivermectin: administration in a single oral dose of 200 µg/kg.
- World Health Organization (WHO) recommendation: DEC given as a single dose, alone or (preferably) in combination with ivermectin as treatment in endemic areas

CHRONIC Rx
- Surgical drainage of hydroceles
- No satisfactory therapy for those patients with chyluria

DISPOSITION
Rarely fatal, but the psychologic impact of limb and scrotal deformities associated with elephantiasis are substantial.

REFERRAL
To a surgeon for management of hydrocele

MISCELLANEOUS

- Studies in endemic areas suggest that filarial-specific IgG1 is associated with amicrofilaremic states highest in children, regardless of sex.
- Levels of IgE and IgG4 increase with age and are associated with increased levels of microfilaremia.

COMMENTS
Individuals who intend to travel or reside in endemic areas should be advised to institute preventive measures such as the use of netting and insect repellents, especially at night.

REFERENCES
Meyrowitsch DW et al: A 15-year follow-up study on bancroftian filariasis in three communities of north-eastern Tanzania, *Ann Trop Med Parasitol* 89(6):665, 1995.

Michael E et al: Re-assessing the global prevalence and distribution of lymphatic filariasis, *Parasitology* 112(part 4):409, 1996.

Noroes J et al: Occurrence of living adult *Wuchereria bancrofti* in the scrotal area of men with microfilaremia, *Trans R Soc Trop Med Hyg* 90(1):55, 1996.

Pani SP, Srividya A: Clinical manifestations of bancroftian filariasis with special reference to lymphedema grading, *Indian J Med Res* 102:114, 1995.

Routh HB, Bhowmik KR: Filariasis, *Dermatol Clin* 12(4):719, 1994.

Weil GJ et al: Parasite antigenemia without microfilaremia in bancroftian filariasis, *Am J Trop Med Hyg* 55(3):333, 1996.

Author: **George O. Alonso, M.D.**

Folliculitis (PTG)

BASIC INFORMATION

DEFINITION
Folliculitis is the inflammation of the hair follicle as a result of infection, physical injury, or chemical irritation.

SYNONYMS
Sycosis barbae

ICD-9-CM CODES
704.8 Other specified diseases of hair and hair follicles

EPIDEMIOLOGY AND DEMOGRAPHICS
- Staphylococcal folliculitis is the most common form of infectious folliculitis; it occurs most commonly in diabetics.
- Sycosis barbae occurs most frequently in men who have commenced shaving.

PHYSICAL FINDINGS
- The lesions generally consist of painful yellow pustules surrounded by erythema; a central hair is present in the pustules.
- Patients with sycosis barbae may initially present with small follicular papules or pustules that increase in size with continued shaving; deep follicular pustules may occur surrounded by erythema and swelling; the upper lip is frequently involved.
- "Hot tub" folliculitis occurs within 1 to 4 days following use of hot tub with poor chlorination, and it is characterized by pustules with surrounding erythema generally effecting torso, buttocks, and limbs (see color plate 8).

ETIOLOGY
- *Staphylococcus* infection (e.g., sycosis barbae), *Pseudomonas aeruginosa* ("hot tub" folliculitis)
- Gram-negative folliculitis (*Klebsiella, Enterobacter, Proteus*) associated with antibiotic treatment of acne
- Chronic irritation of the hair follicle (use of cocoa butter or coconut oil, chronic irritation from workplace)
- Initial use of systemic corticosteroid therapy (steroid acne), eosinophilic folliculitis (AIDS patients), *Candida albicans* (immunocompromised patients)
- Pityrosporum orbiculare

DIAGNOSIS

DIFFERENTIAL DIAGNOSIS
- Pseudofolliculitis barbae (ingrown hairs)
- Acne vulgaris
- Dermatophyte fungal infections
- Keratosis biliaris
- Cutaneous candidiasis
- Superficial fungal infections
- Miliaris

WORKUP
Physical examination and medical history (e.g., use of hot tub: "hot tub" folliculitis; adolescent patients who have started shaving: sycosis barbae; use of occlusive topical steroid therapy: *Staphylococcus* folliculitis).

LABORATORY TESTS
Gram stain is useful to identify the infective organisms in infectious folliculitis and to differentiate infectious folliculitis from noninfectious.

TREATMENT

NONPHARMACOLOGIC THERAPY
- Prevention of chemical or mechanical skin irritation
- Glycemic control in diabetics
- Proper chlorination of hot tubs and spas
- Shaving with a clean razor

ACUTE GENERAL Rx
- Cleansing of the area with chlorhexidine and application of saline compresses to involved area
- Application of 2% mupirocin ointment (Bactroban) for bacterial folliculitis affecting a limited area (e.g., sycosis barbae)
- Treatment of severe cases of *Pseudomonas* folliculitis with ciprofloxacin
- Treatment of *S. aureus* folliculitis with dicloxacillin 250 mg qid for 10 days

CHRONIC Rx
- Chronic nasal or perineal *S. aureus* carriers with frequent folliculitis can be treated with rifampin 300 mg bid for 5 days.
- Mupirocin (Bactroban ointment 2%) applied to nares bid is also effective for nasal carriers.

DISPOSITION
- Most cases of bacterial folliculitis resolve completely with proper treatment.
- Steroid folliculitis responds to discontinuation of steroids.

MISCELLANEOUS

COMMENTS
Patients should be instructed in good personal hygiene and avoidance of sharing razors, towels, and washcloths.

REFERENCES
Bottone VG et al: Pseudomonas aeruginosa folliculitis acquired through use of contaminated sponge: unrecognized potential public health problem, *J Clin Microbiol* 31:480, 1993.

Habif TP: *Clinical dermatology*, ed 3, St Louis, Mosby, 1996.

Author: **Fred. F. Ferri, M.D.**

Food poisoning, bacterial *(PTG)*

BASIC INFORMATION

DEFINITION
Food poisoning is an illness caused by ingestion of food contaminated by bacteria and/or bacterial toxins.

ICD-9-CM CODES
See specific illness.

EPIDEMIOLOGY AND DEMOGRAPHICS
INCIDENCE (IN U.S.):
- Estimated range of 6 to 80 million cases/yr
- Majority of identifiable causes are bacterial

PREDOMINANT AGE: Varies with specific agent

PEAK INCIDENCE: Varies with specific organism
- Summer: *Staphylococcus aureus, Salmonella, Shigella*
- Summer and fall: *Clostridium botulinum, Vibrio parahaemolyticus*
- Spring and fall: *Campylobacter jejuni*
- Winter: *Clostridium perfringens, Yersinia*

NEONATAL INFECTION: Rare but severe with *Shigella*

PHYSICAL FINDINGS
- Any combination of GI symptoms and fever
- Specific organisms suspected on the basis of the incubation period and predominant symptoms, although a great deal of overlap exists
  1. Short incubation period (1 to 6 hr): involve the ingestion of preformed toxin; noninvasive
     a. *S. aureus:* nausea, profuse vomiting, and abdominal cramps common; diarrhea possible, but fever uncommon; usually resolves within 24 hr; foods implicated in outbreaks include meats, mayonnaise, and cream pastries
     b. *B. cereus:* two forms, a short incubation (emetic) form (characterized by vomiting and abdominal cramps in virtually all patients, diarrhea in one third of patients, fever uncommon) and a long incubation *(diarrheal)* form; illness usually mild, resolves within 12 hr; unrefrigerated rice most often implicated as vehicle
  2. Moderate incubation period (8 to 16 hr): involves the in vivo production of toxin; noninvasive
     a. *C. perfringens:* severe crampy abdominal pain and watery diarrhea common; fever and vomiting unlikely; symptoms usually resolving within 24 hr; outbreaks invariably related to cooked meat or poultry that is allowed to cool without refrigeration; most cases in the fall and winter months
     b. *B. cereus:* diarrheal (or long incubation) form most commonly beginning with diarrhea, abdominal cramps, and occasionally vomiting; fever uncommon; usually resolves within 24 hr; the responsible food is usually fried rice
  3. Long incubation period (>16 hr): some toxin-mediated, some invasive
     a. Toxin-producing organisms include:
        (1) *C. botulinum:* should be considered when a diarrheal illness coincides with or precedes paralysis; severity of illness related to the quantity of toxin ingested; characteristic cranial nerve palsies progressing to a descending paralysis; fever usually absent; usually associated with home-canned foods
        (2) Enterotoxigenic *E. coli* (ETEC): most common cause of travelers' diarrhea; after 1- to 2-day incubation period, abdominal cramps and copious diarrhea occur; vomiting and fever uncommon; usually resolves after 3 to 4 days; vehicle usually unbottled water or contaminated salad or ice
        (3) Enterohemorrhagic *E. coli* (EHEC): can cause severe abdominal cramps and watery diarrhea, which may eventually become bloody; bacteria (strain O157:H7) is noninvasive; no fever; illness may be complicated by hemolytic-uremic syndrome; associated with contaminated beef
        (4) *V. cholera:* varies from a mild, self-limited illness to life-threatening cholera; diarrhea, nausea and vomiting, abdominal cramps, and muscle cramps; no fever; severe cases may progress to shock and death within hours of onset; survivors usually have resolution of symptoms in 1 wk; U.S. cases are either imported or result from ingestion of imported food
     b. Invasive organisms include:
        (1) *Salmonella:* associated most often with nontyphoidal strains; incubation period generally 12 to 48 hr; nausea, vomiting, diarrhea, and abdominal cramps typical; fever possible; outbreaks of gastroenteritis related to contaminated poultry, meat, and dairy products
        (2) *Shigella:* asymptomatic infection possible, but some with fever and watery diarrhea that may progress to bloody diarrhea and dysentery; with mild illness, usually self-limited, resolves in a few days; with severe illness, may develop complications; transmission usually from person to person but can occur via contaminated food or water
        (3) *C. jejuni:* the most common food-borne bacterial pathogen; incubation period is about 1 day, then a prodrome of fever, headache, and myalgias; intestinal phase marked by diarrhea associated with fever, malaise, and abdominal pain; diarrhea mild to profuse and bloody; usually resolves in about 7 days, but relapse is possible; associated with undercooked meats and poultry, unpasteurized dairy products, and drinking from freshwater streams

(4) *Y. enterocolitica* and *Y. pseudotuberculosis:* infrequent causes of enteritis in U.S.; children affected more often than adults; fever, diarrhea, and abdominal pain lasting 1 to 3 wk; some with mesenteric adenitis that mimics acute appendicitis; contaminated food or water is usually responsible

(5) *V. parahaemolyticus:* In U.S., most outbreaks in coastal states or on cruise ships during the summer months; incubation period usually <1 day, followed by explosive watery diarrhea in the majority of cases; nausea, vomiting, abdominal cramps, and headache also common; fever less common; usually resolves by 1 wk; related to ingestion of seafood

(6) Enteroinvasive *E. coli* (EIEC): a rare cause of disease in the U.S.; high incidence of fever and bloody diarrhea; may resemble bacillary dysentery

(7) *V. vulnificus:* may cause serious, often fatal illness in persons with chronic liver disease; GI symptoms usually absent, but fever, chills, hypotension, and hemorrhagic skin lesions possible; patients with liver disease at increased risk of developing disease and should avoid eating raw oysters

ETIOLOGY
Classically categorized as either inflammatory (invasive) or noninflammatory:
- Noninflammatory: *B. cereus, S. aureus, C. botulinum, C. perfringens, V. cholera,* enterotoxigenic *E. coli* (ETEC), and enterohemorrhagic *E. coli* (EHEC); toxin-producing organisms that are noninvasive; fecal leukocytes are not seen.
- Inflammatory: *Campylobacter,* enteroinvasive *E. coli* (EIEC), *Salmonella, Shigella, V. parahaemolyticus,* and *Yersinia;* cause disease by invasion of intestinal tissue; fecal leukocytes are seen.

DIAGNOSIS

DIFFERENTIAL DIAGNOSIS
Gastroenteritis caused by viruses (Norwalk or Rotavirus), parasites (*Amoeba histolytica, Giardia lamblia*), or toxins (Ciguatoxins, mushrooms, heavy metals)

LABORATORY TESTS
- Test stool for fecal leukocytes to help narrow the differential diagnosis:
  1. Send stool for culture and for ova and parasites.
  2. Send stool for *C. difficile* toxin in patients with current or recent antibiotic use.
  3. NOTE: Some pathogens are not identified on routine stool culture; laboratory should be advised if *Yersinia, Clostridium botulinum, Vibrio,* or enterohemorrhagic *E. coli (O157:H7) are* suspected.
  4. Finding *B. cereus, C. perfringens,* or *E. coli* in stool is of little value, since these may be part of the normal bowel flora.
- If botulism suspected, send food, serum, and stool for toxin assay.
- Blood cultures are needed for all febrile patients.

TREATMENT

NONPHARMACOLOGIC THERAPY
Adequate rehydration is the mainstay of therapy.

ACUTE GENERAL Rx
- Gastroenteritis caused by the following organisms requires no antimicrobial treatment: *B. cereus, S. aureus, C. perfringens, V. parahaemolyticus, Yersinia,* and enterohemorrhagic and enteroinvasive *E. coli.*
- The usual cause of traveler's diarrhea is enterotoxigenic *E. coli.* Although usually a self-limited illness, antibiotics can shorten the course.
  1. SMX/TMP one DS tab bid for 3 days
  2. Ciprofloxacin 500 mg PO bid for 3 days
- The mainstay of therapy for cholera is fluid replacement. Antibiotics should be given to decrease shedding and duration of illness.
  1. Doxycycline 100 mg PO bid for 3 days
  2. SMX/TMP one DS tab bid for 3 days
- Treatment is not indicated for *Salmonella* gastroenteritis. Patients who are at high risk of developing bacteremia may be treated for 48 to 72 hr (see "Salmonellosis").
- Although shigellosis tends to be a self-limited illness, antibiotics shorten the course of illness and may limit transmission of the illness (see "Shigellosis").
- Those with moderate or severe *Campylobacter* diarrhea may benefit from treatment.
  1. Erythromycin 500 mg PO qid for 5 days
  2. Ciprofloxacin 500 mg PO bid for 5 days
- *V. vulnificus* sepsis should be treated with:
  1. Doxycycline 100 mg IV bid for 2 wk
  2. Ceftazidime 2 g IV q8h for 2 wk
- For suspected botulism, antitoxin should be administered early (see "Botulism").

CHRONIC Rx
Patients with *Salmonella* infections may become carriers and may require treatment (see "Salmonellosis").

DISPOSITION
- Most infections are self-limited and do not require therapy.
- In immunocompromised host or patient with underlying disease, serious complications are possible.
- Postinfectious syndromes are important with some infections:
  1. Reiter's syndrome: *Salmonella, Shigella, Campylobacter, Yersinia;* more common in genetically susceptible host (HLA-B27+)
  2. Guillain-Barré syndrome: *Campylobacter*

REFERRAL
If more than a mild illness

MISCELLANEOUS

COMMENTS
- Grossly underreported and undiagnosed
- All cases to be reported to the local health department

Author: **Maurice Policar, M.D.**

Friedreich's ataxia

BASIC INFORMATION

DEFINITION
Friedreich's ataxia is the term used for the most common of a group of hereditary early-onset ataxias caused by degeneration of multiple spinal cord pathways and peripheral nervous system axons.

ICD-9-CM CODES
334.0 Friedreich's ataxia

EPIDEMIOLOGY AND DEMOGRAPHICS
INCIDENCE (IN U.S.): Not reported
PREVALENCE (IN U.S.): Not reported
PREDOMINANT SEX: Male = Female
PREDOMINANT AGE: Second decade of life
PEAK INCIDENCE: 8 to 15 yr
GENETICS: Autosomal recessive, with gene localized to chromosome 9

PHYSICAL FINDINGS
- Onset of progressive limb and gait ataxia before age 25 yr and absent muscle stretch reflexes in the lower extremity
- With disease progression: dysarthria, areflexia, leg weakness, extensor plantar responses, distal loss of position and vibration sense
- Common findings: scoliosis, distal atrophy, and cardiomyopathy

ETIOLOGY
- Genetic: responsible gene is localized to the centromeric region of chromosome 9.
- Biochemical defect is unknown.

DIAGNOSIS

DIFFERENTIAL DIAGNOSIS
- Hereditary motor and sensory neuropathy type I (Charcot-Marie-Tooth disease type I)
- Abetalipoproteinemia
- Early onset cerebellar ataxia with retained reflexes

WORKUP
- Diagnostic criteria include electrophysiologic documentation of an axonal sensory neuropathy.
- ECG shows widespread T-wave inversion and evidence of left ventricular hypertrophy in 65% of patients.

LABORATORY TESTS
- EMG/NCS
- ECG
- Peripheral smear for acanthocytes
- Lipid profile

IMAGING STUDIES
MRI of the spinal cord may demonstrate atrophy.

TREATMENT

NONPHARMACOLOGIC THERAPY
- Surgical correction of scoliosis and foot deformities in selected patients
- Physical therapy

ACUTE GENERAL Rx
None

CHRONIC Rx
None

DISPOSITION
- Loss of ambulation typically occurs within 15 yr of symptom onset, and 95% are wheelchair bound by age 45 yr.
- Life expectancy is reduced, particularly if heart disease is present.

REFERRAL
- If uncertain about diagnosis
- For genetic counseling (recommended if available)

MISCELLANEOUS

REFERENCES
Johnson WS: Friedreich's ataxia, *Clin Neurosci* 3:33, 1995.
Author: **Michael Gruenthal, M.D., Ph.D.**

Frozen shoulder (PTG)

BASIC INFORMATION

DEFINITION
Frozen shoulder is a condition unique to the shoulder and characterized by pain and restricted passive and active range of motion.

SYNONYMS
Adhesive capsulitis
Periarthritis
Pericapsulitis
Check-rein shoulder

ICD-9-CM CODES
726.0 Adhesive shoulder capsulitis

EPIDEMIOLOGY AND DEMOGRAPHICS
PREVALENT AGE: Over 40 yr
PREVALENT SEX: Females > males

PHYSICAL FINDINGS
- Arm held protectively at the side with apprehension caused by pain
- Varying degrees of deltoid and spinatus atrophy
- Generalized shoulder tenderness
- Restricted active and passive shoulder motion of varying degrees

ETIOLOGY
Unknown

DIAGNOSIS

DIFFERENTIAL DIAGNOSIS
- Secondary causes of shoulder stiffness (prolonged immobilization following trauma or surgery)
- Posterior shoulder dislocation
- Ruptured rotator cuff
- Glenohumeral osteoarthritis
- Rotator cuff inflammation
- Superior sulcus tumor
- Cervical disc disease
- Brachial neuritis
- The differential diagnosis of shoulder pain is described in Table 2-59.

WORKUP
Laboratory and radiographic studies are generally normal.

TREATMENT

NONPHARMACOLOGIC THERAPY
Prevention is important. Shoulder motion should be maintained during those periods of time when the patient may be inactive as a result of illness or injury.

ACUTE GENERAL Rx
- Moist heat, sedation, and analgesics as needed
- A local steroid/lidocaine mixture injected into the subacromial space and joint
- Home exercise program
- Manipulation of shoulder under anesthesia (rarely needed)

DISPOSITION
- The initial stage of pain followed by stiffness may last several months; recovery phase may also last several months; complete recovery is usually the case.
- Recurrence in the same shoulder is rare, although the opposite limb may develop the same symptoms.
- Some patients have mild residual loss of movement but without any significant functional impairment.

REFERRAL
Orthopedic consultation in patients with resistant disease

MISCELLANEOUS

COMMENTS
- "Capsulitis" with an inflammatory infiltrate is not consistently found pathologically.
- Frozen shoulder is increased in patients with diabetes, thyroid disease, and recent cardiopulmonary conditions.
- Some cases present with findings of reflex sympathetic dystrophy.

REFERENCES
Miller MD, Wirth MA, Rockwood CA: Thawing the frozen shoulder: the "patient" patient, *Orthopedics* 19:849, 1996.

Shaffer B, Tibone SE, Kerlan RK: Frozen shoulder: a long-term follow-up, *J Bone Joint Surg* 74(A):738, 1992.

Author: **Lonnie R. Mercier, M.D.**

Gastric cancer

BASIC INFORMATION

DEFINITION
Gastric cancer is an adenocarcinoma arising from the stomach.

SYNONYMS
Stomach cancer
Linitis plastica

ICD-9-CM CODES
451 Malignant neoplasm of stomach

EPIDEMIOLOGY AND DEMOGRAPHICS
- Annual incidence of gastric cancer in the U.S. is 7 cases/100,000 persons. The incidence is much higher in Japan, with rates as high as 80 cases/100,000 persons.
- Most gastric cancers arise in the antrum (35%).
- The incidence of proximal tumors of the cardia and fundus is on the rise.
- Gastric cancer occurs most commonly in male patients >65 yr (70% of patients are >50 yr).
- Incidence of gastric cancer has been declining over the past 30 yr.
- Male: female ratio is 3:2.

PHYSICAL FINDINGS
- Epigastric or abdominal mass (30% to 50%)
- Skin pallor secondary to anemia
- Hard, nodular liver: generally indicates metastatic disease to the liver
- Hemoccult-positive stools
- Ascites, lymphadenopathy, or pleural effusions: may indicate metastasis

ETIOLOGY
Risk factors:
- Chronic *H. pylori* gastritis
- Tobacco abuse, alcohol consumption
- Food additives (nitrosamines), smoked foods, occupational exposure to heavy metals, rubber, asbestos
- Chronic atrophic gastritis with intestinal metaplasia, hypertrophic gastritis, and pernicious anemia

DIAGNOSIS

DIFFERENTIAL DIAGNOSIS
- Gastric lymphoma (5% of gastric malignancies)
- Hypertrophic gastritis
- Peptic ulcer
- Reflux esophagitis

WORKUP
- Upper endoscopy with biopsy will confirm diagnosis.
- Medical history may reveal complaints of postprandial fullness with significant weight loss (70% to 80%), nausea/emesis (20% to 40%), dysphagia (20%), and dyspepsia, usually unrelieved by antacids; epigastric discomfort, usually lessened by fasting and exacerbated by food intake, is also common.

LABORATORY TESTS
- Microcytic anemia
- Hemoccult-positive stools
- Hypoalbuminemia
- Abnormal liver enzymes in patients with metastasis to the liver

IMAGING STUDIES
- Upper GI series with air contrast (90% accurate) if endoscopy is not readily available
- Abdominal CT scan to evaluate for metastasis (70% accurate for regional node metastases)

TREATMENT

ACUTE GENERAL Rx
- Gastrectomy is performed in patients with curative potential (<30% of patients at time of diagnosis).
- Palliative resection may prolong duration and quality of life.
- Chemotherapy (FAM: 5-fluorouracil, adriamycin, and mitomycin C) may provide some palliation; however, it generally does not prolong survival.

DISPOSITION
- 5-yr survival rate of gastric carcinoma is 12% overall.
- 5-yr survival for early gastric cancers (usually detected incidentally with endoscopy in populations where screening is recommended) is >35%.

REFERRAL
Surgical referral for resection

MISCELLANEOUS

COMMENTS
Gastrectomy patients will need vitamin B_{12} replacement. They are also at risk for dumping syndrome and should be advised to ingest frequent, small meals.

REFERENCES
Fuchs CS, Mayer RJ: Gastric carcinoma, *N Engl J Med* 333:22, 1995.
Thompson GB, VanHeeden JA, Sarr MG: Adenocarcinoma of the stomach: are we making progress? *Lancet* 342:713, 1993.

Author: **Fred F. Ferri, M.D.**

Gastritis (PTG)

BASIC INFORMATION

DEFINITION
Histologically, gastritis refers to inflammation in the stomach. Endoscopically, "gastritis" refers to a number of abnormal features such as erythema, erosions, and subepithelial hemorrhages. Gastritis can also be subdivided into erosive, nonerosive, and specific types of gastritis with distinctive features both endoscopically and histologically (see below).

SYNONYMS
Erosive gastritis
Hemorrhagic gastritis
Helicobacter pylori gastritis

ICD-9-CM CODES
535.5 Gastritis (unless otherwise specified)
535.0 Gastritis, acute
535.3 Alcoholic gastritis
535.1 Atrophic (chronic) gastritis
535.4 Erosive gastritis
535.2 Hypertrophic gastritis

EPIDEMIOLOGY AND DEMOGRAPHICS
- Erosive and hemorrhagic gastritis are most commonly seen in patients taking NSAIDs, alcoholics, and critically ill patients (usually on ventilator support).
- *H. pylori* infection with gastritis is believed to be present in 30% to 50% of the population; however, the majority are asymptomatic.
- The prevalence of *H. pylori* infection increases with age from <10% in Caucasians <40 yr old to >50% in patients >50 yr.

PHYSICAL FINDINGS
- Epigastric tenderness in acute alcoholic gastritis (may be absent in chronic gastritis)
- Foul-smelling breath
- Hematemesis ("coffee-ground" emesis)

ETIOLOGY
- Alcohol, NSAIDs, stress (critically ill patients usually on mechanical respiration), hepatic or renal failure, multiorgan failure
- Infection (bacterial, viral)
- Bile reflux, pancreatic enzyme reflux
- Gastric mucosal atrophy, portal hypertension gastropathy
- Irradiation

DIAGNOSIS

DIFFERENTIAL DIAGNOSIS
- Peptic ulcer disease
- GERD
- Nonulcer dyspepsia
- Gastric lymphoma or carcinoma
- Pancreatitis
- Gastroparesis

WORKUP
Patients with gastritis generally present with nonspecific clinical signs and symptoms (e.g., epigastric pain, abdominal tenderness, bloating, anorexia, nausea [with or without vomiting]). Symptoms may be aggravated by eating. Diagnostic workup includes a comprehensive history and endoscopy with biopsy.

LABORATORY TESTS
- Serologic (IgG antibody to *H. pylori*) or breath test (14C and 13C urea breath tests) for *H. pylori*
- Vitamin B_{12} level in patients with atrophic gastritis
- Hct (low if significant bleeding has occurred)

IMAGING STUDIES
Upper GI series is generally insensitive for the detection of gastritis. Gastroscopy with biopsy is the gold standard diagnostic test.

TREATMENT

NONPHARMACOLOGIC THERAPY
- Avoidance of mucosal irritants such as alcohol and NSAIDs
- Life-style modifications with avoidance of tobacco and foods that trigger symptoms

ACUTE GENERAL Rx
- Eradication of infectious agents (e.g., *H. pylori* therapy with omeprazole 40 mg qAM plus clarithromycin 500 mg tid for days 1 through 14, followed by omeprazole 20 mg qAM for days 15 through 28. Alternative regimens include ranitidine bismuth citrate 400 mg (Tritec) bid plus clarithromycin 500 mg tid for days 1 through 14, followed by ranitidine bismuth citrate 400 mg bid for days 15 through 28.
- Prophylaxis and treatment of stress gastritis with sucralfate suspension 1 g orally q4-6h or H_2-receptor antagonists
- Misoprostol (Cytotec) in patients on chronic NSAIDs therapy

CHRONIC Rx
- Misoprostol 100 µg qid in patients receiving chronic NSAIDs
- Avoidance of alcohol, tobacco, and prolonged NSAIDs use
- Surveillance gastroscopy in patients with atrophic gastritis (increased risk of gastric cancer)

DISPOSITION
Prognosis is good with most cases resolving with treatment. Successful eradication of *H. pylori* infection can be achieved in >80% of patients with appropriate therapy.

REFERRAL
- GI referral for endoscopy in selected cases
- Hospitalization of patients with significant bleeding

MISCELLANEOUS

COMMENTS
Patient education explaining the meaning of gastritis, reassuring the patient, and stressing the importance of life-style modifications.

REFERENCES
Fennerty MB: *Helicobacter pylori, Arch Int Med* 154(7):721, 1994.
Kuipers EG et al: Long-term sequelae of *Helicobacter pylori* gastritis, *Lancet* 345:15, 1995.

Author: **Fred F. Ferri, M.D.**

Gastroesophageal reflux disease (PTG)

BASIC INFORMATION

DEFINITION
Gastroesophageal disease (GERD) is a motility disorder characterized primarily by heartburn and caused by the reflux of gastric contents into the esophagus.

SYNONYMS
Peptic esophagitis
Reflux esophagitis
GERD

ICD-9-CM CODES
530.81 Gastroesophageal reflux disease
530.1 Esophagitis
787.1 Heartburn

EPIDEMIOLOGY AND DEMOGRAPHICS
Heartburn (pyrosis) occurs in >60% of adults. Incidence in pregnant women exceeds 80%. Nearly 20% of adults use antacids or OTC H_2-blockers at least once a week for relief of heartburn.

PHYSICAL FINDINGS
- Physical examination: generally unremarkable
- Clinical signs and symptoms: heartburn, dysphagia, sour taste, regurgitation of gastric contents into the mouth
- Chronic cough and bronchospasm
- Chest pain, laryngitis, early satiety, abdominal fullness, and bloating with belching

ETIOLOGY
- Incompetent LES
- Medications that lower LES pressure (calcium channel blockers, β-adrenergic blockers, theophylline, anticholinergics)
- Foods that lower LES pressure (chocolate, yellow onions, peppermint)
- Tobacco abuse, alcohol, coffee
- Pregnancy
- Gastric acid hypersecretion
- Hiatal hernia (controversial) present in >70% of patients with GERD; however, most patients with hiatal hernia are asymptomatic

DIAGNOSIS

DIFFERENTIAL DIAGNOSIS
- Peptic ulcer disease
- Unstable angina
- Esophagitis (from infections such as herpes, *Candida*), medication induced (doxycycline, potassium chloride)
- Esophageal spasm (nutcracker esophagus)
- Cancer of esophagus

WORKUP
- Aimed at eliminating the conditions noted in the differential diagnosis and documenting the type and extent of tissue damage with upper endoscopy
- A clinical algorithm for evaluation of heartburn is described in Fig. 3-37.

LABORATORY TESTS
- 24-hr esophageal pH monitoring and Bernstein test are sensitive diagnostic tests; however, they are not very practical and generally not done. They are useful in patients with atypical manifestations of GERD, such as chest pain or chronic cough.
- Esophageal manometry is indicated in patients with refractory reflux in whom surgical therapy is planned.

IMAGING STUDIES
- Upper GI series can identify ulcerations and strictures; however, it may miss mucosal abnormalities.
- Upper GI endoscopy is useful to document the type and extent of tissue damage in GERD and to exclude potentially malignant conditions such as Barrett's esophagus.

TREATMENT

NONPHARMACOLOGIC THERAPY
- Life-style modifications with avoidance of foods and drugs that decrease LES pressure (e.g., caffeine, β-blockers)
- Avoidance of tobacco and alcohol use
- Elevation of head of bed using blocks
- Avoidance of lying down directly after late or large evening meals

ACUTE GENERAL Rx
- Proton pump inhibitors (omeprazole 20 mg qd or lansoprazole 30 mg qd)
- H_2-blockers (nizatidine 300 mg qhs, famotidine 40 mg qhs, ranitidine 300 mg qhs, or cimetidine 800 mg qhs)
- Antacids (may be useful for relief of mild symptoms, however they are generally ineffective in severe cases of reflux)
- Prokinetic agents (cisapride 10 to 20 mg qid)
- For refractory cases: surgery with Nissen fundoplication

CHRONIC Rx
Life-style modification must be followed lifelong, since this is generally an irreversible condition.

DISPOSITION
- The majority of the patients respond well to therapy.
- Recurrence of reflux is common if treatment is discontinued.

REFERRAL
- GI referral for upper endoscopy is needed when there are concerns about associated PUD, Barrett's esophagus, or esophageal cancer.
- Patients with Barrett's esophagus should undergo surveillance endoscopy with mucosal biopsy every 2 yr or less.

MISCELLANEOUS

COMMENTS
Patient education material can be obtained from Digestive Diseases Clearing House, Suite 600, 1555 Wilson Boulevard, Rosslyn, VA 22209.

REFERENCES
DeVault KR, Castell DO: Guidelines for the diagnosis and treatment of gastroesophageal reflux disease, *Arch Int Med* 135:2165, 1995.

Vigneri S et al: A comparison of five maintenance therapies for reflux esophagitis, *N Engl J Med* 333:1106, 1995.

Author: **Fred F. Ferri, M.D.**

BASIC INFORMATION

DEFINITION
Giardiasis is an intestinal and/or biliary tract infection caused by the protozoal parasite *Giardia lamblia*.

ICD-9-CM CODES
007.1 Giardiasis

EPIDEMIOLOGY AND DEMOGRAPHICS
INCIDENCE (IN U.S.):
- Exact incidence unknown
- Frequently occurs in outbreaks

PREVALENCE (IN U.S.): 4%
PREDOMINANT SEX: Male = female
PREDOMINANT AGE:
- Preschool children, especially if in daycare
- 20 to 40 yr old, especially among sexually-active homosexual men

PEAK INCIDENCE:
- Varies with risk factors, outbreaks
- All age groups affected

GENETICS:
Familial Disposition: Patients with common variable immunodeficiency or X-linked agammaglobulinemia are at increased risk of infection.
Neonatal Infection: Rare; infection is common among preschool children in daycare.

PHYSICAL FINDINGS
- More than 70% with one or more intestinal symptoms (diarrhea, flatulence, cramps, bloating, nausea)
- Fever in <20%
- Malaise, anorexia
- Chronic diarrhea, malabsorption, and weight loss
- GI bleeding is unusual
- Continuous or intermittent symptoms, lasting for weeks
- Of infected patients, 20% to 25% are asymptomatic

ETIOLOGY
Infection is acquired by ingestion of viable cysts of the organism, typically in contaminated water or by fecal-oral contact.

DIAGNOSIS

DIFFERENTIAL DIAGNOSIS
- Other agents of infective diarrhea (amebae, *Salmonella* sp., *Shigella* sp., *Staphylococcus aureus*, *Cryptosporidia*, etc.)
- Noninfectious causes of malabsorption
- Table 2-36 describes the differential diagnosis of infectious diseases in travelers.

WORKUP
Stool specimen (three specimens yield 90% sensitivity) or duodenal aspirate for microscopic examination to establish diagnosis and exclude other pathogens

LABORATORY TESTS
- Serum albumin, vitamin B_{12} levels, and stool fat test to exclude malabsorption
- Serum antibody test if desired for epidemiologic purposes

IMAGING STUDIES
- Not necessary unless biliary obstruction is suspected
- In detection of organism, possible interference by barium in stool from radiographic studies

TREATMENT

NONPHARMACOLOGIC THERAPY
Avoidance of milk products to reduce symptoms of transient lactase deficiency that occur in many patients

ACUTE GENERAL Rx
Adults:
- Metronidazole 250 mg PO three times daily for 7 days (metronidazole avoided in pregnancy) *or*
- Paromomycin 25 to 30 mg/kg/day in three doses for 5 to 10 days

CHRONIC Rx
May require retreatment

DISPOSITION
Reinfection is possible.

REFERRAL
For evaluation by gastroenterologist if malabsorption, weight loss do not resolve with therapy

MISCELLANEOUS

COMMENTS
Travelers to endemic areas (developing world, wilderness areas) should be cautioned to boil drinking water, or if this is impossible, use halogenated water purification tablets.

REFERENCES
Hill DR: Giardiasis: issues in management and treatment, *Infect Dis Clin North Am* 7:503, 1993.

Author: **Joseph R. Masci, M.D.**

Gilbert's disease (PTG)

BASIC INFORMATION

DEFINITION
Gilbert's disease is an autosomal dominant disease characterized by indirect hyperbilirubinemia caused by impaired glucuronyl transferase activity.

SYNONYMS
Gilbert's syndrome

ICD-9-CM CODES
277.4 Gilbert's syndrome

EPIDEMIOLOGY AND DEMOGRAPHICS
- Probable autosomal dominant disease affecting >5% of the U.S. population
- Male:female ratio of 3:1

PHYSICAL FINDINGS
No abnormalities on physical examination other than mild jaundice when bilirubin exceeds 3 mg/dl.

ETIOLOGY
Decreased elimination of bilirubin in bile is caused by inadequate conjugation of bilirubin. Alcohol consumption and starvation diet can increase the bilirubin level.

DIAGNOSIS

DIFFERENTIAL DIAGNOSIS
- Hemolytic anemia
- Liver disease (chronic hepatitis, cirrhosis)
- Crigler-Najjar syndrome

WORKUP
Laboratory evaluation to exclude hemolysis and liver diseases as a cause of the elevated bilirubin level

LABORATORY TESTS
Elevated indirect (unconjugated) bilirubin (rarely exceeds 5 mg/dl)

TREATMENT

ACUTE GENERAL Rx
Treatment is generally unnecessary. Phenobarbital (if clinical jaundice is present) can rapidly decrease serum indirect bilirubin level.

DISPOSITION
Prognosis is excellent. Treatment is generally unnecessary.

REFERRAL
Referral is generally not necessary.

MISCELLANEOUS

COMMENTS
Patients should be reassured about the benign nature of their condition.

REFERENCES
Bosma PJ et al: The genetic basis of the reduced expression of bilirubin UDP-glucuronyl transferase-1 in Gilbert's syndrome, *N Engl J Med* 333:1171, 1995.

Author: **Fred F. Ferri, M.D.**

Gingivitis (PTG)

BASIC INFORMATION

DEFINITION
Gingivitis refers to inflammation of the gums covering the maxilla and mandible.

ICD-9-CM CODES
523.1 Gingivitis

EPIDEMIOLOGY AND DEMOGRAPHICS
PREDOMINANT AGE: Adulthood

PHYSICAL FINDINGS
- Usually painless inflammation
- Possible bleeding with minor trauma such as brushing teeth
- Bluish discoloration of the gums; possible halitosis
- Subgingival plaque on close examination
- In time, detachment of soft tissue from the tooth surface
- Possible long-standing infection leading to destructive periodontal disease that may involve teeth and bones
- Acute necrotizing ulcerative gingivitis (ANUG or "trench mouth"): a dramatic form of gingivitis manifested by acute, painful, inflammation of the gingivae, with bleeding, ulceration, and halitosis
- Possible severe periodontitis in patients with diabetes mellitus or HIV infection and in primary HIV infection (acute retroviral syndrome)
- Pregnancy: sometimes associated with an acute form of gingivitis

ETIOLOGY
- Various organisms found in the environment of plaque; anaerobes are predominant in periodontal disease.
- Improper hygiene and poorly fitting dentures contribute to development of gingivitis.
- Excessive use of tobacco and alcohol predispose individuals to gingival disease.
- Appropriate oral hygiene, such as flossing and tooth brushing, is preventative for the accumulation of bacterial plaque.
- Once plaque is present, adequate hygiene is more difficult.

DIAGNOSIS

DIFFERENTIAL DIAGNOSIS
Gingival hyperplasia, which may be caused by phenytoin or nifedipine

WORKUP
Oral examination

LABORATORY TESTS
Elevated serum glucose in diabetics

IMAGING STUDIES
Radiographs of the teeth and facial bones to reveal extension of infection to these structures

TREATMENT

NONPHARMACOLOGIC THERAPY
Removal of plaque and, at times, debridement of soft tissue

ACUTE GENERAL Rx
- Penicillin VK 500 mg PO qid for 1 to 2 wk *or*
- Clindamycin 300 mg PO qid for 1 to 2 wk

CHRONIC Rx
Periodic evaluation and debridement for extensive or recurrent infection

DISPOSITION
Continued inflammation, leading eventually to destruction of teeth and bone

REFERRAL
To a dentist or oral surgeon

MISCELLANEOUS

COMMENTS
- Presence of periodontal disease is associated with an increased incidence of anaerobic pleuropulmonary infections.
- U.S. Preventive Services Task Force Recommendations for counseling to prevent dental and periodontal disease are described in Section V, Chapter 61.

Author: **Maurice Policar, M.D.**

Glaucoma, chronic open-angle (chronic simple glaucoma)

BASIC INFORMATION

DEFINITION
Chronic open-angle glaucoma refers to optic nerve damage often associated with elevated intraocular pressure; it is a chronic, slowly progressive, usually bilateral disorder associated with visual loss, eye pain, and optic nerve damage.

ICD-9-CM CODES
365.1 Open-angle glaucoma

EPIDEMIOLOGY AND DEMOGRAPHICS
INCIDENCE (IN U.S.): Third most common cause of visual loss (75% to 95% of all glaucomas are open angle.)
PREVALENCE (IN U.S.):
- 15,000,000 Americans may have glaucoma and 1,600,000 have visual field loss.
- 150,000 patients suffer bilateral blindness.
- Disease occurs in 2% of people >40 yr old.
- Prevalence is higher in diabetics, with high myopia, and among older persons.

PREDOMINANT AGE:
- Persons >50 yr old
- Can occur in 30s and 40s

PEAK INCIDENCE: Increases after 40 yr
GENETICS:
- Four to six times higher incidence in blacks than whites
- No clear-cut hereditary patterns but a strong hereditary tendency

PHYSICAL FINDINGS
- High intraocular pressures and large optic nerve cup
- Abnormal visual fields
- Open-angle gonioscopy

ETIOLOGY
- Uncertain hereditary tendency
- Topical steroids
- Trauma
- Inflammatory

DIAGNOSIS

DIFFERENTIAL DIAGNOSIS
- Other optic neuropathies
- Secondary glaucoma from inflammation and steroid therapy

WORKUP
- Intraocular pressure
- Slit lamp examination
- Visual fields
- Gonioscopy

LABORATORY TESTS
Blood sugar

IMAGING STUDIES
- Optic nerve photography
- Fluorescein angiography
- Visual field testing

TREATMENT

ACUTE GENERAL Rx
- β-Blockers (Timolol)
- Diamox or pilocarpine
- Hyperosmotic agents (mannitol)
- Prostaglandins

CHRONIC Rx
At least biannual checks of intraocular pressure

DISPOSITION
Usually followed by ophthalmologist

REFERRAL
Immediately to ophthalmologist

MISCELLANEOUS

COMMENTS
- Early diagnosis and treatment may minimize visual loss.
- Glaucoma is not solely caused by increased intraocular pressure, since approximately 20% of patients with glaucoma have normal intraocular pressure.
- U.S. Preventive Services Task Force Recommendations for screening for glaucoma are described in Section V, Chapter 34.

REFERENCES
Quigley HA: Open-angle glaucoma, *N Engl J Med* 328:1097, 1993
Author: **Melvyn Koby, M.D.**

Glaucoma, primary closed-angle (narrow-angle glaucoma) *(PTG)*

BASIC INFORMATION

DEFINITION
Primary closed-angle glaucoma occurs when elevated intraocular pressure is associated with closure of the filtration angle.

SYNONYMS
Glaucoma
Pupillary block glaucoma

ICD-9-CM CODES
365.2 Primary angle-closure glaucoma

EPIDEMIOLOGY AND DEMOGRAPHICS
INCIDENCE (IN U.S.):
- In 2% to 8% of all patients with glaucoma
- Higher incidence among those with hyperopia

PREDOMINANT SEX: Females > males
PREDOMINANT AGE: 50 to 60 yr
PEAK INCIDENCE: Greater after 50 yr of age
GENETICS: High family history

PHYSICAL FINDINGS
- Hazy cornea
- Narrow angle
- Red eyes
- Pain
- Injection of conjunctiva

ETIOLOGY
Narrow angles with acute closure

DIAGNOSIS

DIFFERENTIAL DIAGNOSIS
- Open angle glaucoma
- Conjunctivitis
- Corneal disease

WORKUP
- Intraocular pressure
- Gonioscopy
- Slit lamp examination
- Visual field examination

LABORATORY TESTS
Blood sugar and CBC (if diabetes or inflammatory disease is suspected)

IMAGING STUDIES
- Fundus photography
- Fluorescein angiography of optic nerve

TREATMENT

NONPHARMACOLOGIC THERAPY
Laser iridotomy early in disease process

ACUTE GENERAL Rx
- IV mannitol
- Pilocarpine
- β-Blockers
- Diamox

CHRONIC Rx
Iridotomy

DISPOSITION
Refer to ophthalmologist immediately.

REFERRAL
This is an emergency—refer immediately to an ophthalmologist.

MISCELLANEOUS

COMMENTS
- After iridotomy, the majority of patients will be totally cured and will need no further medication and have no visual loss.
- U.S. Preventive Services Task Force Recommendations for screening for glaucoma are described in Section V, Chapter 34.

REFERENCES
Chaudhry I, Wong S: Recognizing glaucoma, *Postgrad Med* 99:247, 1996.
Congdon N, Wang F, Tielsch JM: Issues in the epidemiology and population-based screening of primary angle-closure glaucoma, *Surv Ophthalmol* 36:411, 1992.

Author: **Melvyn Koby, M.D.**

Glomerulonephritis, acute (PTG)

BASIC INFORMATION

DEFINITION
Acute glomerulonephritis if an immunologically mediated inflammation primarily involving the glomerulus that can result in damage to the basement membrane, mesangium, or capillary endothelium.

SYNONYMS
Postinfectious glomerulonephritis
Acute nephritic syndrome

ICD-9-CM CODES
583.9 Glomerulonephritis, acute

EPIDEMIOLOGY AND DEMOGRAPHICS
- Over 50% of cases involve children <13 yr old.
- Glomerulonephritis is the most common cause of chronic renal failure (25%).
- IgA nephropathy glomerulonephritis (Berger's disease) is the most common glomerulonephritis worldwide.

PHYSICAL FINDINGS
- Edema (peripheral, periorbital, or pulmonary)
- Joint pains, oral ulcers, malar rash (frequently seen with lupus nephritis)
- Dark urine
- Hypertension
- Findings of palpable purpura in patients with Henoch-Schönlein purpura
- Heart murmurs may indicate endocarditis
- Impetigo, skin pallor, tenderness in the abdomen and/or back, pharyngeal erythema may be present

ETIOLOGY
- Post group A β-hemolytic streptococcus infection (other infectious etiologies including endocarditis and visceral abscess)
- Collagen-vascular diseases (SLE)
- Vasculitis (Wegener's granulomatosis, polyarteritis nodosa)
- Idiopathic glomerulonephritis (membranoproliferative, idiopathic, crescentic, IgA nephropathy)
- Goodpasture's syndrome
- Other cryoglobulinemia (Henoch-Schönlein purpura)
- Drug-induced (gold, penicillamine)

DIAGNOSIS

DIFFERENTIAL DIAGNOSIS
- Cirrhosis with edema and ascites
- CHF
- Acute interstitial nephritis
- Severe hypertension
- Hemolytic uremic syndrome
- SLE, diabetes mellitus, amyloidosis, preeclampsia, sclerodermal renal crisis

WORKUP
- Initial evaluation of suspected glomerulonephritis consists of laboratory testing.
- The approach to the differential diagnosis of suspected glomerular disease is described in Fig. 3-34.

LABORATORY TESTS
- Urinalysis (hematuria, proteinuria, dysmorphic erythrocytes and casts)
- 24-hr urine for protein excretion and creatinine clearance (to document degree of renal dysfunction and amount of proteinuria)
- Streptococcal tests (streptozyme), antistreptolysin O (ASO) quantitative titer (highest in 3 to 5 wk); ASO titer, however, is not related to severity of renal disease, duration, or prognosis
- Additional useful tests depending on the history: ANA (rule out SLE), C3, C4 level, triglycerides, cryoglobulins, hepatitis B and C serologies, ANCA (antineutrophil cytoplasmic antibody), c-ANCA (in suspected cases of Wegener's granulomatosis), p-ANCA found in pauciimmune (lack of immune deposits) idiopathic rapidly progressive glomerulonephritis with or without systemic vasculitis
- Serum BUN and creatinine (elevated in renal failure)
- Hct (decreased in glomerulonephritis), platelet count (thrombocytopenia in cases of lupus nephritis)
- Anti-GBM antibody (in Goodpasture's syndrome)

IMAGING STUDIES
- Chest x-ray examination: pulmonary congestion, Wegener's granulomatosis, and Goodpasture's syndrome
- Renal ultrasound frequently performed (however, not necessary to make diagnosis)
- Echocardiogram in patients with new cardiac murmurs or positive blood cultures to rule out endocarditis and pericardial effusion

- Renal biopsy and light, electron, and immunofluorescent microscopy to confirm diagnosis
- Kidney biopsy: generally reveals a granular pattern in poststreptococcal glomerulonephritis, linear pattern in Goodpasture's syndrome; renal biopsy: although helpful to define the etiology of glomerulonephritis, is generally not indicated
- Immunofluorescence: generally reveals C3; negative immunofluorescence suggests Wegener's granulomatosis, idiopathic crescentic glomerulonephritis, or polyarteritis nodosa

TREATMENT

NONPHARMACOLOGIC THERAPY
- Avoidance of salt if edema or hypertension are present
- Low-protein intake (approximately 0.5 g/kg/day) in patients with renal failure
- Fluid restriction in patients with significant edema
- Avoidance of high-potassium foods

ACUTE GENERAL Rx
- Correction of electrolyte abnormalities (hypocalcemia, hyperkalemia) and acidosis (if present)
- Treatment of streptococcal infection with penicillin (or erythromycin in penicillin-allergic patients)
- Furosemide in patients with significant hypertension and/or edema; hydralazine or nifedipine in patients with hypertension
- Immunosuppressive treatment in patients with heavy proteinuria or rapidly decreasing glomerular filtration rate (high-dose steroids, cyclosporin A, cyclophosphamide); corticosteroids generally not useful in poststreptococcal glomerulonephritis
- Fish oil (n-3 fatty acids) 12 g/day: may prevent or slow down loss of renal function in patients with IgA nephropathy
- Plasma exchange therapy and immunosuppressive drugs (prednisone and cyclophosphamide): effective in Goodpasture's syndrome

CHRONIC RX
- Frequent monitoring of urinalysis, serum creatinine, and blood pressure in the initial 12 mo
- Monitoring for onset of hypertensive retinopathy, encephalopathy
- Aggressive treatment of infections, particularly streptococcal infections
- Dosage adjustment of all renally excreted medications

DISPOSITION
- Prognosis is generally related to histology with excellent prognosis in patients with minimal change glomerulonephritis and focal segmental proliferative glomerulonephritis; 25% to 30% of patients with mesangial IgA disease and membranous glomerulonephritis generally progress to chronic renal failure; >70% of patients with mesangial capillary glomerulonephritis will develop chronic renal failure.
- Generally prognosis is worse in patients with heavy proteinuria, severe hypertension, and significant elevations of creatinine.
- Recovery of renal function occurs within 8 to 12 wk in 95% of patients with poststreptococcal glomerulonephritis.

REFERRAL
- Nephrology consultation
- Surgical referral for biopsy in selected cases

MISCELLANEOUS

COMMENTS
- Anticoagulation to prevent DVT should be considered in patients with a low level of physical activity.
- Monitoring of lipids and aggressive treatment of hyperlipidemias is recommended.
- Close monitoring of side effects of immunosuppressive drugs and complications of corticosteroids is necessary.

REFERENCES
Galla JH: IgA nephropathy, *Kidney Int* 47:377, 1995.
Mason PD, Pulsey CD: Glomerulonephritis: diagnosis and treatment, *Br Med J* 309:1557, 1994.
Short AK et al: Antineutrophil cytoplasmic antibodies and anti-glomerular basement membrane antibodies: two coexisting distinct autoreactivities detectable in patients with rapidly progressive glomerulonephritis, *Am J Kid Dis* 26:439, 1995.

Author: **Fred F. Ferri, M.D.**

Glossitis (PTG)

BASIC INFORMATION

DEFINITION
Glossitis is an inflammation of the tongue that can lead to loss of filiform papillae.

ICD-9-CM CODES
529.0 Glossitis

EPIDEMIOLOGY AND DEMOGRAPHICS
Glossitis is seen more frequently in patients of lower socioeconomic status, malnourished patients, alcoholics, smokers, elderly patients, immunocompromised patients, and patients with dentures.

PHYSICAL FINDINGS
- The appearance of the tongue is variable depending on the etiology of the glossitis. Loss of filiform papillae results in red, smooth-surfaced tongue.
- The tongue may appear pale in patients with significant anemia.
- Pain and swelling of the tongue may be present when glossitis is associated with infections, trauma, or lichen planus.
- Ulcerations may be present in patients with herpetic glossitis, pemphigus, or streptococcal infection.
- Excessive use of mouthwash may result in a "hairy" appearance of the tongue.

ETIOLOGY
- Nutritional deficiencies (vitamin E, riboflavin, niacin, vitamin B_{12}, iron deficiency)
- Infections (viral, candidiasis, TB, syphilis)
- Trauma (generally caused by poorly fitting dentures)
- Irritation of the tongue secondary to toothpaste, medications, alcohol, tobacco, citrus
- Lichen planus, pemphigus vulgaris, erythema multiforme
- Neoplasms

DIAGNOSIS

DIFFERENTIAL DIAGNOSIS
- Infections
- Use of chemical irritants
- Neoplasms
- Skin disorders (e.g., Behçet's syndrome, erythema multiforme)

WORKUP
- Laboratory evaluation to exclude infectious processes, vitamin deficiencies, and systemic disorders
- Biopsy of lesion only when there is no response to treatment

LABORATORY TESTS
- CBC: Decreased Hgb and Hct, low MCV (iron deficiency anemia), elevated MCV (vitamin B_{12} deficiency)
- Vitamin B_{12} level
- 10% KOH scrapings in patients with white patches suspicious for candidiasis

TREATMENT

NONPHARMACOLOGIC THERAPY
Avoidance of primary irritants such as hot foods, spices, tobacco, and alcohol

ACUTE GENERAL Rx
Treatment varies with the etiology of the glossitis.
- Malnutrition with avitaminosis: multivitamins
- Candidiasis: fluconazole 200 mg on day 1, then 100 mg/day for at least 2 wk or nystatin 400,000 U suspension qid for 10 days or 200,000 pastilles dissolved slowly in the mouth four to five times qd for 10 to 14 days
- Painful oral lesions: rinsing of the mouth with 2% lidocaine viscus, 1 to 2 tablespoons q4h PRN; triamcinolone 0.1% applied to painful ulcers PRN for symptomatic relief

CHRONIC Rx
- Life-style changes with elimination of tobacco, alcohol, and other primary irritants
- Dental evaluation for correction of ill-fitting dentures
- Correction of associated metabolic abnormalities such as hyperglycemia from diabetes mellitus

DISPOSITION
Most patients experience prompt improvement with identification and treatment of the cause of the glossitis.

REFERRAL
Surgical referral for biopsy of solitary lesions unresponsive to treatment to rule out neoplasm

MISCELLANEOUS

COMMENTS
If the primary cause of glossitis is not identified or cannot be corrected, enteric nutritional replacement therapy should be considered in malnourished patients.

REFERENCES
Cohen PR et al: Geometric glossitis, *S Med J* 88(12):1231, 1995.
Drinka PJ et al: Nutrition correlates of atrophic glossitis: possible role of vitamin E in papillary atrophy, *J Am Coll Nutr* 12:14, 1993.
Grinspan B et al: Burning mouth syndrome, *Int J Derm* 34:43, 1995.
Author: **Fred F. Ferri, M.D.**

Gonorrhea (PTG)

BASIC INFORMATION

DEFINITION
Gonorrhea is a sexually transmitted bacterial infection with a predilection for columnar and transitional epithelial cells. It commonly manifests as urethritis, cervicitis, or salpingitis. Infection may be asymptomatic. It differs in males and females in course, severity, and ease of recognition.

SYNONYMS
Gonococcal urethritis
Gonococcal vulvovaginitis
Gonococcal cervicitis
Gonococcal Bartholinitis
Clap
GC

ICD-9-CM CODES
098 Gonococcal infections

EPIDEMIOLOGY AND DEMOGRAPHICS
- The disease is common worldwide, affects both sexes, all ages, especially younger adults; highest incidence is in inner-city areas, with an estimated 3,000,000 new cases annually.
- Asymptomatic anterior urethral carriage may occur in 12% to 50% of cases in men.
- Asymptomatic in 50% to 80% of cases in women. Most common dissemination by mucosal passage to fallopian tubes, resulting in PID in 10% to 15% of infected women. Hematogenous spread may result in septic arthritis and skin lesions. Conjunctivitis rarely occurs but may result in blindness if not rapidly treated. Infection can occur in both men and women in oropharynx and anorectally.

PHYSICAL FINDINGS
- Males: purulent discharge from anterior urethra with dysuria appearing 2 to 7 days after infecting exposure. May have rectal infection causing pruritus, tenesmus, and discharge or may be asymptomatic.
- Females: initial urethritis, cervicitis may occur a few days after exposure, frequently mild. In about 20% of cases, uterine invasion occurs after menstrual period with signs and symptoms of endometritis, salpingitis, or pelvic peritonitis. The patient may have purulent discharge, inflamed Skene's or Bartholin's glands.
- Classic presentation of acute gonococcal PID is fever, abdominal and adnexal tenderness, often absence of purulent discharge. Physical examination may be normal if asymptomatic.

ETIOLOGY
Neisseria gonorrhoeae is the gonococcus. Plasmids coding for β-lactamase render some strains resistant to penicillin or tetracycline (PPNG, TRNG). There is an increasing frequency of chromosomally mediated resistance to penicillin, tetracycline, and cefoxitin. In the Far East, high-level resistance to spectinomycin is endemic.

DIAGNOSIS

DIFFERENTIAL DIAGNOSIS
- Nongonococcal urethritis (NGU)
- Nongonococcal mucopurulent cervicitis
- Chlamydia trachomatis

WORKUP
- Diagnosis is dependent on bacteriologic investigation.
- Gram-negative intracellular diplococci are diagnostic in male urethral smears. There is a false-negative rate of 60% to 70% in female cervical or urethral smears. Culture is essential in women.
- U.S. Preventive Services Task Force Recommendations regarding screening for gonorrhea are described in Section V, Chapter 27.

LABORATORY TESTS
- Gonorrhea culture on Thayer-Martin medium (Organism is fastidious, requires aerobic conditions with increased carbon dioxide atmosphere. Incubate ASAP.)
- Serologic testing for syphilis on all patients
- Chlamydia testing on all patients
- Offer of HIV counseling and testing

TREATMENT

ACUTE GENERAL Rx
Uncomplicated urethral, endocervical, or rectal infections:
- Ceftriaxone 125 mg or 250 mg IM
- Alternatives: cefixime 400 mg PO, ciprofloxacin 500 mg PO, ofloxacin 400 mg PO; if infection from source not penicillin-resistant: amoxicillin 3g PO with probenecid 1g

All treatment regimens should include empiric treatment of chlamydial infections (which may be concurrent in up to 45% of GC cases):
- Doxycycline 100 mg PO bid unrelated to meals *or*
- Tetracycline 500 mg PO qid between meals

Pharyngeal infection:
- Ceftriaxone 250 mg IM *or*
- Ciprofloxacin 500 mg PO single dose
- Repeat culture 5 to 7 days later

Pregnant patients:
- Ceftriaxone 250 mg IM plus erythromycin base 500 mg PO qid for 7 days
- Tetracycline and quinolones contraindicated in pregnancy. β-lactam allergic patients should be treated with spectinomycin 2 g IM followed by erythromycin.

DISPOSITION
- Pregnant patients require test of cure; reculture 4 to 7 days after treatment (as do those treated with regimens other than ceftriaxone/doxycycline).
- Treatment failure in nonpregnant patients is rare and test of cure is not required. Rescreening in 1 to 2 mo detects treatment failures and reinfections.
- Sexual partners should all be identified, examined, cultured, and receive presumptive treatment.

REFERRAL
PID requiring hospitalization, disseminated gonococcal infection

MISCELLANEOUS

COMMENTS
- This is a reportable disease.
- U.S. Preventive Services Task Force Recommendations regarding counseling to prevent HIV infection and other STDs is described in Section V, Chapter 62.

REFERENCES
Benenson AS (ed): *Control of communicable diseases in man,* ed 15, Washington, DC, 1990, American Public Health Association.
Drugs for sexually transmitted diseases, *Med Lett Drugs Ther* 37(964):117, 1995.
Moran JS, Levine WC: Drugs of choice for the treatment of uncomplicated gonococcal infections, *Clin Infect Dis* 20(suppl 1): S47, 1995.
Woods GL: Update on laboratory diagnosis of sexually transmitted diseases, *Clin Lab Med* 15(3):665, 1995.

Author: **Eugene Louie-Ng, M.D.**

Goodpasture's syndrome

BASIC INFORMATION

DEFINITION
Goodpasture's syndrome is characterized by idiopathic recurrence of alveolar hemorrhage and rapidly progressive glomerulonephritis. It can also be defined by the triad of glomerulonephritis, pulmonary hemorrhage, and antibody to basement membrane antigens.

ICD-9-CM CODES
446.2 Goodpasture's syndrome

EPIDEMIOLOGY AND DEMOGRAPHICS
- Goodpasture's syndrome affects predominately young white male smokers.
- Male:female ratio is 6:1.
- Goodpasture's syndrome accounts for 5% of all cases of rapidly progressive glomerulonephritis.
- 80% of patients are HLA-BR2 positive.

PHYSICAL FINDINGS
- Dyspnea, cough, hemoptysis
- Skin pallor, fever, arthralgias (may be mild or absent at the time of initial presentation)

ETIOLOGY
Presence of glomerular basement membranes (GBM) antibody deposition in kidneys and lungs with subsequent pulmonary hemorrhage and glomerulonephritis.

DIAGNOSIS

DIFFERENTIAL DIAGNOSIS
- Wegener's granulomatosis
- SLE
- Systemic necrotizing vasculitis
- Idiopathic rapidly progressive glomerulonephritis
- Drug-induced renal pulmonary disease (e.g., penicillamine)

WORKUP
Laboratory evaluation, diagnostic imaging, immunofluorescence studies of renal biopsy

LABORATORY TESTS
- Presence of circulating serum anti-GBM antibodies
- Absence of circulating immunocomplexes, antineutrophils, cytoplasmic antibodies, and cryoglobulins
- Urinalysis revealing microscopic hematuria and proteinuria
- Elevated BUN and creatinine from rapidly progressive glomerulonephritis
- Immunofluorescence studies of renal biopsy material: linear deposits of anti-GBM antibody, often accompanied by C3 deposition
- Anemia from iron deficiency (secondary to blood loss and iron sequestration in the lungs)

IMAGING STUDIES
Chest x-ray examination: fluffy alveolar infiltrates, evidence of pulmonary hemorrhage

TREATMENT

ACUTE GENERAL Rx
- Plasma exchange therapy
- Immunosuppressive therapy with prednisone (1 mg/kg/day) and cyclophosphamide (2 mg/kg/day)
- Dialysis support in patients with renal failure

DISPOSITION
Life-threatening pulmonary hemorrhage and irreversible glomerular damage are the major causes of death.

REFERRAL
- Surgical referral for renal biopsy to guide the management
- Referral of patients with renal failure to dialysis center
- Consideration for renal transplantation in patients with end-stage renal failure

MISCELLANEOUS

REFERENCES
Kelly PT, Haponik EF: Goodpasture's syndrome: molecular and clinical advances, *Medicine* 73: 171, 1994.

Short AK et al: Antineutrophil cytoplasm antibodies and anti-glomerular basement membrane antibodies, two coexisting distinct order activities detectable in patients with rapidly progressive glomerulonephritis, *Am J Kidney Dis* 26:439, 1995.

Author: **Fred F. Ferri, M.D.**

CLINICAL TOPICS   Gout (PTG) 205

BASIC INFORMATION

DEFINITION
Gout is a clinical disorder in which crystals of monosodium urate become deposited in tissue as a result of hyperuricemia. Gout and hyperuricemia can be classified as either primary or secondary if resulting from another disorder.

ICD-9-CM CODES
274.9 Gout

EPIDEMIOLOGY AND DEMOGRAPHICS
PREVALENCE: 3 cases /1000 persons
PREDOMINANT SEX: 95% males, rare in females before menopause
PREDOMINANT AGE: 30 to 50 yr

PHYSICAL FINDINGS
- Usually, initial attack in a single joint or an area of tenosynovium
- Mainly a disease of the lower extremities
- First site of involvement: classically, MP joint of the great toe
- Another common site of acute attack: extensor tenosynovium on the dorsum of the mid-foot
- Severe pain and inflammation, which may be precipitated by exercise, dietary indiscretions, and physical or emotional stress
- Attacks following illness or surgery
- Presence of swelling, heat, redness, and other signs of inflammation (the physical findings simulating cellulitis)
- Exquisite soft-tissue tenderness
- Fever, tachycardia, and other constitutional symptoms
- Eventually, deposits of urate crystals (tophi) in the subcutaneous tissue

ETIOLOGY
- Hyperuricemia and gout develop from excessive uric acid production, a decrease in the renal excretion of uric acid, or both.
- Primary gout results from an inborn error of metabolism and may be attributed to several biochemical defects.
- Secondary hyperuricemia may develop as a complication of acquired disorders (e.g., leukemia) or as a result of the use of certain drugs (e.g., diuretics).

DIAGNOSIS

DIFFERENTIAL DIAGNOSIS
- Pseudogout
- Rheumatoid arthritis
- Osteoarthritis
- Cellulitis
- Infectious arthritis

WORKUP
Hyperuricemia accompanying a typical history of monoarticular acute arthritis is usually sufficient to establish the diagnosis.

LABORATORY TESTS
- Mild leukocytosis
- Elevated ESR
- Hyperuricemia
- Synovial aspirate: usually cloudy and markedly inflammatory in nature; urate crystals in fluid: needle-shaped and birefringent under polarized light

IMAGING STUDIES
- Plain radiography to rule out other disorders
- No typical findings in early gouty arthritis but late disease possibly associated with characteristic punched-out lesions and joint destruction

TREATMENT

NONPHARMACOLOGIC THERAPY
- Modification of diet (avoidance of foods high in purines [e.g., anchovies, organ meat, liver, spinach, mushrooms, asparagus, oatmeal, cocoa, sweet breads]) and life-style
- Treatment for obesity
- Moderation in alcohol intake, no more than two drinks per day
- Hypertension and its management requiring careful assessment and possibly nondiuretic drugs

ACUTE GENERAL Rx
- Quick-acting NSAIDs such as ibuprofen (see Table 7-29)
- Colchicine (given PO or IV)
- Corticosteroids or ACTH for those who are intolerant of NSAIDs or colchicine
- Intraarticular cortisone when oral medication cannot be given
- General measures, such as rest, elevation, and analgesics as needed

CHRONIC Rx
- Prevention is achieved through normalization of serum urate concentration.
- Uricosuric agents (e.g., Probenecid) or xanthine oxidase inhibitors (Allopurinol) are used in patients with recurrent attacks despite adequate dietary restrictions.
- A 24-hr urine collection is useful in deciding which antihyperuremic agent is indicated. Allopurinol is generally used if the uric acid output is >900 mg/day on a regular diet. However, hypouricemic therapy should not be started for at least 2 wk after the acute attack has resolved because it may prolong the acute attack and it can also precipitate new attacks by rapidly lowering the serum uric acid level.
- Urinary uric acid hypoexcretors (<700 mg/day) can be given Probenecid (250 mg bid for 1 wk, then increased to 500 mg bid) to block absorption of uric acid. Probenecid should be started only after the acute attack of gout has completely subsided.
- Colchicine 0.6 mg bid is indicated for acute gout prophylaxis before starting hypouricemic therapy. It is generally discontinued 6 to 8 wk after normalization of serum urate levels. Long-term colchicine therapy (0.6 mg qd or bid) may be necessary in patients with frequent gout attacks despite the use of uricosuric agents.
- Surgery usually limited to excision of large tophi and, occasionally, arthroplasty

DISPOSITION
- Musculoskeletal complications are usually limited to joint disease.
- Surgery intervention may occasionally be indicated.
- Renal disease is the most frequent complication of gout after arthritis; most gouty patients develop renal disease as a result of parenchymal urate deposition but the involvement is only slowly progressive and often has no effect on life expectancy.
- Incidence of urolithiasis is increased, with 80% of calculi being uric acid stones.

REFERRAL
For orthopedic consultation when joint destruction has occurred

MISCELLANEOUS

COMMENTS
- No significant correlation between coronary artery disease and gout
- No indication to treat asymptomatic hyperuricemia
- Acute attacks of gout occasionally associated with normal levels of either acid

REFERENCES
Levinson DJ: Clinical gout and the pathogenesis of hyperuricemia. In McCarthy DJ (ed): *Arthritis and allied conditions*, ed 8, Philadelphia, 1989, Lea and Febiger.
Roubenoff R: Gout and hyperuricemia, *Rheum Dis Clin North Am* 16:539, 1990.
Author: **Lonnie R. Mercier, M.D.**

Granuloma inguinale (PTG)

BASIC INFORMATION

DEFINITION
Granuloma inguinale is caused by a gram-negative bacterium, *Calymmatobacterium granulomatis*, that may be sexually transmitted, possibly by anal intercourse.

SYNONYMS
Donovanosis

ICD-9-CM CODES
099.2 Granuloma inguinale

EPIDEMIOLOGY AND DEMOGRAPHICS
- Rare in the U.S. (<50 cases reported annually) and other developed countries
- Endemic in Australia, India, Caribbean, and Africa
- Can affect both males and females

PHYSICAL FINDINGS
- Indurated nodule is the primary lesion and is usually painless.
- Lesion erodes to granulomatous heaped ulcer, progresses slowly.
- Pathogenic features are as follows:
  1. Large infected mononuclear cell containing many Donovan bodies
  2. Intracytoplasmic location

ETIOLOGY
Calymmatobacterium granulomatis is a gram-negative bacillus that reproduces within PMN, plasma cells, and histiocytes, causing the infected cells to rupture 20 to 30 organisms.

DIAGNOSIS

DIFFERENTIAL DIAGNOSIS
- Carcinoma
- Secondary syphilis: condylomata lata
- Amebiasis: necrotic ulceration
- Concurrent infections

WORKUP
- Check for clinical manifestation:
  1. Lesions bleed easily.
  2. Lesions sharply defined and painless.
  3. Secondary infection may ensue.
  4. Inguinal involvement may cause pseudobuboes.
  5. Elephantiasis can result from obstruction of lymphatics.
  6. Suppuration and sinus formation are rare in female patients.
- Screen for other sexually transmitted diseases.
- Exclude other causes of lesions.
- Obtain stained, crushed prep from lesion.
- A clinical algorithm for evaluation of genital ulcer disease is described in Fig. 3-33.

LABORATORY TESTS
Wright stain: observation of Donovan bodies (intracellular bacteria); organisms in vacuoles within macrophages

TREATMENT

ACUTE GENERAL Rx
- Tetracycline 500 mg, qid × 3 wk
- Chloramphenicol 500 mg, q8h × 3 wk
- Gentamicin 1 mg/kg, bid × 3 wk
- Streptomycin 1 g IM, bid × 3 wk
- Ampicillin 500 g, qid × 12 wk

CHRONIC Rx
If there is a poor initial response, extend treatment. Treatment of relapses is often necessary. Avoid risky sex practices. Do not resume having sex until infection is cleared.

DISPOSITION
Routine annual or semiannual visits

REFERRAL
If response is poor, consider referral to infectious disease specialist.

MISCELLANEOUS

COMMENTS
- Patient education material can be obtained from local and state health clinics and also from ACOG.
- U.S. Preventive Services Task Force Recommendations regarding counseling to prevent HIV infection and other STDs are described in Section V, Chapter 62.

REFERENCES
American College of Obstetricians and Gynecologists: Gonorrhea and Chlamydial infections, *ACOG technical bulletin 190,* Washington, DC, 1994, ACOG.

Author: George T. Danakas, M.D.

Graves' disease (PTG)

BASIC INFORMATION

DEFINITION
Graves' disease is a hypermetabolic state characterized by thyrotoxicosis, diffuse goiter, and infiltrative ophthalmopathy; infiltrative dermopathy is occasionally present.

SYNONYMS
Thyrotoxicosis

ICD-9-CM CODES
242.0 Toxic diffuse goiter

EPIDEMIOLOGY AND DEMOGRAPHICS
INCIDENCE/PREVALENCE: Hyperthyroidism affects 2% of women and 0.2% of men in their lifetimes. Over 80% of these cases are caused by Graves' disease.
PREDOMINANT AGE: Most common before age 50 yr
GENETICS: Increased prevalence of HLA-B8 and HLA-DR3 in Caucasians with Graves' disease

PHYSICAL FINDINGS
- Tachycardia, palpitations, tremor, hyperreflexia
- Goiter, exophthalmos, lid retraction, lid lag
- Increased sweating, brittle nails, clubbing of fingers

ETIOLOGY
Autoimmune etiology: the activity of the thyroid gland is stimulated by the action of T cells, which induce specific B cells to synthesize antibodies against TSH receptors in the follicular cell membrane.

DIAGNOSIS

DIFFERENTIAL DIAGNOSIS
- Anxiety disorder
- Premenopausal state
- Thyroiditis
- Other causes of hyperthyroidism (e.g., toxic multinodular goiter, toxic adenoma)
- Other: metastatic neoplasm, diabetes mellitus, pheochromocytoma

WORKUP
The diagnostic workup includes a detailed medical history followed by laboratory and imaging studies. Patients often present with anxiety, heat intolerance, menstrual dysfunction, increased appetite and weight loss. Elderly patients can have an atypical presentation (apathetic hyperparathyroidism). For additional information, refer to the topic, "Hyperthyroidism."

LABORATORY TESTS
- Increased free thyroxine (T_4) and free triiodothyronine (T_3)
- Decreased TSH
- Presence of thyroid autoantibodies (useful in selected patients to differentiate Graves' disease from toxic nodular goiter)
- A diagnostic approach to thyroid tests is described in Fig. 3-84.

IMAGING STUDIES
24-hr radioactive iodine uptake (RAIU): increased homogeneous uptake

TREATMENT

NONPHARMACOLOGIC THERAPY
Patient education and discussion of therapeutic options

ACUTE GENERAL Rx
- Antithyroid drugs (ATDs) to inhibit thyroid hormone synthesis or peripheral conversion of T_4 to T_3
  1. Propylthiouracil (PTU) 50 to 100 mg q8h or methimazole (Tapazole) 10 to 20 mg q8h for 6 to 24 mo
  2. Side effects: skin rash (3% to 5%), arthralgias, myalgias, granulocytopenia (0.5%); rare side effects: aplastic anemia, hepatic necrosis (PTU), cholestatic jaundice (methimazole)
- Radioactive iodine (RAI)
  1. Treatment of choice for patients > 21 yr of age and younger patients who have not achieved remission after 1 yr of ATD therapy
  2. Contraindicated during pregnancy and lactation
- Surgery: near total thyroidectomy is rarely performed; indications: obstructing goiters despite RAI and ATD therapy, patients who refuse RAI and cannot be adequately managed with ATDs, and pregnant women inadequately managed with ATDs
- Adjunctive therapy: propranolol (20 to 40 mg q6h) to alleviate the β-adrenergic symptoms of hyperthyroidism (tachycardia, tremor); contraindicated in patients with CHF and bronchospasm
- Graves' ophthalmopathy: methylcellulose eye drops to protect against excessive dryness, sunglasses to decrease photophobia, systemic high-dose corticosteroids for severe exophthalmos

CHRONIC Rx
Patients undergoing treatment with ATDs should be seen every 1 to 3 mo until euthyroidism is achieved and every 3 to 4 mo while they remain on ATDs.

DISPOSITION
- ATDs induce sustained remission in <60% of cases.
- The incidence of hypothyroidism post-RAI is >50% within first year and 2%/yr thereafter.
- Complications of surgery include hypothyroidism (28% to 43% after 10 yr), hypoparathyroidism, and vocal cord paralysis (1%).
- Successful treatment of hyperthyroidism requires lifelong monitoring for the onset of hypothyroidism or the recurrence of thyrotoxicosis.

REFERRAL
- Ophthalmology referral for Graves' ophthalmopathy
- Endocrinology referral at the time of diagnosis and during treatment
- Surgical referral in rare cases (see above)
- Hospitalization of all patients with thyroid storm

MISCELLANEOUS

COMMENTS
Information on the diagnosis and treatment of "thyroid storm" and additional information on hyperthyroidism are discussed in Section I of this book.

REFERENCES
Singer PA et al: Treatment guidelines for patients with hyperthyroidism and hypothyroidism, *JAMA* 273:808, 1995.
Wartofsky L: Treatment options for hyperthyroidism, *Hosp Pract* 31:69, 1996.
Author: **Fred F. Ferri, M.D.**

Guillain-Barré syndrome

BASIC INFORMATION

DEFINITION
Guillain-Barré syndrome (GBS) is an acute inflammatory demyelinating polyradiculopathy (AIDP) predominantly affecting motor function.

SYNONYMS
Acute polyneuropathy
Ascending paralysis
GBS

ICD-9-CM CODES
357.0 Guillain-Barré

EPIDEMIOLOGY AND DEMOGRAPHICS
INCIDENCE/PREVALENCE: 1 to 2 cases/100,000 persons annually; incidence increases with age (0.8 cases/100,000 persons at age 18, 3.2 cases/100,000 persons at age 60)
RISK FACTORS: HIV, *Campylobacter jejuni* enteritis, upper respiratory infections, Epstein-Barr viral infection, CMV infection, immunizations, pregnancy, Hodgkin's lymphoma, mycoplasma infections, hepatitis B infections

PHYSICAL FINDINGS
- Symmetric weakness, initially involving proximal muscles, subsequently involving both proximal and distal muscles; difficulty in ambulating, getting up from a chair, or climbing stairs
- Depressed or absent reflexes bilaterally
- Initial manifestations involving the cranial musculature or the upper extremities (e.g., tingling of the hands) in some patients
- Minimal to moderate glove and stocking anesthesia
- Ataxia and pain in a segmental distribution in some patients (caused by involvement of posterior nerve roots)
- Autonomic abnormalities (bradycardia or tachycardia, hypotension, or hypertension)
- Respiratory insufficiency (caused by weakness of intercostal muscles)
- Facial paresis, difficulty swallowing (secondary to cranial nerve involvement)

ETIOLOGY
Infection with *C. jejuni* often precedes GBS and is associated with axonal degeneration, slow recovery, and severe residual disability.

DIAGNOSIS

DIFFERENTIAL DIAGNOSIS
- Neuropathy from heavy metals (lead, arsenic)
- Neuropathy from systemic diseases (uremia, diabetes, amyloidosis, lupus and other collagen-vascular disorders, porphyria)
- Poliomyelitis
- Botulism, diphtheria
- Hysterical paralysis
- Deficiency states (alcoholism, vitamin B_{12}, folic acid)
- Hereditary polyneuropathies

WORKUP
1. Rule out other causes of neuropathy (see above).
2. Lumbar puncture:
   - Typical findings include elevated CSF protein (especially IgG) and presence of few mononuclear leukocytes).
   - Normal values may be seen at the beginning of illness.
   - If the diagnosis is strongly suspected, a repeat lumbar puncture is indicated.
3. Electromyography reveals slowed conduction velocities; prolonged motor, sensory, and F-wave latencies are also present.

LABORATORY TESTS
- CBC may reveal early leukocytosis with left shift.
- Vitamin B_{12} level, folate, and heavy metal screening are indicated only in selected cases.

TREATMENT

NONPHARMACOLOGIC THERAPY
- Close monitoring of respiratory function (frequent measurements of vital capacity and pulmonary toilet), since respiratory failure is the major complication in GBS
- Frequent repositioning of patient to minimize formation of pressure sores
- Prevention of thromboembolism with antithrombotic stockings and SC heparin (5000 U q12h)
- Emotional support and social counseling

ACUTE GENERAL Rx
- Infusion of IV immunoglobulins (0.4 mg/kg/day for 5 days) has replaced plasmapheresis as therapy of choice at many centers. The addition of glucocorticoids (IV methylprednisolone) to IV immunoglobulins is controversial. It may result in additional improvement, but it is often associated with a high frequency of complications.
- Early therapeutic plasma exchange (TPE, plasmapheresis), started within 7 days of onset of symptoms is beneficial in preventing paralytic complications in patients with rapidly progressive disease. It is contraindicated in patients with cardiovascular disease (recent MI, unstable angina), active sepsis, and autonomic dysfunction.
- Mechanical ventilation may be needed if FEV is <12 to 15 ml/kg, vital capacity is rapidly decreasing or is <1000 ml and PaO_2 is <70, or the patient is having significant difficulty clearing secretions and is aspirating.

CHRONIC Rx
- Ventilatory support: may be necessary in 10% to 20% of patients
- Aggressive nursing care to prevent decubiti, infections, fecal impactions, and pressure nerve palsies
- Monitoring and treatment of autonomic dysfunction (bradyarrhythmias or tachyarrhythmias, orthostatic hypotension, systemic hypertension, altered sweating)
- Treatment of back pain and dysesthesia with low-dose tricyclics
- Stress ulcer prevention in patients receiving ventilator support

DISPOSITION
- Mortality is approximately 3%.
- Prognosis for full recovery is very good. Only 15% to 20% of patients may have minor residual motor deficits.

REFERRAL
Tracheostomy may be necessary in patients with prolonged ventilatory support.

MISCELLANEOUS

COMMENTS
Patient education information may be obtained from the Guillain-Barré Foundation International, Box 262, Wynnewood, PA 19096; phone: (610) 667-0131.

REFERENCES
Griffin JW, Ho TW: Guillain-Barré syndromes. In Johnson RT, Griffin JW (eds): *Current therapy in neurologic disease*, ed 5, St Louis, 1996, Mosby.
Rees JH et al: *Campylobacter jejuni* infection and Guillain-Barré syndrome, N Engl J Med 333:1374, 1995.
Author: **Fred F. Ferri, M.D.**

Headache, cluster (PTG)

BASIC INFORMATION

DEFINITION
The term *cluster headache* refers to recurrent episodes of intense, unilateral headache centered around the orbit and lasting 30 to 120 min. Headaches occur in clusters lasting 4 to 12 wk, during which one to three episodes occur per day at predictable times, typically during sleep. The episodes then remit for months to years.

SYNONYMS (all obsolete terms)
Horton's headache
Histaminic cephalgia
Vidian neuralgis
Sphenopalatine neuralgia

ICD-9-CM CODES
346.2 Variants of migraine

EPIDEMIOLOGY AND DEMOGRAPHICS
INCIDENCE (IN U.S.): Unknown
PREVALENCE (IN U.S.): Unknown
PREDOMINANT SEX: Male:female ratio of 10:1
PREDOMINANT AGE: Third to fourth decade, rarely in children
PEAK INCIDENCE: Age 30 yr
GENETICS:
- Unknown
- Association with hazel eye color and "masculine" facial features reported

PHYSICAL FINDINGS
- During attack: conjunctival injection, lacrimation, nasal congestion rhinorrhea, facial sweating, myosis, ptosis, eyelid edema
- Typical avoidance of immobility, with patients pacing, stomping, or running
- Permanent partial Horner's syndrome in 5% of patients; otherwise examination normal

ETIOLOGY
Unknown

DIAGNOSIS

DIFFERENTIAL DIAGNOSIS
- Migraine
- Trigeminal neuralgia
- Arteritis
- Postherpetic neuralgia
- Intracranial mass
- Table 2-29 describes the differential diagnosis of headaches.

WORKUP
- Diagnosis is usually established by characteristic history.
- Imaging studies are sometimes warranted if diagnosis is uncertain.

LABORATORY TESTS
None

IMAGING STUDIES
None, unless history or examination suggests structural etiology.

TREATMENT

NONPHARMACOLOGIC THERAPY
- Avoidance of ethanol and tobacco during clusters
- Surgical ablation of components of the trigeminal nerve in rare instances

ACUTE GENERAL Rx
- Inhalation of 100% oxygen by face mask at 8 to 10 L/min for 15 min often aborts an attack.
- Sumatriptan 6 mg SC or ergotamines may abort an attack or prevent one if given just before a predictable episode.

CHRONIC Rx
Various medications have been tried without great success, although good responses may be obtained in up to 50% of cases. Examples include:
- Prednisone: 30 to 60 mg/day for 1 to 2 wk, then taper
- Lithium: 200 mg tid with frequent monitoring and adjustment to maintain therapeutic serum level
- Verapamil: Up to 240 mg/day as tolerated
- Methysergide: 1 to 2 mg tid; requires familiarity with the potential adverse effects and use of "drug holidays" to decrease risk of fibrosis

DISPOSITION
- Most patients continue to have clusters with variable periods of remission.
- Response to medication is variable.

REFERRAL
- If unfamiliar with potential adverse effects or contraindications of medication
- If surgical opinion is desired for medication failure

MISCELLANEOUS

REFERENCES
Pearce JMS: Cluster headache and its variants, *Postgrad Med* 68:517, 1992.
Author: **Michael Gruenthal, M.D., Ph.D.**

Headache, migraine (PTG)

BASIC INFORMATION

DEFINITION
Migraine headaches are recurrent headaches of variable intensity and duration, often unilateral and associated with nausea and vomiting. Some headaches are preceded by, or associated with, neurologic or mood disturbances.

ICD-9-CM CODES
346 Migraine

EPIDEMIOLOGY AND DEMOGRAPHICS
INCIDENCE (IN U.S.): Females: 22 cases/1000 persons/yr, males: 5 cases/1000 persons/yr
PREVALENCE (IN U.S.): Females: 18%; males: 6%
PREDOMINANT SEX: Female:male ratio of 3:1
PREDOMINANT AGE: >10 yr
PEAK INCIDENCE: Teenage years
GENETICS:
- Familial predisposition, with up to 90% of migraineurs having an affected family member
- Autosomal dominant transmission with incomplete penetrance postulated

PHYSICAL FINDINGS
- Normal between episodes
- During migraine with aura, focal motor or sensory abnormalities possible, but first episode of any headache associated with neurologic deficits requires thorough investigation

ETIOLOGY
- Unknown
- Early theories of primary vascular mechanism have been replaced by proposals that primary neuronal event is responsible.

DIAGNOSIS

DIFFERENTIAL DIAGNOSIS
- Subarachnoid hemorrhage
- Tumor
- Aneurysm
- Arteriovenous malformation
- Meningitis
- Table 2-29 describes the differential diagnosis of headaches.

WORKUP
- Generally no additional investigation is needed with recurrent, typical attacks with typical age of onset, family history, and a normal physical examination.
- Diagnosis is not based on first headache.
- If there is an unusual presentation and/or unexpected findings on examination, investigation for other causes is required.

LABORATORY TESTS
None

IMAGING STUDIES
- Not routinely necessary for typical cases
- If diagnosis uncertain: MRI, MRA, or conventional angiography to detect other causes

TREATMENT

NONPHARMACOLOGIC THERAPY
- Avoid any identifiable provoking factors: caffeine, tobacco, and alcohol may trigger attacks, as may dietary or other environmental precipitants (less common).
- Try biofeedback (effective in some cases).

ACUTE GENERAL Rx
- Medications effective in aborting an attack include nonnarcotic analgesics (NSAIDs, acetaminophen), vasoactive drugs (ergotamine preparations, sumatriptan), and opioids (meperidine, butorphanol nasal spray).
- Early administration improves effectiveness.

CHRONIC Rx
- Medications that provide migraine prophylaxis include β-blockers, calcium channel blockers, antidepressants, anticonvulsants, and serotonin antagonists.
- Prophylactic treatment is generally indicated when headaches occur more than twice a week or when symptomatic treatments are contraindicated or not effective.

DISPOSITION
- After age 30 yr, 40% of patients are migraine free.
- Chronic daily headache is possible, sometimes representing rebound headache caused by overuse of analgesics.

REFERRAL
If uncertain about diagnosis or treatment not effective

MISCELLANEOUS

REFERENCES
Solomon S: Migraine diagnosis and clinical symptomatology, *Headache* 34:S8, 1994.

Author: **Michael Gruenthal, M.D., Ph.D.**

Headache, tension-type (PTG)

BASIC INFORMATION

DEFINITION
Tension headaches are recurrent headaches lasting 30 min to 7 days without nausea or vomiting and with at least two of the following characteristics: pressing or tightening quality, mild or moderate intensity, bilateral, and not aggravated by routine physical activity.

SYNONYMS
Muscle contraction headache
Tension headache
Stress headache
Ordinary headache
Psychomyogenic headache
Psychogenic headache
Essential headache

ICD-9-CM CODES
307.81 Tension headache

EPIDEMIOLOGY AND DEMOGRAPHICS
INCIDENCE (IN U.S.):
- Undetermined
- Believed to be the most common type of headache

PREVALENCE (IN U.S.): Males: 63%/yr; females: 86%/yr
PREDOMINANT SEX: Females > males
PREDOMINANT AGE: >10 yr
PEAK INCIDENCE: Occurs at all ages
GENETICS: Not established

PHYSICAL FINDINGS
No abnormalities

ETIOLOGY
- Unknown
- There is no recent data to support the long-standing belief that these headaches arise from stress or other psychologic factors.
- There is a belief that tension-type headaches and migraine represent two ends of a continuum with similar pathogenesis.

DIAGNOSIS

DIFFERENTIAL DIAGNOSIS
- Migraine
- Cervical spine disease
- Intracranial mass
- Idiopathic intracranial hypertension
- Rebound headache from overuse of analgesics
- Table 2-29 describes the differential diagnosis of headaches.

WORKUP
- Thorough history and physical examination for any new-onset headache
- Imaging studies to rule out intracranial abnormalities

LABORATORY TESTS
No routine tests
ESR in elderly patients suspected of having cranial arteritis

IMAGING STUDIES
CT scan and/or MRI to exclude intracranial pathology as cause of new-onset headaches

TREATMENT

NONPHARMACOLOGIC THERAPY
- Relaxation training
- Biofeedback
- Heat
- Massage
- Ultrasound
- Stretching exercises

ACUTE GENERAL Rx
Nonnarcotic analgesics with limited frequency to prevent drug-induced headache

CHRONIC Rx
- Antidepressants (e.g., amitriptyline 10 to 150 mg hs)
- Trigger point injections
- Occipital nerve blocks

DISPOSITION
Rarely responds fully to treatment

REFERRAL
If uncertain about diagnosis

MISCELLANEOUS

REFERENCES
Silberstein SD: Tension-type headaches, *Headache* 34:S2, 1994.
Author: **Michael Gruenthal, M.D., Ph.D.**

Heart block, complete

BASIC INFORMATION

DEFINITION
In complete heart block, there is complete blockage of all AV conduction. The atria and ventricles have separate, independent rhythms.

SYNONYMS
Third-degree AV block

ICD-9-CM CODES
426.0 Complete heart block

EPIDEMIOLOGY AND DEMOGRAPHICS
Over 100,000 permanent pacemakers are implanted worldwide each year for complete heart block.

PHYSICAL FINDINGS
Physical examination may be normal. Patients may present with the following clinical manifestations:
- Dizziness, palpitations
- Stokes-Adams syncopal attacks
- CHF
- Angina

ETIOLOGY
- Degenerative changes in His-Purkinje system
- Acute anterior wall MI
- Calcific aortic stenosis
- Cardiomyopathy
- Trauma
- Cardiovascular surgery
- Congenital

DIAGNOSIS

DIFFERENTIAL DIAGNOSIS
The differential diagnosis involves only the etiology. ECG will confirm diagnosis.

WORKUP
ECG:
- P waves constantly change their relationship to the QRS complexes.
- Ventricular rate is usually <50 bpm (may be higher in congenital forms).
- Ventricular rate is generally lower than the atrial rate.
- QRS complex is wide.

TREATMENT

ACUTE GENERAL Rx
- Immediate pacemaker insertion unless the patient has congenital third-degree AV block and is completely asymptomatic
- Therapy of underlying etiology

CHRONIC Rx
Patients with permanent pacemakers need regular follow-up and pacemaker monitoring to ensure proper sensing.

DISPOSITION
Prognosis is favorable following insertion of pacemaker and related to the underlying etiology of complete AV block (e.g., MI, cardiomyopathy).

REFERRAL
Referral for implantation of permanent pacemaker

MISCELLANEOUS

COMMENTS
- Patients should be instructed on avoidance of activities that may damage the pacemaker (e.g., contact sports).
- Common environmental causes of pacemaker malformation are electrocautery, transthoracic defibrillation, MRI, extracorporeal shock wave lithotripsy, transcutaneous electrical nerve stimulation, therapeutic radiation, ECT, diathermy, radiofrequency ablation for treatment of tachyarrhythmias.

REFERENCES
Kusumoto SM, Goldschlager N: Cardiac pacing, *New Engl J Med* 334:89, 1996.

Author: **Fred F. Ferri, M.D.**

BASIC INFORMATION

DEFINITION
Second-degree heart block is the blockage of some (but not all) impulses from the atria to the ventricles. There are two types of second-degree AV block:

MOBITZ TYPE I (WENCKEBACH):
- There is a progressive prolongation of the PR interval before an impulse is completely blocked; the cycle repeats periodically.
- Cycle with dropped beat is less than two times the previous cycle.
- Site of block is usually AV node (proximal to the bundle of His).

MOBITZ TYPE II:
- There is a sudden interruption of AV conduction without prior prolongation of the PR interval.
- Site of block is infranodal.

SYNONYMS
Wenckebach block (Mobitz type I block)
Mobitz type II block

ICD-9-CM CODES
426.13 Mobitz type I
426.12 Mobitz type II

EPIDEMIOLOGY AND DEMOGRAPHICS
Mobitz type I block is more common and may occur in individuals with heightened vagal tone or secondary to some medications such as β-blockers or calcium channel blockers.

PHYSICAL FINDINGS
- Patients with Mobitz type I are usually asymptomatic.
- Sudden loss of consciousness without warning (Adams-Stokes attack) can occur in patients with Mobitz type II; however, it is much more common in patients with complete heart block.
- Irregular pulse with dropped beats is present (Mobitz type I).
- Irregular pulse with occasional dropped beats is present (Mobitz type II).

ETIOLOGY
MOBITZ TYPE I:
- Vagal stimulation
- Degenerative changes in the AV conduction system
- Ischemia at the AV nodes (particularly in inferior wall MI)
- Drugs (digitalis, quinidine, procainamide, adenosine, calcium channel blockers, β-blockers)
- Cardiomyopathies
- Aortic regurgitation
- Lyme carditis

MOBITZ TYPE II:
- Degenerative changes in the His-Purkinje system
- Acute anterior wall MI
- Calcific aortic stenosis

DIAGNOSIS

DIFFERENTIAL DIAGNOSIS
The ECG will distinguish between Mobitz type I and Mobitz type II block and other conduction abnormalities.

WORKUP
ECG, 24-hr Holter monitor (selected patients)

MOBITZ TYPE I: ECG shows:
- Gradual prolongation of PR interval leading to a blocked beat
- Shortened PR interval after dropped beat

MOBITZ TYPE II: ECG shows:
- Fixed duration of PR interval
- Sudden appearance of blocked beats

TREATMENT

NONPHARMACOLOGIC THERAPY
Elimination of drugs that may induce AV block

ACUTE GENERAL Rx
MOBITZ TYPE I:
- Treatment generally is not necessary. This type of block is usually transient.
- If symptomatic (e.g., dizziness), atropine 1 mg (may repeat once after 5 min) may be tried to increase AV conduction; if no response, insert temporary pacemaker.
- If block is secondary to drugs (e.g., digitalis), discontinue the drug.
- If associated with anterior wall MI and wide QRS escape rhythm, consider insertion of temporary pacemaker.
- Significant AV block post-MI may be caused by adenosine produced by the ischemic myocardium. These arrhythmias (which may be resistant to conventional therapy such as atropine) may respond to theophylline (adenosine antagonist).

MOBITZ TYPE II:
- Pacemaker insertion is needed, since this type of block is usually permanent and often progresses to complete AV block.

DISPOSITION
Prognosis is good with insertion of pacemaker in patients with Mobitz type II.

REFERRAL
Referral for pacemaker insertion (see "Acute General Rx")

MISCELLANEOUS

COMMENTS
Patients with Mobitz type I should be followed routinely for potential development of high-grade AV block.

REFERENCES
Bertolet BD et al: Theophylline for the treatment of atrioventricular block after myocardial infarction, *Ann Intern Med* 123:509, 1995.
Ferri FF: *Practical guide to the care of the medical patient,* ed 4, St Louis, 1998, Mosby.

Author: Fred F. Ferri, M.D.

Heat exhaustion and heat stroke (PTG)

BASIC INFORMATION

DEFINITION
HEAT EXHAUSTION: An illness resulting from prolonged heavy activity in a hot environment with subsequent dehydration, electrolyte depletion, and rectal temperature >37.8° C.
HEAT STROKE: A life-threatening heat illness characterized by extreme hyperthermia, dehydration, and neurologic manifestations.

SYNONYMS
Heat illness
Hyperthermia

ICD-9-CM CODES
992.0 Heat stroke
992.5 Heat exhaustion

EPIDEMIOLOGY AND DEMOGRAPHICS
Heat exhaustion and stroke occur more frequently in elderly patients, especially those taking diuretics or medications that impair heat dissipation (e.g., phenothiazines, anticholinergics, antihistamines, β-blockers).

PHYSICAL FINDINGS
HEAT EXHAUSTION: Profuse sweating, tachycardia, hypertension, hyperventilation
HEAT STROKE: Elevated body temperature (usually >40° C), delirium, seizures, coma, skin pallor, anhydrosis

ETIOLOGY
- Exogenous heat gain (increased ambient temperature)
- Increased heat production (exercise, infection, hyperthyroidism, drugs)
- Impaired heat dissipation (high humidity, heavy clothing, neonatal or elderly patients, drugs [phenothiazines, anticholinergics, antihistamines, butyrophenones, amphetamines, cocaine, alcohol, β-blockers])

DIAGNOSIS

DIFFERENTIAL DIAGNOSIS
- Infections (meningitis, encephalitis, sepsis)
- Head trauma
- Epilepsy
- Thyroid storm
- Acute cocaine intoxication
- Malignant hyperthermia
- Heat exhaustion can be differentiated from heat stroke by the following:
  1. Essentially intact mental function and lack of significant fever in heat exhaustion
  2. Mild or absent increases in CPK, AST, LDH, ALT in heat exhaustion

WORKUP
- Heat stroke: comprehensive history, physical examination, and laboratory evaluation.
- Heat exhaustion: in most cases, laboratory tests are not necessary for diagnosis.

LABORATORY TESTS
Laboratory abnormalities may include the following:
- Elevated BUN, creatinine, Hct
- Hyponatremia or hypernatremia, hyperkalemia or hypokalemia
- Elevated LDH, AST, ALT, CPK, bilirubin
- Lactic acidosis, respiratory alkalosis (secondary to hyperventilation)
- Myoglobinuria, hypofibrinogenemia, fibrinolysis, hypocalcemia

TREATMENT

NONPHARMACOLOGIC THERAPY
- Treatment of **heat exhaustion** consists primarily of placing the patient in a cool, shaded area and providing rapid hydration and salt replacement.
  1. Fluid intake should be at least 2 L q4h in patients without history of CHF.
  2. Salt replacement can be accomplished by using ¼ teaspoon of salt or two 10-grain salt tablets dissolved in 1 L of water.
  3. If IV fluid replacement is necessary, young athletes can be given normal saline IV (3 to 4 L over 6 to 8 hr); in elderly patients, consider using $D_5 1/2 NS$ IV with rate titrated to cardiovascular status.
- Patients with **heat stroke** should undergo rapid cooling.
  1. Clothing should be removed.
  2. The patient should be placed in a cool, well-ventilated room.
  3. Monitory body temperature q5min.
  4. The goal is to reduce body temperature to 39° C (102.2° F) in 30 to 60 min).
  5. Spray the patient with a cool mist and use fans to enhance air flow over the body (rapid evaporation method).
  6. Immersion of the patient in ice water, stomach lavage with iced saline solution, IV administration of cool fluids, and inhalation of cold air are advisable only when other means for rapid evaporation are not available.
  7. Ice packs should not be used because they increase peripheral vasoconstriction and may induce shivering.
  8. Antipyretics are ineffective because the hypothalamic set point during heat stroke is normal despite increased body temperature.
  9. Immersion in tepid water (15° C, 59° F) is preferred over ice water immersion to minimize risk of shivering.
- Intubate comatose patients and insert Foley catheter.
- Continuous ECG monitoring is recommended.
- Begin IV hydration with NS or lactated Ringer's solution.

ACUTE GENERAL Rx
In addition to the treatment given above, the patient should be monitored and aggressively treated for the following complications:
- Hypotension: vigorous hydration with NS or LR solution
- Convulsions: diazepam 5 to 10 mg IV (slowly)
- Shivering: chlorpromazine 25 to 50 mg IV
- Acidosis: judicious use of bicarbonate (only in severe acidosis)
- Monitoring for evidence of rhabdomyolysis, hepatic, renal, or cardiac failure and treating accordingly

DISPOSITION
Most patients recover completely within 48 hr. Mortality can exceed 30% in patients with prolonged and severe hyperthermia.

MISCELLANEOUS

COMMENTS
Patients should be educated as to the precipitating factors leading to heat illness and should be instructed to acclimatize slowly in warm environments, drink adequate amounts of fluids in warm climate, and limit strenuous activities.

REFERENCES
Aiyer NK et al: Techniques for managing hyperthermia, *J Crit Ill* 10(9):630-640, 1995.
Sandor RP: Heat illness, *Physician Sports Med* 25:35-40, 1997.
Author: **Fred F. Ferri, M.D.**

BASIC INFORMATION

DEFINITION
Hemochromatosis is an autosomal recessive disorder characterized by increased accumulation of iron in various organs (adrenals, liver, pancreas, heart, testes, kidneys, pituitary) and eventual dysfunction of these organs if not treated appropriately.

SYNONYMS
Bronze diabetes

ICD-9-CM CODES
275.0 Hemochromatosis

EPIDEMIOLOGY AND DEMOGRAPHICS
- Hemochromatosis is generally diagnosed in males in their fifth decade.
- Diagnosis in females is generally not made until 10 to 20 yr postmenopause.
- Incidence in Caucasians is approximately 1 in 300 persons.

PHYSICAL FINDINGS
Examination may be normal; patient with advanced case may present with the following:
- Increased skin pigmentation
- Hepatomegaly, splenomegaly, hepatic tenderness, testicular atrophy
- Loss of body hair, peripheral edema, gynecomastia, ascites
- Amenorrhea (25% of females)
- Loss of libido (50% of males)
- Arthropathy

ETIOLOGY
- Autosomal recessive disease with frequent linkage to HLA-A 3, HLA-B 14, and HLA-B 7
- Increased iron absorption despite excessive iron stores, resulting in increased accumulation of iron as hemosiderin

DIAGNOSIS

DIFFERENTIAL DIAGNOSIS
- Hereditary anemias with defect of erythropoiesis
- Cirrhosis
- Repeated blood transfusions

WORKUP
Medical history, physical examination, and laboratory evaluation should be focused on affected organ systems (see "Physical Findings"); liver biopsy is the gold standard for diagnosis; it reveals iron deposition in hepatocytes, bile ducts, and supporting tissues.

LABORATORY TESTS
- Elevated serum ferritin, plasma iron, saturation of transferrin (>50%)
- Elevated AST, ALT, alkaline phosphatase
- Hyperglycemia
- Endocrine abnormalities (decreased testosterone, LH, FSH)
- Measurement of hepatic iron index in liver biopsy specimen can confirm diagnosis

IMAGING STUDIES
CT scan or MRI of the liver is useful to exclude other etiologies and may in some cases show iron overload in the liver.

TREATMENT

NONPHARMACOLOGIC THERAPY
Weekly phlebotomies of 500 ml of blood should be continued for several months until depletion of iron stores is achieved. Subsequent phlebotomies can be performed every 3 to 6 mo depending on Hct and serum iron determinations.

ACUTE GENERAL Rx
Deferoxamine (iron chelating agent) is generally reserved for patients with severe hemochromatosis with diffuse organ involvement (e.g., liver disease, heart disease) and when phlebotomy is not possible. It is administered in a dose of 0.5 to 1 g IM qd or 20 mg SC over a 12- to 24-hr period with a constant infusion pump.

CHRONIC Rx
Phlebotomy on a PRN basis depending on the Hct level; generally, Hct should not exceed 40%.

DISPOSITION
Prognosis is good if phlebotomy is started early (before onset of cirrhosis or diabetes mellitus); women can have the full phenotypic expression of the disease, including cirrhosis, and should also be aggressively treated.

REFERRAL
For liver biopsy if diagnosis is uncertain.

MISCELLANEOUS

COMMENTS
- Patient education material on hemochromatosis can be obtained from the Hemochromatosis Research Foundation, Inc., PO Box 8569, Albany, NY 12208.
- Cirrhotic patients must be periodically monitored (ultrasound or CT scan) because of their increased risk of hepatocellular carcinoma.
- Screening for hemachromatosis in siblings with HLA typing and family members with serum iron studies is recommended.

REFERENCES
Baer DN et al: Hemochromatosis screening in asymptomatic ambulatory men 30 years of age and older, *Am J Med* 98:464, 1995.

Bula J et al: Clinical and biochemical abnormalities in people heterozygous for hemochromatosis, *New Engl J Med* 335:1799, 1996.

Moirand R et al: Clinical features of genetic hemochromatosis in women compared with men, *Ann Intern Med* 127:105, 1997.

Author: **Fred F. Ferri, M.D.**

Hemophilia (PTG)

BASIC INFORMATION

DEFINITION
Hemophilia is a hereditary bleeding disorder caused by low Factor VIII coagulant activity (hemophilia A) or low levels of Factor IX coagulant activity (hemophilia B).

SYNONYMS
Hemophilia A: Classic hemophilia, Factor VIII deficiency hemophilia
Hemophilia B: Christmas disease, Factor IX hemophilia

ICD-9-CM CODES
286.0 Hemophilia A
286.1 Hemophilia B

EPIDEMIOLOGY AND DEMOGRAPHICS
INCIDENCE/PREVALENCE (IN U.S.): Hemophilia A: 100 cases/1,000,000 males, hemophilia B: 20 cases/1,000,000 males
GENETIC FACTORS: Both hemophilias have an X-link recessive pattern of inheritance with only males affected.

PHYSICAL FINDINGS
- Bleeding is most commonly seen in joints (knees, ankles, elbows) resulting in hot, swollen, painful joints and subsequent crippling joint deformity.
- Bleeding can also occur into the muscles and the GI tract.
- Compartment syndromes can occur from large hematomas.
- Hematuria may be present.

ETIOLOGY
- Hemophilia A: low Factor VIII coagulant (VIII:C) activity; can be classified as mild if Factor VIII:C levels are >5%, moderate: levels are 1% to 5%, severe: levels are <1%
- Hemophilia B: low levels of Factor IX coagulant activity
- Both disorders are congenital.
- Spontaneous acquisition of Factor VIII inhibitors (acquired hemophilia) is rare.

DIAGNOSIS

DIFFERENTIAL DIAGNOSIS
- Other clotting factor deficiencies
- Platelet function disorders
- Vitamin K deficiency
- Fig. 3-17 describes a clinical algorithm for evaluation of congenital bleeding disorders. Table 2-10 describes the presumptive diagnosis of common bleeding disorders based on routine screening tests.

WORKUP
Patients with mild hemophilia bleed only in response to major trauma or surgery and may not be diagnosed until young adulthood. Diagnostic workup includes laboratory evaluation (see "Laboratory Tests").

LABORATORY TESTS
- Partial thromboplastin time (PTT) is prolonged.
- Reduced Factor VIII:C level distinguishes hemophilia A from other causes of prolonged PTT.
- Factor VIII antigen, PT, fibrinogen level, and bleeding time are normal.
- Factor IX coagulant activity levels are reduced in patients with hemophilia B.
- Coagulation factor activity measurement is useful to correlate with disease severity: normal range is 50 to 150 U/dl; 5 to 20 U/dl indicates mild disease, 2 to 5 U/dl indicates moderate disease, and <2 U/dl indicates severe disease with spontaneous bleeding episodes.

TREATMENT

NONPHARMACOLOGIC THERAPY
- Avoidance of contact sports
- Patient education regarding their disease; promotion of exercises such as swimming
- Avoidance of aspirin or other NSAIDs
- Orthopedic evaluation and physical therapy evaluation in patients with joint involvement
- Hepatitis vaccination

ACUTE GENERAL Rx
HEMOPHILIA A:
- Infuse Factor VIII concentrates.
- Desmopressin acetate 0.3 µg/kg q24h (causes release of Factor VIII:C) may be used in preparation for minor surgical procedures in mild hemophiliacs.
- Aminocaproic acid (EACA, Amicar) 4 g PO q4h can be given for persistent bleeding that is unresponsive to Factor VIII concentrate or desmopressin.

HEMOPHILIA B:
- Infuse Factor IX concentrates. It is important to remember that Factor IX concentrates contain other proteins that may increase the risk of thrombosis with recurrent use. Therefore Factor IX concentrates must be used only when clearly indicated.
- Daily administration of oral cyclophosphamide and prednisone without empirical Factor VIII therapy is an effective and well tolerated treatment for acquired hemophilia.

CHRONIC Rx
The aim of chronic treatment is to prevent spontaneous bleeding and to prevent excessive bleeding during any surgical intervention.

DISPOSITION
Despite the advent of virally safe blood products and blood treatment programs, nearly 70% of hemophiliacs are HIV-seropositive. Survival is of normal expectancy in HIV-negative patients with mild disease.

REFERRAL
- Outpatient home infusion therapy is preferred. However, significant bleeding episodes will require inpatient treatment for infusions.
- Orthopedic referral may be necessary in patients with severe joint deformity and crippling.

MISCELLANEOUS

COMMENTS
Additional patient education information can be obtained from the National Hemophilia Foundation, 110 Green Street, Room 406, New York, NY 10002.

REFERENCES
Cohen AJ, Kessler CM: Treatment of inherited coagulation disorders, *Am J Med* 99:675, 1995.

Hoyer LW: Hemophilia, *N Engl J Med* 330:38, 1994.

Shaffer L, Phillips M: Successful treatment of acquired hemophilia with oral immunosuppressive therapy, *Ann Intern Med* 127:206, 1997.

Author: **Fred F. Ferri, M.D.**

Hemorrhoids

BASIC INFORMATION

DEFINITION
A hemorrhoid is a varicose dilatation of a vein of the superior or inferior hemorrhoidal plexus, resulting from a persistent increase in venous pressure. External hemorrhoids are below the pectinate line (inferior plexus). Internal hemorrhoids are above the pectinate line (superior plexus).

SYNONYMS
Piles

ICD-9-CM CODES
455.6 Hemorrhoids

EPIDEMIOLOGY AND DEMOGRAPHICS
- Potential for development of symptomatic hemorrhoids in all adults
- Prevalence: estimated 50% of the adult population in the U.S.
- Males = females

PHYSICAL FINDINGS
- Painless bleeding with defecation; bleeding is bright red and staining on toilet paper
- Perianal irritation
- Mucofecal staining of underclothes
- Acute external hemorrhoids: painful, swollen, and often thrombosed
- Prolapse
- Constipation

ETIOLOGY
- Low-fiber, high-fat diet
- Chronic constipation and straining with defecation
- High resting anal sphincter pressures
- Pregnancy
- Obesity
- Rectal surgery (i.e., episiotomy)
- Prolonged sitting
- Anal intercourse

DIAGNOSIS

DIFFERENTIAL DIAGNOSIS
- Fissure
- Abscess
- Anal fistula
- Warts
- Hypertrophied anal papillae
- Rectal prolapse
- Rectal polyp
- Neoplasm

WORKUP
- Inspection
- Digital rectal examination
- Anoscopy
- Sigmoidoscopy

TREATMENT

NONPHARMACOLOGIC THERAPY
- Avoidance of constipation and straining with defecation
- Avoidance of prolonged sitting on toilet
- High-fiber diet (20 to 30 g/day)
- Increased fluid intake (six to eight glasses of water per day)
- Cleaning with mild soap and water after defecation
- Warm soaks or ice to soothe
- Sitz baths

ACUTE GENERAL Rx
- Fiber supplements to provide bulk (psyllium extracts or mucilloids)
- Medicated compresses with witch hazel
- Topical hydrocortisone (1% to 3% cream or ointment)
- Topical anesthetic spray
- Glycerin suppositories
- Stool softeners

CHRONIC Rx
- Rubber-band ligation
- Injection sclerotherapy
- Photocoagulation
- Cryodestruction
- Hemorrhoidectomy
- Anal dilatation
- Laser or cautery hemorrhoidectomy
- Observance for complications: thrombosis, bleeding, infection, anal stenosis or weakness

DISPOSITION
Should resolve, but there is a high rate of recurrence

REFERRAL
To colorectal surgeon for any hemorrhoid that does not respond to conservative therapy

MISCELLANEOUS

COMMENTS
- Patients need to understand the importance of a healthy diet, regular exercise, and rectal hygiene.
- Stress the importance of avoiding prolonged sitting and straining on the toilet.
- Stress the need not to defer the urge to defecate.

REFERENCES
Barnett JL, Raper SE: Anorectal diseases. In Yamada T, Alpers DH, Owyang C: *Textbook of gastroenterology,* ed 2, Philadelphia, 1995, Lippincott.

Beart RW Jr: Common anorectal problems. In Sciarra JJ: *Gynecology and obstetrics,* Philadelphia, 1997, Lippincott.

Author: **Maria A. Corigliano, M.D.**

Hepatic encephalopathy

BASIC INFORMATION

DEFINITION
Hepatic encephalopathy is an abnormal mental status occurring in patients with severe impairment of liver function and consequent accumulation of toxic products not metabolized by the liver.

SYNONYMS
Hepatic coma

ICD-9-CM CODES
572.2 Hepatic encephalopathy

EPIDEMIOLOGY AND DEMOGRAPHICS
INCIDENCE/PREVALENCE: Hepatic encephalopathy occurs in > 30% of all cases of cirrhosis.

PHYSICAL FINDINGS
Hepatic encephalopathy can be classified in stages or grades 1 to 4:
- Grades 1 and 2: mild obtundation
- Grades 3 and 4: stupor to deep coma, with or without decerebrate posturing.

The physical examination in hepatic encephalopathy varies with the stage and may reveal the following abnormalities:
- Skin: jaundice, palmar erythema, spider angiomata, ecchymosis, dilated superficial periumbilical veins (caput medusae) in patients with cirrhosis
- Eyes: scleral icterus, Kayser-Fleischer rings (Wilson's disease)
- Breath: fetor hepaticus
- Chest: gynecomastia in men with chronic liver disease
- Abdomen: ascites, small nodular liver (cirrhosis), tender hepatomegaly (congestive hepatomegaly)
- Rectal examination: hemorrhoids (portal hypertension), guaiac-positive stool (alcoholic gastritis, bleeding esophageal varices, PUD, bleeding hemorrhoids)
- Genitalia: testicular atrophy in males with chronic liver disease
- Extremities: pedal edema from hypoalbuminemia
- Neurologic: flapping tremor-asterixis, obtundation, coma with or without decerebrate posturing

ETIOLOGY
- Precipitating factors in patients with underlying cirrhosis (UGI bleeding, hypokalemia, hypomagnesemia, analgesic and sedative drugs, sepsis, alkalosis, increased dietary protein)
- Acute fulminant viral hepatitis
- Drugs and toxins (e.g., isoniazid, acetaminophen, diclofenac, statins, methyldopa, loratadine, PTU, lisinopril, labetalol, halothane, carbon tetrachloride, erythromycin, nitrofurantoin, troglitazone)
- Reye's syndrome
- Shock and/or sepsis
- Fatty liver of pregnancy
- Metastatic carcinoma, hepatocellular carcinoma
- Other: autoimmune hepatitis, ischemic venoocclusive disease, sclerosing cholangitis, heat stroke, amebic abscesses

DIAGNOSIS

DIFFERENTIAL DIAGNOSIS
- Delirium secondary to medications or illicit drugs
- CVA, subdural hematoma
- Meningitis, encephalitis
- Hypoglycemia
- Uremia
- Cerebral anoxia
- Hypercalcemia
- Metastatic neoplasm to brain
- Alcohol withdrawal syndrome

WORKUP
Exclude other etiologies with comprehensive history (obtained from patient, relatives, and others), physical examination, laboratory and imaging studies. A pertinent history should include exposure to hepatitis, ethanol intake, drug history, exposure to toxins, IV drug abuse, measles or influenza with aspirin use (Reye's syndrome), history of carcinoma (primary or metastatic).

LABORATORY TESTS
- ALT, AST, bilirubin, alkaline phosphatase glucose, calcium, electrolytes, BUN, creatinine, albumin
- CBC, platelet count, PT, PTT
- Serum and urine toxicology screen in suspected medication or illegal drug use
- Blood and urine cultures, urinalysis
- Venous ammonia level
- ABGs

IMAGING STUDIES
CT scan of head may be useful in selected patients to exclude other etiologies.

TREATMENT

NONPHARMACOLOGIC THERAPY
- Identification and treatment of precipitating factors
- Restriction of protein intake (30 to 40 g/day) to reduce toxic protein metabolites

ACUTE GENERAL Rx
REDUCTION OF COLONIC AMMONIA PRODUCTION:
- Lactulose 30 ml of 50% solution qid initially, dose is subsequently adjusted depending on clinical response.
- Neomycin 1 g PO q4-6h or given as a 1% retention enema solution (1 g in 100 ml of isotonic saline solution); neomycin should be used with caution in patients with renal insufficiency; metronidazole may be as effective as neomycin and is not nephrotoxic.
- A combination of lactulose and neomycin can be used when either agent is ineffective alone.

TREATMENT OF CEREBRAL EDEMA:
Cerebral edema is often present in patients with acute liver failure, and it accounts for nearly 50% of deaths. Monitoring intracranial pressure by epidural, intraparenchymal, or subdural transducers and treatment of cerebral edema with mannitol (100 to 200 ml of 20% solution [0.3 to 0.4 g/kg of body weight]) given by rapid IV infusion is helpful in selected patients (e.g., potential transplantation patients).

CHRONIC Rx
- Avoidance of any precipitating factors (e.g., high-protein diet, medications)
- Consideration of liver transplantation in selected patients with progressive or recurrent encephalopathy

DISPOSITION
Prognosis varies with the underlying etiology of the liver failure and the grade of encephalopathy (generally good for grades 1, 2; poor for grades 3, 4).

REFERRAL
The early stages of hepatic encephalopathy can be managed in the outpatient setting, whereas stages 3 or 4 require hospital admission.

MISCELLANEOUS

COMMENTS
Patients not responding to supportive therapy should be evaluated for liver transplantation.

REFERENCES
Koff R: Hepatic encephalopathy. In Noble J (ed): *Textbook of primary care medicine*, ed 2, St Louis, 1996, Mosby.

Lee WM: Acute liver failure, *N Engl J Med* 329:1862, 1993.

Author: **Fred F. Ferri, M.D.**

BASIC INFORMATION

DEFINITION
Hepatitis A is an acute, self-limited infection of liver parenchymal cells caused by the hepatitis A virus (HAV).

SYNONYMS
Infectious hepatitis
Short incubation (15 to 45 days) hepatitis

ICD-9-CM CODES
070.1 Hepatitis A

EPIDEMIOLOGY AND DEMOGRAPHICS
INCIDENCE (IN U.S.):
- 9 to 45 cases/100,000 persons/yr
- Highest rates:
  1. Institutionalized children, adults
  2. Day care centers (infants often not jaundiced; parents infected and more likely to become ill)
  3. Male homosexuals
  4. Exposure to imported apes or chimpanzees
  5. Ingestion of undercooked shellfish (mussels, clams, oysters) from contaminated water or ingestion of water from failed sanitary systems or natural disasters
- Highly contagious

PREVALENCE (IN U.S.):
- Episodic acute disease, generally in point-source outbreaks
- Immunity in 20% to 80% of adult population (70% to 80% of lower and 18% to 30% of middle and upper socioeconomic classes)
- 33% of acute viral hepatitis in U.S.

PREDOMINANT SEX: Equal (but common among male homosexuals)
PREDOMINANT AGE: 2 to 5 yr (associated with day care) and >50 yr
PEAK INCIDENCE:
- Infants infected at day care centers.
- Peak incidence of immunity at >50 yr; possibly reflects childhood infection during endemic HAV.

Neonatal Infection: Subclinical

PHYSICAL FINDINGS
- Often nonspecific
- Often profound anorexia, malaise
- Many asymptomatic cases
- Hepatomegaly (87%), tender RUQ
- Hepatic punch tenderness
- Splenomegaly rare (9%)
- Jaundice, dark urine
- Fever variable (when present, precedes jaundice, rapidly declines after onset of icteric phase)

ETIOLOGY
- Caused by HAV (27 nm picornavirus; single-stranded RNA genome)
- Transmission: fecal-oral route, close contacts, within families
- Rare transmission from infected blood (interleukin-2 and Factor VIII)
- Infection primarily localized to liver
- Rarely causes fulminant hepatitis

DIAGNOSIS

DIFFERENTIAL DIAGNOSIS
ACUTE DISEASE:
- Other hepatitis viruses (B, C, D, E)
- Viral illnesses producing systemic disease, in addition to hepatitis (e.g., yellow fever, EBV, CMV, HIV, rubella, rubeola, coxsackie B, adenovirus, HSV, HZV)
- Nonviral hepatitis (e.g., leptospirosis, toxoplasmosis, alcoholic hepatitis, drug-induced [e.g., acetaminophen, INH], toxic hepatitis [carbon tetrachloride, benzene])

HEPATITIS E:
- Like HAV (fecal-oral spread; short incubation; no chronic disease)
- High mortality (fulminant hepatitis and DIC) in late pregnancy
- Rare in U.S.

WORKUP
- Acute HAV antibody
- Liver function tests
- CBC
- Liver biopsy (fulminant hepatitis)

LABORATORY TESTS
- Diagnosis confirmed by IgM anti-HAV (acute, early convalescent serum).
- IgM present during onset of jaundice; IgG without IgM anti-HAV during acute jaundice suggests remote HAV and another current illness.
- Liver function test:
  1. ALT and AST: usually more than eight times normal (often 1000 U/L) at jaundice onset
  2. Bilirubin: usually five to fifteen times normal
  3. Alkaline phosphatase: minimally elevated (one to three times normal) acutely (may elevate during later cholestasis)
- Albumin and prothrombin time:
  1. Generally normal
  2. If abnormal, possible harbinger of impending hepatic necrosis
- WBC and ESR: generally normal

IMAGING STUDIES
- Rarely useful
- Sonogram (fulminant hepatitis)

TREATMENT

NONPHARMACOLOGIC THERAPY
- Activity as tolerated.
- High-calorie diet (best in AM)

ACUTE GENERAL Rx
- IV therapy: rarely needed (vomiting)
- Avoid hepatically metabolized drugs
- Steroids: not generally helpful; may shorten prolonged cholestasis
- Cholestyramine: occasionally for severe pruritus (cholestasis)
- Liver transplantation: Rarely; recovery in 60% of fulminant hepatitis patients

CHRONIC Rx
No chronic carrier or chronic HAV

DISPOSITION
- Follow-up as outpatient
- Acute disease usually lasting <6 wk
- May have one or two clinical relapses
- Rarely, prolonged (3 to 5 mo) cholestasis (usually if only modest acute SGPT rise)
- Rare (0.1%) fatal fulminant hepatitis
- No chronic hepatitis, cirrhosis, carrier state

REFERRAL
To infectious disease specialist and gastroenterologist for fulminant hepatitis, uncertain etiology, prolonged cholestasis

MISCELLANEOUS

COMMENTS
- Virus in high titer in stool (1 to 2 wk before jaundice, for short time after)
- Rapid fall in transmission following onset of jaundice; highest risk during asymptomatic phase; most fecal excretion of HAV before hospital admission
- Prevention before exposure:
  1. Hygiene; life-style changes
  2. Immune globulin (0.02 ml/kg IM for travel <3 mo to endemic areas)
  3. Inactivated HAV vaccine (90% effective), especially for high-risk groups and caregivers or contacts (universal childhood vaccination being considered; 50% of acute HAV is not associated with high-risk factors)
- Prevention after exposure: immune globulin (0.02 ml/kg IM) given within 2 wk of exposure to HAV; recommended only for close personal contacts (generally not casual office or school exposure or for most hospital personnel exposed to patient)

REFERENCES
Clemens R et al: Clinical experience with an inactivated hepatitis A vaccine, *J Infect Dis* 171(suppl 1): S44, 1995.

Author: Peter Nicholas, M.D.

Hepatitis B (PTG)

BASIC INFORMATION

DEFINITION
Hepatitis B is an acute infection of the liver parenchymal cells caused by the hepatitis B virus (HBV).

SYNONYMS
Serum hepatitis
Long incubation (50 to 180 days) hepatitis

ICD-9-CM CODES
070.3 Hepatitis B

EPIDEMIOLOGY AND DEMOGRAPHICS
INCIDENCE (IN U.S.):
- Approximately 90 cases/100,000 persons/yr
- Highest among IV drug users who share needles, homosexual men, visitors and immigrants from endemic areas, Alaskan natives, patients in institutions for mentally disabled, hemodialysis and hemophiliac patients and their sexual partners, prisoners, medical workers, and infants (perinatal transmission)
- Highly contagious

PREVALENCE (IN U.S.):
- Caucasians: 3%
- Blacks: 14%
- Of 300,000 acute cases yearly, death of 300 (0.1%) as a result of fulminant acute hepatitis, development of chronic HBV in 5% to 10%
- Death of approximately 4000 yearly from chronic disease

PREDOMINANT SEX:
- Predominant in males because of increased IV drug use, homosexuality, and greater likelihood of developing persistent HBV disease.
- Females more frequently terminate in carrier state.

PREDOMINANT AGE: 20 to 45 yr
PEAK INCIDENCE: 30 to 45 yr old, at rates of 5% to 20%

GENETICS:
Neonatal Infection:
- Rare in U.S.
- Transmission from HBV infected mother to neonate is common at birth.
- Infection at early age is common in developing nations, where most primary neonatal disease is mild and anicteric, and persistent disease is common, subclinical, and often leads to hepatocellular carcinoma.

PHYSICAL FINDINGS
- Often nonspecific symptoms
- Profound malaise
- Many asymptomatic cases
- Prodrome:
  1. 15% to 20% serum sickness (urticaria, rash, arthralgia) during early HBsAg
  2. HBsAg-Ab complex disease (arthritis, arteritis, glomerulonephritis)
- Hepatomegaly (87%) with RUQ tenderness
  1. Hepatic punch tenderness
  2. Splenomegaly: rare (10% to 15%)
- Jaundice, dark urine, with occasional pruritus
- Variable fever (when present generally precedes jaundice and rapidly declines following onset of icteric phase)
- Spider angiomata: rare; resolves during recovery
- Rare polyarteritis nodosa, cryoglobulinemia, aplastic anemia

ETIOLOGY
- Caused by hepatitis B virus (42 nm hepadnavirus with an outer surface coat [HBsAg], inner nucleocapsid core [HBcAg; HBeAg]; DNA polymerase; and partially double-stranded DNA genome)
- Transmission by parenteral route (needle use [including tattoos] and injury; unscreened blood products), perinatal, sexual, rare casual contact (saliva), not via urine or feces without GI bleeding
- Infection occurring primarily in liver, where necrosis probably results from cytotoxic T-cell response, direct cytopathic effect of HBcAg (core antigen), high level HBsAg (surface antigen) expression, or coinfection with delta (D) hepatitis virus (RNA delta core within HBsAg envelope)
- Recovery (>90%):
  1. Fulminant hepatitis occurring in <1% (especially if coinfected with hepatitis D); 80% fatal
  2. Unusual (5%) prolonged acute disease for 4 to 12 mo, with recovery
  3. Overall fatality increase with age and viral dose (e.g., transfusions)
- Chronic infection (1% to 2%):
  1. Persistent carrier state without hepatitis (HBsAg+)
  2. Chronic persistent hepatitis [CPH] (clinically well) or chronic active hepatitis [CAH] (HBsAg + HBeAg [e antigen])
  3. Cirrhosis
  4. Hepatocellular carcinoma (especially after neonatal infection)
  5. Chronic infection: more common following low-dose exposure and mild acute hepatitis, with earlier age at infection, in males, or if immunosuppressed

DIAGNOSIS

DIFFERENTIAL DIAGNOSIS
- Acute disease confused with other hepatitis viral diseases (A, C, D, E)
- Any viral illnesses producing systemic disease and hepatitis (e.g., yellow fever, EBV, CMV, HIV, rubella, rubeola, coxsackie B, adenovirus, herpes simplex or zoster)
- Nonviral etiologies of hepatitis (e.g., leptospirosis, toxoplasmosis, alcoholic hepatitis, drug-induced [e.g., acetaminophen, INH], toxic hepatitis [carbon tetrachloride, benzene])

WORKUP
- Acute serum specimen for hepatitis B serology (HBsAg, HBsAb, HBcAb, HBeAg, HBeAb)
- Liver function tests
- CBC
- Liver biopsy: rarely necessary for diagnosis of fulminant viral hepatitis, chronic hepatitis, cirrhosis, carcinoma

LABORATORY TESTS
- Diagnosis of acute HBV infection is best confirmed by IgM HBcAb in acute or early convalescent serum.
  1. Generally, IgM present during onset of jaundice
  2. Coexisting HBsAg
- HBsAb and IgG-HBcAb during acute jaundice are strongly suggestive of remote HBV infection and another etiology for current illness.
- HBsAb alone is suggestive of immunization response.
- With recovery, HBeAg is rapidly replaced by HBeAb in 2 to 3 mo, and HBsAg is replaced by HBsAb in 5 to 6 mo.
- In chronic HBV hepatitis, HBsAg and HBeAg are persistent without corresponding Ab.
- In chronic carrier state, HBsAg is persistent, but HBeAg is replaced by HBeAb.
- HBcAb develops in all outcomes.
- HBeAg correlation with highest infectivity; appearance of HBeAb is herald of recovery.
- Liver function tests:
  1. ALT and AST: usually more than eight times normal (often 1000 U/L) at onset of jaundice (minimal acute ALT/AST rises often followed by chronic hepatitis or hepatocellular carcinoma)
  2. Bilirubin: usually five to fifteen times normal
  3. Alkaline phosphatase: minimally elevated (one to three times normal) acutely
- Albumin and prothrombin time:
  1. Generally normal
  2. If abnormal, possible harbinger of impending hepatic necrosis (fulminant hepatitis)
- WBC and ESR: generally normal

IMAGING STUDIES
- Rarely useful
- Sonogram to document rapid reduction in liver size during fulminant hepatitis or mass in hepatocellular carcinoma

TREATMENT

NONPHARMACOLOGIC THERAPY
- Activity as tolerated
- High-calorie diet preferred; often best tolerated in morning

ACUTE GENERAL Rx
- IV therapy is rarely needed for hydration during severe vomiting.
- Avoid hepatically metabolized drugs.
- No therapeutic measures are beneficial.
- Steroids have not been shown to be helpful, and they may be harmful (increase DNA polymerase activity).

CHRONIC Rx
- Steroids are variably helpful for CAH (HBsAg−, but not HBsAg+).
- Recombinant interferon-alpha often diminishes CAH; variably enduring.
- Ara-A inhibits HBV, but it is toxic.

DISPOSITION
- Follow-up as outpatient
- Acute disease: usually <6 wk
- Rare fatalities (fulminant hepatitis)
- Rare Guillain-Barré
- Possible chronic carrier state, cirrhosis, hepatic carcinoma

REFERRAL
To infectious disease specialist and gastroenterologist for consultation regarding fulminant hepatitis or prolonged cholestasis, for cases of uncertain etiology, or for treatment of chronic hepatitis (CAH)

MISCELLANEOUS

COMMENTS
- Virus and HBsAg in high titers in blood for 1 to 7 wk before jaundice and for a variable time thereafter.
- Transmission is possible during entire period of HBsAg (and especially during HBeAg) in serum.
- Universal precautions should be followed for all contacts with blood or secretions/excretions contaminated with blood.
- Prevention before exposure:
  1. Life-style changes
  2. Meticulous testing of blood supply (although some chronically infected, infectious donors are HBsAg−)
  3. Sterilization via steam or hypochlorite
  4. Hepatitis B vaccine for high-risk groups (>90% effective), given IM in deltoid to induce HBsAb (response should be confirmed), which is protective
  5. Recommendation for universal childhood immunization with doses at birth and 1 mo and 6 mo
- Prevention after exposure:
1. HBV hyperimmune globulin (HBIG) given immediately after needlestick, within 14 days of sexual exposure, or at birth, followed by HBV vaccination
2. Standard immune globulin: nearly as effective as HBIG
- Tables A-7, A-8, and A-9 describe Hepatitis B prophylaxis
- U.S. Preventive Services Task Force Recommendations for screening for Hepatitis B virus infection are described in Section V, Chapter 24.

REFERENCES
Hirschman SZ: Current approaches to viral hepatitis, *Clin Infect Dis* 20:741,1995.

Author: Peter Nicholas, M.D.

Hepatitis C (PTG)

BASIC INFORMATION

DEFINITION
Hepatitis C is an acute liver parenchymal infection caused by hepatitis C virus (HCV).

SYNONYMS
Transfusion-related non-A, B hepatitis
Intermediate incubation (6 to 8 wk; range 15 to 150 days), between hepatitis A and B

ICD-9-CM CODES
070.51 Other viral hepatitis

EPIDEMIOLOGY AND DEMOGRAPHICS
INCIDENCE (IN U.S.):
- 150,000 new cases/yr (37,500, symptomatic; 93,000, later chronic liver disease; 30,700, cirrhosis)
- Approximately 9000 of these ultimately die of HCV infection; most common (40%) cause of nonalcoholic liver disease in U.S.

PREVALENCE (IN U.S.):
- 0.6% among low-risk groups
- 60% to 70% among high-risk groups (transfused hemophiliacs; IV drug users sharing needles)

PREDOMINANT SEX: Equal
PREDOMINANT AGE: 18 to 39 yr (70%)
PEAK INCIDENCE:
- 15 to 40 yr old
- Highly variable among subgroups

GENETICS:
Neonatal Infection: Unlikely

PHYSICAL FINDINGS
- Symptoms: often gradual in onset, milder than hepatitis A or B
- Hepatomegaly, tender RUQ; rare splenomegaly, jaundice, dark urine, but >75% of patients are anicteric with mild symptoms
- Rarely (in chronic HCV hepatitis):
  1. Cryoglobulinemia (II, III)
  2. Immune complex disease (vasculitis, glomerulonephritis, Hashimoto's thyroiditis)

ETIOLOGY
- Caused by HCV (single-stranded RNA togavirus).
- Identified transmission is mostly percutaneous (90%), from IV drug use (50% to 80%), transfusions (90% before screening for HCV; probably 1% now), occupational needlestick exposure (2% to 10% risk), hemodialysis.
- No identifiable risk in about 50% of community-acquired HCV.
- Unlikely sexual (<7%) or perinatal transmission.
- Cytotoxic T lymphocytes and cytokines (interferon-gamma) likely mediate hepatic necrosis; may be enhanced by alcohol.
- Immunity after primary HCV is incomplete; reinfection muted.
- Acute HCV hepatitis (HCVH) is often (75%) asymptomatic.
- Fulminant acute hepatitis is rare (<0.1%), but HCVH causes up to 30% of all fulminant hepatitis cases.
- Persistent infection is common (50% to 70%) following HCVH, resulting in chronic hepatitis (chronic aggressive or chronic persistent hepatitis), often characterized by fluctuating ALT levels; cirrhosis (often asymptomatic, developing in 20% to 50% even after 20 yr); or hepatocellular carcinoma (50% a result of HCV).

DIAGNOSIS

DIFFERENTIAL DIAGNOSIS
- Other hepatitis viruses (A, B, D, E)
- Viral illnesses producing systemic disease, in addition to hepatitis (e.g., yellow fever, EBV, CMV, HIV, rubella, rubeola, coxsackie B, adeno, HSV, HZV)
- Nonviral hepatitis (e.g., leptospirosis, toxoplasmosis, alcoholic hepatitis, drug-induced [e.g., acetaminophen, INH], toxic hepatitis

WORKUP
- Acute hepatitis C antibody
- Liver function tests; CBC
- Liver biopsy: rarely needed for diagnosis of fulminant or chronic viral hepatitis, cirrhosis, or carcinoma

LABORATORY TESTS
- Diagnosis is often by exclusion; it takes 6 wk to 1 yr to develop anti-HCV Ab (6 wk: 70% positive; 6 mo: 90%).
- Anti-HCV Ab detected by ELISA:
  1. False-positive in autoimmune hepatitis; paraproteinemia; up to 50% of screened blood donors
  2. True-positive supported by elevated ALT, ELISA ratio >2 (sample:cutoff); positive neutralizing or immunoblot assay; or HCV-RNA by polymerase chain reaction (PCR)
- HCV-RNA by PCR is detectable before ELISA, but often unavailable.
- Liver function test:
  1. ALT and AST: usually more than eight times normal
  2. Bilirubin: usually five to ten times normal
- Albumin and prothrombin time:
  1. Generally normal
  2. If abnormal, possible harbinger of impending hepatic necrosis
- WBC and ESR are generally normal.

IMAGING STUDIES
- Rarely useful
- Sonogram: rapid liver size reduction during fulminant hepatitis or mass in hepatocellular carcinoma

TREATMENT

NONPHARMACOLOGIC THERAPY
Activity and diet as tolerated

ACUTE GENERAL Rx
- Avoid hepatically metabolized drugs.
- No beneficial therapeutic measures.
- Steroids and Ara-A are not helpful.

CHRONIC Rx
- Steroids and Ara-A are not helpful.
- Recombinant interferon-alpha Rx for 6 mo reduces ALT and HCV viremia (40% to 70% of patients)
- Relapse after treatment: >50%.
- Uncommon 3 to 6 yr remissions.
- Interferon is possibly most useful to patients with fluctuating ALT and active liver disease on biopsy.

DISPOSITION
- Follow-up as outpatient
- Acute disease usually <6 wk (but frequent [>50%] chronic disease)
- Serial ALT levels followed for fluctuation and as a clue for chronicity, since most are asymptomatic, even in chronic disease of <20 yr
- Chronic carrier state, cirrhosis, hepatic carcinoma (>20 yr) more common than with hepatitis A or B

REFERRAL
For consultation with infectious disease specialist and gastroenterologist for fulminant hepatitis; uncertain etiology; or chronic hepatitis

MISCELLANEOUS

COMMENTS
- Follow universal precautions for all contacts with blood or secretions/excretions potentially contaminated with blood.
- Prevention before exposure:
  1. Life-style (IV drug use) change
  2. Testing of blood supply for ALT elevations and HCV Ab (but HCV Ab may develop slowly, producing false-negatives)
  3. Sterilization (steam, hypochlorite)
  4. No vaccine and the prospects are guarded, given failed immunity after natural infection, antigenic variation; immune globulin providing only minimal protection
- Prevention following exposure: immune globulin providing only minimal protection

REFERENCES
Iwarson S et al: Hepatitis C: natural history of a unique infection, *Clin Infect Dis* 20:1361, 1995.

Author: **Peter Nicholas, M.D.**

Hepatorenal syndrome

BASIC INFORMATION

DEFINITION
Hepatorenal syndrome (HRS) is a condition of intense renal vasoconstriction resulting from loss of renal autoregulation occurring as a complication of severe liver disease.

SYNONYMS
Hepatic nephropathy
Oliguric renal failure of cirrhosis
HRS

ICD-9-CM CODES
572.4 Hepatorenal syndrome

EPIDEMIOLOGY AND DEMOGRAPHICS
The probability of HRS in patients with cirrhosis is 18% at 1 yr, and 39% at 5 yr.

PHYSICAL FINDINGS
- Evidence of cirrhosis is usually present: jaundice, spider angiomas, splenomegaly, ascites, fetor hepaticus, pedal edema
- Hepatic encephalopathy: flapping tremor-asterixis, coma
- Tachycardia and bounding pulse
- Oliguria

ETIOLOGY
An exacerbation of end-stage liver disease, HRS may occur after significant reduction of effective blood volume (e.g., paracentesis, GI bleeding, diuretics) or in the absence of any precipitating factors.

DIAGNOSIS

DIFFERENTIAL DIAGNOSIS
- Prerenal azotemia: response to sustained plasma expansion is good (prompt diuresis with volume expansion).
- Acute tubular necrosis: urinary sodium >30, FeNa >1.5%, urinary/plasma creatinine ratio <30, urine-plasma osmolality ratio = 1, urine sediment reveals casts and cellular debris, there is no significant response to sustained plasma expansion.

WORKUP
Patients with acute azotemia and oliguria in the setting of liver disease should undergo laboratory evaluation to differentiate HRS from acute tubular necrosis and volume challenge to differentiate HRS from prerenal azotemia if FeNa <1%.

LABORATORY TESTS
- Obtain serum electrolytes, BUN, creatinine, osmolality, urinalysis, urinary sodium, urinary creatinine, urine osmolality.
- Calculate fractional excretion of sodium (FeNa) (see formula in Appendix).
- In HRS: urinary sodium <10 mEq/L, FeNa <1%, urinary plasma creatinine ratio >30, urinary-plasma osmolality ratio >1.5, urine sediment is unremarkable.

IMAGING STUDIES
Renal ultrasound may be indicated if renal obstruction is suspected.

TREATMENT

NONPHARMACOLOGIC THERAPY
Avoidance of precipitating factors

ACUTE GENERAL Rx
- Volume challenge (to increase mean arterial pressure) followed by large volume paracentesis (to increase cardiac output and decrease renal venous pressure) is recommended to distinguish HRS from prerenal azotemia in patients with FeNa <1%. In patients with prerenal azotemia, the increase in renal perfusion pressure and renal blood flow will result in prompt diuresis; the volume challenge can be accomplished by giving a solution of 100 g of albumin in 500 ml of isotonic saline.
- The only effective treatment of HRS is liver transplantation; low-dose dopamine or ornipressin is used in some liver units to avoid further deterioration of renal function in patients awaiting liver transplantation.

DISPOSITION
Mortality rate exceeds 80%; liver transplantation is the only curative treatment.

REFERRAL
Referral for liver transplantation when indicated (see below)

MISCELLANEOUS

COMMENTS
Liver transplantation may be indicated in otherwise healthy patients (age preferably <65 yr) with sclerosing cholangitis, chronic hepatitis with cirrhosis, or primary biliary cirrhosis; contraindications to liver transplantation are AIDS, most metastatic malignancies, active substance abuse, uncontrolled sepsis, uncontrolled cardiac or pulmonary disease.

REFERENCES
Epstein M: Hepatorenal syndrome: emerging perspectives of pathophysiology and therapy, *J Am Soc Nephrol* 4:1735, 1994.
Roberts LR, Kamath PS: Ascites and hepatorenal syndrome: pathophysiology and management, *Mayo Clin Proc* 71:874, 1996.

Author: **Fred F. Ferri, M.D.**

Herpangina (PTG)

BASIC INFORMATION

DEFINITION
Herpangina is a self-limited upper respiratory tract infection associated with a characteristic vesicular rash on the soft palate.

ICD-9-CM CODES
074.0 Herpangina

EPIDEMIOLOGY AND DEMOGRAPHICS
INCIDENCE (IN U.S.): Unknown
PREVALENCE (IN U.S.): Unknown
PREDOMINANT SEX: Male = female
PREDOMINANT AGE: 3 to 10 yr
PEAK INCIDENCE: Summer outbreaks common

PHYSICAL FINDINGS
- Characterized by ulcerating lesions typically located on the soft palate
- Usually fewer than six lesions that evolve rapidly from a diffuse pharyngitis to erythematous macules and subsequently to vesicles that are moderately painful
- Fever, vomiting, and headache in the first few days of illness but subsiding spontaneously
- Pharyngeal lesions typical for several more days

ETIOLOGY
- Most caused by coxsackie A viruses (A2, A4, A5, A6, A10)
- Occasional cases caused by other viruses

DIAGNOSIS

DIFFERENTIAL DIAGNOSIS
- Herpes simplex
- Bacterial pharyngitis
- Tonsillitis
- Aphthous stomatitis
- Hand-foot-mouth disease

WORKUP
Diagnosis is typically based on characteristic lesions on the soft palate.

LABORATORY TESTS
Viral and bacterial cultures of the pharynx to exclude *Herpes simplex* infection and streptococcal pharyngitis if the diagnosis is in doubt

TREATMENT

- Symptomatic treatment for sore throat
- No antiviral therapy indicated

NONPHARMACOLOGIC THERAPY
Analgesic throat lozenges are helpful in some cases.

ACUTE GENERAL Rx
Antipyretics when indicated

CHRONIC Rx
Self-limited infection

DISPOSITION
- Generally, resolution of symptoms within 1 wk
- Persistence of fever or mouth lesions beyond 1 wk suggestive of an alternative diagnosis (see "Differential Diagnosis")

REFERRAL
For consultation with otolaryngologist or infectious disease specialist if the diagnosis is in doubt

MISCELLANEOUS

COMMENTS
Household outbreaks may occur, especially during the summer months.

Author: **Joseph R. Masci, M.D.**

Herpes simplex (PTG)

BASIC INFORMATION

DEFINITION
Herpes simplex is a viral infection caused by the herpes simplex virus (HSV); HSV-1 is associated primarily with oral infections, whereas HSV-2 causes mainly genital infections; however, each type can infect any site; following the primary infection, the virus enters the nerve endings in the skin directly below the lesions and ascends to the dorsal root ganglia where it remains in a latent stage until it is reactivated.

SYNONYMS
Genital herpes
Herpes labialis
Herpes gladiatorum
Herpes digitalis

ICD-9-CM CODES
054.10 Genital herpes
054.9 Herpes labialis

EPIDEMIOLOGY AND DEMOGRAPHICS
- Over 85% of adults have serologic evidence of HSV-1 infection.
- Most case of eye or digital herpetic infections are caused by HSV-1.
- Frequency of recurrence of HSV-2 genital herpes is higher than HSV-1 oral labial infection.
- The frequency of recurrence is lowest for oral labial HSV-2 infections.
- The incidence of complications from herpes simplex (e.g., herpes encephalitis) is highest in immunocompromised hosts.

PHYSICAL FINDINGS
PRIMARY INFECTION (SEE COLOR PLATE 9):
- Symptoms occur from 3 to 7 days after contact (respiratory droplets, direct contact)
- Constitutional symptoms include low-grade fever, headache and myalgias, regional lymphadenopathy, and localized pain.
- Pain, burning, itching, and tingling last several hours.
- Grouped vesicles usually with surrounding erythema appear and generally ulcerate or crust within 48 hr.
- The vesicles are uniform in size (differentiating it from herpes zoster vesicles that vary in size).
- During the acute eruption the patient is uncomfortable; involvement of lips and inside of mouth may make it unpleasant for the patient to eat; urinary retention may complicate involvement of the genital area.
- Lesions generally last from 2 to 6 wk and heal without scarring.

RECURRENT INFECTION:
- Generally caused by alteration in the immune system; fatigue, stress, menses, local skin trauma, and exposure to sunlight are contributing factors.
- The prodromal symptoms (fatigue, burning and tingling of the affected area) last 12 to 24 hr.
- A cluster of lesions generally evolve within 24 hr from a macule to a papule and then vesicles surrounded by erythema; the vesicles coalesce and subsequently rupture within 4 days, revealing erosions covered by crusts.
- The crusts are generally shed within 7 to 10 days, revealing a pink surface.
- The most frequent location of the lesions is on the vermilion border of the lips (HSV-1), the penile shaft or glans penis and the labia (HSV-2), buttocks (seen more frequently in women), on the fingertips, (herpetic whitlow), and on the trunk (may be confused with herpes zoster).
- Rapid onset of diffuse cutaneous herpes simplex (eczema herpeticum) may occur in certain atopic infants and adults. It is a medical emergency, especially in young infants, and should be promptly treated with acyclovir.
- Herpes encephalitis, meningitis, and ocular herpes can occur in patients with immunocompromised status and occasionally in normal hosts.

ETIOLOGY
HSV-1 and HSV-2 are both DNA viruses.

DIAGNOSIS

DIFFERENTIAL DIAGNOSIS
- Impetigo
- Behçet's syndrome
- Coxsackie virus infection
- Syphilis
- Stevens-Johnson syndrome
- Herpangina
- Aphthous stomatitis
- Varicella
- Herpes zoster

WORKUP
Diagnosis is based on clinical presentation. Laboratory evaluation will confirm diagnosis.

LABORATORY TESTS
- Direct immunofluorescent antibody slide tests will provide a rapid diagnosis.
- Viral culture is the most definitive method for diagnosis; results are generally available in 1 or 2 days; the lesions should be sampled during the vesicular or early ulcerative stage; cervical samples should be taken from the endocervix with a swab.

Herpes simplex (PTG)

- Tzanck smear is a readily available test; it will demonstrate multinucleated giant cells. However, it is not a very sensitive test.
- Pap smear will detect HSV-infected cells in cervical tissue from women without symptoms.
- Serologic tests for HSV: IgG and IgM serum antibodies. Antibodies to HSV occur in 50% to 90% of adults. Routine tests do not discriminate between antibodies that are HSV-1 and HSV-2; the presence of IgM or a fourfold or greater rise in IgG titers indicates a recent infection (convalescent sample should be drawn 2 to 3 wk after the acute specimen is drawn).

TREATMENT

NONPHARMACOLOGIC THERAPY
Application of topical cool compresses with Burow's solution for 15 min four to six times daily may be soothing in patients with extensive erosions on the vulva and penis (decrease edema and inflammation, debridement of crusts and purulent material).

ACUTE GENERAL Rx
- Acyclovir ointment (Zovirax) applied using finger-cot or rubber glove q3-6h (six times daily) for 7 days is useful for the first clinical episode of genital herpes. Severe primary genital infections may be treated with IV acyclovir (5 mg/kg infused at a constant rate over 1 hr q8h for 7 days in patients with normal renal function) or oral acyclovir 200 mg five times daily for 7 to 10 days.
- Valacyclovir caplets (Valtrex) can also be used for the initial episode of genital herpes (1 g bid for 10 days).
- Acyclovir is not indicated for primary or recurrent herpes labialis; however, it is frequently used for this purpose by many physicians.
- Penciclovir 1% cream (Denavir) can be used for recurrent herpes labialis on the lips and face. It should be applied q2h while awake for 4 days. Treatment should be started at the earliest sign or symptom.

CHRONIC Rx
- Recurrent episodes of genital herpes can be treated with acyclovir (200 mg PO five times a day for 5 days, 400 mg PO tid for 5 days or 800 mg PO bid for 5 days, generally started during the prodrome or within 2 days of onset of lesions; famciclovir (Famvir) is also useful for treatment of recurrent genital herpes (dose is 125 mg q12h for 5 days in patients with normal renal function) started at the first sign of symptoms, or valacyclovir (Valtrex) (dose is 500 mg q12h for 5 days in patients with normal renal function).
- Acyclovir-resistant mucocutaneous lesions in patients with HIV can be treated with foscarnet (40 to 60 mg/kg IV q8h in patients with normal renal function); HPMPC has also been reported to be effective in HSV infections resistant to acyclovir or foscarnet.
- Patients with recurrent genital infections may benefit from maintenance acyclovir (600 to 800 mg/day in two or three divided doses) or valacyclovir 500 mg to 1g every 24 hr..

DISPOSITION
Most patients recover from the initial episode or recurrences without complications; immunocompromised hosts are at risk for complications (e.g., disseminated herpes simplex infection, herpes encephalitis).

REFERRAL
- Hospital admission in patients with herpes encephalitis, herpes meningitis and in immunocompromised hosts with diffuse herpes simplex infection
- Ophthalmology referral in patients with suspected ocular herpes

MISCELLANEOUS

COMMENTS
- Provide patient education regarding transmission of HSV.
- Patients should be instructed on the use of condoms for sexual intercourse and on avoiding kissing or sexual intercourse until lesions are crusted.
- Patients should also avoid contact with immunocompromised hosts or neonates while lesions are present.
- Proper hand-washing techniques should be explained.
- Patients with herpes gladiatorum (cutaneous herpes in athletes involved in contact sports) should be excluded from participation in active sports until lesions have resolved.
- For additional information on genital herpes simplex, refer to "Herpes simplex, genital" in Section I.
- U.S. Preventive Services Task Force Recommendations regarding screening for genital herpes simplex are described in Section V, Chapter 30.

REFERENCES
Benedetti JK et al: Frequency and reactivation of nongenital lesions among patients with genital herpes simplex virus, *Am J Med* 8:237, 1995.

Habif TP: *Clinical dermatology*, ed 3, St Louis, 1996, Mosby.

Spruance SL et al: Penciclovir cream for the treatment of herpes simplex labialis: a randomized, multicenter, double-blind placebo-controlled trial, *JAMA* 277:1374, 1997.

Wald A et al: Virologic characteristics of subclinical and symptomatic genital herpes infections, *N Engl J Med* 333:770, 1995.

Author: **Fred F. Ferri, M.D.**

Herpes simplex, genital (PTG)

BASIC INFORMATION

DEFINITION
Herpes simplex infection is a sexually transmitted disease caused by a double-stranded DNA virus. Two forms of infection exist: HSV-1, or oral herpes (15% of genital cases), and HSV-2, or genital herpes.

ICD-9-CM CODES
054.10 Genital herpes

EPIDEMIOLOGY AND DEMOGRAPHICS
INCIDENCE:
- 1% to 2%, with 500,000 new cases/yr
- Antibodies to HSV-1 or HSV-2 in up to 80% of adults

RISK FACTORS:
- Promiscuity
- Highest frequency in 15- to 29-yr-old population
- Associated with other sexually transmitted diseases, such as syphilis, gonorrhea, or chlamydia

GENETICS: No associated genetic predisposition

PHYSICAL FINDINGS
Three separate syndromes, as follows:
- First episode primary:
  1. No antibodies to HSV-1 or HSV-2
  2. Severe local symptoms such as painful bilateral genital ulcers or vesicles, inguinal adenopathy
  3. Constitutional findings of fever, malaise, myalgia
  4. Lesions persisting >16 days, with extragenital symptoms on fingers, buttock, or mouth
- First episode nonprimary:
  1. Presence of antibodies to HSV-1 and HSV-2
  2. Milder clinical course with symptoms similar to those of recurrent disease
- Recurrent herpes:
  1. Shorter duration (5 to 10 days)
  2. Mild symptoms
  3. Unilateral distribution
  4. Few systemic symptoms
  5. Prodrome of itching or burning before lesions appear

ETIOLOGY
Double-stranded DNA virus with a lytic as well as a latent phase

DIAGNOSIS

- Classical appearance of vesicles or ulcers in various stages of development
- Clinical history of recurrent prodromal symptoms and recurrences

DIFFERENTIAL DIAGNOSIS
- Human papilloma virus
- Molluscum contagiosum
- HIV infection
- Fungal infections (candida)
- Bacterial infections (syphilis, chancroid, granuloma inguinale)
- Follicular abscess
- Hydradenitis suppurativa
- Vulvar dystrophies
- Cancer of the vulva

WORKUP
- Clinical history, including a thorough search for other sexually transmitted diseases
- Complete physical examination, including culture of suspected sites
- Possibly antibody screening

LABORATORY TESTS
- Viral culture
  1. Gold standard
  2. Requires 48 to 72 hr in most cases, with a higher chance of a positive culture with more viral load (first episode or early vesicular lesions)
  3. Disease not excluded by a negative culture result
- Tzanck smear
  1. Low sensitivity
  2. Tests for presence of intranuclear inclusions or giant cells
- Immunoperoxidase stains
- Monoclonal antibody, ELISA

TREATMENT

NONPHARMACOLOGIC THERAPY
- Exposure of affected areas to dry environment, avoiding contact of early vesicles with noninfected tissue
- Avoidance of intercourse during outbreak or with prodromal symptoms, with consideration of condom use if there are frequent recurrent episodes

ACUTE GENERAL Rx
- First clinical episode: acyclovir 200 mg PO × 5 for 7 to 10 days or until resolution of symptoms
- Recurrent disease:
  1. Course of recurrence shortened if treatment begun during prodromal phase or within initial phase of disease
  2. Acyclovir 200 mg PO × 5 for 5 days, 400 mg × 3 for 5 days, or 800 mg PO × 2 for 5 days
- Severe disease (encephalitis, pneumonia, or hepatitis):
  1. Requires intravenous treatment
  2. Acyclovir 5 to 10 mg/kg q8h for 7 days

CHRONIC Rx
Suppressive therapy:
- Indicated for patients with >6 recurrences per year
- Acyclovir 200 mg PO three to five times per day or 400 mg PO bid
- Reevaluation after 1 yr of therapy to assess for continued suppression
- May reduce frequency of recurrences by 75%

DISPOSITION
Most cases responsive to initial therapy with acyclovir, but for those with recurrences, suppressive treatment (noted above) is indicated.

REFERRAL
To infectious disease specialist or obstetrician for patients with life-threatening diseases or who are pregnant, especially in third trimester

MISCELLANEOUS

COMMENTS
HSV infection during pregnancy requires consideration of fetus as well as mother:
- Culture of any lesion suspicious for herpes should be performed.
- If active disease is suspected at the time of delivery, C-section may be indicated to decrease chance of neonatal infection.
- U.S. Preventive Services Task Force Recommendations regarding screening for genital herpes simplex are described in Section V, Chapter 30.

REFERENCES
Danakas G, Pietrantoni: *Practical guide to the care of the gynecologic/obstetric patient,* St Louis, 1997, Mosby.
Sweet R, Gibbs R: *Infectious diseases of the female genital tract,* Baltimore, Md, 1995, Williams & Wilkins.

Author: **Scott J. Zuccala, D.O.**

Herpes zoster (PTG)

BASIC INFORMATION

DEFINITION
Herpes zoster is a disease caused by reactivation of the varicella-zoster virus. Following the primary infection (chickenpox) the virus becomes latent in the dorsal root ganglia and reemerges when there is a weakening of the immune system (secondary to disease or advanced age).

SYNONYMS
Shingles

ICD-9-CM CODES
053.9 Herpes zoster

EPIDEMIOLOGY AND DEMOGRAPHICS
- Herpes zoster occurs during lifetime in 10% to 20% of the population.
- There is an increased incidence in immunocompromised patients (AIDS, malignancy), the elderly, and children who acquired chickenpox when younger than 2 mo.

PHYSICAL FINDINGS
- Pain generally precedes skin manifestation by 3 to 5 days and is generally localized to the dermatome that will be affected by the skin lesions.
- Constitutional symptoms are often present (malaise, fever, headache).
- The initial rash consists of erythematous maculopapules generally affecting one dermatome (thoracic region in majority of cases); some patients (<50%) may have scattered vesicles outside of the affected dermatome.
- The initial maculopapules evolve into vesicles and pustules by the third or the fourth day.
- The vesicles have an erythematous base (see color plate 10), are cloudy, and have various sizes (a distinguishing characteristic from herpes simplex in which the vesicles are of uniform size).
- The vesicles subsequently become umbilicated and then form crusts that generally fall off within 3 wk; scarring may occur.
- Pain during and after the rash is generally significant.
- Secondary bacterial infection with *Staphylococcus aureus* or *Streptococcus pyogenes* may occur.
- Regional lymphadenopathy may occur.
- Herpes zoster may involve the trigeminal nerve (most frequent cranial nerve involved); involvement of the geniculate ganglion can cause facial palsy and a painful ear, with the presence of vesicles on the pinna and external auditory canal (Ramsay Hunt syndrome).

ETIOLOGY
Reactivation of varicella virus (human herpesvirus III)

DIAGNOSIS

DIFFERENTIAL DIAGNOSIS
- Rash: herpes simplex and other viral infections
- Pain from herpes zoster: may be confused with acute myocardial infarction, pulmonary embolism, pleuritis, pericarditis, renal colic

LABORATORY TESTS
Laboratory tests are generally not necessary (viral cultures and Tzanck smear will confirm diagnosis in patients with atypical presentation).

TREATMENT

NONPHARMACOLOGIC THERAPY
- Wet compresses (using Burow's solution or cool tap water) applied for 15 to 30 min five to ten times a day are useful to break vesicles and remove serum and crust.
- Care must be taken to prevent any secondary bacterial infection.

ACUTE GENERAL Rx
- Suppression of pain: an approach to herpetic and postherpetic neuralgia is described in Section III, Fig. 3-39.
- Oral antiviral agents can decrease acute pain, inflammation, and vesicle formation when treatment is begun within 48 hr of onset of rash. Treatment options are:
  1. Acyclovir (Zovirax) 800 mg five times a day for 7 days
  2. Valacyclovir (Valtrex) 1000 mg tid for 7 days
  3. Famciclovir (Famvir) 500 mg tid for 7 days
- Immunocompromised patients should be treated with IV acyclovir 500 mg/m^2 or 10 mg/kg q8h in 1-hr infusions for 7 days, with close monitoring of renal function and adequate hydration; vidarabine (continuous 12-hr infusion of 10 mg/kg/day for 7 days) is also effective for treatment of disseminated herpes zoster in immunocompromised hosts.
- Patients with AIDS and transplant patients may develop acyclovir-resistant varicella-zoster; these patients can be treated with foscarnet (40 mg/kg IV q8h) continued for at least 10 days or until lesions are completely healed.
- Capsaicin cream (Zostrix) can be useful for treatment of postherpetic neuralgia. It is generally applied three to five times daily for several weeks.
- Sympathetic blocks (stellate ganglion or epidural) with 0.25% bupivacaine and rhizotomy are reserved for severe cases unresponsive to conservative treatment.
- A clinical algorithm for evaluation and treatment of herpetic and postherpetic neuralgia is described in Fig. 3-39.

DISPOSITION
- The incidence of postherpetic neuralgia increases with age (30% by age of 40 yr, >70% by age 70 yr); acyclovir reduces the risk of postherpetic neuralgia.
- Incidence of disseminated herpes zoster is increased in immunocompromised hosts (e.g., 15% to 50% of patients with active Hodgkin's disease).
- Immunocompromised hosts are also more prone to neurologic complications (mortality rate is 10% to 20% in immunocompromised hosts with disseminated zoster).
- Motor neuropathies occur in 5% of all cases of zoster; complete recovery occurs in >70% of patients.

REFERRAL
- Hospitalization for IV acyclovir in patients with disseminated herpes zoster
- Surgical referral for rhizotomy in patients with severe pain unresponsive to conventional treatment
- Sympathetic blocks in selected patients

MISCELLANEOUS

REFERENCES
Habif TP: *Clinical dermatology*, ed 3, St Louis, 1996, Mosby.

Jackson JL et al: The effect of treating herpes zoster with oral acyclovir in preventing post-herpetic neuralgia: a metaanalysis, *Arch Intern Med* 157:909, 1997.

Tyring S et al: Famciclovir for the treatment of acute herpes zoster: effects on acute disease and postherpetic neuralgia, *Ann Intern Med* 123:89, 1995.

Wood MJ et al: A randomized trial of acyclovir for 7 days or 21 days with and without prednisolone for treatment of acute herpes zoster, *New Engl J Med* 330(13):896, 1994.

Author: **Fred F. Ferri, M.D.**

Histoplasmosis

BASIC INFORMATION

DEFINITION
Histoplasmosis is an infectious disease caused by the fungus *Histoplasma capsulatum*, which is usually asymptomatic and characterized by a primary pulmonary focus with occasional progression to chronic pulmonary histoplasmosis (CPH) or various forms of dissemination. Progressive disseminated histoplasmosis (PDH) may present with a diverse clinical spectrum, including adrenal necrosis, pulmonary and mediastinal fibrosis, and ulcerations of the oropharynx and GI tract. In those patients who are concurrently infected with the human immunodeficiency virus (HIV), it is a defining disease for acquired immunodeficiency syndrome (AIDS).

ICD-9-CM CODES
115.90 Histoplasmosis
115.94 Histoplasmosis with endocarditis
115.91 Histoplasmosis with meningitis
115.93 Histoplasmosis with pericarditis
115.95 Histoplasmosis with pneumonia
115.92 Histoplasmosis with retinitis

EPIDEMIOLOGY AND DEMOGRAPHICS
INCIDENCE (IN U.S.):
- Unknown for acute pulmonary disease
- For CPH, estimated at 1/100,000 cases in endemic areas
- For PDH in immunocompetent adults, estimated at 1/2000 cases of histoplasmosis

PREVALENCE: Unknown
PREDOMINANT SEX: Clinically evident disease is most common in males; male:female ratio of 4:1
PREDOMINANT AGE:
- CPH is most often seen in males >50 yr old with an associated history of COPD.
- Presumed ocular histoplasmosis syndrome (POHS) is most commonly diagnosed between ages of 20 to 40 yr.

PEAK INCIDENCE: Unknown

PHYSICAL FINDINGS
- Conidia are deposited in alveoli, then fungus is converted to a yeast in the initial focus of bronchopneumonia and spreads to regional lymph nodes and other organs, especially liver and spleen, via lymphatics.
- From 7 to 18 days after onset, granulomatous inflammatory response marking host's cellular immunity begins to contain the yeast in the form of discrete granulomas.
- In normal host, fungistasis is achieved slowly as granulomas undergo contraction and, later, fibrosis with frequent calcification.
- With maturation of specific cellular immunity, there is development of delayed-type cutaneous hypersensitivity to *Histoplasma* antigens, usually 3 to 6 wk after exposure.
- Clinical disease manifests in various forms, depending on host cellular immunity and inoculum size:
1. Acute primary pulmonary histoplasmosis
   a. Overwhelming number of patients are asymptomatic.
   b. Most clinically apparent infections manifest by complaints of fever, headache, malaise, pleuritic chest pain, nonproductive cough, and weight loss.
   c. Less than 10%, mainly women, complain of arthralgias, myalgias, and skin manifestations such as erythema multiforme or erythema nodosum.
   d. Acute pericarditis presents in smaller percentage of patients.
   e. On auscultation findings are minimal; hepatosplenomegaly, seen sometimes in adults, is most commonly observed in children.
   f. With particularly heavy exposure, there is severe dyspnea, marked hypoxemia, impending respiratory failure
   g. Most patients are asymptomatic within 6 wk.
2. CPH
   a. Presents insidiously with low-grade fever, malaise, weight loss, cough, sometimes with blood-streaked sputum or frank hemoptysis.
   b. Most patients with cavitary lesions present with associated COPD or chronic bronchitis, masking underlying fungal disease.
   c. Tends to worsen preexisting pulmonary disease and further contribute to eventual respiratory insufficiency.
3. PDH
   a. In both acute and subacute forms constitutional symptoms of fever, fatigue, malaise, and weight loss are common.
   b. Acute form (seen most commonly in infants and children) is distinguished by predominance of respiratory symptoms, fevers consistently >101° F (38.3° C), generalized lymphadenopathy, marked hepatosplenomegaly, and fulminant course resembling septic shock associated with a high fatality rate.
   c. Subacute form is more common in adults and associated with lower temperatures, hepatosplenomegaly, oropharyngeal ulceration, focal organ involvement (including Addison's disease secondary to adrenal destruction, endocarditis, chronic meningitis, and intracerebral mass lesions)
   d. Course of subacute form is relentless, with untreated patient dying within 2 yr.
   e. Chronic PDH is found in adults and marked by gradual, often intermittent, symptoms of weight loss, weakness, easy fatigability; fever only uncommonly and usually of low grade when present; oropharyngeal ulcerations and hepatomegaly and/or splenomegaly in ⅓ of patients.
   f. Less clinical evidence of focal organ involvement in chronic form than in subacute form.
   g. Natural history of chronic form protracted and intermittent, spanning months to years.
- Histoplasmoma
  1. A healed area of caseation necrosis surrounded by a fibrous capsule
  2. Usually asymptomatic
- Mediastinal fibrosis
  1. A rare consequence of a fibroblastic process that encases caseating mediastinal lymph nodes after primary histoplasma bronchopneumonia

2. Progressive fibrosis producing severe retraction, compression, and distortion of mediastinal structures
3. Constriction of the bronchi resulting in bronchiectasis, also esophageal stenosis associated with dysphagia, and superior vena cava syndrome
- POHS
  1. Diagnosis characterized by distinct clinical features, including atrophic choroidal scars and maculopathy in patient with a history suggestive of exposure to the fungus (e.g., residence in an endemic area)
  2. Patient complaints of distortion or loss of central vision without pain, redness, or photophobia
  3. Usually no evidence of systemic infection except for a positive skin reaction to histoplasmin
- In patients with AIDS
  1. Possible presentation as overwhelming infection similar to acute PDH seen in children
  2. Constitutional symptoms: fever, weight loss, malaise, cough, dyspnea
  3. About 10% with cutaneous maculopapular, erythematous eruptions or purpuric lesions on face, trunk, and extremities
  4. Up to 20% with CNS involvement, manifesting as intracerebral mass lesions, chronic meningitis, or encephalopathy
  5. Infrequent oropharyngeal ulceration

ETIOLOGY
- *H. capsulatum* is a dimorphic fungus present in temperate zones and river valleys around the world.
- In U.S., it is highly endemic in southeastern, mid-Atlantic, and central states.
- Exists as mold at ambient temperature and favors surface soil enriched with bird or bat droppings.
- In endemic areas, contaminated dusty soil containing spores (microconidia) may be windswept or otherwise made airborne by sweeping, raking, or bulldozing, and then be inhaled.

DIAGNOSIS

DIFFERENTIAL DIAGNOSIS
- Acute pulmonary histoplasmosis
  1. *Mycobacterium tuberculosis*
  2. Community-acquired pneumonias caused by *Mycoplasma* and *Chlamydia*
  3. Other fungal diseases, such as *Blastomyces dermatitis* and *Coccidioides immitis*
- Chronic cavitary pulmonary histoplasmosis: *M. tuberculosis*
- Yeast forms of histoplasmosis on tissue section: cysts of *Pneumocystis carinii*, which tend to be larger, extracellular, and do not display budding
- Intracellular parasites of *Leishmania* and *Toxoplasma* species: distinguishable by inability to take up methenamine silver
- Histoplasmomas: true neoplasms

WORKUP
- Suspect diagnosis in patients who present with an influenzae-like illness and a history of residence or travel in an endemic area, especially if engaged in occupations (e.g., outside construction or street cleaning) or hobbies (e.g., cave exploring and aviary keeper) that increase the likelihood of exposure to fungal spore.
- Suspect diagnosis in immunosuppressed with remote history of exposure, especially if associated with characteristic calcifications on chest x-ray examination.

LABORATORY TESTS
- Demonstration of organism on culture from body fluid or tissues to make definitive diagnosis
  1. Especially high yield in patients with AIDS
  2. Characteristic oval yeast cells in neutrophils stained with Wright-Giemsa on peripheral smear
  3. Preparations of infected tissue with Gomori's silver methenamine for revealing yeast forms, especially in areas of caseation necrosis
- Serologic tests, including complement-fixing (CF) antibodies and immunodiffusion assays
  1. To establish previous infection and suggest active disease
  2. Possibly limited by inability to distinguish acute disease from remote infection and cross reactivity with other fungi
- Detection of *Histoplasma* antigen in urine: may be influenced by infections with *Blastocystis* and *Coccidioides*
- Skin testing with histoplasmin: useful epidemiologically but essentially useless for diagnosis of acute disease
- In PDH
  1. Pancytopenia
  2. Marked elevations in alkaline phosphatase and alanine aminotransferase (ALT) common
  3. Most evident in acute and subacute forms and to a lesser extent in chronic form
- In chronic meningitis (majority of cases)
  1. CSF pleocytosis with either lymphocytes or neutrophils predominating
  2. Elevated CSF protein levels
  3. Hypoglycorrhachia

IMAGING STUDIES
- Chest x-ray examination in acute pulmonary histoplasmosis
  1. Singular or multiple patchy infiltrates, especially in the lower lung fields
  2. Hilar or mediastinal lymphadenopathy with or without pneumonitis
  3. Diffuse nodular or confluent bilateral miliary infiltrates characteristic of heavier exposure
  4. Infrequent pleural effusions, except when associated with pericarditis
- Chest x-ray examination in histoplasmoma: coin lesion displaying central calcification, ranging from 1 to 4 cm in diameter, predominantly located in the subpleural regions
- Chest x-ray examination in CPH:
  1. Upper lobe disease frequently associated with cavities (thick-walled, secondarily infected with an *Aspergillus* fungus ball)
  2. Preexisting calcifications in the hilum associated with peribronchial streaking extending to the parenchyma

- Chest x-ray examination acute PDH: hilar adenopathy and/or diffuse nodular infiltrates
- CT scan of adrenals to reveal bilateral enlargement and low attenuation centers

TREATMENT

NONPHARMACOLOGIC THERAPY
For life-threatening disease seen in acute disseminated disease or infection in patients with AIDS: supportive therapy with IV fluids

ACUTE GENERAL Rx
- No drug therapy is required for patients with asymptomatic pulmonary disease and most patients with mild symptomatic pulmonary disease.
- Brief course of therapy with ketoconazole 400 mg/day or itraconazole 200 mg/day PO for 3 to 6 wk may be beneficial in some patients with acute pulmonary distress.
- Same therapy appropriate for immunocompetent, mild to moderately symptomatic patients with CPH and subacute and chronic forms of PDH, but duration of therapy is longer, ranging for 6 to 12 mo.
- Use amphotericin B 0.7 to 1 mg/kg IV for 6 to 12 mo in patients hypersensitive or intolerant to azole therapy.
- Do not give immunocompromised patients, especially those with AIDS, ketoconazole as primary therapy for disseminated histoplasmosis.
- Give Amphotericin B for life-threatening disease or continued illness as a result of primary failure or relapse of adequate azole therapy.
  1. For acute pulmonary histoplasmosis associated with acute respiratory distress syndrome (ARDS), acute PDH, and histoplasma meningitis: dose of 0.7 to 1 mg/kg IV >4 hr
  2. End point of therapy for patient with complicated acute pulmonary disease: total dose of 500 mg
  3. End point for patient with acute PDH: total dose 35 mg/kg or 2.5 g total
  4. Concomitant administration of prednisone 60 to 80 mg/day beneficial for severe fungal hypersensitivity complicating acute pulmonary disease
- Endocarditis: surgical treatment is preferable, with excision of infected valve or graft combined with amphotericin for a total dose of 35 mg/kg or 2.5 g
- For pericardial disease:
  1. Antifungal therapy: no apparent benefit
  2. Best managed with NSAIDs
- For POHS:
  1. Antifungal therapy: no apparent benefit
  2. May respond to laser therapy

CHRONIC Rx
In patients with AIDS: lifelong suppressive therapy with either itraconazole, given 200 mg PO qd, or IV amphotericin B at a dose of 50 mg once weekly

DISPOSITION
- Most immunocompetent patients with acute histoplasmosis are asymptomatic.
- For those with chronic or progressive disease, especially if immunocompromised by virtue of disease or medication, outcome and favorable prognosis are dependent on prompt recognition of varied forms of disease and timely administration of appropriate antifungal drugs.

REFERRAL
- For consultation with infectious disease specialist in suspected cases of disseminated disease, especially if immunocompromised
- To a pulmonologist for patients with CPH form because progressive respiratory compromise usually results from chronic infection and underlying COPD
- For consultation with a thoracic surgeon for decompression procedures in patients symptomatic as a consequence of progressive mediastinal fibrosis

MISCELLANEOUS

- *H. capsulatum*, variety *duboisii*, also known as African histoplasmosis, is restricted to Senegal, Nigeria, Zaire, and Uganda.
- Unlike *H. capsulatum*, pulmonary forms of *duboisii* are not seen, and the disease is limited to the skin, soft tissues, and bone.

COMMENTS
- Patients living in endemic areas, especially if immunocompromised, should be advised to take appropriate respiratory precautions when sweeping or disposing of bird waste from rooftop or home aviaries.
- Appropriate respiratory precautions should also be taken when leisure traveling to areas that act as a natural haven for the fungus, such as bat caves.
- Immunocompetent hosts are generally unaware of fungal infection, but the immunocompromised suffer devastating consequences.

REFERENCES
Bradsher RW: Histoplasmosis and blastomycosis, *Clin Infect Dis* 22(suppl 2):S102, 1996.
Kauffman CA: Role of azoles in antifungal therapy, *Clin Infect Dis* 22(suppl 2):S148, 1996.
Marshall JB et al: Mediastinal histoplasmosis presenting with esophageal involvement and dysphagia: case study, *Dysphagia* 10(1):53, 1995.
McKinsey DS et al: Histoplasmosis in Missouri: historical review and current clinical concepts, *Mo Med* 91(1):27, 1994.
Sosa N et al: Histoplasmosis of the central nervous system. Report of two cases and review of the literature, *Rev Med Panama* 21(1-2):18, 1996.
Stobierski MG et al: Outbreak of histoplasmosis among employees in a paper factory—Michigan, 1993, *J Clin Microbiol* 34(5):1220, 1996.
Suzaki A et al: An outbreak of acute pulmonary histoplasmosis among travelers to a bat-inhabited cave in Brazil, *Kansenshogaku Zasshi* 69(4):444, 1995.

Author: **George O. Alonso, M.D.**

HIV infection (PTG)

BASIC INFORMATION

DEFINITION
The human immunodeficiency virus, type 1 (HIV) causes a chronic infection that culminates, usually after several years, in the acquired immunodeficiency syndrome (AIDS).

SYNONYMS
Acquired immunodeficiency syndrome (AIDS) when a patient with HIV infection meets specific diagnostic criteria (see "Acquired Immunodeficiency Syndrome" in Section I)

ICD-9-CM CODES
044.9 HIV, unspecified

EPIDEMIOLOGY AND DEMOGRAPHICS
INCIDENCE (IN U.S.):
- No complete incidence data available.
- Greatest incidence is in metropolitan areas with population >500,000.

PREVALENCE (IN U.S.): Estimated at 1 to 2 million cases.

PREDOMINANT SEX:
- Adults: Most recently, 75% males, 25% females, but is changing toward more women
- Children: male = female

PREDOMINANT AGE: 80% of cases occurring between the ages of 20 and 40 yr

PEAK INCIDENCE: Age 30 to 35 yr

GENETICS:
Familial Disposition: No proven genetic predisposition

Congenital Infection:
- 80% of childhood cases are caused by peripartum infection, which may occur in utero, during delivery, or after delivery via breast-feeding.
- No specific congenital abnormalities are associated with HIV infection, although risk of spontaneous abortion and low birth weight is greater.

Neonatal Infection:
- May occur during delivery or via breast-feeding
- Typically asymptomatic

PHYSICAL FINDINGS
- Signs and symptoms variable with stage of disease
- In acute infection:
  1. May cause a self-limited mononucleosis-like illness characterized by fever, sore throat, lymphadenopathy, headache, and a rash resembling roseola
  2. In a minority of acute cases: frank aseptic meningitis, Bell's palsy, or peripheral neuropathy
- Later in the course of infection, after a prolonged asymptomatic phase: nonspecific symptoms of lymphadenopathy, weight loss, diarrhea, and skin changes including seborrheic dermatitis, localized herpes zoster, or fungal infection
- Advanced disease: characterized by the infections and malignancies associated with the acquired immunodeficiency (see specific disorders).

ETIOLOGY
- RNA retrovirus
- Transmitted by sexual contact, shared needles, blood transfusion, or from mother to child during pregnancy, delivery, or breast feeding
- Primary target of infection: CD4 lymphocyte
- Direct CNS involvement: manifested as encephalopathy, myelopathy, or neuropathy in advanced cases
- Renal failure, rheumatologic disorders, thrombocytopenia, or cardiac abnormalities

DIAGNOSIS

DIFFERENTIAL DIAGNOSIS
- Acute infection: mononucleosis or other respiratory viral infections
- Late symptoms: similar to those produced by other wasting illnesses such as neoplasms, TB, disseminated fungal infection, malabsorption, or depression
- HIV-related encephalopathy: confused with Alzheimer's disease or other causes of chronic dementia; myelopathy and neuropathy possibly resembling other demyelinating diseases such as multiple sclerosis

WORKUP
Diagnosis is established by voluntary testing for antibody to the virus, available through public health laboratories or private facilities.

LABORATORY TESTS
HIV antibody detected by a two-step technique:
- ELISA as a sensitive screening test
- Confirmation of positive ELISA tests with the more specific Western blot technique

TREATMENT

NONPHARMACOLOGIC THERAPY
Maintenance of adequate nutrition

ACUTE GENERAL Rx
- Acute management of opportunistic infections and malignancies (see AIDS-associated disorders, *"Pneumocystis carinii* Pneumonia," "Cryptococcosis," "Tuberculosis," "Toxoplasmosis" elsewhere in this text)
- Acute HIV syndrome:
  1. Treat with combination antiretroviral therapy, consisting of one or more nucleoside agents (zidovudine [AZT], didanosine [DDI], zalcitabine [DDC], lamivudine [3TC]) with or without the addition of a protease inhibitor (ritonavir, indinavir, or saquinavir).
  2. Recommended doses of these drugs and specific combinations are currently being assessed.

CHRONIC Rx
- All HIV-infected patients should be considered candidates for therapy with two or three drug combinations of the agents listed above.
- Specific recommendations are evolving, dictated by clinical and immunologic stage, as well as measurements of viral load.
- Patients with CD4 lymphocyte count <200/mm^3 should be given preventive therapy for *Pneumocystis carinii* pneumonia (PCP) (see "*Pneumocystis carinii* pneumonia").
- Evaluation of chronic diarrhea in patients with HIV is described in Fig. 3-29 and Box 2-33.

DISPOSITION
- Ongoing care consisting of frequent medical evaluations and T-lymphocyte subset analysis
- Long-term care focused on providing up-to-date antiretroviral therapy and prophylaxis of PCP and other opportunistic infections, as well as early detection of complications

REFERRAL
To a physician knowledgeable and experienced in the management of HIV infection and its complications

MISCELLANEOUS

COMMENTS
- Specific treatment regimens are frequently revised, with new therapies rapidly emerging.
- HIV chemoprophylaxis after occupational exposure is described in Table A-10.
- U.S. Preventive Services Task Force Recommendations regarding counseling to prevent HIV infection and other STDs are described in Section V, Chapter 62.

REFERENCES
Carpenter CCJ et al: Antiretroviral therapy for HIV infection in 1997: updated recommendations of the International AIDS Society—USA panel, *JAMA* 277(24):1962, 1997.

Author: **Joseph R. Masci, M.D.**

Hodgkin's disease (PTG)

BASIC INFORMATION

DEFINITION
Hodgkin's disease is a malignant disorder of lymphoreticular origin, characterized histologically by the presence of multinucleated giant cells (Reed-Sternberg cells) usually originating from B lymphocytes in germinal centers of lymphoid tissue.

ICD-9-CM CODES
201.9 Hodgkin's disease, unspecified
201.4 Hodgkin's disease, lymphocyte predominance
201.5 Hodgkin's disease, nodular sclerosis
201.6 Hodgkin's disease, mixed cellularity
201.7 Hodgkin's disease, lymphocyte depletion

EPIDEMIOLOGY AND DEMOGRAPHICS
- There is a bimodal age distribution (15 to 34 yr and >50 yr).
- Concordance for Hodgkin's disease in identical twins suggests a genetic susceptibility underlies Hodgkin's disease in young adulthood.
- The disease is more common in males (in childhood Hodgkin's disease, >80% occurs in males), in Caucasians, and in higher socioeconomic groups.
- Overall incidence of Hodgkin's disease in the U.S. is approximately 4:100,000.

PHYSICAL FINDINGS
- Palpable lymphadenopathy, generally painless
- Most common site of involvement: neck region

ETIOLOGY
Unknown; evidence implicating Epstein-Barr virus remains controversial.

DIAGNOSIS

DIFFERENTIAL DIAGNOSIS
- Non-Hodgkin's lymphoma
- Sarcoidosis
- Infections (e.g., CMV, Epstein-Barr virus, toxoplasma, HIV)
- Drug reaction
- Fig. 3-53 and 3-54 describe clinical algorithms for evaluation of lymphadenopathy.

WORKUP
Symptomatic patients with Hodgkin's disease usually present with the following manifestations:
- Fever and night sweats: fever in a cyclical pattern (days or weeks of fever alternating with afebrile periods) is known as Pel-Epstein fever
- Weight loss, generalized malaise
- Persistent, nonproductive cough
- Pain associated with alcohol ingestion, often secondary to heavy eosinophil infiltration of the tumor sites
- Pruritus
- Others: superior vena cava syndrome and spinal cord compression (rare)

Diagnosis can be made with lymph node biopsy. There are four main **histologic subtypes,** based on the number of lymphocytes, Reed-Sternberg cells, and the presence of fibrous tissue:
1. Lymphocyte predominance
2. Mixed cellularity
3. Nodular sclerosis
4. Lymphocyte depletion

Nodular sclerosis is the most common type and occurs mainly in young adulthood, whereas the mixed cellularity type is more prevalent after age 50 yr.

Staging for Hodgkin's disease follows the **Ann Arbor staging classification.**
- Stage I: Involvement of a single lymph node region
- Stage II: Two or more lymph node regions on the same side of the diaphragm
- Stage III: Lymph node involvement on both sides of diaphragm, including spleen
- Stage IV: Diffuse involvement of external sites
- Suffix A: No systemic symptoms
- Suffix B: Presence of fever, night sweats, or unexplained weight loss of 10% or more body weight over 6 mo
- Suffix X: Indicates bulky disease >⅓ widening of mediastinum or >10 cm maximum dimension of nodal mass on a chest film

Proper **staging** requires the following:
- Detailed history (with documentation of "B symptoms") and physical examination
- Surgical biopsy
- Laboratory evaluation (CBC, sedimentation rate, BUN, creatinine, alkaline phosphatase, liver function studies, albumin, LDH, uric acid)
- Chest x-ray studies (PA and lateral); see Box 2-77 (Section II) for differential diagnosis of mediastinal masses or widening on chest x-ray examination
- Bilateral bone marrow biopsy
- CT scan of the chest (when abnormal findings are noted on chest x-ray examination) and of the abdomen and pelvis to visualize the mesenteric, hepatic, portal and splenic hilar nodes

- Bipedal lymphangiography to define periaortic and iliac lymph node involvement
- Exploratory laparotomy and splenectomy:
  1. Decision to perform staging laparotomy depends on the therapeutic plan; it is generally not indicated in patients who have a large mediastinal mass (these patients will generally be treated with combined chemotherapy and radiation). Staging laparotomy may also not be required in patients with clinical Stage I or unlikely to have abdominal disease (e.g., females with supradiaphragmatic disease).
  2. Exploratory laparotomy and splenectomy may be used for patients with clinical Stage I-IIA or IIB.
  3. It is useful in identifying patients who can be treated with irradiation alone with curative intent.
  4. Polyvalent pneumococcal vaccine should be given prophylactically to all patients before splenectomy (increased risk of sepsis from encapsulated organisms in splenectomized patients).
- Gallium scan

LABORATORY TESTS
See "Workup."

IMAGING STUDIES
See "Workup."

TREATMENT

ACUTE GENERAL Rx
The main therapeutic modalities are radiotherapy and chemotherapy; the indication for each vary with pathologic stage and other factors.

- Stage I and II: radiation therapy alone unless a large mediastinal mass is present (mediastinal to thoracic ratio ≥ 1.3); in the latter case, a combination of chemotherapy and radiation therapy is indicated.
- Stage IB or IIB: total nodal irradiation is often used, although chemotherapy is performed in many centers.
- Stage IIIA: treatment is controversial. It varies with the anatomic substage after splenectomy.
  1. III_1A and minimum splenic involvement: radiation therapy alone may be adequate.
  2. III_2 or III_1A with extensive splenic involvement: there is disagreement whether chemotherapy alone or a combination of chemotherapy and radiation therapy is the preferred treatment modality.
  3. IIIB and IVB: the treatment of choice is chemotherapy with or without adjuvant radiotherapy. Various regimens can be used for combination of chemotherapy; some commonly used regimens are MOPP, MOPP-ABV, ABVD, MOPP-ABVD, MOPP-BAP.

DISPOSITION
- The overall survival at 10 yr is approximately 60%.
- Poor prognostic features include presence of "B symptoms," advanced age, advanced stage at initial presentation, mixed-cellularity, and lymphocyte depletion histology.
- Chemotherapy significantly increases the risk of leukemia.
- The peak in risk of leukemia is seen approximately 5 yr after the initiation of chemotherapy.
- The risk of leukemia is greater for those who undergo splenectomy and for patients with advanced stages of Hodgkin's disease; the risk is unaffected by concomitant radiotherapy.
- Mediastinal irradiation increases the risk of subsequent death from heart disease caused by sclerosis of coronary artery secondary to irradiation. Risk increases with high mediastinal doses, minimal protective cardiac blocking, young age at irradiation, and increased duration of follow-up.
- Both chemotherapy and/or radiation therapy increase the risk of developing secondary solid tumors (e.g., carcinoma of the lung, breast, and stomach).

REFERRAL
- Surgical referral for lymph node biopsy
- Hematology/oncology referral

MISCELLANEOUS

COMMENTS
Young male patients should consider sperm banking before the initiation of therapy.

REFERENCES
Canellos GP et al: Etoposide, vinblastine, and doxorubicin: an active regimen for the treatment of Hodgkin's disease and relapse following MOPP, cancer and leukemia group, *J Clin Oncol* 13:2005, 1995.

Mack TM et al: Concordance for Hodgkin's disease in identical twins suggesting genetic susceptibility to the young adult form of the disease, *New Engl J Med* 332:413, 1995.

Van Leeuwen FE et al: Second cancer risk following Hodgkin's disease: a 20-year follow-up study, *J Clin Oncol* 12:312, 1994.

Author: **Fred F. Ferri, M.D.**

Hookworm (PTG)

BASIC INFORMATION

DEFINITION
Hookworm is a parasitic infection of the intestine caused by helminths.

ICD-9-CM CODES
126.35 Hookworm

EPIDEMIOLOGY AND DEMOGRAPHICS
INCIDENCE (IN U.S.):
- Varies greatly in different areas of the U.S.
- Most common in rural areas of southeastern U.S.
- Increased likelihood in areas of poor sanitation and increased rainfall

PREVALENCE (IN U.S.): Varies from 10% to 90% in regions where it is found

PREDOMINANT AGE: Schoolchildren

PHYSICAL FINDINGS
- Most infections are asymptomatic
- Nonspecific abdominal complaints
- Because these organisms consume host RBCs, symptoms related to iron-deficiency anemia, depending on the amount of iron in the diet and the worm burden
- Fatigue, tachycardia, dyspnea, and high-output failure
- Hypoproteinemia and edema from loss of proteins into the intestinal tract
- Unusual for pulmonary manifestations to occur when the larvae migrate through the lungs
- Skin rash at sites of larval penetration in some individuals without prior exposure

ETIOLOGY
Two species are causative: *Necator americanus* and *Ancylostoma duodenale*. *N. americanus* is the predominant cause of hookworm in U.S.
- Penetration of the skin by the larval form, with subsequent migration via the blood stream to the alveoli, up the respiratory tract, then into the GI tract
- Sharp mouth parts for attachment to intestinal mucosa

DIAGNOSIS

DIFFERENTIAL DIAGNOSIS
- Strongyloidiasis
- Ascariasis
- Table 2-38 describes the differential diagnosis of intestinal helminths.

WORKUP
Examine stool for hookworm eggs.

LABORATORY TESTS
CBC to show hypochromic, microcytic anemia; possible mild eosinophilia and hypoalbuminemia

IMAGING STUDIES
Chest x-ray examination: occasionally shows opacities

TREATMENT

NONPHARMACOLOGIC THERAPY
Prevention of disease by not walking barefoot and improving sanitary conditions

ACUTE GENERAL Rx
- Mebendazole 100 mg PO bid for 3 days
- Iron supplementation possibly helpful

DISPOSITION
Easily treated.

REFERRAL
If diagnosis uncertain

MISCELLANEOUS

COMMENTS
Appropriate disposal of human wastes is important in controlling the disease in areas with a high prevalence of hookworm infestation.

REFERENCES
Grencis RK, BSc Hons, Cooper ES: *Enterobius, Trichuris, Capillaria,* and hookworm including *Ancylostoma caninum*. Gastroenterol Clin North Am 25(3):579, 1996.

Author: **Maurice Policar, M.D.**

Hordeolum (stye)

BASIC INFORMATION

DEFINITION
A hordeolum is an acute inflammatory process affecting the eyelid and arising from the meibomian (posterior) or Zeis (anterior) glands. It is most often infectious and usually caused by *Staphylococcus aureus*.

SYNONYMS
Stye

ICD-9-CM CODES
373.11 External hordeolum
373.12 Internal hordeolum

EPIDEMIOLOGY AND DEMOGRAPHICS
INCIDENCE (IN U.S.): Unknown
PREVALENCE (IN U.S.): Unknown
PREDOMINANT SEX: No gender predilection
PREDOMINANT AGE: May occur at any age
PEAK INCIDENCE: May occur at any age
NEONATAL INFECTION: Rare in the neonatal period

PHYSICAL FINDINGS
- Abrupt onset with pain and erythema of the eyelid
- Localized, tender mass in the eyelid
- May be associated with blepharitis
- External hordeolum: points toward the skin surface of the lid and may spontaneously drain
- Internal hordeolum: can point toward the conjunctival side of the lid and may cause conjunctival inflammation

ETIOLOGY
- 75% to 95% of cases are caused by *S. aureus*.
- Occasional cases are caused by *Streptococcus pneumoniae*, other streptococci, gram-negative enteric organisms, or mixed bacterial flora.

DIAGNOSIS

DIFFERENTIAL DIAGNOSIS
- Eyelid abscess
- Chalazion
- Allergy or contact dermatitis with conjunctival edema
- Acute dacryocystitis
- *Herpes simplex* infection
- Cellulitis of the eyelid

LABORATORY TESTS
- Generally, none are necessary.
- If incision and drainage are performed, specimens should be sent for bacterial culture.

IMAGING STUDIES
None necessary

TREATMENT

NONPHARMACOLOGIC THERAPY
Usually responds to warm compresses

ACUTE GENERAL Rx
- Systemic antibiotics generally not necessary
- In refractory cases, an oral anti-staphylococcal agent (e.g., dicloxacillin 500 mg PO four times daily) possibly helpful
- Topical erythromycin ophthalmic ointment applied to the lid margins two to four times daily until resolution
- Incision and drainage: rarely needed but should be considered for progressive infections

CHRONIC Rx
None necessary

DISPOSITION
- Usually sporadic occurrence
- Possible relapse if resolution is not complete

REFERRAL
- For evaluation by an ophthalmologist if visual acuity or ocular movement is affected or if the diagnosis is in doubt
- For surgical drainage if necessary

MISCELLANEOUS

COMMENTS
Seborrheic dermatitis may coexist with hordeolum.

REFERENCES
O'Brien TP, Green WR: Periocular infections. In Mandell GL, Bennett JE, Dolin R (eds): *Principles and practice of infectious diseases,* ed 4, New York, 1995, Churchill-Livingstone.

Author: **Joseph R. Masci, M.D.**

Human granulocytic ehrlichiosis (PTG)

BASIC INFORMATION

DEFINITION
Human granulocytic ehrlichiosis (HGE) is a zoonotic infection of granulocytes, caused by an *Ehrlichia* species closely related to *E. phagocytophila* and *E. equi*, with multisystem manifestations.

ICD-9-CM CODES
082.8 Other tick-borne rickettsiosis

EPIDEMIOLOGY AND DEMOGRAPHICS
INCIDENCE (IN U.S.): Uncertain; about 150 to 200 cases reported since 1994 from Wisconsin, Minnesota, Massachusetts, Connecticut, Pennsylvania, Rhode Island, and New York; also acquired in Maryland, California, Florida, and Arkansas.
PREVALENCE (IN U.S.): Unknown; definitive serology not available
PREDOMINANT SEX: Uncertain; to date, 78% male
PREDOMINANT AGE: Uncertain; range 6 to 91 yr (median age, 59 yr)
PEAK INCIDENCE:
- Uncertain; probably age 30 to 60 yr
- Occurs throughout the year, with peaks in rural areas during May through July
- More detailed epidemiologic studies needed to define prevalence and incidence parameters

PHYSICAL FINDINGS
- Most common initial symptoms:
  1. Fever (100%)
  2. Chills (98%)
  3. Myalgia (98%)
  4. Headache (85%)
- Tick exposure reported by 90%, tick bites by 73% within a median of 8 days of illness
- Subsequent symptoms
  1. Malaise (98%)
  2. Nausea, vomiting, cough (29%)
  3. Confusion (17%).
- Generally, nonspecific physical examination
- Rash (maculopapular) rare
- Complications:
  1. Hepatitis
  2. Interstitial pneumonitis
  3. Mild azotemia
  4. Anemia

ETIOLOGY
- Obligate intracellular gram-negative bacterium (family *Rickettsiaceae*, genus *Ehrlichia*), closely related (99.8% homology of the 16s rDNA) to *E. phagocytophila* and *E. equi*
- Vector:
  1. Almost certainly tickborne
  2. Strong evidence implicating *Ixodes scapularis (dammini),* which contains *Ehrlichia* in saliva
  3. Possible association with *I. pacificus* in California (experimental vector of *E. equi*)
  4. Tick exposure reported in 90% to 100% of patients, with 65% to 75% reporting tick bite
- Mammalian hosts: deer, horses, dogs, white-footed mice, cattle, sheep, goats
- Precise pathogenesis is unclear, although host inflammatory and immune responses may define final spectrum of disease beyond granulocytes, including hepatitis, interstitial pneumonia, nephritis with mild azotemia, and anemia.
- Recovery is usual outcome, with mortality of approximately 5% (probably higher in untreated patients and lower with early therapy).

DIAGNOSIS

DIFFERENTIAL DIAGNOSIS
- Human monocytic ehrlichiosis (HME)
  1. Caused by *E. chaffeensis* (vector: tick *Amblyomma americanum*, possibly *Dermacentor variabilis*)
  2. Rash more common, sometimes petechial
  3. Morulae in monocytes
- Rocky Mountain spotted fever, Colorado tick fever, Q fever, relapsing fever
- Babesiosis
- Leptospirosis
- Typhus
- Lyme disease
- Legionnaire's disease
- Tularemia
- Typhoid fever, paratyphoid fever
- Brucellosis
- Viral hepatitis
- Enteroviral infections
- Meningococcemia
- Influenza
- Adenovirus pneumonia

WORKUP
- Acute blood samples for Giemsa-stained smears
- CBC
- Prothrombin time
- Acute serum samples for serology
- Chest x-ray examination
- Liver function and renal function tests
- Bone marrow rarely needed

LABORATORY TESTS
- Giemsa-stained smear demonstrating morulae of *Ehrlichia* within granulocytes (in >50% of cases)
- CBC: progressive leukopenia and thrombocytopenia, with nadir near day 7
- Anemia (Hct falls steadily during first few weeks)
- Coagulopathy in severe infections
- Serologic titer (IFA) ≥80, or fourfold increase in titer, to *E. equi* antigen, which resembles the agent of HGE
- Polymerase chain reaction (PCR) to facilitate early diagnosis (not widely available)
- Marrow variable and nonspecific
- Liver function tests to reveal hepatocellular hepatitis (mildly elevated ALT, AST)
- Renal function tests to demonstrate mild azotemia

IMAGING STUDIES
Chest x-ray examination to show interstitial pneumonitis (unusual)

TREATMENT

ACUTE GENERAL Rx
- Immediate therapy to limit extent of acute illness and complications (possibly lifesaving)
- Doxycycline (100 mg PO bid in adults for about 2 to 3 days after defervescence and at least 7 days) recommended on the basis of clinical experience; awaiting therapeutic trials and susceptibility surveys
- Empiric therapy possibly lifesaving

CHRONIC Rx
Probably unnecessary; undefined

DISPOSITION
- Follow-up as outpatient
- Repeat CBC every 2 to 4 wk until normal

REFERRAL
- For consultation with infectious diseases specialist and hematologist in suspected cases
- For coagulopathy
- Although differential diagnosis lengthy and complicated, therapy should not be delayed.

MISCELLANEOUS

COMMENTS
Duration of time tick must be attached to produce illness is uncertain (probably 12 to 24 hr).

REFERENCES
Walker DH: More trouble from ticks, *Hosp Pract* 31:47,1996.
Walker DH, Dumler JS: The emergence of ehrlichioses as human health problems, *Emerg Infect Dis* 2:18,1996.
Author: **Peter Nicholas, M.D.**

Huntington's chorea

BASIC INFORMATION

DEFINITION
Huntington's chorea is an inherited progressive neurodegenerative disorder characterized by choreoathetosis and neuropsychiatric dysfunction associated with pronounced neuronal loss in the caudate nucleus.

SYNONYMS
Huntington's Disease

ICD-9-CM CODES
333.4 Huntington's chorea

EPIDEMIOLOGY AND DEMOGRAPHICS
PREVALENCE (IN U.S.): 4.1 to 5.4 cases/100,000 persons
PREDOMINANT SEX: Female = male
PREDOMINANT AGE: Early adulthood
PEAK INCIDENCE: Late 30s and 40s, with onsets from age 2 to 70 yr
GENETICS: Autosomal dominant; responsible gene an expanded trinucleotide repeat sequence located on the short arm of chromosome 4

PHYSICAL FINDINGS
- Initially, subtle disturbance of oculomotor function, small choreiform movements, or psychiatric dysfunction
- With progression, pronounced choreoathetotic movements, resulting in a characteristically erratic gait
- Juvenile onset variant: cognitive dysfunction, bradykinesia, and rigidity

ETIOLOGY
- Unknown
- Proposed cause: excitatory amino acid transmitter-mediated toxicity

DIAGNOSIS

DIFFERENTIAL DIAGNOSIS
- Drug-induced chorea
- Sydenham's chorea
- Benign hereditary chorea
- Senile chorea
- Wilson's disease
- Neuroacanthocytosis
- Olivopontocerebellar atrophy
- Table 2-32 describes the differential diagnosis of hyperkinetic movement disorders.

WORKUP
Onset of symptoms in an individual with an established family history requires no additional investigation.

LABORATORY TESTS
- Confirm diagnosis by DNA testing.
- If DNA normal, obtain CBC with smear, ESR, electrolytes, serum ceruloplasmin, 24-hr urinary copper excretion, TFT, ANA, VDRL, HIV, and ASO titer.

IMAGING STUDIES
CT scan or MRI scan will show caudate atrophy in more advanced cases.

TREATMENT

NONPHARMACOLOGIC THERAPY
- Supportive counseling
- Physical and occupational therapy
- Home health care
- Genetic counseling

ACUTE GENERAL Rx
None

CHRONIC Rx
- Chorea may be diminished by low doses of neuroleptics (e.g., haloperidol 1 to 10 mg/day).
- Depression with suicidal ideation is common; may improve with tricyclic or SSRI antidepressants.

DISPOSITION
Relentless, progressive course of variable duration leading to progressive disability and death

REFERRAL
If uncertain about diagnosis or management

MISCELLANEOUS

REFERENCES
Furtado S, Suchowersky O: Huntington's disease: recent advances in diagnosis and management, *Can J Neurol Sci* 22:5, 1995.

Author: **Michael Gruenthal, M.D., Ph.D.**

Hydrocephalus, normal pressure

BASIC INFORMATION

DEFINITION
Normal pressure hydrocephalus (NPH) is marked by a clinical triad of gait disturbance, mental deterioration, and urinary incontinence associated with chronic hydrocephalus and normal CSF pressure as measured by routine lumbar puncture.

ICD-9-CM CODES
742.3 Congenital hydrocephalus

EPIDEMIOLOGY AND DEMOGRAPHICS
PREDOMINANT SEX: Males = females
PREDOMINANT AGE: Fourth to sixth decade

PHYSICAL FINDINGS
- Initial symptoms: gait difficulty
- Typical finding: difficulty initiating ambulation, with the appearance that the feet are stuck to the floor ("magnetic gait")
- Cognitive slowing, forgetfulness and inattention without agnosia, aphasia or other "cortical" disturbances
- Later signs: urinary urgency and subsequent incontinence

ETIOLOGY
- Most cases: chronic communicating hydrocephalus (50% idiopathic)
- Other 50%: result from prior subarachnoid hemorrhage, meningitis, trauma, or intracranial surgery

DIAGNOSIS

DIFFERENTIAL DIAGNOSIS
Signs and symptoms are nonspecific and may be seen with any process causing bilateral periventricular white matter lesions.

WORKUP
- Lumbar puncture with accurate opening pressure measurement is essential; elevated opening pressure suggests more acute process, which must be investigated.
- Numerous attempts at establishing a confirming test have been disappointing.
- Clinical response to removal of CSF and isotope cisternography are popular, but lack sensitivity or specificity to confirm the diagnosis or predict improvement from shunting.

LABORATORY TESTS
CSF should be sent for routine fluid analyses to exclude other pathology.

IMAGING STUDIES
CT scan, MRI, and isotope cisternography are popular but unreliable.

TREATMENT

NONPHARMACOLOGIC THERAPY
- Some patients (30% of those with idiopathic NPH and 60% of patients with a known etiology) show significant improvement from shunting.
- There is a better outcome with early shunting, before substantial cognitive decline or incontinence.

ACUTE GENERAL Rx
Shunting in selected patients

REFERRAL
Neurosurgical referral for shunting in appropriate patients.

MISCELLANEOUS

REFERENCES
Vanneste: Three decades of normal pressure hydrocephalus: are we wiser now? *J Neurol Neurosurg Psychiatry* 57:1021, 1994.

Author: **Michael Gruenthal, M.D., Ph.D.**

Hypercholesterolemia (PTG)

BASIC INFORMATION

DEFINITION
Hypercholesterolemia refers to a blood cholesterol measurement >200 mg/dl. A cholesterol level of 200 to 239 mg/dl is considered borderline high, and a level of ≥240 mg/dl is considered to be high a cholesterol measurement.

SYNONYMS
Hypercholesteremia
Hypercholesterinemia
Type II familial hyperlipoproteinemia

ICD-9-CM CODES
272.0 Hypercholesterolemia

EPIDEMIOLOGY AND DEMOGRAPHICS
INCIDENCE/PREVALENCE:
- There are well over 100,000,000 Americans with a total serum cholesterol >200 mg/dl.
- Elevated cholesterol requires drug therapy in about 60 million Americans.
- Incidence of heterozygous familial hypercholesterolemia: about 1:500.
- Incidence of homozygous familial hypercholesterolemia: about 1:1,000,000.
- Prevalence of hypercholesterolemia increases with increasing age.

GENETICS:
- Familial hypercholesterolemia: autosomal dominant disorder
- Familial combined hyperlipidemia: possibly an autosomal dominant disorder
- Multifactorial predilection: apparent in majority of affected individuals

RISK FACTORS:
- Dietary intake
- Genetic predisposition
- Sedentary life-style
- Associated secondary causes

PHYSICAL FINDINGS
- Most patients: no physical findings
- Possible findings particularly in the familial forms
  1. Tendon xanthomas
  2. Xanthelasma
  3. Arcus corneae
  4. Arterial bruits (young adulthood)

ETIOLOGY
Primary
  1. Genetics
  2. Obesity
  3. Dietary intake
Secondary
  1. Diabetes mellitus
  2. Alcohol
  3. Oral contraceptives
  4. Hypothyroidism
  5. Glucocorticoid use
  6. Most diuretics
  7. Nephrotic syndrome
  8. Hepatoma
  9. Extrahepatic biliary obstruction
  10. Primary biliary cirrhosis

DIAGNOSIS

DIFFERENTIAL DIAGNOSIS
No real differential diagnosis; however, consider underlying secondary causes/etiologies for the elevated cholesterol.

LABORATORY TESTS
PRIMARY PREVENTION WITHOUT ATHEROSCLEROSIS:
1. Total cholesterol <200 mg/dl, and the HDL >35: repeat in 5 yr.
2. Cholesterol 200 to 239 mg/dl and the HDL >35: discuss dietary modification, repeat in 1 to 2 yr.
3. Total cholesterol >240 mg/dl or the HDL <35 mg/dl: need a fasting lipid profile (cholesterol, HDL, triglycerides, from which an LDL can be calculated).
4. Fasting lipid profile with LDL <130 mg/dl: dietary guidance and repeat in 5 yr.
5. Fasting lipid profile with LDL 130 to 159 mg/dl (borderline high risk), and less than two risk factors for CAD: diet and exercise modification, with repeat profile in 1 yr.
6. Fasting lipid profile with LDL >160 mg/dl or borderline LDL and two or more risk factors for CAD: need drug therapy.

SECONDARY PREVENTION WITHOUT ATHEROSCLEROSIS:
1. All patients: fasting lipid profile
2. If LDL < 100 mg/dl: instruction on diet and exercise, and repeat annually
3. If LDL > 100 mg/dl: drug therapy required

TREATMENT

NONPHARMACOLOGIC THERAPY
- First line of treatment: dietary therapy
- Dietary modifications
  1. Low-cholesterol, low-fat diet (fat intake to 30% or less of the total caloric intake)
  2. Saturated fats 8% to 10% of total calories
  3. No more than 300 mg/day of cholesterol
- Increased activity with aerobic exercise: encourage 20 to 30 min of aerobic exercise three to four times a week
- Smoking cessation encouraged
- Counseling on CAD risk factors

ACUTE GENERAL Rx
No acute treatment needed

CHRONIC Rx
- In primary prevention: needed for patients with LDL >160 mg/dl or LDL 130 to 159 mg/dl with two or more risk factors for CAD
- In secondary prevention: needed for patients with known CAD and LDL >100 mg/dl
- In primary prevention: considered in patients on dietary therapy with LDL >190 mg/dl with no risk factors, LDL >160 mg/dl with two or more risk factors, or HDL <30 mg/dl
- Medications that can be used:
  1. Bile acid sequestrants (poorly tolerated)
  2. Niacin (poorly tolerated)
  3. HMG-CoA reductase inhibitors ("statins")
  4. Fibric acids
  5. Medication tailored to the patient's lipid profile, life-style, and the medication's side effect profile
- Bile acid sequestrants to lower LDL
- Niacin to lower LDL and triglycerides and raise HDL
- HMG-CoA reductase inhibitors to lower LDL
- Fibric acids work to lower triglycerides more than LDL
- Table 7-25 compares the various lipid-lowering agents.

DISPOSITION
- After initiation of therapy, repeat laboratory tests in 4 to 6 wk, with modifications as necessary.
- Once goal is achieved, lifelong medication and monitoring is needed at least three to four times a year.
- Dietary modification is needed to continue with drug therapy.
- Repeat review for additional CAD risk factors.

MISCELLANEOUS

COMMENTS
U.S. Preventive Services Task Force Recommentdations regarding screening for hypercholesterolemia and other lipid abnormalities are described in Section V, Chapter 2.

REFERENCES
Summary of the second report of the National Cholesterol Education Program (NCEP) expert panel on detection, evaluation, and treatment of high blood cholesterol in adults (Adult Treatment Panel II), *JAMA* 269(13):3015, 1993.

Author: **Beth J. Wutz, M.D.**

Hyperemesis gravidarum

BASIC INFORMATION

DEFINITION
Hyperemesis gravidarum is the persistent nausea and vomiting with onset in the first 20-wk trimester of pregnancy, resulting in weight loss and fluid and electrolyte and acid-base imbalances.

ICD-9-CM CODES
643.1 Hyperemesis gravidarum

EPIDEMIOLOGY AND DEMOGRAPHICS
INCIDENCE: 0.5 to 10 cases /1000 pregnancies
GENETICS: No genetic disposition
RISK FACTORS:
- Multiple pregnancy
- Molar pregnancy
- Previous history of unsuccessful pregnancy
- Nulliparity
- Hyperemesis gravidarum in a prior pregnancy.
- No correlation with race, socioeconomic status, or marital status.

PEAK ONSET: 8 to 12 wk of gestation

PHYSICAL FINDINGS
- Weight loss
- Rapid heart rate
- Fall in blood pressure
- Dry mucous membranes
- Loss of skin elasticity
- Ketotic odor
- In severe cases, Wernicke's encephalopathy as a result of thiamine deficiency

ETIOLOGY
Specific etiology is unknown.

DIAGNOSIS

DIFFERENTIAL DIAGNOSIS
Pancreatitis, cholecystitis, hepatitis, pyelonephritis

WORKUP
Hyperemesis gravidarum is a diagnosis of exclusion. A detailed history and physical examination along with laboratory tests to rule out other causes of vomiting in early pregnancy are indicated.

LABORATORY TESTS
- Urinalysis to document ketonuria and proteinuria
- Urine C&S to rule out pyelonephritis
- Serum electrolytes to rule out electrolyte and acid-base imbalance
- Serum concentration of aminotransferases and bilirubin to rule out hepatitis.
- Serum amylase to rule out pancreatitis
- Free T_4 and TSH (elevated T_4 with suppressed TSH levels present in up to 60% of patients with hyperemesis gravidarum. This biochemical hyperthyroidism usually spontaneously resolves after 18 wk.)

IMAGING STUDIES
- Pelvic ultrasound examination to rule out multiple gestation and molar pregnancy
- Ultrasound of the gallbladder to rule out cholecystitis

TREATMENT

NONPHARMACOLOGIC THERAPY
- Reassurance
- Psychologic support
- Avoidance of foods that trigger nausea
- Frequent small meals once oral intake has resumed

ACUTE GENERAL Rx
- NPO
- Fluid and electrolyte replacement
- Parental vitamin supplementation
- Daily supplementation of thiamine 100 mg IM or IV to prevent Wernicke's encephalopathy
- Antiemetics, such as promethazine (Phenergan) or droperidol (Inapsine), have not been found to be associated with fetal malformations when given in early pregnancy. Promethazine given as a low-dose continuous infusion of 25 mg in each liter of IV fluid has been shown to be very effective in controlling nausea and vomiting.
- Restart oral intake gradually no <48 hr after vomiting has ceased.

CHRONIC Rx
If the above acute therapy does not resolve vomiting and oral intake is not feasible, parenteral hyperalimentation may be necessary.

DISPOSITION
- Untreated hyperemesis gravidarum can result in maternal renal and hepatic damage or death from fluid and electrolyte imbalance.
- Hyperemesis gravidarum with severe weight loss has been associated with lower average birth weight and with CNS malformations in neonates.

REFERRAL
For parenteral hyperalimentation if required

MISCELLANEOUS

COMMENTS
Although the specific etiology of hyperemesis gravidarum is not known, psychogenic causes proposed in older literature have been largely discredited. "Behavioral therapies" for hyperemesis gravidarum are inappropriate.

REFERENCES
Gabbe S, Niebyl J, Simpson J (eds): *Obstetrics: normal and problem pregnancies*, New York, 1996, Churchill Livingstone.
Hod M et al: Hyperemesis gravidarum: a review, *J Reprod Med* 39:605,1994.

Author: **Laurel White, M.D.**

Hyperlipoproteinemia, primary (PTG)

BASIC INFORMATION

DEFINITION
Primary hyperlipoproteinemia refers to a group of genetic disorders of the lipid transport proteins in the blood, which manifests as abnormally elevated levels of cholesterol, triglycerides, or both in the serum of affected patients.

SYNONYMS
Hyperlipidemia

ICD-9-CM CODES
272.4 Hyperlipoproteinemia
272.3 Fredrickson type I
272.0 Fredrickson type IIa
272.2 Fredrickson type IIb, III
272.1 Fredrickson type IV
272.3 Fredrickson type V

EPIDEMIOLOGY AND DEMOGRAPHICS
INCIDENCE:
- Variable depending on the genetic defect
- Spectrum spans the common familial hypercholesterolemia, with an incidence of 1:500, to the rare familial lipoprotein lipase deficiency

PREDOMINANT SEX: None
GENETICS:
- Familial lipoprotein lipase deficiency: autosomal recessive, resulting in an elevation in the plasma chylomicrons and triglycerides
- Familial apoprotein CII deficiency: autosomal recessive, resulting in increased serum chylomicrons, VLDL, and hypertriglyceridemia
- Familial Type 3 hyperlipoproteinemia: single-gene defect requiring contributory factors to manifest
- Familial hypercholesterolemia: autosomal dominant defect of the LDL receptor resulting in an elevated serum cholesterol level and normal triglycerides
- Familial hypertriglyceridemia: common, autosomal dominant defect resulting in elevated VLDL and triglycerides
- Multiple lipoprotein type hyperlipidemia: autosomal dominant, manifesting as isolated hypercholesterolemia, isolated hypertriglyceridemia, or hyperlipidemia
- Polygenic hypercholesterolemia: multifactorial
- Polygenic hyperalphalipoproteinemia: autosomal dominant or polygenic, causing an elevated HDL

PHYSICAL FINDINGS
- Familial lipoprotein lipase deficiency: recurrent bouts of abdominal pain in infancy, eruptive xanthomas, hepatomegaly, splenomegaly, lipemia retinalis
- Familial apoprotein CII deficiency: occasional eruptive xanthomas
- Familial type 3 hyperlipoproteinemia: after age 20 yr see xanthoma striata palmaris or tuberoeruptive xanthomas, xanthelasmas, arterial bruits at a young age, gangrene of the lower extremities at a young age
- Familial hypercholesterolemia: tendon xanthomas, arcus corneae, xanthelasma
- Familial hypertriglyceridemia: associated obesity, with exacerbations can develop eruptive xanthomas
- Multiple lipoprotein type hyperlipidemia: no discerning physical findings
- Polygenic hypercholesterolemia: no discerning physical findings
- Polygenic hyperalphalipoproteinemia: no discerning physical findings

ETIOLOGY
Genetic defects causing lipid abnormalities

DIAGNOSIS

DIFFERENTIAL DIAGNOSIS
Secondary causes of hyperlipoproteinemias:
1. Diabetes mellitus
2. Glycogen storage diseases
3. Lipodystrophies
4. Glucocorticoid use/excess
5. Alcohol
6. Oral contraceptives
7. Renal disease
8. Hepatic dysfunction

WORKUP
- Detailed family history for premature cardiac disease
- Recurrent pancreatitis
- Thorough physical examination

LABORATORY TESTS
- Lipoprotein analysis
- Lipoprotein electrophoresis

TREATMENT

NONPHARMACOLOGIC THERAPY
- Cornerstone of treatment: dietary therapy
- Familial lipoprotein lipase deficiency and familial apoprotein CII deficiency: fat-free diet
- Remainder of cases, except those with polygenic hyperalphalipoproteinemia: fat- and cholesterol-restricted diets

ACUTE GENERAL Rx
No acute treatment needed

CHRONIC Rx
- Familial lipoprotein lipase deficiency, polygenic hyperalphalipoproteinemia, or familial apoprotein CII deficiency: no chronic drug therapy
- Familial type 3 hyperlipoproteinemia: usually responds well to secondary causes being treated and diet therapy; if not, fibric acids may be tried
- Familial hypercholesterolemia: bile acid sequestrants, HMG Co-A reductase inhibitors or niacin
- Familial hypertriglyceridemia: fibric acids
- Multiple lipoprotein type hyperlipidemia: drug therapy aimed at the predominant lipid abnormality noted
- Table 7-25 compares the various lipid-lowering agents.

DISPOSITION
- Those with polygenic hyperalphalipoproteinemia: excellent prognosis for longevity
- Those with familial hypercholesterolemia, familial type 3 hypercholesterolemia, and multiple lipoprotein type hyperlipidemia: even with aggressive treatment, at high risk for accelerated atherosclerosis and CAD

MISCELLANEOUS

COMMENTS
- Patient information is available through the American Heart Association.
- U.S. Preventive Services Task Force Recommendations regarding screening for hyperlipidemia and other lipid abnormalities are described in Section V, Chapter 2.

REFERENCES
Bennett JC, Plum F (eds): *Cecil textbook of medicine,* ed 20, Philadelphia, 1996, WB Saunders.

Author: **Beth J. Wutz, M.D.**

Hyperosmolar coma

BASIC INFORMATION

DEFINITION
Hyperosmolar coma is a state of extreme hyperglycemia, marked dehydration, serum hyperosmolarity, altered mental status, and absence of ketoacidosis.

SYNONYMS
Nonketotic hyperosmolar coma
Hyperosmolar nonketotic state

ICD-9-CM CODES
250.2 Hyperosmolar coma

PHYSICAL FINDINGS
- Evidence of extreme dehydration (poor skin turgor, sunken eyeballs, dry mucous membranes)
- Neurologic defects (reversible hemiplegia, focal seizures)
- Orthostatic hypotension, tachycardia
- Evidence of precipitating factors (pneumonia, infected skin ulcer)

ETIOLOGY
- Infections, 20% to 25% (e.g., pneumonia, UTI, sepsis)
- New or previously unrecognized diabetes (30% to 50%)
- Reduction or omission of diabetic medication
- Stress (MI, CVA)
- Drugs: diuretics (dehydration), phenytoin, diazoxide (impaired insulin secretion)

DIAGNOSIS

DIFFERENTIAL DIAGNOSIS
- Diabetic ketoacidosis
- CVA
- Sepsis
- Myxedema coma
- Metastatic carcinoma
- The differential diagnosis of coma is described in Box 2-26.

WORKUP
- Laboratory evaluation to confirm diagnosis (see "Laboratory Tests") and evaluate precipitating factors
- Admission ECG to evaluate electrolyte abnormalities and rule out myocardial ischemia/infarction as a contributing factor

LABORATORY TESTS
- Hyperglycemia: serum glucose usually >600 mg/dl.
- Hyperosmolarity: serum osmolarity usually >340 mOsm/L.
- Serum sodium: may be low, normal, or high; if normal or high, the patient is severely dehydrated, since an elevated glucose draws fluid from intracellular space decreasing the serum sodium; the corrected sodium can be obtained by increasing the serum sodium concentration by 1.6 mEq/dl for every 100 mg/dl increase in the serum glucose level over normal.
- Serum potassium: may be low, normal, or high; regardless of the initial serum level, the total body loss is approximately 5 to 15 mEq/kg.
- Serum bicarbonate: usually >12 mEq/L (average is 17 mEq/L).
- Arterial pH: usually >7.2 (average is 7.26); both serum bicarbonate and arterial pH may be lower if lactic acidosis is present.
- BUN: azotemia (prerenal) is usually present (BUN generally ranges from 60 to 90 mg/dl).
- Phosphorus: hypophosphatemia (average loss is 70 to 140 mm).
- Calcium: hypocalcemia (average loss is 50 to 100 mEq).
- Magnesium: hypomagnesemia (average loss is 50 to 100 mEq).
- CBC with differential, urinalysis, blood and urine cultures should be performed to rule out infectious etiology.

IMAGING STUDIES
- Chest x-ray examination is useful to rule out infectious process. The initial chest x-ray may be negative if the patient has significant dehydration. Repeat chest x-ray examination after 24 hr if pulmonary infection is suspected.
- CT scan of head should be performed in patients with suspected CVA.

TREATMENT

NONPHARMACOLOGIC THERAPY
- Monitor mental status, vital signs, urine output qh until improved, then monitor q2-4h.
- Monitor electrolytes, renal function, and glucose level (see "Acute General Rx").

ACUTE GENERAL Rx
- Vigorous fluid replacement: infuse 1000 to 1500 ml/hr for the initial 1 to 2 L; then decrease the rate of infusion to 500 ml/hr and monitor urinary output, blood chemistries, and blood pressure; use 0.9% NS if the patient is hypotensive; otherwise use 0.45% NS solution. Slower infusion rate may be used initially in patients with compromised cardiovascular or renal status.
- Replace electrolytes and monitor serum levels frequently (e.g., serum sodium and potassium q2h for the first 12 hr). Serum KCl replacement in patients with normal renal function and adequate urinary output is started when the serum potassium level is <5.2 mEq/L (e.g., 10 mEq KCl/hr if potassium level is 4 to 5.2 mEq/L). Continuous ECG monitoring and hourly measurement of urinary output is recommended.
- Correct hypoglycemia
  1. Vigorous IV hydration will decrease the serum glucose level in most patients by 80 mg/dl/hr; a regular insulin IV bolus is often not necessary.
  2. Low-dose insulin infusion at 1 to 2 U/hr (e.g., 25 U of regular insulin in 250 ml of 0.9% saline solution at 20 ml/hr) until the serum glucose level approaches 300 mg/dl; then the patient is started on regular SC insulin with sliding scale coverage.
  3. Glucose should be monitored q1-2h in the initial 12 hr.

DISPOSITION
Mortality in nonketotic hyperosmolar coma ranges from 20% to 50%.

REFERRAL
Patients with hyperosmolar coma should be admitted to the ICU.

MISCELLANEOUS

COMMENTS
The typical patient presenting with hyperosmolar coma is an elderly or bed-confined diabetic with impaired ability to communicate thirst who is evaluated after an interval of 1 to 2 wk of prolonged osmotic diuresis.

REFERENCES
Ennis ED, Stahl EJ, Kreisberg RA: The hyperosmolar hyperglycemic syndrome, *Diabetes Rev* 2(1):115, 1994.
Lorber D: Nonketotic hypertonicity in diabetes mellitus, *Med Clin North Am* 79(1):39, 1995.
Author: **Fred F. Ferri, M.D.**

Hyperparathyroidism (PTG)

BASIC INFORMATION

DEFINITION
Primary hyperparathyroidism is an endocrine disorder caused by the excessive secretion of parathyroid hormone (PTH) from the parathyroid glands.

ICD-9-CM CODES
252.0 Primary hyperparathyroidism
253.9 Ectopic hyperparathyroidism
588.8 Secondary hyperparathyroidism in chronic renal disease

EPIDEMIOLOGY AND DEMOGRAPHICS
PREVALENCE: 1 case/1000 persons
PREDOMINANT AGE AND SEX: Primary hyperparathyroidism occurs most frequently in postmenopausal women; prevalence in this group may be as high as 3%. The condition is asymptomatic in >50% of patients.
GENETICS: Hyperparathyroidism can occur in conjunction with MEN I or II.

PHYSICAL FINDINGS
Physical examination may be entirely normal. The presence of signs and symptoms varies with the rapidity of development and degree of hypercalcemia. The following abnormalities may be present:
- GI: constipation, anorexia, nausea, vomiting, pancreatitis, ulcers
- CNS: confusion, obtundation, psychosis, lassitude, depression, coma
- GU: nephrolithiasis, renal insufficiency, polyuria, decreased urine-concentrating ability, nocturia, nephrocalcinosis
- Musculoskeletal: myopathy, weakness, osteoporosis, pseudogout, bone pain
- Other: hypertension, metastatic calcifications, band keratopathy (found in medial and lateral margin of the cornea), pruritus

ETIOLOGY
- A single adenoma is found in 80% of patients; 90% of the adenomas are found within one of the parathyroid glands, the other 10% are in ectopic sites (lateral neck, thyroid, mediastinum, retroesophagus).
- Parathyroid gland hyperplasia occurs in 20% of patients.

DIAGNOSIS

DIFFERENTIAL DIAGNOSIS
Other causes of hypercalcemia:
- Malignancy: neoplasms of breast, lung, kidney, ovary, pancreas; myeloma, lymphoma
- Granulomatous disorders (e.g., sarcoidosis)
- Paget's disease
- Vitamin D intoxication, milk-alkali syndrome
- Thiazide diuretics
- Other: familial hypocalciuric hypercalcemia, thyrotoxicosis, adrenal insufficiency, prolonged immobilization, vitamin A intoxication, recovery from acute renal failure, lithium administration, pheochromocytoma, disseminated SLE

WORKUP
- The serum PTH level is the single best test for initial evaluation of confirmed hypercalcemia. The "intact" PTH (iPTH) is the best assay. The iPTH distinguishes primary hyperparathyroidism from hypercalcemia caused by malignancy when the serum calcium level is >12 mg/dl.
- A high level of urinary cyclic AMP is also suggestive of primary hyperparathyroidism.
- Parathyroid hormone-like protein (PLP) is increased in hypercalcemia associated with solid malignancies.
- ECG may reveal shortening of the QT interval secondary to hypercalcemia.
- Fig. 3-41 and 3-42 describe clinical algorithms for evaluation and treatment of hypercalcemia.

LABORATORY TESTS
- Elevated serum calcium level, low serum phosphorus, and normal or elevated alkaline phosphatase
- Elevated urine calcium level (in contrast with very low urinary calcium levels seen in patients with familial hypocalciuric hypercalcemia)
- Possibly elevated serum chloride levels, decreased serum CO_2, hyperchloremic metabolic acidosis

IMAGING STUDIES
- A bone survey may show evidence of subperiosteal bone resorption (suggesting PTH excess). The classic bone disease of primary hyperparathyroidism is *osteitis fibrosa cystica*.
- Bone scan may show hot spots in association with lytic lesions.
- Neck ultrasonography and/or CT scanning with and without contrast are useful to localize the lesion.
- Screen for osteopenia with measurement of bone mineral density in all postmenopausal women.

TREATMENT

NONPHARMACOLOGIC THERAPY
- Unless contraindicated, patients should maintain a high intake of fluids (3 to 5 L/day) and sodium chloride (>400 mEq/day) to increase renal calcium excretion.
- Potential hypercalcemic agents (e.g., thiazide diuretics) should be discontinued.
- Surgery is the only effective treatment for primary hyperparathyroidism. It is generally indicated in all younger patients and patients with complications from hyperthyroidism, such as nephrolithiasis and osteopenia. Asymptomatic elderly patients can be followed conservatively with periodic monitoring of serum calcium level and review of symptoms.

ACUTE GENERAL Rx
Acute severe hypercalcemia (serum calcium >13 mg/dl) or symptomatic patients can be treated with the following:
- Vigorous IV hydration with NS followed by IV furosemide. Use NS with caution in patients with cardiac or renal insufficiency to avoid fluid overload.
- Calcitonin 4 IU/kg q12h is indicated when saline hydration and furosemide are ineffective or contraindicated.
- Biphosphonates (pamidronate, etidronate), mithramycin, and gallium nitrate are also effective for severe hypercalcemia.

CHRONIC Rx
Hormone replacement therapy should be strongly considered in all postmenopausal women with primary hyperparathyroidism.

MISCELLANEOUS

COMMENTS
Patients with hyperparathyroidism should undergo further evaluation for the presence of MEN I or II.

REFERENCES
Grey AB: Effect of hormone replacement therapy on bone mineral density in postmenopausal women with mild primary hyperparathyroidism, *Ann Intern Med* 125:360, 1996.

Author: **Fred F. Ferri, M.D.**

CLINICAL TOPICS   Hypertension   245

BASIC INFORMATION

DEFINITION
Hypertension can be defined as a systolic blood pressure (BP) ≥140 mm Hg and/or diastolic BP >90 mm Hg.

SYNONYMS
Essential hypertension
Idiopathic hypertension
High blood pressure

ICD-9-CM CODES
401.1 Essential hypertension
401.0 Malignant hypertension due to renal artery stenosis
642 Hypertension complicating pregnancy
405.01 Malignant hypertension secondary to renal artery stenosis
437.2 Hypertensive encephalopathy

EPIDEMIOLOGY AND DEMOGRAPHICS
1. Incidence of hypertension in adult population: 10% to 15%
2. Increased incidence in males and in the elderly

PHYSICAL FINDINGS
Physical examination may be entirely within normal limits except for the presence of hypertension. A proper initial physical examination on a hypertensive patient should include the following:
- Measure height and weight.
- Evaluate skin for the presence of cafe-au-lait spots (neurofibromatosis), uremic appearance (CRF), striae (Cushing's syndrome).
- Perform careful funduscopic examination: check for papilledema, retinal exudates, hemorrhages, arterial narrowing, AV compression.
- Examine the neck for carotid bruits, distended neck veins, or enlarged thyroid gland.
- Perform extensive cardiopulmonary examination: check for loud aortic component of S_2, S_4, ventricular lift, murmurs, arrhythmias.
- Check abdomen for masses (pheochromocytoma, polycystic kidneys), presence of bruits over the renal artery (renal artery stenosis), dilation of the aorta.
- Obtain two or more BP measurements separated by 2 min with the patient either supine or seated and after standing for at least 2 min. Measure BP in both upper extremities (if values are discrepant, use the higher value).
- Examine arterial pulses (dilated or absent femoral pulses and BP greater in upper extremities than lower extremities suggests aortic coarctation).
- Note the presence of truncal obesity (Cushing's syndrome) and pedal edema (CHF, nephrosis).
- Perform full neurologic assessment.
- The clinical evaluation should help determine if the patient has primary or secondary (possibly reversible) hypertension, if there is target organ disease present, and if there are cardiovascular risk factors in addition to hypertension.

ETIOLOGY
- Essential (primary) hypertension (90%)
- Renal hypertension (5%)
  1. Renal parenchymal disease (3%)
  2. Renovascular hypertension (<2%)
- Endocrine (4% to 5%)
  1. Oral contraceptives (4%)
  2. Primary aldosteronism (0.5%)
  3. Pheochromocytoma (0.2%)
  4. Cushing's syndrome (0.2%)
- Coarctation of the aorta (0.2%)

DIAGNOSIS

WORKUP
Pertinent history:
- Age of onset of hypertension, previous antihypertensive therapy
- Family history of hypertension, stroke, cardiovascular disease
- Diet, salt intake, alcohol, drugs (e.g., oral contraceptives, NSAIDs, decongestants, steroids)
- Occupation, life-style, socioeconomic status, psychologic factors
- Other cardiovascular risk factors: hyperlipidemia, obesity, diabetes mellitus, carbohydrate intolerance
- Symptoms of secondary hypertension:
  1. Headache, palpitations, excessive perspiration (possible pheochromocytoma)
  2. Weakness, polyuria (consider hyperaldosteronism)
  3. Claudication of lower extremities (seen with coarctation of aorta)

LABORATORY TESTS
- Urinalysis: for evidence of renal disease
- BUN, creatinine: to rule out renal disease
- Serum electrolytes levels: low potassium is suggestive of primary aldosteronism, diuretic use
- Screening for coexisting diseases that may adversely affect prognosis
  1. Fasting serum glucose
  2. Serum cholesterol, HDL, triglycerides, uric acid, calcium
  3. If pheochromocytoma is suspected: 24-hr urine for methanephrines

IMAGING STUDIES
- ECG: check for presence of left ventricular hypertrophy (LVH) with strain pattern.
- Ultrasound of the renal arteries: in suspected renovascular hypertension

TREATMENT

NONPHARMACOLOGIC THERAPY
Life-style modifications:
- Lose weight if overweight.
- Limit alcohol intake to ≤1 oz of ethanol per day.
- Exercise (aerobic) regularly.
- Reduce sodium intake to <100 mmol/day (<2.3 g of sodium).
- Maintain adequate dietary potassium, calcium, and magnesium intake.
- Stop smoking and reduce dietary saturated fat and cholesterol intake for overall cardiovascular health.

ACUTE GENERAL Rx
According to the Sixth Report of the Joint National Committee on Detection, Evaluation, and Treatment of High Blood Pressure:
- Diuretics or β-blockers are preferred initially because a reduction in morbidity and mortality has been demonstrated.
- ACE inhibitors, calcium antagonists, α-1 receptor blockers, and α-β blockers are also effective.
- When selecting drugs, also consider the cost of the medication, metabolic and subjective side-effects, and drug-drug interactions.
- The major advantages and limitations of each class of drugs are described below:
1. Diuretics
   a. Advantages: inexpensive, once per day dosing. Useful in blacks, edema states, CHF, chronic renal disease, elderly patients (decreased incidence of hip fractures in elderly patients)
   b. Disadvantages: significant adverse metabolic effects, increased risk of cardiac arrhythmias, sexual dysfunction, possible adverse effects on lipids and glucose levels.
2. β-Blockers
   a. Advantages: ideal in hypertensive patients with ischemic heart disease or post-MI. Favored in hyperkinetic, young patients (resting tachycardia, wide pulse pressure, hyperdynamic heart).
   b. Disadvantages: adverse effect on quality of life (increased incidence of fatigue, depression, impotence, aggravation of CHF,

Hypertension (PTG)

bronchospasm, hypoglycemia, peripheral vascular disease, adverse effects on lipids, masking of signs and symptoms of hypoglycemia in diabetics; possible increased risk of sudden cardiac death.
3. Calcium antagonists
   a. Advantages: helpful in hypertensive patients with ischemic heart disease. Generally favorable effect on quality of life; can be used in patients with bronchospastic disorders, renal disease, peripheral avascular disease, metabolic disorders, and salt-sensitivity.
   b. Disadvantages: excessive cost; diltiazem and verapamil should be avoided in patients with CHF because of their chronotropic and inotropic effects; pedal edema may occur with nifedipine and amlodipine; constipation can be severe in elderly patients receiving verapamil.
4. ACE inhibitors
   a. Advantages: well tolerated, favorable impact on quality of life; useful in hypertension complicated by CHF; helpful in prevention of diabetic renal disease; effective in decreasing LVH.
   b. Disadvantages: generally more expensive than generic diuretics and β-blockers; cough is a frequent side effect (5% to 20% of patients); hyperkalemia may occur in patient with diabetes or severe renal insufficiency; hypotension may occur in volume-depleted patients.
5. Angiotensin II receptor blockers (ARB)
   a. Advantages: well tolerated, favorable impact on quality of life; useful in patients unable to tolerate ACE inhibitors because of persistent cough; single daily dose.
   b. Disadvantages: excessive cost; hypotension may occur in volume-depleted patients; contraindicated in pregnancy.
6. α-Adrenergic blockers
   a. Advantages: no adverse effect on blood lipids or insulin sensitivity; helpful in BPH.
   b. Disadvantages: frequent postural hypotension; syncope can be avoided by giving an initial low dose at bedtime.

TREATMENT OF RENOVASCULAR HYPERTENSION (RVH): The therapeutic approach varies with the cause of the RVH.
1. Young patients with fibromuscular dysplasia are best treated with percutaneous transluminal renal angioplasty (PTRA).
2. Medical therapy is advisable in elderly patients with atheromatous renal vascular hypertension; useful agents are:
   a. β-Blockers: very effective in patients with elevated plasma renin.
   b. ACE inhibitors: very effective; however, should be avoided in patients with bilateral renal artery stenosis or in patients with solitary kidney and renal stenosis.
   c. Diuretics: often used in combination with ACE inhibitors.
3. Surgical revascularization is generally reserved for atheromatous RVH in patients responding poorly to medical therapy (uncontrolled hypertension, deteriorating renal function).

HYPERTENSION DURING PREGNANCY:
1. Hypertension complicates 5% to 12% of all pregnancies.
2. The American Obstetrical Committee defines blood pressure of 130/80 mm Hg as the upper limit of normal at any time during pregnancy.
3. A rise of 30 mm Hg systolic or 15 mm Hg diastolic is also considered abnormal regardless of the absolute values obtained.
4. Chronic hypertension (occurring before pregnancy) must be distinguished from preeclampsia, since the risk to mother and fetus is much greater in the latter.
5. Treatment of chronic hypertension during pregnancy is as follows:
   a. Initial treatment with conservative measures (proper nutrition, limited physical activity).
   b. When drug therapy is necessary, initiation of one of the following agents—methyldopa, hydralazine, labetalol, or atenolol—is preferred.
   c. ACE inhibitors can cause fetal and neonatal complications; their use should be avoided in pregnancy.
   d. The safety of calcium channel blockers remains unclear.
   e. Diuretics should be used only if there is a specific reason for initiating and maintaining their use (e.g., hypertension associated with severe fluid overload or left ventricular dysfunction).

MALIGNANT HYPERTENSION, HYPERTENSIVE EMERGENCIES, AND HYPERTENSIVE URGENCIES:
- Definitions:
1. **Malignant hypertension** is a potentially life-threatening situation that is secondary to elevated BP.
   a. The rate of BP rise is a critical factor.
   b. The clinical manifestations are grade IV hypertensive retinopathy (exudates, hemorrhages, and papilledema), cardiovascular and/or renal compromise, and encephalopathy.
   c. It requires immediate BP reduction (not necessarily into normal ranges) to prevent or limit target organ disease.
2. **Hypertensive emergencies** are situations that require rapid (within 1 hr) lowering of BP to prevent end-organ damage).
3. **Hypertensive urgencies** are significant BP elevations that should be corrected within 24 hr of presentation.
- Therapy:
The choice of therapeutic agents in malignant hypertension varies with the cause.
1. Nitroprusside is the drug of choice in hypertensive encephalopathy, hypertension and intracranial bleeding, malignant hypertension, hypertension and heart failure, dissecting aortic aneurysm (used in combination with the propanolol); its onset of action is immediate.
2. The following are important points to remember when treating hypertensive emergencies:
   a. Introduce a plan for long-term therapy at the time of the initial emergency treatment.
   b. Agents that reduce arterial pressure can cause the kidney to retain sodium and water; therefore the judicious administration of diuretics should accompany their use.
   c. The initial goal of antihypertensive therapy is not to achieve a normal BP, but rather to gradually reduce the BP; cerebral hyperperfusion may occur if the mean BP is lowered >40% in the initial 24 hr.
3. Hypertensive urgencies can be effectively treated with oral clonidine 0.1 mg q2min (to a maximum of 0.8 mg); sedation is common.

MISCELLANEOUS

COMMENTS
U.S. Preventive Services Task Force Recommendations regarding screening for hypertension are described in Section V, Chapter 3.

REFERENCES
Sixth Report of the Joint National Committee on Detection, Evaluation and Treatment of High Blood Pressure, *Arch Intern Med* 157:2413, 1997.
Hoes AW et al: Diuretics, beta blockers, and the risk of cardiac death in hypertensive patients, *Ann Intern Med* 123:481, 1995.

Author: **Fred F. Ferri, M.D.**

CLINICAL TOPICS Hyperthyroidism 247

BASIC INFORMATION

DEFINITION
Hyperthyroidism is a hypermetabolic state resulting from excess thyroid hormone.

SYNONYMS
Thyrotoxicosis

ICD-9-CM CODES
242.9 Hyperthyroidism
242.0 Hyperthyroidism with goiter
242.2 Hyperthyroidism, multinodular
242.3 Hyperthyroidism, uninodular

EPIDEMIOLOGY AND DEMOGRAPHICS
INCIDENCE/PREVALENCE: Hyperthyroidism affects 2% of women and 0.2% of men in their lifetimes.

PHYSICAL FINDINGS
- Tachycardia (resting rate >90 bpm), palpitations
- Tremor, hyperreflexia
- Increased sweating, warm and moist skin, onycholysis (brittle nails)
- Goiter, bruit over thyroid
- Exophthalmos, lid retraction, lid lag (Graves' ophthalmopathy)
- Clubbing of fingers associated with periosteal new bone formation in other skeletal areas (Graves' acropachy)

ETIOLOGY
- Graves' disease (diffuse toxic goiter): 80% to 90% of all cases of hyperthyroidism
- Toxic multinodular goiter (Plummer's disease)
- Toxic adenoma
- Iatrogenic and factitious
- Transient hyperthyroidism (subacute thyroiditis, Hashimoto's thyroiditis)
- Rare causes: hypersecretion of TSH (e.g., pituitary neoplasms), struma ovarii, ingestion of large amount of iodine in a patient with preexisting thyroid hyperplasia or adenoma (Jod-Basedow phenomenon), hydatidiform mole, carcinoma of thyroid, amiodarone therapy

DIAGNOSIS

DIFFERENTIAL DIAGNOSIS
- Anxiety disorder
- Pheochromocytoma
- Metastatic neoplasm
- Diabetes mellitus
- Premenopausal state

WORKUP
Suspected hyperthyroidism requires laboratory confirmation and identification of its etiology, since treatment varies with its cause. A detailed medical history will often provide clues to the diagnosis and etiology of the hyperthyroidism:
- Patients with hyperthyroidism generally present with the following clinical manifestations: anxiety, irritability, emotional lability, panic attacks, heat intolerance, sweating, increased appetite, diarrhea, weight loss, menstrual dysfunction (oligomenorrhea, amenorrhea); the presentation may be different in elderly patients (see below).
- Patients with Graves' disease may present with the following signs and symptoms of ophthalmopathy: blurring of vision, photophobia, increased lacrimation, double vision, deep orbital pressure.
- Toxic multinodular goiter usually occurs in women >55 yr old and is more common than Graves' disease in the elderly.
- In the elderly the clinical signs of hyperthyroidism may be masked by manifestations of coexisting disease (e.g., new-onset atrial fibrillation, exacerbation of CHF).

LABORATORY TESTS
- Elevated free thyroxine (T_4)
- Elevated free triiodothyronine (T_3): generally not necessary for diagnosis
- Low TSH (unless hyperthyroidism is a result of the rare hypersecretion of TSH from a pituitary adenoma)
- Thyroid autoantibodies useful in selected cases to differentiate Graves' disease from toxic multinodular goiter (absent thyroid antibodies)

IMAGING STUDIES
- 24-hr radioactive iodine uptake (RAIU) is useful to distinguish hyperthyroidism from iatrogenic thyroid hormone synthesis (thyrotoxicosis factitia) and from thyroiditis.
- An overactive thyroid shows increased uptake, whereas a normal underactive thyroid (iatrogenic thyroid ingestion, painless or subacute thyroiditis) shows normal or decreased uptake.
- The RAIU results also vary with the etiology of the hyperthyroidism.
  Graves' disease: increased homogeneous uptake
  Multinodular goiter: increased heterogeneous uptake
  Hot nodule: single focus of increased uptake
- RAIU is also generally performed before the therapeutic administration of radioactive iodine to determine the appropriate dose.

TREATMENT

NONPHARMACOLOGIC THERAPY
Patient education regarding thyroid disease and discussion of the therapeutic options (medications, radioactive iodine, and thyroid surgery)

ACUTE GENERAL Rx
ANTITHYROID DRUGS (THIONAMIDES): Propylthiouracil (PTU) and methimazole (Tapazole) inhibit thyroid hormone synthesis by blocking production of thyroid peroxidase (PTU and methimazole) or inhibit peripheral conversion of T_4 to T_3 (PTU).

1. Dosage: PTU 50 to 100 mg PO q8h; methimazole 10 to 20 mg PO q8h or 30 to 60 mg/day given as a single dose.
2. Antithyroid drugs can be used as the primary form of treatment or as adjunctive therapy before radioactive therapy or surgery or afterward if the hyperthyroidism recurs.
3. Side effects: skin rash (3% to 5% of patients, arthralgias, myalgias, granulocytopenia (0.5%). Rare side effects are aplastic anemia, hepatic necrosis from PTU, cholestatic jaundice from methimazole.
4. When using antithyroid drugs as primary therapy they are usually given for 6 to 24 mo; prolonged therapy may cause hypothyroidism.
5. The use of antithyroid drugs before radioactive iodine therapy is best reserved for patients in whom exacerbation of hyperthyroidism post–radioactive iodine therapy is hazardous (e.g., elderly patients with coronary artery disease or significant coexisting morbidity). In these patients the antithyroid drug can be stopped 2 days before radioactive iodine therapy, resumed 2 days later, and continued for 4 to 6 wk.

RADIOACTIVE IODINE (RAI; ^{131}I):
1. RAI is the treatment of choice for patients >21 yr of age and younger patients who have not achieved remission after 1 yr of antithyroid drug therapy. Radioiodine is also used in hyperthyroidism caused by toxic adenoma or toxic multinodular goiter.
2. Contraindicated during pregnancy (can cause fetal hypothyroidism) and lactation. Pregnancy should be excluded in women of child-bearing age before radioactive iodine is administered.
3. A single dose of radioactive iodine is effective in inducing euthyroid state in nearly 80% of patients.
4. There is a high incidence of post–radioactive iodine hypothyroidism (>50% within first year and 2%/yr thereafter); therefore these patients should be frequently evaluated for the onset of hypothyroidism (see "Chronic Rx.").

SURGICAL THERAPY (SUBTOTAL THYROIDECTOMY):
1. Indicated in obstructing goiters, in any patient who refuses radioactive iodine and cannot be adequately managed with antithyroid medications (e.g., patients with toxic adenoma or toxic multinodular goiter), and in pregnant patients who cannot be adequately managed with antithyroid medication or develop side effects to them.
2. Patients should be rendered euthyroid with antithyroid drugs before surgery.
3. Complications of surgery include hypothyroidism (28% to 43% after 10 yr), hypoparathyroidism, and vocal cord paralysis (1%).
4. Hyperthyroidism recurs post-surgery in 10% to 15% of patients.

ADJUNCTIVE THERAPY: Propanolol alleviates the β-adrenergic symptoms of hyperthyroidism; initial dose is 20 to 40 mg PO q6h; dosage is gradually increased until symptoms are controlled; major contraindications to use of propranolol are CHF and bronchospasm. Diagnosis and treatment of "thyroid storm" is discussed separately in Section I of this book.

CHRONIC Rx

Patients undergoing treatment with antithyroid drugs should be seen every 1 to 3 mo until euthyroidism is achieved and every 3 to 4 mo while they remain on antithyroid therapy. After treatment is stopped, periodic monitoring of thyroid function tests with TSH every 3 mo for 1 yr, then every 6 mo for 1 yr, then annually is recommended.

DISPOSITION
Successful treatment of hyperthyroidism requires lifelong monitoring for the onset of hypothyroidism or the recurrence of thyrotoxicosis.

REFERRAL
- Endocrinology referral is recommended at the time of initial diagnosis and during treatment.
- Surgical referral in selected patients (see "Surgical Therapy" above)
- Hospitalization of all patients with thyroid storm

MISCELLANEOUS

COMMENTS
- Elderly hyperthyroid patients may have only subtle signs (weight loss, tachycardia, fine skin, brittle nails). This form is known as *apathetic hyperthyroidism* and manifests with lethargy rather than hyperkinetic activity. An enlarged thyroid gland may be absent. Coexisting medical disorders (most commonly cardiac disease) may also mask the symptoms. These patients often have unexplained CHF, worsening of angina, or new-onset atrial fibrillation resistant to treatment. See "Graves' Disease" in Section I for additional information on the diagnosis and treatment of Graves' disease.
- Fig. 3-84 illustrates a diagnostic approach to thyroid disease.

REFERENCES
Levetan C, Wartofsky L: A clinical guide to the management of Graves' disease with radioactive iodine, *Endocr Pract* 1:205, 1995.

Singer PA et al: Treatment guidelines for patients with hyperthyroidism and hypothyroidism, *JAMA* 73:808, 1995.

Author: **Fred F. Ferri, M.D.**

Hypoaldosteronism

BASIC INFORMATION

DEFINITION
Hypoaldosteronism is an aldosterone deficiency or impaired aldosterone function.

ICD-9-CM CODES
255.4 Hypoadrenalism

PHYSICAL FINDINGS
- Physical examination may be entirely within normal limits.
- Hypertension may be present in some patients.

ETIOLOGY
- Hyporeninemic hypoaldosteronism: decreased aldosterone production secondary to decreased renin production; the typical patient has renal disease secondary to various factors (e.g., diabetes mellitus, interstitial nephritis, multiple myeloma).
- Hyperreninemic hypoaldosteronism: renin production by the kidneys is intact, the defect is in aldosterone biosynthesis or in the action of angiotensin II. Common causes of this form of hypoaldosteronism are medications (ACE inhibitors, heparin), lead poisoning, aldosterone enzyme defects, and severe illness.

DIAGNOSIS

DIFFERENTIAL DIAGNOSIS
- Pseudohypoaldosteronism: renal unresponsiveness to aldosterone. In this condition, both renin and aldosterone levels are elevated. Pseudohypoaldosteronism can be caused by medications (spironolactone), chronic interstitial nephritis, systemic disorders (SLE, amyloidosis), or primary mineralocorticoid resistance.
- Box 2-63 describes the differential diagnosis of hyperkalemia.

WORKUP
The diagnosis and etiology of hypoaldosteronism can be confirmed with the renin-aldosterone stimulation test:
- Hyporeninemic hypoaldosteronism: low stimulated renin and aldosterone levels
- End-organ refractoriness to aldosterone action: high stimulated renin and aldosterone levels
- Adrenal gland abnormality: high stimulated renin and low aldosterone levels

LABORATORY TESTS
- Increased potassium, normal or decreased sodium
- Hyperchloremic metabolic acidosis (caused by the absence of hydrogen-secreting action of aldosterone)
- Increased BUN and creatinine (secondary to renal disease)
- Hyperglycemia (diabetes mellitus is common in these patients)

TREATMENT

NONPHARMACOLOGIC THERAPY
Low-potassium diet with liberal sodium intake
Avoidance of ACE inhibitors and potassium-sparing diuretics

ACUTE GENERAL Rx
- Judicious use of fludrocortisone (0.05 to 0.1 mg PO qam) in patients with aldosterone deficiency associated with deficiency of adrenal glucocorticoid hormones
- Furosemide 20 to 40 mg qd to correct hyperkalemia of hyporeninemic hypoaldosteronism

DISPOSITION
Prognosis varies with the etiology of hypoaldosteronism and presence of associated disorders.

REFERRAL
Endocrinology referral for renin-aldosterone stimulation test

MISCELLANEOUS

COMMENTS
Treatment of pseudohypoaldosteronism is the same as for hypoaldosteronism; however, effect is limited because of impaired renal sensitivity.

REFERENCES
Noble J (ed): *Primary care medicine*, ed 2, St Louis, 1996, Mosby.
Author: **Fred F. Ferri, M.D.**

Hypothermia (PTG)

BASIC INFORMATION

DEFINITION
Hypothermia is a rectal temperature <35° C (95.8° F). *Accidental hypothermia* is unintentionally induced decrease in core temperature in absence of preoptic anterior hypothalamic conditions.

ICD-9-CM CODES
991.6 Accidental hypothermia
780.9 Hypothermia not associated with low environmental temperature

EPIDEMIOLOGY AND DEMOGRAPHICS
Hypothermia occurs most frequently in the following groups: alcoholics, learning-impaired, patients with cardiovascular, cerebrovascular, or pituitary disorders, those using sedatives or tranquilizers, and elderly patients.

PHYSICAL FINDINGS
- The clinical presentation varies with the severity of hypothermia; shivering may be absent if body temperature is <33.3° C (92° F) or in patients taking phenothiazines.
- Hypothermia may masquerade as CVA, ataxia, or slurred speech, or the patient may appear comatose or clinically dead.
- Physiologic stages of hypothermia:
1. Mild hypothermia (32.2° C to 35° C [90° F to 95° F]): dysarthria, ataxia
2. Moderate hypothermia (28° C to 32.2° C [82.4° F to 90° F]):
   a. Progressive decrease of level of consciousness, pulse, cardiac output, and respiration
   b. Atrial fibrillation, dysrhythmias (increased susceptibility to ventricular tachycardia)
   c. Elimination of shivering mechanism for thermogenesis
3. Severe hypothermia (≤28° C [82.4° F]):
   a. Absence of reflexes or response to pain
   b. Decreased cerebral blood flow, decreased CO_2
   c. Increased risk of ventricular fibrillation or asystole

ETIOLOGY
Exposure to cold temperatures for a prolonged period

DIAGNOSIS

DIFFERENTIAL DIAGNOSIS
- CVA
- Myxedema coma
- Drug intoxication
- Hypoglycemia

LABORATORY TESTS
- ABGs: metabolic and respiratory acidosis; when blood cools, arterial pH increases, Po_2 increases, Pco_2 falls
- Electrolytes: hypokalemia initially, then hyperkalemia with increasing hypothermia
- CBC: elevated Hct (secondary to hemoconcentration), leukopenia, thrombocytopenia (secondary to splenic sequestration)
- Increased blood viscosity, increased clotting time

IMAGING STUDIES
- Chest x-ray examination: generally not helpful; may reveal evidence of aspiration (e.g., intoxicated patient with aspiration pneumonia).
- ECG: prolonged PR, QT, and QRS segments, depressed ST segments, inverted T waves, AV block, hypothermic J waves (Osborn waves) may appear at 25° C to 30° C; characterized by notching of the junction of the QRS complex and ST segments.

TREATMENT

NONPHARMACOLOGIC THERAPY
- Treatment of hypothermia varies with the following:
1. Degree of hypothermia
2. Existence of concomitant diseases (e.g., cardiovascular insufficiency)
3. Patient's age and medical condition (e.g., elderly, debilitated patients vs. young, healthy patients)
- General measures:
1. Secure an airway before warming all unconscious patients; precede endotracheal intubation with oxygenation (if possible) to minimize the risk of dysrhythmias during the procedure.
2. Peripheral vasoconstriction may impede placement of a peripheral intravenous catheter; consider femoral venous access as an alternative to the jugular or subclavian sites to avoid ventricular stimulation.
3. A Foley catheter should be inserted, and urinary output should be monitored and maintained above 0.5 to 1 ml/kg/hr with intravascular volume replacement.

ACUTE GENERAL Rx
- Continuous ECG monitoring of patients is recommended; ventricular arrhythmias can be treated with bretylium; lidocaine is generally ineffective, and procainamide is associated with an increased incidence of ventricular fibrillation in hypothermic patients.
- Correct severe acidosis and electrolyte abnormalities.
- Hypothyroidism, if present, should be promptly treated (refer to "Myxedema Coma").
- If clinical evidence suggests adrenal insufficiency, administer IV methylprednisolone.
- In patients unresponsive to verbal or noxious stimuli or with altered mental status, 100 mg of thiamine, 0.4 mg of naloxone, and 1 ampule of 50% dextrose may be given.
- Warm (104° F to 113° F [40° C to 45° C]), humidified oxygen should also be given if it is available.
- Specific treatment:
1. Mild hypothermia (rectal temperature <32.2° C, [90° F]): passive external rewarming is indicated. Place the patient in a warm room (temperature >21° C [69.8° F]), and cover with insulating material after gently removing wet clothing; recommended rewarming rates vary between 0.5° and 20° C/hr but should not exceed 0.55° C/hr in elderly persons.
2. Moderate to severe hypothermia:
   a. Active core rewarming
   (1) Delivery of heat via fluids: warm GI irrigation (with saline enemas and via NG tube); warm IV fluids (usually D_5NS without potassium) to 104° F to 107.6° F (40° C to 42° C), peritoneal dialysis with dialysate heated to 40.5° C to 42.5° C.
   (2) Inhalation of heated humidified oxygen
   b. Active external rewarming: immersion in a bath of warm water (40° C to 41° C); active external rewarming may produce shock because of excessive peripheral vasodilation. Ideal candidates are previously healthy, young patients with acute immersion hypothermia.
   c. Extracorporeal blood warming with cardiopulmonary bypass appears to be an efficacious rewarming technique in young, otherwise healthy persons.

MISCELLANEOUS

REFERENCES
Bartley B et al: Techniques for managing severe hypothermia, *Gen Crit Ill* 11:123, 1996.
Danzl DS, Pozos RS: Accidental hypothermia, *N Engl J Med* 331:1756, 1994.
Walpoth BH et al: Outcome of survivors of accidental deep hypothermia and circulatory arrest treated with extracorporeal blood warming, *N Engl J Med* 337:1500, 1997.

Author: **Fred F. Ferri, M.D.**

Hypothyroidism (PTG)

BASIC INFORMATION

DEFINITION
Hypothyroidism is a disorder caused by the inadequate secretion of thyroid hormone.

SYNONYMS
Myxedema

ICD-9-CM CODES
244 Acquired hypothyroidism
243 Congenital hypothyroidism
244.1 Surgical hypothyroidism
244.3 Iatrogenic hypothyroidism
244.8 Pituitary hypothyroidism
246.1 Sporadic goitrous hypothyroidism

EPIDEMIOLOGY AND DEMOGRAPHICS
INCIDENCE/PREVALENCE: 1.5% to 2% of women and 0.2% of men
PREDOMINANT AGE: Incidence of hypothyroidism increases with age; among persons older than 60 yr, 6% of women and 2.5% of men have laboratory evidence of hypothyroidism (TSH > twice normal).

PHYSICAL FINDINGS
- Skin: dry, coarse, thick, cool, sallow (yellow color caused by carotenemia); nonpitting edema in skin of eyelids and hands (myxedema) secondary to infiltration of subcutaneous tissues by a hydrophilic mucopolysaccharide substance
- Hair: brittle and coarse; loss of outer one third of eyebrows
- Facies: dulled expression, thickened tongue, thick slow-moving lips
- Thyroid gland: may or may not be palpable (depending on the cause of the hypothyroidism)
- Heart sounds: distant, possible pericardial effusion
- Pulse: bradycardia
- Neurologic: delayed relaxation phase of the DTRs, cerebellar ataxia, hearing impairment, poor memory, peripheral neuropathies with paresthesia
- Musculoskeletal: carpal tunnel syndrome, muscular stiffness, weakness

ETIOLOGY
PRIMARY HYPOTHYROIDISM (THYROID GLAND DYSFUNCTION): The cause of >90% of the cases of hypothyroidism
- Hashimoto's thyroiditis is the most common cause of hypothyroidism after 8 yr of age.
- Idiopathic myxedema (nongoiterous form of Hashimoto's thyroiditis)
- Previous treatment of hyperthyroidism (radioiodine therapy, subtotal thyroidectomy)
- Subacute thyroiditis
- Radiation therapy to the neck (usually for malignant disease)
- Iodine deficiency or excess
- Drugs (lithium, PAS, sulfonamides, phenylbutazone, amiodarone, thiourea)
- Congenital (approximately 1 case/4000 live births)
- Prolonged treatment with iodides

SECONDARY HYPOTHYROIDISM: Pituitary dysfunction, postpartum necrosis, neoplasm, infiltrative disease causing deficiency of TSH

TERTIARY HYPOTHYROIDISM: Hypothalamic disease (granuloma, neoplasm, or irradiation causing deficiency of TRH)

TISSUE RESISTANCE TO THYROID HORMONE: Rare

DIAGNOSIS

Hypothyroid patients generally present with the following signs and symptoms: fatigue, lethargy, weakness, constipation, weight gain, cold intolerance, muscle weakness, slow speech, slow cerebration with poor memory.

DIFFERENTIAL DIAGNOSIS
- Depression
- Dementia from other causes
- Systemic disorders (e.g., nephrotic syndrome, CHF, amyloidosis)

LABORATORY TESTS
- Increased TSH: TSH may be normal if patient has secondary or tertiary hypothyroidism, is receiving dopamine or corticosteroids, or the level is obtained following severe illness
- Decreased free T_4
- Other common laboratory abnormalities: hyperlipidemia, hyponatremia, and anemia
- Increased antimicrosomal and antithyroglobulin antibody titers: useful when autoimmune thyroiditis is suspected as the cause of the hypothyroidism

TREATMENT

NONPHARMACOLOGIC THERAPY
Patient should be educated regarding hypothyroidism and its possible complications. Patients should also be instructed about the need for lifelong treatment and monitoring of their thyroid abnormality.

ACUTE GENERAL Rx
Start replacement therapy with levothyroxine (Synthroid, Levothroid) 25 to 100 μg/day, depending on the patient's age and the severity of the disease. The dose may be increased every 6 to 8 wk, depending on the clinical response and serum TSH level. Elderly patients and patients with coronary artery disease should be started with 12.5 to 25 μg/day (higher doses may precipitate angina). The average maintenance dose of levothyroxine is 1.7 μg/kg/day (100 to 150 μg/day in adults). The elderly may require <1 μg/kg/day, whereas children generally require higher doses (up to 3 to 4 μg/kg/day). Pregnant patients also have increased requirements.

CHRONIC Rx
Periodic monitoring of TSH level is an essential part of treatment. Patients should be evaluated initially with office visit and TSH levels every 6 to 8 wk until the patient is clinically euthyroid and the TSH level is normalized. The frequency of subsequent visits and TSH measurement can then be decreased to every 6 to 12 mo. Pregnant patients should be checked every trimester.

DISPOSITION
Patients generally experience dramatic clinical improvement with appropriate medical therapy.

REFERRAL
Admission to the hospital ICU is recommended in all patients with myxedema coma. Additional information on the diagnosis and treatment of this life-threatening complication of hypothyroidism is available in the topic "Myxedema Coma" in Section I.

MISCELLANEOUS

COMMENTS
- *Subclinical hypothyroidism* occurs in as many as 15% of elderly patients and is characterized by an elevated serum TSH and a normal free T_4 level. Treatment is individualized. Generally, replacement therapy is recommended for all patients with serum TSH >10 mU/L and with presence of goiter or thyroid autoantibodies.
- Fig. 3-84 describes a diagnostic approach to thyroid function tests.

REFERENCES
Bishnoi A, Sachmechi I: Thyroid disease during pregnancy, *Am Fam Physician* 53:215, 1996.
Singer PA et al: Treatment guidelines for patients with hyperthyroidism and hypothyroidism, *JAMA* 273:808, 1995.

Author: **Fred F. Ferri, M.D.**

Idiopathic thrombocytopenic purpura (PTG)

BASIC INFORMATION

DEFINITION
Idiopathic thrombocytopenic purpura (ITP) is a disorder characterized by isolated low platelet count in absence of other causes of thrombocytopenia.

SYNONYMS
ITP
Immune thrombocytopenic purpura
Autoimmune thrombocytopenic purpura

ICD-9-CM CODES
287.3 Idiopathic thrombocytopenic purpura (ITP)

EPIDEMIOLOGY AND DEMOGRAPHICS
PREVALENCE: 5 to 10 cases/100,000 persons
PREDOMINANT SEX: 72% of patients >10 yr old are women; in children, males = females
PREDOMINANT AGE: Children age 2 to 4 yr and young women (70% are <40 yr old)

PHYSICAL FINDINGS
- The physical examination may be entirely normal.
- Patients with severe thrombocytopenia may have petechiae, purpura, epistaxis, or heme-positive stool from GI bleeding.
- Splenomegaly is unusual; its presence should alert to the possibility of other etiologies of thrombocytopenia.
- The presence of dysmorphic features (skeletal anomalies, auditory abnormalities) may indicate a congenital disorder as the etiology of the thrombocytopenia.

ETIOLOGY
Increased platelet destruction caused by autoantibodies to platelet-membrane antigens

DIAGNOSIS

DIFFERENTIAL DIAGNOSIS
- Falsely low platelet count (resulting from EDTA-dependent or cold-dependent agglutinins)
- Viral infections (e.g., HIV, mononucleosis, rubella)
- Drug-induced (e.g., heparin, quinidine, sulfonamides)
- Hypersplenism resulting from liver disease
- Myelodysplastic and lymphoproliferative disorders
- Pregnancy, hypothyroidism
- SLE, TTP, hemolytic-uremic syndrome
- Congenital thrombocytopenias (e.g., Fanconi's syndrome, May-Hegglin anomaly, Bernard-Soulier syndrome)
- Box 2-115 describes the differential diagnosis of thrombocytopenia.

WORKUP
The history should focus on bleeding symptoms and on excluding other potential causes of thrombocytopenia (e.g., medications, alcohol abuse, risk factors for HIV, family history of hematologic disorders). The presentation of ITP is different in children and adults.
- Children generally present with sudden onset of bruising and petechiae from severe thrombocytopenia.
- In adults the presentation is insidious; a history of prolonged purpura may be present; many patients are diagnosed incidentally on the basis of automated laboratories that now routinely include platelet counts.
- Fig. 3-81 describes a diagnostic approach to thrombocytopenia.

LABORATORY TESTS
- CBC, platelet count, and peripheral smear: platelets are decreased but are normal in size or may appear larger than normal. RBCs and WBCs have a normal morphology.
- Additional tests may be ordered to exclude other etiologies of the thrombocytopenia when clinically indicated (e.g., HIV, ANA, TSH, liver enzymes, bone marrow examination).

IMAGING STUDIES
CT scan of abdomen in patients with splenomegaly to exclude other disorders causing thrombocytopenia

TREATMENT

NONPHARMACOLOGIC THERAPY
- Minimize activity to prevent injury or bruising (e.g., contact sports should be avoided).
- Avoid medications that increase the risk of bleeding (e.g., aspirin and other NSAIDs).

ACUTE GENERAL Rx
- Treatment varies with the platelet count and bleeding status.
- Observation and frequent monitoring of platelet count is needed in asymptomatic patients with platelet counts >30,000/mm^3.
- Prednisone 1 to 2 mg/kg qd, continued until the platelet count is normalized then slowly tapered off, is indicated in adults with platelet counts <20,000/mm^3 and those who have counts <50,000/mm^3 and significant mucous membrane bleeding.
- High-dose immunoglobulins (IgG 0.4g/kg/day IV, infused on 3 to 5 consecutive days) or high-dose parenteral glucocorticoids (methylprednisolone 30 mg/kg/day) are used in children with platelet count <20,000/mm^3 and significant bleeding or adults with severe thrombocytopenia or bleeding.
- Platelet transfusion is needed only in case of life-threatening hemorrhage.
- Splenectomy should be considered in adults with platelet count <30,000/mm^3 after 6 wk of medical treatment. In children, splenectomy is generally reserved for persistent thrombocytopenia (>1 yr) and clinically significant bleeding. Appropriate immuni-zations (pneumococcal vaccine in adults and children, *H. influenzae* vaccine, meningococcal vaccine in children) should be administered before splenectomy.

CHRONIC Rx
Frequent monitoring of platelet count and symptom review in patients with chronic ITP

DISPOSITION
- Over 80% of children have a complete remission within a few weeks.
- In adults, the course of the disease is chronic and only 5% of adults have spontaneous remission.
- The principal cause of death from ITP is intracranial hemorrhage (1% of children, 5% of adults).

REFERRAL
- Surgical referral for splenectomy in selected cases (see above)
- Hospitalization in patients with platelet count <20,000/mm^3 who have significant bleeding

MISCELLANEOUS

COMMENTS
In general, patients who have poor response to IV immune globulin are unlikely to have good response to splenectomy.

REFERENCES
George JN et al (American Society of Hematology ITP Practice Guideline Panel): Diagnosis and treatment of idiopathic thrombocytopenic purpura, *Am Fam Physician* 54:2437, 1996.

Law C et al: High-dose IV immune globulin and the response to splenectomy in patients with ITP, *New Engl J Med* 336:1494, 1997.

Author: Fred F. Ferri, M.D.

Impetigo (PTG)

BASIC INFORMATION

DEFINITION
Impetigo is a superficial skin infection generally secondary to *Staphylococcus aureus* and/or *Streptococcus* sp. Common presentations are bullous impetigo (generally secondary to staphylococcal disease) and nonbullous impetigo (secondary to staphylococcal infection and possible staphylococcal infection); the bullous form is caused by an epidermolytic toxin produced at the site of infection.

SYNONYMS
Impetigo vulgaris
Pyoderma

ICD-9-CM CODES
684 Impetigo

EPIDEMIOLOGY AND DEMOGRAPHICS
- Bullous impetigo is most common in infants and children. The nonbullous form is most common in children ages 2 to 5 yr with poor hygiene in warm climates.
- The overall incidence of acute nephritis with impetigo varies between 2% and 5%.

PHYSICAL FINDINGS
- Multiple lesions with golden yellow crusts and weeping areas often found on the skin around the nose, mouth, and limbs (nonbullous impetigo)—see color plate 11.
- Presence of vesicles that enlarge rapidly to form bullae with contents that vary from clear to cloudy; there is subsequent collapse of the center of the bullae; the peripheral area may retain fluid, and a honey-colored crust may appear in the center; as the lesions enlarge and become contiguous with the others, a scaling border replaces the fluid-filled rim (bullous impetigo); there is minimal erythema surrounding the lesions.
- Regional lymphadenopathy is most common with nonbullous impetigo.
- Constitutional symptoms are generally absent.

ETIOLOGY
- *S. aureus* coagulase positive is the dominant microorganism.
- *Str. pyogenes* (group A β-hemolytic streptococci): M-T serotypes of this organism associated with acute nephritis are 2, 49, 55, 57 and 60.

DIAGNOSIS

DIFFERENTIAL DIAGNOSIS
- Acute allergic contact dermatitis
- Herpes simplex infection
- Ecthyma
- Folliculitis
- Eczema
- Insect bites
- Scabies
- Tinea corporis
- Pemphigus vulgaris and bullous pemphigoid
- Chickenpox

WORKUP
Diagnosis is clinical.

LABORATORY TESTS
- Generally not necessary
- Gram stain and C&S to confirm the diagnosis when the clinical presentation is unclear
- Sedimentation rate parallel to activity of the disease
- Increased anti-DNAase B and anti-hyaluronidase
- Urinalysis revealing hematuria with erythrocyte casts and proteinuria in patients with acute nephritis (most frequently occurring in children between 2 and 4 yr of age in the southern part of the U.S.)

TREATMENT

NONPHARMACOLOGIC THERAPY
Remove crusts by soaking with wet cloth compresses (crusts block the penetration of antibacterial creams).

ACUTE GENERAL Rx
- Application of 2% mupirocin ointment (Bactroban) tid for 10 days to the affected area or until all lesions have cleared.
- Oral antibiotics are used in severe cases: commonly used agents are dicloxacillin 250 mg qid for 7 to 10 days, cephalexin 250 mg qid for 7 to 10 days, or azithromycin 500 mg on day 1, 250 mg on days 2 through 5.

CHRONIC Rx
- Impetigo can be prevented by prompt application of mupirocin or triple antibiotic ointment (bacitracin, Polysporin, and neomycin) to sites of skin trauma.
- Patients who are carriers of *S. aureus* in their nares should be treated with mupirocin ointment applied to their nares bid for 5 days.
- Fingernails should be kept short, and patients should be advised not to scratch any lesions to avoid spread of infection.

DISPOSITION
Most cases of impetigo resolve promptly with appropriate treatment. Both bullous and nonbullous forms of impetigo heal without scarring.

REFERRAL
Nephrology referral in patients with acute nephritis

MISCELLANEOUS

COMMENTS
- Patients should be instructed on use of antibacterial soaps and avoidance of sharing of towels and washcloths since impetigo is extremely contagious.
- Children attending day care should be removed until 48 to 72 hr after initiation of antibiotic treatment.

REFERENCES
Bagan R: Impetigo in childhood: changes in epidemiology and new treatments, *Pediatr Ann* 22:235, 1993.
Habif TP: *Clinical dermatology*, ed 3, St Louis, 1996, Mosby.

Author: **Fred F. Ferri, M.D.**

Inappropriate secretion of antidiuretic hormone (PTG)

BASIC INFORMATION

DEFINITION
Inappropriate secretion of antidiuretic hormone (SIADH) is a syndrome characterized by excessive secretion of ADH in absence of normal osmotic or physiologic stimuli (increased serum osmolarity, decreased plasma volume, hypotension).

SYNONYMS
SIADH

ICD-9-CM CODES
276.9 Inappropriate secretion of antidiuretic hormone

EPIDEMIOLOGY AND DEMOGRAPHICS
Nearly 50% of hyponatremia detected in the hospital setting is caused by SIADH.

PHYSICAL FINDINGS
- The patient is generally normovolemic or slightly hypervolemic; edema is absent.
- Delirium, lethargy, and seizures may be present if the hyponatremia is severe or of rapid onset.
- Manifestations of the underlying disease may be evident (e.g., fever from an infectious process or headaches and visual field defects from an intracranial mass).
- Diminished reflexes and extensor plantar responses may occur with severe hyponatremia.

ETIOLOGY
- Neoplasm: lung, duodenum, pancreas, brain, thymus, bladder, prostate, mesothelioma, lymphoma, Ewing's sarcoma
- Pulmonary disorders: pneumonia, TB, bronchiectasis, emphysema, status asthmaticus
- Intracranial pathology: trauma, neoplasms, infections, (meningitis, encephalitis, brain abscess), hemorrhage, hydrocephalus
- Postoperative period: surgical stress, ventilators with positive pressure, anesthetic agents
- Drugs: chlorpropamide, thiazide diuretics, vasopressin, oxytocin, chemotherapeutic agents (vincristine, vinblastine, cyclophosphamide), carbamazepine, phenothiazines, MAO inhibitors, tricyclic antidepressants, narcotics, nicotine, clofibrate, haloperidol
- Other: acute intermittent porphyria, Guillain-Barré syndrome, myxedema, psychosis, delirium tremens, ACTH deficiency (hypopituitarism)

DIAGNOSIS

DIFFERENTIAL DIAGNOSIS
- Hyponatremia associated with hypervolemia (CHF, cirrhosis, nephrotic syndrome)
- Factitious hyponatremia (hyperglycemia, abnormal proteins, hyperlipidemia)
- Hypovolemia associated with hypovolemia (e.g., burns, GI fluid loss)

WORKUP
- Demonstration through laboratory evaluation (see "Laboratory Tests") of excessive secretion of ADH in absence of appropriate osmotic or physiologic stimuli
- Normal thyroid, adrenal, and cardiac function
- No recent or concurrent use of diuretics
- Fig. 3-47 illustrates a diagnostic approach to hyponatremia.

LABORATORY TESTS
- Hyponatremia
- Urinary osmolarity > serum osmolarity
- Urinary sodium usually >30 mEq/L
- Normal BUN, creatinine (indicative of normal renal function and absence of dehydration)
- Decreased uric acid

IMAGING STUDIES
Chest x-ray examination to rule out neoplasm or infectious process

TREATMENT

NONPHARMACOLOGIC THERAPY
Fluid restriction to 500 to 800 ml/day

ACUTE GENERAL Rx
In emergency situations (seizures, coma) SIADH can be treated with combination of hypertonic saline solution (slow infusion of 250 ml of 3% NaCl) and furosemide; this increases the serum sodium by causing diuresis of urine that is more dilute than plasma; the rapidity of correction varies depending on the degree of hyponatremia and if the hyponatremia is acute or chronic; generally the serum sodium should be corrected only halfway to normal in the initial 24 hr and serum sodium should be increased by <0.5 mEq/L/hr.

CHRONIC Rx
- Depending on the underlying etiology, fluid restriction may be needed indefinitely. Monthly monitoring of electrolytes is recommended in patients with chronic SIADH.
- Demeclocycline (Declomycin) 300 to 600 mg PO bid may be useful in patients with chronic SIADH (e.g., secondary to neoplasm), but use with caution in patients with hepatic disease; its side effects include nephrogenic DI and photosensitivity. This medication is expensive (cost to the pharmacist is >$325 for fifty 300 mg tablets).

DISPOSITION
- Prognosis varies depending on the cause. Generally prognosis is benign when SIADH is caused by an infectious process.
- Morbidity and mortality are high (>40%) when serum sodium concentration is <110 mEq/L.

REFERRAL
Hospital admission depending on severity of symptoms and degree of hyponatremia

MISCELLANEOUS

COMMENTS
- Use of hypertonic (3%) saline is contraindicated in patients with CHF, nephrotic syndrome, or cirrhosis
- Too rapid correction of hyponatremia can cause demyelination and permanent CNS damage

REFERENCES
Arieff AI: Management of hyponatremia, Br Med J 307:307, 1993.
Noble J (ed): *Primary care medicine*, ed 2, St Louis, 1996, Mosby.

Author: **Fred F. Ferri, M.D.**

Incontinence (PTG)

BASIC INFORMATION

DEFINITION
Incontinence is the involuntary loss of urine.

ICD-9-CM CODES
788.3 Incontinence
625.6 Stress incontinence
788.33 Mixed stress and urge incontinence
788.32 Male incontinence
788.39 Neurogenic incontinence
307.6 Nonorganic origin

EPIDEMIOLOGY AND DEMOGRAPHICS
INCIDENCE AND PREVALENCE: In the general population between the ages of 15 and 64 yr, 1.5% to 5% of men and 10% to 25% of women will suffer from incontinence. In the nursing home population, 50% of the population suffers some degree of incontinence. Nearly 20% of children through the midteenage years have episodes of urinary incontinence.
CLINICAL, PSYCHOLOGIC, AND SOCIAL IMPACT: Less than 50% of the individuals with incontinence living in the community consult health care providers, preferring to "silently suffer," turning to "home remedies," commercially available absorbent materials, and supportive aids. As their condition worsens they become depressed, sacrifice their independence, suffer from recurrent urinary tract infection and its sequelae, limit their social interaction, refrain from sexual intimacy, and become homebound. In terms of costs, for all ages living in the community, it is estimated that $7 billion is spent for incontinence annually.

MAJOR TYPES OF INCONTINENCE
TRANSIENT INCONTINENCE: Incontinence occurring as a result or reaction to an acute medical problem affecting the lower urinary tract. Many of these problems can be reversed with treatment of the underlying problem.
URGE INCONTINENCE: Involuntary loss of urine associated with an abrupt and strong desire to void. It is usually associated with involuntary detrusor contractions on urodynamic investigation. In *neurologically impaired patients*, the involuntary detrusor contraction is referred to as *detrusor hyperreflexia*. In *neurologically normal patients* the involuntary contraction is called *detrusor instability*.
STRESS INCONTINENCE: The involuntary loss of urine with physical activities that increase abdominal pressure in the absence of a detrusor contraction or an overdistended bladder. Classification of stress incontinence:
Type 0: Complaint of incontinence without demonstration of leakage
Type I: Incontinence in response to stress but little descent of the bladder neck and urethra
Type II: Incontinence in response to stress with >2 cm descent of the bladder neck and urethra
Type III: Bladder neck and urethra wide open without bladder contraction; intrinsic sphincter deficiency, and denervation of the urethra. The most common causes: urethral hypermobility and displacement of the bladder neck with exertion, intrinsic sphincter deficiency from failed antiincontinence surgery, prostatectomy, radiation, cord lesions, epispadias, or myelomeningocele.
OVERFLOW INCONTINENCE: Loss of urine resulting from overdistention of the bladder with resultant "overflow" or "spilling" of the urine. Causes: hypotonic-to-atonic bladder resulting from drug effect, fecal impaction, or neurologic conditions such as diabetes, spinal cord injury, surgery, vitamin B_{12} deficiency. It is also caused by obstruction at the bladder neck and urethra. In this situation, prostatism, prostatic cancer, urethral stenosis, antiincontinence surgery, pelvic prolapse, and detrusor-sphincter-dyssynergia cause the incontinence.
FUNCTIONAL INCONTINENCE: Involuntary loss of urine resulting from chronic impairments of physical and/or cognitive functioning. This is a diagnosis of exclusion. The condition can sometimes be improved or cured by improving the patient's functional status, treating comorbidities, changing medications, reducing environmental barriers, etc.
MIXED STRESS AND URGE INCONTINENCE
SENSORY URGENCY INCONTINENCE: Involuntary loss of urine as a result of decreased bladder compliance and increased intravesical pressures accompanied by severe urgency and bladder hypersensitivity without detrusor overactivity. This is seen with radiation cystitis, interstitial cystitis, eosinophilic cystitis, myelomeningocele, and radical pelvic surgery. Nephropathy can occur as a complication of this vesicoureteral reflux.
SPHINCTERIC INCONTINENCE:
Urethral Hypermobility: The basic abnormality is a weakness of pelvic floor support. Because of this weakness, during increases in abdominal pressure there is rotational descent of the vesical neck and proximal urethra. If the urethra opens concomitantly, stress urinary incontinence ensues. Urethral hypermobility is often present in women who are not incontinent. Its mere presence is not sufficient evidence to make the diagnosis of sphincteric abnormality unless incontinence is shown.
Intrinsic Sphincter Deficiency: There is an intrinsic malfunction of the sphincter itself. It is characterized by an open vesical neck at rest and a low leak point pressure (<65 cm water). Urethral hypermobility and intrinsic sphincter deficiency may coexist in the

same patient. Causes of intrinsic sphincter deficiency are previous pelvic surgery, antiincontinence surgery, urethral diverticulectomy, radical hysterectomy, abdominoperineal resection of the rectum, urethrotomy, Y-V plasty of the vesical neck, myelodysplasia, anterior spinal artery syndrome, lumbosacral disease, aging, and hypoestrogenism.

DIAGNOSIS

HISTORY
- History of present illness, psychosocial factors, congenital disorders, access issues for the physically challenged, neurologic disorders, and disorders pertinent to the urologic tract
- Review of prescription and nonprescription medications
- Voiding diary to assess total voided volume, frequency of micturition, mean volume voided, largest single volume, diurnal distribution, nature and severity of incontinence

WORKUP
- Physical examination including general examination, gait of the patient (neuromuscular deficits), estrogen status, vaginal examination to include the periurethral region, evaluation for cystocele, rectocele, and enterocele
- Pelvic floor strength assessment
- Rectal examination to assess sphincter tone and bulbocavernosus reflex
- Neurologic examination
- Postvoid residual check using bladder scan or catheter

LABORATORY TESTS
Urinalysis, urine culture, urine cytology, BUN, and creatinine.

IMAGING STUDIES
- KUB to assess bony skeleton
- IVP to rule out upper tract abnormalities, developmental anomalies, bladder configuration, and fistula
- Renal ultrasound if dye study is contraindicated

SPECIALIZED STUDIES
Simple cystometrogram, complex urodynamics including leak point pressures and uroflowmetry, endoscopic evaluation, and cystogram

TREATMENT

TRANSIENT INCONTINENCE
Treatment of underlying medical conditions and behavioral therapy to include habit training and timed voiding

URGE INCONTINENCE
Bladder relaxants (i.e., oxybutynin, imipramine), estrogen, biofeedback, Kegel exercises, and surgical removal of obstructing or other pathologic lesions

STRESS INCONTINENCE
- Pelvic floor exercises, Kegel exercises, α-adrenergic agonists (i.e., ephedrine), estrogen, biofeedback.
- For intrinsic sphincter deficiency: bulking agents (i.e., collagen), sling, and artificial sphincter

OVERFLOW INCONTINENCE
Surgical removal of any obstructing lesions, clean intermittent catheterization, and indwelling catheter

FUNCTIONAL INCONTINENCE
Behavioral training to include habit training and timed voiding, incontinence undergarments and pads, external collecting devices, and environmental manipulation

MIXED URGENCY AND STRESS INCONTINENCE
Use of measures recommended in the management of stress and urge incontinence

SENSORY URGENCY
Bladder relaxants (i.e., anticholinergics, muscle relaxants, and tricyclic antidepressants), behavior therapy to include habit training and timed voiding, cystoscopy and hydrodilatation

SPHINCTERIC DEFICIENCY
Urethral bulking agents, sling procedure, artificial sphincter, mechanical clamp, and external collection devices

MISCELLANEOUS

COMMENTS
Other forms of incontinence:
NOCTURNAL ENURESIS: (ICD-9-CM Code: 788.3) Can be caused by sphincter abnormalities and detrusor overactivity; can occur as idiopathic, neurogenic, and with outlet obstruction
POSTVOID DRIBBLE: (ICD-9-CM Code: 599.2) A postsphincteric collection of urine seen with urethral diverticulum and can be idiopathic
EXTRAURETHRAL INCONTINENCE: Enterovesical (ICD-9-CM Codes: 596.1 and 596.2), Urethral (ICD-9-CM Code: 599.1), also known as fistula

REFERENCES
Aliotta, PJ: Urodynamic studies. In Danakas GT, Pietranton, M: *The care of the gynecologic/obstetric patient,* St Louis, 1997, Mosby.

US Department of Health and Human Services, Public Health Service, Agency for Health Care Policy and Research: *Clinical practice guideline: urinary incontinence in adults,* Rockville, Md, 1996, US Department of Health and Human Services.

Author: **Philip J. Aliotta, M.D., M.S.H.A.**

Influenza (PTG)

BASIC INFORMATION

DEFINITION
Influenza is an acute febrile illness caused by infection with influenza type A or B virus.

SYNONYMS
Flu

ICD-9-CM CODES
487.1 Influenza

EPIDEMIOLOGY AND DEMOGRAPHICS:
INCIDENCE (IN U.S.): Annual incidence of influenza-related deaths is approximately 20,000 deaths/year.
PREDOMINANT SEX: Male = female
PREDOMINANT AGE: Attack rates are higher among children than adults, although children are less prone to develop pulmonary complications.
PEAK INCIDENCE: Winter outbreaks lasting 5 to 6 wk

PHYSICAL FINDINGS
- "Classic flu" is characterized by abrupt onset of fever, headache, myalgias, anorexia, and malaise after a 1 to 2 day incubation period.
- Clinical syndromes are similar to those produced by other respiratory viruses, including pharyngitis, common colds, tracheobronchitis, bronchiolitis, croup.
- Respiratory symptoms such as cough, sore throat, and nasal discharge are usually present at the onset of illness but systemic symptoms predominate.
- Elderly patients may experience fever, weakness, and confusion without any respiratory complaints.
- Acute deterioration to status asthmaticus may occur in patients with asthma.
- Influenza pneumonia: rapidly progressive cough, dyspnea, and cyanosis may occur after typical flu onset.

ETIOLOGY
- Variation in the surface antigens of the influenza virus, hemagglutinin (HA) and neuraminidase (NA) leading to infection with variants to which resistance is inadequate in the population at risk
- Transmitted by small-particle aerosols and deposited on the respiratory tract epithelium

DIAGNOSIS

DIFFERENTIAL DIAGNOSIS
- Respiratory syncytial virus, adenovirus, parainfluenza virus infection
- Secondary bacterial pneumonia or mixed bacterial-viral pneumonia

WORKUP
- Virus isolation from nasal or throat swab or sputum specimens is the most rapid diagnostic method in the setting of acute illness.
- Specimens are placed into virus transport medium and processed by a reference laboratory.
- For serologic diagnosis:
  1. Paired serum specimens, acute and convalescent, the latter obtained 10 to 20 days later
  2. Fourfold rises or falls in the titer of antibodies (various techniques) considered diagnostic of recent infection

LABORATORY TESTS
Septic syndrome presentation: CBC, ABG analysis, blood cultures

IMAGING STUDIES
- Chest x-ray examination to demonstrate findings of viral pneumonia: peribronchial and patchy interstitial infiltrates in multiple lobes with atelectasis
- Possible progression to diffuse interstitial pneumonitis

TREATMENT

NONPHARMACOLOGIC THERAPY
- Bed rest
- Hydration

ACUTE GENERAL Rx
- Supportive care: antipyretics—*Avoid aspirin in children because of the association with Reye's syndrome.*
- Antibiotics if bacterial pneumonia is proven or suspected
- Amantadine (100 mg PO twice daily for children >10 yr and adults <65 yr; once daily in patients >65 yr) and rimantadine (same dosing schedule as amantadine)
  1. Further dose adjustments needed with renal insufficiency
  2. Fewer CNS side effects with rimantadine

DISPOSITION
Patients are hospitalized if signs of pneumonia are present.

REFERRAL
Infectious disease and/or pulmonary consultation when influenza pneumonia is suspected

MISCELLANEOUS

COMMENTS
- Prevention of influenza in patients at high risk is an important goal of primary care.
- Vaccines reduce the risk of infection and the severity of illness.
1. Antigenic composition of the vaccine is updated annually.
2. Vaccination should be given at the start of the flu season (October) for the following groups:
   a. Adults ≥65 yr
   b. Adults and children with chronic cardiac or pulmonary disease, including asthma
   c. Adults and children with illness requiring frequent follow-up (e.g., hemoglobinopathies, diabetes mellitus)
   d. Children receiving long-term aspirin therapy
   e. Immunocompromised patients
   f. Household contacts of persons in the above groups
   g. Health-care workers
3. Only contraindication to vaccination is hypersensitivity to hen's eggs.
4. Special efforts should be made to vaccinate high-risk patients younger than 65 yr, only 10% to 15% of whom are vaccinated each year.
- Chemoprophylaxis:
1. Amantadine and rimantadine approved for prophylaxis against influenza A; they are ineffective against influenza B.
2. Consider for:
   a. High-risk patients in whom vaccination is contraindicated
   b. When the available vaccine is known not to include the circulating strain
   c. To provide added protection to immunosuppressed patients likely to have a diminished response to vaccination
   d. In the setting of an outbreak, when immediate protection of unvaccinated or late-vaccinated patients is desired
3. Give for 2 wk in the case of late vaccination and for the duration of the flu season in all other patients.

REFERENCES
Betts RF: Influenza virus. In Mandell GL, Bennett JE, Dolin R (eds.): *Mandell, Douglas, and Bennett's principles and practice of infectious diseases,* New York, 1995, Churchill-Livingstone.
Glezen WP: Influenza: time to prepare for the '96-'97 season, *J Respir Dis* 17(8):643, 1996.

Author: **Claudia L. Dade, M.D.**

Insomnia (PTG)

BASIC INFORMATION

DEFINITION
Insomnia refers to a disturbance of nocturnal sleep patterns that causes adverse daytime consequences.

SYNONYMS
Disorders of initiating and maintaining sleep (DIMS)

ICD-9-CM CODES
780.50 Sleep disturbance, unspecified
780.51 Insomnia with sleep apnea
780.52 Other insomnia

EPIDEMIOLOGY AND DEMOGRAPHICS
INCIDENCE (IN U.S.): 33 cases/100 persons/yr
PREVALENCE (IN U.S.): Up to 33% of the population
PREDOMINANT SEX: More common in women
PREDOMINANT AGE: >60 yr
PEAK INCIDENCE: Affects all age groups, but more common in those >60 yr old.
GENETICS:
- Primary insomnia with childhood onset may be familial.
- No known genetic basis for other causes.

PHYSICAL FINDINGS
- None
- Patients usually complain of:
  a. Difficulty initiating sleep, wakefulness during sleep cycle, or early awakening
  b. Daytime fatigue, drowsiness

ETIOLOGY
- Psychiatric disorders (35%)
- Psychophysiologic (15%)
- Drug and alcohol abuse (12%)
- Periodic leg movements (12%)
- Sleep apnea (6%)
- Medical and toxic conditions (4%)

DIAGNOSIS

DIFFERENTIAL DIAGNOSIS
Insomnia is a symptom that may have numerous underlying causes (see "Etiology").

WORKUP
- Thorough history and examination to identify possible etiology
- Sleep log

LABORATORY TESTS
Nighttime polysomnography in an accredited sleep laboratory may be needed to establish the etiology.

IMAGING STUDIES
None

TREATMENT

NONPHARMACOLOGIC THERAPY
Rules of sleep hygiene may eliminate bad habits and adverse environmental factors.

ACUTE GENERAL Rx
- Transient insomnia: benzodiazepines (see Table 7-14)
- Acute pain: analgesics
- Zolpidem (Ambien), a nonbenzodiazepine agent, 5 to 10 mg qhs may be useful for the short-term treatment of insomnia.

CHRONIC Rx
- Benzodiazepines or antidepressants if appropriate for underlying etiology
- Choice of a particular agent, depending on precise nature of sleep disturbance (see "References" for details)
- Possible tolerance and dependence with prolonged use of benzodiazepines

DISPOSITION
Significant improvements in sleep can be achieved in many cases.

REFERRAL
- If etiology uncertain
- For assessment at a sleep disorders center (recommended)

MISCELLANEOUS

REFERENCES
Rosekind MR: The epidemiology and occurrence of insomnia, *J Clin Psychiatry* 53:4, 1992.
Author: **Michael Gruenthal, M.D., Ph.D.**

BASIC INFORMATION

DEFINITION
Irritable bowel syndrome (IBS) is a chronic functional disorder manifested by alteration in bowel habits and recurrent abdominal pain and bloating.

SYNONYMS
Irritable colon
Spastic colon
IBS

ICD-9-CM CODES
564.1 Irritable colon

EPIDEMIOLOGY AND DEMOGRAPHICS
- IBS occurs in 20% of population of industrialized countries and is responsible for >50% of GI referrals.
- Female:male ratio is 2:1.
- Nearly 50% of patients have psychiatric abnormalities, with anxiety disorders being most common.

PHYSICAL FINDINGS
- Physical examination is generally normal.
- Nonspecific abdominal tenderness and distention may be present.

ETIOLOGY
- Unknown
- Possible abnormal colon motility
- Risk factors: anxiety, depression, personality disorders, history of childhood sexual abuse, and domestic abuse in women

DIAGNOSIS

DIFFERENTIAL DIAGNOSIS
- IBD
- Diverticulitis
- Colon malignancy
- Endometriosis
- PUD
- Biliary liver disease
- Chronic pancreatitis

WORKUP
The clinical presentation of IBS consists of abdominal pain and abnormalities of defecation, which may include loose stools usually after meals and in the morning, alternating with episodes of constipation. Diagnostic workup is aimed primarily at excluding the conditions listed in the differential diagnoses.

LABORATORY TESTS
- Blood work is generally normal. The presence of anemia should alert to the possibility of a colonic malignancy or IBD.
- Testing of stool for ova and parasites should be considered in patients with chronic diarrhea.

IMAGING STUDIES
- Small bowel series and barium enema are normal and not necessary for diagnosis.
- Sigmoidoscopy is generally normal except for the presence of some spasms.

TREATMENT

NONPHARMACOLOGIC THERAPY
- The patient should be encouraged to maintain a high-fiber diet and to eliminate foods that aggravate symptoms.
- Behavioral therapy is also recommended, particularly in younger patients.
- Importance of regular exercise and adequate fluid intake should be stressed.

ACUTE GENERAL Rx
- The mainstay of treatment of IBS is high-fiber diet
- Fiber supplementation with psyllium 1 tablespoon bid or calcium polycarbophil (FiberCon) 2 tablets one to four times daily followed by 8 oz of water may be necessary in some patients.
- Patients should be instructed that there might be some increased bloating on initiation of fiber supplementation, which should resolve within 2 to 3 wk. It is important that patients take these fiber products on a regular basis and not only PRN.
- Antispasmodics-anticholinergics may be useful in refractory cases (e.g., dicyclomine [Bentyl] 10 to 20 mg up to three times daily).
- Patients who appear anxious can benefit from use of sedatives and anticholinergics such as chlordiazepoxide-clidinium (Librax) or fluoxetine (Prozac) 20 mg qd.

CHRONIC Rx
Patient education regarding maintenance of high-fiber diet and elimination of stressors, which can precipitate attacks of IBS

DISPOSITION
Greater than 60% of patients respond successfully to treatment over the initial 12 mo; however, IBS is a chronic relapsing condition and requires prolonged therapy.

REFERRAL
GI referral is recommended in patients with rectal bleeding, fever, nocturnal diarrhea, anemia, weight loss, or onset of symptoms after age 40 yr.

MISCELLANEOUS

COMMENTS
Patients should be reassured that their condition cannot lead to cancer.

REFERENCES
Grossman DA: Diagnosing and treating patients with refractory functional gastrointestinal disorders, *Ann Intern Med* 123:688, 1995.

Author: **Fred F. Ferri, M.D.**

Kaposi's sarcoma (PTG)

BASIC INFORMATION

DEFINITION
Kaposi's sarcoma (KS) is a vascular neoplasm most frequently occurring in AIDS patients. It can be divided in the following 5 subsets:
1. *Classic Kaposi's sarcoma:* most frequently found in elderly Mediterranean males. It consists initially of violaceous macules and papules with subsequent development of plaques and red/purple nodules. Growth is slow, and most of the patients die of unrelated causes.
2. *Epidemic or AIDS-related Kaposi's sarcoma:* most frequently occurs in homosexual men. Lesions are generally multifocal and widespread. Lymphadenopathy may be associated.
3. *Epidemic African Kaposi's sarcoma:* usually affects extremities; nodular form, locally aggressive.
4. *African lymphadenopathic Kaposi's sarcoma:* usually affects children younger than 10 yr.
5. *Immunosuppressive Kaposi's sarcoma:* usually associated with chemotherapy.

SYNONYMS
KS

ICD-9-CM CODES
173.9 Malignant neoplasm of the skin

EPIDEMIOLOGY AND DEMOGRAPHICS
- AIDS-related KS affects >35% of AIDS cases.
- Highest incidence is in homosexual men.

PHYSICAL FINDINGS
- AIDS-related KS: multifocal and widespread red-purple or dark plaques and/or nodules on cutaneous or mucosal surfaces (see color plate 12).
- Generalized lymphadenopathy at the time of diagnosis is present in >50% of patients with AIDS-related KS; the initial lesions have a rust-colored appearance; subsequent progression to red or purple nodules or plaques occurs.
- Most frequently affected areas are the face, trunk, oral cavity, and upper and lower extremities.

ETIOLOGY
A herpesvirus (HHV-8) has been isolated from patients with most forms of KS and is believed to be the causative agent.

DIAGNOSIS

DIFFERENTIAL DIAGNOSIS
- Stasis dermatitis
- Pyogenic granuloma
- Capillary hemangiomas
- Granulation tissue
- Postinflammatory hyperpigmentation
- Cutaneous lymphoma
- Melanoma
- Dermatofibroma
- Hematoma
- Prurigo nodularis

WORKUP
Diagnosis can generally be made on clinical appearance; tissue biopsy will confirm diagnosis.

LABORATORY TESTS
HIV in patients suspected of AIDS

TREATMENT

NONPHARMACOLOGIC THERAPY
Observation is a reasonable option in patients with slowly progressive disease.

ACUTE GENERAL Rx
- Liquid nitrogen cryotherapy can result in complete response in 80% of lesions.
- Interlesional chemotherapy with vinblastine is useful for nodular lesions >1 cm in diameter.
- Radiation therapy is effective in non-AIDS KS and for large tumor masses that interfere with normal function.
- Systemic therapy with interferon is also effective in AIDS-related KS and is often used in combination with AZT.
- Systemic chemotherapy (vinblastine, vincristine) can be used for rapidly progressive disease and for classic and African endemic KS.

DISPOSITION
- Prognosis is poor in AIDS-related KS. Death is often a result of other AIDS-defining illnesses.
- Prognosis is better in African cutaneous KS and classic sarcoma (patients usually die of unrelated causes).

REFERRAL
Surgical referral for biopsy of suspected lesions

MISCELLANEOUS

COMMENTS
Interlesional interferon alfa may be effective in selected patients.

REFERENCES
Foreman KE et al: Propagation of a human herpesvirus from AIDS-associated Kaposi's sarcoma, *N Engl J Med* 336:163, 1997.

Habif TP: *Clinical dermatology*, ed 3, St Louis, 1996, Mosby.

Moore PS, Chang Y: Detection of herpesvirus-like DNA sequences in Kaposi's sarcoma in patients with and without HIV infection, *N Engl J Med* 332:1181, 1995.

Prattner A et al: The therapeutic effect of interlesional interferon in classical Kaposi's sarcoma, *Br J Dermatol* 129:590, 1993.

Author: **Fred F. Ferri, M.D.**

Klinefelter's syndrome (PTG)

BASIC INFORMATION

DEFINITION
Klinefelter's syndrome is a congenital disorder in which a 47,XXY chromosome compliment is associated with hypogonadism.

SYNONYMS
47,XXY Hypogonadism

ICD-9-CM CODES
758.7 Klinefelter's syndrome

EPIDEMIOLOGY AND DEMOGRAPHICS
INCIDENCE: 1 in 400 men
GENETICS: 47,XXY karyotype and occasional 48,XXYY; 48,XXXY; or 49,XXXXY have been reported. The manifestations vary in severity in patients. It is this sex chromosome mosaicism that is thought to account for the variable presentation. Fertility, though very rare, has been reported in men with Klinefelter's syndrome.

PHYSICAL FINDINGS
CLASSIC TRIAD: Small firm testes, azoospermia, and gynecomastia
Prepubertal: Small testes, gonadal volume <1.5 ml is a result of loss of germ cells before puberty.
Postpubertal: Gynecomastia (periductal fat growth) with small, firm, pea-sized testes. Exaggerated growth of the lower extremities results in a decreased crown-to-pubis:pubis-to-floor ratio. There is diminished strength, diminished ability to grow a full beard or mustache, infertility; decreased intellectual development and antisocial behavior are thought to occur with high frequency.

ETIOLOGY
- Several postulated mechanisms: nondisjunction during meiosis and mitosis and anaphase lag during mitosis or meiosis
- Reason: maternal age
  1. The incidence of Klinefelter's rises from 0.6% when the maternal age is 35 yr or less vs. 5.4% when the maternal age is in excess of 45 yr.
  2. It is of interest to note that the extra X chromosome has a paternal origin as often as a maternal origin.

DIAGNOSIS

LABORATORY TESTS
- Decreased serum testosterone
- Increased sex hormone binding globin (acts to further suppress any available free testosterone)
- Increased estradiol (a result of augmented peripheral conversion of testosterone to estradiol)
- Testis biopsy shows azoospermia, hyalinization, and fibrosis of the seminiferous tubules. Mosaics may have focal areas of spermatogenesis and, on rare occasions, a sperm may appear in the ejaculate. It is the extra X chromosome that is the pivotal factor controlling spermatogenesis as well as affecting neuronal function directly leading to the behavioral abnormalities related to decreased IQ.
- Buccal smear: one sex chromatin body

PREPUBERTAL MALE: Gonadotropin levels are normal.
POSTPUBERTAL MALE: Gonadotropin levels are elevated even when the testosterone level is normal.

DISEASE ASSOCIATIONS
Malignancies: Breast cancer (twenty times greater than XY men and 20% the rate of occurrence in women), non-lymphocytic leukemia, lymphomas, marrow dysplastic syndromes, extragonadal germ cell neoplasms
Autoimmune disorders: Chronic lymphocytic thyroiditis, Takayasu arteritis, taurodontism (enlarged molar teeth), mitral valve prolapse, varicose veins, asthma, bronchitis, osteoporosis, and abnormal glucose tolerance testing

TREATMENT

Revolves around three facets of Klinefelter's syndrome:
1. Hypogonadism: androgen replacement in the form of testosterone
2. Gynecomastia: cosmetic surgery
3. Psychosocial problems: androgen therapy and educational support

MISCELLANEOUS

COMMENTS
- Androgen therapy should not be used in the case of severe mental retardation.
- Also, rule out breast and prostate cancer before initiating or continuing androgen therapy.
- Furthermore, androgen therapy will not improve infertility; it may suppress any spermatogenesis that is taking place within the testes.
- Other causes of primary hypogonadism:
  1. Myotonic muscular dystrophy
  2. Sertoli cell only syndrome
  3. Kartagener's syndrome
  4. Anorchia
  5. Acquired hypogonadism

REFERENCES
Jaffe T, Oates RD: Genetic aspects of infertility. In Lipshultz LI, Howards SS (eds): *Infertility in the male,* St Louis, 1997, Mosby.
Plymate SR: Male hypogonadism. In Becker KL (ed): *Principles and practice of endocrinology and metabolism, part VIII, endocrinology of the male,* Philadelphia, 1995, Lippincott.

Author: **Philip J. Aliotta, M.D., M.S.H.A.**

Korsakoff's psychosis

BASIC INFORMATION

DEFINITION
Korsakoff's psychosis involves a disproportionate impairment in memory, relative to other cognitive function, resulting from a thiamine deficiency.

SYNONYMS
Korsakoff's syndrome
Wernicke-Korsakoff syndrome
Alcoholic polyneuritic psychosis

ICD-9-CM CODES
291.1 Alcohol amnestic syndrome

EPIDEMIOLOGY AND DEMOGRAPHICS
INCIDENCE (IN U.S.): Most common in alcoholics
PREVALENCE (IN U.S.): Slightly less than incidence
PREDOMINANT SEX: More common in males
PREDOMINANT AGE: Middle age
PEAK INCIDENCE: Middle age

PHYSICAL FINDINGS
- Impairment of ability to remember new material
- Relatively intact remote memory
- Possible confabulation

ETIOLOGY
Thiamine deficiency, usually in alcoholics

DIAGNOSIS

DIFFERENTIAL DIAGNOSIS
- Brain tumor
- Cerebral anoxia
- Dementia from any cause

WORKUP
Consider in all alcoholics, in malnutrition, and in malabsorption.

LABORATORY TESTS
Thiamine levels can be performed, but treatment is usually given on clinical grounds alone.

IMAGING STUDIES
MRI shows bilateral thalamic and mamillary body lesions in up to 30% of acute cases; ventricular enlargement and cerebral atrophy are common.

TREATMENT

NONPHARMACOLOGIC THERAPY
A supervised environment may be required.

ACUTE GENERAL Rx
Thiamine 100 mg IV or IM, given during Wernicke's phase (disorders of extraocular movements, confusion, and ataxia), is highly effective in preventing Korsakoff's symptoms.

CHRONIC Rx
No cure

DISPOSITION
Patient often must live in protected environment for rest of life.

REFERRAL
If there is doubt about the diagnosis; neuropsychologic tests may be helpful.

MISCELLANEOUS

COMMENTS
- This disease is probably underdiagnosed.
- Give thiamine if the disease is even suspected.

REFERENCES
Heye N et al: Wernicke's encephalopathy—causes to consider, *Intensive Care Med* 20:282, 1994.
Kopelman MD: The Korsakoff syndrome, *Br J Psychiatry* 166:154, 1995.
Author: **William H. Olson, M.D.**

Labyrinthitis (PTG)

BASIC INFORMATION

DEFINITION
Labyrinthitis is an acute onset of vertigo, nausea, and vomiting not associated with auditory or neurologic symptoms.

SYNONYMS
Acute labyrinthitis
Acute vestibular neuronopathy
Viral neurolabyrinthitis

ICD-9-CM CODES
386.3 Labyrinthitis

EPIDEMIOLOGY AND DEMOGRAPHICS
INCIDENCE (IN U.S.): Most common cause of transient vertigo, nausea, and vomiting at any age
PREDOMINANT AGE: Any

PHYSICAL FINDINGS
- Nystagmus
- Nausea
- Vomiting
- Vertigo worsening with head movement
- Abnormal caloric tests
- Normal hearing

ETIOLOGY
Often proceeded 1 wk by an upper respiratory illness

DIAGNOSIS

DIFFERENTIAL DIAGNOSIS
- Cholesteatoma
- Suppurative labyrinthitis
- Labyrinthine fistula
- Benign positional vertigo
- Meniere's syndrome
- Vascular insufficiency
- Drug-induced

WORKUP
- Caloric test
- Careful cranial nerve testing

LABORATORY TESTS
- Routine laboratory tests are generally not helpful.
- CBC with sedimentation rate may be useful in selected patients.

IMAGING STUDIES
None are usually necessary, but enhancement of bony labyrinth can be seen by MRI after injection of contrast material.

TREATMENT

NONPHARMACOLOGIC THERAPY
Reassurance

ACUTE GENERAL Rx
- Compazine or other antiemetics are effective
- Meclizine 12.5 to 25 mg qid

CHRONIC Rx
None necessary

DISPOSITION
Usually not necessary to refer

REFERRAL
If symptoms persist or cranial nerve abnormalities are present

MISCELLANEOUS

COMMENTS
"Labyrinthitis" covers a broad range of diseases; here we refer only to the acute self-limited type.

REFERENCES
Baloh RW, Honrubia V, Jacobson K: Benign positional vertigo: clinical and oculographic features in 240 cases, *Neurology* 37:371, 1987.
Warner EA et al: Dizziness in primary care patients. *J Gen Intern Med* 7:454, 1992.

Author: **William H. Olson, M.D.**

Lactose intolerance (PTG)

BASIC INFORMATION

DEFINITION
Lactose intolerance is the insufficient concentration of lactase enzyme, leading to fermentation of malabsorbed lactose by intestinal bacteria with subsequent production of intestinal gas and various organic acids.

SYNONYMS
Lactase deficiency
Milk intolerance

ICD-9-CM CODES
271.3 Lactose intolerance

EPIDEMIOLOGY AND DEMOGRAPHICS
Nearly 50 million people in the U.S. have partial or complete lactose intolerance. There are racial differences, with <25% of Caucasian adults being lactose intolerant, whereas >85% Asian-Americans and >60% of African-Americans have some form of lactose intolerance.

PHYSICAL FINDINGS
- Abdominal tenderness and cramping, bloating, flatulence
- Diarrhea
- Physical examination: may be entirely within normal limits

ETIOLOGY
- Congenital lactase deficiency: Common in premature infants; rare in full-term infants and generally inherited as a chromosomal recessive trait
- Secondary lactose intolerance: usually a result of injury of the intestinal mucosa (Crohn's disease, viral gastroenteritis, AIDS enteropathy, cryptosporidiosis, Whipple's disease, sprue)

DIAGNOSIS

DIFFERENTIAL DIAGNOSIS
- IBD
- IBS
- Pancreatic insufficiency
- Nontropical and tropical sprue
- Cystic fibrosis

WORKUP
Diagnostic workup includes confirming the diagnosis with hydrogen breath test and excluding other conditions listed in the differential diagnosis that may also coexist with lactase deficiency.

LABORATORY TESTS
- Lactose breath hydrogen test: A rise in breath hydrogen >20 ppm within 90 min of ingestion of 50 g of lactose is positive for lactase deficiency.
- Diarrhea associated with lactase deficiency is osmotic in nature with an osmotic gap and a pH below 6.5.

IMAGING STUDIES
Imaging studies are generally not indicated. A small bowel series may be useful in patients with significant malabsorption.

TREATMENT

NONPHARMACOLOGIC THERAPY
A lactose-free diet generally results in prompt resolution of symptoms.

ACUTE GENERAL Rx
- Addition of lactase (Lactaid tablets) before the ingestion of milk products may prevent symptoms in some patients. However, it is generally not effective for all lactose-intolerant patients.
- Calcium supplementation is recommended to prevent osteoporosis.

CHRONIC Rx
Patient education regarding foods high in lactose, such as milk, cottage cheese, or ice cream, is recommended.

DISPOSITION
Clinical improvement with restriction or elimination of milk products

REFERRAL
GI referral for endoscopic procedures if concomitant GI disorders are suspected

MISCELLANEOUS

COMMENTS
There is great variability in signs and symptoms in patients with lactose intolerance depending on the degree of lactase deficiency.

REFERENCES
Malagelada J: Lactose intolerance, *New Engl J Med* 333:53, 1995.
Author: **Fred F. Ferri, M.D.**

Lambert-Eaton myasthenic syndrome

BASIC INFORMATION

DEFINITION
Lambert-Eaton myasthenic syndrome is a disorder of neuromuscular transmission caused by antibodies directed against presynaptic voltage-gated calcium channels on motor nerve terminals.

SYNONYMS
Eaton-Lambert syndrome

ICD-9-CM CODES
199.1 Malignant neoplasm without specification of site, other

EPIDEMIOLOGY AND DEMOGRAPHICS
INCIDENCE (IN U.S.): Uncertain; estimated at 5 cases/1,000,000 persons/yr
PREVALENCE (IN U.S.): Uncertain; estimated at 400 total cases
PREDOMINANT SEX: Male:female of 2:1
PREDOMINANT AGE: 60 yr
PEAK INCIDENCE: Sixth decade
GENETICS: Predisposition in people with a personal or family history of autoimmune disease

PHYSICAL FINDINGS
- Weakness with diminished or absent muscle stretch reflexes
- Proximal lower extremity muscles affected most
- Ocular and bulbar muscles possibly mildly affected
- Transient strength improvement with brief exercise
- Possible autonomic dysfunction

ETIOLOGY
- Antibodies directed against presynaptic voltage-gated calcium channels are present in most patients.
- The reduction in calcium permeability causes a reduction in acetylcholine release.
- Associated malignancy, usually small cell lung cancer, is present in 50% to 70% of patients.

DIAGNOSIS

DIFFERENTIAL DIAGNOSIS
- Myasthenia gravis
- Polymyositis
- Cachexia

WORKUP
Confirm diagnosis by characteristic electrodiagnostic (EMG/NCS) findings.

LABORATORY TESTS
As needed to screen for an underlying malignancy

IMAGING STUDIES
As needed to screen for an underlying malignancy

TREATMENT

NONPHARMACOLOGIC THERAPY
- Avoid elevated body temperature.
- Treat systemic illnesses promptly.

ACUTE GENERAL Rx
- Anticholinesterase agents (e.g., pyridostigmine 30 to 60 mg q4-6h) may yield some improvement.
- Guanidine hydrochloride: start at 5 to 10 mg/kg/day; may increase up to 30 mg/kg/day in 3-day or longer intervals.
- Plasma exchange or IV immunoglobulins (2 g/kg over 2 to 5 days) often produce significant, temporary improvement.
- Prednisone 60 to 80 mg/day can be gradually tapered over weeks or months to minimal effective dose.
- Azathioprine can be given alone or in combination with prednisone. Give 50 mg/day and increase by 50 mg every 3 days up to 150 to 200 mg/day.

CHRONIC Rx
- Treat underlying malignancy if present.
- Give pharmacotherapy as described in "Acute General Rx."

DISPOSITION
- Gradually progressive weakness leading to impaired mobility
- Possible substantial improvement with successful treatment of underlying malignancy

REFERRAL
To a neurologist (recommended) because of infrequency of this disease and risks associated with some treatments

MISCELLANEOUS

COMMENTS
- Many drugs may worsen weakness and should only be used if absolutely necessary. Included are succinylcholine, d-tubocurarine, quinine, quinidine, procainamide, aminoglycoside antibiotics, β-blockers, and calcium channel blockers.
- Watch for increased weakness when starting any new medication.

REFERENCES
Sanders DB: Lambert-Eaton myasthenic syndrome: pathogenesis and treatment, *Semin Neurol* 14:111, 1994.

Author: **Michael Gruenthal, M.D., Ph.D.**

Laryngitis (PTG)

BASIC INFORMATION

DEFINITION
Laryngitis may be an acute or chronic inflammation of the laryngeal mucous membranes.

SYNONYMS
Laryngotracheitis (although this includes inflammation of the trachea as well as the larynx)

ICD-9-CM CODES
464.0 Acute laryngitis
476.0 Chronic laryngitis

PHYSICAL FINDINGS
ACUTE LARYNGITIS:
- Usually associated with an upper respiratory infection, often the common cold or influenza
- Onset usually characterized by sore throat, cough, nasal congestion, and rhinorrhea, followed by hoarseness and occasionally aphonia
- Larynx with diffuse erythema, edema, and vascular engorgement of the vocal folds, and perhaps mucosal ulcerations
- In young children: subglottis is often affected, resulting in airway narrowing with marked hoarseness, inspiratory stridor, dyspnea, and restlessness
- Respiratory compromise rare in adults

CHRONIC LARYNGITIS:
- Most common physical complaint: hoarseness
- Tends to be indolent, with symptoms lasting for several weeks

ETIOLOGY
ACUTE LARYNGITIS:
- Most often associated with viral infections: influenza virus, rhinovirus, and adenovirus are the most common, but parainfluenza virus, myxovirus, paramyxovirus, coxsackievirus, coronavirus, respiratory syncytial virus, herpesvirus, Epstein-Barr virus, varicella zoster virus, and variola virus are sometimes implicated.
- Superinfection is possible with bacteria such as group A streptococci, *Staphylococcus aureus*, and *Streptococcus pneumoniae*.
- 50% to 55% of adults with laryngitis harbor *Moraxella catarrhalis* in the nasopharynx, compared with 6% to 14% of controls. (NOTE: Laryngeal cultures are not taken, so role of *M. catarrhalis* as causative agent is yet to be determined.)
- *Corynebacterium diphtheriae* is also a cause and may affect both the pharynx and larynx.

CHRONIC LARYNGITIS:
- Results from any of the following: TB, usually through bronchogenic spread; leprosy, from nasopharyngeal or oropharyngeal spread; syphilis, in secondary and tertiary stages; rhinoscleroma, extending from the nose and nasopharynx; actinomycosis; histoplasmosis; blastomycosis; paracoccidioidomycosis; coccidiosis; candidiasis; aspergillosis; sporotrichosis; rhinosporidiosis; and parasitic infections, including leishmaniasis.
- Nonspecific inflammation can occur as a result of exposure to irritants such as tobacco smoke and chemicals, from vocal abuse, and from gastroesophageal reflux.

DIAGNOSIS

DIFFERENTIAL DIAGNOSIS
Young children with signs of airway obstruction:
- Supraglottitis (epiglottitis)
- Laryngotracheobronchitis
- Bacterial tracheitis
- Foreign body aspiration

Adults:
- Hoarseness from streptococcal pharyngitis
- With persistent hoarseness, laryngeal tumors

WORKUP
- History and clinical examination: diagnosis usually apparent
- Laryngeal examination to show physical findings listed above
- Presence of an exudate on mucosa suspicious for diphtheria, streptococcal infection, mononucleosis, candidiasis

LABORATORY TESTS
If etiology other than acute viral infection suspected: laryngeal cultures and biopsies

IMAGING STUDIES
- Not indicated unless evidence of airway compromise
- Plain radiographs of neck, anteroposterior and lateral to differentiate laryngitis from acute laryngotracheobronchitis or supraglottis

TREATMENT

NONPHARMACOLOGIC THERAPY
- Resting the voice
- Inhaling humidified air

ACUTE GENERAL Rx
- Antibiotics and other antimicrobials: indicated only when a specific pathogen is isolated
- Appropriate therapy for gastroesophageal reflux if seen with laryngitis

DISPOSITION
Uncomplicated laryngitis is usually benign, with gradual resolution of symptoms.

REFERRAL
If symptoms persist for >2 wk, to an otorhinolaryngologist for laryngoscopy

MISCELLANEOUS

REFERENCES
Fried MP, Shapiro J: Acute and chronic laryngeal infections. In Paparella MM et al (eds): *Otolaryngology*, ed 3, Philadelphia, 1991, WB Saunders.

Hol C et al: *Moraxella catarrhalis* in acute laryngitis: infection or colonization? *J Infect Dis* 174:636, 1996.

Kamel PL, Hanson D, Kahrilas PJ: Omeprazole for the treatment of posterior laryngitis, *Am J Med* 96:321, 1994.

Kaufman JA: Infectious and inflammatory diseases of the larynx. In Ballenger JJ, Snow JB (eds): *Otorhinolaryngology: head and neck surgery*, ed 15, Media, Pa, 1996, Williams & Wilkins.

Author: **Jane V. Eason, M.D.**

Lead poisoning (PTG)

BASIC INFORMATION

DEFINITION
Lead poisoning refers to multisystem abnormalities resulting from excessive lead exposure.

SYNONYMS
Plumbism

ICD-9-CM CODES
984.0 Lead poisoning

EPIDEMIOLOGY AND DEMOGRAPHICS
- Lead poisoning is most common in children ages 1 to 5 yr (17,000 cases/100,000 persons).
- In 1991 the Center for Disease Control and Prevention lowered the definition of a safe blood lead level to <10 μg/dl of whole blood (a blood lead level of 25 μg/dl was considered acceptable before 1991).
- It is estimated that >15% of preschoolers in the U.S. have a blood lead level >15 μg/dl.

PHYSICAL FINDINGS
- Findings vary with the degree of toxicity. Examination may be normal in patients with mild toxicity.
- Abdominal cramping, constipation, weight loss, tremor, paresthesias and peripheral neuritis, seizures, and coma may occur with severe toxicity.
- Motor neuropathy is common in children with lead poisoning; learning disorders are also frequent.

ETIOLOGY
Chronic repeated exposure to paint containing lead, plumbing, storage of batteries, pottery, lead soldering

DIAGNOSIS

DIFFERENTIAL DIAGNOSIS
- Polyneuropathies from other sources
- Anxiety disorder, attention deficit disorder
- Malabsorption, acute abdomen
- Iron deficiency anemia

WORKUP
Laboratory screening: all U.S. children should be considered to be at risk for lead poisoning and should be screened routinely starting at 1 yr of age for low-risk children and 6 mo of age for high-risk ones.

LABORATORY TESTS
- Venous blood lead level: normal level: <10 μg/dl; levels of 50 to 70 μg/dl: indicative of moderate toxicity, levels >70 μg/dl: associated with severe poisoning
- Mild anemia with basophilic stippling on peripheral smear
- Elevated protoporphyrin levels

IMAGING STUDIES
- Imaging studies are generally not necessary.
- A plain abdominal film can visualize lead particles in the gut.
- "Lead lines" may be noted on x-rays of long bones.

TREATMENT

NONPHARMACOLOGIC THERAPY
Provide adequate amounts of calcium, iron, zinc, and protein in patient's diet.

ACUTE GENERAL Rx
Chelation therapy:
- Succimer (DMSA) 10 mg/kg PO q8h for 5 days then q12h for 2 wk can be used in patient's with levels between 50 and 70 μg/dl.
- Edetate calcium disodium (EDTA) and dimercaprol (BAL) are effective in patients with severe toxicity.
- D-penicillamine (Cuprimine) can also be used for lead poisoning, but it is not FDA approved for this condition.

CHRONIC Rx
- Reduce exposure, remove any potential lead sources.
- Correct iron deficiency and any other nutritional deficiencies.
- Recheck blood lead level 7 to 21 days after chelation therapy.

DISPOSITION
Patients with mild to moderate toxicity generally improve without any residual deficits. The presence of encephalopathy at diagnosis is a poor prognostic sign. Residual neurologic deficits may persist in these patients.

REFERRAL
If exposure to lead is work-related, it should be reported to the Office of the United States Occupational Safety and Health Administration (OSHA).

MISCELLANEOUS

COMMENTS
- Provide patient education regarding ways to prevent or decrease the risk of exposure.
- Screening of household members of affected individuals is recommended.
- Patient education information on lead poisoning can be obtained from Environmental Protection Agency: *Lead in your drinking water*, OPA-87-006, 1988.
- U.S. Preventive Services Task Force Recommendations regarding screening for elevated lead levels in childhood and pregnancy are described in Section V, Chapter 23.

REFERENCES
American Academy of Pediatrics: *Lead poisoning: from screening to primary prevention*, RE 9307, 1993, Committee on Environmental Health, American Academy of Pediatrics.

Landrigan PJ, Todd AC: Lead poisoning, *West J Med* 161:153, 1994.

Author: **Fred F. Ferri, M.D.**

Legg-Calvé-Perthes disease (PTG)

BASIC INFORMATION

DEFINITION
Legg-Calvé-Perthes disease is a self-limited disorder of unknown etiology caused by ischemia of the immature femoral head that leads to bone necrosis and variable amounts of collapse during the reparative process.

SYNONYMS
Coxa plana
Capital femoral osteochondrosis

ICD-9-CM CODES
732.1 Perthes' disease

EPIDEMIOLOGY AND DEMOGRAPHICS
PREVALENCE: 1 case/1300 children
PREDOMINANT SEX: Male:female ratio of 4:1
PREDOMINANT AGE: 3 to 10 yr

PHYSICAL FINDINGS
- Initial complaint: usually a mildly painful limp
- Pain referred down the inner aspect of the thigh to the knee
- Moderate restriction of motion resulting from hip synovitis (abduction and internal rotation are especially limited)
- Pain at the extremes of movement and tenderness over anterior hip joint

ETIOLOGY
Unknown

DIAGNOSIS

DIFFERENTIAL DIAGNOSIS
- Toxic synovitis
- Low-grade septic arthritis
- JRA

WORKUP
Diagnosis is usually based on the physical findings and eventual radiographic findings.

IMAGING STUDIES
- Plain roentgenography to establish the diagnosis
- AP and frog-leg lateral radiographs
- Techmetium bone scanning to assist in making the diagnosis in early cases

TREATMENT

ACUTE GENERAL Rx
- A brief period of bed rest followed by bracing (except in mild cases)
- Bracing possibly required for 2 to 3 yr

DISPOSITION
- Prognosis depends on age of patient and degree of involvement of the femoral head at onset.
- Young patients (under 6 yr) with minimal involvement do well.
- Older patients (over 8 yr) often do poorly.
- A few patients eventually develop degenerative arthritis.

REFERRAL
For orthopedic consultation when diagnosis is suspected

MISCELLANEOUS

REFERENCES
Skaggs DL, Tolo VT: Legg-Calvé-Perthes disease, *J Am Acad Orthop Surg* 4:9, 1996.
Winger DR, Ward WT, Herring JA: Current concepts review: Legg-Calvé-Perthes disease, *J Bone Joint Surg* 73(A) 778, 1991.

Author: **Lonnie R. Mercier, M.D.**

Leptospirosis

BASIC INFORMATION

DEFINITION
Leptospirosis is a zoonosis caused by the spirochete *Leptospira interrogans*.

SYNONYMS
Weil's disease

ICD-9-CM CODES
100.9 Leptospirosis

EPIDEMIOLOGY AND DEMOGRAPHICS
INCIDENCE (IN U.S.):
- 0.05 cases/100,000 persons
- Significant underestimation because of underreporting

PREDOMINANT SEX: Male (4:1)
PREDOMINANT AGE: Teenagers and young adults
PEAK INCIDENCE: Summer months, into the fall
GENETICS:
Neonatal Infection: Can occur

PHYSICAL FINDINGS
ANICTERIC FORM:
- Milder and more common presentation of disease
- A self-limited systemic illness with two stages:
  1. Septicemic stage: presents abruptly with fevers, headache, severe myalgias, rigors, prostration, and sometimes circulatory collapse; conjunctival suffusion is common; skin rash, pharyngitis, lymphadenopathy, hepatomegaly, splenomegaly, or muscle tenderness are possible; lasts about 1 wk with complete resolution usual.
  2. Immune stage: occurs a few days after first stage with similar symptoms; hallmark is aseptic meningitis.

ICTERIC LEPTOSPIROSIS (WEIL'S SYNDROME):
1. Denotes severe cases, with symptoms of hepatic, renal, and vascular dysfunction
2. Biphasic course: persistence of fever, jaundice, and azotemia
3. Complications: oliguria or anuria, hemorrhage, hypotension, vascular collapse

ETIOLOGY
Caused by a spirochete, *L. interrogans*
- Infects a variety of animals, including most mammals
- Specific serotypes associated with different hosts—*pomona* in livestock, *canicola* in dogs, and *icterohaemorrhagiae* in rodents
- Exposure to animal urine or infected water method by which animal penetrates skin or mucous membranes; recent description of cases in inner-city residents are related to exposure to rat urine

DIAGNOSIS

DIFFERENTIAL DIAGNOSIS
- Bacterial meningitis
- Viral hepatitis
- Influenza
- Legionnaire's disease

WORKUP
Culture of blood, CSF, and urine:
- Organism can be isolated from blood or CSF during first 10 days of illness.
- Urine should be cultured after first week and for up to 30 days after onset of illness.

LABORATORY TESTS
- Normal or elevated WBC, at times up to 70,000 mm^3
- Elevated transaminases or bilirubin
- Anemia, azotemia, hypoprothrombinemia in those with icteric illness
- Elevated CK in first phase
- Meningitis in both phases, but aseptic in second phase

IMAGING STUDIES
Chest radiographs to show bilateral nonlobar infiltrates

TREATMENT

NONPHARMACOLOGIC THERAPY
- Supportive
- Observation for dehydration, hypotension, renal failure, hemorrhage

ACUTE GENERAL Rx
- IV Penicillin G 1 million U q4h
- Doxycycline 100 mg PO bid for 7 days
- Vitamin K administration if hypoprothrombinemia present
- Possible Jarisch-Herxheimer reaction when treated with penicillin

DISPOSITION
- Anicteric leptospirosis is self-limited, but administration of antibiotics can decrease severity and duration of symptoms.
- Icteric leptospirosis, even with supportive therapy, has a mortality as high as 10%.

REFERRAL
- If more than mild disease
- If no response to treatment

MISCELLANEOUS

COMMENTS
Significantly underreported illness

REFERENCES
Farr RW: Leptospirosis, *Clin Infect Dis* 21:1, 1995.
Author: **Maurice Policar, M.D.**

Leukemia, acute lymphoblastic

BASIC INFORMATION

DEFINITION
Acute lymphoblastic leukemia (ALL) is characterized by uncontrolled proliferation of abnormal, immature lymphocytes and their progenitors, ultimately replacing normal bone marrow elements.

SYNONYMS
Lymphoid leukemia
ALL

ICD-9-CM CODES
204.0 Acute lymphoblastic leukemia

EPIDEMIOLOGY AND DEMOGRAPHICS
ALL is primarily a disease of children (peak incidence at ages 2 to 10 yr). Median age in adults is 35 to 40 yr; however, incidence increases with age.

PHYSICAL FINDINGS
- Skin pallor, purpura, or easy bruising
- Lymphadenopathy or hepatosplenomegaly
- Fever, bone pain, oliguria, weakness, weight loss, mental status changes

ETIOLOGY
- Unknown; increased risk in patients with a previous use of antineoplastic agents (e.g., chemotherapy of NHL, Hodgkin's disease, ovarian cancer, myeloma)
- Environmental factors (e.g., ionizing radiation), toxins (e.g., benzine)

DIAGNOSIS

DIFFERENTIAL DIAGNOSIS
Acute myeloid leukemia (AML): the distinction between ALL and AML and the classification of the various subtypes are based on the following factors:
- Cell morphology
  1. Lymphoblasts: a high nucleus/cytoplasmic ratio; usually, cytoplasmic granules are not present.
  2. Myeloblasts: abundant cytoplasm; often, cytoplasmic granules (Auer rods) are present.
- Histochemical stains
  1. Peroxidase and Sudan black stains: negative in ALL; useful to distinguish nonlymphoid from lymphoid cells
  2. Chloroacetate esterase: a pink cytoplasmic reaction identifies granulocytes; useful to distinguish granulocytes from monocytes in patients with AML

Lymphoblastic lymphoma
Aplastic anemia
Infectious mononucleosis
Leukemoid reaction to infection
Multiple myeloma

WORKUP
- Laboratory evaluation
- Bone marrow examination (with biopsy, cytochemistry, immunophenotyping, and cytogenetics)
- Lumbar puncture and imaging studies

LABORATORY TESTS
- CBC reveals normochromic, normocytic anemia, thrombocytopenia.
- Peripheral smear will reveal lymphoblasts.
- Initial blood work should also include BUN, creatinine, serum electrolytes, uric acid, LDH.
- Special diagnostic tests include immunophenotyping, cytogenetics, and cytochemistry.
- The French, American, British (FAB) Cooperative Study Group has classified ALL into three groups (L1-L3) based on cell size, cytoplasmic appearance, nucleus shape, and chromatin pattern; the most common form is the L2 type.
- Immunologic classification is on the basis of expression of surface antigens by blast cells: T lineage and B lineage.

IMAGING STUDIES
- Chest radiograph to evaluate for the presence of mediastinal mass
- CT scan or ultrasound of abdomen to assess splenomegaly or leukemic infiltration of abdominal organs

TREATMENT

ACUTE GENERAL Rx
- Emergency treatment is indicated in patients with intracerebral leukostasis. It consists of one or more of the following:
  1. Cranial irradiation of the whole brain in one- or two-dose fractions
  2. Leukapheresis
  3. Oral hydroxyurea (requires 48 to 72 hr to significantly lower the circulating blast count)
- Urate nephropathy can be prevented by vigorous hydration and lowering uric acid level with allopurinol and urine alkalization with acetazolamide.
- Infections must be aggressively treated with broad-spectrum antibiotics.
  1. Any febrile or neutropenic patients must have cultures taken and be properly treated with IV antibiotics.
  2. If evidence of infection persists despite adequate treatment with antibiotics, amphotericin-B may be added to provide coverage against fungal infections (Candida, Aspergillus).
- Correct significant thrombocytopenia (platelet counts <20,000 mm^3) with platelet transfusion.
- Bleeding secondary to DIC is treated with heparin and replacement of clotting factors.
- Induction therapy is intensive chemotherapy to destroy a significant number of leukemic cells and achieve remission; it usually consists of a combination of vincristine (Oncovin), prednisone, L-asparaginase (ELSPAR), and daunorubicin (Cerubidine).
- Consolidation therapy consists of an aggressive course of chemotherapy with or without radiotherapy shortly after complete remission has been obtained. Its purpose is to prolong the remission period or cure. Commonly used agents are VM-26, VP-16, HiDAC.
- Meningeal prophylactic therapy with intrathecal methotrexate with or without cranial irradiation is indicated to prevent meningeal sequestration of leukemic cells.
- The goal of maintenance therapy is to maintain a state of remission. In patients with ALL, intermittent therapy is continued for at least 3 yr with a combination of methotrexate and 6-mercaptopurine (Purinethol).
- Bone marrow transplantation: patients should receive allograft in the first complete remission if they are between ages 20 and 50 yr and have matched a sibling donor.

DISPOSITION
- Prognosis is generally poorer in adult disease compared with childhood disease.
- Five-year leukemia-free survival is <40%.
- The presence of Philadelphia chromosome (Ph$^+$), monosomy 5 and 7, and abnormalities of 11q23 are bad prognostic signs.

MISCELLANEOUS

REFERENCES
Bouchex C et al: Immunophenotype of adult lymphoblastic leukemia, clinical parameters and outcome: an analysis of a prospective trial including 562 tested patients, *Blood* 84:1603, 1994.

Hematology/Oncology Clinics of North America: *Management of acute leukemia*, April 1993.

Author: **Fred F. Ferri, M.D.**

Leukemia, acute myelogenous

BASIC INFORMATION

DEFINITION
Acute myelogenous leukemia (AML) is a disorder characterized by uncontrolled proliferation of primitive myeloid cells (blasts), ultimately replacing normal bone marrow elements.

SYNONYMS
Acute nonlymphoblastic leukemia (ANLL)
Acute nonlymphocytic leukemia
Acute myeloid leukemia
AML

ICD-9-CM CODES
205.0 Acute myelogenous leukemia

EPIDEMIOLOGY AND DEMOGRAPHICS
AML usually affects adults (most patients are 30 to 60 yr old; median age at presentation is 50 yr).

PHYSICAL FINDINGS
Patients generally come to medical attention because of the effects of the cytopenias:
- Anemia manifests with weakness or fatigue.
- Thrombocytopenia can manifest with bleeding, petechiae, and ecchymosis.
- Neutropenia can result in infections and fever.
- Physical examination may reveal skin pallor, bruises, petechiae; abdominal examination may reveal hepatosplenomegaly; peripheral lymphadenopathy may also be present.

ETIOLOGY
Risk factors are previous use of antineoplastic agents, chromosomal abnormalities, ionizing radiation, toxins, immunodeficiency states, and chronic myeloproliferative disorders.

DIAGNOSIS

DIFFERENTIAL DIAGNOSIS
- Acute lymphocytic leukemia
- Leukemoid reaction
- Myelodysplastic syndrome
- Infiltrative diseases of the bone marrow
- Epstein-Barr, other viral infection

LABORATORY TESTS
- CBC reveals anemia, thrombocytopenia.
- Peripheral WBC count varies from $<5000/mm^3$ to $>100,000/mm^3$.
- Additional laboratory findings may include elevated LDH and uric acid levels, decreased fibrinogen, and increased FDP secondary to DIC.
- Cytogenetic abnormalities are common (chromosome 8 is most frequently involved in AML).
- The distinction between ALL and AML and the classification of the various subtypes are based on the following factors:
  1. Cell morphology: myeloblasts reveal abundant cytoplasm; cytoplasmic granules are often present (Auer rods).
  2. Histochemical stains:
     a. Peroxidase and Sudan black stains are negative in ALL.
     b. Chloroacetate esterase: a pink cytoplasmic reaction identifies granulocytes; useful to distinguish granulocytes from monocytes in patients with AML.
- AML is diagnosed by the presence of at least 30% blast cells and positive peroxidase or Sudan black histochemical stain in the bone marrow aspirate.
- The French, American, British (FAB) Cooperative Study Group has classified AML into seven categories (M1-M7) based on the type and percentage of immature cells.

IMAGING STUDIES
- Chest x-ray examination is useful to evaluate for the presence of mediastinal masses.
- CT scan of the abdomen may reveal hepatosplenomegaly or leukemic involvement of other organs.

TREATMENT

ACUTE GENERAL Rx
- Emergency treatment consisting of one or more of the following is indicated in patients with intracerebral leukostasis:
  1. Cranial irradiation
  2. Leukapheresis
  3. Oral hydroxyurea
- Urate nephropathy can be prevented by vigorous hydration and lowering uric acid level with Allopurinol and urine alkalinization with acetazolamide.
- Infections must be aggressively treated with broad-spectrum antibiotics.
- Correct significant thrombocytopenia with platelet transfusions.
- Bleeding secondary to DIC is treated with heparin and replacement of clotting factors.
- Intensive induction chemotherapy to destroy a significant number of leukemic cells and achieve remission usually consists of the following: cytarabine (Cytosar) and daunorubicin. All-trans-retinoic acid is effective for the induction of remission of AML M3 subtype (acute promyelocytic leukemia).
- High-dose cytarabine (ARA-C) (HiDAC) can be used in patients with refractory or relapsed AML. It usually takes 28 to 32 days from the start of therapy to achieve remission. The duration of remission is variable; the median duration of remission in an adult with AML is 1 yr.
- Consolidation therapy consists of an aggressive course of chemotherapy with or without radiation shortly after complete remission has been obtained; its purpose is to prolong the remission period or cure. Complications of consolidation therapy are usually secondary to severe bone marrow suppression (anemia, thrombocytopenia, granulocytopenia).
- Goal of therapy is to maintain a state of remission. Therapy is continued for at least 1 yr; cytarabine and 6-thioguanine are commonly used.
- Autologous bone marrow transplantation is indicated in patients <55 yr without a sibling donor. Allogeneic bone marrow transplantation is generally available to <20% of patients; usually performed only in patients <40 yr old because of higher incidents of GVHD with advancing age.

DISPOSITION
- Remission can be achieved in nearly 80% of patients <55 yr of age. Remission rates are highest in children.
- Cure for allogeneic bone marrow transplantation approaches 60%; cure rates with autologous transplantation are slightly lower.
- Favorable cytogenics are inv (16) (p13;q22) and t(8;21), t(15;17).

MISCELLANEOUS

COMMENTS
The major complication of chemotherapy is profound marrow depression with pancytopenia lasting 3 to 4 wk. Treatment is aimed at RBC and platelet replacement and aggressive monitoring and treatment of suspected infections.

REFERENCES
Mayer RJ et al: Intensive post-remission chemotherapy in adults with acute myeloid leukemia, *New Engl J Med* 331:896, 1994.
Zittoun RA et al: Autologous or allogeneic bone marrow transplantation compared with intensive chemotherapy in acute myelogenous leukemia, *New Engl J Med* 32:217, 1995.

Author: **Fred F. Ferri, M.D.**

Leukemia, chronic lymphocytic (PTG)

BASIC INFORMATION

DEFINITION
Chronic lymphocytic leukemia (CLL) is a lymphoproliferative disorder characterized by proliferation and accumulation of mature appearing neoplastic lymphocytes.

SYNONYMS
CLL

ICD-9-CM CODES
204.1 Leukemia, chronic lymphocytic

EPIDEMIOLOGY AND DEMOGRAPHICS
- Most frequent form of leukemia in western countries (10,000 new cases/yr in U.S.)
- Generally occurs in middle-aged and elderly patients (median age of 65 yr)
- Male:female ratio of 2:1

PHYSICAL FINDINGS
- Lymphadenopathy, splenomegaly, and hepatomegaly in the majority of patients
- Variable clinical presentation according to stage of the disease
- Abnormal CBC: many patients are diagnosed on the basis of laboratory results obtained after routine physical examination
- Some patients come to medical attention because of weakness and fatigue (secondary to anemia) or lymphadenopathy.

ETIOLOGY
Unknown

DIAGNOSIS

DIFFERENTIAL DIAGNOSIS
- Hairy cell leukemia
- Adult T cell lymphoma
- Prolymphocytic leukemia
- Viral infections
- Waldenström's macroglobulinemia

WORKUP
- Laboratory evaluation
- Bone marrow aspirate
- Chromosome analysis

LABORATORY TESTS
- Proliferative lymphocytosis ($\geq$15,000/dl) of well differentiated lymphocytes is the hallmark of CLL.
- There is monotonous replacement of the bone marrow by small lymphocytes (marrow contains $\geq$30% of well differentiated lymphocytes).
- Hypogammaglobulinemia and elevated LDH may be present at the time of diagnosis.
- Anemia or thrombocytopenia, if present, indicates poor prognosis.
- Trisomy-12 is the most common chromosomal abnormality, followed by 14 q+, 13 q, and 11 q; these all indicate a poor prognosis.

STAGING:
- RAI et al divided chronic lymphocytic leukemia into five clinical stages:
  Stage 0 Characterized by lymphocytosis only ($\geq$15,000/mm^3 on peripheral smear, bone marrow aspirate $\geq$40% lymphocytes). The coexistence of lymphocytosis and other factors increases the clinical stage.
  Stage 1 Lymphadenopathy
  Stage 2 Lymphadenopathy/hepatomegaly
  Stage 3 Anemia (Hgb <11 g/mm^3)
  Stage 4 Thrombocytopenia (platelets <100,000/mm^3)
- Another well-known staging system developed by Binet divides chronic lymphocytic leukemia into three stages:
  Stage A Hgb $\geq$10 g/dl, platelets $\geq$100,000/mm^3, and fewer than three areas involved (the cervical, axillary, and inguinal lymph nodes [whether unilaterally or bilaterally]; the spleen; and the liver)
  Stage B Hgb $\geq$10 g/dl, platelets $\geq$100,000/mm^3, and three or more areas involved
  Stage C Hgb <10 g/dl, low platelets (<100,000/mm^3), or both (independently of the areas involved)

IMAGING STUDIES
CT scan of abdomen to evaluate for hepatomegaly and splenomegaly

TREATMENT

NONPHARMACOLOGIC THERAPY
- Treatment goals are relief of symptoms and prolongation of life.
- Observation is appropriate for patients in RAI Stage 0 or Binet Stage A.

ACUTE GENERAL Rx
- Symptomatic patients in RAI Stage I and II or Binet Stage B: chlorambucil; local irradiation for isolated symptomatic lymphadenopathy and lymph nodes that interfere with vital organs
- RAI Stages III and IV, Binet Stage C: chlorambucil chemotherapy with or without prednisone

1. Fludarabine, CAP (cyclophosphamide, adriamycin, prednisone), or CVP (cyclophosphamide, vincristine, prednisone) can be used in patients who respond poorly to chlorambucil.
2. Splenic irradiation can be used in selected for patients with advanced disease.

CHRONIC Rx
Treatment of systemic complications:
- Hypogammaglobulinemia is frequent in CLL and is the chief cause of infections. Immune globulin (250 mg/kg IV every 4 wk) may prevent infections, but has no effect on survival. Infections should be treated with broad-spectrum antibiotics. Patients should be monitored for opportunistic infections.
- Recombinant hematopoietic cofactors (e.g., granulocyte-macrophage colony-stimulating factor and granulocyte colony stimulating factor) may be useful to overcome neutropenia related treatment.
- Erythropoietin may be useful to treat anemia that is unresponsive to other measures.

DISPOSITION
The patient's prognosis is directly related to the clinical stage (e.g., the average survival in patients in RAI Stage 0 or Binet Stage A is >120 mo whereas for RAI Stage 4 or Binet Stage C, it is approximately 30 mo). Overall 5-yr survival is 60%.

MISCELLANEOUS

COMMENTS
Long-term follow-up and frequency of follow-up is generally determined by the pace of the disease.

REFERENCES
Binet JL: Treatment of chronic lymphocytic leukemia, *Clin Hematol* 6:867, 1993.

French Cooperative Group on CL: Multicentre prospective randomized trial of fludarabine versus cyclophosphamide, doxorubicin, and prednisone (CAP) for treatment of advanced stage CLL, *Lancet* 347:1432, 1996.

Rozman C, Montserat E: Chronic lymphocytic leukemia, *New Engl J Med* 333:1052, 1995.

Author: **Fred F. Ferri, M.D.**

BASIC INFORMATION

DEFINITION
Chronic myelogenous leukemia (CML) is a myeloproliferative disorder characterized by abnormal proliferation and accumulation of immature granulocytes. CML is characterized by a chronic phase lasting months to years, followed by an accelerated myeloproliferative phase manifested by poor response to therapy, worsening anemia, or decreased platelet count; the second phase then evolves into a terminal phase (acute transformation), characterized by elevated number of blast cells and numerous complications (e.g., sepsis, bleeding).

SYNONYMS
CML
Chronic granulocytic leukemia

ICD-9-CM CODES
201.1 Chronic myelogenous leukemia

EPIDEMIOLOGY AND DEMOGRAPHICS
CML usually affects middle-aged patients (median age at presentation is 41 yr).

PHYSICAL FINDINGS
- The chronic phase usually reveals splenomegaly; hepatomegaly is not infrequent, but lymphadenopathy is very unusual and generally indicates the accelerated proliferative phase of the disease.
- Common complaints at the time of diagnosis are weakness or discomfort secondary to an enlarged spleen (abdominal discomfort or pain).

ETIOLOGY
Current evidence strongly implicates the chromosome translocation t (9;22) (q34;q11.2) as the cause of chronic granulocytic leukemia.

DIAGNOSIS

DIFFERENTIAL DIAGNOSIS
- Splenic lymphoma
- CLL
- Myelodysplastic syndrome

LABORATORY TESTS
- Elevated WBC count (generally >100,000/mm^3) with broad spectrum of granulocytic forms.
- Bone marrow demonstrates hypercellularity with granulocytic hyperplasia.
- Philadelphia chromosome (which results from the reciprocal translocation between the long arms of chromosomes 9 and 22) is present in >95% of patients with CML; its presence (Ph$^+$) is a major prognostic factor because survival rate of patients with Philadelphia chromosome is approximately eight times better than that of those without it. Some believe that Ph$^+$ defines CML and that those who are Ph$^-$ have another disease.
- Leukocyte alkaline phosphatase (LAP) markedly decreased (used to distinguish CML from other myeloproliferative disorders).
- Anemia and thrombocytosis are often present.
- Additional laboratory results are elevated vitamin B$_{12}$ levels (caused by increased transcobalamin 1 from granulocytes) and elevated blood histamine levels (because of increased basophils).

IMAGING STUDIES
Chest x-ray examination and CT scan of abdomen

TREATMENT

ACUTE GENERAL Rx
The therapeutic approach varies with the clinical phase and the degree of hyperleukocytosis.
- Symptomatic hyperleukocytosis (e.g., CNS symptoms) is treated with leukapheresis and hydroxyurea; allopurinol should be started to prevent urate nephropathy following the rapid lysis of the leukemia cells.
- Cytotoxic chemotherapy with hydroxyurea decreases WBC count and spleen size.
- Persistence of significant thrombocytosis may require treatment with thiotepa or melphalan.
- Long-term treatment of chromosome-positive CML with interferon alfa 2A can induce more karyotypic responses, delay disease progression longer, and prolong survival in patients with Philadelphia chromosome.
- The combination of interferon and cytarabine as compared with interferon alone increases the rate of major cytogenic response and prolongs survival in patients in the chronic phase of CML.
- Allogeneic marrow transplantation (following intense chemotherapy and radiotherapy to destroy residual leukemic cells) is the only curative treatment for CML.
  1. It should be considered in young patients (increased survival in patients <40 yr) with compatible siblings.
  2. Early transplantation is also important for patient's survival.
- Combination chemotherapy with daunorubicin, vincristine, and prednisone can be used for blast crisis.

DISPOSITION
- Survival rate of patients with Philadelphia chromosome is approximately eight times greater than that of those without it.
- Average survival is 3 to 6 yr in the chronic phase.

MISCELLANEOUS

REFERENCES
Italian Cooperative Study Group on CML: Interferon alpha-2A as compared with conventional chemotherapy for the treatment of CML, *New Engl J Med* 330:820, 1994.

Tefferi A et al: Chronic granulocytic leukemia: recent information on pathogenesis, diagnosis, and disease monitoring, *Mayo Clin Proc* 72:445, 1997.

Author: **Fred F. Ferri, M.D.**

Leukemia, hairy cell (PTG)

BASIC INFORMATION

DEFINITION
Hairy cell leukemia is a lymphoid neoplasm characterized by the proliferation of mature B cells with prominent cytoplasmic projections (hairs).

SYNONYMS
Leukemic reticuloendotheliosis

ICD-9-CM CODES
202.4 Hairy cell leukemia

EPIDEMIOLOGY AND DEMOGRAPHICS
PREVALENCE: Occurs predominantly in men between 40 and 60 yr of age
PREDOMINANT SEX: Male:female ratio of 4:1

PHYSICAL FINDINGS
- Usually, splenomegaly (present in >90% of cases) secondary to tumor cell infiltration
- Pallor, ecchymosis, and evidence of infection if the pancytopenia is severe
- Weakness, lethargy, and fatigue
- Infections (resulting from impaired resistance secondary to neutropenia) and easy bruising (secondary to thrombocytopenia) also common

ETIOLOGY
Neoplastic disease of the lymphoreticular system of unknown etiology

DIAGNOSIS

DIFFERENTIAL DIAGNOSIS
- Other forms of leukemia
- Lymphoma
- Viral syndrome

WORKUP
Comprehensive history, physical examination, and laboratory evaluation to confirm the diagnosis

LABORATORY TESTS
- Pancytopenia involving erythrocytes, neutrophils, and platelets is common; anemia is usually present and varies from minimal to severe.
- Hairy cells can account for 5% to 80% of cells in the peripheral blood. The cytoplasmic projections on the cells are redundant plasma membranes.
- Leukemic cells stain positively for tartrate-resistant acid phosphatase (TRAP) stain.
- Bone marrow may result in a "dry tap" (because of increased marrow reticulin).

TREATMENT

NONPHARMACOLOGIC THERAPY
Approximately 8% to 10% of patients are asymptomatic and have minimal splenomegaly and minor cytopenia. They are usually detected on routine laboratory evaluation and do not require initial therapy. They should, however, be frequently monitored for progression of their disease.

ACUTE GENERAL Rx
- Interferon alfa, 2-deoxycoformycin (DCF), and 2-chloro-2 deoxyadenosine (2CAA) are effective treatments.
- 2-Chloro-2 deoxyadenosine (CdA) 0.14 mg/kg qd for 7 days is emerging as the treatment of choice because of its minimal toxicity and its ability to induce complete durable responses with a single course of therapy.
- Splenectomy as the primary treatment has been largely superseded by systemic therapy.

CHRONIC Rx
Patients should be monitored with periodic examination and laboratory tests for progression of their disease.

DISPOSITION
Prognosis has become increasingly favorable with the newer agents. Approximately 90% of patients who are treated have a complete or partial response.

REFERRAL
Hematology consultation is recommended in all patients.

MISCELLANEOUS

COMMENTS
The diagnosis of hairy cell leukemia is occasionally missed and subsequently made by the histopathologist following removal of the spleen for diagnostic purposes.

REFERENCES
Saven A, Piro L: Newer purine analogues for the treatment of hairy cell leukemia, *N Engl J Med* 330:691, 1994.
Author: **Fred F. Ferri, M.D.**

Listeriosis

BASIC INFORMATION

DEFINITION
Listeriosis is a systemic infection caused by the gram-positive aerobic bacterium *Listeria monocytogenes*.

ICD-9-CM CODES
027.0 Listeriosis
771.2 Congenital listeriosis
771.2 Fetal listeriosis
665.4 Suspected fetal damage affecting management of pregnancy

EPIDEMIOLOGY AND DEMOGRAPHICS
INCIDENCE (IN U.S.):
- Listeria meningitis: about 0.7 cases/100,000 persons (fourth most common cause of community-acquired bacterial meningitis in adults)
- Perinatal listeriosis: 8.6 cases/ 100,000 persons
- Nonperinatal listeriosis: 3 cases/ 1,000,000 persons

PREDOMINANT SEX: Pregnant women are more susceptible to *Listeria* bacteremia, accounting for up to one third of reported cases.

PREDOMINANT AGE:
- Pregnant women
- Immunocompromised patients of any age

GENETICS
Congenital Infection:
- With transplacental transmission, syndrome termed *granulomatosis infantisepticum* in neonate
- Characterized by disseminated abscesses in multiple organs, skin lesions, conjunctivitis
- Mortality: 33% to 100%

Neonatal Infection:
- Infant becoming ill after 3 days of age; mother invariably asymptomatic
- Clinical picture of sepsis of unknown origin

PHYSICAL FINDINGS
- Infections in pregnancy
  1. More common in third trimester
  2. Usually present with fever and chills without localizing symptoms or signs of infection
- Meningoencephalitis
  1. More common in neonates and immunocompromised patients, but up to 30% of adults have no underlying condition
  2. In neonates: poor appetite with or without fever possibly only presenting signs
  3. In adults: presentation often subacute, with low-grade fever and personality change as only signs
  4. Focal neurologic signs seen without demonstrable brain abscess on CT scan
- Cerebritis/rhombencephalitis:
  1. Headache and fever may be only presenting complaints.
  2. Progressive cranial nerve palsies, hemiparesis, seizures, depressed level of consciousness, cerebellar signs, respiratory insufficiency may also be seen.
- Focal infections
  1. Ocular infections (purulent conjunctivitis) and skin lesions (granulomatosis infantisepticum) as a result of inadvertent inoculation by laboratory and veterinary personnel
  2. Others: arthritis, prosthetic joint infections, peritonitis, osteomyelitis, organ abscesses, cholecystitis

ETIOLOGY
- Direct invasion of skin and eye has been documented, but mechanism of GI entry is unclear.
- Organism's intracellular life cycle explanatory of:
  1. Importance of cell-mediated immunity in host defense
  2. Increased incidence of infection in neonates, pregnant women, and immunocompromised hosts

DIAGNOSIS

DIFFERENTIAL DIAGNOSIS
- Meningitis caused by other bacteria, mycobacteria, or fungi
- CNS sarcoidosis
- Brain neoplasm or abscess
- Tuberculous and fungal (especially cryptococcal) meningitis
- Cerebral toxoplasmosis
- Lyme disease
- Sarcoidosis

WORKUP
Dictated by age, end-organ involvement, and immune status

LABORATORY TESTS
- Cultures of blood and other appropriate body fluids
- Variable CSF findings, but neutrophils usually predominate
- Organisms uncommonly seen on Gram stain and may be difficult to identify morphologically
- Monoclonal antibodies, polymerase chain reaction, and DNA probe techniques to detect *Listeria* in foods

IMAGING STUDIES
- If focal cerebral involvement suspected: CT scan or MRI
- MRI most sensitive for evaluation of brain stem and cerebellum

TREATMENT

Empiric therapy should be administered when diagnosis is suspected because overall mortality is 23%.

ACUTE GENERAL Rx
- Drugs of choice:
  1. IV Ampicillin 8 to 12 g/day in divided doses
  2. IV Penicillin 12 to 24 million U/day in divided doses
- Continuation of therapy for 2 wk
- Alternative: trimethoprim/ sulfamethoxazole
- Gentamicin added to provide synergy

CHRONIC Rx
Relapses reported, especially in immunocompromised hosts, after 2 wk of therapy

DISPOSITION
Long-term follow-up of immunodeficiency state

REFERRAL
Infectious disease consultation for all patients

MISCELLANEOUS

COMMENTS
- Food-borne cases have been linked to various products: coleslaw, soft cheese, pasteurized milk, vegetables, undercooked chicken, hot dogs.
- Complete decontamination of food products is difficult because *Listeria* is resistant to pasteurization and refrigeration.

REFERENCES
Armstrong D: Listeria monocytogenes. In Mandell GL, Bennett JE, Dolin R (eds): *Principles and practice of infectious diseases,* ed 4, New York, 1995, Churchill Livingstone.

Listeriosis Study Group: Reduction in the incidence of human listeriosis in the United States, *JAMA* 273(14):1118, 1995.

Southwick FS, Purich DL: Intracellular pathogenesis of listeriosis, *N Engl J Med* 334(12):770, 1996.

Author: **Claudia L. Dade, M.D.**

Lumbar disc syndromes (PTG)

BASIC INFORMATION

DEFINITION
Lumbar disc syndromes are diseases resulting from disc disorder, either herniation or degenerative change (spondylosis). Massive disc protrusion may rarely lead to paralysis in the lower extremity, a condition termed *cauda equina syndrome*. Gradual narrowing of the spinal canal (lumbar stenosis), usually from spondylosis, may also cause lower extremity symptoms.

ICD-9-CM CODES
722.10 Lumbar disc displacement
724.02 Lumbar stenosis
344.60 Cauda equina syndrome
721.3 Lumbar spondylosis

EPIDEMIOLOGY AND DEMOGRAPHICS
PREVALENCE:
- Variable
- At least one episode in 80% of adults

PREVALENT AGE:
- Herniation: 20 to 40 yr
- Stenosis: >40 to 50 yr
- Disc symptoms: rare <20 yr

PREVALENT SEX: Approximately equal

PHYSICAL FINDINGS
- Overlapping clinical syndromes that may result:
  1. Mild herniation without nerve root compression
  2. Herniation with nerve root compression
  3. Cauda equina syndrome
  4. Chronic degenerative disease with or without leg symptoms
  5. Spinal stenosis
- Low back pain, often worsened by activity or coughing and sneezing
- Local lumbar or lumbosacral tenderness
- Paresthesias, usually unilateral
- Restricted low back motion
- Increased pain on bending toward affected side
- Weakness and reflex changes
- Sensory examination usually not helpful
- Lumbar stenosis that possibly produces symptoms (pseudoclaudication), which are often misinterpreted as being vascular
- Possibly positive straight leg raising test if nerve root compression is present

ETIOLOGY
Unknown

DIAGNOSIS

DIFFERENTIAL DIAGNOSIS
- Soft-tissue strain/sprain
- Tumor
- Degenerative arthritis of hip

WORKUP
In most cases, the diagnosis can be established on a clinical basis alone.

IMAGING STUDIES
- Plain roentgenograms may be indicated within the first few weeks; they are usually normal in soft disc herniation, but with chronic degenerative disc disease, loss of height of the disc space and osteophyte formation can occur.
- Myelography, CT scanning, and MRI may be indicated in patients whose symptoms do not resolve or when other spinal pathology may be suspected.
- Electrodiagnostic studies may confirm the diagnosis or rule out peripheral nerve disorders.

TREATMENT

NONPHARMACOLOGIC THERAPY
- Short course (3 to 5 days) of bed rest for severe pain; prolonged rest for acute disc herniation with leg pain
- Physical therapy for modalities plus a careful gradual exercise program
- Lumbosacral corset brace during rehabilitation process in conjunction with exercise program

PHARMACOLOGIC THERAPY
- NSAIDs
- "Muscle relaxants" for sedative effect
- Analgesics
- Epidural steroid injection for leg symptoms

DISPOSITION
- Almost all lumbar disc syndromes improve with time.
- Recurrent episodes usually respond to medical management.
- Recovery from the rare paralytic event is often incomplete.

REFERRAL
For orthopedic or neurosurgical consultation for intractable pain or significant neurologic deficit

MISCELLANEOUS

COMMENTS
A clinical algorithm for evaluation of back pain is described in Fig. 3-11.

REFERENCES
Deen HG: Diagnosis and management of lumbar disc disease, *Mayo Clin Proc* 71:283, 1996.
Jensen MC, et al: Magnetic resonance imaging of the lumbar spine in people without back pain, *N Engl J Med* 331:69, 1994.

Author: **Lonnie R. Mercier, M.D.**

Lung neoplasm, primary (PTG)

BASIC INFORMATION

DEFINITION
A primary lung neoplasm is a malignancy arising from lung tissue. The World Health Organization distinguishes twelve types of pulmonary neoplasms. Among them, the major types are *squamous cell carcinoma, adenocarcinoma, small cell carcinoma,* and *large cell carcinoma.* However, the crucial difference in the diagnosis of lung cancer is between small cell and non-small cell types since the therapeutic approach is different. Selective characteristics of lung carcinomas:

ADENOCARCINOMA: Represents 35% of lung carcinomas; frequently located mid lung and periphery; initial metastases are to lymphatics; frequently associated with peripheral scars

SQUAMOUS CELL (EPIDERMOID): 20% to 30% of lung cancers; central location; metastasis by local invasion; frequent cavitation and obstructive phenomena

SMALL CELL (OAT CELL): 20% of lung carcinomas; central location; metastasis through lymphatics; associated with lesion of the short arm of chromosome 3; high cavitation rate

LARGE CELL: 15% to 20% of lung carcinomas; frequently located in the periphery; metastasis to CNS and mediastinum; rapid growth rate with early metastasis

BRONCHOALVEOLAR: 5% of lung carcinomas; frequently located in the periphery; may be bilateral; initial metastasis through lymphatics, hematogenous and local invasion; no correlation with cigarette smoking; cavitation rare

SYNONYMS
Lung cancer

ICD-9-CM CODES
162.9 Malignant neoplasm of bronchus and lung, unspecified

EPIDEMIOLOGY AND DEMOGRAPHICS
- Lung cancer is responsible for >30% of cancer deaths in males and >25% of cancer deaths in females.
- Tobacco smoking is implicated in 85% of cases; second-hand smoke is responsible for approximately 20% of cases.
- There are >180,000 new cases of lung cancer yearly in the U.S., most occurring >age 50 yr (<4% in patients <40 yr of age).

PHYSICAL FINDINGS
- Weight loss, fatigue, fever, anorexia, dysphagia
- Cough, hemoptysis, dyspnea, wheezing
- Chest, shoulder, and bone pain
- Paraneoplastic syndromes:
  1. **Eaton-Lambert syndrome:** myopathy involving proximal muscle groups
  2. Endocrine manifestations: hypercalcemia, ectopic ACTH, SIADH
  3. Neurologic: subacute cerebellar degeneration, peripheral neuropathy, cortical degeneration
  4. Musculoskeletal: polymyositis, clubbing, hypertrophic pulmonary osteoarthropathy
  5. Hematologic or vascular: migratory thrombophlebitis, marantic thrombosis, anemia, thrombocytosis or thrombocytopenia
  6. Cutaneous: acanthosis nigricans, dermatomyositis
- Pleural effusion (10% of patients), recurrent pneumonias (secondary to obstruction), localized wheezing
- Superior vena cava syndrome:
  1. Obstruction of venous return of the superior vena cava is most commonly caused by bronchogenic carcinoma or metastasis to paratracheal nodes.
  2. The patient usually complains of headache, nausea, dizziness, visual changes, syncope, and respiratory distress.
  3. Physical examination reveals distention of thoracic and neck veins, edema of face and upper extremities, facial plethora, and cyanosis.
- **Horner's syndrome:** constricted pupil, ptosis, facial anhydrosis caused by spinal cord damage between C8 and T1 secondary to a superior sulcus tumor (bronchogenic carcinoma of the extreme lung apex); a superior sulcus tumor associated with ipsilateral Horner's syndrome and shoulder pain is known as **"Pancoast" tumor**

ETIOLOGY
- Tobacco abuse
- Environmental agents (e.g., radon) and industrial agents (e.g., ionizing radiation, asbestos, nickel, uranium, vinyl chloride, chromium, arsenic, coal dust)

DIAGNOSIS

DIFFERENTIAL DIAGNOSIS
- Pneumonia
- TB
- Metastatic carcinoma to the lung
- Lung abscess
- Granulomatous disease
- Carcinoid tumor
- Mycobacterial and fungal diseases
- Sarcoidosis
- Viral pneumonitis

The differential diagnosis of solitary pulmonary nodules is described in Section II, Table 2-52.

WORKUP
- Workup includes chest x-ray examination, CT scan of chest, tissue biopsy, or sputum cytology.
- A diagnostic approach to pulmonary nodules is described in Section III, Fig. 3-70.

LABORATORY TESTS
- Cytologic examination of at least three sputum specimens unless a positive cytology is obtained on the first or second specimen (inexpensive test; however, positive yield is low)
- Biopsy of any suspicious lymph nodes (e.g., supraclavicular node)
- Flexible fiberoptic bronchoscopy: brush and biopsy specimens are obtained from any visualized endobronchial lesions
- Transbronchial needle aspiration: done via a special needle passed through the bronchoscope; this technique is useful to sample mediastinal masses or paratracheal lymph nodes
- Transthoracic fine-needle aspiration biopsy with fluoroscopic or CT scan guidance to evaluate peripheral pulmonary nodules
- Mediastinoscopy and anteromedial sternotomy in suspected tumor involvement of the mediastinum
- Pleural biopsy in patients with pleural effusion

IMAGING STUDIES
- Chest x-ray examination:
  1. The radiographic presentation often varies with the cell type (see "Definition").
  2. Pleural effusion, lobar atelectasis, and mediastinal adenopathy can accompany any cell types.
  3. Benign lesions that simulate thoracic malignancy:
     a. Lobar atelectasis: pneumonia, TB, chronic inflammatory disease, allergic bronchopulmonary aspergillosis
     b. Multiple pulmonary nodules: septic emboli, Wegener's granulomatosis, sarcoidosis, rheumatoid nodules, fungal disease, multiple pulmonary AV fistulas
     c. Mediastinal adenopathy: sarcoidosis, lymphoma, primary TB, fungal disease, silicosis, pneumoconiosis, drug-induced (e.g., phenytoin, trimethadione)
     d. Pleural effusion: CHF, pneumonia with parapneumonic effusion, TB, viral pneumonitis, ascites, pancreatitis, collagen-vascular disease

Lung neoplasm, primary (PTG)

- Thoracentesis of pleural effusion and cytologic evaluation of the obtained fluid: may confirm diagnosis
- CT scan of chest: to evaluate mediastinal and pleural extension of suspected lung neoplasms
- Following confirmation of diagnosis, patients should undergo staging:
1. The international staging system is the most widely accepted staging system for non-small cell lung cancer. In this system, stages 1 and 2 include localized tumors for which surgical resection is the preferred treatment. Stage 3 is subdivided into 3A (potentially resectable) and 3B. Stage 4 indicates metastatic disease. The pathologic staging system uses a tumor/nodal involvement/metastasis system.
2. In patients with small cell lung cancer, a more practical accepted staging system is the one developed by the Veterans Administration Lung Cancer Study Group (VALG). This system contains two stages:
   a. Limited stage: disease confined to the regional lymph nodes and to one hemithorax (excluding pleural surfaces)
   b. Extensive stage: disease spread beyond the confines of limited stage disease
3. Pretreatment staging procedures for lung cancer patients, in addition to complete history and physical examination, generally include the following tests:
   a. Chest x-ray examination (PA and lateral), ECG
   b. Laboratory evaluation: CBC, electrolytes, platelets, calcium, phosphorus, glucose, renal and liver functions studies, ABGs, and skin tests for TB
   c. Pulmonary functions studies
   d. CT scan of chest
   e. Mediastinoscopy or anterior mediastinotomy in patients being considered for possible curative lung resection
   f. Biopsy of any accessible suspicious lesions
   g. CT scan of liver and brain; radionuclide scans of bone in all patients with small cell carcinoma of the lung and patients with non-small cell lung neoplasms suspected of involving these organs
   h. Bone marrow aspiration and biopsy only in patients with small cell carcinoma of the lung

TREATMENT

NONPHARMACOLOGIC THERAPY
- Nutritional support
- Avoidance of tobacco or other substances toxic to the lungs
- Supplemental O_2 PRN

ACUTE GENERAL Rx
NON–SMALL CELL CARCINOMA:
- Surgery
  1. Surgical resection is indicated in patients with limited disease (not involving mediastinal nodes, ribs, pleura, or distant sites). This represents approximately 15% to 30% of diagnosed cases.
  2. Preoperative evaluation includes review of cardiac status (e.g., recent MI, major arrhythmias) and evaluation of pulmonary function (to determine if the patient can tolerate any loss of lung tissue). Pneumonectomy is possible if the patient has a preoperative $FEV_1 \geq 2L$ or if the MVV is >50% of predicted capacity.
  3. Preoperative chemotherapy should be considered in patients with more advanced disease (stage 3A) who are being considered for surgery, since it increases the median survival time in patients with non–small cell lung cancer compared with the use of surgery alone.
- Treatment of unresectable non–small carcinoma of the lung:
  1. Radiotherapy can be used alone or in combination with chemotherapy; it is used primarily for treatment of CNS and skeletal metastases, superior vena cava syndrome, and obstructive atelectasis; although thoracic radiotherapy is generally considered standard therapy for stage 3 disease, it has limited effect on survival.
  2. Chemotherapy: various combination regimens are available (e.g., combinations of mitomycin, vinblastine, cisplatin, vindesine, ifosfamide, and paclitaxel; carboplatin, cyclophosphamide, and etoposide are also useful agents); however, the overall results are disappointing.
  3. The addition of chemotherapy to radiotherapy improves survival in patients with locally advanced, unresectable, non–small cell lung cancer. The absolute benefit is relatively small, however, and should be balanced against the increased toxicity associated with the addition of chemotherapy.

TREATMENT OF SMALL CELL LUNG CANCER:
- Limited stage disease: thoracic radiotherapy and chemotherapy (cisplatin and etoposide)
- Extensive stage disease: combination chemotherapy (cisplatin and etoposide or combination regimen of ifosfamide, carboplatin, and oral etoposide or monotherapy with oral etoposide in elderly patients in whom aggressive therapy is not desired)
- Prophylactic cranial irradiation for patients in complete remission to decrease the risk of CNS metastasis

DISPOSITION
- The 5-yr survival of patients with non–small cell carcinoma when the disease is resectable is approximately 30%.
- Median survival time in patients with limited stage disease and small cell lung cancer is 15 mo; in patients with extensive stage disease, it is 9 mo.

REFERRAL
Surgical referral for biopsy and resection (see "Acute General Rx")

MISCELLANEOUS

COMMENTS
Malignant pleural effusions associated with lung cancer are treated with therapeutic thoracentesis and pleurodesis.

REFERENCES
Dholakia S, Rappaport DC: The solitary pulmonary nodule: is it malignant or benign? *Postgrad Med* 99:246, 1996.

McCaughan BC: Primary lung cancer invading the chest wall, *Chest Surg Clin North Am* 4:17, 1994.

Pritchard RS, Anthony SP: Chemotherapy plus radiotherapy compared with radiotherapy alone in the treatment of locally advanced, resectable non–small cell lung carcinoma, *Ann Intern Med* 125:723, 1996.

Author: **Fred F. Ferri, M.D.**

Lyme disease (PTG)

BASIC INFORMATION

DEFINITION
Lyme disease is a multisystem disorder caused by the transmission of a spirochete, *Borrelia burgdorferi*, from a tick. This disease often develops in summer months with the following types of presentation:
Early localized: early Lyme disease, erythema chronicum migrans (ECM); skin rash, often at site of tick bite; possible fever, myalgias 3 to 32 days after tick bite
Early disseminated: days to weeks later; multi-organ system involvement, including CNS, joints, cardiac; related to dissemination of spirochete
Late persistent: months to years after tick exposure; affects central and peripheral nervous system, cardiac, joints

SYNONYMS
Bannworth's syndrome
Acrodermatitis chronica atrophicans

ICD-9-CM CODES
088.8 Lyme disease

EPIDEMIOLOGY AND DEMOGRAPHICS
INCIDENCE (IN U.S.): Geographic variation, 4.4 cases/100,000 persons; reported in 43 states and District of Columbia
PREDOMINANT SEX: Male = female
PREDOMINANT AGE: Median age of 28 yr
PEAK INCIDENCE: May to November

PHYSICAL FINDINGS
- ECM, frequently occurring at site of tick bite, can be followed by annular lesions (secondary).
- Lymphadenopathy, neck pains, pharyngeal erythema, myalgias, hepatosplenomegaly often present early in the disease.
- Patients will complain of malaise, fatigue, lethargy, headache, fever/chills, neck pain, myalgias, back pain.

ETIOLOGY
Borrelia burgdorferi from bite; transmission by the *Ixodes* tick

DIAGNOSIS

Clinical presentation, exposure to ticks in endemic area, and diagnostic testing for antibody response to *B. burgdorferi*

DIFFERENTIAL DIAGNOSIS
- Chronic fatigue/fibromyalgia
- Acute viral illnesses
- Babesiosis
- Ehrlichiosis

WORKUP
- ELISA testing—Western blot
- Immunofluorescent assay
- Early disease often difficult to diagnose serologically secondary to slow immune response
- Culturing of skin lesions (ECM) and polymerase chain reaction (PCR) of skin biopsy and blood to give definitive diagnosis (available only in reference laboratories)

IMAGING STUDIES
- Echocardiogram if conduction abnormalities are present with cardiac involvement
- CT scan, MRI of head for CNS involvement

TREATMENT

- Early Lyme disease
  1. Doxycycline 100 mg bid or amoxicillin 500 mg qid for 21 days (Doxycycline should be avoided in children/pregnant females)
  2. Alternative treatments: cefuroxime axetil 500 mg bid for 21 days, azithromycin 500 mg PO qd for 1 day followed by 250 mg qd for 6 days
- Disseminated infection: 30 days of treatment necessary
- Arthritis: 30 days of doxycycline or amoxicillin plus probenecid (repeated courses of therapy are often needed)
- Neurologic involvement
  1. Parenteral antibiotics
  2. Ceftriaxone 2 g/day for 21 to 28 days
  3. Alternative: cefotaxime 2 g q8h
  4. Alternative: penicillin G 5 million U qid
- Cardiac involvement: IV ceftriaxone or penicillin plus cardiac monitoring
- Other: vaccine therapy under clinical investigation

MISCELLANEOUS

REFERENCES
Lyme disease—United States, 1995, *MMWR* 45:481, 1996.
Sigal LH: The Lyme disease controversy, *Arch Intern Med* 156:1494, 1996.
Steere A: *Borrelia burgdorferi* (Lyme disease, Lyme Borreliosis). In Mandell GL, Bennett JE, Dolin R: *Mandell, Douglas, and Bennett's principles and practice of infectious diseases,* ed 4, New York, 1995, Churchill Livingstone.
Author: **Dennis J. Mikolich, M.D.**

Lymphangitis (PTG)

BASIC INFORMATION

DEFINITION
Lymphangitis refers to the inflammation of lymphatic vessels.

SYNONYMS
Nodular lymphangitis
Sporotrichoid lymphangitis

ICD-9-CM CODES
457.2 Lymphangitis

PHYSICAL FINDINGS
ACUTE LYMPHANGITIS:
- Commonly associated with a bacterial cellulitis
- May or may not recognize site of skin trauma (i.e., laceration, puncture, ulcer)
- In hours to days, distal appearance of erythema, edema, and tenderness, with linear erythematous streaks extending proximally to regional lymph nodes
- Possible lymphadenitis and fever
- Predisposition to group A streptococcal infection of the skin in those with chronic lymphedema and superficial fungal infections (i.e., tinea pedis)

"SPOROTRICHOID" OR "NODULAR" LYMPHANGITIS:
- Includes subcutaneous nodules that develop along the path of involved lymphatics
- Most commonly results from inoculation of the skin of the hand
- Lesions apparent from one to several weeks after inoculation
- Initially, nodular or papular lesion; may ulcerate
- May have frank pus or a serosanguinous discharge
- Systemic complaints uncommon, but infection with certain microorganisms associated with fever, chills, myalgias, and headache

ETIOLOGY
- Acute lymphangitis: usually associated with *Streptococcus pyogenes* (group A *Streptococcus*), but staphylococcal organisms also seen
- Nodular lymphangitis caused by one of several organisms
1. *Sporothrix schenckii*
   a. Most common recognized cause in U.S., usually in the Midwest
   b. Found in soil and plant debris
2. *Nocardia braziliensis:* found in soil
3. *Mycobacterium marinum:* associated with trauma related to water (i.e., aquariums, swimming pools, fish)
4. *Francisella tularensis*
   a. Most often in Midwestern states
   b. Associated with contact with infected mammals (i.e., rabbits) or tick bites

DIAGNOSIS

DIFFERENTIAL DIAGNOSIS
- Nodular lymphangitis
- Insect or snake bites
- Filariasis

WORKUP
- Acute lymphangitis: blood cultures
- Nodular lymphangitis: various stains and cultures of drainage or biopsy specimens of inoculation sites to make definitive diagnosis

LABORATORY TESTS
- WBCs possibly elevated with cellulitis
- Eosinophilia common with helminthic infections

TREATMENT

NONPHARMACOLOGIC THERAPY
Limb elevation

ACUTE GENERAL Rx
- Penicillin possibly sufficient, but 1 wk of dicloxacillin or cephalexin 500 mg PO qid commonly used to ensure antistaphylococcal coverage
- If allergic to penicillin:
  1. Clindamycin 300 mg PO qid for 7 days *or*
  2. Erythromycin 500 mg PO qid for 7 days
- Nodular lymphangitis: specific therapy directed at etiologic agent
- For superficial fungal infections: treatment may be preventive of recurrence of acute lymphangitis

DISPOSITION
- Acute lymphangitis: usually resolves with therapy
- Recurrent attacks: may lead to chronic lymphedema of limb, rarely resulting in elephantiasis nostras (nonfilarial elephantiasis)
- Nodular lymphangitis: usually responds to appropriate therapy

REFERRAL
- If acute lymphangitis is more than a mild disease or involves the face
- If nodular lymphangitis or filariasis is suspected

MISCELLANEOUS

COMMENTS
- Outside of U.S., initial episodes of filariasis caused by *Brugia malayi* resemble acute lymphangitis.
- Chronic lymphedema or elephantiasis result from recurrent episodes.

Author: **Maurice Policar, M.D.**

Lymphedema

BASIC INFORMATION

DEFINITION
Lymphedema is the result of impaired lymph drainage caused by obstruction, injury, or the abnormal development of the lymph vessels that leads to swelling of the extremities.

SYNONYMS
Elephantiasis

ICD-9-CM CODES
457.1 Lymphedema: acquired (chronic), praecox, secondary
457.1 Elephantiasis (nonfilarial)

EPIDEMIOLOGY AND DEMOGRAPHICS
PRIMARY LYMPHEDEMA:
- Found in 1.1/100,000 people <20 yr old.
- Females outnumber males 3.5:1.
- Incidence peaks between ages 12 to 16 yr old.

SECONDARY LYMPHEDEMA: See specific etiology (e.g., filariasis, breast cancer, prostate cancer, etc.)

PHYSICAL FINDINGS
Edema:
- Painless and progressive
  1. Initially, the edema is pitting and smooth; however, with advanced cases, the edema becomes nonpitting (this depends on the extent of fibrosis that has occurred).
  2. Elevation of the leg resolves the swelling in the early stages but not in the advanced stages.
- More often unilateral but depending on the etiology can be bilateral
- Not always restricted to the lower extremities but may involve the genitals, face, or upper extremities (e.g., arm swelling after mastectomy)
- Stemmer's sign (squaring of the toes caused by edema in the digits)
- "Buffalo hump" appearance of the dorsum of the foot
- Loss of the ankle contour, giving a "tree trunk" appearance of the leg

Skin:
- Hard, thick, leathery skin
- Occasional drainage of lymph
- Infections (cellulitis, lymphangitis, onychomycosis)

ETIOLOGY
Primary idiopathic lymphedema (thought to result from developmental abnormalities)
- Congenital lymphedema
  1. Detected at birth; involving one or both extremities, usually the entire leg
  2. May be familial (Milroy's disease)
- Lymphedema praecox
  1. Usually unilateral; occurring in the teenage years
  2. May be familial (Meigs' disease)
- Lymphedema tarda
  1. Usually occurs after the age of 30 yr
- Browse describes a functional classification of the primary lymphedemas:
  1. Distal obliteration (found in 80% of cases)
  2. Proximal obliteration (found in 10% of cases)
  3. Hyperplasia (found in 10% of cases)

Secondary lymphedema
- Malignancy (breast, prostate, lymphoma)
- Inflammation (streptococci, filariasis)
- Trauma
- Radiation with lymph node removal

DIAGNOSIS

DIFFERENTIAL DIAGNOSIS
Exclude other causes of edema (e.g., cirrhosis, nephrosis, CHF, myxedema, hypoalbuminemia, chronic venous stasis, reflex sympathetic dystrophy, obstruction from abdominal or pelvic malignancy).

WORKUP
A detailed history and physical examination should help exclude most of the differential diagnosis.

LABORATORY TESTS
- BUN, Cr, liver function tests, albumin, urine analysis, TFTs are obtained to exclude possible systemic causes of edema.
- Noninvasive venous studies help exclude venous insufficiency.

IMAGING STUDIES
- Lymphoscintigraphy:
  1. Diagnostic image of choice
  2. Sensitivity and specificity of 100% in diagnosing lymphedema
- CT scan: to exclude malignancy leading to obstruction
- Lymphangiography:
  1. Available but rarely used
  2. May be requested by surgeons considering repair or excision of tissue for lymphedema
  3. Difficult to perform; most information can be obtained from the nuclear lymphoscintigram

Lymphedema

TREATMENT

NONPHARMACOLOGIC THERAPY
Reduce leg swelling and size:
- Leg elevation
- Limb massage
- Pneumatic leg compression

Maintain edema-free state:
- Elastic support stockings that are properly fitted according to compression pressure and length are essential to prevent edema from returning.
- Compression pressures are graduated; most of the pressure is distal with less and less pressure from the stockings, moving proximally.
- Compression pressures range from 20 to 30 mm Hg, 30 to 40 mm Hg, 40 to 50 mm Hg, and 50 to 60 mm Hg. Most prefer 40 to 50 mm Hg for lymphedema.
- The length should cover the edematous site. Choices include below the knee, thigh-high, and pantyhose lengths.

ACUTE GENERAL Rx
- Diuretics, including furosemide 40 to 80 mg qd, may aid in reducing leg swelling but should be used only temporarily. Hydrochlorothiazide 25 mg qd can also be used for reducing edema or preventing leg swelling.
- Treat infections, such as lymphangitis (usually caused by group A *Streptococcus*), with penicillin VK 250 mg qid for 10 days or erythromycin 250 mg qid in penicillin-allergic patients. If recurrent episodes of infections occur, many consider prophylaxis with penicillin VK 250 mg qid for 10 days at the beginning of each month. Clotrimazole 1% cream should be applied qd to dried fissured areas in between toes to prevent fungal infections.
- In secondary lymphedema, treating the underlying cause is indicated (e.g., prostate cancer, breast cancer, etc.) If the etiology is filariasis caused by the parasites *Wuchereria bancrofti* or *Brugia malayi*, treatment is diethylcarbamazine citrate (DEC) 5 mg/kg in divided doses for 3 wk.

CHRONIC Rx
Surgery for chronic lymphedema is considered if:
- There is continued increase in leg size despite medical treatment.
- There is impaired leg function.
- There are recurrent infections.
- There is emotional lability secondary to the cosmetic appearance.

Surgical procedures are divided into two types:
- Those performed to improve lymph node drainage (e.g., anastomoses of the lymph system with the venous system)
- Those performed to excise the subcutaneous tissue (e.g., Charles procedure, Thompson's procedure, and the modified Homans' procedure)

DISPOSITION
Lymphedema is a slowly progressive disorder that can lead to significant disfigurement of the extremities or other body parts.

REFERRAL
Consultation with vascular surgeons should be made if medical therapy for leg size reduction fails or if recurrent infections occur.

MISCELLANEOUS

COMMENTS
- It is important to remember that surgery is not a cure.
- Children and adolescents (along with parents and adults) should be encouraged to pursue a normal life, participating in school activities and sports (preferably noncontact, e.g., swimming).
- It should also be remembered that cases of lymphangiosarcomas have been associated, although rarely, with postmastectomy lymphedema.

REFERENCES
Browse N: The diagnosis and management of primary lymphedema, *J Vasc Surg* 3:181,1986.
Rutherford RB: *Vascular surgery*, ed 4, Philadelphia, 1995, WB Saunders.

Author: **Peter Petropoulos, M.D.**

Lymphogranuloma venereum (PTG)

BASIC INFORMATION

DEFINITION
Lymphogranuloma venereum (LGV) is a sexually transmitted, systemic disease caused by *Chlamydia trachomatis*.

SYNONYMS
Tropical bubo
Poradenitis inguinalis
LGV

ICD-9-CM CODES
099.1 Lymphogranuloma venereum

EPIDEMIOLOGY AND DEMOGRAPHICS
- Male:female ratio is 5:1.
- LGV is rare in the U.S. (285 cases reported in 1993).
- LGV is endemic in Africa, India, parts of Southeast Asia, South America, and the Caribbean.

PHYSICAL FINDINGS
Primary stage:
- Primary lesion caused by multiplication of organism at site of infection
- Papule, shallow ulcer
- Herpetiform lesion at site of inoculation (most common)
- Incubation period of 3 to 21 days
- Most common site of lesion in women: posterior wall, fourchette, or vulva
- Spontaneous healing, without scarring

Second stage:
- Inguinal syndrome: characteristic inguinal adenopathy
- Begins 1 to 4 wk after primary lesion
- Syndrome is the most frequent clinical sign of the disease
- Unilateral inguinal adenopathy in 70% of cases
- Symptoms: painful, extensive adenitis (bubo) and suppuration may occur with numerous
- sinus tracts
- "Groove sign" signaling femoral and inguinal node involvement (20%); most often seen in men
- Involvement of deep iliac and retroperitoneal lymph nodes in women may present as a pelvic
- mass

Third stage (anogenital syndrome):
- Subacute: proctocolitis
- Late: tissue destruction or scarring, sinuses, abscesses, fistulas, strictures of perineum, elephantiasis

ETIOLOGY
Chlamydia trachomatis is the causative agent. There are three serotypes: L1, L2, and L3.

DIAGNOSIS

DIFFERENTIAL DIAGNOSIS
Inguinal adenitis, suppurative adenitis, retroperitoneal adenitis, proctitis, schistosomiasis

WORKUP
- Clinical manifestation
- Screening for other STDs
- A clinical algorithm for evaluation of genital ulcer disease is described in Fig. 3-33.

LABORATORY TESTS
- Positive Frei test:
  1. Intradermal Chlamydial antigen
  2. Nonspecific for all *Chlamydia*
  3. No longer available (historical significance only)
- Complement fixation test:
  1. Titer >1:64 in active infection
  2. Convalescent titers no difference
- Cell culture of *Chlamydia*—aspiration of fluctuant node yields highest rates of recovery
- CBC—mild leukocytosis with lymphocytosis or monocytosis
- Elevated sedimentation rate
- VDRL and HIV screening to rule out other STDs

IMAGING STUDIES
- Barium enema: may reveal elongated structure of LGV
- CT scan for retroperitoneal adenitis

TREATMENT

NONPHARMACOLOGIC THERAPY
- Avoid milk and milk products while taking medication.
- Practice sexual abstinence.
- Treat sexual partners.

ACUTE GENERAL Rx
- Doxycycline 100 mg PO bid × 21 days
- Erythromycin base 500 mg PO qid × 21 days
- Sulfisoxazole 500 mg PO qid × 21 days
- Surgical:
  1. Aspirate fluctuant nodes.
  2. Incise and drain abscesses.

CHRONIC Rx
- Longer course of therapy will be needed for chronic or relapsing cases, which may be caused by either reinfection and/or inadequate treatment.
- A rectal stricture will require a colostomy.
- Surgery should be considered only after antibiotic treatment.

DISPOSITION
Good prognosis with early treatment, usually resulting in complete resolution of symptoms.

REFERRAL
Surgical consultation if patient develops obstruction, fistula or rectal stricture. May need referral to plastic surgeon if patient had lymphatic obstruction.

MISCELLANEOUS

COMMENTS
- Pregnant and lactating women should be treated with erythromycin regimen.
- Congenital transmission does not occur, but infection may be acquired through an infected birth canal.
- Patient education materials may be obtained through local and state health clinics.
- U.S. Preventive Services Task Force Recommendations regarding counseling to prevent HIV transmission and other sexually transmitted diseases are described in Section V, Chapter 62.

REFERENCES
Centers for Disease Control: 1993 sexually transmitted diseases treatment guidelines, *MMWR* 42 (RR-14), 1993.
Gugino LJ: Gynecologic infections. In Danakas GT, Pietrantoni M, (eds): *Practical guide to the care of the gynecologic/obstetric patient*, St Louis, 1997, Mosby.

Author: **George T. Danakas, M.D.**

Lymphoma, non-Hodgkin's (PTG)

BASIC INFORMATION

DEFINITION
Non-Hodgkin's lymphoma is a heterogeneous group of malignancies of the lymphoreticular system.

SYNONYMS
NHL

ICD-9-CM CODES
201.9 Lymphoma, non-Hodgkin's

EPIDEMIOLOGY AND DEMOGRAPHICS
- Median age at time of diagnosis: 50 yr
- Sixth most common neoplasm in the U.S.
- Increasing incidence with age

PHYSICAL FINDINGS
- Patients often present with asymptomatic lymphadenopathy.
- Approximately one third of NHL originates extranodally. Involvement of extranodal sites can result in unusual presentations (e.g., GI tract involvement can simulate PUD).
- NHL cases associated with HIV occur predominantly in the brain.
- Pruritus, fever, night sweats, weight loss are less common than in Hodgkin's disease.
- Hepatomegaly and splenomegaly may be present.

DIAGNOSIS

DIFFERENTIAL DIAGNOSIS
- Hodgkin's disease
- Viral infections
- Metastatic carcinoma
- A clinical algorithm for evaluation of lymphadenopathy is described in Fig. 3-53 and 3-54.

LABORATORY TESTS
Initial laboratory evaluation may reveal only mild anemia and elevated LDH and ESR. Proper staging of non-Hodgkin's lymphoma requires the following:
- A thorough history, physical examination, and adequate biopsy
- Routine laboratory evaluation (CBC, ESR, urinalysis, LDH, BUN, creatinine, serum calcium, uric acid, liver function tests, serum protein electrophoresis)
- Chest x-ray examination (PA and lateral)
- Bone marrow evaluation (aspirate and full bone core biopsy)
- CT scan of abdomen and pelvis; CT scan of chest if chest x-ray films abnormal
- Bone scan (particularly in patients with histiocytic lymphoma)
- Depending on the histopathology, the results of the above studies and the planned therapy, some other tests may be performed: gallium scan (e.g., in patients with high-grade lymphomas), liver/spleen scan, lymphangiography, lumbar puncture
- β-2 microglobulin level, serum interleukin level

CLASSIFICATION: The Working Formulation of non-Hodgkin's lymphoma for clinical usage subdivides lymphomas into low grade, intermediate grade, high grade, and miscellaneous.

STAGING: The Ann Arbor classification is used to stage non-Hodgkin's lymphomas (see "Hodgkin's Disease" in Section I). Histopathology has greater therapeutic implications in NHL than in Hodgkin's disease.

IMAGING STUDIES
See "Laboratory Tests."

TREATMENT

ACUTE GENERAL Rx
The therapeutic regimen varies with the histologic type and pathologic stage. Following are the commonly used therapeutic modalities:

LOW-GRADE NHL (e.g., nodular, poorly differentiated):
1. Local radiotherapy for symptomatic obstructive adenopathy
2. Deferment of therapy and careful observation in asymptomatic patients
3. Single agent chemotherapy with cyclophosphamide or chlorambucil and glucocorticoids
4. Combination chemotherapy alone or with radiotherapy: generally indicated only when the lymphoma becomes more invasive, with poor response to less aggressive treatment; commonly used regimens: CVP, CHOP, CHOP-BLEO, COPP, BACOP; addition of recombinant alpha interferon at low doses to chemotherapy prolongs remission duration in patients with low-grade NHL
5. New purine analogs (FLAMP, 2CDA): can be used in salvage treatment of refractory lymphomas

INTERMEDIATE- AND HIGH-GRADE LYMPHOMAS (e.g., diffuse histiocytic lymphoma): Combination chemotherapy regimens (e.g., CHOP, PRO-MACE-CYTABOM, MACOP-B, M-BACOD)
1. High-dose sequential therapy is superior to standard-dose MACOP-B for patients with diffuse large-cell lymphoma of the B-cell type.
2. Dose-modified chemotherapy should be considered for most HIV-infected patients with lymphoma. As compared with treatment with standard doses of cytotoxic chemotherapy (M-BACOD), reduced doses cause significantly fewer hematologic toxic effects yet have similar efficacy in patients with HIV-related lymphoma.
- Granulocyte-colony stimulating factor (G-CSF): may be effective in reducing the risk of infection in patients with aggressive lymphoma undergoing chemotherapy
- Radioimmunotherapy with (^{131}I) anti-B1 antibody therapy for NHL either by itself or in combination with other treatments
- Treatment with high-dose chemotherapy and autologous bone marrow transplant: as compared with conventional chemotherapy, increases event-free and overall survival in patients with chemotherapy-sensitive non-Hodgkin's lymphoma in relapse

DISPOSITION
- Patients with low-grade lymphoma, despite their long-term survival (6 to 10 yr average) are rarely cured, and the great majority (if not all) eventually die of the lymphoma, whereas patients with a high-grade lymphoma may achieve a cure with aggressive chemotherapy.
- Complete remission occurs in 35% to 50% of patients with intermediate- and high-grade lymphoma. Prognostic factors include the histologic subtype, age of patient, and bulk of disease.

MISCELLANEOUS

REFERENCES
Armitage JO: Treatment of non-Hodgkin's lymphoma, *N Engl J Med* 328:1023, 1993.

Kaplan LD et al: Low-dose compared with standard-dose M-BACOD chemotherapy for non-Hodgkin's lymphoma associated with HIV infection, *N Engl J Med* 336:1641, 1997.

Philip T et al: Autologous bone marrow transplantation as compared with salvage chemotherapy in relapses of chemotherapy-sensitive non-Hodgkin's lymphoma, *N Engl J Med* 333:1540, 1995.

Author: **Fred F. Ferri, M.D.**

Macular degeneration

BASIC INFORMATION

DEFINITION
Macular degeneration refers to a group of diseases associated with loss of central vision and damage to the macula. Degenerative changes occur in the pigment, neural, and vascular layers of the macula. The dry macular degeneration is usually ischemic in etiology, and a wet macular degeneration is associated with leakage of fluid from blood vessels.

ICD-9-CM CODES
362.5 Degeneration of macula and posterior pole

EPIDEMIOLOGY AND DEMOGRAPHICS
INCIDENCE (IN U.S.):
- Main cause of blindness in the U.S.
- Increases with age

PREVALENCE (IN U.S.): Varies, but approximately 5% of people <50 yr old have some signs of macular degeneration.

PREDOMINANT SEX: Male = female
PREDOMINANT AGE: >50 yr
PEAK INCIDENCE:
- 75 to 80 yr old
- Dramatic increases in incidence and prevalence with age until approximately 80% of people 75 yr or older have senile macular degeneration.

GENETICS:
- Different syndrome: senile macular degeneration is age-related.
- Several rare neurologic syndromes are associated with macular degeneration.

PHYSICAL FINDINGS
Decreased central vision

ETIOLOGY
- Pigmentary and vascular changes with exudate, edema, and scar tissue development
- Early in course, possible subretinal neovascularization

DIAGNOSIS

DIFFERENTIAL DIAGNOSIS
- Diabetic retinopathy
- Hypertension
- Histoplasmosis
- Trauma

WORKUP
Complete eye examination, including visual field and fluorescein angiography

LABORATORY TESTS
Evaluate for diabetes and other metabolic problems, as well as vascular diseases.

IMAGING STUDIES
None necessary

TREATMENT

NONPHARMACOLOGIC THERAPY
Laser treatment to stop progression of disease

ACUTE GENERAL Rx
Laser treatment

CHRONIC Rx
Repeated laser treatments

DISPOSITION
- Follow closely.
- If vision deteriorates abruptly, refer urgently to an ophthalmologist.

REFERRAL
To ophthalmologist early in the course of the disease if the sight is to be saved

MISCELLANEOUS

COMMENTS
- The vision of only 1 out of 10 people can be saved, but the disease is so devastating that vigorous therapy should be attempted.
- U.S. Preventive Services Task Force Recommendations for screening for visual impairment are described in Section V, Chapter 33.

REFERENCES
Cheraskin E: Macular degeneration: how big is the problem? *J Natl Med Assoc* 84:873, 1992.

Author: **Melvyn Koby, M.D.**

Malaria (PTG)

BASIC INFORMATION

DEFINITION
Malaria is a febrile, flulike illness characterized by fever and chills and caused by one of the four species of the genus *Plasmodium*, which infect human RBCs and produce synchronous lysis.

ICD-9-CM CODES
084.6 Malaria

EPIDEMIOLOGY AND DEMOGRAPHICS
INCIDENCE (IN U.S.):
- Essentially none, although competent mosquito vectors are present (*Anopheles albimanus* in eastern U.S. and *A. freeborni* in western U.S.).
- Transmission is limited by absence of infected humans.
- Transmission at minimal levels, as imported cases of malaria provide the plasmodia for mosquito transmission.
  1. Following return of troops from endemic areas
  2. Following arrival of Southeast Asian refugees

PREVALENCE:
- Essentially none in U.S.
- Possible for approximately 10% of population in hyperendemic areas to be infected at single time

PREDOMINANT AGE: <5 yr old (in Africans)

GENETICS:
Familial Disposition: In sub-Saharan Africa, where *P. falciparum* kills >1,000,000 children annually, survival is enhanced by the selective advantage afforded by sickle cell gene:
- Homozygous (HbSS) sickle cell anemia is often fatal.
- Heterozygous state (HbAS):
  1. Occurs with 25% prevalence
  2. Associated with diminished severe or complicated malaria, compared with normal (HbAA) peers, despite infection (probably caused by parasite growth within distorted SS-RBCs trapped in the hypoxic microvasculature)
- Duffy factor is absent from human RBCs in most of West Africa, conferring resistance to *P. vivax*.
- Other potential protective factors:
  1. Glucose-6-phosphate deficiency
  2. Thalassemia
  3. HLA-Bw53

PHYSICAL FINDINGS
ALL SPECIES:
- Fever (generally daily until synchronization of infection after several weeks, when periodic fevers may result)
- Rigors (especially non-*falciparum* strains)
- Diaphoresis
- Fatigue and malaise
- Nausea, vomiting

P. FALCIPARUM:
- Diarrhea (often bloody)
- Headache
- Seizures
- Coma
- Pulmonary edema
- Cardiogenic shock with hypotension
- Other metabolic complications

OTHER FINDINGS:
- Mild jaundice (from hemolysis)
- Liver tenderness
- Splenomegaly (especially with chronic infection)
- Pulmonary edema
- Nephrotic syndrome
- Uremia

ETIOLOGY
Four species of *Plasmodium*:
1. *P. falciparum*
2. *P. vivax*
3. *P. malariae*
4. *P. ovale*

GEOGRAPHIC DISTRIBUTION:
1. *P. falciparum*
   - Haiti
   - Papua New Guinea
   - Sub-Saharan Africa
   - India
2. *P. vivax*
   - Central America
   - Indian subcontinent
3. *P. vivax* and *P. falciparum*
   - South America
   - Eastern Asia
   - Oceania
4. *P. malariae*
   - Rare
   - Exists in most areas (especially Central and West Africa)
5. *P. ovale*
   - Africa

All are transmitted by the bite of the female anopheline mosquito.

LIFE CYCLE:
- Sporozoites (formed in the mosquito following sexual maturation of ingested gametocytes to produce gametes, and ultimately to zygotes and sporozoites within salivary glands) are injected into humans with mosquito saliva during a bite.
- Sporozoites travel to the human liver via the bloodstream, enter hepatocytes (by binding parasite ligand and circumsporozoite protein), mature to schizonts that rupture and release merozoites into the blood stream, beginning the symptomatic, asexual erythrocytic (RBC) phase.
- Within the liver, an alternative maturation pathway allows some sporozoites of *P. vivax* and *P. ovale* to remain dormant as hypnozoites, which become active 6 to 11 mo later, generating hepatic schizonts, completing the hepatic cycle, producing relapsing malaria.
- After attaching (via the parasite ligands Pv135 or EBA175) to specific RBC surface receptors (Duffy factor or glycophorin A), merozoites enter RBCs, utilize and degrade RBC intracellular proteins (including Hgb, which is reduced to malarial pigment in the parasitic food vacuole) and mature to rings to trophozoites to schizonts (containing multiple merozoites), which rupture, lysing the RBC and releasing merozoites (some of which reenter uninfected RBCs to amplify and perpetuate the infection, while others mature into gametocytes).
- While the gametocytes of *P. vivax*, *P. malariae*, and *P. ovale* appear as similar round forms, the banana-shaped gametocyte of *P. falciparum* is distinctive and diagnostic.

PATHOGENESIS:
- Parasites that evade splenic filtration induce a variety of cellular host defenses, including macrophage activation and release of tumor necrosis factor (TNF) and interleukins (IL 1,6,8).
- Microvascular disease is produced only by *P. falciparum*, resulting from cytoadherence of parasitized RBCs, via knobs that appear on their surface membranes, to endothelial cells (utilizing TNF-alpha-induced host receptor molecules thrombospondin, CD36, ICAM-1, VCAM-1, and ELAM-1), especially in capillaries of brain, kidneys.
- The nondeformable RBCs become sequestered and produce microvascular obstruction, accounting for the severe cerebral, renal, and occasional GI complications of *P. falciparum*, as well as the absence of its mature forms (schizonts, merozoites) on peripheral blood smears, and sheltering from splenic removal.
- Glucose consumption and lactate production (enhanced by the hypoglycemia effects of quinine or quinidine therapy, TNF-alpha, and probably IL-1 and TNF-beta) all contribute to tissue acidosis.
- RBC lysis results from parasite and TNF-alpha effects, and exposes glycosylphosphatidylinositol (GPI) anchors that stimulate TNF-alpha.
- Pulmonary edema may result from TNF-alpha-induced lung damage.
- These events, unique to *P. falciparum*, are consistent with clinical complications (cerebral malaria [seizures, coma], acute renal failure, severe anemia, pulmonary edema, diarrhea, hypoglycemia, lactic acidosis, cardiogenic shock, DIC) accompanying this species.
- *P. malariae* may cause nephrotic syndrome in children.
- *P. vivax* may produce late splenic rupture.

Malaria (PTG)

DIAGNOSIS

DIFFERENTIAL DIAGNOSIS
- Typhoid fever (both produce leukopenia and splenomegaly without localizing symptoms)
- Meningitis
- Pneumonia
- Influenza
- Cerebrovascular accidents
- Dengue
- Leishmaniasis
- Hepatitis
- Gastroenteritis
- Lymphoma
- Miliary tuberculosis

WORKUP
- CBC
- Blood smears for malaria parasites
- Blood cultures to rule out other causes of febrile illness (especially typhoid fever)

LABORATORY TESTS
- Careful, competent examination of Giemsa-stained peripheral blood smears (multiple over 3 days if initial smears are negative) for malarial parasites
1. *P. falciparum*
   a. Produces monotony of ring trophozoites (fine, delicate rings with sparse cytoplasm opposite the dot [nucleus])
   b. Produces heavy (>5%) infestation with many parasitized RBCs of all ages, multiple rings/RBCs, double-chromatin dots/ring, peripheral [applique] adherence of ring to inside of RBC cell membrane
   c. Generally absent schizonts and merozoites
   d. Occasionally diagnostic banana-shaped gametocytes
2. *P. vivax*
   a. Produces rings with thicker cytoplasm opposite the dot (signet shaped)
   b. Produces lighter overall infestation
   c. Produces infection primarily of macrocytes (reticulocytes) and presence of all forms (including schizonts and merozoites)
3. *P. malariae*
   a. Produces band forms (across the equator of the RBC)
   b. Produces rosette-formed schizonts
   c. Appears as *P. vivax*
4. *P. ovale*
   a. Parasitizes senescent RBC with fringed edges
   b. Produces forms similar to *P. vivax*
- Fluorescent staining with Acridine Orange and DNA probes promise efficient and accurate future diagnostic tools.
- Leukopenia is common (its absence argues strongly against malaria as a diagnosis), as is thrombocytopenia, especially with *P. falciparum*.
- Possible associations with *P. falciparum*:
  1. Uremia (elevated creatinine)
  2. Severe anemia
  3. Proteinuria
  4. Hemoglobinuria
  5. Abnormal liver function tests
  6. Evidence of DIC (generally made worse with heparin therapy)
- Serologic testing is of limited value.

IMAGING STUDIES
- Generally not necessary
- Occasionally, brain CT scan to rule out other causes of coma or seizures

TREATMENT

NONPHARMACOLOGIC THERAPY
- DDT is no longer effective in most of the world, as a result of widespread mosquito resistance.
- Particularly in hyperendemic areas (e.g., Africa), increased efforts (especially including DEET repellents and insecticide [pyrethrin]-impregnated bed netting) are focused on diminishing anopheline mosquito exposure to gametocytes.

ACUTE GENERAL Rx
Adults
- Consult infectious disease expert.
- All strains of *P. vivax*, *P. malariae*, and *P. ovale* are sensitive to chloroquine.
- For *P. falciparum*, chloroquine resistance is the rule in most countries, with chloroquine-sensitive strains distributed only in Haiti/Dominican Republic, Central America west and north of the Panama Canal Zone, Paraguay and northern Argentina, Egypt, and the Middle East.
- *P. falciparum* strains are resistant to chloroquine plus Fansidar (sulfapyrimethamine) in Thailand, Myanmar (Burma), Cambodia, the Amazon Basin, and sub-Saharan Africa.
- Strains in Thailand are additionally resistant to mefloquine, leaving only tetracycline as an effective prophylactic agent.
- Chloroquine is effective against RBC phase organisms.
- Primaquine eliminates persistent hepatic-phase forms (only *P. vivax* and *P. ovale*) and gametocytes (which produce no symptoms and need not be treated, except for epidemiologic reasons during massive epidemics).

- Chloroquine and primaquine doses often given in two rather confusing units:
  1. Weight of the compound (chloroquine phosphate or primaquine phosphate)
  2. Lesser weight of the base alone (chloroquine or primaquine)

TREATMENT OF P. VIVAX, P. OVALE:
1. Chloroquine phosphate 1 g (600 mg base) PO at T_o, then 500 mg (300 mg base) at 6, 24, 48 hr (total dose = 2.5 g)
2. Thereafter, primaquine phosphate 26.3 mg (15 mg base) PO qd × 14 days
   a. First dose given on the same day as last dose of chloroquine
   b. May induce severe hemolysis in G_6PD-deficient individuals (test all recipients before treatment)

TREATMENT OF P. MALARIAE AND CHLOROQUINE-SENSITIVE P. FALCIPARUM:
1. Chloroquine phosphate 1 g (600 mg base) PO at T_o, then 500 mg (300 mg base) at 6, 24, 48 hr (total dose 2.5 g)
2. No primaquine needed, since no persistent liver phase exists

TREATMENT OF CHLOROQUINE-RESISTANT P. FALCIPARUM:
1. Quinine sulfate 600 mg (500 mg base) PO tid × 3 to 7 days (10 days if malaria acquired in SE Asia) plus either doxycycline 100 mg PO bid × 7 days, or clindamycin 900 mg PO tid × 5 days. Quinine:
   a. May be difficult to obtain, and tablets may weigh only 260 mg
   b. Causes tinnitus, optic atrophy, delirium, hemolysis, diarrhea
2. Alternative regimen: mefloquine 1250 mg PO in a single dose (25 mg/kg in SE Asia)
   a. Causes GI (abdominal pain, diarrhea), CNS (seizures, psychosis), and cardiac (arrhythmias; do not use if patient on β-blockers) toxicities
   b. Consultation with infectious disease expert
3. Treatment if severely ill:
   a. Quinidine gluconate IV continuous infusion
   b. Loading dose 10 mg/kg over 1 to 4 hr; then maintenance dose 0.02 mg/kg/min by infusion pump for 72 hr or until patient can swallow; then quinine PO to complete 7 day course
   c. Do not use loading dose if patient received quinine, quinidine, or mefloquine in past 24 hr
   d. Contraindication for steroids, as they prolong coma
   e. If no improvement in 24 hr, consider exchange transfusion
   f. Consultation infectious disease expert

PREVENTIVE Rx
Adults
P. FALCIPARUM FROM CHLOROQUINE-SENSITIVE AREAS: See regions above, "Acute General Rx"; *P. vivax, P. malariae, P. ovale*
- Chloroquine phosphate 500 mg (300 mg base [if >70 kg, 5 mg/kg]) PO once weekly
- Begin 1 wk before, and continue 4 wk after exposure
- In highly malarious areas, 100 mg base PO qd

P. FALCIPARUM FROM CHLOROQUINE-RESISTANT AREAS: See regions above, "Acute General Rx"
- Consult infectious disease expert
- Mefloquine 250 mg PO weekly (duration: 1 wk before to 4 wk after exposure) *or*
- Doxycycline 100 mg PO qd (sole effective regimen for Thailand) *or*
- Chloroquine phosphate 500 mg (300 mg base) PO weekly plus proguanil 200 mg PO qd (if >70 kg, 3 mg/kg/day)

DISPOSITION
Follow-up blood smears to confirm cure if resistant *P. falciparum* was possibly the etiologic agent

REFERRAL
To infectious disease expert:
- Species identification requires experience.
- Differential diagnosis is often complex.
- Therapy requires precise knowledge of changing global sensitivity patterns of *P. falciparum* and familiarity with complexities and toxicities of drug therapy.

MISCELLANEOUS

REFERENCES
CDC: *Health information for international travel, 1996-1997*, Atlanta, Ga, 1996, Centers for Disease Control and Prevention, Division of Quarantine.
Author: **Peter Nicholas, M.D.**

Mastoiditis (PTG)

BASIC INFORMATION

DEFINITION
Mastoiditis is inflammation of the mastoid process and air cells, a complication of acute otitis media.

ICD-9-CM CODES
383.00 Mastoiditis, acute or subacute
383.1 Mastoiditis, chronic

EPIDEMIOLOGY AND DEMOGRAPHICS
INCIDENCE (IN U.S.): Markedly decreased since the preantibiotic era
PREDOMINANT SEX: Appears to be more common in males
PREDOMINANT AGE: 2 mo to 18 yr
PEAK INCIDENCE: Early childhood

PHYSICAL FINDINGS
- Most common presenting symptom: pain and tenderness in the postauricular region
- Other findings:
  1. Fever
  2. Postauricular erythema and edema
  3. Protrusion of the pinna inferiorly and anteriorly
  4. Palpable fluctuant mass behind ear if there is a subperiosteal abscess
  5. Tympanic membrane possibly erythematous, perforated, or immobile; walls of the external canal possibly edematous
- Chronic mastoiditis (which follows a long course of recurrent otitis media, treated but never controlled completely):
  1. Possibly none of the above findings are present.
  2. Mastoidectomy often reveals pus and bone destruction.

ETIOLOGY
- Develops as a complication of acute otitis media
- Spread of inflammation in the middle ear to contiguous regions of pneumatization in the temporal bone, including the mastoid air cells
- Possible inflammation and destruction of the adjacent bone and development of subperiosteal abscess
- Most common bacterial isolates:
  1. *Streptococcus pneumoniae*
  2. *Haemophilus influenzae*
  3. *Moraxella catarrhalis*
  4. *Streptococcus pyogenes*
  5. *Staphylococcus aureus*
- Often, multiple organisms in chronic mastoiditis, with predominance of anaerobes and gram-negative bacteria

DIAGNOSIS

DIFFERENTIAL DIAGNOSIS
- Otitis externa
- Malignant otitis externa
- Otitis media
- Labyrinthitis
- Petrositis

WORKUP
Thorough history and physical examination are important in establishing diagnosis.

LABORATORY TESTS
- Fluid for Gram stain and culture may be obtained by myringotomy.
- If there is a perforation in the tympanic membrane with drainage, cultures of this may be taken after carefully cleaning the external canal.

IMAGING STUDIES
- Plain x-rays of the mastoid region may demonstrate clouding or opacification of the mastoid air cells.
- CT scan is the best radiologic modality for evaluating inflammation in this region.
- CT scan can demonstrate early involvement of bone (mastoiditis with bone destruction).
- MRI is more sensitive than CT scan in evaluating soft tissue involvement and is useful in conjunction with CT scan to investigate other complications of mastoiditis.

TREATMENT

NONPHARMACOLOGIC THERAPY
Myringotomy, if the ear is not already draining

ACUTE GENERAL Rx
- Initiated with IV antibiotics directed against the common organisms, with antistaphylococcal activity, or tailored to results of Gram stain and cultures
- Continued until all signs of mastoiditis have resolved
- Directed against enteric gram-negative organisms and anaerobes in chronic mastoiditis
- Indications for mastoidectomy:
  1. Failure to improve after 24 to 72 hr of therapy
  2. Persistent fever
  3. Imminent or overt signs of intracranial complications
  4. Evidence of a subperiosteal abscess in the mastoid bone

DISPOSITION
Proceed with mastoidectomy if the patient fails to respond to antimicrobial therapy.

REFERRAL
- To otolaryngologist:
  1. If diagnosis in doubt
  2. If aural complications present
  3. If surgery may be necessary
- To neurosurgeon if intracranial extension of infection suspected.
  1. Aural complications: bone destruction, subperiosteal abscess, petrositis, facial paralysis, labyrinthitis
  2. Intracranial complications: extradural abscess, lateral sinus thrombophlebitis or thrombosis, subdural abscess, meningitis, brain abscess, otitic hydrocephalus

MISCELLANEOUS

REFERENCES
Carrasco VN, Pillsbury HC, Workman JR: Mastoiditis. In Johnston JT, Yu VL (eds.): *Infectious disease and antimicrobial therapy of the ears, nose and throat*, Philadelphia, 1997, WB Saunders.

Gliklich RE et al: A contemporary analysis of acute mastoiditis, *Arch Otolaryngol Head Neck Surg* 122:135, 1996.

Author: Jane V. Eason, M.D.

Meigs' syndrome

BASIC INFORMATION

DEFINITION
Meigs' syndrome is characterized by the presence of a benign solid ovarian tumor associated with ascites and right hydrothorax that disappear after tumor removal.

ICD-9-CM CODES
620.2 Ovarian mass (unspecified)
220.0 Benign ovarian lesion
789.5 Ascites
511.9 Pleural effusion

EPIDEMIOLOGY AND DEMOGRAPHICS
- Occurs in <1% of ovarian fibromas (associated with approximately .004% of ovarian tumors)
- Most frequently encountered during middle age (average age, approximately 48 yr)

PHYSICAL FINDINGS
- Asymptomatic pelvic mass on bimanual examination
- Intermittent pelvic pain (intermittent torsion)
- Acute pelvic tenderness
- Acute abdominal tenderness
- Abdominal pelvic mass
- Abdominal bloating
- Fluid wave
- Shifting dullness
- "Puddle sign"
- Hyperresonance or flatness to chest percussion, absent tactile and vocal fremitus
- Absent or loud bronchial breath sounds, rales, mediastinal displacement, tracheal shift
- Weight loss and emaciation

ETIOLOGY
- Not specifically known
- Usually associated with "edematous" fibromas (or other benign ovarian solid tumor) in excess of 10 cm
- Plausible that large fibroma with narrow stalk has inadequate lymphatic drainage; when coupled with intermittent torsion, results in back flow transudation into the peritoneal cavity; accumulated peritoneal ascites then passes to the right pleural cavity via lymphatics (overloaded thoracic duct) or via abdominal pleural commutation (i.e., foramen of Bochdalek)

DIAGNOSIS

DIFFERENTIAL DIAGNOSIS
- Abdominal ovarian malignancy
- Various gynecologic disorders:
  1. Uterus: endometrial tumor, sarcoma, leiomyoma ("pseudo-Meigs' syndrome")
  2. Fallopian tube: hydrosalpinx, granulomatous salpingitis, fallopian tube malignancy
  3. Ovary: benign, serous, mucinous, endometrioid, clear cell, Brenner tumor, granulosa, stromal, dysgerminoma, fibroma, metastatic tumor
- Nongynecologic (GI tract or GU tract tumor or pathology) causes of pelvic mass
  1. Ascites
  2. Portal vein obstruction
  3. IVC obstruction
  4. Hypoproteinemia
  5. Thoracic duct obstruction
  6. TB
  7. Amyloidosis
  8. Pancreatitis
  9. Neoplasm
  10. Ovarian hyperstimulation
  11. Pleural effusion
  12. CHF
  13. Malignancy
  14. Collagen-vascular disease
  15. Pancreatitis
  16. Cirrhosis

WORKUP
- Clinical condition characterized by ovarian mass, ascites, and right-sided pleural effusion
- Ovarian malignancy and the other causes (see "Differential Diagnosis") of pelvic mass, ascites, and pleural effusion to be considered
- History of early satiety, weight loss with increased abdominal girth, bloating, intermittent abdominal pain, dyspnea, nonproductive cough

LABORATORY TESTS
- CBC to rule out inflammatory process
- Tumor markers (CA-125, HCG, AFP, CEA) to evaluate malignancy
- Chemical/LFT profile to evaluate metabolic or hepatic involvement

IMAGING STUDIES
- Pelvic sonography (color flow Doppler evaluation of adnexal mass) to evaluate pelvic pathology (CT scan or MRI if etiology indeterminate)
- Chest x-ray examination
- ABG if respiratory compromise

TREATMENT

NONPHARMACOLOGIC TREATMENT
- Informed consent and proper preparation of patient for possible staging laparotomy (TAHBSO, omentectomy, possible bowel resection, pelvic/periaortic lymphadenectomy)
- Bowel prep if considering pelvic malignancy

ACUTE GENERAL Rx
Depending on clinical presentation, size of pelvic mass, amount of ascites, and pleural effusion:
- If pelvic mass <10 cm, minimal ascites/pleural effusion: consider diagnostic open laparoscopy (possible exploratory laparotomy) and salpingo-oophorectomy with removal of ovarian fibroma (tumor).
- If pelvic mass >10 cm, moderate/large amount ascites/pleural effusion: consider pleurocentesis if respiratory compromise (cytology: AFB) and exploratory laparotomy with salpingo-oophorectomy and removal of ovarian fibroma (tumor).
- Treat pelvic malignancy, GI or GU tumor as indicated.

CHRONIC Rx
- Resolution of ascites and right-sided pleural effusion after removal of ovarian fibroma
- No long-term follow-up for benign ovarian fibroma

DISPOSITION
Excellent progress and complete survival is expected.

REFERRAL
To gynecologist or gynecologic oncologist for evaluation and treatment, especially if malignancy considered or encountered

MISCELLANEOUS

REFERENCES
Meigs JV: Fibroma of ovary with ascites and hydrothorax, *Am J Obstet Gynecol* 67:962, 1954.
Nicoll JJ, Cox PJ: Leiomyoma of the ovary with ascites and hydrothorax, *Am J Obstet Gynecol* 161:177, 1989.
Author: **Dennis M. Weppner, M.D.**

Melanoma (PTG)

BASIC INFORMATION

DEFINITION
Melanoma is a skin neoplasm arising from the malignant degeneration of melanocytes. It is classically subdivided in four types:
- Superficial spreading melanoma (70%)
- Nodular melanoma (15% to 20%)
- Lentigo maligna melanoma (5% to 10%)
- Acral lentiginous melanoma (7% to 10%)

SYNONYMS
Malignant melanoma

ICD-9-CM CODES
172.9 Melanoma of the skin, site unspecified

EPIDEMIOLOGY AND DEMOGRAPHICS
- Annual incidence of melanoma is 13 cases/100,000 persons.
- Lifetime risk of cutaneous melanoma for white Americans is 1/90.
- Melanoma is the leading cause of death from skin disease.
- Median age at diagnosis is 53 yr.
- Superficial spreading melanoma occurs most often in young adults on sun-exposed areas.
- Acral lentiginous melanoma is most often found in Asian and African Americans and is not related to sun exposure.
- Death rate for Caucasian men with melanoma is 3/100,000.

PHYSICAL FINDINGS
Variable depending on the subtype of melanoma (see color plate 13):
- *Superficial spreading melanoma* is most often found on the lower legs and arms. It may have a combination of many colors or may be uniformly brown or black.
- *Nodular melanoma* can be found anywhere on the body, but it most frequently occurs on the trunk on sun-exposed areas. It has a dark-brown or red-brown appearance, can be dome shaped or pedunculated; it may resemble a blood blister or hemangioma and may also be amelanotic.
- *Lentigo maligna melanoma* is generally found in older adults in areas continually exposed to the sun and frequently arising from lentigo maligna (Hutchinson's freckle) or melanoma in situ. It might have a complex pattern and variable shape; color is more uniform than in superficial spreading melanoma.
- *Acral lentiginous melanoma* frequently occurs in soles, subungual mucous membranes, and palms in Asian and African Americans (sole of the foot is the most prevalent site).
- The warning signs that the lesion may be a melanoma can be summarized with the ABCD rules:
  A: Asymmetry
  B: Border irregularity
  C: Color variegation
  D: Diameter enlargement (>6 mm)

ETIOLOGY
- UV light is the most important cause of malignant melanoma.
- There is a modest increase in melanoma risk in patients with small nondysplastic nevi and a much greater risk in those with dysplastic lesions.

DIAGNOSIS

DIFFERENTIAL DIAGNOSIS
- Dysplastic nevi
- Solar lentigo
- Vascular lesions
- Blue nevus
- Basal cell carcinoma
- Seborrheic keratosis

WORKUP
Perform excisional biopsy; incisional punch biopsy is sometimes necessary in surgically sensitive areas (e.g., digits, nose).

LABORATORY TESTS
The pathology report should indicate the following:
- Tumor thickness (Breslow microstage)
- Tumor depth (Clark level)
- Mitotic rate
- Radial growth rates vs. vertical growth rate
- Tumor infiltrating lymphocyte
- Histologic regression

TREATMENT

NONPHARMACOLOGIC THERAPY
Avoid excessive sun exposure; liberal use of sunscreens with UVB and UVA protection (recent laboratory data suggest that melanoma is promoted by UVA, therefore UVB sunscreens may not be effective in preventing melanoma).

ACUTE GENERAL Rx
- Initial excision of the melanoma
- Reexcision of the involved area after histologic diagnosis:
  1. The margins of reexcision depend on the thickness of the tumor.
  2. Low-risk or intermediate-risk tumors require excision of 1 to 3 cm.
- Lymph node dissection: recommended in all patients with enlarged lymph nodes.
  1. Elective lymph node dissection remains controversial.
  2. It may be considered in those with a primary melanoma that is between 1 and 4 mm thick (especially in patients <60 yr old).

CHRONIC Rx
Patients with a history of melanoma should be followed with skin examinations every 6 mo or sooner if patient detects any new lesions; the assessments usually consist of medical history, physical examination, chest x-ray examination, and laboratory evaluation.

DISPOSITION
- Prognosis varies with the stage of the melanoma. Five-yr survival related to thickness in mm is as follows: <0.76 mm, 99% survival; 0.6 to 1.49 mm, 85%; 1.5 to 2.49 mm, 84%; 2.5 to 3.9 mm, 70%; >4 mm, 44%.
- The 5-yr survival in patients with distant metastasis is <10%.
- Treatment of advanced disease consists (in addition to surgical excision and lymph node dissection) of chemotherapy, immunotherapy, and radiation therapy.

MISCELLANEOUS

COMMENTS
- There are several computer based programs that can determine the probability of survival based on mitotic rate, thickness, site, tumor infiltrating lymphocytes, sex, regression, and other factors.
- U.S. Preventive Services Task Force Recommendations regarding screening for skin cancer are decribed in Section V, Chapter 12.

REFERENCES
Balch CM et al: Efficacy of an elective regional lymph node dissection of 1- to 4-mm thick melanomas for patients 60 yr of age and younger, *Ann Surg* 224:255, 1996.
Habif TP: *Clinical dermatology*, ed 3, St Louis, 1996, Mosby.
Sim FH et al: Malignant melanoma: Mayo Clinic experience, *Mayo Clin Proc* 72:565, 1997.
Tucker MA et al: Clinically recognized dysplastic nevi: a central risk factor for cutaneous melanoma, *JAMA* 277:1439, 1997.

Author: **Fred F. Ferri, M.D.**

Meniere's disease (PTG)

BASIC INFORMATION

DEFINITION
Meniere's disease is a syndrome characterized by hearing loss, roaring noises in ear, and episodic dizziness associated with nausea and vomiting.

SYNONYMS
Endolymphatic hydrops
Lermoyez's syndrome
Meniere's syndrome or vertigo

ICD-9-CM CODES
386.00 Meniere's disease, syndrome, or vertigo

EPIDEMIOLOGY AND DEMOGRAPHICS
INCIDENCE (IN U.S.): 100 cases/100,000 persons
PREVALENCE (IN U.S.): 15 cases/100,000 persons
PREDOMINANT SEX: Male = female
PREDOMINANT AGE: Adults
PEAK INCIDENCE: 20 to 50 yr
GENETICS: Not known to be genetic

PHYSICAL FINDINGS
- Hearing may be unilaterally decreased.
- Pallor, sweating, and nausea may occur during a severe attack.

ETIOLOGY
- Unknown; viral and autoimmune etiologies have been suggested.
- Associated with endolymphatic hydrops.

DIAGNOSIS

DIFFERENTIAL DIAGNOSIS
- Acoustic neuroma
- Migrainous vertigo
- Multiple sclerosis
- Autoimmune inner ear syndrome
- Otitis media
- Vertebrobasilar disease
- Viral labyrinthitis

WORKUP
- Glycerol test and electrocochleography are used by some ENT specialists.
- A clinical algorithm for evaluation of hearing loss is described in Fig. 3-36.

LABORATORY TESTS
Audiometry suggests cochlear-type hearing loss and unilateral peripheral vestibular hypofunction.

IMAGING STUDIES
MRI to rule out acoustic neuroma, especially if cerebellar or CNS dysfunction is present

TREATMENT

NONPHARMACOLOGIC THERAPY
Limit activity during attacks

ACUTE GENERAL Rx
- Prochlorperazine 5 to 10 mg PO q6h or 25 mg PO bid
- Promethazine 12.5 to 25 mg PO q4-6h
- Diazepam 5 to 10 mg IV/PO for acute attack
- Meclizine 25 mg q6h

CHRONIC Rx
No proven treatment, but diuretics, salt restriction, and avoidance of caffeine are traditional.

DISPOSITION
- Usually followed by ENT specialist
- Usual course of disease consists of alternating attacks and remissions
- Majority of patients can be managed medically. Less than 10% of patients will undergo surgical intervention for persistent incapacitating vertigo.

REFERRAL
If attacks persist

MISCELLANEOUS

COMMENTS
There is no proven medical or surgical therapy.

REFERENCES
Merchant SN, Rauch SD, Nadol JB: Meniere's disease, *Eur Arch Otorhinolaryngol* 252:63, 1995.
Saeed SR, Birzgalis AR, Ramsden RT: Meniere's disease, *Br J Hosp Med* 51:603, 1994.
Shea JJ: Classification of Meniere's disease, *Am J Otol* 14:224, 1993.
Author: **William H. Olson, M.D.**

BASIC INFORMATION

DEFINITION
A meningioma is an intracranial tumor arising from arachnoid cells.

ICD-9-CM CODES
225.2 Cerebral meninges

EPIDEMIOLOGY AND DEMOGRAPHICS
INCIDENCE (IN U.S.): 2 cases/100,000 persons/yr
PREVALENCE (IN U.S.): Not reported
PREDOMINANT SEX: Female:male ratio of 3:2 in adults; female = male in childhood
PREDOMINANT AGE: Males: sixth decade, females: seventh decade
PEAK INCIDENCE: >50 yr of age; rare in childhood
GENETICS: Associated with a missing sequence on chromosome 22

PHYSICAL FINDINGS
- Varies with location and size
- May be asymptomatic
- Seizures and hemiparesis common

ETIOLOGY
- Most are associated with an abnormality on chromosome 22.
- Cranial radiation may be responsible for some cases.
- Trauma and viruses are possible precipitants.

DIAGNOSIS

DIFFERENTIAL DIAGNOSIS
Other well-circumscribed intracranial tumors

WORKUP
Imaging studies followed by surgical removal with histologic confirmation if clinically indicated

IMAGING STUDIES
CT scan with contrast or MRI with contrast

TREATMENT

NONPHARMACOLOGIC THERAPY
Surgical removal if symptomatic

ACUTE GENERAL Rx
- Generally none
- Anticonvulsants to control seizures

CHRONIC Rx
- Radiation therapy may be beneficial in patients with incomplete resections or inoperable tumors.
- Hormonal treatments are under investigation.

DISPOSITION
- Estimated surgical mortality is 7%.
- Long-term outcome is variable, based on location and completeness of resection.

REFERRAL
Neurosurgical consultation for all cases

MISCELLANEOUS

REFERENCES
Black PM: Meningiomas, *Neurosurgery* 32:643, 1993.
Author: **Michael Gruenthal, M.D., Ph.D.**

Meningitis, bacterial

BASIC INFORMATION

DEFINITION
Bacterial meningitis is an inflammation of meninges, increased intracranial pressure, and pleocytosis or increased WBCs in CSF secondary to bacteria in the pia-subarachnoid space and ventricles, leading to neurologic sequelae and abnormalities.

ICD-9-CM CODES
320 Bacterial meningitis

EPIDEMIOLOGY AND DEMOGRAPHICS
INCIDENCE (IN U.S.): 3 cases/100,000 persons
PREDOMINANT SEX: Male = female
PREDOMINANT AGE: All ages, neonate to geriatric

PHYSICAL FINDINGS
- Fever
- Headache
- Neck stiffness, nuchal rigidity, meningismus
- Altered mental state, lethargy
- Vomiting, nausea
- Photophobia
- Seizures
- Coma; lethargy, stupor
- Rash: petechial associated with meningococcal infection
- Myalgia
- Cranial nerve abnormality (unilateral)
- Papilledema
- Dilated, nonreactive pupil(s)
- Posturing: decorticate/decerebrate

ETIOLOGY
Haemophilus influenza is the cause of 45% of cases of meningitis (usually in infants and children <6 yr old). It is associated with sinusitis, otitis media.
- Neonates: group B streptococci, *Escherichia coli*, *Klebsiella* sp., *Listeria monocytogenes*
- Infants through adolescence:
  1. *H. influenza*
  2. *Streptococcus pneumonia*
  3. *Neisseria meningitidis*
- Adults
  1. *S. pneumonia*
  2. *N. meningitidis*
- Elderly
  1. *S. pneumonia*
  2. *N. meningitidis*
  3. *L. monocytogenes*
  4. Gram-negative bacilli

DIAGNOSIS

Diagnostic approach is based on patient presentation and physical examination. Key elements to diagnosis are CSF evaluation and CT scan or MRI if the patient is in a coma or has focal neurologic deficits, pupillary abnormalities, or papilledema.

DIFFERENTIAL DIAGNOSIS
- Endocarditis, bacteremia
- Intracranial tumor
- Lyme disease
- Brain abscess
- Partially treated bacterial meningitis
- Medications
- SLE
- Seizures
- Acute mononucleosis
- Other infectious meningitides
- Neuroleptic malignant syndrome
- Subdural empyema
- Rocky Mountain spotted fever
- Table 2-14 describes CSF abnormalities in various CNS conditions.

WORKUP
CSF examination:
- Opening pressure >100 to 200 mm Hg
- WBC count: <5 to >100
- Neutrophilic predominance: >80%
- Gram stain of CSF: positive in 60% to 90% patients
- CSF protein: >50 mg/dl
- CSF glucose: <40 mg/dl
- Culture: positive in 65% to 90% cases
- CSF bacterial antigen: 50% to 100% sensitivity
- E-test for susceptibility of pneumococcal isolates

LABORATORY TESTS
Blood culturing, WBC with differential, and CSF examination (see "Workup")

IMAGING STUDIES
- CT scan or MRI of head: necessary with increased intracranial pressure, coma, neurologic deficits
- Sinus CT: if sinusitis suspected

TREATMENT

- Empiric therapy may be necessary with IV antibiotic treatment if patient has purulent CSF fluid at time of lumbar puncture, is asplenic, or has signs of DIC/sepsis pending Gram stain and culture results. Therapy after Gram stain pending cultures is recommended for the following age and patient risk groups:
  Neonates: ampicillin plus cefotaxime
  Infants/children: ampicillin or third-generation cephalosporin (plus chloramphenicol if purulent or patient compromised)
  Adults (18 to 50 yr): third-generation cephalosporin
  Older adults (>50 yr): ampicillin plus third-generation cephalosporin
- Penicillin-resistant pneumococcus: because of an increasing incidence of this organism, empiric treatment with ceftriaxone or cefotaxime plus vancomycin (60 mg/kg/day) has been recommended.
- Steroids: dexamethasone 0.15 mg/kg q6h for first 4 days of therapy should be used in adults with bacterial meningitis and mental status changes or acute neurologic phenomenon. Decreased mortality and neurologic sequelae are seen with adjunct therapy.

MISCELLANEOUS

REFERENCES
Girgis NI et al: Dexamethasone treatment for bacterial meningitis in children and adults, *Pediatr Infect Dis J* 8:848, 1989.

Mandell GL, Bennett JE, Dolin R: *Mandell, Douglas, and Bennett's principles and practice of infectious diseases*, ed 4, New York, 1995, Churchill Livingstone.

Paris MM, Ramilo O, McCracken G: Management of meningitis cause by penicillin-resistant *Streptococcus pneumoniae*, *Antimicrob Agents Chemother* 39:2171, 1995.

Quagliarello VJ, Scheld WM: Treatment of bacterial meningitis, *New Engl J Med* 336:712, 1997.

Author: **Dennis J. Mikolich, M.D.**

Meningitis, viral

BASIC INFORMATION

DEFINITION
Viral meningitis is an acute aseptic meningitis usually with lymphocytic pleocytosis and negative CSF stains and cultures.

SYNONYMS
Aseptic meningitis

ICD-9-CM CODES
047.9 Meningitis, aseptic

EPIDEMIOLOGY AND DEMOGRAPHICS
INCIDENCE (IN U.S.): 11 cases/100,000 persons
PREDOMINANT SEX: Male = female
GENETICS: Those with abnormal humoral immunity and agammaglobulinemia have associated difficulty with viral clearance.

PHYSICAL FINDINGS
- Fever
- Headache
- Nuchal rigidity
- Photophobia
- Myalgias
- Vomiting
- Rash
- Diarrhea
- Pharyngitis

ETIOLOGY
- Enterovirus
- Mumps virus
- Arboviruses (enteroviruses)
- Herpes (simplex and zoster)
- HIV
- Lymphocystic choriomeningitis virus
- Adenovirus
- CMV
- Arthropod-borne viruses

DIAGNOSIS

The diagnostic approach is similar to bacterial meningitis (see "Bacterial Meningitis" in Section I); the foremost need is to rule out bacterial meningitis with CSF evaluation. Presentation may be similar to that of meningitis with bacterial involvement.

DIFFERENTIAL DIAGNOSIS
- Bacterial meningitis
- Meningitis secondary to Lyme disease, TB, syphilis, amebiasis, leptospirosis
- Rickettsial illnesses: Rocky Mountain spotted fever
- Migraine headache
- Medications
- SLE
- Acute mononucleosis/Epstein-Barr virus
- Seizures
- Carcinomatous meningitis
- Table 2-14 describes CSF abnormalities in various CSF conditions

WORKUP
CSF examination:
- Usually shows pleocytosis
- Lymphocytic predominance (polys in early stages)
- Opening pressure: 200 to 250 mm Hg
- WBC count: 100 to 1000
- Increased CSF protein
- Decreased or normal CSF glucose
- Negative Gram stain, cultures, CIE, latex agglutination
- No viral cultures routinely available; if patient is suspected of having mumps, serologic testing may be diagnostic; complement fixation used

LABORATORY TESTS
CBC with differential, blood culturing, and CSF examination (see "Workup")

IMAGING STUDIES
CT scan or MRI: if cerebral edema, focal neurologic findings develop

TREATMENT

No specific antiviral therapy for enterovirus, arbovirus, mumps virus, lymphocytic choriomeningitis virus is available.

MISCELLANEOUS

REFERENCES
Mandell GL, Bennett JE, Dolin R: *Mandell, Douglas, and Bennett's principles and practice of infectious diseases,* ed 4, New York, 1995, Churchill Livingstone.

Rice SK et al: Clinical characteristics, management strategies, and cost implications of a statewide outbreak of enterovirus meningitis, *Clin Infect Dis* 20:931, 1995.

Author: **Dennis J. Mikolich, M.D.**

Meningomyelocele

BASIC INFORMATION

DEFINITION
Meningomyelocele is a defective fusion of embryonal tissues in the dorsal region, resulting in a saclike protrusion containing meninges and spinal cord.

SYNONYMS
Meningocele (meninges only)

ICD-9-CM CODES
741.9 Spina bifida without mention of hydrocephalus
741.9 Meningomyelocele

EPIDEMIOLOGY AND DEMOGRAPHICS
INCIDENCE (IN U.S.): 2 cases/1000 births
PREVALENCE (IN U.S.): 50% death if untreated
PREDOMINANT SEX: Male = female
PREDOMINANT AGE: Infancy
PEAK INCIDENCE: Infancy
GENETICS: Autosomal recessive with possible environmental contribution

PHYSICAL FINDINGS
- Evident at birth—a sac protruding in lumbar region
- Usually, paralysis of lower extremity
- Relaxed rectal sphincter
- Constant urinary dribbling

DIAGNOSIS

DIFFERENTIAL DIAGNOSIS
Teratoma

WORKUP
Evaluate for other congenital abnormalities: heart, intestinal malformation, club foot, skeletal deformities.

LABORATORY TESTS
α-Fetoprotein in amniotic fluid or maternal serum

IMAGING STUDIES
- Lumbar x-rays (show spina bifida)
- Cervical spine films (Arnold-Chiari malformation)
- CT scan or MRI to show anatomy more precisely

TREATMENT

NONPHARMACOLOGIC THERAPY
- Surgical reduction
- Control of hydrocephalus
- Management of urinary incontinence
- Correction of deformities
- Counseling of parents

ACUTE GENERAL Rx
Correction within 24 hr of birth is recommended.

CHRONIC Rx
Follow closely for development of hydrocephalus.

DISPOSITION
Usually followed by a team of specialists

REFERRAL
To neurosurgery for evaluation

MISCELLANEOUS

COMMENTS
The decision for vigorous therapy in severely handicapped infants is beset with serious ethical considerations.

REFERENCES
Noctzel MJ: Myelomeningocele: current concepts of management, *Clin Perinatol* 16:311, 1988.
Saskett CK: Spina bifida. I. Physical effects, *Urol Nurs* 13:58, 1983.

Author: **William H. Olson, M.D.**

Menopause (PTG)

BASIC INFORMATION

DEFINITION
Menopause is the occurrence of no menstrual periods for 1 yr after age 40 yr or permanent cessation of ovulation following lost ovarian activity. It is a climacteric reproductive stage of life marked by waxing and waning estrogen levels followed by decreasing ovarian function. Premature ovarian failure and no menstrual periods may also occur because of depletion of ovarian follicles before the age of 40 yr.

SYNONYMS
Change of life
Climacteric ovarian failure

ICD-9-CM CODES
627 Premenopausal menorrhagia
627.2 Menopausal or female climacteric states
627.4 States associated with artificial menopause
716.3 Climacteric arthritis

EPIDEMIOLOGY AND DEMOGRAPHICS
- Average age of menopause in the U.S. is 51 yr.
- Age at which menopause occurs is genetically determined.
- Smokers experience menopause an average of 1.5 yr earlier than nonsmokers.
- More than one third of a woman's life will be spent after menopause.
- Onset of perimenopause is usually in a woman's mid-to-late 40s.
- Approximately 4000 women each day begin menopause.

PHYSICAL FINDINGS
- Atrophic vaginitis, which can cause burning, itching, bleeding, dyspareunia
- Either complete cessation of menses or a period of irregular cycles and diminished or heavier bleeding
- Osteoporosis
- Psychologic dysfunction:
  1. Anxiety
  2. Depression
  3. Insomnia
  4. Nervousness
  5. Irritability
  6. Inability to concentrate
- Sexual changes, decreased libido, dyspareunia
- Urinary incontinence
- Vasomotor symptoms (hot flashes, flushes), night sweats, cardiovascular disease, coronary artery disease, atherosclerosis, headaches, tiredness, and lethargy

ETIOLOGY
- The most common etiology: physiologic, caused by degenerating theca cells that fail to react to endogenous gonadotropins, producing less estrogen; decreased negative feedback in the hypothalamic pituitary access, increased follicle-stimulating hormone (FSH) and luteinizing hormone (LH), which leads to stromal cells that continue to produce androgens as a result of the LH stimulation
- Surgical castration
- Family history of early menopause, cigarette smoking, blindness, abnormal chromosomal karyotype (Turner's syndrome, gonadal dysgenesis), precocious puberty, and left handedness

DIAGNOSIS

DIFFERENTIAL DIAGNOSIS
- Asherman's syndrome
- Hypothalamic dysfunction
- Hypothyroidism
- Pituitary tumors
- Adrenal abnormalities
- Ovarian abnormalities
- Polycystic ovarian syndrome
- Pregnancy
- Ovarian neoplasm
- TB

WORKUP
- If the clinical picture is highly suggestive of menopause, estrogen can be prescribed. If all symptoms resolve, then diagnosis has essentially been made. Before prescribing estrogen, a complete history and physical examination needs to be performed. If a patient has estrogen-dependent malignancy, unexplained abnormal uterine bleeding, history of thrombophlebitis, or acute liver disease, estrogen therapy is contraindicated.
- Progesterone challenge test: progesterone 100 mg is given IM to induce withdrawal bleeding. If no withdrawal bleeding is obtained, it would be safe to assume that there is a hypoestrogenic state present.
- Physical examination, height, weight, blood pressure, breast examination, and pelvic examination are needed.
- Assess risk for coronary artery disease, osteoporosis, cigarette smoking, personal history, history of breast cancer, liver disease, active coagulation disorder, or any unexplained vaginal bleeding.

LABORATORY TESTS
- FSH, LH, and estrogen levels: if the FSH is markedly elevated and the estrogen level is markedly depressed, constitutes laboratory diagnosis of ovarian failure; LH only if polycystic ovarian disease is to be ruled out in a younger patient
- TSH to rule out thyroid dysfunction and prolactin level if patient has symptoms of galactorrhea and if suspicion of pituitary adenoma exists
- A general chemistry profile to check for any systemic diseases
- Pap smear, endometrial biopsy, or D&C in patients who have had irregular periods, intermenstrual or postmenopausal bleeding
- Mammogram

IMAGING STUDIES
- CT scan or MRI of head if pituitary tumor is suspected
- Bone density studies

TREATMENT

NONPHARMACOLOGIC THERAPY
- A balanced diet: low in fat, with total fat intake being <30% of calories; total calories sufficient to maintain body weight or to produce weight loss if that is needed
- Avoidance of smoking, excessive alcohol or caffeine intake
- Exercise: weight-bearing exercise for osteoporosis prevention
- Kegel exercises for strengthening the pelvic floor
- Adequate calcium intake: 1500 mg qd is necessary to maintain zero calcium balance in postmenopausal women

- Change in the ambient temperature (may ameliorate hot flashes and reduce night sweats)
- Vitamin E
- Avoidance of caffeine, alcohol, and spicy foods if they trigger hot flashes
- Vaginal lubricants in order to help with the dyspareunia secondary to vaginal dryness (e.g., Replens, K-Y Jelly, or Gyne-Moistrin cream)

ACUTE GENERAL Rx

Estrogen replacement, which can be done in a variety of forms, including oral estrogen and transdermal estrogen patch.

- Examples of oral estrogen would include conjugated estrogens:
  1. Premarin: start with 0.625 mg qd and increase up to 1.25 mg qd, depending on symptoms.
  2. Estradiol (Estrace): start with 1 mg qd and increase to 2 mg qd; also available in 8.5-mg tablet for patients who experience side effects from the estrogen.
  3. Esterified estrogens (Estratab): start with 0.3 to 1.25 mg qd.
  4. Estropipate (Ogen, Ortho-Est): start with 0.625 mg to 1.25 mg qd.
  5. Esterified estrogen: give 1.25 mg and methyltestosterone 2.5 mg (Estratest) and esterified estrogen 0.625 mg and methyltestosterone 1.25 mg (Estratest HS).
- If the patient has had a hysterectomy for benign disease, estrogen alone is sufficient. However, if she still has her uterus, progestin should be added for its protective effect against endometrial cancer. Medroxyprogesterone acetate (Provera) is the most commonly prescribed progestin. It can be prescribed in a continual daily dose of 2.5 mg or in 5 mg if continual breakthrough bleeding is encountered. This can also be prescribed in a 5-mg cyclic fashion for the first 14 days of the month or in 10-mg tablets for the first 10 days of the month. Patients need to be advised that this generally will cause withdrawal bleeding but in a fairly regular fashion. Continuous hormone replacement therapy is preferred, since after a period of time the patient should be amenorrheic. Patients should be counseled that they may experience some irregular spotting for the first 6 to 9 mo after starting the hormone replacement therapy.
- Transdermal patches can be either estradiol (Estraderm, Vivelle) 0.05 to 0.1 mg applied twice weekly or Climara 0.05 to 0.1 mg used once a week. With these preparations, progesterone should be used in a similar fashion.
- Vaginal creams can be used, and these should be reserved for local therapy of atrophic vaginitis only. Systemic absorption does occur; however, blood levels are unpredictable. Start with a loading dose of 2 to 4 g of estrogen-containing cream nightly for 1 to 2 wk. When symptoms improve, once to twice weekly is adequate maintenance.
- For women in whom estrogen is contraindicated or for those who do not wish to take estrogen, the following regimens can be used:
  1. Depo-Provera 150 mg IM every month (may be helpful in alleviating hot flashes)
  2. Clonidine 0.05 to 0.15 mg qd
  3. Bellergal-S
  4. Fosamax (alendronate sodium) 5 mg qd has recently been approved for prophylactic prevention of osteoporosis. Fosamax should be taken on an empty stomach; wait at least 30 min before ingesting any substance, including liquids, since this decreases its absorption into the body. Fosamax should be swallowed on arising for the day with a full glass of water, 6 to 8 oz, and patients should not lay down for at least 30 min and until after their first food of the day.

CHRONIC Rx

Hormone replacement therapy should be life-long unless the patient develops a contraindication to receiving hormone replacement therapy.

DISPOSITION

If treated, the patient should have resolution of her symptoms, reduced incidence of coronary artery disease, osteoporosis, and, most recently, reduction in the risk of developing Alzheimer's disease. Life-long medical supervision is necessary to monitor adequacy of treatment and prevention of complications. This should include annual Pap smears, pelvic examinations, breast examinations, mammography, and endometrial sampling of any type of abnormal bleeding. If untreated, the vasomotor symptoms will eventually disappear; however, this takes many years, and some women who are in their 80s have experienced hot flashes. Urogenital atrophy will continue to worsen. Osteoporosis and coronary artery disease risks will increase with every passing year.

REFERRAL

Most menopausal women are managed by their gynecologist. However, this condition can be managed adequately with the patient's primary care physician who has an interest in treating menopausal women.

MISCELLANEOUS

COMMENTS

Patient education materials can be obtained through the American College of Obstetricians and Gynecologists, 409 12th Street SW, Washington, DC, 20024, and Menopause News, 2074 Union Street, San Francisco, CA 94123; phone: 1-800-241-MENO, and multiple patient educational brochures are put out by pharmacologic companies.

REFERENCES

Soler M, Danakas G: Menopause. In Danakas G, Pietrontoni M (eds): *Practical guide to the care of the gynecologic-obstetric patient*, St Louis, 1997, Mosby.

Speroff: *Clinical gynecologic endocrinology and infertility*, ed 5, Baltimore, 1994, Williams & Wilkins.

Author: **George T. Danakas, M.D.**

BASIC INFORMATION

DEFINITION
Metatarsalgia refers to pain of the metatarsus, especially of the MTP articulation. This is a nonspecific symptom usually involving the lesser toes.

ICD-9-CM CODES
726.7 Metatarsalgia

PHYSICAL FINDINGS
- Pain beneath the metatarsal heads with ambulation
- Plantar callous formation beneath the metatarsal heads, usually involving one of the middle three toes
- Local tenderness
- Deformity
- Joint stiffness

ETIOLOGY
- Splayfoot
- Osteoarthritis, rheumatoid arthritis
- Freiberg's disease (avascular necrosis of second metatarsal head)
- Cavus foot (high arch)
- Bunion deformity
- Hallux rigidis
- MTP synovitis
- Morton's neuroma
- Often, no obvious cause

DIAGNOSIS

DIFFERENTIAL DIAGNOSIS
See "Etiology."

WORKUP
Underlying cause should always be sought.

LABORATORY TESTS
Rheumatoid factor may be required to rule out rheumatoid synovitis.

IMAGING STUDIES
Plain radiography to determine presence or absence of joint disease or deformity.

TREATMENT

NONPHARMACOLOGIC THERAPY
- Metatarsal bar or pad proximal to heads to redistribute weight
- Extra-depth shoe for contracture or deformity, if present
- Soft orthotic or well-padded liner to diffuse pressure around metatarsal heads
- Relief pads for plantar keratoses
- Soaks and pumice stone abrasion to decrease callous volume
- Rocker bottom shoe for resistant cases

CHRONIC Rx
- NSAIDs
- Intraarticular injection in selected cases with joint involvement

DISPOSITION
Prognosis is variable, depending on etiology.

REFERRAL
Failure to respond to medical management

MISCELLANEOUS

REFERENCES
Mizel MS, Yodlowski, ML: Disorders of the lesser metatarsophalangeal joints, *J Am Acad Orthop Surg* 3:166, 1995.
Author: **Lonnie R. Mercier, M.D.**

Mitral regurgitation (PTG)

BASIC INFORMATION

DEFINITION
Mitral regurgitation (MR) is retrograde blood flow through the left atrium secondary to an incompetent mitral valve. Eventually there is an increase in left atrial and pulmonary pressures with subsequent right ventricular failure.

SYNONYMS
Mitral insufficiency
MR

ICD-9-CM CODES
424.0 Mitral regurgitation

EPIDEMIOLOGY AND DEMOGRAPHICS
The incidence of MR has increased over the past 30 yr; however, this may be because of increasing availability of echocardiography rather than any real increase in this condition.

PHYSICAL FINDINGS
- Hyperdynamic apex, often with palpable left ventricular lift and apical thrill
- Holosystolic murmur at apex with radiation to base or to left axilla; poor correlation between the intensity of the systolic murmur and the degree of regurgitation
- Apical early- to mid-diastolic rumble (rare)

ETIOLOGY
- Papillary muscle dysfunction (as a result of ischemic heart disease)
- Ruptured chordae tendineae
- Infective endocarditis
- Calcified mitral valve annulus
- Left ventricular dilation
- Rheumatic valvulitis
- Primary or secondary mitral valve prolapse
- Hypertrophic cardiomyopathy
- Idiopathic myxomatous degeneration of the mitral valve
- Myxoma
- SLE

DIAGNOSIS

DIFFERENTIAL DIAGNOSIS
- Hypertrophic cardiomyopathy
- Pulmonary regurgitation
- Tricuspid regurgitation
- VSD
- Box 2-21 and Table 2-13 describe the differential diagnosis of heart murmurs.

WORKUP
- Patients with MR generally present with the following symptoms:
  1. Fatigue, dyspnea, orthopnea, frank CHF
  2. Hemoptysis (caused by pulmonary hypertension)
  3. Possible systemic emboli in patients with left atrial mural thrombi associated with atrial fibrillation
- Diagnostic workup consists of echocardiography, ECG, and chest x-ray examination.

IMAGING STUDIES
- Echocardiography: enlarged left atrium, hyperdynamic left ventricle (erratic motion of the leaflet is seen in patients with ruptured chordae tendineae); Doppler electrocardiography will show evidence of MR.
- Chest x-ray study:
  1. Left atrial enlargement (usually more pronounced in mitral stenosis)
  2. Left ventricular enlargement
  3. Possible pulmonary congestion
- ECG:
  1. Left atrial enlargement
  2. Left ventricular hypertrophy
  3. Atrial fibrillation

TREATMENT

NONPHARMACOLOGIC THERAPY
Salt restriction

ACUTE GENERAL Rx
- Medical:
  1. Digitalis (for inotropic effect and to control ventricular response if atrial fibrillation with fast ventricular response is present)
  2. Afterload reduction (to decrease the regurgitant fraction and to increase cardiac output): may be accomplished with nifedipine, hydralazine plus nitrates or ACE inhibitors
  3. Anticoagulants if atrial fibrillation occurs
  4. Antibiotic prophylaxis before dental and surgical procedures (see Boxes A-1, A-2, and A-3 and Tables A-11 and A-12 in Appendix)
- Surgery: generally not recommended unless the patient is significantly symptomatic despite optimal medical therapy; surgery should be considered early in patients with moderate to severe MR and minimal symptoms if there is echocardiographic evidence of rapidly progressive increase in left ventricular end-diastolic and end-systolic dimension (echocardiographic evidence of systolic failure includes end systolic dimension >55 mm and fractional shortening <31%)

DISPOSITION
Prognosis is generally good unless there is significant impairment of left ventricle or significantly elevated pulmonary artery pressures.

REFERRAL
Surgical referral in selected patients (see "Acute General Rx"); emergency surgery may be necessary in patients with MR caused by ruptured chordae tendineae following MI.

MISCELLANEOUS

COMMENTS
Patients should be counseled regarding weight reduction (if obese), avoidance of tobacco, and maintenance of normal (nonstrenuous) activities.

REFERENCES
Carabello BA, Crawford FA: Valvular heart disease, *N Engl J Med* 337:32, 1997.
Fenster MS, Feldman MD: Mitral regurgitation: an overview, *Current Probl Cardiol* 20:193, 1995.

Author: **Fred F. Ferri, M.D.**

Mitral stenosis (PTG)

BASIC INFORMATION

DEFINITION
Mitral stenosis is a narrowing of the mitral valve orifice. The cross section of a normal orifice measures 4 to 6 cm^2. A murmur becomes audible when the valve orifice becomes smaller than 2 cm^2. When the orifice approaches 1 cm^2, the condition becomes critical, and symptoms become more evident.

SYNONYMS
MS

ICD-9-CM CODES
394.0 Mitral stenosis

EPIDEMIOLOGY AND DEMOGRAPHICS
- The occurrence of mitral valve stenosis has decreased worldwide over the past 30 yr (particularly in developed countries) as a result of declining incidence of rheumatic fever.
- The incidence of mitral stenosis is higher in women.

PHYSICAL FINDINGS
- Prominent jugular A waves are present in patients with normal sinus rhythm.
- Opening snap occurs in early diastole; a short (<0.07 second) A$_2$ to opening snap interval indicates severe mitral stenosis.
- Apical middiastolic or presystolic rumble that does not radiate is present.
- Accentuated S$_1$ (because of delayed and forceful closure of the valve) is present.
- If pulmonary hypertension is present, there may be an accentuated P$_2$ and/or a soft, early diastolic decrescendo murmur (Graham-Steell murmur) caused by pulmonary regurgitation (it is best heard along the left sternal border and may be confused with aortic regurgitation).
- A palpable right ventricular heave may be present at the left sternal border.
- Patients with mitral stenosis usually have symptoms of left-sided heart failure: dyspnea on exertion, PND, orthopnea.
- Right ventricular dysfunction (in late stages) may be manifested by peripheral edema, enlarged and pulsatile liver, and ascites.

ETIOLOGY
- Progressive fibrosis, scarring, and calcification of the valve
- Rheumatic fever (still a common cause in underdeveloped countries); heart valves most frequently affected in rheumatic heart disease (in descending order of occurrence): mitral, aortic, tricuspid, and pulmonary
- Congenital defect (parachute valve)
- Rare causes: endomyocardial fibroelastosis, malignant carcinoid syndrome, SLE

DIAGNOSIS

DIFFERENTIAL DIAGNOSIS
- Left atrial myxoma
- Other valvular abnormalities (e.g., tricuspid stenosis, mitral regurgitation)
- Atrial septal defect
- Box 2-21 and Table 2-13 describe the differential diagnosis of heart murmurs.

WORKUP
Physical examination and echocardiography; significant clinical findings:
- Exertional dyspnea initially, followed by orthopnea and PND
- Acute pulmonary edema (may develop after exertion)
- Systemic emboli (caused by stagnation of blood in the left atrium; may occur in patients with associated atrial fibrillation)
- Hemoptysis (may be present as a result of persistent pulmonary hypertension)

IMAGING STUDIES
- Echocardiography:
  1. The characteristic finding on echocardiogram is a markedly diminished E to F slope of the anterior mitral valve leaflet during diastole; there is also fusion of the commissures, resulting in anterior movement of the posterior mitral valve leaflet during diastole (calcification in the valve may also be noted).
  2. Two-dimensional echocardiogram can accurately establish valve area.
- Chest x-ray study:
  1. Straightening of the left cardiac border caused by dilated left atrial appendage
  2. Left atrial enlargement on lateral chest x-ray film (appearing as double density of PA chest x-ray film)
  3. Prominence of pulmonary arteries
  4. Possible pulmonary congestion and edema (Kerley B-lines)
- ECG:
  1. Right ventricular hypertrophy; right axis deviation caused by pulmonary hypertension
  2. Left atrial enlargement (broad notched P waves)
  3. Atrial fibrillation
- Cardiac catheterization to help establish the severity of mitral stenosis and diagnose associated valvular and coronary lesions. Findings on cardiac catheterization include:
  1. Normal left ventricular function
  2. Elevated left atrial and pulmonary pressures

TREATMENT

NONPHARMACOLOGIC THERAPY
Decrease level of activity.

ACUTE GENERAL Rx
- Medical:
  1. If the patient is in atrial fibrillation, control the rate response with digitalis.
  2. If the patient has persistent atrial fibrillation (because of large left atrium), permanent anticoagulation is indicated to decrease the risk of serious thromboembolism.
  3. Treat CHF with diuretics and sodium restriction.
  4. Give antibiotic prophylaxis with dental and surgical procedures (see Boxes A-1, A-2, and A-3 and Tables A-11 and A-12 in Appendix).
- Surgical: valve replacement is indicated when the valve orifice is <0.7 to 0.8 cm^2 or if symptoms persist despite optimal medical therapy; commissurotomy may be possible if the mitral valve is noncalcified and if there is pure mitral stenosis without significant subvalvular disease.
- Percutaneous transvenous mitral valvotomy (PTMV) is becoming the therapy of choice for many patients with mitral stenosis responding poorly to medical therapy, particularly those who are poor surgical candidates and whose valve is not heavily calcified; balloon valvotomy gives excellent mechanical relief, usually resulting in prolonged benefit.

DISPOSITION
- Prognosis is generally good except in patients with chronic pulmonary hypertension.
- Operative mortality rates for mitral valve replacement are 1% to 5% in most institutions.

MISCELLANEOUS

REFERENCES
Carabello BA, Crawford FA: Valvular heart disease, *N Engl J Med* 337:32, 1997.

Author: **Fred F. Ferri, M.D.**

Mitral valve prolapse (PTG)

BASIC INFORMATION

DEFINITION
Mitral valve prolapse (MVP) is the posterior bulging of interior and posterior leaflets in systole.

SYNONYMS
MVP
Mitral click murmur syndrome

ICD-9-CM CODES
424.0 Mitral valve disorders
394.9 Other and unspecified mitral valve diseases

EPIDEMIOLOGY AND DEMOGRAPHICS
- MVP can be found by 2-D echocardiogram in 4% of the general population (females > males).
- Increased incidence is seen with autoimmune thyroid disorders, Ehlers-Danlos syndrome, Marfan's syndrome, pseudoxanthoma elasticum, pectus excavatum, anorexia nervosa, and bulimia.

PHYSICAL FINDINGS
- Usually, young female patient with narrow AP chest diameter, low body weight, low blood pressure
- Mid to late click, heard best at the apex
- Crescendo mid to late diastolic murmur
- Findings accentuated in the standing position

ETIOLOGY
- Myxomatous degeneration of connective tissue of mitral valve
- Congenital deformity of mitral valve and supportive structures
- Secondary to other disorders (e.g., Ehlers-Danlos, pseudoxanthoma elasticum)

DIAGNOSIS

DIFFERENTIAL DIAGNOSIS
- Other valvular abnormalities
- Constrictive pericarditis
- Ventricular aneurysm
- Box 2-21 and Table 2-13 describe the differential diagnosis of heart murmurs.

WORKUP
- Medical history and physical examination: most patients with MVP are asymptomatic; symptoms (if present) consist primarily of chest pain and palpitations.
- Neurologic abnormalities (e.g., TIA or stroke) are rare.
- Workup consists primarily of echocardiography.

IMAGING STUDIES
Echocardiography shows the anterior and posterior leaflets bulging posteriorly in systole.

TREATMENT

NONPHARMACOLOGIC THERAPY
Avoidance of stimulants (e.g., caffeine, nicotine) in patients with palpitations

ACUTE GENERAL Rx
- The empirical use of antiarrhythmic drugs to prevent sudden death in patients with uncomplicated MVP is not advisable; β-blockers may be tried in symptomatic patients (e.g., palpitations, chest pain); they decrease the heart rate, thus decreasing the stretch on the prolapsing valve leaflets.
- Antibiotic prophylaxis for infective endocarditis when undergoing dental, GI, or GU procedures is indicated only in patients with MVP who have a systolic murmur and echocardiographic evidence of mitral regurgitation (see Boxes A-1, A-2, and A-3 and Tables A-11 and A-12 in Appendix).

CHRONIC Rx
Monitoring for complications:
- Bacterial endocarditis (risk is three to eight times that of the general population)
- TIA or stroke secondary to embolic phenomena (from fibrin and platelet thrombi); risk in young patients: <0.05%/yr
- Cardiac arrhythmias (usually supraventricular)
- Sudden death (rare occurrence, most often caused by ventricular arrhythmias)
- Mitral regurgitation (most common complication of MVP)

DISPOSITION
The incidence of complications of MVP is very low (<1%/yr) and generally associated with an increase in mitral leaflet thickness to ≥5 mm; young patients (age <45) with absence of mitral systolic murmur or mitral regurgitation on Doppler echocardiography are at low risk for any complications.

REFERRAL
Surgical referral may be necessary in patients who develop symptomatic progressive mitral regurgitation.

MISCELLANEOUS

COMMENTS
Patient education material may be obtained from the American Heart Association, 7320 Green Mill Avenue, Dallas, TX 75231.

REFERENCES
Carabello BA, Crawford FA: Valvular heart disease, *N Engl J Med* 337:32, 1997.
Zuppiroli, A et al: Natural history of mitral valve prolapse, *Am J Cardiol* 75:1028, 1995.
Author: **Fred F. Ferri, M.D.**

BASIC INFORMATION

DEFINITION
The term *mixed connective tissue disease* describes a set of connective tissue symptoms that sometimes overlap with other known connective tissue diseases (SLE, progressive systemic sclerosis, polymyositis) but whose exact significance remains under debate. The disorder is sometimes referred to as an "overlap syndrome," but many prefer the term *undifferentiated connective tissue disease*.

ICD-9-CM CODES
710.9 Diffuse connective tissue disease

EPIDEMIOLOGY AND DEMOGRAPHICS
PREVALENCE: Approximately 10 to 15 cases/100,000 persons
PREDOMINANT SEX: Female:male ratio of 8:1
PREDOMINANT AGE: 4 to 80 yr

PHYSICAL FINDINGS
- Polyarthritis, polyarthralgia
- Raynaud's phenomenon, hand swelling, or sclerodactyly
- Esophageal hypomotility, myalgia, and muscle weakness
- Other: pericarditis, facial erythema, psychosis

ETIOLOGY
Autoimmune disorder

DIAGNOSIS

DIFFERENTIAL DIAGNOSIS
Other connective tissue disorders (SLE, progressive systemic sclerosis, polymyositis)

WORKUP
- Diagnosis is not well defined.
- Commonly used diagnostic tests are described below.

LABORATORY TESTS
- Rheumatoid factor is often present in low titers.
- If myositis is present, muscle enzyme (CPK) levels increase.
- Positive ANA is often present with a speckled pattern
- ESR is elevated.
- Anti-RNP antibodies may be present.

TREATMENT

- Except for pulmonary and scleroderma-like symptoms, response to corticosteroids is excellent in most cases.
- Rheumatoid symptoms may respond to NSAIDs, but other cases may not even respond to gold or penicillamine.
- Immunosuppressive agents are used on occasion, but the best therapeutic options remain uncertain.

DISPOSITION
- Initially, this disorder was thought to be a mild variant of SLE, sometimes called "benign lupus," with excellent prognosis.
- Further studies suggested, however, that this was not always the case and serious renal, vascular, and neurologic complications were noted.
- Pulmonary involvement is a common clinical manifestation which may even lead to pulmonary hypertension and sometimes death.
- Whether MCTD is a separate entity continues under debate as concepts about the disorder evolve.
- Long-term outcomes remain uncertain.

MISCELLANOUS

COMMENTS
A clinical algorithm for evaluation of a positive ANA titer is described in Fig. 3-7.

REFERENCES
Black C, Isenberg DA: Mixed connective tissue disease—goodbye to all that, *Br J Rheumatol* 31:695, 1992.
Kallenberg CG: Overlapping syndromes, undifferentiated connective tissue disease, and other fibrosing conditions, *Curr Opin Rheumatol* 5:801, 1993.
Mukerji B, Hardin JG: Undifferentiated, overlapping and mixed connective tissue diseases, *Am J Med Sciences* 305:114, 1993.
Author: **Lonnie R. Mercier, M.D.**

Mononucleosis (PTG)

BASIC INFORMATION

DEFINITION
Mononucleosis is a symptomatic infection caused by Epstein-Barr virus.

SYNONYMS
Infectious mononucleosis (IM)

ICD-9-CM CODES
075 Infectious mononucleosis

EPIDEMIOLOGY AND DEMOGRAPHICS
INCIDENCE (IN U.S.): 45 cases/100,000 persons/yr
PREDOMINANT SEX:
- Male = female
- Occurs earlier in females

PREDOMINANT AGE: Most common between the ages of 15 and 24 yr

PHYSICAL FINDINGS
- Incubation period of 1 to 2 mo
- Prodrome
  1. Fever
  2. Chills
  3. Malaise
  4. Anorexia
  5. Lasts several days
- Classic triad
  1. Pharyngitis
  2. Fever
  3. Adenopathy
- Fatigue and malaise prominent
- Pharyngitis usually most severe symptom
- Exudates common
- Lymphadenopathy
  1. Most prominent in cervical region
  2. May be diffuse
- Splenomegaly, most commonly during the second week of illness
- Rash
  1. Uncommon
  2. Occurs in nearly all patients who receive ampicillin
- Can present as fever and adenopathy without pharyngitis
- Complications
  1. May be severe
  2. Uncommon
  3. Tend to resolve completely
- Involvement of other systems
  1. Hematologic
  2. Pulmonary
  3. Cardiac
  4. Nervous
- Splenic rupture rare
- Illness usually self-limited
- Malaise and fatigue may last months before resolving

ETIOLOGY
- Primary infection with Epstein-Barr virus (EBV)
  1. During childhood
     a. Causes little or no symptoms
     b. More common in lower socioeconomic groups
  2. During late adolescence: frequency attributed to the onset of social contact between the sexes
- Transmission
  1. Close personal contact usually necessary for transmission
  2. Transfer via saliva while kissing (responsible for many cases)
  3. Occasionally transmitted by blood transfusion

DIAGNOSIS

DIFFERENTIAL DIAGNOSIS
- Heterophile-negative infectious mononucleosis caused by cytomegalovirus (CMV)
- Bacterial and viral causes of pharyngitis
- Toxoplasmosis
- Acute retroviral syndrome of HIV
- Lymphoma

WORKUP
- Heterophile antibody (Monospot)
- CBC

LABORATORY TESTS
- Commonly, increased WBCs with relative lymphocytosis and neutropenia
- Hallmark: atypical lymphocytes, but not pathognomonic
- Mild thrombocytopenia
- Falling Hct (possible signal of splenic rupture)
- Elevated hepatocellular enzymes and cryoglobulins
- Heterophile antibody:
  1. Measured by the Monospot test
  2. Positive at presentation
  3. May appear later in the course of illness
  4. Negative test repeated if clinical suspicion high
  5. If test negative for 8 wk, other causes likely
  6. Monospot usually positive for 3 to 6 mo, but can last for 1 yr
- Virus-specific antibodies in response to IM
  1. Determination of EBV-specific antibodies is rarely necessary.
  2. Early diagnosis in Monospot negative cases is made by isolating IgM to the viral capsid antigen (VCA) (usually positive during acute illness).

IMAGING STUDIES
Chest radiograph:
- Rarely shows infiltrates
- Possible elevated left hemidiaphragm in cases of splenic rupture

TREATMENT

NONPHARMACOLOGIC THERAPY
- Supportive
- Rest advocated by some, but impact on outcome not clear
- Splenectomy if rupture occurs
- Transfusions for severe anemia or thrombocytopenia

ACUTE GENERAL Rx
- Pharmacologic therapy is not indicated in uncomplicated illness.
- Steroids are suggested in patients who have the following:
  1. Severe thrombocytopenia
  2. Hemolytic anemia
  3. Impending airway obstruction caused by enlarged tonsils
- Prednisone 60 to 80 mg PO is given qd for 3 days, then tapered over 1 to 2 wk.
- There is no role for antiviral agents such as acyclovir.

DISPOSITION
Eventual resolution of all symptoms

REFERRAL
More than mild illness

MISCELLANEOUS

COMMENTS
- Contact sports should be avoided during the first month of illness, since splenic rupture can occur, even in the absence of clinically detectable splenomegaly.
- An extremely rare, chronic form of IM with persistent fevers and other objective findings has been described; this should be differentiated from chronic fatigue syndrome, which is not related to EBV.

Author: **Maurice Policar, M.D.**

CLINICAL TOPICS **Motion sickness (PTG)** 305

BASIC INFORMATION

DEFINITION
Patients with motion sickness suffer perspiration, nausea, vomiting, increased salivation, and generalized malaise in response to movement.

SYNONYMS
Physiologic vertigo

ICD-9-CM CODES
994.6 Motion sickness

EPIDEMIOLOGY AND DEMOGRAPHICS
INCIDENCE (IN U.S.): Common
PREVALENCE (IN U.S.): Common
PREDOMINANT SEX: Male = female
PREDOMINANT AGE: Any age
PEAK INCIDENCE: Any age
GENETICS: Not known to be genetic

PHYSICAL FINDINGS
- Vomiting
- Sweating
- Pallor

ETIOLOGY
- Motion (e.g., amusement rides, rides in automobiles or planes)
- Exacerbated by anxiety, fumes (e.g., industrial pollutants), visual stimuli

DIAGNOSIS

DIFFERENTIAL DIAGNOSIS
- Acute labyrinthitis
- Gastroenteritis
- Metabolic disorders
- Viral syndrome

WORKUP
None necessary in routine case

LABORATORY TESTS
None necessary

IMAGING STUDIES
None necessary

TREATMENT

NONPHARMACOLOGIC THERAPY
- Fixate on far object.
- Cease motion.
- Avoid reading.
- Avoid alcohol.

ACUTE GENERAL Rx
- Scopolamine patches (where available) are effective.
- Over-the-counter oral preparations (e.g., Dramamine) are less effective.
- Meclizine (Antivert) 12.5 to 25 mg q6h may be effective.

CHRONIC Rx
- Rarely chronic
- Symptoms generallly resolve completely with cessation of motion exposure.

DISPOSITION
Follow-up is not needed.

REFERRAL
If another diagnosis is suspected (e.g., purulent ear, fever, cranial nerve abnormalities)

MISCELLANEOUS

COMMENTS
- Many patients with migraine report having severe motion sickness as a child.
- Improved ventilation, avoidance of large meals before travel, semirecumbent sitting, and avoidance of reading while in motion will minimize the risk of motion sickness.

REFERENCES
Bronstein AM: The visual vertigo syndrome, *Acta Otolaryngol Suppl* 520:1, 1995.
Cohen NL: The dizzy patient: update on vestibular disorders, *Med Clin North Am* 75:1251, 1991.
Warner EA et al: Dizziness in the primary care patients, *J Gen Intern Med* 7:454, 1992.

Author: **William H. Olson, M.D.**

Multiple myeloma (PTG)

BASIC INFORMATION

DEFINITION
Multiple myeloma is a malignancy of plasma cells characterized by overproduction of intact monoclonal immunoglobulin or free monoclonal kappa or lambda chains.

SYNONYMS
Plasma cell myeloma

ICD-9-CM CODES
203.0 Multiple myeloma

EPIDEMIOLOGY AND DEMOGRAPHICS
ANNUAL INCIDENCE: 4 cases/100,000 persons (blacks affected twice as frequently as whites)
PREDOMINANT AGE: Peak incidence in the seventh decade at a median age of 69 yr

PHYSICAL FINDINGS
- Pallor and generalized weakness from anemia
- Purpura, epistaxis from thrombocytopenia
- Evidence of infections from impaired immune system
- Bone pain, weight loss
- Swelling on ribs, vertebrae, and other bones

ETIOLOGY
Unknown

DIAGNOSIS

The patient usually comes to medical attention because of one or more of the following:
- Bone pain (back, thorax) or pathologic fractures caused by osteolytic lesions
- Fatigue or weakness because of anemia secondary to bone marrow infiltration with plasma cells
- Recurrent infections as a result of impaired neutrophil function and deficiency of normal immunoglobulins
- Nausea and vomiting caused by constipation and uremia
- Delirium secondary to hypercalcemia
- Neurologic complications, such as spinal cord or nerve root compression, blurred vision from hyperviscosity

DIFFERENTIAL DIAGNOSIS
- Metastatic carcinoma
- Lymphoma
- Bone neoplasms (e.g., sarcoma)
- Monoclonal gammopathy of undetermined significance (MGUS)

LABORATORY TESTS
- Normochromic, normocytic anemia; Rouleaux formation on peripheral smear
- Hypercalcemia
- Elevated BUN, creatinine, uric acid, and total protein
- Proteinuria secondary to overproduction and secretion of free monoclonal kappa or lambda chains (Bence Jones protein)
- Tall homogeneous monoclonal spike (M spike) on protein immunoelectrophoresis (IEP) in approximately 75% of patients; decreased levels of normal immunoglobulins; <2% of patients have nonsecreting myeloma (no increase in immunoglobulins and no light chains in the urine)
- Reduced ion gap, hyponatremia, elevated LDH, serum hyperviscosity
- Bone marrow examination: usually demonstrates nests or sheets of plasma cells, which comprise >30% of the bone marrow, and ≥10% are immature

IMAGING STUDIES
X-ray films of painful areas usually demonstrate punched out lytic lesions or osteoporosis. Bone scans are not useful, since lesions are not blastic.

TREATMENT

NONPHARMACOLOGIC THERAPY
- Prevention of renal failure with adequate hydration and avoidance of nephrotoxic agents and dye contrast studies
- Preservation of ambulation and mobility; physical therapy program for some patients
- Consideration of autologous bone marrow transplantation in younger patients (see "Acute General Rx")

ACUTE GENERAL Rx
Chemotherapy may be withheld until symptoms develop or complications are imminent; frequently used regimen includes:
- Melphalan and prednisone: the rates of response to this treatment range from 40% to 60%. Adding continuous low-dose interferon to standard melphalan-prednisone does not improve response rate or survival; however, response duration and plateau phase duration are prolonged by maintenance therapy with interferon.
- Vincristine, doxorubicin (Adriamycin), and dexamethasone (VAD) can be used in patients not responding or relapsing after treatment with melphalan and prednisone.
- Recent studies report that high-dose chemotherapy (HDCT) with vincristine, melphalan, cyclophosphamide, and prednisone (VMCP) alternating with vincristine, carmustine, doxorubicin, and prednisone (BVAP) combined with bone marrow transplantation improves the response rate, event-free survival, and overall survival in patients with myeloma.
- Current HDCT regimen with autologous stem-cell support achieve complete response in approximately 20% to 30% of patients, with best results seen in good-risk patients, defined as young patients (<50 yr of age) with good performance status, and a low tumor burden (β-2 microglobulin ≤2.5 mg/L).

CHRONIC Rx
- Promptly diagnosis and treat infections.
- Control hypercalcemia and hyperuricemia.
- Control pain with analgesics; radiation therapy and surgical stabilization may also be indicated.
- Treat anemia with epoetin alfa.
- Monthly infusions of pamidronate provide significant protection against skeletal complications and improve the quality of life of patients with advanced multiple myeloma.

DISPOSITION
- The median survival time is approximately 30 mo with standard therapy and depends on the stage of the disease, histologic subtype, and various other factors (e.g., elevated LDH levels, or β2-microglobulin >8 mg/L at the time of diagnosis indicate poor prognosis).
- Prognosis is much better in asymptomatic patients with indolent or smoldering myeloma: median survival time is approximately 10 yr in persons with no lytic bone lesions and a serum myeloma protein concentration <3 g/dl.

MISCELLANEOUS

REFERENCES
Attal M et al: A prospective, randomized trial of autologous bone marrow transplantation and chemotherapy in multiple myeloma, *N Engl J Med* 335:91, 1996.

Nordic Myeloma Study Group: Interferon-alfa 2b added to melphalan-prednisone for initial and maintenance therapy in multiple myeloma, *Ann Intern Med* 124:212, 1996.

Author: **Fred F. Ferri, M.D.**

Multiple sclerosis (PTG)

BASIC INFORMATION

DEFINITION
Multiple sclerosis (MS) is a chronic demyelinating disease of unknown etiology characterized pathologically by zones of demyelinization (plaques) scattered throughout the white matter.

SYNONYMS
MS
Disseminated sclerosis

ICD-9-CM CODES
340 Multiple sclerosis

EPIDEMIOLOGY AND DEMOGRAPHICS
PREVALENCE: 50 to 100 cases/100,000 persons, increasing in higher latitudes
GENETICS: Increased prevalence with haplotypes DR2, DQW1, DQA1, DQB1, A3, and B7 of the major histocompatibility complex
Predominant Age: Young adults (17 to 35 yr)

PHYSICAL FINDINGS
- Visual abnormalities:
  1. Paresis of medial rectus muscle on lateral conjugate gaze (internuclear ophthalmoplegia) and horizontal nystagmus of the adducting eye
  2. Central scotoma, decreased visual acuity (optic neuritis)
  3. Nystagmus
- Abnormalities of reflexes: increased DTRs, positive Hoffmann's and Babinski's signs, decreased abdominal skin reflex, decreased cremasteric reflex
- Lhermitte's sign: flexion of the neck while the patient is lying down elicits an electrical sensation extending bilaterally down the arms, back, and lower trunk
- Charcot's triad: nystagmus, scanning speech, and intention tremor
- Visual disturbances: diplopia, blurred vision, visual loss
- Incoordination: gait impairment, clumsiness of upper extremities
- Other: vertigo, incontinence, loss of sexual function, slurred speech

DIFFERENTIAL DIAGNOSIS
- Systemic disorders: sarcoidosis, SLE, pernicious anemia, vasculitis
- Ruptured intervertebral disc
- Infections: CNS infections, syphilis
- Small cerebral infarctions
- Neoplasms: brain stem, cerebellar, spinal cord
- Other: ALS, syringomyelia, neurofibromatosis, Friedreich's ataxia
- Box 2-91 describes the differential diagnosis of paresthesias.

WORKUP
- Lumbar puncture
  1. In MS the CSF may show increased gamma globulin (mostly IgG, but often IgA and IgM).
  2. Agarose electrophoresis discloses separate discrete "oligoclonal" bands in the gamma region in approximately 90% of patients, including some with normal IgG levels.
  3. Other frequent CSF abnormalities are increased total protein, increased mononuclear WBCs, presence of myelin basic protein (elevated in acute attacks, indicates active myelin destruction).
- Measurement of visual evoked response (VER) to assess nerve fiber conduction (myelin loss or destruction will slow conduction velocity)

IMAGING STUDIES
MRI of the head can identify lesions as small as 3 to 4 mm and is frequently diagnostic in suspected cases; can also be used to assess disease load, activity, and progression; however a normal MRI cannot be used conclusively to exclude MS.

DIAGNOSIS

MS is primarily a clinical diagnosis based on evidence of CNS white matter lesions disseminated in time and space (two distinct episodes of neurologic symptoms affecting two distinct areas of the CNS). The clinical signs vary with the location of the plaques. The following are the more common manifestations:
- Weakness: usually involving the lower extremities; complaints of difficulty ambulating, tendency to drop things, easy fatigability
- Sensory disturbances: numbness, tingling, "pins and needles" sensation

TREATMENT

NONPHARMACOLOGIC THERAPY
Patient education regarding the disease and prognosis and the need for the entire family to accept and understand the disease

ACUTE GENERAL Rx
- Pharmacologic treatment is aimed at ameliorating acute exacerbations with high-dose IV methylprednisolone (5-day course at a dose of 1000 mg/day; an alternative dose is 15 mg/kg/day).
- Interferon-beta-1b (Betaseron) 0.25 mg SC qod can be used to prevent relapses in patients with frequent relapses early in the course of the disease. This medication can, however, cause increased spasticity in many patients. Its use should be limited to relatively young, ambulatory patients who have relapsing-remitting disease.

CHRONIC Rx
- Fatigue is a common complaint; it can be treated with amantadine 100 mg bid. Treatment should continue for 2 to 3 wk before deciding whether it is effective. Pemoline and fluoxetine can also be used when amantadine is not effective.
- Spasticity may be controlled with baclofen or lorazepam.
- Pain is a frequent complaint and can be treated with carbamazepine. Tricyclic antidepressants, misoprostol, and NSAIDs are also effective.
- Depression is frequent and can be treated with antidepressants and referral to a psychiatrist.
- Urinary urgency can be treated with oxybutynin or propantheline.
- Tremor can generally be controlled with clonazepam 0.5 mg bid.

DISPOSITION
The majority of patients experience clinical improvement in weeks to months after the initial manifestations. The disease may be of the exacerbating-remitting type or may follow a chronic progressive course. The average interval from the initial clinical presentation to death is 35 yr. Premature death is usually secondary to infection.

REFERRAL
- Initial neurology referral is recommended in all patients with MS.
- Referral to a physician specializing in rehabilitation or to PT/OT is also recommended following exacerbations.

MISCELLANEOUS

COMMENTS
Additional information on MS can also be obtained from The National Multiple Sclerosis Society, 205 East 42nd Street, New York, NY 10017; phone: (212) 986-3240.

REFERENCES
Lindsey JW, Brod SA, Wolinsky JS: Multiple sclerosis. In Johnson RT, Griffin JW (eds): *Current therapy in neurologic disease*, ed 5, St Louis, 1996, Mosby.
Lublin FD et al: Management of patients receiving interferon beta-1b for multiple sclerosis: report of a consensus conference, *Neurology* 46:12, 1996.
Author: **Fred F. Ferri, M.D.**

Mumps (PTG)

BASIC INFORMATION

DEFINITION
Mumps is a generalized viral infection that is usually characterized by swelling and tenderness of one or both parotid glands. It is caused by mumps virus, a paramyxovirus and member of the *Paramyxoviridae* family.

ICD-9-CM CODES
072.9 Mumps

EPIDEMIOLOGY AND DEMOGRAPHICS
INCIDENCE (IN U.S.):
- About 1600 infections/yr
- More than 150,000 cases/yr before licensure of mumps vaccine in 1967

PREDOMINANT SEX: Males = females
PREDOMINANT AGE: 10 to 14 yr old
PEAK INCIDENCE: Late winter and early spring months
GENETICS:

Congenital Infection:
- First-trimester infection is associated with excessive fetal wastage.
- Second- and third-trimester infection is not associated with increased fetal mortality.

Neonatal Infection:
- Uncommon
- Uncommon in infants <1 yr because of passive immunity conferred by placental transfer of maternal antibody

PHYSICAL FINDINGS
- Prodromal period:
  1. Low-grade fever
  2. Malaise
  3. Anorexia
  4. Headache
- Parotid swelling and tenderness are often first signs of infection.
  1. Progresses over 2 to 3 days, then opposite side may become involved
  2. Unilateral parotitis in 25% of cases
  3. Considerable pain with parotid swelling, causing trismus and difficulty with ingestion and pronunciation
  4. Pain exacerbated by eating or drinking citrus and other acidic foods
  5. Possible fever with parotid swelling, ranging up to 40° C
  6. Parotid swelling usually resolving within 1 wk
- CNS involvement:
  1. May occur from 1 wk before to 3 wk after the onset of parotitis
  2. Meningitis
     a. Occurs in 1% to 10% of persons with mumps parotitis
     b. Symptoms: headache, fever, nuchal rigidity, and vomiting
     c. Full recovery with no sequelae
  3. Encephalitis
     a. May develop early, as a result of direct viral invasion of neurons, or late, around the second week after onset of parotitis, and is a postinfectious demyelinating process
     b. Symptoms: fever, alterations in the level of consciousness, possible seizures, paresis, and aphasia
     c. May result in permanent sequelae or death
  4. Other neurologic complications
     a. Cerebellar ataxia
     b. Transverse myelitis
     c. Guillain-Barré syndrome
- Epididymo-orchitis:
  1. Most common extrasalivary gland complication of mumps in men
  2. Occurs in 30% to 38% of postpubertal males who have mumps
  3. Most often unilateral, but is bilateral in 17% to 38% of males who develop this complication
  4. May precede development of parotitis
  5. May be only manifestation of mumps
  6. Two thirds of cases develop during first week of parotitis
  7. One quarter of cases develop in second week
  8. Symptoms:
     a. Severe pain, swelling, and tenderness of the testes and scrotal erythema
     b. Fever and chills
     c. Fever and severity of testicular involvement parallel
  9. Epididymitis
     a. Precedes orchitis
     b. Occurs in 85% of cases
  10. Testicular atrophy in 50% of cases
  11. Bilateral orchitis possibly resulting in sterility
- Involvement of pancreas and ovaries:
  1. Abdominal pain
  2. Fever
  3. Vomiting
  4. Oophoritis
     a. Occurs in 5% of postpubertal women with mumps
     b. May result in decreased fertility and premature menopause
- Transient renal impairment:
  1. Common
  2. Manifest by hematuria, polyuria, and viruria
- Mastitis: occurs in about 31% of women >15 yr who have mumps
- Joint involvement:
  1. Either polyarthritis or monoarticular arthritis
  2. Infrequently affects adults with mumps
  3. Rarely affects children
  4. Self-limited, with complete resolution
- Deafness:
  1. Most often unilateral and of high frequencies
  2. Most patients recover
  3. Permanent unilateral deafness reported in 1 in 20,000 cases

ETIOLOGY
- Virus is spread via the respiratory route.
- Patients are contagious from 48 hr before to 9 days after parotid swelling.

DIAGNOSIS

DIFFERENTIAL DIAGNOSIS
- Other viruses that may cause parotitis:
  1. Parainfluenza types 1 and 3
  2. Coxsackie viruses
  3. Influenza A
  4. Cytomegalovirus
- Suppurative parotitis:
  1. May result from *Staphylococcus aureus* or gram-negative bacteria
  2. May be differentiated from mumps
     a. Extreme induration, tenderness, and erythema overlying the gland
     b. Ability to express pus from Stensen's duct
- Other conditions that may occur with parotid enlargement or swelling:
  1. Sjögren's syndrome
  2. Leukemia
  3. Sickle cell anemia
  4. Diabetes mellitus
  5. Uremia
  6. Malnutrition
  7. Cirrhosis
- Drugs that cause parotid swelling:
  1. Phenothiazines
  2. Phenylbutazone
  3. Thiouracil
  4. Iodides
- Conditions that cause unilateral parotid swelling:
  1. Tumors
  2. Cysts
  3. Stones
  4. Strictures

WORKUP
- Diagnosis is based on history and physical findings.
- Diagnosis is confirmed by a variety of serologic tests or isolation of the virus.

LABORATORY TESTS
- Diagnosis is confirmed by fourfold rise between acute and convalescent sera, by CF, HAI, ELISA, or neutralization tests.
- Virus can be isolated from the saliva, usually from 2 to 3 days before to 4 to 5 days after the onset of parotitis.

- Virus also can be isolated from CSF in patients with meningitis, during the first 3 days of meningeal findings.
- Virus can be detected in urine during the first 2 wk of infection.
- Viremia is rarely detected.
- WBCs:
  1. May be normal
  2. Possible mild leukopenia with a relative lymphocytosis
  3. Leukocytosis with left shift with extrasalivary gland involvement, such as meningitis, orchitis, or pancreatitis
- Serum amylase:
  1. Elevated in the presence of parotitis
  2. Sometimes elevated without clinical parotitis
  3. May remain elevated for 2 to 3 wk
  4. Elevated in mumps pancreatitis
  5. May be differentiated by isoenzyme analysis
- Mumps meningitis:
  1. CSF WBCs from 10 to 2000 WBC/mm^3, with a predominance of lymphocytes
  2. In 20% to 25% of patients, predominance of polymorphonuclear cells
  3. CSF protein normal or mildly elevated
  4. CSF glucose low, >40 mg/100 ml, in 6% to 30% of patients

TREATMENT

NONPHARMACOLOGIC THERAPY
- Supportive treatment
- Adequate hydration and nutrition

ACUTE GENERAL Rx
- Analgesics and antipyretics to relieve pain and fever
- Narcotic analgesics, along with bed rest, ice packs, and a testicular bridge, to relieve pain associated with mumps orchitis
- IV fluids for patients with frequent vomiting associated with mumps pancreatitis or meningitis

DISPOSITION
Most patients recover without incident.

MISCELLANEOUS

COMMENTS
Prevention:
- Attenuated live mumps virus vaccine has been available since 1967.
  1. Usually given in combination with measles and rubella vaccines
  2. Should be given at 15 mo of age, and again at 5 to 12 yr
  3. Seroconversion in about 98% of infants given the vaccine
  4. Contraindicated in pregnant women and immunocompromised patients
- Infected patients should be isolated until parotid swelling resolves.
- Because virus may be shed before the onset of parotid swelling, isolation possibly not of great value in limiting spread of infection.

REFERENCES
Baum SG, Litman N: Mumps virus. In Mandell GL, Bennett JE, Dolin R (eds): *Principles and practice of infectious diseases,* ed 4, New York, 1995, Churchill Livingstone.

Brunell PA: Mumps. In Rudolph AM, Hoffman JIE, Rudolph CD (eds): *Rudolph's pediatrics,* ed 20, Connecticut, 1996, Appleton & Lange.

Nussinovitch M, Volovitz B, Varsano I: Complications of mumps requiring hospitalization in children, *Eur J Pediatr* 154:732, 1995.

Author: **Jane V. Eason, M.D.**

Munchausen's syndrome

BASIC INFORMATION

DEFINITION
Munchausen's syndrome is marked by the willful, and often active, production of symptoms or feigning of disease, usually associated with exaggerated lying (pseudologia fantastica) and with the apparent purpose of inducing medical testing, procedures, and treatment, or assuming the patient role.

SYNONYMS
Factitious disorder
Munchausen's syndrome
Munchausen by proxy
Deliberate disability
Hospital addiction syndrome
Artifactual illness
Artefaktkrankheit
Dermatitis artefacta
Surreptitious illness

ICD-9-CM CODES
300.19 Factitious disorder

EPIDEMIOLOGY AND DEMOGRAPHICS
INCIDENCE (IN U.S.): Unknown
PREVALENCE (IN U.S.): Unknown
PREDOMINANT SEX: Male:female ratio of 2:1
PREDOMINANT AGE: 30 to 40 yr
PEAK INCIDENCE: 30s
GENETICS: No genetic predisposition known

PHYSICAL FINDINGS
- False complaints or self-inflicted injury or symptoms without clear secondary gain.
- Presentation often acute and dramatic
- Workup usually negative but a predisposing condition often present

ETIOLOGY
- Unknown
- Personality disorders and psychodynamic factors: thought to play a role

DIAGNOSIS

DIFFERENTIAL DIAGNOSIS
- Malingering: a clear secondary gain (e.g., financial gain or avoidance of unwanted duties) is present.
- Somatoform disorders or hypochondriasis: similar presentations, but disorder is not under the patient's control.
- Self-injurious behavior is common in many other psychiatric conditions (e.g., borderline personality disorder, psychoses, or nonfatal suicide attempt as may occur in depression); in those conditions the patients confess the intentional self-harm and describe motivating factors.

WORKUP
- Workup is often dictated by the presenting complaints.
- No specific tests for Munchausen's, although Minnesota Multiphasic Personality Inventory (MMPI) may show an unreliable profile.
- Diagnosis is invariably made when the patient is caught in the act of lying or inducing an injury.

LABORATORY TESTS
No specific tests are required.

TREATMENT

NONPHARMACOLOGIC THERAPY
- Therapy is difficult, since patients nearly always terminate (usually in an angry manner) the physician-patient relationship when discovered.
- Only one case of successful psychiatric therapy exists in the literature.

ACUTE GENERAL Rx
None

DISPOSITION
- Ultimate course is unknown.
- After confronted with their behavior, patients seek other physicians or hospitals.
- Extensive medical workups and exploratory surgery are frequent.

REFERRAL
Always when diagnosis is made

MISCELLANEOUS

REFERENCES
Epstein MS: Munchausen syndrome: case reports and literature overview, *Md Med J* 44:39, 1995.
Folks DG: Munchausen's syndrome and other factitious disorders, *Neurol Clin* 13:267, 1995.
Plassmann R: Munchausen syndromes and factitious diseases, *Psychother Psychosom* 62:7, 1994.
Author: **Rif S. El-Mallakh, M.D.**

Muscular dystrophy

BASIC INFORMATION

DEFINITION
The term *muscular dystrophy* (MD) refers to a group of inherited diseases primarily affecting muscle.

SYNONYMS
Distal MD
Duchenne's MD
Erb's MD
Fascioscapulohumeral disease
Gowers' disease
Landouzy-Dejerine disease
Limb-girdle MD
Myotonic MD
Ocular MD
Oculopharyngeal MD

ICD-9-CM CODES
359 Muscular dystrophies and other myopathies
359.1 Hereditary progressive muscular dystrophy

EPIDEMIOLOGY AND DEMOGRAPHICS
INCIDENCE (IN U.S.): Duchenne's: 1 in 3500 male births
PREVALENCE (IN U.S.): Boys with Duchenne's are usually teens; many other types of dystrophies are possible.
PREDOMINANT SEX: Male (for Duchenne's)
PREDOMINANT AGE:
- Depends on type of dystrophy
- Most commonly diagnosed in children

PEAK INCIDENCE: Childhood (Duchenne's)
GENETICS: Duchenne's: X-linked recessive (Xp21)

PHYSICAL FINDINGS
- Proximal muscle weakness
- Late atrophy
- Contracture of Achilles tendon

ETIOLOGY
Genetic abnormality; specifically, a muscle protein, dystrophin, is absent (Duchenne's dystrophy).

DIAGNOSIS

WORKUP
- Muscle biopsy with histochemistry
- ECG/EMG
- Muscle biopsy with dystrophin analysis

LABORATORY TESTS
- Serum creatine kinase
- Possible DNA analysis

IMAGING STUDIES
Not necessary

TREATMENT

NONPHARMACOLOGIC THERAPY
- Genetic counseling
- Physical therapy

ACUTE GENERAL Rx
None

CHRONIC Rx
- Be alert for development of contractures, respiratory distress, and cardiac complications.
- No cure is known for Duchenne's MD.

DISPOSITION
Usually, follow-up in a MD specialty clinic

REFERRAL
- See "Disposition."
- For family anxiety with the diagnosis

MISCELLANEOUS

COMMENTS
"Muscular dystrophy" refers to many diseases; Duchenne's, limb-girdle, and myotonic dystrophy are the most common, but many other dystrophies have been described if exact diagnosis in doubt.

REFERENCES
Parano E et al: Congenital muscular dystrophies: clinical review and proposed classification, *Pediatr Neurol* 13:97, 1995.

Author: **William H. Olson, M.D.**

Myasthenia gravis (PTG)

BASIC INFORMATION

DEFINITION
Myasthenia gravis (MG) is a disorder of neuromuscular transmission characterized by the presence of a gamma globulin antibody (AChR-ab) directed against the nicotinic acetylcholinic receptor (AChR) of the neuromuscular junction, resulting in postsynaptic response to ACh.

ICD-9-CM CODES
358.0 Myasthenia gravis

EPIDEMIOLOGY AND DEMOGRAPHICS
INCIDENCE (IN U.S.): 2 to 5 cases/yr/1,000,000 persons
PREVALENCE (IN U.S.): 1/20,000 persons
PREDOMINANT SEX: Female > male (3:2) in adults; female = male in elderly
PREDOMINANT AGE: 20 to 40 yr
PEAK INCIDENCE: Female: third decade; male: fifth decade
GENETICS: Increased frequency of HLA-B8, DR3
Familial Predisposition: 5% of adult and juvenile cases
Congenital MG: Autosomal recessive; permanent condition
Neonatal MG: Occurs in 15% to 20% of infants born to mothers with MG. This condition is only temporary and is caused by transplacental passage of AChR-ab. Spontaneous recovery often occurs within 1 mo.

PHYSICAL FINDINGS
- The hallmark of MG is weakness made worse with exercise and improved with rest.
- More than 50% of patients are initially seen with ptosis, ocular muscle weakness, or both.
- Difficulty in chewing, abnormal smile, dysarthria, and dysphagia are also common.
- Pain may occur in fatigued muscles (e.g., neck muscles).
- Clinical manifestations are reproducible with exercise.
- Physical examination may be normal at rest.

ETIOLOGY
Injury of the acetylcholine receptors in the postsynaptic neuromuscular junction on an autoimmune basis (AChR-ab directed against the nicotinic acetylcholinic receptor of the neuromuscular junction)

DIAGNOSIS

DIFFERENTIAL DIAGNOSIS
Polymyositis, multiple sclerosis, chronic fatigue syndrome, myopathies, neurasthenia, polymyositis, cranial nerve lesions, pernicious anemia, thyrotoxic ophthalmopathy

WORKUP
- Improvement of symptoms after use of anticholinesterase medications: Edrophonium chloride (Tensilon), 2 mg IV; useful in MG patients with ocular symptoms; it has rapid onset (30 sec) and short duration of action (5 min). Pyridostigmine bromide (Mestinon), 60 mg PO; has longer duration of action and is often used in patients with generalized symptoms.
- Single-fiber electromyography (SFEMG); highly accurate in confirming MG in suspected patients with normal conventional repetitive stimulation.

LABORATORY TESTS
Elevated level of AChR-ab (present in 90% of patients with generalized MG and 60% of patients with ocular myasthenia): this serological test must be performed only if testing with anticholinesterase drugs supports the diagnosis of MG.
- TSH, free T_4: to rule out thyroid disease (found in 5% to 15% of patients with MG)
- Vitamin B_{12} level to rule out pernicious anemia
- ANA, RF (increased association with SLE, rheumatoid arthritis)

IMAGING STUDIES
CT scan of anterior chest to rule out thymoma (found in 12% of patients with MG)

TREATMENT

NONPHARMACOLOGIC THERAPY
Prevention of exacerbations:
- Avoidance of temperature extremes; prompt treatment of infections, stress reduction
- Avoidance of selected drugs known to provoke exacerbations of MG (penicillamine, aminoglycoside antibiotics, tetracyclines, class I antiarrhythmics)

ACUTE GENERAL Rx
- Cholinesterase inhibitors: pyridostigmine 30 to 60 mg PO q4-6h initially; onset of effects is 30 min, duration 4 h. A longer preparation (Mestinon Timespan, 180 mg) can be given qd or bid; however, absorption may be erratic; major side effects are GI upset and increased salivary and bronchial secretions.
- Corticosteroids: prednisone doses range from 5 mg qod to 100 mg qd, depending on patient response; most patients require steroid therapy indefinitely. Slowly tapering steroids once control is achieved and switching to alternate day doses should be attempted.
- Immunosuppressants: azathioprine (Imuran) 2 to 3 mg/kg/day or cyclosporine 5 mg/kg/day are often used in patients with severe generalized weakness and may reduce the need for corticosteroids. Most patients require lifelong immunosuppressive therapy.
- Plasmaspheresis and leukoplasmapheresis are effective in severely ill patients and preoperatively in thymectomy candidates.

CHRONIC Rx
- Thymectomy is indicated in all patients with thymoma.
- Thymectomy in absence of thymoma is more controversial—generally recommended for MG patients aged 18 (postpubertal) to 50 yr, particularly patients not responding well to medical treatment.
- Drug therapy (cholinesterase inhibitors, corticosteroids, and immunosuppressants) as noted above may be useful.
- Prevent exacerbations (see above).

DISPOSITION
Course of disease is highly variable, with exacerbations and remissions.

REFERRAL
Surgical referral for thymectomy in selected cases (see above).

MISCELLANEOUS

COMMENTS
Patients must be closely monitored for onset of respiratory complications (acute respiratory arrest, aspiration pneumonia, chronic respiratory insufficiency).

REFERENCES
Drachman DB: Mysthemia gravis, *New Engl J Med*, 330:1797, 1994.
Author: **Fred F. Ferri, M.D.**

Myelodysplastic syndromes (PTG)

BASIC INFORMATION

DEFINITION
Myelodysplastic syndromes (MDS) are a group of acquired clonal disorders affecting the hemopoietic stem cells and characterized by cytopenias with hypercellular bone marrow and various morphologic abnormalities in the hemopoietic cell lines. Myelodysplastic syndromes show abnormal (dysplastic) hemopoietic maturation. Marrow cellularity is increased, reflecting an effective hematopoiesis, but inadequate maturation results in peripheral cytopenias. Myelodysplasia encompasses several heterogenous syndromes: refractory anemias, chronic myelomonocytic leukemia (CMML), primary myelodysplasia, secondary myelodysplasia.

SYNONYMS
MDS
Preleukemia
Dysmyelopoietic syndrome

ICD-9-CM CODES
238.7 Myelodysplastic syndrome

EPIDEMIOLOGY AND DEMOGRAPHICS
INCIDENCE (IN U.S.): Approximately 82 cases/100,000 persons/yr
PREDOMINANT AGE: More common in elderly patients, with a median age of >65 yr

PHYSICAL FINDINGS
- Splenomegaly, skin pallor, mucosal bleeding, ecchymosis may be present.
- Patients often present with fatigue.
- Fever, infection, and dyspnea are common.

ETIOLOGY
Unknown

DIAGNOSIS

DIFFERENTIAL DIAGNOSIS
- Hereditary dysplasias (e.g., Fanconi's anemia, Diamond-Blackfan syndrome)
- Vitamin B_{12}/folate deficiency
- Exposure to toxins (drugs, alcohol, chemotherapy)
- Renal failure
- Irradiation
- Autoimmune disease
- Infections (TB, viral infections)
- Paroxysmal nocturnal hemoglobinuria

WORKUP
Diagnostic workup includes laboratory evaluation and bone marrow examination.

LABORATORY TESTS
- Anemia with variable MCV (normal or increased)
- Reduced reticulocyte count (in relation to the degree of anemia)
- Hypogranular or agranular neutrophils
- Thrombocytopenia or normal platelet count
- Hypogranular platelets may be present
- Hypercellular bone marrow, with frequent clonal chromosomal abnormalities

IMAGING STUDIES
Abdominal CT scan may reveal hepatosplenomegaly.

TREATMENT

NONPHARMACOLOGIC THERAPY
RBC transfusions in patients with severe symptomatic anemia

ACUTE GENERAL Rx
- Results of chemotherapy are generally disappointing.
- The role of myeloid growth factors (granulocyte colony-stimulating factor, granulocyte macrophage colony-stimulating factor) is undefined.
- Allogeneic bone marrow transplantation should be considered in patients <65 yr old.

CHRONIC Rx
Monitor for infections, bleeding, and complications of anemia.

DISPOSITION
- Cure rates in young patients with allogeneic bone marrow transplantations approach 30% to 50%.
- The risk of transformation to acute myelogenous leukemia varies with the percentage of blasts in the bone marrow.
- Deletion of chromosomes 5 and 7 is associated with a poor prognosis.

REFERRAL
Hematology referral in all patients with myelodysplastic syndromes

MISCELLANEOUS

COMMENTS
Erythropoietin (epoetin alpha) SC three times weekly may be effective in increasing the Hgb and reducing the RBC transfusion requirement in some patients.

REFERENCES
Lowry PA: Hematologic malignancies. In Noble J (ed): *Primary care medicine*, ed 2, St Louis, 1996, Mosby.
Taylor KM et al: Myelodysplasia, *Curr Opin Oncol* 6:32, 1994.
Author: **Fred F. Ferri, M.D.**

Myocardial infarction

BASIC INFORMATION

DEFINITION
Myocardial infarction (MI) is characterized by necrosis resulting from an insufficient supply of oxygenated blood to an area of the heart.
- *Non–Q wave:* Area of ischemic necrosis is limited to the inner one third to half of myocardial wall.
- *Q wave:* Area of ischemic necrosis penetrates the entire thickness of the ventricular wall.

SYNONYMS
MI
Heart attack
Coronary thrombosis
Coronary occlusion

ICD-9-CM CODES
410.9 Acute myocardial infarction, unspecified site

EPIDEMIOLOGY AND DEMOGRAPHICS
INCIDENCE/PREVALENCE (IN U.S.):
- >500 cases/100,000 persons
- >500,000 MIs in the U.S. yearly
- More prominent in males between the ages of 40 and 65 yr; no predominant sex after age 65 yr

PHYSICAL FINDINGS
Clinical presentation:
- Crushing substernal chest pain usually lasts longer than 30 min.
- Pain is unrelieved by rest or sublingual nitroglycerin or is rapidly recurring.
- Pain radiates to the left or right arm, neck, jaw, back, shoulders, or abdomen and is not pleuritic in character.
- Pain may be associated with dyspnea, diaphoresis, nausea, or vomiting.
- There is no pain in approximately 20% of infarctions (usually in diabetic or elderly patients).

Physical findings:
- Skin may be diaphoretic, with pallor (because of decreased oxygen).
- Rales may be present at the bases of lungs (indicative of CHF).
- Cardiac auscultation may reveal an apical systolic murmur caused by mitral regurgitation secondary to papillary muscle dysfunction; S_3 or S_4 may also be present.
- Physical examination may be completely normal.

ETIOLOGY
- Coronary atherosclerosis
- Coronary artery spasm
- Coronary embolism (caused by infective endocarditis, rheumatic heart disease, intracavitary thrombus)
- Periarteritis and other coronary artery inflammatory diseases
- Dissection into coronary arteries (aneurysmal or iatrogenic)
- Congenital abnormalities of coronary circulation
- MI with normal coronaries (MINC syndrome): more frequent in younger patients and cocaine addicts

DIAGNOSIS

DIFFERENTIAL DIAGNOSIS
See differential diagnosis of chest pain in Section II; Table 2-62 in Section II describes the differential diagnosis of ST-segment elevation.

LABORATORY TESTS
- Serum cardiac enzyme studies: damaged necrotic heart muscle releases cardiac isoenzymes (CK, LDH) into the blood stream in amounts that correlate with the size of the infarct. Electrophoretic fractionation of the enzymes can pinpoint certain isoenzymes (CK-MB and LDH-1) that are more sensitive indicators of MI than total CK or LDH.
- Cardiac troponin levels: cardiac-specific troponin T (cTnT) and cardiac-specific troponin I (cTnI) are new markers for acute MI. Rapid whole blood bedside assays are now available. Increases in serum levels of cTnT and cTnI may occur relatively early after muscle damage and may be present for several days after MI (up to 7 days for cTnI and up to 10 to 14 days for cTnT).
- ECG:
  1. In Q wave infarction, there is development of:
     a. Inverted T waves, indicating an area of ischemia
     b. Elevated ST segment, indicating an area of injury
     c. Q waves, indicating an area of infarction (usually develop over 12 to 36 hr)
  2. In non-Q wave infarction, Q waves are absent, but:
     a. History and myocardial enzyme elevations are compatible with MI.
     b. ECG shows ST segment elevation, depression, or no change followed by T wave inversion.

IMAGING STUDIES
- Chest radiography is useful to evaluate for pulmonary congestion.
- Echocardiography can evaluate wall motion abnormalities and identify mural thrombus or mitral regurgitation, which can occur acutely after MI.

TREATMENT

NONPHARMACOLOGIC THERAPY
- Limit patient's activity: bed rest for the initial 24 hr; if the patient remains stable, gradually increase activity.
- Diet: NPO until stable, then no added salt, low-cholesterol diet.
- Patient education to decrease the risk of subsequent cardiac events (proper diet, cessation of smoking, regular exercise) should be initiated when the patient is medically stable.

ACUTE GENERAL Rx
- Any patient with suspected acute MI should immediately receive the following:
  1. Nasal oxygen: administer at 2 to 4 L/min.
  2. Nitrates: they increase the supply of oxygen by reducing coronary vasospasm and decrease consumption of oxygen by reducing ventricular preload. Sublingual nitroglycerin can be administered immediately on suspicion of MI (unless systolic blood pressure is <90 mm Hg or heart rate is <50 bpm or >100 bpm); IV nitroglycerin can be subsequently used. Nitroglycerin should be used with great caution in patients with inferior wall MI; nitrate usage can result in hypotension because these patients are sensitive to change in preload.
  3. Adequate analgesia: morphine sulfate 2 mg IV q5min PRN can be given for severe pain unrelieved by nitroglycerin.
  4. Aspirin: give 160 to 325 mg orally.
- Thrombolytic therapy: if the duration of pain has been <6 hr, recanalization of the occluded arteries should be attempted with tPA, streptokinase, or APSAC.
  1. All three agents are effective; generally tPA is more efficacious than the others. However, it is much more expensive and its use is associated with higher intracranial bleeding, total stroke, and stroke death rates. When tPA is used, IV heparin is given to increase the likelihood of patency in the infarct-related artery. An IV heparin 5000 U bolus is given at the time of tPA therapy, followed by a continuous infusion of 1000 U/hr (adjusted to keep the APPT at one and a half to two times control for at least 48 hr). In patients receiving streptokinase or APSAC, IV heparin is not indicated, since it does not offer any additional benefit and can result

CLINICAL TOPICS

Myocardial infarction

in increased bleeding complications.
2. Contraindications to thrombolytic therapy and patient selection guidelines are described in Boxes A-16 and A-17 in the Appendix.
- Primary angioplasty (PTCA) may be performed as an excellent alternative to thrombolytic therapy. It is effective, but it is generally not available in community hospitals. Prompt access to emergency coronary artery bypass graft (CABG) surgery is mandatory if primary PTCA is to be undertaken. When primary PTCA is performed, use of IV heparin is recommended.
- β-Adrenergic blocking agents should be given to all patients with evolving acute MI, provided that there are no contraindications (see below). β-Blockers are useful to reduce myocardial oxygen consumption and prevent tachyarrhythmias. Early IV β-blockage (in the initial 24 hr) followed by institution of an oral maintenance regimen is also effective in reducing recurrent infarction and ischemia. Frequently used agents are:
  1. Metoprolol (Lopressor): IV 5 mg q2min × 3 doses, then PO 25 to 50 mg q6h, given 15 min after last IV dose, continued for 48 hr; maintenance dosage is 50 to 100 mg bid.
  2. Atenolol (Tenormin): IV 5 mg over 5 min, repeat in 10 min if initial dose is well tolerated, then start PO dose 10 min after the last IV dose; PO 50 mg qd, increasing to 100 mg as tolerated.
  3. Before using β-blockers, some of the contraindications and side effects (i.e., exacerbation of CHF, exacerbation of asthma, CNS effects, hypertension, bradycardia) must be carefully assessed.
- ACE inhibitors reduce left ventricular dysfunction and dilation and slow the progression of CHF during and after acute MI. They should be initiated within hours of hospitalization, provided that the patient does not have hypotension or a contraindication (bilateral renal stenosis, renal failure or history of angioedema caused by previous treatment with ACE inhibitors).
  1. Commonly used agents are captopril 12.5 mg PO bid, enalapril 2.5 mg bid, or lisinopril 2.5 to 5 mg qd initially, with subsequent titration as needed.
  2. ACE inhibitors may be stopped in patients without complications and no evidence of left ventricular dysfunction after 6 to 8 wk.
  3. ACE inhibitors should be continued indefinitely in patients with impaired left ventricular function (ejection fraction <40%) or clinical CHF.
- Sedation: short-acting benzodiazepines may be useful to minimize anxiety in selected patients.
- Stool softener may be given for constipation.

CHRONIC Rx
Evaluation of post-MI patients:
- Submaximal (low level) treadmill test (can be done 1 to 3 wk after MI) in stable patients without any clinical evidence of significant left ventricular dysfunction or post-MI angina
  1. Useful to assess the patient's functional capacity and formulate an at home exercise program
  2. Helpful to determine the patient's prognosis
- Radionuclide angiography or two-dimensional echocardiography
  1. To evaluate patient's left ventricular ejection fraction
  2. To evaluate ventricular size and segmental wall motion
  3. Echocardiography to rule out presence of mural thrombi in patients with anterior wall infarction; transesophageal echo is preferred if mural thrombosis is suspected
- A 24-hr Holter monitor study to evaluate patients who have demonstrated significant arrhythmias during their hospital stay; selected patients with complex ventricular ectopy may be candidates for programmed electrical stimulation studies and antiarrhythmic therapy and/or implanted defibrillator, depending on the results of these studies

DISPOSITION
The prognosis after MI depends on multiple factors:
- Use of β-blockers: the mortality of patients on a regular regimen of β-blockers is significantly decreased when compared with that of control groups.
- Presence of arrhythmias, frequent ventricular ectopy (≥10/hr), or repetitive forms of ventricular ectopic beats (couplets, triplets) indicates an increased risk (two to three times greater) of sudden cardiac death. New bundle-branch block, Mobitz-II second-degree block, or third-degree heart block also adversely affect outcome.
- Size of infarct: the larger it is, the higher the post-MI mortality rate.
- Site of infarct: inferior wall MI carries a better prognosis than anterior wall MI.
- Type of infarct: although the in-hospital mortality rate is higher for patients with Q wave infarcts, the long-term prognosis for non–Q wave MI may be worse because these patients have a higher incidence of sudden cardiac death after hospital discharge.
- Ejection fraction after MI: the lower the left ventricular ejection fraction, the higher the mortality after MI.
- Presence of post-MI angina indicates a high mortality rate.
- Performance on low-level exercise test: the presence of ST segment changes during the test is a predictor of high mortality during the first year.
- Presence of pericarditis during the acute phase of MI increases mortality at 1 yr.
- Type A behavior (competitive drive, ambitiousness, hostility) is associated with a lower mortality rate after symptomatic MI.
- Thrombolytic and antiplatelet therapy decreases the mortality and increases myocardial perfusion and salvage.
- ACE inhibitors are beneficial after MI (see "Acute General Rx").
- Use of lipid-lowering agents in patients with hyperlipidemia responsive to exercise and dietary restrictions is beneficial.
- Additional poor prognostic factors include the following: cigarette smoking, history of hypertension or prior MI, presence of ST segment depression in acute MI, increasing age, diabetes mellitus, and female sex.

MISCELLANEOUS

COMMENTS
Patient education material regarding MI can be obtained from the American Heart Association, 7320 Green Mill Avenue, Dallas, TX 75231.

REFERENCES
Gusto IIb angioplasty substudy investigators: A clinical trial comparing primary coronary angioplasty with tissue plasminogen activator for acute MI, *N Engl J Med* 336:1621, 1997.

Hennekens CH et al: Adjunctive drug therapy of acute myocardial infarction: evidence from clinical trials, *N Engl J Med* 335:1660, 1996.

Loh E et al: Ventricular dysfunction and the risk of stroke after myocardial infarction, *N Engl J Med* 336:251, 1997.

Peterson et al: Risk and stratification after myocardial infarction, *Ann Intern Med* 126:561, 1997.

Author: **Fred F. Ferri, M.D.**

Myocarditis (PTG)

BASIC INFORMATION

DEFINITION
Myocarditis is an inflammatory condition of the myocardium.

ICD-9-CM CODES
429.0 Myocarditis, nonspecific
391.2 Myocarditis, rheumatic
422.91 Myocarditis, viral (except coxsackie)
074.23 Myocarditis, coxsackie
422.92 Myocarditis, bacterial

EPIDEMIOLOGY AND DEMOGRAPHICS
The incidence of focal myocarditis reported at autopsy is 1% to 7% in asymptomatic patients.

PHYSICAL FINDINGS
- Persistent tachycardia out of proportion to fever
- Faint S_1, S_4 sound on auscultation
- Murmur of mitral regurgitation
- Pericardial friction rub if associated with pericarditis
- Signs of biventricular failure (hypotension, hepatomegaly, peripheral edema, distention of neck veins, S_3)

ETIOLOGY
- Infection
  1. Viral (coxsackie B virus, echovirus, polio virus, adenovirus, mumps, HIV, EBV)
  2. Bacterial (*Staphylococcus aureus, Clostridium perfringens,* diphtheria, and any severe bacterial infection)
  3. Mycoplasma
  4. Mycotic *(Candida,* mucor, *Aspergillus)*
  5. Parasitic *(Trypanosoma cruzi, Trichinella, Echinococcus,* amoeba, toxoplasma)
  6. *Rickettsia rickettsii*
  7. Spirochetal *(Borrelia burgdorferi*—Lyme carditis)
- Rheumatic fever
- Secondary to drugs (e.g., cocaine, emetine, doxorubicin, sulfonamides, isoniazid, methyldopa, amphotericin B, tetracycline, phenylbutazone, lithium, 5-FU, phenothiazines, interferon alpha, tricyclic antidepressants, cyclophosphamides)
- Toxins (carbon monoxide, diphtheria toxin, lead, arsenicals)
- Collagen-vascular disease (SLE, scleroderma, Kawasaki syndrome)
- Sarcoidosis
- Radiation
- Postpartum

DIAGNOSIS

DIFFERENTIAL DIAGNOSIS
- Cardiomyopathy
- Acute myocardial infarction
- Valvulopathies

WORKUP
- Medical history: the clinical presentation of myocarditis is nonspecific and can consist of fatigue, palpitations, dyspnea, precordial discomfort, myalgias.
- Diagnostic workup includes chest x-ray examination, ECG, laboratory evaluation, echocardiogram, and cardiac catheterization (selected patients).

LABORATORY TESTS
- Increased CK (with elevated MB fraction, LDH, and AST secondary to myocardial necrosis)
- Increased ESR (nonspecific but may be of value in following the progress of the disease and the response to therapy)
- Increased WBC (increased eosinophils if parasitic infection)
- Viral titers (acute and convalescent)
- Cold agglutinin titer, ASLO titer, blood cultures
- Lyme disease antibody titer

IMAGING STUDIES
- Chest x-ray examination: enlargement of cardiac silhouette
- ECG: sinus tachycardia with nonspecific ST-T wave changes; interventricular conduction defects and bundle-branch block may be present
  1. Lyme disease and diphtheria cause all degrees of heart block.
  2. Changes of acute MI can occur with focal necrosis.
- Echocardiogram:
  1. Dilated and hypokinetic chambers
  2. Segmental wall motion abnormalities
- Cardiac catheterization and angiography:
  1. To rule out coronary artery disease and valvular disease
  2. A right ventricular endomyocardial biopsy can confirm the diagnosis, although a negative biopsy result does not exclude myocarditis. Recent studies have shown that myocardial biopsy may be unnecessary, since immunosuppression therapy based on biopsy results is generally ineffective.

TREATMENT

NONPHARMACOLOGIC THERAPY
Restrict physical activity (to decrease cardiac work).

ACUTE GENERAL Rx
- Treat underlying cause (e.g., use specific antibiotics for bacterial infection).
- Treat CHF with digitalis, diuretics, ACE inhibitors, and salt restriction.
- If ventricular arrhythmias are present, treat with quinidine or procainamide.
- Provide anticoagulation to prevent thromboembolism.
- Use preload and afterload reducing agents for treating cardiac decompensation.
- Corticosteroid use is contraindicated in early infectious myocarditis; it may be justified in only selected patients with intractable CHF, severe systemic toxicity, and severe life-threatening arrhythmias.
- Immunosuppressive drugs (prednisone with cyclosporin or azathioprine) do not have any significant effect on the prognosis of myocarditis.

DISPOSITION
Nearly 50% of patients with myocarditis will die within 5 yr of diagnosis.

REFERRAL
Consider heart transplant if patient develops intractable CHF.

MISCELLANEOUS

COMMENTS
Many cases of myocarditis resolve spontaneously.

REFERENCES
Brown CA, O'Connoll JB: Myocarditis and idiopathic cardiomyopathy, *Am J Med* 99:309, 1995.
Mason W et al: A clinical trial of immunosuppressive therapy for myocarditis, *N Engl J Med* 333:269, 1995.

Author: **Fred F. Ferri, M.D.**

Myxedema coma

BASIC INFORMATION

DEFINITION
Myxedema coma is a life-threatening complication of hypothyroidism characterized by profound lethargy or coma and usually accompanied by hypothermia.

ICD-9-CM CODES
244.8 Myxedema, pituitary
244.1 Myxedema, primary

PHYSICAL FINDINGS
- Profound lethargy or coma
- Hypothermia (rectal temperature <35 °C [95 °F]); often missed by using ordinary thermometers graduated only to 34.5° C or because the mercury is not shaken below 36° C
- Bradycardia, hypotension (secondary to circulatory collapse)
- Delayed relaxation phase of DTR, areflexia

ETIOLOGY
Decompensation of hypothyroidism secondary to:
- Sepsis
- Exposure to cold weather
- CNS depressants (sedatives, narcotics, antidepressants)
- Trauma, surgery

DIAGNOSIS

DIFFERENTIAL DIAGNOSIS
- Severe depression, primary psychosis
- Drug overdose
- CVA, liver failure, renal failure
- Hypoglycemia, CO_2 narcosis, encephalitis

WORKUP
Diagnosis of hypothyroidism and exclusion of contributing factors (e.g., sepsis, CVA) with laboratory and radiographic studies (see below)

LABORATORY TESTS
- Markedly increased TSH (if primary hypothyroidism), decreased serum free T_4
- CBC with differential, urine and blood cultures to rule out infectious process
- Electrolytes, BUN, creatinine, liver function tests, calcium, glucose
- ABGs to rule out hypoxemia and carbon dioxide retention
- Cortisol level to rule out adrenal insufficiency

IMAGING STUDIES
- CT scan of head in suspected CVA
- Chest x-ray examination to rule out infectious process

TREATMENT

NONPHARMACOLOGIC THERAPY
- Prevent further heat loss; cover the patient but avoid external rewarming because it may produce vascular collapse.
- Support respiratory function; intubation and mechanical ventilation may be required.
- Monitor patients in the ICU.

ACUTE GENERAL Rx
- Give levothyroxine 5 to 8 µg/kg (300 to 500 µg) IV infused over 15 min, then 100 µg IV q24h.
- Glucocorticoids should also be administered until coexistent adrenal insufficiency can be ruled out. Hydrocortisone hemisuccinate 100 mg IV bolus is initially given, followed by 50 mg IV q12h or 25 mg IV q6h until initial plasma cortisol level is confirmed normal.
- IV hydration with D_5NS is used to correct hypotension and hypoglycemia (if present); avoid overhydration and possible water intoxication because clearance of free water is impaired in these patients.
- Rule out and treat precipitating factors (e.g., antibiotics in suspected sepsis).

CHRONIC Rx
Refer to "Hypothyroidism" in Section I.

DISPOSITION
Mortality rate in myxedema coma is 20% to 50%.

REFERRAL
Endocrinology consultation is appropriate in patients with myxedema coma.

MISCELLANEOUS

COMMENTS
If the diagnosis is suspected, initiate treatment immediately without waiting for confirming laboratory results.

REFERENCES
Eng S, Singer PA: Prompt and aggressive therapy for endocrine emergencies, *Contemp Intern Med* 8:27, 1996.
Singer PA et al: Treatment guidelines for patients with hyperthyroidism and hypothyroidism: Standards of Care Committee, American Thyroid Association, *JAMA* 273:808, 1995.

Author: Fred F. Ferri, M.D.

Narcolepsy (PTG)

BASIC INFORMATION

DEFINITION
Narcolepsy is a sleep disorder in which REM sleep occurs suddenly during wakefulness. It is characterized by the tetrad of excessive daytime sleepiness, irresistible sleep attacks, cataplexy, hypnagogic hallucinations, and sleep paralysis.

ICD-9-CM CODES
347 Cataplexy and narcolepsy

EPIDEMIOLOGY AND DEMOGRAPHICS
INCIDENCE (IN U.S.): 1 case/1000 persons/yr; more than fiftyfold increased incidence in families with a positive history
PREVALENCE (IN U.S.): 50 to 60 cases/100,000 persons
PREDOMINANT SEX: Males = females
PREDOMINANT AGE: Second decade
PEAK INCIDENCE: Age 15 to 25 yr
GENETICS: Strong association with HLA-DR2 and HLA-DQw1 antigens

PHYSICAL FINDINGS
- Sleep attacks last from a few seconds to 30 min, during which patients are easily awakened by tactile stimuli.
- Cataplexy, which occurs in 80% of patients, is an abrupt loss of voluntary muscle control precipitated by a strong emotion. Consciousness is preserved.
- Sleep paralysis, which occurs in 60% of patients, is a loss of muscle tone during the transition between sleep and wakefulness. It may be interrupted by tactile stimuli.
- Hypnagogic hallucinations may be experienced during the transition from wakefulness to sleep.

ETIOLOGY
Unknown

DIAGNOSIS

DIFFERENTIAL DIAGNOSIS
- Sleep apnea
- Periodic movements in sleep
- Hypothyroidism
- Sedative drugs
- Encephalopathic states
- Seizures

WORKUP
Nocturnal polysomnography followed by a multiple sleep latency test

LABORATORY TESTS
Some 90% to 95% of patients are HLA-DR2 positive, so a negative test is evidence against the diagnosis, although a positive test does not establish the diagnosis, since HLA-DR2 is found in the normal population.

IMAGING STUDIES
None

TREATMENT

NONPHARMACOLOGIC THERAPY
Short, scheduled daytime naps

ACUTE GENERAL Rx
None

CHRONIC Rx
- For hypersomnolence:
  a. Mehtylphenidate (Ritalin) 10 mg bid initially
  b. Pemoline (Cylert) 37.5 mg/day in the morning initially; increase until desired response is obtained
  c. Dextroamphetamine 10 mg qd initially, increase by 10 mg at weekly intervals to optimal dose.
- For cataplexy:
  a. Clomipramine (Anafranil) 25 mg/day initially
  b. Protriptyline (Vivactil) 5 mg tid initially
  c. Imipramine (Tofranil) 25 to 50 mg/day initially
  d. Desipramine (Norpramine) 10 mg bid initially
  e. Fluoxetine (Prozac) 20 mg qd initially

DISPOSITION
A chronic sleep disorder without periods of remission

REFERRAL
If sleep studies are needed, they should be performed in an accredited sleep disorders laboratory.

MISCELLANEOUS

COMMENTS
True narcolepsy is a relatively rare cause of daytime sleepiness.

REFERENCES
Chaudhary BA, Husain I: Narcolepsy, *J Fam Pract* 36:207, 1993.

Author: **Michael Gruenthal, M.D., Ph.D.**

Nephrotic syndrome (PTG)

BASIC INFORMATION

DEFINITION
Nephrotic syndrome is characterized by high urine protein excretion (>3.5 g per 1.73/m^3 in 24 hr), peripheral edema, and metabolic abnormalities (hypoalbuminemia, hypercholesterolemia).

ICD-9-CM CODES
581.9 Nephrotic syndrome

EPIDEMIOLOGY AND DEMOGRAPHICS
Nephrotic syndrome occurs predominantly in children ages 2 to 6 yr (2 new cases/100,000 persons/yr) and in adults of all ages (3 to 4 new cases/100,000 persons/yr).

PHYSICAL FINDINGS
- Peripheral edema
- Ascites, anasarca
- Hypertension
- Pleural effusion
- Typically patients present with severe peripheral edema, exertional dyspnea, and abdominal fullness secondary to ascites. There is a significant amount of weight gain in most patients.

ETIOLOGY
- Idiopathic (may be secondary to the following glomerular diseases: minimal change disease [nil disease, lipoid nephrosis], focal segmental glomerular sclerosis, membranous nephropathy, membranoproliferative glomerular nephropathy)
- Associated with systemic diseases (diabetes mellitus, SLE, amyloidosis)
- Majority of children with nephrotic syndrome have minimal change disease (this form also associated with allergy, nonsteroidals, and Hodgkin's disease)
- Focal glomerular disease: can be associated with HIV infection, heroin abuse
- Membranous nephropathy: can occur with Hodgkin's lymphoma, carcinomas, SLE, gold therapy
- Membranoproliferative glomerulonephropathy: often associated with upper respiratory infections

DIAGNOSIS

DIFFERENTIAL DIAGNOSIS
- Other edema states (CHF, cirrhosis)
- Primary renal disease (e.g., focal glomerulonephritis, membranoproliferative glomerulonephritis)
- Carcinoma, infections
- Malignant hypertension
- Polyarteritis nodosa
- Serum sickness
- Toxemia of pregnancy

WORKUP
- Diagnostic workup consists of laboratory evaluation. Renal biopsy is generally performed in individuals with persistent proteinuria in whom the etiology of the proteinuria is unclear.
- Box 2-100 describes the differential diagnosis of proteinuria.

LABORATORY TESTS
- Urinalysis reveals proteinuria. The presence of hematuria, cellular casts, and pyuria are suggestive of nephritic syndrome. Oval fat bodies (tubular epithelial cells with cholesterol esters) are also found in the urine in patients with nephrotic syndrome.
- 24-hr urine protein excretion is >3.5 g/1.73 m^3/24 hr.
- Abnormalities of blood chemistries include serum albumin <3 g/dl, decreased total protein, elevated serum cholesterol, azotemia.
- Additional tests in patients with nephrotic syndromes depending on the history and physical examination are ANA, serum and urine immunoelectrophoresis, C3, C4, CH-50.

IMAGING STUDIES
CT scan or ultrasound of kidneys

TREATMENT

NONPHARMACOLOGIC THERAPY
- Bed rest as tolerated, avoidance of nephrotoxic drugs, low-fat diet, fluid restriction in hyponatremic patients; normal protein intake unless urinary protein loss exceeds 10 g/24 hr (some patients may require additional dietary protein to prevent negative nitrogen balance and significant protein malnutrition)
- Strict sodium restriction to help manage peripheral edema
- Close monitoring of patients for development of peripheral venous thrombosis and renal vein thrombosis because of hypercoagulable state secondary to loss of antithrombin III and other proteins involved in the clotting mechanism

ACUTE GENERAL Rx
The mainstay of therapy is treatment of the underlying disorder:
- Minimal change disease generally responds to prednisone 1 mg/kg/day. Relapses can occur when steroids are discontinued. In these individuals, cyclophosphamide and chlorambucil may be useful.
- Focal and segmental glomerulosclerosis: steroid therapy is also recommended. However, response rate is approximately 35% to 40%, and most patients progress to end-stage renal disease within 3 yr.
- Membranous glomerulonephritis: prednisone 2 mg/kg/day may be useful in inducing remission. Cytotoxic agents can be added if there is poor response to prednisone.
- Membranoproliferative glomerulonephritis: most patients are treated with steroid therapy and antiplatelet drugs. Despite treatment, the majority of patients will progress to end-stage renal disease within 5 yr.

CHRONIC Rx
- Patients should be monitored for azotemia and should be aggressively treated for hypertension and hyperlipidemia. Furosemide is useful for severe edema. Anticoagulants may be necessary for thromboembolic events. Prophylactic anticoagulation should be considered in patients with membranous glomerulonephritis.
- Oral vitamin D is useful in the treatment of hypocalcemia (because of vitamin D loss).

REFERRAL
Nephrology consultation is recommended.

MISCELLANEOUS

COMMENTS
Patient education materials can be obtained from the National Kidney Foundation, 30 East 33rd Street, Suite 1100, New York, NY 10016.

REFERENCES
Dorhart EJ, Koomans HA: Understanding nephrotic syndrome: what's new in a decade? *Nephron* 70:1, 1995.

Korbet SM: The management of idiopathic nephrosis in adults including steroid-resistant nephrosis, *Curr Opin Nephrol Hypertens* 4:169, 1995.

Pauker SG, Kopelman RI: Hunting for the cause, how far to go? *N Engl J Med* 328:16, 1993.

Author: **Fred F. Ferri, M.D.**

Neuroblastoma

BASIC INFORMATION

DEFINITION
Neuroblastomas are neural tumors and abnormalities that have cell origins from the neural crest.

ICD-9-CM CODES
194.0 Neuroblastoma, unspecified site

EPIDEMIOLOGY AND DEMOGRAPHICS
INCIDENCE (IN U.S.): 8% of all solid tumors of childhood; 10 cases/1,000,000 children <15
PREDOMINANT SEX: Male:female ratio of 1:1.3
PEAK INCIDENCE: Childhood
PEAK AGE: Infants and children
GENETICS: N-*myc* proto-oncogene; loss of short arm chromosome 1 (1p36) found in some children

PHYSICAL FINDINGS
- Mass in abdomen, neck, or chest
- Spinal cord compression
- Dancing eyes
- Chronic pain
- Ecchymosis around eyes
- Weight loss
- Fever
- Irritability

ETIOLOGY
Tumor arises from neural crest, so gene abnormality is likely.

DIAGNOSIS

DIFFERENTIAL DIAGNOSIS
- Other childhood tumors
- Wilms' tumor

WORKUP
- Careful general physical examination
- Biopsy of tumor when possible
- Staging (Evans classification)
  I. Confined to single organ
  II. Extension beyond organ of origin but not past midline
  III. Extension across midline
  IV. Distant metastases

LABORATORY TESTS
- Urinary catecholamines
- Bone marrow aspiration

IMAGING STUDIES
CT scan or MRI of suspected affected area.

TREATMENT

NONPHARMACOLOGIC THERAPY
Assure patient that there is hope for recovery with aggressive treatment.

ACUTE GENERAL Rx
- Surgery
- Multiagent chemotherapy (e.g., cyclophosphamide, vincristine, dacarbazine, melphalan, doxorubicin, cisplatin)
- Radiotherapy

CHRONIC Rx
- The condition results in either death or cure.
- Overall survival is >40%
- Survival in Stage I is >95%, whereas survival in Stage II is <20%

DISPOSITION
Refer immediately to oncology team.

REFERRAL
If a multidisciplinary team is necessary

MISCELLANEOUS

COMMENTS
Children <1 yr with low-stage disease have 80% chance of survival; those with stage IV have 20% chance of survival.

REFERENCES
Ater JL: Neuroblastoma and brain tumors in childhood, *Am Acad Pediatr Dentistry* 17:4, 1995.
Humpl T: Neuroblastoma, *World J Urol* 13:233, 1995.
Phillip T: Overview of current treatment of neuroblastoma, *Am J Pediatr Hematol/Oncol* 14:97, 1992.

Author: **William H. Olson, M.D.**

Neuroleptic malignant syndrome

BASIC INFORMATION

DEFINITION
Neuroleptic malignant syndrome is an adverse reaction to dopamine-blocking neuroleptics characterized by hyperthermia, muscular rigidity, autonomic dysfunction, and altered consciousness.

SYNONYMS
Malignant hyperthermia

ICD-9-CM CODES
333.92 Neuroleptic malignant syndrome

EPIDEMIOLOGY AND DEMOGRAPHICS
INCIDENCE (IN U.S.): 0.5% to 1% of patients receiving neuroleptics
PREDOMINANT SEX: 2/3> of patients are male.
PREDOMINANT AGE: Young and middle-aged adults
PEAK INCIDENCE: 42 yr
GENETICS:
- Not applicable
- Malignant hyperthermia a familial disorder

PHYSICAL FINDINGS
- "Lead pipe" rigidity
- Hyperthermia (38.6° C to 42.3° C)
- Profuse sweating
- Tachycardia
- Labile BP
- Semicomatose

ETIOLOGY
- History of haloperidol use in 65% of cases
- History of combination drug therapy in 34% of cases
- Rare cases after withdrawal of dopamine agonists

DIAGNOSIS

DIFFERENTIAL DIAGNOSIS
- Heat stroke
- Catatonia
- Similar syndrome: possible complication of anesthesia, thyroid storm, toxins

WORKUP
Careful drug history

LABORATORY TESTS
- Elevated CPK
- Urinary myoglobin
- Leukocytosis
- Electrolytes
- Renal function
- Blood gases
- Drug levels

IMAGING STUDIES
None specific for this disease

TREATMENT

NONPHARMACOLOGIC THERAPY
- Respiratory support
- Careful intake and output monitoring
- Stop all neuroleptic agents

ACUTE GENERAL Rx
- Bromocriptine, a dopamine receptor agonist, is the mainstay of therapy for patients with neuroleptic malignant syndrome. Initial doses of 2.5 to 10 mg are given IV q8h and are increased by 5 mg/day until clinical improvement is seen. The drug should be continued for at least 10 days after the syndrome has been controlled and then tapered slowly.
- Dantrolene therapy is also effective. Initially, patients can be given 0.25 mg/kg IV q6-12h, followed by a maintenance dose up to 3 mg/kg/day. After 2 to 3 days, patients may be given the drug orally (25 to 600 mg/day in divided doses). Oral dantrolene therapy may need to be continued for several days.

CHRONIC Rx
- This is a potentially fatal disease, but most patients recover.
- Mortality rate is currently 10% to 20% despite above therapeutic measures.
- Factors adversely affecting mortality are develpment of renal failure and core temperature >104° (40°C).

DISPOSITION
Monitor closely for future complications of pharmacologic therapy.

REFERRAL
If patient's condition is critical; most patients treated in ICU.

MISCELLANEOUS

COMMENTS
Early detection and diagnosis lead to a more favorable outcome. Treatment is a medical emergency.

REFERENCES
Aiyer MK et al: Techniques for managing severe hyperthermia, *J Crit Illness* 10(9): 630, 1995.
Caroff SN, Mann SC: Neuroleptic malignant syndrome, *Med Clin North Am* 77:185, 1993.
De la Cour J: Neuroleptic malignant syndrome: do we know enough? *J Adv Nurs* 21:897, 1995.

Author: **William H. Olson, M.D.**

Nosocomial infections

BASIC INFORMATION

DEFINITION
Nosocomial infections (NI) are infections acquired as a result of hospitalization, generally after 48 hr of admission.

SYNONYMS
Hospital-acquired infections

EPIDEMIOLOGY AND DEMOGRAPHICS
INCIDENCE (IN U.S.):
- Approximately 1.8 to 4 million yearly in at least 5% of hospitalized patients
- Average extension of hospital stay by 4 days/patient (>6.4 million total days/yr)
- Directly account for 60,000 deaths/yr (indirectly for 80,000 deaths)
- Cost >$10 billion annually
- Similar in large and small hospitals

PREVALENCE (IN U.S.): 2 to 4 million cases/yr

PREDOMINANT SEX:
- Overall, approximately equal
- Elderly women: predominantly nosocomial urinary tract infections

PREDOMINANT AGE:
- Elderly patients (>60 yr old) at highest risk
- High-risk patients who may develop NI at any age:
  1. ICU
  2. Intubation
  3. Chronic lung disease
  4. Renal disease
  5. Comatose
  6. Chronic urethral or vascular catheterization
  7. Malnutrition
  8. Postoperative state

PEAK INCIDENCE: Varies widely with infection site

PHYSICAL FINDINGS
Vary with specific NI

ETIOLOGY
- Bacteria
- Fungi
- Viruses

SOURCES AND MODES OF TRANSMISSION:
1. Patient's own flora
   a. Comprised of resistant organisms acquired during hospitalization
   b. Frequently maintained thereafter by persistent GI colonization
2. Unwashed hands of staff
   a. Physicians
   b. Nurses
3. Invasion of protective defenses (intact skin, respiratory cilia, urinary sphincters, and mucosa)
   a. IV lines
   b. Catheters
   c. Respiratory equipment
   d. Surgical wounds
   e. Scopes and other imaging devices
4. Failure to provide adequate negative pressure, high-volume air flow chambers for respiratory isolation of patients with TB
5. Failure to rapidly identify and provide appropriate care (with isolation or precautions) for patients with communicable diseases
6. Inanimate environment
7. Food
8. Fomites

RISKS AMPLIFIED:
1. Use of broad-spectrum antibiotics
   a. Select highly resistant bacteria
   b. Establish highly resistant bacteria as endemic flora in microenvironments within the hospital
2. Highly vulnerable patients with specific risk factors
   a. Immunosuppression (as a result of therapy, transplantation, AIDS)
   b. Old age
   c. Postsurgery
   d. Prolonged surgery
   e. Chronic lung disease
   f. Ventilator dependence
   g. Antacid therapy
   h. Vascular lines
   i. Hyperalimentation
   j. ICU stay
   k. Recent antibiotic therapy
3. Clustering of seriously ill patients
   a. Often with wounds or drainage of contaminated materials
   b. Intensifying probability of cross-infection

HAND WASHING BETWEEN ALL PATIENT CONTACTS: Single most important method of decreasing NI
1. Regular soap
2. Chlorhexidine for MRSA (Methicillin-resistant *Staphylococcus aureus*) and other resistant gram-positive organisms
3. Iodophor for resistant gram-negative organisms
4. Purpose
   a. Degrease hand surfaces
   b. Wash away oils and associated bacteria
5. Procedure
   a. Lukewarm water
   b. Must include all surfaces
   c. Special attention to areas between fingers and to the dirtier dominant hand (most people reflexively wash their cleaner, nondominant hand more vigorously)

VANCOMYCIN-RESISTANT *ENTEROCOCCUS FAECIUM* (VREF):
1. Highly resistant to most antibiotics
2. Selected by overuse of broad-spectrum antibiotics
   a. Third-generation cephalosporins
   b. Vancomycin
3. Threatens patients in ICUs and other closed environments within hospitals
4. Infections
   a. Highly invasive
   b. Aggressive
   c. Often untreatable
   d. Fatal
5. Control measures
   a. Aggressive isolation of colonized and infected patients
   b. Restraint in using broad-spectrum antibiotics

CLOSTRIDIUM DIFFICILE:
1. Causes diarrhea as a result of pseudomembranous colitis
2. May be transmitted among hospitalized patients
3. Warrants stool (contact) precautions

SURVEILLANCE:
1. Crucial for early identification of infections
   a. Enabling immediate intervention
   b. Education
2. Prospective, concurrent, total hospital surveillance
   a. Provides most complete data
   b. Feasible with sophisticated computerized data collection and analysis
3. Daily plotting of all infections on comprehensive wall maps
   a. Including all beds on all wards
   b. Enhances immediate recognition of microclusters of infections by body site and by organism
   c. Facilitates proper early control of potential outbreaks

DIAGNOSIS

MOST COMMON NI:
- Urinary tract infections (40% to 45%)
- Surgical wound and other soft-tissue infections (25% to 30%)

- Pneumonia (15% to 20%)
- Bacteremia (5% to 12%)

NOSOCOMIAL URINARY TRACT INFECTIONS:
- General associations
  1. Foley catheters
  2. Inappropriate catheter care (including opening catheter junctions)
  3. Female sex
  4. Absence of systemic antibiotics
- Physical findings
  1. Fever
  2. Dysuria
  3. Leukocytosis
  4. Pyuria
  5. Flank or costovertebral angle tenderness
- Usual organisms:
  1. *E. coli*
  2. *Klebsiella*
  3. *Enterobacter*
  4. *Pseudomonas*
  5. *Enterococcus*
- Sepsis in 1% to 3% of nosocomial UTIs
- Approximately 10,000 annual deaths
- Prevention
  1. Meticulous technique during insertion and daily perineal care
  2. Never open the catheter-collection tubing junction
  3. Obtain all specimens using sterile syringe
  4. Substitute intermittent catheterization for Foley catheters
  5. Avoid urine-soaked diapers

NOSOCOMIAL BACTEREMIAS:
- General associations:
  1. IV lines
  2. Arterial lines
  3. CVP lines
  4. Phlebitis
  5. Hyperalimentation
- Fever possibly only presenting sign
- Exit site of all vascular lines carefully evaluated for:
  1. Erythema
  2. Induration
  3. Tenderness
  4. Purulent drainage
- Usual organisms:
  1. *S. aureus*
  2. *Enterococcus*
  3. *Enterobacter*
  4. *Klebsiella*
  5. *Candida* spp.
  6. Occasional coagulase-negative staphylococci
- Phlebitis in 1.3 million patients yearly
- Approximately 10,000 annual deaths from IV sepsis
- Prevention
  1. Meticulous sterile technique during IV insertion
  2. Change needle and lines q72h
  3. Use stainless steel butterfly rather than plastic catheters when feasible
  4. Decrease use of routine IVs (patients would rather drink)

NOSOCOMIAL PNEUMONIAS:
- Rare on hospital wards
- More common in ICUs
- General associations:
  1. Aspiration
  2. Intubation
  3. Altered consciousness
  4. Old age
  5. Chronic lung disease
  6. Postsurgery
  7. Antacids
- Signs of pneumonia common among patients on general wards:
  1. Cough
  2. Sputum
  3. Fever
  4. Leukocytosis
  5. New infiltrate on chest x-ray examination
- Signs more subtle in ICUs, since many patients have purulent sputum because of chronic intubation
  1. Change in sputum character or volume
  2. Small changes on chest x-ray examination
- Usual organisms:
  1. *Klebsiella*
  2. *Acinetobacter*
  3. *Enterobacter*
  4. *Pseudomonas aeruginosa*
  5. *S. aureus*
- Less common organisms:
  1. MRSA
  2. *Legionella, Flavobacterium*
  3. Respiratory syncytial virus (infants)
  4. Adenovirus
- 1% of hospitalized patients affected
- Mortality rate high (40%)
- Prevention
  1. Meticulous sterile technique during suctioning and handling airway
  2. Change tubing q72h
  3. Drain respirator tubing without allowing fluid to return to respirator
  4. Hand washing routinely to prevent colonization of patients and transfer of organisms among patients

NOSOCOMIAL SOFT-TISSUE INFECTIONS:
- Associations
  1. Decubitus ulcers
  2. Surgical wound classification (contaminated or dirty-infected)
  3. Abdominal surgery
  4. Presence of drain
  5. Preoperative length of stay
  6. Duration of surgery >2 hr
  7. Surgeon
  8. Presence of other infection
- Physical findings
  1. Decubitus ulcer with fluctuance at margin or under firm eschar
  2. Erythema extending >2 cm beyond margin of surgical wound
  3. Tenderness
  4. Induration
  5. Erythema
  6. Fluctuance
  7. Purulent drainage
  8. Dehiscence of sutures
- Usual organisms
  1. *S. aureus*
  2. *Enterococcus*
  3. *Enterobacter*
  4. *Acinetobacter*
  5. *E. coli*
- Prevention
  1. Careful skin care and frequent, proper positioning of patient to prevent decubitus ulcer
  2. Meticulous sterile surgical technique
  3. Hand washing to decrease colonization when handling postoperative wound
  4. Limit prophylactic antibiotics to 24 hr perioperatively

5. Double-wrap contaminated dressings (hold in gloved hand and evert gloves over dressings) before disposal

LABORATORY TESTS
- Appropriate to specific NI and specific patient's condition
- Cultures generally indicated for proper confirmation of responsible pathogens
  1. Urine
  2. Blood
  3. Sputum
  4. Soft-tissue infection
- Molecular analysis of nosocomial epidemics
  1. Plasmid fingerprinting
  2. Restriction endonuclease digestion (plasmid and genomic DNA)
  3. Peptide analysis by SDS-PAGE
  4. Immunoblotting
  5. Ribosomal (rRNA) typing
  6. DNA probes
  7. Multilocus enzyme electrophoresis
  8. Restriction fragment length polymorphism (RFLP)
  9. Polymerase chain reaction (PCR)
  10. Provide confirmation of point-source or common strains
  11. Offer occasionally indispensable corroboration of hypotheses reached utilizing classic epidemiology

IMAGING STUDIES
Rarely needed for diagnosis of NI

TREATMENT

ACUTE GENERAL Rx
- Appropriate to etiologic organism:
  1. Antibiotic
  2. Antifungal
  3. Antiviral
- Specific therapy determined after careful consideration of resident flora within the microenvironment in which the patient was hospitalized
1. Empiric therapy
  a. Frequently difficult to accurately fashion
  b. Often undesirable, unless the patient's clinical condition requires urgent treatment
2. Consultation for expert advice regarding antibiotic selection in view of known epidemiologic risks within the hospital
  a. Nosocomial infection control nurses
  b. Hospital epidemiologist
- Avoid unnecessary treatment for organisms that are colonizing but not infecting patients
- Prevention of spread of communicable diseases often requiring Isolation or Precautions
  1. Classic Schema (Strict, Respiratory Isolation and Contact [Skin and Wound] Precautions) being replaced by more streamlined Revised Guidelines (Airborne, Droplet, Contact Isolation Precautions)
  2. Less careful response to some diseases (e.g., hemorrhagic fevers) inadvertently induced by removal of strict isolation category
  3. Universal/Standard Precautions and Body Substance Isolation continue within a new Standard Isolation Precautions Guideline
- Universal Precautions used for all patients during all contacts with blood, body fluids, or secretions
  1. Gloves
  2. Goggles
  3. Impermeable gowns if aerosol or splash is likely
- Consider aggressive isolation to restrict spread of resistant organisms and their plasmids
  1. MRSA
  2. VREF
  3. Highly resistant gram-negative organisms

REFERRAL
- To nosocomial infection control nurses
- To hospital epidemiologist

MISCELLANEOUS

COMMENTS
- Sharps and splash injuries to staff relatively are rare, but nearly all are preventable.
  1. Nurses obtain most injuries
  2. Usual causes:
    a. Needle-sticks
    b. Scalpel and surgical needle injuries
    c. Blood splashes
  3. Prevention
    a. Never recap needles
    b. Needle disposal only in rigid, impermeable plastic containers
    c. Clearly announce instrument passes in operating room or during procedures and use passing trays
    d. Gloves and goggles if aerosol or splash is likely
    e. Never leave needles or other sharp items in beds
    f. Never dispose of sharp items in regular trash bags
  4. Infection control staff should be consulted immediately after exposure to determine need for prophylaxis for Hepatitis B or HIV.
  5. All staff should be immune to hepatitis B (natural or vaccine).
- Fungi previously considered to be contaminants now risks for patients with cancer and organ transplantation
  1. *Candida* spp.
    a. *C. guilliermondi*
    b. *C. krusei*
    c. *C. parapsilosis*
    d. *C. tropicalis*
  2. *Aspergillus* spp.
  3. *Curvularia* spp.
  4. *Bipolaris* spp.
  5. *Exserohilum* spp.
  6. *Alternaria* spp.
  7. *Fusarium* spp.
  8. *Scopulariopsis* spp.
  9. *Pseudallescheria boydii*
  10. *Trichosporon beigelii*
  11. *Malassezia furfur*
  12. *Hensenula* spp.
  13. *Microsporum canis*
- Focused, committed efforts by the entire health care staff continuously directed toward prevention
  1. Each NI addressed as an opportunity to improve the organization and delivery of care
  2. Essential that individual staff members understand that small risks applied to large populations result in a large number of total events (e.g., NI)

REFERENCES
Garner J et al: Guideline for isolation precautions in hospitals, *Inf Control Hosp Epidemiol* 17:53, 1996.
Author: **Peter Nicholas, M.D.**

CLINICAL TOPICS **Obsessive-compulsive disorder** *(PTG)* 325

BASIC INFORMATION

DEFINITION
Obsessive-compulsive disorder (OCD) involves recurrent obsessions (intrusive and inappropriate thoughts, impulses, or images) or compulsions (behaviors or mental acts performed in response to obsessions or rigid application of rules) that consume >1 hr/day or cause impairment or distress.

SYNONYMS
Abortive insanity

ICD-9-CM CODES
F42.8 Obsessive-compulsive disorder (DSM-IV 300.3)

EPIDEMIOLOGY AND DEMOGRAPHICS
PREVALENCE (IN U.S.): 1% to 2% of adults
PREDOMINANT SEX: Approximately equal distribution between sexes.
PREDOMINANT AGE:
- Modal age of onset for females is between 20 and 29 yr.
- Modal age of onset for males is between 6 and 15 yr.
- Condition is chronic.

PEAK INCIDENCE: Mean age of onset is 19.6 yr of age.
GENETICS:
- There is no clear genetic pattern.
- Rate of concordance is higher in monozygotic (33%) vs. dizygotic (7%) twins.
- Rate of disorder is also higher in first-degree relatives of individuals with OCD and Tourette's disorder than the general population.

PHYSICAL FINDINGS
- Persistent and recurrent intrusive and ego-dystonic obsessive ideas, thoughts, impulses, or images that are perceived as alien and beyond one's control.
- Frequent experiencing of obsessions related to contamination (e.g., when using the telephone), excessive doubt (e.g., was the door locked), organization (the need for a particular order), violent impulses (e.g., to yell obscenities in church), or intrusive sexual imagery.
- Obsessions possibly leading to compulsive behaviors (e.g., repeated hand washing, checking, rearranging), or mental tasks (e.g., counting, repeating phrases).
- Obsessions and compulsions almost always accompanied with high anxiety and subjective distress.

ETIOLOGY
- In the past, OCD was seen in context of the psychoanalytic theory in which obsessions and compulsions were viewed as arrest of psychosexual development in the anal stage, perhaps secondary to excessively restrictive or punitive parenting.
- Disorder now seen as a biologic condition closely linked with learning disabilities and Tourette's disorder.
- Serotonergic pathways believed important in some ritualistic instinctual behaviors, with dysfunction of these pathways possibly giving rise to OCD.

DIAGNOSIS

DIFFERENTIAL DIAGNOSIS
- Other psychiatric disorders in which obsessive thoughts occur (e.g., body dysmorphic disorder or phobias).
- Other conditions in which compulsive behaviors are seen (e.g., trichotillomania).
- Major depression, hypochondriasis, and several anxiety disorders with predominant obsessions or compulsions; however, in these disorders the thoughts are not anxiety provoking or are extremes of normal concern.
- Delusions or psychosis, which may be mistaken for obsessive thoughts; distinguished from OCD in that the individual recognizes the ideas are not real.
- Tics and stereotypic movements that appear compulsive but are not driven by the desire to neutralize an obsession.
- Paraphilias or pathologic gambling; distinguished from compulsions in that they are usually enjoyable.

WORKUP
- Careful history leading to diagnosis
- Neurologic examination to rule out concomitant Tourette's or other tic disorder
- In adolescents and children: psychologic testing to reveal learning disabilities

LABORATORY TESTS
No specific tests are indicated.

IMAGING STUDIES
- No specific studies are indicated.
- There have been research reports of reversible abnormalities on PET scans.

TREATMENT

NONPHARMACOLOGIC THERAPY
Behavioral therapies are often quite helpful, but success is often greater for compulsions than for obsessions.

ACUTE GENERAL Rx
None

CHRONIC Rx
- Antidepressants with serotonergic reuptake blockade, including fluoxetine, clomipramine, fluvoxamine, paroxetine, and sertraline (see Table 7-7)
- No response in only 15% of patients
- Indefinite treatment

DISPOSITION
- OCD is a chronic condition with a waxing and waning course.
- Exacerbations are usually associated with stress.
- When untreated, 15% of patients progressively deteriorate in function.

REFERRAL
- If distinction from other psychiatric conditions, particularly delusional disorder, is not clear
- If patient refractory to treatment
- If treatment with antidepressants is problematic (e.g., when comorbid with bipolar illness)

MISCELLANEOUS

REFERENCES
Casey DA: Obsessive-compulsive disorder, *Postgrad Med* 91:171, 1992.
Greist JH: Medication management of obsessive-compulsive disorder, *Today's Ther Trends* 7:29, 1990.
Author: **Rif S. El-Mallakh, M.D.**

Ocular foreign body

BASIC INFORMATION

DEFINITION
The term *ocular foreign body* refers to a foreign body on the surface of the corneal epithelium.

ICD-9-CM CODES
930 Foreign body in external eye

EPIDEMIOLOGY AND DEMOGRAPHICS
INCIDENCE (IN U.S.): Universal, with a predominance in active people
PREDOMINANT SEX: Perhaps slightly more common in men
PREDOMINANT AGE: Childhood through active adult years
PEAK INCIDENCE: Childhood through active adult years

PHYSICAL FINDINGS
Most common foreign bodies:
- Grinding
- Drilling
- Auto mechanics
- Working beneath cars
- Airborne particles blown by fans, etc.

DIAGNOSIS

DIFFERENTIAL DIAGNOSIS
- Corneal abrasion
- Corneal ulceration
- Glaucoma
- Herpes ulcers
- Infection
- Other keratitis

WORKUP
Fluorescein stain, slit lamp examination if no foreign body is found

LABORATORY TESTS
Intraocular pressure to make certain that eye has not been penetrated

IMAGING STUDIES
Occasionally, MRI of the orbits to identify foreign bodies not found by other means

TREATMENT

NONPHARMACOLOGIC THERAPY
Remove foreign body.

ACUTE GENERAL Rx
- Saline irrigation
- Removal of foreign body with moist cotton-tipped applicator after instillation of topical anesthetic drops
- Cycloplegics, antibiotics, and pressure dressing after removal of foreign body

DISPOSITION
If symptoms persist 24 hr after examination, refer to an ophthalmologist.

REFERRAL
To ophthalmology within 24 hr if patient not completely comfortable

MISCELLANEOUS

COMMENTS
Alkaline or acidic chemical foreign bodies can be dangerous and pH test must be performed if either of these are suspected (for all chemical foreign bodies).

REFERENCES
Holt GR, Holt JE: Management of orbital trauma and foreign bodies, *Otolaryngol Clin North Am* 21:35, 1988.
Silverman H, Nunez L: Treatment of common eye emergencies, *Am Fam Physician* 45:2279, 1992.

Author: **Melvyn Koby, M.D.**

Optic atrophy

BASIC INFORMATION

DEFINITION
Optic atrophy refers to the degeneration of the optic nerve, which can have many causes.

SYNONYMS
Bilateral optic atrophy
Unilateral optic atrophy

ICD-9-CM CODES
377.10 Atrophy, optic nerve

EPIDEMIOLOGY AND DEMOGRAPHICS
PREDOMINANT SEX: From head injury, most common in males
PREDOMINANT AGE: 21 to 40 yr
PEAK INCIDENCE: All ages, depending on etiology

PHYSICAL FINDINGS
- At first, the temporal part of optic disc is pale; later it appears "porcelain white."
- Unilateral lesion produces a Marcus-Gunn pupil.
- Decreased visual acuity and central scatoma are noted.

ETIOLOGY
- Optic neuritis
- Ischemia (embolus, temporal arteritis)
- Compression
- Inflammation
- Hereditary
- Toxic metabolic
- Head injury

DIAGNOSIS

DIFFERENTIAL DIAGNOSIS
- Nutritional, toxic, and hereditary causes are usually bilateral.
- Unilateral optic atrophy in a young person is usually MS.
- Postviral atrophy is seen in childhood.

WORKUP
- Skin examination for evidence of phakomatoses
- Visual evoked responses

LABORATORY TESTS
- Depends on suspected etiology: none for trauma, tumor, MS
- Autoimmune diseases: ESR, ANA, etc.

IMAGING STUDIES
MRI with special cuts through orbits to identify compressive lesions or MS

TREATMENT

NONPHARMACOLOGIC THERAPY
None

ACUTE GENERAL Rx
Treat underlying cause (e.g., operation is indicated if tumor is identified.)

CHRONIC Rx
The optic nerve does not regenerate.

DISPOSITION
- Visual loss occurs over weeks to months.
- Usually, follow-up by neurologist or ophthalmologist

REFERRAL
If tumor is found

MISCELLANEOUS

COMMENTS
- Every physician should be able to identify pale optic discs and Marcus-Gunn pupil, which are important in identifying this condition.
- Patient education material can be obtained from the National Eye Institute, Department of Health and Human Services, 9000 Rockville Pike, Bethesda, MD 20892.

REFERENCES
Menon V, Sharma P, Chhabra VK: An etiological profile of optic atrophy, *Acta Ophthalmol* 70:725, 1992.

Author: **William H. Olson, M.D.**

Optic neuritis

BASIC INFORMATION

DEFINITION
Optic neuritis is an inflammation of one or both optic nerves resulting in a temporary reduction of visual function.

SYNONYMS
Optic neuropathy
Optic papillitis
Retrobulbar neuritis

ICD-9-CM CODES
377.3 Optic neuritis

EPIDEMIOLOGY AND DEMOGRAPHICS
INCIDENCE (IN U.S.): Relatively common
PREVALENCE (IN U.S.): Relatively rare
PREDOMINANT SEX: Female
PEAK INCIDENCE: Rare in children and patients >45 yr old
PEAK AGE: 20s and 30s
GENETICS:
- MS more common in patients with certain HLA blood type

PHYSICAL FINDINGS
- Marcus-Gunn pupil (swing flashlight eye to eye—abnormal pupil appears to dilate to direct light)
- Decreased visual acuity
- Visual field abnormalities
- Normal optic disc
- Pain on movement of affected eye

ETIOLOGY
Multiple sclerosis

DIAGNOSIS

DIFFERENTIAL DIAGNOSIS
- Giant cell arteritis
- Ischemic optic atrophy
- Diabetic papillopathy
- Leber's optic neuropathy
- Optic drusen
- Acute papilledema
- Toxic/nutritional optic neuropathy

WORKUP
General physical examination should be normal.

LABORATORY TESTS
- Depends on history
- CBC, ANA, ESR, VDRL
- Possibly HIV testing
- Possibly Lyme disease test
- Possibly sarcoidosis testing (chest x-ray examination, ABS)

IMAGING STUDIES
If MS suspected, MRI may show evidence of other lesions.

TREATMENT

NONPHARMACOLOGIC THERAPY
Assure patient that vision will return.

ACUTE GENERAL Rx
A short course of steroids (e.g., prednisone 1 mg/kg/day for 10 to 14 days, then tapered over 2 wk) may hasten recovery.

CHRONIC Rx
Full visual acuity usually returns in 6 mo.

DISPOSITION
Follow visual acuity weekly until vision improves.

REFERRAL
If patient has other neurologic signs, such as proptosis or tender temporal artery, if onset is gradual, and if vision does not improve after several weeks

MISCELLANEOUS

COMMENTS
- Unilateral optic neuritis is MS until proven otherwise; two thirds of patients will develop MS in 15 yr.
- Patient eduction materials can be obtained from the National Eye Institute, Department of Health and Human Services, 9000 Rockville Pike, Bethesda, MD 20892.

REFERENCES
Newman NJ: Optic neuropathy, *Neurology* 46:315, 1996.
Optic Neuritis Study Group: The clinical profile of optic neuritis, *Arch Ophthalmol* 109:1673, 1991.
Rizzo JF, Lessel S: Optic neuritis and ischemic optic neuropathy, *Arch Ophthalmol* 109:1668, 1991.
Sedwick LA: Optic neuritis, *Neurol Clin* 9:97, 1991.
Author: **William H. Olson, M.D.**

Osgood-Schlatter disease (PTG)

BASIC INFORMATION

DEFINITION
Osgood-Schlatter disease is a painful swelling of the tibial tuberosity that occurs in adolescence.

ICD-9-CM CODES
732.4 Osgood-Schlatter disease

EPIDEMIOLOGY AND DEMOGRAPHICS
PREVALENCE: 4 cases/100 adolescents
PREDOMINANT AGE: 11 to 15 yr (bilateral in 20%)
PREDOMINANT SEX: Male:female ratio of 3:1

PHYSICAL FINDINGS
- Pain at the tibial tubercle that is aggravated by activity, especially stair-walking and squatting
- Tender swelling and enlargement of the tibial tubercle
- Increased pain with knee extension against resistance

ETIOLOGY
- Unknown
- May be traumatically induced inflammation

DIAGNOSIS

DIFFERENTIAL DIAGNOSIS
- Referred hip pain (any child with hip pain should have a thorough clinical hip examination)
- Patellar tendinitis

WORKUP
In most cases, the diagnosis is obvious on a clinical basis.

IMAGING STUDIES
- Lateral roentgenogram of the upper portion of the tibia with the leg slightly internally rotated may reveal variable degrees of separation and fragmentation of the upper tibial epiphysis.
- Occasionally, fragmented area fails to unite to the tibia and persists into adulthood.

TREATMENT

ACUTE GENERAL Rx
- Ice, especially after exercise
- NSAIDs
- Gentle hamstring and quadriceps stretching exercises
- Abstinence from physical activity
- Temporary immobilization in a knee splint for 2 to 4 wk in resistant cases

DISPOSITION
- Prognosis for complete restoration of function and relief from pain is excellent.
- Condition usually heals when the epiphysis closes.
- Complications are rare.
- Symptoms in the adult:
  1. Unusual but prominence of the tibial tubercle is usually permanent
  2. May be more susceptible to local irritation, especially when kneeling
  3. Rarely, nonunion of the epiphyseal fragment, but it is usually asymptomatic
  4. Surgery rarely required

REFERRAL
For orthopedic consultation when diagnosis is uncertain or when symptoms persist

MISCELLANEOUS

REFERENCES
Stanitski CL: Anterior knee pain syndromes in the adolescent, *J Bone Joint Surg* 75(A)1407, 1993.

Author: **Lonnie R. Mercier, M.D.**

Osteoarthritis (PTG)

BASIC INFORMATION

DEFINITION
Osteoarthritis is a joint condition in which degeneration and loss of articular cartilage occurs, leading to pain and deformity. Two forms are usually recognized, primary (idiopathic) and secondary. The primary form may be localized or generalized.

SYNONYMS
Degenerative joint disease
Osteoarthrosis
Arthrosis

ICD-9-CM CODES
715.0 Osteoarthrosis and allied disorders

EPIDEMIOLOGY AND DEMOGRAPHICS
PREVALENCE: 2% to 6% of general population
PREDOMINANT SEX: Female = male
PREDOMINANT AGE: >50 yr

PHYSICAL FINDINGS
- Similar symptoms in most forms: stiffness, pain, and crepitus
- Joint tenderness, swelling
- Decreased range of motion
- Crepitus with motion
- Bony hypertrophy
- Pain with range of motion
- DIP joint involvement possibly leading to development of nodular swellings called Heberden's nodes
- PIP joint involvement possibly leading to development of nodular swellings called Bouchard's nodes

ETIOLOGY
Primary osteoarthritis is of unknown cause. Secondary osteoarthritis may result from a number of disorders including trauma, metabolic conditions, and other forms of arthritis.

DIAGNOSIS

DIFFERENTIAL DIAGNOSIS
- Bursitis, tendinitis
- Radicular spine pain
- Inflammatory arthritides
- Infectious arthritis

WORKUP
- No diagnostic test exists for degenerative joint disease.
- Laboratory evaluation is normal.
- Rheumatoid factor, ESR, CBC, and ANA tests may be required if inflammatory component is present.
- Synovial fluid examination is generally normal.

IMAGING STUDIES
- Roentgenographic evaluation reveals:
  1. Joint space narrowing
  2. Subchondral sclerosis
  3. New bone formation in the form of osteophytes
- When knee is involved, standing AP x-ray

TREATMENT

ACUTE GENERAL Rx
- Rest, restricted use or weight bearing, and heat
- Walking aids such as a cane (often helpful for weight bearing joints)
- Suitable footwear
- Gentle range of motion and strengthening exercise
- Local creams and linaments to provide a counterirritant affect
- Education, reassurance

PHARMACOLOGIC THERAPY
- Mild analgesics for joint pain
- NSAIDs if inflammation is present
- Occasional local corticosteroid injections
- Mild antidepressants, especially at night, if depression is present

DISPOSITION
Progression is not always inevitable, and the prognosis is variable depending on the site and extent of the disease.

REFERRAL
Surgical consultation for patients not responding to medical management

MISCELLANEOUS

COMMENTS
Surgical intervention is generally helpful in degenerative joint disease. Arthroplasty, arthrodesis, and realignment osteotomy are the most common procedures performed.

REFERENCES
Alexander CJ: Osteoarthritis: a review of old myths and current concepts, *Skeletal Radiol* 19:327, 1990.
Altman R et al: Development of criteria for the classification and reporting of osteoarthritis of the knee, *Arthritis Rheum* 29:1039, 1986.
Dieppe P: Drug treatment of osteoarthritis, *J Bone Joint Surg* (B) 673, 1993.
Harris C: Osteoarthritis: how to diagnose and treat the painful joint, *Geriatrics* 48:39, 1993.

Author: **Lonnie R. Mercier, M.D.**

BASIC INFORMATION

DEFINITION
Osteochondritis dissecans is a disorder in which a portion of cartilage and underlying subchondral bone separates from a joint surface and may even become detached.

SYNONYMS
Osteochondrosis
Talar dome fracture: commonly used in describing the lesion of the talus

ICD-9-CM CODES
732.7 Osteochondritis dissecans

EPIDEMIOLOGY AND DEMOGRAPHICS
PREVALENCE: 0.3 cases/1000 persons
PREVALENT AGE: Onset at 10 to 30 yr
PREVALENT SEX: Male:female ratio of 3:1
The most common joint affected is the knee with the lateral surface of the medial femoral condyle the most frequent area involved. The capitellum of the humerus, dome of the talus, shoulder, and hip may also be affected.

PHYSICAL FINDINGS
- Pain, stiffness, and swelling
- Intermittent locking if the fragment becomes detached
- Occasionally palpable loose body
- Tenderness at the site of the lesion
- When the knee is involved, positive Wilson's sign (pain with knee extension and internal rotation)
- Some asymptomatic cases

ETIOLOGY
Unknown

DIAGNOSIS

DIFFERENTIAL DIAGNOSIS
- Acute fracture
- Neoplasm

IMAGING STUDIES
- Plain roentgenography to confirm the diagnosis
- "Tunnel view" helpful in knee cases
- Typical finding: radiolucent, semilunar line outlining the oval fragment of bone (but findings variable, depending on the amount of healing and stability)
- MRI or bone scanning usually not necessary in establishing diagnosis but helpful in determining prognosis and management, especially with regards to the stability of the lesion

TREATMENT

ACUTE GENERAL Rx
- Observation every 4 to 6 mo for patients in whom the lesion is asymptomatic
- Symptomatic patients who are skeletally immature:
  1. Observation with an initial period of non–weight-bearing for 6 to 8 wk
  2. When symptoms subside, gradual resumption of activities

DISPOSITION
- Juvenile cases with open epiphyses have a favorable prognosis.
- Cases developing after skeletal maturity are more likely to develop osteoarthritis.
- Large fragments, especially those in weight-bearing areas, have a more unfavorable prognosis, especially if they involve the lateral femoral condyle.
- Loose body formation and degenerative joint disease are more common when condition develops after age 20 yr.

REFERRAL
For orthopedic consultation:
1. For most adults with unstable lesions
2. If a loose body is present
3. If symptomatic care has failed

MISCELLANEOUS

COMMENTS
- Although inflammation is suggested by the name, it has not been shown to be of significance in this disorder. "Osteochondral lesion" or "osteochondrosis dissecans" may be more appropriate terms to describe these disorders.
- Repetitive trauma with ischemic necrosis is the most likely cause.
- The condition is often bilateral, especially in the knee, which could suggest the possibility of an endocrine or genetic basis.
- This condition should always be considered in the patient whose "sprained ankle" does not improve over the usual course of treatment.

REFERENCES
Cahill BR: Osteochondritis dissecans of the knee: treatment of juvenile and adult forms, *J Am Acad Orthop Surg* 3:237, 1995.
Stone JW: Osteochondral lesions of the talar dome, *J Am Acad Orthop Surg* 4:63, 1996.

Author: **Lonnie R. Mercier, M.D.**

Osteomyelitis (PTG)

BASIC INFORMATION

DEFINITION
Osteomyelitis is an acute or chronic infection of the bone secondary to the hematogenous or contiguous source of infection or direct traumatic inoculation, which is usually bacterial.

SYNONYMS
Bone infection

ICD-9-CM CODES
730.1 Chronic osteomyelitis
730.2 Acute or subacute osteomyelitis

EPIDEMIOLOGY AND DEMOGRAPHICS
PREDOMINANT SEX: Male > female
PREDOMINANT AGE: All ages

PHYSICAL FINDINGS
HEMATOGENOUS OSTEOMYELITIS: Usually occurs in tibia/fibula (children).
- Localized inflammation: often secondary to trauma with accompanying hematoma or cellulitis
- Abrupt fever
- Lethargy
- Irritability
- Pain in involved bone

VERTEBRAL OSTEOMYELITIS: Usually hematogenous.
- Fever: 50%
- Localized pain/tenderness
- Neurologic defects: motor/sensory

CONTIGUOUS OSTEOMYELITIS: Direct inoculation.
- Associated with trauma, fractures, surgical fixation
- Chronic infection of skin/soft tissue
- Fever, drainage from surgical site

CHRONIC OSTEOMYELITIS:
- Bone pain
- Sinus tract drainage, nonhealing ulcer
- Chronic low-grade fever
- Chronic localized pain

ETIOLOGY
- *Staphylococcus aureus*
- *S. aureus* (methicillin-resistant)
- *Pseudomonas aeruginosa*
- Enterobacteriaceae
- *S. pyogenes*
- *Enterococcus*
- *Mycobacteria*
- Fungi
- Coagulase negative staphylococci
- Salmonella (in sickle cell disease)

DIAGNOSIS

DIFFERENTIAL DIAGNOSIS
- Brodie's abscess
- Gaucher's disease
- Bone infarction
- Charcot's joint
- Gout
- Fracture

WORKUP
- ESR, C-reactive protein
- Blood culturing
- Bone culture
- Pathologic evaluation of bone biopsy for acute/chronic changes consistent with necrosis or acute inflammation

IMAGING STUDIES
- Bone x-ray examination
- Bone scan
- Gallium scan
- Indium scan
- MRI (most accurate imaging study)
- Doppler studies: useful in patients with peripheral vascular disease to determine vascular adequacy

TREATMENT

Surgical debridement in biopsy-positive cases will give direction for antibiotic therapy. This will vary with type of osteomyelitis. Duration of therapy is usually 6 wk for acute osteomyelitis, chronic osteomyelitis may need a longer course of medication.
- *S. aureus*: cefazolin IV, nafcillin IV, vancomycin IV (in patient allergic to penicillin)
- *S. aureus* (methicillin resistant): vancomycin IV
- *Streptococcus* sp.: cefazolin or ceftriaxone
- *P. aeruginosa*: piperacillin plus aminoglycoside or ceftazidime plus aminoglycoside
- Enterobacteriaceae: ceftriaxone or fluoroquinolone
- Hyperbaric oxygen therapy: may be useful in treatment of chronic osteomyelitis, especially with associated wound healing
- Surgical debridement of all devitalized bone and tissue
- Immobilization of affected bone (plaster, traction) if bone is unstable
- Bone grafts using a vascularized or open graft may be necessary if the remaining bone is inadequate

MISCELLANEOUS

REFERENCES
Haas DW, McAndrew MP: Bacterial osteomyelitis in adults: evolving considerations in diagnosis and treatment, *Am J Med* 101:550, 1996.

Mader JI, Calhoun J: Osteomyelitis. In Mandell GL, Bennett JE, Dolin R: *Mandell, Douglas, and Bennett's principles and practice of infectious diseases*, ed 4, New York, 1995, Churchill Livingstone.

Author: **Dennis J. Mikolich, M.D.**

CLINICAL TOPICS   Osteoporosis (PTG) 333

BASIC INFORMATION

DEFINITION
Osteoporosis is characterized by a progressive decrease in bone mass that results in increased bone fragility and a higher fracture risk. The various types are as follows:
PRIMARY OSTEOPOROSIS: 80% of women and 60% of men with osteoporosis
- Idiopathic osteoporosis: unknown pathogenesis; may occur in children and young adults
- Type I osteoporosis: may occur in postmenopausal women (age range: 51 to 75 yr); characterized by accelerated and disproportionate trabecular bone loss and associated with vertebral body and distal forearm fractures (estrogen withdrawal effect)
- Type II osteoporosis (involutional): occurs in both men and women >70 yr of age; characterized by both trabecular and cortical bone loss, and associated with fractures of the proximal humerus and tibia, femoral neck, and pelvis

SECONDARY OSTEOPOROSIS: 20% of women and 40% of men with osteoporosis; osteoporosis that exists as a common feature of another disease process, heritable disorder of connective tissue or drug side effect (see "Differential Diagnosis")

ICD-9-CM CODES
733.0 Osteoporosis

EPIDEMIOLOGY AND DEMOGRAPHICS
PREVALENCE (IN U.S.):
- Approximately 25 million men and women
- Twice as common in women
- Results in 1.5 million fractures annually (70% women)
- Osteoporosis-related fractures in 50% women and 20% men >65 yr
- Results: institutionalization, mortality, and costs in excess of $10 billion annually

RISK FACTORS:
- Age: each decade after 40 yr associated with a fivefold increase risk
- Genetics:
  1. Ethnicity (Caucasian/Oriental > black > Polynesian)
  2. Gender (female > male)
  3. Family history
- Environmental factors: poor nutrition, calcium deficiency, physical inactivity, medication (steroids/heparin), tobacco use, ETOH, traumatic injury
- Chronic disease states: estrogen deficiency, androgen deficiency, hyperthyroidism, hypercortisolism, cirrhosis, gastrectomy

PHYSICAL FINDINGS
- Most commonly silent with no signs and symptoms
- Insidious and progressive development of dorsal kyphosis (dowager's hump), loss of height, and skeletal pain typically associated with fracture; other physical findings related to other conditions with associated increased risk for osteoporosis (see "Risk Factors")

ETIOLOGY
- Primary osteoporosis: multifactorial resulting from a combination of factors including nutrition, peak bone mass, genetics, level of physical activity, age of menopause (spontaneous vs. surgical), and estrogen status
- Secondary osteoporosis: associated decrease in bone mass resulting from an identified cause, including endocrinopathies—hypogonadism, hyperthyroidism, hyperparathyroidism, Cushing's syndrome, hyperprolactinemia, acromegaly, diabetes mellitus, gastrointestinal disease, malabsorption, primary biliary cirrhosis, gastrectomy, malnutrition (including anorexia nervosa)

DIAGNOSIS

DIFFERENTIAL DIAGNOSIS
- Malignancy (multiple myeloma, lymphoma, leukemia, metastatic carcinoma)
- Primary hyperparathyroidism
- Osteomalacia
- Paget's disease
- Osteogenesis imperfecta: types I, III, and IV (see also "Epidemiology and Demographics," and "Etiology")

WORKUP
- History and physical examination (20% of women with type I osteoporosis have associated secondary cause), with appropriate evaluation for identified risk factors and secondary causes
- Diagnosis of osteoporosis made by bone mineral density (BMD) determination:
  1. Dual-energy x-ray absorptiometry (DEXA)
  2. Single-energy x-ray
  3. Peripheral dual-energy x-ray
  4. Single photon absorptiometry
  5. Dual photon absorptiometry
  6. Quantitative CT scan
  7. Radiographic absorptiometry

LABORATORY TESTS
- Biochemical profile to evaluate renal and hepatic function, primary hyperparathyroidism, and malnutrition
- CBC for nutritional status and myeloma
- TSH to rule out the presence of hyperthyroidism
- Consideration of 24-hr urine collection for calcium (excess skeletal loss, vitamin D malabsorption/deficiency), creatinine, sodium, and free cortisol (to detect occult Cushing's disease); no need to measure calcitropic hormones unless specifically indicated (PTH, calcitriol, calcitonin)
- Biochemical markers of bone remodeling; may be useful to predict rate of bone loss and/or follow therapy response; specific biochemical markers followed (i.e., 3-mo interval) to document normalization as a response to therapy
  1. High turnover osteoporosis: high levels of resorption markers (lysyl pyridinoline [LP], deoxylysyl pyridinoline [DPD], n-telopeptide of collagen cross-links [NTX], C-telopeptide of collagen cross-links [PICP]) and formation markers (osteocalcin [OCN], bone-specific alkaline phosphatase [BSAP], carboxy-terminal extension peptide of type I procollagen [PICP]); accelerated bone loss responding best to antiresorptive therapy
  2. Low-normal turnover osteoporosis: normal or low levels of the markers of resorption and formation (see "high turnover osteoporosis" above); no accelerated bone loss; responds best to drugs that enhance bone formation

IMAGING STUDIES
- BMD determination (see "Workup") should be performed on all women with determined risk factors and/or associated secondary causes; accepted screening criteria is currently being investigated.
  1. Normal: BMD <1 SD of the young adult reference mean
  2. Osteopenia: BMD <1 to 2.5 SD below the young adult reference mean
  3. Osteoporosis: BMD >2.5 SD below the young adult reference mean
- For patient undergoing treatment: annual BMD to follow response to therapy
- X-ray examination of appropriate part of skeleton to evaluate clinical osteoporotic fracture only

TREATMENT

NONPHARMACOLOGIC THERAPY
Prevention:
- Identification and minimization of risk factors

- Appropriate diagnosis and treatment of secondary causes
- Behavior modification: proper nutrition (dietary calcium >800 mg/day, vitamin D 400 to 800 U/day), physical activity, fracture prevention strategies

ACUTE GENERAL Rx
- Vitamin D supplement: 400 U/day
- Calcium supplement: 1000 to 1500 mg/day
- Estrogen (conjugated equine estrogen or equivalent): 0.3 to 0.625 mg/day
- Progestin: continuous (i.e., 2.5 mg medroxyprogesterone acetate/day or equivalent) or cyclic (i.e., 10 mg medroxyprogesterone acetate days 16 to 25 each month or equivalent) coadministered in nonhysterectomized women
- Alendronate: 10 mg/day on awakening with 8 oz water on empty stomach with no oral intake for at least 30 min
- Synthetic salmon calcitonin: 100 U SC/day or 200 U intranasally/day
- Raloxifene 60 mg qd
- Other FDA approved drugs (without osteoporosis indication) used to treat osteoporosis:
  1. Calcitriol
  2. Etidronate
  3. Thiazide

- BMD baseline obtained before onset of therapy and at 1 yr; decrease of 2% or greater results in dosage adjustment or medication change
- Baseline biochemical markers of remodeling baseline considered; identified high turnover osteoporosis patients rescreened at 3 mo to document marker return to normal

CHRONIC Rx
- Lifelong disorder requiring lifelong attention to behavior modification issues (nutrition, physical activity, fracture prevention strategies) and compliance with pharmacologic intervention
- Continuing need to eliminate high-risk factors where possible and to diagnose and optimally manage secondary causes of osteoporosis

DISPOSITION
Goal for diagnosis and treatment: identification of women at risk, initiation of preventive measures for all women lifelong, institution of treatment modalities that will result in a decrease in fracture risk, and reduction of morbidity, mortality, and unnecessary institutionalization, thereby improving quality of independent life and productivity.

REFERRAL
- To reproductive endocrinologist, endocrinologist, gynecologist, or rheumatologist if unfamiliar with diagnosis and management of osteoporosis.
- If multidisciplinary management is required, to other specialties depending on presence of acute fracture and/or secondary associated disorders

MISCELLANEOUS

COMMENTS
- Patient information is available from American College of Obstetricians and Gynecologists.
- U.S. Preventive Services Task Force Recommendations regarding screening for postmenopausal osteoporosis are described in Section V, Chapter 46.

REFERENCES
Chestnut DH: Osteoporosis. In Hazzard WR et al (eds): *Principles of geriatric medicine and gerontology,* ed 3, New York, 1994, McGraw-Hill.

Hodes RJ: Osteoporosis: emerging research strategies aim at bone biology, risk factors, interventions, *J Am Geriatr Soc* 43(1):75, 1995.

Author: **Dennis M. Weppner, M.D.**

BASIC INFORMATION

DEFINITION
Otitis externa is a term encompassing a variety of conditions causing inflammation and/or infection of the external auditory canal and auricle. There are six subgroups of otitis externa:
- Acute localized otitis externa (furunculosis)
- Acute diffuse bacterial otitis externa (swimmer's ear)
- Chronic otitis externa
- Eczematous otitis externa
- Fungal otitis externa (otomycosis)
- Invasive or necrotizing (malignant) otitis externa

SYNONYMS
See "Definition" above.

ICD-9-CM CODES
381.10 Otitis externa

EPIDEMIOLOGY AND DEMOGRAPHICS
INCIDENCE (IN U.S.):
- Among the most common human disorders
- Affects 3% to 10% of patients seeking otologic care

PREVALENCE (IN U.S.): Diffuse otitis externa (swimmer's ear) is most often seen in swimmers and in hot, humid climates, conditions that lead to retention of moisture in the ear canal.

PREDOMINANT SEX: Male = female

PREDOMINANT AGE
- Occurs at all ages
- Necrotizing otitis externa
  1. Typically occurs in the elderly, diabetics, and other immunocompromised patients
  2. Mean age >65 yr
  3. Some form of glucose intolerance in >90% of adults with infection

PHYSICAL FINDINGS
Acute localized otitis externa (furunculosis):
- Occurs from infected hair follicles, usually in the outer third of the ear canal, forming pustules and furuncles
- Furuncles superficial and pointing or deep and diffuse
- Itching, pain (which often worsens with jaw movement), and tenderness on manipulation of the auricle

Impetigo:
- In contrast to furunculosis, a superficial spreading infection of the ear canal that may also involve the concha and the auricle
- Begins as a small blister that ruptures, releasing straw-colored fluid that dries as a golden crust

Erysipelas:
- Caused by group A *Streptococcus*
- May involve the concha and canal
- May involve the dermis and deeper tissues
- Area of cellulitis, often with severe pain
- Fever, chills, and malaise
- Regional adenopathy

Eczematous otitis externa:
- Stems from a variety of dermatologic problems that can involve the external auditory canal
- Severe itching, erythema, scaling, crusting, and fissuring possible

Acute diffuse otitis externa (swimmer's ear):
- Begins with itching and a feeling of pressure and fullness in the ear that becomes increasingly tender and painful, exacerbated by even slight manipulation of the auricle
- Mild erythema and edema of the external auditory canal, which progresses and narrows the canal lumen
- Minimal serous secretions, which become more profuse and purulent
- Hearing loss possible
- Tympanic membrane may appear dull and infected
- Absence of systemic symptoms such as fever and chills

Otomycosis:
- Chronic superficial infection of the ear canal and tympanic membrane
- In primary fungal infection, major symptom is intense itching
- In secondary infection, in which fungal infection is superimposed on bacterial infection, major symptom is pain
- Fungal growth of a variety of colors

Chronic otitis externa:
- Dry and atrophic canal
- Typically, lack of cerumen
- Itching, often severe, and mild discomfort rather than pain
- Occasionally, mucopurulent discharge
- With time, thickening of the walls of the canal, which causes narrowing of the lumen

Malignant otitis externa:
- Redness, swelling, and tenderness of ear canal
- Classic finding granulation tissue on the floor of the canal and the bone-cartilage junction
- Small ulceration of necrotic soft tissue at bone-cartilage junction
- Most common complaints: pain (often quite severe) and otorrhea
- Lessening of purulent drainage as infection advances
- Facial nerve palsy often the first and only cranial nerve deficit
- Possible involvement of other cranial nerves

ETIOLOGY
- Acute localized otitis externa: *Staphylococcus aureus*
- Impetigo
  1. *S. aureus*
  2. *Streptococcus pyogenes*
- Erysipelas: *Str. pyogenes*
- Eczematous otitis externa
  1. Seborrheic dermatitis
  2. Atopic dermatitis
  3. Psoriasis
  4. Neurodermatitis
- Acute diffuse otitis externa
  1. Swimming
  2. Hot, humid climates
  3. Tightly fitting hearing aids
  4. *Pseudomonas aeruginosa*
  5. *S. aureus*
- Otomycosis
  1. Prolonged use of topical antibiotics and steroid preparations
  2. *Aspergillus*
  3. *Candida*
- Chronic otitis externa: persistent low-grade infection and inflammation
- Malignant otitis externa
  1. Complication of persistent otitis externa
  2. Extends through Santorini's fissures, small apertures at the bone-cartilage junction of the canal, into the mastoid and along the base of the skull
  3. *P. aeruginosa*

DIAGNOSIS

DIFFERENTIAL DIAGNOSIS
- Acute otitis media
- Bullous myringitis
- Mastoiditis
- Foreign bodies
- Neoplasms

WORKUP
Thorough history and physical examination

LABORATORY TESTS
- Cultures from the canal are usually not necessary unless the case refractory to treatment.
- ESR is often quite elevated in malignant otitis externa.

IMAGING STUDIES
- CT scan is the best technique for defining bone involvement and extent of disease in malignant otitis externa.
- MRI is slightly more sensitive in evaluation of soft tissue changes.
- Gallium scans are more specific than bone scans in diagnosing malignant otitis externa.
- Follow-up scans are helpful in determining therapy.

TREATMENT

NONPHARMACOLOGIC THERAPY
- Cleansing and debridement of the ear canal with cotton swabs and hydrogen peroxide or other antiseptic solution allows for a more thorough examination of the ear.
- If the canal lumen is edematous and too narrow to allow adequate cleansing, a cotton wick or gauze strip inserted into the canal serves as a conduit for otic or drops to be drawn into the canal.
- Local heat is useful in treating deep diffuse furunculosis.
- Incision and drainage is indicated in treating superficial pointing furunculosis.

ACUTE GENERAL Rx
Topical medications:
- An acidifying agent, such as acetic acid, applied to inhibit growth of bacteria and fungi
- Topical antibiotics or antifungals, often in combination with the acidifying agent and a steroid preparation
- Topical ophthalmic preparations, which are more neutral and may be easier to tolerate:
  1. Cortisporin otic solution (neomycin sulfate, polymyxin B sulfate, and hydrocortisone 1%)
  2. Chloromycetin otic solution (chloramphenicol 0.5%)
  3. Otic Domeboro solution (acetic acid 2%)
  4. Gentian violet (methylrosaniline chloride 1%, 2%)
  5. TobraDex ophthalmic solution (tobramycin 0.3% and dexamethasone 0.1%)
  6. Garamycin ophthalmic solution (gentamicin 0.3%)
  7. Chloromycetin ophthalmic solution (chloramphenicol 0.25%)
  8. Fungizone lotion (amphotericin B 3%)
- Topical preparations given three to four drops in the ear three to four times daily and continued for 1 to 2 wk

Systemic antibiotics:
- Reserved for severe cases, most often resulting from infection with *P. aeruginosa* or *S. aureus*
- Treatment usually for 10 days with ciprofloxacin 750 mg q12h or ofloxacin 400 mg q12h, or with an antistaphylococcal agent, such as dicloxacillin or cephalexin 500 mg q6h

Pain control:
- May require NSAIDs or opioids
- Topical corticosteroids to reduce swelling and inflammation

Malignant otitis externa:
- Requires prolonged course of therapy until the infection has resolved (6 to 8 wk) with a combination of IV antibiotics (e.g., ceftazidime, piperacillin, or ticarcillin in combination with an aminoglycoside)
- Quinolones early in the course of infection: (e.g., ciprofloxacin 750 mg q12h, orally as a possible alternative to IV therapy or to shorten the course of IV therapy)
- Local debridement

CHRONIC Rx
- Patients prone to recurrent infections may employ some prophylactic measures.
- Swimmers should wear ear plugs and be sure to remove all excess water.

DISPOSITION
Inadequate treatment of otitis externa may cause progression to malignant otitis and mastoiditis.

REFERRAL
To an otolaryngologist:
- Malignant otitis externa
- Treatment response failure
- Severe pain

MISCELLANEOUS

REFERENCES
Bojrab DI, Bruderly TE: External otitis. In Johnson JT, Yu VL, (eds): *Infectious diseases and antimicrobial therapy of the ears, nose and throat*, 1997, WB Saunders.

Mirza N: Otitis externa; management in the primary care office, *Postgrad Med* 99(5):153, 1996.

Author: **Jane V. Eason, M.D.**

BASIC INFORMATION

DEFINITION
Otitis media is the presence of fluid in the middle ear accompanied by signs and symptoms of infection.

SYNONYMS
Acute suppurative otitis media
Purulent otitis media

ICD-9-CM CODES
382.9 Acute or chronic otitis media
381.00 Otitis media with effusion

EPIDEMIOLOGY AND DEMOGRAPHICS
INCIDENCE (IN U.S.):
- In 1990, acute otitis media (AOM) accounted for 24.5 million pediatric examinations.
- The diagnosis of AOM increased from 9.9 million in 1975 to 25.5 million in 1990.
- From 1975 to 1990 office visits for AOM increased threefold for children <2 yr, doubled for children ages 2 to 5, and increased almost double for children ages 6 to 10 yr.

PREDOMINANT SEX: Males
PREDOMINANT AGE: Most commonly a disease of children
- Occurs once in about three fourths of all children
- Occurs three or more times in one third by the age of 3 yr
- Declines with age
- Seen infrequently in adults

PEAK INCIDENCE:
- Between 6 and 36 mo
- Second peak between ages 4 and 6 yr
- Fall, winter, and early spring

GENETICS:
Familial Disposition:
- Native Americans
- Eskimos
- Australian aborigines
- Those with a strong family history

Congenital Infection:
High incidence in children born with midline cleft palates and other craniofacial abnormalities

PHYSICAL FINDINGS
- Fluid in the middle ear along with signs and symptoms of local inflammation
  1. Erythema with diminished light reflex
  2. Retraction and poor motility of the tympanic membrane, which then becomes bulging, convex
- Erythema alone of the tympanic membrane is not a diagnostic criterion for acute otitis media, as it may occur with any inflammation of the upper respiratory tract, crying, or nose blowing.
- Other symptoms:
  1. Otalgia
  2. Otorrhea
  3. Hearing loss
  4. Vertigo
  5. Nystagmus
  6. Tinnitus
  7. Fever
  8. Lethargy
  9. Irritability
  10. Nausea, vomiting
  11. Anorexia
- After an episode of acute otitis media:
  1. Persistence of effusion for weeks or months (termed secretory, serous, or nonsuppurative otitis media)
  2. Fever and ear pain usually absent
  3. Hearing loss possible

ETIOLOGY
- Develops as a consequence of colonization of the nasopharynx by a bacterial pathogen in conjunction with eustachian tube dysfunction (secondary to inflammation and obstruction often following an acute viral infection of the upper respiratory tract)
- May occasionally develop as a result of hematogenous spread or via direct invasion from the nasopharynx
- Most common bacteria isolated:
  1. *Streptococcus pneumoniae* (30% to 40%)
  2. *Haemophilus influenzae* (12% to 27%)
  3. *Moraxella catarrhalis* (20% to 30%)
- Viral causes:
  1. Respiratory syncytial virus
  2. Rhinovirus
  3. Adenovirus
  4. Influenza
  5. *Mycoplasma pneumoniae*
  6. *Chlamydia trachomatis*

Otitis media (PTG)

DIAGNOSIS

DIFFERENTIAL DIAGNOSIS
- Otitis externa
- Referred pain:
  1. Mouth
  2. Nasopharynx
  3. Tonsils
  4. Other parts of the upper respiratory tract

WORKUP
- Thorough observation of the tympanic membrane by pneumatic otoscopy
- Tympanometry
  1. Measures the compliance of the tympanic membrane and middle ear pressure
  2. Detects the presence of fluid
- Acoustic reflectometry
  1. Measures sound waves reflected from the middle ear
  2. Useful in infants >3 mo
  3. Increased reflected sound correlated with the presence of an effusion

LABORATORY TESTS
- Tympanocentesis
  1. Not necessary in most cases as the microbiology of middle ear effusions has been shown to be quite consistent
  2. May be indicated in:
     a. Highly toxic patients
     b. Patients who fail to respond to treatment in 48 to 72 hr
     c. Immunocompromised patients
- Cultures of the nasopharynx: sensitive but not specific

TREATMENT

ACUTE GENERAL Rx
- Amoxicillin is the drug of choice for initial empiric therapy.
- Alternatives for the patient allergic to penicillin:
  1. Azithromycin
  2. Clarithromycin
  3. Trimethoprim-sulfamethoxazole
  4. Combination therapy with erythromycin and sulfisoxazole
- If no history of immediate hypersensitivity to penicillin, cephalosporins:
  1. Cefaclor
  2. Loracarbef
  3. Cefuroxime axetil
  4. Cefprozil
  5. Cefpodoxime
  6. Cefixime
- If cultures obtained, therapy modified according to specific susceptibility patterns of organisms isolated
- Therapy generally continued for 10 to 14 days
- Follow-up examination in 4 wk in patients who respond
- Patients who remain symptomatic on therapy should be reexamined at the completion of therapy to determine the need for additional treatment.

CHRONIC Rx
- Myringotomy and tympanostomy tube placement considered for persistent middle ear effusion unresponsive to medical therapy for ≥3 mo if bilateral, or ≥6 mo unilateral.
- Adenoidectomy, with or without tonsillectomy, often advocated for treatment of recurrent otitis media, although indications for this procedure are controversial.
- Antimicrobial prophylaxis (amoxicillin 20 mg/kg or sulfisoxazole 50 mg/kg qhs) have been shown to be effective in children with recurrent infections.

DISPOSITION
Without proper treatment and follow-up, acute otitis media can become chronic, requiring more invasive treatment procedures.

REFERRAL
To otolaryngologist if:
- Medical treatment failure
- Diagnosis uncertain

MISCELLANEOUS

COMMENTS
Prevention:
- Multiple component conjugate vaccines hold promise for decreasing recurrent episodes of acute otitis media.
- Breast-feeding, bottle-feeding the infant in an upright position, and avoiding tobacco may be useful.

REFERENCES
Bluestone CD: Otitis media. In Johnson JT, Yu VL (eds): *Infectious diseases and antimicrobial therapy of the ears, nose, and throat*, Philadelphia, 1997, WB Saunders.

Cantor RM: Otitis externa and otitis media: a new look at old problems, *Emerg Med Clin North Am* 13(2):445, 1995.

Swanson JA, Hoecker JL: Concise review for primary-care physicians: otitis media in young children, *Mayo Clin Proc* 71:179, 1996.

Author: **Jane V. Eason, M.D.**

Otosclerosis (otospongiosis)

BASIC INFORMATION

DEFINITION
Otosclerosis is a conductive hearing loss secondary to fixation of the stapes resulting in gradual hearing loss. About 15% of cases affect only one ear.

ICD-9-CM CODES
387.9 Otosclerosis

EPIDEMIOLOGY AND DEMOGRAPHICS
INCIDENCE (IN U.S.): Most common cause of hearing loss in young adults
PREVALENCE (IN U.S.): 5 cases/1000 persons
PREDOMINANT SEX: Male:female of 2:1
PREDOMINANT AGE: Symptoms start between 15 and 30 yr, with slowly progressive hearing loss.
PEAK INCIDENCE: Middle age
GENETICS: One half of cases are dominantly inherited.

PHYSICAL FINDINGS
- Tympanic membrane is normal in most cases (tested with tuning fork).
- Bone conduction is greater than air conduction.
- Weber localizes to affected ear.

ETIOLOGY
- A disease where vascular type of spongy bone is laid down
- Unknown

DIAGNOSIS

DIFFERENTIAL DIAGNOSIS
- Hearing loss from any cause: cochlear otosclerosis, polyps, granulomas, tumors, osteogenesis imperfecta, chronic ear infections, trauma
- A clinical algorithm for evaluation of hearing loss is described in Fig. 3-36.

WORKUP
Audiometry

LABORATORY TESTS
None unless infection suspected

IMAGING STUDIES
MRI with specific cuts through inner ear

TREATMENT

NONPHARMACOLOGIC THERAPY
Hearing aid only of temporary use

CHRONIC Rx
Progresses to deafness without surgical intervention

DISPOSITION
Referral to ENT specialist

REFERRAL
To ENT specialist for surgery if moderate hearing loss suspected

MISCELLANEOUS

COMMENTS
- A full ENT evaluation in a young or middle-aged person with hearing loss is mandatory unless cause is obvious (such as trauma or repeated infection).
- U.S. Preventive Services Task Force Recommendations regarding screening for hearing impairment are described in Section V, Chapter 35.

REFERENCES
Emmett J: Physical examination and clinical evaluation of the patient with otosclerosis, *Ontolaryngol Clin North Am* 26:353, 1993.

Author: **William H. Olson, M.D.**

Ovarian cancer (PTG)

BASIC INFORMATION

DEFINITION
Ovarian tumors can be benign, requiring operative intervention but not recurring or metastasizing; malignant, recurring, metastasizing, and having decreased survival, or borderline, having a small risk of recurrence or metastases but generally having a good prognosis.

SYNONYMS
Epithelial ovarian cancer
Germ cell tumor
Sex cord stromal tumor
Ovarian tumor of low malignant potential

ICD-9-CM CODES
183.0 Malignant neoplasm of ovary

EPIDEMIOLOGY AND DEMOGRAPHICS
INCIDENCE: 12.9 to 15.1 cases/100,000 persons; approximately 25,000 new cases annually
PREDOMINANCE: Median age of 61 yr, peaks at age 75 to 79 yr (54/100,000)
GENETICS: Familial susceptibility has been shown with the BRCA1 gene located on 17q12 to 21. This correlates breast-ovarian cancer syndrome.
RISK FACTORS: Low parity, delayed child-bearing, use of talc on the perineum, high-fat diet, fertility drugs (possibly), Lynch II syndrome (nonpolyposis colon cancer, endometrial cancer, breast cancer, and ovarian cancer clusters in first- and second-degree relatives), breast-ovarian familial cancer syndrome, site-specific familial ovarian cancer (NOTE: Use of oral contraceptives appear to have a protective effect)

PHYSICAL FINDINGS
- 60% present with advanced disease
- Abdominal fullness, early satiety, dyspepsia
- Pelvic pain, back pain, constipation
- Pelvic or abdominal mass
- Lymphadenopathy (inguinal)
- Sister Mary Joseph nodule (umbilical mass)

ETIOLOGY
- Can be inherited as site-specific familial ovarian cancer (two or more first-degree relatives have ovarian cancer)
- Breast-ovarian cancer syndrome (clusters of breast and ovarian cancer among first- and second-degree relatives)
- Lynch syndrome
- No family history and unknown etiology in the majority of ovarian cancer cases

DIAGNOSIS

DIFFERENTIAL DIAGNOSIS
- Primary peritoneal cancer
- Benign ovarian tumor
- Functional ovarian cyst
- Endometriosis
- Ovarian torsion
- Pelvic kidney
- Pedunculated uterine fibroid
- Primary cancer from breast, GI tract, or other pelvic organ metastasized to the ovary

WORKUP
- Definitive diagnosis made at laparotomy
- Careful physical and history including family history
- Exclusion of nongynecologic etiologies
- Observation of small, cystic masses in premenopausal women for regression for 2 mo

LABORATORY TESTS
- CBC
- Chemistry profile
- CA-125
- Consider: hCG, Inhibin, AFP, neuron-specific enolase (NSE), and LDH in patients at risk for germ cell tumors

IMAGING STUDIES
- Ultrasound (has not been shown to be effective as a screening mechanism, but is useful in the evaluation of a pelvic mass)
- Chest x-ray examination
- Mammogram
- CT scan to help evaluate extent of disease
- Other studies (BE, MRI, IVP, etc.) as clinically indicated

TREATMENT

NONPHARMACOLOGIC THERAPY
Virtually all cases of ovarian cancer involve surgical exploration. This includes:
- Abdominal cytology
- Total abdominal hysterectomy and bilateral salpingo-oophorectomy (except in early stages where fertility is an issue)
- Omentectomy
- Diaphragm sampling
- Selective lymphadenectomy
- Primary cytoreduction with a goal of residual tumor diameter <2 cm
- Bowel surgery, splenectomy if needed to obtain optimal (<2 cm) cytoreduction

ACUTE GENERAL Rx
- Optimal cytoreduction is generally followed by chemotherapy (except in some early stage disease).
- Cisplatin-based combination chemotherapy is used for Stage II or greater.
- Chemotherapy regimens continue to change as research continues.
- Consider second look surgery when chemotherapy is complete.

CHRONIC Rx
- Physical and pelvic examinations every 3 mo for 2 yr, every 4 mo during third year, then every 6 mo
- CA-125 every visit
- Yearly Pap smear

DISPOSITION
- Overall 5-yr survival rates remain low because of the preponderance of late-stage disease:
  Stage I and II 80% to 100%
  Stage III 15% to 20%
  Stage IV 5%
- Younger patients (<50 yr) in all stages have a considerably better 5-yr survival than older patients (40% vs. 15%).

REFERRAL
- Studies have shown that optimal cytoreduction is most likely to occur in the hands of a gynecologic oncologist.
- Have gynecologic/oncology backup available if suspicious of malignancy.
- Always refer advanced disease.

MISCELLANEOUS

COMMENTS
U.S. Preventive Services Task Force Recommendations for screening for ovarian cancer are described in Section V, Chapter 14.

REFERENCES
Baker TR: Ovarian germ cell tumors. In Piver MS (ed): *Handbook of gynecologic oncology*, ed 2, Boston, 1996, Little, Brown.

Gershenson DM et al: Ovarian intraepithelial neoplasia and ovarian cancer, *Obstet Gynecol Clin North Am* 23(2):475, 1996.

Kristensen GB, Trope G: Epithelial ovarian carcinoma, *Lancet* 349(9045):113, 1997.

Piver MS: Ovarian epithelial cancer. In Piver MS (ed): *Handbook of gynecologic oncology*, ed 2, Boston, 1996, Little, Brown.

Author: **Karen Houck, M.D.**

Ovarian tumor, benign

BASIC INFORMATION

DEFINITION
Benign ovarian neoplasms are clinically indistinguishable from their malignant counterparts. Therefore all persistent adnexal masses must be considered malignant until proven otherwise. Nonneoplastic tumors are as follows:
- Germinal inclusion cyst
- Follicle cyst
- Corpus luteum cyst
- Pregnancy luteoma
- Theca lutein cysts
- Sclerocystic ovaries
- Endometrioma

Neoplastic tumors that are derived from coelomic epithelium are as follows:
- Cystic tumors: serous cystoma, mucinous cystoma, mixed forms
- Tumors with stromal overgrowth: fibroma, adenofibroma, Brenner tumor

Tumors derived from germ cells are dermoids (benign cystic teratomas).

ICD-9-CM CODES
220 Benign neoplasm of ovary

EPIDEMIOLOGY AND DEMOGRAPHICS
- Reproductive years:
  1. Most common benign ovarian neoplasms: serous cystadenoma and benign cystic teratoma
  2. Most common adnexal mass: functional cyst
- Risk of malignancy increases after age 40 yr.
- Infants: adnexal masses are usually follicular cysts secondary to maternal hormone stimulation that regress during first few months of life.
- Childhood:
  1. Adnexal masses are rare.
  2. 8% are malignant.
  3. Almost always dysgerminomas or teratomas (germ cell origin).
  4. Frequency of malignancy is inversely correlated with age.
- Adolescence:
  1. Most common adnexal mass is a functional cyst.
  2. Most common neoplastic ovarian tumor is a benign cystic teratoma.
  3. Solid/cystic adnexal tumors are rare and almost always dysgerminomas or malignant teratomas.

PHYSICAL FINDINGS
- Usually asymptomatic
- Pelvic pain/pressure
- Dyspareunia
- Abdominal pain ranging from mild to severe peritoneal irritation
- Increasing abdominal girth/distention
- Adnexal mass of pelvic examination
- Children: abdominal/rectal mass

ETIOLOGY
- Physiologic
- Endometriosis
- Unknown

DIAGNOSIS

DIFFERENTIAL DIAGNOSIS
- Ovarian torsion
- Malignancy: ovary, fallopian tube, colon
- Uterine fibroid
- Diverticular abscess/diverticulitis
- Appendiceal abscess/appendicitis (especially in children)
- Tubo-ovarian abscess
- Paraovarian cyst
- Distended bladder
- Pelvic kidney
- Ectopic pregnancy
- Retroperitoneal cyst/neoplasm

WORKUP
- Complete history and physical examination
- Pelvic examination/rectovaginal examination to reveal firm, irregular, mobile mass
- Laparoscopy/laparotomy to establish diagnosis

LABORATORY TESTS
- Pregnancy test
- Serum tumor markers:
  1. Cancer antigen 125 (CA 125)
  2. α-Fetoprotein (AFP) (endodermal sinus tumor, immature teratoma)
  3. β Human chorionic gonadotropin (hCG)
  4. Lactic dehydrogenase (LDH) (dysgerminoma)

IMAGING STUDIES
Ultrasound:
- May differentiate adnexal mass from other pelvic masses
- Features that increase risk of malignancy include solid component, papillations, multiple septations/solitary thick septa, ascites, matted bowel, bilaterality, irregular borders
- CT scan with contrast or IVP
- Colonoscopy/barium enema, if symptomatic

TREATMENT

NONPHARMACOLOGIC THERAPY
Repeat pelvic examination for premenopausal women in 4 to 6 wk.

ACUTE GENERAL Rx
Indications for surgery:
- Postmenopausal or premenarchal palpable adnexal mass
- Adnexal mass with suspicious ultrasound features
- Premenopausal woman with persistent cyst >5 cm
- Any adnexal mass >10 cm
- Suspected torsion or rupture

CHRONIC Rx
- Depends on diagnosis
- Possible suppression of formation of new cysts by oral contraceptives

DISPOSITION
Depends on diagnosis

REFERRAL
- If malignancy suspected
- If surgery required

MISCELLANEOUS

COMMENTS
U.S. Preventive Services Task Force Recommendations regarding screening for ovarian cancer are described in Section V, Chapter 14.

REFERENCES
DiSaia PJ, Creasman WT (eds): *Clinical gynecologic oncology,* ed 5, St Louis, 1997, Mosby.

Author: **Maria Elena Soler, M.D.**

Paget's disease of the bone *(PTG)*

BASIC INFORMATION

DEFINITION
Paget's disease of the bone is a nonmetabolic disease of bone characterized by repeated episodes of osteolysis and excessive attempts at repair that results in a weakened bone of increased mass. Monostotic (solitary lesion) and polyostotic (numerous lesions) disease are both described.

SYNONYMS
Osteitis deformans

ICD-9-CM CODES
731.0 Paget's disease (osteitis deformans)

EPIDEMIOLOGY AND DEMOGRAPHICS
PREVALENCE: Localized lesions in 3% of patients >50 yr
PREVALENT AGE: Rare before 40 yr
PREVALENT SEX: Male:female ratio of 2:1

PHYSICAL FINDINGS
- Many lesions are asymptomatic.
- Onset is variable.
- Symptoms result mainly from the effects of complications:
  1. Skeletal pain, especially hip and pelvis
  2. Bowing of long bones, sometimes leading to pathologic fracture
  3. Increased heat of extremity (resulting from increased vascularity)
  4. Skull enlargement and spinal involvement caused by characteristic bone enlargement, which can produce neurologic complications (vision, hearing loss, radicular pain, and cord compression)
  5. Thoracic kyphoscoliosis
  6. Secondary osteoarthritis, especially of hip
  7. Heart failure as a result of chest and spine deformity and blood shunting

ETIOLOGY
Unknown

DIAGNOSIS

DIFFERENTIAL DIAGNOSIS
- Fibrous dysplasia
- Skeletal neoplasm (primary or metastatic)
- Osteomyelitis
- Hyperparathyroidism
- Vertebral hemangioma

LABORATORY TESTS
- Increased serum alkaline phosphatase (SAP)
- Normal serum calcium and phosphorus levels
- Increased urinary excretion of pyridinoline cross-links, although test is expensive and not usually required in routine cases
- Other: bone biopsy only in uncertain cases or if sarcomatous degeneration is suspected

IMAGING STUDIES
- Appropriate radiographs reflect the characteristic radiolucency and opacity.
- Bone scanning usually reflects the activity and extent of the disease.

TREATMENT

ACUTE GENERAL Rx
- Counseling regarding home environment to prevent falls
- Cane for balance and weight-bearing pain

PHARMACOLOGIC THERAPY
- Calcitonin
- Biphosponates
- NSAIDs for pain relief

DISPOSITION
- Many monostotic lesions probably remain asymptomatic.
- Progression of the disease is common.
- Malignant degeneration occurs in <1% of patients and should be considered when there is a sudden increase in pain.
- Sarcomatous change carries a grave prognosis.

REFERRAL
- For dental evaluation if there is involvement of the mandible or maxilla
- For ENT evaluation if there is hearing loss
- For ophthalmologic evaluation if impaired vision
- For orthopedic consultation for assessment of pain in bone or joint

MISCELLANEOUS

COMMENTS
Surgical intervention is often required for neurologic complications or joint symptoms
- Often associated with profuse blood loss
- Elective cases: benefit from preoperative treatment to suppress bone activity and vascularity

REFERENCES
Greenspan A: A review of Paget's disease: radiologic imaging, differential diagnosis and treatment, *Bull Hosp Joint Dis Orth Inst* 51:22, 1991.

Kaplan FS, Singer FR: Paget's disease of bone: pathophysiology diagnosis and management, *J Am Acad Orthop Surg* 3:336, 1995.

Merkow RL, Lane JM: Paget's disease of bone, *Orthop Clin North Am* 21:171, 1990.

Author: **Lonnie R. Mercier, M.D.**

Paget's disease of the breast (PTG)

BASIC INFORMATION

DEFINITION
Paget's disease of the breast is a malignant disease that presents itself as a scaly, sore, eroding, bleeding ulcer of the nipple. Microscopically, typical large clear cells (Paget's cells) with pale and abundant cytoplasm and hyperchromatic nuclei with prominent nucleoli are found in the epidermal layer. Paget's disease is more often associated with primary invasive or in situ carcinoma of the breast.

ICD-9-CM CODES
174.0 Malignant neoplasm of female breast; nipple and areola

EPIDEMIOLOGY AND DEMOGRAPHICS
- Not common
- Found in 1 in 100 to 200 breast cancer patients

PHYSICAL FINDINGS
- Variable
- Itching or burning nipple and/or reported lump
- Very minimal scaly lesion that may bleed when scales are lifted
- Typical ulcer located on nipple with serous fluid weeping or small amount of bleeding coming from it
- Palpable carcinoma in the breast of some patients

ETIOLOGY
- Exact origin unknown
- Possibly migration of either in situ or invasive carcinoma cells in breast to nipple skin to produce Paget's disease

DIAGNOSIS

DIFFERENTIAL DIAGNOSIS
- Chronic dermatitis
- Florid papillomatosis of the nipple or nipple adenoma
- Eczema

WORKUP
- Clinically apparent
- Careful breast examination with diagnosis in mind
- Palpable mass or mammographic lesions in 60% to 70% of patients
- A clinical algorithm for the evaluation of nipple discharge is described in Fig. 3-18.

LABORATORY TESTS
Biopsy of nipple lesion

IMAGING STUDIES
Mammograms to search for possible primary carcinoma

TREATMENT

NONPHARMACOLOGIC THERAPY
- Fewer patients:
  1. Paget's disease of nipple only finding with mammographically negative breast
  2. Consideration of wide excision of nipple with or without radiation
- Other patients: additional invasive or in situ carcinoma recognized
- Either modified mastectomy or breast conservation treatment
- Presence of underlying in situ or invasive carcinoma in mastectomy specimen of majority of patients

ACUTE GENERAL Rx
Systemic adjuvant therapy, depending on extent of invasive carcinoma found

DISPOSITION
- Parallel prognosis to that of breast cancer patient without Paget's disease
- Regular follow-up as in other invasive or in situ carcinoma patients

REFERRAL
At outset, all suspicious nipple lesions should be referred for evaluation and treatment.

MISCELLANEOUS

REFERENCES
Tavassoli, FA: *Pathology of the breast*, New York, 1992, Elsevier.

Author: **Takuma Nemoto, M.D.**

Pancreatitis, acute

BASIC INFORMATION

DEFINITION
Acute pancreatitis is an inflammatory process of the pancreas with intrapancreatic activation of enzymes that may also involve peripancreatic tissue and/or remote organ systems.

ICD-9-CM CODES
577.0 Acute pancreatitis

EPIDEMIOLOGY AND DEMOGRAPHICS
- Acute pancreatitis is most often secondary to biliary tract disease and alcohol.
- Incidence in urban areas is twice that of rural areas (20 cases/100,000 persons in urban areas)
- 20% of patients have necrotizing pancreatitis, the remainder have interstitial pancreatitis.

PHYSICAL FINDINGS
- Epigastric tenderness and guarding; pain usually developing suddenly, reaching peak intensity within 10 to 30 min, severe and lasting several hours without relief
- Hypoactive bowel sounds (secondary to ileus)
- Tachycardia, shock (secondary to decreased intravascular volume)
- Confusion (secondary to metabolic disturbances)
- Fever
- Tachycardia, decreased breath sounds (atelectasis, pleural effusions, ARDS)
- Jaundice (secondary to obstruction or compression of biliary tract)
- Ascites (secondary to tear in pancreatic duct, leaking pseudocyst)
- Palpable abdominal mass (pseudocyst, phlegmon, abscess, carcinoma)
- Evidence of hypocalcemia (Chvostek's sign, Trousseau's sign)
- Evidence of intraabdominal bleeding (hemorrhagic pancreatitis):
  1. Gray-bluish discoloration around the umbilicus (Cullen's sign)
  2. Bluish discoloration involving the flanks (Grey-Turner sign)
- Tender subcutaneous nodules (caused by subcutaneous fat necrosis)

ETIOLOGY
- In >90% of cases: biliary tract disease (calculi or sludge) or alcohol
- Drugs (e.g., thiazides, furosemide, corticosteroids, tetracycline, estrogens, valproic acid, metronidazole, azathioprine, methyldopa, pentamidine, ethacrynic acid, procainamide, sulindac, nitrofurantoin, ACE inhibitors, danazol, cimetidine, piroxicam, gold, ranitidine, sulfasalazine, isoniazid, acetaminophen, cisplatin, opiates, erythromycin)
- Abdominal trauma
- Surgery
- ERCP
- Infections (predominantly viral infections)
- Peptic ulcer (penetrating duodenal ulcer)
- Pancreas divisum (congenital failure to fuse of dorsal or ventral pancreas)
- Idiopathic
- Pregnancy
- Vascular (vasculitis, ischemic)
- Hypolipoproteinemia (types I, IV, and V)
- Hypercalcemia
- Pancreatic carcinoma (primary or metastatic)
- Renal failure
- Hereditary pancreatitis
- Occupational exposure to chemicals: methanol, cobalt, zinc, mercuric chloride, creosol, lead, organophosphates, chlorinated naphthalenes
- Others: scorpion bite, obstruction at ampulla region (neoplasm, duodenal diverticula, Crohn's disease), hypotensive shock

DIAGNOSIS

DIFFERENTIAL DIAGNOSIS
- PUD
- Acute cholangitis, biliary colic
- High intestinal obstruction
- Early acute appendicitis
- Mesenteric vascular obstruction
- DKA
- Pneumonia (basilar)
- Myocardial infarction (inferior wall)
- Renal colic
- Ruptured or dissecting aortic aneurysm

LABORATORY TESTS
Pancreatic enzymes
- Amylase is increased, usually elevated in the initial 3 to 5 days of acute pancreatitis. Isoamylase determinations (separation of pancreatic cell isoenzyme components of amylase) are useful in excluding occasional cases of salivary hyperamylasemia. The use of isoamylase rather than total serum amylase reduces the risk of erroneously diagnosing pancreatitis and is preferred by some as initial biochemical test in patients suspected of having acute pancreatitis.
- Urinary amylase determinations are useful to diagnose acute pancreatitis in patients with lipemic serum, to rule out elevated serum amylase secondary to macroamylasemia, and to diagnose acute pancreatitis in patients whose serum amylase is normal.
- Serum lipase levels are elevated in acute pancreatitis; the elevation is less transient than serum amylase; concomitant evaluation of serum amylase and lipase increases diagnostic accuracy of acute pancreatitis. An elevated lipase-amylase ratio is suggestive of alcoholic pancreatitis.
- Elevated serum trypsin levels are diagnostic of pancreatitis (in absence of renal failure); measurement is made by radioimmunoassay (this test is not readily available in most laboratories).
- Rapid measurement of urinary trypsinogen-2 (if available) is useful in the ER as a screening test for acute pancreatitis in patients with abdominal pain; a negative dipstick test for urinary trypsinogen-2 rules out acute pancreatitis with a high degree of probability, whereas a positive test indicates need for further evaluation.

Additional tests:
- CBC: reveals leukocytosis; Hct may be initially increased secondary to hemoconcentration; decreased Hct may indicate hemorrhage or hemolysis.
- BUN is increased secondary to dehydration.
- Elevation of serum glucose in previously normal patient correlates with the degree of pancreatic malfunction and may be related to increased release of glycogen, catecholamines, glucocorticoid release and decreased insulin release.
- Liver profile: AST and LDH are increased secondary to tissue necrosis; bilirubin and alkaline phosphatase may be increased secondary to common bile duct obstruction. A threefold or greater rise in serum ALT concentrations is an excellent indicator (95% probability) of biliary pancreatitis.
- Serum calcium is decreased secondary to saponification, precipitation, and decreased PTH response.
- ABGs: PaO_2 may be decreased secondary to ARDS, pleural effusion(s); pH may be decreased secondary to lactic acidosis, respiratory acidosis, and renal insufficiency.
- Serum electrolytes: potassium may be increased secondary to acidosis or renal insufficiency, sodium may be increased secondary to dehydration.

IMAGING STUDIES
- Abdominal plain film is useful to distinguish other conditions that may mimic pancreatitis (perforated viscus); it may reveal localized ileus (sentinel loop), pancreatic calcifications (chronic pancreatitis), blurring of left psoas shadow, dilation of transverse colon, calcified gallstones.

- Chest x-ray film may reveal elevation of one or both diaphragms, pleural effusions, basilar infiltrates, plate-like atelectasis.
- Abdominal ultrasonography is useful in detecting gallstones (sensitivity of 60% to 70% for detecting stones associated with pancreatitis). It is also useful for detecting pancreatic pseudocysts; its major limitation is the presence of distended bowel loops overlying the pancreas.
- CT scan is superior to ultrasonography in identifying pancreatitis and defining its extent, and it also plays a role in diagnosing pseudocysts (they appear as a well-defined area surrounded by high density capsule); GI fistulation or infection of a pseudocyst can also be identified by the presence of gas within the pseudocyst. Sequential contrast enhanced CT is useful for detection of pancreatic necrosis. The severity of pancreatitis can also be graded by CT scan.
- ERCP should not be performed during the acute stage of disease unless it is necessary to remove an impacted stone in the ampulla of Vater; patients with severe or worsening pancreatitis but without obstructive jaundice (biliary obstruction) do not benefit from early ERCP and papillotomy.

TREATMENT

NONPHARMACOLOGIC THERAPY
- Bowel rest with avoidance of PO liquids or solids during the acute illness
- Avoidance of alcohol and any drugs associated with pancreatitis

ACUTE GENERAL Rx
General measures:
- Maintain adequate intravascular volume with vigorous IV hydration.
- Patient should remain NPO until clinically improved, stable, and hungry.
- Nasogastric suction is useful in severe pancreatitis to decompress the abdomen in patients with ileus.
- Control pain: oral analgesics may cause spasms of the sphincter of Oddi (meperidine may produce less constriction than other analgesics).
- Correct metabolic abnormalities (e.g., replace calcium and magnesium as necessary).
- TPN may be necessary in prolonged pancreatitis.

Specific measures:
- IV antibiotics should not be used prophylactically; their use is justified if the patient has evidence of septicemia, pancreatic abscess, or pancreatitis secondary to biliary calculi. Appropriate empiric antibiotic therapy should cover:
  1. *B. fragilis* and other anaerobes (cefotetan, cefoxitin, metronidazole, or clindamycin plus aminoglycoside)
  2. *Enterococcus* (ampicillin)
- Surgical therapy has a limited role in acute pancreatitis; it is indicated in the following:
  1. Gallstone-induced pancreatitis: cholecystectomy when acute pancreatitis subsides
  2. Perforated peptic ulcer
  3. Excision or drainage of necrotic or infected foci
- Identification and treatment of complications:
  1. Pseudocyst: round or spheroid collection of fluid, tissue, pancreatic enzymes and blood
     a. Diagnosed by CT scan or sonography
     b. Treatment: CT scan or ultrasound guided percutaneous drainage (with a pigtail catheter left in place for continuous drainage) can be used, but the recurrence rate is high; the conservative approach is to reevaluate the pseudocyst (with CT scan or sonography) after 6 to 7 wk and surgically drain it if the pseudocyst has not decreased in size. Generally pseudocysts <5 cm in diameter are reabsorbed without intervention whereas those >5 cm require surgical intervention after the wall has matured.
  2. Phlegmon: represents pancreatic edema. It can be diagnosed by CT scan or sonography. Treatment is supportive measures, since it usually resolves spontaneously.
  3. Pancreatic abscess: diagnosed by CT scan (presence of bubbles in the retroperitoneum); Gram staining and cultures of fluid obtained from guided percutaneous aspiration (GPA) usually identify bacterial organism. Therapy is surgical (or catheter) drainage and IV antibiotics.
  4. Pancreatic ascites: usually caused by leaking of pseudocyst or tear in pancreatic duct. Paracentesis reveals very high amylase and lipase levels in the pancreatic fluid; ERCP may demonstrate the lesion. Treatment is surgical correction if exudative ascites from severe pancreatitis does not resolve spontaneously.
  5. GI bleeding: caused by alcoholic gastritis, bleeding varices, stress ulceration or DIC
  6. Renal failure: caused by hypovolemia resulting in oliguria or anuria, cortical or tubular necrosis (shock, DIC), or thrombosis of renal artery or vein.
  7. Hypoxia: caused by ARDS, pleural effusion or atelectasis

DISPOSITION
Prognosis varies with the severity of pancreatitis; overall mortality in acute pancreatitis is 5% to 10%; according to Ranson, poor prognostic signs are the following:
- Age >55 yr
- Fluid sequestration >6000 ml
- Laboratory abnormalities on admission: WBC >16,000, blood glucose >200 ml/dl, serum LDH >350 IU/L, AST >250 IU/L
- Laboratory abnormalities during the initial 48 hr: decreased Hct >10% with hydration or Hct <30%, BUN rise >5 mg/dl, serum calcium <8 mg/dl, arterial Po_2 <60 mm Hg, and base deficit >4 mEq/L.

REFERRAL
- Hospitalization is indicated in moderate/severe cases of pancreatitis.
- Surgical consultation is needed in suspected gallstone pancreatitis, perforated peptic ulcer, or presence of necrotic or infected foci.

MISCELLANEOUS

COMMENTS
Additional information on acute pancreatitis can be obtained from the National Digestive Diseases Information Clearinghouse, Box NDDIC, Bethesda, MD 20892.

REFERENCES
Banks PA: Practice guidelines in acute pancreatitis, *Am J Gastroenterol* 92:377, 1997.

Kemppainen E et al: Rapid measurement of urinary trypsinogen-2 as a screening test for acute pancreatitis, *N Engl J Med* 336:1788, 1997.

Ranson JHC: Etiological and prognostic factors in human pancreatitis, *Am J Gastroenterol* 77:633, 1982.

Sternby B et al: What is the best biochemical test to diagnose acute pancreatitis? a prospective clinical study, *Mayo Clin Proc* 71:1138, 1996.

Tanner S et al: Predicting gallstone pancreatitis with laboratory parameters: a meta-analysis, *Am J Gastroenterol* 89:1863, 1994.

Author: Fred F. Ferri, M.D.

Pancreatitis, chronic (PTG)

BASIC INFORMATION

DEFINITION
Chronic pancreatitis is a recurrent or persistent inflammatory process of the pancreas characterized by chronic pain and by pancreatic exocrine and/or endocrine insufficiency.

ICD-9-CM CODES
577.1 Chronic pancreatitis

EPIDEMIOLOGY AND DEMOGRAPHICS
- Chronic pancreatitis occurs in approximately 5 to 10/100,000 persons in industrial countries.
- Male:female ratio is 5:1.

PHYSICAL FINDINGS
- Persistent or recurrent epigastric and LUQ pain, may radiate to the back
- Tenderness over the pancreas, muscle guarding
- Significant weight loss
- Bulky, foul-smelling stools, greasy in appearance
- Epigastric mass (10% of patients)
- Jaundice (5% to 10% of patients)

ETIOLOGY
- Chronic alcoholism
- Obstruction (ampullary stenosis, tumor, trauma, pancreas divisum, annular pancreas)
- Hereditary pancreatitis
- Severe malnutrition
- Idiopathic
- Untreated hyperparathyroidism (hypercalcemia)

DIAGNOSIS

DIFFERENTIAL DIAGNOSIS
- Pancreatic cancer
- PUD
- Cholelithiasis with biliary obstruction
- Malabsorption from other etiologies
- Recurrent acute pancreatitis

WORKUP
Medical history with focus on alcohol use, laboratory tests, diagnostic imaging

LABORATORY TESTS
- Serum amylase and lipase may be elevated (normal amylase levels, however, do not exclude the diagnosis).
- Hyperglycemia, glycosuria, hyperbilirubinemia, and elevated serum alkaline phosphatase may also be present.
- 72-hr fecal fat determination reveals excess fecal fat.
- Bentiromide test or secretin stimulation test can confirm pancreatic insufficiency.

IMAGING STUDIES
- Plain abdominal radiographs may reveal pancreatic calcifications (95% specific for chronic pancreatitis).
- Ultrasound of abdomen may reveal duct dilatation, pseudocyst, calcification, and presence of ascites.
- CT scan of abdomen is useful for the detection of calcifications, to evaluate for ductal dilatation, and for ruling out pancreatic cancer.
- ERCP can be used to evaluate for the presence of dilated ducts, strictures, pseudocysts, and intraductal stones.

TREATMENT

NONPHARMACOLOGIC THERAPY
- Avoidance of alcohol
- Frequent, small-volume, low-fat meals

ACUTE GENERAL Rx
- Avoidance of narcotics if possible (simple analgesics or NSAIDs can be used)
- Treatment of steatorrhea with pancreatic supplements, e.g., Pancrease, Creon, Pancrealipase titrated PRN based on the amount of steatorrhea and patient's weight loss
- Octreotide 200 µg SC tid may be useful for pain secondary to idiopathic chronic pancreatitis
- Treatment of complications (e.g., IDDM)

CHRONIC Rx
- Surgical intervention may be necessary to eliminate biliary tract disease and improve flow of bile into the duodenum by eliminating obstruction of pancreatic duct.
- ERCP with endoscopic sphincterectomy and stone extraction is useful in selected patients.
- Transduodenal sphincteroplasty or pancreaticojejunostomy in selected patients. Surgery should also be considered in patients with intractable pain.

DISPOSITION
- Long-term survival is poor (50% of patients die within 10 yr from chronic pancreatitis or malignancy).
- Prognosis is best in patients with recurrent acute pancreatitis resulting from cholelithiasis, hyperparathyroidism, or stenosis of the sphincter of Oddi.

REFERRAL
GI referral for ERCP, surgical referral in selected patients (see "Chronic Rx").

MISCELLANEOUS

COMMENTS
- Narcotic addiction is frequent.
- Patient education material can be obtained from National Digestive Diseases Information Clearinghouse, Box NDDIC, Bethesda, MD 20892.

REFERENCES
Bruno MJ et al: Maldigestion associated with exocrine pancreatic insufficiency: implications of gastrointestinal physiology and properties of enzyme preparations for cause related and patient-tailored treatment, *Am J Gastroenterol* 90:1383, 1995.

Steer ML et al: Chronic pancreatitis, *N Engl J Med* 332:1282, 1995.

Author: **Fred F. Ferri, M.D.**

Parkinson's disease (PTG)

BASIC INFORMATION

DEFINITION
Parkinson's disease is a progressive neurodegenerative disorder characterized pathologically by cytoplasmic eosinophilic inclusions (Lewy bodies) in neurons of the substantia nigra and locus ceruleus and by depigmentation of the brain stem nuclei.

SYNONYMS
Paralysis agitans

ICD-9-CM CODES
332.0 Idiopathic Parkinson's disease, primary
332.1 Parkinson's disease, secondary

EPIDEMIOLOGY AND DEMOGRAPHICS
INCIDENCE: 40,000 to 50,000 cases/yr
PREVALENCE: 1% of population >60 yr of age

PHYSICAL FINDINGS
Rigidity—increased muscle tone (>20% of patients at initial diagnosis):
- Involves both agonist and antagonist muscle groups
- Widespread resistance to passive movement, which is more prominent at large joints ("cogwheeling" rigidity is noted)

Tremor—resting tremor, with a frequency of 4 to 7 movements/sec (>70% of patients at initial diagnosis):
- Usually noted in the hands and often involves the thumb and forefinger ("pill-rolling" tremor)
- Improves or disappears with purposeful function

Akinesia—inability to initiate or execute a movement:
- Sitting immobile, since even the simple task of getting up from a chair seems impossible
- Face may reveal a marked absence of movement (masked facies); usually open mouth, drooling

Gait disturbance (10% to 20% at initial diagnosis):
- Stooped posture (head bowed, trunk bent forward, shoulders drooped; knees and arms flexed, "soccer goalie stand")
- Difficulty initiating the first step; small shuffling steps that increase in speed (festinating gait) as if the patient is chasing his or her center of gravity (steps become progressively faster and shorter while the trunk inclines further forward)
- Abnormal reflexes
- Palmomental reflex: stroking the palm of the hand near the base of the thumb results in contraction of the ipsilateral mentalis muscle, causing wrinkling of the skin on the chin
- Glabellar reflex: repeated gentle tapping on the glabella evokes blinking of both eyes

Others: orthostatic hypotension, micrographia

ETIOLOGY
Unknown

DIAGNOSIS

There are no formal criteria for making the diagnosis of Parkinson's disease. A presumptive clinical diagnosis can be made based on a comprehensive history and physical examination. The disease often begins insidiously in patients >60 yr of age with resting tremor, generalized slowness and slight loss of motor dexterity. It is important to exclude other conditions that may also present with signs of parkinsonism (see "Differential Diagnosis").

DIFFERENTIAL DIAGNOSIS
- Multisystem degenerative diseases (e.g., striatonigral degeneration, olivopontocerebellar atrophy)
- Alzheimer's disease with extrapyramidal features
- Essential tremor
- Secondary (acquired) parkinsonism:
  1. Iatrogenic (e.g., phenothiazines, butyrophenones)
  2. Postencephalitic (sequela of encephalitis lethargica)
  3. Toxins (e.g., MPTP, manganese, carbon monoxide)
  4. Hypoparathyroidism, hyperparathyroidism
  5. Cerebrovascular disease (Binswanger's disease, basal ganglia lacunae)

WORKUP
Identification of clinical signs and symptoms associated with Parkinson's disease (see "Physical Findings") and elimination of conditions that may mimic it with a comprehensive history, physical examination, and diagnostic imaging

IMAGING STUDIES
CT scan or MRI of head to eliminate conditions that may present with signs of parkinsonism (see "Differential Diagnosis")

TREATMENT

NONPHARMACOLOGIC THERAPY
- Physical therapy, patient education and reassurance, treatment of associated conditions (e.g., depression)
- Avoidance of drugs that can induce or worsen parkinsonism: neuroleptics (especially haloperidol), certain antiemetics (prochlorperazine, trimethobenzamide), metoclo-

pramide, nonselective MAO inhibitors (may induce hypertensive crisis), reserpine, methyldopa

ACUTE GENERAL Rx
Drug therapy should be delayed until symptoms significantly limit the patient's daily activities, since tolerance and side effects to antiparkinsonian agents are common. Medications used in the therapy of Parkinson's disease are discussed under "Chronic Rx."

CHRONIC Rx
- Selegiline (Eldepryl), an inhibitor of MAO B, is favored by many as initial treatment for younger patients with early disease because of its possible neuroprotective effect; usual dose, 5 mg bid with breakfast and lunch. Selegiline also inhibits catabolism of dopamine in the brain and can be added to levodopa in patients experiencing deterioration while taking it. When added to levodopa, a smaller dose should be used (2.5 mg/day) to avoid increasing levodopa toxicity. Concurrent use of fluoxetine or meperidine should be avoided (toxic reaction).
- Levodopa therapy, the cornerstone of symptomatic therapy, is commonly used with a peripheral dopa decarboxylase inhibitor (carbidopa) to minimize side effects (nausea, mood changes, cardiac arrhythmias, postural hypotension). The combination of the two drugs is marketed under the trade name Sinemet; usual starting dose is 25/100 mg tid 1 hr before meals. It is most effective in the first 2 to 5 yr of therapy. Controlled release preparations (Sinemet CR [200 mg levodopa/50 mg of carbidopa, or 100 mg levodopa/25 mg carbidopa] given bid) produce fewer fluctuations in the plasma concentration of levodopa and result in a smoother therapeutic response. Their major problem is slower onset of action. This can be corrected by adding half of the standard Sinemet dose (25/100) with each morning dose of Sinemet CR. Levodopa-induced psychosis, hallucinosis can be treated with clozapine (Clozaril) or risperidone.
- Dopamine receptor agonists are not as potent as levodopa, but they are often used as initial treatment in younger patients to attempt to delay the tolerance and onset of complications (dyskinesias, motor fluctuations) associated with levodopa therapy; these medications are generally expensive and poorly tolerated by elderly patients with cognitive impairment:
  1. Bromocriptine (Parlodel): initial dose, 1.25 mg qhs
  2. Pergolide (Permax): initial dose, 0.05 mg for first 2 days increased by 0.1 mg every third day over next 12 days
- Amantadine (Symmetrel) is an antiviral agent that may increase dopamine in the brain and improve rigidity and bradykinesia; it can be used alone early in the disease or in combination with levodopa; dosage is 100 mg qd (50 mg qd in elderly and renally impaired patients); side effects include delirium and pedal edema.
- Anticholinergics agents are helpful in treating the tremor and drooling in patients with Parkinson's disease and can be used alone or in combination with levodopa; potential side effects (particularly in the elderly) include constipation, urinary retention, memory impairment, and hallucinations:
  1. Trihexyphenidyl (Artane): initial dose, 1 mg PO tid pc
  2. Benztropine (Cogentin): usual dose, 0.5 to 1 mg qd or bid
- Current research involves transplantation of fetal tissues, ventrolateral thalamotomy (for control of tremor, rigidity, dystonia), medial pallidotomy (to control akinesia or "on-off" effects), and development of new synthetic dopamine agonists.

DISPOSITION
Parkinson's disease usually follows a slowly progressive course leading to eventual disability over the course of several years.

REFERRAL
- Neurology consultation is recommended on initial diagnosis of Parkinson's disease.
- Rehabilitation medicine referral to a physiatrist or physical therapist for outpatient physical therapy is recommended for most patients with disabling symptoms.

MISCELLANEOUS

COMMENTS
Additional patient information on Parkinson's disease can be obtained from the National Parkinson Foundation, Inc., 1501 Ninth Avenue NW, Miami, FL 33136; phone: (800) 327-4545.

REFERENCES
Ahlskog JE: Treatment of early Parkinson's disease: are complicated strategies justified? *Mayo Clin Proc* 71:659, 1996.

Alexander GE: Parkinson's disease. In Johnson RT, Griffin JW (eds): *Current therapy in neurologic disease*, ed 5, St Louis, 1996, Mosby.

Author: **Fred F. Ferri, M.D.**

Paroxysmal atrial tachycardia (PTG)

BASIC INFORMATION

DEFINITION
Paroxysmal atrial tachycardia (PAT) is a group of arrhythmias that generally originate as reentrant rhythm from the AV node and are characterized by sudden onset and abrupt termination.

SYNONYMS
PAT
SVT
Supraventricular tachycardia

ICD-9-CM CODES
427.0 Paroxysmal atrial tachycardia

PHYSICAL FINDINGS
- Patient is usually asymptomatic.
- Patient may be aware of "fast" heartbeat.
- Persistent tachycardia may precipitate CHF or hypotension during acute MI.

ETIOLOGY
- Preexcitation syndromes (Wolff-Parkinson-White [WPW] syndrome)
- Atrial septal defect
- Acute MI

DIAGNOSIS

WORKUP
ECG:
- Absolutely regular rhythm at rate of 150 to 220 bpm is present.
- P waves may or may not be seen (the presence of P waves depends on the relationship of atrial to ventricular depolarization).
- Wide QRS complex (>0.12 sec) with initial slurring (delta wave) during sinus rhythm and short PR ≤0.12 sec) is characteristic of WPW syndrome; this syndrome is a result of an accessory AV pathway (bundle of Kent) that preexcites the ventricular muscle earlier than would be expected if the impulse reached the ventricles by way of normal conduction system; arrhythmias associated with WPW are narrow complex SVT, atrial fibrillation and ventricular fibrillation; digoxin and verapamil use should be avoided because they can lead to arrhythmia acceleration through the accessory pathway. Radio frequency catheter ablation of accessory pathways (performed in conjunction with diagnostic electrophysiology testing) is a safe and effective treatment of patients with WPW syndrome.
- A clinical algorithm for the evaluation of narrow-complex tachycardia is described in Fig. 3-79. Evaluation of wide-complex tachycardia is described in Fig. 3-80.

TREATMENT

NONPHARMACOLOGIC THERAPY
- Valsalva maneuver in the supine position is the most effective way to terminate SVT; carotid sinus massage (after excluding occlusive carotid disease) is also commonly used to elicit vagal efferent impulses.
- Synchronized DC shock is used if patient shows signs of cardiogenic shock, angina or CHF.

ACUTE GENERAL Rx
- Adenosine (Adenocard), an endogenous nucleoside, is useful for treatment of paroxysmal SVT, particularly that associated with WPW; it is considered by many the first choice of therapy for treatment of almost all episodes of SVT unresponsive to vagal maneuvers; the dose is 6 mg given as a rapid IV bolus; tachycardia is usually terminated within a few seconds; if necessary, may repeat with 12 mg IV bolus. Contraindications are second or third degree AV block, sick sinus syndrome (SSS), atrial fibrillation, and ventricular tachycardia. Adenosine may cause bronchospasm in asthmatics. Patients receiving theophylline (a competitive antagonist of adenosine receptors) are usually refractory to treatment. Dipyridamole enhances the effect of adenosine; therefore, patients receiving dipyridamole should be started at lower doses.
- Verapamil 5 to 10 mg IV is given over 5 min; if no effect, may repeat in 30 min.
  1. Verapamil should be used cautiously in patients with SVT associated with hypotension.
  2. Slow injection of calcium chloride (10 ml of a 10% solution given over 5 to 8 min before verapamil administration) decreases the hypotensive effect without compromising its antiarrhythmic effect.
- Repeat carotid massage after IV verapamil if SVT persists.
- Metoprolol (5 mg IV Q 2 min up to 15 mg) or esmolol (500 µg/kg IV bolus, then 50 µg/kg/min) may be effective in the treatment of SVT.
- IV digitalization (0.75 to 1 mg slow IV loading)
  1. Repeat carotid massage 30 min later; if not successful, give additional 0.25 mg IV digoxin and repeat carotid sinus massage 1 hr later.
  2. Digoxin should be avoided in patients with WPW syndrome and narrow QRS tachycardia (increased risk of atrial fibrillation during AV reentrant tachycardia).

DISPOSITION
Most patients respond well with resolution of the paroxysmal atrial tachycardia with treatment (see "Acute General Rx").

REFERRAL
Radiofrequency ablation is the procedure of choice in patients with accessory pathways and recurrent symptomatic episodes.

MISCELLANEOUS

COMMENTS
Accessory pathways occur in 0.1% to 0.3% of the general population.

REFERENCES
Ganz LJ, Friedman TL: Supraventricular tachycardia, *N Engl J Med* 332:162, 1995.
Piper LJ, Stanton MS: Narrow QRS complex tachycardias, *Mayo Clin Proc* 70:371, 1995.
Plumb VJ: Catheter ablation of the accessory pathways of the Wolf-Parkinson-White syndrome and its variants, *Prog Cardiovasc Dis* 37:295, 1995.

Author: **Fred F. Ferri, M.D.**

Pediculosis (PTG)

BASIC INFORMATION

DEFINITION
Pediculosis is lice infestation. Humans can be infested with three kinds of lice: *Pediculus capitis* (head louse), *Pediculus corporis* (body louse), and *Phthirus pubis* (pubic, or crab, louse). Lice feed on human blood and deposit their eggs (nits) on the hair shafts (head lice and pubic lice) and along the seams of clothing (body lice). Nits generally hatch within 7 to 10 days. Lice are obligate human parasites and cannot survive off their hosts for longer than 7 to 10 days.

SYNONYMS
Lice

ICD-9-CM CODES
132.9 Pediculosis

EPIDEMIOLOGY AND DEMOGRAPHICS
- There are 6,000,000 to 12,000,000 cases of head lice in the U.S. yearly.
- Lice infestation of the scalp is most common in children (girls > boys).
- Infestation of the eyelashes is most frequently seen in children and may indicate sexual abuse.
- The chance of acquiring pubic lice from one sexual exposure with an infested partner is >90% (most contagious STD known).
- Body lice is most common in conditions of poor hygiene.

PHYSICAL FINDINGS
- Pruritus with excoriation may be caused by hypersensitivity reaction, inflammation from saliva, and fecal material from the lice.
- Nits can be identified by examining hair shafts (see color plate 14).
- The presence of nits on clothes is indicative of body lice.
- Lymphadenopathy may be present (cervical adenopathy with head lice, inguinal lymphadenopathy with pubic lice).
- Head lice is most frequently found in the back of the head and neck, behind the ears.
- Scratching can result in pustules and crusting.
- Pubic lice may affect the hair around the anus.

ETIOLOGY
Lice are transmitted by close personal contact or use of contaminated objects (e.g., combs, clothing, bed linen, hats).

DIAGNOSIS

DIFFERENTIAL DIAGNOSIS
- Seborrheic dermatitis
- Scabies
- Eczema
- Other: pilar casts, trichonodosis (knotted hair), monilethrix
- A clinical evaluation of generalized pruritus is described in Fig. 3-67.

WORKUP
Diagnosis is made by seeing the lice or their nits.

LABORATORY TESTS
Wood's light examination is useful to screen a large number of children: live nits fluoresce, empty nits have a gray fluorescence, nits with unborn louse reveal white fluorescence.

TREATMENT

NONPHARMACOLOGIC THERAPY
- Patients with body lice should discard infested clothes and improve their hygiene.
- Personal items such as combs and brushes should be soaked in hot water for 15 to 30 min.
- Close contacts and household members should also be examined for the presence of lice.

ACUTE GENERAL Rx
The following products are available for treatment of lice:
- Permethrin: available over the counter (1% permethrin [Nix]) or by prescription (5% permethrin [Elimite]); should be applied to the hair and scalp and rinsed out after 10 min. A repeat application is generally not necessary in patients with head lice.
- Lindane 1% (Kwell), pyrethrin S (Rid): available as shampoos or lotions; they are applied to the affected area and washed off in 5 min; treatment should be repeated in 7 to 10 days to destroy hatching nits.
- Eyelash infestation can be treated with the application of petroleum jelly rubbed into the eyelashes three times a day for 5 to 7 days. The application of baby shampoo to the eyelashes and brows three or four times a day for 5 days is also effective. The use of fluorescein drops applied to the lids and eyelashes is also toxic to lice.
- Ivermectin (Mectizan), an antiparasitic drug, given in a single oral dose of 200 µg/kg is effective for head lice resistant to other treatments (currently not FDA approved for pediculosis).

DISPOSITION
Most cases of pediculosis respond promptly with proper treatment. Patients with severe hair matting and dense infestation can be treated with Bactrim or Septra (toxic to the lice); dose is one tablet bid for 3 days, repeated after 7 to 10 days.

MISCELLANEOUS

COMMENTS
- Patients with pubic lice should notify their sexual contacts.
- Parents of patients should also be educated that head lice infestation (unlike body lice) does not indicate poor hygiene.

REFERENCES
Forsman KE: Pediculosis and scabies: what to look for in patients who are crawling with clues, *Postgrad Med* 98:89, 1995.

Habif TP: *Clinical dermatology*, ed 3, St Louis, 1996, Mosby.

Author: Fred F. Ferri, M.D.

BASIC INFORMATION

DEFINITION
Pedophilia is a sexual disorder of at least 6 mo of recurrent, intense, distressing sexual urges and/or fantasies involving prepubescent children.

SYNONYMS
Pedophilia erotica
Acts referred to as child sexual abuse or child molestation
One of the paraphilias

ICD-9-CM CODES
F65.4 (DSM-IV CODES: 302.2)

EPIDEMIOLOGY AND DEMOGRAPHICS
INCIDENCE (IN U.S.): Accurate data is unavailable.
PREVALENCE (IN U.S.): Prevalence of victimization is variable, ranging from 5% to 60% of all adults reporting at least one case of sexual abuse (not necessarily penetration) before age 13 yr.
PREDOMINANT SEX:
- Majority are men: nearly 75% attracted to females exclusively; nearly 25% attracted to males exclusively; small minority attracted to both sexes
- Females: 5% to 20%

PREDOMINANT AGE: No available data
PEAK INCIDENCE:
- No available data
- Usually, onset in adolescence

GENETICS: No genetic factor has been identified.

PHYSICAL FINDINGS
- Often shy, passive, and with social and interpersonal difficulties
- Frequently, has experienced early abuse himself/herself
- Sexually excited by young children and adults with the build that resembles young children
- Do not all act on their sexual fantasies; may occasionally seek help before any sexual acts with children
- Some "belief" among those who actually molest children that their behavior is good for or welcomed by the child

ETIOLOGY
- Etiology is unclear.
- Personal experience with early molestation may be important, but clearly only a minority of molested children develop pedophilia.
- Influence of personality factors is possible.

DIAGNOSIS

DIFFERENTIAL DIAGNOSIS
- Psychosis: may present with unusual ideas or statements that may rarely be confused with pedophilia; but statements or behaviors of psychotic individuals are usually disorganized and relatively short-lived.
- Incest: some is not based in pedophilia, but may instead reflect a dysfunctional family unit.
- Paraphiliac sexual behavior in the setting of another condition such as mental retardation, brain injury, or drug intoxication.

WORKUP
- History is essential for diagnosis; however, most pedophiles are less than forthcoming even to direct questions by a physician.
- Collateral information should be obtained from family members, suspected victims, or legal and social organizations; but even experienced interviewers may be unable to diagnose pedophilia consistently.

LABORATORY TESTS
- Hormone profile (total testosterone, free testosterone, luteinizing hormone, follicle-stimulating hormone, prolactin, and progesterone) is sometimes recommended, but results do not guide diagnosis or treatment.
- If a medical condition with secondary CNS dysfunction is suspected, tailor laboratory investigation accordingly.

IMAGING STUDIES
Only useful if pedophilic behavior is believed to be a consequence of CNS damage (e.g., head trauma or mental retardation), then a head CT scan or MRI may document extent of anatomic damage

TREATMENT

NONPHARMACOLOGIC THERAPY
- Usually obtain treatment under legal coercion after child molestation charge.
- Rarely, may initiate treatment request.
- Behavioral approaches are centered on aversion conditioning in which an aversive stimulus is paired with the pedophilic fantasy; when outcome is measured by repeat child molestation charges, these methods are moderately successful.
- For incestuous adult-child relationships not based in pedophilia intensive family systems investigation and therapy is needed.

ACUTE GENERAL AND CHRONIC Rx
- Castration is an effective method of control of paraphiliac behaviors, including child molestation. However, the irreversibility of the surgery and the subjective aversion to the procedure makes it less than desirable.
- Chemical castration with antiandrogen compounds is more acceptable to the public; although research into the optimal dosage and the efficacy of these compounds is far from complete, they are generally believed to be safe, effective, and reversible.
- Medroxyprogesterone acetate (Provera) can be administered orally (60 mg/day) or in a depot IM form (200 to 400 mg IM once weekly).

DISPOSITION
- Untreated, child molesters are highly likely to be repeat offenders.
- Pedophiles who do not act on their fantasies are likely to continue these fantasies.
- NOTE: Contrary to popular belief, the majority of sexual acts are committed in the absence of alcohol.

REFERRAL
If pedophilia is highly suspected

MISCELLANEOUS

REFERENCES
Ames MA, Houston DA: Legal, social, and biologic definitions of pedophilia, *Arch Sex Behav* 19:333, 1990.
Fuller AK: Child molestation and pedophilia: an overview for the physician, *JAMA* 261:602, 1989.
Lanyon RI: Theory and treatment in child molestation, *J Consult Clin Psychol* 54:176, 1986.

Author: **Rif S. El-Mallakh, M.D.**

Pelvic inflammatory disease (PTG)

BASIC INFORMATION

DEFINITION
Pelvic inflammatory disease (PID) is a spectrum of inflammatory disorders of the upper genital tract including a combination of any of the following:
- Endometritis, salpingitis, tubo-ovarian abscess, or pelvic peritonitis
- Resulting from an ascending lower genital tract infection
- Not related to obstetric or surgical intervention

SYNONYMS
Adnexitis
Pyosalpinx
Salpingitis
Tubo-ovarian abscess

ICD-9-CM CODES
614.9 Unspecified inflammatory disease of female pelvic organs and tissue

EPIDEMIOLOGY AND DEMOGRAPHICS
INCIDENCE/PREVALENCE:
- Estimated 600,000 to 1,000,000 cases annually (U.S.)
- Diagnosed in 2% to 5% of women seen in STD clinics
- Most common cause of female infertility and ectopic pregnancy

RISK FACTORS:
- Adolescent sexually active in females <20 yr old (1:8)
- Previous episode of gonococcal PID
- Multiple sexual partners
- Vaginal douching
- Use of intrauterine device (threefold to fivefold increased risk of developing acute PID)

PHYSICAL FINDINGS
- Lower abdominal pain
- Abnormal vaginal discharge
- Abnormal uterine bleeding
- Dysuria
- Dyspareunia
- Nausea and vomiting (suggestive of peritonitis)
- Fever
- RUQ tenderness (perihepatitis): 5% of PID cases
- Cervical motion tenderness and adnexal tenderness
- Adnexal mass

ETIOLOGY
- *Chlamydia trachomatis*
- *Neisseria gonorrhea*
- Polymicrobial infection—*Escherichia coli, Gardnerella vaginalis, Hemophilus influenza, Mycoplasma hominis*
- *Mycobacterium tuberculosis* (an important cause in developing countries)

DIAGNOSIS

DIFFERENTIAL DIAGNOSIS
- Ectopic pregnancy
- Appendicitis
- Ruptured ovarian cyst
- Endometriosis
- Urinary tract infection (cystitis or pyelonephritis)
- Renal calculus
- Adnexal torsion
- Proctocolitis

WORKUP
DIAGNOSTIC CONSIDERATIONS:
- Clinical diagnosis is difficult and imprecise. A clinical algorithm for the evaluation of pelvic pain in the reproductive-age woman is described in Fig. 3-65; evaluation of vaginal discharge is described in Fig. 3-92.
- Clinical diagnosis of symptomatic PID has a positive predictive value of 65% to 90% when compared with laparoscopy as the standard.
- No single historical, physical, or laboratory finding is both sensitive and specific for the diagnosis of PID.

1998 CDC DIAGNOSTIC CRITERIA FOR PID:
- Empiric treatment is based on the presence of all of the following minimum criteria:
  1. Lower abdominal pain
  2. Adnexal tenderness
  3. Cervical motion tenderness
- Additional criteria to increase the specificity of the diagnosis of PID in women with severe clinical signs:
  1. Oral temperature >38.3° C
  2. Abnormal cervical or vaginal discharge
  3. Elevated ESR
  4. Elevated C-reactive protein
  5. Laboratory documentation of cervical infection with *N. gonorrhoeae* or *C. trachomatis*
- Definitive criteria for diagnosing PID, which are warranted in selected cases:
  1. Laparoscopic abnormalities consistent with PID
  2. Histopathologic evidence of endometritis on biopsy
  3. Transvaginal sonography or other imaging techniques showing thickened fluid-filled tubes with or without free pelvic fluid or tuboovarian complex

LABORATORY TESTS
- Leukocytosis
- Elevated acute phase reactants: ESR >15 mm/hr, C-reactive protein
- Gram stain of endocervical exudate: >30 PMN per high-power field corre-

lates with chlamydial or gonococcal infection
- Endocervical cultures for *N. gonorrhoeae* and *C. trachomatis*
- Fallopian tube aspirate or peritoneal exudate culture if laparoscopy performed
- hCG to rule out ectopic pregnancy

IMAGING STUDIES
Ultrasound to look for adnexal mass

TREATMENT

NONPHARMACOLOGIC THERAPY
- Most patients are treated as outpatients.
- Criteria for hospitalization (1998 CDC) as follows:
  1. Surgical emergencies such as appendicitis cannot be excluded
  2. Tuboovarian abscess
  3. Pregnant patient
  4. Patient is immunodeficient
  5. Severe illness, nausea, or vomiting precluding outpatient management
  6. Patient unable to follow or tolerate outpatient regimens
  7. No clinical response to outpatient therapy

ACUTE GENERAL RX
REGIMENS FOR TREATMENT OF PID RECOMMENDED BY THE CDC 1998:
- Outpatient treatment: Regimen A:
  1. Ofloxacin 400 mg PO bid × 14 days plus metronidazole 500 mg PO bid × 14 days
- Outpatient treatment: Regimen B:
  1. Cefoxitin 2 g IM plus probenecid 1g PO *or*
  2. Ceftriaxone 250 mg IM *or*
  3. Equivalent cephalosporin (ceftizoxime or cefotaxime) plus doxycycline 100 mg PO bid × 10 to 14 days
- Inpatient treatment: Regimen A:
  1. Cefoxitin 2 g IV q12h or cefotetan 2 g IV q6h plus doxycycline 100 mg IV or PO q12h
  2. Continuation of regimen for at least 24 hr after substantial clinical improvement, after which doxycycline 100 mg PO bid is continued for a total of 14 days
- Inpatient treatment: Regimen B:
  1. Clindamycin 900 mg IV q8h plus gentamicin loading dose IV or IM (2 mg/kg of body weight), followed by a maintenance dose (1.5 mg/kg) q8h
  2. Continuation of regimen for at least 24 hr after substantial clinical improvement, after which doxycycline 100 mg PO bid or clindamycin 450 mg PO qid to complete a total of 14 days of therapy

CHRONIC Rx
Hospitalized patients receiving IV therapy:
1. Significant clinical improvement is characterized by defervescence, decreased abdominal tenderness, and decreased uterine, adnexal, and cervical motion tenderness within 3 to 5 days.
2. If no clinical improvement occurs, further diagnostic workup is necessary, including possible surgical intervention.

DISPOSITION
- Long-term sequelae of PID: recurrent PID, chronic pelvic pain, ectopic pregnancy, infertility
- Risk of tubal infertility related to episodes of PID: first episode, 8%; second episode, 20%; third episode, 40%.
- Essential to evaluate and treat male sex partners

REFERRAL
If there is no clinical improvement with outpatient therapy observed within 72 hr, patient should be hospitalized and gynecology consult requested.

MISCELLANEOUS

COMMENTS
- Patient education material is available from local and state health departments or from the American College of Obstetricians and Gynecologists.
- U. S. Preventive Services Task Force Recommendations regarding counseling to prevent HIV infection and other STDs are described in Section V, Chapter 62.

REFERENCES
Centers for Disease Control: 1998 sexually transmitted diseases treatment guidelines, *MMWR* 47(RR-1),1998.
McCormack W: Current concepts: pelvic inflammatory disease, *N Engl J Med* 330(4): 115, 1994.

Author: **George T. Danakas, M.D.**

Peptic ulcer disease (PTG)

BASIC INFORMATION

DEFINITION
Peptic ulcer disease (PUD) is an ulceration in the stomach or duodenum resulting from an imbalance between mucosal protective factors and various mucosal damaging mechanisms (see "Etiology").

SYNONYMS
PUD
Duodenal ulcer (DU)
Gastric ulcer (GU)

ICD-9-CM CODES
536.8 Peptic ulcer disease
531.3 Peptic ulcer, stomach, acute
531.7 Peptic ulcer, stomach, chronic
532.3 Peptic ulcer, duodenum, acute
532.7 Peptic ulcer, duodenum, chronic

EPIDEMIOLOGY AND DEMOGRAPHICS
- Incidence: 250,000 to 500,000 (200,000 to 400,000 DU; 50,000 to 100,000 GU) annually; duodenal ulcer:gastric ulcer ratio is 4:1.
- Anatomic location: >90% of DU occur in the first portion of the duodenum; GU occurs most frequently in the lesser curvature near the incisura angularis.

PHYSICAL FINDINGS
- Physical examination is often unremarkable.
- Patient may have epigastric tenderness, tachycardia, pallor, hypotension (from acute or chronic blood loss), nausea and vomiting (if pyloric channel is obstructed), boardlike abdomen and rebound tenderness (if perforated), and hematemesis or melena (with a bleeding ulcer).

ETIOLOGY
Often multifactorial; the following are common mucosal damaging factors:
- *Helicobacter pylori* infection
- Medications (NSAIDs, glucocorticoids)
- Incompetent pylorus or LES
- Bile acids
- Impaired proximal duodenal bicarbonate secretion
- Decreased blood flow to gastric mucosa
- Acid secreted by parietal cells and pepsin secreted as pepsinogen by chief cells
- Cigarette smoking
- Alcohol

DIAGNOSIS

DIFFERENTIAL DIAGNOSIS
- GERD
- Cholelithiasis syndrome
- Pancreatitis
- Gastritis
- Nonulcer dyspepsia
- Neoplasm (gastric carcinoma, lymphoma, pancreatic carcinoma)
- Angina pectoris, MI, pericarditis
- Dissecting aneurysm
- Other: high small bowel obstruction, pneumonia, subphrenic abscess, early appendicitis

WORKUP
- Comprehensive history and physical examination to exclude other diagnoses. Diagnostic modalities include endoscopy or UGI series. Endoscopy is invasive and more expensive; however, it is preferred for the following reasons:
  1. Highest accuracy (approximately 90% to 95%)
  2. Useful to identify superficial or very small ulcerations
  3. Essential to diagnose gastric ulcers (1% to 4% of gastric ulcers diagnosed as benign by UGI series are eventually diagnosed as gastric carcinoma)
  4. Additional advantages over UGI series include:
     Biopsy of suspicious looking ulcers
     Electrocautery of bleeding ulcers
     Measurement of gastric pH in suspected gastrinoma (e.g., patient with multiple ulcers)
     Diagnosis of esophagitis, gastritis, duodenitis
     Endoscopic biopsy for *H. pylori*

LABORATORY TESTS
- Routine laboratory evaluation is usually unremarkable.
- Anemia may be present in patients with significant GI bleeding.
- *H. pylori* testing via endoscopic biopsy, urea breath test, or specific antibody test is recommended:
  1. Serologic testing for antibodies to *H. pylori* is easy and inexpensive; however, the presence of antibodies demonstrates previous but not necessarily current infection. Antibodies to *H. pylori* can remain elevated for months to years after infection has cleared; therefore antibody levels must be interpreted in light of patient's symptoms and other test results (e.g., PUD seen on UGI series).
  2. The urea breath test documents active infection. The patient ingests a small amount of urea labeled with carbon 13 (^{13}C) or carbon 14. If urease is present (produced by the organism), the urea is hydrolyzed and the patient exhales labeled carbon dioxide that is then collected and measured. This test is more expensive and not as readily available.
  3. Histologic evaluation of endoscopic biopsy samples is currently the gold standard for accurate diagnosis of *H. pylori* infection.
- Additional laboratory evaluation is indicated only in specific cases (e.g., amylase level in suspected pancreatitis, serum gastrin level in suspected Zollinger-Ellison [Z-E] syndrome).

IMAGING STUDIES
Conventional UGI barium studies identify approximately 70% to 80% of PUD; accuracy can be increased to approximately 90% by using double contrast.

TREATMENT

NONPHARMACOLOGIC THERAPY
- Stop cigarette smoking; cigarette smoking increases the risk of PUD, decreases the healing rate, and increases the frequency of recurrence.
- Avoid NSAIDs.
- Special diets have been proved *unrelated* to ulcer development and healing; however, avoid foods that cause symptoms.

ACUTE GENERAL Rx
Eradication of *H. pylori,* when present, can be accomplished with various regimens:
- Omeprazole 40 mg qAM *plus* clarithromycin 500 mg tid for days 1 to 14, followed by omeprazole 20 mg qAM for days 15 to 28 (cost of therapy is $250 to $300, eradication rate is 83%, discontinuation rate because of side effects is 3%).
- Ranitidine bismuth citrate 400 mg (Tritec) bid *plus* clarithromycin 500 mg tid for days 1 to 14, followed by ranitidine bismuth citrate 400 mg bid for days 15 to 28 (cost of therapy is $200 to $250, eradication rate is 84%, discontinuation rate because of side effects is 5%).
- Lansoprazole 30 mg plus clarithromycin 500 mg plus amoxicillin 1 g, all q12h for 14 days; or if allergic or resistant to clarithromycin, lansoprazole 30 mg plus amoxicillin 1 g, both q8h for 14 days.
- Alternate regimens:
  1. Days 1 to 14: metronidazole 250 mg qid, tetracycline 500 mg qid, bismuth 2 tablets qid, ranitidine 300 mg qd (cost of therapy is $60 to $80, eradication rate is 87%, discontinuation rate because of side effects is 20%).
  2. Days 1 to 10: amoxicillin 1 g bid, omeprazole 20 mg bid, clarithromycin 500 mg bid, followed by omeprazole 20 mg qd from days 11 to 28 (cost of therapy $200 to $300, eradication rate 90%, low compliance).

PUD patients testing negative for *H. pylori* should be treated with antisecretory agents:
- Histamine-2 receptor antagonists (H_2RAs): cimetidine, ranitidine, famotidine, and nizatidine are all effective; they are usually given in split dose or at nighttime; refer to Section VII, Table 7-2 for a comparison of these various agents.
- Proton pump inhibitors (PPIs): omeprazole or lansoprazole can also induce rapid healing; they are usually given 30 min before meals; refer to Section VII, Table 7-2 for a comparison of these medications.

Antacids and sucralfate are also effective agents for the treatment and prevention of PUD.

CHRONIC Rx
Maintenance therapy in duodenal ulcer patients is indicated in the following situations:
- Persistent smokers
- Recurrent ulcerations
- Chronic treatment with NSAIDs, glucocorticoids
- Elderly or debilitated patients
- Aggressive or complicated ulcer disease (e.g., perforation, hemorrhage)
- Asymptomatic bleeders

Misoprostol therapy (100 μg qid with food, increased to 200 μg qid if well tolerated) should be considered for the prevention of NSAID-induced gastric ulcers in all patients on long-term NSAID therapy; it is contraindicated in women of childbearing age because of its abortifacient properties. Treatment with high-dose famotidine (40 mg bid) may also reduce the incidence of both gastric and duodenal ulcers in patients with arthritis receiving long-term NSAID therapy.

DISPOSITION
- The recurrence rate for untreated PUD is approximately 60% (>70% in smokers). Treatment decreases the recurrence rate by nearly 30%.
- Patients with recurrent ulcers should be retreated for an additional 8 wk and then placed on maintenance therapy with H_2RAs, PPIs, sucralfate, or antacids.
- An ulcer is considered refractory to treatment if healing is not evident after 8 wk for duodenal ulcers and 12 wk for gastric ulcers. In these patients maximum acid inhibition (e.g., omeprazole 20 mg bid) is preferred over continued therapy with standard antiulcer therapy.
- Eradication of *H. pylori* (when present) is indicated in all patients.
- Screening for Zollinger-Ellison (Z-E) syndrome should also be considered in patients with multiple recurrent ulcers; in patients with Z-E, the serum gastrin level is >1000 pg/ml and the basal acid output is usually >15 mEq/hr.
- Surgery for refractory ulcers is now only rarely performed; it consists of highly selective vagotomy for duodenal ulcers or ulcer removal with antrectomy or hemigastrectomy without vagotomy for gastric ulcers.

REFERRAL
- GI referral for patients requiring endoscopy
- Surgical referral for patients with nonhealing ulcers despite appropriate medical therapy

MISCELLANEOUS

COMMENTS
Patients with gastric ulcers should have repeat endoscopy after 4 to 6 wk of therapy to document healing and test exfoliative cytology for gastric carcinoma.

REFERENCES
Soll AH for the Practice Parameters Committee of the American College of Gastroenterology: Medical treatment of peptic ulcer disease, *JAMA* 275:622, 1996.

Taha AS et al: Famotidine for the prevention of gastric and duodenal ulcers caused by nonsteroidal antiinflammatory drugs, *N Engl J Med* 334:1435, 1996.

Author: **Fred F. Ferri, M.D.**

Pericarditis (PTG)

BASIC INFORMATION

DEFINITION
Pericarditis is the inflammation (or infiltration) of the pericardium associated with a wide variety of causes (see "Etiology").

ICD-9-CM CODES
420.91 Pericarditis

EPIDEMIOLOGY AND DEMOGRAPHICS
- The incidence of acute pericarditis is 2% to 6%.
- Increased incidence in males and adults compared with children.
- Most common cause (>40%) of constrictive pericarditis is idiopathic.

PHYSICAL FINDINGS
- Severe constant pain that localizes over the anterior chest and may radiate to arms and back; it can be differentiated from myocardial ischemia, since the pain intensifies with inspiration and is relieved by sitting up and leaning forward (the pain of myocardial ischemia is not pleuritic).
- Pericardial friction rub is best heard with patient upright and leaning forward and by pressing the stethoscope firmly against the chest; it consists of three short, scratchy sounds:
  1. Systolic component
  2. Diastolic component
  3. Late diastolic component (associated with atrial contraction)
- Cardiac tamponade may be occurring if the following are observed:
  1. Tachycardia
  2. Low blood pressure and pulse pressure
  3. Distended neck veins
  4. Paradoxical pulse

ETIOLOGY
- Idiopathic (possibly postviral)
- Infectious (viral, bacterial, tuberculous, fungal, amebic, toxoplasmosis)
- Collagen-vascular disease (SLE, rheumatoid arthritis, scleroderma)
- Drug-induced lupus syndrome (procainamide, hydralazine)
- Acute MI
- Trauma or posttraumatic
- After MI (Dressler's syndrome)
- After pericardiotomy
- After mediastinal radiation (e.g., patients with Hodgkin's disease)
- Uremia
- Sarcoidosis
- Neoplasm (primary or metastatic)
- Leakage of aortic aneurysm in pericardial sac
- Familial Mediterranean fever
- Rheumatic fever
- Leukemic infiltration
- Other: anticoagulants, amyloidosis, ITP

DIAGNOSIS

DIFFERENTIAL DIAGNOSIS
- Angina pectoris
- Pulmonary infarction
- Dissecting aneurysm
- GI abnormalities (e.g., hiatal hernia, esophageal rupture)
- Pneumothorax
- Hepatitis
- Cholecystitis
- Pneumonia with pleurisy

WORKUP
ECG, laboratory tests, and echocardiogram

LABORATORY TESTS
The following tests may be useful in absence of an obvious cause:
- CBC with differential
- Viral titers (acute and convalescent)
- ESR (not specific but may be of value in following the course of the disease and the response to therapy)
- ANA, rheumatoid factor
- PPD, ASLO titers
- BUN, creatinine
- Blood cultures
- Cardiac isoenzymes (usually normal, but mild elevations of CK-MB may occur because of associated epicarditis)

IMAGING STUDIES
- Echocardiogram to detect and determine amount of pericardial effusion; absence of effusion does not rule out the diagnosis of pericarditis
- ECG: varies with the evolutionary stage of pericarditis
  1. Acute phase: diffuse ST-segment elevations (particularly evident in the precordial leads), which can be distinguished from acute MI by:
     a. Absence of reciprocal ST-segment depression in oppositely oriented leads (reciprocal ST segment depression may be seen in aVR and V1)
     b. Elevated ST segments concave upward
     c. Absence of Q waves
  2. Intermediate phase: return of ST segment to baseline, and T wave inversion in leads previously showing ST-segment elevation
  3. Late phase: resolution of the T wave changes
- Table 2-62 in Section II describes the differential diagnosis of ST-segment elevation.

TREATMENT

NONPHARMACOLOGIC THERAPY
- Limitation of activity until the pain abates
- Patient education regarding potential complications (e.g., cardiac tamponade, constrictive pericarditis)

ACUTE GENERAL Rx
- Antiinflammatory therapy (NSAIDs, e.g., naproxen 500 mg bid, indomethacin 25 to 50 mg tid)
- Prednisone 30 mg bid for severe forms of acute pericarditis (before using prednisone, tuberculous pericarditis must be excluded)
- Codeine 15 to 60 mg PO qid for pain refractory to salicylates, indomethacin, or prednisone
- Close observation of patients for signs of cardiac tamponade

- Avoidance of anticoagulants (increased risk of hemopericardium)

TREATMENT OF UNDERLYING CAUSE:
1. Bacterial pericarditis
   a. Commonly caused by streptococci, meningococci, staphylococci, hemophilus, gram-negative bacteria, anaerobic bacteria
   b. Therapy: systemic antibiotics and surgical drainage of pericardium
2. Fungal pericarditis
   a. Caused by histoplasmosis, coccidioidomycosis, candidiasis, blastomycosis, or aspergillosis
   b. Therapy: IV amphotericin B and drainage of pericardial space (if necessary)
3. Tuberculous endocarditis
   a. Therapy: antituberculous drugs for a minimum of 9 mo; concomitant corticosteroid therapy early in treatment may decrease inflammatory response and improve prognosis.
   b. Pericardiectomy may be necessary 2 to 4 wk after antituberculous drugs have been started.

POTENTIAL COMPLICATIONS FROM PERICARDITIS:
1. Pericardial effusion: the time required for pericardial effusion to develop is of critical importance; if the rate of accumulation is slow, the pericardium can gradually stretch and accommodate a large effusion (up to 1000 ml), whereas rapid accumulation can cause tamponade with as little as 200 ml of fluid.
2. Chronic constrictive pericarditis:
   a. Physical examination reveals jugular venous distention, Kussmaul's sign (increase in jugular venous distention during inspiration as a result of increased venous pulse), pericardial knock (early diastolic filling sound heard 0.06 to 0.1 sec after S_2), clear lungs, tender hepatomegaly, pedal edema, ascites.
   b. Chest x-ray: clear lung fields, normal or slightly enlarged heart, pericardial calcification
   c. ECG: low voltage QRS complex
   d. Echocardiography: may show pericardial thickening or may be normal
   e. Cardiac catheterization: M or W contour of the central venous pattern caused by both systolic (x) and diastolic (y) dips (this differs from cardiac tamponade, which does not display a prominent diastolic descent; in chronic constrictive pericarditis, there is also increased right ventricular and pulmonary arterial pressures)
   f. Therapy: surgical stripping or removal of both layers of the constricting pericardium
3. Cardiac tamponade:
   a. Signs and symptoms: dyspnea, orthopnea, interscapular pain
   b. Physical examination: distended neck veins, distant heart sounds, decreased apical impulse, diaphoresis, tachypnea, tachycardia, Ewart's sign (an area of dullness at the angle of the left scapula caused by compression of the lungs by the pericardial effusion), pulsus paradoxus (decrease in systolic blood pressure >10 mm Hg during inspiration), hypotension, narrowed pulse pressure
   c. Chest x-ray: cardiomegaly (water bottle configuration of the cardiac silhouette may be seen) with clear lungs; the chest x-ray film may be normal when acute tamponade occurs rapidly in the absence of prior pericardial effusion.
   d. ECG reveals decreased amplitude of the QRS complex, variation of the R wave amplitude from beat to beat (electrical alternans). This results from the heart oscillating in the pericardial sac from beat to beat and frequently occurs with neoplastic effusions.
   e. Echocardiography: detects effusions as small as 30 ml; a paradoxical wall motion may also be seen.
   f. Cardiac catheterization: equalization of pressures within chambers of the heart, elevation of right atrial pressure with a prominent x but no significant y descent.
   g. MRI can also be used to diagnose pericardial effusions.
   h. Therapy of pericardial tamponade consists of immediate pericardiocentesis; in patients with recurrent effusions (e.g., neoplasms), placement of a percutaneous drainage catheter or pericardial window draining in the pleural cavity may be necessary. Aspirated fluid should be sent for analysis (protein, LDH, cytology, CBC, Gram stain, AFB stain) and cultures for AFB, fungi, and bacterial C&S.

DISPOSITION
- Complete resolution of pain and other signs and symptoms during the initial 3 wk of therapy
- Recurrence in 10% to 15% of patients within the initial 12 mo
- Recurrent pericarditis in 28% of patients

REFERRAL
- For pericardiocentesis in patients with cardiac tamponade
- For surgical stripping in patients with constrictive pericarditis

MISCELLANEOUS

REFERENCES
Benoff LJ, Schweiter P: Radiation therapy induced cardiac injury, *Am Heart J* 129:1193, 1995.
Sagrista-Sauleda J et al: Purulent pericarditis: review of a 20-year experience in a general hospital, *J Am Coll Cardiol* 22:1661, 1993.

Author: **Fred F. Ferri, M.D.**

Peripheral nerve dysfunction

BASIC INFORMATION

DEFINITION
- *Peripheral neuropathy* is any disorder involving the peripheral nerves.
- *Polyneuropathy (symmetric polyneuropathy)* is a generalized process resulting in widespread and symmetrical effects on the nervous system.
- *Focal or multifocal neuropathy (mononeuropathy, mononeuropathy multiplex)* is the local involvement of one or more individual peripheral nerves.
- *Paresthesias* are spontaneous aberrant sensations (e.g., pins and needles).

ICD-9-CM CODES
356.9 Peripheral nerve neuropathy
355.10 Lower extremity neuropathy
354.11 Upper extremity neuropathy

PHYSICAL FINDINGS
Vary with the etiology of the neuropathy (see below); the following findings may be present:
- Sensory ataxia
- Reduced or absent tendon reflexes
- Muscle weakness and wasting
- Progressive distal weakness and wasting
- Foot and hand deformities
- Neuropathic ulcers and arthropathy with prolonged peripheral neuropathy
- Autonomic neuropathy (postural hypotension, anhidrosis)

ETIOLOGY
HEREDITARY NEUROPATHIES:
- Charcot-Marie-Tooth syndrome
  1. Most common familial motor and sensory abnormality
  2. Foot deformity is common
- Others: Dejerine-Sottas disease, Refsum's disease, Riley-Day syndrome

ACQUIRED NEUROPATHIES:
- Neuropathy associated with systemic disease
  1. Diabetes mellitus: paresthesias of extremities (feet more than hands); the symptoms are symmetric, bilateral, and associated with intense burning pain (particularly at night).
  2. Mononeuropathies involving the cranial nerves III, IV, and VI, intercostal nerves, and femoral nerves are also common. A mononeuropathy involving a segmental nerve of the trunk can cause pain that mimics herpes zoster, but there is no rash.
  3. Myxedema: distal sensory neuropathy manifested by burning sensation and paresthesias of the limbs; delayed relaxation phase of DTR is common.
  4. Uremia: symmetrical distal mixed motor and sensory disturbances
  5. Sarcoidosis: cranial nerve palsies (most common in facial nerve)
  6. Alcohol: pain numbness and weakness of extremities
  7. Neoplasms: sensory and sensorimotor neuropathies
  8. Nutritional deficiencies: thiamine, folic acid, vitamin B_{12}; vitamin B_{12} deficiency affects the posterior and lateral columns of the spinal cord; it manifests with numbness and paresthesias of the extremities, weakness, ataxia, and loss of vibration sense.
- Guillain-Barré neuropathy (see "Guillain-Barré syndrome" in Section I)
- Toxic neuropathies
  1. Drugs: chloramphenicol, lithium, isoniazid, pyridoxine, nitrofurantoin, disulfiram, dapsone, ethionamide, cisplatin, vincristine, metronidazole, gold, hydralazine, amiodarone, phenytoin, penicillamine, indomethacin, amphotericin B, amitriptyline, sulfonamides, colchicine
  2. Toxic chemicals: lead, arsenic, cyanide, thallium, carbon disulfide, mercury, organophosphates, trichloroethylene
- Neuropathies associated with infection: leprosy, herpes zoster, TB, diphtheria, Lyme disease, HIV
- Entrapment neuropathy (e.g., carpal tunnel syndrome)

DIAGNOSIS

DIFFERENTIAL DIAGNOSIS
- Polyradiculopathy
- Combined systems degeneration

WORKUP
- Inquire about the following:
  1. Family history of neuropathies: to rule out hereditary neuropathies
  2. Current and past employment: to rule out exposure to toxic agents
  3. Current or recent medications: to rule out neuropathy secondary to drugs
  4. Any systemic diseases, such as diabetes, renal failure, hypothyroidism, sarcoidosis
  5. Ethanol abuse: to rule out alcoholic neuropathy
  6. Any special diets (e.g., food faddists): to rule out nutritional deficiencies
  7. History of trauma: to rule out compression-entrapment neuropathies
  8. Risk factors for AIDS
  9. History of tick bite or ECM: to rule out Lyme disease
- Electromyography: in neurogenic lesions there are spontaneous fibrillation potentials and positive sharp waves at rest.
- Nerve conduction studies: slowing of motor or sensory conduction velocities and decrease in sensory action potential amplitude may be present.
- Lumbar puncture should be performed in suspected Guillain-Barré syndrome.
- Nerve biopsy may be needed in selected cases.

LABORATORY TESTS
- CBC, glucose, electrolytes, BUN, creatinine, LFTs, calcium, magnesium, phosphate
- ESR, urinalysis
- HIV in patients with risk factors
- Lyme titer in endemic areas or in patients with suggestive history
- TSH level in suspected hypothyroidism
- Vitamin B_{12} and folate levels in suspected nutritional deficiencies
- Heavy metal screening in suspected toxic neuropathy

IMAGING STUDIES
- Chest x-ray examination to rule out sarcoidosis and lung carcinoma
- X-ray study in suspected trauma or peripheral nerve compression

TREATMENT

NONPHARMACOLOGIC THERAPY
- Stop offending agent
- Physical therapy
- Surgical referral for entrapment neuropathy

ACUTE GENERAL Rx
Therapy is tailored to the symptoms and to the causative agents:
- Diffuse pain and paresthesias may be treated with amitriptyline 25 to 75 mg at hs.
- Topical capsaicin (Zostrix) is effective in postherpetic neuralgia.
- Fludrocortisone is useful in autonomic neuropathy with postural hypotension.
- Vitamin B supplements should be used in alcoholic neuropathy.

MISCELLANEOUS

REFERENCES
Johnson RT, Griffin JW (eds): *Current therapy in neurologic disease,* ed 5, St Louis, 1996, Mosby.

Author: Fred F. Ferri, M.D.

Peritonitis, secondary

BASIC INFORMATION

DEFINITION
Peritonitis refers to the acute onset of severe abdominal pain secondary to peritoneal inflammation.

SYNONYMS
Acute abdomen
Surgical abdomen

ICD-9-CU CODES
567.9 Peritonitis

EPIDEMIOLOGY AND DEMOGRAPHICS
Common presentation as a result of diverse etiologies; for example, 5% to 10% of the population have acute appendicitis at some point in their life.

PHYSICAL FINDINGS
- Acute abdominal pain
- Abdominal distension and ascites
- Abdominal rigidity, rebound, and guarding
- Fever, chills
- Exacerbation with movement
- Anorexia, nausea, and vomiting
- Constipation
- Decreased bowel sounds
- Hypotension and tachycardia
- Tachypnea, dyspnea

ETIOLOGY
Although acute peritonitis can be caused by a wide variety of problems, similar clinical presentation is a result of stimulation of pain receptors within the peritoneum by purulent exudates, bleeding, inflammation, or the release of caustic materials such as pancreatic juice, bile, and gastric secretions.

DIAGNOSIS

DIFFERENTIAL DIAGNOSIS
- Postoperative: abscess, sepsis, bowel obstruction, injury to internal organs
- Gastrointestinal: perforated viscous, appendicitis, IBD, infectious colitis, diverticulitis, acute cholecystitis, peptic ulcer perforation, pancreatitis, bowel obstruction
- Gynecologic: ruptured ectopic pregnancy, PID, ruptured hemorrhagic ovarian cyst, ovarian torsion, degenerating leiomyoma
- Urologic: nephrolithiasis, interstitial cystitis
- Miscellaneous: abdominal trauma, penetrating wounds, infections secondary to intraperitoneal dialysis

WORKUP
- Acute peritonitis is mainly a clinical diagnosis based on patient history and physical examination.
- Laboratory and imaging studies (see below) assist in determining the need for and type of intervention.
- If patient is hemodynamically unstable, immediate diagnostic laparotomy should be performed in lieu of adjuvent diagnostic studies.

LABORATORY TESTS
- CBC: leukocytosis, left shift, anemia
- SMA7: electrolyte imbalances, kidney dysfunction
- LFT: ascites secondary to liver disease, cholilithiasis
- Amylase: pancreatitis
- Blood cultures: bacteremia, sepsis
- Peritoneal cultures: infectious etiology
- Blood gas: respiratory vs. metabolic acidosis
- Ascitic fluid analysis: exudate vs. transudate
- Urinalysis and culture: urinary tract infection
- Cervical cultures for gonorrhea and chlamydia
- Urine/serum hCG

IMAGING STUDIES
- Abdominal series: free air secondary to perforation, small or large bowel dilatation secondary to obstruction, identification of fecolith
- Chest x-ray examination: elevated diaphragm, pneumonia
- Pelvic/abdominal ultrasound: abscess formation, abdominal mass, intrauterine vs. ectopic pregnancy, identify free fluid suggestive of hemorrhage or ascites
- CT: mass, ascites

TREATMENT

NONPHARMACOLOGIC THERAPY
- IV hydration to correct dehydration, hypovolemia
- Blood transfusion to correct anemia secondary to hemorrhage
- Nasogastric decompression, especially if obstruction is present
- Oxygen: intubation if necessary
- Bed rest

ACUTE GENERAL Rx
- Surgery to correct underlying pathology, such as controlling hemorrhage, correct perforation, drain abscess, etc.
- Broad-spectrum antibiotics:
  1. Single agent: ceftriaxone 1 to 2 g IV q24h, cefotaxime 1 to 2 g IV q4-6h
  2. Multiple agents:
     a. Ampicillin 2 g IV q4-6h; gentamycin 1.5 mg/kg/day; clindamycin 600 to 900 mg IV q8h
     b. Ampicillin 2 g IV q4-6h; gentamycin 1.5 mg/kg/day; metronidazole 500 mg IV q6-8h
- Pain control: morphine or meperidine as needed (hold until diagnosis confirmed)

DISPOSITION
Dependent on etiology of peritonitis, age of patient, coexisting medical disease, and duration of process before presentation

REFERRAL
Surgical consultation is required in all cases of acute peritonitis.

MISCELLANEOUS

REFERENCES
Schwartz SI, ed: *Principles of surgery,* ed 6, New York, 1994, McGraw-Hill.
Fauci AS et al, eds: *Harrison's principles of internal medicine,* ed 14, New York, 1998, McGraw-Hill.

Author: **Matthew L. Withiam-Leitch M.D., Ph.D.**

Peritonitis, spontaneous bacterial

BASIC INFORMATION

DEFINITION
Spontaneous bacterial peritonitis (SBP) is an inflammatory reaction of the peritoneum secondary to the presence of bacteria or other microorganisms, most commonly associated with alcoholic cirrhosis and ascites in adults.

SYNONYMS
Primary peritonitis
SBP

ICD-9-CM CODES
567.9 Peritonitis

EPIDEMIOLOGY AND DEMOGRAPHICS
PREDOMINANT SEX: Male > female

PHYSICAL FINDINGS
- Acute fever with accompanying abdominal pain/ascites, nausea, vomiting, diarrhea
- In cirrhotic patients, presentation may be subtle with low-grade temperature (100° F) with or without abdominal abnormalities
- In patients with ascites, a heightened degree of awareness is necessary for detection
- Jaundice and encephalopathy
- Deterioration of mental status and/or renal function

ETIOLOGY
- *Escherichia coli*
- *Klebsiella pneumonia*
- *Streptococcus pneumonia*
- *Streptococcus* spp. including *enterococcus*
- *Staphylococcus aureus*
- Anaerobic pathogens: *Bacteroides, Clostridium* organisms
- Other: fungal, mycobacterial, viral

DIAGNOSIS

DIFFERENTIAL DIAGNOSIS
- Appendicitis (in children)
- Perforated peptic ulcer
- Secondary peritonitis
- Peritoneal abscess
- Splenic, hepatic, or pancreatic abscess
- Cholecystitis
- Cholangitis

WORKUP
- Paracentesis and ascitic fluid analysis (see "Laboratory Tests" below) will confirm diagnosis.
- Laparotomy may be life-threatening in end-stage cirrhosis.
- Positive blood cultures in an individual with ascites requires exclusion of a peritoneal source by paracentesis.

LABORATORY TESTS
Ascitic fluid analysis reveals the following:
- Polymorphonuclear (PMN) cell count: >250/mm^3
- Presence of bacteria on Gram stain
- pH: <7.31
- Lactic acid: >32/dl
- Protein: <1 g/dl
- Glucose: >50 mg/dl
- LDH: <225 mU/ml
- Positive culture of peritoneal fluid

IMAGING STUDIES
- Abdominal ultrasound: if there is clinical difficulty in performing paracentesis
- CT scan: to rule out secondary peritonitis (if indicated) and to exclude abscess, mass

TREATMENT

ACUTE GENERAL Rx
Cefotaxime 1 to 2 g IV q8h or ceftriaxone 2 g IV q24h in patients with normal renal function; duration of treatment is generally 7 to 10 days. Oral quinolone therapy (ofloxacin 400 to 800 mg/day) may be an acceptable alternative in selected patients.

PROPHYLAXIS
Give double strength trimethoprim/sulfamethoxazole qd 5 days/wk or ciprofloxacin 750 mg/wk PO. Both have been shown to decrease occurrence of SBP in patients with cirrhosis.

MISCELLANEOUS

REFERENCES
Ho H et al: Prevalence of associated infections in community-acquired spontaneous bacterial peritonitis, *Am J Gastroenterol* 91:735, 1996.

Levison ME, Bush LM: Peritonitis and other intraabdominal infections. In Mandell GL, Bennett JE, Dolin R (eds): *Mandell, Douglas, and Bennett's principles and practice of infectious diseases,* ed 4, New York, 1995, Churchill Livingstone.

Navasa M et al: Randomized comparative study of oral ofloxacin vs. cefotaxime for spontaneous bacterial peritonitis, *Gastroenterol* 111:1011, 1996.

Author: **Dennis J. Mikolich, M.D.**

Pertussis (PTG)

BASIC INFORMATION

DEFINITION
Pertussis is a prolonged bacterial infection of the upper respiratory tract characterized by paroxysms of an intense cough.

SYNONYMS
Whooping cough

ICD-9-CM CODES
033.9 Pertussis

EPIDEMIOLOGY
INCIDENCE (IN U.S.): Approximately 5000 new cases/yr
PREDOMINANT AGE
- 50% in children <1 yr of age
- 20% in children >15 yr of age

PEAK INCIDENCE
- Childhood
- Usually affects children <1 yr of age

PHYSICAL FINDINGS
- Usually begins with a 1- to 2-wk prodrome that resembles a common cold.
- Following this initial phase, increased production of mucus is noted.
- Increased mucus production is followed by an intense, paroxysmal cough, ending with gasps and an inspiratory whoop.
- In some children, cyanosis and anoxia are noted.
- When prolonged, frank exhaustion and even apnea occur.
- Pertussis is characterized by the finding of intense cough with a marked lymphocytosis.
- Improvement during the later stage is possible.
- High fever may be an indication of secondary bacterial pneumonia, which may be a latter complication of pertussis.

ETIOLOGY
Gram-negative rod, *Bordetella pertussis*, which adheres to human cilia

DIAGNOSIS

DIFFERENTIAL DIAGNOSIS
- Croup
- Epiglottitis
- Foreign body aspiration
- Bacterial pneumonia

WORKUP
- Blood cultures
- Chest x-ray examination
- Culture of bacteria, usually from nasopharynx
- Immunofluorescent staining of nasopharyngeal secretions
- ELISA for detection of antibody to pertussis

LABORATORY TESTS
CBC, which usually demonstrates marked lymphocytosis:
1. Up to 18,000 WBC
2. 70% to 80% lymphocytes

IMAGING STUDIES
Chest x-ray examination is of value if secondary bacterial pneumonia is suspected.

TREATMENT

ACUTE GENERAL Rx
- Intensive supportive care:
  1. Adequate hydration
  2. Control of secretions
  3. Maintenance of airway
- Antibiotics are indicated even though their ability to alter the course of the disease is controversial.
  1. Erythromycin 50 mg/kg/day for 14 days
  2. Although unproved, dexamethasone 1 mg/kg/day in 4 doses for severe, life-threatening paroxysms
  3. Ceftriaxone 75 mg/kg/day in 2 doses for broad coverage of secondary bacterial pneumonias
  4. Nafcillin or vancomycin when staphylococcal pneumonia is suspected
- Vaccination is successful in preventing the disease: universal vaccination is advised for all children <7 yr of age.
- Erythromycin is recommended for all close contacts in the household: trimethoprim-sulfa in 2 oral doses per day for those intolerant to erythromycin.

DISPOSITION
Close attention to accepted vaccination schedules is the best prevention.

REFERRAL
To intensive care setting for life-threatening infections:
1. Pulmonologist
2. Infectious disease specialist

MISCELLANEOUS

REFERENCES
Hewlett EL: *Bordetella* species. In Mandell GL, Bennett JE, Dolin R (eds): *Principles and practices of infectious diseases*, ed 4, New York, 1995, Churchill Livingstone.

Author: **Joseph J. Lieber, M.D.**

Pharyngitis/tonsillitis (PTG)

BASIC INFORMATION

DEFINITION
Pharyngitis/tonsillitis is inflammation of the pharynx or tonsils.

SYNONYMS
Sore throat

ICD-9-CM CODES
462 Pharyngitis

EPIDEMIOLOGY AND DEMOGRAPHICS
PREDOMINANT SEX: Equal
PREDOMINANT AGE:
- All ages affected
- Streptococcal pharyngitis most common among school-aged children

PEAK INCIDENCE: Late winter/early spring (group A streptococcal infections)
GENETICS:
Neonatal Infection: Pharyngitis below the age of 3 yr is almost always of viral etiology.

PHYSICAL FINDINGS
- Pharynx:
  1. May appear normal to severely erythematous
  2. Tonsillar hypertrophy and exudates commonly seen but do not indicate etiology
- Viral infection:
  1. Rhinorrhea
  2. Conjunctivitis
  3. Cough
- Bacterial infection, especially group A *Streptococcus*:
  1. High fever
  2. Systemic signs of infection
- Herpes simplex or enterovirus infection: vesicles
- Streptococcal infection:
  1. Rare complications:
     a. Scarlet fever
     b. Rheumatic fever
     c. Acute glomerulonephritis
  2. Extension of infection: tonsillar, parapharyngeal, or retropharyngeal abscess presenting with severe pain, high fever, trismus

ETIOLOGY
- Viruses:
  1. Respiratory syncytial virus
  2. Influenza A and B
  3. Epstein-Barr virus
  4. Adenovirus
  5. Herpes simplex
- Bacteria:
  1. *Streptococcus pyogenes*
  2. *Neisseria gonorrhoeae*
  3. *Arcanobacterium haemolyticum*
- Other organisms:
  1. *Mycoplasma pneumoniae*
  2. *Chlamydia pneumoniae*

DIAGNOSIS

DIFFERENTIAL DIAGNOSIS
- Sore throat associated with granulocytopenia, thyroiditis
- Tonsillar hypertrophy associated with lymphoma

WORKUP
- Throat swab for culture to exclude *S. pyogenes*, *N. gonorrhoeae* (requires specific transport medium)
- Rapid streptococcal antigen test (culture should be performed if rapid test negative)
- Monospot

LABORATORY TESTS
- CBC with differential
  1. May help support diagnosis of bacterial infection
  2. Streptococcal infection suggested by leukocytosis >15,000/mm^3
- Viral cultures, serologic studies rarely needed

IMAGING STUDIES
Seldom indicated

TREATMENT

NONPHARMACOLOGIC THERAPY
- Fluids
- Salt water gargles

ACUTE GENERAL Rx
- Aspirin (acetaminophen in children)
- If streptococcal infection proven or suspected:
  1. Penicillin V 500 mg PO bid for 10 days or benzathine penicillin 1.2 million U IM once (adults)
  2. Erythromycin 500 mg PO bid or 250 mg qid for 10 days if penicillin-allergic
- If gonococcal infection proven or suspected: ceftriaxone 125 mg IM once

CHRONIC Rx
Recurrent streptococcal infections are common and may represent reinfection from other household members.

REFERRAL
- To otolaryngologist:
  1. If peritonsillar or other abscess is suspected
  2. If tonsillar hypertrophy persists
- To infectious diseases expert if unusual pathogen is suspected

MISCELLANEOUS

COMMENTS
Antibiotic therapy should be avoided unless bacterial etiology is suspected or proven, especially in adults.

REFERENCES
Perkins A: An approach to diagnosing the acute sore throat, *Am Fam Physician* 55(1):131, 1997.

Author: **Joseph R. Masci, M.D.**

Pheochromocytoma (PTG)

BASIC INFORMATION

DEFINITION
Pheochromocytomas are catecholamine-producing tumors that originate from chromaffin cells of the adrenergic system. They generally secrete both norepinephrine and epinephrine, but norepinephrine is usually the predominant amine.

SYNONYMS
Paraganglioma

ICD-9-CM CODES
194.0 Pheochromocytoma

EPIDEMIOLOGY AND DEMOGRAPHICS
- Incidence: 0.05% of population; peak incidence in 30s and 40s.
- "Rough" rule of 10: 10% are extraadrenal, 10% are malignant, 10% are familial, 10% occur in children, 10% involve both adrenals, 10% are multiple (other than bilateral adrenal)
- Pheochromocytoma is a feature of two disorders with autosomal dominant pattern of inheritance:
  1. Multiple endocrine neoplasia II
  2. von Hippel-Lindau disease: angioma of the retina, hemangioblastoma of the CNS, renal cell carcinoma, pancreatic cysts, and epididymal cystoadenoma

PHYSICAL FINDINGS
- Hypertension: can be sustained (55%) or paroxysmal (45%).
- Headache (80%): usually paroxysmal in nature and described as "pounding" and severe
- Palpitations (70%): can be present with or without tachycardia
- Hyperhidrosis (60%): most evident during paroxysmal attacks of hypertension
- Physical examination may be entirely normal if done in a symptom-free interval; during a paroxysm the patient may demonstrate marked increase in both systolic and diastolic pressure, profuse sweating, visual disturbances (caused by hypertensive retinopathy), dilated pupils (secondary to catecholamine excess), paresthesias in the lower extremities (caused by severe vasoconstriction), tremor, tachycardia.

ETIOLOGY
Catecholamine-producing tumors that are usually located in the adrenal medulla

DIAGNOSIS

DIFFERENTIAL DIAGNOSIS
- Anxiety disorder
- Thyrotoxicosis
- Amphetamine or cocaine abuse
- Carcinoid
- Essential hypertension

WORKUP
Laboratory evaluation and imaging studies to locate the neoplasm; a diagnostic approach to adrenal mass is described in Section III, Fig. 3-2.

LABORATORY TESTS
- 24-hr urine collection will show increased metanephrines; the accuracy of the 24-hr urinary levels for metanephrines can be improved by indexing urinary metanephrine levels by urine creatinine levels.
- Measurement of plasma metanephrines (normetanephrine and metanephrine) are also useful, since normal plasma concentrations of metanephrines exclude the diagnosis of pheochromocytoma.

IMAGING STUDIES
- Abdominal CT scan is useful in locating pheochromocytomas >0.5" in diameter (90% to 95% accurate).
- MRI: pheochromocytomas demonstrate a distinctive MRI appearance; MRI may become the diagnostic imaging modality of choice.
- Scintigraphy with ^{131}I-MIBG: this norepinephrine analog localizes in adrenergic tissue; it is particularly useful in locating extraadrenal pheochromocytomas.
- Selective vena cava sampling for norepinephrine levels may be useful when diagnostic imaging studies are unsuccessful.

TREATMENT

ACUTE GENERAL Rx
Laparoscopic removal of the tumor (surgical resection for both benign and malignant disease):
1. Preoperative stabilization
   a. Volume expansion is done to prevent postoperative hypotension.
   b. α-Blockade to control hypertension: phenoxybenzamine (Dibenzyline) 10 mg PO bid to qid; metyrosine 250 mg PO qid or prazosin can be used when phenoxybenzamine therapy alone is not effective or not well tolerated.
   c. β-Blockade with propranolol 20 to 40 mg PO q6h (to be used only after α-blockade) is useful to prevent catecholamine-induced arrhythmias and tachycardia.
2. Hypertensive crisis preoperatively and intraoperatively should be controlled with phentolamine (Regitine) 2 to 5 mg IV q1-2h PRN; second drug of choice is nitroprusside used in combination with β-adrenergic blockers.
3. Combination chemotherapy with cyclophosphamide, vincristine, and dacarbazine is effective for advanced malignant pheochromocytoma.

DISPOSITION
- The 5-yr survival rate is approximately 95% with benign disease, 40% for malignant pheochromocytoma (malignancy is determined by metastasis).
- Pheochromocytomas are three times more likely to be malignant in women.

MISCELLANEOUS

COMMENTS
- Screening for pheochromocytoma should be considered in patients with any of the following:
  1. Malignant hypertension
  2. Poor response to antihypertensive therapy
  3. Paradoxical hypertensive response
  4. Hypertension during induction of anesthesia, parturition, surgery, or thyrotropin-releasing hormone testing
  5. Hypertension associated with imipramine or desipramine
  6. Neurofibromatosis (increased incidence of pheochromocytoma)
- All patients with pheochromocytoma should be screened for MEN-II and von Hippel-Lindau disease with pentagastrin test, serum PTH, ophthalmoscopy, MRI of the brain, CT scan of the kidneys and pancreas, and ultrasonography of the testes.

REFERENCES
Lenders JW: Plasma metanephrines in the diagnosis of pheochromocytoma, *Ann Intern Med* 123:101, 1995.

Werbel SF, Ober KP: Pheochromocytoma: update on diagnosis, localization, and management, *Med Clin North Am* 779:131, 1995.

Author: **Fred F. Ferri, M.D.**

Phobias (PTG)

BASIC INFORMATION

DEFINITION
A phobia is severe anxiety that is elicited by a specific object or situation and that often leads to avoidance behavior. The provoking stimuli may be social or performance situations (social phobia) or any other stimulus (specific phobia of animals, natural environments, blood, or situational).

SYNONYMS
Simple phobia (obsolete name for specific phobia)
Phobias named according to the inducing stimulus, e.g., arachnaophobia (fear of spiders), claustrophobia (fear of tight spaces), kneebophobia (fear of knee bending backwards)
Social anxiety disorder (obsolete name for social phobias)

ICD-9-CM CODES
F40.2 Specific phobia (DSM-IV: 300.29)
F40.1 Social phobia (DMS-IV: 300.23)

EPIDEMIOLOGY AND DEMOGRAPHICS
PREVALENCE (IN U.S.):
- For specific phobias, the 1-yr prevalence rate is 9% and the lifetime rates range from 10% to 11.3%.
- For social phobias, prevalence rates of 3% to 13% have been reported, but only about 2% experience a significant degree of impairment to warrant clinical concern or intervention.

PREDOMINANT SEX:
- Females with specific phobias outnumber males.
- Rates vary according to the phobia, e.g., of individuals with animal or nature phobias, 75% to 90% are female; of individuals that fear blood, 55% to 70% are female; of people with situational fears, 75% to 70% are female. Similarly, more women are affected with social phobia; however, men are more likely to present for treatment.

PREDOMINANT AGE:
- Onset of most specific phobias is in childhood.
- Major exceptions: situational phobias, which have two peaks—the first in childhood and the second in the mid-20s.
- Once developed, fears are stable.
- Roots of social phobia may be in childhood, with described shyness or social inhibition, but onset usually in the midteens or into late adulthood; disorder is generally lifelong.

PEAK INCIDENCE:
- Specific phobias: lifelong condition
- Social phobia: may alternate in mid-to-late adulthood

GENETICS: Both specific phobias and social phobia are more common in first-degree relatives than the general population; however, this does not necessarily mean a genetic etiology.

PHYSICAL FINDINGS
- Specific phobias: frequently have other anxiety disorders, particularly panic and agoraphobias; most phobias are associated with sinus tachycardia on exposure to the stimulus, although blood phobias frequently (in 75% of those afflicted) are associated with sinus bradycardia, hypotension, and fainting.
- Social phobias: usually have low self-esteem and fear of evaluation from others; avoid or are fearful of any situation in which others may assess or evaluate them directly or indirectly; concurrent anxiety disorders are common, but these persons are less likely to develop panic than panic disorder patients when challenged with panicogenic lactate infusion or CO_2 inhalation.

ETIOLOGY
- Unknown
- Biologic features probably a relatively small component

DIAGNOSIS

DIFFERENTIAL DIAGNOSIS
- Panic attacks: anxiety symptoms seen in specific phobia may resemble panic attacks, but the stimulus in specific phobias or social phobia is clear whereas panic attacks seem more random.
- Generalized anxiety disorder: difficult to distinguish from social phobia, but in social phobia the cognitive focus is fear of embarrassment or humiliation, whereas in generalized anxiety disorder the focus is more internal on the subjective sensations of discomfort.

WORKUP
- History: usually diagnostic
- Physical examination: to confirm absence of cardiovascular abnormalities (e.g., a chronic sinus arrhythmia)

LABORATORY TESTS
No specific laboratory tests are indicated.

IMAGING STUDIES
If phobias are associated with fainting, a cardiac workup (EEG, Holter) may be indicated.

TREATMENT

NONPHARMACOLOGIC THERAPY
- Treatment of choice for specific phobias is desensitization
- Cognitive-behavioral therapy and other psychotherapeutic approaches are effective.
- Success rates are higher when the phobia is not complicated by other anxiety disorders.
- Social phobia is more problematic to treat because the psychologic difficulties are more pervasive, but cognitive-behavioral therapy and other psychotherapies are quite effective.
- For social phobia, psychotherapy is almost always required, at least as adjunct.

ACUTE GENERAL Rx
- Benzodiazepines: provide rapid, effective relief of anxiety associated with exposure to fearful stimuli
- Alprazolam or lorazepam: both administered sublingually to increase rate of absorption
- β-blockers: given before exposure to the fearful stimulus (e.g., before a public speech); the lipophilic β-blockers are preferred
- Acute management of anxiety symptoms: not advisable in view of chronicity of the symptoms of social phobia

CHRONIC Rx
- If the phobic stimulus is encountered rarely and unexpectedly, benzodiazepines may be appropriate long-term treatment.
- If the phobic stimulus can be anticipated, β-blockers may be appropriate long-term treatment.
- Social phobia is also a chronic condition. Individuals with social phobia often underachieve, drop out of school, avoid seeking work as a result of anxiety about interviews, refrain from dating and remain with family of origin, and are less likely to marry. In addition to this social and occupational dysfunction, these individuals lead very unfulfilled lives.

REFERRAL
If psychotherapy advised

MISCELLANEOUS

REFERENCES
Brown JT, Mulrow CD: The anxiety disorders, *Ann Intern Med* 100:588, 1984.
Authors: **Rif S. El-Mallakh, M.D. and Peggy L. El-Mallakh, B.S.N.**

CLINICAL TOPICS   **Pilonidal disease** 365

BASIC INFORMATION

DEFINITION
A *pilonidal sinus* is a short tract that extends from the skin surface, is most commonly found in the intergluteal fold, and most likely represents a distended hair follicle. An *acute pilonidal abscess*, which consists of pus and a wall of edematous fat, results from rupture of an infected follicle into fat. A chronic pilonidal abscess results when an infected follicle ruptures directly into surround tissues; the wall of a chronic pilonidal abscess consists of fibrous tissue. A *pilonidal cyst* develops from a chronic abscess of long duration as a thin and flat lining of epithelium grows into the cavity from the skin surface.

SYNONYMS
Jeep disease

ICD-9-CM CODES
685.1 Pilonidal cyst

EPIDEMIOLOGY AND DEMOGRAPHICS
INCIDENCE: 26 cases/100,000 persons
PREDOMINANT SEX: Male > female (2.2:1)
AVERAGE AGE OF PRESENTATION: 21 yr
GENETICS: Theory of congenital origin is now disfavored.
RISK FACTORS:
- Male sex
- Caucasian race
- Family predisposition
- Obesity
- Sedentary life-style
- Occupation requiring prolonged sitting
- Local hirsutism
- Poor hygiene
- Increased sweat activity

PHYSICAL FINDINGS
- May manifest as asymptomatic pits or pores in the natal cleft
- Tenderness after physical activity or prolonged sitting
- Acute pilonidal abscess in 20% of patients with pilonidal disease
- Presents as a hot, tender, fluctuant swelling just lateral to the midline over the sacrum that may exude pus through the midline pit
- Chronic pilonidal abscess in 80% of patients with pilonidal disease
- Acute suppuration, tenderness, swelling, and heat
- Infrequently, systemic reaction: occasionally fever, leukocytosis, and malaise

ETIOLOGY
- Currently, thought to be acquired rather than congenital.
- Drilling of hair shed from the perineum or the head into sebaceous or hair follicles in the natal cleft.
- Drilling is facilitated by the friction of the natal cleft.
- Subsequent infection by skin organisms leads to pilonidal abscess.

DIAGNOSIS

DIFFERENTIAL DIAGNOSIS
- Perianal abscess arising from the posterior midline crypt
- Hidradenitis suppurativa
- Carbuncle
- Furuncle
- Osteomyelitis
- Anal fistula
- Coccygeal sinus

WORKUP
- Diagnosis is based on history and physical examination.
- Midline pits present behind the anus overlying the sacrum and coccyx.
- Broken hairs are often seen extruding from the midline pits.
- Insert probe in pilonidal sinus in path away from the anus.
- Complicated anal fistula may be angulating posteriorly before passing into a retrorectal abscess, but thorough examination of the anal cavity usually discloses point of origin.

LABORATORY TESTS
CBC

IMAGING STUDIES
CT scan in advanced recurrent cases

TREATMENT

NONPHARMACOLOGIC THERAPY
Prevention of exacerbations:
1. Local hygiene
2. Avoidance of prolonged sitting position
3. Weight reduction

ACUTE GENERAL Rx
- Procedure of choice for first-episode acute abscess: simple incision and drainage in an outpatient setting
- Cure rate of 76% after 18 mo
- Antibiotics: generally not indicated unless the patient has a medical condition such as rheumatic heart disease or is immunosuppressed

CHRONIC Rx
Elective treatment of pilonidal disease:
1. Minimal surgery
   a. Remove hair from midline pits and shave buttocks.
   b. May use a fine wire brush with local anesthesia to clear the pits and any lateral openings of granulation tissue and hair.
   c. Keep area clean.
2. Opening of sinus tracts
   a. Used when minimal surgery does not control episodes of suppuration.
   b. Pass probe to outline the pilonidal sinus and open tract surgically.
   c. Curette granulation tissue at the base of the sinus and excise edges of the skin.
   d. Keep open granulating wound meticulously clean and allow to heal.
   e. If complete healing does not take place, use a skin graft or advancement flap to close the defect.
3. Excision
   a. This is the treatment of choice for chronic pilonidal disease.
   b. Wide excision of the pilonidal area is performed, including all affected skin and subcutaneous tissues down to the presacral fascia.
   c. Wound is left open, allowed to marsupialize, or closed as a primary procedure.
   d. Give antibiotics for 24 hr (particularly those directed against *Staphylococcus* and *Bacteroides* species).

DISPOSITION
Recurrence rate for excision (most definitive procedure): 1% to 6%

REFERRAL
- Emergency room for incision and drainage for an acute abscess
- To a surgeon for elective treatment or management of chronic or recurrent disease

MISCELLANEOUS

COMMENTS
Because of significant associated morbidity, the elective surgical procedures outlined are performed only after the potential risks vs. benefits are carefully weighed.

REFERENCES
Nyhus LM, RJ Baker, JE Fischer (eds): *Mastery of surgery*, ed 3, vol 2, Boston, 1997, Little, Brown.
Sebastian MW: Pilonidal cysts and sinuses. In Sabiston DC Jr (ed.): *Textbook of surgery: the biologic basis of modern surgical practice*, Philadelphia, 1997, WB Saunders.
Spivak H et al: Treatment of chronic pilonidal disease, *Dis Colon Rectum* 39:1136, 1996.
Author: **Wan J. Kim, M.D.**

Pituitary adenoma

BASIC INFORMATION

DEFINITION
Pituitary adenoma is a benign neoplasm of the anterior lobe of the pituitary that causes symptoms, either by excess secretion of hormones or by a local mass effect as the tumor impinges on other nearby structures (e.g., optic chiasm, hypothalamus, pituitary stalk). Pituitary adenomas are classified by their size, function, and features that characterize their appearance. Microadenomas are <10 mm in size, and macroadenomas are >10 mm in size.

- *Acromegaly* is the disease state characterized by a pituitary adenoma which secretes growth hormone (GH).
- A *prolactinoma* secretes prolactin (PRL).
- *Cushing's disease* is a disease state in which there is hypersecretion of adrenocorticotropic hormone (ACTH).
- *Thytropin-secreting pituitary adenomas* secrete primarily thyroid stimulating hormone (TSH).
- *Nonsecretory pituitary adenomas* are those in which the neoplasm is a space-occupying lesion whose secretory products do not cause a specific disease state.

ICD-9-CM CODES
253 Pituitary adenoma
253.0 Acromegaly
253.1 Prolactinoma

EPIDEMIOLOGY AND DEMOGRAPHICS
CLASSIFICATION (BY HORMONE SECRETED):
PRL only ~35%
No hormone ~30%
GH only ~20%
PRL and GH ~7%
ACTH ~7%
LF/FSH/TSH ~1%
PREVALENCE/INCIDENCE:
Pituitary Adenomas: up to 10% to 15% of all intracranial neoplasms; 3% to 27% autopsy series
Prolactinomas: up to 20% in women with unexplained primary or secondary amenorrhea
Growth Hormone-Secreting Pituitary Adenoma: 50 to 60 cases/1,000,000 persons
Thyrotropin-Secreting Pituitary Adenoma: 2.8% of pituitary adenomas with a slight female:male predominance of 1.7:1
Corticotrophin-Secreting Pituitary Adenomas: Female:male predominance of 8:1

PHYSICAL FINDINGS
PROLACTINOMAS:
- Females:
  1. Galactorrhea
  2. Amenorrhea
  3. Oligomenorrhea with anovulation
  4. Infertility
  5. Estrogen deficiency leading to hirsuitism
  6. Decreased vaginal lubrication
  7. Osteopenia
- Males:
  1. Large tumors more common secondary to delayed diagnosis
  2. Possible impotence or decreased libido or hypogonadism
  3. Galactorrhea rare because males lack the estrogen-dependent breast growth and differentiation

GROWTH HORMONE-SECRETING PITUITARY ADENOMA: Acromegaly
- Coarse facial features
- Oily skin
- Prognathism
- Carpal tunnel syndrome
- Osteoarthritis
- History of increased hat, glove, or shoe size
- Decreased exercise capacity
- Visual field deficits
- Diabetes mellitus

CORTICOTROPIN-SECRETING PITUITARY ADENOMA: Cushing's disease
- Usually presents when the tumor is small (1 to 2 mm)
- 50% of the tumors <5 mm
- Other symptoms:
  1. Truncal obesity
  2. Round facies (moon face)
  3. Dorsocervical fat accumulation (buffalo hump)
  4. Hirsuitism
  5. Acne
  6. Menstrual disorders
  7. Hypertension
  8. Striae
  9. Bruising
  10. Thin skin
  11. Hyperglycemia

THYROTROPIN-SECRETING PITUITARY ADENOMA:
- In males, larger, more invasive, and more rapidly growing tumors that present later in life
- Other symptoms: thyrotoxicosis, goiter, visual impairment

NONSECRETORY PITUITARY ADENOMAS (ENDOCRINE INACTIVE PITUITARY ADENOMA):
- Usually large at the time of diagnosis
- Symptoms:
  1. Bitemporal hemianopia secondary to compression of the optic chiasm
  2. Hypopituitarism secondary to compression of the pituitary gland
  3. Hypogonadism in men and in premenopausal women
  4. Cranial nerve deficits, secondary to extension into the cavernous sinus
  5. Hydrocephalus, secondary to extension into the third ventricle, compressing the foramina of Monro
  6. Diabetes insipidus, secondary to compression of the hypothalamus or pituitary stalk (a rare complication)

ETIOLOGY
Benign neoplasms of epithelial origin

DIAGNOSIS

DIFFERENTIAL DIAGNOSIS
PROLACTINOMA:
- Pregnancy
- Postpartum puerperium
- Primary hypothyroidism
- Breast disease
- Breast stimulation
- Drug ingestion (especially phenothiazines, antidepressants, haloperidol, methyldopa, reserpine, opiates, amphetamines and cimetidine)
- Chronic renal failure
- Liver disease
- Polycystic ovarian disease
- Chest wall disorders
- Spinal cord lesions
- Previous cranial irradiation

ACROMEGALY: Ectopic production of growth hormone–releasing hormone from a carcinoid or other neuroendocrine tumor

CUSHING'S DISEASE:
- Diseases that cause ectopic sources of ACTH overproduction (including small cell carcinoma of the lung, bronchial carcinoid, intestinal carcinoid, pancreatic islet cell tumor, medullary thyroid carcinoma, or pheochromocytoma)
- Adrenal adenomas, adrenal carcinoma
- Nelson's syndrome

THYROTROPIN-SECRETING PITUITARY ADENOMAS: Primary hypothyroidism

NONSECRETORY PITUITARY ADENOMA: Nonneoplastic mass lesions of various etiologies (e.g., infectious, granulomatous, etc.)

WORKUP
PROLACTINOMA: First step: Measurement of basal PRL levels
- Elevated PRL levels are correlated with tumor size
- Levels >200 ng/ml are diagnostic, with levels of 100 to 200 ng/ml being equivocal

- Basal PRL levels between 20 and 100 suggest a microprolactinoma as well as other conditions such as drug ingestion
- Basal level <20 is normal.

ACROMEGALY:
- First screening test is the measurement of the serum IGF-I level
- Follow with an oral glucose tolerance test
- Failure to suppress serum GH to <2 ng/ml with an oral load of 100 g glucose is considered conclusive
- A GHRH level >300 ng/mL is indicative of an ectopic source of GH.

CUSHING'S DISEASE:
- Normal or slightly elevated corticotropin levels ranging from 20 to 200 pg/ml; normal is 10 to 50 pg/mL.
- Levels <10 pg/ml usually indicate an autonomously secreting adrenal tumor
- Levels >200 pg/ml suggest an ectopic corticotropin-secreting neoplasm.
- Cushing's disease is confirmed by demonstration of low-dose dexamethasone, which shows presence of abnormal cortisol suppressibility.
- 24-hr urine collection should demonstrate an increased level of cortisol excretion.

THYROTROPIN-SECRETING PITUITARY ADENOMA:
- Highly sensitive thyrotropin assays, which evaluate the presence of thyrotoxicosis, is one way to detect a thyrotropin-secreting tumor.
- Free alpha subunit is secreted by >80% of tumors with the ratio of the alpha-subunit to thyrotropin >1.
- With central resistance to thyroid hormone, ratio is <1 and the sella is normal.
- Laboratory tests show elevated serum levels of both T_3 and T_4.

NONSECRETORY PITUITARY ADENOMA:
- Visual field testing
- Assessment of the pituitary and organ function to determine if there is hypopituitarism or hypersecretion of hormones (even if the effects of hypersecretion are subclinical)
- TRH to provoke secretion of FSH, LH and LH-beta-subunit; will not elicit response in normal persons
- Exclusion of Klinefelter's syndrome in patient with longstanding primary hypogonadism, elevated gonadotropin levels, and enlargement of the sella

IMAGING STUDIES
- Study of choice: MRI of the pituitary and hypothalamus
  1. When evaluating Cushing's disease, small size at the onset of symptoms noted
- MRI, in this case, only 60% sensitive at best and may yield false positive results
- CT scan only when MRI is unavailable or is otherwise contraindicated

TREATMENT

NONPHARMACOLOGIC THERAPY
SURGERY:
- Selective transsphenoidal resection of the adenoma is the treatment of choice for prolactinoma, acromegaly, Cushing's disease, and thyrotropin-secreting pituitary adenomas, which all tend to be microadenomas at the time of onset of symptoms.
- Macroadenomas, such as the nonsecretory pituitary adenoma, may also be surgically removed, but risk of recurrence is greater with these tumors, and adjunctive therapy such as irradiation may also be necessary.
- Radiotherapy is reserved for patients who have failed surgical treatment and who still experience the symptoms of their adenoma.
- Bilateral adrenalectomy has been done in patients with Cushing's disease on failure of other therapies; complications requiring lifelong hormone replacement or Nelson's syndrome may occur.

RADIOTHERAPY:
- Generally reserved for patients who have failed surgical treatment
- Used with varying degrees of success in all of the different pituitary adenomas

PHARMACOLOGIC THERAPY
PROLACTINOMA:
- Bromocriptime, a dopamine analogue, is generally given orally in divided doses of 1.5 to 10 mg.
- Side effects include orthostatic hypotension, nausea, and dizziness; avoided by beginning with low dose therapy.
- Other compounds under investigation include pergolide mesylate, a long-acting ergot derivative with dopaminergic properties, as well as other nonergot derivatives.

ACROMEGALY:
- Octreotide, a somatostatin analogue, 100 μg SC, is the medical therapy of choice; limited by side effects such as biliary sludge and gallstones, nausea, cramps, steatorrhea, and its parenteral administration
- Bromocriptine 10 to 69 mg PO tid-qid is less effective than octreotide, but has the advantage of oral administration.

CUSHING'S DISEASE:
- Ketoconazole, which inhibits the cytochrome P-450 enzymes involved in steroid biosynthesis, is effective in managing mild to moderate disease in daily oral dosages of 600 to 1200 mg.
- Metyrapone and aminoglutethimide can be used to control hypersecretion of cortisol, but are generally used when preparing a patient for surgery or while waiting for a response to radiotherapy.

THYROTROPIN-SECRETING PITUITARY ADENOMA:
- Ablative therapy with either radioactive iodide or surgery is indicated
- Treatment directed to the thyroid alone may accelerate growth of the pituitary adenoma
- Octreotide has been shown to be effective in doses similar to those used for acromegaly.

NONSECRETORY PITUITARY ADENOMA:
- There is no role for medical therapy at this time
- Surgery and radiotherapy are indicated.

CHRONIC Rx
For all pituitary adenomas:
- Careful follow-up is important. Patients undergoing transsphenoidal microsurgical resection should be seen in 4 to 6 wk to ensure that the adenoma has been completely removed and that the endocrine hypersecretion is resolved.
- If there is good clinical response, patient should be monitored yearly for recurrence and to follow the level of the hypersecreted hormone.
- Patients who have undergone irradiation should have close follow-up with back-up medical therapy because response to radiotherapy may be delayed; incidence of hypopituitarism also increases with time.

MISCELLANEOUS

REFERENCES
Aron DC, Tyrell JB, Wilson CB: Pituitary tumors: current concepts in diagnosis and management, *West J Med* 162:340, 1995.
Chang BW and Newton TH: Hypothalamic and pituitary pathology, *Radiol Clin North Am* 31(5):1147, 1993.
Author: **Candace C. Green, M.D.**

Pityriasis rosea (PTG)

BASIC INFORMATION

DEFINITION
Pityriasis is a common self-limiting skin eruption of unknown etiology.

ICD-9-CM CODES
696.3 Pityriasis rosea

EPIDEMIOLOGY AND DEMOGRAPHICS
- Most cases of pityriasis rosea occur between ages 10 and 35 yr; mean age is 23 yr.
- The incidence of disease is highest in the fall and spring.
- Female:male ratio is 1.5:1.

PHYSICAL FINDINGS
- Initial lesion (herald patch) precedes the eruption by approximately 1 to 2 wk; typically measures 3 to 6 cm; it is round to oval in appearance and most frequently located on the trunk.
- Eruptive phase follows within 2 wk and peaks after 7 to 14 days.
- Lesions are most frequently located in the lower abdominal area. They have a salmon-pink appearance in whites and a hyperpigmented appearance in blacks.
- Most lesions are 4 to 5 mm in diameter; center has a "cigarette paper" appearance; border has a characteristic ring of scale (collarette).
- Lesions occur in a symmetrical distribution and follow the cleavage lines of the trunk (Christmas tree pattern)—see color plate 15.
- The number of lesions varies from a few to hundreds.
- Most patients are asymptomatic; pruritus is the most common symptom.
- History of recent fatigue, headache, sore throat, and low-grade fever is present in approximately 25% of cases.

ETIOLOGY
Unknown, possibly viral (picornavirus)

DIAGNOSIS

DIFFERENTIAL DIAGNOSIS
- Tinea corporis (can be ruled out by potassium hydroxide examination)
- Secondary syphilis (absence of herald patch, positive serologic test for syphilis)
- Psoriasis
- Nummular eczema
- Drug eruption
- Viral exanthem (see Section II, Table 2-21)
- Eczema
- *Lichen planus*
- Tinea versicolor (the lesions are more brown and the borders are not as ovoid)

WORKUP
Presence of herald lesion and characteristic rash are diagnostic. Skin biopsy is generally reserved for atypical cases.

LABORATORY TESTS
Generally not necessary; serologic test for syphilis if clinically indicated

TREATMENT

NONPHARMACOLOGIC THERAPY
The disease is self-limited and generally does not require any therapeutic intervention.

ACUTE GENERAL Rx
- Use calamine lotion or oral antihistamines in patients with significant pruritus.
- Use prednisone tapered over 2 wk in patients with severe pruritus.
- Direct sun exposure or use of ultraviolet light within the first week of eruption is beneficial.

DISPOSITION
- Complete resolution of the rash within 2 to 6 wk
- Recurrence rare (<2% of cases)

MISCELLANEOUS

COMMENTS
Reassure patient that the disease is not contagious and its course is benign.

REFERENCES
Habif TP: *Clinical dermatology,* ed 3, St Louis, 1996, Mosby.
Pierson JC et al: Purpuric pityriasis rosea, *J Am Acad Dermatol* 28:1021, 1993.
Author: **Fred F. Ferri, M.D.**

Pneumonia, aspiration

BASIC INFORMATION

DEFINITION
Aspiration pneumonia is a lung infection caused by bacterial organisms aspirated from nasopharyngeal space.

ICD-9-CM CODES
507.0 Aspiration pneumonia

EPIDEMIOLOGY AND DEMOGRAPHICS
INCIDENCE (IN U.S.):
- Few reliable data
- 20% to 35% of all pneumonias

PREVALENCE (IN U.S.): Unreliable data
PREDOMINANT SEX: Equal
PREDOMINANT AGE: Elderly
PEAK INCIDENCE: Elderly patients in hospitals or nursing homes

PHYSICAL FINDINGS
- Shortness of breath, tachypnea, cough, sputum, fever after vomiting or difficulty swallowing
- Rales, rhonchi, often diffusely throughout lung

ETIOLOGY
Complex interaction of etiologies, ranging from chemical (often acid) pneumonitis following aspiration of sterile gastric contents (generally not requiring antibiotic treatment) to bacterial aspiration

COMMUNITY-ACQUIRED ASPIRATION PNEUMONIA:
- Generally results from predominantly anaerobic mouth bacteria (anaerobic and microaerophilic streptococci, fusobacteria, gram-positive anaerobic non–spore-forming rods) and less common *Bacteroides* species *(melaninogenicus, intermedius, oralis, ureolyticus)*
- Rarely caused by *Bacteroides fragilis* (of uncertain validity in published studies) or *Eikenella corrodens*
- High-risk groups: elderly, alcoholics, IV drug users, patients who are obtunded, those with esophageal disorders, seizures, poor dentition, or recent dental manipulations

HOSPITAL-ACQUIRED ASPIRATION PNEUMONIA:
- Often occurs among elderly patients and others with diminished gag reflex; those with nasogastric tubes, intestinal obstruction, or ventilator support; and especially those exposed to contaminated nebulizers or unsterile suctioning
- High-risk groups: seriously ill hospitalized patients (especially patients with coma, acidosis, alcoholism, uremia, diabetes mellitus, nasogastric intubation, or recent antimicrobial therapy, who are frequently colonized with aerobic gram-negative rods), patients undergoing anesthesia, those with strokes, dementia, swallowing disorders, the elderly, and those receiving antacids or H_2 blockers (but not sucralfate)
- Hypoxic patients receiving concentrated O_2 have diminished ciliary activity, encouraging aspiration
- Causative organisms:
  1. Anaerobes listed previously, although in many studies gram-negative aerobes (60%) and gram-positive aerobes (20%) predominate
  2. *E. coli, P. aeruginosa, S. aureus, Klebsiella, Enterobacter, Serratia,* and *Proteus* spp. *Hemophilus influenzae, S. pneumococcus, Legionella,* and *Acinetobacter* spp. (sporadic pneumonias) in two thirds of cases
  3. Fungi, including *Candida albicans,* in fewer than 1%

DIAGNOSIS

DIFFERENTIAL DIAGNOSIS
- Other necrotizing or cavitary pneumonias (especially tuberculosis, gram-negative pneumonias)
- See "Pulmonary Tuberculosis"

WORKUP
- Chest x-ray examination
- CBC, blood cultures
- Sputum Gram stain and culture
- Consideration of tracheal aspirate

LABORATORY TESTS
- CBC: leukocytosis often present
- Sputum Gram stain
  1. Often useful when carefully prepared immediately after obtaining suctioned or expectorated specimen, examined by experienced observer.
  2. Only specimens with multiple WBCs and rare or absent epithelial cells should be examined.
  3. Unlike nonaspiration pneumonias (e.g. pneumococcal), multiple organisms may be present.
  4. Long, slender rods suggest anaerobes.
  5. Sputum from pneumonia caused by acid aspiration may be devoid of organisms.
  6. Cultures should be interpreted in light of morphology of visualized organisms.

IMAGING STUDIES
- Chest x-ray examination often reveals bilateral, diffuse, patchy infiltrates.
- Aspiration pneumonias of several days or longer duration may reveal necrosis (especially community-acquired, anaerobic pneumonias) and even cavitation with air-fluid levels, indicating lung abscess.

TREATMENT

NONPHARMACOLOGIC THERAPY
- Airway management to prevent repeated aspiration
- Ventilatory support if necessary

ACUTE GENERAL Rx
Acute aspiration of acidic gastric contents without bacteria may not require antibiotic therapy; consult infectious diseases or pulmonary expert.

FOR COMMUNITY-ACQUIRED ANAEROBIC ASPIRATION PNEUMONIA:
- Often successfully treated with penicillin G (12 to 18 million U/day IV), although some *Bacteroides* and *Fusobacterium* spp. may be resistant to penicillin, responding instead to clindamycin 600 mg q8h.
- Treat nursing home aspirations as hospital aspirations in general.

HOSPITAL-ACQUIRED ASPIRATION PNEUMONIA:
- Often responds to vancomycin 15 mg/kg q12h (<2 g/day), plus ceftazidime 1 to 2 g q8-12h, or to imipenem 500 mg q6h, or ampicillin/sulbactam 1.5 to 3 g q6h.
- Knowledge of resident flora in the microenvironment of the aspiration within the hospital is crucial to intelligent antibiotic selection; consult infection control nurses or hospital epidemiologist.
- Confirmed *Pseudomonas* pneumonia should be treated with antipseudomonal β-lactam agent plus an aminoglycoside until antimicrobial sensitivities confirm that less toxic agents may replace aminoglycoside.
- Clindamycin may be added for improved anaerobic coverage.
- Do not use metronidazole alone for anaerobes.

CHRONIC Rx
Generally not indicated, except for lung abscess (usually anaerobic)

DISPOSITION
Repeat chest x-ray examination in 6 to 8 wk.

REFERRAL
For consultation with infectious disease and/or pulmonary experts for patients with respiratory distress, hypoxia, ventilatory support, >1 lobe pneumonia, necrosis or cavitation on x-ray examination, or not responding to antibiotic therapy within 2 to 3 days.

MISCELLANEOUS

Author: Peter Nicholas, M.D.

Pneumonia, bacterial (PTG)

BASIC INFORMATION

DEFINITION
Bacterial pneumonia is an infection involving the lung parenchyma.

ICD-9-CM CODES
486.0 Pneumonia, acute
507.0 Pneumonia, aspiration
482.9 Pneumonia, bacterial
481 Pneumonia, pneumococcal
482.1 Pneumonia, *Pseudomonas*
482.4 Pneumonia, staphylococcal
428.0 Pneumonia, *klebsiella*
482.2 Pneumonia, *hemophilus influenzae*

EPIDEMIOLOGY AND DEMOGRAPHICS
- Incidence of community-acquired pneumonia is 1/100 persons.
- Incidence of nosocomial pneumonia is 8 cases/1000 persons/yr.
- Primary care physicians see an average of 10 cases of pneumonia annually.
- Hospitalization rate for pneumonia is 15% to 20%.
- Most cases of pneumonia occur in the winter months and in elderly patients.

PHYSICAL FINDINGS
- Fever, tachypnea, chills, tachycardia, cough
- Presentation varies with the cause of pneumonia, the patient's age, and clinical situation:
  1. Patients with streptococcal pneumoniae usually present with high fever, shaking chills, pleuritic chest pain, cough, and copious production of purulent sputum.
  2. Elderly or immunocompromised hosts may initially present with only minimal symptoms (e.g., low-grade fever, confusion); respiratory and nonrespiratory symptoms are less commonly reported by older patients with pneumonia.
  3. Generally, auscultation reveals crackles and diminished breath sounds.
  4. Percussion dullness is present if the patient has pleural effusion.

ETIOLOGY
- *Streptococcus pneumoniae*
- *Hemophilus influenzae*
- *Legionella pneumophila* (1% to 5% of adult pneumonias)
- *Klebsiella, Pseudomonas, E. coli*
- *Staphylococcus aureus*
- Pneumococcal infection is responsible for 50% to 75% of community-acquired pneumonias, whereas gram-negative organisms cause >80% of nosocomial pneumonias.
- Predisposing factors are:
  1. COPD: *H. influenzae, S. pneumoniae, Legionella*
  2. Seizures: aspiration pneumonia
  3. Compromised hosts: *Legionella*, gram-negative organisms
  4. Alcoholism: *Klebsiella, S. pneumoniae, H. influenzae*
  5. HIV: *S. pneumoniae*
  6. IV drug addicts with right-sided bacterial endocarditis: *S. aureus*

DIAGNOSIS

DIFFERENTIAL DIAGNOSIS
- Exacerbation of chronic bronchitis
- Pulmonary embolism or infarction
- Lung neoplasm
- Bronchiolitis
- Sarcoidosis
- Hypersensitivity pneumonitis
- Pulmonary edema
- Drug-induced lung injury
- Viral pneumonias
- Fungal pneumonias
- Parasitic pneumonias
- Atypical pneumonia
- Tuberculosis

WORKUP
Laboratory evaluation (in hospitalized patients) and chest x-ray examination

LABORATORY TESTS
- Obtain an adequate sputum specimen for Gram stain and cultures.
  1. An expectorated sputum sample is often inadequate because of many false-positive results (secondary to contamination from oral flora) and many false-negative results; a specimen may be considered adequate if the Gram stain shows >25 PMNs and <10 epithelial cells per low-power field.
  2. Aerosol induction with hypertonic saline solution (3% to 10%) may increase the diagnostic yield of sputum.
  3. The use of fiberoptic bronchoscopy to obtain a sputum sample is generally reserved for critically ill patients responding poorly to initial antimicrobial therapy.
- WBC count is elevated, usually with left shift.
- Blood cultures: positive in approximately 20% of cases of pneumococcal pneumonia.
- ABGs: hypoxemia with partial pressure of oxygen <60 mm Hg while the patient is breathing room air is a standard criterion for hospital admission.
- Direct immunofluorescent examination of sputum (e.g., direct fluorescent antibody [DFA] stain is a highly specific and rapid test for detecting legionella in clinical specimen).
- Quellung reaction (swelling of bacterial capsule when exposed to antibody) is used for diagnosis of streptococcal pneumoniae.

- Serologic testing for HIV is advocated by the CDC for hospitalized patients between the ages of 15 and 54 yr who are treated in hospitals with a high prevalence of AIDS ($\geq$1:1000 discharges).
- Gram stain of sputum:
  1. Lancet-shaped gram-positive cocci indicate streptococcal pneumoniae.
  2. Pleomorphic, small coccobacillary gram-negative organisms indicate *H. influenzae*.
  3. Encapsulated gram-negative bacilli: *K. pneumoniae*

IMAGING STUDIES
Chest x-ray study: findings vary with the stage and type of pneumonia and the hydration of the patient.
- Classically, pneumococcal pneumonia presents with a segmental lobe infiltrate.
- Diffuse infiltrates on chest x-ray can be seen with *L. pneumoniae, M. pneumoniae*, viral pneumonias, *P. carinii*, miliary TB, aspiration, aspergillosis.
- An initial chest x-ray film is also useful to rule out the presence of any complications (pneumothorax, empyema, abscesses).

TREATMENT

NONPHARMACOLOGIC THERAPY
- Avoidance of tobacco use
- Oxygen to maintain partial oxygen pressure in arterial blood >60 mm Hg
- IV hydration, correction of dehydration
- Assisted ventilation in patients with significant respiratory failure

ACUTE GENERAL Rx
- Initial antibiotic therapy should be based on clinical, radiographic, and laboratory evaluation; if the clinical diagnosis is substantiated by an adequate Gram stain, the choice of initial therapy is relatively simple. In otherwise healthy adult patients with community-acquired pneumonia and insidious presentation, erythromycin is the antibiotic of choice. Azithromycin and clarithromycin are also effective.
- In immunocompromised patients with negative Gram stain, the initial antibiotic treatment should be broad spectrum but with emphasis on gram-negative organisms, *Legionella*, and *S. aureus*. In these patients, the following antibiotics should be considered:
  1. Patients with AIDS: high-dose TMP-SMX plus erythromycin or clarithromycin
  2. Neutropenic patients: ticarcillin-piperacillin 3 to 4 g IV q4-6h plus tobramycin 2 mg/kg IV q12h or ceftazidine plus aminoglycoside
  3. Immunocompromised, non-AIDS, nonneutropenic patients (e.g., diabetes mellitus, elderly, COPD): cefuroxime plus aminoglycoside (if pneumonia is hospital or nursing home acquired). Erythromycin should also be considered as part of the initial therapy because of the high prevalence of *Legionella* in immunocompromised hosts.

CHRONIC Rx
Parapneumonic effusion-empyema can be managed with chest tube placement for drainage. Instillation of fibrinolytic agents (streptokinase, urokinase) via the chest tube may be necessary in resistant cases.

DISPOSITION
Most patients respond well to antibiotic therapy. Hospitalization is recommended in immunocompromised patients and patients with hypoxemia with partial pressure oxygen <60 mm Hg while the patient is breathing room air.

REFERRAL
Hospitalization in selected patients (see "Disposition").

MISCELLANEOUS

COMMENTS
Causes of slowly resolving or nonresolving pneumonia:
- Difficult to treat infections: viral pneumonia, legionella, pneumococci, or staphylococci with impaired host response, TB, fungi
- Neoplasm: lung, lymphoma, metastasis
- CHF
- Pulmonary embolism
- Immunologic or idiopathic: Wegener's granulomatosis, pulmonary eosinophilic syndromes, SLE
- Drug toxicity (e.g., amiodarone)

REFERENCES
Bartlet JG, Mundy LM: Community-acquired pneumonia, *N Engl J Med* 333:1618, 1995.

Mandell LA: Community-acquired pneumonias: etiology, epidemiology, and treatment, *Chest* 108:35S, 1995.

Metlay J et al: Influence of age on symptoms at presentation in patients with community-acquired pneumonia, *Arch Intern Med* 157: 1453, 1997.

Niederman MS: Pneumonia: pathogenesis, diagnosis, and management, *Med Clin North Am* 78(5): 1123, 1994.

Author: **Fred F. Ferri, M.D.**

Pneumonia, *Mycoplasma* (PTG)

BASIC INFORMATION

DEFINITION
Mycoplasma pneumonia is an infection of the lung parenchyma caused by *Mycoplasma pneumoniae*.

SYNONYMS
Primary atypical pneumonia
Eaton's pneumonia
Walking pneumonia

ICD-9-CM CODES
483 Mycoplasma pneumonia

EPIDEMIOLOGY AND DEMOGRAPHICS
INCIDENCE (IN U.S.):
- Hard to precisely determine incidence because of difficulty in making the diagnosis, but it is a frequent cause of community-acquired pneumonia.
- Many cases likely resolve without coming to medical attention.
- Incidence is estimated at 1 case/1000 persons/yr.
- Incidence is estimated to at least triple every (approximately) 5 yr during epidemics.

PREVALENCE (IN U.S.):
- Estimated to be present in 1 of 5 patients hospitalized for pneumonia (generally a self-limited disease, so its true prevalence is unknown)
- Estimated to cause 7% of all pneumonias and about half in those aged 5 to 20 yr

PREDOMINANT SEX: Equal distribution

PREDOMINANT AGE:
- Most commonly affected: school-age children and young adults (ages 5 to 20 yr)
- Occurs in older adults as well, especially with household exposure to a young child
- More severe infections in affected elderly patients

PEAK INCIDENCE:
- Some increased incidence in fall to early winter
- Seems more prevalent in temperate climates

GENETICS:
Familial Disposition:
- None known
- May be more severe in patients with sickle cell anemia

Neonatal Infection: Severe respiratory distress, sometimes requiring intubation, attributed to this disease in infants

PHYSICAL FINDINGS
- Nonexudative pharyngitis (common)
- Rhonchi or rales, without evidence of consolidation (common) in lower lung zones
- Associated with bullous myringitis (perhaps no more frequently than in other pneumonias)
- Skin rashes in up to one fourth of patients
  1. Morbilliform
  2. Urticaria
  3. Erythema nodosum (unusual)
  4. Erythema multiforme (unusual)
  5. Stevens-Johnson syndrome (rare)
- Muscle tenderness (<50% of the patients)
- On examination (and confirmed with testing):
  1. Mononeuritis or polyneuritis
  2. Transverse myelitis
  3. Cranial nerve palsies
  4. Meningoencephalitis
- Lymphadenopathy and splenomegaly
- Conjunctivitis

ETIOLOGY
Infection is spread by droplet infection from respiratory tract secretions.

DIAGNOSIS

DIFFERENTIAL DIAGNOSIS
- *Chlamydia pneumoniae*
- *C. psittaci*
- *Legionella* spp.
- *Coxiella burnetii*
- Several viral agents
- Q fever
- *Pneumococcus pneumoniae*
- Pleuritic pain
- Pulmonary embolism/infarction

WORKUP
- Chest x-ray examination
- Thorough history and physical examination
- Laboratory tests
- Evaluation guided by symptoms and findings

LABORATORY TESTS
- WBC:
  1. WBC count >10,000/mm^3 in about a quarter of patients
  2. Differential count nonspecific
  3. Leukopenia rare

- Cold agglutinins:
  1. Detected in about half of the patients
  2. Also may be found in:
     a. Lymphoproliferative diseases
     b. Influenza
     c. Mononucleosis
     d. Adenovirus infections
     e. Occasionally, legionnaires' disease
  3. Titers typically >1:64
     a. May be detectable with bedside testing
     b. Appear between days 5 and 10 of the illness (so may be demonstrable when the patient first presents) and disappear within about 1 mo
- Uncommonly, hemolysis
- Complement fixation testing of paired sera (fourfold rise) in patients with pneumonia and a compatible history:
  1. Considered diagnostic
  2. Not specific for the disease
- Culture of the organism from specimens
  1. Only truly specific test for infection
  2. Technically difficult and done reliably by few laboratories
  3. May require weeks to get results
- Sputum
  1. Often no sputum produced for laboratory testing
  2. When present, Gram-stained specimens show polys without organisms
- Infection occasionally complicated by pancreatitis or glomerulitis
- Disseminated intravascular coagulation is a rare complication.
- Electrocardiographic evidence of pericarditis or myocarditis may be present.

IMAGING STUDIES
- Predilection for lower lobe involvement (upper lobes involved in less than a fourth), with radiographic abnormalities frequently out of proportion to those on physical examination
- Small pleural effusions in about 30% of patients
- Large effusions: rare
- Infiltrates: patchy, unilateral, and with a segmental distribution, although multilobe involvement may be seen
- Evidence of hilar adenopathy on chest films in 20% to 25%
- Rare cases reported:
  1. Associated lung abscess
  2. Residual pneumatoceles
  3. Lobar collapse
  4. Hyperlucent lung syndrome

TREATMENT

ACUTE GENERAL Rx
- Therapy (10 to 14 days) with erythromycin (500 mg qid), azithromycin (500 mg daily), roxithromycin (150 mg bid), or clarithromycin (500 mg bid) is preferred to tetracycline, especially in young children or women of childbearing age.
- Therapy shortens the duration and severity of symptoms and may hasten radiographic clearing, but the disease is self-limiting.

CHRONIC Rx
- Effective antimicrobial therapy does not eliminate the organism from the respiratory secretions, which may be positive for weeks.
- Serum antibody response does not necessarily provide lifelong immunity.
- Chronic symptoms do not occur, although clinical relapses may occur 7 to 10 days following the initial response and may be associated with new areas of infiltration.

DISPOSITION
- Clinical improvement is almost universal within 10 days.
- Infiltrates generally clear within 5 to 8 wk.
- Rare deaths are likely attributable to underlying medical diseases.
- Person-to-person spread can be minimized by avoiding open coughing, especially in enclosed areas.

REFERRAL
- Not responding to treatment
- Severe infection
- Severe extrapulmonary manifestations
- Multilobe involvement accompanied by respiratory embarrassment (very rare)

MISCELLANEOUS

COMMENTS
X-ray resolution complete by 8 wk in about 90% of patients.

REFERENCES
Luby JP: Pneumonia caused by *Mycoplasma pneumoniae*, Clin Chest Med 12:237, 1991.

Author: **Harvey M. Shanies, M.D., Ph.D.**

Pneumonia, *Pneumocystis carinii* (PTG)

BASIC INFORMATION

DEFINITION
Pneumocystis carinii pneumonia is a serious respiratory infection caused by the fungal or protozoal organism *Pneumocystis carinii*.

SYNONYMS
PCP

ICD-9-CM CODES
136.3 *Pneumocystis carinii* pneumonia

EPIDEMIOLOGY AND DEMOGRAPHICS
INCIDENCE (IN U.S.):
- Seen primarily in the setting of acquired immunodeficiency syndrome (AIDS)
- Approximately 11 cases/100 patient-years among HIV-infected patients with CD4 lymphocyte counts <100/mm^3

PREDOMINANT SEX: Equal incidence when corrected for HIV status
PREDOMINANT AGE:
- <2 yr
- 20 to 40 yr

PEAK INCIDENCE: 20 to 40 yr (parallel to AIDS epidemic)
GENETICS:
Neonatal infection:
- Most frequent opportunistic infection among HIV-infected children, occurring in approximately 30%
- Neonatal occurrence unusual

PHYSICAL FINDINGS
- Fever, cough, shortness of breath present in almost all cases
- Lungs frequently clear to auscultation, although rales occasionally present
- Cyanosis and pronounced tachypnea in severe cases
- Hemoptysis unusual

ETIOLOGY
- *Pneumocystis carinii*, recently reclassified as a fungal organism
- Reactivation of dormant infection
- Extrapulmonary involvement rare

DIAGNOSIS

DIFFERENTIAL DIAGNOSIS
- Other opportunistic respiratory infections:
  1. Tuberculosis
  2. Histoplasmosis
  3. Cryptococcosis
- Nonopportunistic infections:
  1. Bacterial pneumonia
  2. Viral pneumonia
  3. Mycoplasmal pneumonia
  4. Legionellosis
- Occurs virtually exclusively in the setting of profound depression of cellular immunity

WORKUP
- Chest x-ray examination
- ABG
- Sputum examination for cysts of PCP and to exclude other pathogens
- Bronchoscopy with bronchoalveolar lavage or lung biopsy for diagnosis if sputum examination is negative or equivocal

LABORATORY TESTS
- ABG monitoring
- Elevated lactate dehydrogenase (LDH) in majority of cases
- HIV antibody test if cause of underlying immune deficiency state is unclear

IMAGING STUDIES
Diffuse uptake on gallium scanning of the lungs is suggestive but not diagnostic.

TREATMENT

NONPHARMACOLOGIC THERAPY
- Supplemental oxygen
- Ventilatory support if needed

ACUTE GENERAL Rx
For confirmed or suspected PCP:
- Trimethoprim-sulfamethoxazole (20 mg/kg trimethoprim and 100 mg/kg sulfamethoxazole qd) PO or IV
- Pentamidine (4 mg/kg IV qd)
- Either regimen with prednisone (40 mg PO bid):
  1. If arterial oxygen pressure <70 mm Hg
  2. If arterial-alveolar oxygen pressure difference >35 mm Hg
  3. Dose tapered to 20 mg bid after 5 days and 20 mg qd after 10 days
- Therapy continued for 3 wk
- Alternative therapies available for patients unable to tolerate conventional therapy:
  1. Dapsone/trimethoprim
  2. Clindamycin/primaquine
  3. Atovaquone
- Alternative therapies should be given in consultation with a physician experienced in the management of PCP.

CHRONIC Rx
- After completion of therapy, lifelong prophylaxis should be maintained with trimethoprim-sulfamethoxazole (one single-strength tablet PO qd or double-strength three times weekly).
- Patients intolerant of this therapy should be treated with dapsone (50 mg PO qd) plus pyrimethamine (50 mg PO weekly) plus leucovorin (25 mg PO weekly).
- Inhaled pentamidine (300 mg monthly by standardized nebulizer) is less effective and reserved for patients intolerant to other forms of prophylaxis.
- Same approach taken to all HIV-infected patients with CD4 lymphocyte counts <200/mm^3 or <20% of the total lymphocyte count because of their high risk of PCP.

DISPOSITION
- Patients should be hospitalized unless infection mild.
- After completion of therapy, long-term ambulatory follow-up is mandatory to provide secondary prevention of PCP (above) and management of the underlying immunodeficiency syndrome.

REFERRAL
To pulmonologist for bronchoscopy if diagnosis cannot be confirmed by sputum examination

MISCELLANEOUS

COMMENTS
All patients, especially those with severe infection or intolerant of conventional therapy, should be followed by a physician experienced in the management of PCP and, if appropriate, in the long-term management of HIV infection or other underlying disease.

REFERENCES
Centers for Disease Control and Prevention: USPHS/IDSA guidelines for the prevention of opportunistic infections in persons infected with human immunodeficiency virus: a summary, *MMWR* 44(RR-8), 1995.

Author: **Joseph R. Masci, M.D.**

CLINICAL TOPICS   Pneumonia, viral (PTG) 375

BASIC INFORMATION

DEFINITION
Viral pneumonia is infection of the pulmonary parenchyma caused by any of a large number of viral agents. The most important viruses are discussed below.

SYNONYMS
Nonbacterial pneumonia
Atypical pneumonia

ICD-9-CM CODES
480.9 Viral pneumonia

EPIDEMIOLOGY AND DEMOGRAPHICS
INCIDENCE (IN U.S.):
- Influenza virus:
  1. 10% to 20% of population in temperate zones infected during 1- to 2-mo epidemics occurring yearly during winter months.
  2. Up to 50% infected during pandemics.
  3. Pneumonia develops in small percentage of infected persons.
- Incidence of other important viral pneumonias is not known precisely.

PREVALENCE (IN U.S.):
- Often related to immune status of the population or presence of an epidemic
- Normal hosts (estimates):
  1. 86% of cases of pneumonia resulting in hospitalization in American adults
  2. 16% of pediatric pneumonias managed as outpatients
  3. 49% of hospitalized infants with pneumonia
- Important problem in hosts with impaired immunity

PREDOMINANT SEX:
- None generally
- Male sex may predispose to more severe respiratory disease in respiratory syncytial virus (RSV) infection

PREDOMINANT AGE:
Influenza:
- Overall incidence greatest at age 5 yr
- Falls with increasing age
- The most serious sequelae in those with chronic medical illnesses, especially cardiopulmonary disease
- Hospitalizations greatest in infants and adults >64 yr of age

RSV:
- Young children (as the major cause of pneumonia)
- Occurs throughout life

Adenoviruses:
- Young children
- Adults, primarily military recruits

Varicella:
- About 16% of adults (not infected in childhood) who contract chickenpox
- Acute varicella during pregnancy more likely to be complicated by severe pneumonia
- 90% of reported varicella pneumonia cases are in adults (highest incidence 20 to 60 yr old)

Measles:
- Young adults and older children who received a single vaccination (5% failure rate)
- Measles during pregnancy more likely to be complicated by pneumonia
- Underlying cardiopulmonary diseases and immunosuppression predispose to serious pneumonia complicating measles
- Before availability of measles vaccine, 90% of pneumonias in those <10 yr
- Currently >1/3 of U.S. patients >14 yr old
- 3% to 50% of measles cases are complicated by pneumonia

CMV:
- Neonatal through adult
- Immunosuppression is key predisposing factor

PEAK INCIDENCE:
Influenza:
- Winter months for influenza A
- Year round for influenza B
- Peak of pneumonia seen weeks into the outbreak of infection

RSV: Winter and spring
Adenovirus: Endemic (military)
Varicella: Spring in temperate zones
Measles: Year round
CMV: Year round

GENETICS:
Familial Disposition:
- Close contact, not genetics, is important in acquisition.
- Congenital anomalies and immunosuppression worsen course of RSV pneumonia.

Congenital Infection:
- CMV is the most common intrauterine infection in the U.S.
- Pneumonia occurs occasionally in infants with symptomatic congenital infection.

Neonatal Infection:
- Severe RSV pneumonia
- Adenovirus pneumonia
  1. 5% to 20% fatality rate
  2. Can lead to residual restrictive or obstructive functional abnormalities
- "Varicella neonatorum"
  1. Disseminated visceral disease including pneumonia
  2. May develop in neonates whose mothers develop peripartum chickenpox
- CMV pneumonia
  1. Generally fatal
  2. Associated with severe cerebral damage in this population

Pneumonia, viral (PTG)

PHYSICAL FINDINGS

INFLUENZA:
- Fever
- Uncomfortable or lethargic appearance
- Prominent dry cough (rarely hemoptysis)
- Flushed integument and erythematous mucous membranes
- Rales or rhonchi

RSV:
- Fever
- Tachypnea
- Prolonged expiration
- Wheezes and rales

ADENOVIRUSES:
- Hoarseness
- Pharyngitis
- Tachypnea
- Cervical adenitis

MEASLES:
- Conjunctivitis
- Rhinorrhea
- Koplik's spots
- Exanthem
- Pneumonitis
  1. May occur as a complication in 3% to 4% of adolescents and young adults
  2. Coincident with rash
  3. May also develop following apparent recovery from measles
- Fever
- Dry cough

VARICELLA:
- Fever
- Maculopapular or vesicular rash
  1. Becomes encrusted
  2. Pneumonia typical 1 to 6 days after rash appears
  3. Pneumonia accompanied by cough, and occasionally hemoptysis
- Few auscultatory abnormalities noted on examination of the lungs

CMV:
- Fever
- Paroxysmal cough
- Occasional hemoptysis
- Diffuse adenopathy when pneumonia occurs posttransfusion

ETIOLOGY
Viral infection can lead to pneumonia in both immunocompetent and immunocompromised hosts.

DIAGNOSIS

DIFFERENTIAL DIAGNOSIS
- Bacterial pneumonia, which frequently complicates (i.e., can follow or be simultaneous with) viral (especially influenza) pneumonia
- Other causes of atypical pneumonia:
  1. *Mycoplasma*
  2. *Chlamydiae*
  3. *Coxiella*
  4. Legionnaires' disease
- ARDS
- Physical findings and associated hypoxemia confused with pulmonary emboli

WORKUP
- Information about the prevalent strain of influenza virus can be obtained from local health departments or from the Centers for Disease Control and Prevention.
- Viral diagnostic tests are usually not necessary once an outbreak has been defined.
- Influenza and other viruses can be cultured from respiratory secretions during the initial few days of the illness (special media and techniques necessary).
- Paired sera antibody titers are also useful.
- Monoclonal antibody tests are available for influenza and other respiratory viruses.
- Measles and adenovirus pneumonia are usually diagnosed clinically.
- Polymerase chain reaction may be able to rapidly detect and identify viral nucleic acid.
- Open lung biopsy is required for definite diagnosis of CMV pneumonia.

LABORATORY TESTS
- Sputum Gram stain (usually produced in scanty amounts) typically shows few polymorphonuclear leukocytes and few bacteria.
- WBC count may vary from leukopenic to modest elevation, usually without a leftward shift.
- Disseminated intravascular coagulation has occasionally complicated adenovirus type 7 pneumonia.
- Multinucleated giant cells on Tzanck preparation of an unroofed vesicular lesion are useful in diagnosing varicella in a patient with an infiltrate (also found in *H. simplex*).
- Severe immunosuppression is associated with symptomatic CMV pneumonia (usually reactivation of latent infection, or in previously seronegative recipients from the donor).
- Hypoxemia may be profound.
- Cultures may be helpful in identifying superinfecting bacterial pathogens.
- When they occur, parapneumonic pleural effusions are exudative.

IMAGING STUDIES
- Chest x-ray examination may demonstrate a spectrum of findings from ill-defined, patchy, or generalized interstitial infiltrates, which can be associated with the acute respiratory distress syndrome (ARDS).
- A localized dense alveolar infiltrate suggests a superimposed bacterial pneumonia.
- Small calcified nodules may develop as a radiographic residual of varicella pneumonia.

TREATMENT

NONPHARMACOLOGIC THERAPY
GENERAL:
- Measures to diminish person-to-person transmission
- Modified bed rest
- Maintenance of adequate hydration
- Possible ventilatory support for severe pneumonia or ARDS

INFLUENZA:
- Yearly prophylactic strain-specific influenza vaccination (only subvirion vaccine should be used in children <13 yr) can be given to prevent infection.
- Live, attenuated influenza vaccines administered by nose drops may be more effective than the injected inactivated viral vaccines now available (under investigation).

RSV:
- Isolation techniques are important in limiting spread of RSV infections.
- Immunoglobulins with a high RSV-neutralizing antibody titer are beneficial in treatment.

ADENOVIRUSES:
- Intestinal inoculation of respiratory adenoviruses have been used to successfully immunize military recruits.
- Although they produce no disease in recipients, the viruses may be shed chronically and may infect others at a later date.
- These vaccines are not available for civilian populations.

VARICELLA:
- Live, attenuated varicella vaccine has been successfully used in clinical trials.
- Varicella-zoster immune globulin should be administered within 4 days of exposure to prevent or modify the disease in susceptible persons.
- Nonimmunized persons exposed to varicella are potentially infectious between 10 and 21 days after exposure.

MEASLES:
- Effective measles vaccine is available:
  1. The vaccine should be administered at 15 mo.
  2. A second dose should be administered at the time of school entry.
- Live, attenuated vaccine or γ-globulin can prevent measles in unvaccinated persons if administered early following exposure.
- Vitamin A given PO for 2 days reduces morbidity and mortality from measles in exposed children.

ACUTE GENERAL Rx
GENERAL: Administer appropriate antibiotics for bacterial superinfections.

INFLUENZA:
- Amantadine and rimantadine (not commercially available) for influenza A. Early use can speed recovery from small airways dysfunction, but whether it influences the development or course of pneumonia is uncertain.
- Amantadine is also effective prophylactically during the time it is administered.
- Aerosolized ribavirin or amantadine may have a role in severe influenza pneumonia but have not been approved for this indication.

RSV: Ribavirin aerosol is effective for severe RSV pneumonia.

ADENOVIRUSES: No effective antiadenovirus agent.

VARICELLA:
- Varicella pneumonia can be treated with IV acyclovir.
- Adults who develop chickenpox should be considered for acyclovir treatment, which may prevent the development of pneumonia.

MEASLES: No effective antimeasles agent.

CMV:
- Acyclovir can prevent CMV infection in renal transplant recipients.
- Ganciclovir and foscarnet, with or without CMV hyperimmune globulin, show promise in the treatment of serious CMV infection, including pneumonia, in compromised hosts.

DISPOSITION
- Supportive therapy is useful.
- Deaths are possible during acute illness.
- Residual functional abnormalities may be persistent, develop into, or predispose to chronic respiratory diseases in later life.
- Morbidity and mortality following most viral pneumonias is increased by bacterial superinfection.

REFERRAL
- Uncertainty about the diagnosis in a compromised host
- Symptoms or findings progressive
- Severe respiratory compromise, diffuse infiltrates, or the development of ARDS

MISCELLANEOUS

COMMENTS
- Influenza spreads by close contact and by small droplets transmitted by cough, which typifies the illness.
- RSV is effectively transmitted by fomites and by direct contact (little by aerosol).
- Varicella is transmitted by direct contact or by aerosol.
- Measles is transmitted by aerosol and possibly by fomites.

REFERENCES
Cate TR: Viral pneumonia in immunocompetent adults. In Niederman MS, Sarosi GA, Glassroth J (eds): *Respiratory infections: a scientific basis for management*, Philadelphia, 1994, WB Saunders.

Author: **Harvey M. Shanies, M.D., Ph.D.**

Poliomyelitis

BASIC INFORMATION

DEFINITION
Poliomyelitis is a symptomatic infection caused by *poliovirus*, which (on rare occasions) may result in paralysis.

SYNONYMS
Polio
Infantile paralysis

ICD-9-CM CODES
045.9 Poliomyelitis

EPIDEMIOLOGY AND DEMOGRAPHICS
INCIDENCE (IN U.S.):
- Approximately 8 cases/yr.
- All cases in the U.S. and western hemisphere are now vaccine-associated (because of oral polio vaccine [OPV]).

PREDOMINANT AGE:
Almost always infants or young children

GENETICS:
Neonatal Infection: Most cases occur in otherwise healthy infants who receive oral polio vaccine, or their contacts.

PHYSICAL FINDINGS
- Exposure of a nonimmune host to poliovirus usually results in asymptomatic infection.
- A small percentage of individuals may have one of three presentations:
  1. Abortive poliomyelitis: a flulike illness
     a. Fever
     b. Malaise
     c. Headache
     d. Sore throat
  2. Nonparalytic poliomyelitis: an aseptic meningitis that correlates with invasion of the CNS
     a. Headache
     b. Neck stiffness
     c. Change in mental status
  3. Paralytic poliomyelitis:
     a. Most commonly affects the lumbar or bulbar regions
     b. Following paralysis, a period of variable degrees of recovery, the majority of which occurs in 2 to 6 mo
     c. Paralysis from involvement of motor neurons in the spinal cord
     d. Flaccid paralysis without sensory defects
     e. Postpolio syndrome late sequela, which may occur many years after the acute illness
     f. Functional deterioration of muscle groups that had recovered from initial paralysis thought to result from failure of reinnervation, which initially was able to restore function to weakened or paralyzed areas

ETIOLOGY
- Virus of genus *Enterovirus*
- Classic endemic and epidemic disease caused by wild-type *poliovirus*
- All cases in U.S. currently caused by a live, attenuated virus in the OPV
  1. Extremely rare complication that occurs in vaccine recipients or their contacts
  2. Paralysis from lower motor neuron damage caused by viral infection

DIAGNOSIS

DIFFERENTIAL DIAGNOSIS
- Guillain-Barré syndrome
- CVA
- Spinal cord compression
- Other enteroviruses:
  1. Aseptic meningitis
  2. Paralysis (rare)

WORKUP
- Isolation of virus:
  1. Stool or a rectal swab
  2. Throat swabs
  3. Rarely CSF
- Paired sera for antibody titer determinations

LABORATORY TESTS
CSF:
- Aseptic meningitis
- Elevated WBCs
- Elevated protein
- Normal glucose

IMAGING STUDIES
MRI may show involvement of anterior horn of the spinal cord.

TREATMENT

NONPHARMACOLOGIC THERAPY
- Maintenance of respiration and hydration
- Early mobilization and exercise once fever subsides

ACUTE GENERAL Rx
- Aimed at reduction of pain and muscle spasm
- No agent to alter the course of disease

CHRONIC Rx
Physical therapy

DISPOSITION
- In the abortive and nonparalytic forms, complete recovery
- Paralytic disease:
  1. Variable degrees of recovery
  2. 80% usually in the first 6 mo following illness

REFERRAL
To an infectious disease consultant

MISCELLANEOUS

COMMENTS
- Risk of disease in recipients of OPV is approximately 1 in 2.5 million.
- Use of inactivated polio vaccine (IPV) is not associated with disease:
  1. Does not confer local (mucosal) immunity
  2. Will not immunize nonvaccinated contacts
  3. Requires boosters
  4. Is given by injection
- Consideration is being given to a regimen combining these two vaccines in a way that might avoid causing polio.
- Cases should be reported to public health agencies.

REFERENCES
Kidd D, Williams AJ, Howard RS: Poliomyelitis, *Postgrad Med J* 853(72):641, 1996.

Author: **Maurice Policar, M.D.**

Polyarteritis nodosa

BASIC INFORMATION

DEFINITION
Polyarteritis nodosa is a vasculitic syndrome involving medium-sized to small arteries, characterized histologically by necrotizing inflammation of the arterial media and inflammatory cell infiltration.

SYNONYMS
Periarteritis nodosa
PAN
Necrotizing arteritis

ICD-9-CM CODES
446.0 Polyarteritis nodosa

EPIDEMIOLOGY AND DEMOGRAPHICS
- Incidence is 1:100,000 annually.
- Male:female ratio is 2:1.
- Increased incidence in patients with hepatitis B surface antigen, hepatitis C virus.

PHYSICAL FINDINGS
- Weight loss, nausea, vomiting
- Testicular pain or tenderness
- Myalgias, weakness, or leg tenderness
- Neuropathy (mononeuritis multiplex), foot drop
- Livedo reticularis, ulceration of digits, abdominal pain after meals, hematemesis, hematochezia, hypertension, asymmetric polyarthritis (tending to involve large joints of lower extremities)
- Fever may be present (polyarteritis nodosa is often a cause of fever of unknown origin)

ETIOLOGY
- Unknown
- Immune complexes have been implicated

DIAGNOSIS

DIFFERENTIAL DIAGNOSIS
Cryoglobulinemia, SLE, infections (e.g., SBE, trichinosis, rickettsia), lymphoma

WORKUP
- Laboratory evaluation, arteriography, and biopsy of small or medium-sized arteries can confirm diagnosis. Clinical manifestations are variable and depend on the arteries involved and the organs affected (e.g., kidney involvement occurs in >80% of cases).
- The presence of any three of the following ten items allows the diagnosis of periarteritis nodosa with a sensitivity of 82% and a specificity of 86%:
  1. Weight loss >4 kg
  2. Livedo reticularis
  3. Testicular pain or tenderness
  4. Myalgias, weakness, or leg tenderness
  5. Neuropathy
  6. Diastolic blood pressure >90 mm Hg
  7. Elevated BUN or creatinine
  8. Positive test for hepatitis B virus
  9. Arteriography revealing small or large aneurysms and focal constrictions between dilated segments
  10. Biopsy of small or medium-sized artery containing WBC

LABORATORY TESTS
- Elevated BUN or creatinine, positive test for hepatitis B virus or hepatitis C
- Elevated ESR, anemia, elevated platelets, eosinophilia, proteinuria, RBC casts in the urine
- Biopsy of small or medium-sized artery of symptomatic sites (muscle, nerve) is >90% specific.

IMAGING STUDIES
Arteriography can be done in patients with negative biopsies or if there are no symptomatic sites. Visceral angiography will reveal aneurysmal dilatation of the renal, mesenteric, or hepatic arteries.

TREATMENT

NONPHARMACOLOGIC THERAPY
Low-sodium diet in hypertensive patients

ACUTE GENERAL Rx
Prednisone 1 to 2 mg/kg/day; cyclophosphamide in refractory cases

CHRONIC Rx
Monitoring for infections and potential complications such as thrombosis, infarction, or organ necrosis

DISPOSITION
The 5-yr survival is <20% in untreated patients. Treatment with corticosteroids increases survival to approximately 50%. Usage of both corticosteroids and immunosuppressive drugs may increase 5-yr survival >80%. Poor prognostic signs are severe renal or GI involvement.

REFERRAL
Surgical referral for biopsy

MISCELLANEOUS

REFERENCES
Fortin PR et al: Prognostic factors in systemic necrotizing vasculitis of the polyarteritis nodosa group: a review of 45 cases, *J Rheumatol* 22:78, 1995.
Guillevin L et al: Prognostic factors in polyarteritis nodosa and Churg-Strauss syndrome, *Medicine* 75:17, 1996.
Lightfoot W et al: The emerging culture of rheumatology criteria for the classification of polyarteritis nodosa, *Arthritis Rheum* 33:1088, 1994.

Author: **Fred F. Ferri, M.D.**

Polycythemia vera (PTG)

BASIC INFORMATION

DEFINITION
Polycythemia vera is a rare hematologic disorder characterized by clonal proliferation of bone marrow progenitors.

SYNONYMS
Primary polycythemia
Vaquez disease

ICD-9-CM CODES
238.4 Polycythemia vera

EPIDEMIOLOGY AND DEMOGRAPHICS
INCIDENCE/PREVALENCE: 0.5 cases/100,000 persons; mean age of onset is 60 yr

PHYSICAL FINDINGS
- Facial plethora, congestion of oral mucosa, ruddy complexion
- Enlargement and tortuosity of retinal veins
- Splenomegaly (found in >75% of patients)

DIAGNOSIS

DIFFERENTIAL DIAGNOSIS
1. **SMOKING:**
   - Polycythemia is secondary to increased carboxyhemoglobin, resulting in left shift in the Hgb dissociation curve.
   - Laboratory evaluation shows increased Hct, RBC mass, erythropoietin level, and carboxyhemoglobin.
   - Splenomegaly is not present on physical examination.
2. **HYPOXEMIA (SECONDARY POLYCYTHEMIA):** Living for prolonged periods at high altitudes, pulmonary fibrosis, congenital cardiac lesions with right-to-left shunts
   - Laboratory evaluation shows decreased arterial oxygen saturation and elevated erythropoietin level.
   - Splenomegaly is not present on physical examination.
3. **ERYTHROPOIETIN-PRODUCING STATES:** Renal cell carcinoma, hepatoma, cerebral hemangioma, uterine fibroids, polycystic kidneys
   - The erythropoietin level is elevated in these patients; the arterial oxygen saturation is normal.
   - Splenomegaly may be present with metastatic neoplasms.
4. **STRESS POLYCYTHEMIA (GAISBÖCK'S SYNDROME, RELATIVE POLYCYTHEMIA):**
   - Laboratory evaluation demonstrates normal RBC mass, arterial oxygen saturation, and erythropoietin level; plasma volume is decreased.
   - Splenomegaly is not present on physical examination.
5. **HEMOGLOBINOPATHIES ASSOCIATED WITH HIGH OXYGEN AFFINITY:** An abnormal oxyhemoglobin-dissociation curve (P50) is present.

WORKUP
The patient generally comes to medical attention because of symptoms associated with increased blood volume and viscosity or impaired platelet function:
- Impaired cerebral circulation resulting in headache, vertigo, blurred vision, dizziness, TIA, CVA
- Fatigue, poor exercise tolerance
- Pruritus, particularly following bathing (caused by overproduction of histamine)
- Bleeding: epistaxis, UGI bleeding (increased incidence of PUD)
- Abdominal discomfort secondary to splenomegaly; hepatomegaly may be present
- Hyperuricemia may result in nephrolithiasis and gouty arthritis

In patients with a presumptive diagnosis of polycythemia vera, the following diagnostic approach is recommended:
- Measure RBC mass by isotope dilution using ^{51}Cr-labeled autologous RBCs; a high value eliminates stress polycythemia.
- Measure arterial saturation; a normal value eliminates polycythemia secondary to smoking.
- Measure erythropoietin level; if elevated, obtain IVP and abdominal CT to rule out renal cell carcinoma.
- The diagnosis of hemoglobinopathy with high affinity is ruled out by a normal oxyhemoglobin dissociation curve.

LABORATORY TESTS
- Elevated RBC count (>6 million/mm^3), elevated Hgb (>18 g/dl in men, >16 g/dl in women), elevated Hct (>54% in men, >49% in women)
- Increased WBC (often with basophilia); thrombocytosis in the majority of patients
- Elevated leukocyte alkaline phosphatase, serum vitamin B$_{12}$, and uric acid levels
- Bone marrow aspiration revealing RBC hyperplasia and absent iron stores

TREATMENT

NONPHARMACOLOGIC THERAPY
Phlebotomy to keep Hgb <15 mg/dl or Hct <45% is the mainstay of therapy.

ACUTE GENERAL Rx
- Hydroxyurea can be used in conjunction with phlebotomy to decrease the incidence of thrombotic events.
- Interferon alfa-2b is also effective in controlling RBC values without significant side effects.
- Myelosuppressive therapy with chlorambucil is effective but not routinely used because of its leukemogenic potential.

CHRONIC Rx
- Patient education regarding need for lifelong monitoring and treatment
- Adjunctive therapy: treatment of pruritus with antihistamines, control of significant hyperuricemia with allopurinol, reduction of gastric hyperacidity with antacids or H$_2$ blockers

DISPOSITION
The median survival time without treatment is 6 to 18 mo following diagnosis; phlebotomy extends the average survival time to 12 yr.

MISCELLANEOUS

COMMENTS
The diagnosis of polycythemia vera requires the following three major criteria or the first two major criteria plus two minor criteria:
- Major criteria
  1. Increased RBC mass (>36 ml/kg in men, >32 ml/kg in women)
  2. Normal arterial oxygen saturation (>92%)
  3. Splenomegaly
- Minor criteria
  1. Thrombocytosis (>400,000/mm^3)
  2. Leukocytosis (>12,000/mm^3)
  3. Elevated leukocyte alkaline phosphatase (>100)
  4. Elevated serum vitamin B$_{12}$ (>900 pg/ml) or vitamin B$_{12}$ binding protein (>2200 pg/ml)

REFERENCES
Gruppo Italiano Studio Policitemia: Polycythemia vera: the natural history of 1213 patients followed for 20 years, *Ann Intern Med* 123:656, 1995.

Silver RT: Interferon alfa 2b: a new treatment for polycythemia vera, *Ann Intern Med* 330:1091, 1993.

Author: **Fred F. Ferri, M.D.**

Polymyalgia rheumatica (PTG)

BASIC INFORMATION

DEFINITION
Polymyalgia rheumatica is a disorder of unknown cause affecting older patients. It is characterized by shoulder and hip stiffness and an elevated erythrocyte sedimentation rate (ESR).

SYNONYMS
Anarthritic rheumatoid syndrome

ICD-9-CM CODES
725.0 Polymyalgia rheumatica

EPIDEMIOLOGY AND DEMOGRAPHICS
PREVALENCE: 1 case/2000 persons >50 yr old
PREDOMINANT SEX: Female:male ratio of 2:1
PREDOMINANT AGE: Rare under age 50 yr; average age of onset: 70 yr

PHYSICAL FINDINGS
- Symptoms are frequently of sudden onset but are often present for months before the diagnosis is made.
- Neck, shoulder, low back, and thigh pain are common complaints.
- Morning stiffness, lasting 2 to 3 hr is typical, and patients often have difficulty getting out of bed.
- Malaise, weight loss, depression, and a low-grade fever are common constitutional symptoms and may suggest systemic inflammation.
- Physical findings are usually limited. Synovitis may be present in peripheral joints and may also be responsible for the proximal girdle symptoms in spite of the fact that they appear to be "muscular" in nature.
- Mild soft-tissue tenderness may be present.
- The temporal arteries should be carefully examined because of the strong relation of polymyalgia rheumatica with temporal or giant cell arteritis.

ETIOLOGY
Unknown

DIAGNOSIS

DIFFERENTIAL DIAGNOSIS
- Rheumatoid arthritis: rheumatoid factor is negative in polymyalgia.
- Polymyositis: enzyme studies are negative in polymyalgia.

WORKUP
The diagnosis of polymyalgia rheumatica is suggested by the following findings:
- Pain and stiffness of pectoral and pelvic musculature
- Patient >50 yr old
- Morning stiffness
- Normal motor strength
- Symptoms for at least 4 to 6 wk
- Elevated ESR (>45)
- Rapid clinical response to low-dose corticosteroid therapy

LABORATORY TESTS
- CBC, ESR, and rheumatoid factor should be performed.
- Mild anemia may be present.

TREATMENT

ACUTE GENERAL Rx
- Prednisone 10 to 20 mg/day is given. The response is often so dramatic that it can be used to confirm the diagnosis. Improvement is usually noted within 24 to 48 hr.
- Steroids are gradually tapered over the next few days as soon as symptoms permit, but small doses (5 mg/day) may be needed for 2 yr.
- NSAIDs may be tried in mild cases.
- Physical therapy is usually unnecessary.

MISCELLANEOUS

COMMENTS
The prognosis is generally favorable. Relapse occasionally occurs in several years, but again responds well to prednisone.

REFERENCES
Chuang T et al: Polymyalgia rheumatica: a 10-year epidemiologic and clinical study, *Ann Intern Med* 97:672, 1982.

Hunder GG: Giant cell arteritis and polymyalgia rheumatica. In Kelley WN et al (eds): Textbook of rheumatology, update 20, Philadelphia, 1996, WB Saunders.

Author: **Lonnie R. Mercier, M.D.**

Posttraumatic stress disorder (PTG)

BASIC INFORMATION

DEFINITION
Posttraumatic stress disorder (PTSD) is an anxiety disorder that arises when an individual has witnessed or experienced a potentially fatal or serious injurious condition during which he or she felt helpless or horrified. After resolution of the event the individual continues to experience the event in the form of flashbacks (reliving the trauma), intrusive recollections, dreams, or physiologic reactivity or psychologic distress in response to cues symbolizing the event. These responses are associated with persistent hyperarousal (e.g., hypervigilance, exaggerated startle, sleep disturbance, irritability, and difficulty concentrating) and avoidance (both physically and cognitively) of stimuli associated with the traumatic event.

SYNONYMS
Soldier's heart
Effort syndrome
Shell shock
Irritable heart
Traumatic neurosis
Survivor syndrome
Concentration camp syndrome
Gross stress reaction (DSM-I published in 1952)

ICD-9-CM CODES
F 43.1 (DSM-IV: 309.81)

EPIDEMIOLOGY AND DEMOGRAPHICS
INCIDENCE (IN U.S.):
Occurs in some 50% of people experiencing a severe life-threatening event (e.g., PTSD was diagnosed in 85% of Nazi concentration camp survivors, 57% of Coconut Grove fire survivors, 67% of WWII prisoners of war, and 50% of Cambodian children subjected to various atrocities).
PREVALENCE (IN U.S.):
- Lifetime prevalence estimates range from 1% to 15% of the American population.
- Prevalence estimates among high-risk populations (e.g., combat veterans or victims of violent crimes) range from 3% to 58%.

PREDOMINANT SEX: No specific gender predisposition has been identified.
PREDOMINANT AGE:
- Development in children is possible, but presentation may be slightly different.
- No predisposing age factors have been identified.

PEAK INCIDENCE: Symptoms may begin immediately after the trauma and peak within 4 to 5 mo of the event.

GENETICS: No specific factors have been identified.

PHYSICAL FINDINGS
- After severe life-threatening event, complaints of derealization, depersonalization, detachment, dissociation, or being dazed, in association with a marked increase in anxiety and arousal
- Within 3 mo, signs of persistent hyperarousal, anxiety, and distressing memories or reexperiences of the traumatic event in most patients; symptoms may be disabling

ETIOLOGY
- There is a "dose-response" relationship between intensity and duration of the stress and severity of PTSD, with duration of the stress the most important factor.
- Man-made disasters cause more intense reactions than natural disasters.
- Premorbid factors (dysthymia, introversion, personality types, alcohol abuse, and family psychiatric history) may predispose to PTSD.
- Symptoms are mediated, in part, by the autonomic nervous system and the hypothalamic-pituitary-adrenal system.

DIAGNOSIS

DIFFERENTIAL DIAGNOSIS
- Diagnosis is made when a dysfunctional response occurs to any stress; so although most people with PTSD technically suffer from an adjustment disorder, the stress to which they are responding is usually extreme.
- Acute stress disorder is similar to PTSD but occurs within the first 4 wk of the stress.
- If symptoms of acute stress disorder persist longer than 4 wk, PTSD is possible.
- Malingering is sometimes difficult to rule out when there is secondary gain.

WORKUP
- History to determine symptoms
- Physical examination to look for signs of autonomic hyperactivity
- NOTE: Only the history is required for diagnosis.

TREATMENT

NONPHARMACOLOGIC THERAPY
- Various forms of individual psychotherapy are effective in reducing severity of symptoms.
- Group therapy is the mainstay treatment for many PTSD victims, particularly in the combat veterans population.

ACUTE GENERAL Rx
- Purely symptomatic and generally aimed at alleviating distress
- Benzodiazepines for reducing the symptoms of anxiety
- β-blockers to alleviate some of the autonomic symptoms
- Sedating antidepressants (e.g., amitriptyline) to treat initial insomnia and suppress nightmares; in low doses may also alleviate daytime anxiety

CHRONIC Rx
- Antidepressants (both tricyclic and serotonin reuptake inhibitor) and nonbenzodiazepine anxiolytic buspirone are mainstay of chronic pharmacologic management.
- Although these agents provide relief, they frequently have persisting residual and often troubling symptoms.
- Alternative approaches:
  1. Monoamine oxidase inhibiting antidepressants
  2. Chronic use of β-blockers or α^2-agonists (e.g., clonidine)
  3. Anticonvulsants such as carbamazepine

DISPOSITION
- Spontaneous remission in 6 mo for nearly half of patients
- Possible chronic symptoms for years
- Predictors of chronic course:
  1. Premorbid psychiatric function
  2. Acute response to stress (e.g., individuals who experience an acute stress disorder immediately after the trauma do better in the long term)

REFERRAL
Since early intervention improves outcome, referral made for all patients to psychotherapy as soon as diagnosis made

MISCELLANEOUS

REFERENCES
Choy T, DeBosset F: Posttraumatic stress disorder: an overview, *Can J Psychiatry* 37:578, 1992.
Gersons BPR, Carlier IVE: Posttraumatic stress disorder: the history of a recent concept, *Br J Psychiatry* 161:742, 1992.

Author: **Rif S. El-Mallakh, M.D.**

BASIC INFORMATION

DEFINITION
Precocious puberty is defined as sexual development occurring before 8 yr of age in males and 9 yr of age in females.

SYNONYMS
Pubertas praecox

ICD-9-CM CODES
259.1 Precocious puberty

EPIDEMIOLOGY AND DEMOGRAPHICS
INCIDENCE: Estimated to be between 1:5000 and 1:10,000
PREDOMINANT SEX: Females > males for the idiopathic variant; for other causes, dependent on the underlying etiology.
GENETICS: The genetics for some of the etiologies of precocious puberty are known.

PHYSICAL FINDINGS
- In females: breast development, pubic hair development, accelerated growth, and menarche
- In males: increase in testicular volume and penile length, pubic hair development, accelerated growth, muscular development, acne, change in voice, and penile erections

ETIOLOGY
- Idiopathic or true: diagnosis of exclusion
- CNS pathology: tumors, hydrocephalus, ventricular cysts, benign lesions
- Severe hypothyroidism
- Posttraumatic head injury
- Genetic disorders: neurofibromatosis, tuberous sclerosis, McCune-Albright syndrome, congenital adrenal hyperplasia
- Gonadal tumors
- Nongonadal tumors: hepatoblastoma
- Exposure to exogenous sex steroids

DIAGNOSIS

DIFFERENTIAL DIAGNOSIS
- Most common diagnoses to consider: premature thelarche and premature adrenarche
- Gonadotropin hormone releasing hormone (GnRH) dependent precocious puberty: idiopathic, CNS tumors, hypothalamic hamartomas, neurofibromatosis, tuberous sclerosis, hydrocephalus, post–acute head injury, ventricular cysts, post–CNS infection
- GnRH independent precocious puberty: congenital adrenal hyperplasia, adrenocortical tumors (males), McCune-Albright syndrome (females), gonadal tumors, ectopic hCG-secreting tumors (chorioblastoma, hepatoblastoma), exposure to exogenous sex steroids, severe hypothyroidism

WORKUP
Thorough history and physical examination is essential to determining if the patient has true precocious puberty. Particular attention should be paid to growth, development, order of appearance of the secondary sexual characteristics, pubertal development in family members, medications, neurologic symptoms, Tanner staging, abdominal and neurologic examination.

LABORATORY TESTS
- GnRH testing will help determine if dependent or independent cause
- Sex hormone studies: LH, FSH, HCG, testosterone (males), estrogen (females)
- T_4, TSH

IMAGING STUDIES
- CT scan or MRI of the brain to evaluate for CNS pathology
- Consideration of pelvic ultrasound in female patients to evaluate for cysts/tumors
- Abdominal imaging with CT scan if intraabdominal pathology suspected

TREATMENT

NONPHARMACOLOGIC THERAPY
- Good communication with the parents is essential to care.
- Psychologic support for the child may be needed with regard to self image and problems with peer acceptance.

ACUTE GENERAL Rx
There is no acute therapy for precocious puberty.

CHRONIC Rx
Therapy depends on the etiology of precocious puberty:
- For true precocious puberty and some CNS lesions, the treatment of choice is leuprolide 0.25 to 0.3 mg/kg with a 7.5 mg minimum IM every 4 wk.
- For other CNS lesions and extragonadal tumors, therapy is dependent on the type of lesion, location of the lesion, and the overall prognosis of the underlying problem.
- For severe hypothyroidism, treatment with thyroid hormone will result in regression of the sexual development. The child will subsequently undergo appropriate pubertal development later in life.
- For familial male gonadotropin-independent precocious puberty, ketoconazole can be used at doses of 600 mg/day divided tid or a combination of testolactone and spironolactone can be used.

DISPOSITION
- For true precocious puberty and some CNS lesions, long-term outcome is usually very good. When drug therapy is instituted, it is continued until a time when further pubertal development is appropriate. It is then discontinued, allowing the child to progress through puberty.
- For other cases, long-term outcomes are dependent on the prognosis of the underlying cause.

REFERRAL
- Initial workup can be instituted by the primary care provider.
- Referral to an endocrinologist is indicated for most children, as they will need long-term management, monitoring, and treatment.

MISCELLANEOUS

REFERENCES
Kulin HE, Muller J: The biological aspects of puberty, *Pediatr Rev* 17(3):75, 1996.
Author: **Beth J. Wutz, M.D.**

Preeclampsia

BASIC INFORMATION

DEFINITION
Preeclampsia involves a triad of hypertension, proteinuria, and edema that develops after the twentieth week of gestation. Mild preeclampsia is defined as a blood pressure of <140/90 mm Hg. Severe preeclampsia is associated with a blood pressure >160/110 mm Hg, proteinuria >5 g in a 24-hr urine collection, oliguria (<400 ml/24 hr), cerebral or visual disturbances, epigastric pain, pulmonary edema, thrombocytopenia, hepatic dysfunction, or severe intrauterine growth retardation.

SYNONYMS
Pregnancy-induced hypertension
Toxemia of pregnancy

ICD-9-CM CODES
642.6 Preeclampsia

EPIDEMIOLOGY AND DEMOGRAPHICS
INCIDENCE: 10% to 14% in primigravidas, 5.7% to 7.3% in multigravida
RISK FACTORS: Increased incidence and severity with multiple gestations, renal or collagen-vascular diseases. Extremes of reproductive age, <20 or >35 yr of age.
GENETICS: Positive correlation with maternal family history. Different paternal gene pool is associated with a decreased risk of recurrence.

PHYSICAL FINDINGS
- Generalized swelling or nondependent edema, possibly manifested by rapid weight gain (>4 lb/wk) even in the absence of edema
- Auscultation of pulmonary rales
- RUQ pain (HELLP syndrome or subcapsular liver hematoma)
- Hyperreflexia or clonus
- Vaginal bleeding (placental abruption)
- Acute or chronic fetal compromise manifested by intrauterine growth restriction or fetal tachycardia with late decelerations, respectively
- Wide range of symptoms attributable to multiorgan system dysfunction, involving hepatic, hematologic, renal, pulmonary, and CNS
- Possibility of severe disease despite "normal" blood pressure readings, so a high index of suspicion must be maintained in high-risk situations

ETIOLOGY
- Exact etiology or toxic substance is unknown.
- Theories:
  1. Imbalance between thromboxane A_2 (vasoconstrictor and platelet aggregator) and prostacyclin (vasodilator)
  2. Abnormal trophoblastic invasion of spiral arteries
  3. Increased sensitivity to angiotensin II by the muscular walls of the arteries.

DIAGNOSIS

DIFFERENTIAL DIAGNOSIS
- Acute fatty liver of pregnancy
- Appendicitis
- Diabetic ketoacidosis
- Gallbladder disease
- Gastroenteritis
- Glomerulonephritis
- Hemolytic uremic syndrome
- Hepatic encephalopathy
- Hyperemesis gravidarum
- Idiopathic thrombocytopenia
- Thrombotic thrombocytopenic purpura
- Nephrolithiasis
- Pyelonephritis
- PUD
- SLE
- Viral hepatitis

WORKUP
- Two blood pressure measurements in lateral recumbent position 6 hr apart, with an absolute pressure >140/90 mm Hg or an increase in 30 mm Hg systolic or 15 mm Hg diastolic from baseline, an increase in the mean arterial pressure (MAP) of 20 mm Hg, or an absolute MAP >105 mm Hg
- Evaluation for proteinuria as defined by >0.1 g/L on urine dipstick or >300 mg protein on a 24-hr urine collection
- Evaluation of fetal status for evidence intrauterine growth restriction, oligohydramnios, alteration in umbilical or uterine artery doppler flow, or acute compromise, such as abruption
- Because of the insidious nature of the disease with potential for multiple organ involvement, complete evaluation for preeclampsia in any pregnant patient presenting with CNS derangement or GI complaints after 20 wk of gestation

- Evaluation for associated conditions such as disseminated intravascular coagulation, hepatic dysfunction, or subcapsular hematoma

LABORATORY TESTS
- High-risk patients: baseline assessment of renal function (24-hr urine collection for protein and creatinine clearance), platelets, BUN, creatinine, liver function tests, and uric acid should be obtained at the first prenatal visit.
- CBC (Hgb, Hct, platelets) may show signs of volume contraction or HELLP syndrome.
- Liver function tests (AST, ALT, LDH) are useful in evaluation for HELLP syndrome or to exclude important differentials.
- Hyperuricemia or increased creatinine may indicate decreasing renal function.
- PT, PTT, and fibrinogen should be checked to rule out disseminated intravascular coagulation.
- Peripheral smear may demonstrate microangiopathic hemolytic anemia.
- Complement levels can be used to differentiate from an acute exacerbation of a collagen-vascular disease.

IMAGING STUDIES
- CT scan of head if atypical presentation of eclampsia, possibility of intracerebral bleed, or prolonged postictal state
- Sonogram of fetus to evaluate for IUGR, amniotic fluid, placenta
- Sonogram of maternal liver if suspect subcapsular hematoma

TREATMENT

NONPHARMACOLOGIC THERAPY
Bed rest in left lateral decubitus position

ACUTE GENERAL Rx
Delivery is the treatment of choice and the only cure for the disease. This must be taken in the context of the gestational age of the fetus, severity of the preeclampsia, and the likelihood of a successful induction and reliability of patient.
- Administer magnesium sulfate 6 g IV loading dose, with 2 to 3 g maintenance or phenytoin at 10 to 15 mg/kg loading dose, then 200 mg IV q8h starting 12 hr after loading dose.
- Hydralazine 10 mg IV, labetalol hydrochloride 20 to 40 mg IV, nifedipine 20 mg SL can be used for acute blood pressure control.
- Continuous fetal monitoring is needed.
- Epidural is anesthesia of choice for pain management in labor or C-section.
- All patients undergoing induction of labor should receive antiseizure medications regardless of severity of disease.

CHRONIC Rx
- Mild preeclampsia <37 wk: close observation for worsening maternal or fetal condition, with delivery at ≥37 wk with favorable cervix or at 40 wk regardless of cervical status.
- Severe preeclampsia: delivery in the presence maternal or fetal compromise, labor, or >34 wk; at 28 to 34 wk consider steroids with close monitoring, and at <24 wk consider termination of pregnancy.
- Aldomet is drug of choice for chronic blood pressure control during pregnancy.

DISPOSITION
Preeclampsia is a progressive and unpredictable disease process; a course of expectancy should be managed with caution. Up to 20% of patients who have seizures are normotensive.

REFERRAL
Obstetric management is indicated because of the insidious nature of the disease, with transfer of all cases <34 wk to a facility with a level three nursery.

MISCELLANEOUS

COMMENTS
Low-dose aspirin 80 mg qd and calcium supplementation 1500 mg qd can be considered in high-risk patients to decrease the risk of recurrence.

REFERENCES
Gabbe S, Niebyl J, Simpson JL: *Obstetrics: normal and problem pregnancies,* ed 3, New York, 1996, Churchill Livingstone.
Sibai B: Hypertension in pregnancy: medical complications during pregnancy, *Obstet Gynecol Clin North Am* 19(4):615, 1992.

Author: Scott J. Zuccala, D.O.

Premenstrual syndrome (PTG)

BASIC INFORMATION

DEFINITION
Premenstrual syndrome (PMS) is a cyclic recurrence during the luteal phase of the menstrual cycle of somatic, affective, and behavioral disturbances that are of sufficient severity to affect interpersonal relationships adversely or interfere with normal activities.

SYNONYMS
PMS

ICD-9-CM CODES
625.4 Premenstrual tension syndromes

EPIDEMIOLOGY AND DEMOGRAPHICS
- PMS is thought to be extremely prevalent, intermittently affecting approximately one third of all premenopausal women.
- Severe cases occur in approximately 2% to 10% of women with PMS.
- Those seeking treatment for PMS are usually in their 30s or 40s.
- The natural history of PMS has not been clearly elucidated.

PHYSICAL FINDINGS
- Diverse and potentially disabling symptoms
- Associated with >150 psychologic, physical, and behavioral symptoms
- Most frequent reason for seeking treatment: emotional symptoms
- Most common emotional symptoms: depression, irritability, anxiety, labile moods, anger, crying easily, sadness, overly sensitive, nervous tension
- Most common physical complaints: headache, bloating, cramps, breast tenderness, migraines, fatigue, weight gain, aches and pains, palpitations
- Most common behavior symptom: food cravings
- Other behavioral symptoms: increased appetite, increased alcohol intake, decreased motivation, decreased efficiency, avoidance of activities, staying home, sleep changes, libido changes, forgetfulness, decreased concentration.

ETIOLOGY
- Etiology remains obscure.
- Because of multifactorial-multiorgan nature of PMS, a single etiologic cause is unlikely.

DIAGNOSIS

DIFFERENTIAL DIAGNOSIS
- A diagnosis of exclusion, so other medical or psychologic disorders should be ruled out.
- Most common disorders are depression or anxiety.

WORKUP
- History
- Physical examination
- Laboratory studies to rule out alternative diagnosis
- If no alternative diagnosis confirms diagnosis of PMS, basal body temperature charting is used to determine if the patient is ovulating:
  1. If not ovulating, it is not PMS.
  2. If ovulating, symptoms should be charted for at least two cycles to determine if the symptoms occur in the luteal phase.
  3. If symptoms are not occurring in the luteal phase, it is not PMS, and further investigation needed.
     a. If symptoms occur in the follicular phase, patient has premenstrual exacerbation of another condition.
     b. If symptoms do not occur in the follicular phase, diagnosis of PMS is confirmed.

LABORATORY TESTS
None available to specifically confirm the diagnosis of PMS

TREATMENT

NONPHARMACOLOGIC THERAPY
- Individualization of the treatment plan to maximize therapeutic response
- Psychosocial intervention:
  1. Education
  2. Stress management
  3. Environmental changes
  4. Adequate rest and sleep
  5. Regular exercise
- Nutritional recommendations:
  1. Regularly eaten well-balanced meals
  2. Adequate amounts of protein, fiber, and complex carbohydrates; low fat
  3. Avoidance of foods that are high in salt and simple sugars; may promote water retention, weight gain, and physical discomfort

4. Avoidance of caffeine-containing beverages; stimulant effects of caffeine may worsen tension, irritability, and insomnia
5. Avoidance of alcohol and illicit drugs; may worsen emotional lability
6. Calcium supplementation (1000 mg/day) to reduce the physical and emotional symptoms
7. Magnesium (360 mg/day) to reduce water retention and the negative affect associated with PMS
8. Pyridoxine (vitamin B_6) 50 mg bid to improve depression, fatigue, and irritability; neurotoxicity observed at higher dosages

ACUTE GENERAL Rx
SUPPRESSION OF OVULATION:
- Oral contraceptives—one pill per day
- Progestin-only oral contraceptive—one pill per day
- Oral micronized progesterone—100 mg qAM and 200 mg qPM on days 17 through 28 of menstrual cycle
- Progestin suppository—200 to 400 mg bid on days 17 through 28 of menstrual cycle
- Medroxyprogesterone (depot)—150 mg IM every 3 mo
- Levonorgestrel implants—surgical insertion every 5 yr
- Transdermal estradiol—one or two 100 µg patches every 3 days
- Danazol—100 to 200 mg/day (ovulation not suppressed at this dose)
- Gonadotropin-releasing hormone (GnRH) agonists—daily by intranasal spray or monthly by depot injection

SUPPRESSION OF PHYSICAL SYMPTOMS:
- Spironolactone—25 to 50 mg bid on days 14 through 28 of menstrual cycle
- Mefenamic acid
  1. For fluid retention: 250 mg tid on days 24 through 28 of cycle
  2. For pain: 500 mg tid on days 19 through 28 of cycle
- Bromocriptine—5 mg/day on days 10 through 26 of cycle
- Danazol—200 mg/day on days 19 through 28 of cycle
- Naproxen (Anaprox)—550 mg bid on days 17 through 28 of cycle; Naprosyn—500 mg bid on days 17 through 28 of cycle.

SUPPRESSION OF PSYCHOLOGIC SYMPTOMS:
- Nortriptyline—50 to 125 mg/day
- Fluoxetine—20 mg/day
- Buspirone—10 mg bid or tid on days 16 through 28 of cycle, then taper drug
- Alprazolam—25 mg tid on days 16 through 28 of cycle, then taper drug
- Fenfluramine—15 mg bid
- Clonidine—0.1 mg bid
- Naltrexone—0.25 mg/day on days 9 through 18 of cycle
- Atenolol—50 mg/day
- Propranolol—20 to 40 mg bid
- Verapamil—100 to 320 mg qd

CHRONIC Rx
- Therapy is largely trial and error, with the goal of providing effective treatment with the safest and most simple therapy.
- For severe intractable PMS: hysterectomy with bilateral oophorectomy; give trial of GnRH therapy or Danazol before surgery.
- Estrogen replacement therapy recommended postoperatively to reduce the risk of osteoporosis, heart disease and genitourinary atrophy.

DISPOSITION
Improved symptoms in 90% of women over time.

REFERRAL
- For counseling with a psychologist or psychiatrist if underlying psychiatric disorder is discovered
- To a gynecologist if surgical therapy is contemplated

MISCELLANEOUS

COMMENTS
Patient educational material is available through most area bookstores and pharmaceutical companies.

REFERENCES
American Psychiatric Association: *Diagnostic and statistical manual of mental disorders*, ed 4, Washington, DC, 1994, American Psychiatric Association.

Danakas GT, Arnold J: Premenstrual syndrome. In Danakas GT, Pietrantoni M (eds): *Practical guide to the care of the gynecologic/obstetric patient*, St Louis, 1997, Mosby.

Parker PH: Premenstrual syndrome, *Am Fam Physician* 50(6):1309, 1994.

Author: **George T. Danakas, M.D.**

Prolactinoma (PTG)

BASIC INFORMATION

DEFINITION
Prolactinomas are monoclonal tumors that secrete prolactin.

ICD-9-CM CODES
253.1 Forbes-Albright syndrome

EPIDEMIOLOGY AND DEMOGRAPHICS
INCIDENCE: Most common pituitary tumor; nearly 30% of all pituitary adenomas secrete enough prolactin to cause hyperprolactinemia.
PREDOMINANT SEX: Microadenomas are more common in women; macroadenomas are more frequent in men.

PHYSICAL FINDINGS
MEN: Decreased facial and body hair, small testicles; may also have decreased libido, impotence, and delayed puberty (caused by decreased testosterone secondary to inhibition of gonadotropin secretion).
WOMEN: Physical examination may be normal; history may reveal amenorrhea, galactorrhea, oligomenorrhea, and anovulation.
BOTH SEXES: Visual field defects and headache may occur depending on size of tumor and its expansion.

ETIOLOGY
Prolactin-secreting pituitary adenomas: microadenomas (<10 mm diameter) or macroadenomas (>10 mm diameter)

DIAGNOSIS

DIFFERENTIAL DIAGNOSIS
Hyperprolactinemia may be caused by the following:
- Drugs: phenothiazines, methyldopa, reserpine, MAO inhibitors, androgens, progesterone, cimetidine, tricyclic antidepressants, haloperidol, meprobamate, chlordiazepoxide, estrogens, narcotics, metoclopramide, verapamil, amoxapine, cocaine, oral contraceptives
- Hepatic cirrhosis, renal failure, primary hypothyroidism
- Ectopic prolactin-secreting tumors (hypernephroma, bronchogenic carcinoma)
- Infiltrating diseases of the pituitary (sarcoidosis, histiocytosis)
- Head trauma, chest wall injury, spinal cord injury
- Polycystic ovary disease, pregnancy, nipple stimulation
- Idiopathic hyperprolactinemia, stress, exercise

WORKUP
- Demonstration of an elevated serum prolactin level:
  1. Normal mean levels are 8 ng/ml in women and 5 ng/ml in men.
  2. Levels >300 ng/ml are virtually diagnostic of prolactinomas.
  3. Prolactin levels can vary with time of day, stress, sleep cycle, and meals. More accurate measurements can be obtained 2 to 3 hr after awakening, preprandially, and when patient is not under distress.
  4. Serial measurements are recommended in patients with mild prolactin elevations.
- TRH stimulation test may be useful in equivocal cases. The normal response is an increase in serum prolactin levels by 100% within 1 hr of TRH infusion; failure to demonstrate an increase in prolactin level is suggestive of pituitary lesion.

IMAGING STUDIES
- MRI with gadolinium enhancement is the procedure of choice in the radiographic evaluation of pituitary disease.
- In absence of MRI, a radiographic diagnosis is best accomplished with a high-resolution CT scanner and special coronal cuts through the pituitary region.

TREATMENT

Management of prolactinomas depends on their size and encroachment on the optic chiasm and other vital structures.

NONPHARMACOLOGIC THERAPY
Pregnancy and breast-feeding should be avoided, since they can encourage tumor growth.

ACUTE GENERAL Rx
- Transsphenoidal resection: the success rate depends on the location of the tumor (entirely intrasellar), experience of neurosurgeon, and size of the tumor (<10 mm in diameter); the recurrence rate may reach 80% within 5 yr. Possible complications of transsphenoidal surgery include transient diabetes insipidus, hypopituitarism, CSF rhinorrhea, and infections (meningitis, wound infection).
- Medical therapy is preferred when fertility is an important consideration.
  1. Bromocriptine (Parlodel): dosage is 2.5 to 10 mg/day; it decreases size of the tumor and generally lowers the prolactin level into the normal range when the initial serum prolactin is <500 ng/ml. Side effects of bromocriptine are nausea, constipation, dizziness, and nasal stuffiness.
  2. Pergolide (Permax) is an alternative medication when bromocriptine is not well tolerated.
  3. Cabergoline (Dostinex) is a newer, longer-acting dopamine agonist that may be more effective and better tolerated than bromocriptine; initial dose is 0.25 mg twice weekly.
- Pituitary irradiation is useful as adjunctive therapy of macroadenomas (>10 mm in diameter) and in patients with persistent hypersecretion following surgery. Potential complications include cranial nerve damage, radionecrosis, and cognitive abnormalities.
- Stereotactic radiosurgery (gamma knife) is a newer modality in the treatment of prolactinomas. A high dose of ionizing radiation is delivered to the tumor through multiple ports. Its advantage is minimal irradiation to surrounding tissues. Proximity of the tumor to the optic chiasm limits this therapeutic modality.

CHRONIC Rx
- Patients on medical therapy require periodic measurement of prolactin levels.
- Evaluation and monitoring of pituitary function is recommended following transsphenoidal surgery.

DISPOSITION
- Transsphenoidal surgery will result in a cure in nearly 50% to 75% of patients with microadenomas and 10% to 20% of patients with macroadenomas.
- Nearly 20% of microprolactinomas resolve during long-term dopamine agonist treatment.

MISCELLANEOUS

COMMENTS
Patients must be monitored for several years after surgery, since up to 50% of microadenomas and nearly 90% of macroadenomas can recur.

REFERENCES
Levy A, Lightman SL: Diagnosis and management of pituitary tumors, *BMJ* 308:1087, 1994.

Saris SC et al: Efficacy of gamma knife radiosurgery for functioning pituitary adenomas, *Progr 2nd Cong Internat Stereotact Radiosurg Soc,* Boston, June 16, 1995, pp 95-96.

Webster J et al: A comparison of cabergoline and bromocriptine in the treatment of hyperprolactinemic amenorrhea, *N Engl J Med* 331:904, 1994.

Author: **Fred F. Ferri, M.D.**

CLINICAL TOPICS Prostate cancer (PTG)

BASIC INFORMATION

DEFINITION AND CLASSIFICATION
Prostate cancer is a neoplasm involving the prostate; various classifications have been developed to evaluate malignant potential and prognosis:
- The degree of malignancy varies with the stage:
  - Stage A: Confined to the prostate, no nodule palpable
  - Stage B: Palpable nodule confined to the gland
  - Stage C: Local extension
  - Stage D: Regional lymph nodes or distant metastases
- In the Gleason classification, histologic patterns are independently assigned numbers 1 to 5 (best to least differentiated). These numbers are added to give a total tumor score:
  1. Prognosis generally good if score is <5.
  2. Score 6 to 10 carries an intermediate prognosis.
  3. Score >10 correlates with anaplastic lesions with poor prognosis.
- Another commonly used classification is the Tumor-Node-Metastasis (TNM) classification of prostate cancer.

ICD-9-CM CODES
185 Malignant neoplasm of prostate

EPIDEMIOLOGY AND DEMOGRAPHICS
- Prostate cancer has surpassed lung cancer as the most common nonskin cancer in men.
- Over 100,000 cases are diagnosed yearly, and nearly 30,000 males die from prostate cancer each year.
- Incidence of prostate cancer increases with age: uncommon <50 yr; 80% of new cases are diagnosed in patients ≥65 yr.
- Average age at time of diagnosis is 72 yr.
- African Americans in the U.S. have the highest incidence of prostate cancer in the world (1 in every 9 males).
- Incidence is low in Asians.
- Approximately 9% of all prostate cancers may be familial.

PHYSICAL FINDINGS
- Generally silent disease until it reaches advanced stages.
- Bone pain and pathologic fractures may be initial symptoms of prostate cancer.
- Local growth can cause symptoms of outflow obstruction.
- Digital rectal examination (DRE) may reveal an area of increased firmness; 10% of patients will have a negative DRE.
- Prostate may be hard, fixed with extension of tumor to the seminal vesicles in advanced stages.

DIAGNOSIS

DIFFERENTIAL DIAGNOSIS
- Benign prostatic hypertrophy
- Prostatitis
- Prostate stones

LABORATORY TESTS
- Measurement of PSA is useful in early diagnosis of prostate cancer and also in monitoring efficacy of therapy. Normal PSA is found in >30% of patients with prostate cancer.
- Prostatic acid phosphatase (PAP) can be used for evaluation of nonlocalized disease.
- Transrectal biopsy and fine needle aspiration of prostate to confirm the diagnosis

IMAGING STUDIES
- Bone scan is useful to evaluate bone metastasis (present or eventually develop in almost 80% of patients).
- CT scan and transrectal ultrasonography may be useful in selected patients to assess extent of prostate cancer. Transrectal prostatic ultrasonography is generally regarded as more sensitive than DRE and useful to guide the biopsy; however, its use as a primary screening test is limited by cost and availability; most useful to detect an occult lesion in patients with elevated PSA but normal digital examination of prostate.

TREATMENT

NONPHARMACOLOGIC THERAPY
Watchful waiting is reasonable in patients with early stage (T-IA) and projected life expectancy <10 yr or in patients with focal and moderately differentiated carcinoma.

ACUTE GENERAL Rx
- Therapeutic approach varies with the following:
  1. Stage of the tumor
  2. Patient's life expectancy
  3. General medical condition
  4. Patient's treatment preference (e.g., patient may be opposed to orchiectomy)
- The optimal treatment of clinically localized prostate cancer is unclear:
  1. Radical prostatectomy is generally performed in patients with localized prostate cancer and life expectancy >10 yr.
  2. Radiation therapy represents an alternative in patients with localized prostate cancer, especially poor surgical candidates or patients with a high-grade malignancy.
- Patients with advanced disease and projected life expectancy <10 yr are candidates for radiation therapy and hormonal therapy (DES, LHRH analogs, antiandrogens, bilateral orchiectomy).
- Recommended treatment of patients with regional metastatic prostate cancer with projected life expectancy ≥10 yr includes radical prostatectomy, radiation therapy, hormonal therapy.
- Adjuvant treatment with GnRH analog goserelin (Zoladex), when started simultaneously with external irradiation, improves local control and survival in patients with locally advanced prostate cancer.

CHRONIC Rx
- Patients should be monitored at 3- to 6-mo intervals with clinical examination, DRE, and PSA for the first year, then every 6 mo for the second year, then yearly if stable.
- Chest x-ray examination, bone scan should be performed yearly or sooner if patient develops symptoms.

DISPOSITION
- Prognosis varies with the stage of the disease (see "Definition") and the Gleason classification (see "Definition").
- The ploidy of the tumor also has prognostic value: prognosis is better with diploid tumor cells, worse with aneuploid tumor cells.
- For grade 1 tumors, the extended 10-yr, disease-specific survival is similar for patients with prostatectomy (94%), radiotherapy (90%), and conservative management (93%); survival rate is better with surgery than with radiotherapy or conservative management in patients with grade 2 or 3 localized prostate cancer.

MISCELLANEOUS

REFERENCES
Bolla M et al: Improved survival in patients with locally advanced prostate cancer treated with radiotherapy and goserelin, *N Engl J Med* 337:295, 1997.
Dearnaley DP, Melia J: Early prostate cancer—to treat or not to treat? *Lancet* 349:892, 1997.

Author: Fred F. Ferri, M.D.

Prostatic hyperplasia, benign

BASIC INFORMATION

DEFINITION
Benign prostatic hyperplasia is the benign growth of the prostate, generally originating in the periureteral and transition zones, with subsequent obstructive and irritative voiding symptoms.

SYNONYMS
BPH
Prostatic hypertrophy

ICD-9-CM CODES
600 Benign prostatic hyperplasia

EPIDEMIOLOGY AND DEMOGRAPHICS
- 80% of men have evidence of benign prostatic hypertrophy by age 80 yr.
- Medical and surgical intervention for problems caused by BPH is required in >20% of males by age 75 yr.
- Transurethral resection of the prostate (TURP) is the tenth most common operative procedure (>400,000/yr in U.S.).
- 10% to 30% of men with BPH have occult prostate cancer.

PHYSICAL FINDINGS
- Digital rectal examination (DRE) reveals enlargement of the prostate.
- Focal enlargement may be indicative of malignancy.
- There is poor correlation between size of prostate and symptoms (BPH may be asymptomatic if it does not encroach on the urethral lumen).
- Most patients with BPH complain of difficulty in initiating urination (hesitancy), decrease in caliber and force of stream; incomplete emptying of bladder often resulting in double voiding (need to urinate again a few minutes after voiding), postvoid "dribbling," and nocturia.

ETIOLOGY
Multifactorial; a functioning testicle is necessary for development of BPH (as evidenced by the absence in males who were castrated before puberty).

DIAGNOSIS

DIFFERENTIAL DIAGNOSIS
- Prostatitis
- Prostate cancer
- Strictures (urethral)
- Medications interfering with the muscle fibers in the prostate and also with bladder function

WORKUP
Symptom assessment (use of American Urological Association Symptom Index for BPH [see Fig. A-2 in Appendix]), laboratory tests, and imaging studies

LABORATORY TESTS
- Prostate specific antigen (PSA): protease secreted by epithelial cells of the prostate; elevated in 30% to 50% of patients with BPH. Testing for PSA increases detection rate for prostate cancer and tends to detect cancer at an earlier stage. However, the PSA test does not discriminate well between patients with symptomatic BPH and those with prostate cancer, particularly if the cancers are pathologically localized and curable. The test may also trigger additional evaluation, including ultrasound biopsy of the prostate. Recent data indicate that asymptomatic men with PSA levels <2 ng/ml do not need annual testing.
- Urinalysis, urine C&S to rule out infection (if suspected)
- BUN and creatinine to rule out postrenal insufficiency

IMAGING STUDIES
- Transrectal ultrasound may be indicated in patients with palpable nodules or significant elevation of PSA. It is also useful to estimate prostate size.
- Uroflowmetry may be used to determine relative impact of obstruction on urine flow. Urethral pressure profile is useful to predict prostatic hypertrophy within the urethral lumen.
- Pressure flow studies, although invasive, are particularly helpful in patients whose history and/or examination suggest primary bladder dysfunction as a cause of symptoms of prostatism. They are also useful in patients for whom a distinction between prostatic obstruction and impaired detrusor contractility may affect the choice of therapy. However, pressure flow studies may not be useful in the workup of the usual patient with symptoms of prostatism.
- Postvoid residual urine measurement has not been proven useful in predicting the need for or response to treatment; may be useful in monitoring the course of the disease in pa-

tients who elect nonsurgical treatment.
- Urethral cystoscopy is an option during later evaluation if invasive treatment is being planned.

TREATMENT

NONPHARMACOLOGIC THERAPY
- Avoidance of caffeine or any other foods that may exacerbate symptoms
- Avoidance of medications that may exacerbate symptoms (e.g., cold and allergy remedies)

ACUTE GENERAL Rx
- Asymptomatic patients with prostate enlargement caused by BPH generally do not require treatment. For those patients who have specific complications from BPH, prostate surgery is usually the most appropriate form of treatment. However, surgery may result in significant complications (e.g., incontinence, infection).
- TURP is the most commonly used surgical procedure for BPH. Transurethral incision of the prostate (TUIP), a procedure almost equivalent in efficacy, is limited to patients whose estimated resection tissue weight would be 30 g or less. TUIP can be performed in an ambulatory setting or during a 1-day hospitalization. Open prostatectomy is typically performed on patients with very large prostates.
- Surgery need not be treatment of last resort for most patients; that is, patients need not undergo other treatments for BPH before they can have surgery. However, recommending surgery on the grounds that a patient's surgical risk will "only increase with age" is generally inappropriate.
- Balloon dilatation of the prostatic urethra is less effective than surgery for relieving symptoms but is associated with fewer complications. It is a reasonable treatment option for patients with smaller prostates and no middle lobe enlargement.
- α-Blockers (e.g., tamsulosin, doxazosin, prazosin, and terazosin) relax smooth muscle of the bladder neck and prostate and can increase peak urinary flow rate. They are useful in patients with mild to moderate symptoms.
- Hormonal manipulation with finasteride (Proscar), a 5α-reductase inhibitor that blocks conversion of testosterone to dihydrotestosterone, can reduce the size of the prostate. Treatment requires 6 mo or more for maximal effect.

CHRONIC Rx
- Avoid medications and foods that exacerbate symptoms.
- Symptomatic improvement occurs in >70% of patients with proper treatment.

DISPOSITION
With appropriate therapy, symptoms improve or stabilize in >70% of patients with BPH.

REFERRAL
Urology referral for patients with severe or intolerable symptoms and for any patient suspected of having prostate cancer (10% to 30% of men with BPH).

MISCELLANEOUS

COMMENTS
Emerging technologies for treating BPH include lasers, coils, stents, thermal therapy, and hyperthermia. Laser prostatectomy appears promising; however, long-term effectiveness has not yet been demonstrated.

REFERENCES
Barry M et al: American Urological Association (AUA) symptoms index for BPH, *J Urol* 148:1549, 1992.

Carter HB et al: Recommended prostate specific antigen testing intervals for the detection of curable prostate cancer, *JAMA* 277:1456, 1997.

Cowles RS et al: A prospective randomized comparison of transurethral resection to visual laser oblation of the prostate for the treatment of benign prostate hyperplasia, *Urology* 46:155, 1995.

Kreder KJ: Combination drug therapy for benign prostatic hyperplasia, *JAMA* 274:359, 1995.

McConnell JD et al: *Benign prostatic hyperplasia: diagnosis and treatment—quick reference guide for clinicians*, AHCPR Publication No 94-0583, Rockville, Md, 1994, Agency for Health Care Policy and Research, Public Health Service, US Department of Health and Human Services.

Wasson JH et al: A comparison of transurethral surgery with watchful waiting for moderate symptoms of benign prostatic hyperplasia, *N Engl J Med* 332:75, 1995.

Author: **Fred F. Ferri, M.D.**

Pruritus ani *(PTG)*

BASIC INFORMATION

DEFINITION
Pruritus ani refers to an intense chronic itching of the anus and perianal skin.

ICD-9-CM CODES
698.0 Pruritus ani

EPIDEMIOLOGY AND DEMOGRAPHICS
- Any age can be affected.
- Occurs in 1% to 5% of the population.
- Male to female predominance of 4:1.

PHYSICAL FINDINGS
- Anal itching
- Anal fissures
- Hemorrhoids
- Excoriations
- Pinworms
- Fecal incontinence

ETIOLOGY
ANORECTAL DISEASES AND FECAL CONTAMINATION:
- Diarrhea
- Anal incontinence
- Hemorrhoids
- Fissures
- Fistulae
- Rectal prolapse
- Malignancy: Bowen's disease, epidermoid cancer, perianal Paget's disease

INFECTIONS:
- Fungal: candidiasis, dermatophytes
- Parasitic: pinworms, scabies
- Bacterial: *Staphylococcus aureus*, erythrasma
- Venereal: herpes gonococcal, syphilis, condyloma acuminatum

LOCAL IRRITANTS:
- Moisture, obesity, excessive perspiration
- Soaps, hygiene products
- Toilet paper: perfumed, dyed
- Underwear: irritating fabrics, detergents
- Anal creams, suppositories
- Dietary: coffee, beer, acidic foods
- Drugs: mineral oil, ascorbic acid, hydrocortisone sodium succinate, quinine, colchicine

DERMATOLOGIC DISEASES:
- Psoriasis
- Atopic dermatitis
- Seborrheic dermatitis

DIAGNOSIS

DIFFERENTIAL DIAGNOSIS
- Allergies
- Anxiety
- Dermatologic conditions
- Infections
- Parasites
- Diabetes mellitus
- Chronic liver disease
- Neoplasia

WORKUP
- Detailed history regarding bowel habits, hygiene, use of perfumed products, and past medical history
- Inspection of perianal area
- Possible biopsy to exclude neoplasia

LABORATORY TESTS
- Chemistry profile
- Urinalysis
- Cultures
- Stool for ova and parasites
- Tape test
- Glucose tolerance test if necessary

TREATMENT

NONPHARMACOLOGIC THERAPY
- Avoidance of tight, nonporous clothing and underclothing
- Discontinuation or curtailment of coffee, beer, citrus fruits, tomatoes, chocolate, and tea
- Cleansing of anal area after bowel movements with a premoistened pad or tissue and avoidance of perfumes and dyes present in toilet paper and soaps
- Avoidance of excessive perspiration
- Aggressive management of fecal leakage or incontinence to avoid soiling of perianal skin

ACUTE GENERAL Rx
- Minimization of frequent loose stools with antidiarrheals and fiber agents if appropriate
- Use of a 1% hydrocortisone cream sparingly bid during the acute phase of pruritus ani but not for >2 wk to avoid atrophy
- Treatment of predisposing factors, such as parasites, diabetes, liver disease, hemorrhoids, and other infections

CHRONIC Rx
- Possible complications: excoriation and secondary bacterial infection; must be treated aggressively
- Long-standing, intractable pruritus ani: good response to intracutaneous injections of methylene blue and other agents

DISPOSITION
- Usually good results with total resolution of symptoms
- In some, persistent and recurrent symptoms

REFERRAL
To colorectal specialist if conservative measures fail

MISCELLANEOUS

REFERENCES
Barnett JL, Raper SE: Anorectal diseases. In Yamada T, Alpers DH, Owyang C (eds): *Textbook of gastroenterology*, ed 2, vol 2, Philadelphia, 1995, Lippincott.

Hanno R, Murphy P: Pruritus ani: classification and management, *Dermatol Clin* 5:81, 1987.

Author: **Maria A. Corigliano, M.D.**

Pruritus vulvae

BASIC INFORMATION

DEFINITION
Pruritus vulvae refers to intense itching of the female external genitalia.

SYNONYMS
Vulvodynia

ICD-9-CM CODES
698.1 Pruritus of genital organs

EPIDEMIOLOGY AND DEMOGRAPHICS
- A female disorder that can affect women at any age
- Young girls: infection is usually causative
- Postmenopausal women: frequently affected because of hypoestrogenic state

PHYSICAL FINDINGS
Constant intense itching or burning of the vulva

ETIOLOGY
- About 50% are caused by monilial infection or trichomoniasis.
- Other infectious causes are herpes simplex, condyloma acuminata, and molluscum contagiosum.
- Other causes:
  1. Infestations with scabies, pediculosis pubis, and pinworms
  2. Dermatoses such as hypertrophic dystrophy, lichen sclerosis, lichen planus, and psoriasis
  3. Neoplasms such as Bowen's disease, Paget's disease, and squamous cell carcinoma
  4. Allergic or chemical dermatitis caused by dyes in clothing or toilet paper, detergents, contraceptive gels, vaginal medications, douches, or soaps
  5. Vulva or vaginal atrophy
- Severe pruritus is probably caused by degeneration and inflammation of terminal nerve fibers.
- Most intense itching occurs with hyperplastic lesions.

DIAGNOSIS

DIFFERENTIAL DIAGNOSIS
- Vulvitis
- Vaginitis
- Lichen sclerosis
- Squamous cell hyperplasia
- Pinworms
- Vulvar cancer

WORKUP
- Inspection of vulva, vagina, and perianal area looking for infection, fissures, ulcerations, induration, or thick plaques
- Must rule out trichomonas, candidiasis, allergy, vitamin deficiencies, diabetes

LABORATORY TESTS
- Wet prep of saline and KOH of vaginal discharge
- Tape test to look for pinworms
- Vaginal cultures
- Biopsy when needed

TREATMENT

NONPHARMACOLOGIC THERAPY
- Keep vulva clean and dry.
- Wear white cotton panties.
- Avoid perfumes and body creams over vulvar area as they can cause irritation.
- Reduce stress.
- Apply wet dressings with aluminum acetate (Burow's) solution frequently.
- Avoid coffee and caffeine-containing beverages, chocolates, tomatoes.
- Sitz baths may be helpful.

ACUTE GENERAL Rx
Need to treat underlying problem:
- Yeast infection: any of the vaginal creams or Diflucan 150 mg one time dose
- *Trichomoniasis* or *Gardnerella vaginitis:* Flagyl 500 mg or 375 mg PO bid for 7 days
- Urinary tract infection: treatment of specific organism
- Estrogen replacement therapy if atrophy is the cause of pruritus
- Pinworms: mebendazole (Vermox) 100 mg one tablet at diagnosis and repeated in 1 to 2 wk; also treat other members in family >2 yr of age
- Squamous cell hyperplasia: local application of corticosteroids
  1. One of the high- or medium-potency corticosteroids (0.025% or 0.01% fluocinolone acetonide or 0.01% triamcinolone acetonide) can be used to relieve itching.
  2. Rub into vulva bid or tid for 4 to 6 wk.
  3. Once itching is controlled, fluorinated steroid can be discontinued and patient can be switched to hydrocortisone preparation.
- Lichen sclerosis: topical 2% testosterone in petrolatum massaged into the vulvar tissue bid or tid

CHRONIC Rx
- If not relieved by topical measures: intradermal injection of triamcinolone (10 mg/ml diluted 2:1 saline) 0.1 ml of the suspension injected at 1-cm intervals and tissue gently massaged
- If symptoms still uncontrollable: SC injection of absolute alcohol 0.1 ml at 1-cm intervals

DISPOSITION
Usually controlled with conservative measures and topical steroids

REFERRAL
To a gynecologist for further workup if conservative measures do not give relief

MISCELLANEOUS

REFERENCES
Berek J: *Novak's gynecology,* ed 12, Baltimore, 1996, Williams & Wilkins.
Meltzer R: Vulvovaginitis. In Sciarra JJ: *Gynecology and obstetrics,* vol 1, Philadelphia, 1994, Lippincott.
Author: **Maria A. Corigliano, M.D.**

Pseudogout (PTG)

BASIC INFORMATION

DEFINITION
Pseudogout is one of the clinical patterns associated with a crystal-induced synovitis resulting from the deposition of calcium pyrophosphate dehydrate crystals in joint hyaline and fibrocartilage. The cartilage deposition is termed *chondrocalcinosis*.

SYNONYMS
Calcium pyrophosphate dehydrate crystal deposition disease (CPDD)
Chondrocalcinosis
Pyrophosphate arthropathy

ICD-9-CM CODES
275.4 Chondrocalcinosis

EPIDEMIOLOGY AND DEMOGRAPHICS
PREVALENCE:
- Uncertain
- Probably similar to gout (3/1000 persons)
- Chondrocalcinosis is present in >20% of all people at age 80 yr, but most are asymptomatic.

PREDOMINANT SEX: Female:male ratio of approximately 1.5:1
PREVALENT AGE: 60 to 70 yr at onset

PHYSICAL FINDINGS
- Symptoms are similar to those of gouty arthritis with acute attacks and chronic arthritis
- Knee joint is most commonly affected
- Swelling, stiffness, and increased heat in affected joint

ETIOLOGY
- Unknown
- Often associated with various medical conditions, including hyperparathyroidism and amyloidosis

DIAGNOSIS

DIFFERENTIAL DIAGNOSIS
- Gouty arthritis
- Rheumatoid arthritis
- Osteoarthritis
- Neuropathic joint

WORKUP
- Variable clinical presentation
- Diagnosis dependent on the identification of CPPD crystals
- The American Rheumatism Association revised diagnostic criteria for CPPD crystal deposition disease (pseudogout) are often used:

1. Criteria
   I. Demonstration of CPPD crystals (obtained by biopsy, necrocopy, or aspirated synovial fluid) by definitive means (e.g., characteristic "fingerprint" by x-ray diffraction powder pattern or by chemical analysis)
   II. (a) Identification of monoclinic and/or triclinic crystals showing either no or only a weakly positive birefringence by compensated polarized light microscopy
   (b) Presence of typical calcifications in roentgenograms
   III. (a) Acute arthritis, especially of knees or other large joints, with or without concomitant hyperuricemia
   (b) Chronic arthritis, especially of knees, hips, wrists, carpus, elbow, shoulder, and metacarpophalangeal joints, especially if accompanied by acute exacerbations; the following features are helpful in differentiating chronic arthritis from osteoarthritis:
      1. Uncommon site—e.g., wrist, MCP, elbow, shoulder
      2. Appearance of lesion radiologically—e.g., radiocarpal or patellofemoral joint space narrowing, especially if isolated (patella "wrapped around" the femur)
      3. Subchondral cyst formation
      4. Severity of degeneration—progressive, with subchondral bony collapse (microfractures), and fragmentation, with formation of intraarticular radiodense bodies
      5. Osteophyte formation—variable and inconstant
      6. Tendon calcifications, especially Achilles, triceps, obturators
2. Categories
   Definite—Criteria I or II (a) plus (b) must be fulfilled.
   Probable—Criteria II(a) or II(b) must be fulfilled.
   Possible—Criteria III(a) or (b) should alert the clinician to the possibility of underlying CPPD deposition.

LABORATORY TESTS
Crystal analysis of the synovidal fluid aspirate to reveal rhomboid-shaped calcium pyrophospate crystals

IMAGING STUDIES
Plain radiographs to reveal the following:
- Stippled calcification in bands running parallel to the subchondral bone margins
- Crystal deposition in menisci, synovium, and ligament tissue; triangular wrist cartilage and symphysis pubis are often affected

TREATMENT

NONPHARMACOLOGIC THERAPY
General measures such as heat, rest, and elevation as needed

ACUTE GENERAL Rx
- NSAIDS (as for gout)
- Colchicine
- Aspiration/steroid injection

DISPOSITION
Structural joint damage may occasionally occur requiring arthroplasty in rare cases.

REFERRAL
For orthopedic consultation for destructive joint changes

MISCELLANEOUS

COMMENTS
As with gout, acute attacks may be triggered by various surgical or medical events.

REFERENCES
Ryan LM, McCarty DJ: Calcium pyrophosphate dihydrate crystal deposition disease. In McCarty DJ, Koopman WJ (eds): *Arthritis and allied conditions*, ed 12, Philadelphia, 1993, Lea and Febiger.

Author: **Lonnie R. Mercier, M.D.**

Pseudomembranous colitis (PTG)

BASIC INFORMATION

DEFINITION
Pseudomembranous colitis is the occurrence of diarrhea and bowel inflammation associated with antibiotic use.

SYNONYMS
Antibiotic-induced colitis

ICD-9-CM CODES
008.45 *Clostridium difficile* pseudomembranous colitis

EPIDEMIOLOGY AND DEMOGRAPHICS
- Cephalosporins are the most frequent offending agent in pseudomembranous colitis because of their high rates of use.
- The antibiotic with the highest incidence is clindamycin (10% incidence of pseudomembranous colitis with its use).

PHYSICAL FINDINGS
- Abdominal tenderness (generalized or lower abdominal)
- Fever
- In patients with prolonged diarrhea, poor skin turgor, dry mucous membranes, and other signs of dehydration may be present

ETIOLOGY
Risk factors for *C. difficile* (the major identifiable agent of antibiotic-induced diarrhea and colitis):
- Administration of antibiotics: can occur with any antibiotic, but occurs most frequently with clindamycin, ampicillin, and cephalosporins
- Prolonged hospitalization
- Abdominal surgery

DIAGNOSIS

The clinical signs of pseudomembranous colitis generally include diarrhea, fever, and abdominal cramps following use of antibiotics.

DIFFERENTIAL DIAGNOSIS
- GI bacterial infections (e.g., *Salmonella, Shigella, Campylobacter, Yersinia*)
- Enteric parasites (e.g., *Cryptosporidium, Entamoeba histolytica*)
- IBD
- Celiac sprue
- Irritable bowel syndrome

WORKUP
- All patients with diarrhea accompanied by current or recent antibiotic use should be tested for *C. difficile* (see "Laboratory Tests").
- Sigmoidoscopy (without cleansing enema) may be necessary when the clinical and laboratory diagnosis is inconclusive and the diarrhea persists.
- In antibiotic-induced pseudomembranous colitis, the sigmoidoscopy will often reveal raised white-yellow exudative plaques adherent to the colonic mucosa.

LABORATORY TESTS
- *C. difficile* toxin can be detected by cytotoxin tissue-culture assay (gold standard for identifying *C. difficile* toxin in stool specimen) and by enzyme-linked immunoassay (EIA) for *C. difficile* toxins A and B.
- Fecal leukocytes (assessed by microscopy or lactoferrin assay) are generally present in stool samples.
- CBC will usually reveal leukocytosis.

IMAGING STUDIES
Abdominal film (flat plate and upright) is useful in patients with abdominal pain or evidence of obstruction on physical examination.

TREATMENT

NONPHARMACOLOGIC THERAPY
- Discontinue offending antibiotic.
- Fluid hydration and correct electrolyte abnormalities.

ACUTE GENERAL Rx
- Metronidazole 250 mg PO qid for 10 to 14 days
- Vancomycin 125 mg PO qid for 10 to 14 days in cases resistant to metronidazole
- Cholestyramine 4 g PO qid for 10 days in addition to metronidazole to control severe diarrhea (avoid use with vancomycin)

CHRONIC Rx
Judicious future use of antibiotics to prevent recurrences (e.g., avoid prolonged antibiotic therapy)

DISPOSITION
Most patients recover completely with appropriate therapy; mortality exceeds 10% in untreated patients.

REFERRAL
Hospital admission and IV hydration in severe cases

MISCELLANEOUS

COMMENTS
Possible complications of pseudomembranous colitis include dehydration, bowel perforation, toxic megacolon, electrolyte imbalance, and reactive arthritis.

REFERENCES
Anand A et al: Epidemiology, clinical manifestations, and outcome of *Clostridium difficile*-associated diarrhea, *Am J Gastroenterol* 89:519, 1994.

Manabe YC et al: *Clostridium difficile* colitis: an efficient clinical approach to diagnosis, *Ann Intern Med* 123:835, 1995.

Author: Fred F. Ferri, M.D.

Psittacosis

BASIC INFORMATION

DEFINITION
Psittacosis is a systemic infection caused by *Chlamydia psittaci*.

SYNONYMS
Ornithosis

ICD-9-CM CODES
073.9 Psittacosis

EPIDEMIOLOGY AND DEMOGRAPHICS
INCIDENCE (IN U.S.):
- 45 cases reported in 1996
- True incidence possibly higher because infections may be subclinical
- Highest incidence among pet owners and people working in contact with birds

PREVALENCE (IN U.S.):
- Low among humans
- Organism carried in 5% to 8% of birds

PREDOMINANT SEX: Equal sex distribution

PREDOMINANT AGE: More common in adults

PEAK INCIDENCE: 30 to 60 yr of age

PHYSICAL FINDINGS
- Incubation period of 5 to 15 days
- Subclinical infection
- Onset abrupt or insidious
- Most common symptoms:
  1. Fever
  2. Myalgias
  3. Chills
  4. Cough
- Most common clinical syndrome: atypical pneumonia with fever, headache, dry cough, and a chest x-ray more dramatically abnormal than the physical examination
- Ranges from mild disease to respiratory failure and death, although this is extremely unusual
- Other clinical presentations:
  1. Mononucleosis-like syndrome
  2. Typhoidal form
- Most frequent physical findings:
  1. Fever
  2. Pharyngeal erythema
  3. Rales
  4. Hepatomegaly
- Less common findings:
  1. Somnolence
  2. Confusion
  3. Relative bradycardia
  4. Pleural rub
  5. Adenopathy
  6. Splenomegaly
  7. Horder's spots (pink blanching maculopapular rash)
- Besides the lungs, other specific end-organ involvement:
  1. Pericarditis
  2. Myocarditis
  3. Endocarditis
  4. Hepatitis
  5. Joints
  6. Kidneys (glomerulonephritis)
  7. CNS

ETIOLOGY
- *Chlamydia psittaci* is an obligate intracellular bacterium.
- Infection is usually spread by the respiratory route from infected birds.
- There is a history of exposure to birds in 85% of patients.
- Strains from turkeys and psittacine birds are most virulent for humans.
- Cows, goats, and sheep are occasionally implicated.

DIAGNOSIS

DIFFERENTIAL DIAGNOSIS
- Legionella
- Mycoplasma
- *Chlamydia pneumoniae* (TWAR)
- Viral respiratory infections
- Bacterial pneumonia
- Typhoid fever
- Viral hepatitis
- Aseptic meningitis
- Fever of unknown origin
- Mononucleosis

WORKUP
- CBC, renal and liver function tests
- Chlamydia serology
- Chest x-ray examination
- Special immunostaining of respiratory secretions

LABORATORY TESTS
- WBC count is normal or slightly elevated.
- Mild liver function abnormalities are common (50%).
- Blood cultures are almost always negative.
- Studies on respiratory secretions:
  1. Direct immunofluorescent antibody (DFA) of respiratory secretions with monoclonal antibodies to chlamydial antigens
  2. Chlamydial LPS (lipopolysaccharide) antigen by enzyme immunoassay (EIA)
  3. Polymerase chain reaction (PCR)
- Serologic studies:
  1. Complement-fixing antibodies
  2. Micro-immunofluorescence
  3. Possible false-negative results and cross-reaction with other chlamydial species with both techniques

IMAGING STUDIES
- Chest x-ray examination is abnormal in 50% to 90% with a variety of patterns.
- Pleural effusions are common.

TREATMENT

NONPHARMACOLOGIC THERAPY
Oxygen supplementation as needed

ACUTE GENERAL Rx
- Tetracycline (500 mg PO qid) *or*
- Doxycycline (100 mg PO bid) *or*
- Erythromycin (500 mg PO qid): less effective

CHRONIC Rx
In the rare cases of endocarditis, combination of heart valve replacement and prolonged antibiotic course may be the treatment of choice.

DISPOSITION
- Mortality low (0.7%)
- Poor prognostic factors:
  1. Advanced age
  2. Leukopenia
  3. Severe hypoxemia
  4. Renal failure
  5. Confusion
  6. Multilobe pulmonary involvement
- Possible reinfection

REFERRAL
- To infectious disease expert:
  1. Complicated atypical pneumonia or other end-organ involvement
  2. Suspicion of an outbreak
- To pulmonologist for diagnostic bronchoscopy

MISCELLANEOUS

COMMENTS
- Hospitalized patients do not require specific isolation precautions.
- Any confirmed or suspected case of psittacosis should be reported to public health authorities.

REFERENCES
Schlossberg D: Chlamydia psittaci (psittacosis). In Mandell GL, Bennett JE, Dolin R (eds): *Principles and practice of infectious diseases,* New York, 1995, Churchill Livingstone.

Verweij PE et al: Severe human psittacosis requiring artificial ventilation: case report and review, *Clin Infect Dis* 20:440, 1995.

Author: **Michele Halpern, M.D.**

Psoriasis (PTG)

BASIC INFORMATION

DEFINITION
Psoriasis is a chronic skin disorder, characterized by excessive proliferation of keratinocytes resulting in the formation of thickened scaly plaques, itching, and inflammatory changes of the epidermis and dermis. The various forms of psoriasis include guttate, pustular, and arthritic variants.

ICD-9-CM CODES
696.0 Psoriasis, arthritic, arthropathic
696.1 Psoriasis, any type except arthropathic

EPIDEMIOLOGY AND DEMOGRAPHICS
- Psoriasis affects 1% to 3% of the world's population.
- There is a strong association between psoriasis and HLA B13, B17, and B27 (pustular psoriasis).
- Peak age of onset is bimodal (adolescents and at 60 yr of age).
- Men and women are equally affected.

PHYSICAL FINDINGS
- Chronic plaque psoriasis generally manifests with symmetric, sharply-demarcated, erythematous, silver-scaled patches affecting primarily the intergluteal folds, elbows, scalp, fingernails, toenails and knees (see color plate 16).
- Psoriasis can also develop at the site of any physical trauma (sunburn, scratching). This is known as Koebner's phenomenon.
- Nail involvement is common (pitting of the nail plate), resulting in hyperkeratosis, onychodystrophy with onycholysis.
- Pruritus is variable.
- Joint involvement can result in sacroiliitis and spondylitis.
- Guttate psoriasis is generally preceded by streptococcal pharyngitis and manifests with multiple drop-like lesions on the extremities and the trunk.

ETIOLOGY
- Unknown
- Familial clustering (genetic transmission with a dominant mode with variable penetrants)

DIAGNOSIS

DIFFERENTIAL DIAGNOSIS
- Contact dermatitis
- Atopic dermatitis
- Stasis dermatitis
- Tinea
- Nummular dermatitis
- Candidiasis
- Mycoses fungoides
- Cutaneous SLE
- Secondary and tertiary syphilis
- Drug eruption

WORKUP
- Diagnosis is clinical.
- Skin biopsy is rarely necessary.

LABORATORY TESTS
Generally not necessary for diagnosis

TREATMENT

NONPHARMACOLOGIC THERAPY
- Sunbathing generally leads to improvement.
- Eliminate triggering factors (e.g., stress, certain medications [e.g., lithium, β-blockers, antimalarials]).

ACUTE GENERAL Rx
Therapeutic options vary according to the extent of disease.
- Patients with limited disease (>20% of the body) can be treated with the following:
  1. Topical steroids: disadvantages are brief remissions, expense, and decreased effect with continued use.
  2. Calcipotriene (Dovonex): effective for moderate plaque psoriasis; adults should comb the hair, apply solution to the lesions, and rub it in, avoiding uninvolved skin; disadvantages are its cost and potential burning and skin irritation.
  3. Tar products (Estar, LCD, psori-Gel) can be used overnight and are most effective when combined with UVB light (Goeckerman regimen).
  4. Anthralin (Drithocreme): useful for chronic plaques, can result in purple/brown staining; best used with UVB light.
  5. Other useful measures include tape or occlusive dressing, UVB and lubricating agents, interlesional steroids.
- Therapeutic options for persons with generalized disease (affecting >20% of the body):
  1. UVB light exposure three times a week.
  2. PUVA (psoralen plus ultraviolet A) is effective for generalized disease. However, many treatments are required, necessitating frequent office visits, and it may be associated with increased risk of skin cancer.
- Systemic treatments include methotrexate 25 mg every week for severe psoriasis. Etretinate (Tegison) (a synthetic retinoid) is most effective for palmar-plantar pustular psoriasis. Dose is 0.5 to 1 mg/kg/day. It can cause liver enzyme and lipid abnormalities and is teratogenic.
- Cyclosporine is also affective in severe psoriasis; however, relapses are common.

CHRONIC Rx
See "Acute General Rx."

DISPOSITION
The course of psoriasis is chronic, and the disease may be refractory to treatment.

REFERRAL
- Dermatology referral is recommended in all patients with generalized disease.
- Hospital admission may be necessary for severe diffuse or poorly responsive psoriasis. The Goeckerman regimen combines daily application of tar with UVB exposure and can result in prolonged remissions.

MISCELLANEOUS

COMMENTS
Psoriasis is more emotionally than physically disabling for most patients. Counseling may be indicated, particularly when it affects younger patients.

REFERENCES
Habif TP: *Clinical dermatology,* ed 3, St Louis, 1996, Mosby.
Highton A et al: Calcipotriene ointment for psoriasis: a safety and efficacy study, *J Am Acad Dermatol* 32:67, 1995.

Author: **Fred F. Ferri, M.D.**

Pulmonary edema

BASIC INFORMATION

DEFINITION
Cardiogenic pulmonary edema is a life-threatening condition caused by severe left ventricular decompensation.

SYNONYMS
Cardiogenic pulmonary edema

ICD-9-CM CODES
428.1 Acute pulmonary edema with heart disease

PHYSICAL FINDINGS
- Dyspnea with rapid, shallow breathing
- Diaphoresis, perioral and peripheral cyanosis
- Pink, frothy sputum
- Moist, bilateral pulmonary rales
- Increased pulmonary second sound, S_3 gallop (in association with tachycardia)
- Bulging neck veins

ETIOLOGY
Increased pulmonary capillary pressure secondary to:
- Acute myocardial infarction
- Exacerbation of CHF
- Valvular regurgitation
- Ventricular septal defect
- Severe ischemia
- Mitral stenosis
- Other: cardiac tamponade, endocarditis, myocarditis, arrhythmias, cardiomyopathy

DIAGNOSIS

DIFFERENTIAL DIAGNOSIS
- Noncardiogenic pulmonary edema
- Pulmonary embolism
- Exacerbation of asthma
- Exacerbation of COPD
- Sarcoidosis
- Pulmonary fibrosis
- Viral pneumonitis and other pulmonary infections

LABORATORY TESTS
ABGs: respiratory and metabolic acidosis, decreased Pa_{O_2}, increased Pc_{O_2}, low pH. NOTE: The patient may initially show respiratory alkalosis secondary to hyperventilation in attempts to maintain Pa_{O_2}.

IMAGING STUDIES
- Chest x-ray examination:
  1. Pulmonary congestion with Kerley B lines; fluffy perihilar infiltrates in the early stages; bilateral interstitial alveolar infiltrates
  2. Pleural effusions
- Echocardiogram:
  1. Useful to evaluate valvular abnormalities, diastolic vs. systolic dysfunction
  2. Can aid in differentiation of cardiogenic vs. noncardiogenic pulmonary edema
  3. Can also estimate pulmonary capillary wedge pressure and rule out presence of myxoma or atrial thrombus
- Right heart catheterization (selected patients): cardiac pressures and cardiogenic pulmonary edema reveal increased PADP and PCWP ≥25 mm Hg)

TREATMENT

NONPHARMACOLOGIC THERAPY
Patients should be placed in a sitting position with legs off the side of the bed to improve breathing and decrease venous return.

ACUTE GENERAL Rx
All the following steps can be performed concomitantly:
- 100% oxygen by face mask: check ABGs; if marked hypoxemia or severe respiratory acidosis, intubate the patient and place on a ventilator. Positive end expiratory pressure (PEEP) increases functional capacity and improves oxygenation.
- Furosemide 40 to 100 mg IV bolus to rapidly establish diuresis and decrease venous return through its venodilator action; may double the dose in 30 min if no effect.
- Vasodilator therapy:
  1. Nitrates: particularly useful if the patient has concomitant chest pain.
     a. Nitroglycerin: 150 to 600 µg sublingual PRN may be given immediately on arrival.
     b. 2% nitroglycerin ointment: 1 to 3 inches out of the tube applied continuously; absorption may be erratic.
     c. IV nitroglycerin: 100 mg in 500 ml of D_5W solution; start at 6 µg/min (2 ml/hr).
  2. Nitroprusside: useful for afterload reduction in hypertensive patients with decreased cardiac index (CI).
     a. Increases the CI and decreases left ventricular filling pressure.
     b. Vasodilator and diuretic therapy should be tailored to achieve PCWP ≤18 mm Hg, RAP ≤8 mm Hg, systolic blood pressure >90 mm Hg, SVR >1200 Dynes/sec cm^5. The use of nitroprusside in patients with acute MI is controversial because it may intensify ischemia by decreasing the blood flow to the ischemic left ventricular myocardium.
- Morphine: 3 to 10 mg IV/SC/IM initially. May repeat q15min PRN. It decreases venous return, anxiety and systemic vascular resistance (Naloxone should be available at bedside to reverse the effects of morphine if respiratory depression occurs). Morphine may induce hypotension in volume depleted patients.
- Dobutamine: parenteral inotropic agent of choice in severe cases of cardiogenic pulmonary edema. It can be administered at a dosage of 2.5 to 10 µg/kg/min IV. IV phosphodiesterase inhibitors (amrinone, milrinone) may be useful in refractory cases.
- After load reduction with ACE inhibitors (e.g., IV enalaprilat 1 mg given over 2 hr) in patients that are not hypotensive is also useful in the treatment of cardiogenic pulmonary edema.
- Aminophylline: useful only if patient has concomitant severe bronchospasm.
- Digitalis: limited use in acute pulmonary edema caused by MI, but it is useful in pulmonary edema resulting from atrial fibrillation or flutter with a fast ventricular response.
- Acute cardiogenic pulmonary edema caused by IHSS must be treated with IV normal saline solution and negative inotropic agents such as verapamil and β-blockers.

DISPOSITION
Mortality for cardiogenic pulmonary edema is approximately 60% to 80%.

MISCELLANEOUS

REFERENCES
Annane D et al: Placebo-controlled randomized, double-blind study of IV enalaprilat efficacy and safety in acute cardiogenic pulmonary edema, *Circulation* 94:1316, 1996.

Groppa MB et al: Acute cardiogenic pulmonary edema, *Clin Chest Med* 15:501, 1994.

Author: **Fred F. Ferri, M.D.**

CLINICAL TOPICS   Pulmonary embolism   399

BASIC INFORMATION

DEFINITION
Pulmonary embolism (PE) refers to the lodging of a thrombus or other embolic material from a distant site in the pulmonary circulation.

SYNONYMS
Pulmonary thromboembolism
PE

ICD-9-CM CODES
415.1 Pulmonary embolism and infarction

EPIDEMIOLOGY AND DEMOGRAPHICS
- 650,000 cases of PE occur each year; 50,000 result in death (increased incidence in women and with advanced age).
- More than 90% of pulmonary emboli originate in the deep venous system of the lower extremities.
- Pulmonary thromboembolism is associated with >200,000 hospitalizations each year in the U.S.
- 8% to 10% of victims of PE die within the first hour.

PHYSICAL FINDINGS
- Most common symptom: dyspnea
- Chest pain: may be nonpleuritic or pleuritic (infarction)
- Syncope (massive PE)
- Fever, diaphoresis, apprehension
- Hemoptysis, cough
- Evidence of DVT may be present (e.g., swelling and tenderness of extremities)
- Cardiac examination: may reveal tachycardia, increased pulmonic component of S_2, murmur of tricuspid insufficiency, right ventricular heave, right-sided S_3
- Pulmonary examination: may demonstrate rales, localized wheezing, friction rub
- Most common physical finding: tachypnea

ETIOLOGY
- Thrombus, fat, or other foreign material
- Risk factors for PE:
  1. Prolonged immobilization
  2. Postoperative state
  3. Trauma to lower extremities
  4. Estrogen-containing birth control pills
  5. Prior history of DVT or PE
  6. CHF
  7. Pregnancy and early puerperium
  8. Visceral cancer (lung, pancreas, alimentary and genitourinary tracts)
  9. Trauma, burns
  10. Advanced age
  11. Obesity
  12. Hematologic disease (e.g., antithrombin III deficiency, protein C deficiency, protein S deficiency, lupus anticoagulant, polycythemia vera, dysfibrinogenemia, paroxysmal nocturnal hemoglobinuria, factor V Leiden mutation)
  13. COPD, diabetes mellitus

DIAGNOSIS

DIFFERENTIAL DIAGNOSIS
- Myocardial infarction
- Pericarditis
- Pneumonia
- Pneumothorax
- Chest wall pain
- GI abnormalities (e.g., peptic ulcer, esophageal rupture, gastritis)
- CHF
- Pleuritis
- Anxiety disorder with hyperventilation
- Pericardial tamponade

WORKUP
- Lung scan or pulmonary angiogram will confirm the diagnosis.
- Compressive duplex ultrasonography of lower extremities may be useful in patients with "low-probability" lung scan and high clinical suspicion (see "Imaging Studies").

LABORATORY TESTS
- ABGs generally reveal decreased Pa_{O_2} and Pa_{CO_2} and increased pH; normal results do not rule out PE.
- Alveolar-arteriolar (A-a) oxygen gradient, a measure of the difference in oxygen concentration between alveoli and arterial blood, is a more sensitive indicator of the alteration in oxygenation than Pa_{O_2}; it can easily be calculated using the information from ABGs (see Box A-14 in Appendix); a normal A-a gradient among patients without history of PE or DVT makes the diagnosis of PE unlikely.

IMAGING STUDIES
- Chest x-ray film may be normal; suggestive findings include elevated diaphragm, pleural effusion, dilation of pulmonary artery, infiltrate or consolidation, abrupt vessel cut-off or atelectasis. A wedge-shaped consolidation in the middle and lower lobes is suggestive of a pulmonary infarction and is known as "Hampton's hump."
- Lung scan and arteriography:
  1. A normal lung scan rules out PE.
  2. A ventilation perfusion mismatch is suggestive of PE, and a lung scan interpretation of high probability is confirmatory.
  3. If the clinical suspicion of PE is high and the lung scan is interpreted as low probability, moderate probability or indeterminate, a pulmonary arteriogram is indi-

400 Pulmonary embolism

cated; a positive arteriogram confirms diagnosis; a positive compressive duplex ultrasonography for DVT obviates the need for an arteriogram, since treatment with IV anticoagulants is indicated in these patients; the overall sensitivity of compressive ultrasonography for DVT in patients with PE is 29%, specificity 97%; adding ultrasonography in patients with a nondiagnostic lung scan prevents 9% of angiographies; however, this improvement in efficacy is achieved at the cost of unnecessary anticoagulant therapy in 26% of patients who have false-positive ultrasonography results.
4. The term *low probability lung scan* is misleading and should be changed to *nondiagnostic lung scan* in patients with inadequate cardiorespiratory reserve (i.e., pulmonary edema, right ventricular failure, hypotension, syncope, acute tachyarrhythmia, abnormal spirometry [FEV_1 sec <1 or VC < 1.5 L] or abnormal arterial blood gases [Po_2 <50 mm Hg or Pco_2 >45 mm Hg]), since mortality rate directly attributed to PE is high (>7%) despite erroneous low probability result on lung scan in these patients.

- Gadolinium-enhanced magnetic resonance angiography of the pulmonary arteries has a high sensitivity and specificity for the diagnosis of PE; this new technique shows promise as a noninvasive method of diagnosing PE without the need for ionizing radiation or iodinated contrast material.
- ECG: frequent abnormalities are sinus tachycardia, S-I, Q-III T-III pattern, S-I, S-II, S-III pattern, T wave inversion in V_1 to V_6, acute RBBB, new onset A-fibrillation, ST segment depression in lead II, right ventricular strain.

TREATMENT

NONPHARMACOLOGIC THERAPY
Correction of risk factors (see "Etiology") to prevent future PE

ACUTE GENERAL Rx
- Heparin by continuous infusion for at least 5 days; many experts recommend a larger initial IV heparin bolus (15,000 to 20,000 U) to block platelet aggregation and thrombi and subsequent release of vasoconstrictive substances.
- Thrombolytic agents (urokinase, tPA, streptokinase): provide rapid resolution of clots; thrombolytic agents are the treatment of choice in patients with massive PE who are hemodynamically unstable and with no contraindication to their use; patients with right ventricular wall motion abnormalities on echocardiography may also be candidates for thrombolytic therapy.
- Long-term treatment is generally carried out with warfarin therapy started on day 1 or 2 and given in a dose to maintain the INR at 2 to 3.
- If thrombolytics and anticoagulants are contraindicated (e.g., GI bleeding, recent CNS surgery, recent trauma) or if the patient continues to have recurrent PE despite anticoagulation therapy, vena caval interruption is indicated by transvenous placement of a Greenfield vena caval filter.
- Acute pulmonary artery embolectomy may be indicated in a patient with massive pulmonary emboli and refractory hypotension.

CHRONIC Rx
Elimination of risk factors (see "Etiology") and monitoring of warfarin dose with INR on a routine basis

DISPOSITION
- Mortality can be reduced to <10% by rapid and effective treatment.
- Mortality from recurrent pulmonary emboli is 8% with effective treatment and >30% in patients with untreated pulmonary emboli.

REFERRAL
Acute pulmonary embolectomy in selected patients (see "Acute General Rx")

MISCELLANEOUS

COMMENTS
- The duration of oral anticoagulant treatment is 6 mo in patients with reversible risk factors and indefinitely in patients with persistence of risk factors that caused the initial PE.
- Patients should be educated about the need for compliance with long-term anticoagulation therapy.

REFERENCES
Becker RC, Ansell J: Antithrombotic therapy: an abbreviated reference for clinicians, *Arch Intern Med* 155:149, 1995.

Goldhaber SV: Pulmonary embolism: epidemiology, pathophysiology, diagnosis, and management, *Chest* 107:1S, 1995.

Hull D et al: The low probability lung scan: a need to change nomenclature, *Arch Intern Med* 155:1845, 1995.

Meaney J et al: Diagnosis of pulmonary embolism with magnetic resonance angiography, *N Engl J Med* 336:1422, 1997.

Turkstra F et al: Diagnostic utility of ultrasonography of leg veins in patients suspected of having PE, *Ann Intern Med* 126:775, 1997.

Author: **Fred F. Ferri, M.D.**

Pyelonephritis (PTG)

BASIC INFORMATION

DEFINITION
Pyelonephritis is an infection, usually bacterial in origin, of the upper urinary tract.

SYNONYMS
Acute pyelonephritis
Pyonephrosis
Renal carbuncle
Lobar nephronia
Acute bacterial nephritis

ICD-9-CM CODES
590.81 Pyelonephritis
599.0 Urinary tract infection
595.9 Cystitis

EPIDEMIOLOGY AND DEMOGRAPHICS
INCIDENCE (IN U.S.): Extremely common
PREDOMINANT SEX: Female
PREDOMINANT AGE:
- Sexually active years in women
- Usually >50 yr of age in men

PEAK INCIDENCE: See above.
GENETICS:
Congenital Infection: Congenital urologic structural disorders may predispose to infections at an early age.

PHYSICAL FINDINGS
- Fever
- Rigors
- Chills
- Flank pain
- Dysuria
- Polyuria
- Hematuria
- Toxic feeling and appearance
- Nausea and vomiting
- Headache
- Diarrhea
- Physical examination notable
  1. Costovertebral angle tenderness
  2. Exquisite flank pain

ETIOLOGY
- Gram-negative bacilli such as *E. coli* and *Klebsiella* species in more than 95% of cases
- Other more unusual gram-negative organisms, especially if instrumentation of the urinary system has occurred
- Resistant gram-negative organisms or even fungi in hospitalized patients with indwelling catheters
- Gram-positive organisms such as enterococci
- *Staphylococcus aureus:* presence in urine indicates hematogenous origin
- Viruses: rarely, but these are usually limited to the lower tract

DIAGNOSIS

DIFFERENTIAL DIAGNOSIS
- Nephrolithiasis
- Appendicitis
- Ovarian cyst torsion or rupture
- Acute glomerulonephritis
- PID
- Endometritis
- Other causes of acute abdomen
- Perinephric abscess
- Hydronephrosis

WORKUP
- No workup in sexually active women
- Poorly responding infections, especially with azotemia and frank bacteremia
  1. Renal sonogram
  2. IVP
  3. To assess for underlying urologic pathology such as hydronephrosis
- Urologic imaging studies in all young men and boys
- Prostate assessment in older men

LABORATORY TESTS
- CBC with differential
- Renal panel
- Blood cultures
- Urine cultures
- Urinalysis
- Gram stain of urine
- Urgent renal sonography if obstruction or closed space infection suspected

TREATMENT

ACUTE GENERAL Rx
- Hospitalization for:
  1. Toxic patients
  2. Complicated infections
  3. Diabetes
  4. Suspected bacteremia
- Keep patients well hydrated.
- IV fluids are indicated for those unable to take adequate amounts of liquids.
- Give antipyretics such as acetaminophen when necessary.
- Antibiotic therapy should be initiated after cultures are obtained.
  1. Oral trimethoprim-sulfa DS (bid for 10 days) or ciprofloxacin (500 mg orally bid for 10 days): adequate for stable patients who can tolerate oral medications
  2. Trimethoprim-sulfa or ciprofloxacin IV for more toxic patients
  3. Ceftazidime 1 g IV q6-8h
  4. Aminoglycosides such as gentamicin (2 mg/kg IV load followed by 1 mg/kg IV q8h adjusted for renal function) added but nephrotoxic especially in diabetics with azotemia
  5. Vancomycin 1 g IV q12h to cover gram-positive cocci such as enterococci or staphylococcus
  6. Ampicillin 1 to 2 g IV q4-6h to cover enterococci, but an aminoglycoside is needed for synergy
  7. Oral ampicillin or amoxicillin: no longer adequate for therapy of gram-negative infections because of resistance
- Prompt drainage with nephrostomy tube placement for obstruction
- Surgical drainage of large collections of pus to control infection
- Diabetic patients, as well as those with indwelling catheters, are especially prone to complicated infections and abscess formation.

CHRONIC Rx
- Repair underlying structural problems, especially when renal function is compromised.
  1. Reflux
  2. Obstruction
  3. Nephrolithiasis should be considered
- Patients with diabetes mellitus and indwelling urinary catheters are at particular risk of severe and complicated infections.
- When possible, remove catheters.

REFERRAL
- To surgeon: surgical correction of underlying urologic problems, such as reflux and hydronephrosis
- To pediatrician: in young children, prompt correction of reflux to avoid recurrent infections as well as loss of renal function
- To internist: aggressive metabolic as well as urologic evaluation and treatment for patients with nephrolithiasis

MISCELLANEOUS

REFERENCES
Sobel JD, Kaye D: Urinary tract infections. In Mandell GL, Dolin R, Bennett JE (eds): *Principles and practices of infectious diseases,* ed 4, New York, 1995, Churchill Livingstone.

Author: **Joseph J. Lieber, M.D.**

Rabies

BASIC INFORMATION

DEFINITION
Rabies is a fatal illness caused by the rabies virus and transmitted to humans by the bite of an infected animal.

SYNONYMS
Hydrophobia

ICD-9-CM CODES
071 Rabies

EPIDEMIOLOGY AND DEMOGRAPHICS
INCIDENCE (IN U.S.): Approximately 2 cases/yr
PREDOMINANT SEX: Men (70% of cases)
PREDOMINANT AGE: <16 yr and >55 yr

PHYSICAL FINDINGS
- Incubation period of 10 to 90 days
  1. Shorter with bites of the face
  2. Longer if extremities involved
- Prodrome
  1. Fever
  2. Headache
  3. Malaise
  4. Pain or anesthesia at exposure site
  5. Sore throat
  6. GI symptoms
  7. Psychiatric symptoms
- Acute neurologic period, with objective evidence of CNS involvement
  1. Extreme hyperactivity and bizarre behavior alternating with periods of relative calm
  2. Hallucinations
  3. Disorientation
  4. Seizures
  5. Paralysis may occur
  6. Spasm of the pharynx and larynx, accompanied by severe pain, caused by drinking
  7. Fear elicited by seeing water
  8. Paralysis
  9. Coma
- Possible death from respiratory arrest

ETIOLOGY
- Rabies virus
- Cases in U.S. are associated with:
  1. Bats
  2. Raccoons
  3. Foxes
  4. Skunks
- Imported cases are usually associated with dogs.
- Unusual acquisition:
  1. Via corneal transplantation
  2. Via aerosol transmission in laboratory workers and spelunkers

DIAGNOSIS

DIFFERENTIAL DIAGNOSIS
- Delirium tremens
- Tetanus
- Hysteria
- Psychiatric disorders
- Other viral encephalitides
- Guillain-Barré syndrome
- Poliomyelitis

WORKUP
- Rabies antibody
  1. Serum
  2. CSF
- Viral isolation
  1. Saliva
  2. CSF
  3. Serum
- Rabies fluorescent antibody: skin biopsy from the hair-covered area of the neck
- Characteristic eosinophilic inclusions (Negri bodies) in infected neurons

LABORATORY TESTS
See "Workup."

TREATMENT

NONPHARMACOLOGIC THERAPY
- Isolation of the patient to prevent transmission to others
- Supportive therapy (although this has not been shown to change outcome except in three cases in which the patients had received prophylaxis before onset of symptoms)

ACUTE GENERAL Rx
- No beneficial therapy
- Emphasis placed on prophylaxis of potentially exposed individuals as soon as possible following an exposure:
  1. Thorough wound cleansing
  2. Both active and passive immunization is most effective when used within 72 hr of exposure
- Vaccinations:
  1. Human diploid cell vaccine (HDCV) or rhesus monkey diploid cell vaccine (RVA), 1 ml IM (deltoid) on days 0, 3, 7, 14, and 28
  2. Human rabies hyperimmune globulin, 20 IU/kg, half the dose infiltrated around the wound, the rest given as an IM injection in the gluteal area
- Preexposure prophylaxis using HDCV or RVA (1 ml IM days 0, 7, and 21 or 28) in individuals at high risk for acquisition:
  1. Veterinarians
  2. Laboratory workers working with rabies virus
  3. Spelunkers
  4. Visitors to endemic areas

DISPOSITION
Virtually always fatal

REFERRAL
- To infectious disease consultant
- To local health authorities

MISCELLANEOUS

COMMENTS
- Most cases in U.S. are caused by:
  1. Wild animal bites (bats)
  2. Dog bites occurring outside U.S.
  3. Some unknown exposure
- Rare cases can be transmitted by mucous membrane contact of aerosolized virus.
- Box A-15 describes bite wound guidelines.

REFERENCES
Sang E et al: Antemortem diagnosis of human rabies, *J Fam Pract* 43:83, 1996.

Author: **Maurice Policar, M.D.**

Ramsay Hunt syndrome

BASIC INFORMATION

DEFINITION
Ramsay Hunt syndrome is a localized herpes zoster infection involving the seventh nerve and geniculate ganglia, resulting in hearing loss, vertigo, and facial nerve palsy.

SYNONYMS
Herpes zoster oticus
Geniculate herpes
Herpetic geniculate ganglionitis

ICD-9-CM CODES
053.11 Ramsay Hunt syndrome

EPIDEMIOLOGY AND DEMOGRAPHICS
PREDOMINANT SEX: Equal sex distribution
PREDOMINANT AGE:
- Increasingly common with advancing age
- Rare in childhood

PHYSICAL FINDINGS
- Characteristic vesicles:
  1. On pinna
  2. In external auditory canal
  3. In distribution of the facial nerve and, occasionally, adjacent cranial nerves
- Facial paralysis on the involved side

ETIOLOGY
Reactivation of dormant infection with varicella zoster virus following primary varicella (usually in childhood)

DIAGNOSIS

- Usually made by recognition of the clinical features detailed above
- Viral culture and/or microscopic examination of specimens taken from active vesicles

DIFFERENTIAL DIAGNOSIS
- Herpes simplex
- External otitis
- Impetigo
- Enteroviral infection
- Bell's palsy of other etiologies
- Acoustic neuroma (before appearance of skin lesions)
- The differential diagnosis of headache and facial pain is described in Box 2-52.

WORKUP
If the diagnosis is in doubt, confirmation of varicella zoster virus infection should be sought.

LABORATORY TESTS
- Viral culture of specimens of vesicular fluid and scrapings of the vesicle base
- Tzanck preparation, which may reveal multinucleated giant cells
- Direct immunofluorescent staining of scrapings

IMAGING STUDIES
MRI may demonstrate enhancement of the facial and vestibulocochlear nerves before appearance of vesicles.

TREATMENT

ACUTE GENERAL Rx
- Prednisone (40 mg PO for 2 days; 30 mg for 7 days; followed by tapering course) is recommended by some authors.
- Acyclovir (800 mg PO five times qd for 10 days) may hasten healing.
- Analgesics should be used as indicated.

CHRONIC Rx
- Amitriptyline is effective in some cases of postherpetic pain.
- Narcotic analgesics may occasionally be necessary.

DISPOSITION
Recurrences are unusual.

REFERRAL
To otolaryngologist: patients with persistent facial paralysis for potential surgical decompression of the facial nerve

MISCELLANEOUS

COMMENTS
Immunodeficiency states, particularly infection with the human immunodeficiency virus (HIV) should be considered in:
- Younger patients
- Severe cases
- Patients with a history of specific risk behavior

REFERENCES
Kuo MJ et al: Early diagnosis and treatment of Ramsay Hunt syndrome: the role of magnetic resonance imaging, *J Laryngol Otol* 109(8):777, 1995.

Author: **Joseph R. Masci, M.D.**

Raynaud's phenomenon (PTG)

BASIC INFORMATION

DEFINITION
Raynaud's phenomenon is a vasospastic disorder usually affecting the digital arteries precipitated by exposure to cold temperatures or emotional distress and manifesting in a triphasic discoloration of the fingers or toes.

SYNONYMS
Primary Raynaud's phenomenon or Raynaud's disease
Secondary Raynaud's phenomenon

ICD-9-CM CODES
443.0 Raynaud's syndrome, Raynaud's disease, Raynaud's phenomenon (secondary)
785.4 If gangrene present

EPIDEMIOLOGY AND DEMOGRAPHICS
- Raynaud's phenomenon (either primary [idiopathic] or secondary [see "Etiology"]) is found in 5% to 20% of the population.
- Primary Raynaud's phenomenon is more common than secondary Raynaud's and usually occurs in women more often than men (4:1) and in the young (<40 yr of age) compared with the old.
- Between 5% to 15% of patients thought to have primary Raynaud's will develop a secondary cause (commonly scleroderma or CREST syndrome).

PHYSICAL FINDINGS
- The classic manifestation is the triphasic color response to cold exposure:
  1. Pallor of the digit resulting from vasospasm.
  2. Blue discoloration (cyanosis) secondary to desaturated venous blood.
  3. Red (rubor) along with pain and paresthesia when vasospasm resolves and blood returns to the digit.
- Color changes are well delineated, symmetrical, and usually bilateral.
- Fingertips are most often involved, but feet, ears, and nose can be affected.
- Ulcerations and rarely gangrene may occur.
- Secondary Raynaud's phenomenon may be associated with typical findings of the underlying disease (e.g., sclerodactyly and telangiectasia in CREST syndrome).

ETIOLOGY
- Primary Raynaud's phenomenon is generally referred to as *Raynaud's disease* when no cause can be found.
- Secondary Raynaud's phenomenon has many causes:
  1. CREST syndrome (calcinosis, Raynaud's phenomenon, esophageal dysmotility, sclerodactyly, and telangiectasia)
  2. Scleroderma
  3. Mixed connective tissue disease, polymyositis, and dermatomyositis
  4. SLE
  5. Rheumatoid arthritis
  6. Thromboangiitis obliterans (Buerger's disease)
  7. Drug induced (β-blockers, ergotamine, methysergide, vinblastine, bleomycin, oral contraceptives)
  8. Polycythemia, cryoglobulinemia, and certain vasculitides
  9. Carpal tunnel syndrome
  10. Tools causing vibration

DIAGNOSIS

- The diagnosis of Raynaud's phenomenon can be made by a history of well demarcated digit discoloration induced by cold exposure and a physical examination looking for possible secondary causes.
- The digit triphasic color changes can sometimes be induced in the office by placing the hand in an ice bath.
- Color photos and questionnaires may be useful in assisting in the diagnosis (see "References" below).

DIFFERENTIAL DIAGNOSIS
See "Etiology."

WORKUP
- Once the diagnosis of Raynaud's phenomenon is established, differentiating primary from secondary is helpful in treatment and prognosis. History and physical examination usually make this distinction, whereas certain laboratory studies may predict secondary causes (see "Laboratory Tests").
- A test available but not commonly used is the nailfold microscopy; if positive, may be associated with certain collagen-vascular diseases.

LABORATORY TESTS
- CBC, electrolytes, BUN, Cr, ESR, ANA, urinalysis should be included in the initial evaluation.
- If the history, physical examination, and initial laboratory tests suggest a possible secondary cause, specific serologic testing (e.g., anticentromere antibodies, anti-Scl 70, cryoglobulins, complement testing, and protein electrophoresis) may be indicated.

IMAGING STUDIES

- Chest x-ray examination may be helpful if a secondary cause, such as scleroderma, is suggested.
- Barium swallow may be helpful if CREST syndrome is suspected.
- Angiography is rarely needed for Raynaud's phenomenon but may be helpful in diagnosing Buerger's disease as a possible etiology.

TREATMENT

NONPHARMACOLOGIC THERAPY

- Avoid medications that may precipitate Raynaud's phenomenon (see "Etiology").
- Avoid cold exposure. Use warm gloves, hats, and garments during the winter months or before going into cold environments (e.g., air conditioned rooms).
- Avoid stressful situations.
- Avoid nicotine, caffeine, and over-the-counter decongestants.

ACUTE GENERAL Rx

- Typically, patients with Raynaud's phenomenon respond well to nonpharmacologic measures.
- Medications should be used if the above mentioned treatment does not work.
- Goal is to prevent digital ulcers and gangrene.
- Medications commonly used are described in "Chronic Rx."

CHRONIC Rx

- Calcium channel blockers are the most effective treatment for Raynaud's phenomenon.
  1. Nifedipine is most often prescribed at a dose of 10 to 20 mg 30 min before going outside. If symptoms occur with long duration, nifedipine XL 30 mg to 90 mg PO qd is effective.
  2. If side effects occur with nifedipine, other calcium-blockers can be used (e.g., diltiazem 30 mg qid and gradually increased to a maximum dose of 120 mg qid). Felodipine 2.5 mg qd up to 10 mg qd can also be used.
  3. Verapamil has not been shown to be effective with Raynaud's phenomenon.
- Prazosin 1 mg bid up to 4 mg bid has been effective with Raynaud's phenomenon.
- Reserpine and guanethidine, although effective, have a high side effect profile.
- Other agents that have been tried with limited results include aspirin, pentoxifylline, captopril, and topical nitrates.
- IV prostaglandins, although not available in the U.S., may be promising in severe secondary Raynaud's phenomenon.

DISPOSITION

The prognosis of patients with Raynaud's phenomenon depends on the etiology.

- Primary Raynaud's phenomenon is fairly benign, usually remaining stable and controlled with nonpharmacologic medical treatment.
- Patients with secondary Raynaud's phenomenon, specifically those with scleroderma, CREST syndrome, and thromboangiitis obliterans, may develop severe ischemic digits with ulceration, gangrene, and autoamputation.

REFERRAL

- Rheumatology consult is indicated if secondary collagen-vascular disease is diagnosed.
- Vascular surgery consult is indicated if ulcers, gangrene, or threatened digit loss is noted.

MISCELLANEOUS

COMMENTS

Most patients with Raynaud's phenomenon can be managed by the primary care provider; however, it is important to differentiate primary from secondary forms. Secondary forms may become manifest as far out as 10 yr from the diagnosis of Raynaud's phenomenon. Periodic follow-up visits and reassessment to exclude secondary forms is important toward future treatment options and outcome.

REFERENCES

Adee AC: Managing Raynaud's phenomenon: a practical approach, *Am Fam Physician* 47(4):823, 1993.

Bacharach JM, Olin JW: Raynaud's phenomenon, *Heart Dis Stroke* 3:255, 1994.

Bolster MB, Maricq HR, Lee RL: Office evaluation and treatment of Raynaud's phenomenon, *Cleve Clin J Med* 62(1):51, 1995.

Wigley FM: Raynaud's phenomenon, *Rheum Dis Clin North Am* 22(4):765, 1996.

Author: **Peter Petropoulos, M.D.**

Reiter's syndrome (PTG)

BASIC INFORMATION

DEFINITION
Reiter's syndrome is one of the seronegative spondyloarthropathies, so called because serum rheumatoid factor is not present in these forms of inflammatory arthritis. Reiter's syndrome is an asymmetric polyarthritis that affects mainly the lower extremities and is associated with one or more of the following:
- Urethritis
- Cervicitis
- Dysentery
- Inflammatory eye disease
- Mucocutaneous lesions

SYNONYMS
Reiter's disease
Reactive arthritis
Seronegative spondyloarthropathy

ICD-9-CM CODES
099.3 Reiter's syndrome

EPIDEMIOLOGY AND DEMOGRAPHICS
INCIDENCE (IN U.S.): 0.0035% annually of men <50 yr
PREDOMINANT SEX: Male
PREDOMINANT AGE: 20 to 40 yr
PEAK INCIDENCE: Most common in the third decade
GENETICS:
Familial Disposition: Strongly associated with HLA-B27 (63% to 96%)

PHYSICAL FINDINGS
- Polyarthritis
  1. Affecting the knee and ankle
  2. Commonly asymmetric
- Heel pain and Achilles tendinitis, especially at the insertion of the Achilles tendon
- Plantar fasciitis
- Large effusions
- Dactylitis or "sausage toe"
- Urethritis
- Uveitis or conjunctivitis; uveitis can progress to blindness without treatment
- Keratoderma blennorrhagica
  1. Hyperkeratotic lesions on soles of the feet, toes, penis, hands
  2. Closely resembles psoriasis
- Aortic regurgitation similar to that seen in ankylosing spondylitis

ETIOLOGY
- Epidemic Reiter's syndrome following outbreaks of dysentery has been well described.
- Genetically susceptible, HLA-B27 positive individuals are at risk for developing Reiter's syndrome following infection with certain pathogens:
  1. Salmonella
  2. Shigella
  3. *Yersinia enterocolitica*
  4. *Chlamydia trachomatis*
  5. Molecular mimicry mechanism suspected
- Symptom complex indistinguishable from Reiter's syndrome has been described in association with HIV infection.

DIAGNOSIS

DIFFERENTIAL DIAGNOSIS
- Ankylosing spondylitis
- Psoriatic arthritis
- Rheumatoid arthritis
- Gonococcal arthritis-tenosynovitis
- Rheumatic fever

WORKUP
- X-ray examination of affected joints
- Synovial fluid examination and culture
- Careful examination of eyes and skin
- Cultures for gonococcus (urethral, cervical, stool)

LABORATORY TESTS
- Elevated but nonspecific ESR
- No specific laboratory tests to diagnose Reiter's syndrome

IMAGING STUDIES
Plain radiographs:
- Juxtaarticular osteopenia of affected joints
- Erosions and joint space narrowing in more advanced disease
- Periostitis and reactive new bone formation at the insertions of the Achilles tendon and the plantar fascia
- Sacroiliitis:
  1. Unilateral or bilateral
  2. Indistinguishable from ankylosing spondylitis
- Vertebral bridging osteophytes

TREATMENT

NONPHARMACOLOGIC THERAPY
Physical therapy to maintain range of motion of the back and other joints

ACUTE GENERAL Rx
- Flares treated NSAIDs such as indomethacin (25 to 50 mg orally, three times qd)
- Enteric or urethral infection should be treated with appropriate antibiotic coverage.
- Uveitis should be treated with steroid eye drops in consultation with an ophthalmologist.
- Achilles tendinitis and plantar fasciitis should be treated with injections of methylprednisolone (40 to 80 mg).
- Sulfasalazine (2 to 3 g orally, twice qd) may be effective.
- Careful monitoring for the following is essential:
  1. GI toxicity
  2. Hypersensitivity
  3. Bone marrow suppression
- Persistent and uncontrolled disease should be managed with cytotoxic drugs (methotrexate, azathioprine) in consultation with a rheumatologist

CHRONIC Rx
Chronic disease is best managed by a team approach with the collaboration of a rheumatologist or other experienced physician and physical therapist.

DISPOSITION
- Recurrences are frequent, even with treatment.
- Long-term sequelae:
  1. Persistent polyarthritis
  2. Chronic back pain
  3. Heel pain
  4. Progressive iridocyclitis
  5. Aortic regurgitation

REFERRAL
- To ophthalmologist if uveitis is suspected
- To rheumatologist if arthritis and tendinitis fail to improve rapidly after a course of NSAIDs

MISCELLANEOUS

COMMENTS
- Infection with HIV is associated with particularly severe cases of Reiter's syndrome.
- HIV testing is recommended, especially if risk factors such as unprotected sexual activity or IV drug use are identified.

REFERENCES
Hughes RA, Keat AL: Reiter's syndrome and reactive arthritis: a current view, *Semin Arthritis Rheum* 24(3):190, 1994.
Lin WY, Wang SJ, Jan JL: Evaluation of arthritis in Reiter's disease by bone scintigraphy and radiography, *Clin Rheumatol* 14(4):441, 1995.
Author: **Deborah L. Shapiro, M.D.**

Renal failure, acute (PTG)

BASIC INFORMATION

DEFINITION
Acute renal failure (ARF) is the rapid impairment in renal function resulting in retention of products in the blood that are normally excreted by the kidneys.

SYNONYMS
ARF

ICD-9-CM CODES
584.9 Acute renal failure, unspecified

EPIDEMIOLOGY AND DEMOGRAPHICS
- ARF requiring dialysis develops in 5/100,000 persons annually.
- >10% of ICU patients develop ARF.
- >40% of hospital ARF is iatrogenic.

PHYSICAL FINDINGS
- Peripheral edema
- Skin pallor, ecchymoses
- Oliguria (however, patients can have nonoliguric renal failure)
- Delirium, lethargy, myoclonus, seizures
- Back pain, fasciculations, muscle cramps
- Tachypnea, tachycardia
- Weakness, anorexia, generalized malaise, nausea

ETIOLOGY
- Prerenal: inadequate perfusion caused by hypovolemia, CHF, cirrhosis, sepsis
- Postrenal: outlet obstruction from prostatic enlargement, ureteral obstruction (stones), bilateral renal vein occlusion
- Intrinsic renal: glomerulonephritis, acute tubular necrosis, drug toxicity, contrast nephropathy

DIAGNOSIS

DIFFERENTIAL DIAGNOSIS
Refer to "Etiology."

WORKUP
Laboratory evaluation to quantify degree of abnormality; radiographic studies to exclude prerenal and postrenal factors

LABORATORY TESTS
- Elevated serum creatinine: the rate of rise of creatinine is approximately 1 mg/dl/day in complete renal failure.
- Elevated BUN: BUN/creatinine ratio is >20:1 in prerenal azotemia, postrenal azotemia, and acute glomerulonephritis; it is <20:1 in acute interstitial nephritis and acute tubular necrosis.
- Electrolytes (potassium, phosphorus) are elevated; bicarbonate level and calcium are decreased.
- CBC may reveal anemia because of decreased erythropoietin production, hemoconcentration, or hemolysis.
- Urinalysis may reveal the presence of hematuria (GN), proteinuria (nephrotic syndrome), casts (e.g., granular casts in ATN, RBC casts in acute GN, WBC casts in acute interstitial nephritis), eosinophiluria (acute interstitial nephritis).
- Urinary sodium and urinary creatinine should also be obtained in order to calculate the fractional excretion of sodium (FE_{Na}) (refer to Appendix). The fractional excretion of sodium is <1 in prerenal failure, >1 in intrinsic renal failure.
- Urinary osmolarity is 250 to 300 mOsm/kg in ATN, <400 mOsm/kg in postrenal azotemia, and >500 mOsm/kg in prerenal azotemia and acute glomerulonephritis.
- Additional useful studies are blood cultures for patients suspected of sepsis, liver function studies, immunoglobulins and protein electrophoresis in patients suspected of myeloma, creatinine kinase in patients with suspected rhabdomyolysis.
- Renal biopsy may be indicated in patients with intrinsic renal failure when considering specific therapy; major uses of renal biopsy are differential diagnosis of nephrotic syndrome, separation of lupus vasculitis from other vasculitis and lupus membranous from idiopathic membranous, confirmation of hereditary nephropathies on the basis of the ultrastructure, diagnosis of rapidly progressing glomerulonephritis, separation of allergic interstitial nephritis from ATN, separation of primary glomerulonephritis syndromes.

IMAGING STUDIES
- Chest x-ray examination is useful to evaluate for CHF and for pulmonary renal syndromes (Goodpasture's syndrome, Wegener's granulomatosis).
- Ultrasound of kidneys is used to evaluate for kidney size (useful to distinguish ARF from CRF) and to evaluate for the presence of obstruction.
- Anterograde and/or retrograde pyelogram can be used for ruling out obstruction; useful in patients at high risk of obstruction.

TREATMENT

NONPHARMACOLOGIC THERAPY
- Dietary modification to supply adequate calories while minimizing accumulation of toxins; appropriate control of fluid balance
- Daily weight
- Modifications of dosage of renally excreted drugs

ACUTE GENERAL Rx
Treatment is variable with etiology of ARF:
- Prerenal: IV volume expansion in hypovolemic patients
- Intrinsic renal: discontinuation of any potential toxins and treatment of condition causing the renal failure
- Postrenal: removal of obstruction

CHRONIC Rx
- Monitoring of renal function and electrolytes
- Prevention of further insults to the kidneys with proper hydration, especially before contrast studies and avoidance of nephrotoxic agents

DISPOSITION
Prognosis is variable depending on the etiology of the renal failure, degree of renal failure, multiorgan involvement, and patient's age.

REFERRAL
- Nephrology consultation is recommended in renal failure.
- Surgical consult may be necessary in patients with obstruction.

MISCELLANEOUS

COMMENTS
- Patient education material can be obtained from the National Kidney and Neurologic Disease Information Clearinghouse, Box NKUDIC, Bethesda, MD 20893.
- Booklet entitled *What everyone should know about kidneys and kidney disease* is available from the National Kidney Foundation, Inc., 30 East 33rd Street, New York, NY 10016.
- Serum, radiographic, and urinary abnormalities in renal failure are described in Tables 2-54 and 2-55.

REFERENCES
Abuel JG: Diagnosing vascular causes of renal failure, *Ann Intern Med* 123:601, 1995.
Conger JD: Interventions in clinical acute renal failure: what are the data? *Am J Kidney Dis* 26:565, 1995.

Author: Fred F. Ferri, M.D.

Renal failure, chronic (PTG)

BASIC INFORMATION

DEFINITION
Chronic renal failure (CRF) is a progressive decrease in renal function (>3 mo in duration) with subsequent accumulation of waste products in the blood (which are normally excreted by the kidneys), electrolyte abnormalities, and anemia.

SYNONYMS
CRF

ICD-9-CM CODES
585 Chronic renal failure

EPIDEMIOLOGY AND DEMOGRAPHICS
- In the U.S., >150,000/yr receive treatment for end-stage renal disease.
- Each year nearly 2/10,000 persons develop end-stage CRF.

PHYSICAL FINDINGS
- Skin pallor, ecchymoses
- Edema
- Hypertension
- Emotional lability and depression
- The clinical presentation varies with the degree of renal failure and its underlying etiology. Common symptoms are generalized fatigue, nausea, anorexia, pruritus, insomnia, taste disturbances.

ETIOLOGY
- Polycystic kidney disease
- Glomerulonephropathies (primary, secondary)
- Tubular interstitial nephritis (e.g., drug hypersensitivity, analgesic nephropathy), obstructive nephropathies (e.g., nephrolithiasis, prostatic disease)
- Vascular diseases (renal artery stenosis, hypertensive nephrosclerosis)

DIAGNOSIS

DIFFERENTIAL DIAGNOSIS
- See "Etiology."
- CRF is primarily distinguished from ARF by the duration (progression over several months).
- Sonographic evaluation of the kidneys reveals smaller kidneys with increased echogenicity in CRF.

WORKUP
- Laboratory evaluation and imaging studies
- Kidney biopsy: generally not performed in patients with small kidneys or with advanced disease

LABORATORY TESTS
- Elevated BUN, creatinine, creatinine clearance
- Urinalysis: may reveal proteinuria, RBC casts
- Serum chemistry: elevated BUN and creatinine, hyperkalemia, hyperuricemia, hypocalcemia, hyperphosphatemia, hyperglycemia, decreased bicarbonate
- Special studies: serum and urine immunoelectrophoresis (in suspected multiple myeloma), ANA (in suspected SLE)

IMAGING STUDIES
Ultrasound of kidneys to measure kidney size and to rule out obstruction

TREATMENT

NONPHARMACOLOGIC THERAPY
- Provide adequate nutrition and calories.
- Restrict sodium and potassium (2 g/day).
- Adjust drug doses to correct for prolonged half-lives.
- Restrict fluid if significant edema is present.
- Protein restriction (40 g/day) may slow deterioration of renal function; however, recent studies have not confirmed this benefit.
- Initiate hemodialysis or peritoneal dialysis (see "Acute General Rx").
- Kidney transplantation in selected patients.

ACUTE GENERAL Rx
- Initiation of dialysis
  1. Urgent indications: uremic pericarditis, neuropathy, neuromuscular abnormalities, CHF, hyperkalemia, seizures
  2. Judgmental indications: creatinine clearance 10 to 15 ml/min; progressive anorexia, weight loss, reversal of sleep pattern, pruritus, uncontrolled fluid gain with hypertension and signs of CHF
- Erythropoietin for anemia: 2000 to 3000 U three times a week IV/SC to maintain Hct 30% to 33%
- Diuretics for significant fluid overload (loop diuretics are preferred)
- Correction of hypertension with ACE inhibitors (avoid in patients with significant hyperkalemia)
- Correction of electrolyte abnormalities (e.g., calcium chloride, glucose, sodium polystyrene sulfonate for hyperkalemia), sodium bicarbonate in patients with severe metabolic acidosis
- Control of renal osteodystrophy with calcium supplementation and vitamin D

CHRONIC Rx
Routine monitoring of renal function, Hct, and electrolytes

DISPOSITION
- Prognosis is influenced by comorbidity of multisystem diseases.
- Kidney transplantation in selected patients improves survival. The 2-yr kidney graft survival rate for living related donor transplantations is >80%, whereas the 2-yr graft survival rate for cadaveric donor transplantation is approximately 70%.

REFERRAL
- Referral to nephrologist
- Vascular consult for placement of AV shunt in hemodialysis patients

MISCELLANEOUS

COMMENTS
- Additional information on patient education can be obtained from the National Kidney and Urological Diseases Information Clearinghouse, Box NKUDIC, Bethesda, MD 20893 and from the National Kidney Foundation, Inc., 30 East 33rd Street, New York, NY 10016.
- Serum, radiographic, and urinary abnormalities in renal failure are described in Tables 2-54 and 2-55.

REFERENCES
Mashio G et al: The effect of the angiotensin converting enzyme inhibitor benazepril on the progression of chronic renal insufficiency, N Engl J Med 34:939, 1996.

Modification of Diet and Renal Disease Study Group: Dietary protein restriction, blood pressure control, and the progression of polycystic kidney disease, J Am Soc Nephrol 5:2037, 1995.

Author: **Fred F. Ferri, M.D.**

Renal tubular acidosis

BASIC INFORMATION

DEFINITION
Renal tubular acidosis (RTA) is a disorder characterized by inability to excrete H^+ or inadequate generation of new HCO_3^-. There are four types of renal tubular acidosis:
- Type I (classic, distal RTA): abnormality in distal hydrogen secretion resulting in hypokalemic hyperchloremic metabolic acidosis
- Type II (proximal RTA): defect in proximal bicarbonate reabsorption resulting in hypokalemic hyperchloremic metabolic acidosis
- Type III (RTA of glomerular insufficiency): normokalemic hyperchloremic metabolic acidosis as a result of impaired ability to generate sufficient NH_3 in the setting of decreased glomerular filtration rate (<30 ml/min). This type of RTA is described in older textbooks and is considered by many not to be a distinct entity.
- Type IV (hyporeninemic hypoaldosteronemic RTA): aldosterone deficiency or antagonism resulting in decreased distal acidification and decreased distal sodium reabsorption with subsequent hyperkalemic hyperchloremic acidosis

SYNONYMS
RTA

ICD-9-CM CODES
588.8 Renal tubular acidosis

EPIDEMIOLOGY AND DEMOGRAPHICS
RTA type IV affects mostly adults whereas RTA type I and II are more frequent in children.

PHYSICAL FINDINGS
- Examination may be normal.
- Poor skin turgor may be present from dehydration.
- Muscle weakness and muscle aches from hypokalemia may occur.
- Low back pain and bone pain may be present in patients with abnormalities of calcium metabolism (RTA II).
- There is failure to thrive in children (RTA II).

ETIOLOGY
- Type I RTA: primary biliary cirrhosis and other liver diseases, medications (amphotericin, nonsteroidals), SLE, Sjögren's syndrome
- Type II RTA: Fanconi's syndrome, primary hyperparathyroidism, multiple myeloma, medications (acetazolamide)
- Type IV RTA: Diabetes mellitus, sickle cell disease, Addison's disease, urinary obstruction

DIAGNOSIS

DIFFERENTIAL DIAGNOSIS
- Diarrhea with significant bicarbonate loss
- Other causes of metabolic acidosis
- Respiratory acidosis

WORKUP
Detection of hyperchloremic metabolic acidosis with ABGs and serum electrolytes and evaluation of potential causes (see "Etiology")

LABORATORY TESTS
- ABGs reveal metabolic acidosis; serum potassium is low in RTA types I and II, normal in type III, and high in type IV.
- Minimal urine pH is >5.5 in RTA type I, <5.5 in types II, III, and IV.
- Urinary anion gap is 0 or positive in all types of RTA.
- Additional useful studies include serum calcium level and urine calcium.
- Anion gap is normal.
- PTH measurement is useful in patients suspected of primary hyperparathyroidism (may be associated with type II RTA).

IMAGING STUDIES
- Plain abdominal radiography is useful to evaluate for nephrocalcinosis.
- Renal sonogram can be used to evaluate renal size or presence of stones.
- IVP in patients with nephrocalcinosis or nephrolithiasis.

TREATMENT

ACUTE GENERAL Rx
- Type I and type II are treated with oral sodium bicarbonate (1 to 2 mEq/kg/day in RTA I, 2 to 4 mEq/kg/day in RTA type II) titrated to correct acidosis.
- Potassium supplementation is needed in hypokalemic patients.
- Type IV RTA can be treated with furosemide to lower elevated potassium levels and sodium bicarbonate to correct significant acidosis. Fludrocortisone 100 to 300 µg/day can be used to correct mineralocorticoid deficiency.

CHRONIC Rx
- Frequent monitoring of potassium levels in type IV RTA
- Monitoring for bone disease in RTA type II
- Monitoring for nephrocalcinosis and nephrolithiasis in RTA type I

DISPOSITION
Prognosis varies with the presence of associated conditions (see "Etiology").

MISCELLANEOUS

COMMENTS
Patient education material can be obtained from the National Kidney and Urologic Diseases Information Clearinghouse, Box NKUDIC, Bethesda, MD 20893.

REFERENCES
Arieff, AI: Managing metabolic acidosis: update of the sodium bicarbonate controversy, *J Crit Ill* 8:224, 1993.
Kurtzman, MA: Disorders of distal acidification, *Kidney Int* 38:720, 1990.
Author: **Fred F. Ferri, M.D.**

Respiratory distress syndrome, acute

BASIC INFORMATION

DEFINITION
The acute respiratory distress syndrome (formerly called the "adult respiratory distress syndrome") (ARDS) is characterized by acute diffuse infiltrative lung lesions with resulting interstitial and alveolar edema, severe hypoxemia, and respiratory failure. The definition of ARDS includes the following three components:
1. A ratio of PaO_2 to FiO_2 ≤200 regardless of the level of PEEP.
2. The detection of lateral pulmonary infiltrates on frontal chest x-ray.
3. Pulmonary artery wedge pressure (PAWP) ≤18 mm Hg or no clinical evidence of elevated left atrial pressure on the basis of chest radiograph or other clinical data.

SYNONYMS
ARDS
Adult respiratory distress syndrome

ICD-9-CM CODES
518.82 Acute respiratory distress syndrome

EPIDEMIOLOGY AND DEMOGRAPHICS
In the U.S. there are 36,000 ARDS cases/yr.

PHYSICAL FINDINGS
- Signs and symptoms:
  1. Dyspnea
  2. Chest discomfort
  3. Cough
  4. Anxiety
- Physical examination
  1. Tachypnea
  2. Tachycardia
  3. Hypertension
  4. Coarse crepitations of both lungs
  5. Fever may be present if infection is the underlying etiology.

ETIOLOGY
- Sepsis (>40% of cases)
- Aspiration: near drowning, aspiration of gastric contents (>30% of cases)
- Trauma (>20% of cases)
- Multiple transfusions, blood products
- Drugs (e.g., overdose of morphine, methadone, heroin, reaction to nitrofurantoin)
- Noxious inhalation (e.g., chlorine gas, high O_2 concentration)
- Postresuscitation
- Cardiopulmonary bypass
- Pneumonia
- Burns
- Pancreatitis
- A history of chronic alcohol abuse significantly increases the risk of developing ARDS in critically ill patients

DIAGNOSIS

DIFFERENTIAL DIAGNOSIS
- Cardiogenic pulmonary edema
- Viral pneumonitis
- Lymphangitic carcinomatosis

WORKUP
- Chest x-ray examination
- ABGs
- Hemodynamic monitoring
- Bronchoalveolar lavage (selected patients)

LABORATORY TESTS
- ABGs:
  1. Initially: varying degrees of hypoxemia, generally resistant to supplemental oxygen
  2. Respiratory alkalosis, decreased P_{CO_2}
  3. Widened alveolar-arterial gradient
  4. Hypercapnia as the disease progresses
- Bronchoalveolar lavage:
  1. The most prominent finding is an increased number of polymorphonucleocytes.
  2. The presence of eosinophilia has therapeutic implications, since these patients respond to corticosteroids.
- Blood and urine cultures

IMAGING STUDIES
Chest x-ray examination:
- The initial chest radiogram might be normal in the initial hours after the precipitating event.
- Bilateral interstitial infiltrates are usually seen within 24 hr; they often are more prominent in the bases and periphery.
- "White out" of both lung fields can be seen in advanced stages.

Hemodynamic monitoring:
- Hemodynamic monitoring can be used for the initial evaluation of ARDS (in ruling out cardiogenic pulmonary edema) and its subsequent management.
- Although no dynamic profile is diagnostic of ARDS, the presence of pulmonary edema, a high cardiac output, and a low PAWP are characteristic of ARDS.
- It is important to remember that partially treated intravascular volume overload and flash pulmonary edema can have the hemodynamic features of ARDS; filling pressures can also be elevated by increased intrathoracic pressures or with fluid administration; cardiac function can be depressed by acidosis, hypoxemia, or other factors associated with sepsis.

TREATMENT

NONPHARMACOLOGIC THERAPY
Ventilatory support: mechanical ventilation is generally necessary to maintain adequate gas exchange; assist-control is generally preferred initially with the following ventilator settings:
- FiO_2 1.0 (until a lower value can be used to achieve adequate oxygenation).
- Tidal volume: conventional tidal volume (10 to 5 ml/kg of body weight) can be used in ARDS; however, recent evidence shows that it may be detrimental to patients with ARDS; the American College of Chest Physicians has recommended that the alveolar (plateau) should not exceed 35 cm H_2O, which in ARDS corresponds to a tidal volume of <5 ml/kg. Recently, a new strategy of mechanical ventilation, the "open lung approach" has been shown to have better oxygenation and tendency toward decreased mortality in patients with ARDS.
- PEEP <5 cm H_2O in order to increase lung volume and keep alveoli open.
- Inspiratory flow: 60 L/min.
- Ventilatory rate: high ventilatory rates of 20 to 25 breaths/min are often necessary in patients with ARDS because of their increased physiologic dead space and smaller lung volumes. Patients must be monitored for excessive intrathoracic gas trapping ("auto-PEEP" or "intrinsic-PEEP") that can depress cardiac output.

ACUTE GENERAL Rx
Identify and treat precipitating conditions:
- Blood and urine cultures and trial of antibiotics in presumed sepsis (routine administration of antibiotics in all cases of ARDS is not recommended)
- Prompt repair of bone fractures in patients with major trauma
- Bowel rest and crystalloid resuscitation in pancreatitis
- Fluid management: optimal fluid and hemodynamic management of patients with ARDS is patient-specific; generally, administration of crystalloids is recommended if a downward trend in pulmonary capillary wedge pressures (PCWP) is associated with diminished cardiac index, resulting in prerenal azotemia, oliguria, and relative tachycardia; on the other hand, if PCWP increases with little or no change in cardiac index, one should begin diuretic therapy and use low dose dopamine (2 to 4 µg/kg/min) to maintain natriuresis and support adequate renal flow.
- Positioning the patient: changes in position can improve oxygenation by improving the distribution of perfusion to ventilated lung regions; repositioning (lateral decubitus positioning) should be attempted in patients with hypoxemia that is not responsive to other medical interventions.
- Corticosteroids: routine use of corticosteroids in ARDS is not recommended; corticosteroids may be beneficial in patients with many eosinophils in the bronchoalveolar lavage fluid; systemic infections should be ruled out or adequately treated before administration of corticosteroids.
- Nutritional support: nutritional support is necessary to maintain adequate colloid oncotic pressure and intravascular volume.
- Tracheostomy: tracheostomy is warranted in patients requiring >2 wk of mechanical ventilation; discussion regarding tracheostomy should begin with patient (if alert and oriented) and family members/legal guardian, after 5 to 7 days of ventilatory support.

DISPOSITION
- Prognosis for ARDS varies with the underlying cause.
- Overall mortality varies between 40% and 60%.

REFERRAL
Surgical referral for tracheostomy (see "Acute General Rx").

MISCELLANEOUS

COMMENTS
DVT prophylaxis and stress ulceration prophylaxis are recommended.

REFERENCES
Bernard GR et al: The American-European consensus conference on ARDS: definitions, mechanisms, relevant outcomes, and the clinical trial coordination, *Am J Respir Crit Care Management* 149:818, 1994.

Kollef MH, Schuster DP: The acute respiratory distress syndrome, *N Engl J Med* 332:27, 1995.

Author: **Fred F. Ferri, M.D.**

Retinal detachment (PTG)

BASIC INFORMATION

DEFINITION
Retinal detachment is a retinal separation where the inner or neural layer of the retina separates from the pigment epithelial layer and results from numerous causes.

SYNONYMS
Inflammatory lesions of choroid
Uveitis
Tumor
Vascular lesions
Congenital disorders

ICD-9-CM CODES
361 Retinal detachment and defects

EPIDEMIOLOGY AND DEMOGRAPHICS
INCIDENCE (IN U.S.):
- 0.02% of the population
- Particularly common in patients with high myopia of 5 diopters or more

PREVALENCE (IN U.S.): Busy ophthalmologist may see 1 or 2 acute retinal detachments per month
PREDOMINANT SEX: None
PREDOMINANT AGE:
- Congenital in younger patients
- Usually trauma in patients 30 to 40 yr and older
- High myopia a predisposition

PEAK INCIDENCE: Incidence increases with increasing age or increasing myopia.

PHYSICAL FINDINGS
Elevation of retina and vessels associated with tears in the retina, with fluid, and/or with hemorrhage beneath the retina and changes in the vitreous.

ETIOLOGY
- Trauma
- Tears in the retina
- Uveitis
- Fluid accumulation beneath the retina
- Tumors
- Scleritis
- Inflammatory disease
- Diabetes
- Collagen-vascular disease
- Vascular abnormalities

DIAGNOSIS

DIFFERENTIAL DIAGNOSIS
- Detachment
- Hemorrhage
- Tumors

WORKUP
- Full eye examination
- Fluorescein angiography
- Visual fields
- Ultrasonography to show the retinal detachment or tumors beneath it
- Medical workup only when inflammation or systemic disease considered

LABORATORY TESTS
Usually not necessary

IMAGING STUDIES
B scan of the eye

TREATMENT

NONPHARMACOLOGIC THERAPY
Immediate surgery

ACUTE GENERAL Rx
- Early surgery to repair the detachment
- Treatment of the underlying disorder

CHRONIC Rx
Occasionally steroids or other treatment of underlying disease is indicated.

DISPOSITION
- Make an immediate referral to an ophthalmologist.
- Early intervention improves outcomes.

REFERRAL
Immediately

MISCELLANEOUS

COMMENTS
If treated early, most patients will recover a substantial portion of their vision.

REFERENCES
Cavallerano AA: Retinal detachment, *Optom Clin* 2:25, 1992.
Dolan BJ: Traumatic retinal detachment, *Optom Clin* 3:67, 1993.
Author: **Melvyn Koby, M.D.**

Retinal hemorrhage

BASIC INFORMATION

DEFINITION
In a retinal hemorrhage, blood accumulates in the retinal and subretinal areas.

SYNONYMS
Pseudoxanthomylastica
Coat's disease
Retinal trauma
High altitude retinopathy

ICD-9-CM CODES
362.81 Retinal hemorrhage

EPIDEMIOLOGY AND DEMOGRAPHICS
INCIDENCE (IN U.S.): Busy ophthalmologist sees one or two cases a month.
PREDOMINANT AGE: Degenerative disease in older patients
PEAK INCIDENCE:
- Children—associated primarily with trauma and hematologic disorders
- Increases with age

PHYSICAL FINDINGS
- Hemorrhage within the retina or subretinal area
- Evidence of retinal tears, tumors, and inflammation

ETIOLOGY
- Diabetes
- Hypertension
- Trauma
- Inflammation
- Tumors
- Subretinal neovascularization
- Associated with diabetes and aging

DIAGNOSIS

DIFFERENTIAL DIAGNOSIS
- Evaluate patients for local and systemic diseases.
- Either venous or arterial occlusion may cause retinal hemorrhage, and such occlusion is associated with atherosclerotic or heart disease, so look for these.
- Rule out malignant melanoma, trauma, hypertensive cardiovascular disease.

WORKUP
Complete general physical examination

LABORATORY TESTS
- Minimum: CBC, sedimentation rate, and complete blood chemistries
- Fluorescin
- Angiography
- Visual field testing

IMAGING STUDIES
Usually not necessary

TREATMENT

NONPHARMACOLOGIC THERAPY
Laser or treatment of underlying disorder

ACUTE GENERAL Rx
- Laser is often indicated.
- Steroids may be indicated, depending on etiology.
- Treat underlying disease.
- Repair damage if from trauma.

CHRONIC Rx
Laser if hemorrhage is recurrent

DISPOSITION
Consider this an emergency.

REFERRAL
- Immediate referral to an ophthalmologist
- An emergency, with early treatment significantly affecting outcome

MISCELLANEOUS

COMMENTS
- Vision may return substantially.
- Complete recovery dependent on amount of scar tissue formed.

REFERENCES
Dul MW: Optic nerve trauma, *Optom Clin* 3:91, 1993.
Kaur B, Taylor D: Retinal haemorrhages, *Arch Dis Child* 65:1369, 1990.

Author: **Melvyn Koby, M.D.**

Retinitis pigmentosa

BASIC INFORMATION

DEFINITION
Retinitis pigmentosa is a generalized retinal pigment degeneration associated with a variety of inheritance patterns resulting in decreased vision. A simple recessive pattern is most severe. It may be associated with some rare neurologic syndromes.

ICD-9-CM CODES
362.74 Retinitis pigmentosa, pigmentary retinal dystrophy

EPIDEMIOLOGY AND DEMOGRAPHICS
PREVALENCE (IN U.S.): 1 in 4000 people
PREDOMINANT SEX: Depends on inheritance
PREDOMINANT AGE: 60 yr
PEAK INCIDENCE:
- Recessive incidence: in the 20s
- Dominant form: in the 40s

GENETICS:
- 19% dominant
- 19% recessive
- 8% X-linked
- 46% not known to be genetically related (mutations)
- 8% undetermined cause

PHYSICAL FINDINGS
- Deposition of retinal pigment in midperiphery and centrally in the retina with a pale optic nerve and narrowing of blood vessels
- Possible cataracts and macular edema

ETIOLOGY
Usually hereditary

DIAGNOSIS

DIFFERENTIAL DIAGNOSIS
- Syphilis
- Old inflammatory scars
- Old hemorrhage
- Diabetes
- Toxic retinopathies (phenothiazines, chloroquine)

WORKUP
- Electrophysiologic studies
- Dark adaptation studies
- Visual fields

LABORATORY TESTS
- Usually not necessary
- VDRL, glucose (selected patients)

IMAGING STUDIES
Usually not necessary

TREATMENT

NONPHARMACOLOGIC THERAPY
None

CHRONIC Rx
- No proven effective therapy
- Sometimes vitamin E or vitamin A may be helpful

DISPOSITION
Disease may be either mild or severe, but if the patient is expected to progress to total blindness, counseling and early education are important.

REFERRAL
To ophthalmologist to confirm diagnosis

MISCELLANEOUS

COMMENTS
- The spiderweb-like appearance of macular degeneration should not be confused with the extra pigments sometimes seen in dark-skinned individuals.
- Patient education material can be obtained from the Retinitis Pigmentosa Foundation Fighting Blindness, 1401 Mt. Royal Avenue, 4th Floor, Baltimore, MD 21217.

REFERENCES
Berson EL: Retinitis pigmentosa, *Invest Ophthalmol Vis Sci* 34:1659, 1993.

Author: **Melvyn Koby, M.D.**

Retinoblastoma

BASIC INFORMATION

DEFINITION
Retinoblastoma is an inherited, highly malignant congenital neoplasm arising from the neural layers of the retina.

ICD-9-CM CODES
190.5 Retinoblastoma, malignant neoplasm of eyes, retina

EPIDEMIOLOGY AND DEMOGRAPHICS
INCIDENCE (IN U.S.): 1 in every 23,000 to 34,000 births
PREDOMINANT AGE: 8 mo
PEAK INCIDENCE:
- 6 to 13 mo
- 72% diagnosed by 3 yr of age
- 90% diagnosed by 4 yr of age

GENETICS:
- Gene mutation or an autosomal dominant gene with 80% to 95% penetration
- 5% mutations

PHYSICAL FINDINGS
- White pupils
- White elevated retinal masses
- Strabismus
- Glaucoma
- Uveitis

ETIOLOGY
Genetic

DIAGNOSIS

DIFFERENTIAL DIAGNOSIS
- Strabismus
- Retinal detachment
- Uveitis
- Other tumors
- Glaucoma
- Endophthalmitis

WORKUP
Ophthalmologic examination

IMAGING STUDIES
- MRI: may show calcifications in retina
- Ultrasonography: good delineation of mass

TREATMENT

NONPHARMACOLOGIC THERAPY
- Surgical enucleation of the eye
- Radiation and chemotherapy

ACUTE GENERAL Rx
Not applicable

CHRONIC Rx
Not applicable

DISPOSITION
Usually treated by an ophthalmologist/oncologist

REFERRAL
To oncologist/ophthalmologist

MISCELLANEOUS

COMMENT
With early aggressive treatment, some patients may survive.

REFERENCES
Blach LE et al: Trilateral retinoblastoma—incidence and outcome: a decade of experience, *Int J Radiat Oncol Biol Phys* 29:729, 1994.

Author: **Melvyn Koby, M.D.**

Retinopathy, diabetic

BASIC INFORMATION

DEFINITION
Diabetic retinopathy is an eye abnormality associated with diabetes and consisting of microaneurysms, punctate hemorrhages, white and yellow exudates, flame hemorrhages, and neovascular vessel growth.

SYNONYMS
NPDR—Nonproliferative diabetic retinopathy
PDR—Proliferative (advanced) diabetic retinopathy

ICD-9-CM CODES
250.5 Diabetes with ophthalmic manifestations
362.1 Retinopathy, diabetic, background
362.02 Retinopathy, diabetic, proliferative

EPIDEMIOLOGY AND DEMOGRAPHICS
INCIDENCE (IN U.S.):
- Affects 11 million persons
- A leading cause of blindness in people 20 to 70 yr old
- 5000 new cases annually

PREVALENCE (IN U.S.): Prevalence of retinopathy increases with duration of diabetes. Found in 18% of people diagnosed with diabetes for 3- to 4-yr duration and in up to 80% of diabetics with a diagnosis of 15 yr or more.
PREDOMINANT SEX: Male = female
PREDOMINANT AGE: 30 yr or older
PEAK INCIDENCE: Begins after 10 yr of onset of diabetes
GENETICS: Diabetes is usually hereditary.

PHYSICAL FINDINGS
- See "Definition"
- Microaneurysms
- Hemorrhages
- Exudates
- Macular edema
- Neovascularization
- Retinal detachment
- Hemorrhages in the vitreous

ETIOLOGY
Associated with diabetes mellitus

DIAGNOSIS

DIFFERENTIAL DIAGNOSIS
- Retinal inflammatory diseases
- Tumor
- Trauma
- Arteriosclerotic vascular disease

WORKUP
Fluorescein angiogram

LABORATORY TESTS
Those appropriate for diabetes mellitus

TREATMENT

NONPHARMACOLOGIC THERAPY
Laser treatment

ACUTE GENERAL Rx
- Laser therapy
- Vitrectomy
- Repair of retinal detachment

CHRONIC Rx
Repeated laser treatments may be necessary.

DISPOSITION
- Retinal examination should be performed on all routine medical visits.
- Prognosis is improved with early diagnosis and treatment.

REFERRAL
If diabetic retinopathy is severe enough to interfere with vision, follow-up is best done by an ophthalmologist.

MISCELLANEOUS

COMMENTS
- Early laser treatment of severe, nonproliferative and proliferative retinopathy may minimize complications and visual loss.
- Patient education information can be obtained from the American Academy of Ophthalmology (655 Beach Street, San Francisco, CA 94109-1336) and from the American Diabetes Association (1-800-232-3472).

REFERENCES
Davis MD: Diabetic retinopathy, *Diabetes Care* 15:1844, 1992.
Fukuda M: Classification and treatment of diabetic retinopathy, *Diabetes Res Clin Pract* 24(S):S171, 1994.
Smith SC: Diabetic retinopathy, *Ophthalmic Nursing* 27:745, 1992.
Author: **Melvyn Koby, M.D.**

Rh incompatibility

BASIC INFORMATION

DEFINITION
Rh incompatibility is when there is an absence of the D antigen on maternal RBCs and its presence on fetal RBCs causes risk of Rh isoimmunization.

ICD-9-CM CODES
656.1 Rh incompatibility

EPIDEMIOLOGY AND DEMOGRAPHICS
INCIDENCE:
- The absence of the D antigen (Rh$^-$ blood type) occurs in 15% of Caucasians, 8% of African Americans, and virtually no Asians or Native Americans. If the father's blood type not known, the chance that an Rh$^-$ pregnant woman is bearing an Rh$^+$ fetus is about 60%.
- Of those pregnancies complicated by Rh incompatibility, the risk of maternal isoimmunization to the D antigen is about 8% for each ABO compatible pregnancy *if no prophylaxis is given.*
- Maternal-fetal ABO incompatibility is somewhat protective against Rh isoimmunization.

GENETICS: Five major loci determine Rh status: C, D, E, c, e. The presence of the D antigen results in an Rh$^+$ individual. Its absence results in an Rh$^-$ individual. Of Rh$^+$ fathers, 45% are homozygotes, 55% are heterozygotes. For homozygous Rh$^+$ fathers, the probability of an Rh$^+$ offspring is 100%. The probability for heterozygotes is about 50%.

RISK FACTORS FOR ISOIMMUNIZATION:
- Antepartum: fetal-to-maternal transfusion
- Intrapartum: fetal-to-maternal transfusion, spontaneous abortion, ectopic pregnancy, abruption placentae, abdominal trauma, chorionic villus sampling, amniocentesis, percutaneous umbilical blood sampling (PUBS), external cephalic version, manual removal of the placenta, therapeutic abortion, autologous blood product administration

PHYSICAL FINDINGS
None

ETIOLOGY
The initial response to D antigen exposure is production if IgM (MW 900,000) that does not cross the placenta. With a repeated exposure, IgG (MW 160,000) is produced. IgG can cross the placenta and enter the fetal circulation, producing hemolysis in the fetus. This may produce erythroblastosis fetalis or hemolytic disease in the newborn with resulting in antepartum or neonatal death or neurologic damage to the fetus because of hyperbilirubinemia and kernicterus.

DIAGNOSIS

DIFFERENTIAL DIAGNOSIS
None

LABORATORY TESTS
ABO and Rh blood type and an antibody screen as part of the initial prenatal profile
1. If antibody screen negative:
- Repeat antibody screen at 28 wk gestation.
- Obtain neonatal blood type after delivery.
- If Rh incompatibility is confirmed by the neonatal blood type, a Kleihauer-Betke or Rosette test should be performed to determine the amount of fetomaternal transfusion in the following high-risk circumstances: abruptio placentae, placenta previa, cesarean delivery, intrauterine manipulation, manual removal of the placenta.
2. If anti-D antibody screen is positive:
- Maternal indirect Coombs' test is needed to determine antibody titer.
- Determine paternal Rh status and zygosity.
- If father is heterozygous, PUBS or amniotic fluid is needed to determine fetal Rh status.

IMAGING STUDIES
Ultrasound evaluation can diagnose hydrops fetalis, but it cannot predict it.

TREATMENT

NONPHARMACOLOGIC THERAPY
None

PREVENTION OF D ISOIMMUNIZATION
- Give 50 µg of D immunoglobulin: after spontaneous or induced abortion or ectopic pregnancy <13 wk gestation
- Give 300 µg of D immunoglobulin (protects against 30 ml of fetal blood):
  1. After spontaneous or induced abortion >13 wk gestation, amniocentesis, CVS, PUBS, external cephalic version or other intrauterine manipulation
  2. As antepartum prophylaxis at 28 wk gestation
  3. At delivery if the neonate is D- or Du-positive
  4. If Kleihauer-Betke or Rosette test confirms >30 ml of fetal red blood in maternal circulation, additional D immunoglobulin is indicated. Confirm adequacy of therapy by a maternal indirect Coombs' test 48 to 72 hr after Rh immune globulin is given.

MANAGEMENT OF D ISOIMMUNIZED PREGNANCIES
- Serial amniocentesis for assessment of OD$_{450}$ after 25 wk gestation with interpretation of the Delta OD$_{450}$ according to criteria established by Liley
- PUBS if ultrasonographic evidence of hydrops, rising zone II Delta OD$_{450}$ values on amniocentesis, maternal history of a severely affected child
- Intrauterine exchange transfusion if severe anemia is documented remote from term
- Initiation of steroids for lung maturation at 28 wk in severely affected pregnancies with delivery at lung maturity
- Delivery as soon as lung maturation is achieved in mild to moderately affected pregnancies

DISPOSITION
Survival of nonhydropic infants is 90%. Of infants with hydrops, 82% survive.

REFERRAL
Refer all Rh isoimmunized pregnancies to a tertiary care center before 18 to 20 wk gestation.

MISCELLANEOUS

REFERENCES
Duerbeck NB, Seeds JW: Rhesus immunization in pregnancy: a review, *Obstet Gynecol Surv* 48:801, 1993.
Gollin YG, Copel JA: Management of the Rh-sensitized mother, *Clin Perinatol* 22:545, 1995.

Author: **Laurel M. White, M.D.**

Rhabdomyolysis (PTG)

BASIC INFORMATION

DEFINITION
Rhabdomyolysis is the dissolution or disintegration of muscle, which causes membrane lysis and leakage of muscle constituents, resulting in the excretion of myoglobin in the urine.

ICD-9-CM CODES
728.89 Rhabdomyolysis

EPIDEMIOLOGY AND DEMOGRAPHICS
PREDOMINANT AGE: Rare in children

PHYSICAL FINDINGS
- Variable muscle tenderness
- Weakness
- Muscular rigidity
- Fever
- Altered consciousness
- Muscle swelling
- Malaise
- Dark urine

ETIOLOGY
- Exertion (exercise-induced)
- Electrical injury
- Drug-induced (haloperidol)
- Compartment syndrome
- Multiple trauma
- Limb ischemia
- Reperfusion after revascularization procedures for ischemia
- Extensive surgical (spinal) dissection
- Tourniquet ischemia
- Prolonged static positioning during surgery
- Infectious and inflammatory myositis
- Metabolic myopathies

DIAGNOSIS

DIFFERENTIAL DIAGNOSIS
Fig. 3-24 describes a clinical algorithm for the evaluation of CPK elevation.

LABORATORY TESTS
- Screening for myoglobinuria with a simple urine dipstick test using orthotoluidine or benzidine
- Increased CPK
- Hyperkalemia
- Hypocalcemia
- Hyperphosphatemia
- Increased urinary myoglobin
- Pigmented granular casts
- Hyperuricemia

TREATMENT

ACUTE GENERAL Rx
- Aggressive IV fluid replacement to prevent acute renal failure
- Treatment of electrolyte imbalances

DISPOSITION
The condition is easily treatable, but early diagnosis and management are necessary to avoid renal failure, which occurs in 30% of cases.

MISCELLANEOUS

COMMENTS
A clinical algorithm for the evaluation of muscle cramps and aches is described in Fig. 3-57.

REFERENCES
Better OS, Stein JH: Early management of shock and prophylaxis of acute renal failure, *N Engl J Med* 332:825, 1990.

Lachiewicz PF, Latimer HA: *Rhabdomyolysis* following total hip arthroplasty, *J Bone Joint Surg* 73(B):576, 1991.

Levenson JL: Neuroleptic malignant syndrome, *Am J Psychiatry* 142:1137, 1985.

Author: **Lonnie R. Mercier, M.D.**

Rheumatic fever (PTG)

BASIC INFORMATION

DEFINITION
Rheumatic fever is a multisystem inflammatory disease that occurs in the genetically susceptible host after a pharyngeal infection with group A streptococci.

SYNONYMS
Acute rheumatic fever
Rheumatic carditis

ICD-9-CM CODES
390; 716.9 Rheumatic fever

EPIDEMIOLOGY AND DEMOGRAPHICS
INCIDENCE (IN U.S.):
- 0.1% to 3% in patients with untreated streptococcal pharyngitis
- Higher incidence of streptococcal pharyngitis with:
  1. Crowding
  2. Poverty
  3. Young age

PREDOMINANT AGE:
- Age 5 to 15 yr for first attack
- Possible relapses later

PEAK INCIDENCE: School-age children
GENETICS:
Familial Disposition: Predisposition to the disease is likely to be genetically determined.

PHYSICAL FINDINGS
- Acute streptococcal pharyngitis, which may be subclinical and not reported by the patient
- After latent period of 1 to 5 wk (average, 19 days), acute rheumatic attack
- Patient is febrile, with a migratory polyarthritis of knees, ankles, wrists, elbows; typically severe for 1 wk, remits by 3 to 4 wk.
- Carditis
  1. New heart murmur
     a. Mitral regurgitation
     b. Aortic insufficiency
     c. Diastolic mitral murmur
  2. Cardiomegaly
  3. CHF
  4. Pericardial friction rub or effusion
- Rarely, pancarditis is severe and fatal.
- Subcutaneous nodules can be palpated over extensor tendon surfaces or bony prominences, such as the skull.
- Chorea (Sydenham's chorea) is characterized by rapid involuntary movements affecting all muscles.
  1. Muscular weakness
  2. Emotional lability
  3. Rarely seen after adolescence and almost never in adult males
- Erythema marginatum
  1. Evanescent, pink, well-demarcated spreading to trunk and proximal extremities
  2. Not specific
- Arthralgias (joint pain without swelling)
- Abdominal pain

ETIOLOGY
- Group A streptococci not recovered from tissue lesions.
- Does not occur in the absence of a streptococcal antibody response.
- Immunologic cross-reactivity between certain streptococcal antigens and human tissue antigens, suggests an autoimmune etiology.
- Both initial attacks and recurrences can be completely prevented by prompt treatment of streptococcal pharyngitis with penicillin.

DIAGNOSIS

DIFFERENTIAL DIAGNOSIS
- Rheumatoid arthritis
- Juvenile rheumatoid arthritis (Still's disease)
- Bacterial endocarditis
- Systemic lupus
- Viral infections
- Serum sickness

WORKUP
- "Jones Criteria (revised) for Guidance in the Diagnosis of Rheumatic Fever" published by the American Heart Association:
  1. Two major criteria
  2. One major and two minor criteria if supported by evidence of an antecedent group A streptococcal infection
     a. Increased titer of antistreptococcal antibodies such as ASO
     b. Positive throat culture
     c. Recent scarlet fever
- Minor criteria
  1. Previous rheumatic fever or rheumatic heart disease
  2. Fever
  3. Arthralgia
  4. Increased acute-phase reactants
     a. ESR
     b. C-reactive protein
     c. Leukocytosis
  5. Prolonged P-R interval

LABORATORY TESTS
- Throat cultures are usually negative.
- Streptococcal antibody tests are more useful in establishing the diagnosis.
  1. Peak at the beginning of the attack
  2. Can document a recent streptococcal infection
- ASO (anti-streptolysin O) titers peak:
  1. 4 to 5 wk after a streptococcal throat infection
  2. During the second or third week of illness
- Anti-DNase B (Streptozyme) is also commonly used but is less reliable.
- High-titer streptococcal antibodies:
  1. Are supportive of diagnosis, but not proof
  2. Should be interpreted in the context of clinical criteria

IMAGING STUDIES
- Chest x-ray to assess heart size
- Echocardiogram:
  1. To evaluate murmurs
  2. To rule out pericardial effusion

TREATMENT

ACUTE GENERAL Rx
- Course of penicillin to eradicate throat carriage of group A streptococci
- Arthralgia or arthritis without carditis: aspirin 40 mg/lb/day for 2 wk, followed by 20 mg/lb/day for 4 to 6 wk
- Carditis and heart failure:
  1. Prednisone 40 to 60 mg/day
  2. IV corticosteroids, such as methylprednisolone, 10 to 40 mg/day for severe carditis

CHRONIC Rx
Secondary prevention (prevention of recurrences):
- Monthly treatment with benzathine penicillin 1.2 million U IM
- Erythromycin in patients with penicillin allergy

DISPOSITION
- Damage of heart valves because of fibrosis
  1. Late sequela of recurrent attacks
  2. Frequent cause of valvular heart disease in developing countries
- May progress to heart failure

REFERRAL
To cardiologist for management of severe carditis

MISCELLANEOUS

REFERENCES
Bronze MS, Dale JB: The re-emergence of serious group A streptococcal infections and acute rheumatic fever, *Am J Med Sci* 311(1):41, 1996.

Dajain A et al: Treatment of acute streptococcal pharyngitis and prevention of rheumatic fever: a statement for health professionals, *Pediatrics* 96(4):758, 1995.

Author: **Deborah L. Shapiro, M.D.**

Rhinitis, allergic (PTG)

BASIC INFORMATION

DEFINITION
Allergic rhinitis is an IgE-mediated hypersensitivity response to nasally inhaled allergens.

SYNONYMS
Hay fever
IgE-mediated rhinitis

ICD-9-CM CODES
477.9 Allergic rhinitis

EPIDEMIOLOGY AND DEMOGRAPHICS
- Allergic rhinitis affects approximately 10% of the U.S. population.
- Mean age of onset is 8 to 12 yr.

PHYSICAL FINDINGS
- Pale or violaceous mucosa of the turbinates caused by venous engorgement (this can distinguish it from erythema present in viral rhinitis)
- Nasal polyps
- Lymphoid hyperplasia in the posterior oropharynx with cobblestone appearance
- Erythema of the throat, conjunctival and scleral injection
- Clear nasal discharge
- Clinical presentation: usually consists of sneezing, nasal congestion, cough, postnasal drip, loss of or alteration of smell, and sensation of plugged ears

ETIOLOGY
- Pollens in the springtime, ragweed in fall, grasses in the summer
- Dust in house, mites
- Smoke or any irritants
- Perfumes, detergents, soaps
- Emotion, changes in atmospheric pressure or temperature

DIAGNOSIS

DIFFERENTIAL DIAGNOSIS
- Infections (sinusitis; viral, bacterial, or fungal rhinitis)
- Rhinitis medicamentosa (cocaine, sympathomimetic nasal drops)
- Vasomotor rhinitis (e.g., secondary to air pollutants)
- Septal obstruction (e.g., deviated septum), nasal polyps, nasal neoplasms
- Systemic diseases (e.g., Wegener's granulomatosis, hypothyroidism [rare])
- Table 2-57 describes the differential diagnosis of chronic rhinitis.

WORKUP
- Workup is often unnecessary if the diagnosis is apparent.
- Allergy testing can be performed using skin testing or radioallergosorbent (RAST) testing.
- Examination of nasal smears for the presence of neutrophils to rule out infectious causes and the presence of eosinophils (suggestive of allergy) may be useful in selected patients.

LABORATORY TESTS
See "Workup."

IMAGING STUDIES
Sinus films only when sinusitis is suspected

TREATMENT

NONPHARMACOLOGIC THERAPY
- Maintain allergen-free environment by covering mattresses and pillows, eliminating animal products, and removing dust collecting fixtures.
- Use of air purifiers and dust filters is helpful.
- Maintain humidity in the environment below 50% to prevent dust mites and mold.
- Use air conditioners, especially in the bedroom.
- Remove pets in patients with suspected sensitivity to animal allergens.

ACUTE GENERAL Rx
- Use antihistamines (see Table 7-10 in Section VII).
- Topical nasal steroids are very effective if the patients are instructed on proper use and informed that improvement might not occur for at least 1 wk after initiation of therapy. Commonly available inhalers are:
  1. Beclomethasone dipropionate (Beconase AQ): one to two sprays in each nostril bid
  2. Fluticasone (Flonase): initially two sprays in each nostril qd or one spray in each nostril bid, decreasing to one spray in each nostril qd based on response
  3. Flunisolide (Nasalide): initially two sprays in each nostril bid
  4. Budesonide (Rhinocort): two sprays in each nostril bid or four sprays in each nostril qAM

CHRONIC Rx
- Cromolyn sodium (Nasalcrom): one spray to each nostril three to four times daily can be used for prophylaxis (mast cell stabilizer).
- Immunotherapy is generally reserved for patients responding poorly to the above treatments.

DISPOSITION
Most patients experience significant relief with avoidance of allergens and proper use of medications.

REFERRAL
Allergy testing in patients with severe symptoms that are unresponsive to therapy or when the diagnosis is uncertain

MISCELLANEOUS

COMMENTS
Drug interactions must be considered when using terfenadine or astemizole, since concomitant use of erythromycin, ketoconazole, clarithromycin, and itraconazole can result in QT prolongation and arrhythmias.

REFERENCES
Meltzer EO et al: A pharmacologic continuum in the treatment of rhinorrhea: the clinician as economist, *J Allergy Clin Immunol* 95:1147, 1995.

Noble SL, Forbes RC, Woodbridge HB: Allergic rhinitis, *Am Fam Physician* 51:837, 1995.

Author: **Fred F. Ferri, M.D.**

Rickets

BASIC INFORMATION

DEFINITION
Rickets is a systemic disease of infancy and childhood in which mineralization of growing bone is deficient as a result of abnormal calcium, phosphorus, or vitamin D metabolism. *Osteomalacia* is the same condition in the adult. *Renal osteodystrophy* is a term used to describe a similar condition in patients with chronic kidney disease. Certain forms of the disorder may respond only to high doses of vitamin D and are referred to as *vitamin D–resistant rickets* (VDRR).

ICD-9-CM CODES
268.0 Active rickets
275.3 Vitamin D–resistant rickets
588.0 Renal rickets (renal osteodystrophy)
268.2 Osteomalacia

PHYSICAL FINDINGS
The child with classic rickets usually develops a number of specific abnormalities:
- Softening of the skull bones (craniotabes) early in the disorder
- Enlargement of the ribs at the costochondral junctions, producing the "rachitic rosary"
- Limb deformities and epiphyseal swelling
- Height below normal range
- Irritability and easy fatigability
- Pigeon breast deformity and an indentation of the lower ribcage at the insertion of the diaphragm, sometimes referred to as Harrison's groove; possible decrease in thoracic volume, resulting in diminished pulmonary ventilation

Physical findings in the adult with osteomalacia are more subtle:
- Possible malaise and bone pain
- Many patients presumed to have osteoporosis but may also have osteomalacia

ETIOLOGY
- Deficiency states
  1. True classic vitamin D–deficient rickets (VDDR) is rare in western society.
  2. Absorption of vitamin D, however, may be blocked in several GI disorders.
  3. Similar disorders may also prevent absorption of calcium and phosphorus, but in the absence of these other diseases, deficiencies of calcium and phosphorus are also rare.
- Acquired or inherited renal tubular abnormalities that cause resorptive defects and result in rickets and osteomalacia; syndromes include classical vitamin D–resistant rickets (probably the most common form of rickets seen in general practice)
- Chronic renal failure:
  1. Can produce renal rickets or renal osteodystrophy
  2. Results in the retention of phosphate

DIAGNOSIS

DIFFERENTIAL DIAGNOSIS
- Osteoporosis
- Hyperparathyroidism
- Hyperthyroidism

LABORATORY TESTS
- Requires a high degree of interest because many of the conditions are so similar that only a complicated laboratory evaluation may establish the diagnosis
- BUN, creatinine, alkaline phosphatase, calcium, and phosphorus levels in any patient suspected of having metabolic bone disease

IMAGING STUDIES
- In rickets:
  1. Characteristic radiographic changes in the ends of growing long bones caused by the lack of calcification of the cartilage matrix
  2. Typically widening and irregularity of the epiphyseal plate
- Radiographs in the adult with osteomalacia:
  1. More subtle and often confused with osteoporosis
  2. Possible pseudofractures (Looser's zones) where major arteries cross bone
  3. Insufficiency compression deformities in the vertebral bodies

TREATMENT

- Because of the complex nature of many of these disorders, a qualified endocrinologist and nephrologist should be consulted for treatment.
- The need for orthopedic intervention is rare.
- Surgical care is indicated for slipped capital femoral epiphysis, which is fairly common in renal rickets.
- Deformity may require bracing.

MISCELLANEOUS

REFERENCES
Key LL, Bell NH: Osteomalacia and disorders of vitamin D metabolism. In Stein J (ed): *Internal medicine*, ed 4, St Louis, 1994, Mosby.

Mankin HJ: Rickets, osteomalacia, and renal osteodystrophy, *J Bone Joint Surg* 56A:101, 1974.

Mankin HJ: Rickets, osteomalacia, and renal osteodystrophy: an update, *Orthop Clin North Am* 21 (1):81, 1990.

Author: **Lonnie R. Mercier, M.D.**

Rosacea (PTG)

BASIC INFORMATION

DEFINITION
Rosacea is a chronic skin disorder characterized by papules and pustules affecting the face and often associated with flushing and erythema.

SYNONYMS
Acne rosacea

ICD-9-CM CODES
695.3 Rosacea

EPIDEMIOLOGY AND DEMOGRAPHICS
- Onset often between age 30 and 50 yr
- More common in people of Celtic origin
- Female:male ratio of 3:1

PHYSICAL FINDINGS
- Facial erythema, presence of papules, pustules, and telangiectasia (see color plate 17)
- Excessive facial warmth and redness
- Comedones are absent (unlike acne)

ETIOLOGY
- Unknown
- Hot drinks, alcohol, and sun exposure may accentuate the erythema by causing vasodilation of the skin.

DIAGNOSIS

DIFFERENTIAL DIAGNOSIS
- Drug eruption
- Acne vulgaris
- Contact dermatitis
- SLE
- Carcinoid flush
- Idiopathic facial flushing
- Seborrheic dermatitis

WORKUP
Diagnosis is based on clinical findings.

LABORATORY TESTS
Not indicated

TREATMENT

NONPHARMACOLOGIC THERAPY
- Avoid alcohol, excessive sun exposure, and hot drinks of any type.
- Use of mild, nondrying soap is recommended; local skin irritants should be avoided.

ACUTE GENERAL Rx
- Systemic antibiotics: tetracycline 250 mg qid until symptoms diminish, then taper off; erythromycin and doxycycline are also effective.
- Minocycline 50 to 100 mg qd should be used only in resistant cases, since this medication is very expensive.
- Isotretinoin (Accutane) 0.5 to 1 mg/kg/day in two divided doses for 15 to 20 wk can be used for refractory rosacea.
- Topical therapy with metronidazole aqueous gel (MetroGel) applied bid is effective as initial therapy for mild cases or following the use of oral antibiotics.

CHRONIC Rx
See "Acute General Rx."

DISPOSITION
Rosacea is often resistant to initial treatment and recurrent.

MISCELLANEOUS

COMMENTS
Patients with resistant cases may have *Demodex folliculorum* mite infestation or tinea infection (diagnosis can be confirmed with potassium hydroxide examination); the role of *D. folliculorum* in rosacea is unclear. These mites can sometimes be found in large numbers in the lesions; however, their numbers do not generally decline with treatment.

REFERENCES
Habif TP: *Clinical dermatology*, ed 3, St Louis, 1996, Mosby.
Thiboutot DM: Acne rosacea, *Am Fam Physician* 50:1691, 1994.

Author: **Fred F. Ferri, M.D.**

Rotator cuff syndrome (PTG)

BASIC INFORMATION

DEFINITION
Rotator cuff syndrome refers to a spectrum of afflictions involving the tendons of the rotator cuff (primarily the supraspinatus), ranging from simple strains and tendinitis to complete rupture with cuff-tear arthropathy.

SYNONYMS
Impingement syndrome
Painful arc syndrome
Internal derangement of the subacromial joint
Supraspinatus syndrome

ICD-9-CM CODES
726.10 Rotator cuff syndrome
727.61 Rotator cuff rupture

EPIDEMIOLOGY AND DEMOGRAPHICS
PREVALENCE: 5% to 10% of the general population
PREDOMINANT AGE: Uncommon under 20 yr of age
PREDOMINANT SEX: More common in males than females

PHYSICAL FINDINGS
- Pain, often at night
- Rotator cuff tenderness
- Referred pain down deltoid, especially with abduction between 70 and 120 degrees ("the painful arc")
- Weakness in abduction or forward flexion
- Increased pain with overhead activities
- Atrophy in longstanding cases of complete tear
- Positive "drop-arm" test

ETIOLOGY
- Microtrauma from repetitive use
- Abnormally shaped acromion
- Shoulder instability
- Worsening of process by the overhead throwing motion

DIAGNOSIS

DIFFERENTIAL DIAGNOSIS
- Shoulder instability
- Degenerative arthritis
- Cervical radiculopathy
- Avascular necrosis
- Suprascapular nerve entrapment
- The differential diagnosis of shoulder pain is described in Fig. 2-59.

WORKUP
- In chronic tendinitis, clinical findings similar to those seen in partial rupture
- Even with complete rupture, may have full, active range of motion in shoulder

IMAGING STUDIES
- Plain radiography to rule out other causes of shoulder pain; special views (if needed) to detect abnormally shaped acromion
- Shoulder arthrogram to diagnose full-thickness rotator cuff tear
- Ultrasonography to diagnose full-thickness rotator cuff tears
- MRI to evaluate full- or partial-thickness tears, chronic tendinitis, and other causes of shoulder pain

TREATMENT

ACUTE GENERAL Rx
- Rest to avoid overhead activity
- Ice or heat for comfort
- Carefully supervised program of stretching and strengthening
- Medication: NSAIDs, subacromial corticosteroid injection

DISPOSITION
- All forms are likely to respond to nonsurgical management.
- Even many complete rotator cuff tears have minimal pain and little loss of function.

REFERRAL
For orthopedic consultation in cases that fail to respond to medical management or in which rotator cuff tear is suspected

MISCELLANEOUS

COMMENTS
- There is considerable disagreement regarding the likelihood of recovery once a rotator cuff tear has developed.
- Indications for surgery vary among surgeons.

REFERENCES
Bigliane LU et al: Rotator cuff disorders: evaluation and treatment. In Iannotti JP (ed): *Am Acad Orthop Surgeons Monograph Series*, Park Ridge, Ill, 1991.
Author: **Lonnie R. Mercier, M.D.**

Salmonellosis (PTG)

BASIC INFORMATION

DEFINITION
Salmonellosis is an infection caused by one of several serotypes of *Salmonella*.

SYNONYMS
Typhoid
Typhoid fever
Enteric fever

ICD-9-CM CODES
003.0 Salmonellosis

EPIDEMIOLOGY AND DEMOGRAPHICS
INCIDENCE (IN U.S.):
- Estimated 1,000,000 cases/yr of nontyphoidal salmonellosis
- Approximately 500 cases of *S. typhi* infections reported each year
- Largest outbreak: 200,000 persons who ingested contaminated milk

PREDOMINANT AGE:
- <20 yr old
- >70 yr old
- Highest rates of infection in infants, especially neonates

PEAK INCIDENCE: Summer and fall
GENETICS:
Neonatal Infection: Highly susceptible to infection with nontyphoidal *Salmonella*

PHYSICAL FINDINGS
- Infections
  1. Localized to GI tract (gastroenteritis)
  2. Systemic (typhoid fever)
  3. Localized outside of GI tract
- Gastroenteritis
  1. Accounts for majority of disease in humans
  2. Incubation period: generally 12 to 48 hr
  3. Nausea
  4. Vomiting
  5. Diarrhea
  6. Abdominal cramps
  7. Fever
  8. Bacteremia
     a. Uncommon
     b. Occurs mostly in the immunocompromised host or those with underlying conditions
  9. Self-limited illness lasting 3 or 4 days
  10. Colonization of GI tract persistent for months, especially in those treated with antibiotics
- Typhoid fever
  1. Incubation period of few days to several months, usually several weeks
  2. Prolonged fever
  3. Myalgias
  4. Headache
  5. Cough
  6. Sore throat
  7. Malaise
  8. Anorexia
  9. Abdominal pain
  10. Hepatosplenomegaly
  11. Diarrhea or constipation early in the course of illness
  12. Rose spots (faint, maculopapular, blanching lesions) sometimes seen on chest or abdomen
- Untreated disease
  1. Fever lasting 1 to 2 mo
  2. Main complication of untreated disease: GI bleeding caused by perforation from ulceration of Peyer's patches in the ileum
  3. Rare complications:
     a. Mental status changes
     b. Shock
  4. Relapse rate of approximately 10%
- Infections outside GI tract
  1. Can occur in virtually any location.
  2. Rare.
  3. Usually occur in patients with underlying diseases.
  4. Endovascular infections are caused by seeding of atherosclerotic plaques or aneurysms.
  5. Endocarditis is a rare complication.
  6. Hepatic or splenic abscesses in patients with underlying disease in these organs.
  7. Urinary tract infections in patients with renal TB or schistosomiasis.
  8. *Salmonellae* are a frequent cause of gram-negative meningitis in neonates.
  9. Osteomyelitis in children with hemoglobinopathies may be caused by these organisms.

ETIOLOGY
- More than 2000 serotypes of *Salmonella* exists, but only a few cause disease in humans.
- Some found only in humans are the cause of enteric fever.
  1. *S. typhi*
  2. *S. paratyphi*
- Some responsible for gastroenteritis and frequently isolated from raw meat and poultry and uncooked or undercooked eggs
  1. *S. typhimurium*
  2. *S. enteritidis*
- *S. choleraesuis* is a prototype organism that causes extraintestinal nontyphoidal disease; however, any serotype associated with this illness
- Transmission generally via ingestion of contaminated food or drink
- Outbreaks of gastroenteritis related to contaminated poultry, meat, and dairy products
- Typhoid fever is a systemic illness caused by serotypes exclusive to humans
  1. Acquisition by ingestion of food or water contaminated by other humans
  2. Most cases in U.S. are:
     a. Acquired during foreign travel
     b. Acquired by ingestion of food prepared by chronic carriers, many of whom have acquired the organism outside of U.S.

DIAGNOSIS

DIFFERENTIAL DIAGNOSIS
- Other causes of prolonged fever:
  1. Malaria
  2. TB
  3. Brucellosis
  4. Amebic liver abscess

- Other causes of gastroenteritis:
  1. Bacterial: *Shigella, Yersinia, Campylobacter*
  2. Viral: Norwalk virus, rotavirus
  3. Parasitic: *Amoeba histolytica, Giardia lamblia*
  4. Toxic: enterotoxigenic *E. coli, Clostridium difficile*

WORKUP
- Typhoid fever
  1. Cultures of blood, stool, urine; repeat if initially negative.
  2. Blood cultures are more likely to be positive early in the course of illness.
  3. Stool and urine cultures are more commonly positive in the second and third week of illness.
  4. Highest yield with bone marrow biopsy cultures:
     a. 90% positive
     b. Usually not necessary
  5. Serology using Widal's test is helpful in retrospect, showing a fourfold increase in convalescent titers.
- Gastroenteritis: stool cultures
- Extraintestinal localized infection:
  1. Blood cultures
  2. Cultures from the site of infection

LABORATORY TESTS
- Neutropenia is common.
- Transaminitis is possible.
- Culture to grow organism: blood, body fluids, biopsy specimens

IMAGING STUDIES
- Radiographs of bone may be suggestive of osteomyelitis.
- CT scan or sonogram of abdomen:
  1. May reveal hepatic or splenic abscesses
  2. May reveal aortic aneurysm

TREATMENT

NONPHARMACOLOGIC THERAPY
Adequate hydration and electrolyte replacement in persons with diarrhea

ACUTE GENERAL Rx
- Typhoid fever:
  1. Ciprofloxacin 500 mg PO bid or 400 mg IV bid for 14 days
  2. Ceftriaxone 2 g IV qd for 14 days
  3. If sensitive, may switch therapy to SMX/TMP 1 to 2 DS tabs PO bid or amoxicillin 2 g PO q8h to complete 14 days
  4. Dexamethasone 3 mg IV initially, followed by 1 mg IV q6h for eight doses for patients with shock or mental status changes
- Gastroenteritis:
  1. Usually not indicated for gastroenteritis alone because this illness usually self-limited
  2. May prolong the carrier state
  3. Prophylactic treatment for patients who are at high risk of developing complications from bacteremia
     a. Neonates
     b. Patients with hemoglobinopathies
     c. Patients with atherosclerosis
     d. Patients with aneurysms
     e. Patients with prosthetic devices
     f. Immunocompromised patients
  4. Treatment can be oral or parenteral, with the same regimens used for typhoid, but only for 48 to 72 hr
- Intravascular infections require 6 wk of parenteral therapy.

CHRONIC Rx
- Carrier states are possible in those with typhoid fever.
- More common in persons >60 yr of age and in persons with gallstones.
- Usual site of colonization is the gallbladder.
- Treatment should be considered for those with persistently positive stool cultures and for food-handlers.
- Suggested regimens for eradication of carrier state:
  1. Ciprofloxacin 500 mg PO bid for 4 wk
  2. SMX/TMP one to two DS tabs PO bid for 6 wk (if susceptible)
  3. Amoxicillin 2 g PO q8h for 6 wk (if susceptible)
- Cholecystectomy may be required in carriers with gallstones who fail medical therapy.
- Prolonged course of oral therapy or lifetime suppression for:
  1. Patients with AIDS who have chronic infection
  2. Patients with AIDS who relapse after therapy

DISPOSITION
- Typhoid fever
  1. Treated patients usually respond to therapy; small percentage of chronic carriers.
  2. Untreated patients may have serious complications.
- Gastroenteritis
  1. Usually self-limited
  2. May be recurrent or persistent in AIDS patients

REFERRAL
- If gastroenteritis is persistent or recurrent
- If there is evidence of extraintestinal infection
- For typhoid fever
- For chronic carriers

MISCELLANEOUS

COMMENTS
- Quinolones should not be used in children or pregnant women.
- Infections should be reported to local health departments.

Author: **Maurice Policar, M.D.**

Sarcoidosis (PTG)

BASIC INFORMATION

DEFINITION
Sarcoidosis is a chronic systemic granulomatous disease of unknown cause, characterized histologically by the presence of nonspecific, noncaseating granulomas.

SYNONYMS
Boeck's sarcoid

ICD-9-CM CODES
135.0 Sarcoidosis

EPIDEMIOLOGY AND DEMOGRAPHICS
- Incidence in U.S.: 10.9/100,000 whites, 35.5/100,000 blacks
- Increased incidence in females and patients 20 to 40 yr old
- Presents most commonly in the winter and early spring months

PHYSICAL FINDINGS
- Clinical manifestations often vary with the stage of the disease and degree of organ involvement; patients may be asymptomatic, but a chest x-ray film may demonstrate findings consistent with sarcoidosis (see "Imaging Studies").
- Frequent manifestations:
  1. Pulmonary manifestations: dry, nonproductive cough, dyspnea, chest discomfort
  2. Constitutional symptoms: fatigue, weight loss, anorexia, malaise
  3. Visual disturbances: blurred vision, ocular discomfort, conjunctivitis, iritis, uveitis
  4. Dermatologic manifestations: erythema nodosum, macules, papules, subcutaneous nodules, hyperpigmentation
  5. Myocardial disturbances: arrhythmias, cardiomyopathy
  6. Splenomegaly, hepatomegaly
  7. Rheumatologic manifestations: arthralgias, arthritis
  8. Neurologic and other manifestations: cranial nerve palsies, diabetes insipidus, meningeal involvement, parotid enlargement

DIAGNOSIS

DIFFERENTIAL DIAGNOSIS
- TB
- Lymphoma
- Hodgkin's disease
- Metastases
- Pneumoconioses
- Enlarged pulmonary arteries
- Infectious mononucleosis
- Lymphangitic carcinomatosis
- Idiopathic hemosiderosis
- Alveolar cell carcinoma
- Pulmonary eosinophilia
- Hypersensitivity pneumonitis
- Fibrosing alveolitis
- Collagen disorders
- Parasitic infection

Table 2-28 in Section II describes the differential diagnosis of granulomatous disorders; a classification of granulomatous disorders is described in Box 2-48 in Section II.

WORKUP
- Chest x-ray examination and biopsy
- Biopsy should be done on accessible tissues suspected of sarcoid involvement (conjunctiva, skin, lymph nodes); bronchoscopy with transbronchial biopsy is the procedure of choice in patients without any readily accessible site.

LABORATORY TESTS
Laboratory abnormalities:
- Hypergammaglobulinemia
- Liver function test abnormalities
- Hypercalcemia, hypercalciuria (secondary to increased GI absorption, abnormal vitamin D metabolism, and increased calcitriol production by sarcoid granuloma)
- Cutaneous anergy to trichophyton, candida, mumps, and tuberculin
- Angiotensin-converting enzyme (ACE): elevated in approximately 60% of patients with sarcoidosis; nonspecific and generally not useful in following the course of the disease
- Bronchoalveolar lavage may be useful to evaluate the cellularity of the lavage fluid; however, overall it has been disappointing as a predictor of the course of the disease.

IMAGING STUDIES
- Chest x-ray film: adenopathy of the hilar and paratracheal nodes is a frequent finding; parenchymal changes may also be present, depending on the stage of the disease (stage I, normal x-ray; stage I, bilateral hilar adenopathy; stage II, stage I plus pulmonary infiltrate; stage III, pulmonary infiltrate without adenopathy).
- PFTs: may be normal or may reveal a restrictive pattern and/or obstructive pattern.
- Gallium-67 scan: will localize in areas of granulomatous infiltrates; however, it is not specific. The "panda" sign (localization in the lacrimal and salivary glands, giving a "panda" appearance to the face) is suggestive of sarcoidosis.

TREATMENT

ACUTE GENERAL Rx
- Corticosteroids remain the mainstay of therapy (e.g., prednisone 40 mg qd for 8 to 12 wk with gradual tapering of the dose to 10 mg qod over a 8 to 12 mo); corticosteroids should be considered in patients with severe symptoms (e.g., dyspnea, chest pain), hypercalcemia, ocular, CNS or cardiac involvement and progressive pulmonary disease.
- Patients with progressive disease refractory to corticosteroids may be treated with methotrexate.
- Hydroxychloroquine is effective for chronic disfiguring skin lesions.

CHRONIC Rx
- Closely monitor patients receiving steroids.
- Immunosuppressants (e.g., methotrexate, hydroxychloroquine) should be reserved for resistant cases.

DISPOSITION
The majority of patients with sarcoidosis have spontaneous remission within 2 yr and do not require any treatment. Their course can be followed by periodic clinical evaluation, chest x-ray studies, and PFTs.

REFERRAL
Ophthalmologic examination is indicated in all patients with suspected sarcoidosis, since ocular findings (iridocyclitis, uveitis, conjunctivitis, and keratopathy) are found in >25% of documented cases.

MISCELLANEOUS

COMMENTS
Approximately 15% to 20% of patients with lung involvement advance to irreversible lung impairment (bronchiectasis, cavitation, progressive fibrosis, pneumothorax, and respiratory failure). Death from pulmonary failure occurs in 5% to 7% of patients with sarcoidosis.

REFERENCES
DeRemee RA: Sarcoidosis, *Mayo Clin Proc* 70:177, 1995.
Newman LS et al: Sarcoidosis, *New Engl J Med* 336:1223, 1997.

Author: Fred F. Ferri, M.D.

BASIC INFORMATION

DEFINITION
Scabies is a contagious disease caused by the mite *Sarcoptes scabiei*.

ICD-9-CM CODES
133.0 Scabies

EPIDEMIOLOGY AND DEMOGRAPHICS
- Scabies is generally acquired by sleeping with or in the bedding of infested individuals.
- It is generally associated with poor living conditions and is also common in hospitals and nursing homes.

PHYSICAL FINDINGS
- Primary lesions are caused when the female mite burrows within the stratum corneum, laying eggs within the tract she leaves behind; burrows (linear or serpiginous tracts) end with a minute papule or vesicle.
- Primary lesions are most commonly found in the web spaces of the hands (see color plate 18), wrists, buttocks, scrotum, penis, breasts, axillae, and knees.
- Secondary lesions result from scratching or infection.
- Intense pruritus, especially nocturnal, is common; it is caused by an acquired sensitivity to the mite or fecal pellets and is usually noted 1 to 4 wk after the primary infestation.
- Examination of the skin may reveal burrows, tiny vesicles, excoriations, inflammatory papules.
- Widespread and crusted lesions (Norwegian or crusted scabies) may be seen in elderly and immunocompromised patients.

ETIOLOGY
Human scabies is caused by the mite *Sarcoptes scabiei*, var. hominis.

DIAGNOSIS

DIFFERENTIAL DIAGNOSIS
- Pediculosis
- Atopic dermatitis
- Flea bites
- Seborrheic dermatitis
- Dermatitis herpetiformis
- Contact dermatitis
- Nummular eczema
- Syphilis
- Other insect infestation
- The differential diagnosis of pruritus is described in Box 2-101.
- A clinical algorithm for the evaluation of generalized pruritus is described in Fig. 3-67.

WORKUP
Diagnosis is made on the clinical presentation and on the demonstration of mites, eggs, or mite feces.

LABORATORY TESTS
- Microscopic demonstration of the organism, feces, or eggs: a drop of mineral oil may be placed over the suspected lesion before removal; the scrapings are transferred directly to a glass slide; a drop of potassium hydroxide is added and a cover slip is applied.
- Skin biopsy is rarely necessary to make the diagnosis.

TREATMENT

NONPHARMACOLOGIC THERAPY
Clothing, underwear, and towels used in the 48 hr before treatment must be laundered.

ACUTE GENERAL Rx
- Following a warm bath or shower, Lindane (Kwell, Scabene) lotion should be applied to all skin surfaces below the neck (can be applied to the face if area is infested); it should be washed off 8 to 12 hr after application. Repeat application 1 wk later is usually sufficient to eradicate infestation.
- Pruritus generally abates 24 to 48 hr after treatment, but it can last up to 2 wk; oral antihistamines are effective in decreasing postscabietic pruritus.
- Topical corticosteroid creams may hasten the resolution of secondary eczematous dermatitis.
- If the patient is a resident of an extended care facility, it is important to educate the patients, staff, family, and frequent visitors about scabies and the need to have full cooperation in treatment. Scabicide should be applied to all patients, staff, and frequent visitors, whether symptomatic or not; symptomatic family members of staff and visitors should also receive treatment.
- Permethrin 5% cream (Elimite) is also effective with usually one treatment; it should be massaged into the skin from head to soles of feet; remove 8 to 14 hr later by washing. If living mites are present after 14 days, retreat.
- Crotamiton 10% cream (Eurax) is another effective agent; it should be applied to the entire cleansed body from chin down; reapply after 48 hr; change clothing and bed linen the next day and bathe after 48 hr.

DISPOSITION
- Most patients respond well to treatment.
- Refractory cases usually are seen with immunocompromised hosts or patients with underlying skin diseases.

MISCELLANEOUS

COMMENTS
- Lindane is potentially neurotoxic and should be avoided in infants and pregnant women (permethrin is safe and effective in these situations).
- Sexual partners should be notified and treated.

REFERENCES
Habif TP: *Clinical dermatology*, ed 3, St Louis, 1996, Mosby.
Moore P: Diagnosing and treating scabies, *Practitioner* 238:632, 1994.
Author: **Fred F. Ferri, M.D.**

Schizophrenia (PTG)

BASIC INFORMATION

DEFINITION
Schizophrenia is diagnosed when an individual has experienced at least 1 mo of hallucinations, delusions, thought disorder, or catatonia and at least 6 mo of decreased function and negative symptoms (avolition, anhedonia, social isolation, affective flattening).

SYNONYMS
Dementia praecox

ICD-9-CM CODES
F 20.x (DSM Code: 295.X)

EPIDEMIOLOGY AND DEMOGRAPHICS
PREVALENCE: World: 0.2% to 2%, U.S.: 1%
PREDOMINANT SEX: Males have a more severe illness and therefore skew the gender distribution toward higher in males; however, distribution is probably equal.
PREDOMINANT AGE:
- Age of onset of psychotic symptoms is in the early 20s for males and late 20s for females.
- Age of onset of the negative symptoms is usually earlier (midteenage years).

PEAK INCIDENCE: 20 to 40 yr
GENETICS:
- First-degree relatives of schizophrenics have ten times greater chance of becoming schizophrenic than the general population.
- Discordant rates among identical twins are higher than expected with simple inheritance pattern.
- Associations with several chromosomes have been described, but none have been replicated.
- Evidence exists that triplet nucleotide repeat expansion (such as seen with Huntington's disease) may play a role in inheritance of the disease.

PHYSICAL FINDINGS
- Best defined as a dementing illness beginning in early life and progressing slowly throughout the lifetime.
- Initial "negative" symptoms of adolescence—cognitive decline, social withdrawal and awkwardness, loss of motivation and pleasure, and loss of emotional expressiveness—begin after a period of normal development.
- In early adulthood, positive symptoms of psychosis and thought disturbance occur; psychotic symptoms then wax and wane throughout life; treatment ameliorates positive symptoms but generally does little for negative ones.
- Greatest chunk of occupational and social desirability is secondary to negative symptoms.

ETIOLOGY
- Unknown
- Basic distinction of whether this is a degenerative or a developmental condition is not settled.
- Loss of cortical tissue has been established in a series of landmark studies of discordant identical twins.
- Major hypothesis: generation of the mesocortical pathways produce the hypofrontality and negative symptoms, along with a compensatory hyperactivation of the mesolimbic pathways, which produce the positive symptoms of psychosis.

DIAGNOSIS

DIFFERENTIAL DIAGNOSIS
- Any medical condition, medicinal, or substance of abuse that can affect brain homeostasis and cause psychosis: distinguished from schizophrenia by their relatively brief course and the alteration in mental status that could suggest an underlying delirium
- Other neurologic conditions (e.g., Huntington's) that have psychosis as the initial presentation
- Other psychiatric disorders: source of greatest confusion
- Mood disorders with psychosis: indistinguishable from schizophrenia cross-sectionally, but have a longitudinal course that includes full recovery
- Delusional disorder: has nonbizarre delusions and lacks the thought disturbance, hallucinations, and negative symptoms of schizophrenia
- Autism in the adult: has an early age of onset and lacks significant hallucinations or delusions

WORKUP
- History and physical examination to aid in determining if psychosis is secondary or primary
- Neurologic examination to uncover soft neurologic signs (clumsy, cortical thumb, loss of fine motor movements) common in schizophrenia

LABORATORY TESTS
- No laboratory tests are specific for schizophrenia.
- Laboratory examinations (chemistry profile, blood count, sedimentation rate, toxicology screen, and urinalysis) are geared toward excluding a primary medical condition.

IMAGING STUDIES

- CT scan or MRI of brain during initial workup; repeated if the course of the illness varies from expected
- Sometimes EEG to reveal slowing when psychosis is secondary to an encephalopathy
- Chest x-ray examination during initial workup to rule out a primary medical condition

TREATMENT

NONPHARMACOLOGIC THERAPY

- Significant social support is required by most schizophrenic patients; available support services are grossly inadequate and schizophrenia patients comprise nearly one third of all homeless individuals. They usually require help with basic social, occupational, and interactive skills.
- For schizophrenic patients that continue to live with their families, relapse rates are related to the degree of emotionality in the family (i.e., schizophrenics living in families with high expressed emotion levels relapse with greater rates), so family interventions can sometimes reduce morbidity.
- Traditional psychotherapy is usually not useful in schizophrenia, but supportive psychotherapy may reduce suicide rate.

ACUTE GENERAL Rx

- Acute psychosis is usually adequately controlled by antipsychotic agents.
- Mainstay of therapy are traditional neuroleptics (e.g., haloperidol, perphenazine, fluphenazine, chlorpromazine), and the newer atypical antipsychotics (e.g., risperidone, olanzapine, clozapine), which usually block dopamine and can cause a parkinsonian state; antiparkinsonian drugs (benztropine, amantadine) can frequently ameliorate these side effects.
- Sedatives (benzodiazepines, and to a lesser degree, barbiturates) can be used transiently if there is an agitated state.

CHRONIC Rx

- Compliance is long-term focus of treatment; relapse rates are quite high in noncompliant patients. Antipsychotic agents usually must be continued at the same doses that controlled psychosis. For noncompliant patients, depot preparations that are given biweekly or monthly can be used.
- Antiparkinsonian agents may also need to be continued chronically.
- Tardive dyskinesia (choreoathetoid movements of the muscles of tongue, face, and occasionally other muscle groups) can occur in as many as 30% of patients with chronic use of the neuroleptics.
- The negative symptoms of schizophrenia can resemble depression. Additionally, depressive disorders may occur in schizophrenic patients. Antidepressant treatment of the negative symptoms is usually without effect. However, antidepressants can improve the symptoms of a discrete comorbid depressive episode.
- Mood stabilizers, such as lithium, valproate, or carbamazepine, are of little use unless there is a comorbid impulse control disorder.
- Substance abuse is a major problem in more than one third of schizophrenics. Unfortunately, these patients do poorly in traditional substance abuse treatment programs. Specialized "dual diagnosis" programs with highly structured aftercare are required.

DISPOSITION

- The positive symptoms of as many as 20% to 30% of schizophrenic patients do not respond to available treatments. A much higher fraction relapse as a result of poor compliance.
- The negative symptoms are responsible for the 50% to 70% of cases in which deterioration in occupational and social function continues.
- More than 10% of patients will complete suicide.

REFERRAL

- If hospitalization is required
- If patient is noncompliant
- If patient is resistant to treatment

MISCELLANEOUS

REFERENCES

Andreasen NC: Symptoms, signs, and diagnosis of schizophrenia, *Lancet* 346:477, 1995.

Carpenter WT Jr, Buchanan RW: Schizophrenia, *N Engl J Med* 330:681, 1994.

Weinberger DR: Implications of normal brain development for the pathogenesis of schizophrenia, *Arch Gen Psychiatry* 44:660, 1987.

Author: **Rif S. El-Mallakh, M.D. and Peggy L. El-Mallakh, B.S.N.**

Scleritis

BASIC INFORMATION

DEFINITION
Scleritis is inflammation of the sclera.

SYNONYMS
Anterior scleritis
Diffuse nodular, necrotizing scleritis
Scleromalacia perforans

ICD-9-CM CODES
379.0 Scleritis and episcleritis

EPIDEMIOLOGY AND DEMOGRAPHICS
INCIDENCE (IN U.S.): Busy ophthalmologist may see one or two cases a year
PREVALENCE (IN U.S.): Relatively rare
PREDOMINANT SEX: 61% women
PREDOMINANT AGE: 52 yr
PEAK INCIDENCE: Increases with increasing age

PHYSICAL FINDINGS
- Deep, boring eye pain
- Photophobia
- Tearing
- Conjunctival injection
- Thinning of the sclera

ETIOLOGY
- Inflammatory
- Allergic
- Toxic

DIAGNOSIS

DIFFERENTIAL DIAGNOSIS
- Most common causes are rheumatoid arthritis and collagen-vascular disease.
- Occasionally, there are allergic, infectious, or traumatic causes.
- Conjunctivitis, iritis, and episcleritis should be considered in the differential diagnosis.

WORKUP
- Fluorescein angiography
- Eye examination
- Visual field examination
- Workup for autoimmune disease

LABORATORY TESTS
- Usually not necessary
- RF, ANA, ESR may be useful

IMAGING STUDIES
Usually not necessary; CT scan of orbit may be useful in selected patients

TREATMENT

NONPHARMACOLOGIC THERAPY
- Patching
- Bandage lenses
- Surgery if thinning of the sclera is severe

ACUTE GENERAL Rx
- Steroids (topical, periocular, and systemic)
- Cycloplegic drops
- NSAIDs (see Table 7-29)
- Other immunosuppressive drugs

CHRONIC Rx
- Systemic steroids can be given for the underlying disease.
- Local steroids may be helpful.

DISPOSITION
Urgent referral to ophthalmologist

REFERRAL
If not referred to an ophthalmologist early, patients may develop uveitis and other complications.

MISCELLANEOUS

COMMENTS
An ominous diagnosis because these patients often have other severe underlying debilitating disease processes.

REFERENCES
Legmann A, Foster CS: Noninfectious necrotizing sclerosis, *Int Ophthalmol Clin* 36(1):73, 1996.
Sainz de la Maza M, Jabbur NS, Foster CS: An analysis of therapeutic decisions for scleritis, *Ophthalmology* 100:1372, 1993.
Sainz de la Maza M, Jabbur NS, Foster CS: Severity of scleritis and episcleritis, *Ophthalmology* 101:389, 1994.
Author: **Melvyn Koby, M.D.**

BASIC INFORMATION

DEFINITION
Scoliosis is a lateral curvature of the spine in the upright position, usually 10 degrees or greater. Scoliosis may be classified as either structural (fixed, nonflexible) or nonstructural (flexible, correctable).

ICD-9-CM CODES
737.30 Idiopathic scoliosis
737.39 Paralytic scoliosis
754.2 Congenital scoliosis
724.3 Sciatic scoliosis
737.43 Associated with neurofibromatosis

EPIDEMIOLOGY AND DEMOGRAPHICS (IDIOPATHIC FORM)
PREVALENCE: 4 cases/1000 persons
PREVALENT AGE:
- Onset is variable.
- Most curves are found in adolescents (age 11 yr and over).

PREDOMINENT SEX: Females > male (7:1)

PHYSICAL FINDINGS
- Record patient age (in years plus months) and height.
- Perform neurologic examination to rule out neuromuscular disease.
- Inspect the shoulders and iliac crests to determine if they are level.
- Palpate the spinous processes to determine their alignment.
- Have the patient bend forward symmetrically at the waist with the arms hanging free (Adams' position); observe from the back or front to detect abnormal spine rotation.

ETIOLOGY
- 90% unknown, usually referred to as idiopathic (genetic)
- Congenital spine deformity
- Neuromuscular disease
- Leg length inequality
- Local inflammation or infection
- Acute pain (disc disease)

Curves of an idiopathic nature or those accompanying congenital deformity or neuromuscular disease are those associated with structural changes. The nonstructural types (leg length discrepancy, inflammation, or acute pain) disappear when the offending disorder is corrected.

DIAGNOSIS

WORKUP
Curvatures associated with congenital spine abnormalities, neuromuscular disease, and the other less common forms of scoliosis can usually be identified by history or associated radiographic or physical findings.

IMAGING STUDIES
- Diagnosis of idiopathic scoliosis is confirmed by a standing roentgenogram of the spine.
- Severity of the curve is measured in degrees, usually by the Cobb method.

TREATMENT

ACUTE GENERAL Rx
- Treatment or correction of cause if curve is nonstructural
- Early detection is key in treating genetic curve
- Regular observation for curves <20 degrees
- Bracing for idiopathic curves of 20 to 40 degrees to prevent progression
- Surgery for idiopathic curves >40 degrees in immature patient

DISPOSITION
- The larger the curve at detection, the greater the chance of progression.
- Progression is more common in young children who are beginning their growth spurt.
- Curves in females are more likely to progress.
- Curves <20 degrees will improve spontaneously more than 50% of the time.
- Failure to diagnose and treat these curves may produce progressive deformity, pain, and cardiopulmonary compromise.
- Spinal deformities >50 degrees in adults may progress and eventually become painful.

REFERRAL
For orthopedic consultation if structural curve is present

MISCELLANEOUS

COMMENTS
- Congenital scoliosis has a high incidence of cardiac and urinary tract abnormalities.
- U.S. Preventive Services Task Force Recommendations regarding screening for adolescent idiopathic scoliosis are described in Section V, Chapter 47.

REFERENCES
Edmonson AS: Scoliosis. In Crenshaw AH (ed): *Campbell's operative orthopedics*, ed 8, St Louis, 1992, Mosby.
Lonstein JE: Natural history and school screening for scoliosis, *Orthop Clin North Am* 19:227, 1988.
Peterson LE, Nachemson AL: Prediction of progression of the curve in girls who have adolescent idiopathic scoliosis of moderate severity, *J Bone Joint Surg* 77(A):823, 1995.
Weinstein SL: Adolescent idiopathic scoliosis: prevalence and natural history, *Am Acad Orthop Surg Lect* 38:115, 1989.

Author: **Lonnie R. Mercier, M.D.**

Seizure disorder, absence (PTG)

BASIC INFORMATION

DEFINITION
Absence seizures are a type of generalized nonconvulsive seizure characterized by brief loss of consciousness (typically ≤15 sec) associated with a 3-sec generalized spike and slow wave EEG pattern, followed by abrupt return to full consciousness.

SYNONYMS
Petit mal seizures (obsolete)

ICD-9-CM CODES
345.0 Generalized nonconvulsive epilepsy

EPIDEMIOLOGY AND DEMOGRAPHICS
INCIDENCE (IN U.S.): 11 case/100,000 persons from ages 1 through 10 yr, rare after age 14 yr
PREVALENCE (IN U.S.): 6.5 cases/1000 persons for all types of epilepsy
PREDOMINANT SEX: Female:male ratio of 2:1
PREDOMINANT AGE: 1 to 10 yr
PEAK INCIDENCE: 5 to 10 yr
GENETICS: Clear genetic predisposition; undetermined mode of inheritance

PHYSICAL FINDINGS
- Findings are normal between seizures in children with typical absence epilepsy.
- During seizure, patient typically appears awake but abruptly ceases ongoing activity and does not respond to or recall stimuli.
- More prolonged episodes may be associated with automatisms and therefore mistaken for complex partial seizures.

ETIOLOGY
- Unknown
- Experimental data: seizures arise from impaired regulation of rhythmic thalamic discharges

DIAGNOSIS

DIFFERENTIAL DIAGNOSIS
- Complex partial seizures
- Fatigue
- Daydreaming
- Psychogenic unresponsiveness
- Table 2-20 describes the differential diagnosis of epilepsy.

WORKUP
- EEG is the most powerful tool for identification of this seizure type.
- In the vast majority of untreated individuals, vigorous hyperventilation for 3 to 5 min provokes characteristic EEG finding.

LABORATORY TESTS
None

IMAGING STUDIES
None needed for typical presentation

TREATMENT

NONPHARMACOLOGIC THERAPY
- Avoid sleep deprivation.
- Some patients are photosensitive.

ACUTE GENERAL Rx
Not indicated for individual seizures

CHRONIC Rx
- Drug of choice is ethosuximide. Initial dose for adults and children >6 yr is 500 mg/day.
- Sodium valproate is also effective.
- Table 7-6 compares various anticonvulsant medications.

DISPOSITION
- Favorable prognosis in typical childhood absence epilepsy without other seizure types
- Excellent response to medication
- Subsidence of seizures with advancing age in 70% to 90% of patients

REFERRAL
If uncertain about diagnosis

MISCELLANEOUS

COMMENTS
- Absence seizures may be mistakenly diagnosed as complex partial seizures on the basis of clinical descriptions. The EEG is essential for making this distinction.
- Administering other anticonvulsants (particularly carbamazepine or phenytoin) to patients with typical absence epilepsy may exacerbate seizures.
- Patient education information can be obtained from the Epilepsy Foundation of America, 4351 Garden City Drive, Landover, MD 20785; phone: (800) EFA-1000.

REFERENCES
Devinsky O: Seizure disorders, *Clin Symp* 46(1):2, 1994.
Author: **Michael Gruenthal, M.D., Ph.D.**

CLINICAL TOPICS — **Seizure disorder, generalized tonic-clonic** *(PTG)* 433

BASIC INFORMATION

DEFINITION
Generalized tonic-clonic seizure disorder is marked by paroxysmal hypersynchronous neuronal activity involving both cerebral hemispheres and resulting in loss of consciousness and tonic muscle contraction followed by rhythmic clonic contractions.

SYNONYMS
All obsolete:
Grand mal seizure
Major motor seizure

ICD-9-CM CODES
345.1 Generalized convulsive epilepsy

EPIDEMIOLOGY AND DEMOGRAPHICS
INCIDENCE (IN U.S.): 10 cases/100,000 persons/yr between ages 10 and 65 yr; higher in older age groups
PREVALENCE (IN U.S.): 6.5 cases/1000 persons for all types of epilepsy
PREDOMINANT SEX: Males slightly higher than females
PREDOMINANT AGE: 80 yr
PEAK INCIDENCE: >65 yr old
GENETICS: Genetic predisposition exists for many of the primary generalized epilepsies; mode of transmission varies with the particular epilepsy syndrome.

PHYSICAL FINDINGS
- Generally normal
- Possible focal deficits in patients with secondary generalized tonic-clonic seizures, depending on underlying etiology

ETIOLOGY
- Seizures are a symptom of an underlying abnormality affecting the CNS, not a disease.
- In idiopathic generalized tonic-clonic seizures, the postulated inherited cellular abnormality remains undetermined.
- Secondary (symptomatic) generalized tonic-clonic seizures may result from several underlying causes, including inborn errors of metabolism, acquired metabolic abnormalities, CNS infection, and neuronal migration abnormalities.
- Secondary generalized tonic-clonic seizures (i.e., with partial onset) may be caused by tumors, infection, trauma, vascular malformations, or genetic predisposition.

DIAGNOSIS

DIFFERENTIAL DIAGNOSIS
- Syncope
- Psychogenic events

WORKUP
New-onset seizures: a detailed history and physical examination with the goal of determining the underlying etiology

LABORATORY TESTS
- Serum glucose and electrolytes
- Additional blood studies as indicated by history and physical examination
- EEG: most valuable diagnostic tool for identifying seizure type and predicting the likelihood of recurrence

IMAGING STUDIES
- Generally not necessary in well-documented cases of idiopathic generalized tonic-clonic seizures
- MRI: modality of choice if history, examination, or EEG suggest partial (focal) onset

TREATMENT

NONPHARMACOLOGIC THERAPY
Avoid sleep deprivation or environmental precipitants (e.g., photosensitive epilepsy).

ACUTE GENERAL Rx
- Individual seizures lasting <5 min generally require no acute pharmacologic intervention.
- See "Status Epilepticus" in Section I for management of recurrent seizures.

CHRONIC Rx
- A single seizure with an identifiable and easily correctable provoking factor (e.g., hyponatremia) does not warrant long-term use of anticonvulsants.
- If there is significant risk of recurrence or more than one unprovoked seizure, treatment is indicated.
- The appropriate medication depends on several factors. In general, sodium valproate is the drug of choice for patients >4 yr of age with idiopathic generalized tonic-clonic epilepsy.
- Refer to Table 7-6 for a comparison of various anticonvulsants.

DISPOSITION
- Varies with underlying etiology
- Excellent outcome for most patients with idiopathic generalized tonic-clonic seizures

REFERRAL
If uncertain about diagnosis or seizure type

MISCELLANEOUS

REFERENCES
Devinsky O: Seizure disorders, *Clin Symp* 46(1):2, 1994.
Author: **Michael Gruenthal, M.D., Ph.D.**

Seizure disorder, partial (PTG)

BASIC INFORMATION

DEFINITION
In partial seizure disorder, seizures occur in which the onset of abnormal electrical activity is confined to one hemisphere. Clinical manifestations may involve sensory, motor, autonomic, or psychic symptoms. Consciousness may be preserved (simple partial seizures) or impaired (complex partial seizures).

SYNONYMS
All obsolete:
Minor motor seizures
Jacksonian seizures
Psychomotor seizures

ICD-9-CM CODES
345.5 Partial epilepsy, without mention of impairment of consciousness

EPIDEMIOLOGY AND DEMOGRAPHICS
INCIDENCE (IN U.S.): 20 cases/100,000 persons through age 65 yr, then rises sharply
PREVALENCE (IN U.S.): 6.5 cases/1000 persons for all types of epilepsy
PREDOMINANT SEX: Males slightly higher than females
PREDOMINANT AGE: >60 yr
PEAK INCIDENCE: >65 yr
GENETICS: Most acquired, but several distinct inherited syndromes have been identified.

PHYSICAL FINDINGS
Range from normal to focal neurologic deficits, depending on underlying cause

ETIOLOGY
- Seizures are a symptom of an underlying abnormality affecting the CNS, not a disease.
- Partial-onset seizures may be caused by underlying disorders, including stroke, tumor, infection, trauma, vascular malformations or genetic factors.

DIAGNOSIS

DIFFERENTIAL DIAGNOSIS
- Migraine
- TIA
- Presyncope
- Psychogenic phenomena
- Table 2-20 describes the differential diagnosis of epilepsy.

WORKUP
Because partial seizures are manifestations of an underlying focal CNS disturbance that must be identified if possible, imaging studies, preferably MRI, are essential.

LABORATORY TESTS
EEG is the most powerful tool for localization of the seizure focus.

IMAGING STUDIES
- MRI with contrast: modality of choice because of its high sensitivity for stroke, tumor, abscess, atrophy, and vascular malformations
- CT scan without contrast if hemorrhage is suspected

TREATMENT

NONPHARMACOLOGIC THERAPY
Avoid sleep deprivation.

ACUTE GENERAL Rx
- Individual seizures lasting <5 min generally require no acute pharmacologic intervention.
- For management of recurrent seizures, see "Status Epilepticus" in Section I.

CHRONIC Rx
Carbamazepine or phenytoin are common first-line therapeutic agents (see Table 7-6).
- Sodium valproate may also be effective.
- For each patient, choice is influenced by factors such as effectiveness, cost, adverse effects, and ease of administration.

DISPOSITION
- Determined by underlying cause
- Approximately 70% of patients controlled with medication

REFERRAL
If uncertain about diagnosis or patient fails to respond to appropriate medication

MISCELLANEOUS

COMMENTS
Patient education information can be obtained from the Epilepsy Foundation of America, 4351 Garden City Drive, Landover, MD 20785; phone: (800) EFA-1000.

REFERENCES
Devinsky O: Seizure disorders, *Clin Symp* 46(1):2, 1994.

Author: **Michael Gruenthal, M.D., Ph.D.**

Seizures, febrile (PTG)

BASIC INFORMATION

DEFINITION
A febrile seizure is a single tonic or tonic-clonic seizure without focal features, lasting <15 min, provoked by a fever from a source outside the CNS.

SYNONYMS
Benign febrile seizure

ICD-9-CM CODES
780.3 Convulsions

EPIDEMIOLOGY AND DEMOGRAPHICS
INCIDENCE (IN U.S.): Not reported
PREVALENCE (IN U.S.): 2% to 4% in children <5 yr of age
PREDOMINANT SEX: Male = female
PREDOMINANT AGE: 18 to 22 mo
PEAK INCIDENCE: 6 mo to 5 yr; 90% occur by age 3 yr
GENETICS:
- Family history increases risk two to three times.
- Mode of inheritance is unknown.

PHYSICAL FINDINGS
- Typically occur early in the course of an illness when temperature is rising.
- Most commonly associated with a viral upper respiratory infection.
- Physical and neurologic examination and developmental history may be normal.

ETIOLOGY
Unknown

DIAGNOSIS

DIFFERENTIAL DIAGNOSIS
- Epilepsy
- Meningitis
- Encephalitis
- Intracranial mass

WORKUP
- Typical presentation: child between 6 mo and 5 yr with a family history of simple febrile seizures; no further evaluation is usually required.
- Atypical presentations: seizures lasting >15 min, focal features or recurrent seizures with an interval of <24 hr; requires investigation.

LABORATORY TESTS
- Signs or symptoms of intracranial infection require CSF examination.
- Atypical presentation may warrant EEG, toxicology screening, assessment of electrolytes, etc., depending on history and examination findings.

IMAGING STUDIES
- Typical presentation: not needed.
- Atypical presentation: may warrant CT scan or MRI, depending on history and examination findings.

TREATMENT

NONPHARMACOLOGIC THERAPY
- Avoid excessive clothing.
- Encourage fluids.
- Apply tepid sponge bath to control fever.

ACUTE GENERAL Rx
- Antipyretics
- Possibly rectal diazepam in some instances of recurrent febrile seizures

CHRONIC Rx
- Prophylactic treatment with anticonvulsants is not indicated in children with typical benign febrile seizures.
- Use anticonvulsants prophylactically for other presentations of seizures associated with fever.

DISPOSITION
- Risk of recurrent benign febrile seizures is 30% up to the age of 5 yr.
- Risk of subsequent epilepsy is estimated at 1% to 2.5%.
- Available data: there is no risk reduction with prophylactic anticonvulsants.

REFERRAL
If uncertain about diagnosis or with atypical presentation

MISCELLANEOUS

REFERENCES
Smith MC: Febrile seizures: recognition and management, *Practical Therapeutics* 47:933, 1994.

Author: **Michael Gruenthal, M.D., Ph.D.**

Septicemia

BASIC INFORMATION

DEFINITION
Septicemia is a systemic illness caused by general bacterial infection and characterized by evidence of infection, fever or hypothermia, hypotension, and evidence of end-organ compromise.

SYNONYMS
Sepsis
Sepsis syndrome
Systemic inflammatory response syndrome
Septic shock

ICD-9-CM CODES
038.9 Sepsis
038.40 Sepsis, gram-negative bacteremia
038.1 Sepsis, *Staphylococcus*

EPIDEMIOLOGY AND DEMOGRAPHICS
INCIDENCE (IN U.S.):
- Exact incidence is unknown
- Approximately 300,000 cases of gram-negative bacteremia among hospitalized patients each year
- Complicates a minority of bacteremia cases and may occur in the absence of documented bacteremia

PREDOMINANT SEX: Male = female
PREDOMINANT AGE:
- Neonatal period
- Patients >70 yr of age

GENETICS:
Familial Disposition: A great variety of congenital immunodeficiency states and other inherited disorders may predispose to septicemia.
Neonatal Infection: Incidence is high in neonatal period.

PHYSICAL FINDINGS
- Fever or hypothermia
- Hypotension
- Tachycardia
- Tachypnea
- Altered mental status
- Bleeding diathesis
- Skin rashes
- Symptoms that reflect primary site of infection: urinary tract, GI tract, CNS, respiratory tract

ETIOLOGY
- Disseminated infection with a great variety of bacteria:
  1. Gram-negative bacteria
  2. *E. coli*
  3. *Klebsiella* spp.
  4. *Pseudomonas aeruginosa*
  5. *Proteus* spp.
  6. *Staphylococcus aureus*
  7. *Streptococcus* spp.
  8. *Neisseria meningitidis*
- Less common infections:
  1. Fungal
  2. Viral
  3. Rickettsial
  4. Parasitic
- Activation of coagulation, complement, and kinin cascades with release of a variety of vasoactive endogenous mediators
- Predisposing host factors:
  1. General medical condition
  2. Age
  3. Immunosuppressive therapy
  4. Recent surgery
  5. Granulocytopenia
  6. Hyposplenism
  7. Diabetes
  8. Instrumentation

DIAGNOSIS

DIFFERENTIAL DIAGNOSIS
- Cardiogenic shock
- Acute pancreatitis
- Pulmonary embolism
- Systemic vasculitis
- Toxic ingestion
- Exposure-induced hypothermia
- Fulminant hepatic failure
- Collagen-vascular diseases

WORKUP
- Evaluation should focus on identifying a specific pathogen and localizing the site of primary infection.
- Hemodynamic, metabolic, coagulation disorders should be carefully characterized.
- Intensive monitoring, including the use of central venous or Swan-Ganz catheters, may be necessary.

LABORATORY TESTS
- Cultures of blood and examination and culture of sputum, urine, wound drainage, stool, CSF
- CBC with differential, coagulation profile
- Routine chemistries, liver function tests
- ABGs
- Urinalysis

IMAGING STUDIES
- Chest x-ray examination
- Other radiographic and radioisotope procedures according to suspected site of primary infection

TREATMENT

NONPHARMACOLOGIC THERAPY
- Tissue oxygenation: oxygen saturation maintained as high as possible; early mechanical ventilation
- Focal infection drained if possible

ACUTE GENERAL Rx
- Blood pressure support
  1. IV hydration
  2. Therapy with pressors (e.g., dopamine) if mean blood pressure of 70 to 75 mm Hg cannot be maintained by hydration alone
- Correction of acidosis
  1. IV bicarbonate
  2. Mechanical ventilation
- Antibiotics
  1. Directed at the most likely sources of infection
  2. Should generally provide broad coverage of gram-positive and gram-negative bacteria
  3. Typical regimens:
     a. For hospital-acquired septicemia (pending culture results): vancomycin plus ceftazidime, imipenem, aztreonam, or an aminoglycoside
     b. For community-acquired infection in the absence of granulocytopenia: above or single-drug therapy with third generation cephalosporin
     c. For infection in the granulocytopenic host: above or dual gram-negative coverage (e.g., cephalosporin and aminoglycoside)

CHRONIC Rx
- Adjust antibiotic therapy on the basis of culture results.
- In general, continue therapy for a minimum of 2 wk.

DISPOSITION
All patients with suspected septicemia should be hospitalized and given access to intensive monitoring and nursing care.

REFERRAL
- To infectious diseases expert
- To physician experienced in critical care

MISCELLANEOUS

COMMENTS
Mortality rises quickly if antibiotic therapy is not instituted promptly and metabolic derangements are not treated aggressively.

REFERENCES
Bone RC: The sepsis syndrome: definition and general approach to management, *Clin Chest Med* 17(2):175, 1996.
Ognibene FP: Hemodynamic support during sepsis, *Clin Chest Med* 17(2):279, 1996.

Author: **Joseph R. Masci, M.D.**

BASIC INFORMATION

DEFINITION
Sheehan's syndrome is a state of hypopituitarism resulting from an infarct of the pituitary secondary to postpartum hemorrhage or shock, causing partial or complete loss of the anterior pituitary hormones (i.e., ACTH, FSH, LH, GH, PRL, TSH) and their target organ functions.

ICD-9-CM CODES
253.2 Sheehan's syndrome

EPIDEMIOLOGY AND DEMOGRAPHICS
INCIDENCE: 1 case per 10,000 deliveries (perhaps more rare in the U.S.)
PREDOMINANT SEX: Affects only females
RISK FACTORS:
- Hypovolemic shock
- Type I (insulin-dependent) diabetes mellitus (secondary to microvascular disease)
- Sickle cell anemia (secondary to occlusion of the small vessels in the pituitary)

ONSET OF SYMPTOMS: Average delay of 5 to 7 yr between onset of symptoms and diagnosis of disease.

PHYSICAL FINDINGS
- Failure of lactation
- Infertility
- Failure to resume menses after delivery
- Failure to regrow shaved pubic or axillary hair
- Skin depigmentation (including areola)
- Rapid breast involution
- Superinvolution of the uterus
- Hypothyroidism
- Adrenal cortical insufficiency
- Diabetes insipidus (rare)

ETIOLOGY
- Compromise of the blood supply to the low-pressure pituitary sinusoidal system may occur with postpartum hemorrhage or shock, resulting in pituitary infarct and/or necrosis.
- It is hypothesized that locally released factors may mediate vascular spasm of the pituitary blood supply.
- Severity of postpartum hemorrhage does not always correlate with the presence of Sheehan's syndrome.

DIAGNOSIS

DIFFERENTIAL DIAGNOSIS
- Chronic infections
- HIV
- Sarcoidosis
- Amyloidosis
- Rheumatoid disease
- Hemachromatosis
- Metastatic carcinoma
- Lymphocytic hypophysitis

WORKUP
- Target gland deficiency should be investigated by measuring levels of ACTH, FSH, LH, TSH (which may be normal or low), and T_4. Cortisol and estradiol (which may be low) should also be measured.
- Provocative testing of pituitary hormone reserves (e.g., metyrapone test, insulin tolerance test and cosyntropin test): normal, subnormal, or delayed responses may suggest the presence of islands of pituitary cells that no longer have the support of the hypothalamic-portal circulation.
- Measurement of IGF-I to screen for GH deficiency: subnormal levels suggest decreased GH.
- Impaired prolactin response to TRH or dopamine antagonist stimulation is frequently found.
- During pregnancy, adjustments must be made in interpreting both hormone levels and responses to various stimuli because of normal physiologic changes.

IMAGING STUDIES
- Study of choice: MRI of the pituitary
  1. Sella turcica partially or totally empty
  2. Rules out mass lesion
- CT scan of the pituitary when MRI is unavailable or contraindicated

TREATMENT

ACUTE GENERAL Rx
- Acute form can be lethal, presenting with hypotension, tachycardia, failure to lactate, and hypoglycemia.
- A high degree of suspicion is required with any woman who has undergone postpartum hemorrhage and shock.
- Intravenous corticosteroids and fluid replacement should be given initially
- Diagnosis is confirmed with a full endocrinological workup as noted above.
- Thyroid hormone is replaced as L-thyroxin in doses of 0.1 to 0.2 mg qd.

CHRONIC Rx
- With late onset disease (symptoms of general hypopituitarism, such as oligomenorrhea or amenorrhea, vaginal atrophic changes, and loss of libido): a full endocrinological workup and replacement of the appropriate hormones are needed.
- With symptoms of adrenal insufficiency: corticosteroids should be given.
  1. A maintenance dose of cortisone acetate or prednisone may be given.
  2. Since adrenal production of cortisol is not entirely dependent on ACTH, replacement of mineralocorticoids is rarely necessary.
  3. Stress doses of glucocorticoids should be administered during surgery or during labor and delivery.

DISPOSITION
Patients who receive early diagnosis and adequate hormonal replacement may expect favorable outcomes, including subsequent pregnancy.

REFERRAL
Patients should have yearly examinations by endocrinologist.

MISCELLANEOUS

REFERENCES
Chang BW, Newton TH: Hypothalamic and pituitary pathology, *Radiol Clin North Am* 31(5):1147, 1993.
Prager D, Braunstein GD: Pituitary disorders during pregnancy, *Endocrinol Metab Clin North Am* 24(1):1, 1995.
Author: **Candace C. Green, M.D.**

Shigellosis (PTG)

BASIC INFORMATION

DEFINITION
Shigellosis is an inflammatory disease of the bowel caused by one of several species of *Shigella*. It is the most common cause of bacillary dysentery in the U.S.

SYNONYMS
Bacillary dysentery

ICD-9-CM CODES
004.9 Shigellosis

EPIDEMIOLOGY AND DEMOGRAPHICS
INCIDENCE (IN U.S.): Approximately 15,000 cases/yr
PREDOMINANT SEX: Male homosexuals at increased risk
PREDOMINANT AGE: Young children
PEAK INCIDENCE: Summer
GENETICS:
Neonatal Infection: Rare but severe

PHYSICAL FINDINGS
- Possibly asymptomatic
- Mild illness that is usually self-limited, resolving in a few days
- Fever
- Watery diarrhea
- Bloody diarrhea
- Dysentery (abdominal cramps, tenesmus, and numerous, small-volume stools with blood, mucus, and pus)
- Descending intestinal tract illness, reflecting infection of small bowel first and then the colon
- Severe disease is more common in children and elderly
- Complications of severe illness:
  1. Seizures
  2. Megacolon
  3. Intestinal perforation
  4. Death
- Extraintestinal manifestations are rare
- Bacteremia described in patients with AIDS
- Hemolytic-uremic syndrome: usually occurs as the initial illness seems to be resolving
- Reactive arthritis, sometimes as part of Reiter's syndrome

ETIOLOGY
- *Shigella*
  1. *S. flexneri*
  2. *S. dysenteriae*
  3. *S. sonnei*
  4. *S. boydii*
- *S. sonnei* is the most commonly isolated species in the U. S., and it usually causes a mild watery diarrhea.
- Direct person-to-person transmission is thought to be the most common route.
- Contaminated food or water may transmit disease.

DIAGNOSIS

DIFFERENTIAL DIAGNOSIS
- May mimic any bacterial or viral gastroenteritis
- Dysentery also caused by *Entamoeba histolytica*
- Bloody diarrhea may resemble disease caused by enterotoxigenic *E. coli*

LABORATORY TESTS
- Total WBCs may be low, normal, or high.
- Stool should be cultured from fresh samples, since the yield is increased by processing the specimen soon after passage.
- Serology is available but rarely useful.
- Polymerase chain reaction may be diagnostic.
- Fecal leukocyte preparation may show WBCs.

IMAGING STUDIES
Abdominal radiographs may suggest megacolon or perforation in rare severe cases.

TREATMENT

NONPHARMACOLOGIC THERAPY
- Adequate hydration
- Electrolyte replacement

ACUTE GENERAL Rx
Antibiotics:
- To shorten course of illness
- To limit transmission of illness
- SMX/TMP, one DS tablet PO bid for 5 days
- Ciprofloxacin 500 mg PO bid for 5 days

DISPOSITION
- Most disease is self-limited.
- Severe illness may be fatal.

REFERRAL
For severe illness or complications

MISCELLANEOUS

COMMENTS
- *Shigella* is one cause of "gay bowel syndrome."
- Illness is worsened by agents that decrease intestinal motility.

REFERENCES
Arnell B et al: *Shigella sonnei* outbreak associated with contaminated drinking water—Island Park, Idaho, 1995, *MMWR* 45:229, 1996.

Author: **Maurice Policar, M.D.**

BASIC INFORMATION

DEFINITION
Sialadenitis is an inflammation of the salivary glands.

ICD-9-CM CODES
527.2 Sialadenitis

EPIDEMIOLOGY AND DEMOGRAPHICS
Parotid or submandibular glands are most frequently affected.

PHYSICAL FINDINGS
- Pain and swelling of the affected salivary gland
- Increased pain with meals
- Erythema, tenderness at the duct opening
- Purulent discharge from duct orifice
- Induration and pitting of the skin with involvement of the masseteric and submandibular spatial planes in severe cases

ETIOLOGY
- Ductal obstruction is generally secondary to a mucus plug caused by stasis of saliva with increased viscosity with subsequent stasis and infection.
- Most frequent infecting organisms are *Staphylococcus aureus*, *Pseudomonas*, *Enterobacter*, *Klebsiella*, enterococci, *Proteus*, and *Candida* spp.
- Sjögren's syndrome, trauma, radiation therapy, chemotherapy, dehydration, and chronic illness are predisposing factors.

DIAGNOSIS

DIFFERENTIAL DIAGNOSIS
- Salivary gland neoplasm
- Ductal stricture
- Sialolithiasis
- Decreased salivary secretion secondary to medications (e.g., amitriptyline, diphenhydramine, anticholinergics)

WORKUP
- Generally not necessary.
- Ultrasound or CT scan in patients not responding to medical treatment (see "Imaging Studies").

LABORATORY TESTS
- Generally not indicated.
- CBC with differential may reveal leukocytosis with left shift.

IMAGING STUDIES
- Ultrasound or CT scan may be needed in patients not responding to medical therapy.
- Sialography should not be performed during the acute phase.

TREATMENT

NONPHARMACOLOGIC THERAPY
- Massage of the gland: may express pus and relieve some of the pressure
- Rehydration
- Warm compresses
- Oral cavity irrigations

ACUTE GENERAL Rx
- Amoxicillin clavulanate (Augmentin) 500 to 875 mg or cefuroxime (Ceftin) 250 mg bid should be given bid for 10 days. Clindamycin is an alternative choice in patients allergic to penicillin.
- IV antibiotics (e.g., cefoxitin, nafcillin) can be given in severe cases.

DISPOSITION
Complete recovery unless the patient has underlying obstruction (e.g., ductal stricture, tumor, or stone)

REFERRAL
- ENT referral for nonresolving cases despite appropriate antibiotic therapy
- Salivary gland incision and drainage may be necessary in resistant cases

MISCELLANEOUS

COMMENTS
Prevention of dehydration will decrease the risk of sialadenitis.

REFERENCES
Schweitzer VG: Oral cavity and salivary gland disease. In Noble JN (ed): *Primary care medicine*, ed 2, St Louis, 1996, Mosby.

Author: **Fred F. Ferri, M.D.**

Sinusitis (PTG)

BASIC INFORMATION

DEFINITION
Sinusitis is inflammation of the mucous membrane lining of one or more of the paranasal sinuses. Chronic sinusitis usually results from failure of resolution of acute sinusitis.

ICD-9-CM CODES
473.9 Sinusitis (accessory) (nasal) (hyperplastic) (nonpurulent) (purulent) (chronic)
461.9 Acute sinusitis

EPIDEMIOLOGY AND DEMOGRAPHICS
INCIDENCE (IN U.S.): Seems to correlate with the incidence of upper respiratory tract infections
PEAK INCIDENCE:
Fall, winter, spring; September through March

PHYSICAL FINDINGS
- Mucopurulent nasal secretions in nasal passages
  1. Purulent nasal and postnasal discharge lasting >10 days
  2. Facial tightness or pressure
  3. Nasal obstruction
  4. Headache
- Erythema, swelling, and tenderness over infected sinus in a small proportion of cases
  1. Diagnosis cannot be excluded by absence of such findings.
  2. Findings are not common compared with positive sinus aspirates.
- Intermittent low-grade fever in about half of adults with acute bacterial sinusitis
- Toothache: common complaint when dental infection is the origin of maxillary sinusitis
- Periorbital cellulitis and excessive tearing with ethmoid sinusitis
  1. Orbital extension of infection: chemosis, proptosis, impaired extraocular movements
- Characteristics of acute sinusitis in children with upper respiratory tract infections:
  1. Persistence of symptoms
  2. Cough
  3. Bad breath
- Symptoms of chronic sinusitis (variable; may or may not be present):
  1. Nasal or postnasal discharge
  2. Fever
  3. Facial pain or pressure
  4. Headache

ETIOLOGY
- Acute viral infection:
  1. Infection with the common cold or influenza
  2. Mucosal edema and sinus inflammation
  3. Impeding drainage of thick secretions
  4. Subsequent entrapment of bacteria
     a. Multiplication of bacteria
     b. Secondary bacterial infection
- Other predisposing factors:
  1. Tumors
  2. Polyps
  3. Foreign bodies
  4. Congenital choanal atresia
  5. Other entities that cause obstruction of sinus drainage
  6. Allergies
  7. Asthma
- Dental infections lead to maxillary sinusitis.
- Viruses recovered alone or in combination with bacteria (in 16% of cases):
  1. Rhinovirus
  2. Coronavirus
  3. Adenovirus
  4. Parainfluenza virus
  5. Influenza virus
  6. Respiratory syncytial virus
- 50% to 75% of cases are caused by *Streptococcus pneumoniae* or unencapsulated strains of *H. influenzae*
- Remaining cases:
  1. Mixed anaerobic infections: *Bacteroides, Peptostreptococcus, Fusobacterium* spp., others
  2. *Moraxella catarrhalis*
  3. α-Hemolytic streptococci
  4. *S. pyogenes*
  5. *S. aureus*
- Infection polymicrobial in approximately one third of cases
- Anaerobic infections:
  1. Usually associated with dental infections
  2. Uncommon in children
- *Chlamydia pneumoniae*:
  1. Recovery not well documented
  2. Role in acute infection unclear
- Fungal pathogens isolated with increasing frequency:
  1. *Aspergillus*
  2. *Pseudallescheria*
  3. *Sporothrix*
  4. Phaeohyphomycoses
  5. Hyalohyphomycoses
  6. Zygomycetes
- Nosocomial infections:
  1. *S. aureus*
  2. *Pseudomonas aeruginosa*
  3. *Klebsiella pneumoniae*
  4. *Enterobacter* spp.
  5. *Proteus mirabilis*
  6. Generally occur in:
     a. Patients who have nasogastric tubes
     b. Immunocompromised patients
     c. Patients with cystic fibrosis
- Organisms typically isolated in chronic sinusitis:
  1. *S. aureus*
  2. *Streptococcus pneumoniae*
  3. *Haemophilus influenzae*
  4. *P. aeruginosa*
  5. Anaerobes

DIAGNOSIS

DIFFERENTIAL DIAGNOSIS
Acute upper respiratory infection: upper respiratory symptoms persisting >10 days should raise suspicion of acute sinusitis.

WORKUP
- Transillumination:
  1. Diagnosis of frontal and maxillary sinusitis
  2. Cannot be used to detect infection of the ethmoid and sphenoid sinuses
  3. Complete opacity in a previously normal sinus correlated with probability of active infection
  4. Dullness (decreased light transmission) less helpful in determining active infection
- Standard four-view sinus radiographs:
  1. Correlated with bacterial cultures of sinus aspirates in adults suspected of having acute sinusitis

2. Clouding
3. Opacification
4. Air-fluid levels
5. Mucosal thickening
6. Far less sensitive than CT scanning
- CT scans:
  1. Much more sensitive than plain radiographs in detecting acute changes and disease in the sinuses
  2. Cannot distinguish viral from bacterial etiology in the absence of an air-fluid level
- Endoscopy:
  1. Visualizes secretions coming from the ostium of the infected sinus
  2. Endoscopic collection of samples for bacterial culture not shown to compare with those collected by sinus puncture because of contamination with nasal flora
- Sinus puncture:
  1. Gold standard for collecting samples for bacterial culture
  2. Indications: suspected intracranial extension, treatment failures, nosocomial sinusitis

TREATMENT

NONPHARMACOLOGIC THERAPY
- Humidification to promote good drainage of the sinuses
- Surgical drainage:
  1. If intracranial or orbital complications are suspected
  2. If frontal and sphenoid sinusitis
  3. If chronic sinusitis recalcitrant to medical therapy
- Surgical debridement to treat fungal sinusitis

ACUTE GENERAL Rx
- Sinus drainage:
  1. Nasal vasoconstrictors, such as phenylephrine nose drops, 0.25% or 0.5%
  2. Topical decongestants: should not be used for >3 or 4 days to avoid rebound nasal congestion
  3. Systemic decongestants
  4. Topical or systemic corticosteroids:
     a. Intranasal beclomethasone twice daily
     b. Short-course oral prednisone
     c. Few controlled studies to support their efficacy
- Appropriate antimicrobial therapy for acute bacterial sinusitis
  1. Empiric therapy selected based on the well-established list of common pathogens
  2. Bactrim double strength twice daily
  3. Cefuroxime axetil 250 mg q12h
  4. Amoxicillin/clavulanate 500/125 mg q8h
  5. Loracarbef 400 mg q12h
  6. Cefixime 200 mg q12h
  7. Ampicillin and ampicillin-like drugs: not recommended
     a. Prevalence of β-lactamase producing strains of *H. influenzae* and *M. catarrhalis*
  8. 14-day course
  9. No treatment response:
     a. Tetracycline to cover the possibility of *Chlamydia pneumoniae*
     b. Parenteral vancomycin to cover the possibility of resistant pneumococci and staphylococci
  10. Hospitalization and IV antibiotics: may be required for severe infection and suspected intracranial complications
  11. Surgical debridement
  12. Antifungal therapy in complicated cases and immunocompromised patients

CHRONIC Rx
- Broad-spectrum antibiotics that cover both aerobes and anaerobes
- Duration of therapy: not well established (range from 3 to 6 wk)
- Adjunctive therapy
  1. Nasal and oral corticosteroids:
     a. Nasal steroid sprays: Beconase AQ, Vancenase AQ, 2 sprays bid for 3 to 6 wk or Nasacort 2 sprays qd
     b. Short-course oral prednisone 20 to 40 mg qd for 3 to 5 days, then taper
  2. Topical and oral decongestants:
     a. Oxymetazoline 2 sprays bid, 5 days on, 3 days off for 3 to 6 wk
     b. Pseudoephedrine 30 mg qid
     c. Phenylpropanolamine for 3 to 6 wk
  3. Antihistamines and sodium cromoglycate to control allergic responses
  4. Mucolytics, such as guaifenesin, to decrease viscosity of secretions and promote drainage
  5. Humidification and nasal irrigations to promote drainage
- Surgical intervention for patients who fail to respond to medical therapy

DISPOSITION
Appropriate management of acute sinusitis is important to avoid progression to chronic sinusitis.

REFERRAL
- To infectious disease specialist if there is failure to respond to initial therapy
- To otorhinolaryngologist:
  1. Failure to respond to initial therapy
  2. Intracranial or orbital involvement is suspected
  3. Fungal infection is suspected

MISCELLANEOUS

REFERENCES
Brook I: Microbiology and management of sinusitis, *J Otolaryngol* 25(4):249, 1996.

Guarderas JC: Rhinitis and sinusitis: office management, *Mayo Clin Proc* 71(9):882, 1996.

Gwaltney JM: Management of acute sinusitis in adults. In Johnson JT, Yu VL (eds): *Infectious diseases and antimicrobial therapy of the ears, nose and throat*, Philadelphia, 1997, WB Saunders.

Stankiewicz J: Chronic sinusitis. In Johnson JT, Yu VL (eds): *Infectious diseases and antimicrobial therapy of the ears, nose, and throat*, Philadelphia, 1997, WB Saunders.

Author: **Jane V. Eason, M.D.**

Sjögren's syndrome (PTG)

BASIC INFORMATION

DEFINITION
Sjögren's syndrome (SS) is an autoimmune disorder characterized by lymphocytic and plasma cell infiltration and destruction of salivary and lacrimal glands with subsequent diminished lacrimal and salivary gland secretions.
- *Primary:* dry mouth (xerostomia) and dry eyes (xerophthalmia) develop as isolated entities.
- *Secondary:* associated with other disorders.

SYNONYMS
SS
Sicca syndrome

ICD-9-CM CODES
710.2 Sjögren's syndrome

EPIDEMIOLOGY AND DEMOGRAPHICS
INCIDENCE/PREVALENCE: 1 case/2500 persons; secondary SS is just as common and can affect up to one third of SLE patients and nearly 20% of RA patients.
PREDOMINANT AGE: Peak incidence is in the sixth decade.
PREDOMINANT SEX: Female > male

PHYSICAL FINDINGS
- Dry mouth with dry lips (cheilosis), erythema of tongue and other mucosal surfaces, carious teeth
- Dry eyes (conjunctival injection, decreased luster, and irregularity of the corneal light reflex)
- Possible salivary gland enlargement
- Purpura (nonthrombocytopenic, hyperglobulinemic, vasculitic) may be present
- Evidence of associated conditions (e.g., RA or other connective disease, lymphoma, hypothyroidism, COPD, trigeminal neuropathy, chronic liver disease, polymyopathy)

ETIOLOGY
Autoimmune disorder

DIAGNOSIS

DIFFERENTIAL DIAGNOSIS
- Medication-related dryness (e.g., anticholinergics)
- Age-related exocrine gland dysfunction
- Mouth breathing
- Anxiety
- Other: sarcoidosis, primary salivary hypofunction, radiation injury, amyloidosis

WORKUP
Workup involves the demonstration of the following criteria for diagnosis of primary and secondary Sjögren's syndrome:
PRIMARY:
- Symptoms and objective signs of ocular dryness:
  1. Schirmer's test: <8 mm wetting per 5 min
  2. Positive rose bengal or fluorescein staining of cornea and conjunctiva to demonstrate keratoconjunctivitis sicca
- Symptoms and objective signs of dry mouth:
  1. Decreased parotid flow using Lashley cups or other methods
  2. Abnormal biopsy result of minor salivary gland (focus score >2 based on average of four assessable lobules)
- Evidence of systemic autoimmune disorder:
  1. Elevated titer of rheumatoid factor >1:320
  2. Elevated titer of ANA >1:320
  3. Presence of anti-SS A (Ro) or anti-SS B (La) antibodies

SECONDARY:
- Characteristic signs and symptoms of SS (described in "Physical Findings" above)
- Clinical features sufficient to allow a diagnosis of RA, SLE, polymyositis, or scleroderma

LABORATORY TESTS
- Positive ANA (>60% of patients) with autoantibodies anti-SS A and anti-SS B may be present.
- Additional laboratory abnormalities may include elevated ESR, anemia (normochromic, normocytic), abnormal liver function studies, elevated serum β-2 microglobulin levels, rheumatoid factor.

TREATMENT

NONPHARMACOLOGIC THERAPY
- Adequate fluid replacement
- Proper oral hygiene to reduce the incidence of caries

ACUTE GENERAL Rx
- Use artificial tears frequently.
- Therapy of associated conditions (e.g., RA, SLE, lymphoma): refer to Section I in this book for specific therapy of these topics.

CHRONIC Rx
Periodic dental and ophthalmology evaluations to screen for complications

DISPOSITION
Prognosis is variable and depends on the presence of associated conditions.

MISCELLANEOUS

COMMENTS
Unusual presentations of SS may occur in association with polymyalgia rheumatica, chronic fatigue syndrome, FUO, and inflammatory myositis.

REFERENCES
Fox IR: Sjögren's syndrome. In Stein JH (ed): *Internal medicine,* ed 5, St Louis, 1997, Mosby.
Vivino FB, Katz WA: Sjögren's syndrome: clinical picture and diagnostic tests, *J Musculoskeletal Med* 40, March 1995.
Author: Fred F. Ferri, M.D.

Sleep apnea, obstructive (PTG)

BASIC INFORMATION

DEFINITION
Obstructive sleep apnea refers to upper airway occlusion usually accompanied by oxygen desaturation occurring repeatedly during sleep.

SYNONYMS
Sleep apnea syndrome

ICD-9-CM CODES
780.53 Sleep apnea with hypersomnia
780.51 Sleep apnea with hyposomnia
780.57 Sleep apnea with sleep disturbance
306.1 Psychogenic apnea

EPIDEMIOLOGY AND DEMOGRAPHICS
Obstructive sleep apnea occurs most frequently in obese, middle-aged men (4%) and women (2%).

PHYSICAL FINDINGS
- History of snoring and excessive daytime somnolence
- Obesity with body mass >20% of normal
- Memory impairment, inability to concentrate, personality changes
- Examination of oropharynx may reveal narrowing secondary to large tonsils, pendulous uvula, excessive soft tissue, prominent tongue.
- Patient's bed partner usually reports loud, cyclical snoring, disrupted sleep with repetitive awakenings, thrashing movements of extremities during sleep.
- Decreased libido and depression
- Systemic hypertension

ETIOLOGY
Narrowing of upper airway secondary to:
- Obesity
- Macroglossia
- Tonsillar hypertrophy
- Micrognathia
- Hypothyroidism
- Use of alcohol or sedatives at bedtime

DIAGNOSIS

DIFFERENTIAL DIAGNOSIS
- Narcolepsy
- Psychiatric: depression
- CHF
- COPD
- GERD
- Seizure disorder
- Parasomnias

Fig. 3-76 in Section III describes the diagnostic approach to sleep disorders

WORKUP
- Medical history should include questions about snoring, since essentially all patients with obstructive sleep apnea snore when they sleep; other important signs of sleep apnea are daytime somnolence and higher frequency of accidents (automobile or work-related).
- Sleep apnea can be confirmed by polysomnography: patient with sleep apnea has >15 apneic episodes per hour with desaturation of at least 4% by oximetry. Syndrome can be ruled out by normal overnight oximetry test or if saturation of oxygen level is <90%, <1% for a total sleep time.

LABORATORY TESTS
- TSH level is indicated in suspected hypothyroidism.
- CBC generally reveals erythrocytosis.

IMAGING STUDIES
Radiography of soft tissues in the neck in patients with suspected anatomic abnormalities

TREATMENT

NONPHARMACOLOGIC THERAPY
- Weight loss
- Avoidance of sedating medications and alcohol
- Elimination of the supine sleeping position
- Nighttime treatment with continuous positive airway pressure (CPAP) to overcome desaturation
- An oral appliance that attaches to the upper teeth and pushes the mandible forward enlarging the upper airway is also available as an initial treatment for mild obstructive sleep apnea

ACUTE GENERAL Rx
Patients that are unresponsive to CPAP and weight loss may be candidates for surgical therapy:
- Uvulopalatopharyngoplasty (UPPP, both standard and laser-assisted [LAUP]) in patients with significant obstruction of retropalatal airway
- Nasal septoplasty in patients with nasoseptal deformity
- Tracheostomy: reserved for life-threatening cases that are unresponsive to other treatments

CHRONIC Rx
See "Acute General Rx."

DISPOSITION
- Most patients improve with weight loss and CPAP.
- Overall success rate for UPPP is about 40%.
- Pharmacologic therapy with protriptyline 10 to 20 mg PO qhs can provide improvement in a limited number of patients.

REFERRAL
Surgical referral for patients unresponsive to weight loss and CPAP

MISCELLANEOUS

COMMENTS
Additional information on sleep apnea can be obtained from the American Sleep Disorders Associations, 1610 14th Street, NW, Suite 300, Rochester, MN 55901-2205.

REFERENCES
Douglas NJ, Thomas S, Jan MA: Clinical value of polysomnography, *Lancet* 339:347, 1992.
National Heart, Lung, and Blood Institute Working Group on Sleep Apnea: Sleep apnea: is your patient at risk? *Am Fam Physician* 53(1): 247, 1996.
Odens ML, Fox CH: Adult sleep apnea syndromes, *Am Fam Physician* 52:859, 1995.
Presberg KW: Respiratory failure. In Noble J (ed): *Primary care medicine,* ed 2, St Louis, 1996, Mosby.
Strollo PJ Jr, Rogers RM: Obstructive sleep apnea, *N Engl J Med* 334:99, 1996.
Author: **Fred F. Ferri, M.D.**

Somatization disorder

BASIC INFORMATION

DEFINITION
Somatization disorder refers to a pattern of recurring multiple somatic complaints that begin before the age of 30 yr and persist over several years. Patients complain of multiple sites of pain (a minimum of four), GI symptoms (a minimum of two), a sexual or reproductive symptom, and a pseudoneurologic symptom. These cannot be explained by a medical condition or are in excess to expected disability from a coexisting medical condition.

SYNONYMS
Briquet's syndrome
Nonorganic physical symptoms
Medically unexplained symptoms
Functional somatic symptoms

ICD-9-CM CODES
300.81 Somatization disorder

EPIDEMIOLOGY AND DEMOGRAPHICS
PREVALENCE (IN U.S.): Lifetime rates of 0.25% to 2% in women, <0.2% in men
PREDOMINANT SEX:
- Women are more commonly affected in the U.S.
- Males of other cultures (e.g., Greece and Puerto Rico) are more commonly affected.

PREDOMINANT AGE: By definition, onset occurs before age 30 yr.
PEAK INCIDENCE: Typically before age 25 yr
GENETICS:
- Genetic and environmental factors may be involved.
- There is a high risk of associated substance abuse or antisocial personality disorder.

PHYSICAL FINDINGS
- Typical patient is unmarried, non-white, poorly educated, and from rural setting.
- Onset is frequently in the teens; course is marked by frequent, unexplained, and frequently disabling pain and physical complaints.
- Patient frequently undergoes multiple procedures and seeks treatment from multiple physicians.
- Patient meets criteria for at least one other psychiatric condition, most commonly substance abuse disorders and personality disorders (antisocial disorder is the most common); anxiety and depressive disorders are also common.

ETIOLOGY
- Believed to be the physical expression of psychologic distress
- May be more common in individuals without sufficient verbal or intellectual capacity to communicate psychologic distress, individuals with alexithymia (inability to describe emotional states), or individuals from cultural backgrounds that consider emotional distress as an undesirable weakness
- Some aspects of somatization behavior possibly learned from somatizing patients

DIAGNOSIS

DIFFERENTIAL DIAGNOSIS
- Undifferentiated somatoform disorder (ICD-10 F45.1, DMS-IV 300.81): one or more physical complaints that cannot be explained by a medical condition is present for at least 6 mo (NOTE: Somatization is more severe and less common).
- Conversion disorder: there is an alteration or loss of voluntary motor or sensory function with demonstrable physical cause and related to a psychologic stress or a conflict (NOTE: With multiple complaints, the diagnosis of conversion is not made).
- Pain disorder: distinguished from somatization disorder by the presence of other somatic complaints.
- Munchausen's (factitious disorder) and malingering: the psychologic basis of the complaints in somatization disorder are not conscious as in factitious disorder (Munchausen's) and malingering, in which symptoms are produced intentionally.

WORKUP
- Rule out a general medical condition.
- If somatization is suspected on the basis of a history of repeated, multiple, unexplained complaints, restraint in ordering tests is recommended.

LABORATORY TESTS
No specific laboratory tests are required.

IMAGING STUDIES
No specific imaging studies are required.

TREATMENT

NONPHARMACOLOGIC THERAPY
- Legitimize patient's complaints; when this is not done, there is frequently an increase in complaints and associated disability.
- Minimize diagnostic investigation and symptomatic treatment.
- Set attainable treatment goals.
- Treat coexisting psychiatric conditions.

ACUTE GENERAL Rx
- No specific pharmacologic therapy is available.
- Antidepressants may be useful for coexisting anxiety and depression.

CHRONIC Rx
- A trusting relationship based on mutual respect between the patient and the physician is the best long-term treatment.
- If there is coexisting anxiety or depression, chronic use of antidepressants may be warranted.

DISPOSITION
A chronic condition with frequent exacerbations

REFERRAL
If therapy is required and the patient has the psychologic mindedness to participate

MISCELLANEOUS

REFERENCES
Ford CV: Dimensions of somatization and hypochondriasis, *Neurol Clin* 13:253, 1995.
Noyes R Jr, Holt CS, Kathol RG: Somatization: diagnosis and management, *Arch Fam Med* 4:790, 1995.
Author: **Rif S. El-Mallakh, M.D.**

Spinal cord compression

BASIC INFORMATION

DEFINITION
Spinal cord compression is the neurologic loss of spine function. Lesions may be complete or incomplete and develop gradually or acutely. Incomplete lesions often present as distinct syndromes, as follows:
- Central cord syndrome
- Anterior cord syndrome
- Brown-Sequard syndrome
- Conus medullaris syndrome
- Cauda equina syndrome

ICD-9-CM CODES
344.89 Brown-Sequard syndrome
344.60 Cauda equina syndrome
336.8 Conus medullaris syndrome
　　　Other lesions listed by site

PHYSICAL FINDINGS
Clinical features reflect the amount of spinal cord involvement:
- Motor loss and sensory abnormalities
- Babinski testing usually positive
- Clonus
- Gradual compression, often manifested by progressive difficulty walking, clonus with weight bearing, and involuntary spasm; development of sensory symptoms; bladder dysfunction (late)
- Central cord syndrome: results in a variable quadriparesis with the upper extremities more severely involved than the lower extremities; some sensory sparing
- Anterior cord syndrome: results in motor, pain, and temperature loss below the lesion
- Brown-Sequard syndrome:
  1. Spinal cord syndrome caused by injury to either half of the spinal cord and resulting in the loss of motor function, position, vibration, and light touch on the affected side
  2. Pain and temperature sense lost on the opposite side
- Conus medullaris syndrome: results in variable motor loss in the lower extremities with loss of bowel and bladder function
- Cauda equina syndrome: typical low back pain, weakness in both lower extremities, saddle anesthesia, and loss of voluntary bladder and bowel control

ETIOLOGY
- Trauma
- Tumor
- Infection
- Inflammatory processes
- Degenerative disc conditions with spinal stenosis
- Acute disc herniation
- Cystic abnormalities

DIAGNOSIS

DIFFERENTIAL DIAGNOSIS
- See "Etiology."
- Box 2-90 describes the differential diagnosis of paraplegia.

WORKUP
- Spinal cord compression: requires an immediate referral for radiographic and neurologic assessment
- Results usually unremarkable unless infectious or inflammatory causes suspected

IMAGING STUDIES
- Depend on the suspected etiology
- MRI usually required

TREATMENT

Urgent surgical decompression is usually indicated as soon as the etiology is established.

DISPOSITION
Important indicators regarding prognosis (see Leventhal in references):
- The greater the distal motor and sensory sparing, the greater the expected recovery.
- When a plateau of recovery is reached, no further improvement is expected.

REFERRAL
Immediate referral for radiographic and neurologic evaluation and treatment in all suspected cases of spinal cord compression

MISCELLANEOUS

REFERENCES
Kostuik JP et al: Cauda equina syndrome and lumbar disc herniation, *J Bone Joint Surg* 68(A)386, 1986.
Leventhal MR: Fractures, dislocations, and fracture-dislocations of spine. In Crenshaw AH (ed): *Campbell's operative orthopaedics,* ed 8, St Louis, 1992, Mosby, 1992.

Author: **Lonnie R. Mercier, M.D.**

Spontaneous miscarriage

BASIC INFORMATION

DEFINITION
Fetal loss before wk 20 of pregnancy, calculated from the patient's last menstrual period or the delivery of a fetus weighing <500 g. *Early loss* is before menstrual wk 12, while *late loss* refers to losses from 12 to 20 wk.
Miscarriage can also be classified as incomplete (partial passage of fetal tissue through partially dilated cervix), **complete** (spontaneous passage of all fetal tissue), **threatened** (uterine bleeding without cervical dilation or passage of tissue), **inevitable** (bleeding with cervical dilation without passage of fetal tissue), and **missed abortion** (intrauterine fetal demise without passage of tissue).
Recurrent miscarriage involves three or more spontaneous pregnancy losses before wk 20.

ICD-9-CM CODES
634.0 Spontaneous abortion

SYNONYMS
Abortion

EPIDEMIOLOGY AND DEMOGRAPHICS
INCIDENCE: 15% to 20% of clinically recognized pregnancies, with 80% of miscarriages occurring in the first trimester
RISK FACTORS: Prior pregnancy history (risk after live birth = 5%, prior pregnancy aborted = 20% subsequent risk) is the most significant risk factor. Vaginal bleeding, especially >3 days, carries with it a 15% to 20% chance of miscarriage.

GENETICS:
- Distribution of abnormal karyotypes: autosomal trisomy (50%), monosomy 45,X (20%), triploidy (15%), tetraploidy (10%), structural chromosomal abnormalities (5%).
- With two or more spontaneous miscarriages, a karyotype should be performed to evaluate for balanced translocation, which has 80% risk for abortion, and if the pregnancy is carried to term has 3% to 5% risk for unbalanced karyotype.
- After 9 wk, the later in gestation, the greater the chance of a normal karyotype.

PHYSICAL FINDINGS
- Profuse bleeding and cramping has a higher association with miscarriage than bleeding without cramping, which is more consistent with a threatened miscarriage.
- Cervical dilation with history or finding of fetal tissue at cervical os may be present.
- In cases of missed abortion, uterine size may be smaller than menstrual dating, in contrast to molar gestation, where size may be greater than dates.

ETIOLOGY
- In a general overview the etiology can be classified in terms of maternal (environmental) and fetal (genetic) factors, with the majority of miscarriages being related to genetic or chromosomal causes.
- Causes: uterine anomalies (unicornuate uterus risk = 50%, bicornuate or septae uterus, risk = 25% to 30%), incompetent cervix (iatrogenic or congenital, associated with 20% of midtrimester losses), diethylstilbestrol exposure in utero (T-shaped uterus), submucous leiomyomas, intrauterine adhesions or synechiae, luteal phase or progesterone deficiency, autoimmune disease such as anticardiolipin antibodies, uncontrolled diabetes mellitus, HLA associations between mother and father, infections such as TB, chlamydia, ureaplasma, smoking and alcohol use, irradiation, and environmental toxins

DIAGNOSIS

DIFFERENTIAL DIAGNOSIS
- Normal pregnancy
- Hydatidiform molar gestation
- Ectopic pregnancy
- Dysfunctional uterine bleeding
- Pathologic endometrial or cervical lesions

WORKUP
- Because of the potential for morbid maternal sequelae, all patients with bleeding in the first trimester should have an evaluation for possible ectopic pregnancy.
- Prior pregnancy history will guide the workup, such that if there are three early, prior, pregnancy losses a workup and treatment for recurrent miscarriage should begin before next conception, or if there is a strong history for second trimester loss, then consideration for cerclage should be given.
- Many of the treatments require preconceptual therapy, including control of disease processes, such as

diabetes, and thus a careful workup can begin after the prior pregnancy loss, but before conception.

LABORATORY TESTS
- Type and antibody screen is used to evaluate for the need for Rh immune globulin.
- In circumstances in which an ectopic gestation is considered, quantitative serum hCG can be used with transvaginal sonogram to assign a level of risk. 2000 mIU/ml (third reference standard) is the discriminatory zone above which an intrauterine gestational sac should be demonstrated.
- During the preconception period, Hgb A1C, anticardiolipin antibody, lupus anticoagulant, karyotyping, endometrial biopsy with progesterone level, and cervical cultures or serum antibodies can be checked for suspected disease processes.
- Progesterone level <5 mg/dl indicates nonviable gestation vs. >25 mg/dl, which confers a good prognosis.

IMAGING STUDIES
Transabdominal or transvaginal sonogram can be used in combination with menstrual dating and serum quantitative hCG to document pregnancy location, fetal heart presence, gestational sac size, adnexal pathology and, if used serially, can help confirm a missed abortion.

TREATMENT

NONPHARMACOLOGIC THERAPY
Depending on the patient's clinical status, desire to continue the pregnancy, and certainty of the diagnosis, expectancy can be considered. In pregnancies <6 wk or >14 wk, complete expulsion of fetal tissue occurs and surgical intervention such as dilation and curettage (D&C) can be avoided.

ACUTE GENERAL Rx
- **Incomplete miscarriage** between 6 and 14 wk can be associated with large amounts of blood loss, and thus these patients should undergo D&C.
- In the cases of **missed abortion,** if fetal demise has occurred >6 wk before or gestational age is >14 wk, there is an increased risk of hypofibrinogenemia with disseminated intravascular coagulation, and thus D&C should be performed early in the disease course.
- **Threatened abortions** may be managed expectantly, watching for signs of cervical dilation or sonographic evidence of missed abortion. Hormonal therapy, such as progesterone, is contraindicated during this time as it may increase the chance of missed abortion.
- If surgical intervention is required, preoperative use of 40 U of oxytocin (Pitocin) in 1000-ml lactated Ringer's solution may be used to decrease amount of bleeding and shorten the operative time.
- Postoperatively all patients undergoing a D&C should receive antibiotics (doxycycline 100 mg bid for 7 days), methylergonovine (Methergine) 0.2 mg q6h for four doses, and Motrin or NSAIDs PRN for pain.
- Preoperative laminaria is useful in cases a nondilated or primigravida cervices.
- In all cases of first or second trimester bleeding in Rh-negative patients, Rh immune globulin 300 μg should be given to prevent Rh sensitization.

CHRONIC Rx
Expectancy may be considered for those pregnancies <6 menstrual weeks depending on the clinical situation and the patients desire.

DISPOSITION
In most cases it is important to document the resolution of the pregnancy, either in terms of a pathology specimen from a D&C, or documentation of decreasing quantitative hCGs. If the pathology report does not confirm a miscarriage or the quantitative hCG values plateaus or rises postevacuation, the diagnosis of ectopic or molar gestation must be examined.

REFERRAL
In cases of ectopic gestation, incomplete or missed abortion, surgical evacuation of the uterus and possible laparoscopic evaluation of the adnexa should be undertaken by qualified personnel.

MISCELLANEOUS

REFERENCES
Herbst AL et al: *Comprehensive gynecology,* ed 2, St Louis, 1992, Mosby.
Warburton D: Reproductive loss: how much is preventable? *N Engl J Med* 316:158, 1987.

Author: **Scott J. Zuccala, D.O.**

Sporotrichosis

BASIC INFORMATION

DEFINITION
Sporotrichosis is a granulomatous disease caused by *Sporothrix schenckii*.

ICD-9-CM CODES
117.1 Sporotrichosis

EPIDEMIOLOGY AND DEMOGRAPHICS
PREDOMINANT SEX: Male in pulmonary sporotrichosis
PREDOMINANT AGE: 30 to 60 yr of age in pulmonary sporotrichosis
GENETICS:
Neonatal Infection: At least one case of transmission from the cheek lesion of the mother to the skin of the infant has been reported.

PHYSICAL FINDINGS
- Cutaneous disease
  1. Arises at the site of inoculation
  2. Initial lesion usually located on the distal part of an extremity, although any area may be affected, including the face
  3. Variable incubation period of approximately 3 wk once introduced into the skin
  4. Granulomatous reaction provoked
  5. Lesion becomes papulonodular, erythematous, elastic, variable in size
  6. Subsequently nodule becomes fluctuant, undergoes central necrosis, breaks down, discharges mucoid pus from which fungus may be isolated
  7. Indolent ulcer with raised erythematous or violaceous borders
  8. Secondary lesions:
     a. Develop along superficial lymphatic channels
     b. Evolve in the same manner as the primary lesion, with subsequent inflammation, induration and suppuration
- Fixed, or plaque form
  1. Erythematous verrucous, ulcerated or crusted lesions
  2. Does not spread locally
  3. Does not involve lymphatic vessels
  4. Rarely undergoes spontaneous resolution
  5. More often persists for years without systemic symptoms and within a setting of normal laboratory examinations
- Osteoarticular involvement
  1. Most common extracutaneous form
  2. Usually presents as monoarticular arthritis
  3. Left untreated, may progress to:
     a. Synovitis
     b. Osteitis
     c. Periostitis
     d. All involving elbows, knees, wrists, and ankles
  4. Joint inflamed
     a. Associated with an effusion
     b. Painful on motion
- Early pulmonary disease
  1. Usually associated with a paucity of clinical findings
     a. Low-grade fever
     b. Cough
     c. Fatigue
     d. Malaise
     e. Weight loss
  2. Untreated
     a. Cavitary pulmonary disease
     b. Frank pulmonary dysfunction
  3. Meningitis uncommon
     a. Except perhaps in the immunocompromised patient
     b. Presents with few signs or symptoms of neurologic involvement
  4. Few reported cases
     a. Infection of the ocular adnexa
     b. Endophthalmitis without antecedent trauma
     c. Infection of the testes and epididymis

ETIOLOGY
- *Sporothrix schenckii*
  1. Global in distribution
  2. Often isolated from soil, plants, and plant products
  3. Majority of case reports from tropical and subtropical regions of the Americas
- Occupational or recreational exposure
  1. Hay
  2. Straw
  3. Sphagnum moss
  4. Timber
  5. Thorny plants (e.g., roses and barberry bushes)
- Animal contact
  1. Armadillos
  2. Cats
  3. Squirrels
- Human-to-human transmission
- Tattooing

DIAGNOSIS

DIFFERENTIAL DIAGNOSIS
- Fixed, or plaque, sporotrichosis
  1. Bacterial pyoderma
  2. Foreign body granuloma
  3. Tularemia
  4. Anthrax
  5. Other mycoses: blastomycosis, chromoblastomycosis
- Lymphocutaneous sporotrichosis
  1. *Nocardia brasiliensis*
  2. *Leishmania brasiliensis*
  3. Atypical mycobacterial disease: *M. marinum*, *M. kansasii*
- Pulmonary sporotrichosis
  1. Pulmonary TB
  2. Histoplasmosis
  3. Coccidioidomycoses
- Osteoarticular sporotrichosis
  1. Pigmented villonodular synovitis
  2. Gout
  3. Rheumatoid arthritis
  4. Infection with *M. tuberculosis*
  5. Atypical mycobacteria: *M. marinum*, *M. kansasii*, *M. avium-intracellulare*
- Meningitis
  1. Histoplasmosis
  2. Cryptococcosis
  3. TB

WORKUP
- The diagnosis should be considered in individuals who are occupationally exposed to soil, decaying plant matter, and thorny plants (gardeners, horticulturists, farmers) who present with chronic nonhealing ulcers or lesions with or without associated arthritis or pulmonary symptoms.
- Diagnosis is made by culture:
  1. Pus
  2. Joint fluid
  3. Sputum
  4. Blood
  5. Skin biopsy
- Isolation of the fungus from any site is considered diagnostic of infection.
- Saprophytic colonization of the respiratory tract has been described.
- A positive blood culture may indicate infection in an immunocompromised host.
- Increasingly sensitive laboratory culturing systems may detect the fungus in the normal host.
- Biopsy specimens are diagnostic if characteristic cigar-shaped, round, oval, or budding yeast forms are seen.

- Despite special staining, the yeast may remain difficult to detect unless multiple sections are examined.
- No standard method of serologic testing is available.
- Previously described techniques have been hampered by the presence of antibody in the absence of infection.

LABORATORY TESTS
- CBCs and serum chemistries are generally normal.
- Elevated ESR is seen with extracutaneous disease.
- CSF analysis in meningeal disease reveals:
  1. Lymphocytic pleocytosis
  2. Elevated protein
  3. Hypoglycorrhachia

IMAGING STUDIES
- Chest x-ray examination: unilateral or bilateral upper lobe cavitary or noncavitary lesions
- Radiographic findings of affected joints:
  1. Loss of articular cartilage
  2. Periosteal reaction
  3. Periarticular osteopenia
  4. Cystic changes

TREATMENT

NONPHARMACOLOGIC THERAPY
Local heat and prevention of bacterial superinfection in cutaneous or plaque form

ACUTE GENERAL Rx
CUTANEOUS AND LYMPHOCUTANEOUS SPOROTRICHOSIS:
- Use saturated solution of potassium iodide (SSKI) 5 to 10 drops PO tid or 1.5 ml PO tid, gradually increasing to 40 to 50 drops PO tid or 3 ml PO tid after meals
- Maximum tolerated dose should be continued until cutaneous lesions have resolved, approximately 6 to 12 wk.
- Adjunctive therapy with heat is useful and occasionally curative.
- Side effects:
  1. Nausea
  2. Anorexia
  3. Diarrhea
  4. Parotid or lacrimal gland hypertrophy
  5. Acneiform rash
- Itraconazole at doses of 100 to 200 mg/day is effective if iodide therapy is unsuccessful, poorly tolerated, or contraindicated because of drug hypersensitivity
- Because of its increased cost, itraconazole should not be first line therapy for cutaneous disease.

OSTEOARTICULAR SPOROTRICHOSIS:
- Parenteral amphotericin B, total course of 2 to 2.5 g or more results in cure in approximately two thirds of cases.
- Relapses are common.
- Isolates of *Sporothrix schenckii* are resistant to amphotericin B.
- Intraarticular administration of amphotericin B and surgical debridement have been used but without clearly defined efficacy.
- Itraconazole:
  1. Effective
  2. Less toxic than amphotericin B
  3. Better tolerated than ketoconazole
  4. Appropriate initial chemotherapy (although not FDA approved)
  5. 200 to 600 mg qd in divided doses bid, for the first 6 mo with 200 mg given qd thereafter for an extended, and as yet undefined, time period
  6. Absence of relapses at 68 mo have been documented when doses of at least 200 mg/day administered for 24 mo.

NONCAVITARY PULMONARY DISEASE:
- SSKI
- Amphotericin B
- For advanced or cavitary disease:
  1. Surgical resection
  2. Perioperative administration of amphotericin B
- Azoles:
  1. High relapse rate
  2. Slow response to therapy

MENINGITIS:
- Amphotericin B alone or in combination with 5-fluorocytosine
- No data on the use of azoles

CHRONIC Rx
For lymphocutaneous and visceral disease, therapy with itraconazole 200 mg/day for periods of 24 mo or greater

DISPOSITION
- Prognosis for cutaneous disease is good.
- Prognosis is less satisfactory for extracutaneous disease, especially if associated with abnormal immunologic states or other underlying systemic diseases.

REFERRAL
To surgeon; with an established diagnosis of pulmonary sporotrichosis, cavitary lesions require resection of involved tissue

MISCELLANEOUS

COMMENTS
- In patients with underlying immunosuppression (e.g., hematologic malignancy or infection with HIV), progression of the initial infection may develop into multifocal extracutaneous sporotrichosis.
- In this subset of patients, dissemination of cutaneous lesions is accompanied by hematogenous spread to lungs, bone, mucous membranes, CNS
- Osteoarticular and pulmonary manifestations predominate with the development of polyarticular arthritis and osteolytic bone lesions.
- In the absence of therapy, the infection is ultimately fatal.
- Patients with underlying immunosuppressive states should be carefully evaluated even when presenting with single cutaneous lesions.
- Diagnostic modalities should include:
  1. Radiographic examination of chest
  2. Technetium pyrophosphate bone scan
  3. Culture of synovial fluid, blood, skin lesion(s)

REFERENCES
Badley AD, Van Scoy RE: Long term follow-up of multifocal osteoarticular sporotrichosis treated with itraconazole, *Clin Infect Dis* 23:394, 1996.

Kauffman CA: Role of azoles in antifungal therapy, *Clin Infect Dis* 22(suppl 2):S148, 1996.

Kauffman CA et al: Treatment of lymphocutaneous and visceral sporotrichosis with fluconazole, *Clin Infect Dis* 22:46, 1996.

Rios-Fabra A et al: Fungal infection in Latin American countries, *Infect Dis Clin North Am* 8(1):129, 1994.

Author: **George O. Alonso, M.D.**

Squamous cell carcinoma

BASIC INFORMATION

DEFINITION
Squamous cell carcinoma (SCC) is a malignant tumor of the skin arising in the epithelium.

SYNONYMS
SCC
Skin cancer

ICD-9-CM CODES
173.9 Skin neoplasm, site unspecified

EPIDEMIOLOGY AND DEMOGRAPHICS
- SCC is the second most common cutaneous malignancy.
- Incidence is highest in lower latitudes (e.g., southern U.S., Australia).
- Male:female ratio is 2:1.
- Incidence increases with age and sun exposure.
- Average age at diagnosis is 66 yr.

PHYSICAL FINDINGS
- SCC commonly affects scalp, back of hands, superior surface of the pinna, and the lip.
- The lesion may have a scaly, erythematous macule or plaque.
- Telangiectasia, central ulceration may also be present (see color plate 19).

ETIOLOGY
Risk factors include UVB radiation and immunosuppression (renal transplant recipients have a threefold increased risk).

DIAGNOSIS

DIFFERENTIAL DIAGNOSIS
- Keratoacanthomas
- Actinic keratosis

WORKUP
Diagnosis is made with biopsy.

TREATMENT

ACUTE GENERAL Rx
- Electrodesiccation and curettage for small SCCs.
- Tumors thinner than 4 mm can be managed by simple local removal.
- Lesions between 4 and 8 mm thick or those with deep dermal invasion should undergo excision.
- Tumors penetrating the dermis can be treated with several modalities, including excision and Mohs' surgery, radiation therapy, and chemotherapy.
- Metastatic SCC can be treated with chemotherapy using 13-*cis*-retinoic acid and interferon α-2A.

DISPOSITION
- Survival is related to size, location, degree of differentiation, immunologic status of the patient, depth of invasion, and presence of metastases.
- Patients whose tumors penetrate through the dermis or exceed 8 mm in thickness are at the risk of recurrence.
- Tumors on the scalp, forehead, ears, nose, and lips also carry a higher risk.
- SCCs originating in the lip and pinna metastasize in 10% to 20% of cases.

REFERRAL
Oncology referral for metastatic SCC

MISCELLANEOUS

COMMENTS
- SCC arising in areas of prior radiation, thermal injury, and areas of chronic ulcers or chronic draining sinuses are more aggressive and have a higher frequency of metastases than those originating in actinic damaged skin.
- U.S. Preventive Services Task Force Recommendations regarding screening for skin cancer are described in Section V, Chapter 12.

REFERENCES
Habif, TP: *Clinical dermatology*, ed 3, St Louis, 1996, Mosby.
Lawrence N, Cottel WI: Squamous cell carcinoma of skin with perineural invasion, *J Am Acad Dermatol* 31:30, 1994.
Author: **Fred F. Ferri, M.D.**

Status epilepticus

BASIC INFORMATION

DEFINITION
The term *status epilepticus* refers to >30 min of: (1) continuous seizure activity or (2) two or more sequential seizures without full recovery of consciousness between seizures.

ICD-9-CM CODES
345.3 Grand mal status

EPIDEMIOLOGY AND DEMOGRAPHICS
INCIDENCE (IN U.S.): 61 cases/100,000 persons/yr
PREDOMINANT SEX: Male = female
PREDOMINANT AGE: >60 yr
PEAK INCIDENCE: <1 yr and >60 yr
GENETICS: Familial predisposition is rare.

PHYSICAL FINDINGS
- Findings depend on underlying etiology and duration.
- Convulsive seizures may evolve into subtle face or eye movements or into an appearance of coma despite ongoing electrographic seizure activity.

ETIOLOGY
- Stroke
- Systemic infection
- Low antiepileptic drug levels
- Remote CNS insult

DIAGNOSIS

DIFFERENTIAL DIAGNOSIS
- Coma
- Encephalopathic states
- Psychogenic unresponsiveness

WORKUP
Because convulsive and complex partial status epilepticus are emergencies with substantial morbidity and mortality, treatment must be early and aggressive, not postponed until an etiology is determined.

LABORATORY TESTS
- While treatment is being initiated: glucose, electrolytes, BUN, ABG, drug levels, CBC, UA
- Lumbar puncture in children with fever and adults suspected to have meningitis

IMAGING STUDIES
Unless the etiology is known, CT scan is recommended as soon as possible after seizures have been controlled.

TREATMENT

NONPHARMACOLOGIC THERAPY
- Give oxygen by nasal cannula.
- Maintain blood pressure.
- Maintain body temperature.
- Monitor ECG.
- Obtain IV access.

ACUTE GENERAL Rx
- Thiamine 100 mg IV and glucose 50 mg D_{50} by IV push (2 ml/kg D_{25} in children) unless hyperglycemic
- Lorazepam 0.1 mg/kg IV at 2 mg/min
- If seizures persist, fosphenytoin 20 mg/kg IV at 150 mg/min (if not available use phenytoin at up to 50 mg/min as tolerated)
- If seizures persist, phenobarbital 20 mg/kg IV at 100 mg/min; will likely require intubation
- If seizures persist, emergency neurologic consultation

CHRONIC Rx
- A single episode with an identifiable and easily correctable provoking factor (e.g., hyponatremia) does not warrant long-term use of anticonvulsants.
- Treatment is indicated if there is significant risk of recurrence (e.g., known epilepsy, brain lesion, epileptiform EEG abnormalities).
- Table 7-6 compares the various anticonvulsant drugs.

DISPOSITION
- Favorable if status is treated promptly and no acute brain lesion is present
- Overall mortality of 22%; higher in the elderly (38%) and substantially lower in children (2.5%)

REFERRAL
If seizures do not respond to initial management as outlined

MISCELLANEOUS

COMMENTS
- Because of varied clinical presentations of status epilepticus, there are no clinical grounds of certainty that seizures have stopped unless the patient regains full consciousness.
- EEG provides definitive information about seizure cessation. If available, use of EEG in the management of status epilepticus is recommended highly.

REFERENCES
Working Group on Status Epilepticus: Treatment of convulsive status epilepticus, *JAMA* 270:854, 1993.
Author: **Michael Gruenthal, M.D., Ph.D.**

Stevens-Johnson syndrome (PTG)

BASIC INFORMATION

DEFINITION
Stevens-Johnson syndrome (SJS) is a severe vesiculobullous form of erythema multiforme affecting skin, mouth, eyes, and genitalia.

SYNONYMS
SJS
Herpes iris
Febrile mucocutaneous syndrome

ICD-9-CM CODES
695.1 Stevens-Johnson syndrome

EPIDEMIOLOGY AND DEMOGRAPHICS
- SJS affects predominantly children and young adults.
- Male:female ratio is 2:1.

PHYSICAL FINDINGS
- The cutaneous eruption is generally preceded by vague, nonspecific symptoms of low-grade fever and fatigue occurring 1 to 14 days before the skin lesions. Cough is often present. Fever may be high during the active stages.
- Bullae generally occur on the conjunctiva, mucous membranes of the mouth, nares, genital regions.
- Corneal ulcerations may result in blindness.
- Ulcerative stomatitis results in hemorrhagic crusting.
- Flat, atypical target lesions or purpuric maculae may be distributed on the trunk or be widespread (see color plate 20).
- The pain from oral lesions may compromise fluid intake and result in dehydration.
- Thick, mucopurulent sputum and oral lesions may interfere with breathing.

ETIOLOGY
- Drugs (e.g., phenytoin, penicillins, phenobarbital, sulfonamides) are the most common cause.
- Upper respiratory tract infections (e.g., *Mycoplasma pneumoniae*), and herpes simplex viral infections have also been implicated in SJS.

DIAGNOSIS

DIFFERENTIAL DIAGNOSIS
- Toxic erythema (drugs or infection)
- Pemphigus
- Pemphigoid
- Urticaria
- Hemorrhagic fevers
- Serum sickness
- *Staphylococcus* scalded-skin syndrome
- Behçet's syndrome

WORKUP
- Diagnosis is generally based on clinical presentation and characteristic appearance of the lesions.
- Skin biopsy is generally reserved for when classic lesions are absent and diagnosis is uncertain.

LABORATORY TESTS
CBC with differential, cultures in cases of suspected infection

IMAGING STUDIES
Chest x-ray examination may show patchy changes in patients with pulmonary involvement.

TREATMENT

NONPHARMACOLOGIC THERAPY
- Withdrawal of any potential drug precipitants
- Careful skin nursing to prevent secondary infection

ACUTE GENERAL Rx
- Treatment of associated conditions, (e.g., acyclovir for herpes simplex virus infection, erythromycin for mycoplasma infection)
- Antihistamines for pruritus
- Treatment of the cutaneous blisters with cool, wet Burow's compresses
- Relief of oral symptoms by frequent rinsing with lidocaine (xylocaine viscous)
- Liquid or soft diet with plenty of fluids to ensure proper hydration
- Treatment of secondary infections with antibiotics
- Corticosteroids: use remains controversial; when used, prednisone 20 to 30 mg bid until new lesions no longer appear, then rapidly tapered
- Topical steroids: may use to treat papules and plaques; however, should not be applied to eroded areas
- Vitamin A: may be used for lacrimal hyposecretion

DISPOSITION
- Prognosis varies with severity of disease. It is generally good in patients with limited disease; however, mortality may approach 10% in patients with extensive involvement.
- Oral lesions may continue for several months.
- Scarring and corneal abnormalities may occur in 20% of patients.

REFERRAL
- Hospital admission in a unit used for burn care is recommended in severe cases.
- Urethral involvement may necessitate catheterization.
- Ocular involvement should be monitored by an ophthalmologist.

MISCELLANEOUS

COMMENTS
Risk of recurrence of SJS is 30% to 40%.

REFERENCES
Cote D et al: Clinical pathological relation of erythema multiforme and Stevens-Johnson syndromes, *Arch Dermatol* 131:1268, 1995.
Habif TP: *Clinical dermatology,* ed 3, St Louis, 1996, Mosby.
Author: **Fred F. Ferri, M.D.**

BASIC INFORMATION

DEFINITION
Strabismus is a condition of the eyes in which the visual axes of the eyes are not straight in the primary position or where the eyes do not follow each other in the different positions of gaze.

SYNONYMS
Esotropia
Exotropia
Restrictive eye movement

ICD-9-CM CODES
378.9 Strabismus

EPIDEMIOLOGY AND DEMOGRAPHICS
INCIDENCE (IN U.S.): 2% of all children
PREDOMINANT SEX: None
PREDOMINANT AGE: Birth to 5 yr of age
PEAK INCIDENCE: Childhood
GENETICS: None known

PHYSICAL FINDINGS
Conjugate gaze loss in both eyes with the eyes focusing independently

ETIOLOGY
- Most cases are congenital.
- Rarely, there is neurologic disease or severe refractive errors.

DIAGNOSIS

DIFFERENTIAL DIAGNOSIS
- Refractive errors
- CNS tumors
- Orbital tumors
- Brain and CNS dysfunction

WORKUP
- Eye examination
- Visual field refraction

LABORATORY TESTS
Generally not needed

IMAGING STUDIES
Necessary only if other neurologic findings are found

TREATMENT

NONPHARMACOLOGIC THERAPY
- Glasses
- Patching
- Prisms

CHRONIC Rx
- Glasses
- Alternate eye-patching
- Surgery

DISPOSITION
- The earlier the condition is treated, the more likely it is that the child will have normal vision in both eyes.
- After age 5 yr, visual loss is usually permanent.

REFERRAL
- If surgery is contemplated
- To an ophthalmologist for management (usually)

MISCELLANEOUS

COMMENTS
- If properly treated, this easily recognizable and treatable condition results in normal vision.
- If not treated, this condition will result in blindness in one eye.

REFERENCES
Campos ED: Update on strabismus and amblyopia, *Acta Ophthalmol Suppl* 214:17, 1995.
Author: Melvyn Koby, M.D.

Subarachnoid hemorrhage

BASIC INFORMATION

DEFINITION
Subarachnoid hemorrhage is mechanical disruption of an intracranial portion of the vascular system resulting in entry of blood into the subarachnoid space.

ICD-9-CM CODES
430 Subarachnoid hemorrhage

EPIDEMIOLOGY AND DEMOGRAPHICS
INCIDENCE (IN U.S.): 6 to 28 cases/100,000 persons/yr
PREDOMINANT SEX: Males > females in persons <40 yr of age; then female:male ratio of 3:2 in persons >40 yr old
PREDOMINANT AGE: >50 yr
PEAK INCIDENCE: 50 to 60 yr
GENETICS:
- Familial predisposition to multiple aneurysms
- Increased incidence in some inherited systemic diseases

PHYSICAL FINDINGS
- Patients typically present with abrupt onset of a severe headache of maximal intensity ("the worse headache of my life"), accompanied by nuchal rigidity, nausea, and vomiting.
- Transient loss of consciousness occurs in 45% of patients.
- Focal neurologic deficits may be present.
- Funduscopic examination may reveal subhyaloid hemorrhage.

ETIOLOGY
- Two thirds of cases: rupture of saccular ("berry") aneurysms
- Others: fusiform, mycotic, traumatic, dissecting and tumor-related aneurysms

DIAGNOSIS

DIFFERENTIAL DIAGNOSIS
- Intraparenchymal hemorrhage
- Meningitis

WORKUP
- CT scan without contrast is initial test of choice, with a sensitivity of about 90%.
- If CT scan is negative or unavailable, do lumbar puncture.

LABORATORY TESTS
CSF analysis for cell counts and xanthochromia

IMAGING STUDIES
CT scan followed by cerebral angiography if hemorrhage is confirmed

TREATMENT

NONPHARMACOLOGIC THERAPY
- Intubation as necessary
- Bed rest

ACUTE GENERAL Rx
- Short-acting analgesics (e.g., morphine 1 to 4 mg IV)
- Sedation (e.g., midazolam 1 to 5 mg IV)
- Stool softeners

CHRONIC Rx
- Seizure prophylaxis (phenytoin 15 to 20 mg/kg IV)
- Vasospasm prophylaxis (nimodipine 60 mg PO q4h)
- BP control (e.g., labetalol 10 to 40 mg IV q30min)

DISPOSITION
Approximately 35% early mortality, 45% at 1 mo

REFERRAL
Transfer as soon as possible to a facility with neurosurgical care.

MISCELLANEOUS

COMMENTS
About 20% of patients experience warning signs within 3 mo before aneurysm rupture, including moderate or severe headache ("sentinel headache"), dizziness, nausea and vomiting, transient motor or sensory deficits, loss of consciousness, or visual disturbances.

REFERENCES
Miller J, Diringer M: Management of aneurysmal subarachnoid hemorrhage, *Neurol Clin* 13:451, 1995.

Author: **Michael Gruenthal, M.D., Ph.D.**

Suicide (PTG)

BASIC INFORMATION

DEFINITION
Suicide refers to the successful and unsuccessful attempts to kill one's self.

SYNONYMS
Self-murder

ICD-9-CM CODES
Categorized by method (e.g., poisoning)

EPIDEMIOLOGY AND DEMOGRAPHICS
INCIDENCE (IN U.S.):
- 11.4 cases/100,000 persons; 1.4% of total deaths
- 18.8/100,000 men
- 4.3/100,000 women

PREDOMINANT AGE: Increases with age, e.g. 13.1 cases/100,000 persons aged 15 to 24 yr; 16.9 cases/100,000 persons aged 65 to 74 yr; and 23.5 cases/100,000 persons aged 75 to 84 yr

PEAK INCIDENCE: >65 yr of age

GENETICS:
- Biologic factors may increase the risk of suicide directly (e.g., by increasing impulsivity), or indirectly (e.g., by predisposing to a mental illness).
- Family history of suicide is associated with suicidal behavior.

PHYSICAL FINDINGS
Methods used in attempted (unsuccessful) suicides differ from those used in completed suicides.
- Overdose used in >70% of attempted suicides. Cutting of wrists or other parts of the body is the second most common form.
- About 60% of completed suicides are accomplished with firearms. Hanging is the second most common method for completed suicides. Suffocation (e.g., carbon monoxide) and overdose are also relatively common forms of completing suicide.
- Several risk factors are usually present concurrently, including a psychiatric illness such as depression or anxiety, middle-age or advanced age, white race, male gender, a recent divorce or separation, comorbid substance abuse particularly when intoxicated, previous history of suicide attempts, fatal plan (e.g., firearms or hanging), history of violence, and family history of suicide. Concurrent chronic physical illness increases the risk for suicide greatly (e.g., the risk for suicide among AIDS or renal dialysis patients is nearly thirty times that of the general population).

ETIOLOGY
- Individuals with a mental or a substance abuse disorder are responsible for >90% of all suicides.
- The co-occurrence of more than one condition (e.g., depression and alcohol abuse) greatly increases the risk of suicide.
- Hopelessness is a strong predictor of suicide potential.

DIAGNOSIS

DIFFERENTIAL DIAGNOSIS
- Some disorders are associated with self-injurious behavior that is not suicidal. Borderline personality disorder, e.g., manifests with self-mutilation without active suicidal intent. Eating disorders are harmful and may be fatal, but death is never the goal.
- Some suicidal behavior is intended as a "call for help." In these situations the individual usually designs the suicide so that they will be discovered before significant damage has been done.

WORKUP
- Suicidal patients present in one of four ways:
  1. Covert suicidal ideation
  2. Overt suicidal ideation
  3. After a suicide attempt
  4. Dead from a suicide attempt
- Covert suicidal ideation occurs in patients primarily with multiple vague physical complaints, depression, anxiety, or substance abuse.
- As part of the history, the physician must directly inquire into the presence of suicidal ideation.
- The co-occurrence of multiple psychiatric problems, substance abuse, and multiple physical problems increases the risk.

TREATMENT

NONPHARMACOLOGIC THERAPY
- Major immediate intervention: placement of the patient in a safe environment (usually hospitalization in a psychiatric unit or a medical unit with continuous observation)
- Long-term: psychotherapy aimed at factors that underlie the decision to pursue suicide or at the risk factors contributing to suicidal behavior
- Substance abuse treatment (e.g., AA, NA) when substance abuse is present

ACUTE GENERAL Rx
- Benzodiazepines are useful in reducing the extreme anxiety and dysphoria in a suicidal patient; however, these agents are depressive and should be used only when patient is in safe environment.
- Antipsychotics can be used if psychosis is present (e.g., voices telling patient to hurt themselves).
- Mood stabilizers and antidepressants should be started in the acute setting but may have up to a 2-wk latency period.

CHRONIC Rx
- Therapy should be aimed at the underlying condition (e.g., antidepressants for depression, anxiolytics or antidepressants for anxiety, ongoing substance abuse treatment for substance abuse history, or psychotherapy for chronic low self-esteem, hopelessness).
- In elderly, loneliness and medical disability are major reasons for suicide and therefore major targets for intervention.

DISPOSITION
- Prior suicide attempt is the best predictor for completed suicides (i.e., patients who attempt suicide once are at high risk for completing suicide in the future).
- Conditions associated with suicide (e.g., depression, physical ailments) are usually chronic and recurring.

REFERRAL
If patient is acutely suicidal and requires protection in hospital

MISCELLANEOUS

COMMENTS
U.S. Preventive Services Task Force Recommendations regarding screening for suicide risk are described in Section V, Chapter 50.

REFERENCES
Buzan RD, Meissberg MP: Suicide: risk factors and therapeutic considerations in the emergency department, *J Emer Med* 10:335, 1992.

Moscicki EK: Epidemiology of suicidal behavior, *Suicide Life Threat Behav* 25:22, 1995.

Author: **Rif S. El-Mallakh, M.D.**

Syncope (PTG)

BASIC INFORMATION

DEFINITION
Syncope is the temporary loss of consciousness resulting from an acute global reduction in cerebral blood flow.

ICD-9-CM CODES
720.2 Syncope

EPIDEMIOLOGY AND DEMOGRAPHICS
- Syncope accounts for 3% to 5% of emergency room visits.
- 30% of the adult population will experience at least one syncopal episode during their lifetime.
- Incidence of syncope is highest in elderly men and young women.

PHYSICAL FINDINGS
- Blood pressure: if low, consider orthostatic hypertension; if unequal in both arms (difference >20 mm Hg), consider subclavian steal or dissecting aneurysm. (NOTE: Blood pressure and heart rate should be recorded in the supine, sitting, and standing positions.)
- Pulse: if patient has tachycardia, bradycardia, or irregular rhythm, consider dysrhythmia.
- Mental status: if patient is confused after the "syncopal episode," consider postictal state.
- Heart: if there are murmurs present suggestive of AS or IHSS, consider syncope secondary to left ventricular outflow obstruction; if there are JVD and distal heart sounds, consider cardiac tamponade.
- Carotid sinus pressure: can be diagnostic if it reproduces symptoms and other causes are excluded; a pause >3 sec or a systolic BP drop >50 mm Hg without symptoms or <30 mm Hg with symptoms when sinus pressure is applied separately on each side for <5 sec is considered abnormal. This test should be avoided in patients with carotid bruits or cerebrovascular disease; ECG monitoring, IV access, and bedside atropine should be available when carotid sinus pressure is applied.

ETIOLOGY
- Vasovagal (vasodepressor)
  1. Psychophysiologic (panic disorders, hysteria)
  2. Visceral reflex
  3. Carotid sinus
  4. Glossopharyngeal neuralgia
  5. Reduction of venous return caused by Valsalva maneuver, cough, defecation, or micturition
- Orthostatic hypotension
  1. Hypovolemia
  2. Antihypertensive drugs
  3. Neurogenic, idiopathic
  4. Pheochromocytoma
  5. Systemic mastocytosis
- Cardiac
  1. Reduced cardiac output
     a. Left ventricular outflow obstruction (aortic stenosis, hypertrophic cardiomyopathy)
     b. Obstruction to pulmonary flow (pulmonary embolism, pulmonic stenosis, primary pulmonary hypertension)
     c. MI with pump failure
     d. Cardiac tamponade
     e. Mitral stenosis
  2. Dysrhythmias or asystole
     a. Extreme tachycardia (>160 to 180 bpm)
     b. Severe bradycardia (<30 to 40 bpm)
     c. Sick sinus syndrome
     d. AV block (second- or third-degree)
     e. Ventricular tachycardia or fibrillation
     f. Long QT syndrome
     g. Pacemaker malfunction
- Cardiovascular
  1. Vertebrobasilar TIA, spasm
  2. Subclavian steal
  3. Basilar migraine
  4. Colloid cyst of the third ventricle
- Other causes
  1. Mechanical reduction of venous return (atrial myxoma, valve thrombus)
  2. Not related to decreased blood flow: hypoxia, hypoglycemia, anemia, hyperventilation, seizure disorder, drug or alcohol abuse

DIAGNOSIS

DIFFERENTIAL DIAGNOSIS
See "Workup."

WORKUP
- Sudden loss of consciousness: consider cardiac arrhythmias, vertebrobasilar TIA.
- Gradual loss of consciousness: consider orthostatic hypotension, vasodepressor syncope, hypoglycemia.
- Patient's activity at the time of syncope:
  1. Micturition, coughing, defecation: consider syncope secondary to decreased venous return.
  2. Turning head while shaving: consider carotid sinus syndrome.
  3. Physical exertion in a patient with murmur: consider aortic stenosis.
  4. Arm exercise: consider subclavian steal syndrome.
  5. Assuming an upright position: consider orthostatic hypotension.

- Associated events:
  1. Chest pain: consider MI, pulmonary embolism.
  2. Palpitations: consider dysrhythmias.
  3. History of aura, incontinence during episode, and transient confusion after syncope: consider seizure disorder.
  4. Psychological stress: syncope may be vasovagal.
- Review current medications, particularly antihypertensive drugs.

LABORATORY TESTS
- CBC to rule out anemia, infection
- Electrolytes, BUN, creatinine, magnesium, calcium to rule out electrolyte abnormalities and evaluate fluid status
- ECG to rule out arrhythmias; may be diagnostic in 5% to 10% of patients
- ABGs to rule out pulmonary embolus, hyperventilation (when suspected)

IMAGING STUDIES
- Echocardiogram is useful in patients with a heart murmur to rule out AS, IHSS, or atrial myxoma.
- If seizure is suspected, CT scan of the head and EEG are indicated.
- If pulmonary embolism is suspected, ventilation-perfusion scan should be done.
- If arrhythmias are suspected, a 24-hr Holter monitor and admission to a telemetry unit is appropriate; loop recorders that can be activated after syncopal episode and retrieve information about the cardiac rhythm during the preceding 4 min add considerable diagnostic yield in patients with unexplained syncope.
- Evaluate drug and alcohol levels when suspecting toxicity.

- Cardiac isoenzymes should be obtained if the patient gives a history of chest pain before the syncopal episode.
- Electrophysiologic studies may be indicated in patients with structural heart disease and/or recurrent syncope.

TILT TABLE TESTING:
- Useful to support a diagnosis of neurocardiogenic syncope.
- Indicated in patients with recurrent episodes of unexplained syncope.
- It is performed by keeping the patient in an upright posture on a tilt table with footboard support. The angle of the tilt table varies from 60 to 80 degrees. The duration of upright posture during tilt table testing varies from 25 to 45 min. Pharmacologic provocation with graded isoproterenol infusions can be used in selected patients.
- The hallmarks of neural cardiogenic syncope are severe hypotension associated with a paradoxical bradycardia after a period of symptomatic excitation. The diagnosis of neurocardiogenic syncope is likely if upright-tilt testing without the infusion of isoproterenol reproduces these hemodynamic changes in <15 min and causes presyncope or syncope.

TREATMENT

NONPHARMACOLOGIC THERAPY
- Ensure proper hydration.
- Eliminate medications that may induce hypotension.

ACUTE GENERAL Rx
- Varies with the underlying etiology of syncope (e.g., pacemaker in patients with syncope secondary to complete heart block).
- Metoprolol or isopropamide may be useful in the treatment of neurocardiogenic syncope.

DISPOSITION
Prognosis varies with the age of the patient and the etiology of the syncope. Generally:
- Benign prognosis (very low, 1-yr morbidity) in patients:
  1. Age <30 yr and having noncardiac syncope
  2. Age <70 yr and having vasovagal/psychogenic syncope or syncope of unknown cause
- Poor prognosis (high mortality and morbidity) in patients with cardiac syncope

REFERRAL
Hospital admission in elderly patients without a prior history of syncope or unknown etiology of their syncope and in any patients suspected of having cardiac syncope.

MISCELLANEOUS

COMMENTS
The etiology of syncope is identified in <50% of cases during the initial evaluation.

REFERENCES
Abboud FM: Neural cardiogenic syncope, *N Engl J Med* 328:11, 1993.
Kapoor WN: Workup and management of patients with syncope, *Med Clin North Am* 79:1153, 1995.
Linzer M et al: Diagnosing syncope, *Ann Int Med* (part I) 126:989, (part II) 127:76, 1997.

Author: **Fred F. Ferri, M.D.**

Syphilis (PTG)

BASIC INFORMATION

DEFINITION
Syphilis is a sexually transmitted treponemal disease, acute and chronic, characterized by primary skin lesion, secondary eruption involving skin and mucous membranes, long periods of latency, and late lesions of skin, bone, viscera, CNS, and cardiovascular system.

SYNONYMS
Lues

ICD-9-CM CODES
097.9 Syphilis, acquired unspecified

EPIDEMIOLOGY AND DEMOGRAPHICS
- Widespread, primarily involving ages 20 to 35 yr. Racial differences in incidence are related to social factors. Usually more prevalent in urban areas. Estimated annual incidence of 90,000 cases in the U.S. Increase in incidence in the late 1980s to 1990s, likely related to illicit drug use and prostitution. Increase occurred primarily in lower socioeconomic groups.
- Communicability is indefinite and variable. Communicable during primary, secondary, and latent mucocutaneous lesions in up to first 4 yr of latency. Most probable congenital transmission occurs in early maternal syphilis. Adequate penicillin treatment ends infectivity within 24 to 48 hr.

PHYSICAL FINDINGS
PRIMARY SYPHILIS: Characteristic lesion is a painless chancre on genitalia, mouth, or anus; atypical primary lesions may occur. Usually appears 3 wk after exposure and may spontaneously involute.

SECONDARY SYPHILIS:
- Localized or diffuse mucocutaneous lesions and generalized lymphadenopathy. Common to have constitutional symptoms, flulike symptoms. May begin about 4 to 6 wk after appearance of primary lesion. Manifestations may resolve in 1 wk to 12 mo.
- 60% to 80% of patients have maculopapular lesions on their palms and soles.
- Condylomata latum intertriginous papules form at areas of friction and moisture such as the vulva.
- 21% to 58% have mucocutaneous or mucosal lesions (pharyngitis, tonsillitis, "mucous patch" lesion on oral and genital mucosa).

EARLY LATENT (<1 YR): Generally asymptomatic.

LATE LATENT (>1 YR):
- Characterized by gummas (nodular, ulcerative lesions) that can involve the skin, mucous membranes, skeletal system, and viscera.
- Manifestations of cardiovascular syphilis include aortitis, aneurysm, or aortic regurgitation.
- Neurosyphilis may be asymptomatic or symptomatic. Tabes dorsalis, meningovascular syphilis, general paralysis of the insane. Iritis, choroidoretinitis, and leukoplakia may also occur.

ETIOLOGY
- *Treponema pallidum,* a spirochete
- Spread by sexual intercourse or by intrauterine transfer

DIAGNOSIS

DIFFERENTIAL DIAGNOSIS
- Other genitoulcerative diseases such as herpes, chancroid.
- See Fig. 3-33 for a clinical algorithm for the evaluation of genital ulcer disease.

WORKUP
Confirmation is primarily through laboratory diagnosis.

LABORATORY TESTS
- Dark-field microscopy of fluid from lesion to look for treponeme
- Serologic testing, both nontreponemal (VDRL, RPR) and treponemal (FTA, MHA)
- Lumbar puncture for CSF VDRL in patients with evident of latent syphilis

TREATMENT

ACUTE GENERAL Rx
- Early (primary, secondary, early latent): penicillin G benzathine 2.4 million U IM × 1 or doxycycline 100 mg PO bid × 14 days
- Late (late latent, cardiovascular, gumma): penicillin G benzathine 2.4 million U IM every week × 3 wk or doxycycline 100 mg PO bid × 4 wk
- Neurosyphilis: penicillin G 2 to 4 million U IV q4h × 10 to 14 days or penicillin G procaine 2.4 million U IM qd plus probenecid 500 mg qid, both for 10 to 14 days
- Congenital syphilis: penicillin G 50,000 U/kg IM or IV q8-12h × 10 to 14 days OR penicillin G procaine 50,000 U/kg IM qd × 10 to 14 days
- Tetracyclines are contraindicated in pregnancy. If pregnant and penicillin-allergic, must be desensitized.

DISPOSITION
- Repeat quantitative nontreponemal tests at 3, 6, and 12 mo. Pregnancy requires monthly tests until delivery.
- If a fourfold increase in titer occurs, if initial high titer fails to drop by fourfold within a year, or persistent signs, retreatment may be indicated. Use treatment regimen for late syphilis.
- Pregnant women without a fourfold drop in titer in a 3-mo period need to be retreated.
- Cases should be reported to local or state health department for referral, follow-up, and partner notification.

REFERRAL
- Pregnant and possible congenital syphilis
- Pregnant and allergic to penicillin, with need to be desensitized
- Late latent syphilis with serious CNS, cardiovascular, or other organ system compromise

MISCELLANEOUS

COMMENTS
- Jarisch-Herxheimer reaction (fever, myalgia, tachycardia, hypotension) may occur within 24 hr of treatment.
- One third of untreated patients will develop CNS and/or cardiovascular sequelae.
- Up to 80% of those treated during late stages will remain seropositive indefinitely.
- Treponemal tests will remain positive even after adequate therapy.
- U.S. Preventive Services Task Force Recommendations regarding screening for syphilis are described in Section V, Chapter 26.

REFERENCES
Benenson AS (ed): *Control of communicable diseases in man,* ed 15, Washington, DC, 1990 American Public Health Association.

Drugs for sexually transmitted diseases, *Med Lett Drug Ther* 37(964): 117, Dec 1995.

Rolfs RT: Treatment of syphilis—1993, *Clin Infect Dis* 20 (suppl 1): S23, 1995.

Woods GL: Update on laboratory diagnosis of sexually transmitted diseases, *Clin Lab Med* 15(3):665, 1995.

Author: **Eugene J. Louie-Ng, M.D.**

Syringomyelia

BASIC INFORMATION

DEFINITION
Syringomyelia is a disease of the spine characterized by the formation of fluid-filled cavities within the spinal cord, sometimes extending into the brain stem.

ICD-9-CM CODES
336.0 Syringomyelia

PHYSICAL FINDINGS
- Often a history of birth injury exists.
- Onset is usually insidious, with symptoms often not beginning until the third or fourth decade.
- Cervical spine is the most commonly affected area.
  1. Intrinsic hand atrophy, weakness, and anesthetic sensory loss may develop.
  2. The latter may lead to unnoticed burns or other injuries in the hand.
  3. Loss of pain and temperature sensation may occur, but tactile sense in the upper extremity is preserved.
  4. Sharp testing elicits no pain, but patient often perceives the sharpness of the object.
  5. A Charcot joint in the shoulder or elbow may develop.
- Reflexes are absent in the upper extremity.
- Spasticity and hyperreflexia are present in the lower extremity.
- Scoliosis is common.
- Nystagmus and Horner's syndrome may also occur.
- Trophic skin changes eventually develop in many cases.

ETIOLOGY
- Cause is unknown, but condition is thought to result from obstruction of the outlet of the fourth ventricle, often associated with a Chiari I malformation, which causes fluid to be diverted down the central cord.
- Syrinxes later in life may be the result of trauma or an intramedullary tumor.

DIAGNOSIS

DIFFERENTIAL DIAGNOSIS
- ALS
- MS
- Spinal cord tumor
- Tabes dorsalis
- Progressive spinal muscular atrophy

IMAGING STUDIES
- Plain radiographs usually reveal widening of the bony canal in the region of involvement.
- Bony anomalies are often present at the base of the skull and at the C1-C2 spinal segments.
- Myelography and other imaging studies are recommended.

TREATMENT

Drainage and operative repair of any bony anomalies is undertaken, often with decompression laminectomy of C1 and C2.

DISPOSITION
- Condition is slowly progressive in most cases, but course may be quite variable, ranging from death in a few months to slow incapacitation over several years: progression may halt at any time.
- Surgical intervention often stops progression, but frequently does not lead to improvement in neurologic findings.

REFERRAL
For neurosurgical consultation when diagnosis is suspected

MISCELLANEOUS

REFERENCES
Kramer KM, Levine AM: Posttraumatic syringomyelia, *Clin Orthop* 334:190, 1997.

Logue V: Compressive lesions at the foramen magnum. In Ruge D, Wiltse L (eds): *Spinal disorders, disagnosis, and treatment,* Philadelphia, 1977, Lea & Febiger.

Williams B: Orthopedic features in the presentation of syringomyelia, *J Bone Joint Surg* 61(B):314, 1979.

Author: **Lonnie R. Mercier, M.D.**

Systemic lupus erythematosus (PTG)

BASIC INFORMATION

DEFINITION
Systemic lupus erythematosus (SLE) is a chronic multisystemic disease characterized by production of autoantibodies and protean clinical manifestations.

SYNONYMS
SLE

ICD-9-CM CODES
710.0 Systemic lupus erythematosus

EPIDEMIOLOGY AND DEMOGRAPHICS
PREVALENCE: 20 cases/100,000 persons
PREDOMINANT SEX: Female:male ratio of 7:1
PREDOMINANT AGE: 20 to 45 yr (childbearing years)

PHYSICAL FINDINGS
- Skin: erythematous rash over the malar eminences, generally with sparing of the nasolabial folds (butterfly rash), alopecia, raised erythematous patches with subsequent edematous plaques and adherent scales (discoid lupus), leg, nasal, or oropharyngeal ulcerations, livedo reticularis, pallor (from anemia), petechiae (from thrombocytopenia)
- Joints: tenderness, swelling, or effusion generally involving peripheral joints
- Cardiac: pericardial rub (in patients with pericarditis), heart murmurs (if endocarditis or valvular thickening or dysfunction)
- Other: fever, conjunctivitis, dry eyes, dry mouth (sicca syndrome), oral ulcers, abdominal tenderness, decreased breath sounds (pleural effusions)

ETIOLOGY
Unknown

DIAGNOSIS

DIFFERENTIAL DIAGNOSIS
- Other connective tissue disorders (e.g., RA, MCTD, progressive systemic sclerosis)
- Metastatic neoplasm
- Infection

WORKUP
The diagnosis of SLE can be made by demonstrating the presence of any four or more of the following criteria of the American Rheumatism Association:
1. Butterfly rash
2. Discoid rash
3. Photosensitivity (particularly leg ulcerations)
4. Oral ulcers
5. Arthritis
6. Serositis (pleuritis, pericarditis)
7. Renal disorder (persistent proteinuria >0.5 g/day or 3+ if quantitation not performed, cellular casts)
8. Neurologic disorder (seizures, psychosis [in absence of offending drugs or metabolic derangement])
9. Hematologic disorder:
   a. Hemolytic anemia with reticulocytosis
   b. Leukopenia (<4000/mm^3 total on two or more occasions)
   c. Lymphopenia (<1500/mm^3 on two or more occasions)
   d. Thrombocytopenia (<100,000/mm^3 in the absence of offending drugs)
10. Immunologic disorder:
    a. Positive SLE cell preparation
    b. Anti-DNA (presence of antibody to native DNA in abnormal titer)
    c. Anti-Sm (presence of antibody to Smith nuclear antigen)
    d. False-positive STS known to be positive for at least 6 mo and confirmed by negative TPI or FTA tests
11. ANA: an abnormal titer of ANA by immunofluorescence or equivalent assay at any time in the absence of drugs known to be associated with "drug-induced lupus" syndrome

LABORATORY TESTS
Suggested initial laboratory evaluation of suspected SLE:
- Immunologic evaluation: ANA, anti-DNA antibody, anti-Sm antibody
- Other laboratory tests: CBC with differential, platelet count (Coombs' test if anemia detected), urinalysis (24-hr urine collection for protein if proteinuria is detected), PTT and anticardiolipin antibodies in patients with thrombotic events, BUN, creatinine to evaluate renal function

IMAGING STUDIES
- Chest x-ray examination for evaluation of pulmonary involvement (e.g., pleural effusions, pulmonary infiltrates)

- Echocardiogram to screen for significant valvular heart disease (present in 18% of patients with SLE); echocardiography can identify a subset of lesions (valvular thickening and dysfunction) other than verrucous (Libman-Sacks) endocarditis that are prone to hemodynamic deterioration

TREATMENT

NONPHARMACOLOGIC THERAPY
Patients with photosensitivity should avoid sunlight and use high-factor sunscreen.

ACUTE GENERAL Rx
- Joint pain and mild serositis are generally well controlled with NSAIDs; antimalarials are also effective (e.g., hydroxychloroquine [Plaquenil]).
- Cutaneous manifestations can be treated with topical corticosteroids and antimalarials.
- Renal disease: prednisone can be used for patients with mesangial and mild focal proliferative glomerulonephritis, whereas patients with diffuse proliferative or severe focal proliferative glomerulonephritis are candidates for immunosuppressive therapy (e.g., high-pulsed doses of cyclophosphamide given at monthly intervals).
- CNS involvement: treatment generally consists of corticosteroid therapy; however, its efficacy is uncertain, and it is generally reserved for organic brain syndrome. Anticonvulsants and antipsychotics are also indicated in selected cases; headaches are treated symptomatically.
- Hemolytic anemia: treatment of Coombs'-positive hemolytic anemia consists of high doses of corticosteroids; nonhemolytic anemia (secondary to chronic disease) does not require specific therapy.
- Thrombocytopenia: initial treatment consists of corticosteroids. In patients with poor response to steroids, encouraging results have been reported with the use of danazol, vincristine, and immunoglobulins; splenectomy generally does not cure the thrombocytopenia of SLE, but it may be necessary as an adjunctive in managing selected cases.
- Infections are common because of compromised immune function secondary to SLE and the use of corticosteroids, cytotoxic, and antimetabolite drugs; pneumococcal bacteremia is associated with high mortality rate.

CHRONIC Rx
Close monitoring for exacerbation of the disease and for potential side effects from medications (corticosteroids, cytotoxic agents) with frequent laboratory evaluation and office visits

DISPOSITION
- Most patients with lupus experience remissions and exacerbations.
- The leading cause of death in SLE is infection (one third of all deaths); active nephritis causes approximately 18% of deaths and CNS disease causes 7% of deaths; the survival rate is 75% over the first 10 yr. Blacks and Hispanics generally have a worse prognosis.
- Renal histologic studies and evaluation of renal function are useful in determining disease activity and predicting disease outcome (e.g., serum creatinine levels >3 mg/dl or evidence of diffuse proliferative involvement on renal biopsy are poor prognostic factors).

REFERRAL
- Rheumatology consultation in all patients with SLE
- Hematology consultation in patients with significant hematologic abnormalities (e.g., severe hemolytic anemia or thrombocytopenia)
- Nephrology consultation in patients with significant renal involvement

MISCELLANEOUS

COMMENTS
Patient information on lupus can be obtained from the Lupus Foundation of America, Inc., No. 4 Research Place, Suite 180, Rockville, MD 20850-3226; phone: (800) 558-0121.

REFERENCES
Boumpas DT et al: Systemic lupus erythematosus: emerging concepts, *Ann Intern Med* (part I) 122:940; (part II) 123:42, 1995.

Tan E et al: The 1982 revised criteria for the classification of systemic lupus erythematosus, *Arthritis Rheum* 25:1271, 1982.

Author: **Fred F. Ferri, M.D.**

Tabes dorsalis

BASIC INFORMATION

DEFINITION
Tabes dorsalis is a form of tertiary neurosyphilis characterized by paroxysmal pain, particularly in the abdomen and legs, ataxia caused by posterior-column dysfunction, and Argyll-Robertson pupils. Charcot's joint may also be present, indicating severe degenerative osteoarthritis.

SYNONYMS
Locomotor ataxia
Posterior spinal sclerosis
Tabetic neurosyphilis

ICD-9-CM CODES
094.0 Tabes dorsalis, ataxia, locomotor

EPIDEMIOLOGY AND DEMOGRAPHICS
INCIDENCE (IN U.S.): Rare, but increasing with AIDS
PREVALENCE (IN U.S.): Rare; more common with AIDS epidemic
PREDOMINANT SEX: Male
PREDOMINANT AGE: 50 yr or older
PEAK INCIDENCE: 50 to 60 yr

PHYSICAL FINDINGS
- Argyll-Robertson pupil (reacts poorly to light but well to accommodation)
- Loss of position and vibration at ankles (wide-based gait; inability to walk in the dark)
- Loss of deep pain sensation
- Degenerative joint disease, especially in knees

ETIOLOGY
Infectious *(T. pallidum)*

DIAGNOSIS

DIFFERENTIAL DIAGNOSIS
- Combined system disease (vitamin B_{12} deficiency)
- Spinal cord neoplasm

WORKUP
Thorough neurologic examination

LABORATORY TESTS
- Lumbar puncture for VDRL and FTA-ABS
- Serum studies

IMAGING STUDIES
Not necessary if diagnosis confirmed

TREATMENT

NONPHARMACOLOGIC THERAPY
None

ACUTE GENERAL Rx
Procaine penicillin 2 to 4 million U IM qd, along with 500 mg of probenecid PO qid, both for 14 days. Some experts also recommend subsequent administration of 2 to 4 million U of benzathine penicillin IM every week for 3 wk.

CHRONIC Rx
- Refer to rehabilitation center for physical therapy.
- Analgesics, carbamazepine, or steroids may help "lightning" pain.

DISPOSITION
Follow closely until CSF reverts to normal.

REFERRAL
If a spinal cord tumor persists

MISCELLANEOUS

COMMENTS
- Many of the symptoms—degenerative joint disease, lightning pains—persist after treatment.
- U.S. Preventive Services Task Force Recommendations regarding screening for syphilis are described in Section V, Chapter 26.

REFERENCES
Hahn RD: Tabes dorsalis with special reference to primary optic atrophy, *Br J Venereal Dis* 33:139, 1957.
Luxon LM: Neurosyphilis, *Int J Dermatol* 14:310, 1980.
Author: **William H. Olson, M.D.**

BASIC INFORMATION

DEFINITION
Four species of adult tapeworm may infect humans as the definitive host: *Taenia saginatum* (beef tapeworm), *Taenia solium* (pork tapeworm), *Diphyllobothrium latum* (fish tapeworm), and *Hymenolepis nana*. In addition, *T. solium* may infect humans in its larval form (cysticercosis), and several animal tapeworms (see "Echinococcosis" in Section I) may cause infection in an analogous manner.

SYNONYMS
Cysticercosis (larval infection by *T. solium*)

ICD-9-CM CODES
123.9 Tapeworm infestation

EPIDEMIOLOGY AND DEMOGRAPHICS
INCIDENCE (IN U.S.):
- Diagnosed primarily in immigrants
- Varies widely by country of origin and dietary practices

PREVALENCE (IN U.S.):
- *T. saginata:* <0.1%
- *D. latum:* <0.05%
- *T. solium:* <0.1%
- *H. nana:* sporadic, often in setting of outbreak

PREDOMINANT SEX: Equal sex distribution

PREDOMINANT AGE:
- *T. saginata, T. solium, D. latum:* 20 to 39 yr of age
- *H. nana* in setting of institution outbreaks: children

PHYSICAL FINDINGS
- Adult worms
  1. Attach to bowel mucosa
  2. Feed and grow
  3. Cause minimal or no symptoms or sequelae
- Cysticercosis
  1. Mass lesions of brain (neurocysticercosis), soft tissue, viscera
  2. Neurocysticercosis may cause seizures, hydrocephalus
- Prolonged infection with *D. latum*
  1. Vitamin B_{12} deficiency
  2. Megaloblastic anemia

ETIOLOGY
TAPEWORM:
- Adult worm resides in small or large bowel; proglottids and eggs passed in stool.
- Eggs are ingested by the animal intermediate host.
- Eggs hatch into larvae.
- Larvae disseminate largely in skeletal muscle, brain, viscera.
- Humans eat infected beef *(T. saginata)*, infected pork *(T. solium)*, or infected fish *(D. latum)*.
- Larvae mature into adults within the GI lumen.
- *H. nana* infection is acquired by ingesting eggs in human or rodent feces.

CYSTICERCOSIS:
- Humans ingest eggs of *T. solium* in food contaminated with human feces that contain the eggs.
- Eggs hatch into larvae in gut.
- Larvae disseminate widely through tissues (particularly soft tissue and CNS) forming cystic lesions containing either viable or nonviable larvae.

DIAGNOSIS

DIFFERENTIAL DIAGNOSIS
Table 2-38 describes the differential diagnosis of intestinal helminths.

WORKUP
- Stool examination for eggs or proglottids (tapeworm)
- Cerebral CT scan (neurocysticercosis)
- Serum antibody (neurocysticercosis)

IMAGING STUDIES
- Tapeworm: incidental finding on upper GI series
- Neurocysticercosis:
  1. Cerebral cysts are readily demonstrated by CT scan or MRI.
  2. Calcified lesions are an incidental finding.

TREATMENT

ACUTE GENERAL Rx
- All patients with intestinal tapeworm infections should be treated with a single oral dose of praziquantel.
  1. *T. solium:* 5 mg/kg
  2. *T. saginata:* 20 mg/kg
  3. *D. latum:* 10 mg/kg
  4. *H. nana:* 25 mg/kg
- Therapy that may be considered for symptomatic cysticercosis:
  1. May regress spontaneously
  2. Surgery
  3. Albendazole 15 mg/kg PO qd in three doses for 28 days
  4. Praziquantel 50 mg/kg PO qd in three doses for 15 days
- Therapy contraindicated with:
  1. Ocular infections
  2. Cerebral infections in which local inflammation caused by destruction of the parasite may cause significant damage

CHRONIC Rx
- Retreatment if required
- Avoidance of undercooked pork, meat, or fish
- Cysticercosis: proper hand washing, proper disposal of human waste

DISPOSITION
- Neurologic follow-up for patients with neurocysticercosis
- Ophthalmologic follow-up for patients with ocular involvement

REFERRAL
Patients treated for neurocysticercosis should be evaluated by a physician experienced in managing this infection if possible.

MISCELLANEOUS

COMMENTS
T. solium is the most dangerous of the tapeworms because of the potential for cysticercosis by means of autoinfection.

REFERENCES
Drugs for parasitic infections, *Med Lett Drug Ther* 35:1, Dec 1993.

Author: **Joseph R. Masci, M.D.**

Tarsal tunnel syndrome (PTG)

BASIC INFORMATION

DEFINITION
Tarsal tunnel syndrome is a rare entrapment neuropathy that develops as a result of compression of the posterior tibial nerve in the tunnel formed by the flexor retinaculum behind the medial malleolus of the ankle.

ICD-9-CM CODES
355.5 Tarsal tunnel syndrome

EPIDEMIOLOGY AND DEMOGRAPHICS
PREVALENCE: Unknown
PREDOMINANT SEX: Female = male

PHYSICAL FINDINGS
- Neuritic symptoms along the course of the posterior tibial nerve in the sole and heel
- Swelling over tarsal tunnel
- Possible positive Tinel's sign
- Possible reproduction of symptoms with sustained eversion of hindfoot or digital compression of tunnel
- Sensory and motor changes unusual

ETIOLOGY
Space-occupying lesions (ganglia, varicosities, lipomata, synovial hypertrophy)

DIAGNOSIS

DIFFERENTIAL DIAGNOSIS
- Plantar fasciitis
- Peripheral neuropathy
- Proximal radiculopathy
- Local tendinitis
- Peripheral vascular disease
- Morton's neuroma

ELECTRICAL STUDIES
Electrodiagnostic testing is often inconclusive. Delayed sensory conduction or increased motor latency may be seen.

TREATMENT

- NSAIDs
- Immobilization
- Medial heel wedge or orthotic to minimize heel eversion
- Local steroid injection into tunnel

REFERRAL
For surgical decompression if needed

MISCELLANEOUS

REFERENCES
Cimino WR: Tarsal tunnel syndrome: review of the literature, *Foot Ankle* 11:47, 1990.
Radin EL: Tarsal tunnel syndrome, *Clin Orthop* 181:167, 1983.
Takakura Y et al: Tarsal tunnel syndrome: causes and results of operative treatment, *J Bone Joint Surg* 73(B):125, 1991.

Author: **Lonnie R. Mercier, M.D.**

CLINICAL TOPICS — Temporal arteritis 465

BASIC INFORMATION

DEFINITION
Temporal arteritis is a systemic segmental granulomatous inflammation predominantly involving the arteries of the carotid system in patients >50 yr; however, it can involve any large- or medium-sized arteries.

SYNONYMS
Giant cell arteritis
Cranial arteritis

ICD-9-CM CODES
446.5 Temporal arteritis

EPIDEMIOLOGY AND DEMOGRAPHICS
PREVALENCE: 200 cases/100,000 persons
INCIDENCE: 17 to 23.3 new cases/100,000 persons >50 yr

PHYSICAL FINDINGS
- Tenderness, decreased pulsation, and nodulation of temporal arteries
- Visual disturbances: visual field cuts, diplopia, amaurosis fugax, ophthalmoplegia
- Diminished or absent pulses in upper extremities

ETIOLOGY
Vasculitis of unknown etiology

DIAGNOSIS

DIFFERENTIAL DIAGNOSIS
- Other vasculitic syndromes
- Primary amyloidosis
- TIA, CVA
- Infections
- Occult neoplasm, multiple myeloma

WORKUP
Temporal arteritis can present with the following clinical manifestations:
- Headache, often associated with marked scalp tenderness
- Constitutional symptoms (fever, weight loss, anorexia, fatigue)
- Polymyalgia syndrome (aching and stiffness of the trunk and proximal muscle groups)
- Visual disturbances, intermittent claudication of jaw and tongue on mastication

The presence of any three of the following five items allows the diagnosis of temporal arteritis with a sensitivity of 94% and a specificity of 91%:
- Age of onset >50 yr
- New-onset or new type of headache
- Temporal artery tenderness or decreased pulsation on physical examination
- Westergren ESR >50 mm/hr
- Temporal artery biopsy with vasculitis and mononuclear cell infiltrate or granulomatous changes. NOTE: Because of the presence of "skip lesions" in the artery, the biopsy segment of the temporal artery should be at least 2 cm long.

LABORATORY TESTS
- Elevated ESR (usually >50 mm/hr; however, a normal ESR does not exclude the diagnosis)
- Mild-to-moderate normochromic normocytic anemia, elevated platelets
- Liver function test abnormalities (most common: elevation of alkaline phosphatase)

IMAGING STUDIES
- Temporal arteritis is associated with a markedly increased risk for the development of aortic aneurysm, which is often a late complication and may cause death.
- Patients with a history of temporal arteritis may benefit from an annual radiograph of the chest, including a lateral view, and an examination that includes palpation of the abdominal aorta.
- Color duplex ultrasonography of the temporal arteries reveals a dark halo (which may be caused by edema of the artery wall) in patients with temporal arteritis. Patients with typical clinical signs and a halo on ultrasonography may be started on treatment without performing a temporal artery biopsy.

TREATMENT

ACUTE GENERAL Rx
- In stable patients without significant ocular involvement, therapy is usually started with prednisone 40 to 60 mg/day in divided doses, continued for a few weeks until symptoms resolve and ESR returns to normal. If the ESR remains normal, prednisone can be reduced by 5 mg every other week until a dose of 20 mg/day is reached. Subsequent dose reductions should be by 2.5 mg/day every 2 to 4 wk. When the total dose reaches 5 mg/day, reduction should be by 1 mg every 2 to 4 wk as tolerated. Usual duration of prednisone treatment is 6 mo to 2 yr.
- In very ill patients and those with significant ocular involvement (e.g., visual loss in one eye) rapid aggressive treatment with large doses of IV steroids (e.g., IV Solu-Medrol 1000 mg qd for 3 days before starting oral prednisone) is indicated to provide optimal protection to the uninvolved eye and offer any chance of recovery of the involved eye.

CHRONIC Rx
Patients should be instructed and monitored regarding the potential toxicity from prednisone (e.g., hypertension, diabetes, cataracts, dyspepsia, osteoporosis, psychosis). A baseline bone-density study in female patients is recommended.

DISPOSITION
Prognosis is generally good; complete blindness is rare with treatment.

REFERRAL
- Surgical referral for biopsy of temporal artery
- Ophthalmology referral in patients with visual disturbances and following initiation of corticosteroid therapy

MISCELLANEOUS

COMMENTS
The decision to continue tapering prednisone or to resume it after it has been discontinued should not be based solely on the sedimentation rate but on the clinical picture. A rising ESR in a clinically asymptomatic patient with normal Hct should raise suspicion for alternate explanations (e.g., infections, neoplasms).

REFERENCES
Evans JM, O'Fallon WM, Hunder GG: Increased incidence of aortic aneurysm and dissection in giant cell (temporal) arteritis, Ann Intern Med 122:502, 1995.
Flynn JA, Hellmann DB: Giant cell arteritis and cerebral vasculitis. In Johnson RT, Griffin JW (eds): Current therapy in neurologic disease, ed 5, St Louis, 1996, Mosby.
Schmidt WA et al: Color duplex ultrasonography in the diagnosis of temporal arteritis, N Engl J Med 337:1336, 1997.

Author: **Fred F. Ferri, M.D.**

Tetanus

BASIC INFORMATION

DEFINITION
Tetanus is a life-threatening illness manifested by muscle rigidity and spasms, which is caused by a neurotoxin (tetanospasmin) produced by *Clostridium tetani*.

ICD-9-CM CODES
037 Tetanus

EPIDEMIOLOGY AND DEMOGRAPHICS
INCIDENCE (IN U.S.): 48 to 64 cases reported annually since 1986
PREDOMINANT AGE: >60 yr of age
GENETICS:
Neonatal Infection:
- Rare in U.S.
- Among the leading causes of neonatal mortality in many parts of the world (caused by infection of the umbilical cord stump)

PHYSICAL FINDINGS
- Trismus ("lockjaw")
- Risus sardonicus (peculiar grin), characteristic grimace that results from contraction of the facial muscles
- Generalized muscle spasms causing severe pain and, at times, respiratory compromise and death
- Rigid abdominal muscles, flexed arms, and extended legs
- Autonomic dysfunction several days after onset of illness
- Leading cause of death: fluctuations in heart rate and blood pressure
- Usually, absence of fever
- Localized tetanus
  1. Rigidity of muscles near the injury
  2. Weakness as a result of lower motor neuron injury
  3. May be self-limited and resolve spontaneously
  4. More often progresses to generalized tetanus
  5. Cephalic tetanus:
     a. May occur with head injuries
     b. Can manifest as cranial nerve dysfunction

ETIOLOGY
- *C. tetani* is a gram-positive, spore-forming bacillus that resides primarily in the soil.
- Majority of cases are caused by punctures and lacerations.
- Toxin is elaborated from organisms in a contaminated wound.
- Local symptoms are caused by inhibition of neurotransmitter at presynaptic sites.
  1. Over the next 2 to 14 days, the toxin travels up the neurons to the CNS, where it acts on inhibitory neurons to prevent neurotransmitter release.
  2. Unopposed motor activity results in tonic contractions of muscles.

DIAGNOSIS

DIFFERENTIAL DIAGNOSIS
- Strychnine poisoning
- Dystonic reaction caused by neuroleptic agents
- Local infection (dental or masseter muscle) causing trismus
- Severe hypocalcemia
- Hysteria

WORKUP
- Positive wound culture is not helpful in diagnosis.
- Isolation of organism is possible in patients without the illness.

LABORATORY TESTS
- Usually, normal blood counts and chemistries
- Toxicology of serum and urine to rule out strychnine poisoning

TREATMENT

NONPHARMACOLOGIC THERAPY
- Monitoring in a hospital ICU: keep surroundings dark and quiet
- Intubation or tracheostomy caused by severe laryngospasm
- Debridement of wound

ACUTE GENERAL Rx
- Human tetanus immunoglobulin (HTIg) 500 U via IM injection
- Tetanus toxoid (Td) 0.5 ml by IM injection at a different site
- Metronidazole 500 mg IV q6h, or penicillin G 1 million U IV q4h for 10 days
- IV diazepam to control muscle spasms
- Neuromuscular blockade if necessary

CHRONIC Rx
- Supportive care
- Possible mechanical ventilation
- Minimal external stimuli
- Control of heart rate and blood pressure:
  1. Labetalol for sympathetic hyperactivity
  2. Pacemaker for sustained bradycardia
  3. Physical therapy once spasms subside

DISPOSITION
Full recovery over weeks to months if complications can be avoided

REFERRAL
- To emergency department
- To infectious disease specialist

MISCELLANEOUS

COMMENTS
- Illness is preventable.
- Boosters of tetanus toxoid (Td) should be given every 10 yr to maintain immune status.
- Passive as well as active immunization (HTIg + Td) should be given for patients with tetanus-prone wounds who have not been adequately immunized in the previous 5 yr.

REFERENCES
Sanford JP: Tetanus—forgotten but not gone, *N Engl J Med* 332:812, 1995.

Author: **Maurice Policar, M.D.**

Therapeutic insemination (frozen donor semen)

BASIC INFORMATION

DEFINITION
Insemination is a therapeutic intervention designed to overcome defects preventing achieving proper concentration of functional sperm cells in the vicinity of the egg.

SYNONYMS
Artificial insemination

ICD-9-CM CODES
606.0 Irreversible azoospermia
Husband's carrier status for genetic disease such as:
303.1 Tay Sachs
286.0 Hemophilia
333.4 Huntington's disease
758.9 Chromosomal abnormalities
773.0 Severe Rh disease
608.89.1 Husband's sperm frozen before orchidectomy
606.8 Husband's sperm frozen before radiation or chemotherapy

ETIOLOGY
See "ICD-9-CM Codes" above.

DIAGNOSIS

DIFFERENTIAL DIAGNOSIS
See "ICD-9-CM Codes" above.

WORKUP
Male: refer to urologist, ascertain that azoospermia is indeed irreversible. Individuals that were considered intractable in the recent past can now produce pregnancies with intracytoplasmic sperm injections (ICSI), even with cells obtained by testicular biopsy. Such an option should be offered to the patient before recommending a donor.

LABORATORY TESTS
- Testing of both partners for hepatitis, HIV, and other STD is recommended before donor inseminations.
- Female: as described in the topic, "Therapeutic Insemination (Husband/Partner)" for general infertility workup.

IMAGING STUDIES
As described in the topic, "Therapeutic Insemination (Husband/Partner)" for general infertility workup.

TREATMENT

NONPHARMACOLOGIC THERAPY
SPERM SOURCE: *Use of fresh donor semen is no longer acceptable.* Semen is obtained from state-certified "sperm banks" adhering to the proper routines of donor screening for genetic and infectious diseases, and quarantining the sperm for at least 6 mo. Sperm can be shipped from the bank in the containers that will maintain the sample in a frozen state for 48 hr. After this time the sample has to be transferred to another liquid nitrogen storage tank.
SPERM PREPARATION: Sperm is removed from the liquid nitrogen and allowed to thaw at room temperature, or is thawed per sperm bank instructions. Refer to "Therapeutic Insemination (Husband/Partner)" in Section I for insemination techniques. If sperm supply is not limited and the woman's age is not a factor (<35 yr), simple applications of thawed semen to the external cervical os are usually undertaken first.

DISPOSITION
In healthy women <34 yr of age, fecundity of approximately 10% per cycle can be expected. Fertility is age dependent. After 12 cycles, expect 75% pregnancy for women <34 yr of age.

MISCELLANEOUS

COMMENTS
- Risks: infections with STDs, including AIDS, although rare, have been reported as a result of donor semen insemination.
- Caution: observe laws applicable in the state and obtain proper consents.
- Caution: before declaring the male azoospermic, centrifuge the semen and examine sediment; several sperm cells missed on "plain" microscopic examination may suffice for ICSI.

REFERENCES
Speroff L et al: *Clinical gynecologic endocrinology and infertility*, ed 5, Baltimore, 1994, Williams & Wilkins.

Author: **John M. Wieckowski, M.D., Ph.D.**

Therapeutic insemination (husband/partner)

BASIC INFORMATION

DEFINITION
Insemination is a therapeutic intervention designed to overcome defects preventing achieving proper concentration of functional sperm cells in the vicinity of the egg.

SYNONYMS
Artificial insemination

ICD-9-CM CODES
628.9 Infertility (female unspecified)
606.9 Infertility (male unspecified)
302.7 Sexual/erectile dysfunction
625.1 Vaginismus
752.6 Hypospadia
792.2 Asthenospermia
606.1 Oligospermia

EPIDEMIOLOGY AND DEMOGRAPHICS
Approximately 15% of couples experience infertility

ETIOLOGY
MALE:
- Hypospadia: congenital
- Sexual/erectile dysfunction: psychologic, vascular, neurogenic
- Asthenospermia: idiopathic, varicocele, status postvasectomy reversal, environmental (toxins, heavy metals, heat exposure, trauma to testicles)
- Antisperm antibodies, unknown, trauma to testicles, vasectomy

FEMALE:
- Cervical mucus hostility: unknown, infection
- Antisperm antibodies, unknown
- Idiopathic infertility: unknown

DIAGNOSIS

DIFFERENTIAL DIAGNOSIS
- Diagnosis of infertility is established by a history of 1 yr of unprotected intercourse without conception.
- Establish male vs. female infertility, or combined.
- Male: rule out congenital abnormalities, varicocele, endocrine defects.
- Female: rule out ovulatory dysfunction, tubal factors, uterine defects, endometriosis.

WORKUP
- Male routine: urologic examination, semen analysis
- Specialized (if indicated): sonography, vasogram, Doppler studies, testicular biopsy
- Female routine: gynecologic examination, establish ovulatory pattern by basal body temperature or endometrial biopsy
- Postcoital test
- Specialized (if indicated): diagnostic/therapeutic laparoscopy

LABORATORY TESTS
- Male routine: semen analysis; specialized (if indicated): antisperm antibodies, endocrine studies, testicular biopsy
- Female routine: blood type, rubella immunity, hepatitis immunity
- Selectively (>35 yr or as indicated by history): day 3 of the cycle, test FSH, LH, and estradiol to rule out occult ovarian failure, polycystic ovarian syndrome (LH/FSH inversion); androgen levels if hirsutism present; prolactin level if galactorrhea; thyroid studies if clinically indicated; anti-*Chlamydia* antibodies if tubal damage suspected or history of IUD use

IMAGING STUDIES
- Hysterosalpingogram: rule out hydrosalpinx, salpingitis isthmica nodosa, intramural tubal polyps, intrauterine synechiae, or polyps
- Pelvic sonography: in midcycle to rule out myomas, endometrial polyps, endometrial hypoplasia, ovarian pathology (cysts, endometriomas), or confirm dominant follicle formation
- Pituitary MRI if tumor suspected

TREATMENT

NONPHARMACOLOGIC THERAPY
Type of insemination depends on the nature of the fertility defect and varies in depth to which the sperm cells are delivered into the female genital tract. The following types of inseminations may be done:
- Cervical and endocervical insemination
- Intrauterine insemination
- Intratubal insemination
- Cul-de-sac insemination
- Intrafollicular insemination
- In vitro fertilization (IVF)
- IVF with intracytoplasmic sperm injection (ICSI)

Only the cervical and intrauterine inseminations can be done in a primary care setting.

CERVICAL AND INTRACERVICAL INSEMINATION: This method is indicated when normal coital sperm delivery to the cervix is prevented (e.g., coital dysfunction and hypospadia).

Semen Preparation: None; whole semen is used.

Technique: Semen is delivered to the external os or endocervical canal using a syringe with soft tipped cannula. Cervical cap, which prolongs the contact of semen with the cervix, can be used to overcome high semen viscosity.

Therapeutic insemination (husband/partner)

INTRAUTERINE INSEMINATION (IUI):
This method is used for the following reasons (listed in order of decreasing effectiveness):
- Cervical mucus hostility caused by poor mucus production or quality (idiopathic or iatrogenic, such as status postcervical conization, laser treatment, etc.)
- Antisperm antibodies
- Empirical treatment for unexplained infertility
- Mild male factor defects, such as oligospermia, high semen viscosity, high or low seminal volume

Semen preparation: Seminal fluid should not be introduced into the uterine cavity. Sperm cells have to be separated from the seminal fluid by the process of sperm "washing," and resuspended in a protein-containing medium (5% to 10% serum or synthetic serum substitute), to endow the cells with proper motility. Method that can be used without the necessity of having incubator involves centrifugation of semen through a density gradient and resuspending the pellet in the protein-containing medium. Media for the above procedures, with or without antibiotics, are commercially available from several sources.

Technique: Internal cervical os is negotiated with one of the various commercially available "insemination catheters" and the "washed" sperm suspension is delivered to the endometrial cavity. Timing: basal body temperature graphs, cervical mucus observation, testing of urine for LH surge, or serial sonography are often used for detecting ovulation. Cervical insemination should be performed within 24 hr before anticipated ovulation. Timing of IUI should be within a few hours of ovulation, preferably before it. It is usually performed at 40 hr after the ovulation-inducing hCG injection.

ACUTE GENERAL Rx
- Clomiphene citrate (Clomid, Serophene) is commonly used to correct ovulatory defects. It is given in doses of 50 to 200 mg qd, on days 5 through 9 after the onset of progesterone withdrawal bleeding. The higher the dose of clomiphene necessary to induce ovulation, the lower the pregnancy chance. Prolonged use of clomiphene may adversely affect the endometrium and cervical mucus.
- Tamoxifen (Nolvadex) 10 to 20 mg qd given on days 5 through 9 as described above is also a mild ovulation-inducing agent that improves endometrial formation and cervical mucus.
- Human chorionic gonadotropin (hCG, Pregnyl, Profasi, APL) can be used to trigger ovulation when the dominant follicle size reaches 20 mm diameter.
- Use of injectable FSH (Humegon, Fertinex) preparations is not advisable in primary care setting.

DISPOSITION
Majority of conceptions should occur within the first 6 mo of inseminations. In healthy young women a 15% to 25% pregnancy rate per cycle can be expected. The great variety of results reported in the literature indicates that the practitioner's skill in performing ovarian stimulations and sperm preparation plays a significant role in the outcome.

REFERRAL
To specialist if:
- No result after six cycles of inseminations
- Ovulatory dysfunction does not promptly respond to a low-dose (50 to 100 mg of clomiphene citrate)
- Woman's age >35 yr: efficiency of treatment becomes critical
- Poor semen parameters
- Pelvic pathology needs correction

MISCELLANEOUS

COMMENTS
- Risks of insemination: flare-up of unsuspected pelvic infection, ovarian overstimulation with gonadotropins, multifetal pregnancy.
- Caution: if sperm is in limited supply (semen frozen before orchidectomy) or woman's age is an issue, a thorough fertility evaluation is indicated to make sure that no valuable time or valuable semen is wasted. If fertility defects are found, they should be corrected, or IVF should be offered.
- IVF combined with ICSI is the ultimate insemination technique and delivers pregnancy rates of 20% to 40% per cycle.

REFERENCES
Speroff L et al: *Clinical gynecologic endocrinology and infertility,* ed 5, Baltimore, 1994, Williams & Wilkins.

Author: **John M. Wieckowski, M.D., Ph.D.**

Thoracic outlet syndrome

BASIC INFORMATION

DEFINITION
Thoracic outlet syndrome is the term used to describe a condition producing upper extremity symptoms thought to result from neurovascular compression at the thoracic outlet. Three types are described based on the point of compression: (1) cervical rib and scalenus syndrome, in which abnormal scalene muscles or the presence of a cervical rib may cause compression, (2) the costoclavicular syndrome, in which compression may occur under the clavicle, and (3) the hyperabduction syndrome, in which compression may occur in the subcoracoid area.

ICD-9-CM CODES
353.0 Thoracic outlet syndrome

EPIDEMIOLOGY AND DEMOGRAPHICS
PREVALENCE: Varies from source to source; presence of cervical ribs in 0.5% to 1% of population (50% bilateral), but most are asymptomatic
PREDOMINANT AGE: Rare under 20 yr of age
PREDOMINANT SEX: Female > male (3.5:1)

PHYSICAL FINDINGS
- Symptoms and signs are related to the degree of involvement of each of the various structures at the level of the first rib.
- True venous or arterial involvement is rare.
- Diagnosis is most often used in the consideration of neural pain affecting the arm, which would suggest involvement of the brachial plexus.
  1. *Arterial compression:* pallor, paresthesias, diminished pulses, coolness, digital gangrene, and a supraclavicular bruit or mass
  2. *Venous compression:* edema and pain; thrombosis causing superficial venous dilatation about the shoulder
  3. *"True" neural compression:* lower trunk (C8,T1) findings with intrinsic weakness and diminished sensation to the finger and small fingers and ulnar aspect of the forearm
  4. Possible supraclavicular tenderness
  5. Provocative tests (Adson's, Wright's): may reproduce pain but are of disputed usefulness

ETIOLOGY
- Congenital cervical rib or fibrous extension of cervical rib
- Abnormal scalene muscle insertion
- Drooping of shoulder girdle resulting from generalized hypotonia or trauma
- Narrowed costoclavicular interval as a result of downward and backward pressure on shoulder (sometimes seen in individuals who carry heavy backpacks)
- Acute venous thrombosis with exercise (effort thrombosis)
- Bony abnormalities of first rib
- Abnormal fibromuscular bands

DIAGNOSIS

DIFFERENTIAL DIAGNOSIS
- Carpal tunnel syndrome
- Cervical radiculopathy
- Brachial neuritis
- Ulnar nerve compression
- Reflex sympathetic dystrophy
- Superior sulcus tumor

WORKUP
Except for venous or arterial pathology, no ancillary diagnostic tests are reliable for diagnostic confirmation.

IMAGING STUDIES
- Arteriography or venography when vascular pathology is strongly suspected clinically
- Cervical spine radiographs to rule out cervical disc disease
- Chest film to rule out lung tumor
- EMG, NCV studies to rule out carpal tunnel syndrome, cervical radiculopathy

TREATMENT

ACUTE GENERAL Rx
- Sling for pain relief
- Physical therapy: modalities plus shoulder girdle strengthening exercises
- Postural reeducation
- NSAIDs

DISPOSITION
- Surgery: generally successful for vascular disorders
- Nonsurgical treatment: often successful for patients with pain as the primary symptom

REFERRAL
For vascular surgery consultation when venous or arterial impairment is present

MISCELLANEOUS

COMMENTS
- True thoracic outlet syndrome is probably an uncommon condition.
- Diagnosis is often used to describe a wide variety of clinical symptoms.
- Considerable disagreement exists regarding the frequency of this disorder.

REFERENCES
Fechter JD, Kuschner SH: Review: the thoracic outlet syndrome, *Orthopedics* 16:1243, 1993.
Leffert RD: Thoracic outlet syndrome, *J Am Acad Orthop Surg* 2:317, 1994.
Wilborn AJ: The thoracic outlet syndrome is over-diagnosed, *Arch Neurol* 47:328, 1990.

Author: **Lonnie R. Mercier, M.D.**

Thromboangiitis obliterans (Buerger's disease)

BASIC INFORMATION

DEFINITION
Thromboangiitis obliterans (Buerger's disease) is an occlusive inflammatory disease of the small- to medium-size arteries of the upper and lower extremities.

SYNONYMS
Buerger's disease
Presenile gangrene

ICD-9-CM CODES
443.1 Thromboangiitis obliterans (Buerger's disease)

EPIDEMIOLOGY AND DEMOGRAPHICS
- From 1947 to 1986 the incidence of thromboangiitis obliterans at the Mayo Clinic has fallen from 104 cases/100,000 patients to 12.6 cases/100,000 patients.
- The prevalence of thromboangiitis obliterans is higher in Japan, India, and Southeast Asia when compared with the U.S.
- Thromboangiitis obliterans is rare in women, with only 24 histologic cases reported until 1987.
- The disease typically occurs before the age of 50 yr and is found predominantly in men who smoke.

PHYSICAL FINDINGS
- Paresthesia, coldness, skin ulcers, gangrene, along with pain at rest or with walking (claudication)
- Prolonged capillary refill with dependent rubor
- Necrotic skin ulcers at the tips of the digits
- Pathognomonic migratory thrombophlebitis

ETIOLOGY
- Unknown
- The remarkable feature is the close association between tobacco smoking and disease exacerbation. If abstinence from tobacco is adhered to, thromboangiitis obliterans takes a favorable course. If smoking is continued, the disease progresses, leading to gangrene and small-digit amputations.
- There is some thought of a genetic predisposition because the prevalence is higher in the Far East.

DIAGNOSIS

DIFFERENTIAL DIAGNOSIS
Thromboangiitis obliterans must be distinguished from arteriosclerotic peripheral vascular disease by the criteria mentioned in "Workup."

WORKUP
The diagnosis of thromboangiitis obliterans is made on:
- Clinical criteria
  1. Peripheral vascular disease occurring predominantly in men before the age of 50 yr
  2. Typically, affects the arms and the legs and not just the lower extremities as arteriosclerosis does
  3. Found solely in tobacco smokers, with improvement in those who abstain
  4. Associated with migratory thrombophlebitis
  5. No other atherosclerotic risk factors (e.g., diabetes, cholesterol, or hypertension)
- Angiographic criteria (see "Imaging Studies" below)
- Pathologic criteria (see reference, Lie JT, 1988): fresh inflammatory thrombus within both small- and medium-size arteries and veins, along with giant cells around the thrombus.

IMAGING STUDIES
- Noninvasive vascular studies help differentiate proximal occlusive disease characteristic of arteriosclerosis from distal disease typical of thromboangiitis obliterans.
- Angiography findings in thromboangiitis obliterans include:
  1. Involvement of distal small- and medium-size vessels.
  2. Occlusions are segmental, multiple, smooth, and tapered.
  3. Collateral circulation gives a "tree root" or "spider leg" appearance.
  4. Both upper and lower extremities are involved.

TREATMENT

NONPHARMACOLOGIC THERAPY
Abstaining from smoking is the only way to stop the progression of the disease. Medical and surgical treatments will prove to be futile if the patient continues to smoke. Exacerbation of ischemic ulcers are directly related to tobacco use.

ACUTE GENERAL Rx
- The goal of medical treatment is to provide relief of ischemic pain and healing of ischemic ulcers. If the patient does not completely abstain from tobacco, medical measures will not be helpful.
- Prostaglandin vasodilator therapy given IV or intraarterially provides some relief of pain but does not change the course of the disease.
- Epidural anesthesia and hyperbaric oxygen has a vasodilator effect and has been shown to aid in pain relief from ischemic ulcers.

CHRONIC Rx
- Surgical bypass procedures and sympathectomy, as with medical treatment, will not be efficacious unless the patient stops smoking.
- Surgical bypass may be difficult because the occlusions of thromboangiitis obliterans are distal. Nevertheless if successfully done, this can lead to rapid healing of ischemic ulcers.
- Sympathectomy leads to increased flow by decreasing the vasoconstriction of distal vessels and has been shown to aid in the healing and relief of pain from ischemic ulcers.
- Debridement must be done on necrotic ulcers if needed.
- Amputation is frequently required for gangrenous digits; however, below knee or above knee amputations are rarely necessary.

DISPOSITION
The course of thromboangiitis obliterans can be dramatically changed by the cessation of tobacco smoking. If the patient continues to smoke, recurrent exacerbation of ischemic ulcers, necrosis, and gangrene leading to small digit amputations will be inevitable.

REFERRAL
Vascular surgical consultation is recommended in any young smoker with claudication and ischemic ulcers, especially if both the upper and lower extremities are involved.

MISCELLANEOUS

COMMENTS
Smoking cessation is mandatory. In individuals who quit smoking, prognosis is markedly improved.

REFERENCES
Lie JT: Thromboangiitis obliterans (Buerger's disease) revisited, *Pathol Annu* 23:27, 1988.
Shionoya S: Buerger's disease (Thromboangiitis obliterans). In Rutherford RB: *Vascular surgery*, ed 4, Philadelphia, 1995, WB Saunders.

Author: **Peter Petropoulos, M.D.**

Thrombophlebitis, superficial

BASIC INFORMATION

DEFINITION
Superficial thrombophlebitis is inflammatory thrombosis in subcutaneous veins.

SYNONYMS
Phlebitis

ICD-9-CM CODES
451.0 Thrombophlebitis, superficial

EPIDEMIOLOGY AND DEMOGRAPHICS
- 20% of superficial thrombophlebitis cases are associated with occult DVT.
- Catheter-related thrombophlebitis incidence is 100:100,000.

PHYSICAL FINDINGS
- Subcutaneous vein is palpable, tender; tender cord is present with erythema and edema of the overlying skin and subcutaneous tissue.
- Induration, redness, and tenderness are localized along the course of the vein. This linear appearance rather than circular appearance is useful to distinguish thrombophlebitis from other conditions (cellulitis, erythema nodosum).
- There is no significant swelling of the limb (superficial thrombophlebitis generally does not produce swelling of the limb).
- Low-grade fever may be present. High fever and chills are suggestive of septic phlebitis.

ETIOLOGY
- Trauma to preexisting varices
- Intravenous cannulation of veins (most common cause)
- Abdominal cancer (e.g., carcinoma of pancreas)
- Infection (*Staphylococcus* is the most common pathogen)
- Hypercoagulable state
- DVT

DIAGNOSIS

DIFFERENTIAL DIAGNOSIS
- Lymphangitis
- Cellulitis
- Erythema nodosum
- Panniculitis
- Kaposi's sarcoma

WORKUP
Laboratory evaluation to exclude infectious etiology and imaging studies to rule out DVT in suspected cases.

LABORATORY TESTS
CBC with differential, blood cultures, culture of IV catheter tip (when secondary to intravenous cannulation)

IMAGING STUDIES
- Serial ultrasound or venography in patients with suspected DVT
- CT scan of abdomen in patients with suspected malignancy (Trousseau syndrome: recurrent migratory thrombophlebitis)

TREATMENT

NONPHARMACOLOGIC THERAPY
- Warm, moist compresses
- It is not necessary to restrict activity; however, if there is extensive thrombophlebitis, bed rest with the leg elevated will limit the thrombosis and improve symptoms.

ACUTE GENERAL Rx
- NSAIDs to relieve symptoms
- Treatment of septic thrombophlebitis with antibiotics with adequate coverage of *Staphylococcus*
- Ligation and division of the superficial vein at the junction to avoid propagation of the clot in the deep venous system when the thrombophlebitis progresses toward the junction of the involved superficial vein with deep veins

DISPOSITION
Clinical improvement within 7 to 10 days

REFERRAL
Surgical referral in selected cases (see "Acute General Rx")

MISCELLANEOUS

COMMENTS
- Patients with positive cultures should be evaluated and treated for endocarditis.
- Septic thrombophlebitis is more common in IV drug addicts.

REFERENCES
Samlaskie CT, James WD: Superficial thrombophlebitis: primary hypercoagulable states, *J Am Acad Dermatol* 22:975, 1990.

Author: **Fred F. Ferri, M.D.**

Thrombosis, deep vein

BASIC INFORMATION

DEFINITION
Deep vein thrombosis (DVT) is the development of thrombi in the deep veins of the extremities or pelvis.

SYNONYMS
DVT
Deep venous thrombophlebitis

ICD-9-CM CODES
451.1 Thrombosis of deep vessels of lower extremities
451.83 Thrombosis of deep veins of upper extremities
541.9 Deep vein thrombosis of unspecified site

EPIDEMIOLOGY AND DEMOGRAPHICS
Annual incidence in urban population is 1.6 cases/1000 persons.

PHYSICAL FINDINGS
- Pain and swelling of the affected extremity
- In lower extremity DVT, leg pain on dorsiflexion of the foot (Homans' sign)
- Physical examination may be unremarkable

ETIOLOGY
The etiology is often multifactorial (prolonged stasis, coagulation abnormalities, vessel wall trauma). The following are risk factors for DVT:
- Prolonged immobilization (≥3 days)
- Postoperative state
- Trauma to pelvis and lower extremities
- Birth control pills, high-dose estrogen therapy
- Visceral cancer (lung, pancreas, alimentary tract, GU tract)
- Age >60 yr
- Prior history of thromboembolic disease
- Hematologic disorders (e.g., antithrombin III deficiency, protein C deficiency, protein S deficiency, lupus anticoagulant, dysfibrinogenemias, anticardiolipin antibody, hyperhomocystinemia, concurrent homocystinuria, and factor V Leiden mutation)
- Pregnancy and early puerperium
- Obesity, CHF
- Surgery, fracture, or injury involving lower leg or pelvis
- Surgery requiring >30 min of anesthesia
- Gynecologic surgery (particularly gynecologic cancer surgery)

DIAGNOSIS

DIFFERENTIAL DIAGNOSIS
- Postphlebitic syndrome
- Superficial thrombophlebitis
- Ruptured Baker's cyst
- Cellulitis, lymphangitis, Achilles tendinitis
- Hematoma
- Muscle or soft tissue injury, stress fracture
- Varicose veins, lymphedema
- Arterial insufficiency

WORKUP
The clinical diagnosis of DVT is inaccurate. Pain, tenderness, swelling, or color changes are not specific for DVT. Commonly used diagnostic tests are described below. An initial negative test on compression ultrasonography should be repeated after 3 to 5 days (if the clinical suspicion of DVT persists) in order to detect propagation of any thrombosis to the proximal veins.

LABORATORY TESTS
- Laboratory tests are not specific for DVT. Baseline PT (INR), PTT, and platelet count should be obtained on all patients before starting anticoagulation.
- Laboratory evaluation of young patients with DVT, patients with recurrent thrombosis without obvious causes, and those with a family history of thrombosis should include protein S, protein C, fibrinogen, antithrombin III level, lupus anticoagulant, anticardiolipin antibodies, factor V Leiden, and plasma homocysteine levels.

IMAGING STUDIES
- Contrast venography is the "gold standard" for evaluation of DVT of the lower extremity. It is, however, invasive and painful. Additional disadvantages are the increased risk of phlebitis, new thrombosis, renal failure, and hypersensitivity reaction to contrast media; it also gives poor visualization of deep femoral vein in the thigh and internal iliac vein and its tributaries.
- Compression ultrasonography is generally preferred as the initial study because it is noninvasive and can be repeated serially (useful to monitor suspected acute DVT); it offers good sensitivity for detecting proximal vein thrombosis (in the popliteal or femoral vein). Its disadvantages are poor visualization of deep iliac and pelvic veins and poor sensitivity in isolated or nonocclusive calf vein thrombi.

TREATMENT

NONPHARMACOLOGIC THERAPY
- Initial bed rest for 1 to 4 days followed by gradual resumption of normal activity
- Patient education on anticoagulant therapy and associated risks

ACUTE GENERAL Rx
- IV heparin for 4 to 7 days followed by warfarin therapy
- Close monitoring of PTT and platelets while on heparin and of INR when started on warfarin
- Monitoring for significant bleeding (GI, hematuria)
- Fixed-dose, SC low-molecular-weight heparin is also effective for initial management of DVT and allows outpatient treatment.

CHRONIC Rx
- The optimal duration of anticoagulant therapy varies with the cause of DVT and the patient's risk factors:
  1. Therapy for 6 wk is generally satisfactory in patients with reversible risk factors.
  2. Anticoagulation for 6 mo is recommended for patients with idiopathic venous thrombosis.
  3. Indefinite anticoagulation is necessary in patients with DVT associated with active cancer; long-term anticoagulation is also indicated in patients with inherited thrombophilia and those with recurrent episodes of idiopathic DVT.

REFERRAL
Hematology consultation in patients with suspected hereditary coagulopathy

MISCELLANEOUS

COMMENTS
Prophylaxis of DVT is recommended in all patients at risk (e.g., low-molecular-weight heparin after major trauma, postsurgery of hip and knee; gradient elastic stockings alone or in combination with intermittent pneumatic compression [IPC] boots following neurosurgery).

REFERENCES
Ginsberg JS: Management of venous thromboembolism, *N Engl J Med* 335:1816, 1996.
Hirsh J: The optimal duration of anticoagulant therapy for venous thrombosis, *N Engl J Med* 332:1710, 1995.
Kearon C et al: Noninvasive diagnosis of deep vein thrombosis, *Ann Intern Med* 128:663, 1998.

Author: **Fred F. Ferri, M.D.**

Thrombotic thrombocytopenic purpura

BASIC INFORMATION

DEFINITION
Thrombotic thrombocytopenic purpura (TTP) is a rare disorder characterized by thrombocytopenia (often accompanied by purpura) and microangiopathic hemolytic anemia; neurologic impairment, renal dysfunction, and fever may also be present.

SYNONYMS
TTP

ICD-9-CM CODES
446.6 Thrombotic thrombocytopenic purpura

EPIDEMIOLOGY AND DEMOGRAPHICS
- TTP primarily affects females between 10 and 50 yr of age.
- Frequency is 3.7 cases/yr/1,000,000 persons.

PHYSICAL FINDINGS
- Purpura (secondary to thrombocytopenia)
- Jaundice, pallor (secondary to hemolysis)
- Mucosal bleeding
- Fever
- Fluctuating levels of consciousness (secondary to thrombotic occlusion of the cerebral vessels)

ETIOLOGY
The exact cause of TTP remains unknown. Recent studies reveal that there is platelet aggregation as a result of abnormalities in circulating von Willebrand factor caused by endothelial injury.

DIAGNOSIS

DIFFERENTIAL DIAGNOSIS
- DIC
- Malignant hypertension
- Vasculitis
- Eclampsia or preeclampsia
- Hemolytic-uremic syndrome (typically encountered in children, often following a viral infection)
- Gastroenteritis as a result of a serotoxin-producing serotype of *Escherichia coli*
- Medications: ticlopidine, penicillin, antineoplastic chemotherapeutic agents, oral contraceptives

WORKUP
- A comprehensive history, physical examination, and laboratory evaluation will usually confirm the diagnosis.
- The disease often begins as a flulike illness ultimately followed by clinical and laboratory abnormalities.
- See Fig. 3-81 for a clinical algorithm for the evaluation of thrombocytopenia.

LABORATORY TESTS
- Severe anemia and thrombocytopenia
- Elevated BUN and creatinine
- Evidence of hemolysis: elevated reticulocyte count, indirect bilirubin, LDH, decreased haptoglobin
- Urinalysis: hematuria (red cells and red cell casts in urine sediment) and proteinuria
- Peripheral smear: severely fragmented RBCs (schistocytes)
- No laboratory evidence of DIC (normal FDP, fibrinogen)

TREATMENT

ACUTE GENERAL Rx
- Plasmapheresis with fresh frozen plasma (FFP) replacement; cryosupernatant may be substituted for FFP in patients who fail to respond to this treatment. Daily plasma exchange is generally performed until hemolysis has ceased and the platelet count has normalized.
- Corticosteroids (prednisone 1 to 2 mg/kg/day) may be effective alone in patients with mild disease or may be administered concomitantly with plasmapheresis plus plasma exchange with FFP.
- Vincristine has been used in patients refractory to plasmapheresis.
- Use of antiplatelet agents (ASA, dipyridamole) is controversial.
- Platelet transfusions are contraindicated except in severely thrombocytopenic patients with documented bleeding.
- Splenectomy is performed in refractory cases.

CHRONIC Rx
- Relapsing TTP may be treated with plasma exchange.
- Splenectomy done while the patients are in remission has been used in some centers to decrease the frequency of relapse in TTP.

DISPOSITION
- Survival of patients with TTP currently exceeds 80% with plasma exchange therapy.
- Relapse occurs in 20% to 40% of patients who have TTP in remission.

REFERRAL
Surgical referral for splenectomy in selected patients (see "Acute General Rx" and "Chronic Rx")

MISCELLANEOUS

COMMENTS
Thrombotic microangiopathy can also be associated with administration of cyclosporine, mitomycin C, and HIV infection.

REFERENCES
Bennett CL et al: Thrombotic thrombocytopenic purpura associated with ticlopidine, *Ann Intern Med* 128:541, 1998.

Crowther M et al: Splenectomy done during hematologic remission to prevent relapse in patients with thrombotic thrombocytopenic purpura, *Ann Intern Med* 125:294, 1996.

Shumak KH, Rock GA, Nair RC: Late relapses in patients successfully treated for thrombotic thrombocytopenic purpura: Canadian Apheresis Group, *Ann Intern Med* 122:569, 1996.

Author: **Fred F. Ferri, M.D.**

Thyroid carcinoma (PTG)

BASIC INFORMATION

DEFINITION
Thyroid carcinoma is a primary neoplasm of the thyroid. There are four major types of thyroid carcinoma: papillary, follicular, anaplastic, and medullary.

SYNONYMS
Papillary carcinoma of thyroid
Follicular carcinoma of thyroid
Anaplastic carcinoma of thyroid
Medullary carcinoma of thyroid

ICD-9-CM CODES
193 Malignant neoplasm of thyroid

EPIDEMIOLOGY AND DEMOGRAPHICS
- Thyroid cancer is the most common endocrine cancer, with an annual incidence of 14,000 new cases in the U.S. and about 1100 deaths.
- Female:male ratio is 3:1.
- Most common type (50% to 60%) is papillary carcinoma.
- Median age at diagnosis: 45 to 50 yr.

PHYSICAL FINDINGS
- Presence of thyroid nodule
- Hoarseness and cervical lymphadenopathy
- Painless swelling in the region of the thyroid

ETIOLOGY
- Risk factors: prior neck irradiation
- Multiple endocrine neoplasia II (medullary carcinoma)

DIAGNOSIS

DIFFERENTIAL DIAGNOSIS
- Multinodular goiter
- Lymphocytic thyroiditis
- Ectopic thyroid

WORKUP
The workup of thyroid carcinoma includes laboratory evaluation and diagnostic imagining. However, diagnosis is confirmed with fine-needle aspiration (FNA) or surgical biopsy. The characteristics of thyroid carcinoma vary with the type:
- Papillary carcinoma
  1. Most frequently occurs in women during second or third decades.
  2. Histologically, psammoma bodies (calcific bodies present in papillary projections) are pathognomonic; they are found in 35% to 45% of papillary thyroid carcinomas.
  3. Majority are not papillary lesions but mixed papillary follicular carcinomas.
  4. Spread is via lymphatics and by local invasion.
- Follicular carcinoma
  1. More aggressive than papillary carcinoma.
  2. Incidence increases with age.
  3. Tends to metastasize hematogenously to bone, producing pathologic fractures.
  4. Tends to concentrate iodine (useful for radiation therapy).
- Anaplastic carcinoma
  1. Very aggressive neoplasm.
  2. Two major histologic types: small cell (less aggressive, 5-yr survival approximately 20%) and giant cell (death usually within 6 mo of diagnosis).
- Medullary carcinoma
  1. Unifocal lesion: found sporadically in elderly patients.
  2. Bilateral lesions: associated with pheochromocytoma and hyperparathyroidism; this combination is known as MEN-II and is inherited as an autosomal dominant disorder.

LABORATORY TESTS
- Thyroid function studies are generally normal. TSH, T_4, and serum thyroglobulin levels should be obtained before thyroidectomy in patients with confirmed thyroid carcinoma.
- Increased plasma calcitonin assay in patients with medullary carcinoma (tumors produce thyrocalcitonin).

IMAGING STUDIES
- Thyroid scanning with iodine-123 or technetium-99m can identify hypofunctioning (cold) nodules, which are more likely to be malignant. However, warm nodules can also be malignant.
- Thyroid ultrasound can detect solitary solid nodules that have a high risk of malignancy. However, a negative ultrasound does not exclude diagnosis of thyroid carcinoma.
- FNA biopsy is the best method to assess a thyroid nodule (refer to "Thyroid nodule" in Section I).

TREATMENT

ACUTE GENERAL Rx
- Papillary carcinoma
  1. Total thyroidectomy is indicated if the patient has:
     a. Extrapyramidal extension of carcinoma
     b. Papillary carcinoma limited to thyroid but a positive history of irradiation to the neck
     c. Lesion >2 cm
  2. Lobectomy with isthmectomy may be considered in patients with intrathyroid papillary carcinoma <2 cm and no history of neck or head irradiation; most follow surgery with suppressive therapy with thyroid hormone because these tumors are TSH responsive. The accepted practice is to suppress serum TSH concentrations to <0.1 µU/mL.
  3. Radiotherapy with iodine-131 (after total thyroidectomy), followed by thyroid suppression therapy with triiodothyronine can be used in metastatic papillary carcinoma.
- Follicular carcinoma
  1. Total thyroidectomy followed by TSH suppression as noted above
  2. Radiotherapy with iodine-131 followed by thyroid suppression therapy with triiodothyronine is useful in patients with metastasis.
- Anaplastic carcinoma
  1. At diagnosis, this neoplasm is rarely operable; palliative surgery is indicated for extremely large tumor compressing the trachea.
  2. Management is usually restricted to radiation therapy or chemotherapy (combination of doxorubicin, cisplatin, and other antineoplastic agents); these measures rarely provide significant palliation.
- Medullary carcinoma
  1. Thyroidectomy should be performed.
  2. Patients and their families should be screened for pheochromocytoma and hyperparathyroidism.

DISPOSITION
Prognosis varies with the type of thyroid carcinoma: 5-yr survival approaches 80% for follicular carcinoma and is approximately 5% with anaplastic carcinoma.

MISCELLANEOUS

COMMENTS
- Family members of patients with medullary carcinoma should be screened; DNA analysis for the detection of mutations in the RET gene structure permits the identification of MEN IIA gene carriers.
- U.S. Preventive Services Task Force Recommendations regarding screening for thyroid cancer are described in Section V, Chapter 18.

REFERENCES
Moley JF: Medullary thyroid cancer, *Surg Clin North Am* 75:405, 1995.
Schlumberger MJ: Papillary and follicular thyroid carcinoma, *N Engl J Med* 338:297, 1998.

Author: **Fred F. Ferri, M.D.**

Thyroid nodule (PTG)

BASIC INFORMATION

DEFINITION
A thyroid nodule is an abnormality found on physical examination of the thyroid gland; nodules can be benign (70%) or malignant.

ICD-9-CM CODES
241.0 Nodule, thyroid

EPIDEMIOLOGY AND DEMOGRAPHICS
- Thyroid nodules can be found in 50% of autopsies; however, only 1 in 10 are palpable.
- Malignancy is present in 5% to 30% of palpable nodules.
- Incidence of thyroid nodules increases after 45 yr of age. They are found more frequently in women.
- History of prior head and neck irradiation increases the risk of thyroid cancer.
- Increased likelihood that nodule is malignant: nodule increasing in size or >2 cm, regional lymphadenopathy, fixation to adjacent tissues, age <40 yr, male sex.

PHYSICAL FINDINGS
- Palpable, firm, and nontender nodule in the thyroid area should be suspicious for carcinoma. Signs of metastasis are regional lymphadenopathy, inspiratory stridor.
- Signs and symptoms of thyrotoxicosis can be found in functioning nodules.

ETIOLOGY
- History of prior head and neck irradiation
- Family history of pheochromocytoma, carcinoma of the thyroid, and hyperparathyroidism (medullary carcinoma of the thyroid is a component of MEN-II)

DIAGNOSIS

DIFFERENTIAL DIAGNOSIS
- Thyroid carcinoma
- Multinodular goiter
- Thyroglossal duct cyst
- Epidermoid cyst
- Laryngocele
- Nonthyroid neck neoplasm
- Branchial cleft cyst

WORKUP
- Fine-needle aspiration (FNA) biopsy is the best diagnostic study; the accuracy can be >90%, but it is directly related to the level of experience of the physician and the cytopathologist interpreting the aspirate.
- FNA biopsy is less reliable with thyroid cystic lesions; surgical excision should be considered for most thyroid cysts not abolished by aspiration.
- A diagnostic approach to nodular thyroid disease is described in Section III, Fig. 3-83.

LABORATORY TESTS
- TSH, T_4, and serum thyroglobulin levels should be obtained before thyroidectomy in patients with confirmed thyroid carcinoma on FNA biopsy.
- Serum calcitonin at random or after pentagastrin stimulation is useful when suspecting medullary carcinoma of the thyroid.
- Serum thyroid autoantibodies (see "Thyroiditis" in Section I) are useful when suspecting thyroiditis.

IMAGING STUDIES
- Thyroid ultrasound is done in some patients to evaluate the size of the thyroid and the number, composition (solid vs. cystic), and dimensions of the thyroid nodule; solid thyroid nodules have a higher incidence of malignancy, but cystic nodules can also be malignant.
- The introduction of high-resolution ultrasonography has made it possible to detect many nonpalpable nodules (incidentalomas) in the thyroid (found at autopsy in 30% to 60% of cadavers). Most of these lesions are benign. For most patients with nonpalpable nodules that are incidentally detected by thyroid imaging, simple follow-up neck palpation is sufficient.
- Thyroid scan with technetium-99m pertechnetate:
  1. Classifies nodules as hyperfunctioning (hot), normally functioning (warm), or nonfunctioning (cold); cold nodules have a higher incidence of malignancy; the differential diagnosis of cold thyroid nodules is described in Section II, Box 2-116.
  2. Scan has difficulty evaluating nodules near the thyroid isthmus or at the periphery of the gland.
  3. Normal tissue over a nonfunctioning nodule might mask the nodule as "warm" or normally functioning.
- Both thyroid scan and ultrasound provide information about the risk of malignant neoplasia based on the characteristics of the thyroid nodule, but their value in the initial evaluation of a thyroid nodule is limited because neither one provides a definite tissue diagnosis.

TREATMENT

ACUTE GENERAL Rx
- Evaluation of results of FNA
  1. Normal cells: may repeat biopsy during present evaluation or reevaluate patient after 3 to 6 mo of suppressive therapy (l-thyroxine, 100 to 200 μg PO qd)
     a. Failure to regress indicates increased likelihood of malignancy
     b. Reliance on repeat needle biopsy is preferable to routine surgery for nodules not responding to thyroxine.
  2. Malignant cells: surgery
  3. Hypercellularity: thyroid scan
     a. Hot nodule: 131-I therapy if the patient is hyperthyroid
     b. Warm or cold nodule: surgery (rule out follicular adenoma vs. carcinoma)

DISPOSITION
Variable with results of FNA biopsy. Refer to "Thyroid carcinoma" in Section I for prognosis in patients with malignant nodules diagnosed with biopsy.

REFERRAL
Surgical referral for FNA biopsy

MISCELLANEOUS

COMMENTS
Surgery is indicated in hard or fixed nodule, presence of dysphagia or hoarseness, and rapidly growing solid masses regardless of "benign" results on FNA.

REFERENCES
LaRosa GL et al: Levothyroxine and iodine are both effective for treating benign solitary solid cold nodules of the thyroid, *Ann Intern Med* 122:1, 1995.

Schlinkert RT et al: Factors that predict malignant thyroid lesions when fine-needle aspiration is "suspicious for follicular neoplasm," *Mayo Clin Proc* 72:913, 1997.

Tan GH, Gharib H: Thyroid incidentalomas: management approaches to a nonpalpable nodule discovered incidentally on thyroid imaging, *Ann Intern Med* 126:226, 1997.

Author: **Fred F. Ferri, M.D.**

Thyroiditis (PTG)

BASIC INFORMATION

DEFINITION
Thyroiditis is an inflammatory disease of the thyroid. It is a multifaceted disease with varying etiology, different clinical characteristics (depending on the stage) and distinct histopathology. Thyroiditis can be subdivided into three common types (Hashimoto's, subacute, silent) and two rare forms (suppurative, Riedel's). To add to the confusion, there are various synonyms for each form, and there is no internationally accepted classification of autoimmune thyroid disease.

SYNONYMS
Hashimoto's thyroiditis: chronic lymphocytic thyroiditis, chronic autoimmune thyroiditis
Subacute thyroiditis: granulomatous thyroiditis, de Quervain's thyroiditis
Silent thyroiditis: lymphocytic thyroiditis, painless thyroiditis, postpartum thyroiditis
Suppurative thyroiditis: acute thyroiditis, bacterial thyroiditis
Riedel's thyroiditis: invasive fibrous thyroiditis

ICD-9-CM CODES
245.2 Hashimoto's thyroiditis
245.1 Subacute thyroiditis
245.9 Silent thyroiditis
245.0 Suppurative thyroiditis
245.3 Riedel's thyroiditis

PHYSICAL FINDINGS
- Hashimoto's: patients may have signs of hyperthyroidism (tachycardia, diaphoresis, palpitations, weight loss) or hypothyroidism (fatigue, weight gain, delayed reflexes) depending on the stage of the disease. Usually there is diffuse, firm enlargement of the thyroid gland; thyroid gland may be also be of normal size (atrophic form with clinically manifested hypothyroidism).
- Subacute: exquisitely tender, enlarged thyroid, fever; signs of hyperthyroidism are initially present; signs of hypothyroidism can subsequently develop.
- Silent: clinical features are similar to subacute thyroiditis except for the absence of tenderness of the thyroid gland (painless thyroiditis).
- Suppurative: patient is febrile with severe neck pain, focal tenderness of the involved portion of the thyroid, erythema of the overlying skin.
- Riedel: slowly enlarging hard mass in the anterior neck; often mistaken for thyroid cancer; signs of hypothyroidism occur in advanced stages.

ETIOLOGY
- Hashimoto's: autoimmune disorder that begins with the activation of CD4 (helper) T-lymphocytes specific for thyroid antigens. The etiologic factor for the activation of these cells is unknown.
- Subacute: possibly postviral; usually follows a respiratory illness; it is not considered to be a form of autoimmune thyroiditis.
- Silent: autoimmune thyroiditis; it frequently occurs postpartum.
- Suppurative: infectious etiology, generally bacterial, although fungi and parasites have also been implicated; it often occurs in immunocompromised hosts or following a penetrating neck injury.
- Riedel's: fibrous infiltration of the thyroid; etiology is unknown.

DIAGNOSIS

DIFFERENTIAL DIAGNOSIS
- The hyperthyroid phase of Hashimoto's, subacute, or silent thyroiditis can be mistaken for Graves' disease.
- Riedel's thyroiditis can be mistaken for carcinoma of the thyroid.
- Subacute thyroiditis can be mistaken for infections of the oropharynx and trachea or for suppurative thyroiditis.
- Factitious hyperthyroidism can mimic silent thyroiditis.

WORKUP
- The diagnostic workup includes laboratory and radiologic evaluation to rule out other conditions that may mimic thyroiditis (see "Differential Diagnosis") and to differentiate the various forms of thyroiditis.
- The patient's medical history may be helpful in differentiating the various types of thyroiditis (e.g., presentation following childbirth is suggestive of silent (postpartum, painless) thyroiditis; occurrence following a viral respiratory infection suggests subacute thyroiditis; history of penetrating injury to the neck indicates suppurative thyroiditis).

LABORATORY TESTS
- TSH, free T_4: may be normal, or indicative of hypo- or hyperthyroidism depending on the stage of the thyroiditis.
- WBC with differential: increased WBC with "shift to the left" occurs with subacute and suppurative thyroiditis.
- Antimicrosomal antibodies: detected in >90% of patients with Hashimoto's thyroiditis and 50% to 80% of patients with silent thyroiditis.
- Serum thyroglobulin levels are elevated in patients with subacute and silent thyroiditis; this test is nonspecific but may be useful in monitoring the course of subacute thyroiditis and distinguishing silent thyroiditis from factitious hyperthyroidism (low or absent serum thyroglobulin level).

IMAGING STUDIES
24-hr radioactive iodine uptake (RAIU) is useful to distinguish Graves' disease (increased RAIU) from thyroiditis (normal or low RAIU).

TREATMENT

ACUTE GENERAL Rx
- Treat hypothyroid phase with levothyroxine 25 to 50 µg/day initially and monitor serum TSH initially every 6 to 8 wk.
- Control symptoms of hyperthyroidism with β-blockers (e.g., propranolol 20 to 40 mg PO q6h).
- Control pain in patients with subacute thyroiditis with NSAIDs. Prednisone 20 to 40 mg qd may be used if NSAIDs are insufficient, but it should be gradually tapered off over several weeks.
- Use IV antibiotics and drain abscess (if present) in patients with suppurative thyroiditis.

DISPOSITION
- Hashimoto's thyroiditis: long-term prognosis is favorable; most patients will recover their thyroid function.
- Subacute thyroiditis: permanent hypothyroidism occurs in 10% of patients.
- Silent thyroiditis: 6% of patients will have permanent hypothyroidism.
- Suppurative thyroiditis: there is usually full recovery following treatment.
- Riedel's thyroiditis: hypothyroidism occurs when fibrous infiltration involves the entire thyroid.

REFERRAL
Surgical referral in patients with compression of adjacent neck structures and in some patients with suppurative thyroiditis

MISCELLANEOUS

REFERENCES
Dayan CM, Daniels GH: Chronic autoimmune thyroiditis, *N Engl J Med* 335:99, 1996.
Smallridge RC: Postpartum thyroid dysfunction: a frequently undiagnosed endocrine disorder, *Endocrinologist* 6:46, 1996.

Author: **Fred F. Ferri, M.D.**

Thyrotoxic storm

BASIC INFORMATION

DEFINITION
Thyrotoxic storm is the abrupt and severe exacerbation of thyrotoxicosis.

ICD-9-CM CODES
242.9 Thyrotoxic storm
242.0 With goiter
242.2 Multinodular
242.3 Adenomatous
242.8 Thyrotoxicosis factitia

PHYSICAL FINDINGS
- Goiter
- Tremor, tachycardia, fever
- Warm, moist skin
- Lid lag, lid retraction, proptosis
- Altered mental status (psychosis, coma, seizures)
- Other: evidence of precipitating factors (infection, trauma)

ETIOLOGY
- Major stress (e.g., infection, MI, DKA) in an undiagnosed hyperthyroid patient
- Inadequate therapy in a hyperthyroid patient

DIAGNOSIS

The clinical presentation is variable. The patient may present with the following signs and symptoms:
- Fever
- Marked anxiety and agitation, psychosis
- Hyperhidrosis, heat intolerance
- Marked weakness and muscle wasting
- Tachyarrhythmias, palpitations
- Diarrhea, nausea, vomiting
- Elderly patients may have a combination of tachycardia, CHF, and mental status changes

DIFFERENTIAL DIAGNOSIS
- Psychiatric disorders
- Alcohol or other drug withdrawal
- Pheochromocytoma
- Metastatic neoplasm

WORKUP
- Laboratory evaluation to confirm hyperthyroidism (elevated free T_4, decreased TSH)
- Evaluation for precipitating factors (e.g., ECG and cardiac enzymes in suspected MI, blood and urine cultures to rule out sepsis)
- Elimination of disorders noted in the differential diagnosis (e.g., psychiatric history, evidence of drug and alcohol abuse)

LABORATORY TESTS
- Free T_4, TSH
- CBC with differential
- Blood and urine cultures
- Glucose
- Liver enzymes
- BUN, creatinine
- Serum calcium
- CPK

IMAGING STUDIES
Chest x-ray examination to exclude infectious process, neoplasm, CHF in suspected cases

TREATMENT

NONPHARMACOLOGIC THERAPY
- Nutritional care: replace fluid deficit aggressively (daily fluid requirement may reach 6 L); use solutions containing glucose and add multivitamins to the hydrating solution.
- Monitor for fluid overload and CHF in the elderly and in those with underlying cardiovascular or renal disease.
- Treat significant hyperthermia with cooling blankets.

ACUTE GENERAL Rx
- Inhibition of thyroid hormone synthesis
  1. Administer propylthiouracil (PTU) 300 to 600 mg initially (PO or via NG tube), then 150 to 300 mg q6h.
  2. If the patient is allergic to PTU, use methimazole (Tapazole) 80 to 100 mg PO or PR followed by 30 mg PR q8h.
- Inhibition of stored thyroid hormone
  1. Iodide can be administered as sodium iodine 250 mg IV q6h, potassium iodide (SSKI) 5 gtt PO q8h, or Lugol's solution, 10 gtt q8h. It is important to administer PTU or methimazole 1 hr *before* the iodide to prevent the oxidation of iodide to iodine and its incorporation in the synthesis of additional thyroid hormone.
  2. Corticosteroids: dexamethasone 2 mg IV q6h or hydrocortisone 100 mg IV q6h for approximately 48 hr is useful to inhibit thyroid hormone release, impair peripheral conversion of T_3 from T_4, and to provide additional adrenocortical hormone to correct deficiency (if present).
- Suppression of peripheral effects of thyroid hormone
  1. β-Adrenergic blockers: Administer propranolol 80 to 120 mg PO q4 to 6h. Propranolol may also be given IV 1 mg/min for 2 to 10 min under continuous ECG and blood pressure monitoring. β-Adrenergic blockers must be used with caution in patients with CHF or bronchospasm. Cardioselective β-blockers (e.g., esmolol, or metoprolol) may be more appropriate for patients with bronchospasm, but these patients must be closely monitored for exacerbation of bronchospasm because these agents lose their cardioselectivity at high doses.
- Control of fever with acetaminophen 325 to 650 mg q4h; avoidance of aspirin because it displaces thyroid hormone from its binding protein
- Digitalization of patients with CHF and atrial fibrillation (these patients may require higher than usual digoxin doses)
- Treatment of any precipitating factors (e.g., antibiotics if infection is strongly suspected)

CHRONIC Rx
Refer to "Hyperthyroidism" in Section I.

DISPOSITION
Patients with thyrotoxic crisis should be treated and appropriately monitored in the ICU.

REFERRAL
Endocrinology referral is appropriate in patients with thyrotoxic crisis.

MISCELLANEOUS

COMMENTS
If the diagnosis is strongly suspected, therapy should be started immediately without waiting for laboratory confirmation.

REFERENCES
Eng S, Singer PA: Prompt and aggressive therapy for endocrine emergencies, *Contemp Med* 8:27, 1996.
Franklyn JA: The management of hyperthyroidism, *N Engl J Med* 330:1731, 1994.
Tietgens ST, Leinung MC: Thyroid storm, *Med Clin North Am* 79:169, 1995.
Author: **Fred F. Ferri, M.D.**

Tinea corporis (PTG)

BASIC INFORMATION

DEFINITION
Tinea corporis is a dermatophyte fungal infection caused by the genera *Trichophyton* or *Microsporum*.

SYNONYMS
Ringworm
Body ringworm
Tinea circinata

ICD-9-CM CODES
110.5 Tinea corporis

EPIDEMIOLOGY AND DEMOGRAPHICS
- The disease is more common in warm climates.
- There is no predominant age or sex.

PHYSICAL FINDINGS
- Annular lesions with an advancing scaly border; the margin is slightly raised, reddened, and may be pustular.
- The central area becomes hypopigmented and less scaly as the active border progresses outward (see color plate 21).
- The trunk and legs are primarily involved.

ETIOLOGY
Trichophyton rubrum is the most common pathogen.

DIAGNOSIS

DIFFERENTIAL DIAGNOSIS
- Pityriasis rosea
- Erythema multiforme
- Psoriasis
- SLE
- Syphilis
- Nummular eczema
- Eczema
- Granuloma annulare

WORKUP
Diagnosis is usually made on clinical grounds. It can be confirmed by direct visualization under the microscope of a small fragment of the scale using wet mount preparation and potassium hydroxide solution; dermatophytes appear as translucent branching filaments (hyphae) with lines of separation appearing at irregular intervals.

LABORATORY TESTS
- Microscopic examination of hyphae.
- Culture is usually not necessary.

TREATMENT

NONPHARMACOLOGIC THERAPY
Effected areas should be kept clean and dry.

ACUTE GENERAL Rx
- Various creams are effective:
  1. Miconazole 2% cream (Monistat-Derm) applied bid for 2 wk
  2. Clotrimazole 1% cream (Mycelex) applied and gently massaged into the affected areas and surrounding areas bid for up to 4 wk
  3. Naftifine 1% cream (Naftin) applied qd
  4. Econazole 1% (Spectazole) applied qd
- Nonsystemic therapy is reserved for severe cases; commonly used agents:
  1. Ketoconazole (Nizoral), 200 mg qd
  2. Itraconazole (Sporanox), 100 to 200 mg qd for 2 to 4 wk
  3. Griseofulvin (Fulvicin, Grisactin, Gris-Peg), 250 to 500 mg bid.

DISPOSITION
Majority of cases resolve without sequelae within 3 to 4 wk of therapy.

REFERRAL
Dermatology referral in patients with persistent or recurrent infections

MISCELLANEOUS

REFERENCES
Habif TP: *Clinical dermatology,* ed 3, St Louis, 1996, Mosby.
Pariser DM et al: Double blind comparison of itraconazole and placebo in the treatment of tinea corporis and tinea cruris, *J Am Acad Dermatol* 31:232, 1994.

Author: **Fred F. Ferri, M.D.**

Tinea cruris (PTG)

BASIC INFORMATION

DEFINITION
Tinea cruris is a dermatophyte fungal infection of the groin.

SYNONYMS
Jock itch
Ringworm

ICD-9-CM CODES
110.3 Tinea cruris

EPIDEMIOLOGY AND DEMOGRAPHICS
- Most common during the summer months.
- Men are affected more frequently than women.

PHYSICAL FINDINGS
- Erythematous plaques have a half-moon shape and a scaling border.
- The acute inflammation tends to move down the inner thigh and usually spares the scrotum; in severe cases the fungus may spread onto the buttocks.
- Itching may be severe.
- Red papules and pustules may be present.
- An important diagnostic sign is the advancing well-defined border with a tendency toward central clearing (see color plate 22).

ETIOLOGY
- Dermatophytes of the genera *Trichophyton, Epidermophyton,* and *Microsporum*
- Transmission from direct contact (e.g., infected persons, animals)

DIAGNOSIS

DIFFERENTIAL DIAGNOSIS
- Intertrigo
- Psoriasis
- Seborrheic dermatitis
- Erythrasma
- Candidiasis
- Tinea versicolor

WORKUP
Diagnosis is based on clinical presentation and demonstration of hyphae microscopically using potassium hydroxide.

LABORATORY TESTS
- Microscopic examination
- Cultures are generally not necessary

TREATMENT

NONPHARMACOLOGIC THERAPY
- Keep infected area clean and dry.
- Use of boxer shorts is preferred to regular underwear.

ACUTE GENERAL Rx
- Drying powders (e.g., Miconazole nitrate [Zeasorb AF]) may be useful in patients with excessive perspiration.
- Various topical antifungal agents are available: miconazole (Lotrimin), terbinafine (Lamisil), sulconazole nitrate (Exelderm), betamethasone dipropionate/clotrimazole (Lotrisone).
- Oral antifungal therapy is generally reserved for cases unresponsive to topical agents; frequently used agents are: griseofulvin microsize (Grifulvin V) 250 to 500 mg bid for 1 to 2 wk, itraconazole (Sporanox) 100 mg/day for 2 to 4 wk, or ketoconazole (Nizoral) 200 mg qd.

DISPOSITION
Most cases respond promptly to therapy with complete resolution within 2 to 3 wk.

MISCELLANEOUS

REFERENCES
Habif TP: *Clinical dermatology,* ed 3, St Louis, 1996, Mosby.
Pariser DM et al: Double blind comparison of itraconazole and placebo in the treatment of tinea corporis and tinea cruris, *J Am Acad Dermatol* 31:232, 1994.
Author: **Fred F. Ferri, M.D.**

Tinea versicolor (PTG)

BASIC INFORMATION

DEFINITION
Tinea versicolor is a fungal infection of the skin caused by the yeast *Pityrosporum orbiculare (Malassezia furfur)*.

SYNONYMS
Pityriasis versicolor

ICD-9-CM CODES
111.0 Tinea versicolor

EPIDEMIOLOGY AND DEMOGRAPHICS
- Increased incidence in adolescence and young adulthood
- More common during the summer (hypopigmented lesions are more evident when the skin is tanned)

PHYSICAL FINDINGS
- Most lesions begin as multiple small, circular macules of various colors.
- The macules may be darker or lighter than the surrounding normal skin and will scale with scraping.
- Most frequent site of distribution is trunk.
- Facial lesions are more common in children (forehead is most common facial site).
- Eruption is generally of insidious onset and asymptomatic.
- Lesions may be hyperpigmented in blacks.
- Lesions may be inconspicuous in fair-complexioned individuals, especially during the winter.
- Most patients will become aware of the eruption when the involved areas will not tan (see color plate 23).

ETIOLOGY
The infection is caused by the lipophilic yeast *P. orbiculare* (round form) and *P. ovale* (oval form); these organism are normal inhabitants of the skin flora; factors that favor their proliferation are pregnancy, malnutrition, immunosuppression, oral contraceptives, and excess heat and humidity.

DIAGNOSIS

DIFFERENTIAL DIAGNOSIS
- Vitiligo
- Pityriasis alba
- Secondary syphilis
- Pityriasis rosea
- Seborrheic dermatitis

WORKUP
Diagnosis is based on clinical appearance; identification of hyphae and budding spores (spaghetti and meatballs appearance) with microscopy will confirm diagnosis.

LABORATORY TESTS
Microscopic examination using potassium hydroxide will confirm diagnosis when in doubt.

TREATMENT

NONPHARMACOLOGIC THERAPY
Sunlight accelerates repigmentation of hypopigmented areas.

ACUTE GENERAL Rx
- Topical treatment: selenium sulfide 2.5% suspension (Selsun or Exsel) applied daily for 10 min for 7 consecutive days results in a cure rate of 80% to 90%.
- Antifungal topical agents (e.g., miconazole, ciclopirox, clotrimazole) are also effective but generally expensive.
- Oral treatment is generally reserved for resistant cases. Effective agents are ketoconazole (Nizoral) 200 mg qd for 5 days, or single 400-mg dose (cure rate >80%), fluconazole (Diflucan), 400 mg given as a single dose (cure rate >70% at 3 wk after treatment) or itraconazole 200 mg/day for 5 days.

DISPOSITION
The prognosis is good, with death of the fungus usually occurring within 3 to 4 wk of treatment; however, recurrence is common.

MISCELLANEOUS

COMMENTS
Patients should be informed that the hypopigmented areas will not disappear immediately after treatment, and that several months may be necessary for the hypopigmented areas to regain their pigmentation.

REFERENCES
Habif TP: *Clinical dermatology*, ed 3, St Louis, 1996, Mosby.
Lesher J: Recent developments in antifungal therapy, *Dermatol Clin* 14:163, 1996.

Author: **Fred F. Ferri, M.D.**

Torticollis

BASIC INFORMATION

DEFINITION
Torticollis is a contraction or contracture of the muscles of the neck that occurs and causes the head to be tilted to one side. It is usually accompanied by rotation of the chin to the opposite side with flexion. Usually it is a symptom of some underlying disorder. This term is often used incorrectly in cases when the torticollis may simply be positional.

SYNONYMS
Twisted neck
"Wry neck"

ICD-9-CM CODES
723.5 Spastic (intermittent) torticollis
754.1 Congenital muscular (sternocleidomastoid)
300.11 Hysterical
714.0 Rheumatoid
333.83 Spasmodic

PHYSICAL FINDINGS
- Congenital muscular torticollis:
  1. Palpable soft tissue "mass" in the sternocleidomastoid shortly after birth
  2. Mass gradually subsides, leaving a shortened, contracted sternocleidomastoid muscle
  3. Head characteristically tilted toward the side of the mass and rotated in the opposite direction
  4. Facial asymmetry and other secondary changes persisting into adulthood
- Spasmodic torticollis:
  1. "Spasms" in the cervical musculature; may be bilateral and uncontrollable
  2. Head often tilted toward the affected side
- Findings in other cases will depend on etiology.

ETIOLOGY
Torticollis has been attributed to over 50 different causes:
- Localized fibrous shortening of unknown cause involving the sternocleidomastoid, leading to the condition termed *congenital muscular torticollis*
- Spasmodic torticollis: of uncertain etiology, possibly a variant of dystonia musculorum deformans
- Infection, specifically pharyngitis, tonsillitis, retropharyngeal abscess
- Miscellaneous rare causes: congenital musculoskeletal deformities, trauma, inflammation from rheumatoid arthritis, vestibular disturbances, posterior fossa tumor, syringomyelia, neuritis of spinal accessory nerve, and drug reactions

DIAGNOSIS

DIFFERENTIAL DIAGNOSIS
- Usually involves separating each disorder from the others
- Acquired positional disorders (e.g., ocular disturbances, acute disc herniation)

WORKUP
- Workup is dependent on the clinical situation
- Laboratory studies are usually not helpful unless infection or rheumatoid disease is suspected.
- Fig. 3-58 describes a clinical algorithm for the evaluation and therapy of neck pain.

IMAGING STUDIES
- Plain radiographs in cases of trauma or to rule out congenital abnormalities
- MRI in appropriate cases
- Electrodiagnostic studies: only rarely indicated to rule out neurologic causes

TREATMENT

- Congenital muscular torticollis: gentle stretching exercises carried out by the parent
- Spasmodic torticollis: physical therapy, psychotherapy, cervical braces, biofeedback, and pain control
- Other forms: treated according to etiology

DISPOSITION
- Most patients with congenital muscular torticollis respond well to conservative treatment.
- Spasmodic torticollis is often resistant to normal conservative treatment.
- Prognosis of other forms of torticollis is dependent on etiology.

REFERRAL
- Torticollis often requires a multidisciplinary approach unless the etiology is obvious.
- Children usually do not require any specific studies; however, an orthopedic consultation is recommended.

MISCELLANEOUS

REFERENCES
Duane DD: Spasmodic torticollis, *Adv Neurol* 49:135, 1988.
Kahn ML, Davidson R, Brummond DS: Acquired torticollis in children, *Orthop Rev* 20:667, 1991.
Kiwak KJ: Establishing an etiology for torticollis, *Postgrad Med* 75:127, 1984.

Author: **Lonnie R. Mercier, M.D.**

Tourette's syndrome (PTG)

BASIC INFORMATION

DEFINITION
The onset of Tourette's syndrome is in childhood, with axial motor (body or facial) tics or vocal tics (barking or coprolalia).

SYNONYMS
Gilles de la Tourette syndrome
Motor-verbal tic disorder

ICD-9-CM CODES
307.23 Gilles de la Tourette disorder

EPIDEMIOLOGY AND DEMOGRAPHICS
INCIDENCE (IN U.S.): Chronic, nonfatal disease
PREVALENCE (IN U.S.): 5 to 10 cases/10,000 persons
PREDOMINANT SEX: Male:female ratio of 9:1
PREDOMINANT AGE: <21 yr of age
PEAK INCIDENCE: Lifetime
GENETICS: Autosomal dominant, but variability in symptoms

PHYSICAL FINDINGS
- Vocal tics (clearing of throat, repetitive short phrases, e.g., "You bet," swearing [coprolalia])
- Axial tics (grimacing, blinking, head jerking)
- Tics that wax, wane (worse with emotional stress), and change over lifetime

ETIOLOGY
Genetic, associated with obsessive-compulsive disorder (OCD).

DIAGNOSIS

DIFFERENTIAL DIAGNOSIS
- Other idiopathic tic disorders
- Sydenham's chorea
- Transient tic disorders
- Head trauma
- Drug intoxication
- Postinfectious encephalitis

WORKUP
Clinical observation to confirm diagnosis

LABORATORY TESTS
No definitive laboratory tests

IMAGING STUDIES
CT scan and MRI of brain is normal.

TREATMENT

NONPHARMACOLOGIC THERAPY
Multidisciplinary: parents, teachers, psychologists, school nurses (educational)

ACUTE GENERAL Rx
- Dopamine blocking agents may be used to reduce severity of tics (e.g., haloperidol 0.25 mg PO qhs initially).
- Clonidine 0.05 mg PO qd initially may be effective in patients with attention deficit disorder (ADD).
- Fluoxetine 20 mg PO qd initially is useful in patients with obsessive-compulsive symptoms.

CHRONIC Rx
Low-dose dopamine blocking neuroleptic agents only if tics interfere with activities of daily living

DISPOSITION
- Usually live relatively normal life if psychologic consequences of tic avoided.
- More than 30% of patients develop OCD or ADD.

REFERRAL
To neurologist to confirm initial diagnosis

MISCELLANEOUS

COMMENTS
- Once thought rare, now recognized as common because of recognition of milder forms.
- Patient education may be obtained from the Tourette's Syndrome Association (TSA), 4240 Bell Blvd., Bayside, NY, 11361-2864; phone: (800) 237-0717.

REFERENCES
Hyde TM: Tourette's syndrome: a model neuropsychiatric disorder, *JAMA* 273:498, 1995.
Author: **William H. Olson, M.D.**

Toxic shock syndrome (PTG)

BASIC INFORMATION

DEFINITION
Toxic shock syndrome is an acute febrile illness resulting in multiple organ system dysfunction caused most commonly by a bacterial exotoxin. Disease characteristics also include hypotension, vomiting, myalgia, watery diarrhea, vascular collapse, and an erythematous sunburn-like cutaneous rash that desquamates during recovery.

ICD-9-CM CODES
040.89 Toxic shock syndrome

EPIDEMIOLOGY AND DEMOGRAPHICS
- Case reported incidence peak: 14 cases/100,000 menstruating women/yr in 1980; has since fallen to >1 case/100,000 persons
- Occurs most commonly between ages 10 and 30 yr in healthy, young menstruating white females
- Case fatality ratio of 3%

ETIOLOGY
- Menstrually associated TSS: 45% of cases associated with tampons, diaphragm, or vaginal sponge use
- Nonmenstruating associated TSS: 55% of cases associated with puerperal sepsis, postcesarean section endometritis, mastitis, wound or skin infection, insect bite, pelvic inflammatory disease, and postoperative fever
- Causative agent: S. aureus infection of a susceptible individual (10% of population lacking sufficient levels of antitoxin antibodies), which liberates the disease mediator TSST-1 (exotoxin)
- Other causative agents: coagulase-negative streptococci producing enterotoxins B or C, and exotoxin A producing group A β-hemolytic streptococci

PHYSICAL FINDINGS
- Fever ($\geq 38.9°$ C)
- Diffuse macular erythrodermatous rash that desquamates 1 to 2 wk after disease onset in survivors
- Orthostatic hypotension
- GI symptoms: vomiting, diarrhea, abdominal tenderness
- Constitutional symptoms: myalgia, headache, photophobia, rigors, altered sensorium, conjunctivitis, arthralgia
- Respiratory symptoms: dysphagia, pharyngeal hyperemia, strawberry tongue
- Genitourinary symptoms: vaginal discharge, vaginal hyperemia, adnexal tenderness
- End-organ failure
- Severe hypotension and acute renal failure
- Hepatic failure
- Cardiovascular symptoms: DIC, pulmonary edema, ARDS, endomyocarditis, heart block

DIAGNOSIS

DIFFERENTIAL DIAGNOSIS
- Staphylococcal food poisoning
- Septic shock
- Mucocutaneous lymph node syndrome
- Scarlet fever
- Rocky Mountain spotted fever
- Meningococcemia
- Toxic epidermal necrolysis
- Kawasaki's syndrome
- Leptospirosis
- Legionnaire's disease
- Hemolytic uremic syndrome
- Stevens-Johnson syndrome
- Scalded skin syndrome
- Erythema multiforme
- Acute rheumatic fever

WORKUP
Broad-spectrum syndrome with multi-organ system involvement and variable but acute clinical presentation, including the following:
1. Fever $\geq 38.1°$ C
2. Classic desquamating (1 to 2 wk) rash
3. Hypotension/orthostatic SBP 90 or less
4. Syncope
5. Negative throat/CSF cultures
6. Negative serologic test for Rocky Mountain spotted fever, rubeola, and leptospirosis
7. Clinical involvement of three or more of the following:
   a. Cardiopulmonary: ARDS, pulmonary edema, endomyocarditis, second- or third-degree AV block
   b. CNS: altered sensorium without focal neurologic findings
   c. Hematologic: thrombocytopenia (PLT <100 k)
   d. Liver: elevated liver function test results
   e. Renal: WBCs per HPF 5, negative urine cultures, azotemia, and increased creatinine double normal
   f. Mucous membrane involvement: vagina, oropharynx, conjunctiva
   g. Musculoskeletal: myalgia, increased CPK double normal
   h. GI: vomiting, diarrhea

LABORATORY TESTS
- Pan culture (cervix/vagina, throat, nasal passages, urine, blood, CSF, wound) for *Staphylococcus, Streptococcus*, or other pathogenic organisms
- Electrolytes to detect hypokalemia, hyponatremia
- CBC with differential and clotting profile for anemia (normocytic/normochromic), thrombocytopenia, leukocytosis, coagulopathy, and bacteremia

- Chemistry profile to detect decreased protein, increased AST, increased ALT, hypocalcemia, elevated BUN/creatinine, hypophosphatemia, increased LDH, increased CPK
- Urinalysis to detect WBC (>5/HPF), proteinemia, microhematuria
- ABGs to assess respiratory function and acid-base status
- Serologic tests considered for Rocky Mountain spotted fever, rubeola, and leptospirosis

IMAGING STUDIES
- Chest x-ray examination to evaluate pulmonary edema
- ECG to evaluate arrhythmia
- Sonography/CT scan/MRI considered if pelvic abscess or TOA suspected

TREATMENT

NONPHARMACOLOGIC THERAPY
- For optimal outcome: high index of suspicion and early and aggressive supportive management in an ICU setting
- Aggressive fluid resuscitation (maintenance of circulating volume, CO, SBP)
- Thorough search for a localized infection or nidus: incision and drainage, debridement, removal of tampon or vaginal sponge
- Central hemodynamic monitoring, Swan-Ganz catheter and arterial line for surveillance of hemodynamic status and response to therapy
- Foley catheter to monitor hourly urine output
- Possible MAST trousers as temporary measure
- Acute ventilator management if severe respiratory compromise
- Renal dialysis for severe renal impairment
- Surgical intervention for indicated conditions (i.e., ruptured TOA, wound abscess, mastitis)

ACUTE GENERAL Rx
- Isotonic crystalloid (normal saline solution) for volume replacement following "7-3" rule
- Electrolyte replacement (K^+, Ca^+)
- PRBC/coagulation factor replacement/FFP to treat anemia or D&C
- Vasopressor therapy for hypotension refractory to fluid volume replacement (i.e., dopamine beginning at 2 to 5 µg/kg/min)
- Naloxone infusion (i.e., 0.5 mg/kg/hr) to improve SBP by blocking endogenous endorphin effects
- Parenteral antibiotic therapy; β-lactamase resistant antibiotic (methicillin, nafcillin, or oxacillin) initiated early
- Broad-spectrum antibiotic added if concurrent sepsis suspected
- Tetracycline added if considering Rocky Mountain spotted fever

CHRONIC Rx
- Severely ill patient: may require prolonged hospitalization and supportive management with gradual recovery and/or sequelae from severe end-organ involvement (ARDS or renal failure requiring dialysis)
- Majority of patients: complete recovery
- Early late-onset complications (within 2 wk):
  1. Skin desquamation
  2. Impaired digit sensation
  3. Denuded tongue
  4. Vocal cord paralysis
  5. ATN
  6. ARDS
- Late-onset complications (after 8 wk):
  1. Nail splitting/loss
  2. Alopecia
  3. CNS sequelae
  4. Renal impairment
  5. Cardiac dysfunction
- Recurrent TSS:
  1. More common in menstrually related cases
  2. Less common in patient treated with β-lactamase resistant anti-staphylococcal antibiotics
  3. Patients with history of TSS: if suspect signs and symptoms occur, should have high index of suspicion and low threshold for evaluation and treatment

PREVENTION
- Avoidance of tampons or use of low-absorbancy tampons only (<4 hr in situ) and alternate with napkins
- Education for patients concerning signs and symptoms of TSS
- Avoidance of tampons for patients with history of TSS

DISPOSITION
- Complete recovery for most patients
- Long-term management of early- and late-onset complications for minority of patients

REFERRAL
- For multidisciplinary management, involving primary physician, gynecologist, internist, infectious disease specialist, and other supportive care specialists
- To tertiary level hospital

MISCELLANEOUS

COMMENTS
Patient information available from American College of Gynecologists and Obstetricians.

REFERENCES
Sweet RL, Gibbs RS: *Infectious disease of the female genital tract,* ed 2, Baltimore, 1990, Williams & Wilkins.
Toxic shock syndrome—United States 1970-1982, *MMWR* 31:201, 1982.

Author: **Dennis M. Weppner, M.D.**

Toxoplasmosis (PTG)

BASIC INFORMATION

DEFINITION
Toxoplasmosis is an infection caused by the protozoal parasite *Toxoplasma gondii*.

ICD-9-CM CODES
130.9 Toxoplasmosis

EPIDEMIOLOGY AND DEMOGRAPHICS
INCIDENCE (IN U.S.):
- Increases with age
- Increases with certain activities
  1. Slaughterhouse workers
  2. Cat owners
- Increases with certain geographic locations: high prevalence of cats

INCIDENCE (IN U.S.): 3% to 70% of healthy adults

PREDOMINANT SEX: Equal gender distribution

PREDOMINANT AGE:
- Infancy (congenital infection)
- Prevalence increases with age

PEAK INCIDENCE: Temperate climates

GENETICS:

Congenital Infection:
- Incidence and severity vary with the trimester of gestation during which the mother acquired infection.
  1. 10% to 25% (first trimester)
  2. 30% to 54% (second trimester)
  3. 60% to 65% (third trimester)
- Congenital infection occurring in the first trimester is the most severe.
- 89% to 100% of infections in the third trimester are asymptomatic.
- Risk to the fetus is not correlated with symptoms in the mother.

PHYSICAL FINDINGS
- Acquired (immunocompetent host)
  1. 80% to 90% asymptomatic
  2. Adenopathy (usually cervical)
  3. Fever
  4. Myalgias
  5. Malaise
  6. Sore throat
  7. Maculopapular rash
  8. Hepatosplenomegaly
  9. Chorioretinitis rare
- Acquired (in patients with AIDS)
  1. 89% of symptomatic cases
     a. Encephalitis
     b. Intracerebral mass lesions
  2. Pneumonitis
  3. Chorioretinitis
  4. Other end-organ
- Acquired (immunocompromised patients)
  1. Encephalitis
  2. Myocarditis (especially in heart transplant patients)
  3. Pneumonitis
- Ocular infection in the immunocompetent host
  1. Congenital infection
  2. Blurred vision
  3. Photophobia
  4. Pain
  5. Loss of central vision if macula involved
  6. Focal necrotizing retinitis
  7. Typically presents in second or third decade
- Congenital
  1. Results from acute infection acquired by the mother within 6 to 8 wk before conception or during gestation
  2. Usually, asymptomatic mother
  3. No sign of disease
  4. Chorioretinitis
  5. Blindness
  6. Epilepsy
  7. Psychomotor or mental retardation
  8. Intracranial calcifications
  9. Hydrocephalus
  10. Microcephaly
  11. Encephalitis
  12. Anemia
  13. Thrombocytopenia
  14. Hepatosplenomegaly
  15. Lymphadenopathy
  16. Jaundice
  17. Rash
  18. Pneumonitis
  19. Most infected infants are asymptomatic at birth

ETIOLOGY
- *Toxoplasma gondii*
  1. Ubiquitous intracellular protozoan
  2. Present worldwide
  3. Cat is definitive host
- Human infection
  1. Ingestion of oocysts shed by cats
  2. Ingestion of meat containing tissue cysts
  3. Vertical transmission

DIAGNOSIS

DIFFERENTIAL DIAGNOSIS
- Lymphadenopathy
  1. Infectious mononucleosis
  2. CMV mononucleosis
  3. Cat-scratch disease
  4. Sarcoidosis
  5. Tuberculosis
  6. Lymphoma
  7. Metastatic cancer
- Cerebral mass lesions in immunocompromised host
  1. Lymphoma
  2. Tuberculosis
  3. Bacterial abscess
- Pneumonitis in immunocompromised host
  1. *Pneumocystis carinii* pneumonia
  2. Tuberculosis
  3. Fungal infection
- Chorioretinitis
  1. Syphilis
  2. Tuberculosis
  3. Histoplasmosis (competent host)
  4. CMV
  5. Syphilis
  6. Herpes simplex
  7. Fungal infection
  8. Tuberculosis (AIDS patient)
- Myocarditis
  1. Organ rejection in heart transplant recipients
- Congenital infection
  1. Rubella
  2. CMV
  3. Herpes simplex
  4. Syphilis
  5. Listeriosis
  6. Erythroblastosis fetalis
  7. Sepsis

WORKUP
- Acute infection, immunocompetent host
  1. CBC
  2. *Toxoplasma* serology (IgG, Ig) in serial blood specimens 3 wk apart
  3. Lymph node biopsy if diagnosis uncertain
- Immunocompromised host
  1. CNS symptoms
     a. Cerebral CT scan or MRI if CNS symptoms present
     b. Spinal tap, if safe
     c. Brain biopsy if no response to empirical therapy
  2. Ocular symptoms
     a. Funduscopic examination
     b. Serologic studies
     c. Rarely, vitreous tap
  3. Pulmonary symptoms
     a. Chest x-ray examination
     b. Bronchoalveolar lavage
     c. Transbronchial or open lung biopsy
  4. Myocarditis
     a. Cardiac enzymes
     b. Electrocardiogram
     c. Endomyocardial biopsy for definitive diagnosis
- Toxoplasmosis in pregnancy
  1. Initial maternal screening with IgM and IgG
     a. If negative, mother at risk of acute infection and should be retested monthly
     b. If both IgG and IgM positive, obtain IgA and IgE ELISA, AC/HS test
     c. IgA and IgE ELISA, AC/HS test elevated in acute infection
     d. Ig high for 1 yr or more
     e. IgG repeated 3 to 4 wk later to determine if titer is stable
  2. Acute maternal infection not excluded or documented
     a. Fetal blood sampling (for culture, Ig, IgA, IgE)
     b. Amniotic fluid PCR
  3. Fetal ultrasound every other week if maternal infection documented
- Congenital toxoplasmosis
  1. Placental histology
  2. Specific IgM or IgA in infant's blood

LABORATORY TESTS
- Antibody studies
  1. More than one test necessary to establish diagnosis of acute toxoplasmosis
  2. IgM antibody
     a. Appears 5 days into infection
     b. Peaks at 2 wk
     c. Falls to low level or disappears within 2 mo
     d. May persist at low levels for 1 yr or more
  3. Antibody not measurable
     a. Ocular toxoplasmosis
     b. Reactivation
     c. Immunocompromised hosts
  4. IgA ELISA, IgE ELISA, and IgE ASAGA
     a. More sensitive tests
     b. Disappear more rapidly than Ig, establishing diagnosis of acute infection
  5. IgG antibody
     a. Appears 1 to 2 wk after infection
     b. Peaks at 6 to 8 wk
     c. Gradually declines over months to years

IMAGING STUDIES
- Chest x-ray examination if pulmonary involvement suspected
- Cerebral CT scan or MRI if encephalitis suspected

TREATMENT

NONPHARMACOLOGIC THERAPY
- Selected cases of ocular infection
  1. Photocoagulation
  2. Vitrectomy
  3. Lentectomy
- Selected cases of congenital cerebral infection
  1. Ventricular shunting

ACUTE GENERAL Rx
- Acute infection, immunocompetent host
  1. No treatment, unless severe and persistent symptoms or vital organ damage
- Acute infection, immunocompromised host, non-AIDS
  1. Treat even if asymptomatic
  2. Duration
     a. Until 4 to 6 wk after resolution of all signs and symptoms
     b. Usually 6 mo or longer
- Reactivated infection, immunocompromised host, non-AIDS
  1. Treat if symptomatic
- Acute or reactivated infection, AIDS
  1. Treat in all cases
  2. Induction course
     a. 3 to 6 wk
     b. Maintenance therapy continued for life
  3. Empiric therapy
     a. AIDS with positive IgG
     b. Multiple ring-enhancing lesions on cerebral CT scan or MRI
     c. Response seen by day 7 in 71% and day 14 in 91%
- Ocular infection
  1. Treat in all cases
  2. Therapy continued for 1 mo or longer if needed
  3. Response seen in 70% within 10 days
  4. Retreat as needed
  5. Steroids may be indicated
  6. Surgical treatment in selected cases
- Treatment regimens
  1. Pyrimethamine 100 to 200 mg loading dose once PO, then 25 mg PO qd (50 to 75 mg in AIDS) *plus*
  2. Leucovorin 10 to 20 mg PO qd *plus*
  3. Sulfadiazine 1 to 1.5 g PO q6h
- Acute infection in pregnancy
  1. Treat immediately
  2. Risk of fetal infection reduced by 60% with treatment
     a. First trimester
        i. Spiramycin 3 g PO qd in two to four divided doses
        ii. Sulfadiazine 4 g PO qd in four divided doses
     b. Second and third trimester
        i. Sulfadiazine as above *plus*
        ii. Pyrimethamine 25 mg PO qd *plus*
        iii. Leucovorin 5 to 15 mg PO qd
        iv. Spiramycin as above
- Congenital infection
  1. Sulfadiazine 50 mg/kg PO bid *plus*
  2. Pyrimethamine 2 mg/kg PO for 2 days, then 1 mg/kg PO, three times weekly *plus*
  3. Leucovorin 5 to 20 mg PO three times weekly
  4. Minimum duration of treatment: 12 mo

CHRONIC Rx
- Maintenance therapy in AIDS patients because of the high risk (80%) of relapse
  1. Pyrimethamine 25 mg PO qd
  2. Sulfadiazine 500 mg PO qid
  3. Leucovorin 10 to 20 mg PO qd

DISPOSITION
- Prognosis
  1. Excellent in the immunocompetent host
  2. Good in ocular infection (although relapses are common)
- Treatment of acute infection in pregnancy
  1. Reduces incidence and severity of congenital toxoplasmosis
- Treatment of congenital infection
  1. Improvement in intellectual function
  2. Regression of retinal lesions
- AIDS
  1. 70% to 95% response to therapy

REFERRAL
- To infectious disease expert:
  1. Immunocompromised hosts
  2. Pregnant women
  3. Difficulty in making a diagnosis or deciding on treatment
- To pediatric infectious disease expert:
  1. Congenital infection
- To obstetrician:
  1. Pregnant seronegative mother
  2. Acute seroconversion
- To ophthalmologist:
  1. Congenital infection
  2. Any case of ocular infection

MISCELLANEOUS

COMMENTS
- Prevention of toxoplasmosis is most important in seronegative pregnant women and immunocompromised hosts.
- Patient instructions:
  1. Cook meat to 66° C.
  2. Cook eggs.
  3. Do not drink unpasteurized milk.
  4. Wash hands thoroughly after handling raw meat.
  5. Wash kitchen surfaces that come in contact with raw meat.
  6. Wash fruits and vegetables.
  7. Avoid contact with materials potentially contaminated with cat feces.

REFERENCES
Beaman MH et al: Toxoplasma gondii. In Mandell GL, Bennett JE, Dolin R (eds): *Mandell, Douglas, and Bennett's principles and practice of infectious diseases,* ed 4, New York, 1995, Churchill Livingstone.

Montoya JG, Remington JS: Toxoplasmic chorioretinitis in the setting of acute acquired toxoplasmosis, *Clin Infect Dis* 23: 277, 1996.

Remington JS, McLeod R, Desmonts G: Toxoplasmosis. In Remington JS, Klein JO (eds): *Infectious diseases of the fetus and newborn infant,* ed 4, Philadelphia, 1995, WB Saunders.

Author: **Michele Halpern, M.D.**

Tracheitis (PTG)

BASIC INFORMATION

DEFINITION
Bacterial tracheitis is an acute infectious disease affecting the trachea and large conducting airways. Tracheal inflammation may be caused by a large number of inhaled stimuli, but bacterial infection is a life-threatening illness associated with viscous purulent secretions and subglottic edema.

SYNONYMS
Bacterial tracheobronchitis
Pseudomembranous croup
Membranous laryngotracheobronchitis

ICD-9-CM CODES
464.10 Tracheitis

EPIDEMIOLOGY AND DEMOGRAPHICS
INCIDENCE (IN U.S.):
- Uncommon
- May be the most common cause of acute upper airway obstruction requiring admission to pediatric ICUs

PREDOMINANT SEX: Boys > girls in one series

PREDOMINANT AGE:
- 1 mo to 8 yr
- Almost all <13 yr (most <3 yr)

PEAK INCIDENCE: Three fourths of cases reported in winter months

GENETICS: Down syndrome is a possible predisposing factor.

Congenital Infection: Some cases found in those with anatomic abnormalities of the upper airways.

PHYSICAL FINDINGS
- Croupy or "brassy" cough
- Inspiratory stridor (frequent)
- Wheezing (unusual)
- Fever (often >102° F)
- Thick, purulent secretions expectorated
  1. Minority of patients expectorate "rice-like" pellets.
  2. Most patients are unable to mobilize secretions.
     a. Become inspissated
     b. Form pseudomembranes

ETIOLOGY
- *Staphylococcus aureus*
- *Haemophilus influenzae*
- β-Hemolytic streptococcal infection
- Secondary to viral infections of the respiratory tract
  1. Primary influenza
  2. RSV
  3. Parainfluenza
- Many cases follow measles
  1. Especially when accompanied by chest radiographic infiltrates
  2. Sometimes fatal outcome

DIAGNOSIS

DIFFERENTIAL DIAGNOSIS
- Viral croup
- Epiglottitis
- Diphtheria
- Necrotizing herpes simplex infection in the elderly
- CMV in immunocompromised patients
- Invasive *Aspergillosis* in immunocompromised patients

WORKUP
- Direct laryngoscopy
  1. Typical secretions
     a. May form pseudomembranes
     b. Airway obstruction
  2. Normal epiglottis rules out epiglottitis
  3. Possible subglottic edema

LABORATORY TESTS
- WBC is sometimes elevated.
- On differential, left shift is almost universal.
- Gram stain and culture of tracheal secretions confirm diagnosis.
- Blood cultures are positive in a minority.

IMAGING STUDIES
- Lateral x-ray examination of neck
  1. Normal epiglottis
  2. Vague density or a "dripping candle" appearance of tracheal mucosa
     a. Secretions
     b. Pseudomembranes
- Films
  1. Not diagnostic
  2. Should not be performed on patients in acute respiratory distress, since severe or fatal upper airways obstruction can develop suddenly
- Pneumonic infiltrates frequent
- Atelectasis
  1. Unusual
  2. May involve an entire lung

TREATMENT

NONPHARMACOLOGIC THERAPY
- Aggressive maintenance of a patent airway
  1. Laryngoscopy or bronchoscopy used diagnostically and therapeutically to strip away pseudomembranes
  2. Voluminous and tenacious secretions suctioned from the underlying friable mucosa
     a. May extend from between the vocal cords to the main carina
     b. Larger channels of rigid instruments for more effective suctioning
- Prevention of complete large airway obstruction
  1. Nasotracheal intubation
  2. Humidification of inspired gas
  3. Frequent saline instillation and suctioning
  4. Intubation with general anesthesia, performed in the operating room, is preferred by some
- Ventilatory support necessary
- Initial management in ICU

ACUTE GENERAL Rx
- Antibiotic therapy
  1. Start immediately
  2. Continue for 2 wk
- Initial therapy
  1. β-Lactamase producing *H. influenzae*
  2. β-Lactamase producing staphylococci
- Oral therapy is usually sufficient after 5 or 6 days of IV administration

DISPOSITION
- Most patients are extubated in 5 to 6 days after initiating antibiotic therapy.
- Anoxic encephalopathy is reported in 7% of survivors.

REFERRAL
Suspected diagnosis

MISCELLANEOUS

COMMENTS
- Infants are at increased risk of airway obstruction because of the small transverse area of the upper airway.
- Presence of pneumonia and a staphylococcal etiology are thought to worsen prognosis.
- Reported complications:
  1. Toxic shock syndrome
  2. Persistent postextubation stridor
  3. Pneumothorax
  4. Volu-trauma

REFERENCES
Penn RL: Upper airways infections. In George RB et al (eds): *Current pulmonology and critical care medicine*, Chicago, 1996, Mosby.

Author: **Harvey M. Shanies, M.D., Ph.D.**

Transfusion reaction, hemolytic

BASIC INFORMATION

DEFINITION
Hemolytic transfusion reaction is an acute intravascular hemolysis caused by mismatches in the ABO system. It is caused by complement fixing Ig and IgG antibodies to group A and B RBCs. Hemolytic transfusion reactions can also be caused by minor antigen systems; however, they are usually less severe. In delayed serologic transfusion reactions, hemolysis with hemoglobinemia is unusual; in these delayed reactions the only manifestations may be the development of a newly positive Coombs' test and fever.

ICD-9-CM CODES
999.8 Other transfusion reaction

EPIDEMIOLOGY AND DEMOGRAPHICS
Acute intravascular hemolysis occurs in <1 in 50,000 transfusions.

PHYSICAL FINDINGS
- Hypotension
- Pain at the infusion site
- Fever, tachycardia, chest or back pain, dyspnea
- Often, severe reactions occur in surgical patients under anesthesia who are unable to give any warning signs

ETIOLOGY
Most fatal hemolytic reactions are caused by clerical errors and mislabeled specimens.

DIAGNOSIS

DIFFERENTIAL DIAGNOSIS
- Bacterial contamination of blood
- Hemoglobinopathies

WORKUP
The transfusion must be stopped immediately. The blood bank must be notified and the donor transfusion bag must be returned to the blood bank along with a freshly drawn posttransfusion specimen.

LABORATORY TESTS
- Positive Coombs' test, elevated BUN, creatinine, and bilirubin
- Hemoglobinuria (wine-colored urine), hemoglobinemia (pink plasma)
- Decreased Hct, decreased serum haptoglobin

TREATMENT

NONPHARMACOLOGIC THERAPY
- Stop transfusion immediately. Test anticoagulated blood from the recipient for the presence of free Hgb in the plasma.
- Monitor vital signs.

ACUTE GENERAL Rx
- Vigorous IV hydration to maintain urine flow at >100 ml/hr until hypotension is corrected and hemoglobinuria clears. IV furosemide may be necessary to maintain adequate renal flow.
- The addition of mannitol may prevent renal damage (controversial).
- Monitor for the presence of DIC.
- Use of IV steroids is controversial.

DISPOSITION
Mortality exceeds 50% in severe transfusion reactions.

MISCELLANEOUS

COMMENTS
Hemolysis caused by minor antigen systems is generally less severe and may be delayed 5 to 10 days after transfusion.

REFERENCES
Dodd, RY: Adverse consequences of blood transfusions: quantitative risk estimates. In Nance ST (ed): *Blood supply: risks, perceptions, and prospects for the future*, Bethesda, Md, 1994, American Association of Blood Banks.

Forrara JLM: The febrile platelet reaction: a cytokine shower, *Transfusion* 35:89, 1995.

Vamvakas EC et al: The differentiation of delayed hemolytic and delayed serologic transfusion reaction: incidence and predictors of hemolysis, *Transfusion* 35:26, 1995.

Author: **Fred F. Ferri, M.D.**

Transient ischemic attack (PTG)

BASIC INFORMATION

DEFINITION
The term *transient ischemic attack* (TIA) refers to a transient focal neurologic deficit caused by cerebrovascular compromise that typically lasts <60 min but always <24 hr and is followed by a full recovery of function.

SYNONYMS
TIA

ICD-9-CM CODES
435.9 Unspecified transient cerebral ischemia

EPIDEMIOLOGY AND DEMOGRAPHICS
INCIDENCE (IN U.S.): 49 cases/100,000 persons/yr
PREDOMINANT SEX: Males > females
PREDOMINANT AGE: >60 yr
PEAK INCIDENCE: >60 yr
GENETICS:
- There is no distinct genetic etiology.
- Family history is a risk factor.

PHYSICAL FINDINGS
- During an episode, neurologic abnormalities are confined to discrete vascular territory.
- Typical carotid territory symptoms are ipsilateral monocular visual disturbance, contralateral homonomous hemianopsia, contralateral hemimotor or sensory dysfunction, and language dysfunction (dominant hemisphere) alone or in combination.
- Typical vertebrobasilar territory symptoms are binocular visual disturbance, vertigo, diplopia, dysphagia, dysarthria, and motor or sensory dysfunction involving the ipsilateral face and contralateral body.

ETIOLOGY
Multiple, including emboli from extracranial or intracranial sources.

DIAGNOSIS

DIFFERENTIAL DIAGNOSIS
- Seizures
- Hypoglycemia
- Labyrinthine disease
- Migraine
- Mass lesions
- Box 2-85 describes the differential diagnosis of focal neurologic deficits.

WORKUP
- Thorough history and physical examination
- Ancillary investigations aimed at identifying the etiology

LABORATORY TESTS
- CBC
- Platelet count
- PT
- PTT
- ESR
- Glucose
- VDRL
- Lipid profile
- Urinalysis
- Chest x-ray examination
- ECG
- Other tests as dictated by suspected etiology

IMAGING STUDIES
- Head CT scan to exclude hemorrhage
- MRI if mass lesion suspected
- Noninvasive vascular studies and echocardiography if cardiac source is suspected
- 24-hr Holter monitoring if history suggests arrhythmia
- Four-vessel cerebral angiogram if considering carotid endarterectomy

TREATMENT

NONPHARMACOLOGIC THERAPY
- Carotid endarterectomy for carotid territory TIA associated with an ipsilateral stenosis of 70% to 99%
- Modification of risk factors

ACUTE GENERAL Rx
- Depends on etiology
- Acute anticoagulation possibly beneficial in patients with documented cardiogenic emboli

CHRONIC Rx
- No data support the use of long-term anticoagulation in the management of TIA, although subpopulations may emerge in which this is found to be more effective than antiplatelet therapy.
- Antiplatelet agents (aspirin, ticlopidine) significantly reduce the risk of stroke and myocardial infarction in patients with TIA.
- No significant benefit of high-dose aspirin (up to 1500 mg/day) has been conclusively found over lower doses (75 mg to 325 mg/day).

DISPOSITION
- Stroke risk is 4.4% in the first month and 11.6% in the first year.
- The annual risk of myocardial infarction is 2.4%.
- One-year and 3-yr survival rates are 98% and 94%, respectively.

REFERRAL
If uncertain about diagnosis or management

MISCELLANEOUS

REFERENCES
Scheinberg P: Transient ischemic attacks: an update, *J Neurol Sci* 101:133, 1991.
Author: **Michael Gruenthal, M.D., Ph.D.**

Trichinosis (PTG)

BASIC INFORMATION

DEFINITION
Trichinosis is an infection by one of various species of *Trichinella*.

ICD-9-CM CODES
124 Trichinosis

EPIDEMIOLOGY AND DEMOGRAPHICS
INCIDENCE (IN U.S.): <100 cases/yr
GENETICS:
Congenital Infection:
- Abrupt delivery of stillbirths in infected pregnant women
- Vertical infection of the fetus

PHYSICAL FINDINGS
- Symptoms
  1. May vary widely depending on the time from ingestion of contaminated meat and on worm burden
  2. Most persons asymptomatic
- Enteral phase
  1. Correlates with penetration of ingested larvae into the intestinal mucosa
  2. May last from 2 to 6 wk
  3. Mild, transient diarrhea and nausea
  4. Abdominal pain
  5. Diarrhea or constipation
  6. Vomiting
  7. Malaise
  8. Low-grade fevers
- Migratory or parenteral phase
  1. In the intestine, maturation and mating
  2. Newborn larvae
     a. Penetrate into lymphatic and blood vessels
     b. Migrate to muscles where they penetrate into muscle cells, enlarge, coil, and develop a cyst wall
  3. Patients may present with
     a. Fever
     b. Myalgias
     c. Periorbital or facial edema
     d. Headache
     e. Skin rash
     f. Other symptoms caused by the penetration of tissues by the newborn migrating larva
  4. Peak in symptoms 2 to 3 wk after infection, then slowly subside
- Severe complications
  1. Brain damage by granulomatous inflammation or occlusion of arteries
  2. Cardiac involvement
  3. Can lead to death

ETIOLOGY
- The nematode responsible for this illness is an obligate intracellular parasite belonging to the genus *Trichinella*.
- It is one of the most ubiquitous parasites in the world and may be found in virtually all warm-blooded animals.
- Infection in humans occurs by the ingestion of contaminated animal meat that is raw or partially cooked and contains viable cysts.
- Most cases are now related to the consumption of poorly processed pork or wild game (bear, wild boar, cougar, and walrus).

DIAGNOSIS

DIFFERENTIAL DIAGNOSIS
- Different presentations have different differential diagnoses.
- Early illness may resemble gastroenteritis.
- Later symptoms may be confused with:
  1. Measles
  2. Dermatomyositis
  3. Glomerulonephritis
- The differential diagnosis of nematode tissue infections is described in Table 2-47 of Section II.

WORKUP
- Antibody assay of serum is usually positive by approximately 2 wk after infection.
- Muscle biopsy is used to detect the larva in muscle tissue if diagnosis unclear; best done by placing the tissue between two slides.

LABORATORY TESTS
- CBC: leukocytosis with prominent eosinophilia
- ESR: usually normal
- Elevation of muscle enzymes common (i.e., CPK, aldolase)

IMAGING STUDIES
Soft tissue radiographs may show calcified cyst walls.

TREATMENT

NONPHARMACOLOGIC THERAPY
Bed rest for myalgias

ACUTE GENERAL Rx
- No clinical evidence that treatment alters the course of infection in symptomatic individuals
- Thiabendazole to treat persons within 24 hr of ingesting contaminated meat, at the dose of 25 mg/kg/day for 1 wk
- Salicylates to decrease muscle discomfort
- Steroids in critically ill patients

DISPOSITION
- Most symptoms subside over time.
- Reports of long-term sequelae:
  1. Myalgias
  2. Headaches
- Occasionally, death occurs.

REFERRAL
Diagnosis uncertain

MISCELLANEOUS

COMMENTS
- Prevention by thorough cooking of meats
- Inadequate to smoke, cure, or dry meats

REFERENCES
Stack PS: Trichinosis—still a public threat, *Postgrad Med* 7:137, 1995.
Vollbrect A et al: Outbreak of trichinellosis associated with eating cougar jerky—Idaho, 1995, *MMWR* 45:205, 1996.

Author: **Maurice Policar, M.D.**

Trichomoniasis (PTG)

BASIC INFORMATION

DEFINITION
Trichomoniasis is a sexually transmitted disease that often coexists with other STDs.

SYNONYMS
Trick

ICD-9-CM CODES
131.00 Urogenital trichomoniasis
131.01 Trichomonial vulvovaginitis
131.9 Trichomoniasis, unspecified

EPIDEMIOLOGY AND DEMOGRAPHICS
- Trichomoniasis is responsible for 25% of all cases of clinically evident vaginitis.
- Incidence or prevalence is as follows:
  1. 5% family planning clinics
  2. 25% gynecology clinics
  3. 75% prostitutes
- Pathogenesis is uncertain for the disease.
- Both males and females can be affected, but more females are symptomatic.
- The disease is associated with preterm labor and premature rupture of membranes.

PHYSICAL FINDINGS
- Profuse, malodorous vaginal discharge
- Postcoital bleeding
- Dysuria
- Cervical "strawberry patches"
- Vaginal mucosal erythema
- Labial erythema
- Males: may be asymptomatic or complain of dysuria, urethral discharge, or (rarely) epididymitis

ETIOLOGY
Trichomoniasis vaginalis is the etiologic agent. It is an anaerobic flagellated protozoan. Humans are its only hosts. Having multiple sexual partners is a major risk factor. Incubation period is 5 to 28 days.

DIAGNOSIS

DIFFERENTIAL DIAGNOSIS
- Bacterial vaginosis
- Vulvovaginal candidiasis
- Mucopurulent cervicitis
- Chemical vaginitis
- Male-chlamydial urethritis

WORKUP
- Clinical manifestations
- Laboratory diagnosis

LABORATORY TESTS
- pH >5
- Wet mount: motile trichomonads, PMNs; diagnostic 80%
- Culture for *T. vaginalis* in rare circumstances of treatment failures

TREATMENT

NONPHARMACOLOGIC THERAPY
- Evaluate all sexual contacts and treat
- No sexual activity until completed course of treatment
- No alcohol consumption while on medication
- Screen for other STDs

ACUTE GENERAL Rx
- Metronidazole 2 g PO, single dose
- Metronidazole 500 mg bid × 7 days
- Metronidazole 375 mg bid × 7 days

CHRONIC Rx
If treatment fails, retreat with metronidazole 500 mg bid × 7 days. If treatment fails repeatedly, treat with metronidazole 2 g PO daily × 3 to 5 days; consider culture for possible resistant strain of *T. vaginalis;* evaluate sex partner.

DISPOSITION
No follow-up is necessary if patient becomes asymptomatic. Counsel patient to practice safe sex by using condoms and have a monogamous relationship.

REFERRAL
If treatment repeatedly fails, consider infectious disease consult.

MISCELLANEOUS

COMMENTS
- Patient education material can be obtained from local and state health departments or from ACOG, 409 12th St., SW, Washington, DC 20024-2188
- U.S. Preventive Services Task Force Recommendations regarding counseling to prevent HIV infections and other STDs is described in Section V, Chapter 62.

REFERENCES
Centers for Disease Control: 1998 sexually transmitted diseases treatment guidelines, *MMWR* 44(RR-1),1998.
Faro S: Review of vaginitis, *Infect Dis Obstet Gynecol* 1:158, 1993.
Author: **George T. Danakas, M.D.**

BASIC INFORMATION

DEFINITION
Trigeminal neuralgia is paroxysmal brief but intense lancinating pain in the distribution of one or more divisions of the trigeminal nerve. Pain may occur spontaneously but is often provoked by mild sensory stimuli. Involvement of the second and third divisions is common.

SYNONYMS
Tic douloureux

ICD-9-CM CODES
350.1 Trigeminal neuralgia

EPIDEMIOLOGY AND DEMOGRAPHICS
INCIDENCE (IN U.S.):
- Females: 5.9 cases/100,000 persons/yr
- Males: 3.4 cases/100,000 persons/yr

PREVALENCE (IN U.S.): 155/1,000,000 persons
PREDOMINANT SEX: Females > males
PREDOMINANT AGE: >50 yr
PEAK INCIDENCE: Sixth to seventh decade
GENETICS: Family clustering rarely occurs

PHYSICAL FINDINGS
- Primary (idiopathic) cases: none
- Secondary (symptomatic) cases: possibly a fixed sensory loss in the distribution of the affected trigeminal nerve, as well as involvement of adjacent cranial nerves
- Multiple sclerosis in 3% of patients

ETIOLOGY
- Symptomatic cases: lesions in the vicinity of the nerve or nucleus, such as cerebellopontine angle tumors
- Some "idiopathic" cases: vascular compression of root of trigeminal nerve

DIAGNOSIS

DIFFERENTIAL DIAGNOSIS
- Dental pathology
- Posterior fossa masses
- Vascular malformations
- The differential diagnosis of headache and facial pain is described in Box 2-52.

WORKUP
MRI scans (CT scan with thin posterior fossa cuts if MRI not available) for all patients to exclude mass lesions

LABORATORY TESTS
None

IMAGING STUDIES
See "Workup."

TREATMENT

NONPHARMACOLOGIC THERAPY
In refractory cases, surgical options, including percutaneous radiofrequency gangliolysis and microvascular decompression

ACUTE GENERAL Rx
None, episodes are too brief

CHRONIC Rx
- Carbamazepine is the treatment of choice, providing relief to at least 75% of patients. Begin with 100 mg bid and increase gradually as tolerated using a tid regimen.
- If carbamazepine is not tolerated or effective, use baclofen. Start at 5 mg tid and gradually increase as tolerated to a total daily dose of 80 mg.
- Additional options are phenytoin, valproate, gabapentin, clonazepam, and pimozide.

DISPOSITION
Spontaneous remissions occur after months to years.

REFERRAL
If uncertain about diagnosis or surgical treatment is necessary

MISCELLANEOUS

COMMENTS
Since prolonged remission may occur, drug tapering at yearly intervals is recommended.

REFERENCES
Mauskop A: Trigeminal neuralgia (tic douloureux), *J Pain Symptom Management* 8:148, 1993.

Author: **Michael Gruenthal, M.D., Ph.D.**

Tropical sprue

BASIC INFORMATION

DEFINITION
Tropical sprue is a malabsorption syndrome occurring primarily in tropical regions, including Puerto Rico, India, and Vietnam.

SYNONYMS
"Tropical enteropathy" refers to a subclinical form of tropical sprue.

ICD-9-CM CODES
579.1 Tropical sprue

EPIDEMIOLOGY AND DEMOGRAPHICS
Tropical sprue is endemic in tropical regions, the Middle East, the Far East, the Caribbean, and India.

PHYSICAL FINDINGS
- Diffuse, nonspecific abdominal tenderness and distention
- Low-grade fever
- Glossitis, cheilosis, hyperkeratosis, hyperpigmentation

ETIOLOGY
- Unknown
- Possible link to infection with unknown agent

DIAGNOSIS

The clinical features of tropical sprue include anorexia, diarrhea, weight loss, abdominal pain, and steatorrhea; these symptoms can develop in expatriates even several months after emigrating to temperate regions.

DIFFERENTIAL DIAGNOSIS
- Celiac disease
- Parasitic infestation
- Inflammatory bowel disease
- Other causes of malabsorption (e.g., Whipple's disease)

WORKUP
- Diagnostic workup includes a comprehensive history (especially travel history), physical examination, laboratory evidence of malabsorption (see below), and jejunal biopsy; the biopsy results are nonspecific, with blunting, atrophy, and even disappearance of the villi and subepithelial lymphocytic infiltration.
- A clinical algorithm for the evaluation of malabsorption is described in Fig. 3-56.

LABORATORY TESTS
- Megaloblastic anemia (>50% of cases)
- Vitamin B_{12} deficiency, folate deficiency
- Steatorrhea, abnormal D-xylose absorption

IMAGING STUDIES
GI series with small bowel follow-through may reveal coarsening of the jejunal folds.

TREATMENT

NONPHARMACOLOGIC THERAPY
Monitoring of weight and calorie intake

ACUTE GENERAL Rx
- Folic acid therapy (5 mg bid for 2 wk followed by a maintenance dose of 1 mg tid) will improve anemia and malabsorption in over two thirds of patients.
- Tetracycline 250 mg qid for 4 to 6 wk in individuals who have returned to temperate zones, up to 6 mo in patients in endemic areas; ampicillin 500 mg bid for at least 4 wk in patients intolerant to tetracycline
- Correction of vitamin B_{12} deficiency: vitamin B_{12} 1000 µg IM weekly for 4 wk, then monthly for 3 to 6 mo
- Correction of other nutritional deficiencies (e.g., calcium, iron)

DISPOSITION
Complete recovery with appropriate therapy

REFERRAL
GI referral for jejunal biopsy

MISCELLANEOUS

COMMENTS
Additional patient education information can be obtained from National Digestive Diseases Information Clearinghouse, Box NDDIC, Bethesda, MD 20892; phone: (301) 654-3810.

REFERENCES
Klipstein FA: Tropical sprue in travelers and expatriates living abroad, *Gastroenterology* 80:590, 1981.

Mandell GL (ed): *Principles and practice of infectious diseases,* ed 4, New York, 1995, Churchill Livingstone.

Stein JH (ed): *Internal medicine,* ed 5, St Louis, 1997, Mosby.

Author: **Fred F. Ferri, M.D.**

CLINICAL TOPICS   Tuberculosis, miliary   495

BASIC INFORMATION

DEFINITION
Miliary tuberculosis (TB) is an infection of extrapulmonary (potentially multiple) sites, caused by the bacterium *Mycobacterium tuberculosis*.

SYNONYMS
Extrapulmonary TB
Disseminated TB

ICD-9-CM CODES
018.94 Miliary tuberculosis

EPIDEMIOLOGY AND DEMOGRAPHICS
INCIDENCE (IN U.S.):
- Approximately 4000 new cases annually (1.5 cases/100,000 population), comprising an increasing proportion of total TB cases.
- >18% of all TB cases have extrapulmonary TB.
- >38% of AIDS patients with TB have disseminated disease, often with concurrent pulmonary and extrapulmonary active sites. (See "Pulmonary tuberculosis" in Section I.)

PREVALENCE (IN U.S.):
- Undetermined
- Highest prevalence
  1. AIDS patients
  2. Minorities
  3. Children
  4. Foreign-born persons

PREDOMINANT SEX:
- No specific predilection
- Male predominance in AIDS, shelters, and prisons reflected in disproportionate male TB incidence

PREDOMINANT AGE: Predominantly among 24-to-45-yr-olds

PEAK INCIDENCE: HIV-positive patients, regardless of age

PHYSICAL FINDINGS
- See also "Etiology"
- Common symptoms
  1. Fever
  2. Night sweats
  3. Weight loss
- Symptoms referable to individual organ systems may predominate
  1. Meninges
  2. Pericardium
  3. Liver
  4. Kidney
  5. Bone
  6. GI tract
  7. Lymph nodes
  8. Serous spaces
     a. Pleural
     b. Pericardial
     c. Peritoneal
     d. Joint
  9. Skin
- Adrenal insufficiency possible
- Pancytopenia
  1. With fever and weight loss *or*
  2. Without other localizing symptoms or signs *or*
  3. With only splenomegaly
- TB hepatitis
  1. Tender liver
  2. Obstructive enzymes (alkaline phosphatase) elevated out of proportion to minimal hepatocellular enzymes (SGOT, SGPT) and bilirubin
- TB meningitis
  1. Gradual-onset headache
  2. Minimal meningeal signs
  3. Malaise
  4. Low-grade fever (may be absent)
  5. Sudden stupor or coma
  6. Cranial nerve VI palsy
- TB pericarditis
  1. Effusions resembling TB pleurisy
- Skeletal TB
  1. Large joint arthritis (with effusions resembling TB pericarditis)
  2. Bone lesions (especially ribs)
  3. Pott's disease
     a. TB spondylitis, especially of lower thoracic spine
     b. Paraspinous TB abscess
     c. Possible psoas abscess
     d. Frequent cord compression (often relieved by steroids)
- Genitourinary TB
  1. Renal TB
     a. Papillary necrosis
     b. Destruction of renal pelvis
     c. Strictures of upper third of ureters
     d. Hematuria
     e. Pyuria with misleading bacterial cultures
     f. Preserved renal function
  2. TB orchitis or epididymitis
     a. Scrotal mass
     b. Draining abscess
  3. Chronic prostatic TB
- Gastrointestinal TB
  1. Diarrhea
  2. Pain
  3. Obstruction
  4. Bleeding
  5. Especially common with AIDS
  6. Bowel lesions
     a. Circumferential ulcers
     b. Short strictures
     c. Calcified granulomas
     d. TB mesenteric caseous adenitis
     e. Abscess, but rare fistula formation
     f. Often difficult to distinguish from granulomatous bowel disease
- TB peritonitis
  1. Fluid resembles TB pleurisy
  2. PPD often negative
  3. Tender abdomen
  4. Doughy peritoneal consistency, often with ascites
  5. Peritoneal biopsy indicated for diagnosis
- TB lymphadenitis (scrofula)
  1. May involve all node groups
  2. Common adenopathies
     a. Cervical
     b. Supraclavicular
     c. Axillary
     d. Retroperitoneal
  3. Biopsy generally needed for diagnosis
  4. Surgical resection of nodes may be necessary
  5. Especially common with AIDS
- Cutaneous TB
  1. Skin infection from autoinoculation or dissemination
  2. Nodules or abscesses
  3. Tuberculids (possibly allergic reactions)
  4. Erythema nodosum
- Miscellaneous presentations
  1. TB laryngitis
  2. TB otitis
  3. Ocular TB
     a. Choroidal tubercles
     b. Iritis
     c. Uveitis
     d. Episcleritis
  4. Adrenal TB
  5. Breast TB

ETIOLOGY
- See also "Pulmonary tuberculosis" in Section I.
- *Mycobacterium tuberculosis* (Mtb), a slow-growing, aerobic, non-spore-forming, nonmotile bacillus
- Humans are the only reservoir for Mtb.
- Pathogenesis:
  1. AFB (Mtb) are ingested by macrophages in alveoli, then transported to regional lymph nodes where spread is contained.
  2. Some AFB reach the bloodstream and disseminate widely.
  3. Immediate active disseminated disease may ensue or a latent period may develop.
  4. During latent period, T-cell immune mechanisms contain infection in granulomas until later reactivation occurs as a result of immunosuppression or other undefined factors in conjunction with reactivated pulmonary TB or alone.
- Extrapulmonary TB is possible from contiguous spread.
  1. From pulmonary foci
  2. From mucosal spread (e.g., to GI tract or larynx) of large numbers of Mtb organisms from pulmonary secretions
- Rapid local progression and dissemination may occur in infants, with devastating illness before PPD conversion occurs.

Tuberculosis, miliary

DIAGNOSIS

DIFFERENTIAL DIAGNOSIS
- Widespread sites of possible dissemination associated with myriad differential diagnostic possibilities
- Lymphoma
- Typhoid fever
- Brucellosis
- Other tumors
- Collagen-vascular disease

WORKUP
- Sputum for AFB stains and culture
- Chest x-ray examination
- PPD (may be negative) (See "Pulmonary tuberculosis" in Section I)
- Biopsy
  1. Bone marrow
  2. Node
  3. Peritoneal
  4. Pericardial
  5. Bone
- Imaging studies
  1. Bone
  2. Renal
  3. Nodes
  4. Liver

LABORATORY TESTS
- Sputum for AFB stains and culture, especially with abnormal chest x-ray examination (See "Pulmonary tuberculosis" in Section I)
  1. AFB stain–negative sputum may grow Mtb subsequently
- Gastric aspirates, especially in HIV-negative patients
- CBC
  1. Variable values
     a. WBC low, normal, or elevated (including leukemoid reaction: >50,000)
     b. Normocytic, normochromic anemia
  2. Rarely helpful diagnostically
- ESR usually elevated
- Bone marrow biopsy in difficult-to-diagnose cases, especially without localizing signs
- TB meningitis
  1. CSF
     a. WBC: 0 to 1500 (polys early; lymphs later)
     b. Moderately elevated protein
     c. Glucose often only modestly depressed
  2. AFB smears usually negative (although Mtb may eventually grow)
  3. Tuberculomas (small, round lesions) seen on CT scan or MRI of brain (which may also reveal typical basilar arachnoiditis)
- TB pleurisy
  1. Pleural fluid
     a. 1000 to 2000 WBC (polys early; lymphs late)
     b. Protein up to 2.5 g
     c. Glucose rarely <20
     d. pH generally <7.3
  2. Pleural fluid AFB smears generally negative
  3. Pleural biopsy more likely diagnostic
  4. Diagnosis crucial, since TB pleurisy often resolves spontaneously, but heralds later severe TB disease elsewhere

IMAGING STUDIES
- Chest x-ray examination (may or may not be positive) (See "Pulmonary tuberculosis" in Section I)
- CT scan or MRI of brain
  1. Tuberculoma
  2. Basilar arachnoiditis
- Barium studies of bowel

TREATMENT

NONPHARMACOLOGIC THERAPY
- Bed rest during acute phase of treatment
- High-calorie, high-protein diet to reverse malnutrition and enhance immune response to TB
- Isolation in negative-pressure rooms with high-volume air replacement and circulation (with health care provider wearing proper protective 0.5- to 1-micron filter respirators)
  1. Until three consecutive sputum AFB smears are negative, if pulmonary disease coexists
  2. Isolation not required for closed-space TB infections

ACUTE GENERAL Rx
- See "Pulmonary tuberculosis" in Section I.
- More rapid response to chemotherapy by disseminated TB foci than cavitary pulmonary TB.
- Treatment for 6 mo with INH plus rifampin plus PZA.
  1. Treatment for 12 mo often required for bone and renal TB.
  2. Prolonged treatment often required for CNS and pericardial.
  3. Prolonged treatment often required for all disseminated TB in infants.
- Compliance (rigid adherence to treatment regimen) is the chief determinant of success.
  1. Supervised DOT is recommended for all patients.
  2. Supervised DOT is mandatory for unreliable patients.
- Steroids are often helpful additions to TB treatment to prevent constrictive pericarditis with ascites.

CHRONIC Rx
- Generally not indicated beyond treatment described above
- Prolonged treatment supervised by ID expert required in a few complicated infections caused by resistant organisms

DISPOSITION
- Monthly follow-up by physician experienced in TB treatment
- Confirm sensitivity testing, and alter treatment appropriately (see "Pulmonary tuberculosis" in Section I)

REFERRAL
- To infectious-disease expert for:
  1. HIV-positive patient
  2. Patient with suspected drug-resistant TB
  3. Patients previously treated for TB
  4. Patients whose fever has not decreased and sputum (if positive) has not converted to negative in 2 to 4 wk
  5. Patients with overwhelming pulmonary or extrapulmonary tuberculosis
- To pulmonary, orthopedic, or GI physicians for examinations or biopsy

MISCELLANEOUS

COMMENTS
- All contacts (especially close household contacts and infants) should be properly tested for PPD conversions >3 mo following exposure.
- Those with positive PPD should be evaluated for active TB and properly treated or given prophylaxis.
- U.S. Preventive Services Task Force Recommendations regarding screening for tuberculous infection are described in Section V, Chapter 25.

REFERENCES
Centers for Disease Control and Prevention, Division of Tuberculosis Elimination: *Core curriculum on tuberculosis,* ed 3, Atlanta, 1994, Centers for Disease Control and Prevention. (Order via CDC Fax Information: 404-332-4565).

Centers for Disease Control: Tuberculosis morbidity—United States, 1995, *MMWR* 45:365, 1996.

Drugs for tuberculosis, *Med Lett Drugs Ther* 37:767, 1995.

Hass DW: Current and future applications of polymerase chain reaction for *Mycobacterium tuberculosis, Mayo Clin Proc* 71:311, 1996.

Author: Peter Nicholas, M.D.

Tuberculosis, pulmonary (PTG)

BASIC INFORMATION

DEFINITION
Pulmonary tuberculosis (TB) is an infection of the lung and, occasionally, surrounding structures, caused by the bacterium *Mycobacterium tuberculosis*.

SYNONYMS
TB

ICD-9-CM CODES
011.9 Pulmonary tuberculosis

EPIDEMIOLOGY AND DEMOGRAPHICS

INCIDENCE (IN U.S.):
- Approximately 10 cases/100,000 persons
- >90% of new cases each year from reactivated prior infections
- 9% newly infected
- Only 10% of patients with PPD conversions (higher [8%/yr] in HIV-positive patients) will develop TB, most within 1 to 2 yr
- Two thirds of all new cases in racial and ethnic minorities
- 80% of new cases in children in racial and ethnic minorities
- Occurs most frequently in geographic areas and among populations with highest AIDS prevalence
  1. Urban blacks and Hispanics between 25 and 45 yr old
  2. Poor, crowded urban communities
- Nearly 36% of new cases from new immigrants

PREVALENCE (IN U.S.):
- Estimated 10 million people infected
- Varies widely among population groups

PREDOMINANT SEX:
- No specific predilection
- Male predominance in AIDS, shelters, and prisons reflected in disproportionate male incidence

PREDOMINANT AGE:
- 24 to 45 yr old
- Childhood cases common among minorities
- Nursing home outbreaks among elderly

PEAK INCIDENCE:
- Infancy
- Teenage years
- Pregnancy
- Elderly
- HIV-positive patients, regardless of age, at highest risk

GENETICS:
- Populations with widespread low native resistance have been intensely infected when initially exposed to TB.
- Following elimination of those with least native resistance, incidence and prevalence of TB tend to decline.

PHYSICAL FINDINGS
- See "Etiology"
- Primary pulmonary TB infection generally asymptomatic
- Reactivation pulmonary TB
  1. Fever
  2. Night sweats
  3. Cough
  4. Hemoptysis
  5. Scanty nonpurulent sputum
  6. Weight loss
- Progressive primary pulmonary TB disease: same as reactivation pulmonary TB
- TB pleurisy
  1. Pleuritic chest pain
- Rare massive, suffocating, fatal hemoptysis secondary to erosion of pulmonary artery within a cavity (Rasmussen's aneurysm)
- Chest examination
  1. Not specific
  2. Usually underestimates extent of disease
  3. Rales accentuated following a cough (posttussive rales)

ETIOLOGY
- *Mycobacterium tuberculosis* (Mtb), a slow-growing, aerobic, non-spore-forming, nonmotile bacillus, with a lipid-rich cell wall
  1. Lacks pigment
  2. Produces niacin
  3. Reduces nitrate
  4. Produces heat-labile catalase
  5. Mtb staining, acid-fast and acid-alcohol fast by Ziehl-Neelsen method, appearing as red, slightly bent, beaded rods 2 to 4 microns long (acid fast bacilli [AFB]), against a blue background
  6. Polymerase chain reaction (PCR) to detect <10 organisms/ml in sputum (compared with the requisite 10,000 organisms/ml for AFB smear detection)
  7. Culture
     a. Growth on solid media (Lowenstein-Jensen; Middlebrook 7H11) in 2 to 6 wk
     b. Growth in liquid media (BACTEC, utilizing a radioactive carbon source for early growth detection) often in 9 to 16 days
     c. Enhanced in a 5% to 10% carbon dioxide atmosphere
  8. DNA fingerprinting (based on restriction fragment length polymorphism [RFLP])
     a. Facilitates immediate identification of Mtb strains in early growing cultures
     b. False-negatives possible if growth suboptimal
  9. Humans are the only reservoir for Mtb
  10. Transmission
      a. Facilitated by close exposure to high-velocity cough (unprotected by proper mask or respirators) from patient with AFB-positive sputum and cavitary lesions, producing aerosolized droplets containing AFB, which are inhaled directly into alveoli
      b. Occurs within prisons, nursing homes, and hospitals
- Pathogenesis
  1. AFB (Mtb) ingested by macrophages in alveoli, then transported to regional lymph nodes where spread is contained
  2. Some AFB may reach bloodstream and disseminate widely
  3. Primary TB (asymptomatic, minimal pneumonitis in lower or midlung fields, with hilar lymphadenopathy) essentially an intracellular infection, with multiplication of organisms continuing for 2 to 12 wk after primary exposure, until cell-mediated hypersensitivity (detected by positive skin test reaction to tuberculin purified protein derivative [PPD]) matures, with subsequent containment of infection
  4. Local and disseminated AFB thus contained by T-cell mediated immune responses
     a. Recruitment of monocytes
     b. Transformation of lymphocytes with secretion of lymphokines
     c. Activation of macrophages and histiocytes
     d. Organization into granulomas, where organisms may survive within macrophages (Langhans' giant cells), but within which multiplication essentially ceases (95%) and from which spread is prohibited
  5. Progressive primary pulmonary disease
     a. May immediately follow the asymptomatic phase
     b. Necrotizing pulmonary infiltrates
     c. Tuberculous bronchopneumonia
     d. Endobronchial TB
     e. Interstitial TB
     f. Widespread miliary lung lesions
  6. Postprimary TB pleurisy with pleural effusion
     a. Develops after early primary infection, although often before conversion to positive PPD
     b. Results from pleural seeding from a peripheral lung lesion

c. May produce a large (sometimes hemorrhagic) exudative effusion (with polymorphonuclear cells early, rapidly replaced by lymphocytes), frequently without pulmonary infiltrates
d. Generally resolves without treatment
e. Portends a high risk of subsequent clinical disease, and therefore must be diagnosed and treated early (pleural biopsy and culture) to prevent future catastrophic TB illness
f. May result in disseminated extrapulmonary infection
7. Reactivation pulmonary TB
a. Occurs months to years following primary TB
b. Preferentially involves the apical posterior segments of the upper lobes and superior segments of the lower lobes
c. Associated with necrosis and cavitation of involved lung, hemoptysis, chronic fever, night sweats, weight loss
8. Reinfection TB
a. May mimic reactivation TB
b. Ruptured caseous foci and cavities, which may produce endobronchial spread
9. Mtb in both progressive primary and reactivation pulmonary TB
a. Intracellular (macrophage) lesions (undergoing slow multiplication)
b. Closed caseous lesions (undergoing slow multiplication)
c. Extracellular, open cavities (undergoing rapid multiplication)
d. INH and rifampin cidal in all three sites
e. PZA especially active within acidic macrophage environment
f. Extrapulmonary reactivation disease also possible
10. Rapid local progression and dissemination in infants with devastating illness before PPD conversion occurs
11. Most symptoms (fever, weight loss, anorexia) and tissue destruction (caseous necrosis) from cytokines and cell-mediated immune responses
12. Mtb has no important endotoxins or exotoxins
13. Granuloma formation related to tumor necrosis factor (TNF) secreted by activated macrophages

DIAGNOSIS

DIFFERENTIAL DIAGNOSIS
- Necrotizing pneumonia (anaerobic, gram-negative)
- Histoplasmosis
- Coccidioidomycosis
- Melioidosis
- Interstitial lung diseases (rarely)
- Cancer
- Sarcoidosis
- Silicosis
- Paragonimiasis
- Rare pneumonias
  1. *Rhodococcus equi* (cavitation)
  2. *Bacillus cereus* (50% hemoptysis)
  3. *Eikenella corrodens* (cavitation)

WORKUP
- Sputum for AFB stains
- Chest x-ray examination
- PPD
  1. Recent conversion from negative to positive within 3 mo of exposure is highly suggestive of recent infection.
  2. Single positive PPD is not helpful diagnostically.
  3. Negative PPD never rules out acute TB.
  4. Be certain that positive PPD does not reflect "booster phenomenon" (prior positive PPD may become negative after several years and return to positive only after second repeated PPD; repeat second PPD within 1 wk), which thus may mimic skin-test conversion.
  5. Positive PPD reaction is determined as follows:
     a. Induration after 72 hr of 0.1 ml intradermal injection of 0.1 ml of 5 TU-PPD
     b. 5-mm induration if HIV-positive, close contact of active TB, fibrotic chest lesions
     c. 10-mm induration if in high medical risk groups (immunosuppressive disease or therapy, renal failure, gastrectomy, silicosis, diabetes), foreign-born high-risk group (Southeast Asia, Latin America, Africa, India), low socioeconomic groups, IV drug addict, prisoner, health care worker
     d. 15-mm induration if low risk
  6. Anergy antigen testing (using mumps, *Candida*, tetanus toxoid) may identify patients who are truly anergic to PPD and these antigens, but results are often confusing.
  7. Patients with TB may be selectively anergic only to PPD.
  8. Positive PPD indicates prior infection but does not itself confirm active disease.

LABORATORY TESTS
- Sputum for AFB stains and culture
  1. Induced sputum if patient not coughing productively
- Sputum from bronchoscopy if high suspicion of TB with negative expectorated induced sputum for AFB
  1. Positive AFB smear is essential before or shortly after treatment to ensure subsequent growth for definitive diagnosis and sensitivity testing
  2. Consider lung biopsy if sputum negative, especially if infiltrates are predominantly interstitial
- AFB stain–negative sputum may grow Mtb subsequently
- Gastric aspirates reliable, especially in HIV-negative patients
- CBC
  1. Variable values
     a. WBC: low, normal or elevated (including leukemoid reaction: >50,000)
     b. Normocytic, normochromic anemia often
  2. Rarely helpful diagnostically
- ESR usually elevated
- Thoracentesis
  1. Exudative effusion
     a. Elevated protein
     b. Decreased glucose
     c. Elevated WBC (polymorphonuclear leukocytes early, replaced later by lymphocytes)
     d. May be hemorrhagic
  2. Pleural fluid usually AFB-negative
  3. Pleural biopsy often diagnostic
  4. Culture pleural biopsy tissue for AFB
- Bone marrow biopsy is often diagnostic in difficult-to-diagnose cases, especially miliary tuberculosis

IMAGING STUDIES
- Chest x-ray examination
  1. Primary infection reflected by calcified peripheral lung nodule with calcified hilar lymph node
  2. Reactivation pulmonary TB
     a. Necrosis
     b. Cavitation (especially on apical lordotic views)
     c. Fibrosis and hilar retraction
     d. Bronchopneumonia
     e. Interstitial infiltrates
     f. Miliary pattern
     g. Many of above may also accompany progressive primary TB
  3. TB pleurisy
     a. Pleural effusion, often rapidly accumulating and massive

Tuberculosis, pulmonary (PTG)

4. TB activity not established by single chest x-ray examination
5. Serial chest x-ray examinations are excellent indicators of progression or regression

TREATMENT

NONPHARMACOLOGIC THERAPY
- Bed rest during acute phase of treatment
- High-calorie, high-protein diet to reverse malnutrition and enhance immune response to TB
- Isolation in negative-pressure rooms with high-volume air replacement and circulation, with health care provider wearing proper protective 0.5- to 1-micron filter respirators, until three consecutive sputum AFB smears are negative

ACUTE GENERAL Rx
- Compliance (rigid adherence to treatment regimen) chief determinant of success
  1. Supervised directly observed therapy (DOT) recommended for all patients and mandatory for unreliable patients
- Preferred adult regimen: DOT
  1. Isoniazid (INH) 15 mg/kg (max 900 mg) + rifampin 600 mg + ethambutol (EMB) 30 mg/kg (max 2500 mg) + pyrazinamide (PZA) (2 g [<50 kg]; 2.5 g [51 to 74 kg]; 3 g [>75 kg]) thrice weekly for 6 mo
  2. Alternative, more complicated DOT regimens
- Short-course daily therapy: adult
  1. HIV-negative patient: 6 mo total therapy (2 mo INH 300 mg + rifampin 600 mg + EMB 15 mg/kg (max 2500 mg) + PZA (1.5 g [<50 kg]; 2 g [51 to 74 kg]; 2.5 g [>75 kg]) daily and until smear negative and sensitivity confirmed; then INH+ rifampin daily × 4 mo)
  2. HIV-positive patient: 9 mo total therapy (2 mo INH + rifampin + EMB + PZA daily until smear negative and sensitivity confirmed; then INH + rifampin qd × 7 mo)
  3. Continue treatment at least 3 mo following conversion to negative cultures
- Drug resistance (often multiple drug resistance [MDRTB]) increased by:
  1. Prior treatment
  2. Acquisition of TB in developing countries
  3. Homelessness
  4. AIDS
  5. Prisoners
  6. IV drug addicts
  7. Known contact with MDRTB
- Never add single drug to failing regimen
- Never treat TB with fewer than two to three drugs or two to three new additional drugs
- Monitor for clinical toxicity (especially hepatitis)
  1. Patient and physician awareness that anorexia, nausea, RUQ pain, and unexplained malaise require immediate cessation of treatment
  2. Evaluation of liver function tests
     a. Minimal SGOT/SGPT elevations without symptoms generally transient and not clinically significant
- Preventive treatment for PPD conversion only (infection without disease)
  1. Must be certain that chest x-ray examination is negative and patient has no symptoms of TB
  2. INH 300 mg daily for 6 to 12 mo; at least 12 mo if HIV-positive
  3. Most important groups:
     a. HIV-positive
     b. Close contact of active TB
     c. Recent converter
     d. Old TB on chest x-ray examination
     e. IV drug addict
     f. Medical risk factor
     g. High-risk foreign country
     h. Homeless
- Infants generally given prophylaxis immediately if recent contact of active TB (even if infant PPD negative), then retested with PPD in 3 mo (continuing INH if PPD becomes positive and stopping INH if PPD remains negative)
- Chronic, stable PPD (several years) given INH prophylaxis generally only if patient is <35 yr old
  1. INH toxicity may outweigh benefit
  2. Individualize decision
- Preventive therapy for suspected INH-resistant organisms is unclear

CHRONIC Rx
- Generally not indicated beyond treatment described above
- Prolonged treatment, supervised by ID expert, in a few very complicated infections caused by resistant organisms

DISPOSITION
- Monthly follow-up by physician experienced in TB treatment
- Confirm sensitivity testing and alter treatment appropriately
- Frequent sputum samples until culture is negative
- Confirm chest x-ray regression at 2 to 3 mo

REFERRAL
- To infectious disease expert for:
  1. HIV-positive patient
  2. Patient with suspected drug-resistant TB
  3. Patients previously treated for TB
  4. Patients whose fever has not decreased and sputum has not converted to negative in 2 to 4 wk
  5. Patients with overwhelming pulmonary or extrapulmonary tuberculosis
- To pulmonologist for bronchoscopy or pleural biopsy

MISCELLANEOUS

COMMENTS
- All contacts (especially close household contacts and infants) should be properly tested for PPD conversions during 3 mo following exposure.
- Those with positive PPD should be evaluated for active TB and properly treated or given prophylaxis.
- U.S. Preventive Services Task Force Recommendations regarding screening for tuberculosis are described in Section V, Chapter 25.

REFERENCES
Centers for Disease Control and Prevention, Division of Tuberculosis Elimination: *Core curriculum on tuberculosis,* ed 3, Atlanta, 1994, Centers for Disease Control and Prevention. (Order via CDC Fax Information: 404-332-4565).

Centers for Disease Control: Tuberculosis morbidity—United States, 1995, *MMWR* 45:365, 1996.

Drugs for tuberculosis, *Med Lett Drugs Ther* 37:767, 1995.

Hass DW: Current and future applications of polymerase chain reaction for *Mycobacterium tuberculosis, Mayo Clin Proc* 71:311, 1996.

Author: **Peter Nicholas, M.D.**

Tularemia

BASIC INFORMATION

DEFINITION
Tularemia is a systemic infection primarily of animals, and occasionally humans, caused by the bacterium *Francisella tularensis*.

SYNONYMS
Rabbit fever
Deer-fly fever
Market men's disease (U.S.)
Wild hare disease
Ohara's disease (Japan)
Water-rat trapper's disease (Russia)

ICD-9-CM CODES
021.9 Tularemia

EPIDEMIOLOGY AND DEMOGRAPHICS
INCIDENCE (IN U.S.):
- 0.05 to 0.15 cases/100,000 persons
- Varies greatly among states
- Most cases (55%)
  1. Arkansas
  2. Oklahoma
  3. Missouri
- Fewer cases
  1. Texas
  2. Oklahoma
- Total reported cases/yr = about 200

PREVALENCE (IN U.S.):
- Varies widely
- Most commonly affected:
  1. Laboratory workers
  2. Farmers
  3. Veterinarians
  4. Sheep workers
  5. Hunters
  6. Trappers
  7. Meat handlers

PREDOMINANT SEX: Male
PREDOMINANT AGE: >30 yr
PEAK INCIDENCE: Summer

PHYSICAL FINDINGS
- 2- to 5-day incubation period (range 1 to 21 days)
- Fever
- Chills
- Headache
- Myalgias
- Diarrhea
- Vomiting
- Cough (pulmonic form)
- Relative bradycardia (40% of patients)
- Ulceroglandular (UG) tularemia
  1. 80% of cases
  2. Follows skin inoculation
     a. Papule
     b. Sharp ulcer with necrotic base (absent in 20%)
     c. Large, tender regional lymph nodes
  3. Pharyngeal variant
     a. Exudative pharyngitis
     b. Ulceration
     c. Occasional membrane
  4. Adenopathy
     a. Rabbit-associated is predominantly axillary
     b. Tickborne is predominantly inguinal
- Oculoglandular (OG) tularemia
  1. 0% to 5%
  2. Follows eye inoculation
     a. Conjunctivitis
     b. Regional adenopathy
- Pulmonic tularemia
  1. High mortality
  2. May coexist with other forms
  3. Nonproductive cough
  4. Bilateral rales
  5. Consolidation
  6. Pleuritic chest pain
  7. Hemoptysis rare
- Typhoidal form
  1. 5% to 30%
  2. Often concomitant with pulmonic form
  3. Fever
  4. Malaise
  5. Sore throat
  6. Abdominal discomfort
  7. Diarrhea
  8. Myalgias
  9. Absence of skin lesions
  10. Absence of adenopathy
  11. Hepatomegaly
  12. Splenomegaly
- Secondary skin rash
  1. Maculopapular
  2. Urticarial
  3. Erythema nodosum (especially in pulmonic form)
  4. Erythema multiforme

ETIOLOGY
- Gram-negative coccobacilli, *Francisella tularensis*
  1. Two biogroups
     a. *F. tularensis* biogroup *tularensis* Type A (North America; most virulent)
     b. *F. tularensis* biogroup *palaearctica* Type B (Asia, Europe > North America; less virulent)
  2. Encapsulated strains are more virulent
  3. Overall mortality <5%
- Most frequent during June to August
- Predominantly a disease of Northern Hemisphere
  1. 30° to 71° latitude
  2. Absent in United Kingdom
- Ecology
  1. Infection of rabbits
  2. Infection of rodents
     a. Squirrels
     b. Muskrats
     c. Beaver
- Human infection
  1. Insect bite
  2. Contact with contaminated animal (usually rabbit) products
  3. Contact with contaminated water
- Vectors
  1. Blood-feeding arthropods
     a. Ticks in Rocky Mountain states
  2. Biting flies
     a. California
     b. Southwest
  3. Most common tick vectors in U.S.
     a. Dog tick (*Dermacentor variabilis*)
     b. Wood tick (*D. andersoni*)
     c. Lone Star tick (*Amblyomma americanum*) (organism present in tick feces, saliva)
     d. Deer flies
  4. Most childhood disease in U.S. from tick bites
- Pathogenesis
  1. Primary infection (required dose: cutaneous much less than ingestion)
  2. Papule
     a. Develops locally over 3 to 5 days after cutaneous inoculation
     b. Followed by ulceration, spreading to lymph nodes, and dissemination (also via bacteremia)
  3. Granulomas (some caseating)
  4. Cell-mediated immunity required for recovery
  5. Antibodies not completely protective
  6. Pulmonic form
     a. May follow inhalation (often occupational)
     b. May follow hematogenous spread
  7. Pleural effusion usually lymphocytic; granulomas on biopsy
- Complications
  1. Disseminated suppurative adenitis
  2. Intravascular coagulation
  3. Hepatitis with jaundice
  4. Renal failure
  5. Rhabdomyolysis
  6. Rarely, meningitis (lymphocytic)
  7. Incidence of the following is decreased owing to antibiotic therapy:
     a. Osteomyelitis
     b. Encephalitis
     c. Splenic rupture

DIAGNOSIS

DIFFERENTIAL DIAGNOSIS
- UG form
  1. Pyogenic bacterial infections
  2. Cat-scratch disease
  3. Disseminated bacillary angiomatosis
  4. Syphilis
  5. Chancroid
  6. Lymphogranuloma venereum
  7. Tuberculosis
  8. Other mycobacteria
  9. Toxoplasmosis
  10. Sporotrichosis
  11. Rat-bite fever

Tularemia

12. Anthrax
13. Plague
14. Diphtheria
15. Streptococcal pharyngitis
16. Mononucleosis
17. Adenovirus
- OG form
  1. Cat-scratch disease
  2. Adenovirus conjunctivitis
  3. Syphilis
  4. Herpes simplex conjunctivitis
- Pulmonic form
  1. Tuberculosis
  2. *Mycoplasma*
  3. *Legionella*
  4. Q fever
  5. Psittacosis
  6. Mycoses
- Typhoidal form
  1. Typhoid fever
  2. Brucellosis
  3. *Legionella*
  4. Rickettsioses
  5. Malaria
  6. Endocarditis
  7. Histoplasmosis

WORKUP
- Cultures
  1. Blood
  2. Sputum
  3. Skin
  4. See warning under "Laboratory Tests"
- Serum for serology
- Chest x-ray examination
- Skin or other biopsy for fluorescent staining
- Liver function tests
- Renal function tests

LABORATORY TESTS
- CBC
  1. Usually nonspecific
  2. Thrombocytopenia common
  3. ESR variable
- Cultures
  1. Pose extreme danger to laboratory personnel; warn laboratory upon submission
  2. Often unsuccessful except on extremely supportive media containing cystine, thioglycolate, or Thayer-Martin; CO_2 atmosphere
- Serology
  1. More sensitive; especially ELISA, hemagglutination
  2. Both IgM and IgG may persist >10 yr
     a. Need serial rising titers for confirmation
     b. Cross-reaction with *Brucella, Yersinia, Proteus OX19*, heterophile titers
- Direct fluorescent antibody staining of tissue is definitive
- Severe disease
  1. Myoglobinuria
  2. Elevated CPK
  3. Hyponatremia
  4. Elevated creatinine
  5. Hepatitis with elevated ALT
  6. Decreased fibrinogen
  7. Elevated fibrin split products

IMAGING STUDIES
- Chest x-ray examination
  1. Lobar, apical, or miliary infiltrates
  2. Hilar adenopathy
  3. Pleural effusion
  4. Rare cavitation

TREATMENT

ACUTE GENERAL Rx
- Streptomycin is drug of choice (at least 7.5 to 10 mg/kg IM q12h × 7 to 14 days)
- Gentamicin is a suitable alternative
- For meningitis:
  1. Streptomycin plus chloramphenicol
  2. Failures reported with:
     a. Ceftriaxone
     b. Imipenem
     c. Quinolones
- Higher relapse rates with:
  1. Tetracycline
  2. Chloramphenicol (bacteriostatic)

CHRONIC Rx
Surgical drainage is required for chronic suppurative adenitis.

DISPOSITION
Careful follow-up until adenopathy, pneumonitis, pleural effusions, meningitis completely resolve

REFERRAL
- To infectious disease specialist for all aspects of diagnosis and treatment
- To surgeon for suppurative adenitis, empyema drainage

MISCELLANEOUS

COMMENTS
- Prevention
  1. Avoid exposure
     a. Skinning or handling animals with bare hands (use masks, eyecovers, gloves)
  2. Thoroughly cook wild game before ingestion
  3. Avoid tick and deer-fly exposure
     a. Repellents
     b. Clothing fitting tightly at wrists and ankles
- Person-to-person transmission does not occur
- Live attenuated vaccine
  1. Usually prevents typhoidal form
  2. Modifies but does not prevent other forms
- Streptomycin probably effective for postexposure prophylaxis following definite exposure (e.g., laboratory accidents)
- Considerable protective immunity induced by natural disease

Author: Peter Nicholas, M.D.

Turner's syndrome

BASIC INFORMATION

DEFINITION
Turner's syndrome refers to a pattern of malformation characterized by short stature, ovarian hypofunction, loose nuchal skin, and cubitus valgus as described by Turner in 1938. An associated 45,X chromosome constitution was recognized by Ford et al in 1959.

SYNONYMS
All obsolete:
Ullrich-Turner syndrome
Bonnevie-Ullrich-Turner syndrome

ICD-9-CM CODES
758.6 Syndrome, Turner's

EPIDEMIOLOGY AND DEMOGRAPHICS
INCIDENCE: 1 case out of every 2500 to 5000 live births

PHYSICAL FINDINGS
- Turner's phenotype is recognizable at any point on the developmental spectrum.
- In spontaneous abortuses the most common sex chromosome abnormality detected (45,X chromosome constitution) is found in 75% of affected individuals and accounts for 20% of such cases.
- In fetuses, it is suspected because of such ultrasonographic manifestations as thickening of the nuchal folds, frank nuchal cystic hygromas, or mild shortness of the femora at midtrimester.
- In infants:
  1. At birth may display loose nuchal skin (pterygium colli) and edema on the dorsa of hands and feet
  2. Canthal folds reflecting midface hypoplasia and redundant skin in the periorbital region
  3. Nipples appearing widely spaced
  4. Heart and cardiovascular system: murmur of aortic stenosis or bicuspid aortic valve or diminished femoral pulses suggestive of aortic coarctation
  5. Renal ultrasonography: renal ectopia such as pelvic kidney or horseshoe kidneys
- In older children:
  1. Slow linear growth
  2. Short stature—may be improved with growth hormone therapy
  3. Delayed or absent menses—secondary sex characteristics possibly normalized with estrogen replacement therapy
  4. Intelligence is often normal, but delays in spatial perception or visual motor integration are commonly observed; frank mental retardation is rare

ETIOLOGY
- Phenotype caused by absence of the second sex chromosome, whether X or Y
- 45,X chromosome constitution in about 50% of affected individuals
- Other chromosome aberrations (40% of cases): isochromosome Xq (46,X,i(Xq)) or mosaicism (XX/X)
- With deletions involving the short (or "p") arm of the X chromosome: short stature but little ovarian hypofunction
- Deletions involving Xq13-q27: ovarian failure
- Usually a deficiency of paternal contribution of sex chromosome, reflecting paternal nondisjunction

DIAGNOSIS

DIFFERENTIAL DIAGNOSIS
- Noonan syndrome, an autosomal dominantly inherited disorder also characterized by loose nuchal skin, midface hypoplasia, canthal folds, and stenotic cardiac valvular defects and affecting both males and females equally; also have normal chromosome constitutions
- Other conditions in the differential diagnosis of loose skin, whether or not associated with edema:
  1. Fetal hydantoin syndrome (loose nuchal skin, midface hypoplasia, distal digital hypoplasia)
  2. Disorders of chromosome constitution (trisomy 21, tetrasomy 12p mosaicism)
  3. Congenital lymphedema (Milroy edema)

WORKUP
- Giemsa banded karyotype to confirm clinical diagnosis
- Once diagnosis is established: cardiologic consultation for evaluation for cardiac valvular abnormalities or aortic coarctation
- Renal ultrasonography
- Endocrine evaluations in older patients with short stature or amenorrhea
- Psychometrics to document known or suspected learning disabilities

LABORATORY TESTS
- As noted, routine Giemsa banded karyotype on peripheral lymphocytes to confirm the clinical impression in all suspected cases of Turner's syndrome
- Recognition of associated medical problems, such as hypergonadotropic hypogonadism or autoimmune thyroiditis prompting periodic evaluation of these potential areas

IMAGING STUDIES
- Echocardiogram
- Renal ultrasonography
- Abdominal ultrasonography for evaluation of ovarian and uterine size and morphology
- MRI of brain (especially in cases with known or suspected neurologic impairment)
- Radiographs (for evaluation of carpal/metacarpal abnormalities, radioulnar synostosis)
- Bone age (for evaluation of short stature)

TREATMENT

Recognition of the multisystem involvement of Turner's syndrome necessitates multiple medical specialists working in concert with the primary care provider to maximize and improve outcome while minimizing unnecessary or redundant testing.

NONPHARMACOLOGIC THERAPY
General medical care guided by normal medical standards with special attention paid to identifying such age-related problems as developmental delays, learning disabilities, slow growth, or amenorrhea.

ACUTE GENERAL Rx
Specific treatment geared to the specific medical problem (e.g., cardiac or renal dysfunction)

CHRONIC Rx
- Estrogen replacement therapy in early adolescence
- Some benefit from recombinant human growth hormone therapy

REFERRAL
- To geneticist: clinical diagnosis, differential diagnosis, recurrence risk counseling, cytogenetic tests
- To endocrinologist (pediatric): evaluation of short stature, estrogen or growth hormone replacement therapy
- To cardiologist

MISCELLANEOUS

COMMENTS
- Although newer studies are optimistic regarding outcomes, previous reports suffered from retrospective observations, case reports, and ascertainment bias, contributing to a generally poor interaction between physician and patient.
- Affected individuals and families often benefit from the contemporary experiences and expertise of members of genetic support groups. The Turner Syndrome Association (phone: 612-379-3607 or 800-365-9944; Internet: http://www.turner-syndrome-us.org) and the Alliance of Genetic Support Groups (phone: 800-336-4363; Internet: http://medhelp.org/www/agsg.htm) are valuable resources.

REFERENCES
Jones KL: *Smith's recognizable patterns of malformation,* ed 5, Philadelphia, 1997, WB Saunders.

Rosenfeld RG, Grumbach MM (eds): *Turner's syndrome,* New York, 1989, Marcel Dekker.

Rosenfeld RG et al: Recommendations for diagnosis, treatment, and management of individuals with Turner's syndrome, *Endocrinologist* 4:351, 1994.

Author: **Luther K. Robinson, M.D.**

Typhoid fever

BASIC INFORMATION

DEFINITION
Typhoid fever is a systemic infection caused by *Salmonella typhi*.

SYNONYMS
Typhoid
Enteric fever

ICD-9-CM CODES
002.0 Typhoid fever

EPIDEMIOLOGY AND DEMOGRAPHICS
INCIDENCE (IN U.S.): Approximately 500 cases of *S. typhi* infections are reported annually.

PHYSICAL FINDINGS
- Incubation period of a few days to several weeks
- Usual manifestations
  1. Prolonged fever
  2. Myalgias
  3. Headache
  4. Cough
  5. Sore throat
  6. Malaise
  7. Anorexia, at times with abdominal pain and hepatosplenomegaly
  8. Diarrhea or constipation may occur early in the course of illness.
  9. Rose spots, which are faint, maculopapular, blanching lesions, may sometimes be seen on the chest or abdomen.
- In the untreated patient, fever may last 1 to 2 mo. The main complication of untreated disease is GI bleeding as a result of perforation from ulceration of Peyer's patches in the ileum. Mental status changes and shock are rare complications. The relapse rate is approximately 10%.

ETIOLOGY
- *Salmonella typhi*
- *S. paratyphi*
- *S. typhi* or *S. paratyphi* found only in humans
- Acquisition of disease by ingestion of food or water contaminated by other humans
- In the U.S., most cases are acquired either during foreign travel or by ingestion of food prepared by chronic carriers, many of whom acquired the organism outside of the U.S.

DIAGNOSIS

DIFFERENTIAL DIAGNOSIS
- Malaria
- Tuberculosis
- Brucellosis
- Amebic liver abscess

WORKUP
- Blood, stool, and urine cultures are helpful.
- Cultures should be repeated if initially negative.
- Blood cultures are more likely to be positive early in the course of illness.
- Stool and urine cultures are more commonly positive in the second and third week of illness.
- Bone marrow biopsy cultures are 90% positive, although this procedure is usually not necessary.
- Serology using Widal test is helpful in retrospect, showing a fourfold increase in convalescent titers.

LABORATORY TESTS
- Neutropenia is common.
- Transaminitis is possible.
- Culture:
  1. Blood
  2. Body fluids
  3. Biopsy specimens

TREATMENT

ACUTE GENERAL Rx
- Ciprofloxacin 500 mg PO bid or 400 mg IV bid for 14 days
- Ceftriaxone 2 g IV qd for 14 days
- If organism sensitive
  1. SMX/TMP, 1 to 2 DS tabs PO bid or
  2. Amoxicillin, 2 g PO q8h to complete 14 days
- Dexamethasone, 3 mg IV initially, followed by 1 mg IV q6h for 8 doses for patients with shock or mental status changes

CHRONIC Rx
- Carrier states possible
- More common in age >60 yr and in persons with gallstones
- Usual site of colonization: gallbladder
- Treatment in those with persistently positive stool cultures and in food-handlers
- Suggested regimens for eradication of carrier state
  1. Ciprofloxacin 500 mg PO bid for 4 wk
  2. SMX/TMP 1 to 2 tabs PO bid for 6 wk (if susceptible)
  3. Amoxicillin, 2 g PO q8h for 6 wk (if susceptible)
- Cholecystectomy possibly required in carriers with gallstones who fail medical therapy

DISPOSITION
- Treated patients usually respond to therapy, with a small percentage becoming chronic carriers.
- The relapse rate is approximately 10%.
- Untreated patients may have serious complications.

REFERRAL
- Failure of therapy
- Chronic carrier

MISCELLANEOUS

COMMENTS
- Oral and parenteral vaccines are available for travelers to areas of high risk.
- Vaccines are about 70% effective.
- Immunity wanes after several years.
- Parenteral preparations are accompanied by frequent side effects:
  1. Pain at injection site
  2. Fever
  3. Malaise
  4. Headaches

Author: **Maurice Policar, M.D.**

BASIC INFORMATION

DEFINITION
Ulcerative colitis is a chronic inflammatory bowel disease of undetermined etiology.

SYNONYMS
Inflammatory bowel disease (IBD)
Idiopathic proctocolitis

ICD-9-CM CODES
556.9 Ulcerative colitis

EPIDEMIOLOGY AND DEMOGRAPHICS
INCIDENCE: 50 to 150 cases/100,000 persons; most common between age 14 and 38 yr

PHYSICAL FINDINGS
- Abdominal distention and tenderness
- Bloody diarrhea
- Fever, evidence of dehydration
- Evidence of extraintestinal manifestations may be present: liver disease, sclerosing cholangitis, iritis, uveitis, episcleritis, arthritis, erythema nodosum, pyoderma gangrenosum, aphthous stomatitis

DIAGNOSIS

DIFFERENTIAL DIAGNOSIS
- Crohn's disease
- Bacterial infections
  1. Acute: *Campylobacter, Yersinia, Salmonella, Shigella, Chlamydiae, Escherichia coli, Clostridium difficile*, gonococcal proctitis
  2. Chronic: Whipple's disease, TB, enterocolitis
- Irritable bowel syndrome
- Protozoal and parasitic infections (amebiasis, giardiasis, cryptosporidium)
- Neoplasm (intestinal lymphoma, carcinoma of colon)
- Ischemic bowel disease
- Diverticulitis
- Celiac sprue, collagenous colitis, radiation enteritis, endometriosis, gay bowel syndrome

WORKUP
Patients with ulcerative colitis often present with bloody diarrhea accompanied by tenesmus, fever, dehydration, weight loss, anorexia, nausea, and abdominal pain. Diagnostic workup includes:
- Comprehensive history, physical examination
- Laboratory and radiographic studies
- Sigmoidoscopy to establish the presence of mucosal inflammation: typical endoscopic findings in ulcerative colitis are friable mucosa, diffuse, uniform erythema replacing the usual mucosal vascular pattern, and pseudopolyps; rectal involvement is invariably present if the disease is active

LABORATORY TESTS
- Anemia, high sedimentation rate (in severe colitis) is common.
- Potassium, magnesium, calcium, albumin may be decreased.
- Antineutrophil cytoplasmic antibodies (ANCA) with a perinuclear staining pattern (pANCA) can be found in >45% of patients; there is an increased frequency in treatment-resistant left-sided colitis, suggesting a possible association between these antibodies and a relative resistance to medical therapy in patients with ulcerative colitis.

IMAGING STUDIES
Air-contrast barium enema may reveal continuous involvement (including the rectum), pseudopolyps, decreased mucosal pattern, and fine superficial ulcerations.

TREATMENT

NONPHARMACOLOGIC THERAPY
- Correct nutritional deficiencies; TPN with bowel rest may be necessary in severe cases; folate supplementation may reduce the incidence of dysplasia and cancer in chronic ulcerative colitis.
- Avoid oral feedings during acute exacerbation to decrease colonic activity; a low-roughage diet may be helpful in *early* relapse.
- Psychotherapy is useful in most patients. Referral to self-help groups is also important because of the chronicity of the disease and the young age of the patients.

ACUTE GENERAL Rx
The therapeutic options vary with the degree of disease (mild, severe, fulminant) and areas of involvement (distal, extensive):
- Mild or moderate disease can be treated with an oral aminosalicylate (e.g., sulfasalazine 500 mg PO bid initially, increased qd or qod by 1 g until therapeutic doses of 4 to 6 g/day are achieved; distal colitis can be treated with mesalamine (5-aminosalicylic acid) enemas 4 g (60 ml) at hs or steroid retention enemas.
- Severe disease usually responds to oral corticosteroids (e.g., prednisone 40 to 60 mg/day); corticosteroid suppositories or enemas are also useful for distal colitis.
- Fulminant disease generally requires hospital admission and parenteral corticosteroids (e.g., IV hydrocortisone 100 mg q6h); when bowel movements have returned to normal and the patient is able to eat normally, oral prednisone is resumed. IV cyclosporine can also be used in severe refractory cases; renal toxicity is a potential complication.
- Surgery is indicated in patients who fail to respond to intensive medical therapy. Colectomy is usually curative in these patients and also eliminates the high risk of developing adenocarcinoma of the colon (10% to 20% of patients develop it after 10 yr with the disease); newer surgical techniques allow for the preservation of the sphincter.

CHRONIC Rx
- Colonoscopic surveillance and multiple biopsies should be instituted approximately 10 yr after diagnosis because of the increased risk of colon carcinoma.
- Erythropoietin is useful in patients with anemia refractory to treatment with iron and vitamins.

DISPOSITION
The clinical course is variable, 15% to 20% of patients will eventually require colectomy; >75% of patients treated medically will experience relapse.

REFERRAL
- GI consultation for initial diagnostic sigmoidoscopy/colonoscopy in suspected cases
- Surgical referral for patients with severe disease unresponsive to medical therapy

MISCELLANEOUS

COMMENTS
Additional patient information on ulcerative colitis can be obtained from National Foundation for Ileitis and Colitis, 444 Park Avenue South, 11th floor, New York, NY 10016-7374, phone: (800) 343-3637.

REFERENCES
Hanauer SB: Inflammatory bowel disease, *N Engl J Med* 334:841, 1996.
Sandborn WJ et al: Association of antineutrophil cytoplasmic antibodies with resistance to treatment of left-sided ulcerative colitis: result of a pilot study, *Mayo Clin Proc* 71:431, 1996.

Author: **Fred F. Ferri, M.D.**

Urethritis, gonococcal (PTG)

BASIC INFORMATION

DEFINITION
Gonococcal urethritis (GCU) is the inflammation of the urethra.

ICD-9-CM CODES
597.80 Urethritis, unspecified
098.20 Gonococcal

EPIDEMIOLOGY AND DEMOGRAPHICS
- The major single specific etiology of acute urethritis is *Neisseria gonorrhoeae*, producing GCU. Urethritis of all other etiologies is called nongonococcal urethritis (NGU).
- NGU is twice as common as GCU in the U.S. NGU is the most common STD syndrome occurring in men, accounting for 6 million office visits annually. NGU is more frequently encountered in higher socioeconomic groups. GCU is more common in homosexual males than heterosexual males with acute urethritis.

GONOCOCCAL URETHRITIS: *Gonococcus* is a gram-negative, kidney-shaped diplococcus with flattened opposed margins. The urethra is the most common site of infection in all men. In heterosexual men, the pharynx is infected in 7%, and in homosexual men, the pharynx is infected in 40% and the rectum in 25%. A single episode of intercourse with an infected partner carries a transmission risk of 20% for males; female partners of an infected male will contract the disease 80% of the time.

Symptoms of Gonococcal Urethritis: Urethral discharge and dysuria are the most common symptoms. There is complaint of urethral itching. Prostatic involvement can cause frequency, urgency, and nocturia. It can involve the epididymis through spreading down the vas deferens, causing acute epididymitis.

Incubation Period: 3 to 10 days. Without treatment urethritis persists for 3 to 7 wk, with 95% of men becoming asymptomatic after 3 mo. Asymptomatic GCU is asymptomatic in up to 60% of contacts.

Signs of Gonococcal Urethritis: Yellow-brown discharge, meatal edema, urethral tenderness to palpation. Rectal bleeding with pus is seen with gonococcal proctitis. Periurethritis leading to urethral stenosis can occur. Disseminated infection can occur. Tenosynovitis and arthritis can occur. Rarely, hepatitis, myocarditis, endocarditis, and meningitis can occur.

DIAGNOSIS

DIFFERENTIAL DIAGNOSIS
- NGU
- Herpes simplex virus

LABORATORY TESTS
- Calcium alginate or rayon swab on a metal shaft (NOT cotton tipped swabs, which are bactericidal) of the urethra should be done anywhere from 2 to 4 hr after voiding to prevent bacterial washout with voiding.
- Cultures of the pharynx and rectum when indicated.
- Gram staining should be done. Modified Thayer-Martin media is used.
- On examination of the urethral smear, the presence of small numbers of PMNs provides objective evidence of urethritis. The complete absence of PMNs on a urethral smear argues against urethritis. If in addition to the PMNs there are gram-negative, intracellular diplococci, the diagnosis of gonorrhea is established.

TREATMENT

NONPHARMACOLOGIC THERAPY
BEHAVIORAL MANAGEMENT: Avoid intercourse until cure has been attained and sexual partners have been evaluated and treated.

ACUTE GENERAL Rx
FOR UNCOMPLICATED URETHRAL, CERVICAL, AND RECTAL GCU: Ceftriaxone 125 mg IM + doxycycline 100 mg bid × 7 days. Alternative therapy: ciprofloxacin 500 mg PO × 1 day; ofloxacin 400 mg PO × 1 day (all of these to be followed by 7 days of doxycycline 100 mg PO bid).

FOR EPIDIDYMITIS: Ceftriaxone 250 mg IM followed by doxycycline 100 mg PO bid × 10 days. Alternative therapy: ofloxacin 300 mg PO bid × 10 days.

CHRONIC Rx
POSTGONOCOCCAL URETHRITIS (PGU): Reinfection is the most common cause of recurrence. Repeat swab and culture of the urethra, pharynx, and rectum (where applicable) is mandatory. Persistence of PMNs with the absence of gram-negative intracellular diplococci suggests a diagnosis of postgonococcal urethritis. This occurs when GCU is treated with a regimen that is ineffective against coincident chlamydial infection; it represents NGU following GCU. The syndrome should be treated as NGU. Persistence of *N. gonorrhoeae* by smear or culture requires treatment for *N. gonorrhoeae*.

MISCELLANEOUS

COMMENTS
- CAUTION: Tetracyclines and fluoroquinolones are **contraindicated** in pregnancy. *Chlamydia* infection in pregnancy can be treated with amoxicillin 500 mg PO tid for 7 days or with clindamycin 450 mg PO tid for 10 days.
- **Posttreatment cultures are required.**
- U.S. Preventive Services Task Force Recommendations regarding screening for gonorrhea are described in Section V, Chapter 27. Recommendations regarding counseling to prevent HIV infection and other STDs are described in Section V, Chapter 62.

REFERENCES
Berger RE, Rothman I: Sexually transmitted diseases in males. In Tanagho EA, McAninch JW (eds): *Smith's general urology*, Norwalk, Conn, 1995, Appleton & Lange.

Jernigan JA, Rein MF: Sexually transmitted diseases. In Reese RE, Betts RF (eds): *Practical approach to infectious diseases*, Boston, 1996, Little, Brown.

Author: **Philip J. Aliotta, M.D., M.S.H.A.**

Urethritis, nongonococcal (PTG)

BASIC INFORMATION

DEFINITION
Nongonococcal urethritis is urethral inflammation caused by any of several organisms.

SYNONYMS
NGU

ICD-9-CM CODES
099.40 Nongonococcal
099.41 Chlamydial

EPIDEMIOLOGY AND DEMOGRAPHICS
- Occurrence is 50% in STD clinics.
- Most commonly affects men in higher socioeconomic class, affecting heterosexual men more frequently than homosexual men.
- NGU carries a greater morbidity than GCU.

ETIOLOGY
- Most common agent is *Chlamydia* spp., an obligate intracellular parasite possessing both DNA and RNA, replicating by binary fission. It causes 20% to 50% of NGU cases. Two species exist:
  1. *Chlamydia psittaci*
  2. *Chlamydia trachomatis* with its 15 serotypes
     a. Serotypes A-C cause hyperendemic blinding trachoma.
     b. Serotypes D-K cause genital tract infection.
     c. Serotypes L1-L3 cause lymphogranuloma venereum.
- Other causes of NGU: ureaplasma urealyticum causing 15% to 30% of the cases of NGU, *Trichomonas vaginalis*, and herpes simplex virus. The cause of 20% of the cases of NGU has not been identified.
- Asymptomatic infection occurs in 28% of the contacts of women with chlamydial cervical infection.

Incubation Period: 2 to 35 days.
Symptoms: Dysuria, whitish-to-clear urethral discharge, and urethral itching. The onset of symptoms in NGU is less acute than GCU.
Signs: Whitish-to-clear urethral discharge, meatal edema, and erythema. Infected women manifest pyuria and can present as acute urethral syndrome.
Complications: Epididymitis in heterosexual men, may be linked to causing nonbacterial prostatitis; proctitis in homosexual men; and Reiter's syndrome.

DIAGNOSIS

DIFFERENTIAL DIAGNOSIS
- GCU
- Herpes simplex virus
- Trichomoniasis

LABORATORY TESTS
- Requires demonstration of urethritis and exclusion of infection with *N. gonorrhoeae*.
- The appearance of PMNs on urethral smear confirms the diagnosis of urethritis. Because chlamydia is an intracellular parasite of the columnar epithelium, the best specimen for culture is an endourethral swab taken from an area 2 to 4 cm inside the urethra. The organism can only be grown in tissue culture, which is expensive.
- New techniques have been developed and are useful in making the diagnosis: nucleic acid hybridization, enzyme-linked immunosorbent assay (ELISA), and direct immunofluorescence.
- For culture, a dacron-tipped swab is used; avoid calcium alginate or cotton swabs.

TREATMENT

Because it is impossible to differentiate among the common etiologies of NGU, the condition is treated syndromically, including in the initial treatment regimen those drugs effective against the common causative agents.
- Recommended: doxycycline 100 mg PO bid for 7 days
- Other drugs: tetracycline 500 mg PO qid for 7 days
- Alternative regimens: azithromycin 1000 mg as a single dose, erythromycin 500 mg PO qid for 7 days, ofloxacin 300 mg PO bid for 7 days

MISCELLANEOUS

COMMENTS
- CAUTION: Tetracyclines and fluoroquinolones are **contraindicated** in pregnancy. *Chlamydia* infection in pregnancy can be treated with amoxicillin 500 mg PO tid for 7 days or with clindamycin 450 mg PO tid for 10 days.
- **Posttreatment cultures are required.**

REFERENCES
Berger RE, Rothman I: Sexually transmitted diseases in males. In Tanagho EA, McAninch JW (eds): *Smith's general urology,* Norwalk, Conn, 1995, Appleton & Lange.

Jernigan JA, Rein MF: Sexually transmitted diseases. In Reese RE, Betts RF (eds): *Practical approach to infectious diseases,* Boston, 1996, Little, Brown.

Author: **Philip J. Aliotta, M.D., M.S.H.A.**

Urinary tract infection (PTG)

BASIC INFORMATION

DEFINITION
Urinary tract infection (UTI) is a term that encompasses a broad range of clinical entities that have in common a positive urine culture. A conventional threshold is growth of >100,000 colony-forming units per ml from a midstream-catch urine sample. In symptomatic patients, a smaller number of bacteria (between 100 and 10,000 colony-forming units per ml of midstream urine) is recognized as an infection.

SYNONYMS
UTI

ICD-9-CM CODES
595.0 Acute cystitis
595.3 Trigonitis
595.2 Chronic cystitis
590.1 Acute pyelonephritis
590.0 Chronic pyelonephritis
590.8 Nonspecific pyelonephritis

CLASSIFICATION
FIRST INFECTION: The first documented UTI; tends to be uncomplicated and is easily treated.
UNRESOLVED BACTERIURIA: UTI in which the urinary tract is not sterilized during therapy. Main causes are bacterial resistance, patient noncompliance with medication, resistance, mixed bacterial infection, rapid reinfection, azotemia, and infected stones.
BACTERIAL PERSISTENCE: UTI in which the urine cultures become sterile during therapy but a persistent source of infection from a site within the urinary tract that was excluded from the high urinary concentrations gives rise to reinfection by the same organism. Causes: infected stone, chronic bacterial prostatitis, atrophic infected kidney, vesicovaginal or enterovesical fistulas, obstructive uropathy, infected pyelocaliceal diverticula, infected ureteral stump following nephrectomy, infected necrotic papillae from papillary necrosis, infected urachal cysts, infected medullary sponge kidney, urethral diverticula and foreign bodies.
REINFECTION: UTI in which a new infection occurs with new pathogens at variable intervals after a previous infection has been eradicated.

EPIDEMIOLOGY AND DEMOGRAPHICS
INCIDENCE:
In Neonates: More common in boys as a result of anatomic abnormalities.
In Preschool Children: More common in girls (4.5% vs. 0.5% for boys).
In Adulthood: More common in women, with a 1% to 3% prevalence in nonpregnant women. In pregnancy at 12 wk, the incidence of asymptomatic bacteriuria is similar to nonpregnant women, at 2% to 10%. However, 70% to 80% of women with asymptomatic bacteriuria develop acute pyelonephritis, especially in the second and third trimester and suffer a pyelonephritic recurrence rate of 10%. In adults, 65 yr and older, at least 10% of men and 20% of women have bacteriuria.
PATHOGENESIS:
- Four major pathways:
  1. Ascending from the urethra
  2. Lymphatic
  3. Hematogenous
  4. Direct extension from another organ system.
- Other risk factors: neurologic diseases, renal failure, diabetes; anatomic abnormalities: bladder outlet obstruction, urethral stricture, vesicoureteral reflux, fistula, urinary diversion, megacystis, and infected stones; age; pregnancy; instrumentation, poor patient compliance, poor hygiene, infrequent voider, diaphragm contraceptives, tampon use, douches, and catheters
- Once bacteria reach the urinary tract three factors determine whether the infection occurs:
  1. Virulence of the microorganism
  2. Inoculum size
  3. Adequacy of the host defense mechanisms.
- These factors also determine the anatomic level of the UTI.

Urinary Pathogens: In >95% of UTIs the infecting organism is a member of the *Enterobacteriaceae, Pseudomonas aeruginosa,* enterococci, or, in young women, *Staphylococcus saprophyticus.* In contrast, the organisms that commonly colonize the distal urethra and skin of both men and women and the vagina of women are *Staphylococcus epidermidis, Diphtheroids, Lactobacilli, Gardnerella vaginalis,* and a variety of anaerobes that rarely cause UTI. Generally, the isolation of two or more bacterial species from a urine culture signifies a contaminated specimen, unless the patient is being managed with a indwelling catheter, urinary diversion, or has a chronic complicated infection.

Defense mechanisms against cystitis: Low pH and high osmolarity, mucopolysaccharide glycosaminoglycan protective layer, normal bladder that empties completely and has no incontinence, and the presence of estrogen.

PHYSICAL FINDINGS

- UTI presentation is inconsistent and cannot be relied upon to diagnose UTI accurately or to localize the site of infection. Patients complain of:
  1. Urinary frequency, urgency
  2. Dysuria
  3. Urge incontinence
  4. Suprapubic pain
  5. Gross or microscopic hematuria
- When negative cultures are associated with significant pyuria, vaginal discharge, or hematuria, infections with *Chlamydia trachomatis, Neisseria gonorrhoeae,* and *Trichomonas vaginalis* should be considered.
- Acute pyelonephritis (PN) presents with fever, flank or abdominal pain, chills, malaise, vomiting, and diarrhea. It is these systemic symptoms that distinguish pyelonephritis from cystitis. Complications of acute pyelonephritis are renal abscess, perinephric abscess, emphysematous pyelonephritis, and pyonephrosis.

DIAGNOSIS

DIFFERENTIAL DIAGNOSIS
- Interstitial cystitis
- Vaginitis
- Urethritis (gonococcal, nongonococcal, trichomonas)
- Frequency-urgency syndrome, prostatitis (acute and chronic)
- Obstructive uropathy
- Infected stones
- Fistulas
- Papillary necrosis
- Vesicoureteral reflux

LABORATORY TESTS
- Urinalysis with microscopic evaluation of clean-catch urine for bacteria and pyuria
- Urine C&S
- CBC with differential (shows leukocytosis)
- Antibody-coated bacteria are seen with pyelonephritis

IMAGING STUDIES
- Warranted only if renal infection or genitourinary abnormality is suspected
- KUB, VCUG, renal sonogram, IVP, CT scan, and nuclear scan
- Specialty examination: cystoscopy with occasional retrograde pyelography to rule out obstructive uropathy; stenting the obstruction possibly required

TREATMENT

NONPHARMACOLOGIC THERAPY
- Hot sitz baths, anticholinergics, urinary analgesics
- For pyelonephritis: bed rest, analgesics, antipyretics, and IV hydration

ACUTE GENERAL Rx
- Conventional therapy of 7 days; short-term therapy of 1, 3, or 5 days.
- Agents of choice: amoxicillin/clavulanate, cephalosporins, fluoroquinolones, nitrofurantoin, and trimethoprim with sulfonamide.
- For pyelonephritis: hospitalization until afebrile and stable, then at home via home care agency with IV antibiotic comprised of aminoglycoside plus cephalosporin × 1 wk followed by oral agents (based on sensitivity) for 2 wk. Moderate forms of pyelonephritis have been successfully treated with fluoroquinolone therapy for 21 days, without requiring hospitalization. Most importantly, complicating factors like obstructive uropathy or infected stones must be identified and treated.

MISCELLANEOUS

COMMENTS
- **Asymptomatic bacteriuria:** occurs in both anatomically normal and abnormal urinary tracts. This can clear spontaneously, persist, or lead to symptomatic kidney infection. Treatment is recommended in patients with vesicoureteral reflux, stones, obstructive uropathy, parenchymal renal disease, diabetes mellitus, and pregnant or immunocompromised patients.
- **Pregnancy:** 20% to 40% of pregnant women with untreated bacteriuria develop pyelonephritis. This is associated with prematurity and low-birth-weight infants. Confirmed significant bacteriuria should be treated with an aminopenicillin and cephalosporin.
- **Recurrent UTI:** caused by an unresolved infection, vaginal colonization of the originally infecting organism, or reinfection with a new strain. Management of recurrent UTI includes continuous antibiotic prophylaxis, intermittent self-treatment and postcoital prophylaxis. Prophylaxis is recommended for women who experience two or more symptomatic UTIs over a 6-mo period or three or more episodes over a 12-mo period.
- **Causes of recurrent pyelonephritis:** inadequate initial therapy, reflux, neurogenic bladder, obstruction, stone disease, diabetes, analgesic abuse, nephrosclerosis, cystic disease, sickle cell disease.

REFERENCES
Fowler, JE Jr: Urinary tract infections in women, *Urol Clin North Am* 13:673, 1986.

Meares EM Jr: Nonspecific infections of the genitourinary tract. In McAninch JW, Tanagho EA (eds): *Smith's general urology,* Norwalk, Conn, 1996, Appleton & Lange.

Schaeffer AJ: Infections of the urinary tract. In Walsh PC et al (eds): *Campbell's urology,* Philadelphia, 1992, WB Saunders.

Author: **Philip J. Aliotta, M.D., M.S.H.A.**

Urolithiasis (PTG)

BASIC INFORMATION

DEFINITION
Urolithiasis is the presence of calculi within the urinary tract. The five major types of urinary stones are calcium oxalate (>50%), calcium phosphate (10% to 20%), uric acid (8%), struvite (15%), and cystine (3%).

SYNONYMS
Nephrolithiasis
Renal colic

ICD-9-CM CODES
592.9 Urinary calculus

EPIDEMIOLOGY AND DEMOGRAPHICS
- Urinary stone disease afflicts 250,000 to 750,000 Americans/yr.
- Male:female ratio is 4:1. After the sixth decade, the ratio is 1.5:1.
- Incidence of symptomatic nephrolithiasis is greatest during the summer (resulting from increased humidity and temperatures with increased risk of dehydration and concentrated urine).
- Calcium oxalate or mixed calcium oxalate/calcium phosphate stones account for 70% of urolithiasis.

PHYSICAL FINDINGS
Stones may be asymptomatic or may cause the following signs and symptoms from obstruction:
- Sudden onset of flank tenderness
- Nausea and vomiting
- Patient in constant movement, attempting to lessen his pain (patients with an acute abdomen are usually still because movement exacerbates the pain)
- Pain may be referred to the testes or labium (progression of stone down the urinary ureter)
- Fever and chills accompanying the acute colic if there is superimposed infection
- Pain may radiate anteriorly over to the abdomen and result in intestinal ileus

ETIOLOGY
- Increased absorption of calcium in the small bowel: type I absorptive hypercalciuria (independent of calcium intake)
- Increased dietary calcium: type II absorptive hypercalciuria
- Increased vitamin D synthesis (e.g., secondary to renal phosphate loss: type III absorptive hypercalciuria)
- Renal tubular malfunction with inadequate reabsorption of calcium and resulting hypercalciuria
- Hyperparathyroidism with resulting hypercalcemia
- Elevated uric acid level (metabolic defects, dietary excess)
- Chronic diarrhea (e.g., inflammatory bowel disease) with increased oxalate absorption
- Type I (distal tubule) renal tubular acidosis (<1% of calcium stones)
- Chronic hydrochlorothiazide treatment
- Chronic infections with urease-producing organisms (e.g., *Proteus, Providencia, Pseudomonas, Klebsiella*)
- Abnormal excretion of cystine
- Chemotherapy for malignancies

DIAGNOSIS

DIFFERENTIAL DIAGNOSIS
- Urinary tract infection
- Pyelonephritis
- Diverticulitis
- Pelvic inflammatory disease
- Ovarian pathology
- Factitious (drug addicts)
- Appendicitis
- Small bowel obstruction
- Ectopic pregnancy
- The differential diagnosis of obstructive uropathy is described in Section II, Box 2-118.

WORKUP
- Laboratory and imaging studies. Stone analysis should be performed on recovered stones.
- Fig. 3-59 is a clinical algorithm for evaluation of nephrolithiasis.

LABORATORY TESTS
- Urinalysis: hematuria may be present; however, its absence does not exclude urinary stones. Evaluation of urinary pH is of value in identification of type of stone (pH >7.5 is associated with struvite stones, whereas pH <5 generally is seen with uric acid or with cystine stones.

- Urine C&S should be obtained in all patients.
- Serum chemistries should include calcium, electrolytes, phosphate, and uric acid.
- Additional tests: 24-hr urine collection for calcium, uric acid, phosphate, oxalate and citrate excretion are generally reserved for patients with recurrent stones.

IMAGING STUDIES
- Plain films of the abdomen can identify radioopaque stones (calcium, uric acid stones).
- Renal sonogram may be helpful.
- IVP demonstrates the size and location of the stone, as well as degree of obstruction.
- Unenhanced helical CT scan does not require contrast media and can visualize the calculus (identified by the "rim sign" or "halo" representing the edematous ureteral wall around the stone).

TREATMENT

NONPHARMACOLOGIC THERAPY
- Increase in water or other fluid intake (doubling of previous fluid intake unless patient has a history of CHF or fluid overload)
- Low-calcium diet in patients with type II absorptive hypercalciuria
- Sodium restriction (to decrease calcium excretion), decreased protein intake to 1 g/kg/day (to decrease uric acid, calcium and oxalate excretion)
- Increase in bran (may decrease bowel transit time with increased binding of calcium and subsequent decrease in urinary calcium)

ACUTE GENERAL Rx
- Pain control (use of narcotics is generally indicated because of the severity of pain)
- Specific therapy tailored to the stone type:
  1. Uric acid calculi: control of hyperuricemia with allopurinol 100 to 300 mg/day; increase urinary pH with potassium citrate, 10-mEq tablets tid
  2. Calcium stones:
     a. HCTZ 25 to 50 mg qd in patients with type I absorptive hypercalciuria
     b. Decrease bowel absorption of calcium with cellulose phosphate 10 g/day in patients with type I absorptive hypercalciuria
     c. Orthophosphates to inhibit vitamin B synthesis in patients with type III absorptive hypercalciuria
  3. Potassium citrate supplementation in patients with hypocitraturic calcium nephrolithiasis
  4. Purine dietary restrictions or allopurinol in patients with hyperuricosuric calcium nephrolithiasis
  5. Surgical treatment in patients with severe pain unresponsive to medication and patients with persistent fever or nausea or significant impediment of urine flow:
     a. Ureteroscopic stone extraction
     b. Extracorporeal shock wave lithotripsy (ESWL) for most renal stones

CHRONIC Rx
Maintenance of proper hydration and dietary restrictions (see "Acute General Rx").

DISPOSITION
- >50% of patients will pass the stone within 48 hr.
- Stones will recur in approximately 50% of patients within 5 yr if no medical treatment is provided.

REFERRAL
Urology referral in complicated or recurrent urolithiasis; most patients with small uncomplicated ureteral or renal calculi can be followed as outpatient, whereas patients with persistent vomiting, suspected UTI, pain unresponsive to oral analgesics, or obstructing calculus associated with solitary kidney should be admitted

MISCELLANEOUS

COMMENTS
- Early identification and aggressive treatment of urinary tract infections is indicated in all patients with struvite stones.
- Alkalinization of urine (pH >7.5 with penicillamine) is useful in patients with recurrent cystine stones.

REFERENCES
Gault MH et al: Bacteriology of urinary tract stones, *J Urol* 153:1164, 1995.
Heneghan JP et al: Soft tissue "rim" sign in the diagnosis of ureteral calculi with use of unenhanced helical CT, *Radiology* 202:709, 1997.
Kupin WL: A practical approach to nephrolithiasis, *Hosp Prac* 30:57, 1995.
Parivar F et al: The influence of diet on urinary stone disease, *J Urol* 155:432, 1996.

Author: Fred F. Ferri, M.D.

Urticaria

BASIC INFORMATION

DEFINITION
Urticaria is a pruritic rash involving the epidermis and the upper portions of the dermis, resulting from localized capillary vasodilation and followed by transudation of protein-rich fluid in the surrounding tissue and manifesting clinically with the presence of hives.

SYNONYMS
Hives
Wheals

ICD-9-CM CODES
708.8 Other unspecified urticaria

EPIDEMIOLOGY AND DEMOGRAPHICS
- At least 20% of the population will have 1 episode of hives during their lifetime.
- Incidence is increased in atopic patients.
- The etiology of chronic urticaria (hives lasting longer than 6 wk) is determined in only 5% to 20% of cases.

PHYSICAL FINDINGS
- Presence of elevated, erythematous, or white nonpitting plaques that change in size and shape over time; they generally last a few hours and disappear without a trace.
- Annular configuration with central pallor (see color plate 24).

ETIOLOGY
- Foods (e.g., shellfish, eggs, strawberries, nuts)
- Drugs (e.g., penicillin, aspirin, sulfonamides)
- Systemic diseases (e.g., SLE, serum sickness, autoimmune thyroid disease, polycythemia vera)
- Food additives (e.g., salicylates, benzoates, sulfites)
- Infections (viral infections, fungal infections, chronic bacterial infections)
- Physical stimuli (e.g., pressure urticaria, exercise-induced, solar urticaria, cold urticaria)
- Inhalants (e.g., mold spores, animal danders, pollens)
- Contact (nonimmunologic) urticaria (e.g., caterpillars, plants)
- Other: hereditary angioedema, urticaria pigmentosa, pregnancy, cold urticaria, hair bleaches, chemicals, saliva, cosmetics, perfumes, pemphigoid, emotional stress

DIAGNOSIS

DIFFERENTIAL DIAGNOSIS
- Erythema multiforme
- Erythema marginatum
- Erythema infectiosum
- Urticarial vasculitis
- Herpes gestationis
- Drug eruption
- Multiple insect bites
- Bullous pemphigoid
- The differential diagnosis of urticaria is also described in Section II, Box 2-119.

WORKUP
- It is useful to determine whether hives are acute or chronic; a medical history focused on various etiologic factors is necessary before embarking on extensive laboratory testing.
- A diagnostic approach to chronic urticaria is described in Section III, Fig. 3-91.

LABORATORY TESTS
- CBC with differential
- Stool for ova and parasites in patients with suspected parasitic infestations
- ANA, ESR, TSH, liver function tests, eosinophil count are indicated only in selected patients

TREATMENT

NONPHARMACOLOGIC THERAPY
- Remove suspected etiologic agents (e.g., stop aspirin and all nonessential drugs), restrict diet (e.g., elimination of tomatoes, nuts, eggs, shellfish).
- Elimination of yeast should be attempted in patients with chronic urticaria (*Candida albicans* sensitivity may be a factor in patients with chronic urticaria).

ACUTE GENERAL Rx
- Oral antihistamines: use of nonsedating antihistamines (e.g., loratadine [Claritin] 10 mg qd or cetirizine [Zyrtec] 10 mg qd) is preferred over first-generation antihistamines (e.g., hydroxyzine, diphenhydramine).
- Doxepin (a tricyclic antidepressant) 25 to 75 mg qhs may be effective in patients with chronic urticaria.
- Oral corticosteroids should be reserved for refractory cases (e.g., prednisone 20 mg qd or 20 mg bid).

CHRONIC Rx
Use of nonsedating antihistamines, doxepin and/or oral corticosteroids (see "Acute General Rx")

DISPOSITION
- Most cases of urticaria resolve within 6 wk.
- Only 25% of patients with a history of chronic urticaria are completely cured after 5 yr.

REFERRAL
Referral to allergist in patients with chronic urticaria

MISCELLANEOUS

COMMENTS
Local treatment (e.g., starch baths or Aveeno baths) may be helpful in selected patients; however, local treatment is generally not rewarding.

REFERENCES
Greaves MW: Chronic urticaria, *N Engl J Med* 332:1767, 1995.
Habif TP: *Clinical dermatology,* ed 3, St Louis, 1996, Mosby.
Author: **Fred F. Ferri, M.D**

BASIC INFORMATION

DEFINITION
Uterine malignancy includes tumors from the endometrium (discussed elsewhere in this text) and sarcomas. Uterine sarcoma is an abnormal proliferation of cells originating from the mesenchymal, or connective tissue, elements of the uterine wall.

SYNONYMS
Leiomyosarcomas
Endometrial stromal sarcoma
Malignant mixed mullerian tumors
Adenosarcomas

ICD-9-CM CODES
182.0 Malignant neoplasm of body of uterus, corpus uteri, except isthmus
182.1 Malignant neoplasm of body of uterus, isthmus
182.8 Malignant neoplasm of body of uterus, other specified sites of body of uterus

EPIDEMIOLOGY AND DEMOGRAPHICS
PREVALENCE: Uterine sarcoma accounts for 4.3% of all cancers of the uterine corpus.
INCIDENCE: 17.1 cases/1,000,000 females
MEAN AGE AT DIAGNOSIS: The age at diagnosis is variable. Mean age at diagnosis is 52 yr old.

PHYSICAL FINDINGS
- Abnormal vaginal bleeding is the most common symptom.
- May also present as pelvic pain or pressure and pelvic mass on examination.
- May appear as tumor protruding through the cervix.
- Vaginal discharge may also be a presenting symptom.

ETIOLOGY
- The exact etiology is unknown.
- Prior pelvic radiation is a risk factor for sarcoma.
- Black women may be at higher risk.

DIAGNOSIS

DIFFERENTIAL DIAGNOSIS
Leiomyoma

WORKUP
Diagnosis is made histologically by biopsy for abnormal bleeding.

LABORATORY TESTS
Chest radiography, CT scans, and MRI are used to evaluate spread.

IMAGING STUDIES
- Chest radiography is usually done as routine preoperative testing.
- CT scans and MRI are good for assessing tumor spread once diagnosis is made.

TREATMENT

NONPHARMACOLOGIC THERAPY
- Surgery excision is the mainstay of treatment.
- Adjuvant radiotherapy may improve pelvic disease control, but it does not improve survival.
- Chemotherapeutic agents have produced only partial and short-term responses.

DISPOSITION
- Survival varies with each type of sarcoma.
- Five-year survival for leiomyosarcoma ranges from 48% for stage I to 0% for stage IV.
- Five-year survival for malignant mixed mesodermal tumor ranges from 36% for stage I to 6% for stage IV.

REFERRAL
Uterine sarcoma should be managed by a gynecologic oncologist and radiation oncologist.

MISCELLANEOUS

COMMENTS
U.S. Preventive Services Task Force Recommendations for counseling to prevent gynecologic cancers are described in Section V, Chapter 66.

REFERENCES
Berek JS, Hacker NF: *Practical gynecologic oncology,* Baltimore, 1994, William & Wilkins.
Hoskins WJ, Perez CA, Young RC: *Principles and practice of gynecologic oncology,* Philadelphia, 1997, Lippencott-Raven.
Levenback CF, Tortolero-Luna G, Pandey DK et al: Uterine sarcoma, *Obstet Gynecol Clin North Am* 23(2):457, 1996.
Morrow CP, Curtin JP, Townsend DE: *Synopsis of gynecologic oncology,* New York, 1993, Churchill Livingston.
Piver MS: *Handbook of gynecologic oncology,* Boston, 1996, Little Brown.
Shingleton HM et al: *Gynecologic oncology: current diagnosis and treatment,* Philadelphia, 1996, WB Saunders.
Author: Yukio Sonoda, M.D.

Uterine myomas (PTG)

BASIC INFORMATION

DEFINITION
Uterine myomas are discrete nodular tumors that vary in size and number and that may be found subserosal, intramucosal, or submucosal within the uterus or may also be found in the cervix, broad ligament, or on a pedicle.

SYNONYMS
Leiomyomas, fibroids

ICD-9-CM CODES
218.9 Leiomyomas, fibroids

EPIDEMIOLOGY AND DEMOGRAPHICS
- Estimated presence in at least 20% of all reproductive age women.
- The most common benign uterine tumor.
- More common in African-American than in white women.
- Asymptomatic fibroids may be present in 40% to 50% of women >40 yr of age.
- May occur singly but are often multiple.
- Fewer than one half of all fibroids are estimated to produce symptoms.
- Frequently diagnosed incidentally on pelvic examination.
- There is increased familial incidence.
- Potential to enlarge during pregnancy, as well as to regress after menopause.
- Infrequent primary cause of infertility in <3% of infertile patients.

PHYSICAL FINDINGS
- Enlarged, irregular uterus on pelvic examination.
- Presenting symptoms:
  1. Menorrhagia (most common)
  2. Chronic pelvic pain (dysmenorrhea, dyspareunia, pelvic pressure)
  3. Acute pain (torsion of pedunculated myoma, infarction and degeneration)
  4. Urinary symptoms (frequency from bladder pressure, partial ureteral obstruction, complete ureteral obstruction)
  5. Rectosigmoid compression with constipation or intestinal obstruction
  6. Prolapse through cervix of pedunculated submucous tumor
  7. Venous stasis of lower extremities
  8. Polycythemia
  9. Ascites

ETIOLOGY
Unknown. It is suggested that myomas arise from a single neoplastic smooth muscle cell in the myometrium. Malignant degeneration of preexisting leiomyoma is extremely uncommon (<0.5%).

DIAGNOSIS

DIFFERENTIAL DIAGNOSIS
Leiomyosarcoma, ovarian mass (neoplastic, nonneoplastic, endometrioma), inflammatory mass, pregnancy

WORKUP
- Complete pelvic examination, rectovaginal examination, Pap test.
- Estimation of size of mass in centimeters.
- Endometrial sampling may be indicated (biopsy or D&C) when abnormal bleeding and pelvic mass present.
- If urinary symptoms are prominent, cystometry, cystoscopy to rule out bladder lesions, IVP to rule out impingement on urinary system.

LABORATORY TESTS
- Pregnancy test
- Pap smear
- CBC, ESR
- Fecal occult blood

IMAGING STUDIES
- Pelvic ultrasound (transvaginal may have higher diagnostic accuracy) is useful.
- CT scan is helpful in planning treatment if malignancy is strongly suspected.
- Hysteroscopy may provide direct evidence of intrauterine pathology or submucous leiomyoma that distort uterine cavity.

TREATMENT

Management should be based on primary symptoms and may include observation with close follow-up, temporizing surgical therapies, medical management, or definitive surgical procedures.

NONSURGICAL Rx
- Patient observation and follow-up with periodic repeat pelvic examinations to ensure that tumors are not growing rapidly.
- GnRH agonist use results in 40% to 60% reduction in uterine volume. Hypoestrogenism, reversible bone loss, hot flushes associated with use. Limit to short-term use and consider low-dose hormonal replacement to minimize hypoestrogenic effects.
- Regrowth occurs in about 50% of women treated a few months after cessation.
- Indications for GnRH:
  1. Fertility preservation in women with large myomas before attempting conception or preoperative myectomy treatment.
  2. Anemia treatment to normalize hemoglobin before surgery.
  3. Women approaching menopause to avoid surgery.
  4. Preoperative for large myomas to make vaginal hysterectomy, hysteroscopic resection/ablation, or laparoscopic destruction more feasible.
  5. Women with medical contraindications for surgery.
  6. Personal or medical indications for delaying surgery.
- Progestational agents may also result in decrease in uterine size and amenorrhea, allowing iron therapy to treat anemia with limited success.

SURGICAL Rx
- Indications
  1. Abnormal uterine bleeding with anemia, refractory to hormonal therapy
  2. Chronic pain with severe dysmenorrhea, dyspareunia, or lower abdominal pressure/pain
  3. Acute pain, torsion, or prolapsing submucosal fibroid
  4. Urinary symptoms or signs such as hydronephrosis
  5. Rapid uterine enlargement premenopausal or any postmenopausal increase in size
  6. Infertility with leiomyoma as only finding
  7. Enlarged uterus with compression symptoms or discomfort
- Procedures
  1. Hysterectomy (definitive procedure), abdominal myomectomy (to preserve fertility), vaginal myomectomy for prolapsed pedunculated submucous fibroid, hysteroscopic resection

REFERRAL
Consultation with gynecologic oncologist if suspicion of malignancy

MISCELLANEOUS

REFERENCES
Berek J, Adashi E, Hillard P: *Novak's gynecology,* ed 12, 1996, Baltimore, Williams & Wilkins.
Herbst et al: *Comprehensive gynecology,* ed 2, St Louis, 1992, Mosby.
Author: **Eugene J. Louie-Ng, M.D.**

Uterine prolapse (PTG)

BASIC INFORMATION

DEFINITION
Uterine prolapse refers to the protrusion of the uterus into or out of the vaginal canal. In a *first-degree uterine prolapse*, the cervix is visible when the perineum is depressed. In a *second-degree uterine prolapse*, the uterine cervix has prolapsed through the vaginal introitus, with the fundus remaining within the pelvis proper. In a *third-degree uterine prolapse* (i.e., *complete uterine prolapse, uterine procidentia*), the entire uterus is outside the introitus.

SYNONYMS
Genital prolapse
Uterine descensus
Pelvic organ prolapse

ICD-9-CM CODES
618.8 Genital prolapse
618. 1 Uterine descensus
618.8 Pelvic organ prolapse

EPIDEMIOLOGY AND DEMOGRAPHICS
Most prevalent in postmenopausal multiparous women.
RISK FACTORS:
- Pregnancy
- Labor
- Vaginal childbirth
- Obesity
- Chronic coughing
- Constipation
- Pelvic tumors
- Ascites
- Strenuous physical exertion
- Caucasian race

GENETICS: Increased incidence in women with spina bifida occulta.

PHYSICAL FINDINGS
- Pelvic pressure
- Bearing-down sensation
- Bilateral groin pain
- Sacral backache
- Coital difficulty
- Protrusion from vagina
- Spotting
- Ulceration
- Bleeding
- Examination of patient in lithotomy, sitting, and standing positions and before, during, and after a maximum Valsalva effort
- Erosion or ulceration of the cervix possible in the most dependent area of the protrusion

ETIOLOGY
- Vaginal childbirth and chronic increases in intraabdominal pressure leading to detachments, lacerations, and denervations of the vaginal support system
- Further weakening of pelvic support system by hypoestrogenic atrophy
- Some cases from congenital or inherited weaknesses within the pelvic support system
- Neonatal uterine prolapse mostly coexistent with congenital spinal defects

DIAGNOSIS

DIFFERENTIAL DIAGNOSIS
Occasionally, elongated cervix; body of the uterus remains undescended

WORKUP
- Diagnosis is based on history and physical examination.
- If erosion or ulceration of the cervix is present, a Pap smear followed by a cervical biopsy should be performed if indicated.
- If urinary symptoms are significant, further urodynamic workup is indicated, looking for concurrent cystourethrocele, cystocele, enterocele, or rectocele.

LABORATORY TESTS
Urine culture

IMAGING STUDIES
Ultrasound if concurrent fibroids need further evaluation

TREATMENT

NONPHARMACOLOGIC THERAPY
- Prophylactic measures
  1. Diagnosis and treatment of chronic respiratory and metabolic disorders
  2. Correction of constipation
  3. Weight control, nutrition, and smoking cessation counseling
  4. Teaching of pelvic muscle exercises
- Supportive pessary therapy
  1. Ring-type pessary useful for first- or second-degree prolapse
  2. Gellhorn pessary preferred for more advanced prolapse
  3. Use of pessaries in conjunction with continuous hormone replacement therapy, unless contraindicated
  4. Perineorrhaphy under local anesthesia possibly needed to support the pessary if the vaginal outlet is very relaxed

ACUTE GENERAL Rx
- Patients who are only infrequently symptomatic: insertion of a tampon or diaphragm for temporary relief when prolonged standing is anticipated
- Neonatal uterine prolapse: simple digital reduction or the use of a small pessary

CHRONIC Rx
- Hormone replacement therapy at the time of menopause helps preserve tissue strength, maintain elasticity of the vagina, and contributes to the durability of surgical repairs.
- Gold standard for therapy is vaginal hysterectomy.
- Vaginal apex should be well suspended, but a prophylactic sacrospinous ligament fixation is not routinely required.
- If occult enterocele present, McCall culdoplasty performed.
- If vaginal approach to hysterectomy is contraindicated, abdominal hysterectomy is performed; vaginal apex likewise well supported.
- Colpocleisis is favored for the elderly patient who is sexually inactive or is a highrisk patient from a surgical point of view; can be done rapidly under local anesthesia with mild sedation if necessary.
- For symptomatic women who desire childbearing: management with pessaries or pelvic muscle exercises is recommended; if surgical correction is required, transvaginal sacrospinous fixation is the preferred method.
- Other surgical options are sling operations and sacral cervicopexy.

DISPOSITION
If untreated, uterine prolapse progressively worsens.

REFERRAL
To a gynecologist if pessary fitting or surgical intervention is needed

MISCELLANEOUS

COMMENTS
Surgery contraindicated in mild or asymptomatic uterine prolapse because the patient will seldom benefit from the operation although exposed to its risks.

REFERENCES
American College of Obstetricians and Gynecologists: Pelvic organ prolapse, *ACOG Tech Bull 214,* Washington, DC, 1995, ACOG.
de Mola JRL, Carpenter SE: Management of genital prolapse in neonates and young women, *Obstet Gynecol Surv* 51: 253, 1996.
Morley GW: Treatment of uterine and vaginal prolapse, *Clin Obstet Gynecol* 39:959, 1996.

Author: **Wan J. Kim, M.D.**

Uveitis

BASIC INFORMATION

DEFINITION
Uveitis is inflammation of the uveal tract, including the iris, ciliary body, and choroid. It may also involve other closed structures such as the sclera, retina, and vitreous humor.

SYNONYMS
Anterior uveitis
Posterior uveitis
Acute or chronic uveitis
Granulomatous or nongranulomatous uveitis

ICD-9-CM CODES
364.3 Unspecified iridocyclitis, uveitis

EPIDEMILOGY AND DEMOGRAPHICS
INCIDENCE (IN U.S.): Common; busy ophthalmologist will see two or more cases per week
PREVALENCE (IN U.S.): 17cases/100,000 persons
PREDOMINANT SEX: None
PREDOMINANT AGE: 38 yr
PEAK INCIDENCE: Middle age or older

PHYSICAL FINDINGS
- Photophobia
- Blurred visual acuity
- Irregular pupil
- Hazy cornea
- Abnormal cells and flare in anterior chamber or vitreous humor

ETIOLOGY
- Conjunctival injection
- Ciliary flush
- Keratitic precipitates (precipitates on the cornea)
- Hazy vitreous
- Retinal inflammation
- Iris nodules
- Glaucoma

DIAGNOSIS

DIFFERENTIAL DIAGNOSIS
- Glaucoma
- Conjunctivitis
- Retinal detachment
- Retinopathy
- Keratitis
- Scleritis
- Episcleritis

WORKUP
- Associated with arthritis, syphilis, tuberculosis, granulomatous disease, collagen-vascular disease, allergies, AIDS, sarcoid, Behçet's disease, histoplasmosis, and toxoplasmosis
- Slit lamp examination, indirect ophthalmoscopy

LABORATORY TESTS
- CBC
- Laboratory tests for specific inflammatory causes cited above in "Workup" (e.g., ANA, ESR, VDRL, PPD, Lyme titer)

IMAGING STUDIES
- Chest x-ray examination in suspected sarcoidosis, TB, histoplasmosis
- Sacroiliac x-ray examination in suspected ankylosing spondylitis

TREATMENT

NONPHARMACOLOGIC THERAPY
Treat the underlying disease.

ACUTE GENERAL Rx
- Cycloplegic drops (cyclopentolate [Cyclogyl]) or cystoplegic agents (homatropine hydrobromide [Optic] 1gtt q3-4h while awake) and topical steroids (prednisone acetate 1% 1gtt qh during day, PRN at night until favorable response, then q4-6h); avoid topical corticosteroids in infectious uveitis
- Antibiotics when infection is suspected
- Systemic steroids if appropriate for the underlying disease

CHRONIC Rx
Topical steroids and cycloplegics

DISPOSITION
Urgent referral to ophthalmologist

REFERRAL
- Eye problem should be followed early on by an ophthalmologist.
- Underlying medical disease should be treated by the primary care physician.

MISCELLANEOUS

COMMENTS
- In 90% of cases, the condition is idiopathic.
- Associated causes are found approximately 10% of the time, usually chronic and recurrent.

REFERENCES
Anglade E, Whitcup SM: The diagnosis and management of uveitis, *Drugs* 49:213, 1995.
Barrsma GS: The epidemiology and genetics of endogenous uveitis: a review, *Curr Eye Res* 11:1, 1992.
Simmons CA, Mathews D: Prevalence of uveitis: a retrospective study, *J Am Optom Assoc* 64:386, 1993.

Author: **Melvyn Koby, M.D.**

Vaginal bleeding during pregnancy

BASIC INFORMATION

DEFINITION
Bleeding per vagina at any time during pregnancy must be regarded as abnormal and is associated with an increased likelihood of pregnancy complications.

SYNONYMS
Hemorrhage

ICD-9-CM CODES
634.9 Spontaneous abortion
633.9 Ectopic pregnancy
630/631 Molar pregnancy
622.7 Cervical polyps
180.9/180.0/180.8 Cervical dysplasia/cancer
616.0 Cervicitis
616.10 Vulvovaginitis
184.0 Vaginal cancer
644.2 Premature labor term labor
641.1 Placenta previa
641.2 Placental abruption

EPIDEMIOLOGY AND DEMOGRAPHICS
- Common in U.S.; 20% to 25% of patients have vaginal spotting/bleeding in first trimester; of those, miscarriage occurs in 50%.
- Occurs in women of childbearing age.
- 1% to 2% of all pregnancies in the U.S. are ectopic.
- After one ectopic pregnancy, the chance of another is 7% to 15%.
- Ectopic pregnancy is the leading cause of maternal mortality in the first trimester.
- Average reported frequency for placental abruption is about 1 in 150 deliveries (0.3%).
- Incidence of placenta previa is <1 in 200 deliveries (0.5%).

PHYSICAL FINDINGS
- Bleeding: ranges from scant to life-threatening with hemodynamic instability
- Color: brown to bright red
- Can be painless or painful (cramps, back pain, severe abdominal pain)
- Fetal compromise: ranges from none to fetal demise

ETIOLOGY
- Influenced by gestational age
- Vaginal
- Cervical
- Uterine

DIAGNOSIS

DIFFERENTIAL DIAGNOSIS
- Any gestational age:
  1. Cervical lesions: polyps, decidual reaction, neoplasia
  2. Vaginal trauma
  3. Cervicitis/vulvovaginitis
  4. Postcoital trauma
  5. Bleeding dyscrasias
- Gestation <20 wk:
  1. Spontaneous abortion
  2. Presence of intrauterine device
  3. Ectopic pregnancy
  4. Molar pregnancy
  5. Implantation bleeding
  6. Low-lying placenta
- Gestation >20 wk:
  1. Molar pregnancy
  2. Placenta previa
  3. Placental abruption
  4. Vasa previa
  5. Marginal separation of the placenta
  6. Bloody show at term
  7. Preterm labor
- Box 2-120 describes the differential diagnosis of vaginal bleeding in pregnancy.

WORKUP
- Gestation <20 wk (Fig. 3-12 describes a clinical algorithm for evaluation of vaginal bleeding in early pregnancy.)
  1. Pelvic examination
  2. Culdocentesis
  3. Laparoscopy
  4. Laparotomy
- Gestation >20 wk:
  1. Ultrasound to locate placenta before pelvic examination
  2. If placenta previa, no speculum or bimanual examination
  3. If preterm labor, appropriate evaluation done

LABORATORY TESTS
- Urine pregnancy test: if positive, get quantitative β human chorionic gonadotropin (hCG)
  1. Early pregnancy: follow serially every 48 hr
  2. Normal pregnancy: hCG doubles approximately every 48 hr
  3. Spontaneous abortion: hCG levels will fall
  4. Ectopic pregnancy: hCG level will rise inappropriately
  5. Molar pregnancy: hCG level is extremely high
- CBC
- Blood type and screen (Rh negative patients need RhoGAM)
- Coagulation profile (useful in missed abortion and abruption)
- Cervical cultures/wet mount
- Pap smear for cervical malignancy; caution with biopsy, since cervix can bleed extensively

IMAGING STUDIES
Ultrasound:
- 5 to 6 wk: gestational sac (transvaginally; hCG >2500 mIU/ml (third IS) or >1000 mIU/ml (second IS)
- 8 to 9 wk: fetal cardiac activity
- Molar pregnancy: characteristic cluster of cysts
- Location of placenta
- Degree of placental separation: difficult to assess

TREATMENT

NONPHARMACOLOGIC THERAPY
- Pelvic rest: no coitus, douching, or tampons
- Bed rest, if >20 wk
- Counseling: genetic, bereavement

ACUTE GENERAL Rx
- Hemodynamic stabilization
- Emergency D&C, laparotomy, or cesarean section as necessary

CHRONIC Rx
Depends on diagnosis

DISPOSITION
Depends on diagnosis

REFERRAL
- If patient is unstable and needs emergency Ob/Gyn management and/or surgery
- If patient has diagnosis of ectopic or molar pregnancy, since immediate surgical treatment is indicated
- Perinatal consultation for high risk pregnancy

MISCELLANEOUS

REFERENCES
Cunningham FG, MacDonald PC, Gant NF (eds): *Williams' obstetrics*, ed 20, Norwalk, Conn, 1997, Appleton & Lange.

Author: **Maria Elena Soler, M.D.**

Vaginal malignancy

BASIC INFORMATION

DEFINITION
Vaginal malignancy is an abnormal proliferation of vaginal epithelium demonstrating malignant cells below the basement membrane.

SYNONYMS
Squamous cell carcinoma of the vagina
Adenocarcinoma of the vagina
Melanoma of the vagina
Sarcoma of the vagina

ICD-9-CM CODES
184.0 Vagina, vaginal neoplasm

EPIDEMIOLOGY AND DEMOGRAPHICS
PREVALENCE: Vaginal cancer is the second rarest gynecologic cancer. It comprises 2% of malignancies of the female genital tract.
INCIDENCE: 0.42 cases/100,000 persons
MEAN AGE AT DIAGNOSIS: Predominantly a disease of menopause. Mean age at diagnosis is 60 yr old.

PHYSICAL FINDINGS
- Majority of cases are asymptomatic.
- Postmenopausal vaginal bleeding and/or vaginal discharge are the most common symptoms.
- May also present as pelvic pain or pressure, dyspareunia, dysuria, malodor, or postcoital bleeding.
- May present as a vaginal lesion or abnormal Pap smear.

ETIOLOGY
- The exact etiology is unknown.
- Vaginal intraepithelial neoplasia is thought to be a precursor for squamous cell carcinoma of the vagina.
- Chronic pessary use has been associated with vaginal malignancy.
- Prior pelvic radiation may be a risk factor.
- Clear-cell adenocarcinoma is related to in utero diethylstilbestrol exposure.

DIAGNOSIS

DIFFERENTIAL DIAGNOSIS
- Extension from other primary carcinoma
- Vaginitis

WORKUP
- Diagnosis is made histologically by biopsy.
- Colposcopy and biopsy should follow suspicious Pap smear.
- Cystoscopy, proctosigmoidoscopy, chest radiography, IV urography, and barium enema may be used for clinical staging.
- CT scan and MRI are being used to evaluate spread.

IMAGING STUDIES
- Chest radiography, intravenous urography, and barium enema are used for staging.
- CT scan and MRI are good for assessing tumor spread.

TREATMENT

NONPHARMACOLOGIC THERAPY
- Radiation therapy is the mainstay of treatment.
- Stage I tumors that are small and confined to the posterior, upper third of the vagina may be treated with radical surgery.
- Other stages require a whole-pelvis, interstitial, and/or intracavitary radiation therapy.
- Chemotherapy is used in conjunction with radiotherapy in rare select cases.

DISPOSITION
Five-year survival ranges from 80% for stage I to 17% for stage IV.

REFERRAL
Vaginal cancer should be managed by a gynecologic oncologist and radiation oncologist.

MISCELLANEOUS

COMMENTS
U.S. Preventive Services Task Force Recommendations regarding counseling to prevent gynecologic cancers are described in Section V, Chapter 64.

REFERENCES
Berek JS, Hacker NF: *Practical gynecologic oncology,* Baltimore, 1994, William & Wilkins.
Hoskins WJ, Perez CA, Young RC: *Principles and practice of gynecologic oncology,* Philadelphia, 1997, Lippencott-Raven.
Morrow CP, Curtin JP, Townsend DE: *Synopsis of gynecologic oncology,* New York, 1993, Churchill Livingston.
Piver MS: *Handbook of gynecologic oncology,* Boston, 1996, Little Brown.
Shingleton HM et al: *Gynecologic oncology: current diagnosis and treatment,* Philadelphia, 1996, WB Saunders.
Wharton JT et al: Vaginal intraepithelial neoplasia and vaginal cancer, *Obstet Gynecol Clin North Am* 23(2):325,1996.
Author: **Yukio Sonoda, M.D.**

Vaginismus

BASIC INFORMATION

DEFINITION
Vaginismus refers to the involuntary spasm of the vaginal, introital, and/or levator ani muscles, preventing penetration or causing painful intercourse.

ICD-9-CM CODES
300.11 Hysterical vaginismus
306.51 Psychogenic or functional vaginismus
625.1 Reflex vaginismus

EPIDEMIOLOGY AND DEMOGRAPHICS
PREVALENCE: Affects approximately 1/200 women
INCIDENCE: Estimated at about 11.7% to 42% of women presenting to sexual dysfunction clinics
RISK FACTORS: Any previous sexual trauma, including incest or rape
PREDOMINANT SEX: Affects only females

PHYSICAL FINDINGS
- Fear of pain with coitus
- Dyspareunia
- Orgasmic dysfunction

ETIOLOGY
- Learned conditioned response to real or imagined painful vaginal experience (e.g., traumatic speculum examination, incest, rape)
- Vaginitis
- PID
- Endometriosis
- Anatomic anomalies
- Atrophic vaginitis
- Mucosal tears
- Inadequate lubrication
- Focal vulvitis
- Painful hymenal tags
- Scarring secondary to episiotomy
- Skin disorders
- Topical allergies
- Postherpetic neuralgia

DIAGNOSIS

WORKUP
- Thorough history (including sexual history)
- Careful pelvic examination
- Behavioral therapy

TREATMENT

NONPHARMACOLOGIC THERAPY
- Deconditioning the response by systematic self-administered progressive dilation techniques using fingers or dilators
- Behavioral and/or psychosexual therapy

ACUTE GENERAL Rx
- Botulinum toxin therapy given locally has been shown to relieve the perineal muscle spasms associated with vaginismus, allowing resumption of intercourse.
  1. Acts by preventing neuromuscular transmission, causing muscle weakness
  2. Considered experimental treatment for vaginismus at this time
- Cause should be determined by history and explained to the patient so that she understands the mechanics of the muscle spasms.
- Patient must be motivated to desire painless vaginal insertion for such reasons as pleasurable coitus, tampon insertion, or gynecologic examination.
- Patient (and her partner) must be willing to patiently undergo the process of systematic desensitization and counseling.

DISPOSITION
A high percentage of successfully treated patients

REFERRAL
To a gynecologist or sex therapist

MISCELLANEOUS

COMMENTS
- May uncover early sexual abuse or an aversion to sexuality in general
- To American Association of Sex Educators, Counselors and Therapists, 11 Dupont Circle, NW, Washington, DC, 20036.
- To Sex Information and Education Council of the U.S. (SIECUS), 85th Avenue, New York, NY 10022.

REFERENCES
Brin MF, Vapnek JM: Treatment of vaginismus with botulinum toxin injections, *Lancet* 349:pp, 1997.
Caplan HS: An effective clinical approach to vaginismus—putting the patient in charge, *West J Med* 149(6):769, 1988.
Scholl GM: Prognostic variables in treating vaginismus, *Obstet Gynecol* 72(2):231, 1988.

Author: **Candace C. Green, M.D.**

Vaginosis, bacterial (PTG)

BASIC INFORMATION

DEFINITION
Bacterial vaginosis (BV) is a gray homogeneous, odorous vaginal discharge of a polymicrobial nature.

SYNONYMS
Gardnerella vaginalis vaginitis
Haemophilus vaginalis vaginitis
Corynebacterium vaginalis vaginitis
Nonspecific vaginitis

ICD-9-CM CODES
616.10 Vaginitis, bacterial

EPIDEMIOLOGY AND DEMOGRAPHICS
- Most common vaginal infection
- Various studies by Thomason et al revealed that BV is present in:
  1. 16% of private patients
  2. 10% to 25% of obstetric clinic patients
  3. 38% to 64% of STD clinic patients
- *Gardnerella*, *Mycoplasma*, and *Mobiluncus* are harbored in the urethra of male partners; however, male partners are asymptomatic. Therefore treating them does not decrease the recurrence rates.

PHYSICAL FINDINGS
- Most patients are asymptomatic.
- Gray vaginal discharge is evident at introitus, typically homogeneous and adherent to vaginal mucosa.
- Pruritus occurs in only 13% of cases.
- Offensive vaginal odor, which is accentuated after coitus or during and immediately after menses.

ETIOLOGY AND PATHOGENESIS
- *Gardnerella vaginalis* is detected in 40% to 50% of vaginal secretions.
  1. Marked decrease in hydrogen peroxide-producing lactobacilli, with increase in vaginal pH.
  2. Anaerobes become predominant and produce amines.
- Such amines when alkalinized by semen, menstrual blood, the use of alkaline douches or the addition of 10% KOH, will volatilize, or break down, causing the unpleasant "fishy" odor.
- In bacterial vaginosis:
  1. Bacteroides (anaerobes) species are present in 1000 times the usual concentration.
  2. *Gardnerella vaginalis* species are present in 100 times normal.
  3. Anaerobic streptococci are present in 10 times normal.
  4. *Mycoplasma hominis* are present in increased concentration.
- Bacterial vaginosis is associated with PID, cystitis, and postoperative vaginal cuff infections.
- High concentration of bacteria in bacterial vaginosis may weaken the chorioamnionic membrane and lead to their subsequent rupture.
- Bacterial injury to lysosomes in the fetal membranes releases phospholipase A_2 and initiates the production of prostaglandins to cause uterine contraction.

DIAGNOSIS

- Thin, homogeneous discharge with a consistency that is not flocculent or curd-like
- Vaginal pH of >4.5
- Clue cells on saline wet mounts
- True clue cells are epithelial cells with obscured borders as a result of stippling with bacteria
- Cultures for anaerobes are unnecessary
- No diagnostic value in demonstrating *Gardnerella vaginalis* in vaginal secretions
- Gram stain of vaginal secretions used to reveal a true clue cell and abnormal mixed and numerous bacteria

TREATMENT

- Association of bacterial vaginosis with preterm labor, chorioamnionitis, and premature rupture of membranes in pregnant women dictates treatment.
- 2% clindamycin cream administered vaginally, one applicator (approximately 6 to 7 ml) nightly for 7 nights, is the primary mode of treatment in both pregnant and nonpregnant patients, with a short-term cure of 93%.
- Metronidazole vaginal gel 0.75% has similar advantages.
- Metronidazole 500 mg PO bid $\times$ 7 days has a short-term cure rate of 95%.
- Single 2-g dose of metronidazole is also used with a short-term cure rate of 86%, but the relapse rate is significantly higher.
- Augmentin (amoxicillin and clavulanic acid) 500 mg PO tid $\times$ 7 days has a cure rate of 85%.
- Asymptomatic nonpregnant patients with persistent infection should be treated.
- Women with bacterial vaginosis who are scheduled for hysterectomy may benefit from treatment.
- Recommended not to treat male sexual partners unless the patient has persistent or recurrent symptoms.

MISCELLANEOUS

REFERENCES
Meltzer RM: Vulvovaginitis. In Sciarra J: *Gynecology and obstetrics*, vol l, Philadelphia, 1995, Lippencott.

Sweet RL, Gibbs RS: *Infectious diseases of the female genital tract*, Baltimore, 1990, Williams & Wilkins.

Thomason JL, Gelbart SM, Broekhuizen FF: Office and clinical laboratory diagnosis of vulvovaginal infections: an overview. In Horowitz BJ, March, P-A (eds): *Vaginitis and vaginosis*, New York, 1991, Wiley-Liss.

Author: **Jeffrey Constantine, M.D.**

Varicose veins

BASIC INFORMATION

DEFINITION
Varicose veins are dilated networks of the subcutaneous venous system that result from valvular incompetence.

SYNONYMS
Chronic venous insufficiency
Stasis skin changes

ICD-9-CM CODES
454.9 VARICOSE VEINS

EPIDEMIOLOGY AND DEMOGRAPHICS
PREVALENCE:
- Approximately 30% of adults, with increasing incidence with age
- Increased incidence during pregnancy, especially with advanced maternal age

GENETICS:
- Familial tendency
- Evidence for dominant, recessive, and multifactorial types of inheritance

PREDOMINANT SEX: Female > male

RISK FACTORS:
- Advancing age
- Prolonged standing
- Pregnancy
- Obesity
- Use of oral contraceptives

PHYSICAL FINDINGS
- Dull ache, burning, or cramping in leg muscles
- Worsening discomfort with standing, warm temperatures, or menses
- Tortuous dilatation of superficial veins
- Edema
- Varicose ulcer, sometimes with superficial infection
- Dermatitis pigmentation

ETIOLOGY
- Normally, blood flow directed from the superficial venous system to the deep venous system via communication of perforating vessels
- Best thought of as "venous hypertension"
- Valvular incompetence in perforator veins of lower extremity leading to reverse flow of fluid from high-pressure deep venous system to low-pressure superficial venous system, resulting in dilatation of superficial veins, leg edema, and pain
- Rarely associated with deep vein thrombophlebitis
- Exacerbated by restrictive clothing

DIAGNOSIS

DIFFERENTIAL DIAGNOSIS
Conditions that can lead to superficial venous stasis other than primary valvular insufficiency include:
- Arterial occlussive disease
- Diabetes
- Deep vein thrombophlebitis
- Peripheral neuropathies
- Unusual infections
- Carcinoma

WORKUP
- Mainly a clinical diagnosis
- Arterial studies to rule out arterial insufficiency before initiating therapy for venous insufficiency

LABORATORY TESTS
Not useful

IMAGING STUDIES
Duplex ultrasound
- Gold standard for evaluation of varicose veins
- Quantitation of flow through venous valves under direct vizualization
- Allows precise anatomic identification of source of venous reflux

TREATMENT

NONPHARMACOLOGIC THERAPY
- Leg elevation and rest
- Graded compression stockings: used early in morning before edema accumulates and removed before going to bed
- Weight loss
- Avoidance of occlusive clothing

ACUTE GENERAL Rx
- For associated stasis dermatitis: topical corticosteroids
- Treatment of secondary infection with appropriate antibiotics

CHRONIC Rx
- Sclerotherapy: injection of 1% to 3% solution of sodium tetradecyl sulphate
- Surgery: indications include the following.
  1. Persistent varicosities with conservative treatment
  2. Failed sclerotherapy
  3. Previous or impending bleeding from ulcerated varicosities
  4. Disabling pain
  5. Cosmetic concerns
- Surgical methods include (must be combined with compressive therapy):
  1. Saphenous vein ligation
  2. Ligation of incompetent perforating veins
  3. Saphenous vein stripping with or without avulsion of varicosities
  4. Ambulatory "miniphlebectomies: avulsion of superficial varicosities with saphenous vein stripping

DISPOSITION
A chronic condition where a combination of compressive and surgical therapy can adequately control varicosites

REFERRAL
- To dermatologist for dermatitis complications
- To surgeon for failed conservative management

MISCELLANEOUS

REFERENCES
Goldman et al: Diagnosis and treatment of varicose veins: a review, *J Am Acad Dermatol* 31:393, 1994.

Author: **Matthew L. Withiam-Leitch, M.D., Ph.D.**

von Willebrand's disease (PTG)

BASIC INFORMATION

DEFINITION
Von Willebrand's disease is a congenital disorder of hemostasis characterized by defective or deficient von Willebrand factor (vWF). There are several subtypes of von Willebrand's disease. The most common type (80% of cases) is type I, which is caused by a quantitative decrease in von Willebrand factor; type IIA and type IIB are results of qualitative protein abnormalities; type III is a rare autosomal recessive disorder characterized by a near complete quantitative deficiency of vWF.

SYNONYMS
Pseudohemophilia

ICD-9-CM CODES
286.4 von Willebrand's disease

EPIDEMIOLOGY AND DEMOGRAPHICS
- Autosomal dominant disorder
- Most common inherited bleeding disorder
- Occurs in >100/1,000,000 persons

PHYSICAL FINDINGS
- Generally normal physical examination
- Mucosal bleeding (gingival bleeding, epistaxis) and GI bleeding may occur
- Easy bruising
- Postpartum bleeding, bleeding postsurgery or dental extraction, menorrhagia

ETIOLOGY
Quantitative or qualitative deficiency of vWF (see "Definition")

DIAGNOSIS

DIFFERENTIAL DIAGNOSIS
- Platelet function disorders, clotting factor deficiencies
- A clinical algorithm for evaluation of congenital bleeding disorders is described in Fig. 3-17

WORKUP
- Laboratory evaluation (see "Laboratory Tests")
- Initial testing includes PTT (increased), platelet count (normal), and bleeding time (prolonged)
- Subsequent tests include vWF level (decreased), factor VIII:C (decreased), and ristocetin agglutination (increased in type II B)

LABORATORY TESTS
- Normal platelet number and morphology
- Prolonged bleeding time
- Decreased factor VIII coagulant activity
- Decreased von Willebrand factor antigen or ristocetin cofactor
- Normal platelet aggregation studies
- Type II A von Willebrand can be distinguished from type I by absence of ristocetin cofactor activity and abnormal multimer
- Type IIB von Willebrand is distinguished from type I by abnormal multimer

TREATMENT

NONPHARMACOLOGIC THERAPY
- Avoidance of aspirin and other NSAIDs
- Evaluation for likelihood of bleeding (with measurement of bleeding time) before surgical procedures

ACUTE GENERAL Rx
- Desmopressin acetate (DDAVP) is useful to release stored vWF from endothelial cells. It is used to cover minor procedures and traumatic bleeding in mild type I von Willebrand's disease. Dose is 0.3 μg/kg in 100 ml of normal saline solution IV infused >20 min. DDAVP is also available as a nasal spray (dose of 150 μg spray administered to each nostril) as a preparation for minor surgery and management of minor bleeding episodes. DDAVP is not effective in type IIA von Willebrand's and is potentially dangerous in type IIB (increased risk of bleeding and thrombocytopenia).
- In patients with severe disease, replacement therapy in the form of cryoprecipitate is the method of choice. The standard dose is 1 bag of cryoprecipitate per 10 kg of body weight.
- Factor VIII concentrate rich in vWF (Humate-P, Armour) is useful to correct bleeding abnormalities.
- Life-threatening hemorrhage unresponsive to therapy with cryoprecipitate or factor VIII concentrate may require transfusion of normal platelets.

DISPOSITION
Prognosis is very good; most patients have minor bleeding complications and are able to lead a normal life.

MISCELLANEOUS

REFERENCES
Ruggeri ZM: von Willebrand's disease and the mechanisms of platelet function, *Ciba Found Symp* 189:35, 1995.
Sadler JE, Gralnick HR: Commentary: a new classification for von Willebrand disease, *Blood* 84:676, 1994.

Author: Fred F. Ferri, M.D.

Vulvar cancer

BASIC INFORMATION

DEFINITION
Vulvar cancer is an abnormal cell proliferation arising on the vulva exhibiting malignant potential. The majority is of squamous cell origin; however, other types include adenocarcinoma, basal cell carcinoma, sarcoma, and melanoma.

SYNONYMS
Squamous cell carcinoma of the vulva
Basal cell carcinoma of the vulva
Adenocarcinoma of the vulva
Melanoma of the vulva
Bartholin gland carcinoma
Verrucous carcinoma of the vulva
Vulvar sarcoma

ICD-9-CM CODES
184.4 Vulvar neoplasm

EPIDEMIOLOGY AND DEMOGRAPHICS
PREVALENCE: Vulvar cancer is uncommon. It comprises 4% of malignancies of the female genital tract.
INCIDENCE: 1.8 cases/100,000 persons
MEAN AGE AT DIAGNOSIS: Predominantly a disease of menopause. Mean age at diagnosis is 65 yr.

PHYSICAL FINDINGS
- Vulvar pruritus or pain is present.
- May produce a malodor or discharge or present as bleeding.
- Raised lesion, may have fleshy, ulcerated, leukoplakic, or warty appearance; may have multifocal lesions.
- Lesions are usually located on labia majora, but may be seen on labia minora, clitoris, and perineum.
- The lymph nodes of groin may be palpable.

ETIOLOGY
- The exact etiology is unknown.
- Vulvar intraepithelial neoplasia has been reported in 20% to 30% of invasive squamous cell carcinoma of the vulva, but the malignant potential is unknown.
- Human papillomavirus is found in 30% to 50% of vulvar carcinoma, but its exact role is unclear.
- Chronic pruritus, wetness, industrial wastes, arsenicals, hygienic agents, and vulvar dystrophies have been implicated as causative agents.

DIAGNOSIS

DIFFERENTIAL DIAGNOSIS
- Lymphogranuloma inguinale
- Tuberculosis
- Vulvar dystrophies
- Vulvar atrophy
- Paget's disease

WORKUP
- Diagnosis is made histologically by biopsy.
- Thorough examination of the lesion and assessment of spread.
- Possible colposcopy of adjacent areas.
- Cytologic smear of vagina and cervix.
- Cystoscopy and proctosigmoidoscopy may be necessary.

IMAGING STUDIES
- Chest radiography
- CT scan and MRI for assessing local tumor spread

TREATMENT

NONPHARMACOLOGIC THERAPY
- Treatment is individualized depending on the stage of the tumor.
- Stage I tumors with <1 mm stromal invasion are treated with complete local excision without groin node dissection.
- Stage I tumors with >1 mm stromal invasion are treated with complete local excision with groin node dissection.
- Stage II require radical vulvectomy with bilateral groin node dissection.
- Advanced stage disease may require the addition of radiation and chemotherapy to the surgical regimen.

DISPOSITION
Five-year survival ranges from 90% for stage I to 15% for stage IV.

REFERRAL
Vulvar cancer should be managed by a gynecologic oncologist and radiation oncologist.

MISCELLANEOUS

COMMENTS
U.S. Preventive Services Task Force Recommendations regarding counseling to prevent gynecologic cancers is described in Section V, Chapter 64.

REFERENCES
Berek JS, Hacker NF: *Practical gynecologic oncology,* Baltimore, 1994, William & Wilkins.
Edwards CL et al: Vulvar intraepithelial neoplasia and vulvar cancer, *Obstet Gynecol Clin North Am* 23(2):295,1996.
Hoskins WJ, Perez CA, Young RC: *Principles and practice of gynecologic oncology,* Philadelphia, 1997, Lippencott-Raven.
Morrow CP, Curtin JP, Townsend DE: *Synopsis of gynecologic oncology,* New York, 1993, Churchill Livingston.
Piver MS: *Handbook of gynecologic oncology,* Boston, 1996, Little, Brown.
Author: **Yukio Sonoda, M.D.**

Vulvovaginitis, bacterial

BASIC INFORMATION

DEFINITION
Bacterial vulvovaginitis is inflammation affecting the vagina, only rarely affecting vulva, caused by anaerobic and aerobic bacteria.

SYNONYMS
Bacterial vaginosis
Gardnerella vaginalis
Haemophilus vaginalis
Corynebacterium vaginalis

ICD-9-CM CODES
616.10 Vulvovaginitis

EPIDEMIOLOGY AND DEMOGRAPHICS
- Most prevalent form of vaginal infection of reproductive age women in the U.S.
- 32% to 64% in patients visiting STD clinics
- 12% to 25% in other clinic populations
- 10% to 26% in patients visiting obstetric clinics

PHYSICAL FINDINGS
- >50% of all women may be without symptoms.
- Unpleasant, fishy, or musty vaginal odor in about 50% to 70% of all patients. Odor exacerbates immediately after intercourse or during menstruation.
- Vaginal discharge is increased.
- Vaginal itching and irritation occurs.

ETIOLOGY
- Synergistic polymicrobial infection characterized by an overgrowth of bacteria normally found in the vagina
- Anaerobics: *Bacteroids* spp., *Peptostreptococcus* spp., *Mobiluncus* spp.
- Facultative anaerobes: *Gardnerella vaginalis, Mycoplasma hominis*
- Concentration of anaerobic bacteria increase 100 to 1000 times normal
- Lactobacilli are absent or greatly reduced

DIAGNOSIS

DIFFERENTIAL DIAGNOSIS
- Fungal vaginitis
- Trichomonas vaginitis
- Atrophic vaginitis
- Cervicitis

WORKUP
- Pelvic examination
- Speculum examination
- Normal saline slide of discharge
- Amsel criteria for diagnosis (three of four should be present):
  1. pH >4.5
  2. Clue cells (epithelial cells covered with bacteria) on saline solution slide
  3. Positive whiff test on 10% KOH
  4. Homogeneous, white, adherent discharge

LABORATORY TESTS
Culture not useful

TREATMENT

ACUTE GENERAL Rx
- Metronidazole 500 mg PO bid × 7 days, >90% cure rate
- Metronidazole 2 g PO × 1 day, 67% to 92% cure rate
- Metronidazole gel 5 g, intravaginal bid × 5 days
- Clindamycin 2% cream 5 g, intravaginal qd × 7 days

CHRONIC Rx
Clindamycin 300 mg PO bid × 7 days; cure rate similar to those achieved with metronidazole

DISPOSITION
- Reevaluate if not cured with treatment
- Recurrence fairly common

REFERRAL
Refer to obstetrician/gynecologist for recurrence or pregnant patient with bacterial vaginosis

MISCELLANEOUS

COMMENTS
Treating sexual partners has failed to demonstrate a benefit.

REFERENCES
Eschenbach et al: Diagnosis and clinical manifestations of bacterial vaginosis, *Am J Obstet Gynecol* 158:819, 1988.

Graves WL et al: Clindamycin versus metronidazole in the treatment of bacterial vaginosis, *Obstet Gynecol* 72:799, 1988.

Herbst A et al: *Comprehensive gynecology*, ed 2, St Louis, 1992, Mosby.

Martius et al: Relationship of vaginal lactobacillus species, cervical chlamydia trachomatis, and bacterial vaginosis to preterm birth, *Obstet Gynecol* 71:89, 1988.

Reed BD, Eyler A: Vaginal infections: diagnosis and management, *Am Fam Physician* 47(8):1805, 1993.

Scott JR et al: *Danforth's obstetrics and gynecology*, ed 7, 1994, JB Lippincott.

Sobel JD, Vaginitis in adult women, *Obstet Gynecol Clin North Am* 17:851, 1990.

Speigel CA et al: Anaerobic bacteria in nonspecific vaginitis, *N Engl J Med* 303:601, 1980.

Author: **Won S. Lee, M.D.**

Vulvovaginitis, estrogen deficient

BASIC INFORMATION

DEFINITION
Estrogen deficient vulvovaginitis is the irritation and/or inflammation of the vulva and vagina because of progressive thinning and atrophic changes secondary to estrogen deficiency.

SYNONYMS
Atrophic vaginitis

ICD-9-CM CODES
616.10 Vulvovaginitis

EPIDEMIOLOGY AND DEMOGRAPHICS
- Seen most often in postmenopausal women
- Average age of menopause is 52 yr
- In 1990, there were 36 million women 50 yr of age or older

PHYSICAL FINDINGS
- Thinning of pubic hair, labia minora and majora
- Decreased secretions from the vestibular glands with vaginal dryness
- Regression of subcutaneous fat
- Vulvar and vaginal itching
- Dyspareunia
- Dysuria and urinary frequency
- Vaginal spotting

ETIOLOGY
Estrogen deficiency

DIAGNOSIS

DIFFERENTIAL DIAGNOSIS
- Infectious vulvovaginitis
- Squamous cell hyperplasia
- Lichen sclerosis
- Vulva malignancy
- Vaginal malignancy
- Cervical and endometrial malignancy

WORKUP
- Pelvic examination
- Speculum examination
- Pap smear
- Possible endometrial biopsy if bleeding

LABORATORY TESTS
FSH and estradiol: generally after menopause, estradiol <15 pg and FSH >40 mIU/ml

TREATMENT

ACUTE GENERAL Rx
- Premarin 0.625 mg PO qd
- Estrace 1 mg PO qd
- Estraderm patch 0.05 mg × 2 per week
- If uterus present
  1. Estrogen + 2.5 mg PO Provera qd or
  2. Estrogen + 10 mg PO Provera × 10 days each mo
- Supplement PO estrogen with conjugated estrogen vaginal cream intravaginally:
  1. 2 to 4 g/day × 2 wk
  2. 1 to 2 g/day × 2 wk
  3. 1 to 2 g × 3 days/wk

CHRONIC Rx
See "Acute General Rx." May discontinue vaginal estrogen cream once symptoms alleviate.

DISPOSITION
The symptoms should be improved with the therapy. Caution for vaginal bleeding if uterus present.

REFERRAL
To obstetrician/gynecologist if vaginal bleeding

MISCELLANEOUS

REFERENCES
ACOG Technical Bulletin: *Hormone replacement therapy,* No 166, Washington, DC, 1992, ACOG.

Herbst A et al: *Comprehensive gynecology,* ed 2, St Louis, 1992, Mosby.

Sale PB: Genitourinary infection in older women, *J Obstet Gynecol Neonatal Nurs* 24(8):769, 1995.

Scott JR et al: *Danforth's obstetrics and gynecology,* ed 7, Philadelphia, 1994, JB Lippincott.

Author: Won S. Lee, M.D.

Vulvovaginitis, fungal (PTG)

BASIC INFORMATION

DEFINITION
Fungal vulvovaginitis is the inflammation of vulva and vagina caused by *Candida* spp.

SYNONYMS
Monilial vulvovaginitis

ICD-9-CM CODES
112.1 Vulvovaginitis, monilial

EPIDEMIOLOGY AND DEMOGRAPHICS
- Second most common cause of vaginal infection.
- Approximately 13 million people were affected in 1990.
- 75% of women will have at least one episode during their child-bearing years, and approximately 40% to 50% of these will experience a second attack.
- No symptoms in 20% to 40% of women who have positive cultures.

PHYSICAL FINDINGS
- Intense vulvar and vaginal pruritus
- Edema and erythema of vulva
- Thick, curd-like vaginal discharge
- Adherent, dry, white, curdy patches attached to vaginal mucosa

ETIOLOGY
- *Candida albicans* is responsible for 80% to 95% of vaginal fungal infections.
- *Candida tropicals* and *Torulopsis glabrata* are the most common non-albicans *Candida* species that can induce vaginitis.

PREDISPOSING HOST FACTORS
- Pregnancy
- Oral contraceptives (high-estrogen)
- Diabetes mellitus
- Antibiotics
- Immunosuppression
- Tight, poorly ventilated, nylon underclothing with increased local perineal moisture and temperature

DIAGNOSIS

DIFFERENTIAL DIAGNOSIS
- Bacterial vaginosis
- *Trichomonas* vaginitis
- Atrophic vaginitis

WORKUP
- Pelvic examination
- Speculum examination
- Hyphae or budding spores on 10% KOH preparation

LABORATORY TESTS
Culture, especially recurrence for identification

TREATMENT

ACUTE GENERAL Rx
- Cure rate of the various azole derivatives 85% to 90%; little evidence of superiority of one azole agent over the other
- Cure rate of polyene (Nystatin) cream and suppositories, 75% to 80%
- Miconazole 200-mg suppository (Monistat 3), one suppository × 3 or 2% vaginal cream (Monistat 7), one applicator full intravaginally qhs × 7
- Clotrimazole 200-mg vaginal tablet, one tablet intravaginally qhs × 3 or 100 mg vaginal tablet (Gyne-Lotrimin, Mycelex-G) one tablet intravaginally qhs × 7, or 1% vaginal cream intravaginally qhs × 7
- Butoconazole 2% cream (Femstat) one applicator intravaginally qhs × 3
- Terconazole 80-mg suppository or 0.8% vaginal cream (Terazol 3), one suppository or one applicator intravaginally qhs × 3 or 0.4% vaginal cream (Terazol 7), one applicator intravaginally qhs × 7
- Tioconazole 6.5% ointment (Vagistat), one applicator intravaginally × 1
- Fluconazole (Diflucan) 150 mg PO × 1

CHRONIC Rx
- Resistance or recurrence
  1. 14- to 21-day course of 7 day regimens mentioned in "Acute General Rx"
  2. Fluconazole (Diflucan) 150 mg PO × 1
  3. Ketoconazole (Nizoral) 200 mg PO bid × 5 to 14 days
  4. Itraconazole (Sporanox) 200 mg PO qd × 3 days
  5. Boric acid 600-mg capsule intravaginally bid × 14 days
- Prophylactic regimens
  1. Clotrimazole one 500-mg vaginal tablet each month
  2. Ketoconazole 200 mg PO bid × 5 days each month
  3. Fluconazole 150 mg PO × 1 each month
  4. Miconazole 100-mg vaginal tablet × 2 weekly

DISPOSITION
- Approximately 40% of adult women experience more than one lifetime episode of fungal vulvovaginitis.
- If symptoms do not resolve completely with treatment, or if they recur within a 2- to 3-mo period, further evaluation is indicated.
- Reexamination and possibly culture is necessary.

REFERRAL
To obstetrician/gynecologist for recurrence

MISCELLANEOUS

COMMENTS
Treatment of sexual partner is not recommended.

REFERENCES
Eschenbach DA, Hiller SL: Advances in diagnostic testing for vaginitis and cervicitis, *J Reprod Med* 34(suppl 18):555, 1989.
Herbst A et al: *Comprehensive gynecology*, ed 2, St Louis, 1992, Mosby.
Reed BD, Eyler A: Vaginal infection: diagnosis and management, *Am Fam Physician* 47(8):1805, 1993.
Scott JR et al: *Danforth's obstetrics and gynecology*, ed 7, Philadelphia, 1994, JB Lippincott.
Sobel JD: Candidal vulvovaginitis, *Clin Obstet Gynecol* 36(1):153, 1993.

Author: **Won S. Lee, M.D.**

Vulvovaginitis, prepubescent

BASIC INFORMATION

DEFINITION
Prepubescent vulvovaginitis is an inflammatory condition of vulva and vagina.

ICD-9-CM CODES
616.10 Vulvovaginitis

EPIDEMIOLOGY AND DEMOGRAPHICS
- Most common gynecologic problem of the premenarcheal female.
- Prepubertal girl is susceptible to irritation and trauma because of the absence of protective hair, labial fat pads, and the lack of estrogenization with atrophic vaginal mucosa.
- Symptoms of vulvovaginitis and introital irritation and discharge account for 80% to 90% of gynecologic visits.
- Nonspecific etiology in approximately 75% of children with vulvovaginitis.
- Majority of vulvovaginitis in children involves a primary irritation of the vulva with secondary involvement of the lower one third of the vagina.

PHYSICAL FINDINGS
- Vaginal discharge may be foul smelling and bloody
- Pruritus of vulva, vagina, or perineum
- Dysuria
- Irritation and erythema of vulva or vagina

ETIOLOGY
- Bacterial infections
- Protozoal infections
- Mycotic infections
- Viral infections
- Poor hygiene
- Foreign body
- Sexual abuse
- Allergic substance
- Masturbation
- Trauma

DIAGNOSIS

DIFFERENTIAL DIAGNOSIS
- Physiologic leukorrhea
- Foreign body
- Bacterial vaginosis
- Gonorrhea
- Fungal vulvovaginitis
- Trichomonas vulvovaginitis
- Sexual abuse
- Pinworms

WORKUP
- Pelvic, genital examination
- Speculum examination
- Rectal examination
- KOH and normal saline preparation of discharge

LABORATORY TESTS
- Urinalysis to rule out UTI and diabetes
- Cultures including STDs

TREATMENT

NONPHARMCOLOGIC THERAPY
- Avoid tight clothing
- Perineal hygiene
- Avoid irritant chemicals
- Reassurance

ACUTE GENERAL Rx
- Group A B *Streptococcus* and *Streptococcus pneumoniae*: penicillin V potassium 125 to 250 mg PO qid × 10 days
- *Chlamydia trachomatis*: erythromycin 50 mg/kg/day PO × 10 days
  1. Children >8 yr of age, doxycycline 100 mg bid PO × 7 days
- *Neisseria gonorrhoeae*: ceftriaxone 125 mg IM × 1 day
  1. Children >8 yr of age should also be given doxycycline 100 mg bid PO × 7 days
- *Staphylococcus aureus*: amoxicillin-clavulanate 20 to 40 mg/kg/day PO × 7 to 10 days
- *Haemophilus influenzae*: amoxicillin 20 to 40 mg/kg/day PO × 7 days
- *Trichomonas*: metronidazole 125 mg (15 mg/kg/day) tid PO × 7 to 10 days
- Pinworms: mebendazole 100-mg tablet chewable, repeat in 2 wk

CHRONIC Rx
See "Referral."

DISPOSITION
Further education:
- Young child: hygiene
- Adolescent: pregnancy prevention and "safe sex"

REFERRAL
- To obstetrician/gynecologist
- To pediatrician

MISCELLANEOUS

REFERENCES
Herbst A et al: *Comprehensive gynecology*, ed 2, St Louis, 1992, Mosby.
Scott JR et al: *Danforth's obstetrics and gynecology*, ed 7, Philadelphia, 1994, Lippincott.
Stevenson L, Brooke DS: Vulvovaginitis in the prepubertal child, *J Pediatr Health Care* 9(5):227, 1995.
Vandeven AM, Emans SJ: Vulvovaginitis in the child and adolescent, *Pediatr Rev* 14(4):141, 1993.

Author: Won S. Lee, M.D.

Vulvovaginitis, trichomonas (PTG)

BASIC INFORMATION

DEFINITION
Trichomonas vulvovaginitis is the inflammation of vulva and vagina caused by *Trichomonas* spp.

SYNONYMS
Trichomonas vaginalis

ICD-9-CM CODES
131.01 Vulvovaginitis, trichomonal

EPIDEMIOLOGY AND DEMOGRAPHICS
- Acquired through sexual contact
- Diagnosed in:
  1. 50% to 75% of prostitutes
  2. 5% to 15% of women visiting gynecology clinics
  3. 7% to 32% of women in STD clinics
  4. 5% of women in family planning clinics
- Asymptomatic in approximately 50% of women and 90% of men

PHYSICAL FINDINGS
- Profuse, yellow, malodorous vaginal discharge and severe vaginal itching
- Vulvar itching
- Dysuria
- Dyspareunia
- Intense erythema of the vaginal mucosa
- Cervical petechiae ("strawberry cervix")

ETIOLOGY
Single cell parasite known as *trichomonad*

RISK FACTORS
- Multiple sexual partners
- History of previous STDs
- Coexistent infection with *Neisseria gonorrhoeae* or other STDs

DIAGNOSIS

DIFFERENTIAL DIAGNOSIS
- Bacterial vaginosis
- Fungal vulvovaginitis
- Cervicitis
- Atrophic vulvovaginitis

WORKUP
- Pelvic examination
- Speculum examination
- Mobile trichomonads seen on normal saline preparation: 70% to 90% sensitivity when symptomatic
- Elevated pH (>5) of vaginal discharge
- A large number of inflammatory cells on normal saline preparation

LABORATORY TESTS
- Culture (modified Diamond media): 90% sensitivity
- Direct enzyme immunoassay
- Fluorescein-conjugated monoclonal antibody test

TREATMENT

NONPHARMACOLOGIC THERAPY
Condom use

ACUTE GENERAL Rx
Metronidazole (Flagyl) 2 g PO × 1 or 500 mg PO bid × 7 days

CHRONIC Rx
Metronidazole, 500 mg PO bid × 14 days or 2 g PO qd × 3 days accompanied by:
- Metronidazole gel (MetroGel-Vaginal), 5 g intravaginally bid × 5 days *or*
- Povidone-iodine suppository (Betadine), one suppository intravaginally bid × 14 to 28 days *or*
- Clotrimazole 100 mg vaginal tablet (Gyne-Lotrimin, Mycelex-G), one tablet intravaginally qhs × 7 nights

DISPOSITION
Trichomonas is considered an STD; therefore treatment of the sexual partner is necessary.

REFERRAL
To obstetrician/gynecologist for recurrence and pregnancy

MISCELLANEOUS

REFERENCES
Herbst A et al: *Comprehensive gynecology*, ed 2, St Louis, 1992, Mosby.
Reed BD, Dyle A: Vaginal infections: diagnosis and management, *Am Fam Physician* 47(8):1805, 1993.
Rein M, Muller M: *Trichomonas vaginalis* and trichomoniasis. In Holmes KK (ed): *Sexually transmitted diseases*, ed 2, New York, 1990, McGraw-Hill.
Schmid GP et al: Evaluation of six media for the growth of trichomonas vaginalis from vaginal secretions, *J Clin Microbiol* 27:1230, 1989.
Thomason, JL, Gelbart SM: *Trichomonas vaginalis*, Obstet Gynecol 74(3):536, 1989.

Author: Won S. Lee, M.D.

BASIC INFORMATION

DEFINITION
Warts are benign epidermal neoplasms caused by human papilloma virus (HPV).

SYNONYMS
Verruca vulgaris (common warts)
Verruca plana (flat warts)
Condyloma acuminatum (venereal warts)
Verruca plantaris (plantar warts)
Mosaic warts (cluster of many warts)

ICD-9-CM CODES
0.78.10 Viral warts
0.79.19 Veneral wart (external genital organs)

EPIDEMIOLOGY AND DEMOGRAPHICS
- Common warts occur most frequently in children and young adults.
- Anogenital warts are most common in young, sexually active patients.
- Common warts are longer lasting and more frequent in immunocompromised patients (e.g., lymphoma, AIDS, immunosuppressive drugs).
- Plantar warts occur most frequently at points of maximal pressure (over the heads of the metatarsal bones or on the heels).

PHYSICAL FINDINGS
- Common warts have an initial appearance of a flesh-colored papule with a rough surface; they subsequently develop a hyperkeratotic appearance with black dots on the surface (thrombosed capillaries); they may be single or multiple and are most common on the hands (see color plate 25).
- Warts obscure normal skin lines (important diagnostic feature). Cylindrical projections from the wart may become fused together forming a mosaic pattern.
- Flat warts generally are pink or light yellow, slightly elevated, and often found on the forehead, back of hands, mouth and beard area; they often occur in lines corresponding to trauma (e.g., a scratch); are often misdiagnosed (particularly when present on the face) and inappropriately treated with topical corticosteroids.
- Filiform warts have a fingerlike appearance with various projections; they are generally found near the mouth, beard, or periorbital and paranasal regions.
- Plantar warts are slightly raised and have a roughened surface; they may cause pain when walking; as they involute, small hemorrhages (caused by thrombosed capillaries) may be noted.
- Genital warts are generally pale pink with several projections and a broad base. They may coalesce in the perineal area to form masses with a cauliflower-like appearance.
- Genital warts on the cervical epithelium can produce subclinical changes that may be noted on Pap smear or colposcopy.

ETIOLOGY
Human papilloma virus infection; >60 types of viral DNA have been identified. Transmission of warts is by direct contact.

DIAGNOSIS

DIFFERENTIAL DIAGNOSIS
- Molluscum contagiosum
- Condyloma lata
- Acrochordon (skin tags) or seborrheic keratosis
- Epidermal nevi
- Hypertrophic actinic keratosis
- Squamous cell carcinomas
- Acquired digital fibrokeratoma
- Varicella zoster virus in patients with AIDS
- Recurrent infantile digital fibroma
- Plantar corns (may be mistaken for plantar warts)

WORKUP
- Diagnosis is generally based on clinical findings.
- Suspicious lesions should be biopsied.

LABORATORY TESTS
Colposcopy with biopsy of patients with cervical squamous cell changes

TREATMENT

NONPHARMACOLOGIC THERAPY
- Importance of use of condoms to reduce transmission of genital warts should be emphasized.
- Watchful waiting is an acceptable option in the treatment of warts, since many warts will disappear without intervention over time.
- Plantar warts that are not painful do not need treatment.

ACUTE GENERAL Rx
- Common warts:
  1. Application of topical salicylic acid 17% (e.g., Duofilm). Soak area for 5 min in warm water and dry. Apply thin layer once or twice daily for up to 12 wk, avoiding normal skin. Bandage.
  2. Liquid nitrogen, electrocautery are also excellent methods of removal.
  3. Blunt dissection can be used in large lesions or resistant lesions.
- Filiform warts: surgical removal is necessary.
- Flat warts: generally more difficult to treat.
  1. Tretinoin cream applied at HS over the involved area for several weeks may be effective.
  2. Application of liquid nitrogen
  3. Electrocautery
  4. 5-Fluorouracil cream (Efudex 5%) applied once or twice a day for 3 to 5 wk is also effective. Persistent hyperpigmentation may occur following Efudex use.
- Plantar warts:
  1. Salicylic acid therapy (e.g., Occlusal-HP). Soak wart in warm water for 5 min, remove loose tissue, dry. Apply to area, allow to dry, reapply. Use once or twice daily; maximum 12 wk. Use of 40% salicylic acid plasters (Mediplast) is also a safe, nonscarring treatment; it is particularly useful in treating mosaic warts covering a large area.
  2. Blunt dissection is also a fast and effective treatment modality.
  3. Laser therapy can be used for plantar warts and recurrent warts; however, it leaves open wounds that require 4 to 6 wk to fill with granulation tissue.
  4. Interlesional bleomycin is also effective but generally reserved for when all other treatments fail.
- Genital warts:
  1. Can be effectively treated with 20% podophyllin resin in compound tincture of benzoin applied with a cotton tip applicator by the treating physician.
  2. Podofilox (Condylox 0.5% gel) is now available for application by the patient. Local adverse effects include pain, burning, and inflammation at the site.
  3. Cryosurgery with liquid nitrogen delivered with a probe or as a spray is effective for treating smaller genital warts.
  4. Carbon dioxide laser can also be used for treating primary or recurrent genital warts (cure rate >90%).
  5. Imiquimod (Aldara) cream, 5% is a new patient-applied immune response modifier effective in the treatment of external genital and perianal warts (complete clearing of genital warts in >70% of females and >30% of males in 4 to 16 wk. Sexual contact should be avoided while the cream is on the skin.

DISPOSITION
- Warts can be effectively treated with the above noted modalities, with complete resolution in the majority of patients; however, recurrence rate is high.
- Cervical carcinomas and precancerous lesions in women are associated with genital papilloma virus infection.
- Squamous cell anal cancer is also associated with a history of genital warts.

REFERRAL
- Dermatology referral in warts resistant to conservative therapy
- Surgical referral in selected cases
- STD counseling in patients with anogenital warts

MISCELLANEOUS

COMMENTS
Subungual and periungual warts are generally more resistant to treatment. Dermatology referral for cryosurgery is recommended in resistant cases.

REFERENCES
Drake LA et al: Guidelines for care of warts: human papilloma virus: Canadian guidelines of care, *J Am Acad Dermatol* 32:98, 1995.

Habif TP: *Clinical dermatology,* ed 3, St Louis, 1996, Mosby.

Kipchener KC: The role of HPV in the genesis of cervical cancer, *Cancer Treatment Res* 70:29, 1994.

Sterling J: Treating the troublesome wart, *Practitioner* 239:44, 1995.

Vittorio CC, Schiffman MH, Weinstock MA: Epidemiology of human papillomaviruses, *Dermatol Clin* 13:561, 1995.

Author: **Fred F. Ferri, M.D.**

Wegener's granulomatosis (PTG)

BASIC INFORMATION

DEFINITION
Wegener's granulomatosis is a multisystem disease generally consisting of the classic triad of:
1. Necrotizing granulomatous lesions in the upper or lower respiratory tracts
2. Generalized focal necrotizing vasculitis involving both arteries and veins
3. Focal glomerulonephritis of the kidneys

"Limited forms" of the disease can also occur and may evolve into the classic triad; Wegener's granulomatosis can be classified using the "ELK" classification, which identifies the three major sites of involvement: *E,* ears, nose, and throat or respiratory tract; *L,* lungs; *K,* kidneys.

ICD-9-CM CODES
446.4 Wegener's granulomatosis

EPIDEMIOLOGY AND DEMOGRAPHICS
- The incidence of Wegener's granulomatosis is 0.5 cases/100,000 persons.
- Mean age of onset is 40 yr.

PHYSICAL FINDINGS
- Clinical manifestations often vary with the stage of the disease and degree of organ involvement.
- Frequent manifestations are:
  1. Upper respiratory tract: chronic sinusitis, chronic otitis media, mastoiditis, nasal crusting, obstruction and epistaxis, nasal septal perforation, nasal lacrimal duct stenosis, saddle nose deformities (resulting from cartilage destruction)
  2. Lung: hemoptysis, multiple nodules, diffuse alveolar pattern
  3. Kidney: renal insufficiency, glomerulonephritis
  4. Skin: necrotizing skin lesions
  5. Nervous system: mononeuritis multiplex, cranial nerve involvement
  6. Joints: monarthritis or polyarthritis (nondeforming), usually affecting large joints
  7. Mouth: chronic ulcerative lesions of the oral mucosa, "mulberry" gingivitis
  8. Eye: proptosis, uveitis, episcleritis, retinal and optic nerve vasculitis

ETIOLOGY
Unknown

DIAGNOSIS

DIFFERENTIAL DIAGNOSIS
- Other granulomatous lung diseases (e.g., lymphomatoid granulomatosis, Churg-Strauss syndrome, necrotizing sarcoid granulomatosis, bronchocentric granulomatosis, sarcoidosis); Table 2-28 in Section II describes the differential diagnosis of granulomatous disorders
- Neoplasms
- Goodpasture's syndrome
- Bacterial or fungal sinusitis
- Midline granuloma
- Viral infections

WORKUP
Chest x-ray examination, laboratory evaluation, PFTs, and tissue biopsy

LABORATORY TESTS
- Positive test for cytoplasmic pattern of ANCA (c-ANCA)
- Anemia, leukocytosis
- Urinalysis: may reveal hematuria, RBC casts and proteinuria
- Elevated serum creatinine, decreased creatinine clearance
- Increased ESR, positive rheumatoid factor, and elevated C-reactive protein may be found.

IMAGING STUDIES
- Chest x-ray film: may reveal bilateral multiple nodules, cavitated mass lesions, pleural effusion (20%).
- PFTs: useful in detecting stenosis of the airways.
- Biopsy of one or more affected organs should be attempted; the most reliable source for tissue diagnosis is the lung. Lesions in the nasopharynx (if present) can be easily biopsied.

TREATMENT

NONPHARMACOLOGIC THERAPY
- Ensure proper airway drainage.
- Give nutritional counseling.

ACUTE GENERAL Rx
- Prednisone 60 to 80 mg/day, and cyclophosphamide 2 mg/kg are generally effective and are used to control clinical manifestations; once the disease comes under control, prednisone is tapered and cyclophosphamide is continued.
- TMP-SMX therapy may represent a useful alternative in patients with lesions limited to the upper and/or lower respiratory tracts in absence of vasculitis or nephritis. Treatment with TMP-SMX (160 mg/800 mg bid) also reduces the incidence of relapses in patients with Wegener's granulomatosis in remission.

DISPOSITION
Five-year survival with aggressive treatment is approximately 80%; without treatment 2-yr survival is <20%.

REFERRAL
Surgical referral for biopsy

MISCELLANEOUS

COMMENTS
- Methotrexate (20 mg/wk) represents an alternative to cyclophosphamide in patients who do not have immediately life-threatening disease.
- C-ANCA levels should not dictate changes in therapy, since they correlate erratically with disease activity.

REFERENCES
Roo JK et al: The role of antineutrophil cytoplasmic antibodies (C-ANCA) testing in the diagnosis of Wegener's granulomatosis, *Ann Intern Med* 123:925, 1995.

Steleman CA et al: Trimethoprim-sulfamethoxazole for the prevention of relapses of Wegener's granulomatosis, *N Engl J Med* 335:16, 1996.

Author: **Fred F. Ferri, M.D.**

Wernicke's encephalopathy

BASIC INFORMATION

DEFINITION
Wernicke's encephalopathy is marked by an acute onset of extraocular muscle disorder associated with confusion and ataxia as a result of thiamin disturbance.

SYNONYMS
Wernicke-Korsakoff syndrome or psychosis

ICD-9-CM CODES
265.1 Wernicke's encephalopathy, disease, or syndrome

EPIDEMIOLOGY AND DEMOGRAPHICS
INCIDENCE (IN U.S.): Highest incidence in alcoholics
PREVALENCE (IN U.S.): Highest prevalence in alcoholics
PREDOMINANT SEX: Male most common
PEAK INCIDENCE: Early adulthood and upward
PEAK AGE: Adults
GENETICS: None proved

PHYSICAL FINDINGS
- Almost any disturbance of extraocular motility from nystagmus to paralysis
- Mental confusion
- Ataxia from cerebellar dysfunction
- Peripheral neuropathy

ETIOLOGY
Thiamin deficiency

DIAGNOSIS

DIFFERENTIAL DIAGNOSIS
- Give all patients with the triad 100 mg thiamin immediately.
- Consider other diagnoses (such as multiple sclerosis) if symptoms do not dramatically improve in 12 hr.

WORKUP
When suspected, treat immediately.

LABORATORY TESTS
- CBC
- Serum chemistries

IMAGING STUDIES
- MRI shows bilateral thalamic and mammillary body lesions in some cases.
- CT scan may show cerebral atrophy from chronic alcoholism.

TREATMENT

NONPHARMACOLOGIC THERAPY
Alcoholics Anonymous

ACUTE GENERAL Rx
- 100 mg thiamin IV or IM
- Prophylactic treatment for delirium tremens

CHRONIC Rx
Attempt to treat alcoholism.

DISPOSITION
Enter substance abuse program after acute phase.

REFERRAL
If symptoms do not resolve after thiamin therapy

MISCELLANEOUS

COMMENTS
The syndrome may occur in malnutrition, malabsorption states, and in patients on prolonged IV therapy without vitamins.

REFERENCES
Heye N et al: Wernicke's encephalopathy—causes to consider, *Intensive Care Med* 20:282, 1994.
Kopelman MD: The Korsakoff syndrome, *Br J Psychiatry* 166:154, 1995.

Author: **William H. Olson, M.D.**

CLINICAL TOPICS Yellow fever 533

BASIC INFORMATION

DEFINITION
Yellow fever is an infection, primarily of the liver, with systemic manifestations caused by the yellow fever virus (YFV).

ICD-9-CM CODES
060.9 Yellow fever

EPIDEMIOLOGY AND DEMOGRAPHICS
INCIDENCE (IN U.S.):
- None
- Approximate attack rates of 3% in Africa and Amazon

PREVALENCE (IN U.S.):
- None
- Endemic areas: 20% of population

PREDOMINANT SEX: In Africa and Amazon, male agricultural workers
PREDOMINANT AGE: 20 to 40 yr
PEAK INCIDENCE: Variable with outbreaks

PHYSICAL FINDINGS
- Clinical illness with jaundice in about 5% to 20% of infections
- Most subclinical
- Onset sudden after incubation period of 3 to 6 days
- Viremic (early) phase
  1. Fever, chills
  2. Severe headache
  3. Lumbosacral pain
  4. Myalgias
  5. Nausea
  6. Severe malaise
  7. Conjunctivitis
  8. Relative bradycardia
- After brief recovery, toxic phase:
  1. Jaundice
  2. Oliguria
  3. Albuminuria
  4. Hemorrhage (especially hematemesis)
  5. Encephalopathy
  6. Shock
  7. Acidosis

ETIOLOGY
- Yellow fever virus (*L. flavus*)
  1. Prototype Flavivirus
  2. Infects primarily hepatic cells
  3. Replication
     a. Exclusively intracellular and intracytoplasmic
     b. Primarily in the endoplasmic reticulum
  4. Late in infection, cytopathic effects (antibody- and cell-mediated) produce pathology
- Vector
  1. *Aedes aegypti* (urban)
  2. *Aedes* spp., *Haemagogus* (especially in Amazon) mosquitos (sylvan)
  3. Primary hosts humans and simian species
  4. Virus maintained in mosquito ova during dry season
  5. Sylvan cycle interrupted by humans: agriculture, forest clearing
- Geographic distribution
  1. South America and Africa, in countries between +15 and −15 degrees latitude
  2. Not in Asia
- Recent increase in epidemics in Africa (especially Nigeria)
  1. Several hundred thousand cases between 1987-1991
  2. Fatality rate approximately 20% in jaundiced patients
  3. Death between days 7 to 10
- Pathogenesis
  1. Unclear
  2. Probably involves Kupffer cell, followed by hepatocyte infection
  3. Renal failure accompanied by viral antigen in glomeruli
  4. Shock and lactic acidosis accompanied by release of vasoactive mediators from liver, nodes, spleen
  5. Myocarditis contributes to shock and collapse
  6. Hemorrhage
     a. Decreased synthesis of clotting factors
     b. Disseminated intravascular coagulation
  7. Encephalopathy secondary to cerebral edema

DIAGNOSIS

DIFFERENTIAL DIAGNOSIS
- Viral hepatitis
- Leptospirosis
- Malaria
- Typhoid fever
- Hemorrhagic Fevers (HF) with jaundice
  1. Dengue (HF)
  2. Rift Valley fever
  3. Crimean-Congo (HF)

WORKUP
- CBC
- Liver function tests
- Serum for serology (YFV, viral isolation)
- Coagulation studies
  1. Prothrombin time
  2. Fibrinogen
  3. Fibrin split products
- Liver biopsy contraindicated (death from bleeding)

LABORATORY TESTS
- CBC
  1. Generally nonspecific
  2. Mild leukopenia
  3. Thrombocytopenia
  4. Anemia
- Liver function tests
  1. Mildly to severely abnormal ALT, AST
- Elevated creatinine and BUN
- Coagulation studies
  1. Normal *or*
  2. Demonstrate abnormal prothrombin time *or*
  3. Reveal disseminated intravascular coagulation (DIC)
- Terminal hypoglycemia
- Specific diagnosis confirmed by viral isolation from blood
- Serologic diagnosis
  1. Viral antigen in serum (ELISA)
  2. Viral RNA by PCR
  3. IgM by:
     a. Antibody-capture ELISA
     b. Hemagglutination inhibition
     c. Complement fixation
     d. Neutralization assays
  4. Appear within 5 to 7 days
     a. IgM
     b. HI
     c. N Ab
  5. Appear within 7 to 14 days
     a. CF Ab
  6. Rising Ab confirmed by paired sera
  7. CF persists up to 1 yr

TREATMENT

ACUTE GENERAL Rx
- Treatment symptomatic
- Acetaminophen (headache and fever)
- Antacids, cimetidine (GI bleeding)
- Blood transfusion, volume replacement for hemorrhage and shock
- Dialysis for renal failure
- No clearly useful antiviral agents

DISPOSITION
Follow-up until hepatic, renal, CNS disease resolved

REFERRAL
To infectious diseases expert for accurate diagnosis and management

MISCELLANEOUS

COMMENTS
- Yellow fever is preventable.
- Live, attenuated yellow fever vaccine gives long-lasting immunity in >90% of recipients.
- Vaccination contraindicated in:
  1. Infants <6 mo (postvaccinal encephalitis)
  2. Immunosuppressed patients
  3. Pregnant women (congenital infection may result, although generally without adverse effects on fetus)
  4. Patients with egg hypersensitivity

Author: **Peter Nicholas, M.D.**

SECTION II

Differential Diagnosis, Etiology, and Classification of Common Signs and Symptoms

ABDOMINAL DISTENTION

> **BOX 2-1 Abdominal Distention**
>
> **Nonmechanical Obstruction**
> Excessive intraluminal gas
> Intraabdominal infection
> Trauma
> Retroperitoneal irritation (renal colic, neoplasms, infections)
> Vascular insufficiency (thrombosis, embolism)
> Mechanical ventilation
> Extraabdominal infection (sepsis, pneumonia, empyema, osteomyelitis of spine)
> Metabolic/toxic (hypokalemia, uremia, lead poisoning)
> Chemical irritation (perforated ulcer, bile, pancreatitis)
> Peritoneal inflammation
> Severe pain, pain medications
>
> **Mechanical Obstruction**
> Neoplasm (intraluminal, extraluminal)
> Adhesions, endometriosis
> Infection (intraabdominal abscess, diverticulitis)
> Gallstones
> Foreign body, bezoars
> Pregnancy
> Hernias
> Volvulus
> Stenosis at surgical anastomosis, radiation stenosis
> Fecaliths
> Inflammatory bowel disease
> Hematoma
> Other: parasites, superior mesenteric artery (SMA) syndrome, pneumatosis intestinalis, annular pancreas, Hirschsprung's disease, intussusception, meconium

ABDOMINAL PAIN, BY LOCATION

> **BOX 2-2 Abdominal Pain, by Location**
>
> **Diffuse**
> Early appendicitis
> Aortic aneurysm
> Gastroenteritis
> Intestinal obstruction
> Diverticulitis
> Peritonitis
> Mesenteric insufficiency or infarction
> Pancreatitis
> Inflammatory bowel disease
> Irritable bowel
> Mesenteric adenitis
> Metabolic: toxins, lead poisoning, uremia, drug overdose, DKA, heavy metal poisoning
> Sickle cell crisis
> Pneumonia (rare)
> Trauma
> Urinary tract infection, PID
> Other: acute intermittent porphyria, tabes dorsalis, periarteritis nodosa, Henoch-Schönlein purpura, adrenal insufficiency
>
> **Epigastric**
> Gastric: PUD, gastric outlet obstruction, gastric ulcer
> Duodenal: PUD, duodenitis
> Biliary: cholecystitis, cholangitis
> Hepatic: hepatitis
> Pancreatic: pancreatitis
> Intestinal: high small bowel obstruction, early appendicitis
> Cardiac: angina, MI, pericarditis
> Pulmonary: pneumonia, pleurisy, pneumothorax
> Subphrenic abscess
> Vascular: dissecting aneurysm
>
> **Suprapubic**
> Intestinal: colon obstruction or gangrene, diverticulitis, appendicitis
> Reproductive system: ectopic pregnancy, mittelschmerz, torsion of ovarian cyst, PID, salpingitis, endometriosis, rupture of endometrioma
> Cystitis, rupture of urinary bladder
>
> **Right Upper Quadrant (RUQ)**
> Biliary: calculi, infection, inflammation, neoplasm
> Hepatic: hepatitis, abscess, hepatic congestion, neoplasm, trauma
> Gastric: PUD, pyloric stenosis, neoplasm, alcoholic gastritis, hiatal hernia
> Pancreatic: pancreatitis, neoplasm, stone in pancreatic duct or ampulla
> Renal: calculi, infection, inflammation, neoplasm, rupture of kidney
> Pulmonary: pneumonia, pulmonary infarction, right-sided pleurisy
> Intestinal: retrocecal appendicitis, intestinal obstruction, high fecal impaction
> Cardiac: myocardial ischemia (particularly involving the inferior wall), pericarditis
> Cutaneous: herpes zoster
> Trauma
> Fitz-Hugh–Curtis syndrome (perihepatitis)
>
> **Left Upper Quadrant (LUQ)**
> Gastric: PUD, gastritis, pyloric stenosis, hiatal hernia
> Pancreatic: pancreatitis, neoplasm, stone in pancreatic duct or ampulla
> Cardiac: MI, angina pectoris
> Splenic: splenomegaly, ruptured spleen, splenic abscess, splenic infarction
> Renal: calculi, pyelonephritis, neoplasm
> Pulmonary: pneumonia, empyema, pulmonary infarction
> Vascular: ruptured aortic aneurysm
> Cutaneous: herpes zoster
> Trauma
> Intestinal: high fecal impaction, perforated colon
>
> **Periumbilical**
> Intestinal: small bowel obstruction or gangrene, early appendicitis
> Vascular: mesenteric thrombosis, dissecting aortic aneurysm
> Pancreatic: pancreatitis

Continued

BOX 2-2 Abdominal Pain, by Location—cont'd

Periumbilical—cont'd
Metabolic: uremia, DKA
Trauma

Right Lower Quadrant (RLQ)
Intestinal: acute appendicitis, regional enteritis, incarcerated hernia, cecal diverticulitis, intestinal obstruction, perforated ulcer, perforated cecum, Meckel's diverticulitis
Reproductive: ectopic pregnancy, ovarian cyst, torsion of ovarian cyst, salpingitis, tuboovarian abscess, mittelschmerz, endometriosis, seminal vesiculitis
Renal: renal and ureteral calculi, neoplasms, pyelonephritis
Vascular: leaking aortic aneurysm
Psoas abscess
Trauma
Cholecystitis

Left Lower Quadrant (LLQ)
Intestinal: diverticulitis, intestinal obstruction, perforated ulcer, inflammatory bowel disease, perforated descending colon, inguinal hernia, neoplasm, appendicitis
Reproductive: ectopic pregnancy, ovarian cyst, torsion of ovarian cyst, tuboovarian abscess, mittelschmerz, endometriosis; seminal vesiculitis
Renal: renal or ureteral calculi, pyelonephritis, neoplasm
Vascular: leaking aortic aneurysm
Psoas abscess
Trauma

ABDOMINAL PAIN, POORLY LOCALIZED

BOX 2-3 Causes of Poorly Localized Acute Abdominal Pain

Extraabdominal

Metabolic
DKA, acute intermittent porphyria, hyperthyroidism, hypothyroidism, hypercalcemia, hypokalemia, uremia, hyperlipidemia, hyperparathyroidism

Hematologic
Sickle cell crisis, leukemia or lymphoma, Henoch-Schönlein purpura

Infectious
Infectious mononucleosis, Rocky Mountain spotted fever, acquired immunodeficiency syndrome (AIDS), streptococcal pharyngitis (in children), herpes zoster

Drugs and Toxins
Heavy metal poisoning, black widow spider bites, withdrawal syndromes, mushroom ingestion

Referred Pain
Pulmonary: pneumonia, pulmonary embolism, pneumothorax
Cardiac: angina, myocardial infarction, pericarditis, myocarditis
Genitourinary: prostatis, epididymitis, orchitis, testicular torsion
Musculoskeletal: rectus sheath hematoma

Functional
Somatization disorder, malingering, hypochondriasis, Munchausen syndrome

Intraabdominal
Early appendicitis, gastroenteritis, peritonitis, pancreatitis, abdominal aortic aneurysm, mesenteric insufficiency or infarction, intestinal obstruction, volvulus, ulcerative colitis

From Rosen P et al (eds): *Emergency medicine: concepts and clinical practice,* St Louis, 1997, Mosby.

ABDOMINAL PAIN, BY AGE GROUPS

BOX 2-4 Common Causes of Acute Abdominal Pain by Age Groups

Infancy
GI
Acute gastroenteritis
Appendicitis
Intussusception
Volvulus
Meckel's diverticula
Other
   Colic
   Trauma

Childhood
GI
Acute gastroenteritis
Appendicitis
Constipation
Cholecystitis, acute
   Intestinal obstruction
Pancreatitis
Neoplasm
Inflammatory bowel disease
Other
   Functional abdominal pain
   Pyelonephritis
   Pneumonia
   DKA
   Heavy metal poisoning
   Sickle cell crisis
   Trauma

Adolescence
GI
Acute gastroenteritis
Appendicitis
Inflammatory bowel disease
Peptic ulcer disease
Cholecystitis
Neoplasm
Other
   Functional abdominal pain
   Pelvic inflammatory disease
   Pregnancy
   Pyelonephritis
   Renal stone
   Trauma

From Rosen P et al (eds): *Emergency medicine: concepts and clinical practice,* St Louis, 1997, Mosby.

ABDOMINAL PAIN, IN PREGNANCY

TABLE 2-1 Differential Diagnosis of Abdominal Pain in Pregnancy

DIAGNOSIS	GESTATIONAL AGE	COMMENTS
Gynecologic		
Miscarriage	<20 wk; 80% <12 wk	Ultrasonography to confirm location
Septic abortion	<20 wk	Fever, uterine tenderness
Ectopic pregnancy	<14 wk	Must always consider in first trimester until IUP confirmed
Corpus luteum cyst rupture	<12 wk	Sudden focal peritoneal pain; no fever
Ovarian torsion	Especially <24 wk	Large ovary; ischemic pain
PID	<12 wk	Very rare
Chorioamnionitis	>16 wk	Tender uterus, fever; amniocentesis reveals WBCs
Abruptio placentae	>16 wk	Focal uterine tenderness, fetal distress, variable bleeding; possible DIC
Nongynecologic		
Appendicitis	Throughout	Guarding may be less prominent; location changes
Cholecystitis	Throughout	Confirm with sonography
Hepatitis	Throughout	Confirm with LFTs
Pyelonephritis	Throughout	Flank pain, fever, positive catheterized urinalysis
Preeclampsia	>20 wk	Hypertension, proteinuria, edema; RUQ pain

From Rosen P et al (eds): *Emergency medicine: concepts and clinical practice,* St Louis, 1992, Mosby.

ABORTION, RECURRENT

> **BOX 2-5 Potential Causes of Recurrent Abortion**
>
> Parental chromosomal abnormalities
> Congenital anatomic abnormalities
>   Incomplete müllerian fusions or septum resorption defects
>   DES exposure
>   Uterine artery abnormalities
> Acquired anatomic abnormalities
>   Uterine synechiae (adhesions)
>   Uterine fibroids
>   Endometriosis
> Endocrinologic abnormalities
>   Luteal phase insufficiency
> Hypothyroidism
> Diabetes mellitus
> Maternal infections
>   Cervical mycoplasma, ureaplasma, and chlamydia
> Other causes
>   Heavy metal and chemical exposures
>   Chronic medical illness
>   Thrombocytosis
> Immunologic phenomena
>   Allogenic immunity
>   Autoimmunity

From Carlson KJ et al: *Primary care of women,* St Louis, 1995, Mosby.
DES, Diethylstilbestrol.

ACIDOSIS, ANION GAP

Anion gap acidosis → Dipstick urine for ketones

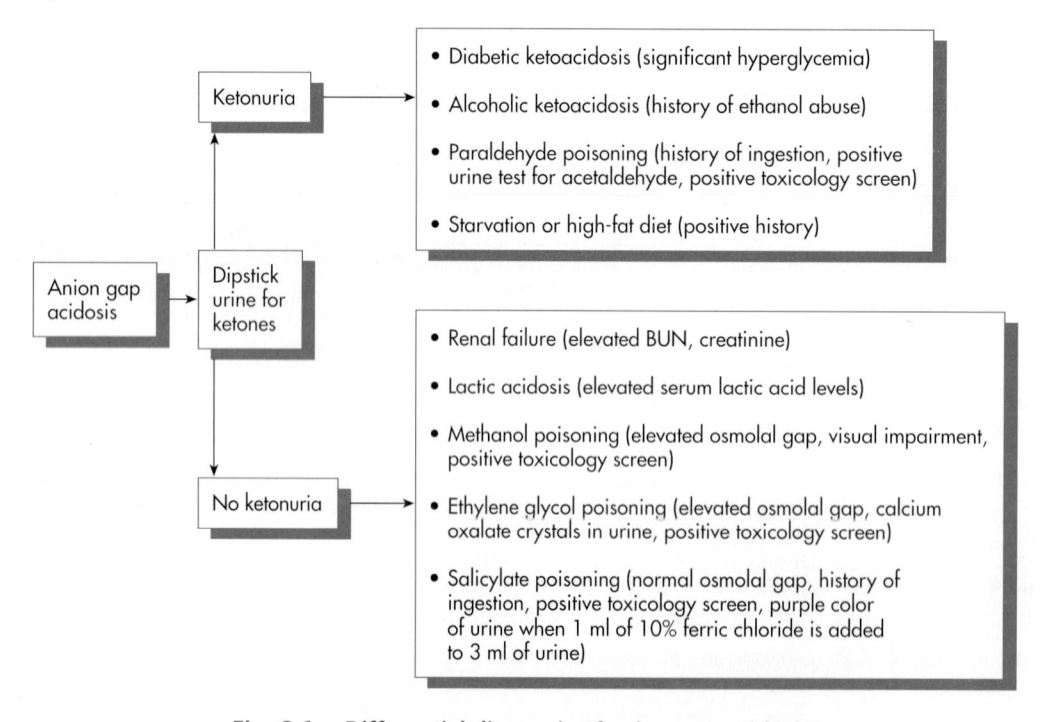

Ketonuria:
- Diabetic ketoacidosis (significant hyperglycemia)
- Alcoholic ketoacidosis (history of ethanol abuse)
- Paraldehyde poisoning (history of ingestion, positive urine test for acetaldehyde, positive toxicology screen)
- Starvation or high-fat diet (positive history)

No ketonuria:
- Renal failure (elevated BUN, creatinine)
- Lactic acidosis (elevated serum lactic acid levels)
- Methanol poisoning (elevated osmolal gap, visual impairment, positive toxicology screen)
- Ethylene glycol poisoning (elevated osmolal gap, calcium oxalate crystals in urine, positive toxicology screen)
- Salicylate poisoning (normal osmolal gap, history of ingestion, positive toxicology screen, purple color of urine when 1 ml of 10% ferric chloride is added to 3 ml of urine)

Fig. 2-1 Differential diagnosis of anion gap acidosis.

ACIDOSIS, LACTIC

BOX 2-6 Etiology of Lactic Acidosis

Tissue Hypoxia
Shock (hypovolemic, cardiogenic, endotoxic)
Respiratory failure (asphyxia)
Severe CHF
Severe anemia
Carbon monoxide or cyanide poisoning

Associated with Systemic Disorders
Neoplastic diseases (e.g., leukemia, lymphoma)
Liver or renal failure
Sepsis
Diabetes mellitus
Seizure activity
Abnormal intestinal flora (D-lactic acidosis)
Alkalosis
HIV

Secondary to Drugs or Toxins
Salicylates
Ethanol, methanol, ethylene glycol
Fructose and sorbitol
Biguanides (phenformin, metformin [usually occurring in patients with renal insufficiency])
Isoniazid
Streptozocin

Hereditary Disorders
G_6PD deficiency and others

ACIDOSIS, METABOLIC

BOX 2-7 Metabolic Acidosis

1. Metabolic acidosis with increased anion gap (AG acidosis)
   a. Lactic acidosis
   b. Ketoacidosis (diabetes mellitus, ethanol intoxication, starvation)
   c. Uremia (chronic renal failure)
   d. Ingestion of toxins (paraldehyde, methanol, salicylate, ethylene glycol)
   e. High-fat diet (mild acidosis)
2. Metabolic acidosis with normal anion gap (hyperchloremic acidosis)
   a. Renal tubular acidosis (including acidosis of aldosterone deficiency)
   b. Intestinal loss of bicarbonate (diarrhea, pancreatic fistula)
   c. Carbonic anhydrase inhibitors (e.g., acetazolamide)
   d. Dilutional acidosis (as a result of rapid infusion of bicarbonate-free isotonic saline)
   e. Ingestion of exogenous acids (ammonium chloride, methionine, cystine, calcium chloride)
   f. Ileostomy
   g. Ureterosigmoidostomy
   h. Drugs: amiloride, triamterene, spironolactone, beta blockers

ACIDOSIS, RESPIRATORY

BOX 2-8 Causes of Respiratory Acidosis

Disorders of ventilatory control
  Central nervous system
    Depression of respiratory center
      Anesthetics
      Drug intoxication
      Primary central hypoventilation
      Myxedema
      Oxygen therapy in chronic hypercapnic patients
      Sleep
  Peripheral neuromuscular disease
    Disorders of peripheral nerves
      Spinal cord injury
      Phrenic nerve palsy
      Guillain-Barré syndrome
      Myasthenia gravis
      Paralytic agents
      Botulism
Disorders of muscle
  Myositis, myopathy, muscular dystrophies
  Fatigue in hypokalemia, hypophosphatemia
  Fatigue in obstructive airways disease
Disorders of pulmonary function
  Restrictive lung disease
    Kyphoscoliosis
    Flail chest
  Airways obstruction
    Upper airways obstruction (trachea, larynx, bronchi)
    Asthma and chronic obstructive pulmonary disease
Shunts
  Congenital heart disease with left-to-right shunt
  Intrapulmonary shunt
    Arteriovenous malformation
    Severe pneumonia, large emboli
Errors of ventilator management

From Stein JH (ed): *Internal medicine,* ed 4, St Louis, 1994, Mosby.

ADRENAL MASSES

BOX 2-9 Adrenal Masses

Unilateral Adrenal Masses
Functional Lesions
Adrenal adenoma
Adrenal carcinoma
Pheochromocytoma
Primary aldosteronism, adenomatous type

Nonfunctional Lesions
Adrenal adenoma
Adrenal carcinoma
Ganglioneuroma
Myelolipoma
Hematoma
Adrenolipoma
Metastasis

Bilateral Adrenal Masses
Functional Lesions
ACTH-dependent Cushing's syndrome
Congenital adrenal hyperplasia
Pheochromocytoma
Conn's syndrome, hyperplastic variety
Micronodular adrenal disease
Idiopathic bilateral adrenal hypertrophy

Nonfunctional Lesions
Infection (tuberculosis, fungi)
Infiltration (leukemia, lymphoma)
Replacement (amyloidosis)
Hemorrhage
Bilateral metastases

From Stein JH (ed): *Internal medicine,* ed 5, St Louis, 1998, Mosby.

ALKALOSIS, METABOLIC

BOX 2-10 Metabolic Alkalosis

1. Chloride-responsive (urinary chloride <15 mEq/L)
   a. Vomiting
   b. Nasogastric suction
   c. Diuretics
   d. Post–hypercapnic alkalosis
   e. Stool losses (laxative abuse, cystic fibrosis, villous adenoma)
   f. Massive blood transfusion
   g. Exogenous alkali administration

2. Chloride-unresponsive (urinary chloride >15 mEq/L)
   a. Hyperadrenocorticoid states (Cushing's syndrome, primary hyperaldosteronism, secondary mineralocorticoidism [licorice, chewing tobacco])
   b. Hypomagnesemia
   c. Hypokalemia
   d. Bartter's syndrome

ALKALOSIS, RESPIRATORY

BOX 2-11 Causes of Respiratory Alkalosis

Hypoxemia
  Most pulmonary disease
  Organic heart disease
    Congenital heart disease with right-to-left shunts
    Congestive heart failure
  Altitude
Stimulation of respiratory center
  Drugs
    Salicylates
    Catecholamines
    Theophylline
    Doxapram
  Progesterone excess
    Pregnancy
    Cirrhosis
  CNS disease
    Subarachnoid hemorrhage
    Disease of respiratory center
    Cheyne-Stokes respirations
  Fever
  Sepsis
  Anxiety
Stimulation of peripheral pulmonary receptors
  Pneumonia
  Asthma
  Embolism
  Pulmonary edema
  Pulmonary fibrosis
  Pleural disease
Errors of ventilator management

From Stein JH (ed): *Internal medicine,* ed 4, St Louis, 1994, Mosby.

ALOPECIAS

TABLE 2-2 Differential Diagnosis of Alopecias

DISEASE	HISTORY	PHYSICAL	LABORATORY	MANAGEMENT
Scarring Alopecias				
Congenital (aplasia cutis)	Present at birth	Alopecia Ulceration occasionally	None	Plastic surgery
Tinea capitis with inflammation (kerion)	Pruritic, scaly patches Pain and tenderness	Alopecia, scales Boggy patches Pustules	KOH positive Fungal culture	Oral antifungals
Bacterial folliculitis	Pruritic pustules	Pustules, papules Some alopecia	Gram's stain Bacterial culture	Antibiotics
Discoid lupus erythematosus	Pruritus occasionally Lesions other than scalp common	Erythema Scaly thick plaques Pigmentation	Skin biopsy DIF occasionally	Topical steroids Intralesional steroids Antimalarial agents
Lichen planopilaris	Pruritus occasionally	Alopecia Peripheral erythema Follicular accentuation	Skin biopsy	Topical steroids Intralesional steroids
Folliculitis decalvans	Rare Asymptomatic alopecia, inflammation	Patchy alopecia Follicular erythema at periphery	Skin biopsy	No effective Rx
Neoplasm	Asymptomatic alopecia	Evidence of tumor on the scalp	Skin biopsy	Treat tumor
Trauma	Traction, excessive hair treatments	Distribution where traction is most severe	None	Eliminate trauma
Nonscarring Alopecia *Breakage of Hairs*				
Cosmetic treatment	Frequent or excessive hair Rx	Broken hairs	None	Eliminate trauma
Tinea capitis	Pruritic scaly patches	Erythema, scales	KOH positive Fungal culture	Oral antifungals
Structural hair shaft disease	Unmanageable hair Childhood onset usual	Kinky hair Broken hairs	Microscopic hair examination	No effective Rx
Trichotillomania (hair pulling)	Children Frequently no history	Hair loss in irregular, bizarre pattern	Skin biopsy in difficult to diagnose cases	Counseling Behavior modification Clomipramine

Continued

TABLE 2-2 Differential Diagnosis of Alopecias—cont'd

DISEASE	HISTORY	PHYSICAL	LABORATORY	MANAGEMENT
Nonscarring Alopecia—cont'd				
Breakage of Hairs—cont'd				
Anagen arrest	Chemotherapy Radiation Rx Rapid fallout	Widespread shedding	None	Self-correcting
Shedding by Roots				
Telogen effluvium (telogen arrest)	Occurs 3 months after physical insult	Diffuse alopecia or thinning	Hair pull >5-10 hairs Forced hair pull analysis for anagen:telogen ratio	Reassurance Correct any identified causes Eliminate offending drug
Alopecia areata	Asymptomatic patches of alopecia	Round patches Noninflammatory May be diffuse	Skin biopsy in difficult cases	Topical steroids Intralesional steroids Induce contact dermatitis (DNCB) Ultraviolet therapy
Thinning without Increased Shedding				
Androgenetic alopecia (male pattern balding)	Gradual thinning	Men: temporal and vertex Women: thinning over crown area	None usually Skin biopsy occasionally Rule out other causes	Topical minoxidil Hair transplant

From Noble J (ed): *Primary care medicine,* ed 2, St Louis, 1996, Mosby.
DIF, Direct immunofluorescence; *DNCB,* dinitrochlorobenzene.

AMENORRHEA

TABLE 2-3 Differential Diagnosis of Amenorrhea

SITE OF ABNORMAL FUNCTION	DISORDER	PRIMARY OR SECONDARY AMENORRHEA	GONADOTROPHIN LEVELS	ESTRADIOL LEVELS	CLINICAL FINDINGS	CONFIRMATORY TESTS
Uterus or outflow tract	Müllerian anomalies or agenesis	Primary	LH, FSH normal	Normal	May have cyclic pelvic pain	
	Testicular feminization	Primary	LH increased, FSH normal	Increased	Minimal body hair, good breast development, blind vagina	Elevated testosterone karyotype
	Uterine synechiae (Asherman's syndrome)	Secondary	LH, FSH normal	Normal	History of instrumentation or infection	Hysteroscopy or hysterosalpingogram
Ovary	Turner's syndrome (or mosaic)	Primary; sometimes secondary in mosaic form	FSH increased	Decreased	Short stature, webbed neck, shield chest, cardiac abnormalities and hypothyroidism (mosaics may be atypical)	Karyotype
	Premature ovarian failure	Secondary	FSH increased	Decreased	May have history of autoimmune disorder	

Continued

TABLE 2-3 Differential Diagnosis of Amenorrhea—cont'd

SITE OF ABNORMAL FUNCTION	DISORDER	PRIMARY OR SECONDARY AMENORRHEA	GONADOTROPHIN LEVELS	ESTRADIOL LEVELS	CLINICAL FINDINGS	CONFIRMATORY TESTS
	Resistant ovary syndrome	Primary	FSH increased	Decreased		
Pituitary gland	Prolactinoma	Secondary	FSH, LH decreased or normal	Decreased	May have galactorrhea	Prolactin, cranial imaging
	Other tumors	Secondary	FSH, LH decreased or normal	Decreased	Signs of Cushing's syndrome or acromegaly	Urine free cortisol, growth hormone, cranial imaging
	Pituitary infarction	Secondary	FSH, LH decreased or normal	Decreased	Usually occurs postpartum	
Hypothalamus	Hypothalamic amenorrhea	Primary or secondary	FSH, LH decreased or normal	Decreased	Sometimes associated with stress, exercise, weight loss, chronic illness	
	Pituitary tumors	Primary or secondary	FSH, LH decreased or normal	Decreased	May manifest headache, visual symptoms	Cranial imaging
	Traumatic: head injury or irradiation	Secondary	FSH, LH decreased or normal	Decreased	History of head trauma or cranial irradiation	
Other	Polycystic ovarian syndrome	Secondary	Increased LH:FSH ratio	Decreased or normal	Signs of androgen excess	Testosterone, dehydroepiandrosterone sulfate, ultrasound

From Carlson KJ et al: *Primary care of women*, St Louis, 1995, Mosby.
LH, Luteinizing hormone; *FSH*, follicle-stimulating hormone.

AMNESIA

BOX 2-12 Causes of Amnesia

Cerebrovascular events
  Hippocampal lesions
  Thalamic lesions
  Basal forebrain lesions
Wernicke-Korsakoff syndrome
Head trauma
Hypoxia
Hypoglycemia

Herpes simplex encephalitis
Degenerative diseases
  Alzheimer's disease
  Pick's disease
  Huntington's disease
  Creutzfeldt-Jakob disease
Transient global amnesia
Neoplasms

Limbic encephalitis
Postsurgery
  Bilateral temporal lobectomy
  Bilateral fornix section
  Mammillary body surgery
  Cingulectomy

From Stein JH (ed): *Internal medicine*, ed 4, St Louis, 1994, Mosby.

ANDROGEN RESISTANCE SYNDROMES

TABLE 2-4 Androgen Resistance Syndromes

	EXTERNAL PHENOTYPE	INTERNAL PHENOTYPE	KARYOTYPE	INHERITANCE	SERUM TESTOSTERONE	SERUM ESTRADIOL	LH	FSH	PATHOGENESIS
5-Alpha-reductase deficiency	Female genitalia at birth; variable virilization at expected time of puberty	Testes, epididymides, vasa deferentia present	46,XY	Autosomal recessive	Normal	Normal	Normal or slightly increased	Normal	Inability to form dihydrotestosterone
Complete testicular feminization	Female external genitalia with a blind-ending vagina, female habitus and breast development, paucity of axillary and pubic hair	Testes present, absent wolffian and müllerian derivatives	46,XY	X-linked recessive	Normal or high male plasma levels	Higher than in normal men	Elevated	Normal	*Androgen receptor defects* — Absent +++, Qualitatively abnormal +, Decreased amount +
Incomplete testicular feminization	Female habitus and breast development, normal axillary and pubic hair, clitoromegaly, and partial fusion of the labioscrotal folds	Testes present, underdeveloped wolffian duct derivatives	46,XY	X-linked recessive	Normal or high	Higher than in normal men	Elevated	Normal	++ +
Reifenstein syndrome	Male with perineoscrotal hypospadias, normal axillary and pubic hair	Testes and wolffian duct structure present, varying in degree of male development	46,XY	X-linked recessive	Normal or high	Higher than in normal men	Elevated	Normal	+ ++
Infertile male syndrome		Testes with oligospermia or azoospermia	46,XY	Probably X-linked	Normal	Higher than in normal men	Elevated (usually)	Normal	++ ++

From Moore WT, Eastman RC: *Diagnostic endocrinology*, ed 2, St Louis, 1996, Mosby.
+, Frequency; *FSH*, follicle-stimulating hormone; *LH*, lutenizing hormone.

ANEMIA, IRON DEFICIENCY

TABLE 2-5   Differential Diagnosis of Iron Deficiency: Clinical and Laboratory Features

HISTORY/PHYSICAL EXAMINATION	IRON	TOTAL IRON-BINDING CAPACITY	FERRITIN	SMEAR	RED CELL DISTRIBUTION WIDTH	MARROW IRON
Iron Deficiency						
Bleeding				Microcytosis		Absent
Pica	↓	↑	↓	Hypochromia	↑	
Angular cheilosis				Pencil shapes		
Koilonychia						
Dysphagia						
Anemia of Chronic Disease						
Chronic infection or inflammation	↓	↓	↑	RBC normal (¼ microcytosis)	Normal	↑ (In reticuloendothelial system, not RBC precursors)
Thalassemia Trait						
Family history	Normal/↑	Normal	↑	Microcytosis		
Splenomegaly (±)				Targets Hypochromia	Normal	↑

From Carlson KJ et al: *Primary care of women,* St Louis, 1995, Mosby.
RBC, Red blood cells.

ANEMIA, MEGALOBLASTIC

BOX 2-13   Megaloblastic Anemias

I. Etiopathophysiologic classification of cobalamin (Cbl) deficiency
   A. Nutritional Cbl deficiency (insufficient Cbl intake) vegetarians, vegans, breast-fed infants of mothers with pernicious anemia
   B. Abnormal intragastric events (inadequate proteolysis of food Cbl), atrophic gastritis, partial gastrectomy with hypochlorhydria
   C. Loss/atrophy of gastric oxyntic mucosa (deficient IF molecules), total or partial gastrectomy, pernicious anemia (PA), caustic destruction (lye)
   D. Abnormal events in small bowel lumen
      1. Inadequate pancreatic protease (R-Cbl not degraded, Cbl not transferred to IF)
         (a.) Insufficiency of pancreatic protease—pancreatic insufficiency
         (b.) Inactivation of pancreatic protease—Zollinger-Ellison syndrome
      2. Usurping of luminal Cbl (inadequate Cbl binding to IF)
         (a.) By bacteria—stasis syndromes (blind loops, pouches of diverticulosis, strictures, fistulas, anastomoses); impaired bowel motility (scleroderma, pseudo-obstruction), hypogammaglobulinemia
         (b.) By *Diphyllobothrium latum*
   E. Disorders of ileal mucosa/IF receptors (IF-Cbl not bound to IF receptors)
      1. Diminished or absent IF receptors—ileal bypass/resection/fistula
      2. Abnormal mucosal architecture/function—tropical/nontropical sprue, Crohn's disease, TB ileitis, infiltration by lymphomas, amyloidosis
      3. IF-/post IF-receptor defects—Immerslund-Gräsbeck syndrome, TC II deficiency
      4. Drug-induced effects (slow K, biguanides, cholestyramine, colchicine, neomycin, PAS)
   F. Disorders of plasma Cbl transport (TCII-Cbl not delivered to TC II receptors)
      1. Congenital TC II deficiency, defective binding of TC II-Cbl to TC II receptors (rare)
   G. Metabolic disorders (Cbl not utilized by cell)
      1. Inborn enzyme errors (rare)
      2. Acquired disorders: (Cbl oxidized to cob[III]alamin)—N_2O inhalation
II. Etiopathophysiologic classification of folate deficiency
   A. Nutritional causes
      1. Decrease dietary intake—poverty and famine (associated with kwashiorkor, marasmus), institutionalized individuals (psychiatric/nursing homes), chronic debilitating disease/goat's milk (low in folate), special diets (slimming), cultural/ethnic cooking techniques (food folate destroyed) or habits (folate-rich foods not consumed)

IF, Intrinsic factor; *TC,* transcobalamin.

Continued

BOX 2-13 Megaloblastic Anemias—cont'd

2. Decreased diet and increased requirements
   a. *Physiologic:* pregnancy and lactation, prematurity, infancy
   b. *Pathologic:* intrinsic hematologic disease (autoimmune hemolytic disease), drugs, malaria; hemoglobinopathies (SS, thalassemia), RBC membrane defects (hereditary spherocytosis, paroxysmal nocturnal hemoglobinopathy); abnormal hematopoiesis (leukemia/lymphoma, myelodysplastic syndrome, agnogenic myeloid metaplasia with myelofibrosis); infiltration with malignant disease; dermatologic (psoriasis)
B. Folate malabsorption
   1. With normal intestinal mucosa
      a. Some drugs (controversial)
      b. Congenital folate malabsorption (rare)
   2. With mucosal abnormalities—tropical and nontropical sprue, regional enteritis
C. Defective cellular folate uptake—familial aplastic anemia (rare)
D. Inadequate cellular utilization
   1. Folate antagonists (methotrexate)
   2. Hereditary enzyme deficiencies involving folate
E. Drugs (multiple effects on folate metabolism)—alcohol, sulfasalazine, triamterine, pyrimethamine, trimethoprim-sulfamethoxazole, diphenylhydantoin, barbiturates
F. Acute folate deficiency
III. Miscellaneous megaloblastic anemias (not caused by Cbl or folate deficiency)
A. Congenital disorders of DNA synthesis (rare)—orotic aciduria, Lesch-Nyhan syndrome, congenital dyserythropoietic anemia
B. Acquired disorders of DNA synthesis
   1. Thiamine-responsive megaloblastosis (rare)
   2. Malignancy—erythroleukemia
      —refractory sideroblastic anemias
      —*all* antineoplastic drugs that inhibit DNA synthesis
   3. Toxic—alcohol

From Stein JH (ed): *Internal medicine*, ed 4, St Louis, 1994, Mosby.

ANERGY, CUTANEOUS

BOX 2-14 Causes of Cutaneous Anergy

I. Immunologic
   A. Acquired
      1. Acquired immunodeficiency syndrome (AIDS)
      2. Acute leukemia
      3. Carcinoma
      4. Chronic lymphocytic leukemia
      5. Hodgkin's disease
      6. Non-Hodgkin's lymphoma
   B. Congenital
      1. Ataxia telangiectasia
      2. Di George's syndrome
      3. Nezelof's syndrome
      4. Severe combined immunodeficiency
      5. Wiskott-Aldrich syndrome
II. Infections
   A. Bacterial
      1. Bacterial pneumonia
      2. Brucellosis
   B. Disseminated mycotic infections
   C. Mycobacterial
      1. Lepromatous leprosy
      2. Miliary and active tuberculosis
   D. Viral
      1. Varicella
      2. Hepatitis
      3. Influenza
      4. Infectious mononucleosis
      5. Measles
      6. Mumps
III. Immunosuppressive medications
   A. Cyclophosphamide
   B. Methotrexate
   C. Rifampin
   D. Systemic corticosteroids
IV. Other
   A. Alcoholic cirrhosis
   B. Anemia
   C. Biliary cirrhosis
   D. Burns
   E. Crohn's disease
   F. Diabetes
   G. Malnutrition
   H. Old age
   I. Pregnancy
   J. Pyridoxine deficiency
   K. Rheumatic disease
   L. Sarcoidosis
   M. Sickle cell anemia
   N. Surgery
   O. Uremia

From Stein JH (ed): *Internal medicine*, ed 4, St Louis, 1994, Mosby.

ANISOCORIA

> **BOX 2-15 Anisocoria**
>
> Mydriatic or miotic drugs
> Prosthetic eye
> Inflammation (keratitis, iridocyclitis)
> Infections (herpes zoster, syphylis, meningitis, encephalitis, TB, diphtheria, botulism)
> Subdural hemorrhage
> Cavernous sinus thrombosis
> Intracranial neoplasm
> Cerebral aneurysm
> Glaucoma
> CNS degenerative diseases
> Internal carotid ischemia
> Toxic polyneuritis (alcohol, lead)
> Adie's syndrome
> Horner's syndrome
> Diabetes mellitus
> Trauma
> Congenital

ARTHRITIS, AXIAL SKELETON

TABLE 2-6 Arthritis of the Axial Skeleton

	INTERVERTEBRAL DISK SPACE NARROWING	VACUUM PHENOMENA	INTERVERTEBRAL DISK SPACE CALCIFICATION	BONE OUTGROWTHS	APOPHYSEAL JOINT EROSION	APOPHYSEAL JOINT ANKYLOSIS	ATLANTOAXIAL SUBLUXATION
Rheumatoid arthritis	+	−	−	−	+	±	+
Psoriatic arthritis, Reiter's syndrome	±	−	−	Paravertebral ossification	±	±	+
Ankylosing spondylitis	±	−	±	Syndesmophytes	+	+	+
Juvenile rheumatoid arthritis	+	−	±	−	+	+	+
Degenerative disease of the nucleus pulposus	+	+	−	−	−	−	−
Spondylosis deformans	−	−	−	Osteophytes	−	−	−
Diffuse idiopathic skeletal hyperostosis	−	−	±	Flowing anterolateral ossification	−	−	−
Alkaptonuria	+	+	+	Syndesmophytes (rare)	−	−	−
Infection	+	−	−	−	−	−	−

From Stein JH (ed): *Internal medicine*, ed 4, St Louis, 1994, Mosby.
+, Common presentation; ±, uncommon; −, rare or absent.

ARTHRITIS, CRYSTAL-INDUCED

TABLE 2-7 Comparison of Crystal-Induced Arthritides

CRYSTAL-INDUCED ARTHRITIS	CHARACTERISTICS OF CRYSTALS (FROM JOINT ASPIRATION)	COMMONLY INVOLVED JOINTS	COMMENTS AND THERAPY
Gouty arthritis	Monosodium urate crystals	First metatarsophalangeal, ankles, midfoot	See Section I
Calcium pyrophosphate deposition disease (pseudogout)	Calcium pyrophosphate dihydrate crystals Rhomboid or polymorphic-shaped, weakly positive, birefringent crystals	Knees, wrists	X-ray films of involved joint may reveal linear calcifications (chondrocalcinosis) on articular cartilage Possible associated conditions must be ruled out: Hyperparathyroidism Hypothyroidism Hemochromatosis Hypomagnesemia Therapy: NSAIDs, joint immobilization, intraarticular steroids
Hydroxyapatite arthropathy	Calcium hydroxyapatite crystals Crystals from nonbirefringent clumps with synovial fluid when placed on slide Diagnosis often requires electron microscopy because of small size of the crystals	Knees, hips, shoulders	Usually affects younger patients than the other crystal-induced arthritides Therapy: NSAIDs, joint immobilization, intraarticular steroids
Calcium oxalate–induced arthritis	Calcium oxalate crystals Bipyramidal-shaped, positive birefringent crystals	DIP, PIP joints of hands	Often seen in dialysis patients taking large doses of ascorbic acid (metabolized to oxalate) Therapy: NSAIDs, joint immobilization, intraarticular steroids

ARTHRITIS, MONOARTICULAR AND OLIGOARTICULAR

BOX 2-16 **Differential Diagnosis of Acute Monoarticular and Oligoarticular Arthritis**

Septic arthritis
Crystalline-induced arthritis
    Gout
    Pseudogout (calcium pyrophosphate arthropathy)
    Hydroxyapatite and other basic calcium/phosphate crystals
    Calcium oxalate

Traumatic joint injury
Hemarthrosis
Monoarticular or oligoarticular flare of an inflammatory polyarticular rheumatic disease (rheumatoid arthritis, psoriatic arthritis, Reiter's syndrome, systemic lupus erythematosus)

From Noble J (ed): *Primary care medicine*, ed 2, St Louis, 1996, Mosby.

ARTHRITIS, POLYARTICULAR

TABLE 2-8 Causes of Polyarthritis: Inflammatory Joint Diseases

	COURSE			DISTRIBUTION	
CAUSE	ACUTE	INTERMITTENT	CHRONIC	SYMMETRIC	ASYMMETRIC
Rheumatoid arthritis*		±	+	+	±
Systemic lupus erythematosus*		±	±	+	
Other connective tissue diseases		±	±	+	
Crystal deposition diseases		±	+	+	±
Neisserial infection	+			±	+
Hepatitis B	+		±	+	
Rubella	+			+	
Lyme arthritis	±	+	±		+
Bacterial endocarditis	+			+	±
Rheumatic fever	+			+	±
Erythema nodosum	+	±		+	±
Sarcoidosis	+	+	±	+	+
Hypersensitivity to serum or drugs	+	±		+	±
Henoch-Schönlein purpura	+			±	+
Relapsing polychondritis	±	+	±	+	+
Juvenile (rheumatoid) polyarthritis	±	±	+	+	+
Hypertrophic pulmonary osteoarthropathy	±		+	+	
Ankylosing spondylitis*		±	+	±	+
Reiter's disease*	±	±	±	±	+
Enteropathic arthropathy*	±	+	±	±	+
Psoriatic arthritis*		±	+	+	+
Reactive arthritis	+	±	±	±	+
Behçet's disease	±	+	±		+
Familial Mediterranean fever	±	+	±		+
Whipple's disease	±	+	±	±	+
Palindromic rheumatism	±	+		±	+

From Stein JH (ed): *Internal medicine,* ed 5, St Louis, 1998, Mosby.
+, Most common; ±, less common.
*The most important diagnoses.

ASCITES

> **BOX 2-17 Ascites**
>
> Hypoalbuminemia: nephrotic syndrome, protein-losing gastroenteropathy, starvation
> Cirrhosis
> Hepatic congestion: CHF, constrictive pericarditis, tricuspid insufficiency, hepatic vein obstruction (Budd-Chiari syndrome), inferior vena cava or portal vein obstruction
> Peritoneal infections: TB and other bacterial infections, fungal diseases, parasites
> Neoplasms: primary hepatic neoplasms, metastases to liver or peritoneum, lymphomas, leukemias, myeloid metaplasia
> Lymphatic obstruction: mediastinal tumors, trauma to the thoracic duct, filariasis
> Ovarian disease: Meigs' syndrome, struma ovarii
> Chronic pancreatitis or pseudocyst: pancreatic ascites
> Leakage of bile: bile ascites
> Urinary obstruction or trauma: urine ascites
> Myxedema
> Chylous ascites

ATAXIA

> **BOX 2-18 Ataxia**
>
> Vertebral-basilar artery ischemia
> Diabetic neuropathy
> Tabes dorsalis
> Vitamin B_{12} deficiency
> Multiple sclerosis and other demyelinating diseases
> Meningomyelopathy
> Cerebellar neoplasms, hemorrhage, abscess, infarct
> Nutritional (Wernicke's encephalopathy)
> Paraneoplastic syndromes
> Parainfectious: Guillain-Barré syndrome, acute ataxia of childhood and young adults
> Toxins: phenytoin, alcohol, sedatives, organophosphates
> Wilson's disease (hepatolenticular degeneration)
> Hypothyroidism
> Myopathy
> Cerebellar and spinocerebellar degeneration: ataxia/telangiectasia, Friedreich's ataxia
> Frontal lobe lesions: tumors, thrombosis of anterior cerebral artery, hydrocephalus
> Labyrinthine destruction: neoplasm, injury, inflammation, compression
> Hysteria
> AIDS

BACK PAIN

TABLE 2-9 Differential Diagnosis of Common Low Back Pain Syndromes

CLINICAL ENTITY	HISTORY	PHYSICAL EXAMINATION	SUPPORTING STUDIES
Mechanical low back pain	Pain in back, buttocks ± thigh; may be severe Onset after new or unusual exertion No history of major trauma, systemic infection or malignancy Relief of pain in supine position	Paravertebral tenderness/spasm Scoliosis or loss of lumbar lordosis common No neurologic signs	None necessary
Herniated intervertebral disk	Acutely, pain in back is severe and lancinating Antecedent flexion strain injury or trauma Sciatica Relief of pain in supine position with hip flexed Bilateral weakness with bowel and/or bladder dysfunction may be present with massive central disk prolapse With chronic disk herniation, pain, usually dull, may be confined to leg	Striking paravertebral tenderness/spasm with splinting in awkward postures Signs of radicular irritation/injury usually present in acute setting	MRI, CT, or myelogram Electromyography may provide supporting documentation of level of denervation
Referred visceral or vascular pain	Patient writhes in discomfort, with no relief in any position Pain may occur in waves	Abdominal findings usually predominate Fever or incipient shock often present	Imaging studies directed at abdomen and retroperitoneum may visualize aortic aneurysm or abnormality of viscera (e.g., ureteral calculus, pancreatitis, etc.)
Metastatic malignancy (or multiple myeloma)	Unremitting or progressive pain at rest Known or suspected malignancy Weight loss, fever, or other systemic symptoms History of weakness, bowel and/or bladder dysfunction may be present	Tender spinous process at level of involvement Variable neurologic findings, up to full paraplegia	Standard radiographs may reveal destructive bony lesions Radionuclide bone scan sensitive for metastatic carcinoma but not for myeloma Epidural impingement of spinal cord or roots best delineated by MRI, myelography, and/or CT Erythrocyte sedimentation rate elevated

Continued

TABLE 2-9 Differential Diagnosis of Common Low Back Pain Syndromes—cont'd

CLINICAL ENTITY	HISTORY	PHYSICAL EXAMINATION	SUPPORTING STUDIES
Epidural abscess, vertebral osteomyelitis, or septic diskitis	Unremitting or progressive pain at rest Fever Drug abuse, diabetes mellitus, immunosuppression Suspected or known systemic infection Previous spinal or genitourinary surgery History of weakness, bowel and/or bladder dysfunction may be present	Tender spinous process at level of involvement Variable neurologic findings, up to full paraplegia Stigmata of systemic infection	Standard radiographs may reveal destructive bony lesions Radionuclide scans may suggest abscess Blood cultures often positive MRI probably best imaging modality to delineate extent of lesion and neural impingement Erythrocyte sedimentation rate elevated
Ankylosing spondylitis	Insidious onset Progressive morning back pain and stiffness over several months Relief with exercise Age at onset ≤40 yr	Painful or ankylosed sacroiliac joints Reduced mobility of spine Reduced chest wall expansion Possible associated uveitis	Sacroiliac joints and lumbosacral spine ankylosed on standard radiographs Erythrocyte sedimentation rate elevated HLA-B27 confirmatory Uveitis may be confirmed on ophthalmologic examination
Reactive spondyloarthropathies	As with ankylosing spondylitis Antecedent urethritis, rash, or colitis	As with ankylosing spondylitis Conjunctivitis, balanitis, urethritis, and/or keratoderma blennorrhagicum Psoriasis	As with ankylosing spondylitis Bowel studies may reveal infectious or idiopathic inflammatory bowel disease Infectious urethritis may be confirmed
Spinal stenosis	Back pain may vary from severe to absent Pseudoclaudication often prominent, often involving L4 root (anterior thigh) Pain worsens during the day, is aggravated by standing and relieved by rest Weakness, bladder and/or bowel dysfunction may be present	Neurologic findings vary, but often there is evidence of impairment at multiple spinal levels Findings of osteoarthritis may be prominent	Standard radiographs generally show extensive vertebral osteophytes and degenerative disk disease Imaging with MRI or CT ± myelography supports diagnosis if neurologic and imaging findings are concordant

From Noble J (ed): *Primary care medicine*, ed 2, St Louis, 1996, Mosby.
CT, Computed tomography; *MRI*, magnetic resonance imaging.

BLEEDING DISORDERS

TABLE 2-10 Presumptive Diagnosis of Common Bleeding Disorders Based on Routine Screening Tests

PLATELET COUNT	BLEEDING TIME	PT	PTT	TT	MISCELLANEOUS	PRESUMPTIVE PROBLEM
↓	N-↑	N	N	N		Thrombocytopenia
N	↑	N	N	N		Platelet function defect or vascular defect
N	↑	N	↑	N	↓ VIII$_e$, ↓ VIII$_{ag}$, ↓ VIII$_{vWF}$	von Willebrand's disease
N	N	↑	N	N		Extrinsic pathway defect (VII)
N	N	N	↑	N		Intrinsic pathway defect (VIII, IX, XI, XII, prekallikrein, high molecular weight kininogen, inhibitor)
N	N	↑	↑	N		Common pathway or multiple pathway defects excluding fibrinogen
N	N	↑	↑	↑	High levels of FDP	Fibrinogen deficiency or dysfunction, vitamin K deficiency, liver disease, primary fibrinolysis
↓	N-↑	↑	↑	↑	High levels of FDP	DIC
N	N	N	N	N	Positive clot solubility	XIII deficiency

From Noble J (ed): *Primary care medicine*, ed 2, St Louis, 1996, Mosby.
N, Normal; ↓, decreased; ↑, increased; *FDP*, fibrin(ogen) degradation products; *DIC*, disseminated intravascular coagulation.

BLEEDING, GASTROINTESTINAL: BY LOCATION

BOX 2-19 Gastrointestinal Bleeding, by Location

Upper GI Bleeding (Originating Above the Ligament of Treitz)

Oral or pharyngeal lesions: swallowed blood from nose or oropharynx
Swallowed hemoptysis
Esophageal: varices, ulceration, esophagitis, Mallory-Weiss tear, carcinoma, trauma
Gastric: peptic ulcer (including Cushing and Curling's ulcers), gastritis, angiodysplasia, gastric neoplasms, hiatal hernia, gastric diverticulum, pseudoxanthoma elasticum, Rendu-Osler-Weber syndrome
Duodenal: peptic ulcer, duodenitis, angiodysplasia, aortoduodenal fistula, duodenal diverticulum, duodenal tumors, carcinoma of ampulla of Vater, parasites (e.g., hookworm), Crohn's disease
Biliary: hematobilia (e.g., penetrating injury to liver, hepatobiliary malignancy, endoscopic papillotomy)

Lower GI Bleeding (Originating Below the Ligament of Treitz)

Small Intestine

Ischemic bowel disease (mesenteric thrombosis, embolism, vasculitis, trauma)
Small bowel neoplasm: leiomyomas, carcinoids
Hereditary hemorrhagic telangiectasia (Rendu-Osler-Weber syndrome)
Meckel's diverticulum and other small intestine diverticula
Aortoenteric fistula
Intestinal hemangiomas: blue rubber-bleb nevi, intestinal hemangiomas, cutaneous vascular nevi
Hamartomatous polyps: Peutz-Jeghers syndrome (intestinal polyps, mucocutaneous pigmentation)
Infections of small bowel: tuberculous enteritis, enteritis necroticans
Volvulus
Intussusception
Lymphoma of small bowel, sarcoma, Kaposi's sarcoma
Irradiation ileitis
AV malformation of small intestine
Inflammatory bowel disease
Polyarteritis nodosa
Other: pancreatoenteric fistulas, Schönlein-Henoch purpura, Ehler-Danlos syndrome, systemic lupus erythematosus, amyloidosis, metastatic melanoma

Colon

Carcinoma (particularly left colon)
Diverticular disease
Inflammatory bowel disease
Ischemic colitis
Colonic polyps
Vascular abnormalities: angiodysplasia, vascular ectasia
Radiation colitis
Infectious colitis
Uremic colitis
Aortoenteric fistula
Lymphoma of large bowel
Hemorrhoids
Anal fissure
Trauma, foreign body
Solitary rectal/cecal ulcers
Long-distance running

BLEEDING, GASTROINTESTINAL: DIAGNOSTIC CONSIDERATIONS BY AGE

TABLE 2-11 Gastrointestinal Hemorrhage: Diagnostic Consideration by Age

INFANT (<3 MO)	TODDLER (<2 YR)	PRESCHOOLER (<5 YR)	SCHOOL-AGE CHILD (>5 YR)
Upper Gastrointestinal Bleeding			
Swallowed maternal blood	Esophagitis	Esophagitis	Esophagitis
Gastritis	Gastritis	Gastritis	Gastritis
Ulcer, stress	Ulcer	Ulcer	Ulcer
Bleeding diathesis	Pyloric stenosis	Esophageal varices	Esophageal varices
Foreign body (NG tube)	Mallory-Weiss syndrome	Foreign body	Mallory-Weiss syndrome
Vascular malformation	Vascular malformation	Mallory-Weiss syndrome	Inflammatory bowel disease*
Duplication	Duplication	Hemophilia	Hemophilia
		Vascular malformation	Vascular malformation
Lower Gastrointestinal Bleeding			
Swallowed maternal blood	Anal fissure	Infectious colitis*	Infectious colitis*
Infectious colitis*	Infectious colitis*	Anal fissure	Inflammatory bowel disease*
Milk allergy	Milk allergy	Polyp	Pseudomembranous enterocolitis*
Bleeding diathesis*	Colitis	Intussusception*	Polyp
Intussusception*	Intussusception*	Meckel's diverticulum	Hemolytic-uremic syndrome
Midgut volvulus*	Meckel's diverticulum	Henoch-Schönlein purpura*	Hemorrhoid
Meckel's diverticulum	Polyp	Hemolytic uremic syndrome*	
Necrotizing enterocolitis (NEC)*	Duplication	Inflammatory bowel disease*	
	Hemolytic uremic syndrome*	Pseudomembranous enterocolitis*	
	Inflammatory bowel disease*		
	Pseudomembranous enterocolitis*		

From Barkin RM, Rosen P: *Emergency pediatrics: a guide to ambulatory care*, ed 4, St Louis, 1994, Mosby.
*Commonly associated with systemic illness involving multiple organ systems either primarily or secondarily.

BREAST MASS

BOX 2-20 Differential Diagnosis of Breast Mass

Inflammatory disease
  Acute bacterial mastitis
  Chronic mastitis
  Fat necrosis

Mammary dysplasia (benign breast disease)
  Adenosis
  Cystic disease
  Duct ectasia

Benign tumors
  Fibroadenoma
  Papilloma
Malignant tumors

From Stein JH (ed): *Internal medicine*, ed 4, St Louis, 1994, Mosby.

DIFFERENTIAL DIAGNOSIS

BULLOUS DISEASES

TABLE 2-12 Differential Diagnosis of Selected Bullous Diseases

DISEASE	HISTORY	PHYSICAL	LABORATORY	MANAGEMENT
Bullous Pemphigoid (BP)				
BP	Elderly population; intense pruritus; tense bullae; hives common	Widespread bullae; urticarial lesions; distribution not diagnostic	Skin biopsy; DIF linear IgG along basement membrane	Systemic oral corticosteroids; occasionally azathioprine or cyclophosphamide
Cicatricial pemphigoid	Elderly; mucous membranes and conjunctivae	Erosive blisters on mucous membranes and conjunctivae; skin lesions in 20%	Skin biopsy; DIF	Corticosteroids; tetracyclines
Herpes gestationis	Pregnancy; intense pruritus; hives and blisters	Urticaria; vesicles and bullae	Skin biopsy; DIF	Resolves after delivery; may require systemic corticosteroids
Epidermolysis bullosa acquisita (EBA)	Adult onset; skin fragility and blisters, extensor areas; pruritus	Bullae and vesicles; erosions; healed areas with scars and milia	Skin biopsy, DIF similar to BP; differentiation requires split skin DIF	Corticosteroids; immunosuppressive agents; difficult to treat
Dermatitis herpetiformis (DH)	Intense pruritus; extensor areas; GI symptoms occasionally	Grouped (herpetiforme) vesicles; elbows, knees, back, buttocks	Skin biopsy; DIF; GI if diarrhea	Dapsone; gluten-free diet
Linear IgA bullous dermatosis	Pruritus; any age; vesicles and bullae	May be similar to DH or BP	Skin biopsy; DIF	Corticosteroids; immunosuppressive agents
Pemphigus Vulgaris				
Pemphigus vulgaris	Widespread erosions: oral lesions	Oral and cutaneous bullae and erosions	Skin biopsy; DIF; indirect IF	Systemic corticosteroids: immunosuppressive agents; gold
BP	Elderly; intense pruritus; blisters	Bullae widespread; urticaria common	Skin biopsy; DIF	Corticosteroids
Cicatricial pemphigoid	Elderly; mucous membranes and conjunctivae	Bullae, erosions, and scarring on mucous membranes and conjunctivae	Skin biopsy; DIF	Systemic corticosteroids: tetracyclines
Erythema multiforme (oral)	Oral mucosal lesions; painful	Oral erosions; may have target lesions on skin	Skin biopsy occasionally helpful; DIF to exclude pemphigus	Supportive; eliminate or treat underlying cause
Erosive lichen planus	Oral mucosal and tongue lesions	Erosions; white lacy mucosal changes	Skin biopsy helpful; DIF to exclude pemphigus	Topical and systemic steroids; retinoids; cyclosporin
Pemphigus Foliaceus				
Pemphigus foliaceus	Widespread crusted erosions; adult onset	Crusted plaques	Skin biopsy; DIF	Systemic corticosteroids
Impetigo	Crusted lesions; face; children	Crusted plaques; honey crusts; serous oozing	Culture	Antibiotics
Paraneoplastic Pemphigus				
Paraneoplastic pemphigus	Erosions; mucous membranes; associated malignancy	Oral and cutaneous erosions	Skin biopsy; DIF	Treat malignancy; systemic corticosteroids; immunosuppressive agents
Erythema multiforme (major Stevens-Johnson syndrome)	Mouth, conjunctivae, ears, and widespread; drug, viral infection	Erosions on mucous membranes; target lesions on skin	Skin biopsy	Supportive; treat or eliminate underlying cause

Adapted from Noble J (ed): *Primary care medicine*, ed 2, St Louis, 1996, Mosby.
DIF, Direct immunofluorescence.

CARDIAC MURMURS

> **BOX 2-21 Cardiac Murmurs**
>
> **Systolic**
> Mitral regurgitation (MR)
> Tricuspid regurgitation (TR)
> Ventricular septal defect (VSD)
> Aortic stenosis (AS)
> Idiopathic hypertrophic subaortic stenosis (IHSS)
> Pulmonic stenosis (PS)
> Innocent murmur of childhood
> Coarctation of aorta
> Mitral valve prolapse (MVP)
>
> **Diastolic**
> Aortic regurgitation (AR)
> Atrial myxoma
> Mitral stenosis (MS)
> Pulmonary artery branch stenosis
> Tricuspid stenosis (TS)
> Graham Steell murmur (diastolic decrescendo murmur heard in severe pulmonary hypertension)
> Pulmonic regurgitation (PR)
> Severe MR
> Austin Flint murmur (diastolic rumble heard in severe AR)
> Severe VSD and patent ductus arteriosus
>
> **Continuous**
> Patient ductus arteriosus
> Pulmonary AV fistula

TABLE 2-13 Response of Selected Murmurs to Physiologic Intervention

CARDIAC MURMUR	ACCENTUATION	DECREASE	CARDIAC MURMUR	ACCENTUATION	DECREASE
Systolic			**Diastolic**		
AS	Valsalva release Sudden squatting Passive leg raising	Handgrip Valsalva Standing	AR MR	Sudden squatting Isometric handgrip Exercise	
IHSS	Valsalva strain Standing	Handgrip Squatting Leg elevation		Left lateral position Isometric handgrip Coughing	
MR	Sudden squatting Isometric handgrip	Valsalva Standing	TS	Inspiration Passive leg raising	Expiration
PS	Valsalva release	Expiration			
TR	Inspiration Passive leg raising	Expiration			

CEREBROSPINAL FLUID ABNORMALITIES

TABLE 2-14 CSF Abnormalities in Various CNS Conditions

	APPEARANCE	GLUCOSE (MG/DL)	PROTEIN (MG/DL)	CELL COUNT (CELLS/MM^3) AND CELL TYPE	PRESSURE (MM HG)
Normal	Clear	50-80	20-45	<6 Lymphocytes	100-200
Acute bacterial meningitis	Cloudy	↓↓	↑↑	↑↑ PMN	↑↑
Aseptic (viral) meningitis	Clear/cloudy	N	↑	↑, Usually mononuclear cells May be PMN in early stages	N/↑
Hemorrhage	Bloody/xanthochromic	N/↓	↑	↑↑ RBC	↑
Neoplasm	Clear/xanthochromic	N/↓	N/↑	N/↑ Lymphocytes	↑↑
Tuberculous meningitis	Cloudy	↓	↑	↑ PMN (early) ↑ Lymphocytes (later)	↑
Fungal meningitis	Clear/cloudy	↓	↑	↑ Monocytes	↑
Neurosyphilis	Clear/cloudy	N	↑	↑ Monocytes	N/↑
Guillain-Barré syndrome	Clear/cloudy	N	↑↑	N/↑ Lymphocytes	N

↑, Increased; ↑↑, markedly increased; ↓, decreased; ↓↓, markedly decreased; N, normal; PMN, polymorphonucleocytes; RBC, red blood cells.

CESTODE TISSUE INFECTIONS

TABLE 2-15 Cestode Tissue Infections

SPECIES	EPIDEMIOLOGY	TRANSMISSION	MAJOR CLINICAL PRESENTATION	DIAGNOSIS	TREAMTENT
Taenia solium (cysticercosis)	Worldwide	Ingestion of eggs or autoinfection from tapeworm	Seizures, focal neurologic symptoms, hydrocephalus	Serology, characteristic CT scan of head, radiograph of soft tissues	Albendazole 5 mg/kg tid for 8-28 days, repeated as necessary or praziquantel 20 mg/kg tid for 15 days; both treatments with or without steroids
Echinococcus granulosus (hydatid disease)	Sheep- and cattle-raising areas of world	Association with dogs, ingestion of contaminated dog excreta	Single mass in liver or lungs, anaphylactic shock after blunt trauma	Characteristic abdominal CT scan, serology	Surgery or surgery and/or albendazole 400 mg bid for 28 days, repeated as necessary or albendazole plus praziquantel†
Echinococcus multilocularis	Northern latitudes; North America, Europe, and Asia	Associated with infected animals or ingestion of food contaminated with dog excreta	Alveolar mass in liver	Characteristic abdominal CT scan, serology	Surgery or surgery plus albendazole*† 400 mg bid for 28 days

From Stein JH (ed): *Internal medicine*, ed 5, St Louis, 1998, Mosby.
CT, Computed tomography; tid, three times a day; bid, twice a day.
*Considered an investigational drug for this indication by the US Food and Drug Administration.
†Effectiveness not clearly established.

CHEST PAIN IN CHILDREN

> **BOX 2-22 Cardiac and Noncardiac Causes of Chest Pain in Children**
>
> Cardiac
>   I. Congenital cardiac structural diseases
>   A. Obstruction of the outflow tract of the left ventricle
>   B. Mitral valve prolapse
>   C. Anomalous origin of the coronary artery (from the pulmonary artery)
>   D. Cardiomyopathy
>   II. Dysrhythmias
>   A. Supraventricular tachycardia
>   B. Ventricular ectopy or tachycardia
>   III. Acquired cardiopulmonary diseases
>   A. Inflammation of myocardium, pericardium— viral, bacterial, rheumatic
>   B. Coronary arteritis, Kawasaki's syndrome, systemic lupus erythematosus
>   C. Pulmonary embolism
>   D. Local tumor, inflammation, toxin related (cocaine)
>
> Noncardiac
>   I. Psychogenic
>   A. Hyperventilation
>   B. Depression
>   C. Conversion reaction
>   II. Rib cage
>   A. Costochondritis
>   B. Muscle-skeletal trauma and strains
>   C. Mastalgia
>   D. Pleuritis, bronchitis, bronchospasm
>   E. Pneumothorax
>   III. Gastrointestinal
>   A. Gastroesophageal reflux
>   B. Peptic ulcer

From Rosen P et al (eds): *Emergency medicine: concepts and clinical practice,* St Louis, 1992, Mosby.

CHEST PAIN, NONPLEURITIC

> **BOX 2-23 Nonpleuritic Chest Pain**
>
> Cardiac: myocardial ischemia/infarction, myocarditis
> Esophageal: spasm, rupture, esophagitis, ulceration, neoplasm, achalasia, diverticula, foreign body
> Referred pain from subdiaphragmatic GI structures
>   Gastric and duodenal: hiatal hernia, neoplasm, PUD
>   Gallbladder and biliary: cholecystitis, cholelithiasis, impacted stone, neoplasm
>   Pancreatic: pancreatitis, neoplasm
> Dissecting aortic aneurysm
> Pain originating from skin, breasts, and musculoskeletal structures: herpes zoster, mastitis, cervical spondylosis
> Mediastinal tumors: lymphoma, thymoma
> Pulmonary: neoplasm, pneumonia, pulmonary embolism/infarction
> Psychoneurosis
> Chest pain associated with mitral valve prolapse

CHEST PAIN, PLEURITIC

> **BOX 2-24 Pleuritic Chest Pain**
>
> Cardiac: pericarditis, postpericardiotomy/Dressler's syndrome
> Pulmonary: pneumothorax, hemothorax, embolism/infarction, pneumonia, empyema, neoplasm, bronchiectasis, TB, carcinomatous effusion
> GI: liver abscess, pancreatitis, Whipple's disease with associated pericarditis or pleuritis
> Subdiaphragmatic abscess
> Pain originating from skin and musculoskeletal tissues: costochondritis, chest wall trauma, fractured rib, interstitial fibrositis, myositis, strain of pectoralis muscle, herpes zoster, soft tissue and bone tumors
> Collagen-vascular diseases with pleuritis
> Psychoneurosis
> Familial Mediterranean fever (FMF)

CLUBBING

> **BOX 2-25 Clubbing**
>
> Pulmonary neoplasm (lung, pleura)
> Other neoplasm (GI, liver, Hodgkin's, thymus)
> Pulmonary infectious process (empyema, abscess, bronchiectasis, TB, chronic pneumonitis)
> Extrapulmonary infectious process (subacute bacterial endocarditis, intestinal TB, bacterial or amebic dysentery)
> Pneumoconiosis
> Cystic fibrosis
> Sarcoidosis
> Cyanotic congenital heart disease
> Endocrine (Graves' disease, hyperparathyroidism)
> Inflammatory bowel disease
> Sprue
> Chronic liver disease
> Congenital heart disease
> Idiopathic
> Hereditary (pachydermoperiostitis)
> Chronic trauma (jackhammer operators, machine workers)

COAGULOPATHY, CONGENITAL

TABLE 2-16 Congenital Disorders of Blood Coagulation

COAGULATION FACTOR	INHERITANCE	INCIDENCE (PER MILLION)	BLEEDING SYMPTOMS	ABNORMAL SCREENING TESTS	BIOLOGIC HALF-LIFE OF PROTEIN (HR)	TREATMENT
I (fibrinogen)	Autosomal recessive	1	Umbilical bleeding at birth, posttrauma hemorrhage	PT, PTT, TT	100	Cryoprecipitate
II (prothrombin)	Autosomal recessive	1	Similar to hemophilia	PT, PTT	72	FFP, rarely prothrombin complex concentrates
V	Autosomal recessive	1	Similar to hemophilia	PT, PTT	24	FFP, possibly platelet concentrates
VII	Autosomal recessive	1	Similar to hemophilia	PT	4-6	VII concentrates
VIII (hemophilia)	Sex-linked recessive	100 (milder disease is much more common)	Hemarthrosis, hematoma, bruising, severe postoperative bleeding	PTT	12	VIII concentrates
vWf (von Willebrand's factor)	Autosomal dominant or recessive	Probably as frequent as hemophilia A	Epistaxis, gingival bleeding, bruising, menorrhagia, severe postoperative bleeding	PTT	4-6, for correction of bleeding time	DDAVP, WF-rich VII concentrates

Continued

TABLE 2-16 Congenital Disorders of Blood Coagulation—cont'd

COAGULATION FACTOR	INHERITANCE	INCIDENCE (PER MILLION)	BLEEDING SYMPTOMS	ABNORMAL SCREENING TESTS	BIOLOGIC HALF-LIFE OF PROTEIN (HR)	TREATMENT
IX (hemophilia B)	Sex-linked recessive	20	Identical to hemophilia	PT, PTT	24	IX concentrates
X	Autosomal recessive	1	Similar to hemophilia	PT, PTT	50	FFP, rarely prothrombin complex concentrates
XI	Autosomal recessive	1	Mild; however, severe postoperative hemorrhage can occur	PTT	60	FFP, level of 25% adequate for hemostasis
XII	Autosomal recessive	1	None	PTT	60	None
XIII	Autosomal recessive	1	Umbilical bleeding at birth, posttrauma hemorrhage, poor wound healing	—	120	FFP monthly, since level of 2% is adequate for hemostasis
Alpha$_2$ antiplasmin	Autosomal recessive	Unknown	Similar to hemophilia	—	Unknown	FFP
Plasminogen activator inhibitor (PAI-I)	Unknown	Unknown	Severe postoperative and posttrauma bleeding	—	Unknown	EACA
Passovoy	Autosomal dominant	Unknown	Similar to factor XI	PTT	Unknown	FFP

From Stein JH (ed): *Internal medicine*, ed 5, St Louis, 1998, Mosby.
FFP, Fresh-frozen plasma; *PT*, prothrombin time; *PTT*, partial thromboplastin time; *TT*, thrombin (clotting) time; *DDAVP*, I-deamino-8-D-arginine vasopressin; *EACA*, ϵ-aminocaproic acid.

COMA

BOX 2-26 Common Differential Diagnoses of Coma

Bihemispheric dysfunction
  Functional
    Metabolic
      Hypoxia*
      Hypoglycemia*
      Hepatic dysfunction (hyperammonemia)
      Uremia
      Hyponatremia, hypernatremia
      Hyperglycemic hyperosmolar nonketotic coma
      Hypothyroidism (myxedema coma)
    Toxic
      Drug overdose
        Drugs of abuse: narcotics, barbiturates, benzodiazepines, etc.
        Therapeutic drugs: anticholinergics, tricyclics, etc.
    Infectious
      Meningitis/meningoencephalitis
    Others
      Nonconvulsive status epilepticus
  Structural
    Infarction
      Bilateral hemispheric infarcts
    Mass lesions
      Bilateral hemispheric
      Unilateral or bilateral hemispheric with elevated intracranial pressure* or local mass effect
Brainstem dysfunction
  Functional
  Structural
    Infarction
    Mass lesion
Mimics
  Organic
    Bilateral pontine infarcts ("locked-in" syndrome)
    Neuromuscular weakness
      Acute inflammatory demyelinating polyneuropathy
      Myasthenia gravis
      Botulism
      Drug-induced neuromuscular blockade
  Psychiatric
    Malignant catatonia
    Psychogenic unresponsiveness

From Johnson RT, Griffin JW: *Current therapy in neurologic disease*, ed 5, St Louis, 1997, Mosby.
*These possibilities need to be treated immediately.

CONSTIPATION

> **BOX 2-27 Constipation**
>
> Intestinal obstruction
>   Fecal impaction
>   GI neoplasm
>   Gallstone ileus
>   Adhesions
>   Volvulus
>   Intussusception
>   Inflammatory bowel disease
>   Diverticular disease
>   Strangulated femoral hernia
>   Tuberculous stricture
>   Ameboma
>   Hematoma of bowel wall secondary to trauma or anticoagulants
> Poor dietary habits: insufficient bulk in diet, inadequate fluid intake
> Change from daily routine: travel, hospital admission, physical inactivity
> Acute abdominal conditions: renal colic, salpingitis, biliary colic, appendicitis
> Hypercalcemia or hypokalemia, uremia
> Irritable bowel syndrome, pregnancy, anorexia nervosa, depression
> Painful anal conditions: hemorrhoids, fissure, stricture
> Decreased intestinal peristalsis: old age, spinal cord injuries, myxedema, diabetes, multiple sclerosis, parkinsonism, and other neurologic dieases
> Drugs: codeine, morphine, antacids with aluminum, verapamil, anticonvulsants, anticholinergics, disopyramide, cholestyramine, iron supplements
> Hirschsprung's disease, meconium ileus, congenital atresia in infants

COUGH

> **BOX 2-28 Cough**
>
> Infectious process (viral, bacterial)
> Postinfectious
> "Smoker's cough"
> Rhinitis (allergic, vasomotor, postinfectious)
> Asthma
> Exposure to irritants (noxious fumes, smoke, cold air)
> Drug-induced (especially ACE inhibitors, β blockers)
> GERD
> Interstitial lung disease
> Lung neoplasms
> Lymphomas, mediastinal neoplasms
> Bronchiectasis
> Cardiac (CHF, pulmonary edema, mitral stenosis, pericardial inflammation)
> Recurrent aspiration
> Inflammation of larynx, pleura, diaphragm, mediastinum
> Cystic fibrosis
> Anxiety
> Other: pulmonary embolism, foreign body inhalation, aortic aneurysm, Zenker's diverticulum, osteophytes

CUTANEOUS SIGNS OF INTERNAL MALIGNANCY

TABLE 2-17 Cutaneous Reactions to Internal Malignancy

DISEASE	HISTORY	PHYSICAL	MALIGNANCY
Acanthosis nigricans	Thickening of skin on hands and intertriginous areas	Hyperpigmented, velvety hyperkeratotic changes	Gastric carcinoma
Acquired hypertrichosis lanuginosa	Increased hair on face or other areas	Fine hypertrichosis; face common	Lymphoma
Acquired ichthyosis	Thickening, scaling on palms, soles, or other areas	Hyperkeratotic changes	Lymphoma
Bazex's syndrome (hyperkeratosis paraneoplastica)	Thickening of skin on nose, hands, feet	Focal hyperkeratotic plaques	Squamous cell carcinoma in the upper respiratory tract
Dermatomyositis	Muscle weakness; photoaccentuated dermatitis	Erythema, telangiectasia, atrophy, Gottron's papules, heliotrope rash (eyelids)	Multiple associated malignancies have been reported
Erythema gyratum repens	Rare; pruritus, scaling	Characteristic swirls of erythema, scaling	Lung carcinoma
Erythroderma	Rapid-onset total erythema	Erythema, some scaling	Cutaneous T-cell lymphoma
Flushing	Episodic head and neck flushing	Erythema (transient)	Carcinoid
Necrolytic migratory erythema (NME)	Periorificial shallow erosions; sore tongue; weight loss	Superficial blisters and erosions, perioral, perineal; glossitis	Glucagonoma
Herpes zoster	Pain and blisters; pain may precede lesions by 72 hr	Dermatomal; vesicles, papules, pustules	Any malignancy; immunosuppression
Leser-Trélat sign (multiple seborrheic keratoses)	Rapid onset of large numbers of asymptomatic small lesions	Multiple (>100) small to medium seborrheic keratoses	Breast carcinoma; GI carcinomas
Migratory thrombophlebitis	Painful swelling on an extremity; occasionally generalized hypercoagulability	Firm, linear, cordlike lesions involving superficial vessels	Visceral carcinomas, prostate carcinoma
Pruritus	Total body pruritus; sometimes worse after shower	No primary skin findings	Multiple malignancies; lymphomas
Pyoderma gangrenosum	Enlarging painful ulcers	Pustules, ulcerations; erythematous rolled edge	Leukemia, lymphoma; adenocarcinoma
Sweet's syndrome (acute febrile neutrophilic dermatosis)	High fever; malaise, arthralgias; skin rash	Erythematous nodules, plaques; lesions are tender; arthritis	Hematologic; AML most common
Urticaria	Pruritic hives	Urticaria	Multiple

From Noble J (ed): *Primary care medicine*, ed 2, St Louis, 1996, Mosby.

CUTANEOUS ERUPTIONS, DRUG-INDUCED

BOX 2-29 Drug-induced Cutaneous Eruptions

Acneiform eruptions
  ACTH
  Bromides
  Corticosteroids
  Cyanocobalamin (vitamin B_{12})
  Dactinomycin
  Iodides
  Isoniazid (INH)
  Lithium
  Oral contraceptives
  Phenytoin
Alopecia
  Allopurinol
  Amphetamines
  Anticoagulants (coumarin, heparin)
  Antithyroid drugs (carbimazole, thiouracil)
  Chemotherapeutic agents
  Heavy metals
  Hypocholesterolemic drugs
  Levodopa
  Oral contraceptives
  Propranolol
  Retinoids
Eczematous eruptions (topical sensitizer/systemic medication)
  Ampicillin
  Chlorbutanol/chloral hydrate
  Diphenhydramine (Caladryl/Benadryl)
  Disulfiram (Antabuse)
  Ethylenediamine/aminophylline, antihistamines
  Iodine/iodides
  Neomycin sulfate/streptomycin, kanamycin
  Para-amino aromatic benzenes/para-aminobenzoic acid, sulfonamides, tolbutamide
  Penicillin
Erythema multiforme
  Allopurinol
  Barbiturates
  Chlorpropamide
  Griseofulvin
  Hydantoins
  Nonsteroidal antiinflammatory agents (meclofenamate, piroxicam, sulindac)
  Penicillin
  Phenothiazines
  Sulfonamides
  Thiazide diuretics
Erythema nodosum
  Bromides
  Codeine
  Iodides
  Oral contraceptives
  Penicillin
  Salicylates
  Sulfonamides
Exanthematous eruptions
  Allopurinol
  Antibiotics
  Anticonvulsants
  Barbiturates
  Benzodiazepines
  Captopril
  Chloropropamide
  Gold salts
  Isoniazid
  Nonsteroidal antiinflammatory agents (meclofenamate, naproxen, phenylbutazone, piroxicam)
  Para-aminosalicylic acid
  Penicillamine
  Phenothiazines
  Quinidine
  Thiazide diuretics
Exfoliative dermatitis
  Allopurinol
  Carbamazepine
  Gold salts
  Hydantoins
  Isoniazid
  Para-aminosalicylic acid
  Phenindione
  Phenylbutazone
  Streptomycin
  Sulfonamides
Fixed drug eruptions
  Allopurinol
  Barbiturates
  Chlordiazepoxide
  Nonsteroidal antiinflammatory agents (naproxen, phenacetin, phenylbutazone, salicylates, sulindac, tolmatin)
  Phenolphthalein
  Sulfonamides
  Tetracycline
Leukocytoclastic vasculitis
  Allopurinol
  Cimetidine
  Gold salts
  Hydantoins
  Nonsteroidal antiinflammatory agents (ibuprofen, meclofenamate, piroxicam)
  Phenothiazine
  Sulfonamides
  Thiazide diuretics
  Thiouracils
Lichenoid and lichen planus–like eruptions
  Antimalarials (chloroquine, hydroxychloroquine, quinacrine)
  Captopril
  Chlordiazepoxide
  Hydroxyurea
  Para-aminosalicylic acid
  Penicillamine
  Quinidine
  Thiazide diuretics
Photosensitivity eruptions
  Griseofulvin
  Nonsteroidal antiinflammatory agents
  Phenothiazines
  Sulfonamides
  Sulfonylureas
  Tetracycline
  Thiazide diuretics
Toxic epidermal necrolysis
  Allopurinol
  Aminopenicillins
  Anticonvulsant agents
  Imidazole antifungal agents
  Nonsteroidal antiinflammatory agents (oxicam derivatives)
  Sulfonamides
  Tetracycline
Urticaria
  Enzymes (L-asparaginase)
  Indomethacin
  Opiates
  Penicillin and related antibiotics
  Salicylates
  Sulfonamides
  X-ray contrast media

From Stein JH (ed): *Internal medicine*, ed 5, St Louis, 1998, Mosby.

CYANOSIS

> **BOX 2-30 Cyanosis**
>
> Congenital heart disease with right-to-left shunt
> Pulmonary embolism
> Hypoxia
> Pulmonary edema
> Pulmonary disease (oxygen diffusion and alveolar ventilation abnormalities)
> Hemoglobinopathies
> Decreased cardiac output
> Vasospasm
> Arterial obstruction
> Pulmonary AV fistulas

DELIRIUM

> **BOX 2-31 Differential Diagnosis of Delirium**
>
> **Toxic Etiologies**
> Steroids
> Lithium
> Salicylates
> Anticholinergics
> Sympathomimetics (cocaine, amphetamines)
> Phencyclidine
> Mushrooms containing muscimol and ibutinic acid: *Amanita pantherina, Amanita muscaria*
> Monoamine oxidase inhibitors
> Solvents
> Carbon monoxide
> Sedative-hypnotic withdrawal
>
> **Metabolic Etiologies**
> Sodium disorders
> Hypoglycemia
> Hypercarbia
> Hypoxia, severe anemia
> Calcium disorders
> Uremia
> Thyrotoxicosis
> Hepatic encephalopathy
> Hypertensive encephalopathy
> Shock
> Sepsis
>
> **Infectious and Inflammatory Etiologies**
> Meningoencephalitis
> Meningitis
> Vasculitis
>
> **Neurologic and Neurosurgical Abnormalities**
> Cerebrovascular accident
> Subarachnoid hemorrhage
> Subdural and epidural hematoma
> Frontal contusion
> Postictal state
> Temporal lobe seizures

From Rosen P et al (eds): *Emergency medicine: concepts and clinical practice,* St Louis, 1997, Mosby.

DEMENTIA

TABLE 2-18 Causes of Dementia

DISEASE	LABORATORY AIDS TO DIAGNOSIS	DISEASE	LABORATORY AIDS TO DIAGNOSIS
Primary Neurologic Disease		**Toxic Encephalopathies**	
Alzheimer's disease and senile dementia	—	Alcohol-related dementia	Alcohol level, aspartate aminotransferase, mean corpuscular volume (MCV)
Pick's disease	CT or MRI, SPECT	Heavy metals (lead, arsenic, mercury)	24-hr urine collection
Huntington's disease	CT or MRI	Dialysis dementia	—
Progressive supranuclear palsy	—	Psychiatric drugs	Blood levels where available
Olivopontocerebellar degeneration	MRI	Barbiturates, bromides, benzodiazepines, phenothiazines, haloperidol, lithium, especially certain combinations (e.g., thioridazine/lithium, haloperidol/methyldopa)	Urine toxicology screening
Parkinsonism	—		
Brain tumors	CT with contrast or MRI		
Multiple sclerosis	CSF γ-globulin, oligoclonal banding, basic myelin protein, evoked potentials		
Wilson's disease	Serum ceruloplasmin, urinary copper, slit-lamp examination for Kayser-Fleischer rings	Drugs used in general medicine Analgesics, antihypertensives, antidiabetic agents, digitalis preparations, cimetidine, methyldopa, propranolol, reserpine, OTC medications	
Ceroid lipofuscinosis	Brain biopsy		
Vascular Disease			
Multiinfarct dementia	MRI		
Lacunar state	CT or MRI		
Binswanger encephalopathy	CT or MRI	**Infectious-inflammatory**	
Cerebral vasculitis (as in systemic lupus)	Erythrocyte sedimentation rate, specific antibodies (e.g., antinuclear antibody)	General paralysis	Blood and CSF tests for syphilis
Traumatic CNS Lesions		Chronic basilar meningitis (with/without hydrocephalus)	—
Multiple contusions	MRI	Fungal (especially cryptococcal)	CSF cryptococcal antigen and fungal cultures
Dementia pugilistica ("punch-drunk" syndrome)	—	Syphilitic	Blood and CSF tests for syphilis
Chronic subdural hematoma	CT or MRI	Sarcoid	Angiotensin-converting enzyme level, lymph node biopsy
Normal-pressure Hydrocephalus		Carcinomatous-leukemic	CSF cytology
Idiopathic or following meningitis or subarachnoid hemorrhage	CT or MRI, isotope cisternography, high-volume lumbar puncture	Whipple disease of brain	Brain biopsy, periodic acid–Schiff staining of CSF cells, small bowel biopsy
Seizures		Creutzfeldt-Jakob disease	EEG, brain biopsy
Nonconvulsive status	EEG	Brain abscess	CT with contrast or MRI
Metabolic Disturbances		Progressive multifocal leukoencephalopathy	MRI
Anoxia-hypoxia	Arterial blood gases	Limbic encephalitis	Search for occult carcinoma (usually small cell carcinoma of lung)
Chronic hypercapnea	Arterial blood gases		
Hyperammonemic encephalopathy	Liver function studies, serum-ammonia, CSF glutamine	AIDS encephalopathy	HIV antibodies
Chronic electrolyte-calcium or acid-base imbalance	Serum Na, K, Cl, CO_2, Ca, pH, alkaline phosphatase	**Psychiatric**	
Endocrine dysfunction, hypothyroidism, apathetic form of hyperthyroidism, Cushing's disease, Addison's disease	Thyroid-stimulating hormone, timed serum cortisol levels	Pseudodementia of depression	Neuropsychologic testing Dexamethasone suppression test
Vitamin B_{12} deficiency	Serum B_{12} level, methylmalonic acid	Sensory deprivation	Hearing/vision testing
Thiamine or niacin deficiency	—		
Azotemia	Serum creatinine, blood urea nitrogen		

From Noble J (ed): *Primary care medicine*, ed 2, St Louis, 1996, Mosby.
CT, Computed tomography; *MRI*, magnetic resonance imaging; *SPECT*, single photon emission computed tomography; *CSF*, cerebrospinal fluid; *EEG*, electroencephalography.

DERMATITIS

TABLE 2-19 Differential Diagnosis of Dermatitis

DIAGNOSIS	HISTORY	PHYSICAL EXAMINATION	LABORATORY	MANAGEMENT

Atopic dermatitis	Onset by age 5 yr
	Family Hx of atopy
	Pruritus
	Exacerbating factors
	Coexistent hay fever, asthma
		Flexural distribution
		Lichenification
		Papules, erythema
		Pustules if secondary *Staphylococcus*
			Routine: none
			Consider:
			  culture/pustule
			  IgE
				Topical corticosteroids
				Control environment
				Antihistamines
				Emollients

Contact dermatitis Irritant type	Predisposing Hx of atopy Frequent water exposure Solvents Job description	Hands commonly Erythema, scale, fissuring	None	Topical steroid ointments Protect from wet exposures Gloves Emollients

Allergic type	Rapid onset
	Pruritus
	Exposures:
	  Plants
	  Cosmetics
		Erythema, vesicles, oozing
		Location corresponds to exposure
			None	Wet to dry dressings
				Topical or systemic corticosteroids
				Identify and avoid allergen

Stasis dermatitis	Gradual onset Distal legs Previous history Varicosities, leg trauma, etc.	Erythema Pigmentation Edema Fibrosis	None	Acute: steroid ointments Long-term: compression, leg elevation, emollient ointments
Xerotic dermatitis	Winter Low humidity Frequent baths Soap use Pretibial common	Patchy, erythema, scale Extensor areas Spares folds	None	Decrease soap and water exposure Liberal use of thick emollients, especially after bath Steroids short-term prn
Dyshidrosis	Pruritic papules and vesicles on hands Recurrent	Papules and small vesicles on hands	None Exclude fungus with KOH Exclude allergen	Systemic or topical steroids Antibiotics
Nummular dermatitis	Gradual onset Pruritic Frequent history Exposure to drying	Round patches Erythema Scaling occasional Oozing occasional	None KOH to exclude fungus	Steroid ointments Tar cream, gel Ultraviolet light

From Noble J (ed): *Primary care medicine*, ed 2, St Louis, 1996, Mosby.

DIARRHEA, DRUG-INDUCED

BOX 2-32 **Drugs Associated with Diarrhea**

Laxatives (e.g., cascara sagrada, bisacodyl, phenolphthalein, ricinoleic acid, lactulose)
Magnesium-containing antacids
Antibiotics: clindamycin, lincomycin, ampicillin, cephalosporin; may be associated with *Clostridium difficile* toxin and pseudomembranes
Antiarrhythmic drugs: quinidine, propranolol
Digitalis

Antihypertensive drugs: guanethidine, propranolol
Potassium supplements
Artificial sweeteners: sorbitol, mannitol
Chenodeoxycholic acid
Cholestyramine*
Sulfasalazine
Anticoagulants

From Stein JH (ed): *Internal medicine*, ed 4, St Louis, 1994, Mosby.
*In patients with extensive ileal resection, bile salt depletion can result in malabsorption and diarrhea.

DIARRHEA IN PATIENTS WITH AIDS

BOX 2-33 Causes of Diarrhea in Patients with AIDS

FREQUENCY	ORGANISM
Most common	*Cryptosporidium*
	Cytomegalovirus
Common	*Entamoeba histolytica* (probably comensual, not causative)
	Giardia lamblia
	Mycobacterium avium-intracellularae
	Salmonella spp., especially *tymphimurium*
	Aeromonas hydrophilia
	Microsporidia
	Astrovirus/picobirnavirus
	Clostridium difficile
Less common	*Campylobacter jejuni*
	Viruses—herpes simplex, rotovirus, adenovirus, Norwalk agent
	Cyclospora
Rare	*Isospora belli*
	Enteromonas hominis
	Strongyloides stercoralis
	Blastocystis hominis
	Shigella spp.
	Yersinia enterocolitica

From Rosen P et al (eds): *Emergency medicine: concepts and clinical practice*, St Louis, 1997, Mosby.

DIZZINESS

BOX 2-34 Differential Diagnosis of Dizziness

1. Vertigo

ACUTE	RECURRENT	POSITIONAL
Vertebrobasilar event	Ménière's disease	Benign positional vertigo
Toxic (illness or drug)	Migraine	Postinfectious
Infectious	Hypothyroid	Posttrauma
Trauma	Multiple sclerosis	Cervical
Tumor	Seizure	Central causes
Seizure	Syphilis	
	Vertebrobasilar transient ischemic attacks	

2. Presyncope (Impending Faint)

Orthostasis or near syncope
Hyperventilation

3. Imbalance

Medication toxicity
Multiple sensory impairments
Cervical spine disease
Muscle weakness, unstable joints
Neurologic disease (previous stroke, cerebellar degeneration, peripheral neuropathy, myelopathy, parkinsonism)

4. Ill-defined Lightheadedness

Medications, visual disorders, previous stroke
Hyperventilation, psychiatric disorders
Carbon monoxide exposure

From Yoshikawa TT, Cobbs EL, Brummel-Smith K: *Practical ambulatory geriatrics*, St Louis, 1997, Mosby.

DYSPHAGIA

BOX 2-35 Causes of Dysphagia

Neuromuscular Causes of Dysphagia

Vascular
Cerebrovascular accident

Immunologic (Presumed)
Dermatomyositis
Polymyositis
Myasthenia gravis
Scleroderma
Multiple sclerosis

Infectious
Poliomyelitis
Diphtheria
Botulism
Rabies
Tetanus
Sydenham's chorea

Metabolic
Lead poisoning
Magnesium deficiency

Other
Thyrotoxic myopathy
Parkinson's disease
Amyotrophic lateral sclerosis
Myotonic dystrophy
Oculopharyngeal muscular dystrophy
Familial dysautonomia
Brain tumor
Diabetic neuropathy

Obstructive Causes of Dysphagia
Carcinoma
Hypertrophic cervical spurs
Goiter
Vascular anomalies (dysphagia lusoria)
Foreign bodies
Esophageal webs
Esophageal ring (Schatzki's ring)
Achalasia
Esophageal stricture
Zenker's diverticulum
Aortic aneurysm
Left atrial enlargement
Benign tumors
Inflamatory lesions (tonsillitis, etc.)
Foreign body

From Rosen P et al (eds): *Emergency medicine: concepts and clinical practice,* St Louis, 1997, Mosby.

DYSPNEA

BOX 2-36 Causes of Dyspnea

Increased Drive to Breathe

Lung Reflexes
Congestive heart failure
Pulmonary edema
  Cardiogenic
    Noncardiogenic (e.g., high-altitude illness)
Adult respiratory distress syndrome
Pneumonia and other pulmonary infections
Pulmonary embolism
Myocardial infarction
Aspiration
Toxic gas inhalation
Atelectasis
Valvular heart disease
Pulmonary vascular disease
Cardiomyopathy
Pulmonary contusion
Decompression illness
Sickle cell disease
Fat embolism
Amniotic fluid embolism
Collagen vascular diseases
Goodpasture's syndrome
Wegener's granulomatosis and other pulmonary vasculitides
Eosinophilic granuloma

Chemical Stimulation
Hypoxemia
  Congenital heart disease
  Pulmonary arteriovenous fistulae
Hypercapnia
Acidemia
Increased metabolic rate
  Fever
  Hyperthyroidism

Hemodynamic Stimulation
Shock
Cardiac dysrhythmia
Cardiac tamponade
Anemia
Myocarditis
Low cardiac output syndrome
Peripheral arteriovenous fistulae
Cerebral cortex
Anxiety
Hyperventilation syndrome

Impedance of Ventilation

Increased Airways Resistance
Asthma
Chronic obstructive pulmonary disease
  Emphysema
  Chronic bronchitis
Upper airway obstruction
Bronchiectasis
Cystic fibrosis

Intrapulmonary Restriction
Interstitial lung diseases
Pneumoconioses
Sarcoidosis
Interstitial fibrosis
Thoracic neoplasms

Extrapulmonary Restriction
Pleural effusion
Pneumothorax
Hemothorax
Open pneumothorax
Empyema
Flail chest
Ascites
Obesity
Pregnancy
Kyphoscoliosis
Ankylosing spondylitis
Pectus excavatum

Neuromuscular Insufficiency
Respiratory muscle paralysis
Diaphragmatic paralysis
Polyneuropathy
Guillain-Barré syndrome
Myasthenia gravis
Polymyositis
Poliomyelitis
Botulism
Hypokalemia
Coral snake bite
Tick paralysis

From Rosen P et al (eds): *Emergency medicine: concepts and clinical practice,* St Louis, 1992, Mosby.

DYSURIA

BOX 2-37 Differential Diagnosis of Dysuria

I. Urinary tract infection
   A. Enterobacteriaceae
   B. Gram-positive organisms
   C. *Chlamydia trachomatis*
   D. *Mycobacterium tuberculosis*
II. Vaginitis
   A. Fungi (*Candida albicans*)
   B. Bacterial
      1. *Gardnerella vaginalis* (*Haemophilus vaginalis*)
      2. *Neisseria gonorrhoeae*
      3. *Treponema pallidum* (endourethral chancre)
      4. *Chlamydia trachomatis*
   C. Protozoa (*Trichomonas vaginalis*)
III. Genital infection
   A. Herpes simplex (genitalis)
   B. Condyloma accuminatum
   C. Paraurethral glands
IV. Estrogen deficiency
V. Interstitial cystitis (Hunner's ulcer)
VI. Reiter's syndrome
VII. Chemical irritants
   A. Douches
   B. Deodorant aerosols
   C. Contraceptive jellies
   D. Bubble bath
VIII. Impedance to flow
   A. Urethral caruncle or diverticula
   B. Meatal stenosis or stricture
   C. Transient urethral edema
   D. Chronic fibrosis after trauma
   E. Impaired synergy: bladder contraction and sphincter relaxation
IX. Regional disease
   A. Crohn's disease
   B. Diverticulitis
   C. Cervical radium implant
X. Bladder tumor

From Stein JH (ed): *Internal medicine*, ed 4, St Louis, 1994, Mosby.

EDEMA, GENERALIZED

BOX 2-38 Causes of Generalized Edema

I. Common causes
   A. Congestive heart failure
   B. Cirrhosis of the liver
   C. Nephrotic syndrome
   D. Acute "nephritic" syndrome
   E. Pregnancy
      1. Normal pregnancy
      2. Toxemia of pregnancy
   F. Idiopathic edema
II. Unusual causes
   A. Arteriovenous fistulas
   B. Hypothyroidism
   C. Diabetes mellitus
      1. Associated with microangiopathy (rare)
      2. Associated with insulin treatment of ketoacidosis
   D. Drugs
      1. Nonsteroidal antiinflammatory drugs
      2. Estrogens
      3. Vasodilator antihypertensive drugs
      4. Hyperstimulation syndrome secondary to menotropins (Pergonal)

From Stein JH (ed): *Internal medicine*, ed 4, St Louis, 1994, Mosby.

EDEMA OF LOWER EXTREMITIES

BOX 2-39 Edema of Lower Extremities

CHF (right-sided)
Hepatic cirrhosis
Nephrosis
Myxedema
Lymphedema
Pregnancy
Abdominal mass: neoplasm, cyst
Venous compression from abdominal aneurysm
Varicose veins
Bilateral cellulitis
Bilateral thrombophlebitis
Venous thrombosis
Retroperitoneal fibrosis

ELEVATED HEMIDIAPHRAGM

> **BOX 2-40 Elevated Hemidiaphragm**
>
> Neoplasm (bronchogenic carcinoma, mediastinal neoplasm, intrahepatic lesion)
> Substernal thyroid
> Infectious process (pneumonia, empyema, TB, subphrenic abscess, hepatic abscess)
> Atelectasis
> Idiopathic
> Eventration
> Phrenic nerve dysfunction (myelitis, myotonia, herpes zoster)
> Trauma to phrenic nerve or diaphragm (e.g., surgery)
> Aortic aneurysm
> Intraabdominal mass
> Pulmonary infarction
> Pleurisy
> Radiation therapy
> Rib fracture

EPILEPSY

TABLE 2-20 Differential Diagnosis of Epilepsy

DISORDER	UNLIKE EPILEPSY	LIKE EPILEPSY
Syncope	Premonitory symptoms Precipitating factors Diffuse fading vision	Myoclonic jerks or tonic stiffening, on occasion
Transient ischemic attack	No "march" of symptoms No jerks, twitches No loss of consciousness, amnesia Brain stem symptoms	Focal EEG slowing Normal examination between attacks
Migraine	Prominent headache Preserved consciousness	Focal symptoms Focal EEG slowing
Hypoglycemia	Temporal relationship to fasting Initial sympathetic discharge	Focal symptoms and EEG slowing Loss of consciousness Postictal headache, confusion
Paroxysmal vertigo	Preserved consciousness Monosympatomatic spells Auditory, vestibular abnormalities	Severe temporary disability
Narcolepsy	Cataplexy Appropriate sleep behavior with attacks	Hallucinations Inappropriate, unpredictable timing of attacks
Psychogenic spells	Event-related Stressful context Lack of autonomic features Lack of incontinence	Dramatic convulsive behavior

From Stein JH (ed): *Internal medicine*, ed 4, St Louis, 1994, Mosby.

EPISTAXIS

> **BOX 2-41 Epistaxis**
>
> Trauma
> Medications (nasal sprays, NSAIDs, anticoagulants, antiplatelets)
> Nasal polyps
> Cocaine use
> Coagulopathy (hemophilia, liver disease, DIC, thrombocytopenia)
> Systemic disorders (hypertension, uremia)
> Infections
> Anatomic malformations
> Rhinitis
> Nasal polyps
> Local neoplasms (benign and malignant)
> Desiccation
> Foreign body

EOSINOPHILIA

> **BOX 2-42 Causes of Significant Peripheral Blood Eosinophilia**
>
> **Helminthic Parasites**
> *Ascaris lumbricoides* (invasive larval stage)
> Hookworms (invasive larval stage)
> *Strongyloides stercoralis* (initial infection and autoinfection)
> Trichinosis
> Filariasis
> *Echinococcus granulosus* and *E. multilocularis*
> *Toxocara* species
> Animal hookworms
> *Angiostrongylus cantonensis* and *A. costaricensis*
> Schistosomiasis
> Liver flukes
> *Fasciolopis buski*
> Anisakiasis
> *Capillaria philippinensis*
> *Paragonimus westermani*
> "Tropical eosinophilia" (unidentified microfilariae)
>
> **Other Infections/Infestations**
> Pulmonary aspergillosis
> Severe scabies
>
> **Allergies**
> Asthma
> Hay fever
> Drug reactions
> Atopic dermatitis
>
> **Autoimmune and Related Disorders**
> Polyarteritis nodosa
> Necrotizing vasculitis
> Eosinophilic fasciitis
> Pemphigus
>
> **Neoplastic Diseases**
> Hodgkin's disease
> Mycosis fungoides
> Chronic myelocytic leukemia
> Eosinophilic leukemia
> Polycythemia vera
> Mucin-secreting adenocarcinomas
>
> **Immunodeficiency States**
> Hyperimmunoglobulin E with recurrent infection
> Wiscott-Aldrich syndrome
>
> **Other**
> Addison's disease
> Inflammatory bowel disease
> Dermatitis herpetiformis
> Toxic/chemical syndrome
> Eosinophilic myalgia syndrome, tryptophan, toxic oil syndrome
> Hypereosinophilic syndrome (unknown etiology)

From Noble J (ed): *Primary care medicine*, ed 2, St Louis, 1996, Mosby.

EXANTHEMS

TABLE 2-21 Exanthems

DISEASE	AGE	PRODROME	SKIN MORPHOLOGY	DISTRIBUTION	OTHER FINDINGS	DIAGNOSIS
Measles	Infants Young adults	Fever, URI, conjunctivitis	Erythematous macules—papules become confluent	Face first Moves down over entire body	Koplik's spots, cough, photophobia, adenopathy	Clinical; acute/convalescent hemagglutinin serology
Rubella	Adolescents Young adults	Fever, malaise, cough	Rose-pink macules and papules Not confluent	Face first Moves downward	Forschheimer spots Postauricular adenopathy Headache	Rubella hemagglutinin inhibition or complement fixation titers acute/convalescent
Erythema infectiosum (fifth disease) (parvovirus B19)	5-15 yr	None or mild fever, malaise	Slapped red cheeks Reticulate erythema or maculopapular Not pruritic	Face—red cheeks Arm/legs reticulate	Rash waxes-wanes several weeks Arthritis; aplastic anemia	IgM antibody
Roseola exanthem HHV 6	6 mo-3 yr	High fever 3-5 days, then rash	Rose-pink, maculopapular Appears after fever resolves	Neck, trunk with little involvement of face Lasts only hours to few days	Cervical and postauricular adenopathy Human herpesvirus-6 may cause neonatal hepatitis	Clinical
Varicella chickenpox	1-14 yr	Fever, malaise	Vesicles (often umbilicated) or red base Very pruritic	Generalized involvement Lesions leave scars	Oral lesions Pneumonia in older patients	Tzanck viral culture
Enterovirus (coxsackie, ECHO)	Children	Fever, URI	Variable—maculopapular, petechial, vesicular	Generalized or acral (hand-foot-mouth)	Fever, myocarditis, meningitis, pleurodynia, mouth ulcers	Clinical, viral culture
Adenovirus	5 mo-5 yr	Fever, URI	Maculopapular, morbilliform, rubelliform, petechial roseolalike	Generalized	Fever, URI, conjunctivitis	Viral culture Acute/convalescent titer

DIFFERENTIAL DIAGNOSIS
Exanthems

Epstein-Barr virus (infectious mononucleosis)	Children Adolescents	Fever, sore throat	Maculopapular, morbilliform, urticarial, erythema multiformelike	Trunk Extremities	Cervical adenopathy Hepatosplenomegaly	Mono spot Acute/convalescent EBV nuclear Ag titers
Kawasaki disease	6 mo-6 yr	Fever, eye irritation	Papular, morbilliform, scarletiniform Commonly desquamates as clears	Generalized with palm, sole, and perineal accentuation	Conjunctivitis cheilitis, glossitis, adenopathy, peripheral edema, coronary artery abnormalities	Clinical
Staphylococcal scalded skin (staphylococcus toxin)	Neonates, infants		Sudden onset, tender, red rash that exfoliates leaving raw surfaces Nikolsky's sign	Generalized	Fever, conjunctivitis	Culture of coagulase + staphylococcus from systemic site Not skin
Scarlet fever (β streptococcus toxin)	School age	Fever, sore throat, malaise, headache	Diffuse, erythema with "sandpaper" texture Exfoliative as rash clears	Generalized, circumoral pallor Pastia's lines	Pharyngitis, palate perlèche, abdominal pain, strawberry tongue	Throat culture ↑ASO titer
Staphylococcal scarlet fever (exfoliative toxin)	School age		Tender, red, erythroderma with sandpaper quality Does not desquamate		No pharyngitis	Negative throat culture No ASO ↑
Meningococcemia	<2 yr	Malaise, fever, URI	Papules, petechiae, large areas of purpura, purpurafulminans	Trunk, extremities, soles, palms	High fever, meningismus, shock	Blood culture, spinal tap
Rocky Mountain fever (rickettsii)	Any age	Fever, malaise	Maculopapular, petechial rash	Acral areas first; trunk later	CNS, pulmonary, and cardiac involvement	Serology Weil-Felix test

From Noble J (ed): *Primary care medicine*, ed 2, St Louis, 1996, Mosby.
URI, Upper-respiratory infection.

EYE PAIN

BOX 2-43   Eye Pain

Foreign body	Ingrown lashes	Cerebral neoplasm
Herpes zoster	Orbital or periorbital cellulitis/abscess	Entropion
Trauma	Sinusitis	Retrobulbar neuritis
Conjunctivitis	Headache	UV light
Iritis	Glaucoma	Dry eyes
Iridocyclitis	Inflammation of lacrimal gland	Irritation or inflammation from eye drops, dust, cosmetics, etc.
Uveitis	Tic douloureux	
Blepharitis	Cerebral aneurysm	

FACIAL PAIN

TABLE 2-22   Facial Pain

	LOCATION	NATURE	TIMING	ASSOCIATED PHYSICAL FINDINGS
Tic douloureaux	V2, then V2-V3; rarely V1	Triggered	Brief jabs	None
Geniculate neuralgia	Ear	Not often triggered	Brief jabs, or long duration	Vesicles in ear, VII palsy, ± VIII findings
Glossopharyngeal neuralgia	Tonsillar fosa, ear	Triggered	Brief jabs	Episodes of syncope
Postherpetic neuralgia	One or more adjacent cranial or cervical nerves	Burning	Constant	Healed skin lesions, sensory loss, or hyperpathia
Posttraumatic neuralgia	Usually one cranial or cervical nerve	Burning, aching	Constant	Sensory disturbances
Cluster headache	Retro-orbital, cheek, temple	Boring, deep, intense	Attacks of 30-120 min	Lacrimation, ptosis, rhinorrhea
"Lower-half headache"	Orbit, nose, cheek, mastoid; may spread to neck and arm	Boring, deep, intense	Attacks lasting 1 or more hr	Sometimes flushing, lacrimation, rhinorrhea
Carotidynia	One side of neck	Deep, aching	Several days	Tender carotid in neck
Atypical facial pain	Cheek, jaw, entire face	Aching, may be bizarre	Constant	Emotional disturbance

From Stein JH (ed): *Internal medicine*, ed 4, St Louis, 1994, Mosby.

FACIAL PARALYSIS

BOX 2-44   Etiology of Facial Paralysis

Infection
  Bacterial
    Otitis media
    Mastoiditis
    Chronic suppurative otitis media (especially with cholesteatoma)
    Meningitis
    "Malignant otitis media"
    Lyme disease
  Viral
    Infectious mononucleosis
    Herpes zoster
    Varicella
    Rubella
    Mumps
  Mycobacterial
    Tuberculous meningitis
    Leprosy
  Miscellaneous
    Syphilis
    Malaria
Trauma
  Temporal bone fracture
  Facial lacerations
  Surgical
Neoplasm
  Malignant
    Squamous cell carcinoma
    Basal cell and adenocystic tumors
    Leukemia
    Parotid neoplasms
    Metastatic tumors
  Benign
    Vestibular schwannoma
    Congenital cholesteatoma
    Facial nerve neuroma
Immunologic
  Guillain-Barré syndrome
  Reaction to tetanus antiserum
  Periarteritis nodosa
Metabolic
  Pregnancy
  Hypothyroidism
  Diabetes mellitus

From Noble J (ed): *Primary care medicine*, ed 2, St Louis, 1996, Mosby.

FEVER AND RASH

DIFFERENTIAL DIAGNOSIS — Fever and rash

TABLE 2-23 Identification of Life-threatening Diseases Associated with Fever and Rash

DISEASE	HISTORY	CHARACTERISTICS OF RASH	DISTRIBUTION OF RASH	ASSOCIATED CLINICAL FINDINGS	DIAGNOSTIC AIDS
Rocky Mountain spotted fever	Tick exposure (75%) May-September occurrence in temperate-zone states. Heaviest endemic area: middle Atlantic states and Southeast	Initial maculopapular petechiae appearing on second to sixth febrile day and usually painless.	Begins on wrists, ankles, forearms, spreading within 6-8 hr to palms, soles, trunk	Prodrome of fever, headache, myalgias. Hyponatremia, normal to slightly increased WBC, thrombocytopenia, hypoalbuminemia	Biopsy of involved skin with immunofluorescence and other serologic tests. Serology: Complement-fixation more sensitive and more specific than Weil-Felix agglutination.
Meningococcemia*	Tends to occur in late winter, early spring. Outbreaks in military recruits, crowded living conditions	*Acute:* May be maculopapular initially. Small petechiae with irregular borders ("smudging"), at times with vesicular or grayish ulcer. Painful. May coalesce. *Chronic:* Maculopapules, petechial vesicles, or pustules; tender nodules.	*Acute:* Extremities and trunk in random fashion. *Chronic:* Extremities, particularly over joints	*Acute:* Meningitis, disseminated intravascular coagulation, shock, acidosis. *Chronic:* Rash appears with recurrent cycles of fever over 2-3 months	*Acute:* Aspiration of center of skin lesions for Gram's stain, culture (up to 60% positive). Blood cultures. Cerebrospinal fluid culture and Gram's stain. *Chronic:* Blood culture usually positive during febrile episode. Biopsy findings resemble leukocytoclastic angiitis.
Disseminated gonococcal infection	Incidence higher in women than in men. Young, sexually active. Onset often related to menstruation	Pustules on erythematous base most characteristic. Also, macules, papules, pustules, and bullae less commonly.	Over extremities, with relative sparing of face and trunk; usually few (5-40) lesions	Migratory polyarthralgia, tenosynovitis, septic arthritis	Gram's stain of lesion. Blood, joint fluid culture (50%) prove diagnosis. Cervical, rectal, throat cultures support diagnosis.
Staphylococcal septicemia	Nosocomial: indwelling catheters, pacemakers, dialysis shunts, wound infections. Drug abuse	Pustules, purulent purpura, subcutaneous nodules, infarcts.	Widespread, with infracts having predilection for distal extremities	Endocarditis, with valvular incompetence, meningitis, multiple-organ involvement	Aspiration of lesions for Gram's stain culture. Blood, cerebrospinal fluid (where indicated) cultures. Teichoic acid antibody suggestive of deep-seated infection.
Pseudomonas septicemia	Hospitalized patients, especially with neutropenia or burns	*Vesicles:* Isolated or in small clusters rapidly becoming hemorrhagic.	Random	Generally extremity toxic, with fever; septic picture	Aspiration of lesion for Gram's stain, culture.

Continued

TABLE 2-23 Identification of Life-threatening Diseases Associated with Fever and Rash—cont'd

DISEASE	HISTORY	CHARACTERISTICS OF RASH	DISTRIBUTION OF RASH	ASSOCIATED CLINICAL FINDINGS	DIAGNOSTIC AIDS
		Ecthyma gangrenosum: Round, indurated, ulcerated painless lesion with central gray eschar.	Axillary or anogenital area, thigh		Cultures of blood, urine, sputum, etc.
		Maculopapular lesion: Small erythematous lesion resembling "rose spots." Gangrenous cellulitis.	Trunk Localized		
Candida septicemia	Broad-spectrum antibiotics, leukemia, immunosuppression, hyperalimentation, cardiac surgery	Multiple discrete pink maculopapular lesions 2-5 mm in diameter.	Trunk and extremities	Toxic state; associated ophthalmitis, esophagitis, cystitis	Punch biopsy of lesion with stains for fungus. Buffy coat of blood. Blood cultures (definitive diagnosis). Examination and culture of stool, urine, sputum (supportive of diagnosis with multiple-site involvement). Barium or endoscopic examination of esophagus.
Infective endocarditis	Indwelling catheters, pacemakers, dialysis shunts, valvular heart disease, prosthetic valves, intravenous drug abuse, preceding dental or surgical manipulations	*Petechiae*: often in small groups. *Osler's nodes*: pea-sized, tender, erythematous nodules. *Janeway's lesions*: small erythematous or hemorrhagic macules.	Conjunctivae, palate, upper chest, distal extremities Pads of fingers and toes Palms and soles	Heart murmur, valvular imcompetence, metastatic abscesses, infracts, Roth's spots, splenomegaly, hematuria, glomerulonephritis, etc.	Serology not yet reliable. Blood cultures (3-5 sets). Echocardiogram. Circulating immune complexes.

DIFFERENTIAL DIAGNOSIS — Fever and rash

Toxic shock syndrome	Young female predominance 1-4 days prodrome of fever, myalgias, arthralgias, and diarrhea Onset during or soon after menses (has also been reported in men and unassociated with menses in women)	Erythroderma: Seen at presentation. Diffuse, blanching, macular (deep-red "sunburned" appearance). Resolves within 3 days, followed 5-12 days later by desquamation, most commonly of hands and feet. Mucosal hyperemia: pharynx, conjunctivae, vagina.	Diffuse, hands and feet predominantly	Fever, severe hypotension, multisystem involvement (gastrointestinal, muscular, renal, hepatic, hematologic, CNS)	Clinical criteria. See Section I. Negative serology for RMSF, leptospirosis, measles. Identification of toxin producing strain of S. aureus.
Lyme disease	From endemic areas—Northeast, Midwest (Minnesota/Wisconsin), and West (California/Oregon) Usually begins in summer	Erythema chronicum migrans: Expanding annular erythema (median diameter 15 cm) from central macule or papule. Secondary annular lesions seen.	Commonly, thigh, groin, axilla. Any site can be involved.	Fever, chills, malaise, myalgias, lymphadenopathy Late (weeks to months) CNS, cardiac, and joint involvement	Primarily history and clinical criteria. Organism can be cultured (difficult, special media). Serology.

From Stein JH (ed): Internal medicine, ed 4, St Louis, 1994, Mosby.
*Acute syndrome may occasionally be caused by Haemophilus influenzae and Streptococcus pneumoniae, especially in splenectomized patients.

FEVER OF UNKNOWN ORIGIN

BOX 2-45 Etiologies of Prolonged Fever of Unknown Origin

Infection

Bacterial

Endocarditis
Sinusitis
Mastoiditis
Occult abscess
Pyelonephritis
Tuberculosis
Adenitis

Viral

Infectious mononucleosis
Cytomegalovirus
Hepatitis A, B, or C

Chlamydial

Lymphogranuloma venereum
Psittacosis

Mycoplasmal, Fungal

Cysticercosis
Blastomycosis
Histoplasmosis

Rickettsial

Q fever
Rocky Mountain spotted fever

Parasitic

Malaria
Toxoplasmosis

Collagen Vascular

Juvenile rheumatoid arthritis
Lupus erythematosus
Ulcerative colitis
Regional enteritis
Vasculitis
Rheumatic fever

Malignancy

Leukemia
Lymphoma
Neuroblastoma
Wilms' tumor

Drug-Induced Fever

Antibiotics
Antituberculous agents
Anticonvulsants
Propylthiouracil
Quinidine
Procainamide
Serum sickness

Miscellaneous

Kawasaki disease
AIDS
Serial infections
CNS/hypothalamic
Environmental
Factitious
Familial dysautonomia
Thyrotoxicosis
Pulmonary embolus

From Rosen P et al (eds): *Emergency medicine: concepts and clinical practice,* St Louis, 1997, Mosby.

FLUSHING

BOX 2-46 Differential Diagnosis of Flushing

Physiologic Flushing

Menopause
Ingestion of monosodium glutamate (Chinese restaurant syndrome)
Ingestion of hot drinks

Drugs

Alcohol (with or without disulfiram, metronidazole, or chlorpropamide)
Diltiazem
Nifedipine
Nicotinic acid
Levodopa
Bromocriptine
Thyrotropin-releasing hormone
Amyl nitrate

Neoplastic Disorders

Carcinoid syndrome
VIPoma* syndrome
Medullary carcinoma of the thyroid
Systemic mastocytosis
Basophilic chronic myelocytic leukemia
Renal cell carcinoma

Agnogenic Flushing

From Moore WT, Eastman RC: *Diagnosis endocrinology,* ed 2, St Louis, 1996, Mosby.
*VIPoma, Vasoactive intestinal peptide-secreting tumor.

FUNGAL INFECTIONS IN THE CENTRAL NERVOUS SYSTEM

TABLE 2-24 Common Fungal Infections of the Central Nervous System (CNS)

ORGANISM	HOST FACTORS	COMMON NEUROLOGIC PRESENTATION	OTHER NEUROLOGIC PRESENTATION	COMMENT

Molds
  Aspergillus species
  Mucorales
  P. boydii
  Fusarium
  S. griseus
	Immunocompromised (defective neutrophil function, e.g., cytotoxic chemotherapy recipients)
	Injection drug use
	Acidosis
	Near drowning
		Rhinocerebral syndrome
		Strokelike syndrome
		Inflammatory mass
			Meningitis	Diabetics are predisposed to rhinocerebral syndrome caused by Mucorales
				Cytotoxic agents predispose to Aspergillus
				Desferoximine predisposes to Mucorales

Cryptococcus species C. neoformans	Immunocompromised (defective T-cell function, HIV infection, corticosteroid use, inherited immune defects) Normal host	Meningitis	Cryptococcoma	Acute meningitis more common in immunosuppressed patients; more indolent course in immunocompetent persons Cryptococcus has high predilection for CNS involvement

Candida species
  C. albicans
  C. tropicalis
  C. parapsilosis
  T. glabrata
  C. krusei
	Immunocompromised (defective neutrophil function)
	Inherited immune defects
	Cytotoxic agents
	Injecting drug use
	Corticosteroid use
	Intravenous catheters
	Broad-spectrum antibiotics
	Prematurity
		Meningitis
		Abscess
			Infarct	Community-acquired pathogens

Dimorphic fungi
  B. dermatitidis
  P. brasilienssis
  H. capsulatum
  C. immitis
  S. schenckii
	Normal host
	Immunocompromised (defective T-cell function)
		Meningitis
		Abscess
				Community-acquired pathogens
				C. immitis has increased predilection for CNS

Dematiacious fungi
  X. bantiana
  Bipolaris species
  Exerohilum species
  Curvularia species
  F. pedrosi
  R. obovoideum
	Normal host
	Immunocompromised
		Abscess	Meningitis	Community-acquired pathogens

From Johnson RT, Griffin JW: *Current therapy in neurologic disease*, ed 5, St Louis, 1997, Mosby.

GALACTORRHEA

TABLE 2-25 Causes of Galactorrhea

CAUSES	MECHANISM
Prolonged suckling	Reduction in PIF from hypothalamus
Drugs (isoniazid, phenothiazines, reserpine derivatives, amphetamines, and tricyclic antidepressants)	Depletion of dopamine or blocked dopamine receptors
Major stressors (surgery, trauma)	Inhibition of hypothalamic PIF
Hypothyroidism	TRH acts as prolactin-releasing factor
Pituitary tumors	Secretion of prolactin; tumor may compress pituitary and decrease products of other hormones

From Noble J (ed): *Primary care medicine,* ed 2, St Louis, 1996, Mosby.

GAY BOWEL SYNDROME

TABLE 2-26 Clinical Features of Gay Bowel Syndrome

DISEASE	SIGNS AND SYMPTOMS	DIAGNOSIS	TREATMENT
Anorectal gonorrhea	Creamy rectal discharge, constipation, pain	Culture of *Neisseria* on selective medium	Procaine penicillin, 4.8 million U IM, plus 1 g probenecid orally or Spectinomycin, 2 g IM
Herpes simplex infection	Extreme rectal pain and tenderness, bloody discharge; discrete on sigmoidoscopy	Viral isolation from stool, discharge, or acute and convalescent sera	Acyclovir, 5 mg/kg IV q8h
Anorectal syphilis	Mild or no symptoms	Darkfield examination of ulcer, serologic testing	Benzathine penicillin, 2.4 million U IM (single dose) or Tetracycline, 500 mg qid for 15 days
Ambebiasis	Diarrhea with mucus or blood; diffuse proctitis with scattered ulcers at sigmoidoscopy	Motile trophozoites or cysts in stool, serologic studies	Metronidazole, 750 mg qid for 10 days
Lymphogranuloma venereum	Diarrhea, discharge; diffuse proctitis at sigmoidoscopy	Granulomas in rectal biopsy or stool	Tetracycline, 500 mg PO qid for 2-3 wk

From Noble J (ed): *Primary care medicine,* ed 2, St Louis, 1996, Mosby.

GENITAL LESIONS

TABLE 2-27 Differential Diagnosis of Genital Lesions

MORPHOLOGY	NUMBER	DISTRIBUTION	SURFACE	BASE	EDGE
Ulcers	Single (55%) or multiple	Penis, labia, cervix	Clean	Indolent	Indurated
	Single	Penis	Purulent	Inflamed	Ragged
	Single	Penis, labia	Beefy red, granulation tissue	Friable	Serpiginous
	Single	Penis, labia	Eroded papule	Benign	Benign
	Multiple	Penis, vulva, thigh, cervix, grouped	Clean	Clean, all same size	
	Multiple (30%) or single (70%)	Penis, vulva, thigh	Necrotic	Variable size, ragged	Erythema
Papules	Single	Penis, labia	Clean or small erosion	Benign	Undermined erythema
	Multiple	One or more rows behind corona	Clean	Benign	Benign
	Multiple	Penis, labia, vagina, often grouped	Verrucous	Benign	Benign
	Multiple	Penis, labia, pubic hair, thighs, buttocks	Umbilicated, with tiny plug	Benign	Benign
	Multiple	Disseminated, palms, soles	Coppery	Benign	
	Multiple	Penis, labia, thighs, buttocks, wrists, and ankles	Crusted		Linear tracks may be seen
Vesicles	Multiple	Penis, labia, thighs, cervix, grouped	Umbilicated	Erythema	
Crusts	Multiple	Grouped		Erythema	
	Multiple	Disseminated		Erythema may be present	
Erythema	Patches	Glans, shaft of penis, labia, vulva	Intense erythema		Satellite lesions

MORPHOLOGY	PAIN	ADENOPATHY	INCUBATION PERIOD	SUGGESTED DIAGNOSIS
Ulcers	Mild (30%)	Moderate	<21 days (up to 90 days)	Syphilis
	Mild to severe	Mild or absent	<24 hr	Human bite, other trauma
		Inguinal granulomas	1-12 wk	Donovanosis
	Lesion often goes entirely unnoticed	Moderate, but usually appears after lesion resolves	2 wk	Lymphogranuloma venereum
	Severe: prodome of paresthesia	Moderate, tender	3-7 days, recurrent	Herpes genitalis
	Moderate	Moderate, tender	2-5 days	Chancroid
Papules			2 wk	Early lymphogranuloma venereum
				Pearly penile papules
			3-30 wk	Veneral warts
			2-26 wk	Molluscum contagiosum
	Occasional, mild	Prominent	6-12 wk	Secondary syphilis
	Intense pruritus	Rare superinfected excoriation	4 wk	Scabies
Vesicles	Mild	Moderate, tender	2-5 days	Herpes genitalis
Crusts	Mild	Mild	2-5 days	Healing herpes genitalis
	Pruritus	Mild or absent	4 wk	Scabies
Erythema	Pruritus		Undefined	Candidiasis

From Stein JH (ed): *Internal medicine,* ed 4, St Louis, 1994, Mosby.

GOITER

BOX 2-47 Goiter

Thyroiditis
Toxic multinodular goiter
Graves' disease
Medications (PTU, methimazole, sulfonamides, sulfonylureas, ethionamide, amiodarone, lithium, etc.)
Iodine deficiency
Sarcoidosis, amyloidosis
Defective thyroid hormone synthesis
Resistance to thyroid hormone

GRANULOMATOUS DISORDERS

BOX 2-48 Classification of Granulomatous Disorders

Infections
Fungi
  Histoplasma
  Coccidioides
  Blastomyces
  Sporothrix
  Aspergillus
  Cryptococcus

Protozoa
  Toxoplasma
  Leishmania

Metazoa
  Toxocara
  Schistosoma

Spirochetes
  T. pallidum
  T. pertunue
  T. carateum

Mycobacteria
  M. tuberculosis
  M. leprae
  M. kanasasii
  M. marinum
  M. avian
  Bacille Calmette-Guérin (BCG) vaccine

Bacteria
  Brucella
  Yersinia

Other Infections
  Cat scratch
  Lymphogranuloma

Neoplasia
  Carcinoma
  Reticulosis
  Pinealoma
  Dysgerminoma
  Seminoma
  Reticulum cell sarcoma
  Malignant nasal granuloma

Chemicals
  Beryllium
  Zirconium
  Silica
  Starch

Immunologic Aberrations
  Sarcoidosis
  Crohn's disease
  Primary biliary cirrhosis
  Wegener's granulomatosis
  Giant-cell arteritis
  Peyronie's disease
  Hypogammaglobulinemia
  Systemic lupus erythematosus
  Lymphomatoid granulomatosis

  Histiocytosis X
  Hepatic granulomatous disease
  Immune complex disease
  Rosenthal-Melkersson syndrome
  Churg-Strauss allergic granulomatosis

Leukocyte Oxidase Defect
  Chronic granulomatous disease of childhood

Extrinsic Allergic Alveolitis
  Farmer's lung
  Bird fancier's
  Mushroom worker's
  Suberosis (cork dust)
  Bagassosis
  Maple bark stripper's
  Paprika splitter's
  Coffee bean
  Spatlese lung

Other Disorders
  Whipple's disease
  Pyrexia of unknown origin
  Radiotherapy
  Cancer chemotherapy
  Panniculitis
  Chalazion
  Sebaceous cyst
  Dermoid
  Sea urchin spine injury

From Schwarz MI, King TE: *Interstitial lung disease*, ed 2, St Louis, 1993, Mosby.

GRANULOMATOUS LUNG DISEASE

TABLE 2-28 Differential Diagnosis of Granulomatous Lung Diseases

FEATURE	WEGENER'S GRANULOMATOSIS — CLASSIC	WEGENER'S GRANULOMATOSIS — LIMITED	LYMPHOMATOID GRANULOMATOSIS	CHURG-STRAUSS SYNDROME	NECROTIZING SARCOID GRANULOMATOSIS	BRONCHOCENTRIC GRANULOMATOSIS — ASTHMA	BRONCHOCENTRIC GRANULOMATOSIS — NO ASTHMA	SARCOIDOSIS
Sex	M/F	Equal	Affects men slightly more frequently	Same	Same	Same	Same	Same
Decade of incidence	50s	50s	30s–50s	50s	30s and 40s	30s	60s	30s and 40s
Presentation	Sinusitis Rhinorrhea Epistaxis	+	Cough Dyspnea Hemoptysis Arthralgia	Bronchitis Asthma Pneumonia	Fever Cough Pleurisy Malaise	Asthma	Cough Pleurisy Dyspnea	Insignificant symptoms
Ulcerated nose and nasal sputum	+	+	–	–	–	Bronchiectasis Bronchial obstruction Eosinophilia	–	Only when associated with lupus pernio and SURT
Saddle nose								
Chest radiograph opacities	+	+	+	+	+	Particularly in upper lobes		+
Cavitation	++	+	+	Infiltration	+	Pulmonary fibrosis	–	Infiltration
Hilar adenopathy	–	–	–	–	–	–	–	+

Continued

TABLE 2-28 Differential Diagnosis of Granulomatous Lung Disease

FEATURE	WEGENER'S GRANULOMATOSIS CLASSIC	WEGENER'S GRANULOMATOSIS LIMITED	LYMPHOMATOID GRANULOMATOSIS	CHURG-STRAUSS SYNDROME	NECROTIZING SARCOID GRANULOMATOSIS	BRONCHOCENTRIC GRANULOMATOSIS ASTHMA	BRONCHOCENTRIC GRANULOMATOSIS NO ASTHMA	SARCOIDOSIS
Kidneys	Glomerulonephritis in 85%	−	Renal vasculitis	−	−	−	−	Nephrocalcinosis
Ocular	+	−	−	−	−	+	+	−
Allergy	±	±	−	−	−	±	−	+
Skin lesions	+	−	+	+	−	−	−	−
CNS	+	−	+	Rare	Rare	−	−	+
Cardiac	+	−	−	−	−	−	−	+
Characteristics	↑ESR ↑ANCA	−	−	Eosinophilia	−	Hypersensitivity to aspergillus Eosinophilia	−	Increased SACE
Granulomas	±	±	Very rare	Infrequent	Always	+	+	Always
Vasculitis	++	++	Always	Always	++	±	±	Inconspicuous
Necrosis	Prominent and resemble infarcts	−	Prominent	Prominent	Prominent	+	+	Inconspicuous
Treatment	Cyclophosphamide	Cyclophosphamide Azathioprine	Cyclophosphamide Azathioprine	Steroids, azathioprine	Steroids, azathioprine	Corticosteroids		Steroids Azathiprine
Prognosis	Poor		Poor	Poor	Good	Good		Good

From Schwarz MI, King TE: *Interstitial lung disease*, ed 2, St Louis, 1993, Mosby.
+, Present; ++, prominent; −, absent; ±, inconspicuous; ESR, erythrocyte sedimentation rate; SACE, serum angiotensin-converting enzyme; ANCA, antineutrophil cycloplasmic antibody; SURT, sarcoidosis of upper respiratory tract.

GROIN PAIN IN ACTIVE PEOPLE

BOX 2-49 Differential Diagnosis of Groin Pain in Active People

Musculoskeletal
Avascular necrosis of the femoral head
Avulsion fracture (lesser trochanter, anterior superior iliac spine, anterior inferior iliac spine)
Bursitis (iliopectineal, trochanteric)
Entrapment of the ilioinguinal or iliofemoral nerve*
Gracilis syndrome
Muscle tear (adductors, iliopsoas, rectus abdominis, gracilis, sartorius, rectus femoris)
Myositis ossificans of the hip muscles
Osteitis pubis
Osteoarthritis of the femoral head
Slipped capital femoral epiphysis
Stress fracture of the femoral head or neck and pubis
Synovitis

Hernia-related
Avulsion of the internal oblique muscle in the conjoined tendon
Defect at the insertion of the rectus abdominis muscle
Direct inguinal hernia
Femoral ring hernia
Indirect inguinal hernia
Inguinal canal weakness

Urologic
Epididymitis
Fracture of the testis
Hydrocele
Kidney stone
Posterior urethritis
Prostatis
Testicular cancer
Torsion of the testis
Urinary tract infection
Varicocele

Gynecologic
Ectopic pregnancy
Ovarian cyst
Pelvic inflammatory disease
Torsion of the ovary
Vaginitis

Lymphatic Enlargement in Groin

From Swain R, Snodgrass: Managing groin pain, *Physician Sportsmedicine* 23:56, 1995.
*Usually postoperative.

GYNECOMASTIA

BOX 2-50 Differential Diagnosis of Gynecomastia

Physiologic
Newborns
Puberty
Aging
Refeeding

Pathologic
Testosterone deficiency
Congenital anorchia
Klinefelter's syndrome
Defects in the structure or function of androgen receptors
  Complete (testicular feminization syndrome)
  Partial (Reifenstein, Lubs, Rosewater, and Dreyfus syndromes)
Defects in androgen synthesis

Primary Gonadal Failure
Viral orchitis, trauma, castration, granulomatous disease, varicocele

Secondary Hypogonadism

Increased Estrogen Production
Increased testicular estrogen secretion
HCG-producing tumor (especially lung, liver, and kidney cancer), testicular tumor, bronchogenic carcinoma, gastrointestinal tumors, ectopic choriocarcinomas
True hermaphroditism
Estrogen-producing adrenal tumor

Increased Peripheral Conversion
Adrenal disease, liver disease (alcohol), starvation, thyrotoxicosis

Increase in Peripheral Aromatose Activity
Heredity, obesity

Increased Prolactin Level
Pituitary tumors (prolactinoma)
Drugs that deplete catecholamine or catecholamine antagonists—sulpiride, phenothiazine, methyldopa, reserpine, tricyclic antidepressant, metoclopramide

Drugs
Initiating or terminating exogenous androgens
Estrogen and estrogenlike substances (estradiol, diethylstilbestrol, digitalis)
Estrogen precursors—testosterone enanthate, testosterone propionate
GH therapy with elevated serum IGF-I level
Drugs that enhance endogenous estrogen formation—hCG, clomiphene
Drugs that inhibit testosterone synthesis and/or action, such as ketoconazole, alkylating agents, spironolactone, cimetidine, aminoglutethimide, flutamide, cyproterone
Others: amiodarone, busulfan, captopril, ethionamide, isoniazid, D-penicillamine, phenytoin, diazepam, marijuana, heroin, omeprazole, ranitidine, enalapril, nifedipine, verapamil

Idiopathic

From Moore WT, Eastman RC: *Diagnostic endocrinology*, ed 2, St Louis, 1996, Mosby.
GH, Growth hormone; *hCG*, human chorionic gonadotropin; *IGF*, insulinlike growth factor.

HALITOSIS

> **BOX 2-51 Halitosis**
>
> Tobacco use
> Alcohol use
> Dry mouth (mouth breathing, insufficient fluid intake)
> Foods (onion, garlic, meats, nuts)
> Diseases of the mouth or nose (infections, cancer, inflammation)
> Medications (antihistamines, antidepressants)
> Systemic disorders (diabetes, uremia)
> GI disorders (esophageal diverticuli, hiatal hernia, GERD)
> Sinusitis
> Pulmonary disorders (bronchiectasis, pneumonia, neoplasms, TB)

HEADACHE

TABLE 2-29 Clinical Characteristics of Common Headaches

	TENSION	MIGRAINE	SINUSITIS	MASS LESION
Pain				
Location	Bilateral (frontal, occipital, bandlike)	Unilateral (but not always on same side)	Bifrontal (may be unilateral)	Unilateral (always on same side) or bilateral
Character	Pressure	Throbbing	Pressure	Pressure
Severity	Mild to moderate	Moderate to severe	Moderate	Progressively worse as mass expands
Time of occurrence	Late in day or any time	Morning or any time	Worse in morning	Constant (may be intermittent early in course)
Frequency	Several times per week	Less than weekly	Daily until resolved	Constant
Aura	No	Sometimes	No	No
Precipitants	Stress	Bright lights, menstruation, alcohol	None	None but pain aggravated by Valsalva-type provocation
Alleviating factors	Relxation, sleep	Reclining in dark room, migraine-specific drug	Decongestants, antihistamines, antibiotics	None
Associated symptoms	None or stress related	Vomiting, photophobia	Nasal stuffiness or dripping, epistaxis	Projectile vomiting, neurologic symptoms
Age at onset	Any age	10-30 yr	Any age	Any age for primary brain tumor, older for metastatic brain tumor
Gender	Both	Majority female	Both	Both
Family history	Sometimes	Often	No	No
Chronicity	Several months to years	Several months to years	Acute except in allergic rhinitis (may be seasonal)	Progressive

From Wachtel T, Stein M: *Practical guide to the care of the ambulatory patient,* St Louis, 1995, Mosby.

HEADACHES AND FACIAL PAIN

BOX 2-52　A Classification of Headaches and Facial Pain

I. Vascular headaches
  A. Migraine
    1. Migraine with headaches and inconspicuous neurologic features
       a. *Migraine without aura* ("common migraine")
    2. Migraine with headaches and conspicuous neurologic features
       a. With transient neurologic symptoms
          (1) *Migraine with typical aura* ("classical migraine")
          (2) *Sensory, basilar,* and *hemiplegic migraine*
       b. With prolonged or permanent neurologic features ("complicated migraine")
          (1) *Ophthalmoplegic migraine*
          (2) *Migrainous infarction*
    3. Migraine without headaches but with conspicuous neurologic features ("migraine equivalents")
       a. Abdominal migraine
       b. *Benign paroxysmal vertigo of childhood*
       c. *Migraine aura without headache* ("isolated auras," transient migrainous accompaniments)
  B. Cluster headaches
    1. *Episodic cluster headache* ("cyclic cluster headaches")
    2. *Chronic cluster headaches*
    3. *Chronic paroxysmal hemicrania*
  C. Other vascular headaches
    1. Headaches of reactive vasodilatation (fever, drug-induced, postictal, hypoglycemia, hypoxia, hypercarbia, hyperthyroidism).
    2. *Headaches associated with arterial hypertension*
       a. Chronic severe hypertension (diastolic > 120 mm Hg)
       b. Paroxysmal severe hypertension (pheochromocytoma, some coital headaches)
    3. Headaches caused by cranial arteritis
       a. *Giant cell arteritis* ("temporal arteritis")
       b. Other vasculitides
II. Headaches associated with demonstrable muscle spasm
  A. Headache caused by posturally induced or paralesional muscle spasm
    1. Headaches of sustained or impaired posture (e.g., prolonged close work, driving)
    2. Headaches associated with cervical spondylosis and other diseases of cervical spine
    3. Myofascial pain dysfunction syndrome *(headache or facial pain associated with disorders of teeth, jaws, and related structures, or "TMJ syndrome")*
  B. Headaches caused by psychophysiologic muscular contraction ("muscle contraction headaches," or *tension-type headache associated with disorder of pericranial muscles*)
III. Headaches and facial pain without demonstrable physical substrate
  A. Headaches of uncertain etiology
    1. "Tension headaches" *(tension-type headache unassociated with disorder of pericranial muscles)*
    2. Some forms of posttraumatic headache
  B. Psychogenic headaches (e.g., hypochondriacal, conversional, delusional, malingered)
  C. Facial pain of uncertain etiology ("atypical facial pain")
IV. Combined tension-migraine headaches
  A. Episodic migraine superimposed on chronic tension headaches
  B. Chronic daily headaches
    1. Associated with analgesic and/or ergotamine overuse ("rebound headaches")
    2. Not associated with drug overuse
V. Headaches and head pains caused by diseases of eyes, ears, nose, sinuses, teeth, or skull
VI. Headaches caused by meningeal inflammation
  A. Subarachnoid hemorrhage
  B. Meningitis and meningoencephalitis
  C. Others (e.g., meningeal carcinomatosis)
VII. Headaches associated with altered intracranial pressure ("traction headaches")
  A. Increased intracranial pressure
    1. Intracranial mass lesions (neoplasm, hematoma, abscess, etc.)
    2. Hydrocephalus
    3. Benign intracranial hypertension
    4. Venous sinus thrombosis
  B. Decreased intracranial pressure
    1. Post–lumbar puncture headaches
    2. Spontaneous hypoliquorrheic headaches
VIII. Headaches and head pains caused by cranial neuralgias
  A. Presumed irritation of superficial nerves
    1. Occipital neuralgia
    2. Supraorbital neuralgia
  B. Presumed irritation of intracranial nerves
    1. Trigeminal neuralgia ("tic douloureux")
    2. Glossopharyngeal neuralgia

From Stein JH (ed): *Internal medicine,* ed 4, St Louis, 1994, Mosby.

HEARING LOSS, ACUTE

> **BOX 2-53 Common Causes of Sudden Hearing Loss**
>
> **Infectious**
> Mumps
> Measles
> Influenza
> Herpes simplex
> Herpes zoster
> Cytomegalovirus
> Mononucleosis
> Syphilis
>
> **Vascular**
> Macroglobulinemia
> Sickle cell disease
> Berger's disease
> Leukemia
>
> Polycythemia
> Fat emboli
> Hypercoagulable states
>
> **Metabolic**
> Diabetes
> Pregnancy
> Hyperlipoproteinemia
>
> **Conductive**
> Cerumen impaction
> Foreign bodies
> Otitis media
> Otitis externa
> Barotrauma
> Trauma
>
> **Medications**
> Aminoglycosides (gentamicin, theomycin, vancomycin, kanamycin, streptomycin)
> Loop diuretics (furosemide, ethacrynic acid)
> Antineoplastics
> Salicylates
>
> **Neoplasm**
> Acoustic neuroma

From Rosen P et al (eds): *Emergency medicine: concepts and clinical practice,* ed 4, St Louis, 1998, Mosby.

HEMATURIA

> **BOX 2-54 Hematuria**
>
> Use the mnemonic TICS:
>
> **T** (trauma): below to kidney, insertion of Foley catheter or foreign body in urethra, prolonged and severe exercise, very rapid emptying of overdistended bladder
> (tumor): hypernephroma, Wilms' tumor, papillary carcinoma of the bladder, prostatic and urethral neoplasms
> (toxins): turpentine, phenols, sulfonamides and other antibiotics, cyclophosphamide, NSAIDs
>
> **I** (infections): glomerulonephritis, TB, cystitis, prostatitis, urethritis, *Schistosoma haematobium,* yellow fever, blackwater fever
> (inflammatory processes): Goodpasture's syndrome, periarteritis, postirradiation
>
> **C** (calculi): renal, ureteral, bladder, urethra
> (cysts): simple cysts, polycystic disease
> (congenital anomalies): hemangiomas, aneurysms, AVM
>
> **S** (surgery): invasive procedures, prostatic resection, cystoscopy
> (sickle cell disease and other hematologic disturbances): hemophilia, thrombocytopenia, anticoagulants
> (somewhere else): bleeding genitals, factitious (drug addicts)

HEMIPARESIS/HEMIPLEGIA

> **BOX 2-55 Hemiparesis/hemiplegia**
>
> Cerebrovascular accident
> Transient ischemic attack
> Cerebral neoplasm
> Multiple sclerosis or other demyelinating disorder
> CNS infection
> Migraine
> Subdural hematoma
> Vasculitis
> Todd's paralysis
> Epidural hematoma
> Metabolic (hyperosmolar state, electrolyte imbalance)
> Psychiatric disorders
> Congenital disorders
> Leukodystrophies

HEMOPTYSIS

> **BOX 2-56 Hemoptysis**
>
> **Cardiovascular**
> Pulmonary embolism/infarction
> Left ventricular failure
> Mitral stenosis
> AV fistula
> Severe hypertension
> Erosion of aortic aneurysm
>
> **Pulmonary**
> Neoplasm (primary or metastatic)
> Infection
>   Pneumonia: *Streptococcus pneumoniae, Klebsiella pneumoniae, Staphylococcus aureus, Legionella pneumophila*
>   Bronchiectasis
>   Abscess
>   TB
>   Bronchitis
>   Fungal infections (aspergillosis, coccidiodomycosis)
> Parasitic infections (amebiasis, ascariasis, paragonimiasis)
> Vasculitis: Wegener's granulomatosis, Churg-Strauss syndrome, Henoch-Schönlein purpura
> Goodpasture's syndrome
> Trauma (needle biopsy, foreign body, right heart catheterization, prolonged and severe cough)
> Cystic fibrosis, bullous emphysema
> Pulmonary sequestration
> Pulmonary AV fistula
> SLE
> Idiopathic pulmonary hemosiderosis
> Drugs: aspirin, anticoagulants, penicillamine
> Pulmonary hypertension
> Mediastinal fibrosis
>
> **Other**
> Epistaxis, trauma
> Laryngeal bleeding (laryngitis, laryngeal neoplasm)
> Hematologic disorders (clotting abnormalities, DIC, thrombocytopenia)

HEPATOMEGALY

> **BOX 2-57 Hepatomegaly**
>
> **Frequent Jaundice**
> Infectious hepatitis
> Toxic hepatitis
> Carcinoma: liver, pancreas, bile ducts, metastatic neoplasm to liver
> Cirrhosis
> Obstruction of common bile duct
> Alcoholic hepatitis
> Biliary cirrhosis
> Cholangitis
> Hemochromatosis with cirrhosis
>
> **Infrequent Jaundice**
> Congestive heart failure
> Amyloidosis
> Liver abscess
> Sarcoidosis
> Infectious mononucleosis
> Alcoholic fatty infiltration
> Lymphoma
> Leukemia
> Budd-Chiari syndrome
> Myelofibrosis with myeloid metaplasia
> Familial hyperlipoproteinemia type 1
> Other: amebiasis, hydatid disease of liver, schistosomiasis, kala-azar *(Leishmania donovani)*, Hurler's syndrome, Gaucher's disease, kwashiorkor

HIP PAIN IN CHILDREN AND ADULTS

BOX 2-58 Causes of Hip Pain in Children and Adults

Trauma
Fractured proximal femur
Fractured acetabulum
Fractured pelvis
Dislocated hip or prosthesis
Referred pain from knee injury

Infection
Septic hip
Osteomyelitis of proximal femur
Tuberculous synovitis
Referred pain from septic knee or osteomyelitis of distal femur or proximal tibia

Neoplasm
Primary or secondary neoplasm
　Leukemia

Hematologic Conditions
Hemophilia
Sickle cell crisis

Connective Tissue Disorders
Acute rheumatic fever
Juvenile rheumatoid arthritis
Henoch-Schönlein purpura
Other arthritides
Osteoarthritis

Other Causes
Slipped capital femoral epiphysis
Aseptic necrosis
Transient synovitis
Femoral hernia

From Rosen P et al (eds): *Emergency medicine: concepts and clinical practice*, St Louis, 1997, Mosby.

HIRSUTISM AND HYPERTRICHOSIS

BOX 2-59 Differential Diagnosis of Excess Hair in Women

Hirsutism (Increased Sexual Hair)
Most Common
Polycystic ovary syndrome
Idiopathic hirsutism
Medications
　Danazol for endometriosis
　Androgenic oral contraceptives (norgestrel)
Hyperprolactinemia
Hyperthecosis

Less Common
Congenital adrenal hyperplasia
Ovarian tumors
　Sertoli-Leydig cell tumors
　Granulosa-theca cell tumors
　Other tumors that stimulate ovarian stroma
Adrenal tumors
　Cushing's disease
　Other tumors of the adrenal cortex
Severe insulin resistance syndromes

Hypertrichosis (Increased Total Body Hair)—Rare
Drugs
Dilantin
Streptomycin
Hexachlorobenzene
Penicillamine
Diazoxide
Minoxidil
Cyclosporine

Systemic Illness
Hypothyroidism
Anorexia nervosa
Malnutrition
Porphyria
Dermatomyositis

From Carlson KJ et al: *Primary care of women*, St Louis, 1995, Mosby.

HOARSENESS

> **BOX 2-60 Hoarseness**
>
> Allergic rhinitis
> Infections (laryngitis, epiglottitis, tracheitis, croup)
> Vocal cord polyps
> Voice strain
> Irritants (tobacco smoke)
> Vocal cord trauma (intubation, surgery)
> Neoplastic involvement of vocal cord (primary and metastatic)
> Neurologic abnormalities (multiple sclerosis, amyotrophic lateral sclerosis, parkinsonism)
> Endocrine abnormalities (puberty, menopause, hypothyroidism)
> Other (laryngeal webs or cysts, psychogenic, muscle tension abnormalities)

HYPERCALCEMIA, LABORATORY DIFFERENTIAL DIAGNOSIS

TABLE 2-30 Laboratory Differential Diagnosis of Hypercalcemia

DIAGNOSIS	Ca	PO₄	PTH	25(OH)D	1,25(OH)₂D	cAMP	TmP/GFR	Ca	COMMENTS
Primary hyperparathyroidism	↑	N/↓	↑	N	N/↑	↑	↓	↑	Parathyroid adenoma most common
MEN I									Parathyroid hyperplasia; also includes pituitary and pancreatic neoplasms
MEN IIa									Parathyroid hyperplasia; also includes medullary thyroid carcinoma and pheochromocytoma
MEN IIb									Parathyroid disease uncommon, primarily medullary thyroid carcinoma and pheochromocytoma
FHH	↑	N	N/↑	N	N	N/↑	N/↓	↓↓	Autosomal dominant inheritance; hypercalcemia present within first decade; benign
Malignancy									
Solid tumor—humoral	↑	N/↓	↓	N	N	↑	↓	↑↑	Primarily epidermoid tumors; PTH-related protein(s) is mediator
Solid tumor—osteolytic	↑	N/↑	↓	N	N	↓	↑	↑↑	
Lymphoma	↑	N/↑	↓	N/↓	↑	↓	↑	↑↑	
Granulomatous disease	↑	N/↑	↓	N/↓	↑↑	↓	↑	↑↑	Sarcoid most common etiology
Vitamin D intoxication	↑	N/↑	↓	↑↑	N	↓	↑	↑↑	
Hyperthyroidism	↑	N	↓	N	N	N	N	↑↑	Plasma concentrations of T₄ and/or T₃ are elevated

From Moore WT, Eastman RC: *Diagnostic endocrinology*, ed 2, St Louis, 1996, Mosby.
Ca, Calcium; *cAMP*, cyclic adenosine monophosphate; *GFR*, glomerular filtration rate; *FHH*, familial hypocalciuric hypercalcemia; *MEN*, multiple endocrine neoplasia; *25(OH)D*, 25 hydroxyvitamin D; *PO₄*, phosphate; *PTH*, parathormone; *T₃*, triiodothyronine; *T₄*, thyroxine; *TmP*, renal threshold for phosphorus.

HYPERCAPNIA

> **BOX 2-61 Causes of Persistent Hypercapnia**
>
> 1. With normal lungs:
>   a. CNS disturbances (e.g., cerebrovascular disease, Parkinson's disease, encephalitis)
>   b. Metabolic alkalosis
>   c. Myxedema
>   d. Primary alveolar hypoventilation (Ondine's curse)
>   e. Spinal cord lesions
> 2. Diseases of the chest wall (e.g., kyphoscoliosis, ankylosing spondylitis)
> 3. Neuromuscular disorders (e.g., myasthenia gravis, Guillain-Barré syndrome, amyotrophic lateral sclerosis, acid maltase disease, muscular dystrophy, poliomyelitis)
> 4. Chronic obstructive pulmonary disease

From Stein JH (ed): *Internal medicine,* ed 4, St Louis, 1994, Mosby.

HYPERCOAGULABLE STATES

> **BOX 2-62 Hypercoagulable States**
>
> Suspect when unusual, recurrent thromboses or thromboembolism in a young person with no predisposing factors (e.g., surgery)
>
> **Hereditary Disorders**
>
> *Protein C Deficiency (Vitamin K–Dependent Clot Inhibitor)*
>
> Heterozygous autosomal dominant transmission
> Prevalence of 1 in 300 individuals
> Dx by functional and immunoassay of protein C
> Causes disease in newborns, skin necrosis, purpura
> Responsible for up to 10% of thromboses in <45 years of age
>
> *Protein S Deficiency (Vitamin K–Dependent Clot Inhibitor)*
>
> Codominant autosomal transmission
> Prevalence of 1 in 15,000 individuals
> Dx by functional and immunoassay of protein S
> Responsible for 5% to 8% of thromboses in patients <45 years of age
> Often starts in the early teen years
>
> *Antithrombin III (Inhibits Final Coagulation Cascade)*
>
> Autosomal dominant transmission
> Measure antithrombin III levels, Dx if <60% of normal
> Responsible for 2% to 4% of thromboses in patients <45 years of age
> Often starts in early childhood
>
> *Dysfibrinogenemia*
>
> Can be inherited or spontaneous mutation
> Prolonged thrombin time suggests this disorder
>
> **Acquired Disorders**
>
> *IgG Antiphospholipid Antibodies*
>
> Responsible for spontaneous abortion, arterial and venous thrombi
> Lupus anticoagulant present
> PTT that is prolonged and does not correct with a 1:1 mix suggests the Dx
>
> *Malignancy*
>
> Increased platelet adhesion
> Procoagulant factors involved
>
> *Other Conditions*
>
> Surgery, trauma, estrogens, pregnancy, renal disease, sepsis, varicose veins, CHF, myeloproliferative disorder

From Driscoll CE et al: *The family practice desk reference,* ed 3, St Louis, 1996, Mosby.

HYPERINSULINISM

TABLE 2-31 Differential Diagnosis of Hyperinsulinism

| | POSTABSORPTIVE VENOUS PLASMA GLUCOSE <45 MG/DL ||||
	INSULIN	C PEPTIDE	INSULIN ANTIBODIES	OTHER
Exogenous hyperinsulinism	↑	↓†	+	
Endogenous hyperinsulinism				
Insulinoma	↑	↑	—	↑ Proinsulin
Sulfonylurea	↑	↑	—	Positive sulfonylurea assay
Autoimmune hypoglycemia				
Antibodies to insulin	↑↑↑*	↓†	+	
Antibodies to insulin receptor	↑	?	—	Insulin receptor antibodies present; associated autoimmune disorder

From Stein JH (ed): *Internal medicine*, ed 5, St Louis, 1998, Mosby.
*Insulin antibodies artifactually increase insulin levels measured by double-antibody radioimmunoassay.
†Free C-peptide levels are low, but total C-peptide levels may not be because of cross reactivity with antibody-bound proinsulin.

HYPERKALEMIA

BOX 2-63 Causes of Hyperkalemia

I. Pseudohyperkalemia
  A. Hemolysis of sample
  B. Thrombocytosis
  C. Leukocytosis
  D. Laboratory error
II. Increased potassium intake and absorption
  A. Potassium supplements (oral and parenteral)
  B. Dietary—salt substitutes
  C. Stored blood
  D. Potassium-containing medications
III. Impaired renal excretion
  A. Acute renal failure
  B. Chronic renal failure
  C. Tubular defect in potassium secretion
    1. Renal allograft
    2. Analgesic nephropathy
    3. Sickle cell disease
    4. Obstructive uropathy
    5. Interstitial nephritis
    6. Chronic pyelonephritis
    7. Potassium-sparing diuretics
    8. Miscelaneous (lead, systemic lupus erythematosus, pseudohypoaldosteronism)
  D. Hypoaldosteronism
    1. Primary (Addison's disease)
    2. Secondary
      a. Hyporeninemic hypoaldosteronism (type IV RTA)
      b. Congenital adrenal hyperplasia
      c. Drug-induced
        i. Nonsteroidal antiinflammatory medications
        ii. ACE inhibitors
        iii. Heparin
        iv. Cyclosporine
IV. Transcellular shifts
  A. Acidosis
  B. Hypertonicity
  C. Insulin deficiency
  D. Drugs
    1. Beta-blockers
    2. Digitalis toxicity
    3. Succinylcholine
  E. Exercise
  F. Hyperkalemic periodic paralysis
V. Cellular injury
  A. Rhabdomyolysis
  B. Severe intravascular hemolysis
  C. Acute tumor lysis syndrome
  D. Burns and crush injuries

From Rosen P et al (eds): *Emergency medicine: concepts and clinical practice*, ed 4, St Louis, 1998, Mosby.

HYPERKINETIC MOVEMENT DISORDERS

TABLE 2-32 Hyperkinetic Movement Disorders

DISORDER	CLINICAL MANIFESTATIONS	DIFFERENTIAL DIAGNOSIS	TESTS	TREATMENT
Chorea, choreoathetosis, tardive dyskinesia	Continuum of abnormal involuntary movements; jerky, nonrhythmic, semipurposive, predominantly in limbs; may affect head, neck, trunk; lips and tongue may participate (buccolingual dyskinesia); often mixed with writhing (choreoathetosis)	Drug-induced Phenothiazines L-Dopa Phenytoin Cocaine Amphetamines Tricyclics Oral contraceptives	Urine toxic screen	Withdrawal of toxic drug Symptomatic treatment: clonazepam: 0.5 mg bid up to 4-16 mg/day Haloperidol: 0.5-1.0 mg tid up to 5-15 mg/day
		Liver failure	Liver function tests	Treatment of hepatic encephalopathy
		Wilson's disease: dyskinesia accompanied by dystonia, cerebellar ataxia, dysarthria, proximal limb tremor, emotional lability	Slit-lamp examination for Kayser-Fleischer rings; serum ceruloplasmin, serum copper	Penicillamine
		Thyrotoxicosis	Serum thyroxine, TSH	Antithyroid drugs
		Polycythemia	Hematocrit	Phlebotomy
		Systemic lupus erythematosus	Antinuclear antibody	Steroids
		Sydenham's chorea	—	Symptomatic
		Huntington's chorea	Brain CT/MRI, DNA analysis	Symptomatic
Hemiballismus	Large, flinging, ballistic limb movements; predominates in arm or leg	Lacunar CVA in vicinity of subthalamic nuclei in basal ganglia; other focal lesions: metastases and toxoplasmosis (in AIDS)	Brain CT/MRI	Therapy of underlying lesion Symptomatic treatment same as for chorea
Focal dystonia	Spasmodic torticollis	Idiopathic	Clinical	Anticholinergics (high dose): trihexyphenidyl (Artane), 2 mg bid up to 10-40 mg/day Benzodiazepines: clonazepam as above; diazepam, 5 mg bid up to 20-60 mg/day Botulin A toxin: focal injections Surgery: peripheral muscle denervation

DIFFERENTIAL DIAGNOSIS — Hyperkinetic movement disorders

Spasmodic dysphonia (laryngeal) Essential blepharospasm: dystonia of obicularis oculi muscle is principal feature; if accompanied by dystonia of facial, tongue, and neck muscles, called Meige's syndrome	Idiopathic Idiopathic	Botulin A toxin: injection into vocal muscles Clonazepam as above Botulin A toxin: injection into appropriate muscles
Segmental and generalized dystonia — May affect different segments of body or be generalized or multifocal	Idiopathic Hereditary Drug induced: Phenothiazines L-Dopa Calcium channel blockers Wilson's disease Diurnal dystonia: childhood-onset (Segawa disease type) may have parkinsonian features	Symptomatic treamtent: anticholinergics, clonazepam Baclofen: 10 mg bid up to 50-100 mg/day Carbamazepine: 100 mg bid up to 600-1200 mg/day — — — Same as for chorea Familial — Penicillamine plus symptomatic treatment Dramatic response to L-Dopa Carbidopa/L-Dopa: 25/100 mg bid or tid
Acute dystonic reaction — May be segmental or generalized with oculogyric crisis, torticollis, tongue protrusion, opisthotonus; children more susceptible	Drug-induced Prochlorperazine Metoclopramide	Benztropine (Cogentin): 1-2 mg IM Diphenhydramine: 50 mg IM
Paroxysmal dystonia — Kinesigenic: brief attacks of dystonia triggered by sudden movements	Idiopathic or familial	Carbamazepine: 100-200 mg tid Phenytoin: 100 mg tid
Nonkinesigenic dystonia: prolonged paroxysm of dystonia unrelated to activity	Idiopathic or familial	Carbamazepine, clonazepam Acetazolamide (Diamox): 250 mg tid

From Noble J (ed): *Primary care medicine*, ed 2, St Louis, 1996, Mosby.
TSH, Thyroid-stimulating hormone; *CT*, computed tomography; *MRI*, magnetic resonance imaging; *DNA*, deoxyribonucleic acid; *CVA*, cerebrovascular accident; *AIDS*, acquired immunodeficiency syndrome.

HYPERMAGNESEMIA

BOX 2-64 Causes of Hypermagnesemia

I. Decreased renal excretion
   A. Renal failure—glomerular filtration rate less than 30 ml/min
   B. Hyperparathyroidism
   C. Hypothyroidism
   D. Addison's disease
   E. Lithium intoxication
   F. Familial hypocalciuric hypercalcemia
II. Other causes: usually in association with decrease in glomerular filtration rate
   A. Endogenous loads
     1. Diabetic ketoacidosis
     2. Severe tissue injury—burns
   B. Exogenous loads
     1. Gastrointestinal
        a. Magnesium-containing laxatives and antacids
        b. High-dose vitamin D analogs
     2. Parenteral: management of toxemia of pregnancy

From Stein JH (ed): *Internal medicine,* ed 5, St Louis, 1998, Mosby.

HYPERVENTILATION

BOX 2-65 Causes of Persistent Hyperventilation

Fibrotic lung disease
Metabolic acidosis (e.g., diabetes, uremia)
CNS disorders (midbrain and pontine lesions)
Hepatic coma
Salicylate intoxication
Fever
Psychogenic (e.g., anxiety)

From Stein JH (ed): *Internal medicine,* ed 4, St Louis, 1994, Mosby.

HYPOCALCEMIA, LABORATORY DIFFERENTIAL DIAGNOSIS

TABLE 2-33 Laboratory Differential Diagnosis of Hypocalcemia

	PLASMA TESTS					URINE TESTS				
DIAGNOSIS	Ca	PO₄	PTH	25(OH)D	1,25(OH)₂D	cAMP	cAMP AFTER PTH	TmP/GFR	TmP/GFR AFTER PTH	Ca	COMMENTS
Hypoparathyroidism	↓	↑	N/↓	N	↓	↓	↑↑	↑	↓↓	N/↓	Deficiency of PTH
Pseudohypoparathyroidism Type I	↓	↑	↑↑	N	↓	↓	NC	↑	↑	N/↓	Resistance to PTH; patients may have Albright's hereditary osteodystrophy and resistance to multiple hormones
Type II	↓	N	↑↑	N	↓	↓	↑	↑	↑	N/↓	Renal resistance to cAMP
Vitamin D deficiency	↓	N/↓	↑↑	↓↓	N/↓	↑	↑	↑	↑	↓↓	Deficient supply (e.g., nutrition) or absorption (e.g., pancreatic insufficiency) of vitamin D
Vitamin D–dependent rickets Type I	↓	N/↓	↑↑	N	↓	↑		↑		↓↓	Deficient activity of renal 25(OH)D-1α-hydroxylase
Type II	↓	N/↓	↑↑	N	↑↑	↑		↑		↓↓	Resistance to 1,25(OH)₂D

From Moore WT, Eastman RC: *Diagnostic endocrinology*, ed 2, St Louis, 1996, Mosby.
Ca, Calcium; *cAMP*, cyclic adenosine monophosphate; *GFR*, glomerular filtration rate; *FHH*, familial hypocalciuric hypercalcemia; *MEN*, multiple endocrine neoplasia; *NC*, no change or small increase; *(OH)D*, hydroxycalciferol D; *PO₄*, phosphate; *PTH*, parathyroid hormone; *T₃*, triiodothyronine; *T₄*, thyroxine; *TmP*, renal threshold for phosphorus.

HYPOGLYCEMIA SYNDROMES, TEST RESULTS

TABLE 2-34 Hypoglycemia Syndromes, Test Results

CASE		GLUCOSE (MG/DL)	INSULIN (µU/ML, <6 µU/ML)	TOTAL CPR (NG/ML, <0.9 NG/ML)	FREE CPR (NG/ML, <0.9 NG/ML)	IA	SULFONYLUREA ASSAY HPLC	GCMS
1	Insulinoma	35	10	2	2	Absent	Absent	—
2	Factitious insulin	39	5067	0.56	—	Present	Absent	—
3	Factitious insulin	25	4600	4.41	0.65	Present	Absent	—
4	Factitious sulfonylurea	35	25	9	9	Absent	Present	Present
5	Pseudofactitious sulfonylurea (insulinoma)	27	7	2.4	—	Absent	Present	Absent

From Moore WT, Eastman RC: *Diagnostic endocrinology*, ed 2, St Louis, 1996, Mosby.
CPR, C-peptide immunoreactivity; *GCMS*, gas chromatography mass spectroscopy; *HPLC*, high-performance liquid chromatography; *IA*, antiinsulin antibodies; —, not done.

HYPOGONADISM

> **BOX 2-66** **Causes of Hypogonadism**
>
> ### Primary (Hypergonadotropic) Hypogonadism
> Gonadal defects
>   Genetic defect
>   Klinefelter's syndrome
>   Myotonic dystrophy
>   Polyglandular autoimmune disease
>   Other genetic syndromes
>   Anatomic defect (including castration)
>   Defect caused by toxins
>   Drugs (cytotoxins and spironolactone)
>   Radiation
>   Alcohol
>   Viral orchitis (mumps most common)
> Hormone resistance
>   Androgen insensitivity
>   Luteinizing hormone insensitivity
>
> ### Secondary (Hypogonadotropic) Hypogonadism
> Organic causes
>   Panhypopituitarism
>   Idiopathic
>   Pituitary or hypothalamic tumor
>   Miscellaneous
>   Granulomatous disease
>   Vasculitis
>   Hemochromatosis
>   Infarction
>   Trauma
>   Hyperprolactinemia
>   Isolated gonadotropin deficiency
>   Kallmann's syndrome variants
>   Idiopathic hypothalamic hypogonadism
>   Isolated deficiency of luteinizing hormone or follicle-stimulating hormone
>   Genetic disorder
>   Prader-Willi syndrome
>   Laurence-Moon-Biedl syndrome
>   Systemic disorder
>   Chronic disease
>   Nutritional deficiency or starvation
>   Massive obesity
>   Drugs
>   Glucocorticoids
> Constitutional cause (delayed puberty)

From Bagatell CJ, Bremner WJ: Androgens in men, uses and abuses, *N Engl J Med* 334:707-714, 1996.

HYPOKALEMIA

> **BOX 2-67 Causes of Hypokalemia**
>
> I. Decreased intake
>   A. Decreased dietary potassium
>   B. Impaired absorption of potassium
>   C. Clay ingestion
>   D. Kayexalate
> II. Increased loss
>   A. Renal
>   1. Hyperaldosteronism
>   a. Primary
>   1. Conn's syndrome
>   2. Adrenal hyperplasia
>   b. Secondary
>   1. CHF
>   2. Cirrhosis
>   3. Nephrotic syndrome
>   4. Dehydration
>   c. Bartter's syndrome
>   2. Glycyrrhizic acid (licorice, chewing tobacco)
>   3. Excessive adrenal corticosteroids
>   a. Cushing's syndrome
>   b. Steroid therapy
>   c. Adrenogenital syndrome
>   4. Renal tubular defects
>   a. Renal tubular acidosis
>   b. Obstructive uropathy
>   c. Salt-wasting nephropathy
>   5. Drugs
>   a. Diuretics
>   b. Aminoglycosides
>   c. Mannitol
>   d. Amphotericin
>   e. Cisplantin
>   f. Carbenicillin
>   B. Gastrointestinal
>   1. Vomiting
>   2. Nasogastric suction
>   3. Diarrhea
>   4. Malabsorption
>   5. Ileostomy
>   6. Villous adenoma
>   7. Laxative abuse
>   C. Increased losses from the skin
>   1. Excessive sweating
>   2. Burns
> III. Transcellular shifts
>   A. Alkalosis
>   1. Vomiting
>   2. Diuretics
>   3. Hyperventilation
>   4. Bicarbonate therapy
>   B. Insulin
>   1. Exogenous
>   2. Endogenous response to glucose
>   C. β_2-Agonists (albuterol, terbutaline, epinephrine)
>   D. Hypokalemia periodic paralysis
>   1. Familial
>   2. Thyrotoxic
> IV. Miscellaneous
>   A. Anabolic state
>   B. IV hyperalimentation
>   C. Treatment of megaloblastic anemia
>   D. Acute mountain sickness

From Rosen P et al (eds): *Emergency medicine: concepts and clinical practice,* ed 4, St Louis, 1998, Mosby.

HYPOMAGNESEMIA

BOX 2-68　Causes of Hypomagnesemia

Alcoholic abuse

Diuretic use

Renal losses
Acute and chronic renal failure
Postobstructive diuresis
Acute tubular necrosis
Chronic glomerulonephritis
Chronic pyelonephritis
Interstitial nephropathy
Renal transplantation

GI losses
Chronic diarrhea
Nasogastric suctioning
Short bowel syndrome

Protein calorie malnutrition
Bowel fistula
Total parenteral nutrition
Acute pancreatitis

Endocrine
Diabetes mellitus
Hyperaldosteronism
Hyperthyroidism
Hyperparathyroidism
Acute intermittent porphyria

Pregnancy

Drugs
Aminoglycosides
Amphotericin
β-Agonists
Cisplatin
Cyclosporine
Diuretics
Foscarnet
Pentamidine
Theophylline

Congenital disorders
Familial hypomagnesemia
Maternal diabetes
Maternal hypothyroidism
Maternal hyperparathyroidism

From Rosen P et al (eds): *Emergency medicine: concepts and clinical practice,* ed 4, St Louis, 1998, Mosby.

IMPOTENCE

BOX 2-69　Causes of Impotence

Psychogenic
Primary or secondary

Endocrine
Hypothalamic-pituitary-testicular axis
Thyroid: hyperthyroidism, hypothyroidism
Hyperprolactinemia
Diabetes mellitus
Cushing's syndrome

Vascular
Arterial insufficiency
Venous leakage
Arteriovenous malformation
Local trauma

Medications

Neurogenic
Peripheral neuropathy: autonomic or sensory neuropathy
Spinal cord: trauma, tumor
Central nervous system: stroke, multiple sclerosis, temporal lobe epilepsy
Neurotransmitters

Systemic Illness
Renal failure
Chronic obstructive pulmonary disease
Cirrhosis of liver
Myotonia dystrophy

Peyronie's Disease

Prostatectomy

Multiple Causes

From Moore WT, Eastman RC: *Diagnostic endocrinology,* ed 2, St Louis, 1996, Mosby.

INFECTIOUS DISEASES IN COMPROMISED HOST

TABLE 2-35 Patterns of Infection in Patients with Impaired Host Defense Mechanisms

HOST DEFENSE MECHANISM IMPAIRED	CAUSE OF IMPAIRMENT	SITE OF INFECTION	COMMON INFECTING AGENTS
I. Anatomic and physiologic barriers to infection		Recurrent at site of abnormality	
A. Skin	Dermatitis Burns IV catheters	Skin → blood	Staphylococci, streptococci, GNR
B. Skull	Skull fracture Cerebrospinal fluid leak	Meninges	Depends on site of leak: predominantly pneumococci but occasionally staphylococci or GNR if a dermal sinus is present
C. Mucociliary elevator	Alcohol Smoking Endotracheal tube Obstruction Immotile cilia (Kartagener's syndrome)	Bronchi, lungs	Colonizing flora
D. Gastric acid	Surgery, pernicious anemia, antacids	Intestine	*Salmonella* *Mycobacterium tuberculosis* Cholera
E. Intestinal motility or mucosal barrier	Blind loop syndrome, obstruction, tumor	Intestine → blood	Colonizing flora (*Streptococcus bovis*, clostridia, usually in the presence of a colonic neoplasm)
F. Urinary tract	Obstruction Catheterization Stones	Upper or lower urinary tract → blood	*Escherichia coli* "Urea splitters": *Proteus, Providencia*
G. Lymphatics	Obstruction	Lymphangitis	Group A streptococci
II. Immunologic barriers to infection			
A. Antibody IgG		Blood, meninges, bronchopulmonary tree, sinuses, ears, intestine	Encapsulated bacteria* Enteroviruses *Giardia lamblia* *Pneumocystis carinii*
IgM IgA	Acquired or inherited	Blood Bronchopulmonary tree, sinuses	Meningococci, GNR Colonizing flora
B. Complement	Acquired or inherited	Blood, meninges, bronchopulmonary tree, sinuses, ears	Encapsulated bacteria* Disseminated gonococcal infection

C. Cell-mediated immunity	Acquired or inherited	Lungs, meninges, gastrointestinal tract	Bacteria
			  Listeria
			  M. tuberculosis
			  Atypical mycobacteria
			Viruses
			  Herpes simplex
			  Cytomegalovirus
			  Varicella zoster (shingles)
			Fungi
			  Candida
			  Cryptococcus
			Protozoa
			  P. carinii
			  Toxoplasma gondii
			  Cryptosporidium

TABLE 2-35 Patterns of Infection in Patients with Impaired Host Defense Mechanisms—cont'd

HOST DEFENSE MECHANISM IMPAIRED	CAUSE OF IMPAIRMENT	SITE OF INFECTION	COMMON INFECTING AGENTS
D. Phagocytic function			
1. Neutrophils			
Deficient numbers ($<500/mm^3$)	Neoplasia Cytotoxic chemotherapy Autoimmune neutropenia	Skin, soft tissue, lung, blood	Staphylococci, GNR, *Candida*, *Aspergillus*
Defective function	Chronic granulomatous disease	Skin, soft tissue, lung, blood, bone, liver	Staphylococci, GNR, *Nocardia*, *Candida*, *Aspergillus*
	Job's (hyperimmunoglobulinemia E) syndrome	Skin, soft tissue	Staphylococci
	Chediak-Higashi syndrome	Skin, soft tissue	Staphylococci
	Myeloperoxidase deficiency	Lung	*Candida*
2. Reticuloendothelial function	Asplenia Hemoglobinopathies	Blood	Encapsulated bacteria*
	Cirrhosis	Blood	GNR

From Stein JH (ed): *Internal medicine,* ed 5, St Louis, 1998, Mosby.
GNR, gram-negative rods; IgA, IgG, and IgM, immunoglobulins A, G, and M.
Streptococcus pneumoniae, Haemophilus influenzae, Neisseria meningitidis.

INFECTIOUS DISEASES IN TRAVELERS

TABLE 2-36 Infectious Disease in Travelers Categorized According to Approximate Time After Exposure When Patients are Likely to Present with Evidence of Disease

3 DAYS OR LESS	3 TO 28 DAYS	1 TO 6 MO	6 TO 18 MO	SEVERAL YR
Cholera	Amebiasis	Amebiasis	Amebiasis	Amebiasis
Diarrhea from *Campylobacter, E. coli,* or *Vibrio* sp.	Bartonellosis	Ascariasis	Ascariasis	Chagas' disease, chronic phase
Plague	Brucellosis	Bartonellosis	Clonorchiasis	Clonorchiasis
Salmonellosis	Chagas' disease, acute phase	Brucellosis	Cutaneous leishmaniasis	
Shigellosis	Dengue fever	Chagas' disease, acute phase	Fascioliasis	Hookworm infection
Viral gastroenteritis	Diarrhea from *Campylobacter*	Clonorchiasis	Fasciolopsiasis	Mucocutaneous leishmaniasis
	Giardiasis	Cutaneous leishmaniasis	Loiasis	Paragonimiasis
	Hemorrhagic fevers	Fascioliasis	Malaria	Schistosomiasis, chronic
	Hepatitis A	Fasciolopsiasis	Onchocerciasis	Strongyloidiasis
	Leptospirosis	Hepatitis A	Paragonimiasis	Tapeworm infection
	Malaria	Hepatitis B	Sleeping sickness	Tropical sprue
	Meningococcal disease	Hookworm disease	Strongyloidiasis	
	Paragonimiasis	Kala-azar	Tropical sprue	
	Plague	Malaria		
	Polio	Paragonimiasis		
	Relapsing fever	Relapsing fever		
	Sleeping sickness	Schistosomiasis, acute		
	Tularemia	Sleeping sickness		
	Typhoid fever	Strongyloidiasis		
	Typhus	Tropical sprue		

From Stein JH (ed): *Internal medicine,* ed 4, St Louis, 1994, Mosby.

INSOMNIA IN THE ELDERLY

TABLE 2-37 Causes of Insomnia in Elderly Persons

	INSOMNIA			
CAUSE	SLEEP ONSET PROBLEMS	NIGHTTIME AWAKENINGS	EARLY AWAKENINGS	EXCESSIVE DAYTIME SLEEPINESS
Advanced sleep phase syndrome			++++*	
Central sleep apnea		++		++
Dementia	++	++++	+	+++
Depression	++	+	++++	+
Fibromyalgia		++		+++
Hypnotic-dependent sleep disorder	++++	++		++
Inadequate sleep hygiene	+++			+
Narcolepsy		+		++++
Obstructive sleep apnea		++		++++
Pain	++	+++	+	+
Parkinsonism and movement disorders	++	++		
Periodic leg movements of sleep		+++		+++
Psychophysiologic insomnia	++++			+
REM behavioral disorder		±		
Restless leg syndrome	++++			+
Sleep bruxism		++		+
Sleep-related asthma		++		
Sleep-related gastroesophageal reflux		++		+

From Yoshikawa TT, Cobbs EL, Brummel-Smith K: *Ambulatory geriatric care,* St Louis, 1993, Mosby.
*Range of involvement: +, minimal involvement; ++++, major involvement.

INTESTINAL HELMINTHS

TABLE 2-38 Intestinal Helminths

FAMILY	SPECIES	TRANSMISSION	MAJOR CLINICAL PRESENTATION	EOSINOPHILIA	DIAGNOSIS (ADULTS)	TREATMENT
Strictly Intestinal Helminths						
Nematode	*Enterobius vermicularis* (pinworm)	Fecal-oral	Perianal pruritus	No	Cellophane tape applied to rectum	Mebendazole 100 mg once (repeat in 2 wk) or pyrantel pamoate 11 mg/kg (max, 1 g), or albendazole 400 mg/kg once
Nematode	*Trichuris trichiura* (whipworm)	Fecal-oral	Diarrhea, rectal prolapse	No	Stool O&P	Albendazole* 400-600 µg/hg once or 400 mg/hg daily for 3 days, or mebendazole 100 mg bid for 3 days
Cestode	*Taenia saginata* (beef tapeworm)	Ingestion of raw beef	Passage of proglottids	No	Proglottid in stool	Niclosamide 2 g once or praziquantel* 5-10 mg/kg once
Cestode	*Taenia solium* (pork tapeworm)	Ingestion of raw pork	Passage of proglottids	No (yes in cysticercosis)	Stool O&P for intestinal infection	Praziquantel 5-10 mg/kg once for intestinal infection
Cestode	*Diphyllobothrium latum* (fish tapeworm)	Ingestion of raw fish	Vitamin B_{12} deficiency	No	Stool O&P	Same as for *T. saginata*
Cestode	*Hymenolepsis nana* (dwarf tapeworm)	Fecal-oral	Diarrhea, dizziness in children	Yes	Stool O&P	Praziquantel 25 mg/kg once
Trematode	*Fasciolopsis buski*	Ingestion of raw water chestnuts or bamboo	Diarrhea, intestinal or biliary obstruction	Yes	Stool O&P	Praziquantel 25 mg/kg tid for 1 day or niclosamide 2 g once
Trematode	*Heterophyes heterophyes*	Ingestion of raw fish	Diarrhea, abdominal pain	Yes	Stool O&P	Praziquantel 25 mg/kg tid for 1 day
Trematode	*Metagonimus yokogawai*	Ingestion of raw fish	Diarrhea	Yes	Stool O&P	Praziquantel 25 mg/kg tid for 1 day
Trematode	*Echinostoma ilocanum*	Ingestion of raw fish	Diarrhea	Yes	Stool O&P	Praziquantel* 25 mg/kg tid for 1 day
Nematode	*Ascaris lumbricoides* (giant roundworm)	Fecal-oral	PIE, intestinal or biliary	During migration, obstruction	Stool O&P	Mebendazole 100 mg PO bid for 3 days or albendazole* 400 µg/kg once or pyrantel pamoate 11 mg/kg once

Continued

TABLE 2-38 Intestinal Helminths—cont'd

FAMILY	SPECIES	TRANSMISSION	MAJOR CLINICAL PRESENTATION	EOSINOPHILIA	DIAGNOSIS (ADULTS)	TREATMENT
Nematode	*Ancylostoma duodenale* (hookworm)	Skin penetration	PIE, iron deficiency anemia, dermatitis	During migration	Stool O&P	Mebendazole 100 mg PO bid for 3 days, albendazole 400 µg/kg once, or pyrantel pamoate* 11 mg/kg (max, 1 g) for 3 days
Nematode	*Necator duodenale* (hookworm)	Skin penetration	PIE, iron deficiency anemia, dermatitis	During migration	Stool O&P	Same as for *A. duodenale*
Nematode	*Strongyloides stercoralis*	Skin penetration	PIE, diarrhea, malabsorption Hyperinfection syndrome	Yes	Stool O&P	Thiabendazole 25 mg/kg bid for 2 days, 5 days for disseminated infection, or albendazole*† 400 mg daily for 3 days, or ivermectin* 200 µg/kg/day for 1-2 days

From Stein JH (ed): *Internal medicine*, ed 5, St Louis, 1998, Mosby.
O&P, Ova and parasites; *PO*, orally; *bid*, twice a day; *tid*, three times a day.
*Considered an investigational drug by the US Food and Drug Administration.
†Should be considered experimental treatment.

INTESTINAL PSEUDO-OBSTRUCTION

BOX 2-70 Classification of Intestinal Pseudo-obstruction

I. "Primary" (idiopathic intestinal pseudo-obstruction)
  A. Hollow visceral myopathy
    1. Familial
    2. Sporadic
  B. Neuropathic
    1. Abnormal myenteric plexus
    2. Normal myenteric plexus
II. Secondary
  A. Scleroderma
  B. Myxedema
  C. Amyloidosis
  D. Muscular dystrophy
  E. Hypokalemia
  F. Chronic renal failure
  G. Diabetes mellitus
  H. Drug toxicity caused by
    1. Anticholinergics
    2. Opiate narcotics
  I. Ogilvie's syndrome

From Stein JH (ed): *Internal medicine*, ed 4, St Louis, 1994, Mosby.

JAUNDICE

BOX 2-71 Jaundice

Predominance of Direct (Conjugated) Bilirubin

Extrahepatic obstruction:
  Common duct abnormalities: calculi, neoplasm, stricture, cyst, sclerosing cholangitis
  Metastatic carcinoma
  Pancreatic carcinoma, pseudocyst
  Ampullary carcinoma
Hepatocellular disease: hepatitis, cirrhosis
Drugs: estrogens, phenothiazines, captopril, methyltestosterone, labetalol
Cholestatic jaundice of pregnancy

Hereditary disorders: Dubin-Johnson syndrome, Rotor's syndrome
Recurrent benign intrahepatic cholestasis

Predominance of Indirect (Unconjugated) Bilirubin

Hemolysis: hereditary and acquired hemolytic anemias
Inefficient marrow production
Impaired hepatic conjugation: chloramphenicol, pregnanediol
Neonatal jaundice
Hereditary disorders: Gilbert's syndrome, Crigler-Najjar syndrome

JUGULAR VENOUS DISTENTION

BOX 2-72 Jugular Venous Distention

Right-sided heart failure
Cardiac tamponade
Constrictive pericarditis
Goiter
Tension pneumothorax
Pulmonary hypertension
Cardiomyopathy (restrictive)
Superior vena cava syndrome
Valsalva
Right atrial myxoma
Chronic obstructive pulmonary disease

KNEE PAIN

TABLE 2-39 Selected Causes of Knee Pain

DISORDER	EPIDEMIOLOGY	HISTORY	PHYSICAL EXAMINATION	DIAGNOSTIC TESTS	DIFFERENTIAL DIAGNOSIS	MANAGEMENT
Gout	Middle age, elderly, overproducers of urate, transplant patients	Acute onset of pain, often with previous attack in first MTP	Warmth, erythema, effusion, exquisite tenderness	High synovial WBC, urate crystals seen under polarizing microscope, "rat bite" erosions on radiograph	Rheumatoid arthritis, spondylitis, other crystal-induced arthropathy, infection	NSAIDs, colchicine, local corticosteroid injection acutely, allopurinol or uricosuric long-term
Pseudogout	Elderly, patients with metabolic disorders such as hypothyroidism, hypomagnesemia, ochronosis, hemochromatosis, Wilson's disease, hyperparathyroidism	Acute onset of pain, if metabolic disease, systemic complaints	Similar to gout	High synovial WBC, calcium pyrophosphate crystals seen under polarizing microscope, chondrocalcinosis on radiograph; if clinically indicated, serum iron studies, magnesium, phosphate, calcium, ceruloplasmin, thyroid studies	Gout, rheumatoid arthritis, spondylitis, infection	NSAIDs, colchicine, local corticosteroid injection acutely, daily colchicine as prophylaxis against further attacks
Rheumatoid arthritis	Age varies, usually female	Morning stiffness, involvement of joints of the hand, multiple joint involvement, fatigue, multiple attacks	Warmth, erythema with effusion, if long-standing "boggy" synovium, symmetrical involvement of joints, decreased ROM	High synovial WBC, RF often positive, elevated ESR, anemia, consistent with chronic disease, bone erosions on radiographs	Crystal-induced arthropathy, spondylitis, infection	NSAIDs, local corticosteroid injection, second-line agents such as methotrexate and gold
Spondyloarthropathy (reactive arthritis, Reiter's syndrome)	Young adults, male predominance; patients with associated disorders such as IBD, psoriasis, *Chlamydia*, *Yersinia*, or *Shigella* infection, ankylosing spondylitis; acute or subacute onset of pain, often associated with low back pain and pain in other joints, may have a component of morning stiffness, may have systemic complaints related to underly-	Acute or subacute onset of pain, often associated with low back pain and pain in other joints, may have a component of morning stiffness, may have systemic complaints related to underlying condition	Warmth, erythema, with effusion; may have "boggy" synovium if disease is long-standing; may have evidence of underlying disease, such as oral ulcers, rash, nail changes, decreased ROM of spine	High synovial WBC, erosions on radiograph, sacroiliitis on radiograph, squaring of vertebral bodies, syndesmophytes	Rheumatoid arthritis, crystal-induced arthritis, infection	NSAIDs, local corticosteroid injection, sulfasalazine, methotrexate

DIFFERENTIAL DIAGNOSIS   Knee pain   611

Gonococcal infection	Young adults predominantly, but any age if sexually active	Acute onset of symptoms, may complain of GU symptoms, recent menses, general malaise	Warmth, erythema, with very large tense effusion, decreased ROM, maculopapular rash over trunk, fever, urethral or cervical discharge, arthritis of other joints, tenosynovitis	High synovial WBC, positive culture for Gc from GU tract, blood, or synovial fluid	Rheumatoid arthritis, spondylitis, crystal-induced arthropathy, nongonococcal infection, Lyme disease	Ceftriaxone or penicillin G for sensitive strains
Nongonococcal infection	IV drug abusers, severely debilitated, patients prone to fulminant sepsis or endocarditis	Acute onset of severe pain, swelling, redness, decreased ROM, may have associated systemic symptoms, may have arthritis in other joints	Warmth, erythema, effusion, decreased ROM, signs of source for bacteremia (e.g., pneumonia, UTI, etc.)	Very high synovial WBC, positive synovial or blood culture or Gram's stain, high ESR, elevated peripheral blood WBC, periosteal elevation on radiograph suggests concomitant osteomyelitis	Rheumatoid arthritis, spondylitis, crystal-induced arthritis, gonococcal infection	IV antibiotic therapy guided by Gram's stain, culture results, and sensitivities; drain with needle aspiration or arthroscopically, ROM exercises, and analgesics
Lyme disease	Those who have traveled to or live in endemic areas	Subacute onset of symptoms, swelling, warmth, decreased ROM, pain, history of ECM skin lesion(s), Bell's palsy, other painful joints	Warmth, erythema, effusion, may have "boggy" synovium	Lyme titers, synovial fluid culture rarely positive, radiographs may eventually show erosions	Rheumatoid arthritis, spondylitis, gonococcal and other nongonococcal infection, crystal-induced arthropathy	IV penicillin G or ceftriaxone
Fracture	Any age, risk factors include steroid use, osteoporosis or other causes, metastatic malignancy	History of trauma, sudden-onset pain, swelling, warmth	Swelling, tenderness over affected area, pain on weight bearing, decreased ROM	Bloody synovial fluid, may show fat droplets under polarizing microscopy, fracture seen on radiograph, bone scan may detect stress fractures inapparent on radiograph	Meniscal tear, ligamentous tear, hemophilia, PVNS, anticoagulant therapy	Splinting to protect against additional neurovascular injury, reduction, and casting
Ligamentous injury	Young adults, athletes	Trauma with pivoting or hyperextension, feeling of "giving way," acute pain and swelling	Swelling, point tenderness medial or lateral joint line, positive anterior or posterior drawer sign, medial or lateral laxity depending on ligament disrupted	Bloody or serosanguineous noninflammatory synovial fluid, radiographs to rule out fracture, MRI reveals high T_2 signal in area of ligamentous tear	Meniscal tear, fracture, hemophilia, PVNS, anticoagulant therapy	Analgesics, knee immobilizer, orthopedic consultation for possible surgical repair for complete tears in patients who are active

Continued

612 Knee pain — DIFFERENTIAL DIAGNOSIS

TABLE 2-39 Selected Causes of Knee Pain—cont'd

DISORDER	EPIDEMIOLOGY	HISTORY	PHYSICAL EXAMINATION	DIAGNOSTIC TESTS	DIFFERENTIAL DIAGNOSIS	MANAGEMENT
Meniscal tear	Two groups: elderly with OA and young adults, athletes	Acute or subacute onset of pain, locking, painful popping	Swelling, tenderness over the lateral or medial joint line, positive McMurray's test	Bloody or serosanguineous synovial fluid, radiograph to rule out fracture, MRI, arthrography, or arthroscopy diagnostic	Fracture, ligamentous tear, hemophilia, PVNS, anticoagulant therapy, worsening osteoarthritis	Initial conservative (rest, NSAIDs); if unsuccessful, orthopedic referral for arthroscopic debridement, or total knee replacement if concomitant severe osteoarthritis
Osteonecrosis/avascular necrosis	Any age, patients with sickle cell anemia, chronic steroid use, alcoholism, decompression illness, trauma, SLE, dyslipoproteinemia	Acute onset of pain, swelling, rest pain, increased pain with weight bearing	Swelling, tenderness, decreased ROM	Area of subchondral collapse appears after weeks on plain radiograph, MRI most sensitive for AVN before subchondral collapse	Tumor, fracture, osteomyelitis, osteoarthritis, meniscal tear	Initial conservative (non-weight bearing, NSAIDs, analgesics); if unsuccessful, tibial osteotomy, hemiarthroplasty, or total knee replacement
Osgood-Schlatter syndrome	Young adolescents	Pain at the inferior aspect of the patella, subacute to chronic onset	Tenderness to palpation, occasionally swelling in region of tibial tubercle	None	Fracture, tendinitis of patellar tendon, tumor, osteomyelitis	Reassurance, analgesics
Chondromalacia	Young active persons, either gender	Subacute onset of patellar pain, worse walking stairs, little pain at rest	Reproduction of pain on pressing patella against femoral condyles	Synovial fluid noninflammatory, sunrise radiograph may reveal irregularity of articulating surface of patella	Tendinitis, bursitis, meniscal injury	Quadriceps isometric strengthening exercises, NSAIDs, or pure analgesics
Anserine bursitis	Middle age, elderly with OA, young active patients	Subacute onset of pain localized to the posteromedial aspect of the knee	Point tenderness over anserine bursa, rarely palpable swelling	None	Osteoarthritis, medial meniscus injury	NSAIDs, local heat, local corticosteroid injection
Prepatellar bursitis	Those who kneel on hard surfaces, especially carpenters, plumbers, roofers, carpet layers	Subacute onset of pain in prepatellar area, swelling, erythema, desquamation or purulent discharge suggests septic bursitis	Tenderness, erythema, fluctuant swelling of bursa anterior to patella, knee flexion may be limited but full extension possible without increased pain	Bursal aspirate, culture, Gram's stain, crystal search	Cellulitis, gouty bursitis, hemobursa, septic bursitis, patellar fracture, fat necrosis, erythema nodosum	If septic: antibiotics, repeated needle aspiration for drainage; if nonseptic: NSAIDs, local heat, activity modification

DIFFERENTIAL DIAGNOSIS — Knee pain

Osteoarthritis	Middle-aged, elderly, athletes, obese, those with prior knee trauma	Progressive, slowly increasing pain, stiffness, decreased ROM over years, "cracking" of joint, no rest pain unless very advanced arthritis, short-lived morning stiffness (minutes)	Decreased ROM, swelling, crepitation, bony prominence	Synovial fluid noninflammatory, osteophyte formation, subchondral cysts, sclerosis, joint space narrowing seen on radiograph	Inflammatory arthritis, meniscal tear, anserine bursitis, secondary forms of osteoarthritis: hemochromatosis, Wilson's disease, ochronosis, gout, acromegaly, hypothyroidism, hyperparathyroidism	Analgesics or NSAIDs, quadriceps strengthening exercises, weight loss if appropriate, use of cane. Consider surgical intervention (tibial osteotomy or total knee replacement) for unremitting pain
Synovial chondromatosis	Wide age range, either gender	Slowly progressing pain, swelling, stiffness	Swelling with effusion, diffuse tenderness	Multiple calcific densities and effusion on plain radiograph, noncalcified chondral bodies may only be apparent on MRI, arthrography, or arthroscopy	Other synovial tumors, inflammatory arthritis, pigmented villonodular synovitis, avascular necrosis with loose osteochondral fragments	Surgical synovectomy, total knee replacement if advanced disease with articular cartilage destruction
Pigmented villonodular synovitis	Young adults	Recurrent knee pain and swelling	Erythema, swelling, limited ROM, and tenderness	Synovial fluid reddish brown, noninflammatory; effusion or soft tissue swelling, joint space narrowing, and erosions may be seen on plain radiograph MRI suggestive, synovial biopsy definitive	Inflammatory arthritis, recurrent hemorrhage, synovial chondromatosis	Surgical synovectomy or radiation synovectomy
Malignancy	Metastatic cancer most common, primary bone and soft tissue sarcomas less likely, leukemia, lymphoma, and myeloma	Slowly worsening pain, swelling, stiffness, prominent night pain is suggestive	Decreased ROM, diffuse tenderness, effusion	Synovial fluid with lymphocytic predominance, tumor cells sometimes seen, periosteal disruption or lytic bone lesions on plain radiograph; MRI defines bone and soft tissue involvement; biopsy if no known primary	Inflammatory arthritis, benign tumors, osteomyelitis	Primary tumors: surgical excision or amputation, adjuvant chemotherapy or radiation therapy. Metastatic tumors: radiation therapy for pain control, other treatment based on type of malignancy

From Noble J (ed): *Primary care medicine*, ed 2, St Louis, 1996, Mosby.
MTP, Metatarsophalangeal joint; *WBC*, white blood cell; *NSAIDs*, nonsteroidal antiinflammatory drugs; *ROM*, range of motion; *RF*, rheumatoid factor; *ESR*, erythrocyte sedimentation rate; *IBD*, inflammatory bowel disease; *GU*, genitourinary; *GC*, gonococci; *UTI*, urinary tract infection; *ECM*, erythema chronicum migrans; *PVNS*, pigmented villonodular synovitis; *OA*, osteoarthritis; *SLE*, systemic lupus erythematosus; *AVN*, avascular necrosis.

LEG CRAMPS, NOCTURNAL

BOX 2-73 Nocturnal Leg Cramps

Diabetic neuropathy
Medications
Electrolyte abnormalities (hypokalemia, hyponatremia, hypoglycemia, hypocalcemia, hyperkalemia, hypermagnesemia)
Respiratory alkalosis
Uremia
Hemodialysis
Peripheral nerve injury
ALS
Alcohol use
Heat cramps
Vitamin B_{12} deficiency
Hyperthyroidism
Contractures
DVT
Peripheral vascular insufficiency

LEG PAIN WITH EXERCISE

TABLE 2-40 Differential Diagnosis of Leg Pain with Exercise

	SEX	AGE	FREQUENCY	CAUSE	PULSES
Arteriosclerosis obliterans	M > F	Seventh decade	Very common	Occluded or stenosed large or medium size arteries; lower extremity involvement	Abnormal
Neurogenic	M = F	Sixth-seventh decade	Common	Spinal cord compression or ischemia	Normal
Thromboangiitis obliterans	M >> F	Third-fourth decade	Rare	Vasculitis of medium to small arteries; upper and lower extremity involvement	Abnormal; loss of ulnar pulse
Adventitial cysts	M > F	Fourth decade	Rare	Unknown	Usually normal
Popliteal artery entrapment syndrome	M > F	Third-fourth decade	Rare	Abnormal origin of muscles	Usually normal
Venous claudication	M = F	Any age	Rare	Iliofemoral thrombophlebitis	Normal
McArdle syndrome	M = F	Any age	Rare	Deficient muscle phosphorylases	Normal
Shin splints	M = F	Any age	Common	Swollen anterior tibial muscle	Normal

From Noble J (ed): *Primary care medicine*, ed 2, St Louis, 1996, Mosby.

LEG ULCERS

> **BOX 2-74 Differential Diagnosis of Leg Ulcers**
>
> **Vascular**
> - Arterial
>   - Arteriosclerosis
>   - Thromboangiitis obliterans
>   - Cholesterol emboli
>   - Hypertension
>   - Arteriovenous malformation
> - Venous
>   - Superficial varicosities
>   - Deep venous thrombosis
>   - Incompetent perforators
> - Lymphatics (elephantiasis nostra)
>
> **Vasculitis**
> - Small vessel
>   - Hypersensitivity vasculitis (leukocytoclastic vasculitis)
>   - Lupus erythematosus
>   - Rheumatoid arthritis
>   - Scleroderma
>   - Livedo vasculitis (atrophie blanche)
>   - Pyoderma gangrenosa
>   - Antiphospholipid antibodies (anticardiolipin or lupus anticoagulant)
> - Medium and large vessel
>   - Polyarteritis nodosa
>   - Nodular vasculitis
>
> **Hematologic**
> - Sickle cell anemia
> - Spherocytosis
> - Thalassemia
> - Polycythemia rubra vera
> - Leukemia
> - Dysproteinemias
>   - Cryoglobulinemia
>   - Cold agglutinin disease
>   - Macroglobulinemia
> - Deficiencies of coagulation inhibitors
>   - Protein C and S deficiency
>
> **Infectious**
> - Fungus
>   - Blastomycosis
>   - Coccidiomycosis
>   - Histoplasmosis
>   - Sporotrichosis
> - Bacterial
>   - Furuncle
>   - Ecthyma
>   - Ecthyma gangrenosum
>   - Septic emboli
>   - Pseudomonas
>   - Mycobacterial (typical and atypical)
> - Protozoal
>   - Leishmaniasis
>
> **Metabolic**
> - Diabetes
>   - Necrobiosis lipoidica diabeticorum
> - Gout
> - Gaucher's disease
> - Prolidase deficiency
> - Calcinosis cutis
> - Localized bullous pemphigoid
>
> **Tumors**
> - Basal cell carcinoma
> - Squamous cell carcinoma
> - Melanoma
> - Kaposi's sarcoma
> - Metastatic tumors
> - Lymphoproliferative
> - Cutaneous T-cell lymphoma (mycoses fungoides)
>
> **Trauma**
> - Insect bites
> - Pressure
> - Cold injury (frostbite, lupus pernio)
> - Radiation dermatitis
> - Burns
> - Factitial
>
> **Neuropathic**
> - Diabetic trophic ulcers
> - Tabes dorsalis
> - Syringomyelia
>
> **Drug**
> - Halogens
> - Methotrexate
> - Coumarin necrosis
> - Ergotism
> - Hydroxyurea
>
> **Panniculitis**
> - Weber-Christian disease
> - Pancreatic fat necrosis
> - α_1 Antitrypsinase deficiency

From Noble J (ed): *Primary care medicine*, ed 2, St Louis, 1996, Mosby.

LIVER DISEASE IN PREGNANCY

TABLE 2-41 Characteristics of Liver Diseases in Pregnancy

DISEASE	SYMPTOMS	JAUNDICE	TRIMESTER	INCIDENCE IN PREGNANCY	LABORATORY VALUES*	ADVERSE EFFECTS
Hyperemesis gravidarum	Nausea, vomiting	Mild	1 or 2	0.3%-1.0%	Bilirubin <4 mg/dl, ALT <200 U/L	Low birth weight
Intrahepatic cholestasis of pregnancy	Pruritus	In 20%-60%, 1-4 wk after pruritus starts	2 or 3	0.1%-0.2% in US	Bilirubin <6 mg/dl, ALT <300 U/L, increased bile acids	Stillbirth, prematurity, bleeding, fetal mortality 3.5%
Biliary tract disease	Right upper quadrant pain, nausea, vomiting, fever	With CBD obstruction	Any	Unknown	If CBD stone, increased bilirubin and GGT	Unknown
Drug-induced hepatitis	None or nausea, vomiting, pruritus	Early (in cholestatic hepatitis)	Any	Unknown	Variable	Unknown
Acute fatty liver of pregnancy	Upper abdominal pain, nausea, vomiting, confusion late in disease	Common	3	0.008%	ALT <500 U/L low glucose, DIC in >75%, increased bilirubin and ammonia late in disease	Increased maternal mortality (≤20%) and fetal mortality (13%-18%)
Preeclampsia and eclampsia	Upper abdominal pain, edema, hypertension, mental status changes	Late, 5%-14%	2 or 3	5%-10%	ALT <500 U/L (unless infarction), proteinuria, DIC in 7%	Increased maternal mortality (~1%)
HELLP syndrome	Upper abdominal pain, nausea, vomiting, malaise	Late, 5%-14%	3	0.1% (4%-12% of women with preeclampsia)	ALT <500 U/L platelets <100,000/mm^3, hemolysis, increased LDH, DIC in 20%-40%	Increased maternal mortality (1%-3%) and fetal mortality (35%)
Viral hepatitis	Nausea, vomiting, fever	Common	Any	Same as general population	ALT greatly increased (>500 U/L), increased bilirubin, DIC rare	Maternal mortality increased with hepatitis E

From Knox TA, Olans LB: Liver disease in pregnancy, *N Engl J Med* 335:569-576, 1996.
ALT, Alanine aminotransferas; *CBD,* common bile duct; *DIC,* disseminated intravascular coagulation; *GGT,* γ-glutamyltranspeptidase; *LDH,* lactate dehydrogenase.
*To convert bilirubin values to micromoles per liter, multiply by 17.1.

LIVER FUNCTION TESTS IN LIVER DISEASE

TABLE 2-42 Liver Function Test Patterns in Hepatobiliary Disorders and Jaundice

TYPE OF DISORDER	BILIRUBIN	AMINOTRANSFERASES	ALKALINE PHOSPHATASE	ALBUMIN	GLOBULIN	PROTHROMBIN TIME
Hemolysis	Normal to 5 mg/dl	Normal	Normal	Normal	Normal	Normal
Gilbert's syndrome	85% due to indirect fractions No bilirubinuria					
Acute hepatocellular necrosis (viral and drug hepatitis, hepatotoxins, acute heart failure)	Both fractions may be elevated Peak usually follows aminotransferases Bilirubinuria	Elevated, often >500 IU ALT ≥ AST	Normal to <3 times normal elevation	Normal	Normal	Usually normal; if > 5 sec above control and not corrected by parenteral vitamin K, suggests poor prognosis
Chronic hepatocellular disorders	Both fractions may be elevated Bilirubinuria	Elevated, but usually <300 IU	Normal to <3 times normal elevation	Often decreased	Increased gamma globulin	Often prolonged Fails to correct with parenteral vitamin K
Alcoholic hepatitis Cirrhosis	Both fractions may be elevated Bilirubinuria	AST/ALT >2 suggests alcoholic hepatitis or cirrhosis	Normal to <3 times normal elevation	Often decreased	Increased IGA and increased gamma globulin	
Intrahepatic cholestasis Obstructive jaundice	Both fractions may be elevated Bilirubinuria	Normal to moderate elevation Rarely >500 IU	Elevated, often >4 times normal elevation	Normal, unless chronic	Gamma globulin normal Beta globulin may be increased	Normal If prolonged, will correct with parenteral vitamin K
Infiltrative diseases (tumor, granulomata); partial bile duct obstruction	Usually normal	Normal to slight elevation	Elevated, often >4 times normal elevation Fractionate, or confirm liver origin with 5'-nucleotidase, γ-glutamyl transpeptidase	Normal	Usually normal Gamma globulin may be increased in granulomatous disease	Normal

From Stein JH (ed): *Internal medicine*, ed 4, St Louis, 1994, Mosby.

LYMPHADENOPATHY

> **BOX 2-75 Lymphadenopathy**
>
> **Generalized**
>
> AIDS
> Lymphoma: Hodgkin's disease, non-Hodgkin's lymphoma
> Leukemias, reticuloendotheliosis
> Infectious mononucleosis, CMV, and other viral infections
> Diffuse skin infection: generalized furunculosis, multiple tick bites
> Parasitic infections: toxoplasmosis, filariasis, leishmaniasis, Chagas disease
> Serum sickness
> Collagen vascular diseases (RA, SLE)
> Dengue (arbovirus infection)
> Sarcoidosis and other granulomatous diseases
> Drugs: isoniazid, hydantoin derivatives, antithyroid and antileprosy drugs
> Secondary syphilis
> Hyperthyroidism, lipid storage diseases
>
> **Localized**
>
> Any of the causes of generalized lymphadenopathy
> Draining lymphatics from local infection: infected furuncle, throat infection, dental abscess, lymphogranuloma venereum, brucellosis, parasitic infections, cat-scratch disease
> Neoplasm
> TB (scrofula)

LYMPHOCYTE ABNORMALITIES IN PERIPHERAL BLOOD

TABLE 2-43 Differential Diagnosis of Abnormal Lymphocytes in Peripheral Blood

LYMPHOCYTE TYPE	USUAL DISEASE ASSOCIATION	CYTOLOGIC FEATURES	LABORATORY FEATURES	CLINICAL FEATURES
Small lymphocyte	Chronic lymphocytic leukemia	B-cell surface markers with low concentration of surface immunoglobulin, CD5 antigen	Hypogammaglobulinemia in 50%; positive direct Coombs' test in 15%; on node biopsy, diffuse, well-differentiated lymphocytic infiltrate	Elderly adults; presentation runs gamut from asymptomatic with lymphocytosis only to bulky disease with adenopathy, splenomegaly, and "packed" bone marrow
Atypical lymphocyte	Infectious mononucleosis, other viral illnesses	Suppressor T-cell markers	Heterophil agglutinin; positive serology for Epstein-Barr virus, cytomegalovirus, toxoplasma, HBsAg	Pharyngitis, fever, adenopathy, rash, splenomegaly, palatal petechiae, jaundice
Plasmacytoid lymphocyte	Waldenström's macroglobulinemia	Cytoplasmic IgM, periodic acid–Schiff (PAS) positivity	IgM paraprotein, rouleaux, cryoglobulins	Adenopathy, splenomegaly, absence of bone lesions, hyperviscosity syndrome, cryopathic phenomena
Lymphoblast	Acute lymphoblastic leukemia (ALL)	Terminal transferase positivity, common ALL antigen, B- or T-precursor markers	Anemia, granulocytopenia, thrombocytopenia, hyperuricemia, diffuse bone marrow infiltration	Peak incidence in childhood, acute onset, bone pain frequent
Lymphosarcoma cell	Lymphocytic lymphoma	B-cell surface markers with high concentration of monoclonal surface immunoglobulin	Nodular or diffuse, poorly differentiated lymphocytic lymphoma on node biopsy, patchy, peritrabecular bone marrow involvement	Middle-aged to older adults, generalized adenopathy, constitutional symptoms
Sézary cell	Cutaneous lymphomas	T-lymphocyte surface markers	Skin biopsy is diagnostic	Exfoliative erythroderma, cutaneous plaques or tumors
Hairy cell	Hairy cell leukemia	B-lymphocyte markers, cytoplasmic projections, tartrate-resistant acid phosphatase, interleukin-2 receptors, CD11 antigen	Pancytopenia	Middle-aged males, moderate to marked splenomegaly without adenopathy
Prolymphocyte	Prolymphocytic leukemia	B-cell surface markers with high concentration of surface immunoglobulin, CD5 negative	Marked lymphocytosis (frequently >100 × 10^9/L)	Elderly adults, massive splenomegaly, minimum adenopathy, poor response to therapy

From Stein JH (ed): *Internal medicine*, ed 5, St Louis, 1998, Mosby.

MALABSORPTIVE DISORDERS

> **BOX 2-76** Classification of Malabsorptive Disorders (with Comments on Occurrence and Associated Abnormalities)
>
> I. Inadequate mixing of food with bile salts and lipase—mild chemical steatorrhea common, but clinical steatorrhea uncommon. Actual diarrhea uncommon. Anemia in approximately 15%-35%; most often iron deficiency, rarely megaloblastic.
>   A. Pyloroplasty
>   B. Subtotal and total gastrectomy (occasional megaloblastic anemias reported)
>   C. Gastrojejunostomy
> II. Inadequate lipolysis—lack of lipase or normal stimulation of pancreatic secretion. Steatorrhea only in far-advanced pancreatic destruction, and diarrhea even less often.
>   A. Cystic fibrosis of the pancreas
>   B. Chronic pancreatitis
>   C. Cancer of the pancreas or ampulla of Vater
>   D. Pancreatic fistula
>   E. Severe protein deficiency
>   F. Vagus nerve section
> III. Inadequate emulsification of fat—lack of bile salts. Clinical steatorrhea uncommon, sometimes occurs in very severe cases. Usually no diarrhea.
>   A. Obstructive jaundice
>   B. Severe liver disease
> IV. Primary absorptive defect—small bowel
>   A. Inadequate length of normal absorptive surface; unusual complication of surgery
>   1. Surgical resection
>   2. Internal fistula
>   3. Gastroileostomy
>   B. Obstruction of mesenteric lymphatics (rare)
>   1. Lymphoma
>   2. Hodgkin's disease
>   3. Carcinoma
>   4. Whipple's disease
>   5. Intestinal tuberculosis
>   C. Inadequate absorptive surface resulting from extensive mucosal disease; except for *Giardia* infection and regional enteritis, most of these diseases are uncommon; steatorrhea only if there is extensive bowel involvement
>   1. Inflammatory
>   a. Tuberculosis
>   b. Regional enteritis or enterocolitis (diarrhea very common)
>   c. *Giardia lamblia* infection (diarrhea common; malabsorption rare)
>   2. Neoplastic
>   3. Amyloid disease
>   4. Scleroderma
>   5. Pseudomembranous enterocolitis (diarrhea frequent)
>   6. Radiation injury
>   7. Pneumatosis cystoides intestinalis
>   D. Biochemical dysfunction of mucosal cells
>   1. "Gluten-induced" (steatorrhea and diarrhea very common)
>   a. Celiac disease (childhood)
>   b. Nontropical sprue (adult)
>   2. Enzymatic defect
>   a. Disaccharide malabsorption (diarrhea a frequent symptom)
>   b. Pernicious anemia (deficiency of gastric "intrinsic factor")
>   3. Cause unknown; uncommon except for tropical sprue (which is common only in the tropics)
>   a. Tropical sprue (diarrhea and steatorrhea common)
>   b. Severe starvation
>   c. Diabetic visceral neuropathy
>   d. Endocrine and metabolic disorder (e.g., hypothyroidism)
>   e. Zollinger-Ellison syndrome (diarrhea common; steatorrhea may be present)
>   f. Miscellaneous
> V. Malabsorption associated with altered bacterial flora (diarrhea fairly common)
>   1. Small intestinal blind loops, diverticula, anastomoses (rare)
>   2. Drug (oral antibiotic) administration (infrequent but not rare)

From Ravel R: *Clinical laboratory medicine,* ed 6, St Louis, 1995, Mosby.

MEDIASTINAL MASSES OR WIDENING ON CHEST X-RAY

BOX 2-77 Mediastinal Masses or Widening on Chest X-ray

Lymphoma: Hodgkin's disease and non-Hodgkin's lymphoma
Sarcoidosis
Vascular: aortic aneurysm, ectasia or tortuosity of aorta or bronchocephalic vessels
Carcinoma: lungs, esophagus
Esophageal diverticula
Hiatal hernia
Prominent pulmonary outflow tract: pulmonary hypertension, pulmonary embolism, right-to-left shunts
Trauma: mediastinal hemorrhage
Pneumomediastinum

Lymphadenopathy caused by silicosis and other pneumoconioses
Leukemias
Infections: tuberculosis, viral (rare), *Mycoplasma* (rare), fungal, tularemia
Substernal thyroid
Thymoma
Teratoma
Bronchogenic cyst
Pericardial cyst
Neurofibroma, neurosarcoma, ganglioneuroma

METASTATIC NEOPLASMS

BOX 2-78 Metastatic Neoplasms

BONE	BRAIN	LIVER	LUNG
Breast	Lung	Colon	Breast
Lung	Breast	Stomach	Colon
Prostate	Melanoma	Pancreas	Kidney
Thyroid	GU tract	Breast	Testis
Kidney	Colon	Lymphomas	Stomach
Bladder	Sinuses	Bronchus	Thyroid
Endometrium	Sarcoma	Lung	Melanoma
Cervix	Skin		Sarcoma
Melanoma	Thyroid		Choriocarcinoma

MICROPENIS

BOX 2-79 Causes of Micropenis

Hypogonadotropic Hypogonadism (Hypothalamic or Pituitary Deficiencies)

Kallman syndrome: autosomal dominant; associated with hyposmia
Prader-Willi syndrome: hypotonia, mental retardation, obesity, small hands and feet
Rud syndrome: hyposomia, icthyosis, mental retardation
De Morsier syndrome (septo-optic dysplasia): hypopituitarism, hypoplastic optic discs, absent septum pellucidum

Hypergonadotropic Hypogonadism

Primary testicular defect: disorders of testicular differentiation or inborn errors of testosterone synthesis

Klinefelter syndrome
Other X polysomies (i.e., XXXXY, XXXY)
Robinow syndrome: brachymesomelic dwarfism, dysmorphic facies

Partial Androgen Insensitivity

Idiopathic

Defective morphogenesis of the penis

From Moore WT, Eastman RC: *Diagnostic endocrinology,* ed 2, St Louis, 1996, Mosby.

MIOSIS

> **BOX 2-80 Miosis**
>
> Medications (morphine, pilocarpine, etc.)
> Neurosyphilis
> Congenital
> Iritis
> CNS pontine lesion
> CNS infections
> Cavernous sinus thrombosis
> Inflammation/irritation of cornea or conjunctiva

MUSCLE WEAKNESS

> **BOX 2-81 Causes of Muscle Weakness**
>
> I. Primary proximal weakness
>   A. Muscle
>   1. Endocrine: hyperthyroidism, hypothyroidism, subacute thyroiditis, hyperparathyroidism, acromegaly, Addison's disease (acute adrenal insufficiency), primary aldosteronism, steroid myopathy (Cushing's syndrome; iatrogenic), and male hypogonadism
>   2. Metabolic: diabetes mellitus, insulin-induced hypoglycemia, glycogen storage diseases (acid maltase deficiency, muscle phosphorylase deficiency, muscle phosphofructokinase deficiency), lipid storage disease (carnitine deficiency), and alcoholic myopathy
>   3. Muscular dystrophies: limb-girdle, Duchenne's, Becker's
>   4. Inflammatory myopathies: polymyositis, dermatomyositis, other collagen vascular diseases including rheumatoid arthritis, sarcoidosis, human immunodeficiency virus
>   5. Hypercalcemia, hypophosphatemia, hypokalemia, and hyperkalemia of any cause
>   6. Drug induced: colchine, chloroquine, cimetidine, amidarone, beta blockers, D-penicillamine, cyclosporin
>   B. Neuromuscular junction: myasthenia gravis, Eaton-Lambert, botulism, organophosphate poisoning
>   C. Peripheral nerve: diabetic proximal neuropathy, Guillain-Barré syndrome, acute intermittent porphyria, tick paralysis, and arsenic poisoning
>   D. Anterior horn cell: poliomyelitis, chronic spinal muscular atrophy
> II. Primary distal weakness
>   A. Muscle: myotonic dystrophy
>   B. Peripheral nerve: beriberi, diphtheria, lead, porphyrins, carcinomatous neuropathy, chronic progressive demyelinating neuropathy, peroneal muscle atrophy (Charcot-Marie-Tooth), Guillain-Barré syndrome, Refsum's disease, compressive lesions (root, plexus, nerve)
>   C. Anterior horn cell: poliomyelitis, motor neuron disease
> III. Generalized weakness
>   A. Decreased cardiac output (mitral stenosis, tricuspid stenosis, mitral regurgitation)
>   B. Acute infectious diseases and chronic infectious diseases such as tuberculosis, brucellosis, and trichinosis
>   C. Chronic glomerulonephritis and other causes of uremia, including generalized rhabdomyolysis
>   D. Pernicious anemia (and other anemias)
>   E. Hepatitis
>   F. Neurosyphilis
>   G. Psychiatric illnesses such as depression
>   H. Multiple sclerosis
>   I. Mitochondrial myopathy (genetic, zidovudine)
>   J. L-Tryptophan (eosinophilia-myalgia)

From Stein JH (ed): *Internal medicine*, ed 4, St Louis, 1994, Mosby.

MYDRIASIS

> **BOX 2-82 Mydriasis**
>
> Coma
> Medications (cocaine, atropine, epinephrine, etc.)
> Glaucoma
> Cerebral aneurysm
> Ocular trauma
> Head trauma
> Optic atrophy
> Cerebral neoplasm

MYELOPATHY AND MYELITIS

> **BOX 2-83 Causes of Myelopathy and Myelitis**
>
> Inflammatory
>   Infectious
>   Bacterial: spirochetal, tuberculous
>   Viral: poliomyelitis; herpes HTLV, HIV, zoster; rabies
>   Other: rickettsial, fungal, parasitic
>   Noninfectious
>   Idiopathic transverse myelitis, multiple sclerosis
> Toxic/metabolic
>   Arsenic
>   Pernicious anemia
>   Pellagra
>   Diabetes mellitus
>   Chronic liver disease
> Trauma
>   Spinal fracture/dislocation
>   Stab/bullet wound
>   Herniated nucleus pulposus
> Compression
>   Spinal neoplasm
>   Cervical spondylosis
>   Extramedullary hematopoiesis
>   Epidural abscess
>   Epidural hematoma
> Vascular
>   Arteriovenous malformation
>   Periarteritis nodosa
>   Lupus erythematosus
>   Dissecting aortic aneurysm
> Physical agents
>   Electrical injury
>   Irradiation
> Neoplastic
>   Spinal cord tumors
>   Paraneoplastic myelopathy

From Stein JH (ed): *Internal medicine,* ed 4, St Louis, 1994, Mosby.

NAIL DISORDERS

TABLE 2-44 Differential Diagnosis of Nail Disorders

CONDITION	PE/HISTORY	LABORATORY	MANAGEMENT
Onychomycosis	Hyperkeratosis of nail bed, yellow-brown discoloration, onycholysis. Usually chronic.	KOH positive Culture positive	Systemic or topical antifungal therapy
Paronychia, acute	Red, warm, tender nail. Often follows injury to nail fold.	Positive bacterial culture, usually *Staphylococcus*	Systemic antibiotic
Paronychia, chronic	Boggy, swollen, red, inflamed nail folds. Usually occurs in people who have wet-work jobs.	Pus is KOH positive and culture positive for *C. albicans*	Anticandida therapy, topical or systemic
Psoriasis	Usually associated with cutaneous psoriasis. Pitting, onycholysis, splinter hemorrhages, nail bed hyperkeratosis.	KOH negative	Topical or intralesional steroids
Lichen planus	Pitting and ridging early. Can eventuate in scarring and pterygium formation.	KOH negative	Systemic, topical, or intralesional steroids
Melanoma	Pigmented band in the nail that widens or darkens.	Biopsy nail bed or matrix depending on site of pigment	Wide excision
SCC	Hyperkeratosis, onycholysis.	Biopsy lesion	Excision, sometimes Mohs' surgery
Habit tic	Usually thumbs, horizontal parallel lines on nail plate. History of manipulating nail folds.	KOH negative	Explain cause to patient; occasionally wrapping nail
Mucous cyst	Occurs on proximal nail fold and over DIP joint.	Mucin expressed from punctured lesion	Excision, repeated liquid N_2, intralesional cortisone

From Noble J (ed): *Primary care medicine*, ed 2, St Louis, 1996, Mosby.

NAUSEA AND VOMITING

BOX 2-84 **Causes of Nausea and Vomiting**

Infections (viral, bacterial)
Intestinal obstruction
Metabolic (uremia, electrolyte abnormalities, DKA, acidosis, etc.)
Severe pain
Anxiety, fear
Psychiatric disorders (bulimia, anorexia nervosa)
Pregnancy
Medications (NSAIDs, erythromycin, morphine, codeine, aminophylline, chemotherapeutic agents, etc.)
Withdrawal from substance abuse (drugs, alcohol)
Head trauma
Vestibular or middle ear disease
Migraine headache
CNS neoplasms
Radiation sickness
Peptic ulcer disease
Carcinoma of GI tract
Reye's syndrome
Eye disorders
Abdominal trauma

NECK MASS

TABLE 2-45 Differential Diagnosis of Nonneoplastic Inflammatory Etiologies of a Neck Mass

ETIOLOGY	PATIENT CHARACTERISTICS, SIGNS, AND SYMPTOMS	TESTING STRATEGIES AND FINDINGS	TREATMENT
Adenopathy secondary to peritonsillar abscess	Sore throat Dysphagia Odynophagia Malaise Fever Drooling "Hot potato" voice Trismus Deviation of uvula Bulging of palate Fluctuance in peritonsillar region	Needle aspiration of peritonsillar space	Incision and drainage Antibiotics Hydration
Retropharyngeal abscess	Neck mass often not discrete Usually in pediatric age group Fever Malaise Dysphagia	Lateral neck x-ray Axial CT	Incision and drainage (after careful endotracheal intubation) in the OR Antibiotics
Parapharyngeal abscess	Spiking fever Rigors Malaise Trismus Dysphagia Odynophagia Aphasia Drooling Torticollis Neck rigidity and pain Paresthesias	Leukocytosis Anemia CT scan with contrast	IV antibiotics Hydration Incision and drainage
Salivary gland infections	Gland enlargement and tenderness ↑ Pain with eating Mucopurulent discharge from duct (if suppuration) Patients often elderly, dehydrated	X-ray for sialolith CT, if abscess suspected (Radionuclide scanning) (Sialogram)	Hydration Bland diet Analgesics Bed rest Antistaphylococcal antibiotics Warm compresses Gentle massage Surgical incision and drainage, if suppuration Gland excision for chronic/recurrent sialoadenitis or sialolithiasis

Jugular vein thrombus	Neck swollen, diffuse, usually tender
	Often H/O indwelling catheter (IJ or subclavian)
	If *suppurative* thrombophlebitis:
	  Overlying erythema
	  ↑ Tenderness
	  Malaise
	  Fever
		CT with contrast or duplex Doppler ultrasound
		(Angiography)
			Broad-spectrum antibiotics
			Hydration
			Supportive care
			Anticoagulants controversial
			Vein ligation if septic emboli

Mononucleosis	Mild and nonspecific URI
	80% have triad:
	  Sore throat
	  Fever
	  Lymphadenopathy
	Fatigue sometimes marked
		CBC with differential
		Atypical lymphocytes
		Monospot
		Heterophile antibodies
		↑ Serum liver enzymes
			Supportive care:
			  Hydration
			  Bed rest
			(?) Antibiotics
			Steroids for prolonged or severe cases

TABLE 2-45 Differential Diagnosis of Nonneoplastic Inflammatory Etiologies of a Neck Mass—cont'd

ETIOLOGY	PATIENT CHARACTERISTICS, SIGNS, AND SYMPTOMS	TESTING STRATEGIES AND FINDINGS	TREATMENT

	Exudative adenotonsillitis
	  Yellowish white
	  Confluent
	Adenopathy
	  Usually bilateral
	  Commonly posterior triangle
	  Tender
	  Can grow to impressive sizes
	Palatal petechiae
	Nonallergic rash to ampicillin
	Hepatosplenomegaly
			Endotracheal intubation or tonsillectomy if airway compromised

CMV	Mild URI sxs Similar to EBV, but less severe No exudative pharyngitis	Negative heterophile antibody Serologic test for CMV (+)	Supportive care

Tuberculosis	Nodes usually painless
	  Usually nonerythematous
	  Usually enlarging
	  Multiple (66%)
	  Posterior (70%)
	Overlying skin indurated and slightly brown
	Sinus tracts may open in skin
		Smear or pathologic examination of node or drainage
		Culture
			Systemic antituberculosis medication

Atypical mycobacterium	Unilateral cervical lymphadenitis, most commonly submandibular
	Skin erythematous
	  Usually nontender
	  Usually not warm
	  Changes in color from red to lilac pink
	Minimal systemic findings
	Not associated with pulmonary disease
		PPD negative or weakly positive	Surgical excision of infected nodes without antimicrobial chemotherapy

AIDS	Opportunistic infections Hairy leukoplakia Kaposi's sarcoma Candidiasis Verrucae Giant aphthous stomatitis	ELISA Western blot Helper/suppressor T-cell ratios	Treatment of underlying disease Biopsy of nodes if neoplasm suspected

Toxoplasmosis	Common cold sxs
	Asymptomatic or mildly tender posterior triangle adenopathy
	Nodes usually confined to one side
	  May fluctuate in size
	  Do not suppurate or develop fistulae
		Fluorescent antibody test
		Compliment fixation test
		Hemagglutination
		Sabin-Feldman dye test
			Sulfonamides
			Pyrimethamine

Actinomyces	Neck mass: not true lymphadenitis Blue Rubbery Nontender Central loculation Discharge of water material	Curettage and culture	High-dose penicillin G IV 4-6 wk followed by 12 mo of oral penicillin
Cat-scratch disease	Mild clinical symptoms Regional lymphadenopathy	Serologic test for *Rochalimaea henseale*	Supportive care

Patient characteristics in parentheses are less commonly seen; those testing strategies in parentheses are unnecessary in many patients.
H/O, History of; *IJ*, internal jugular; *URI*, upper respiratory tract infection; *sxs*, symptoms; *CBC*, complete blood count; *PPD*, purified protein derivative; *ELISA*, enzyme-linked immunosorbent assay; *FTA-ABS*, fluorescent treponemal antibody absorption.

TABLE 2-46 Differential Diagnosis of Congenital Anomalies Presenting as a Neck Mass

ANOMALY	PATIENT CHARACTERISTICS, SIGNS, SYMPTOMS	TESTING STRATEGIES AND FINDINGS	TREATMENT
Syphilis	Cervical adenopathy	FTA-ABS	Penicillin
Tularemia	See Section I	See Section I	See Section I
Brucellosis	See Section I	See Section I	See Section I
Leptospirosis	See Section I	See Section I	See Section I

Thyroglossal duct cyst	Most patients <30 yr
	Midline mass
	  Usually inferior to hyoid
	  Soft
	  Retraction of cyst on protrusion of tongue is pathognomonic
			Surgical excision
			Antibiotics if infection

Branchial apparatus anomalies	Usually present in childhood
	  Usually diagnosed by age 30 yr
	Mass
	  Along anterior border of SCM
	  Between ear canal and clavicle
	  Smooth
	  Fluctuant
	  Nontender
	  Ill-defined margins
	  Varies in size (associated with URIs)
		Needle aspiration results in decompression
		Thin or mucopurulent fluid
			Surgical excision

Cystic hygroma	Multiloculated cystic masses
	90% diagnosed before age 2 yr
	Often enlarge during URIs
	  (Airway compromise)
	Transilluminate
		CT scan
		May have visible cysts
		(Aspiration → clear yellow fluid)
			Excision if:
			  Functional impairment
			  Recurrent infection
			  Severe cosmetic deformity

Hemangioma	Most diagnosed by age 6 mo
	Proliferate during first year
	  (Airway obstruction)
	  (High-output cardiac failure)
		CT scan	Surgical excision if:
			  No regression by age 5 yr
			  Impending complications

Dermoid cysts	Midline masses
	  Smooth
	  Not attached to larynx or hyoid
	  Doughy consistency
	  Commonly found in 20s
			Surgical excision

Teratomas	Mass
	  Irregular
	  Firm
	  Lateral
			Surgical excision

Laryngoceles	Very soft, compressible mass ↑ Size with Valsalva's maneuver Laryngeal component		Surgical excision (Antibiotics if infection)
Ranula	Soft, compressible mass Associated with sublingual gland	CT scan (Salivary amylase)	Surgical excision

From Noble J (ed): *Primary care medicine,* ed 2, St Louis, 1996, Mosby.
SCM, Sternocleidomastoid muscle; *URI,* upper respiratory tract infection.

NEMATODE TISSUE INFECTIONS

TABLE 2-47 Nematode Tissue Infections

SPECIES	EPIDEMIOLOGY	TRANSMISSION	MAJOR CLINICAL PRESENTATION	DIAGNOSIS	TREATMENT
Wuchereria bancrofti (lymphatic filariasis)	Tropics, subtropics	Mosquito	Lymphatic obstruction	Night blood	Diethylcarbamazine (DEC),* 50 mg first day, 50 mg tid second day, 100 mg tid third day, 2 mg/kg tid for 20 days; or ivermectin, †,‡,§ 400 μg/kg; or albendazole, †,‡,§ 400 mg for 21 days
Brugia malayi (lymphatic filariasis)	South and Southeast Asia	Mosquito	Lymphatic obstruction	Night blood	Same as for *W. bancrofti*
Onchocerca volvulus (river blindness)	Central and South America	Blackfly	Dermatitis blindness	Skin snips	Ivermectin,§ 150 μg/kg once every 3 to 12 mo or every 4 mo
Loa loa (eyeworm)	West and Central Africa	Deerfly, horsefly	Calabar swellings	Day or night blood samples	DEC or ivermectin†‡§ as for *W. bancrofti*
Tropical pulmonary eosinophilia (TPE)	All the above areas	Unknown	Eosinophilia pneumonitis	Serology and clinical picture	DEC, 2 mg/kg tid for 7-10 days; ivermectin or albendazole†,‡,§ as for *W. bancrofti*
Dracunculiasis medinensis (guinea worm)	Africa	Step-in wells	Painful boil in legs	Visualization of worm	Niridazole,† 25 mg/kg for 10 days, or metronidazole,† 250 mg tid for 10 days
Trichinella spiralis	Worldwide	Raw meat	Fever, myalgias, periorbital edema	Serology, muscle biopsy	Thiabendazole,‡ 25 mg/kg for 5 days (max, 3 g/day), or mebendazole,†‡ 200-400 mg tid for 3 days, 400-500 mg tid for 10 days, or albendazole,†‡ 400 mg bid for 10 days, and ?steroids
Angiostrongylus cantonensis	Southeast Asia, Pacific Islands	Raw mollusks or crustaceans	Eosinophilia, meningitis	Clinical picture	Surgical removal
Angiostrongylus costaricensis	Same as above	Same as above	Same as above	Same as above	Surgical removal; mebendazole, 100 mg bid for 5 days, or ?thiabendazole,†‡ 25 mg/kg tid for 3 days
Gnathostoma spinigerum	Thailand, Japan	Raw fish	Eosinophilia, meningitis, subcutaneous swellings	Serology	Surgical removal; mebendazole, ‡ 200 mg every 3 hr for 6 days
Anisakis species	Japan, Scandinavia	Raw fish	Benign stomach "tumor"	Endoscopy with biopsy, serology	Surgical removal
Visceral larva migrans	Worldwide	Ingestion of soil (pica)	Fever, abdominal pain, optic involvement, diarrhea	Serology	Albendazole, 400 mg bid for 3-5 days, or thiabendazole, 25 mg/kg bid for 5 days (max, 3g/day), or DEC,† 2 mg/kg bid for 10 days, or mebendazole,† 100-200 for 5 days, all with steroids‡
Cutaneous larva migrans	Worldwide	Skin penetration	Creeping eruption	Clinical picture	Thiabendazole, topically or 50 mg/kg/day (max, 3 g/day) for 2-5 days, or albendazole, 200 mg bid for 3 days or ivermectin,†§ 150-200 μg/hg once
Strongy-loidosis	Worldwide, immuno-suppressor	Fecal-oral	Gram-negative bacteremia, multiple organ involvement	Stool ova and parasites, tissue biopsy	Thiabendazole, 25 mg/kg bid for 2 days, 5 days for dissemination; or albendazole, 400 mg/day for 3 days,†,§ or ivermectin, 200 μg/kg/day for 1-2 days†,§

From Stein JH (ed): *Internal medicine,* ed 5, St Louis, 1998, Mosby.
tid, Three times a day; *bid,* twice a day.
*May precipitate severe reactions in infected individuals.
†Considered an investigational drug by the US Food and Drug Administration.
‡Effectiveness not clearly established.
§Not available in the United States.

NEUROLOGIC DEFICIT, FOCAL

BOX 2-85 Causes of Acute Focal Neurologic Deficit

Traumatic: intracranial, intraspinal
  Subdural hematoma
  Intraparenchymal hemorrhage
  Epidural hematoma
  Traumatic hemorrhagic necrosis
Infectious
  Brain abscess
  Epidural and subdural abscesses
  Meningitis
Neoplastic
  Primary CNS tumors
  Metastatic tumors
  Syringomyelia
Vascular
  Thrombosis
  Embolism
  Spontaneous hemorrhage: AVM, aneurysm, hypertensive
Metabolic
  Hypoglycemia
  B_{12} deficiency
  Postseizure
  Hyperosmolar nonketotic
Other
  Migraine
  Bell's palsy
  Psychogenic

From Rosen P et al (eds): *Emergency medicine: concepts and clinical practice,* ed 4, St Louis, 1998, Mosby.

NEUROLOGIC DEFICIT, MULTIFOCAL

BOX 2-86 Causes of Multifocal Neurologic Deficit

Acute disseminated encephalomyelitis
  Postviral or postimmunization
Infectious encephalomyelitis
  Poliovirus, enteroviruses, arbovirus, herpes zoster, Epstein-Barr virus
Granulomatous encephalomyelitis
  Sarcoid
Autoimmune
  Systemic lupus erythematosus
Other
  Familial spinocerebellar degenerations

From Rosen P et al (eds): *Emergency medicine: concepts and clinical practice,* ed 4, St Louis, 1998, Mosby.

NEUROPATHIES

TABLE 2-48 Diseases Associated with Different Types of Neuropathy

	AIDP	CIDP	AXONAL SMP	MN	MNMP	PLEX	SMALL
Metabolic							
Diabetes			+	+	+	+	+
Acromegaly*			+	+ (CTS)			
Hypothyroidism*		+	+	+ (CTS)			
Infectious							
AIDS*	+	+	+		+		
Leprosy			+		+		
Lyme disease	+		+	+	+		
Connective Tissue							
SLE*	+		+		+		
Rheumatoid arthritis			+	+	+		
Sjögren's syndrome			+		+		
Periarteritis nodosa*			+		+		
Wegener's granulomatosis*			+		+		
Cranial arteritis*			+		+		
Churg-Strauss syndrome			+		+		
Cryoglobulinemia			+		+		
Hypersensitivity angiitis			+		+		
Idiopathic							
Sarcoidosis*			+		+		

From Stein JH (ed): *Internal medicine*, ed 5, St Louis, 1998, Mosby.
AIDP, Acute inflammatory demyelinating polyneuropathy; *CIDP*, chronic idiopathic demyelinating polyradiculoneuropathy; *axonal SMP*, axonal sensorimotor polyneuropathy; *MN*, mononeuropathy; *MNMP*, mononeuropathy multiplex; *plex*, plexopathy; *small*, small-fiber polyneuropathy; *CTS*, carpal tunnel syndrome; *AIDS*, acquired immunodeficiency syndrome; *SLE*, systemic lupus erythematosus.
*Central nervous system manifestations may be present.

NYSTAGMUS

BOX 2-87 **Nystagmus**

Medications (meperidine, barbiturates, phenytoin, phenothiazines, etc.)
Multiple sclerosis
Congenital
Neoplasm (cerebellar, brain stem, cerebral)
Labyrinthine or vestibular lesions
CNS infections
Optic atrophy
Other: Arnold-Chiari malformation, syringobulbia, chorioretinitis, meningeal cysts

PANCYTOPENIA

> **BOX 2-88** **Causes of Pancytopenia**
>
> 1. Pancytopenia with hypocellular bone marrow
>   a. Acquired aplastic anemia
>   b. Constitutional aplastic anemia
>   c. Exposure to chemical or physical agents, including ionizing irradiation and chemotherapeutic agents
>   d. Some hematologic malignancies, including myelodysplasia and aleukemic leukemia
> 2. Pancytopenia with normal or increased cellularity of hematopoietic origin
>   a. Some hematologic malignancies, including myelodysplasia, and some leukemias, lymphomas, and myelomas
>   b. Paroxysmal nocturnal hemoglobinuria
>   c. Hypersplenism
>   d. Vitamin B_{12}, folate deficiencies
>   e. Overwhelming infection
> 3. Pancytopenia with bone marrow replacement
>   a. Tumor metastatic to marrow
>   b. Metabolic storage diseases
>   c. Osteopetrosis
>   d. Myelofibrosis

From Stein JH (ed): *Internal medicine*, ed 4, St Louis, 1994, Mosby.

PAPILLEDEMA

> **BOX 2-89** **Papilledema**
>
> CNS infections (viral, bacterial, fungal)
> Medications (lithium, cisplatin, corticosteroids, tetracycline, etc.)
> Head trauma
> CNS neoplasm (primary or metastatic)
> Pseudotumor cerebri
> Cavernous sinus thrombosis
> SLE
> Sarcoidosis
> Subarachnoid hemorrhage
> Carbon dioxide retention
> Arnold-Chiari malformation and other developmental or congenital malformations
> Orbital lesions
> Central retinal vein occlusion
> Hypertensive encephalopathy
> Metabolic abnormalities

PARAPLEGIA

> **BOX 2-90** **Paraplegia**
>
> Trauma: penetrating wounds to motor cortex, fracture-dislocation of vertebral column with compression of spinal cord or cauda equina, prolapsed disk, electrical injuries
> Neoplasm: parasagittal region, vertebrae, meninges, spinal cord, cauda equina, Hodgkin's disease, NHL, leukemic deposits, pelvic neoplasms
> Multiple sclerosis and other demyelinating disorders
> Mechanical compression of spinal cord, cauda equina, or lumbosacral plexus: Paget's disease, kyphoscoliosis, herniation of intervertebral disk, spondylosis, ankylosing spondylitis, rheumatoid arthritis, aortic aneurysm
> Infections: spinal abscess, syphilis, TB, poliomyelitis, leprosy
> Thrombosis of superior sagittal sinus
> Polyneuritis: Guillain-Barré syndrome, diabetes, alcohol, beri-beri, heavy metals
> Heredofamilial muscular dystrophies
> ALS
> Congenital and familial conditions: syringomyelia, myelomeningocele, myelodysplasia
> Hysteria

PARESTHESIAS

BOX 2-91 Paresthesias

Multiple sclerosis
Nutritional deficiencies (thiamin, vitamin B_{12}, folic acid)
Compression of spinal cord or peripheral nerves
Medications (isoniazid, lithium, nitrofurantoin, gold, cisplatin, hydralazine, amitriptyline, sulfonamides, amiodarone, metronidazole, dapsone, disulfiram, chloramphenicol, etc.)
Toxic chemicals (lead, arsenic, cyanide, mercury, organophosphates, etc.)
Diabetes mellitus
Myxedema
Alcohol
Sarcoidosis
Neoplasms
Infections (HIV, Lyme disease, herpes zoster, leprosy, diphtheria)
Charcot-Marie-Tooth syndrome and other hereditary neuropathies
Guillain-Barré neuropathy

PELVIC MASS

BOX 2-92 Differential Diagnosis of Pelvic Masses

Benign

Ovarian

Simple cyst (follicle or corpus luteum)
Hemorrhagic cyst
Cystadenoma
Endometrioma
Teratoma
Other benign tumors: papilloma, fibroma

Nonovarian

Leiomyoma
Paraovarian cyst
Hydrosalpinx
Tuboovarian abscess
Ectopic pregnancy
Intrauterine pregnancy

Diverticulitis
Appendiceal abscess
Peritoneal inclusion cyst

Malignant

Ovarian

Epithelial ovarian carcinoma
Germ cell tumors of the ovary
Borderline tumors

Nonovarian

Leiomyosarcoma
Endometrial cancer
Carcinoma of fallopian tube
Colorectal carcinoma

From Carlson KJ et al: *Primary care of women,* St Louis, 1995, Mosby.

PELVIC PAIN

BOX 2-93 Causes of Chronic Pelvic Pain

Gynecologic Disorders

Primary dysmenorrhea
Endometriosis
Adenomyosis
Adhesions
Fibroids
Retained ovary syndrome after hysterectomy
Previous tubal ligation
Chronic pelvic infection

Musculoskeletal Disorders

Myofascial pain syndrome

Gastrointestinal Disorders

Irritable bowel syndrome
Inflammatory bowel disease

Urinary Tract Disorders

Interstitial cystitis
Nonbacterial urethritis

From Carlson KJ et al: *Primary care of women,* St Louis, 1995, Mosby.

PHOTOSENSITIVITY

TABLE 2-49   Photosensitivity: Differential Considerations

	HISTORY	MORPHOLOGY AND PHYSICAL EXAMINATION	LABORATORY	MANAGEMENT
PML	26-year-old woman: onset with extreme sun exposure; delayed onset 6-8 hr postexposure, lasts 7-10 days; pruritic	Papules, vesicles, or plaques; distribution includes face, neck, dorsal arms	Biopsy: superficial and deep mononuclear cell infiltrate	Topical corticosteroids oral corticosteroids, β-carotene, PUVA, Trisoralen, antimalarial
Solar urticaria	Hives appear immediately with sun exposure, last 1-4 hr; pruritic	Uriticaria appearing in sun-exposed areas	MED testing with UVA and UVB may reproduce lesions; biopsy: superficial perivascular mononuclear cell infiltrates	Antihistamines, UVB/UVA hardening, PUVA, oral corticosteroids
Phototoxic	Sunburn appears after minimal exposure; patient may have used new oral medications	Sunburn erythema with sharp cutoffs at non-exposed areas		Discontinue offending agent; oral corticosteroids; PUVA if becomes chronic
Photoallergic	Itchy dermatitis with sun exposure; patient may have used new topical product or oral medication	Eczematous dermatitis; may spread somewhat into non-sun-exposed areas	Reduced MED to UVA; biopsy: spongiosis in epidermis; superficial and deep mononuclear cell infiltrate	Same as above; topical corticosteroids
PCT	Estrogen or alcohol intake; history of skin fragility or blisters on hands	Vesicles and bullae on dorsal hands that heal with scarring and milia; mottled hypopigmentation of face; hyperpigmentation of the periorbital area	Biopsy: subepidermal bullae; increased uroporphyrin I and 7-carboxyl porphyrin III in urine; increased isocoproporphyrin in feces	Phlebotomy—500 ml/wk until clinical clearing occurs
SLE	Sunburn persists days or weeks with no further exposure; rash in butterfly distribution across nose; drugs associated with lupuslike syndrome	Long-lasting sunburn reaction; plaques in butterfly distribution of smaller area	Biopsy: positive ANA; positive Ro antigen; dif-band of fluorescent material at dermal epidermal junction	Chloroquine 125 to 250 mg twice weekly

From Noble J (ed): *Primary care medicine*, ed 2, St Louis, 1996, Mosby.
PML, Polymorphous light eruption; *PCT*, porphyria cutanea tarda; *SLE*, systemic lupus erythematosus; *MED*, minimum erythema dose.

PLEURAL EFFUSIONS

BOX 2-94   **Pleural Effusions**

Exudative

Neoplasm: bronchogenic carcinoma, breast carcinoma, mesothelioma, lymphoma, ovarian carcinoma, multiple myeloma, leukemia, Meigs' syndrome
Infections: viral pneumonia, bacterial pneumonia, *Mycoplasma*, TB, fungal and parasitic diseases
Trauma
Collagen vascular diseases: SLE, RA, scleroderma, polyarteritis, Wegener's granulomatosis
Pulmonary infarction
Pancreatitis
Postcardiotomy/Dressler's syndrome
Drug-induced lupus erythematosus (hydralazine, procainamide)
Postabdominal surgery
Ruptured esophagus
Chronic effusion secondary to congestive failure

Transudative

CHF
Hepatic cirrhosis
Nephrotic syndrome
Hypoproteinemia from any cause
Meigs' syndrome

PLEURAL EFFUSIONS, DRUG-INDUCED

BOX 2-95 Drugs That Can Cause a Pleural Effusion

Drugs that induce SLE (diphenylhydantion, hydralazine, isoniazid, procainamide)
Sclerosing agents for esophageal varices
Chemotherapeutic agents (e.g., procarbazine, methotrexate)
Tocolytics used for premature labor
Bromocriptine
Dantrolene
Methysergide
L-Tryptophan
Nitrofurantoin
Amiodarone

From Noble J (ed): *Primary care medicine,* ed 2, St Louis, 1996, Mosby.

POLYCYTHEMIAS

TABLE 2-50 Differential Diagnosis of Relative Erythrocytosis, Secondary Erythrocytosis, and Polycythemia Vera

EXAMINATION	RELATIVE ERYTHROCYTOSIS	SECONDARY ERYTHROCYTOSIS	POLYCYTHEMIA VERA
RBC mass	N	I	I
Plasma volume	D	N or I	N or I
Granulocytes	N	N	N or I
Platelets	N	N	N or I
Serum vitamin B_{12}	N	N	I
Transcobalamin 1	N	N	I
Serum iron	N	N	Usually D
Leukocyte alkaline phosphatase	N	N	N or I
Arterial oxygen saturation	N	N or D	N
Bone marrow	N	Erythroid hyperplasia	Panhyperplasia
Erythropoietin	N	I	N or D
Splenomegaly	Absent	Absent	Usually present

From Noble J (ed): *Primary care medicine,* ed 2, St Louis, 1996, Mosby.
N, Normal; *D,* decreased; *I,* increased.

POLYNEUROPATHY, DRUG-INDUCED

BOX 2-96 Drugs that Cause Polyneuropathy

Drugs in oncology
  Vincristine
  Procarbazine
  Cisplatin
  Mesonidazole
  Metronidazole (Flagyl)
  Taxol
Drugs in infectious diseases
  Isoniazid
  Nitrofurantoin

Dapsone
ddC (dideoxy-cytidine)
ddI (dideoxyinosine)
Drugs in cardiology
  Hydralazine
  Perhexiline maleate
  Procainamide
  Disopyramide
Drugs in rheumatology
  Gold salts
  Chloroquine

Drugs in neurology and psychiatry
  Diphenylhydantoin
  Glutethimide
  Methaqualone
Miscellaneous
  Disulfiram (Antabuse)
  Vitamin: pyridoxine (megadoses)

From Noble J (ed): *Primary care medicine,* ed 2, St Louis, 1996, Mosby.

POLYNEUROPATHY, SYMMETRIC

> **BOX 2-97** A Classificaton of Chronic Symmetric Polyneuropathies
>
> Acquired neuropathies
>   Toxic
>   Drugs
>   Industrial toxins
>   Heavy metals
>   Abused substances
>   Metabolic/endocrine
>   Diabetes
>   Chronic renal failure
>   Hypothyroidism
>   Polyneuropathy of critical illness
>   Nutritional deficiency
>   Vitamin B_{12} deficiency
>   Alcoholism
>   Vitamin E deficiency
>   Paraneoplastic
>   Carcinoma
>   Lymphoma
>   Plasma cell dyscrasia
>   Myeloma, typical, atypical, and solitary forms
>   Primary systemic amyloidosis
>   Idiopathic chronic inflammatory demyelinating polyneuropathies
>   Polyneuropathies associated with peripheral nerve autoantibodies
>   AIDS
> Inherited neuropathies
>   Neuropathies with biochemical markers
>   Refsum disease
>   Bassen-Kornzweig disease
>   Tangier disease
>   Metachromatic leukodystrophy
>   Krabbe's disease
>   Adrenomyeloneuropathy
>   Fabry's disease
>   Neuropathies without biochemical markers or systemic involvement
>   Hereditary motor neuropathy
>   Hereditary sensory neuropathy
>   Hereditary sensorimotor neuropathy

From Noble J (ed): *Primary care medicine,* ed 2, St Louis, 1996, Mosby.

POLYURIA

> **BOX 2-98** Polyuria
>
> Diabetes mellitus
> Diabetes insipidus
> Primary polydipsia (compulsive water drinking)
> Hypercalcemia
> Hypokalemia
> Postobstructive uropathy
> Diuretic phase of renal failure
> Drugs: diuretics, caffeine, lithium
> Sickle cell trait or disease, chronic pyelonephritis (failure to concentrate urine)
> Anxiety, cold weather

POPLITEAL SWELLING

> **BOX 2-99** Popliteal Swelling
>
> Phlebitis (superficial)
> Lymphadenitis
> Trauma: fractured tibia or fibula, contusion, traumatic neuroma
> Deep vein thrombosis
> Ruptured varicose vein
> Baker's cyst
> Popliteal abscess
> Osteomyelitis
> Ruptured tendon
> Aneurysm of popliteal artery
> Neoplasm: lipoma, osteogenic sarcoma, neurofibroma, fibrosarcoma

PROTEINURIA

> **BOX 2-100 Proteinuria**
>
> Nephrotic syndrome as a result of primary renal diseases
> Malignant hypertension
> Malignancies: multiple myeloma, leukemias, Hodgkin's disease
> CHF
> Diabetes mellitus
> SLE, rheumatoid arthritis
> Sickle cell disease
> Goodpature's syndrome
> Malaria
> Amyloidosis, sarcoidosis
> Tubular lesions: cystinosis
> Functional (after heavy exercise)
> Pyelonephritis
> Pregnancy
> Constrictive pericarditis
> Renal vein thrombosis
> Toxic nephropathies: heavy metals, drugs
> Radiation nephritis
> Orthostatic (postural) proteinuria
> Benign proteinuria: fever, heat or cold exposure

PRURITUS

> **BOX 2-101 Pruritus**
>
> Dry skin
> Drug eruption, fiber glass exposure
> Scabies
> Skin diseases
> Myeloproliferative disorders: mycosis fungoides, Hodgkin's lymphoma, multiple myeloma, polycythemia vera
> Cholestatic liver disease
> Endocrine disorders: diabetes mellitus, thyroid disease, carcinoid, pregnancy
> Carcinoma: breast, lung, gastric
> Chronic renal failure
> Iron deficiency
> AIDS
> Neurosis
> Sjögren's syndrome

PUBERTY, DELAYED

BOX 2-102 Causes of Delayed Puberty

I. Normal or low serum gonadotropin levels
   A. Constitutional delay in growth and development
   B. Hypothalamic and/or pituitary disorders
      1. Isolated deficiency of growth hormone
      2. Isolated deficiency on Gn-RH
      3. Isolated deficiency of LH and/or FSH
      4. Multiple anterior pituitary hormone deficiencies
      5. Associated with congenital anomalies: Kallmann's syndrome; Prader-Willi syndrome; Laurence-Moon-Biedl syndrome; Friedreich's ataxia
      6. Trauma
      7. Postinfection
      8. Hyperprolactinemia
      9. Postirradiation
      10. Infiltrative disease (histiocytosis)
      11. Tumor
      12. Autoimmune hypophysitis
      13. Idiopathic
   C. Functional
      1. Chronic endocrinologic or systemic disorders
      2. Emotional disorders
      3. Drugs: cannabis

II. Increased serum gonadotropin levels
   A. Gonadal abnormalities
      1. Congenital
         a. Gonadal dysgenesis
         b. Klinefelter's syndrome
         c. Bilateral anorchism
         d. Resistant ovary syndrome
         e. Myotonia dystrophy in males
         f. 17-Hydroxylase deficiency in females
         g. Galactosemia
      2. Acquired
         a. Bilateral gonadal failure resulting from trauma or infection or after surgery, irradiation, or chemotherapy
         b. Oophoritis: isolated or with other autoimmune disorders
III. Uterine or vaginal disorders
   A. Absence of uterus and/or vagina
   B. Testicular feminization: complete or incomplete androgen insensitivity

From Moore WT, Eastman RC: *Diagnostic endocrinology*, ed 2, St Louis, 1996, Mosby.
FSH, Follicle-stimulating hormone; *Gn-RH*, gonadotropin-releasing hormone; *LH*, luteinizing hormone.

PUBERTY, PRECOCIOUS

BOX 2-103 Causes of Precocious Puberty

Central nervous system tumors
   Neurofibroma
   Hamartoma
   Pinealoma
   Astrocytoma
   Fibrous dysplasia
   Ganglioneuroma
   Ependymoma
Steroid-producing neoplasms
   Adrenal adenoma
   Adrenal carcinoma
   Gonadal neoplasms
Gonadotropin-producing neoplasms
   Teratoma
      Gonadal
      Pineal
      Mediastinal
   Hepatoblastoma
Exogenous hormones (iatrogenic)
   Steroids
   Gonadotropins
   Drugs
Familial (testotoxicosis)
Mutation of luteinizing hormone receptor
Adrenocorticotropic hormone–producing neoplasm
Hypothyroidism, primary
Cushing's disease
Congenital adrenal hyperplasia
   21-Hydroxylase deficiency
   11-Hydroxylase deficiency
Idiopathic isosexual precocious puberty
McCune-Albright syndrome
   Polyostotic fibrous dysplasia

From Moore WT, Eastman RC: *Diagnostic endocrinology*, ed 2, St Louis, 1996, Mosby.

PULMONARY FUNCTION ABNORMALITIES

TABLE 2-51 PFT Abnormalities in Common Disorders

DISORDER	FVC	FEV₁	FEV₁/FVC	RV	TLC	DIFFUSING CAPACITY
Asthma	↓	↓	↓	↑	N/↑	N
COPD	N/↓	↓	↓	↑	N/↑	N/↓
Kyphoscoliosis	↓	↓	N/↑	N/↓	↓	N
Interstitial fibrosis	↓	↓	N/↑	↓	↓	↓

From Ferri FF: *Practical guide to the care of the medical patient*, ed 3, St Louis, 1995, Mosby.
↓, Decreased; ↑, increased; *COPD*, chronic obstructive pulmonary disease; *N*, normal; *FVC*, forced vital capacity; *FEV₁*, forced expiratory volume in 1 sec; *RV*, residual volume; *TLC*, total lung capacity.

PULMONARY LESIONS

BOX 2-104 **Pulmonary Lesions**

Tuberculosis
Legionallea pneumonia
Mycoplasma pneumonia
Viral pneumonia
Pneumocystis carinii
Hypersensitivity pneumonitis
Aspiration pneumonia
Fungal disease (aspergillosis, histoplasmosis)
ARDS associated with pneumonia
Psittacosis
Sarcoidosis
Septic emboli
Metastatic cancer
Multiple pulmonary emboli
Rheumatoid nodules

PULMONARY NODULE, SOLITARY

TABLE 2-52 Causes of Solitary Pulmonary Nodules

CAUSE	RANGE OF REPORTED INCIDENCE (%)	CAUSE	RANGE OF REPORTED INCIDENCE (%)
Malignant tumors		Granulomas–cont'd	
Bronchogenic carcinoma	16-52	Coccidioidomycosis	2-14
Bronchial adenoma (certain cell types seen benign and have benign courses)	1-2	Cryptococcosis	0-1
		Miscellaneous	
Metastatic carcinoma	1-10	Bronchogenic cyst	1-3
Benign tumors	5-12	Arteriovenous malformation	0-1
Hamartoma	1-2	Bronchopulmonary sequestration	0-1
Fibroma	0-1	Sclerosing hemangioma	0-1
Granulomas		Intrapulmonary lymph node	0-1
Histoplasmosis	5-38		
Tuberculosis	10-15		

From Stein JH (ed): *Internal medicine*, ed 4, St Louis, 1994, Mosby.

PURPURA

> **BOX 2-105 Purpura**
>
> Trauma
> Septic emboli, atheromatous emboli
> DIC
> Thrombocytopenia
> Meningococcemia
> Rocky Mountain spotted fever
> Hemolytic-uremic syndrome
> Viral infection: echo, coxsackie
> Scurvy
> Other: left atrial myxoma, cryoglobulinemia, vasculitis, hyperglobulinemic purpura

RECTAL PAIN

> **BOX 2-106 Rectal Pain**
>
> Anal fissure
> Thrombosed hemorrhoid
> Anorectal abscess
> Foreign bodies
> Fecal impaction
> Endometriosis
> Neoplasms (primary or metastatic)
> Pelvic inflammatory disease
> Inflammation of sacral nerves
> Compression of sacral nerves
> Prostatitis
> Other: proctalgia fugax, uterine abnormalities, myopathies, coccygodynia

RED EYE

TABLE 2-53 Differential Diagnosis of Red Eye

ASPECT	ACUTE CONJUNCTIVITIS	ACUTE IRITIS	ACUTE GLAUCOMA	CORNEAL ULCER OR TRAUMA
Redness	Diffuse	Circumcorneal	Diffuse	Diffuse
Vision	Normal	Slightly blurred	Markedly blurred	Blurred
Discharge	Large	None	None	Watery or purulent
Pain	None	Moderate	Severe	Moderate to severe
Cornea	Clear	Anterior chamber may be cloudy	Cloudy	Opacity, fluorescein positive
Pupil size	Normal	Small	Dilated	Normal or small if secondary iritis
Pupil light response	Normal	Poor	Poor	Normal
Intraocular pressure	Normal	Normal	Increased	Normal
Therapy	Antibiotics	Atropine, cortisone	Pilocarpine, Diamox, surgery	Antibiotics
Prognosis	3-5 days	Definitive treatment needed to avoid serious complications		

From Driscoll CE et al: *The family practice desk reference*, ed 3, St Louis, 1996, Mosby.

RENAL CYSTIC DISEASES

TABLE 2-54   Features of Renal Cystic Diseases

	CORTEX AND MEDULLA				MEDULLA	
	SIMPLE	ACQUIRED	POLYCYSTIC DOMINANT	POLYCYSTIC RECESSIVE	SPONGE KIDNEY	MEDULLARY CYSTIC
Prevalence	Common	>50% of dialysis patients	1:1500-1:1000	Rare	1:5000-1:1000	Rare
Symptoms	Rare	Occasional	Common	Common	Occasional	Common
Inherited	No	No	Yes	Yes	Unknown	Dominant and recessive forms
Kidney size	Normal	Small to large	Large	Large	Normal	Small
Hypertension	Rare	Variable	Common	Common	Rare	Rare
Hematuria	Occasional	Occasional	Common	Occasional	Rare (except with stones)	Rare
Associated conditions						
Azotemia	No	Always	Common	Common	Rare	Common
Liver disease	No	No	40%-60%	100%	No	No
Arterial aneurysm	No	No	10%	No	No	No
Differential diagnosis	Tumor Diverticula of renal pelvis	ADPKD Simple cysts Hippel-Lindau disease	ARPKD Tuberous sclerosis Multiple simple cysts	ADPKD Medullary sponge kidney	Medullary cystic kidney Renal tubular acidosis Idiopathic nephrocalcinosis	End-stage renal disease Medullary sponge kidney

From Stein JH (ed): *Internal medicine,* ed 5, St Louis, 1998, Mosby.
ADPKD, Autosomal dominant polycystic kidney disease; ARPKD, autosomal recessive polycystic kidney disease.

RENAL FAILURE, SERUM AND RADIOGRAPHIC ABNORMALITIES

TABLE 2-55   Serum and Radiographic Abnormalities in Renal Failure

	PRERENAL	POSTRENAL (ACUTE)	INTRINSIC RENAL (ACUTE)	INTRINSIC RENAL (CHRONIC)
BUN	↑10:1 > Cr	↑ 20-40/day	↑ 20-40/day	Stable, ↑ varies with protein intake
Serum creatinine	N/moderate ↑	↑ 2-4/day	↑ 2-4/day	Stable ↑ (production equals excretion)
Serum potassium	N/moderate ↑	↑ varies with urinary volume	↑↑ (particularly when patient is oliguric) ↑↑↑ with rhabdomyolysis	Normal until end stage, unless tubular dysfunction (type 4 RTA)
Serum phosphorus	N/moderate ↑	Moderate ↑ ↑↑ with rhabdomyolysis	↑ Poor correlation with duration of renal disease	Becomes significantly elevated when serum creatinine level surpasses 3 mg/dl
Serum calcium	N	N/↓ with PO_4^{-3} retention	↓ (poor correlation with duration of renal failure)	Usually ↓
Renal size				
By ultrasound	N/↑	↑ and dilated calyces	N/↑	↓ and with ↑ echogenicity
FE_{Na}*	<1	<1 → >1	>1	>1

From Grant J. In Ferri FF: *Practical guide to the care of the medical patient,* ed 3, St Louis, 1995, Mosby.
↑, Increase; ↓, decrease; N, normal; ↑↑, large increase, U, urine; P, plasma; Na, sodium; Cr, creatinine.
*$FE_{Na} = U_{Na}/P_{Na}U_{Cr}/P_{Cr} \times 100$.

RENAL FAILURE, URINARY ABNORMALITIES

TABLE 2-56 Urinary Abnormalities in Renal Failure

	PRERENAL	POSTRENAL (ACUTE)	INTRINSIC RENAL (ACUTE)	INTRINSIC RENAL (CHRONIC)
Urinary volume	↓	Absent-to-wide fluctuation	Oliguric or nonoliguric	1000 ml + until end stage
Urinary creatinine	↑ (U/P Cr ±40)	↓ (U/P Cr ±20)	↓ (U/P Cr <20)	↓ (U/P Cr <20)
Osmolarity	↑ (±400 mOsm/kg)	(<350 mOsm/kg)	(<350 mOsm/kg)	(<350 mOsm/kg)
Degree of proteinuria	Minimum	Absent	Varies with cause of renal failure: Modest with ATN Nephrotic range common with acute glomerulopathies, usually <2 g/24 hr with interstitial disease*	Varies with cause of renal disease (from 1-2 g/d to nephrotic range)
Urinary sediment	Negative, or occasional hyaline cast	Negative or hematuria with stones or papillary necrosis Pyuria with infectious prostatic disease	ATN: muddy brown Interstitial nephritis: lymphocytes, eosinophils (in stained preparations), and WBC casts RPGN: RBC casts Nephrosis: oval fat bodies	Broad casts with variable renal "residual" acute findings

From Grant J. In Ferri FF: *Practical guide to the care of the medical patient*, ed 3, St Louis, 1995, Mosby.

↑, Increased; ↓, decreased; *U/P*, urine/plasma; clearance = $\dfrac{\text{Urinary concentration} \times \text{Urinary volume}}{\text{Plasma concentration}}$; *Cr*, creatinine.

*Except NSAID-induced allergic interstitial nephritis with concomitant "nil disease."

RESPIRATORY FAILURE, HYPOVENTILATORY

BOX 2-107 Causes of Hypoventilatory Respiratory Failure

Abnormal Respiratory Capacity (Normal Respiratory Workloads)

Acute depression of central nervous system (CNS)
 Various causes
Chronic central hypoventilation syndromes
 Obesity-hypoventilation syndrome
 Sleep apnea syndrome
 Hypothyroidism
 Shy-Drager syndrome (multisystem atrophy syndrome)
Acute toxic paralysis syndromes
 Botulism
 Tetanus
 Toxic ingestion or bites
 Organophosphate poisoning
Neuromuscular disorders (acute and chronic)
 Myasthenia gravis
 Guillain-Barré syndrome
 Drugs
 Amyotrophic lateral sclerosis
 Muscular dystrophies
 Polymyositis
Spinal cord injury
Traumatic phrenic nerve paralysis

Abnormal Pulmonary Workloads

Chronic obstructive pulmonary disease (COPD)
 Chronic bronchitis
 Asthmatic bronchitis
 Emphysema
Asthma and acute bronchial hyperreactivity syndromes
Upper airway obstruction
Interstitial lung diseases

Abnormal Extrapulmonary Workloads

Chronic thoracic cage disorders
 Severe kyphoscoliosis
 After thoracoplasty
 After thoracic cage injury
Acute thoracic cage trauma and burns
Pneumothorax
Pleural fibrosis and effusions
Abdominal processes

From Noble J (ed): *Primary care medicine*, ed 2, St Louis, 1996, Mosby.

DIFFERENTIAL DIAGNOSIS

RHINITIS, CHRONIC

TABLE 2-57 Classification and Therapy of Chronic Rhinitis

DIAGNOSTIC CLASSIFICATION	DIFFERENTIAL CLINICAL FINDINGS	NASAL CYTOLOGY	ALLERGY SKIN TESTS	PHARMACOLOGIC THERAPY	NONPHARMACOLOGIC THERAPY
I. Inflammatory rhinitis					
A. Eosinophilic allergic rhinitis	Onset typically in, but not limited to, childhood Sneezing, nasal itching, clear rhinorrhea, ocular symptoms Pale, swollen nasal mucosa Specific allergen precipitants (historically) Associated atopic disorders	↑ Eosinophils with or without ↑ basophils and/or mast cells	Positive and correlate with history	Antihistamines Antihistamine-decongestant combinations Intranasal corticosteroids Intranasal cromolyn	Antigen avoidance Immunotherapy
1. Seasonal	Hay fever Typically spring, summer, fall Extended asymptomatic intervals common				
2. Perennial	Typically daily Usually triggered by animals, dust mites, mold				
B. Eosinophilic nonallergic rhinitis	Onset in adulthood (usually) Perennial symptoms Prominent pale mucosal edema Aspirin may increase symptoms Anosmia common Frequent polyps and/or sinus disease	↑ Eosinophils with or without ↑ basophils and/or mast cells	Negative or coincidental (not correlated with history)	Antihistamine-decongestant combinations Intranasal corticosteroids Oral corticosteroids (for severe cases)	Saline lavage Exercise
C. Primary nasal mastocytosis	Onset adulthood (usually)	↑ Mast cells	Negative or coincidental	Intranasal corticosteroids	

Continued

TABLE 2-57 Classification and Therapy of Chronic Rhinitis—cont'd

DIAGNOSTIC CLASSIFICATION	DIFFERENTIAL CLINICAL FINDINGS	NASAL CYTOLOGY	ALLERGY SKIN TESTS	PHARMACOLOGIC THERAPY	NONPHARMACOLOGIC THERAPY
	Perennial rhinorrhea and congestion May be associated with migraine headaches or asthma Nonspecific precipitants frequent			Intranasal cromolyn Systemic oral corticosteroids (for severe cases)	
D. Nasal polyps	Severe obstruction Anosmia Polyps on physical examination Sinus involvement common				Polypectomy with or without submucous resection Ethmoidectomy
1. Eosinophilic	Incidence, 85% Uncommon in children Seromucous secretion Associated with aspirin sensitivity, intrinsic asthma Role of allergy doubtful Steroid responsive	↑ Eosinophils with or without ↑ basophils and/or mast cells	Negative or coincidental	Intranasal corticosteroids Oral corticosteroids	
2. Neutrophilic	Incidence, 15% Purulent secretions Associated with cystic fibrosis, Kartagener's triad, ciliary disturbances, sinusitis, immune deficiency Steroid unresponsive	↑ Neutrophils with or without bacteria	Negative or coincidental	Antibiotics	
E. Neutrophilic nasopharyngitis or sinusitis	Prominent postnasal drip Frequent sinus pain or tenderness Purulent secretions in nose and throat Infection characteristic	↑ Neutrophils with prominent bacteria	Negative or when positive may be related to underlying allergic rhinitis	Control underlying rhinitis/polyps (if present) Topical decongestants (short courses) Antibiotic courses (2 to 3 weeks)	Saline lavage Sinus irrigation Sinus surgery (especially ethroidectomy with or without sphenoidectomy)

DIFFERENTIAL DIAGNOSIS

Rhinitis 645

	Sinus films frequently abnormal (sinusitis) May complicate eosinophilic rhinitis or polyps or occur with immune deficiencies, foreign bodies, or trauma or without demonstrable cause		Possibly oral decongestants Sometimes longer-term antibiotics Possibly mucoevacuants Sometimes oral corticosteroids, plus antibiotics
F. Atrophic rhinitis	Severe nasal obstruction Physiologically patent nasal passages Associated with aging, too extensive nasal tissue extirpation, Wegener's granulomatosis	Unremarkable unless infected	Antibiotics when appropriate Saline lavage Lubricants (petrolatum) Surgical transplantation
II. Noninflammatory rhinitis			
A. Rhinitis medicamentosa			
1. Topical	Obstruction (most prominent symptom) Associated with local sympathomimetric abuse	Unremarkable (usually)	Discontinue topical decongestants Intranasal corticosteroid Oral corticosteroids (for severe cases) Saline lavage Exercise
2. Systemic	Current antihypertensive therapy, oral decongestant (rare), β agonist, birth control pills	Negative or related to underlying disorder	Consider reducing dosage or discontinuing (if possible) or switching to alternate effective medication or therapy Intranasal corticosteroids

Continued

TABLE 2-57 Classification and Therapy of Chronic Rhinitis—cont'd

DIAGNOSTIC CLASSIFICATION	DIFFERENTIAL CLINICAL FINDINGS	NASAL CYTOLOGY	ALLERGY SKIN TESTS	PHARMACOLOGIC THERAPY	NONPHARMACOLOGIC THERAPY
B. Vasomotor instability	Nonspecific hypersensitivity of nasal mucosal vasculature and glands apparently related to local autonomic nervous system imbalance	Unremarkable	Unrelated	Possibly oral decongestants Intranasal ipratropium for prominent rhinorrhea	Saline lavage Exercise Avoid precipitants
1. Associated with systemic conditions	Thyroid disorders Pregnancy			Correct disorder (if possible)	
2. Idiopathic vasomotor rhinitis (primary vasomotor instability)	Most common in young adult women				Exercise essential
III. Structurally related rhinitis	Frequent history of nasal trauma Unilateral obstruction Abnormality diagnosed on physical examination	Unremarkable	Unrelated		Surgery (including laser)

From Stein JH (ed): *Internal medicine*, ed 4, St Louis, 1994, Mosby.

SHORT STATURE

TABLE 2-58 Differential Diagnosis of Short Stature

TYPE OF GROWTH PATTERN	CHRONOLOGIC AGE, HEIGHT AGE, AND BONE AGE	GROWTH RATE	DIFFERENTIAL DIAGNOSIS
Intrinsic short stature	CA = BA > HA*	Normal range†	Familial short stature Intrauterine growth retardation Chromosomal anomalies, especially Turner's syndrome or one of its variants Bone dysplasias Dysmorphic syndromes Secondary to spinal irradiation
	CA > BA > HA		Constitutional delay in growth and puberty with familial short stature Intrauterine growth retardation Chromosomal anomalies
Delayed growth	CA > BA = HA	Normal range†	Constitutional delayed growth and puberty Chronic disorders Malnutrition

Acquired growth failure	CA > HA ≥ BA	Subnormal	Endocrinopathies
			  Growth hormone deficiency
			    Non–growth hormone deficient, GH-responsive growth failure (biologic inactive GH or GH and/or somatomedin-C resistance)
			Hypothyroidism
			Cushing's syndrome
			Sex hormone deficiency after 10 years of age
			Severe chronic organic diseases
			Severe malnutrition
			Psychosocial short stature

	CA > HA ≥ BA	Subnormal	Hypopituitarism Hypothyroidism

From Moore WT, Eastman RC: *Diagnostic endocrinology,* ed 2, St Louis, 1996, Mosby.
*BA, Bone age; CA, chronologic age; GH, growth hormone; HA, height age.
†Slightly subnormal growth rate may occur occasionally.

SHOULDER PAIN

TABLE 2-59 Shoulder Pain: Diagnosis, Evaluation, and Treatment

ENTITY	CHARACTER OF PAIN AND HISTORY	PHYSICAL FINDINGS	X-RAY FINDINGS	TREATMENT
Glenohumeral osteoarthritis	Dull, aching, not severe	Crepitus, decreased ROM	Degenerative changes of joint	Conservative*
Rotator cuff injury	Chronic pain, history of weakness in arm elevation	Pain in active abduction between 70-100 degrees; positive "drop arm" sign	Normal or degenerative changes of greater tuberosity	Surgery if total, otherwise conservative*
Bicipital tendinitis	Pain, anterior shoulder; radiates to biceps and forearm; limited abduction	Tender to palpation in bicipital groove; pain on resisted elbow flexion or wrist supination	Irregularity of bicipital groove (requires special views); X-ray findings are usually normal	Conservative* plus steroid injection over bicipital groove
Adhesive capsulitis (frozen shoulder)	Pain and stiffness often follows prior shoulder condition (i.e., prolonged immobility)	Restricted active and passive ROM, all planes	Localized osteopenia; otherwise normal	Prevention: early mobilization of shoulder injuries; steroid injection plus conservative*, active and passive ROM
Calcific tendinitis/subacromial bursitis	Sudden, severe, diffuse pain, radiates to deltoid; cannot sleep on side; greater prevalence in diabetics	Severe pain on active abduction; tender over upper deltoid and teres major	Fluffy calcific deposit in supraspinatus tendon or other rotator cuff tendons	Conservative*; treat pain; intrabursal steroid injection; rest, but mobilize as soon as possible
Thoracic outlet syndrome	Pain in shoulder and/or arm, plus fullness or numbness	Decreased sensation, muscle weakness, decreased radial pulse; positive Adson's maneuver (decreased pulse plus reproduces symptoms)	Cervical rib on chest x-ray film	Postural training; surgery if recurrent
Referred shoulder pain	Many types, usually diffuse and vague; consider neck, arm, hand pain	Examination of shoulder should be normal; increased by neck motion	Normal	Diagnose underlying cause, (e.g., nerve root compression, lung/pleural disease, MI, subphrenic abscess)
Impingement syndrome	Pain has gradual onset; increased pain with activity	Pain with elevation, loss of forward flexion and internal rotation	Normal	Rest from offending activity; NSAIDs; subacromial steroid injection
Fibrositis	Aching pain in muscles between shoulder and neck; aggravated by stress or cold	Diffuse tenderness, some trigger points of pain		Reassurance, warm modalities, NSAIDs

From Driscoll CE et al: *The family practice desk reference*, ed 3, St Louis, 1996, Mosby.
*Conservative treatment: sling, ASA, or NSAIDs; cold packs for acute; hot packs for chronic pendulum qid.

SKIN LESIONS, PRIMARY

BOX 2-108 Primary Skin Lesions

DESCRIPTION	DIFFERENTIAL DIAGNOSIS

Macule

A circumscribed flat discoloration, that may be brown, blue, red, or hypopigmented

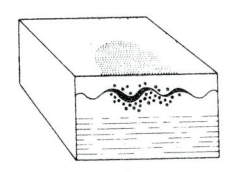

Brown
   Becker's nevus
   Café-au-lait spot
   Erythrasma
   Fixed drug eruption
   Freckle
   Junction nevus
   Lentigo
   Lentigo maligna
   Melasma
   Photoallergic drug eruption
   Phototoxic drug eruption
   Stasis dermatitis
   Tinea nigra palmaris
Blue
   Ink (tattoo)
   Maculae caeruleae (lice)
   Mongolian spot
   Ochronosis

Red
   Drug eruptions
   Juvenile rheumatoid arthritis
     (Still's disease)
   Rheumatic fever
   Secondary syphilis
   Viral exanthems
Hypopigmented
   Idiopathic guttate hypomelanosis
   Piebaldism
   Postinflammatory (psoriasis)
   Radiation dermatitis
   Nevus anemicus
   Tinea versicolor
   Tuberous sclerosis
   Vitiligo

Pustule

A circumscribed collection of leukocytes and free fluid that varies in size

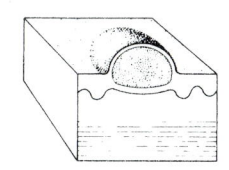

Acne
Candidiasis
Dermatophyte infection
Dyshidrosis
Folliculitis
Gonococcemia
Hidradenitis suppurativa

Herpes simplex
Herpes zoster
Impetigo
Psoriasis
Pyoderma gangrenosum
Rosacea
Varicella

Vesicle

A circumscribed collection of free fluid up to 0.5 cm in diameter

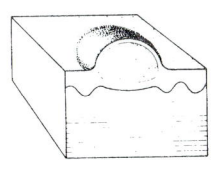

Benign familial chronic pemphigus
Cat-scratch disease
Chicken pox
Dermatitis herpetiformis
Eczema (acute)
Erythema multiforme
Herpes simplex

Herpes zoster
Impetigo
Lichen planus
Pemphigus foliaceus
Porphyria cutania tarda
Scabies

Bulla

A circumscribed collection of free fluid more than 0.5 cm in diameter

Fixed drug eruption
Herpes gestationis
Lupus erythematosus
Pemphigus

Bullae in diabetics
Bullous pemphigoid
Cicatricial pemphigoid
Epidermolysis bullosa acquisita

Wheal

A firm edematous plaque resulting from infiltration of the dermis with fluid; it is transient and may last only a few hours

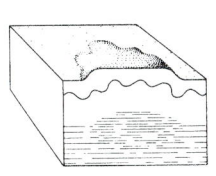

Angioedema
Dermographism
Hives
Insect bites
Urticaria pigmentosa (mastocytosis)

Continued

BOX 2-108 Primary Skin Lesions—cont'd

DESCRIPTION	DIFFERENTIAL DIAGNOSIS

Papule

An elevated solid lesion up to 0.5 cm in diameter; color varies; papules may become confluent and form plaques

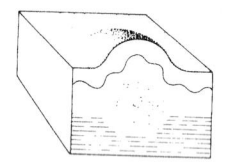

Flesh colored, yellow, or white
- Adenoma sebaceum
- Basal cell epithelioma
- Closed comedone (acne)
- Flat warts
- Granuloma annulare
- Lichen nitidus
- Lichen sclerosis et atrophicus
- Molluscum contagiosum
- Milium
- Nevi (dermal)
- Neurofibroma
- Pearly penile papules
- Pseudoxanthoma elasticum
- Sebaceous hyperplasia
- Skin tags
- Syringoma

Brown
- Dermatofibroma
- Keratosis follicularis
- Melanoma
- Nevi
- Seborrheic keratosis
- Urticaria pigmentosa
- Warts

Red
- Acne
- Atopic dermatitis
- Cholinergic urticaria
- Chondrodermatitis nodularis chronica helicis
- Eczema
- Folliculitis
- Insect bites
- Keratosis pilaris
- Leukocytoclastic vasculitis
- Miliaria
- Polymorphic light eruption
- Psoriasis
- Pyogenic granuloma
- Scabies
- Urticaria

Blue or violaceous
- Angiokeratoma
- Blue nevus
- Lichen planus
- Lymphoma
- Kaposi's sarcoma
- Melanoma
- Mycosis fungoides
- Venous lake

Plaque

A circumscribed, elevated, superficial, solid lesion more than 0.5 cm in diameter, often formed by the confluence of papules

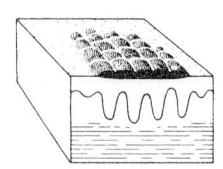

Eczema
Mycosis fungoides
Papulosquamous (papular and scaling)
- Discoid lupus erythematosus
- Lichen planus
- Pityriasis rosea
- Psoriasis
- Seborrheic dermatitis
- Syphilis (secondary)
- Tinea corporis
- Tinea versicolor

Nodule

A circumscribed, elevated, solid lesion more than 0.5 cm in diameter; a large nodule is referred to as a tumor

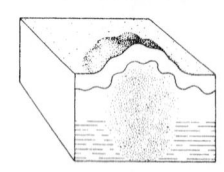

Basal cell epithelioma
Erythema nodosum
Furuncle
Hemangioma
Kaposi's sarcoma
Keratoacanthoma
Lipoma
Lymphoma
Melanoma

Metastatic carcinoma
Mycosis fungoides
Neurofibromatosis
Prurigo nodularis
Sporotrichosis
Squamous cell carcinoma
Warts
Xanthoma

From Habif TP: *Clinical dermatology, a color guide to diagnosis and therapy,* ed 2, St Louis, 1990, Mosby.

SKIN LESIONS, SECONDARY

BOX 2-109 Secondary Skin Lesions

DESCRIPTION	DIFFERENTIAL DIAGNOSIS

Scale
Exceeds dead epidermal cells that are produced by abnormal keratinization and shedding

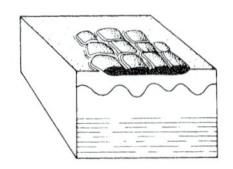

Fine to stratified
   Eczema craquele
   Ichthyosis (quadrangular)
   Lupus erythematosus (carpet tack)
   Pityriasis rosea (collarette)
   Psoriasis (silvery)
   Scarlet fever (fine on trunk)
   Seborrheic dermatitis (greasy)
   Syphilis (secondary)
   Tinea (dermatophytes)
   Tinea versicolor
   Xerosis (dry skin)
Scaling in sheets
   Scarlet fever (hands and feet)
   Staphylococcal scalded skin syndrome

Crust
A collection of dried serum and cellular debris; a scab

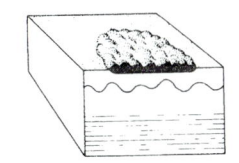

Acute eczematous inflammation
Atopic (face)
Impetigo (honey colored)
Pemphigus foliaceus
Tinea capitis

Erosion
A focal loss of epidermis; it does not penetrate below dermal-epidermal junction and therefore heals without scarring

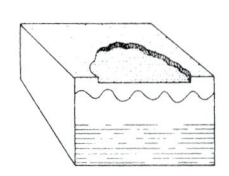

Candidiasis
Dermatophyte infection
Eczematous diseases
Intertrigo
Perlèche
Senile skin
Toxic epidermal necrolysis
Vesiculobullous diseases

Ulcer
A focal loss of epidermis and dermis; it heals with scarring

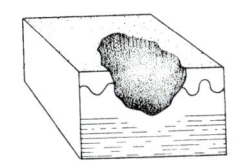

Aphthae
Chancroid
Decubitus
Factitial
Ischemic
Necrobiosis lipoidica diabeticorum
Neoplasms
Pyoderma gangrenosum
Radiodermatitis
Syphilis (chancre)
Stasis ulcers

Continued

BOX 2-109 Secondary Skin Lesions—cont'd

DESCRIPTION	DIFFERENTIAL DIAGNOSIS
Fissure A linear loss of epidermis and dermis with sharply defined nearly vertical walls 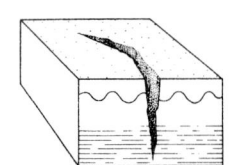	Chapping (hands, feet) Eczema (fingertip) Intertrigo Perlèche
Atrophy A depression in skin resulting from thinning of epidermis or dermis 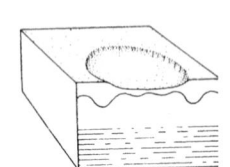	Aging Dermatomyositis Discoid lupus erythematosus Lichen sclerosis et atrophicus Morphea Necrobiosis lipoidica diabeticorum Radiodermatitis Striae Topical and intralesional steroids
Scar An abnormal formation of connective tissue implying dermal damage; when following injury or surgery, it is initially thick and pink but with time becomes white and atrophic 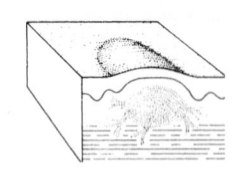	Acne Burns Herpes zoster Hidradenitis suppurativa Porphyria Varicella

From Habif TP: *Clinical dermatology, a color guide to diagnosis and therapy,* ed 2, St Louis, 1990, Mosby.

SKIN LESIONS, SPECIAL

TABLE 2-60 Special Skin Lesions

DESCRIPTION	DIFFERENTIAL DIAGNOSIS
Excoriation An erosion caused by scratching; often linear	—
Comedone A plug of sebaceous and keratinous material lodged in the opening of a hair follicle; the follicular orifice may be dilated (blackhead) or narrowed (whitehead) or closed (comedone)	—
Milia Small superficial keratin cysts with no visible openings	—
Cyst A circumscribed lesion having a wall and a lumen; the lumen may contain fluid or solid matter	—
Burrow A narrow, elevated, tortuous channel produced by a parasite	—
Lichenification An area of thickened epidermis induced by scratching; the skin lines are accentuated so the surface looks like a washboard	—

Telangiectasia
Dilated superficial blood vessels
	Actinically damaged skin
	Adenoma sebaceum
	Ataxia-telangiectasia
	Basal cell carcinoma
	Bloom's syndrome
	CRST syndrome
	Hereditary hemorrhagic telangiectasia
	Keloid
	Lupus erythematosus
	Necrobiosis lipoidica diabeticorum
	Of the proximal nail fold
	  Dermatomyositis
	  Lupus erythematosus
	  Scleroderma
	Poikiloderma
	Radiodermatitis
	Rosacea
	Scleroderma
	Vascular spiders
	  Pregnancy
	  Cirrhosis
	Xeroderma pigmentosum

Petechia Circumscribed deposits of blood less than 0.5 cm in diameter **Purpura** A circumscribed deposit of blood greater than 0.5 cm in diameter	Gonococcemia Leukocytoclastic vasculitis Meningococcemia Platelet abnormalities Progressive pigmentary purpura Rocky Mountain spotted fever Scurvy Senile (traumatic)

From Habif PF: *Clinical dermatology, a color guide to diagnosis and therapy*, ed 2, St Louis, 1990, Mosby.

SPHEROCYTOSIS

BOX 2-110 Causes of Spherocytosis

ABO hemolytic disease of newborn
Acute transfusion reactions (especially ABO type)
Hereditary spherocytosis
Transfused stored bank blood
Autoimmune hemolytic anemia
Thermal injury, especially in first 24 hr

Physical RBC injury (as a component of microangiopathic hemolytic anemia)
Toxins (*Clostridium welchii* sepsis and certain snake venoms)
Hereditary elliptocytosis (10%-20% of cases)
Occasionally in severe Heinz body hemolytic anemias

From Ravel R: *Clinical laboratory medicine*, ed 6, St Louis, 1995, Mosby.

SPLENOMEGALY

BOX 2-111 Causes of Splenomegaly

Infections
  Subacute bacterial endocarditis
  Brucellosis
  Infectious mononucleosis, cytomegalovirus
  Tuberculosis
  Parasites
    Malaria
    Schistomiasis
    Kala-azar
    Other
  Sepsis
Immune disorders
  Systemic lupus erythematosus
  Sarcoidosis
  Rheumatoid arthritis (Felty's syndrome)
Hematologic disorders
  Hemolytic anemias, acute and chronic
  Immune thrombocytopenic purpura

Lymphomas
Leukemias
Myeloproliferative diseases
Metastatic diseases
Infiltrative splenomegaly
  Lipid storage disease
  Amyloidosis
  Diabetic lipemia
  True cysts
    Epithelial
    Endothelial
    Dermoids, lymphangiomyomatosis, hydatid
Vascular congestion
  Congestive heart failure
  Portal hypertension secondary to cirrhosis
  Splenic vein obstruction
  Budd-Chiari syndrome

From Noble J (ed): *Primary care medicine*, ed 2, St Louis, 1996, Mosby.

SPONDYLOARTHROPATHIES

> **BOX 2-112** **Differential Diagnosis for Spondyloarthropathies**
>
> Axial arthritis
>   Discogenic back pain
>   Osteoarthritis
>   Facet disease
>   Diffuse idiopathic hypertrophic osteoarthropathy
>   Osteoarthritis of sacroiliac joints
>   Osteitis condensans ilii
>   Infection (sacroiliitis)
>   Tuberculosis, brucellosis*
>   Bacteremia from intravenous drug abuse
>   Others
>   Whipple's disease*
>   Behçet's syndrome*
>   Relapsing polychondritis
>   Secondary hyperparathyroidism
> Peripheral arthritis
>   Other inflammatory arthritides
>   Rheumatoid arthritis
>   Crystals
>   Infections
>   *Borrella burgdorferi* (Lyme disease)
>   Gonacoccal
>   Poststreptococcal, acute rheumatic fever*
>   HIV
>   Chronic fungal or tuberculous
>   Noninflammatory arthritides
>   Osteoarthritis, particularly inflammatory osteoarthritis
>   Mechanical derangement
>   Synovial neoplasia
>   Pigmented villonodular synovitis*
>   Osteogenic sarcoma*
>   Synovial osteochondromatosis*
>   Others
>   Sarcoidosis
> Axial and peripheral arthritis
>   Osteoarthritis
>   Rheumatoid arthritis
>   Whipple's disease*
>   Behçet's syndrome*
>   Relapsing polychondritis*
>   Familial Mediterranean fever*

From Noble J (ed): *Primary care medicine,* ed 2, St Louis, 1996, Mosby.
*Rare occurrences.

SPONDYLOARTHROPATHIES, SERONEGATIVE

TABLE 2-61 Comparison of Seronegative Spondyloarthropathies

SPONDYLOARTHROPATHY	ANKYLOSING SPONDYLITIS	REITER'S SYNDROME	PSORIATIC ARTHRITIS	ARTHRITIS ASSOCIATED WITH GI DISEASE

Characteristics and presentation	Insidious onset of constant back pain lasting longer than 3 mo in patient less than 40 yr of age
	Pain and stiffness are improved by exercise; patients often walk around at night to gain relief from nocturnal back pain
	Associated with anterior uveitis (25%), aortitis (5%)
		Arthritis usually follows episode of urethritis
		Eye involvement: bilateral conjunctivitis, uveitis, keratitis, retinitis
		Dermatitis: usually painless mucocutaneous lesions on glans penis and mouth, hyperkeratotic lesions on palms and soles (keratoderma blenorrhagicum)
			Arthritis usually involves DIP joints, often resulting in "sausage" digits
			
			Skin lesions usually precede arthritis
			Nail changes (pitting) often accompany psoriatic arthritis
				Occurs with:
				  Whipple's disease (up to 90% of patients) Crohn's disease (20%)
				  After interstinal bypass
				  Ulcerative colitis (10%)
				  Remission of underlying disorder usually results in complete remission of the arthritis
				May be associated with erythema nodosum, pyoderma gangrenosum, anterior uveitis

Association with HLA-B27	Strong association	Strong association	No significant association	No significant association except in patients with inflammatory bowel disease and sacroiliitis
Characteristic radiographic patterns of spine	Radiographs of spine initially show straightening of lumbar part of spine; in advanced disease, diffuse syndesmophyte formation may result in fusion of entire spine (bamboo spine)	Unlike ankylosing spondylitis, distribution of syndesmophytes is asymmetrics and non-marginal	Similar to Reiter's syndrome	Radiographic evaluation may be normal or may reveal sacroiliitis
Peripheral arthritis	Oligoarticular Hips, shoulder	Oligoarticular Asymmetric Lower extremities	DIP joints Usually asymmetric and oligoarticular but can be variable	Large joints (knees, ankles) Symmetric
Therapy	NSAIDs, physical therapy	Joint immobilization, NSAIDs Topical corticosteroids for conjunctivitis, corticosteroid therapy, physical therapy	Treat skin disease NSAIDs Methotrexate Gold therapy	Treat underlying disorder Sulfasalazine (Azulfidine) for sacroiliitis associated with inflammatory bowel disease

ST SEGMENT ELEVATION

TABLE 2-62 Differential Diagnosis of ST Segment Elevation (by Degree, Morphology, and Associated Findings)*

	MYOCARDIAL ISCHEMIA	EARLY REPOLARIZATION	ACUTE (SIMPLE) PERICARDITIS
ST elevation (over 5 mm)	+	0	0
Reciprocal ST depression	+	±	±
Convex ST	+	0	±
Concave ST	+	+	+
Prominent T (over 5 mm)	+	+	0
Same lead ST elevation and T depression	+	±	±
Pathologic Q waves	+	0	0
Special findings	Atrioventricular block	0	Electrical alternans

From Rosen P et al (eds): *Emergency medicine: concepts and clinical practice,* St Louis, 1992, Mosby.
*Only positive findings are classified; negative findings do not exclude ischemia or pericarditis; +, often found; ±, not often found or restricted to certain leads; 0, reliably absent.

SWOLLEN LIMB

TABLE 2-63 Differential Diagnosis of the Swollen Limb

	PAIN	INFLAMMATORY SIGNS	VARICOSE VEINS	NONINVASIVE VENOUS STUDIES	CLUES TO DIAGNOSIS
Thrombophlebitis	+	+	±	+	Acute onset of swelling
Lymphedema	Usually absent	0	0	Negative	Gradual onset of swelling
Postphlebitic syndrome	+	±	+	Negative	Stasis pigmentation, subcutaneous tissue induration
Ruptured popliteal synovial membrane	+	+	0	Negative	Fluid in the knee joint, history of arthritis
Ruptured calf	+	+	0	Negative	Ecchymoses around ankle, tender knot in muscle, sudden onset during exercise—may feel a pop
Myositis ossificans	+	+	0	Negative	Indurated area in thigh with localized swelling; positive bone scan

From Noble J (ed): *Primary care medicine,* ed 2, St Louis, 1996, Mosby.

SYNOVIAL FLUID ABNORMALITIES

TABLE 2-64 Classification and Interpretation of Synovial Fluid Analysis

GROUP	DISEASES	APPEARANCE	VISCOSITY	MUCIN CLOT	WBC/MM³	%PMN	GLUCOSE (MG/DL) (BLOOD-SYNOVIAL FLUID)	PROTEIN (G/DL)
Normal	—	Clear	↑	Firm	<200	<25	<10	<2.5
I (noninflammatory)	Osteoarthritis, aseptic necrosis, traumatic arthritis, erythema nodosum, osteochondritis dissecans	Clear, yellow (may be xanthochromic if traumatic arthritis)	↑	Firm	↑ Up to 10,000	<25	<10	<2.5
II (inflammatory)	Crystal-induced arthritis, rheumatoid arthritis, Reiter's syndrome, collagen vascular disease, psoriatic arthritis, serum sickness, rheumatic fever	Clear, yellow, turbid	↓	Friable	↑↑ Up to 100,000	40-90	<40	>2.5
III (septic)	Bacterial (staphylococcal, gonococcal, TB)	Turbid	↓/↑	Friable	↑↑↑ Up to 5,000,000	40-100	20-100	>2.5

PMN, Polymorphonuclear leukocytes; ↑, elevated; ↑↑, markedly high; ↓, decreased. Note that there is considerable overlap in the numbers listed above.

TALL STATURE

BOX 2-113 **Causes of Tall Stature**

Constitutional (familial or genetic)—most common cause
Endocrine causes
    Growth hormone excess—gigantism
    Sexual precocity (tall as children, short as adults)
        True sexual precocity
        Pseudosexual precocity
    Androgen deficiency
        Klinefelter's syndrome
        Bilateral anorchism
Genetic causes
    Klinefelter's syndrome
    Syndromes of XYY, XXYY
Miscellaneous syndromes and disorders
    Cerebral gigantism or Sotos' syndrome: prominent forehead, hypertelorism, high arched palate, dolichocephaly, mental retardation, large hands and feet, and premature eruption of teeth. Large at birth, with most rapid growth in first 4 years of life.

Marfan's syndrome: disorder of mesodermal tissues, subluxation of the lenses, arachnodactyly, and aortic aneurysm.
Homocystinuria: same phenotype as Marfan's syndrome.
Obesity: tall as infants, children, and adolescents.
Total lipodystrophy: large hands and feet, generalized loss of subcutaneous fat, insulin-resistant diabetes mellitus, and hepatomegaly.
Beckwith-Wiedemann syndrome: neonatal tallness, omphalocele, macroglossia, and neonatal hypoglycemia.
Weaver-Smith syndrome: excessive intrauterine growth, mental retardation, megalocephaly, widened bifrontal diameter, hypertelorism, large ears, micrognathia, camptodactyly, broad thumbs, and limited extension of elbows and knees.
Marshall-Smith syndrome: excessive intrauterine growth, mental retardation, blue sclerae, failure to thrive, and early death.

From Moore WT, Eastman RC: *Diagnostic endocrinology*, ed 2, St Louis, 1996, Mosby.

TESTICULAR SIZE VARIATIONS

> **BOX 2-114 Causes of Variations in Testicular Size**
>
> **Small Testes**
> Hypothalamic-pituitary dysfunction
>   Gonadotropin deficiency
>   Growth hormone deficiency
> Normal variant
> Primary hypogonadism
>   Autoimmune destruction, chemotherapy, cryptorchidism, irradiation, Klinefelter syndrome, orchiditis, testicular regression syndrome, torsion, trauma
>
> **Large Testes**
> Adrenal rest tissue
> Compensatory
> Fragile X syndrome
> Idiopathic
> Tumor

From Moore WT, Eastman RC: *Diagnostic endocrinology,* ed 2, St Louis, 1996, Mosby.

THROMBOCYTOPENIA

> **BOX 2-115 Major Causes of Thrombocytopenia**
>
> I. Decreased platelet production
>   A. Megakaryocyte hypoplasia
>   1. Aplastic anemia
>   2. Myelofibrosis
>   3. Leukemia
>   4. Marrow invasion by metastatic tumor, granulomas
>   5. Viral infection
>   6. Radiation myelosuppression
>   7. Toxic agents, drugs, antineoplastic chemotherapy
>   B. Ineffective thrombopoiesis
>   1. Vitamin B$_{12}$ deficiency
>   2. Folate deficiency
> II. Splenic sequestration, hypersplenism
> III. Increased platelet destruction
>   A. Non-immune-mediated platelet destruction
>   1. Disseminated intravascular coagulation (DIC)
>   2. Prosthetic intravascular devices
>   3. Extracorporeal circulation
>   4. Thrombotic thrombocytopenic purpura (TTP)
>   B. Immune-mediated platelet destruction
>   1. Drug-induced immune thrombocytopenia
>   2. Alloimmune thrombocytopenia
>   a. Neonatal
>   b. Posttransfusion purpura
>   3. Autoimmune thrombocytopenia
>   a. Idiopathic thrombocytopenic purpura (ITP)
>   b. Secondary to rheumatic diseases, infections, lymphoproliferative disorders

From Stein JH (ed): *Internal medicine,* ed 4, St Louis, 1994, Mosby.

THYROID NODULE, COLD

> **BOX 2-116 Differential Diagnosis of the Cold Thyroid Nodule**
>
> **Common Causes**
> Follicular adenoma—with or without cystic/hemorrhagic degeneration
> Hyperplastic nodule
> Thyroiditis—subacute, "silent," or chronic (rarely acute)
> Thyroid carcinoma—papillary, follicular, or anaplastic
> Colloid cyst
> Previous surgery
>
> **Rare Causes**
> Hemiagenesis
> Primary thyroid lymphoma
> Medullary thyroid carcinoma
> Branchiogenic cyst
> Parathyroid adenoma, carcinoma, or cyst
> Malignancy metastatic to thyroid
> Tuberculoma
> Amyloidosis
> Postradiation fibrosis
> Marine-Lenhart syndrome

From Moore WT, Eastman RC: *Diagnostic endocrinology,* ed 2, St Louis, 1996, Mosby.

TREMATODE TISSUE INFECTIONS

TABLE 2-65 Trematode Tissue Infections

SPECIES	EPIDEMIOLOGY	TRANSMISSION	LOCATION OF ADULT WORMS	MAJOR CLINICAL PRESENTATION	DIAGNOSIS	TREATMENT
Schistosoma spp.						
S. mansoni	Africa, South America, Middle East, Caribbean	Contact with fresh water	Mesenteric vasculature	Portal hypertension hepatosplenomegaly	Stool O&P, rectal snips	Praziquantel, 20 mg/kg bid for 1 day, or praziquantel, 40 mg/kg once, or oxamniquine, 10 mg/kg bid for 1 day
S. japonicum	China, Philippines, Indonesia	Contact with fresh water	Mesenteric vasculature	Same as for S. mansoni plus seizures	Same as for S. mansoni	Praziquantel, 20 mg/kg tid for 1 day
S. mekongi	Thailand, Laos, Cambodia	Contact with fresh water	Mesenteric vasculature	Same as for S. japonicum	Same as for S. mansoni	Praziquantel, 20 mg/kg tid for 1 day
S. haematobium	Africa, Middle East	Contact with fresh water	Vesical venules	Hematuria, hydronephrosis, carcinoma of bladder	Urine O&P	Praziquantel, 20 mg/kg bid for 1 day, or praziquantel 40 mg/kg once
Clonorchis sinensis	Japan, China, Korea	Raw fish	Biliary tree	Cholangitis, portal hypertension, cholangiocarcinoma	Stool O&P	Praziquantel,* 25 mg/kg tid for 2 days
Fasciola hepatica	Worldwide where sheep are raised	Raw watercress	Bile ducts, liver tissue	Right upper quadrant pain and fever, biliary obstruction, hepatic fibrosis	Stool O&P serology	Albendazole* 10 mg/kg for 7 days or bithionol,† 30-50 mg/kg every other day for 15 days
Paragonimus westermani	Orient, India, Central Africa	Raw crab	Lungs	Cough, sputum production, resembling tuberculosis	Sputum, stool O&P	Praziquantel,* 25 mg/kg tid for 2 days, or bithionol† as for F. hepatica
Opisthorchis viverrini	Europe, Asia, Southeast Asia	Raw freshwater fish	Biliary tree	Same as for C. sinensis	Stool O&P	Praziquantel,* 25 mg/kg tid for 1 wk

From Stein JH (ed): *Internal medicine*, ed 5, St Louis, 1998, Mosby.
Tid, Three times a day; *bid,* twice a day; *O&P,* ova and parasites.
*Considered an investigational drug by the US Food and Drug Administration.
†Available only from the Centers for Disease Control and Prevention in the United States.

TREMOR

BOX 2-117 Tremor

Tremor present at rest
  Parkinsonism
  CNS neoplasms
  Tardive dyskinesia
Postural tremor (present during maintenance of a posture)
  Essential senile tremor

Action tremor (present with movement)
  Anxiety
  Medications (bronchodilators, caffeine, corticosteroids, lithium, etc.)
  Endocrine disorders (hyperthyroidism, pheochromocytoma, carcinoid)
  Withdrawal from substance abuse

UROPATHY, OBSTRUCTIVE

BOX 2-118 Causes of Obstructive Uropathy

I. Intrinsic Causes
  A. Intraluminal
    1. Intratubular deposition of crystals (uric acid, sulfas)
    2. Stones
    3. Papillary tissue
    4. Blood clots
  B. Intramural
    1. Functional
      a. Ureter (ureteropelvic or ureterovesical dysfunction)
      b. Bladder (neurogenic): spinal cord defect or trauma, diabetes, multiple sclerosis, Parkinson's disease, cerebrovascular accidents
      c. Bladder neck dysfunction
    2. Anatomic
      a. Tumors
      b. Infection, granuloma
      c. Strictures

II. Extrinsic Causes
  A. Originating in the reproductive system
    1. Prostate: benign hypertrophy or cancer
    2. Uterus: pregnancy, tumors, prolapse, endometriosis
    3. Ovary: abscess, tumor, cysts
  B. Originating in the vascular system
    1. Aneurysms (aorta, iliac vessels)
    2. Aberrant arteries (ureteropelvic junction)
    3. Venous (ovarian veins, retrocaval ureter)
  C. Originating in the gastrointestinal tract: Crohn's disease, pancreatitis, appendicitis, tumors
  D. Originating in the retroperitoneal space
    1. Inflammations
    2. Fibrosis
    3. Tumor, hematomas

From Stein JH (ed): *Internal medicine,* ed 4, St Louis, 1994, Mosby.

URTICARIA

BOX 2-119 Etiologic Classification of Urticaria

Foods
  Fish, shellfish, nuts, eggs, chocolate, strawberries, tomatoes, pork, cow's milk, cheese, wheat, yeast
Food additives
  Salicylates, benzoates, penicillin, dyes such as tartrazine
Drugs
  Penicillin, aspirin, sulfonamides; also drugs that cause nonimmunologic release of histamine (e.g., morphine, codeine, polymyxin, dextran, curare, quinine)
Infections
  Chronic bacterial infections (e.g., sinus, dental, chest, gallbladder, urinary tract), fungal infections (dermatophytosis, candidiasis), viral infections (viral hepatitis, infectious mononucleosis, coxsackie), protozoal and helminth infections (intestinal worms, malaria)
Inhalants
  Pollens, mold spores, animal danders, house dust, aerosols, volatile chemicals
Internal disease
  Serum sickness, systemic lupus erythematosus, hyperthyroidism, carcinomas, lymphomas, juvenile rheumatoid arthritis (Still's disease), leukocytoclastic vasculitis, polycythemia vera (acne urticata—urticarial papule surmounted by a vesicle), rheumatic fever
Physical stimuli (the physical urticarias)
  Dermographism, pressure urticaria, cholinergic urticaria, solar urticaria, cold urticaria, urticarias induced by heat, vibration, water (aquagenic)
Nonimmunologic contact urticaria
  Plants (nettles), animals (caterpillars, jellyfish), medications (cinnamic aldehyde, compound 48/80, dimethyl sulfoxide)
Immunologic or uncertain mechanism contact urticaria
  Ammonium persulfate used in hair bleaches, chemicals, foods, textiles, wood, saliva, cosmetics, perfumes
Skin diseases
  Urticaria pigmentosa (mastocytosis), dermatitis herpetiformis, pemphigoid, amyloidosis
Pregnancy
Genetic, autosomal dominant (all rare)
  Hereditary angioedema, cholinergic urticaria with progressive nerve deafness and amyloidosis of the kidney, familial cold urticaria, vibratory urticaria

From Habif PF: *Clinical dermatology, a color guide to diagnosis and therapy,* ed 2, St Louis, 1990, Mosby.

VAGINAL BLEEDING ABNORMALITIES

TABLE 2-66 Differential Diagnosis: Abnormal Vaginal Bleeding

FACTORS	DIAGNOSIS
General	Trauma
	Neoplasia
Specific to Reproductive Cycle	
Pregnancy	
First trimester	Miscarriage
	Ectopic implantation
Third trimester	Placenta previa
	Placental abruption
	Premature labor
Ovulatory Cycles Present	Shortened follicular luteal phase
	Anatomic lesion
	Endometrial polyps
	Cervical polyps
	Adenomyosis
	Fibroids
	Systemic disease
	Coagulopathies
	Intrauterine device
	Cervical cancer
	Sarcomas
	Pelvic inflammatory disease
Anovulatory Cycles	Immature hypothalamic regulation
	Polycystic ovary syndrome
	Perimenopausal changes
	Endometrial hyperplasia
	Endometrial carcinoma
	Postmenopausal hormone replacement
	Dysfunctional uterine bleeding (no pelvic organ disease or systemic disorder)
	Endometriosis

From Carlson KJ et al: *Primary care of women,* St Louis, 1995, Mosby.

VAGINAL BLEEDING, PREGNANCY

BOX 2-120 Differential Diagnosis of Abnormal Vaginal Bleeding in Pregnant Women

FIRST TRIMESTER	THIRD TRIMESTER
Implantation bleeding	Placenta previa
Abortion	Placenta abruption
Threatened	Premature labor
Complete	Choriocarcinoma
Incomplete	
Missed	
Ectopic pregnancy	
Neoplasia	
Hydatidiform mole	
Cervix	

From Carlson KJ et al: *Primary care of women,* St Louis, 1995, Mosby.

VAGINITIS

TABLE 2-67 Differential Diagnosis of Vaginitis

	SYMPTOMS	VOLUME OF DISCHARGE	APPEARANCE OF DISCHARGE	WET MOUNT	pH	CULTURE
Normal vagina	None	4-6 cm^3/day	Clear, white	Squamous epithelial cells	<4.5	Normal vaginal flora
Bacterial vaginosis	Asymptomatic, irritation	Increased	Homogeneous, gray	NS: clue cells KOH: amine odor	>4.5	Nondiagnostic
Candida vaginitis	Pruritus, burning	Usually increased	Cottage cheese–like, white	KOH: pseudohyphae	4-5	90% sensitive
Trichomonas vaginitis	Pruritus	Increased	Frothy, green or gray	NS: trichomonads, increased polyps	>4.5	95% sensitive
Atrophic vaginitis	Irritation, pruritus, dyspareunia	None or increased	Watery, yellow or green	Increased polys	>4.5	Normal vaginal flora
Cytolytic vaginosis	Burning, irritation, dyspareunia	Increased	Clumpy, white	Cytolysis of squamous epithelial cells	>4.5	Nondiagnostic

From Carlson KJ et al: *Primary care of women*, St Louis, 1995, Mosby.
NS, Normal saline-solution; *KOH*, potassium hydroxide 10% solution; *polys*, polymorphonuclear leukocytes.

VASCULITIC SYNDROMES

TABLE 2-68 Classification of Vasculitic Syndromes

CLINICAL SYNDROME	PREDOMINANT VESSELS AFFECTED
Takayasu arteritis	Large arteries (aorta and primary branches)
Giant-cell (temporal) arteritis	Large and medium-sized arteries (aorta, primary and secondary branches)
Thromboangiitis obliterans (Buerger's disease)	Medium-sized and small muscular arteries (diverse distributions and locations)
Kawasaki disease	
Polyarteritis nodosa	
Allergic angiitis and granulomatosis (Churg-Strauss syndrome)	
Vasculitis in rheumatic disease (e.g., rheumatoid arthritis, Behçet's syndrome)	
Granulomatous angiitis of CNS	
Wegener's granulomatosis	
Vasculitis associated with malignancy (e.g., hairy-cell leukemia)	
Hypersensitivity vasculitis (e.g., serum sickness, drug reactions)	Small vessels (arterioles, capillaries, venules)
Henoch-Schönlein purpura	
Mixed cryoglobulinemia	
Hypocomplementemic urticarial vasculitis	
Cutaneous vasculitis associated with other diseases (e.g., biliary cirrhosis, ulcerative colitis)	

From Stein JH (ed): *Internal medicine*, St Louis, 1984, Mosby.

VENTRICULAR FAILURE

> **BOX 2-121 Ventricular Failure**
>
> | LEFT VENTRICULAR FAILURE | RIGHT VENTRICULAR FAILURE | BIVENTRICULAR FAILURE |
> |---|---|---|
> | Systemic hypertension | Valvular heart disease (mitral stenosis) | Left ventricular failure |
> | | | Cardiomyopathy |
> | Valvular heart disease (AS, AR, MR) | Pulmonary hypertension | Myocarditis |
> | Cardiomyopathy, myocarditis | Bacterial endocarditis (right-sided) | Arrhythmias |
> | | | Anemia |
> | Bacterial endocarditis | Right ventricular infarction | Thyrotoxicosis |
> | MI | | AV fistula |
> | IHSS | | Paget's disease |
> | | | Beri-beri |

VERTIGO

> **BOX 2-122 Vertigo**
>
> **Peripheral**
>
> Otitis media
> Acute labyrinthitis
> Vestibular neuronitis
> Benign positional vertigo
> Meniere's disease
> Ototoxic drugs: streptomycin, gentamycin
> Lesions of the eighth nerve: acoustic neuroma, meningioma, mononeuropathy, metastatic carcinoma
> Mastoiditis
>
> **CNS or Systemic**
>
> Vertebrobasilar artery insufficiency
> Posterior fossa tumor or other brain tumors
> Infarction/hemorrhage of cerebral cortex, cerebellum, or brain stem
> Basilar migraine
> Metabolic: drugs, hypoxia, anemia, fever
> Hypotension/severe hypertension
> Multiple sclerosis
> CNS infections: viral, bacterial
> Temporal lobe epilepsy
> Arnold-Chiari malformation, syringobulbia
> Psychogenic: ventilation, hysteria

DIFFERENTIAL DIAGNOSIS   **Visual field defects** 665

VISUAL FIELD DEFECTS

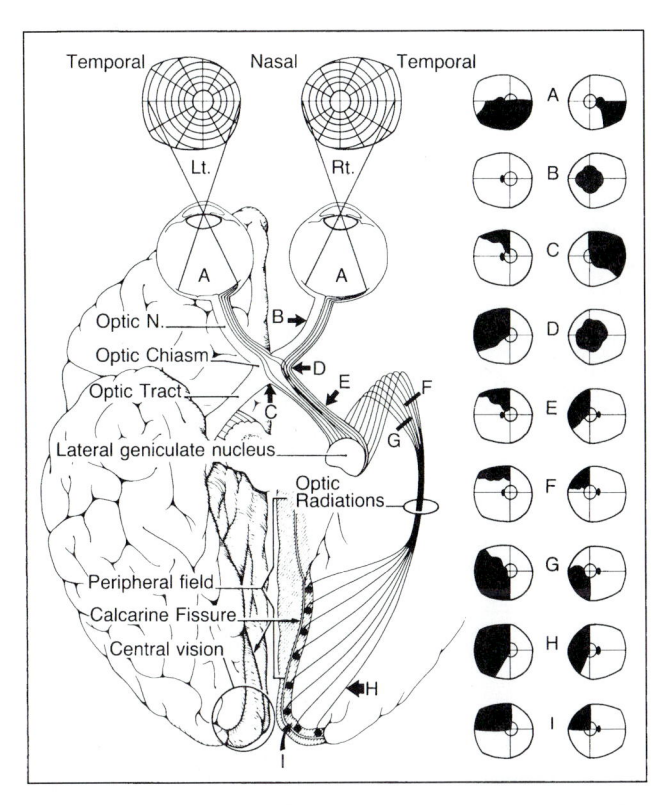

Fig. 2-2 **A,** Two examples of *altitudinal visual field defects* that could be caused either by occlusion of a superior branch of the central retinal artery or by an episode of ischemic optic neuropathy involving the superior optic disc. On the left is a large field defect involving both lower quadrants. On the right the injury is more limited, and the defect involves only the temporal quadrant, but it connects with the blind spot and does not go to fixation or have a border at the vertical meridian. **B,** A *central scotoma* in the visual field of the right eye caused by a lesion of the right optic nerve. **C,** *Bitemporal hemianopia* caused by a lesion of the optic chiasm. The asymmetry is typical of chiasmal field defects until a late stage, when the hemianopia may be complete in both eyes. **D,** *Junctional scotoma,* that is, a central scotoma on the side of a lateral chiasmal lesion with a temporal hemianopia in the visual field of the opposite eye. **E,** Markedly incongruous *homonymous hemianopia* seen with a lesion of the optic tract. **F,** *Homonymous superior quadrantanopia* seen with lesions of the optic radiations in the temporal lobe. **G,** *Homonymous inferior quadrantanopia* seen with lesions of the superior optic radiations in the low parietal or parietotemporal lobe junction. **H,** *Congruous homonymous hemianopia* seen with lesions either of the optic radiations close to their termination or of the calcarine cortex itself. **I,** *Precise inferior quadrantanopia* seen if an occipital lobe lesion involves just the superior bank of the calcarine cortex. (From Stein JH (ed): *Internal medicine,* ed 4, St Louis, 1994, Mosby.)

VISUAL LOSS

> **BOX 2-123 Visual Loss**
>
> Cataracts
> Presbyopia
> Diabetic retinopathy
> Glaucoma
> Corneal degeneration or opacity
> Central retinal artery occlusion
> Macular degeneration
> Temporal arteritis
> Hysteria
> CNS neoplasm
> Cerebral aneurysm
> Optic neuritis (inflammatory, multiple sclerosis)
> Methanol ingestion
> Multiple sclerosis
> Head or eye trauma

VOMITING

> **BOX 2-124 Vomiting**
>
> GI disturbances
>   Obstruction: esophageal, pyloric, intestinal
>   Infections: viral or bacterial enteritis, viral hepatitis, food poisoning
>   Pancreatitis
>   Appendicitis
>   Biliary colic
>   Peritonitis
>   Perforated bowel
>   Diabetic gastroparesis
>   Other: gastritis, PUD, IBD, GI tract neoplasms
> Drugs: morphine, digitalis, cytotoxic agents, bromocriptine
> Severe pain: MI, renal colic
> Metabolic disorders: uremia, acidosis/alkalosis, hyperglycemia, DKA, thyrotoxicosis
> Trauma: blows to the testicles, epigastrium
> Vertigo
> Reye's syndrome
> Increased intracranial pressure
> CNS disturbances: trauma, hemorrhage, infarction, neoplasm, infection, hypertensive encephalopathy, migraine
> Radiation sickness
> Vomiting associated with pregnancy
> Motion sickness
> Bulimia, anorexia nervosa
> Psychogenic: emotional disturbances, offensive sights or smells
> Severe coughing
> Pyelonephritis

WEIGHT GAIN

> **BOX 2-125 Weight Gain**
>
> Sedentary life-style
> Fluid overload
> After discontinuation of tobacco abuse
> Endocrine disorders: hypothyroidism, hyperinsulinism associated with maturity-onset diabetes mellitus, Cushing's syndrome, hypogonadism, insulinoma, hyperprolactinemia, acromegaly
> Medications: nutritional supplements, oral contraceptives, glucocorticoids, etc.
> Anxiety disorders with compulsive eating
> Laurence-Moon-Biedl syndrome, Prader-Willi syndrome, other congenital diseases
> Hypothalamic injury (rare; <100 cases reported in medical literature)

WEIGHT LOSS

> **BOX 2-126** **Causes of Weight Loss**
>
> I. Weight loss with normal to increased food intake associated with unimpaired appetite
>   A. Insulin-dependent diabetes mellitus
>   B. Thyrotoxicosis
>   C. Pheochromocytoma
>   D. Carcinoid
>   E. Malabsorption and maldigestion
>   F. Intestinal parasite infestation
>   G. Diencephalic syndrome
>   H. Malignancy (uncommon)
>   I. Luft's syndrome
> II. Weight loss with normal or decreased food intake
>   A. Impaired appetite that in some cases may be coupled with an increased caloric requirement
>   1. Malignancy
>   2. Psychiatric disorders (including anorexia nervosa)
>   3. AIDS
>   4. Liver disease
>   5. Addison's disease
>   6. Uremia
>   7. Chronic infection
>   8. Chronic lung disease
>   9. Chronic inflammatory disease
>   10. Cardiac cachexia
>   11. Diabetic neuropathic cachexia
>   12. Hypothalamic tumor (very rare)
>   B. Unimpaired appetite but decrease of food intake secondary to other factors
>   1. Gastric ulcer
>   2. Duodenal ulcer with outlet obstruction
>   3. Postgastrectomy syndrome
>   4. Regional enteritis
>   5. Ulcerative colitis
>   6. Food faddism
>   7. Social isolation

From Stein JH (ed): *Internal medicine*, ed 5, St Louis, 1998, Mosby.

WHEEZING

> **BOX 2-127** **Wheezing**
>
> Asthma
> COPD
> Interstitial lung disease
> Infections: pneumonia, bronchitis, bronchiolitis, epiglottitis
> Cardiac asthma
> GERD with aspiration
> Foreign body aspiration
> Pulmonary embolism
> Anaphylaxis
> Obstruction airway: neoplasm, goiter, edema or hemorrhage from trauma, aneurysm, congenital abnormalities, strictures, spasm
> Carcinoid syndrome

SECTION III

Clinical Algorithms

PLEASE NOTE: These algorithms are designed to assist clinicians in the evaluation and treatment of patients. They may not apply to all patients with a particular condition and are not intended to replace a clinician's individual judgment.

CLINICAL ALGORITHMS **Abdominal pain** 671

ABDOMINAL PAIN

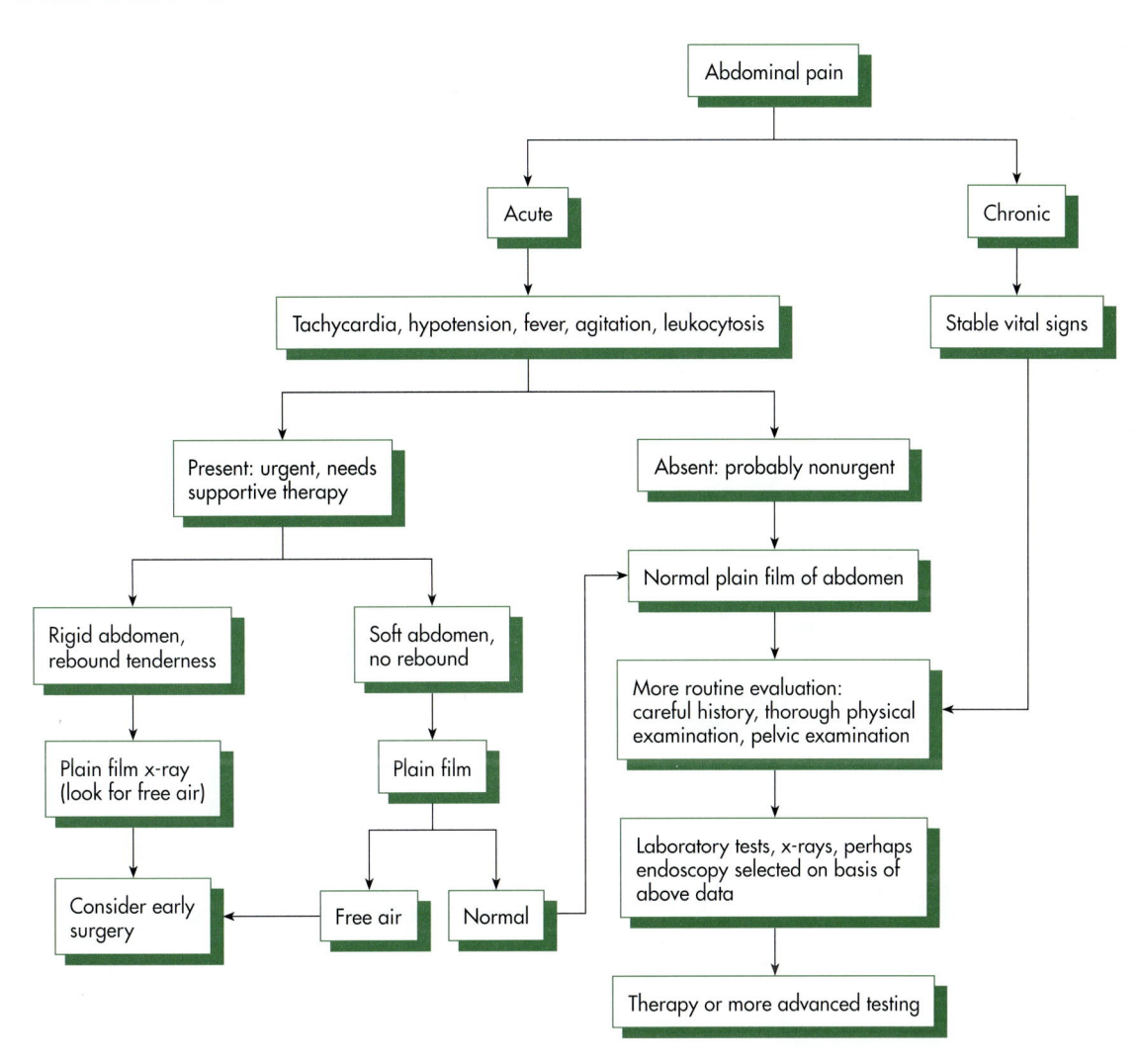

```
                          Abdominal pain
                         /              \
                      Acute            Chronic
                        |                 |
     Tachycardia, hypotension,      Stable vital signs
     fever, agitation, leukocytosis
         /              \
  Present: urgent,     Absent: probably nonurgent
  needs supportive              |
  therapy                  Normal plain film of abdomen
    /         \                   |
 Rigid       Soft abdomen,   More routine evaluation:
 abdomen,    no rebound      careful history, thorough
 rebound         |           physical examination,
 tenderness   Plain film     pelvic examination
    |          /    \              |
 Plain film  Free   Normal   Laboratory tests, x-rays,
 x-ray (look  air            perhaps endoscopy selected
 for free air)               on basis of above data
    |                              |
 Consider early            Therapy or more advanced testing
 surgery
```

Fig. 3-1 **Evaluation of patients with abdominal pain.** (From Stein JH [ed]: *Internal medicine,* ed 5, St Louis, 1998, Mosby.)

ADRENAL MASS

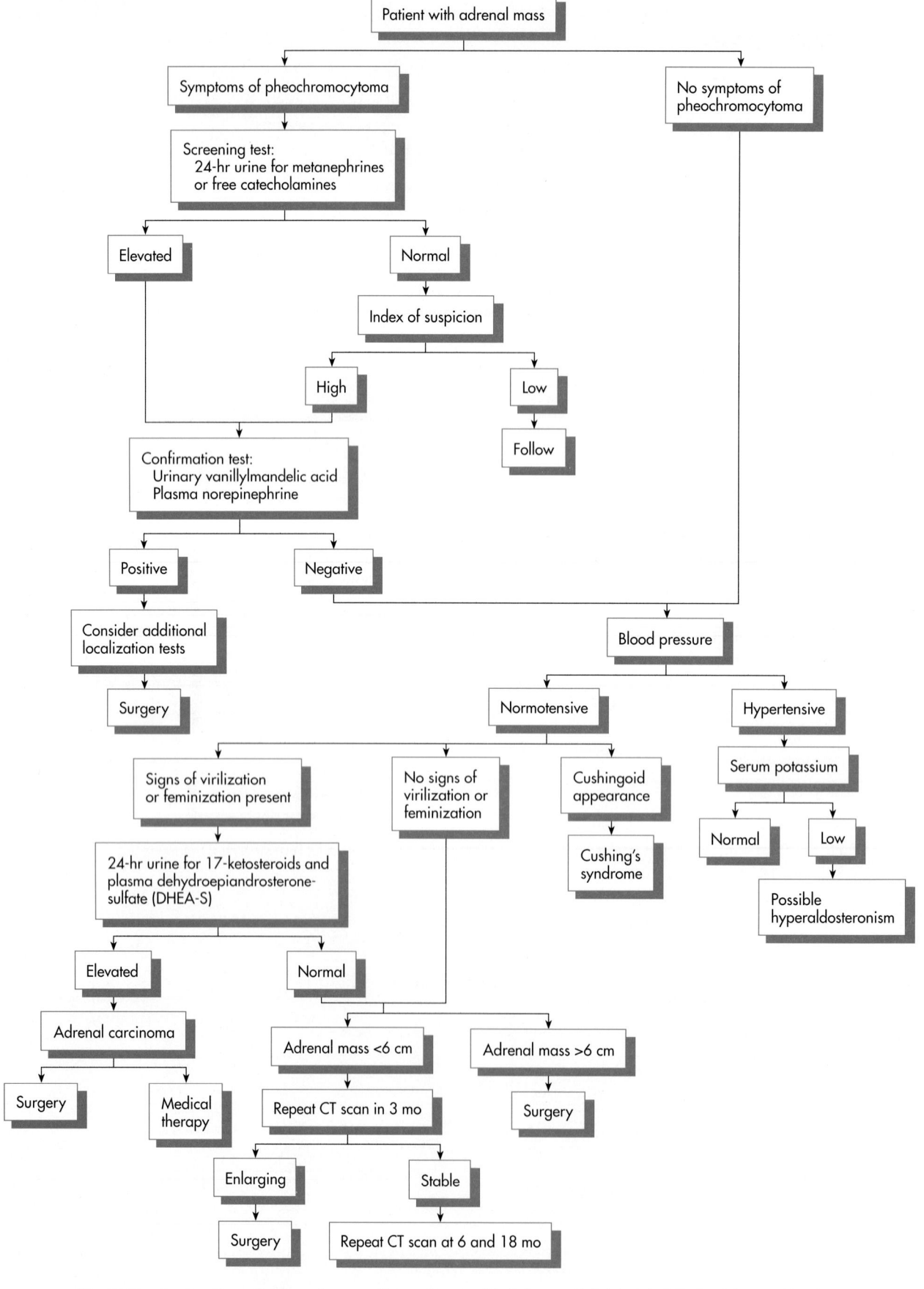

Fig. 3-2 **Evaluation of adrenal mass.** (From Greene HL, Johnson WP, Maricic MJ: *Decision making in medicine,* St Louis, 1993, Mosby.)

AMENORRHEA

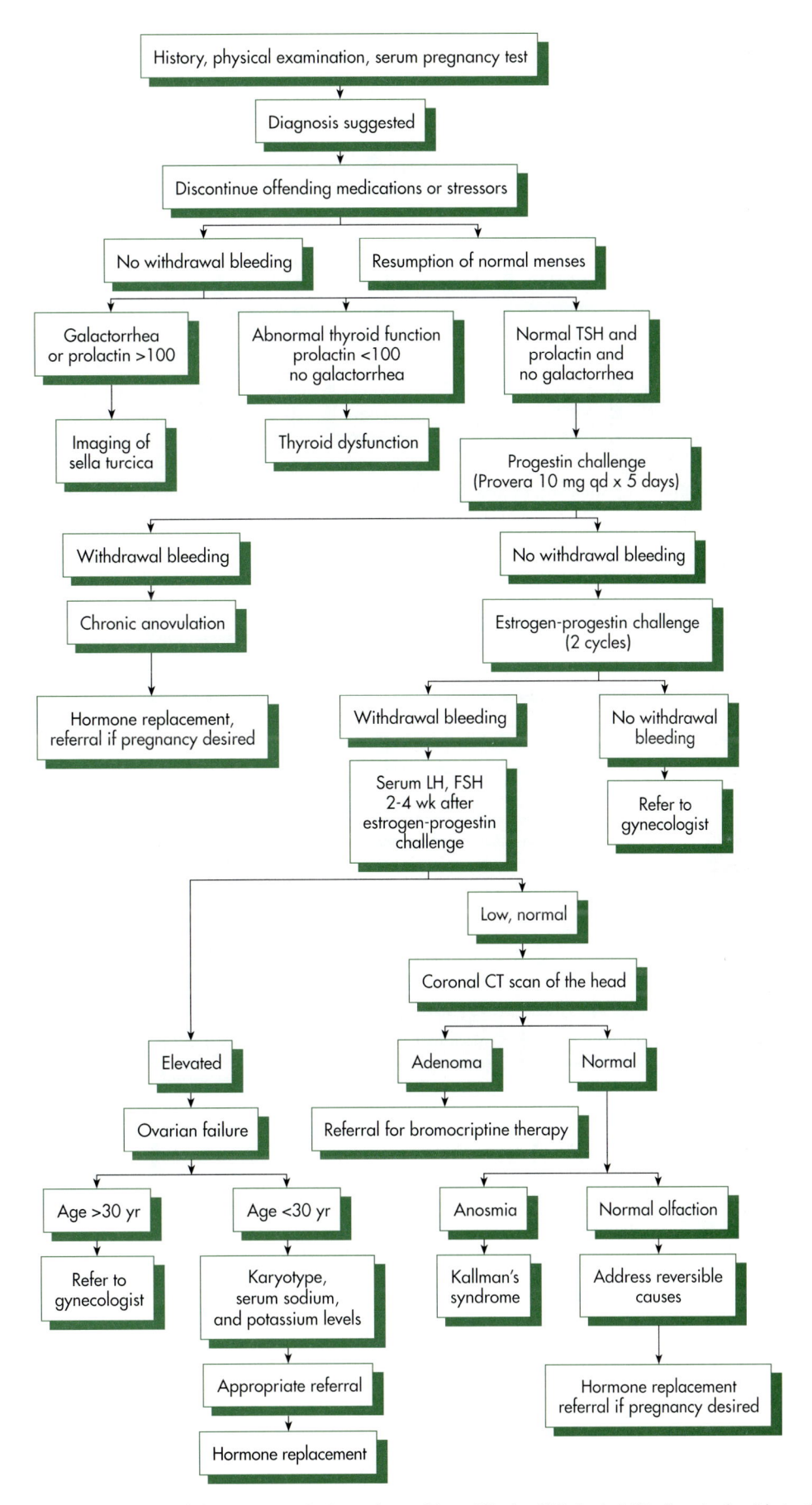

Fig. 3-3 Evaluation of the amenorrheic patient. (From Wachtel TJ, Stein MD: *Practical guide to the care of the ambulatory patient,* St Louis, 1995, Mosby.)

ANEMIA

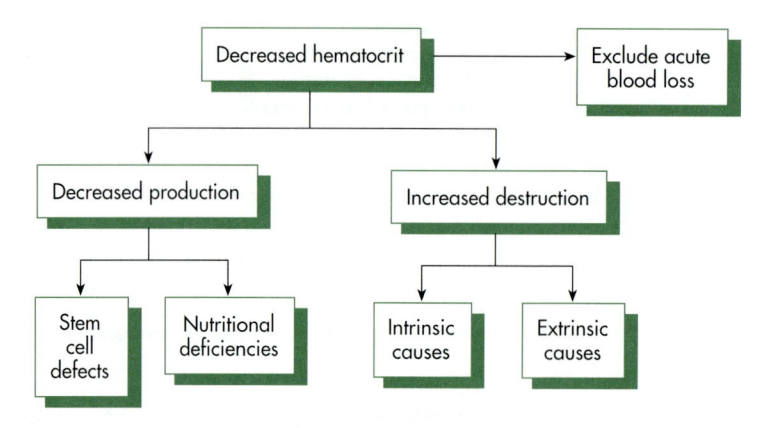

Fig. 3-4 Simplified classification of anemias. (From Stein JH (ed): *Internal medicine*, ed 4, St Louis, 1994, Mosby.)

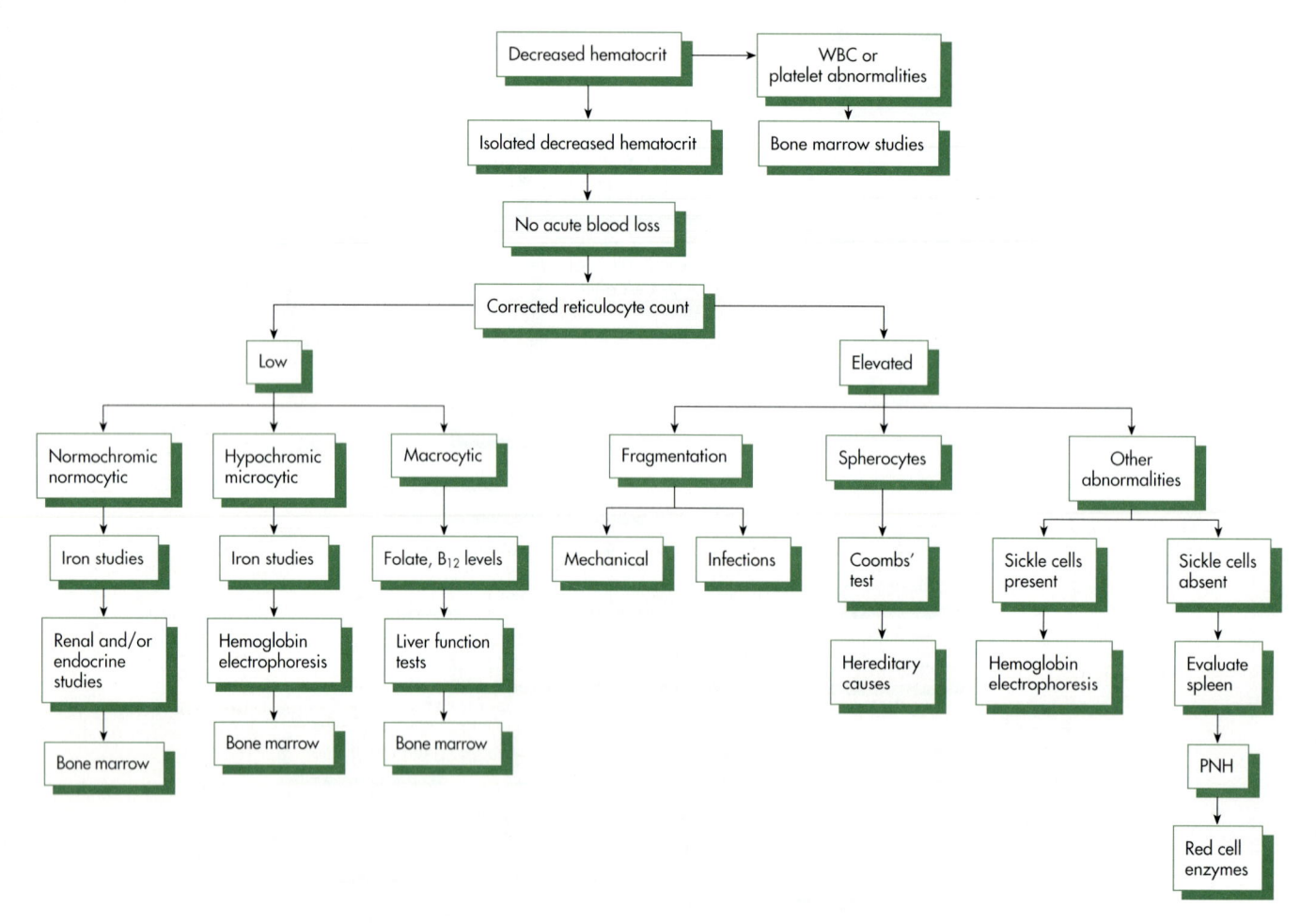

Fig. 3-5 Evaluation of a patient with a low hematocrit. (From Stein JH [ed]: *Internal medicine*, ed 4, St Louis, 1994, Mosby.)

ANOREXIA

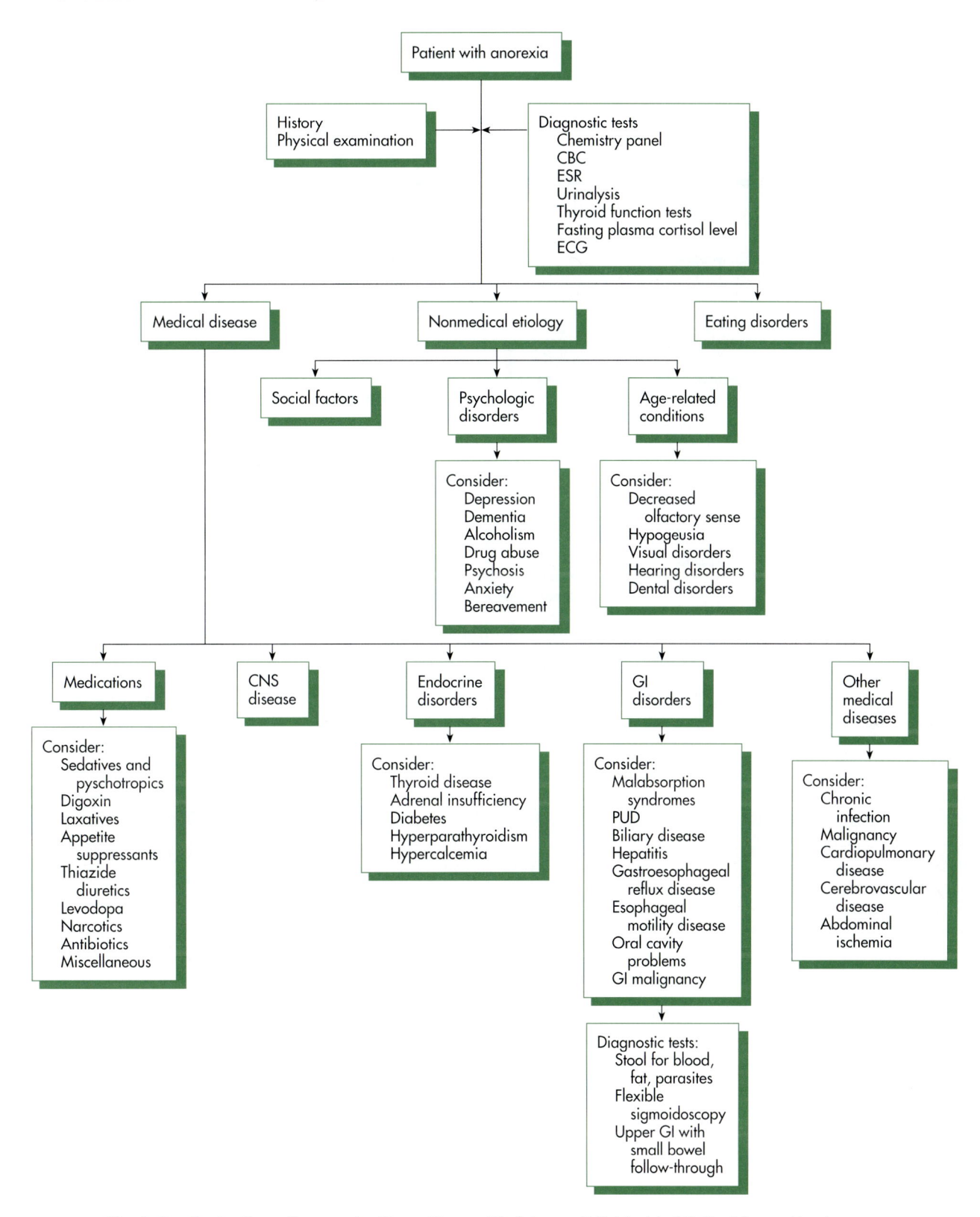

Fig. 3-6 Evaluation of anorexia. (From Greene HL, Johnson WP, Maricic MJ: *Decision making in medicine*, St Louis, 1993, Mosby.)

ANTINUCLEAR ANTIBODY ABNORMALITY

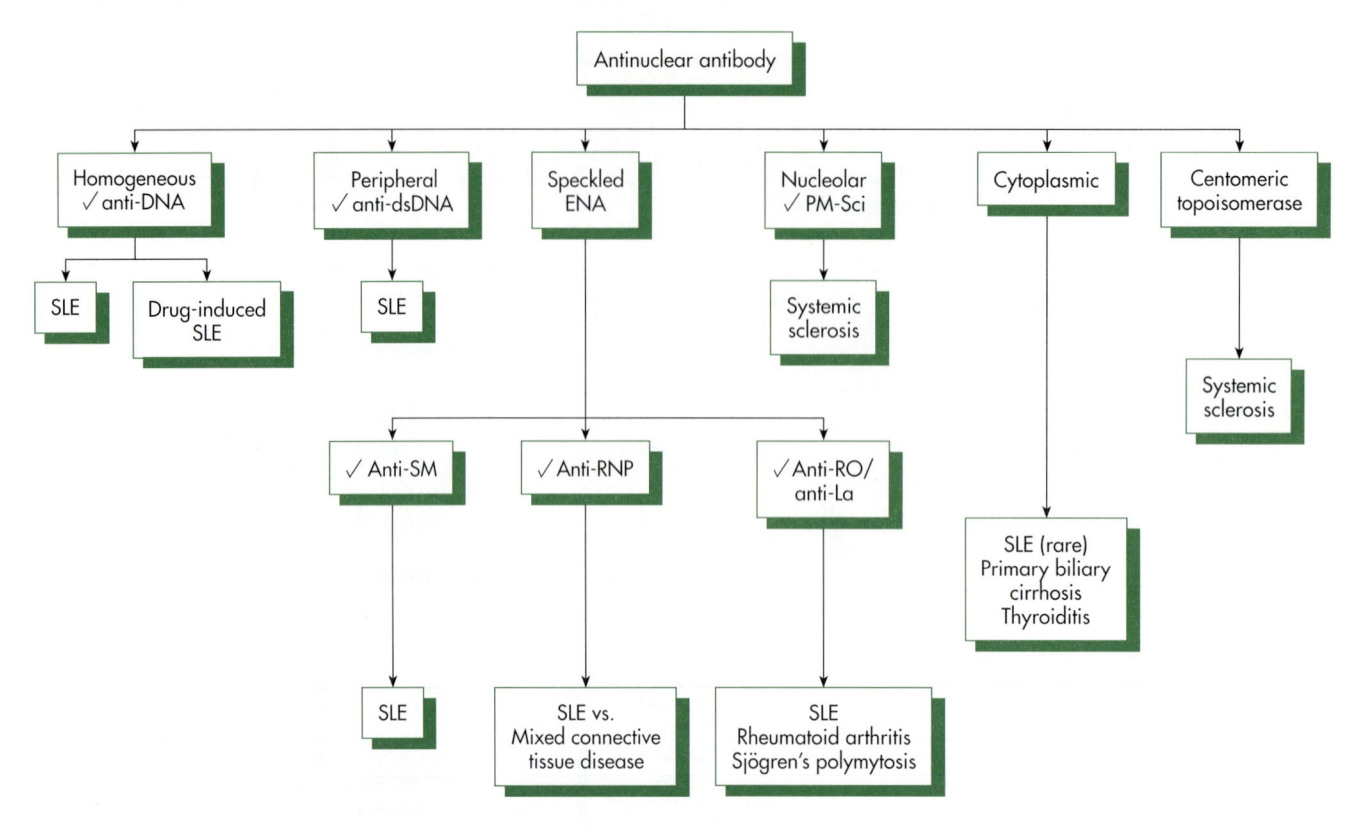

```
                        ┌─────────────────────┐
                        │ Antinuclear antibody │
                        └──────────┬──────────┘
        ┌──────────┬───────────┬───┴────────┬───────────┬────────────┐
   Homogeneous  Peripheral   Speckled    Nucleolar   Cytoplasmic  Centomeric
   ✓ anti-DNA  ✓ anti-dsDNA    ENA       ✓ PM-Sci                topoisomerase
        │           │           │           │            │            │
    ┌───┴───┐       │           │           │            │            │
   SLE  Drug-      SLE          │       Systemic      SLE (rare)   Systemic
       induced                  │       sclerosis    Primary biliary sclerosis
        SLE                     │                      cirrhosis
                    ┌───────────┼───────────┐         Thyroiditis
                 ✓ Anti-SM  ✓ Anti-RNP  ✓ Anti-RO/
                                         anti-La
                    │           │           │
                   SLE       SLE vs.       SLE
                          Mixed connective Rheumatoid arthritis
                          tissue disease   Sjögren's polymytosis
```

Fig. 3-7 Diagnostic tests and diagnoses to consider from ANA pattern. (From Carlson KJ et al: *Primary care of women,* St Louis, 1995, Mosby.)

ARTHRALGIA LIMITED TO ONE OR FEW JOINTS

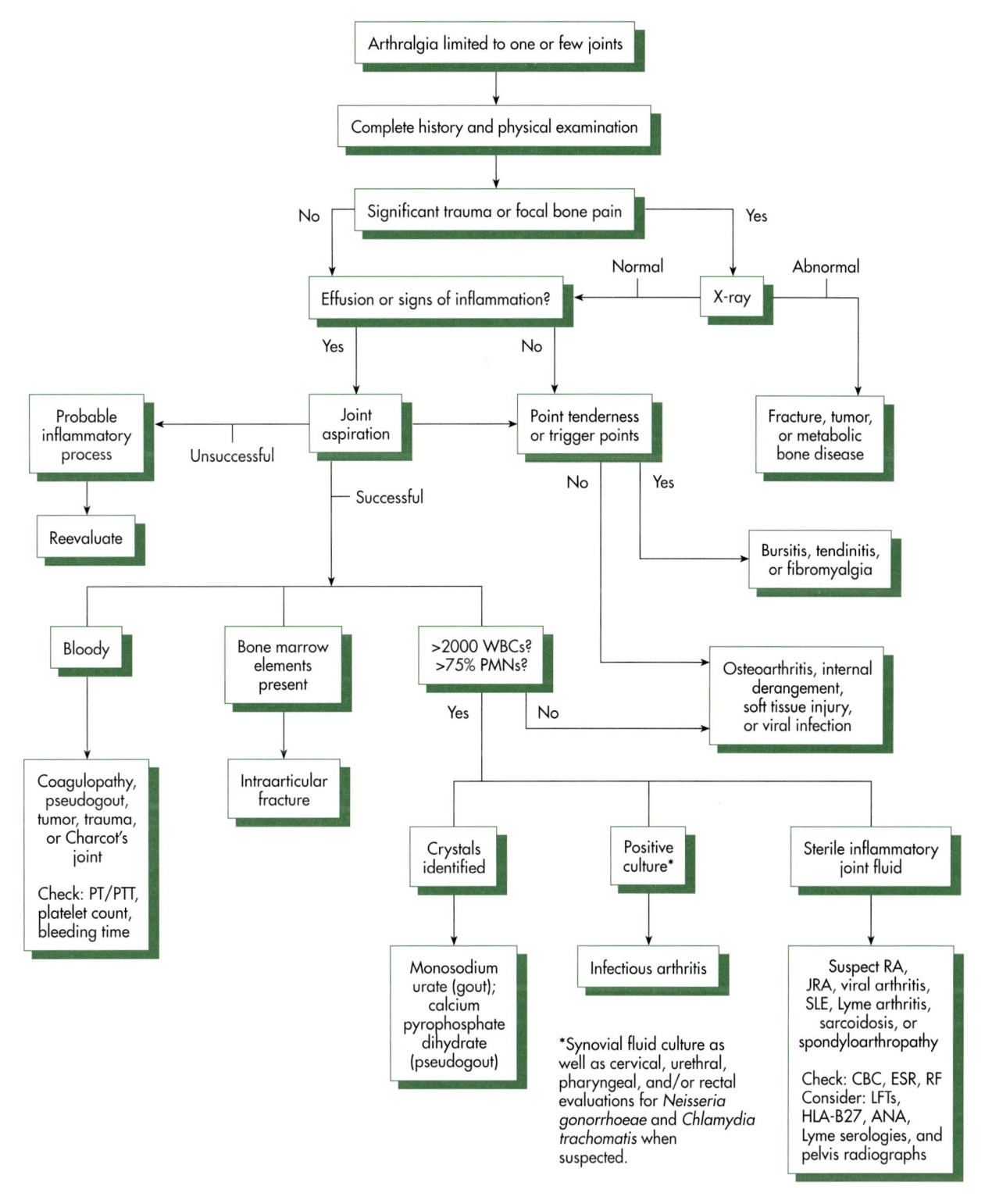

Fig. 3-8 A diagnostic approach to arthralgia in a few joints. ANA, Antinuclear antibodies; JRA, juvenile rheumatoid arthritis; LFTs, liver function tests; PMNs, polymorphonuclear neutrophilis; PT, prothrombin time; PTT, partial thromboplastin time; RA, rheumatoid arthritis; RE, rheumatoid facto; SLE, systemic lupus erythematosus. (Adapted with permission from American College of Rheumatology Ad Hoc Committee on Clinical Guidelines: Guidelines for the initial evaluation of the adult patient with acute musculoskeletal symptoms, *Arthritis Rheum* 39:1-8, 1996.)

678 Ascites

CLINICAL ALGORITHMS

ASCITES

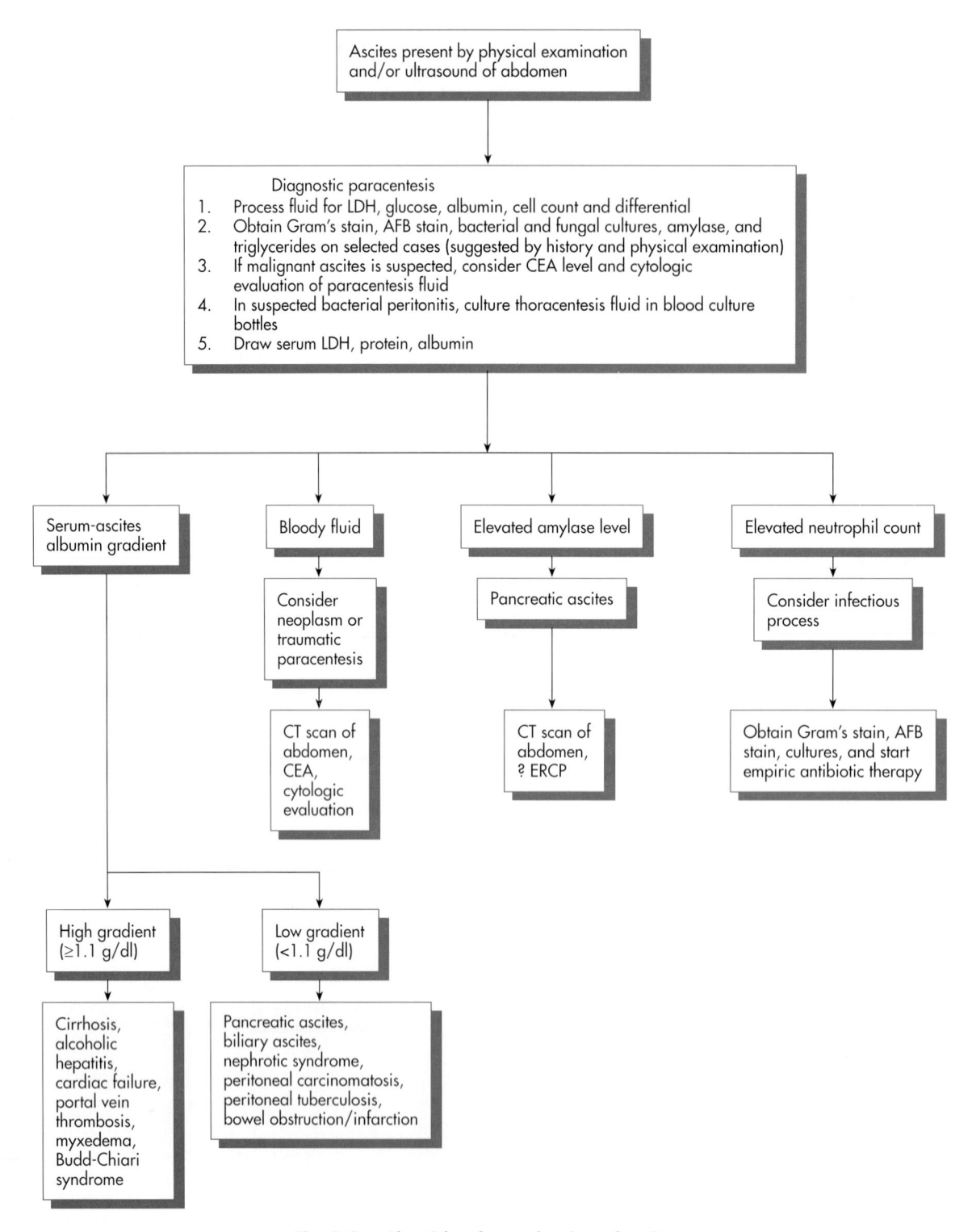

Ascites present by physical examination and/or ultrasound of abdomen

↓

Diagnostic paracentesis
1. Process fluid for LDH, glucose, albumin, cell count and differential
2. Obtain Gram's stain, AFB stain, bacterial and fungal cultures, amylase, and triglycerides on selected cases (suggested by history and physical examination)
3. If malignant ascites is suspected, consider CEA level and cytologic evaluation of paracentesis fluid
4. In suspected bacterial peritonitis, culture thoracentesis fluid in blood culture bottles
5. Draw serum LDH, protein, albumin

↓

- **Serum-ascites albumin gradient**
- **Bloody fluid** → Consider neoplasm or traumatic paracentesis → CT scan of abdomen, CEA, cytologic evaluation
- **Elevated amylase level** → Pancreatic ascites → CT scan of abdomen, ? ERCP
- **Elevated neutrophil count** → Consider infectious process → Obtain Gram's stain, AFB stain, cultures, and start empiric antibiotic therapy

From Serum-ascites albumin gradient:
- **High gradient (≥1.1 g/dl)** → Cirrhosis, alcoholic hepatitis, cardiac failure, portal vein thrombosis, myxedema, Budd-Chiari syndrome
- **Low gradient (<1.1 g/dl)** → Pancreatic ascites, biliary ascites, nephrotic syndrome, peritoneal carcinomatosis, peritoneal tuberculosis, bowel obstruction/infarction

Fig. 3-9   Algorithm for evaluation of ascites.

ASYSTOLE

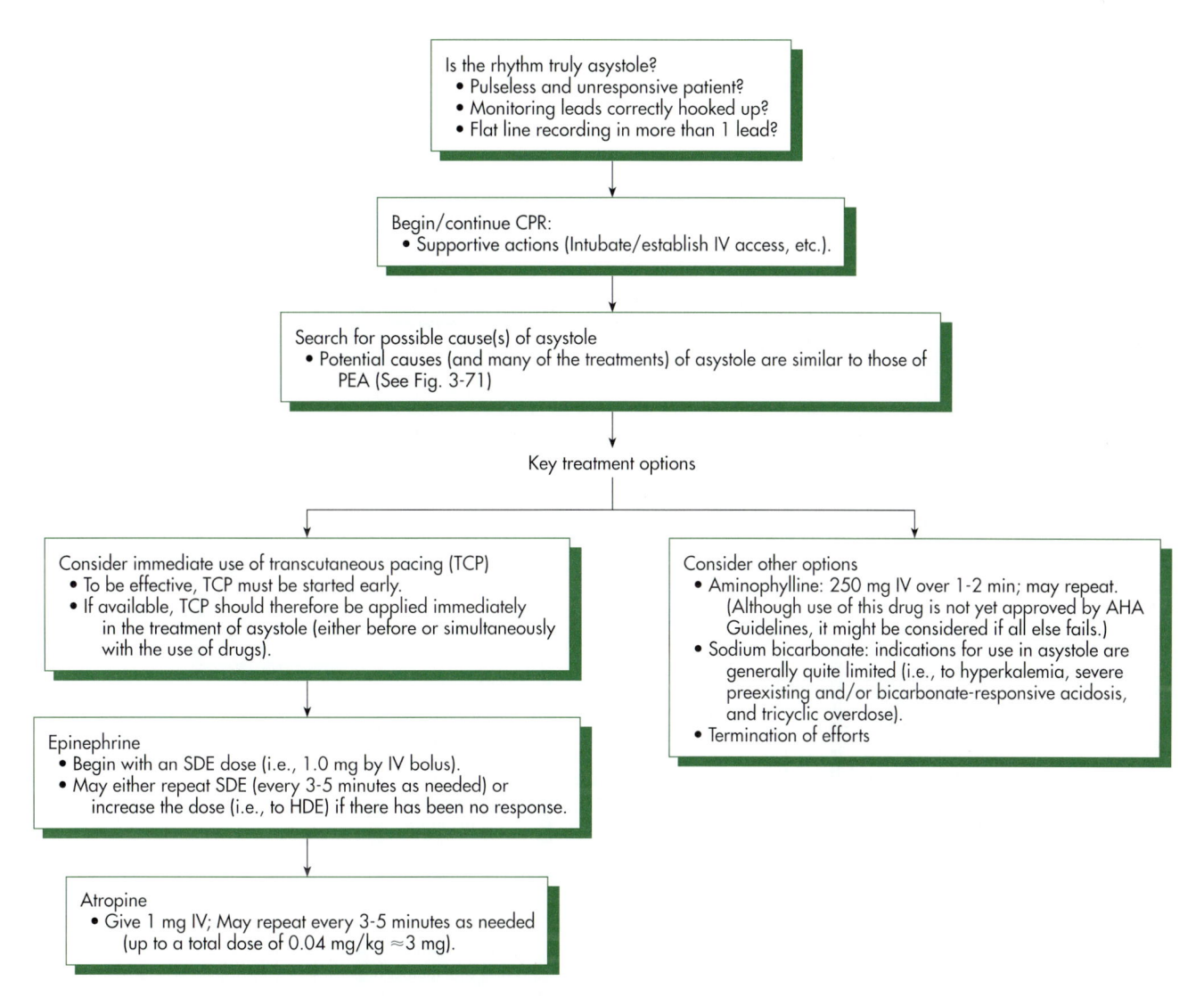

Is the rhythm truly asystole?
- Pulseless and unresponsive patient?
- Monitoring leads correctly hooked up?
- Flat line recording in more than 1 lead?

Begin/continue CPR:
- Supportive actions (Intubate/establish IV access, etc.).

Search for possible cause(s) of asystole
- Potential causes (and many of the treatments) of asystole are similar to those of PEA (See Fig. 3-71)

Key treatment options

Consider immediate use of transcutaneous pacing (TCP)
- To be effective, TCP must be started early.
- If available, TCP should therefore be applied immediately in the treatment of asystole (either before or simultaneously with the use of drugs).

Epinephrine
- Begin with an SDE dose (i.e., 1.0 mg by IV bolus).
- May either repeat SDE (every 3-5 minutes as needed) or increase the dose (i.e., to HDE) if there has been no response.

Atropine
- Give 1 mg IV; May repeat every 3-5 minutes as needed (up to a total dose of 0.04 mg/kg ≈ 3 mg).

Consider other options
- Aminophylline: 250 mg IV over 1-2 min; may repeat. (Although use of this drug is not yet approved by AHA Guidelines, it might be considered if all else fails.)
- Sodium bicarbonate: indications for use in asystole are generally quite limited (i.e., to hyperkalemia, severe preexisting and/or bicarbonate-responsive acidosis, and tricyclic overdose).
- Termination of efforts

Fig. 3-10   Asystole. (Adapted from Grauer K, Cavallaro D: *ACLS: Rapid review and case scenarios,* ed 4, St Louis, 1996, Mosby and from American Heart Association ACLS Textbook, 1994.)

BACK PAIN

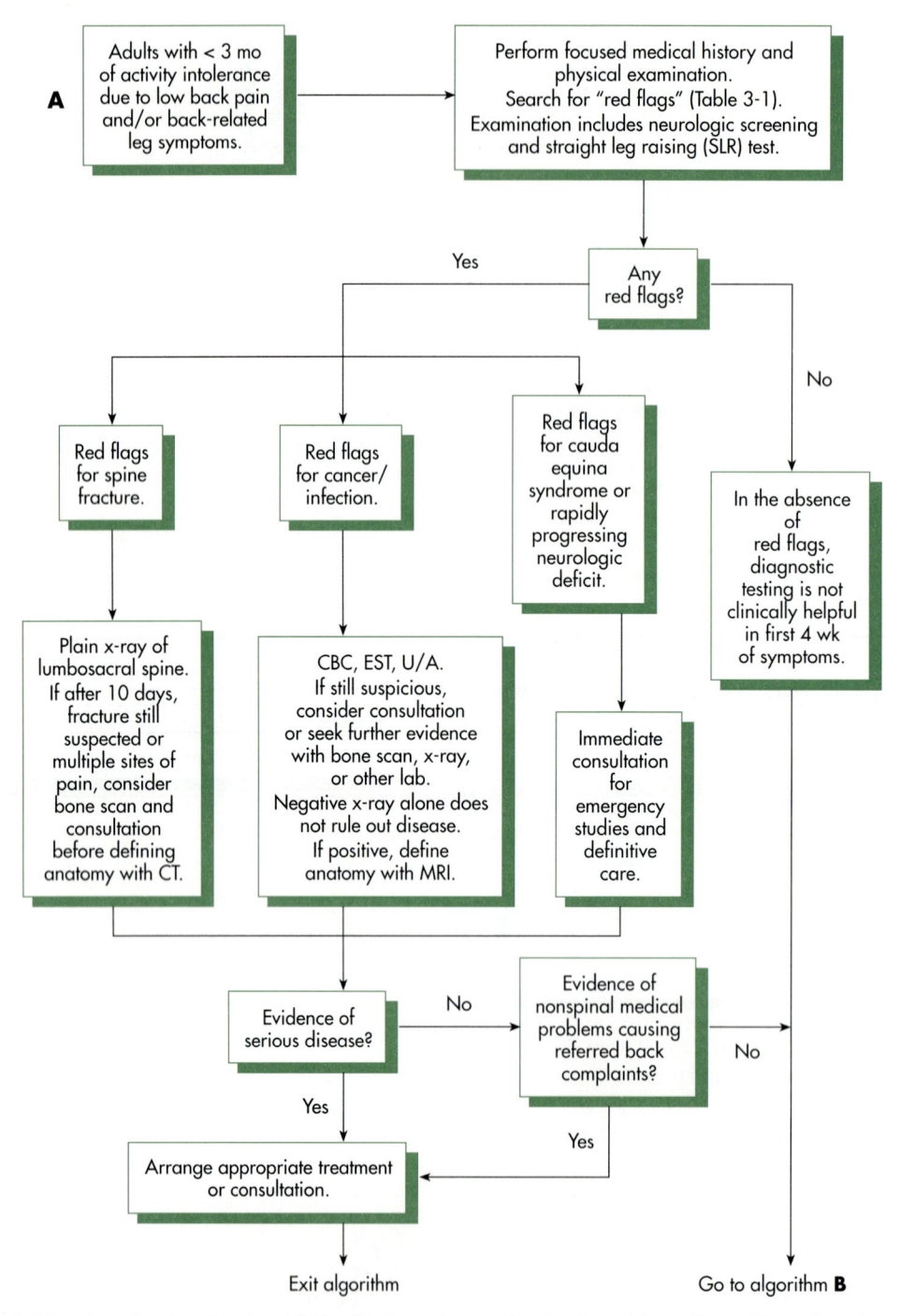

Fig. 3-11 Low back pain. **A,** Initial evaluation of acute low back problem. (From Bigos S et al: *Acute low back problems in adults,* Clinical Practice Guideline, Quick Reference Guide Number 14, Rockville, MD, US Department of Health and Human Services, Public Health Service, Agency for Health Care Policy and Research, AHCPR Pub No 95-0643, Dec 1994.)

BACK PAIN—cont'd

TABLE 3-1 **Red Flags for Potentially Serious Conditions**

POSSIBLE FRACTURE	POSSIBLE TUMOR OR INFECTION	POSSIBLE CAUDA EQUINA SYNDROME
From Medical History		
Major trauma, such as vehicle accident or fall from height.	Age over 50 or under 20 yr.	Saddle anesthesia.
Minor trauma or even strenuous lifting (in older or potentially osteoporotic patient).	History of cancer.	Recent onset of bladder dysfunction, such as urinary retention, increased frequency, or overflow incontinence.
	Constitutional symptoms, such as recent fever or chills or unexplained weight loss.	Severe or progressive neurologic deficit in the lower extremity.
	Risk factors for spinal infection: recent bacterial infection (e.g., urinary tract infection); IV drug abuse; or immune suppression (from steroids, transplant, or HIV).	
	Pain that worsens when supine; severe nighttime pain.	
From Physical Examination		
		Unexpected laxity of the anal sphincter.
		Perianal/perineal sensory loss.
		Major motor weakness: quadriceps (knee extension weakness); ankle plantar flexors, evertors, and dorsiflexors (foot drop).

BACK PAIN—cont'd

B Initial visit

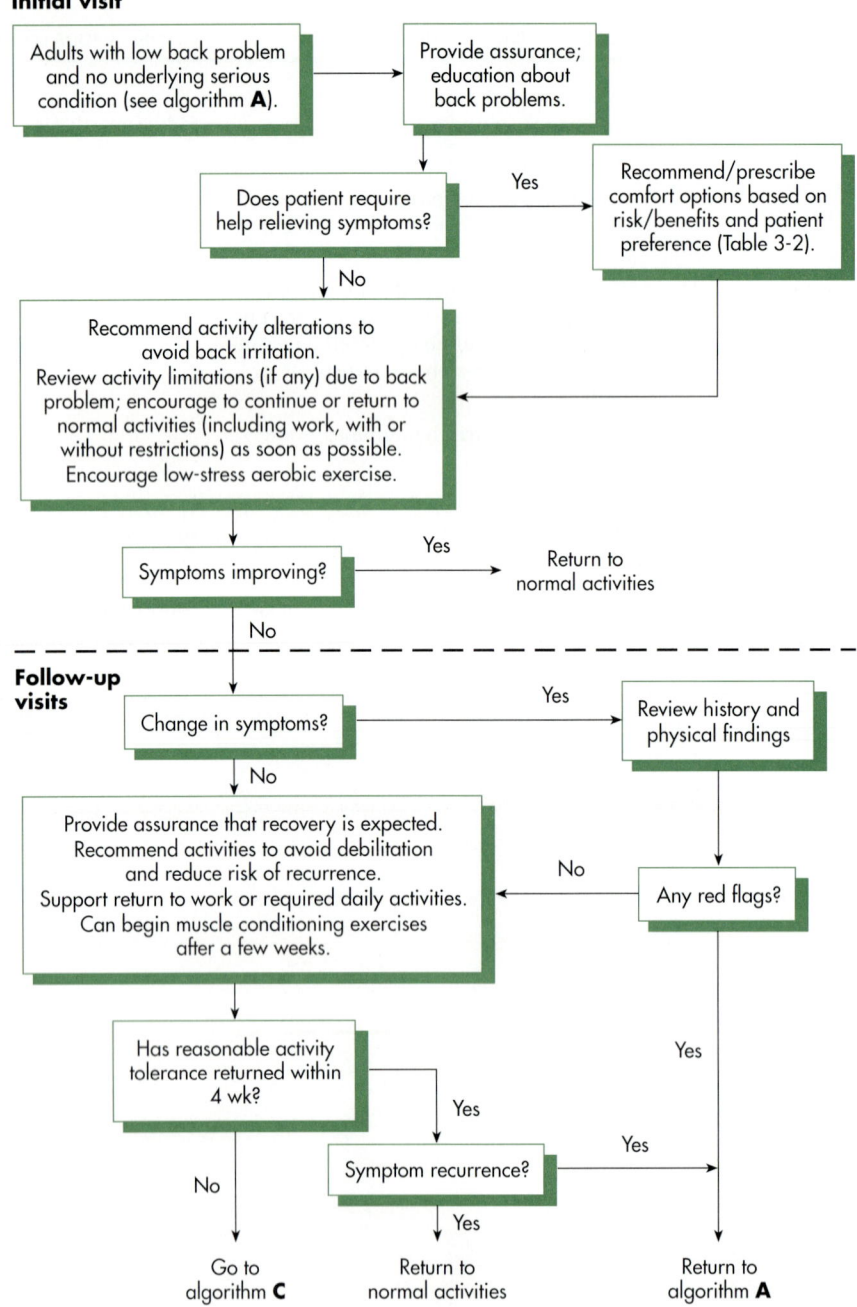

Fig. 3-11—cont'd **B**, Treatment of acute low back problem on initial and follow-up visits.

BACK PAIN—cont'd

TABLE 3-2 Symptom Control Methods

RECOMMENDED		
Nonprescription Analgesics		
Acetaminophen (safest)		
NSAIDs (aspirin,* ibuprofen*)		
Prescribed Pharmaceutical Methods	**Prescribed Physical Methods**	
Nonspecific Low Back Symptoms and/or Sciatica	*Nonspecific Low Back Symptoms*	*Sciatica*
Other NSAIDs*	Manipulation (in place of medication or a shorter trial if combined with NSAIDs)	
Options		
Nonspecific Low Back Symptoms and/or Sciatica	*Nonspecific Low Back Symptoms*	*Sciatica*
Muscle relaxants†,‡,§	Physical agents and modalities† (heat or cold modalities for home programs only)	Manipulation (in place of medication or a shorter trial if combined with NSAIDs)
Opioids	Shoe insoles†	Physical agents and modalities† (heat or cold modalities for home programs only)
		Few days' rest§
		Shoe insoles†

*Aspirin and other NSAIDs are not recommended for use in combination with one another due to the risk of GI complications.
†Equivocal efficacy.
‡Significant potential for producing drowsiness and debilitation; potential for dependency.
§Short course (few days only) for severe symptoms.

Back pain

BACK PAIN—cont'd

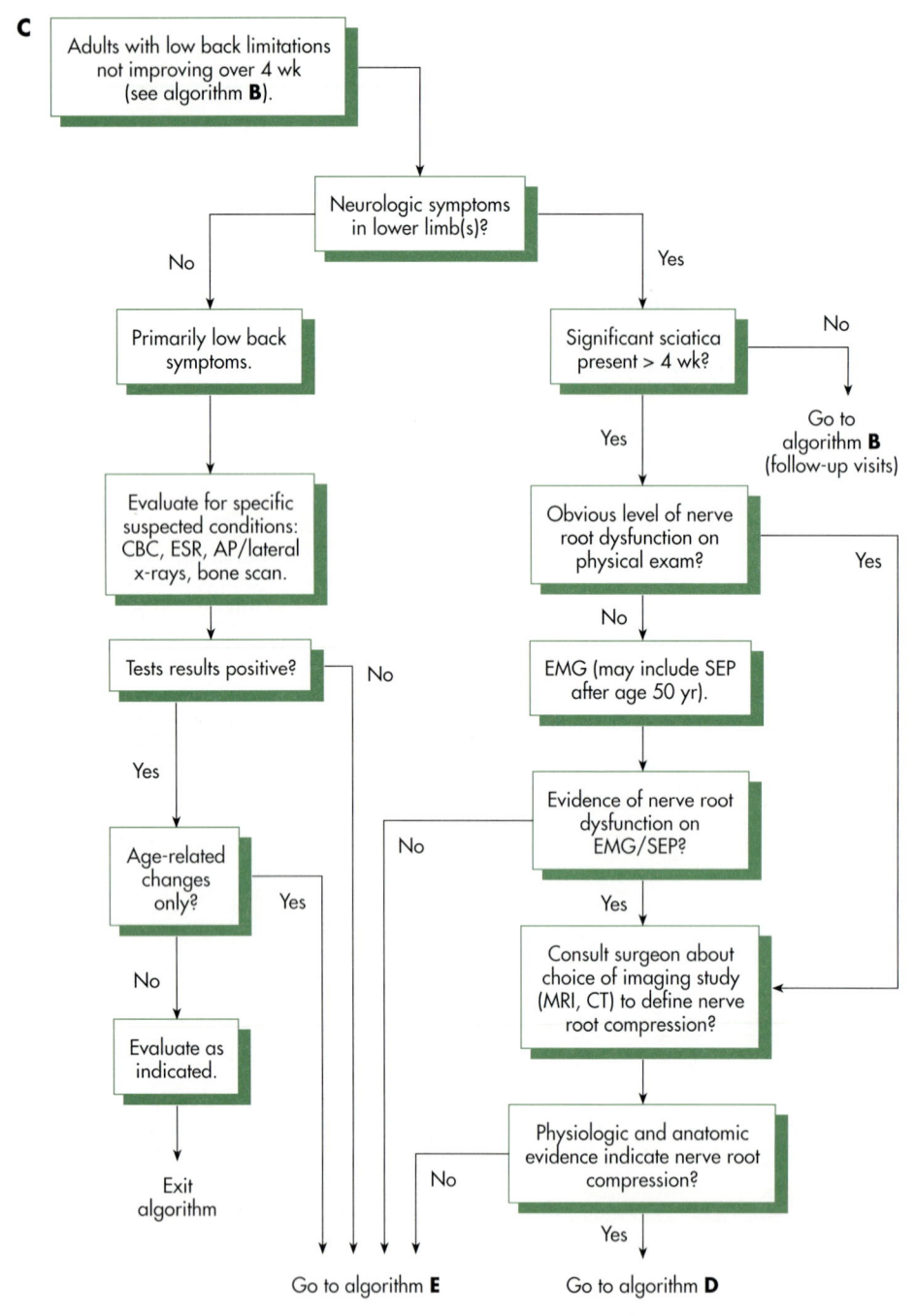

Fig. 3-11—cont'd   C, Evaluation of the slow-to-recover patient (symptoms >4 wks)

BACK PAIN—cont'd

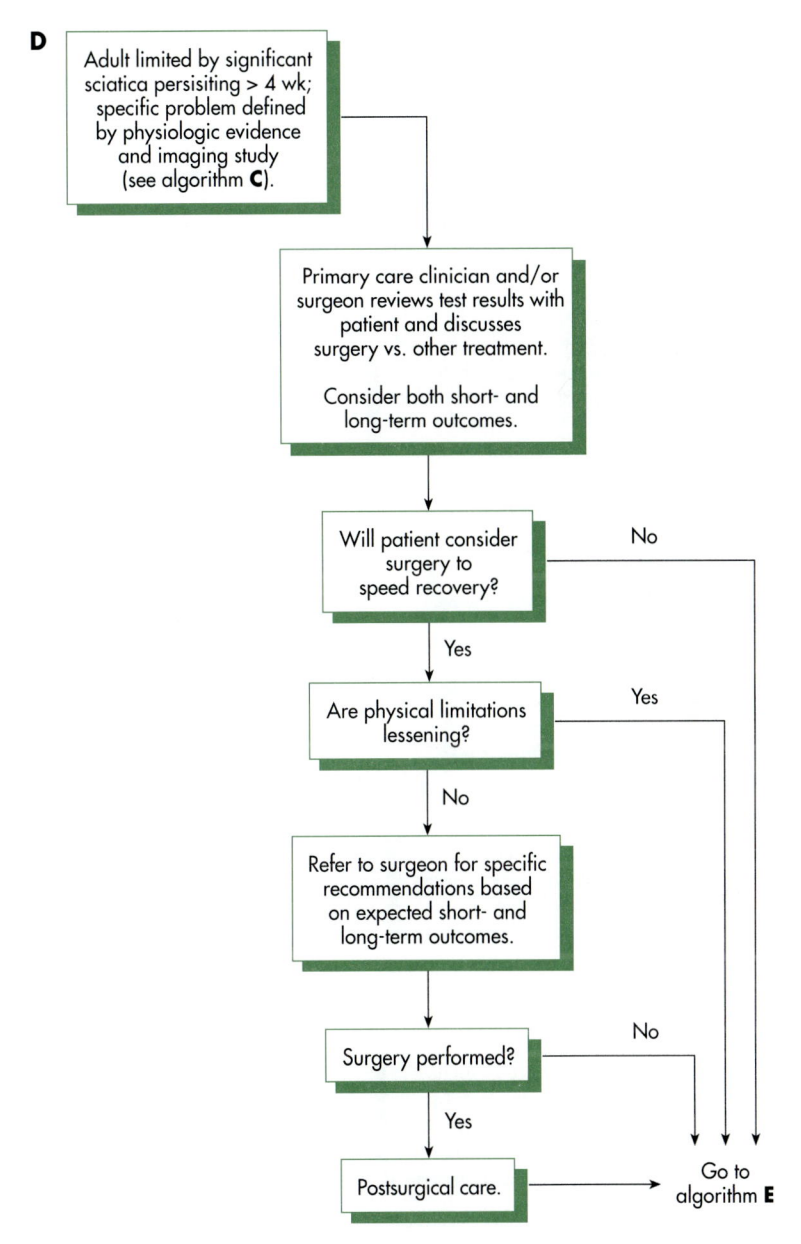

D Adult limited by significant sciatica persisiting > 4 wk; specific problem defined by physiologic evidence and imaging study (see algorithm **C**).

↓

Primary care clinician and/or surgeon reviews test results with patient and discusses surgery vs. other treatment. Consider both short- and long-term outcomes.

↓

Will patient consider surgery to speed recovery? — No → Go to algorithm **E**

↓ Yes

Are physical limitations lessening? — Yes → Go to algorithm **E**

↓ No

Refer to surgeon for specific recommendations based on expected short- and long-term outcomes.

↓

Surgery performed? — No → Go to algorithm **E**

↓ Yes

Postsurgical care. → Go to algorithm **E**

Fig. 3-11—cont'd   **D**, Surgical considerations for patients with persistent sciatica.

Back pain

BACK PAIN—cont'd

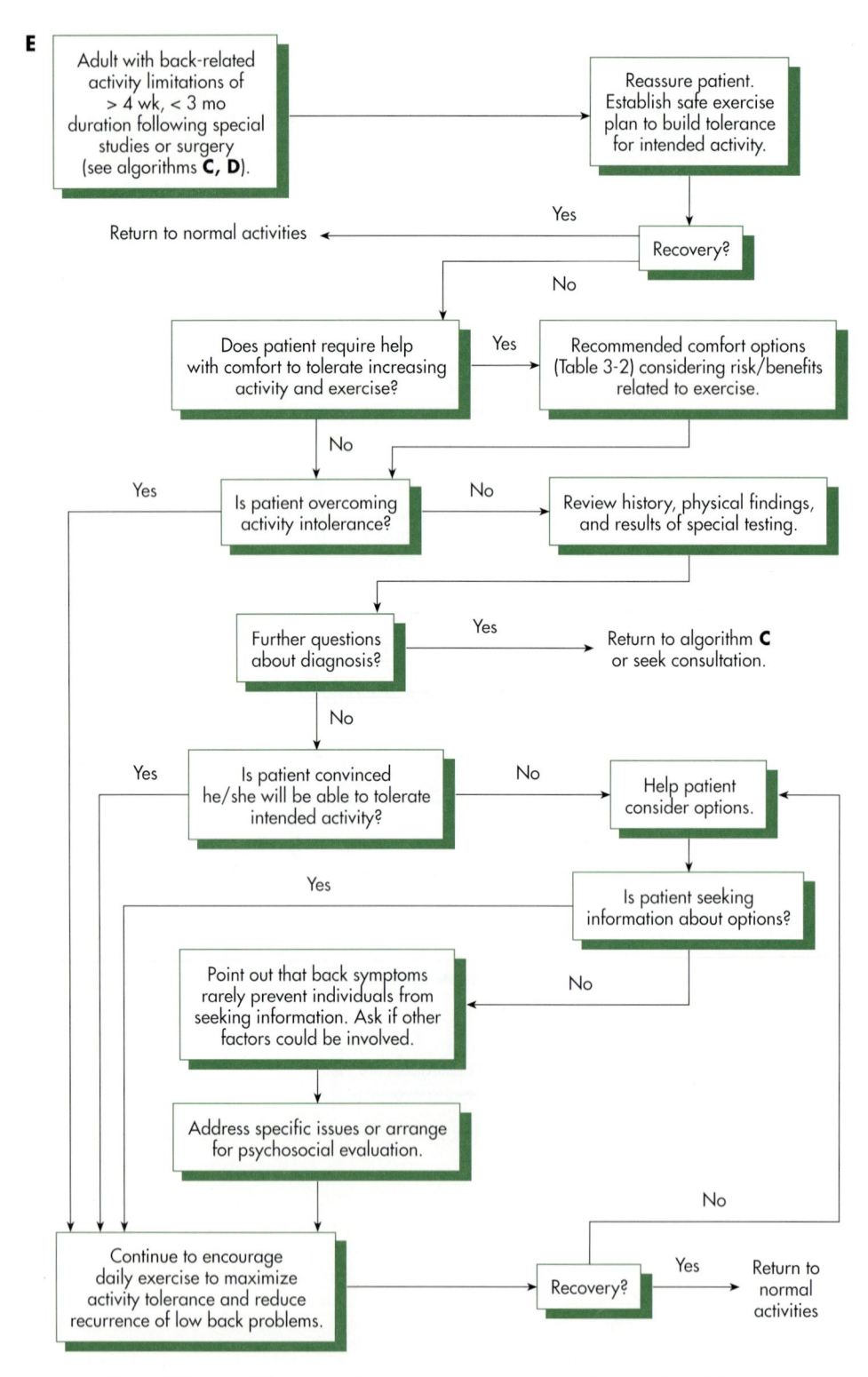

E Adult with back-related activity limitations of > 4 wk, < 3 mo duration following special studies or surgery (see algorithms **C, D**).

→ Reassure patient. Establish safe exercise plan to build tolerance for intended activity.

Recovery?
- Yes → Return to normal activities
- No ↓

Does patient require help with comfort to tolerate increasing activity and exercise?
- Yes → Recommended comfort options (Table 3-2) considering risk/benefits related to exercise.
- No ↓

Is patient overcoming activity intolerance?
- Yes ←
- No → Review history, physical findings, and results of special testing.

Further questions about diagnosis?
- Yes → Return to algorithm **C** or seek consultation.
- No ↓

Is patient convinced he/she will be able to tolerate intended activity?
- Yes ←
- No → Help patient consider options.

Is patient seeking information about options?
- Yes ↑
- No → Point out that back symptoms rarely prevent individuals from seeking information. Ask if other factors could be involved.

Address specific issues or arrange for psychosocial evaluation.

Continue to encourage daily exercise to maximize activity tolerance and reduce recurrence of low back problems.

Recovery?
- Yes → Return to normal activities
- No ↑

Fig. 3-11—cont'd   **E,** Further management of acute low back problem.

CLINICAL ALGORITHMS Bleeding 687

BLEEDING, EARLY PREGNANCY

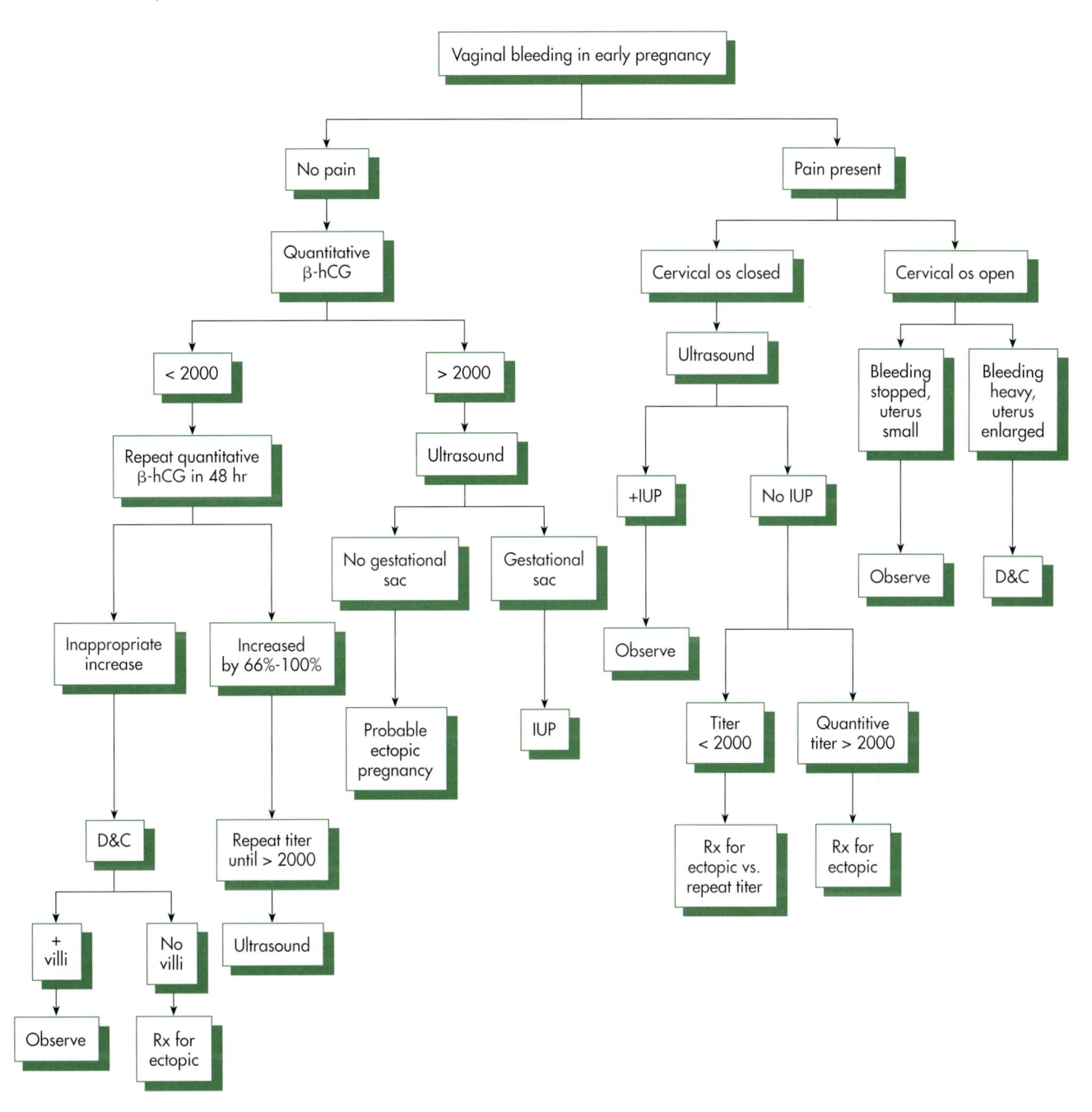

Fig. 3-12 Diagnosis of vaginal bleeding in early pregnancy. *IUP*, Intrauterine pregnancy; *B-hCG*, β-human chorionic gonadotropin; *D&C*, dilation and curettage. (From Carlson KJ et al: *Primary care of women,* St Louis, 1995, Mosby.)

BLEEDING, GASTROINTESTINAL

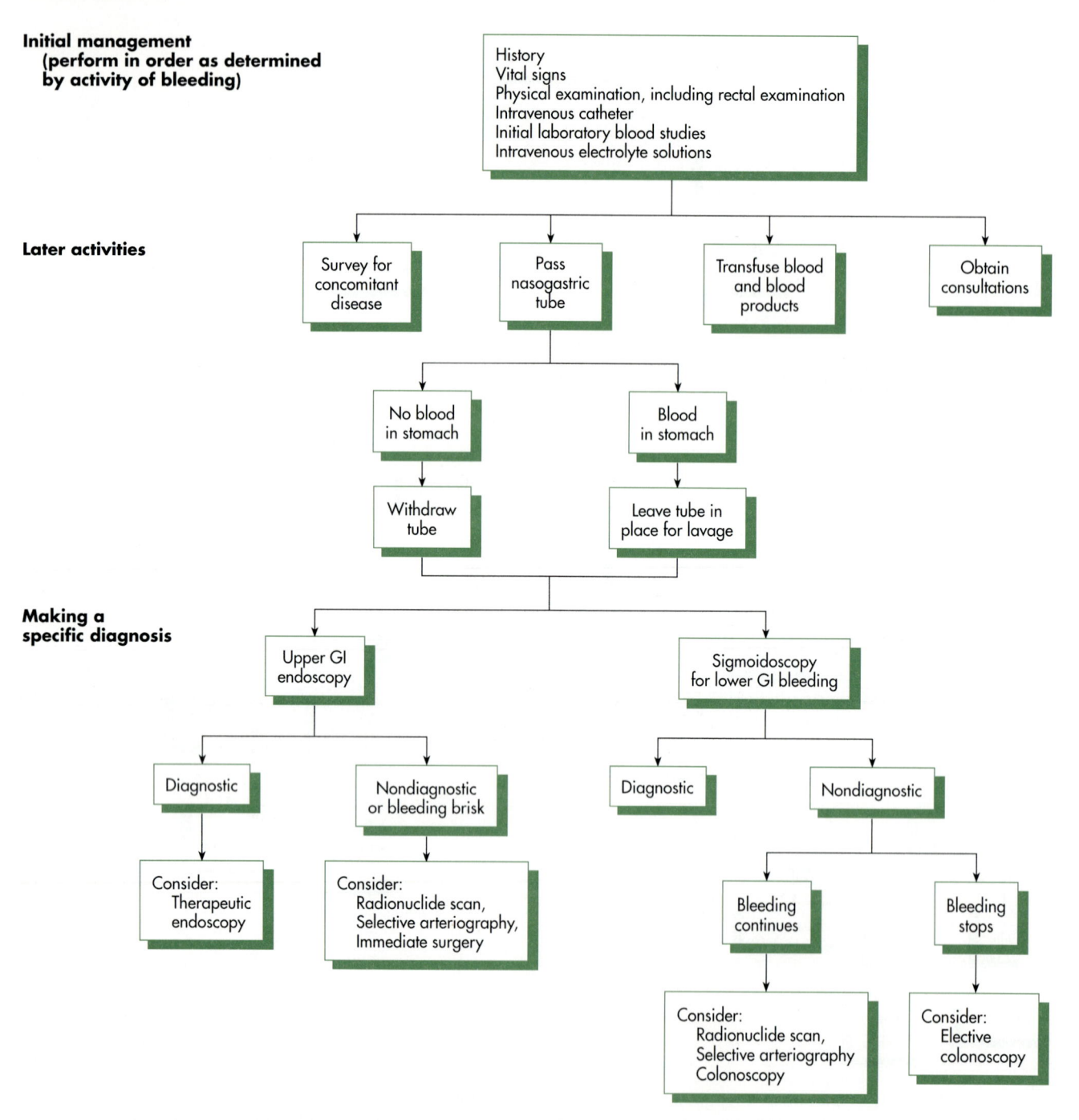

Initial management
(perform in order as determined by activity of bleeding)

- History
- Vital signs
- Physical examination, including rectal examination
- Intravenous catheter
- Initial laboratory blood studies
- Intravenous electrolyte solutions

Later activities

- Survey for concomitant disease
- Pass nasogastric tube
  - No blood in stomach → Withdraw tube
  - Blood in stomach → Leave tube in place for lavage
- Transfuse blood and blood products
- Obtain consultations

Making a specific diagnosis

- Upper GI endoscopy
  - Diagnostic → Consider: Therapeutic endoscopy
  - Nondiagnostic or bleeding brisk → Consider: Radionuclide scan, Selective arteriography, Immediate surgery
- Sigmoidoscopy for lower GI bleeding
  - Diagnostic
  - Nondiagnostic
    - Bleeding continues → Consider: Radionuclide scan, Selective arteriography, Colonoscopy
    - Bleeding stops → Consider: Elective colonoscopy

Fig. 3-13 Management of acute gastrointestinal bleeding. (From Stein JH [ed]: *Internal medicine*, ed 5, St Louis, 1998, Mosby.)

BLEEDING, VAGINAL

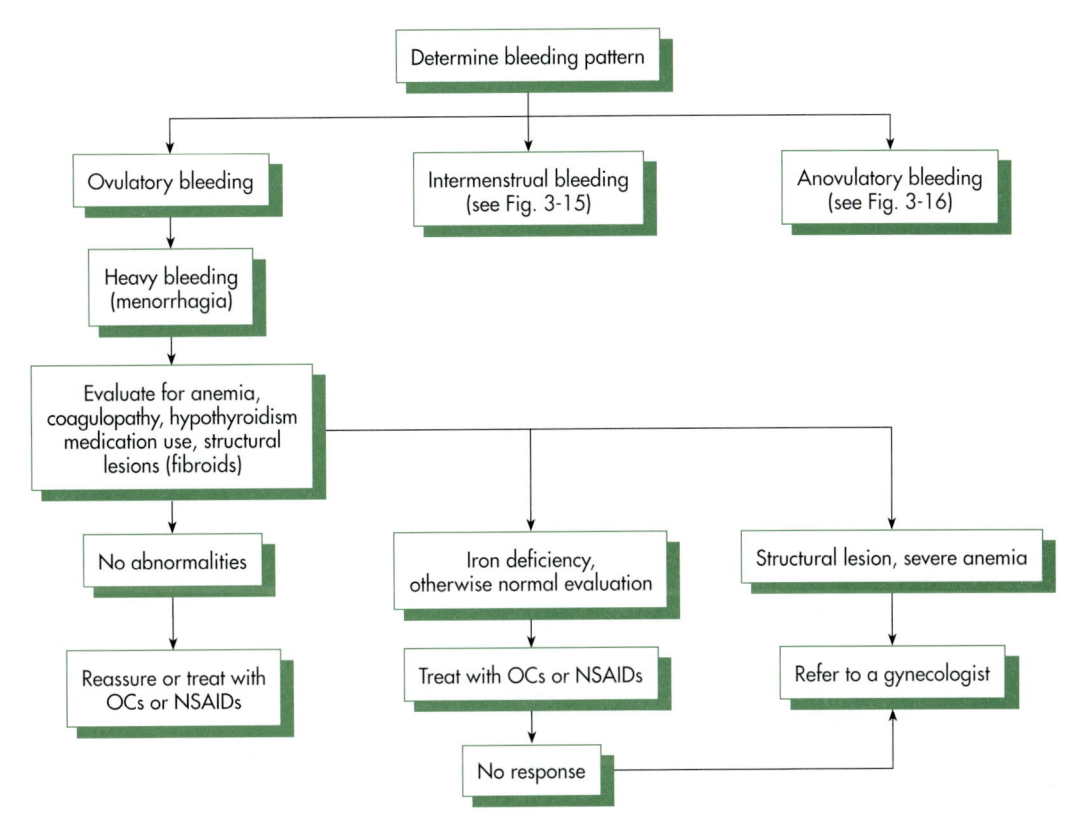

Fig. 3-14 Evaluation of ovulatory bleeding. *OCs,* Oral contraceptives; *NSAIDs,* nonsteroidal anti-inflammatory drugs. (From Appleby J, Henderson M, Wathen PI: Management of abnormal menstrual bleeding, *Intern Med,* Sept:17-36, 1996, copyright Medical Economics Company.)

BLEEDING, VAGINAL—cont'd

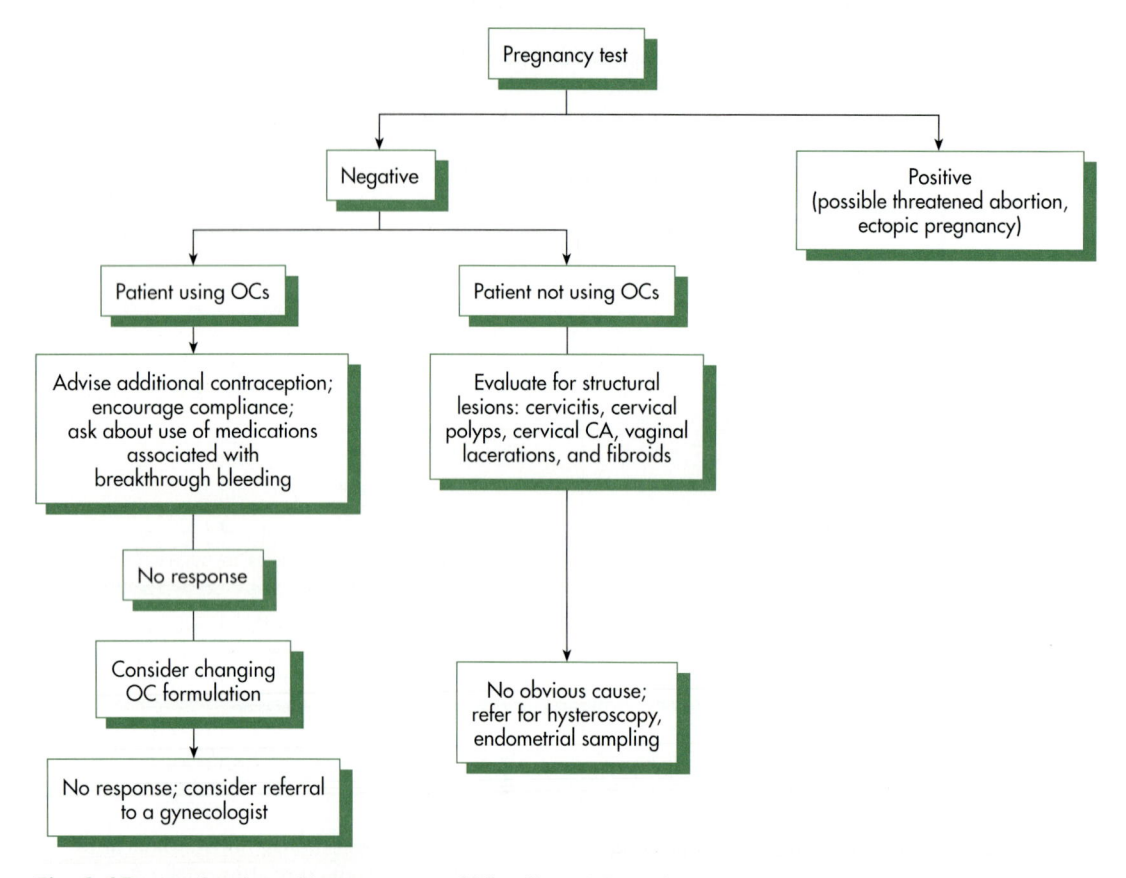

Fig. 3-15 **Evaluation of intermenstrual bleeding.** *OCs,* oral contraceptives; *CA,* cancer. (From Appleby J, Henderson M, Wathen PI: Management of abnormal menstrual bleeding, *Intern Med,* Sept:17-36, 1996, copyright Medical Economics Company.)

CLINICAL ALGORITHMS

BLEEDING, VAGINAL—cont'd

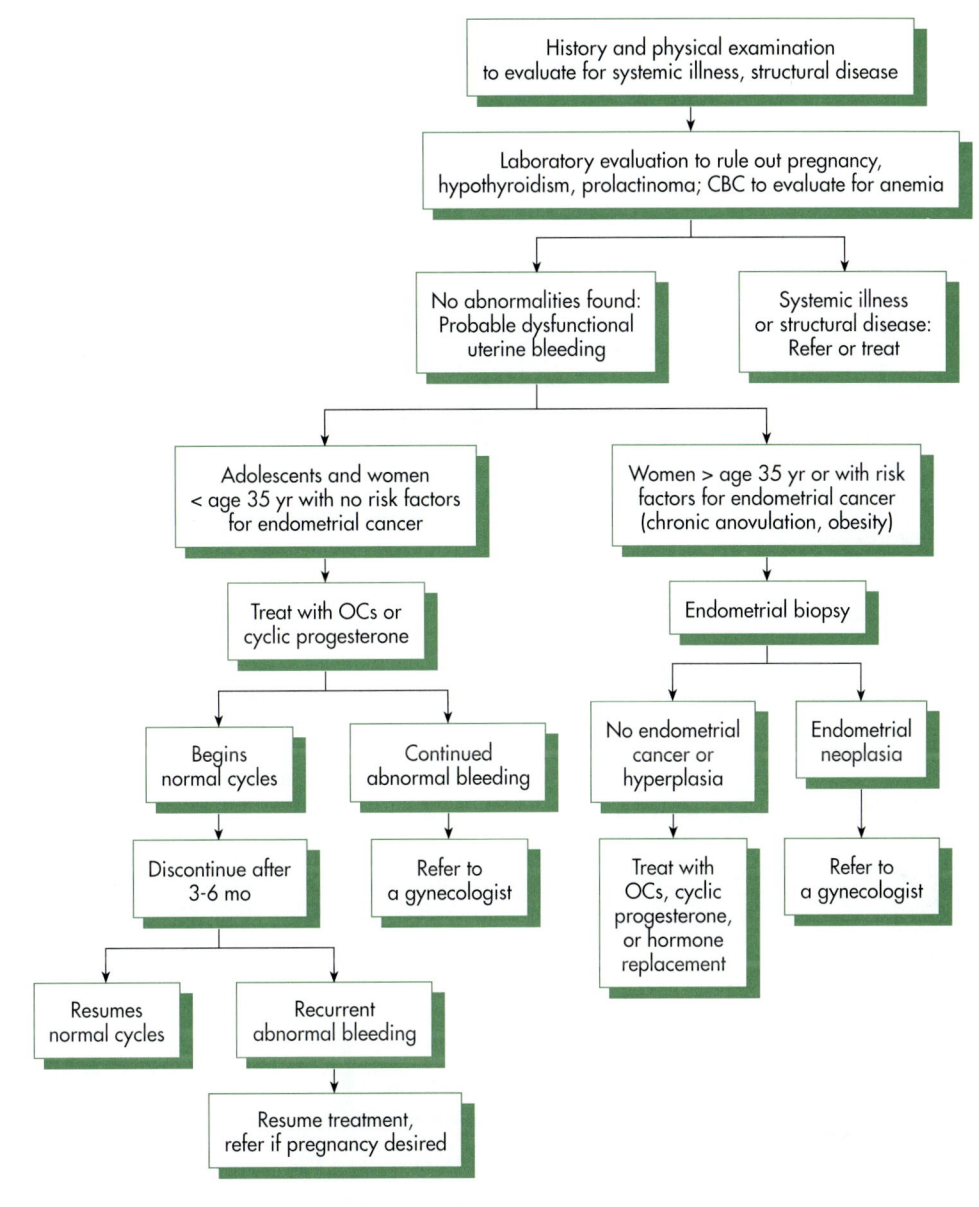

Fig. 3-16 Evaluation of anovulatory bleeding. *CBC,* complete blood count; *OCs,* oral contraceptives. (From Appleby J, Henderson M, Wathen PI: Management of abnormal menstrual bleeding, *Intern Med,* Sept:17-36, 1996, copyright Medical Economics Company.)

BLEEDING DISORDER, CONGENITAL

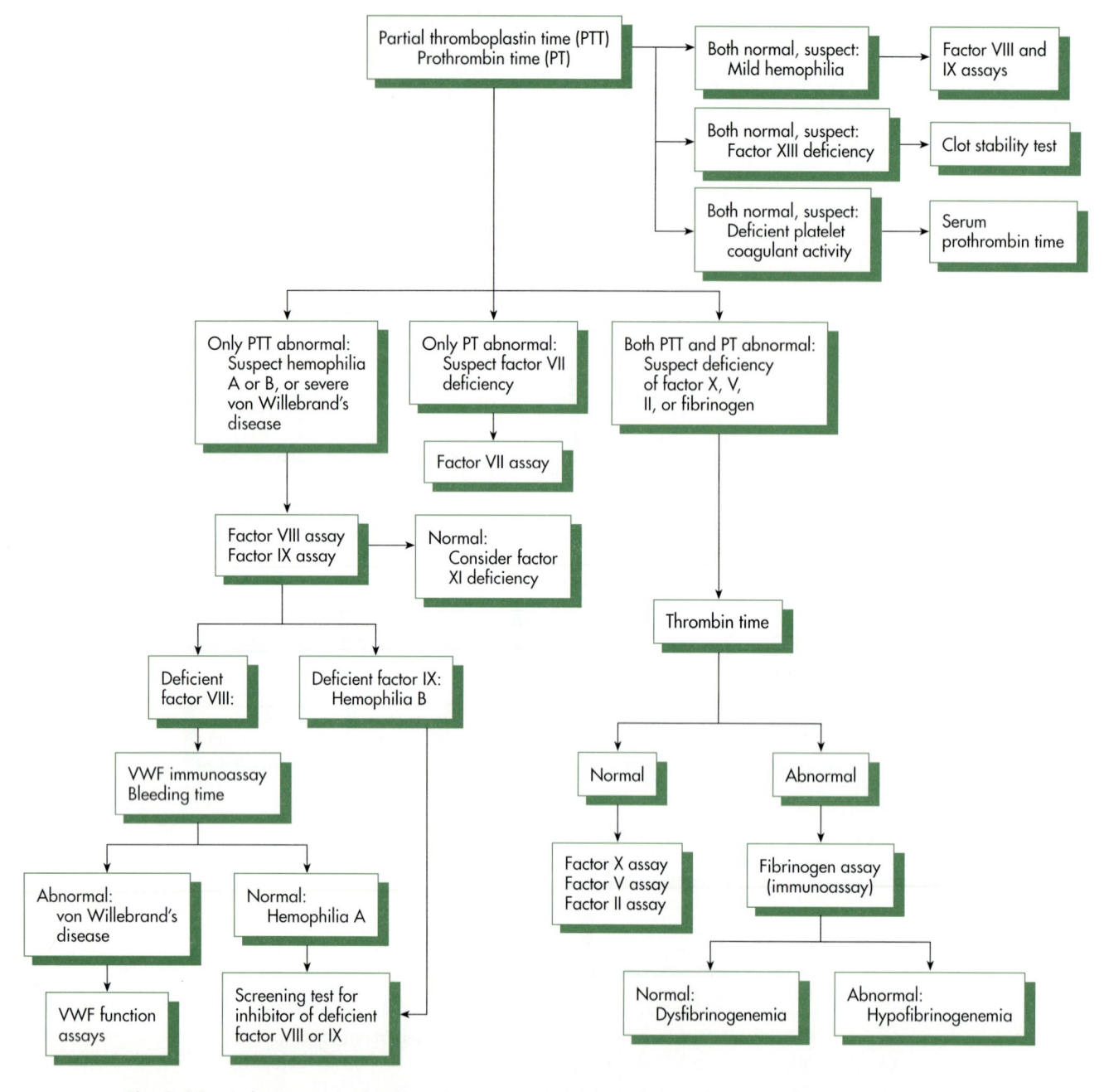

Fig. 3-17 Laboratory evaluation of a patient with a bleeding disorder in whom the history and physical examination suggest a congenital coagulation disorder. (From Stein JH [ed]: *Internal medicine,* ed 4, St Louis, 1994, Mosby.)

BREAST, NIPPLE DISCHARGE EVALUATION

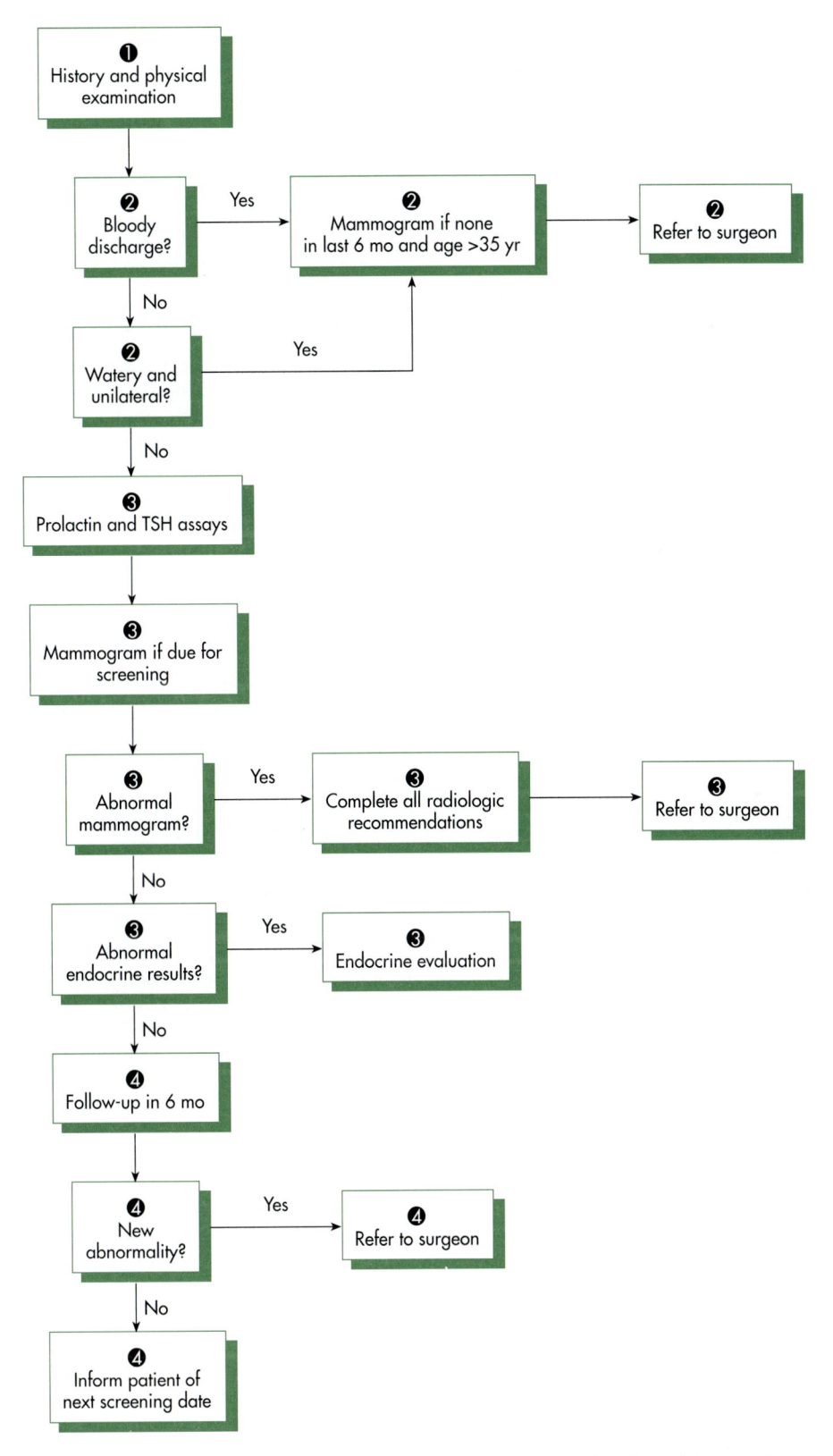

Fig. 3-18 **Breast cancer screening and evaluation.** (From Institute for Clinical Systems Integration, Minneapolis: Breast cancer screening and evaluation guidelines, *Postgrad Med* 100:182-187, 1996.)

Continued

Fig. 3-18—cont'd

1 **History and physical examination.*** Patients who present with a complaint of nipple discharge should be evaluated with breast-related history taking and a physical examination. History taking is aimed at uncovering and characterizing any other breast-related symptom. A risk assessment should also be undertaken for identified risk factors, including patient age over 50 years, any past personal history of breast cancer, history of hyperplasia on previous breast biopsies, and family history of breast cancer in first-degree relatives (mother, sister, daughter). Physical examination should include inspection of the breast for any evidence of ulceration or contour changes and inspection of the nipple for Paget's disease. Palpation should be performed with the patient in both the upright and the supine positions to determine the presence of any palpable mass.

2 **Bloody discharge?** If the discharge appears frankly bloody, the patient should be referred to a surgeon for evaluation. At the time of referral, a mammogram of the involved breast should be obtained if the patient is over 35 years of age and has not had a mammogram within the preceding 6 months. Similarly, patients with a watery, unilateral discharge should be referred to a surgeon for evaluation and possible biopsy.

3 **Endocrine tests. Mammogram.** If the discharge appears frankly milky or is bilateral, serum prolactin and serum thyroid-stimulating hormone (TSH) assays should be performed to rule out the presence of an endocrinologic basis for the symptoms. At the time of that visit, a mammogram should also be performed if the patient is due for routine mammographic screening according to the recommended intervals. A patient with an abnormal mammogram should be further evaluated radiologically to better characterize the lesion and then be referred to a surgeon if appropriate. Make certain that all recommended additional views, ultrasound examinations, and follow-up studies have been obtained before referral to a surgeon. Should the mammogram appear normal, results of the assays for TSH and prolactin should be reviewed. If the results are abnormal, the patient should undergo appropriate evaluation for etiology, either by a primary care physician or by an endocrinologist.

4. **Six-month follow-up results.** If results of the mammogram and the endocrinologic screening studies are normal, the patient should return for a follow-up visit in 6 months to ensure that there has been no specific change in the character of the discharge, such as development of frank bleeding or Paget's disease, that would warrant surgical evaluation. If the evaluation at that follow-up visit fails to reveal any palpable or visible abnormalities, the patient should be returned to the routine screening process with studies performed at the recommended intervals.

---

*ICSI healthcare guidelines are designed to assist clinicians by providing an analytic framework for the evaluation and treatment of patients. They are not intended either to replace a clinician's judgment or to establish a protocol for all patients with a particular condition. A guideline will rarely establish the only approach to a problem. In addition, guidelines are "living documents" that are expected to be imperfect and are subject to annual review and revision.

ICSI is a nonprofit organization that provides healthcare quality improvement services to 20 medical groups affiliated with HealthPartners in central and southern Minnesota and western Wisconsin. The guidelines are developed through a process that involves physicians, nurses, and other healthcare professionals from beginning to end, and healthcare purchasers are included in decision making. To order any of the over 40 guidelines ICSI has developed, contact the ICSI Publications Fulfillment Center, in care of the ARDEL Group, 6518 Walker St., Suite 150, Minneapolis, MN 55426; 612-927-6707.

CLINICAL ALGORITHMS   Breast   695

BREAST, RADIOLOGIC EVALUATION

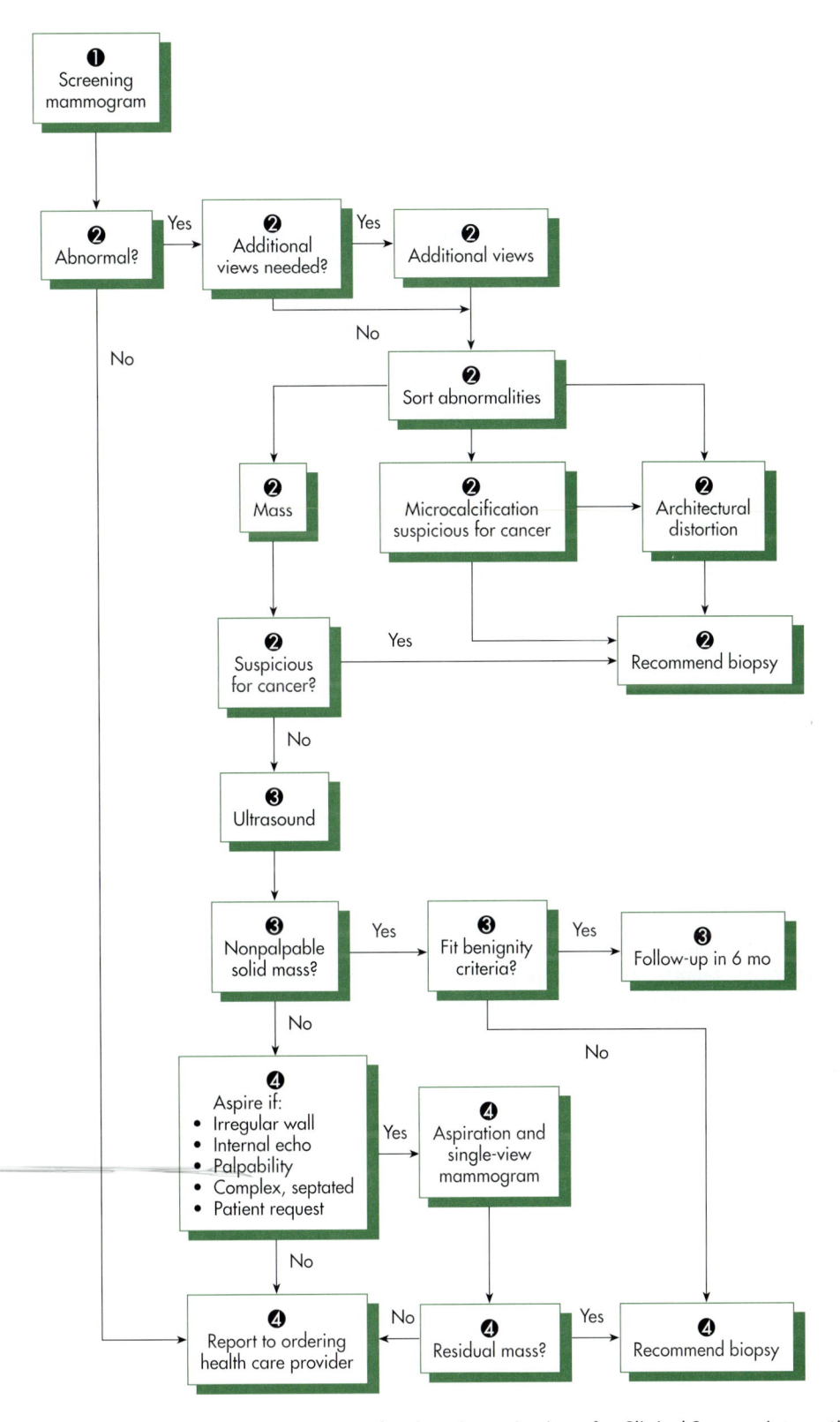

Fig. 3-19 Breast cancer screening and evaluation. (From Institute for Clinical Systems Integration, Minneapolis: Breast cancer screening and evaluation guidelines, *Postgrad Med* 100:182-187, 1996.)

Continued

Fig. 3-19—cont'd

1 **Screening mammogram.*** Patients are most commonly referred to a radiologist for screening mammography. Occasionally, however, patients are referred for diagnostic mammography on the basis of symptoms or findings on breast exam. In the event of an abnormal finding on the mammogram, complete evaluation under the direction of a radiologist is recommended. It is the responsibility of the radiologist to complete the radiologic assessment so that the best possible characterization of the abnormality can be provided in an expeditious fashion to the primary care physician who ordered the original study. Any recommendations for referral to a surgeon for possible biopsy should be made directly to the primary care physician. The ultimate responsibility to make the referral will rest with the primary care physician.

2 **Abnormal mammogram. Sorting abnormalities. Suspicious for cancer?** On obtaining an abnormal finding on a mammogram, the radiologist determines whether further mammographic images are required for completion of the evaluation process. This may include a repeated image of the involved breast at 6 months to document stability of a low-risk, probably benign lesion. Alternatively, spot compression, magnification, or both may be necessary to obtain further characterization of indeterminate breast lesions. These additional studies should be done with the radiologist present to reduce the risk of patient recall for further studies necessary to evaluate the same lesion.

On completion of these views, each and every abnormality uncovered for each independent lesion of the breast studied should be sorted according to the nature of the abnormality. The radiologist should classify the lesion as representing either suspicious microcalcifications, architectural distortion, or a soft-tissue mass. For any lesions identified as demonstrating microcalcifications that suggest cancer, biopsy will be recommended. It is up to the primary care physician to make the referral to a surgeon for biopsy. If a soft-tissue mass is identified on the mammogram, it should be studied further to determine its relative risk for malignancy. Any suspect lesions identified as having associated microcalcifications, architectural distortion, or interval growth when compared with the previous mammogram should likewise be referred to a surgeon for possible biopsy.

3 **Ultrasound results.** When the mass is not immediately suggestive of cancer, an ultrasound should be performed to determine whether the lesion is solid. A solid mass should be further characterized for its level of benignity according to three criteria:
- Size less than 15 mm
- Three or fewer lobulations
- More than 50% of the margin of the lesion appearing well circumscribed in any view

Patients who have lesions that fit all three criteria may be observed and then evaluated with a 6-month follow-up study. Any lesion that does not fit all three criteria for benignity should be characterized as indeterminate, and biopsy should be considered. Likewise, any solid mass that is palpable should be referred to a surgeon for possible open biopsy. Finally, any lesion that appears to be new since the last screening mammogram should be considered for biopsy.

4 **Aspiration and results.** If the ultrasound of the soft tissue mass demonstrates that it is a cystic lesion, the cyst should be further categorized by the criteria listed in the algorithm: irregular wall, as seen on ultrasonography; internal echoes; complex, septated appearance; and palpability within the region of the ultrasound-proven cyst. A positive finding for any of these criteria would be an indication for ultrasound-directed aspiration of the cyst. Aspiration should also be offered if the patient requests it.

After cyst aspiration, a single-view mammogram should be obtained to demonstrate complete resolution of the lesion. If the lesion is sufficiently complex, a cyst pneumogram may be performed. Should any residual mass be present or if the cyst pneumogram findings are abnormal, biopsy should be recommended. If, on the other hand, the mass is a simple cyst that does not fit any of the previously listed criteria, the patient should be returned to the screening process, and completion of this evaluation should be reported to the ordering health care provider.

---

*ICSI healthcare guidelines are designed to assist clinicians by providing an analytic framework for the evaluation and treatment of patients. They are not intended either to replace a clinician's judgment or to establish a protocol for all patients with a particular condition. A guideline will rarely establish the only approach to a problem. In addition, guidelines are "living documents" that are expected to be imperfect and are subject to annual review and revision.

ICSI is a nonprofit organization that provides healthcare quality improvement services to 20 medical groups affiliated with HealthPartners in central and southern Minnesota and western Wisconsin. The guidelines are developed through a process that involves physicians, nurses, and other healthcare professionals from beginning to end, and healthcare purchasers are included in decision making. To order any of the over 40 guidelines ICSI has developed, contact the ICSI Publications Fulfillment Center, in care of the ARDEL Group, 6518 Walker St., Suite 150, Minneapolis, MN 55426; 612-927-6707.

CLINICAL ALGORITHMS   Breast   697

BREAST, ROUTINE SCREEN OR PALPABLE MASS EVALUATION

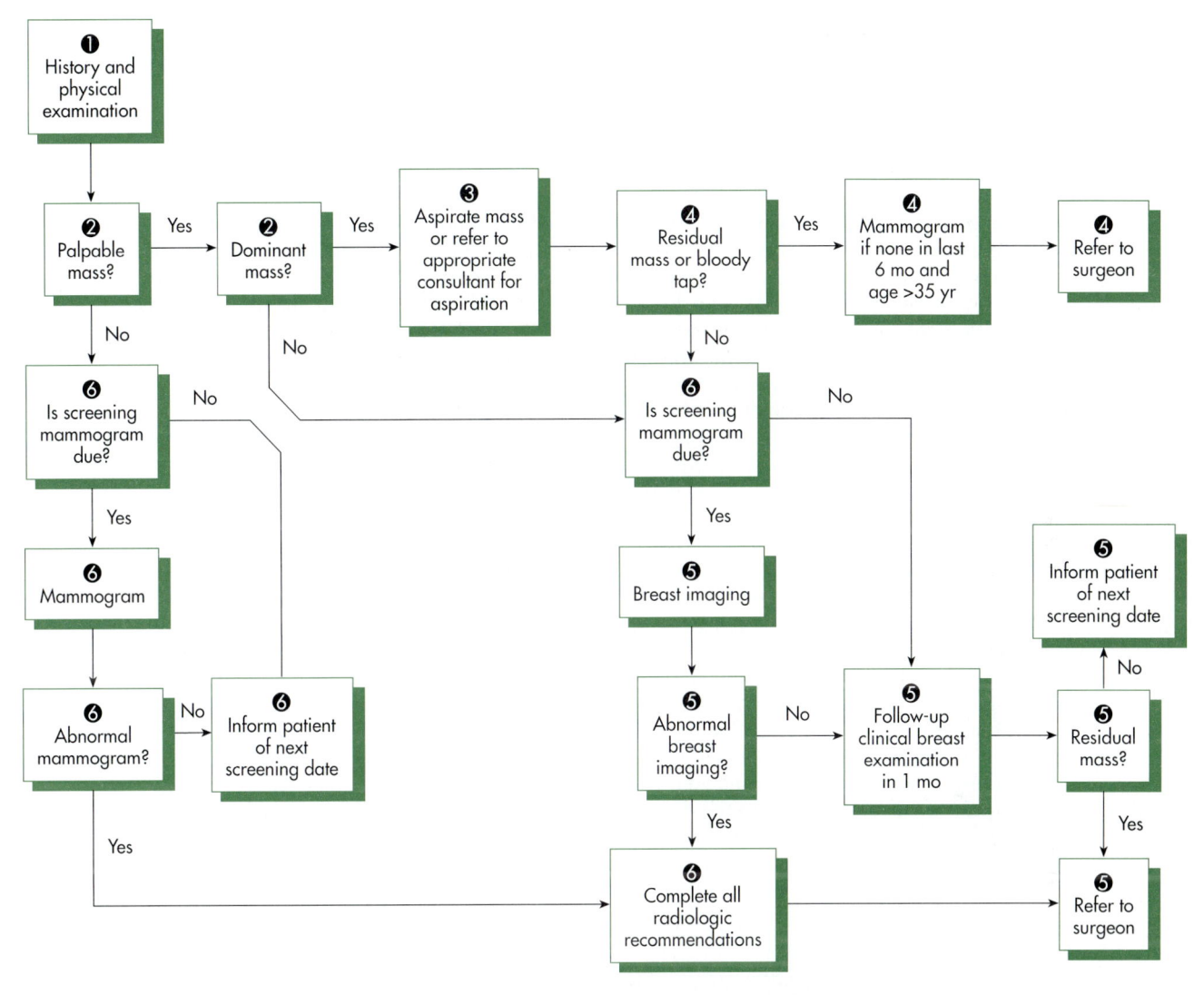

Fig. 3-20 Breast cancer screening and evaluation. (From Institute for Clinical Systems Integration, Minneapolis: Breast cancer screening and evaluation guidelines, Postgrad Med 100:182-187, 1996.)

1 **History and physical examination.*** Primary care evaluation is initiated with history taking aimed at uncovering and characterizing any breast-related symptom. A risk assessment should also be undertaken for identified risk factors, including patient age over 50 years, any past personal history of breast cancer, history of hyperplasia on previous breast biopsies, and family history of breast cancer in first-degree relatives (mother, sister, daughter). Physical examination should include inspection of the breast for any evidence of ulceration or contour changes and inspection of the nipple for Paget's

Continued

---

*ICSI healthcare guidelines are designed to assist clinicians by providing an analytic framework for the evaluation and treatment of patients. They are not intended either to replace a clinician's judgment or to establish a protocol for all patients with a particular condition. A guideline will rarely establish the only approach to a problem. In addition, guidelines are "living documents" that are expected to be imperfect and are subject to annual review and revision.

ICSI is a nonprofit organization that provides healthcare quality improvement services to 20 medical groups affiliated with HealthPartners in central and southern Minnesota and western Wisconsin. The guidelines are developed through a process that involves physicians, nurses, and other healthcare professionals from beginning to end, and healthcare purchasers are included in decision making. To order any of the over 40 guidelines ICSI has developed, contact the ICSI Publications Fulfillment Center, in care of the ARDEL Group, 6518 Walker St., Suite 150, Minneapolis, MN 55426; 612-927-6707.

Fig. 3-19—cont'd

disease. Palpation should be performed with the patient in both the upright and supine positions to determine the presence of any palpable mass.

2 **Palpable mass? Dominant mass?** A dominant mass is a palpable finding that is discrete and clearly different from the surrounding parenchyma. If a palpable mass is identified, it should be determined whether it represents a dominant (i.e., discrete) mass, which requires immediate evaluation. The primary care physician should attempt to aspirate any dominant mass because a simple cyst may be uncovered, in which case aspiration completes the evaluation process.

3 **Aspirate mass or refer for aspiration.** Aspiration of a dominant palpable mass should be performed by the primary care physician or by the appropriate consultant. The breast skin is prepped with alcohol. Then, with the lesion immobilized by the nonoperating hand, an 18- to 25-gauge needle mounted on a 10 cc syringe is directed to the central portion of the mass for a single attempt at aspiration. Successful aspiration of a simple cyst would yield a nonbloody fluid with complete resolution of the dominant mass. Typical watery fluid may be discarded. However, cyst fluid that is bloody or unusually tenacious should be examined cytologically.

4 **Residual mass or bloody tap? Mammogram if none in last 6 months. Refer to surgeon.** Should the mass remain after the attempt at aspiration or should frank blood be aspirated during the process, the presence of a malignant process cannot be ruled out. Patients with a residual mass or bloody tap should be referred to a surgeon for possible biopsy. Before the referral, a mammogram should be obtained for any patient over age 35 years who has not had a mammogram within the preceding 6 months. In patients 35 years and under, obtaining any other breast-imaging studies should be left to the discretion of the surgeon or radiologist.

5 **Is screening mammogram due? Breast imaging. Follow-up clinical breast examination. Refer to surgeon.** Should physical examination demonstrate a palpable mass that is not clearly a discrete and dominant mass, its size, location, and character should be documented in anticipation of a follow-up examination. A screening mammogram should be obtained if one has not been done within the recommended interval. If no mammogram is required or if a required mammogram demonstrates no abnormality, a follow-up examination in 1 month is indicated. Should any residual mass be identified, the patient should be referred to a surgeon for possible biopsy. Patients with a persisting nondominant palpable mass that does not resolve within 1 month and those with any recurring cystic mass should be referred for surgical evaluation. If no mass is apparent at the time of the follow-up examination, the patient should then be informed of the appropriate date for her next screening examination, according to the recommended intervals

6 **Screening mammogram and results.** After completion of the physical examination, the appropriateness of a routine screening mammogram should be determined. If a mammogram is done, the radiologist should provide the results to the primary care physician for reporting to the patient. Should any abnormalities be uncovered, it will be the responsibility of the radiologist to complete any additional imaging studies required for the complete radiographic characterization of the lesion. The radiologist should make certain that all recommended additional views, follow-up studies, and ultrasound examinations have been completed before referral to a surgeon.

However, it is important that the primary care physician who ordered the mammogram review the results of these studies to understand fully the opinion of the radiologist and to ensure that all recommendations of the radiologist have been completed. Should the radiologist recommend that surgical consultation is warranted, it will be the responsibility of the primary care physician to establish this referral.

NOTE: *The importance of communication between the surgical consultant and the primary care physician cannot be overstated. Biopsy results should be reported both to the surgeon and to the primary care physician. More important, patients who do not require biopsy after surgical consultation should be returned to the routine screening process. This process is under the supervision of the primary care physician. Therefore it is absolutely necessary for the primary care physician to know when the patient reenters the routine screening population. In the event that new symptoms arise during the screening interval, the patient should be evaluated by the primary care physician using the primary care evaluation process of this guideline.*

CODE STATUS DETERMINATION BEFORE CARDIAC ARREST

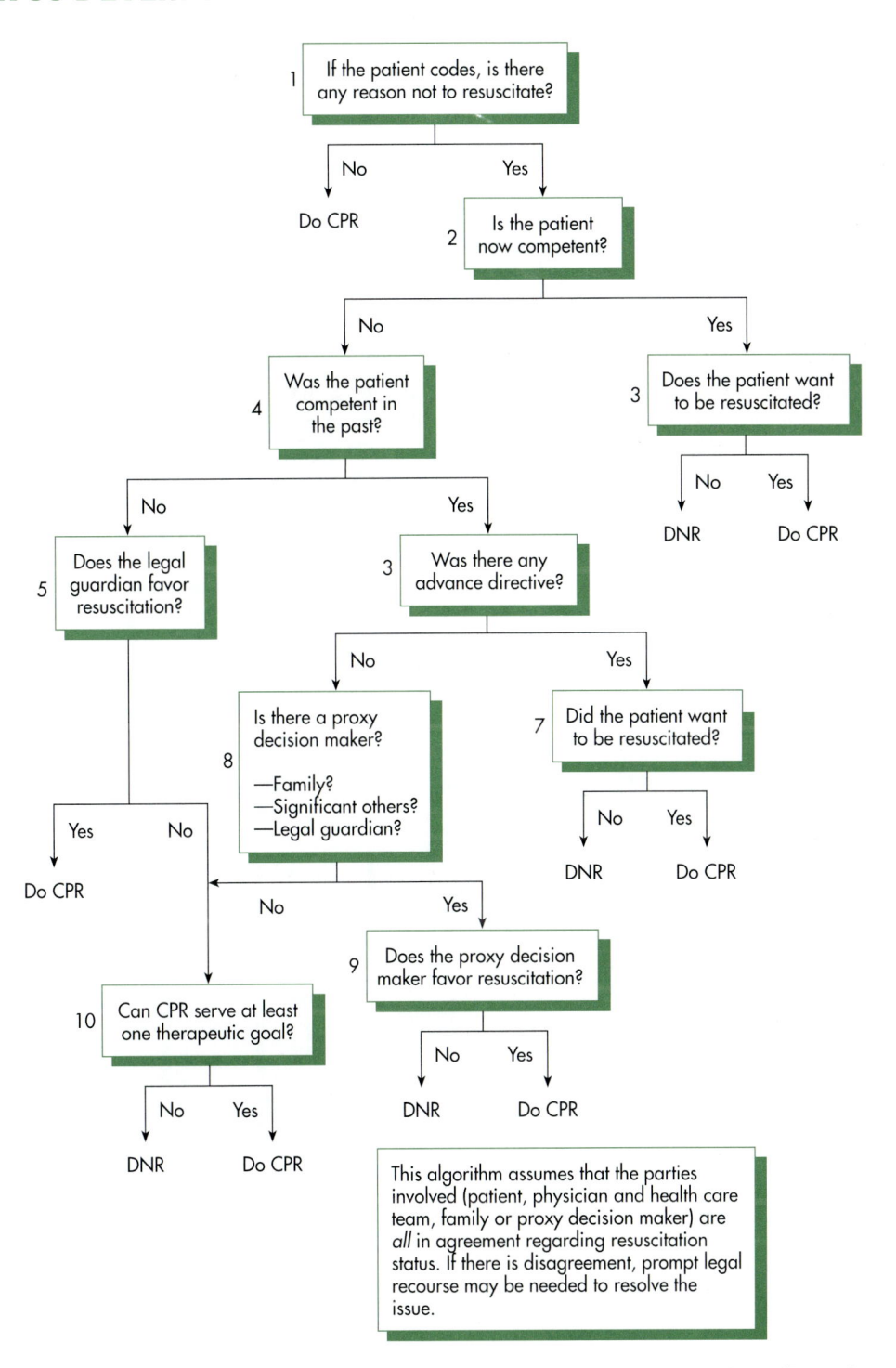

Fig. 3-21 Determination of code status *before the arrest*. *DNR,* Do not resuscitate. (From Grauer K, Cavallaro D [eds]: *ACLS certification preparation,* St Louis, 1993, Mosby.)

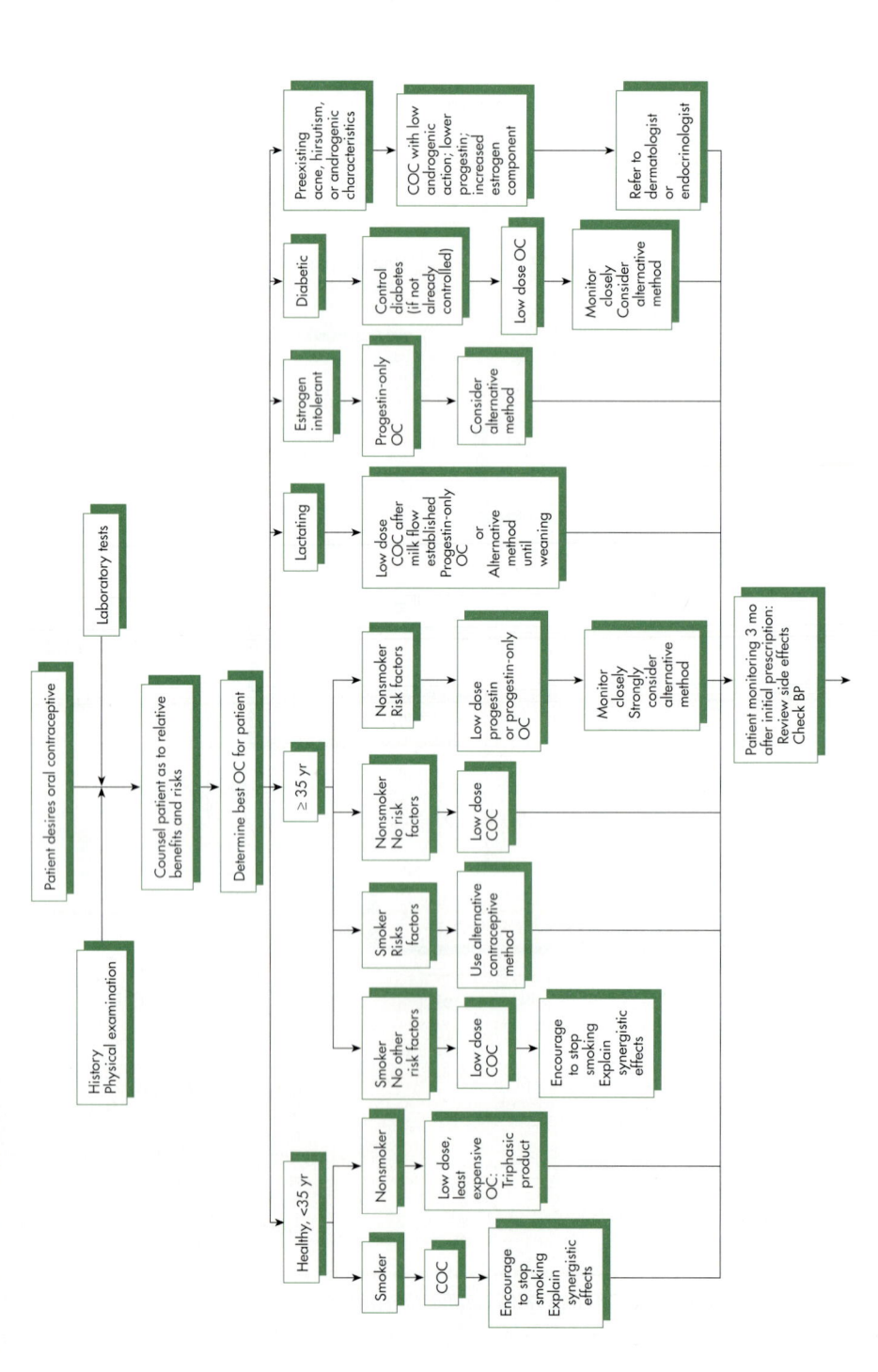

Contraceptive use

CONTRACEPTIVE USE, ORAL

Patient desires oral contraceptive
→ History, Physical examination
→ Laboratory tests
→ Counsel patient as to relative benefits and risks
→ Determine best OC for patient

Healthy, <35 yr
- Nonsmoker → Low dose, least expensive OC; Triphasic product
- Smoker → COC → Encourage to stop smoking; Explain synergistic effects

≥ 35 yr
- Smoker No other risk factors → Low dose COC → Encourage to stop smoking; Explain synergistic effects
- Smoker Risks factors → Use alternative contraceptive method
- Nonsmoker No risk factors → Low dose COC
- Nonsmoker Risk factors → Low dose progestin or progestin-only OC → Monitor closely; Strongly consider alternative method

Lactating → Low dose COC after milk flow established; Progestin-only OC or Alternative method until weaning

Estrogen intolerant → Progestin-only OC → Consider alternative method

Diabetic → Control diabetes (if not already controlled) → Low dose OC → Monitor closely; Consider alternative method

Preexisting acne, hirsutism, or androgenic characteristics → COC with low androgenic action; lower progestin; increased estrogen component → Refer to dermatologist or endocrinologist

→ Patient monitoring 3 mo after initial prescription: Review side effects; Check BP

CLINICAL ALGORITHMS

Contraceptive use 701

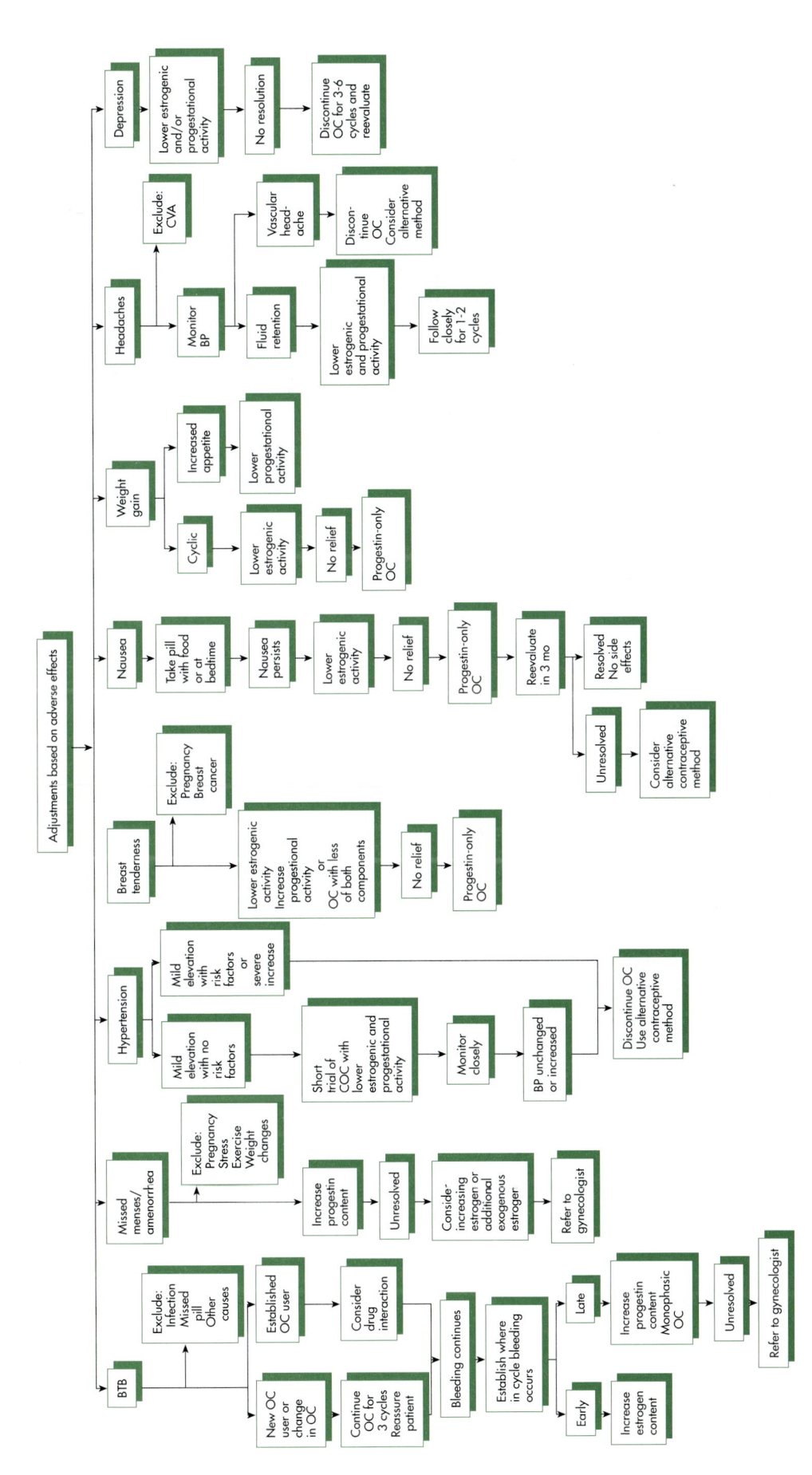

Fig. 3-22 **Contraceptive use.** (From Robles TA: Use of oral contraceptives. In Greene HL, Johnson WP, Maricic MJ [eds]: *Decision making in medicine*, St Louis, 1993, Mosby.)

COUGH, CHRONIC

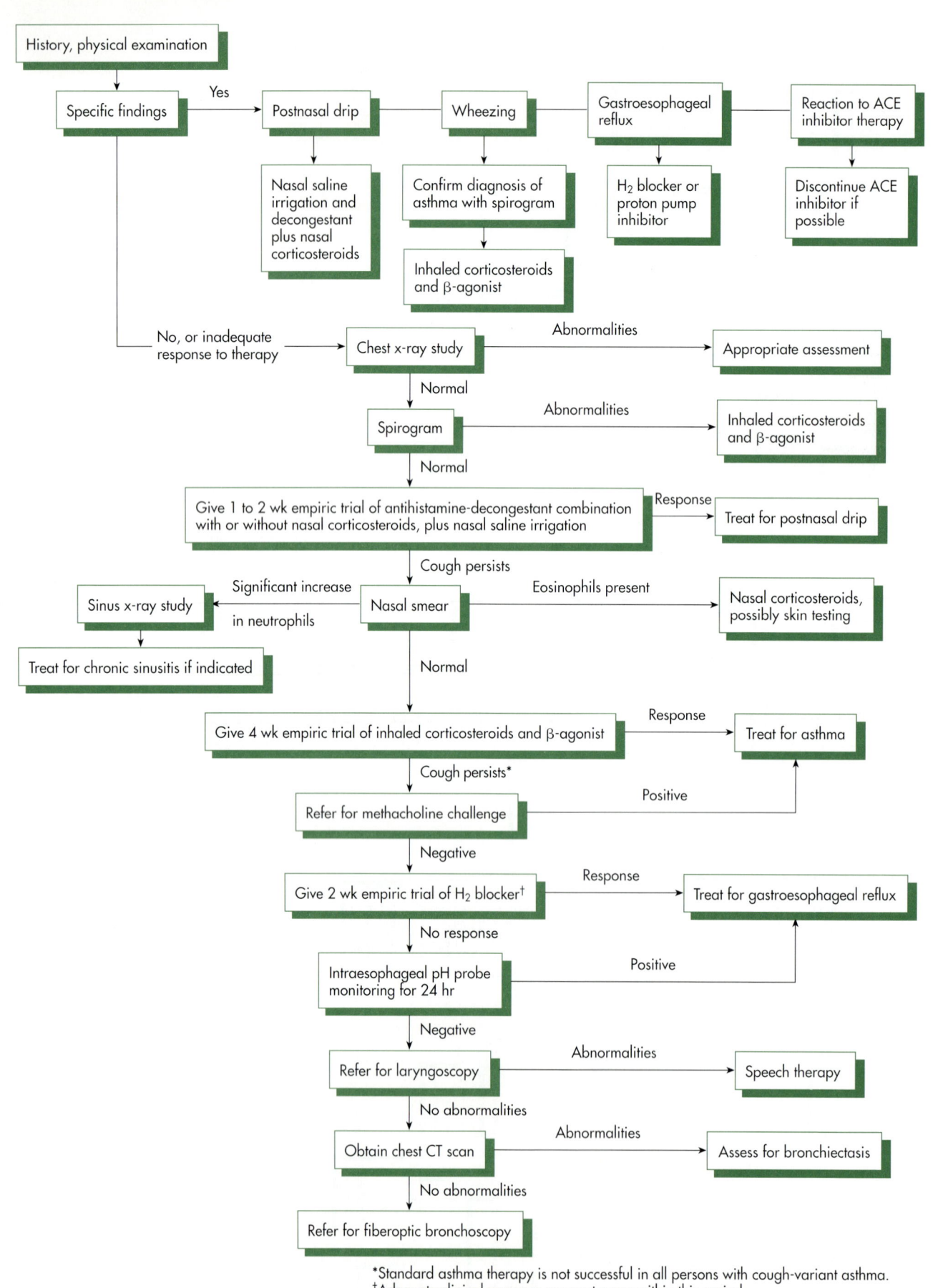

Fig. 3-23 Investigation and management of chronic cough. (From Newman KB, Milgrom H: Chronic cough: a step-by-step diagnostic work-up, *Consultant*, Oct, 1537-1542, 1995.)

*Standard asthma therapy is not successful in all persons with cough-variant asthma.
†Adequate clinical response may not occur within this period.

CREATINE KINASE ELEVATION

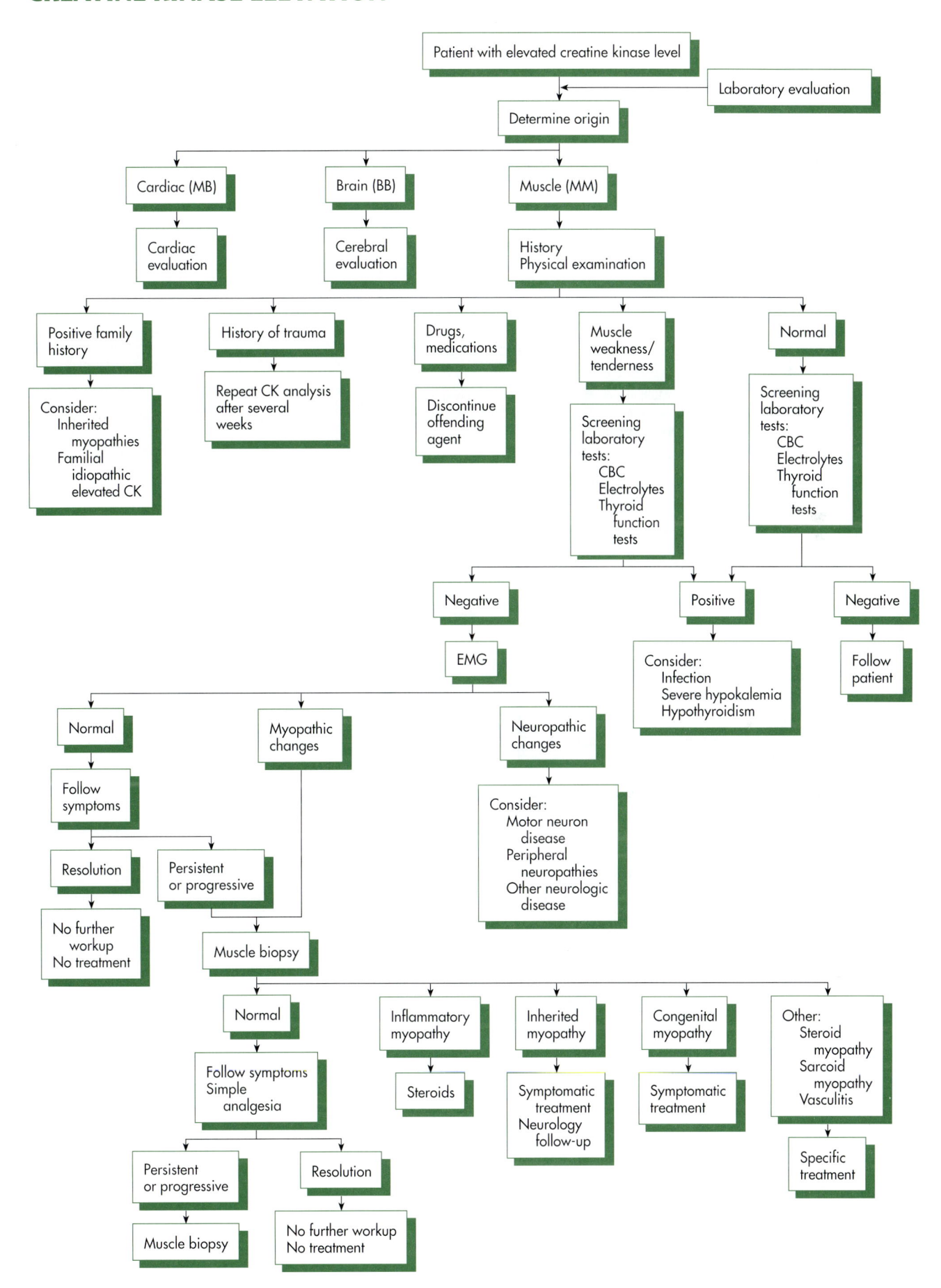

Fig. 3-24 Evaluation of creatine kinase elevation. (From Greene HL, Johnson WP, Maricic MJ: *Decision making in medicine,* St Louis, 1993, Mosby.)

DEMENTIA

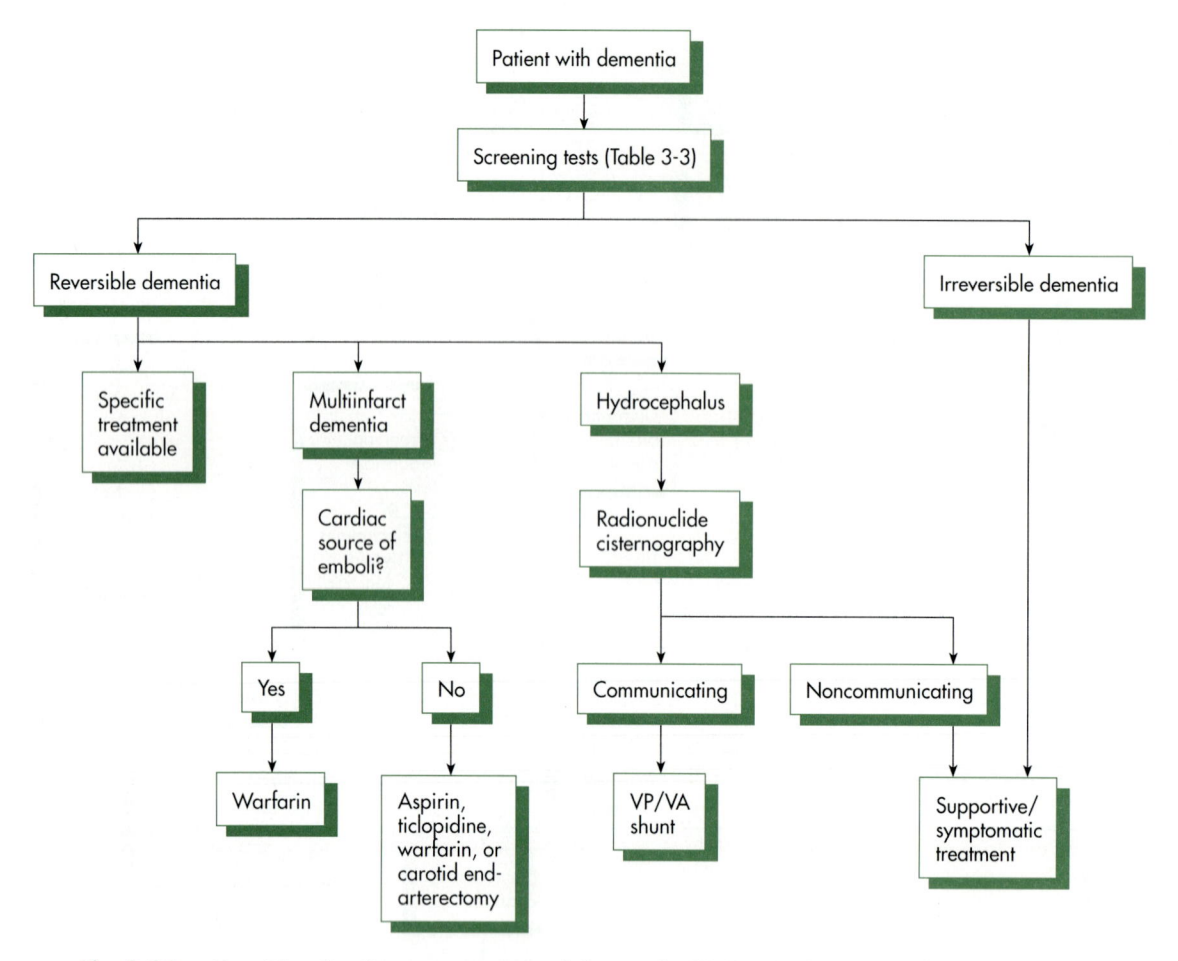

Fig. 3-25 Algorithm for the management of dementia. *VP,* Ventriculoperitoneal; *VA,* ventriculoatrial.

DEMENTIA—cont'd

TABLE 3-3 Screening Tests for Diagnosis of Dementia

TEST	RATIONALE	REMARKS
Blood Test		
Complete blood count	Assess general nutritional status	
Serum B_{12} level	Exclude vitamin B_{12} deficiency	Schilling's test if B_{12} level is low
TSH + free T_4 *or* TSH + FTI	Exclude primary and secondary hypothyroidism	
HIV serology	Exclude HIV infection	Perform only if indicated; consent from patient required
Cerebrospinal Fluid		
Cell count/protein level	Exclude chronic meningitis	Perform only if indicated
Cytology	Exclude carcinomatous meningitis	Perform only if indicated
VDRL	Exclude neurosyphilis	Perform only if indicated; check serum TPHA and HIV serology if CSF VDRL is positive
CT Scan/MRI of the Brain	Identify infarcts and white matter changes; exclude presence of neoplasm, demyelinating disease, and hydrocephalus; location of atrophy may suggest the diagnosis (e.g., parahippocampal atrophy in Alzheimer's disease, frontotemporal atrophy in Pick's disease)	
Electroencephalogram	Exclude metabolic encephalopathies; useful if Creutzfeldt-Jakob disease or status epilepticus is suspected	Perform only if indicated
Neuropsychologic Evaluation	Help to characterize pattern of cognitive impairment, which may aid in the classification of dementia; rule out pseudodementia from depression	

From Johnson RT, Griffin JW: *Current therapy in neurologic disease*, ed 5, St Louis, 1997, Mosby.
TSH, Thyroid-stimulating hormone; *FTI*, free thyroxine index; *HIV*, human immunodeficiency virus; *VDRL*, Veneral Disease Research Laboratory test; *TPHA*, *Treponema pallidum* hemagglutination assay; *CSF*, cerebrospinal fluid; *CT*, computed tomography; *MRI*, magnetic resonance imaging.

706 Developmental delay

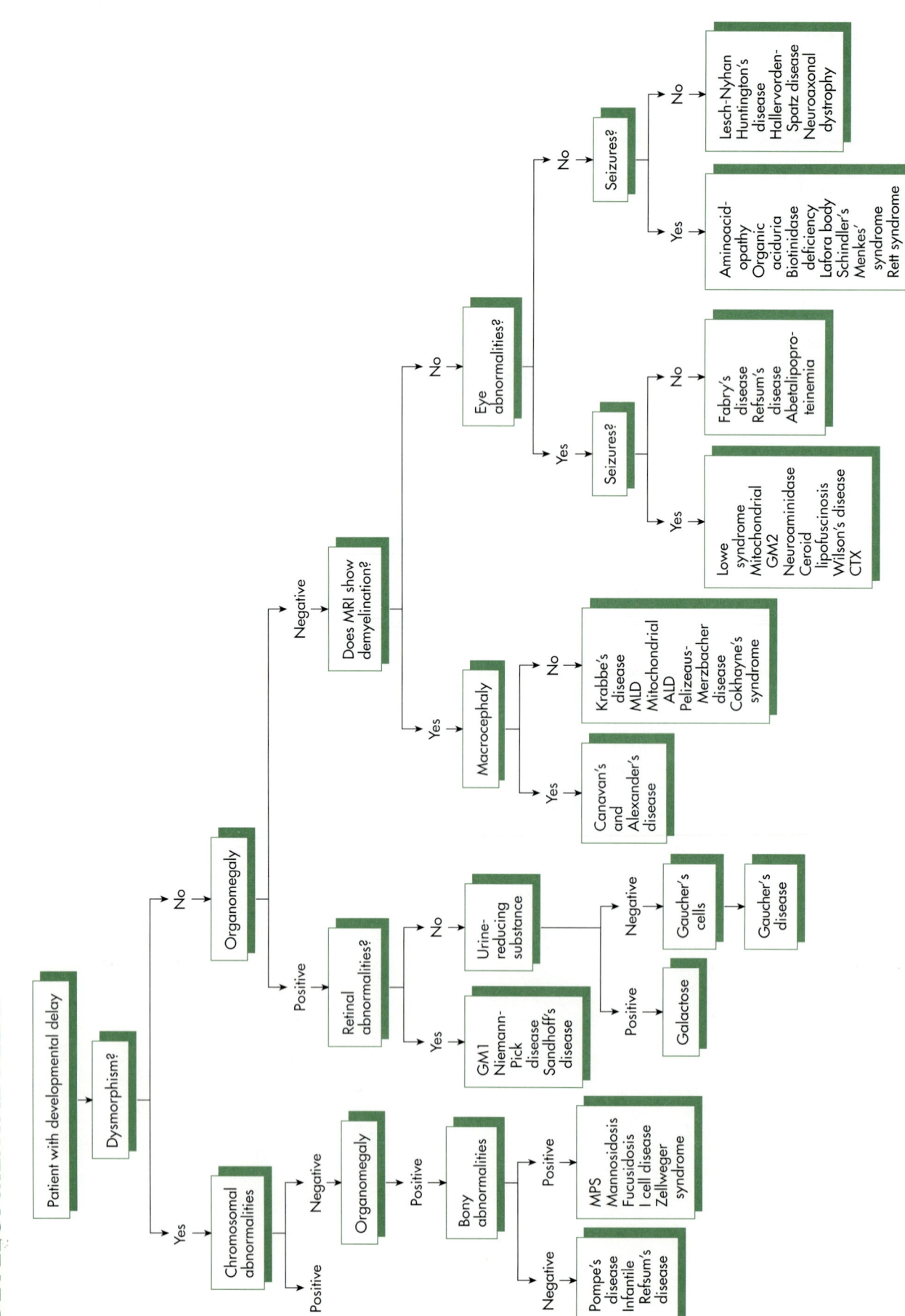

Fig. 3-26 Workup for developmental delay. *MRI,* Magnetic resonance imaging; *MPS,* mucopolysaccharidosis; *MLD,* metachromatic leukodystrophy; *ALD,* adrenoleukodystrophy; *CTX,* cerebrotendinous xanthomatosis. (From Johnson RT, Griffin JW: *Current therapy in neurologic disease,* ed 5, St Louis, 1997, Mosby.)

DIARRHEA, ACUTE

1. Physical examination

Hydrate as necessary

2. Stool examination

Inflammatory cells

Present: suggests mucosal disease
a. IBD
b. Invasive bacterial infections (such as *Shigella* spp., *Salmonella* spp., amebiasis, *Campylobacter*)
Absent: suggests viral gastroenteritis, toxin (*Staphylococcus*, *E. coli*, *Aeromonas*, or *Plesiomonas* spp.), or drug-related diarrhea or IBS

Ova and parasites

Blood: if present, consider:
a. IBD
b. Bacterial infections:
   Salmonella spp.
   Shigella spp.
   Amebiasis
   Campylobacter
   Clostridium difficile toxin
   E. coli O157:H7

3. Culture stool

Positive culture result

Treat appropriately, except for *Salmonella* infections in which treatment may prolong the carrier state

Negative culture result

See step 5 in Fig. 3-28

Flexible sigmoidoscopy

Abnormal mucosa

a. Pseudomembranes: check for *C. difficile* toxin: treat with vancomycin, bacitracin, or metronidazole
b. Ulcerations/granularity
   (1) Proctitis only: culture for *Chlamydia trachomatis*, *Neisseria gonorrhoeae*; Gram's stain and culture urethra and pharynx; biopsy as in (2)
   (2) More extensive: culture; biopsy to look for ameba, granulomas, or nonspecific finding of IBD

Normal mucosa

Wait for culture results

Negative stool culture result

Inflammatory cells in stool

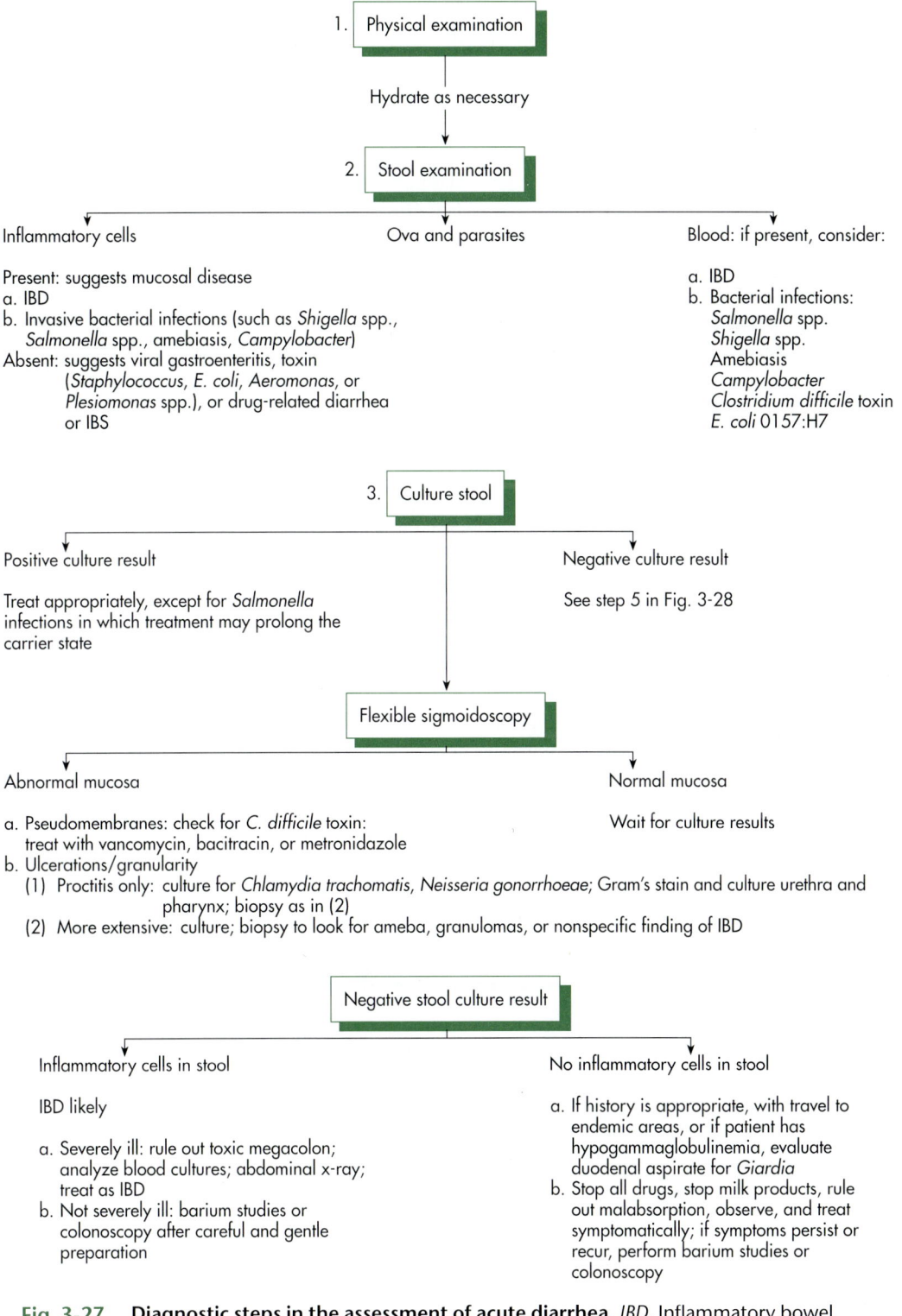

IBD likely

a. Severely ill: rule out toxic megacolon; analyze blood cultures; abdominal x-ray; treat as IBD
b. Not severely ill: barium studies or colonoscopy after careful and gentle preparation

No inflammatory cells in stool

a. If history is appropriate, with travel to endemic areas, or if patient has hypogammaglobulinemia, evaluate duodenal aspirate for *Giardia*
b. Stop all drugs, stop milk products, rule out malabsorption, observe, and treat symptomatically; if symptoms persist or recur, perform barium studies or colonoscopy

Fig. 3-27 Diagnostic steps in the assessment of acute diarrhea. *IBD*, Inflammatory bowel disease; *IBS*, irritable bowel syndrome. (From Stein JH [ed]: *Internal medicine,* ed 5, St Louis, 1998, Mosby.)

DIARRHEA, CHRONIC

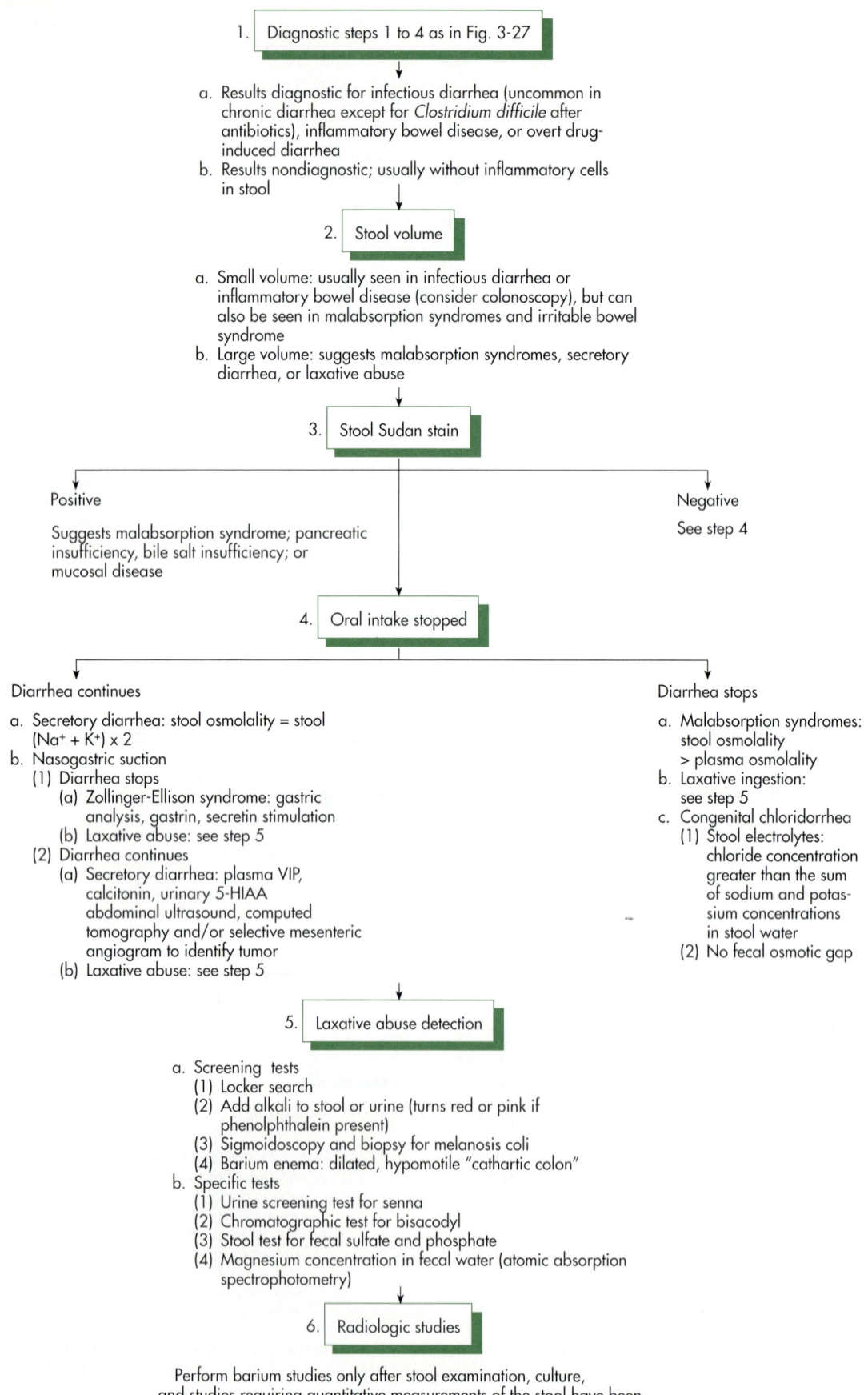

1. Diagnostic steps 1 to 4 as in Fig. 3-27
   a. Results diagnostic for infectious diarrhea (uncommon in chronic diarrhea except for *Clostridium difficile* after antibiotics), inflammatory bowel disease, or overt drug-induced diarrhea
   b. Results nondiagnostic; usually without inflammatory cells in stool

2. Stool volume
   a. Small volume: usually seen in infectious diarrhea or inflammatory bowel disease (consider colonoscopy), but can also be seen in malabsorption syndromes and irritable bowel syndrome
   b. Large volume: suggests malabsorption syndromes, secretory diarrhea, or laxative abuse

3. Stool Sudan stain

   Positive
   Suggests malabsorption syndrome; pancreatic insufficiency, bile salt insufficiency; or mucosal disease

   Negative
   See step 4

4. Oral intake stopped

   Diarrhea continues
   a. Secretory diarrhea: stool osmolality = stool $(Na^+ + K^+) \times 2$
   b. Nasogastric suction
      (1) Diarrhea stops
         (a) Zollinger-Ellison syndrome: gastric analysis, gastrin, secretin stimulation
         (b) Laxative abuse: see step 5
      (2) Diarrhea continues
         (a) Secretory diarrhea: plasma VIP, calcitonin, urinary 5-HIAA abdominal ultrasound, computed tomography and/or selective mesenteric angiogram to identify tumor
         (b) Laxative abuse: see step 5

   Diarrhea stops
   a. Malabsorption syndromes: stool osmolality > plasma osmolality
   b. Laxative ingestion: see step 5
   c. Congenital chloridorrhea
      (1) Stool electrolytes: chloride concentration greater than the sum of sodium and potassium concentrations in stool water
      (2) No fecal osmotic gap

5. Laxative abuse detection
   a. Screening tests
      (1) Locker search
      (2) Add alkali to stool or urine (turns red or pink if phenolphthalein present)
      (3) Sigmoidoscopy and biopsy for melanosis coli
      (4) Barium enema: dilated, hypomotile "cathartic colon"
   b. Specific tests
      (1) Urine screening test for senna
      (2) Chromatographic test for bisacodyl
      (3) Stool test for fecal sulfate and phosphate
      (4) Magnesium concentration in fecal water (atomic absorption spectrophotometry)

6. Radiologic studies

   Perform barium studies only after stool examination, culture, and studies requiring quantitative measurements of the stool have been completed.

Fig. 3-28 **Diagnostic approach to the patient with chronic diarrhea.** *VIP,* Vasoactive intestinal polypeptide; *5-HIAA,* 5-hydroxyindoleacetic acid. (From Stein JH [ed]: *Internal medicine,* ed 5, St Louis, 1998, Mosby.)

DIARRHEA, CHRONIC, IN PATIENTS WITH HIV INFECTION

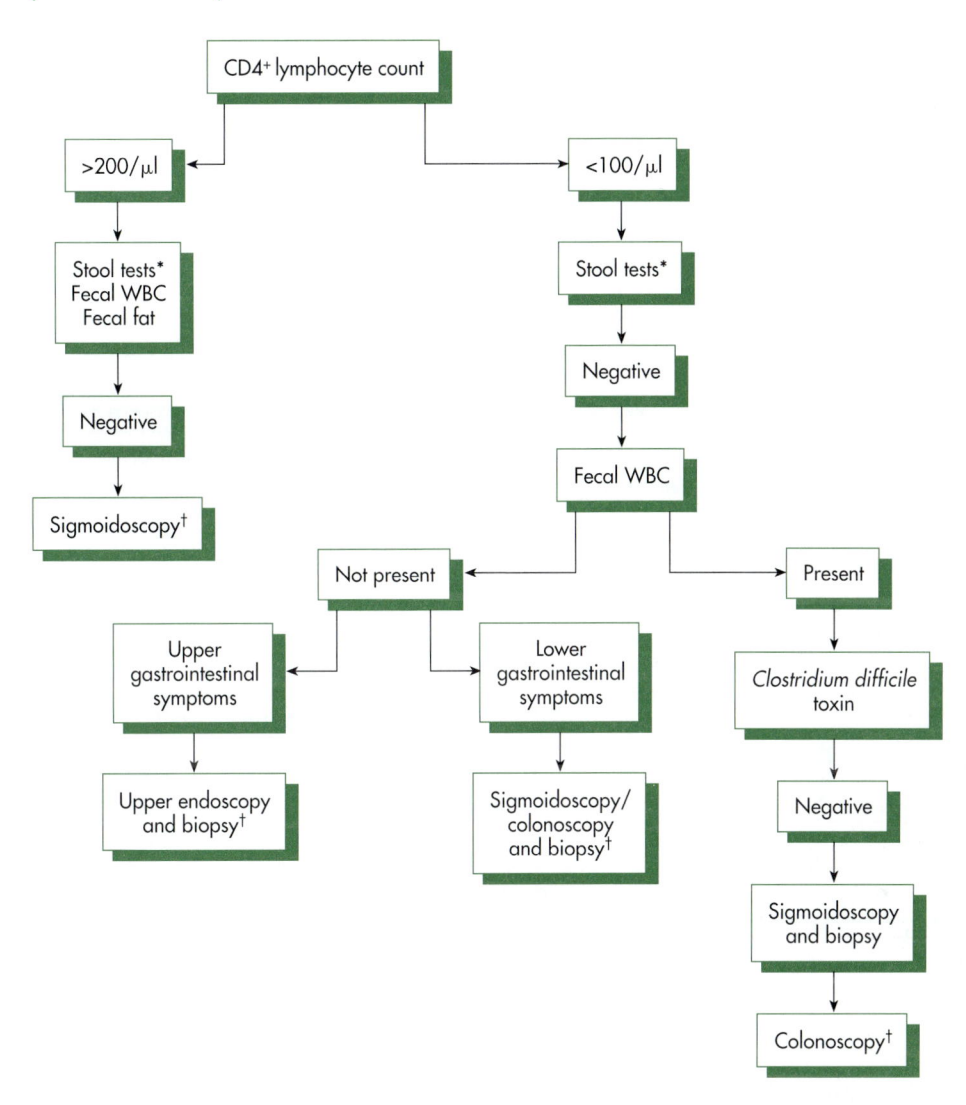

Fig. 3-29 Approach to evaluating chronic diarrhea in patients with HIV infection. (From Wilcox CM: Diarrhea: a difficult problem in patients infected with human immunodeficiency virus, Gastrointest Dis Today 5:9, 1996.)

TABLE 3-4 Common Gastrointestinal Pathogens Associated With HIV Infection

PATHOGEN	CD4+ CELLS/μL	STOOL VOLUME AND FREQUENCY	ABDOMINAL PAIN	WEIGHT LOSS	FEVER	FECAL LEUKOCYTES
Cytomegalovirus*	<100	Mild to moderate	++	++	++	+
Cryptosporidiosis	<100	Moderate to severe	−	++	−	−
Microsporidiosis	<100	Mild to moderate	−	+	−	−
Mycobacterium avium complex†	<100	Mild to moderate	+	+++	+++	−

From Wilcox CM: Diarrhea: a difficult problem in patients infected with human immunodeficiency virus, Gastrointest Dis Today 5:9, 1996.
+++, Very common; ++, frequent; +, can occur; −, absent.
*Can have proctitis symptoms when involving the distal colon.
†Typical presentation is fever and wasting; diarrhea is usually secondary.

EDEMA, GENERALIZED

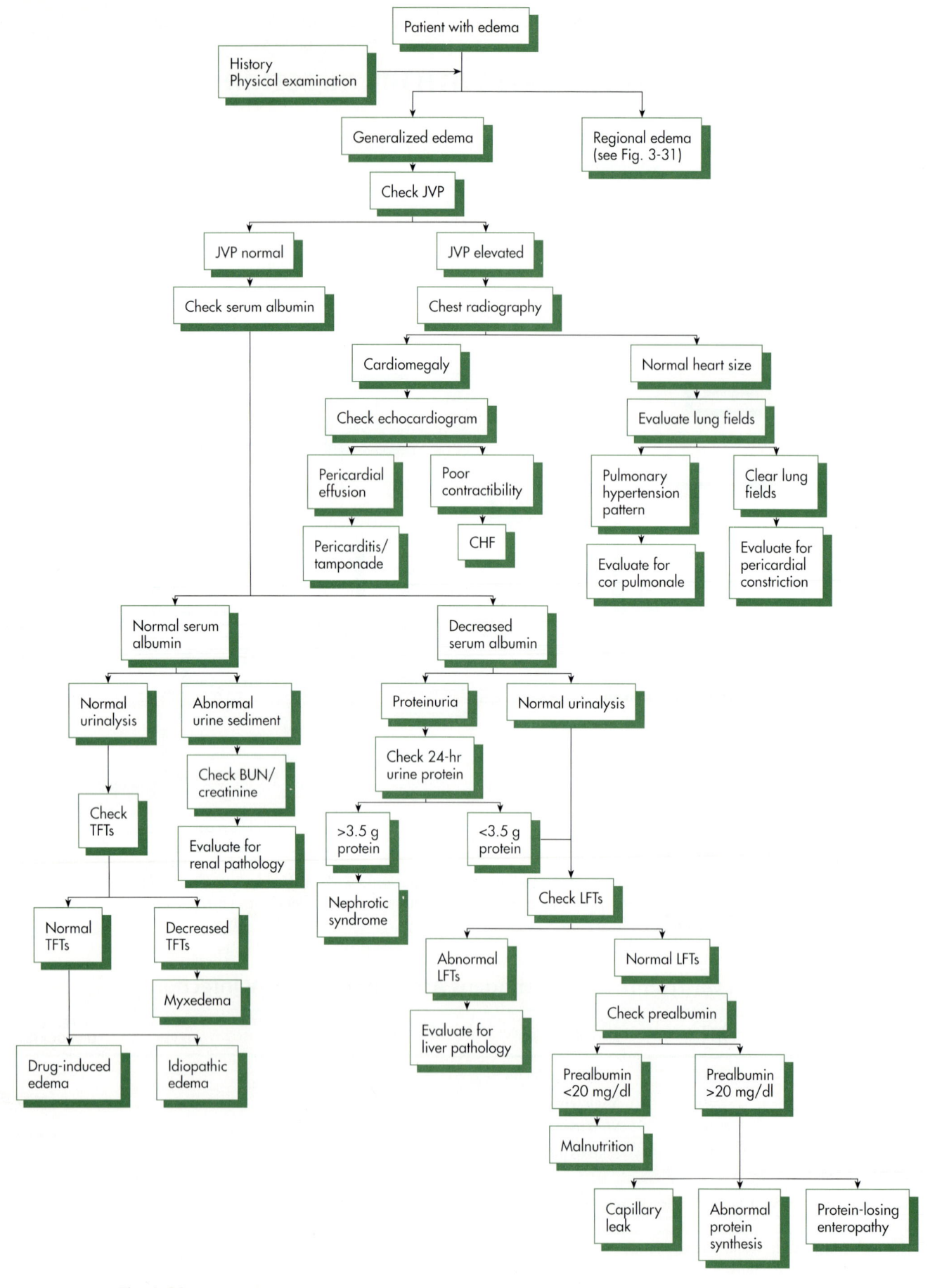

Fig. 3-30 Evaluation of generalized edema. *TFT,* Thyroid function tests; *LFT,* liver function tests; *JVP,* jugular venous pressure. (From Greene HL, Johnson WP, Maricic MJ: Decision making in medicine, St Louis, 1993, Mosby.)

CLINICAL ALGORITHMS

EDEMA, REGIONAL

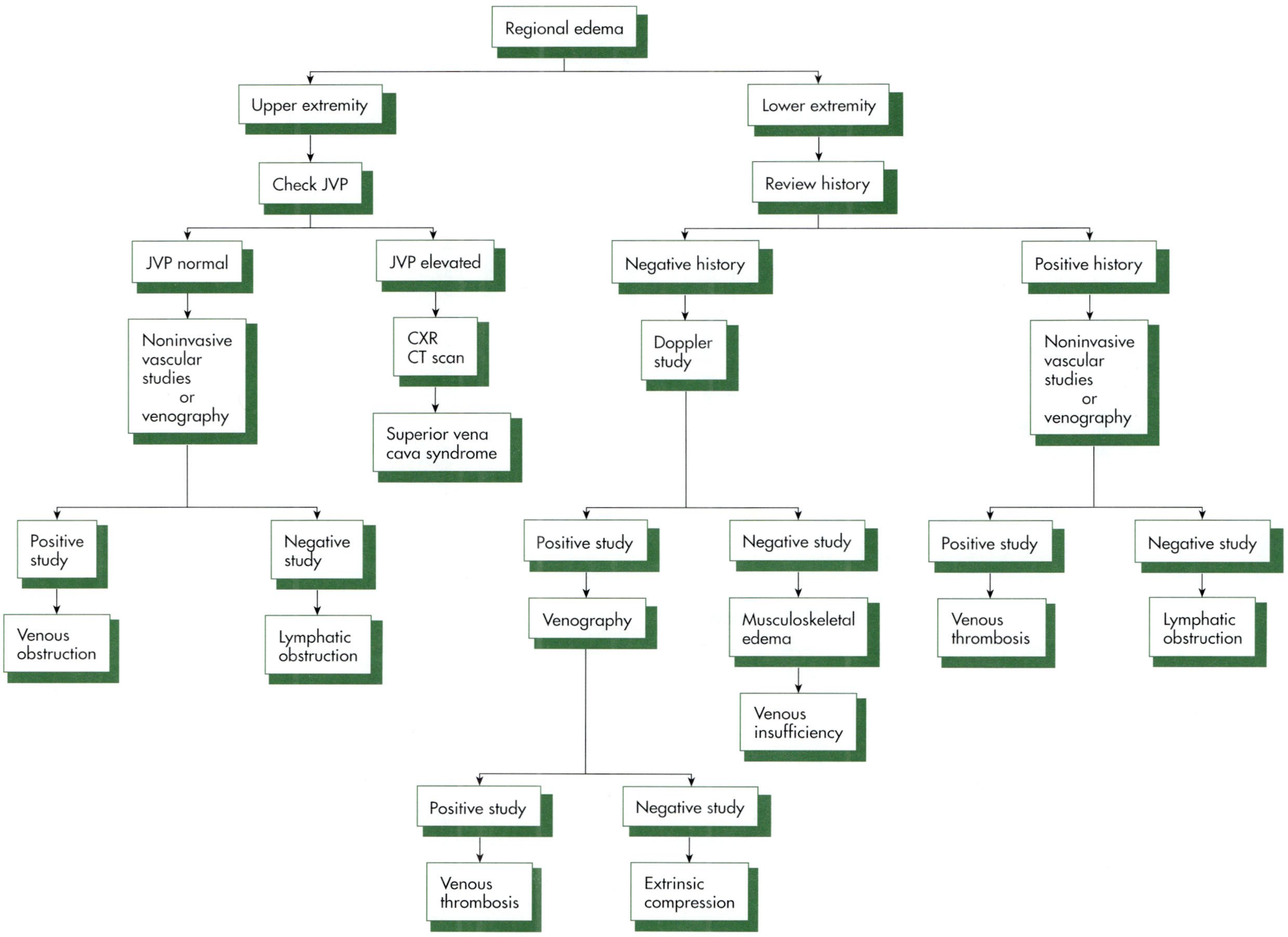

Fig. 3-31 Evaluation of regional edema. (From Greene HL, Johnson WP, Maricic MJ: *Decision making in medicine*, St Louis, 1993, Mosby.)

FECAL OCCULT BLOOD EVALUATION

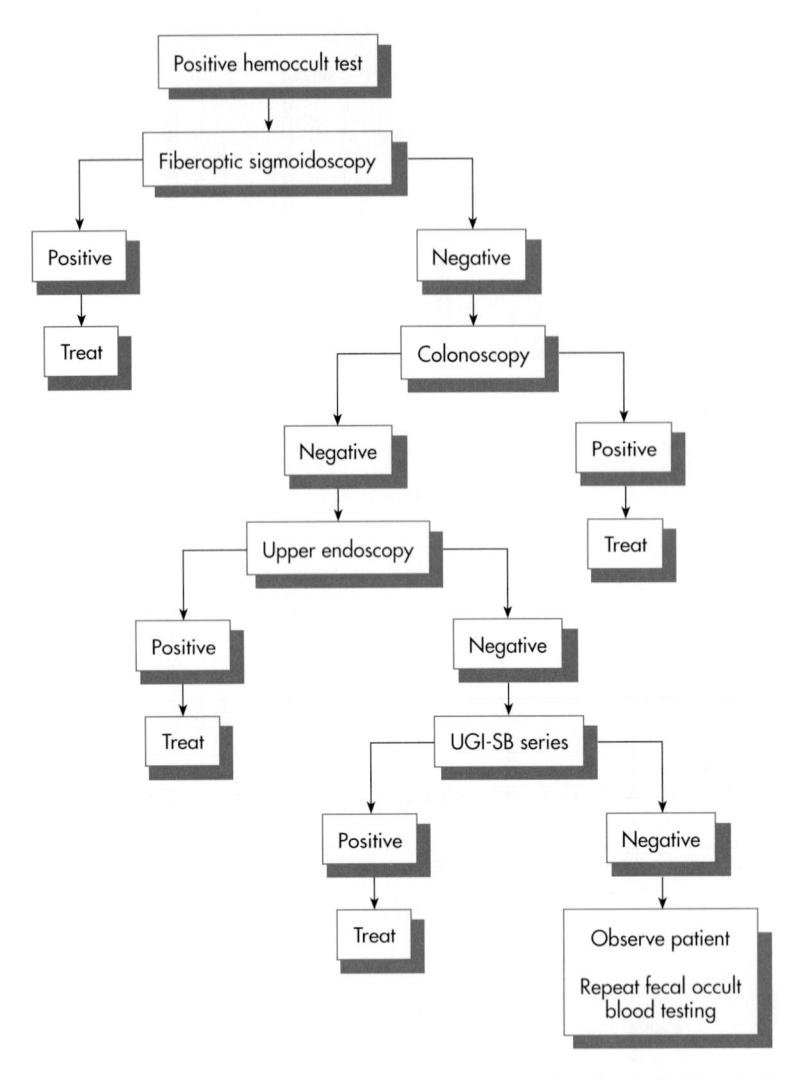

Fig. 3-32 Evaluation of asymptomatic patients with positive fecal occult blood. (From Ferri FF: *Practical guide to the care of the medical patient,* ed 3, St Louis, 1995, Mosby.)

GENITAL ULCER DISEASE

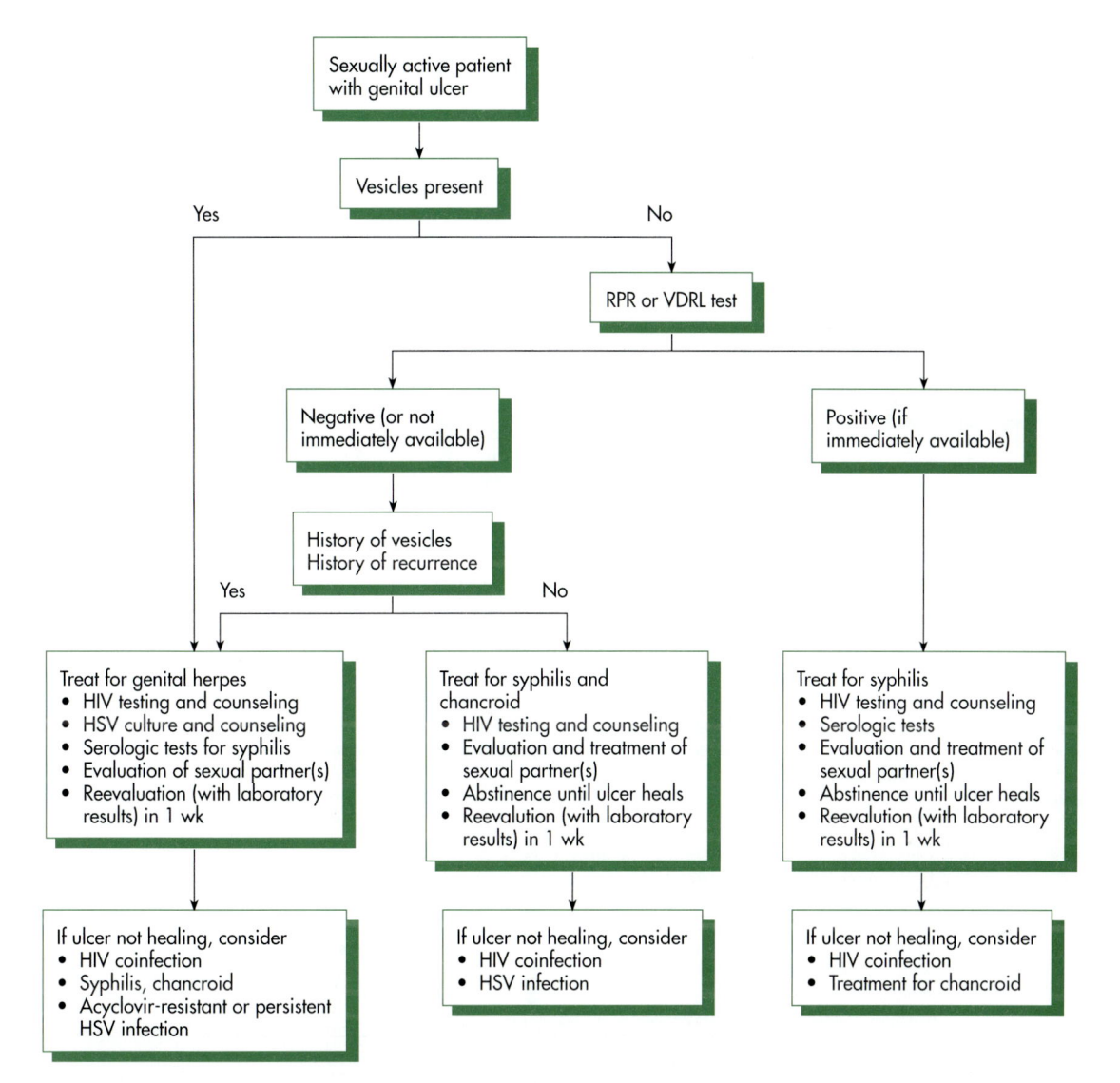

```
                    Sexually active patient
                    with genital ulcer
                              │
                              ▼
                       Vesicles present
         Yes ─────────────────┴───────────────── No
          │                                       │
          │                                       ▼
          │                                RPR or VDRL test
          │                          ┌────────────┴────────────┐
          │                          ▼                         ▼
          │                  Negative (or not          Positive (if
          │                  immediately available)    immediately available)
          │                          │                         │
          │                          ▼                         │
          │                  History of vesicles               │
          │                  History of recurrence             │
          │              Yes ─────┴───── No                    │
          │               │             │                      │
          ▼               ▼             ▼                      ▼
```

Treat for genital herpes
- HIV testing and counseling
- HSV culture and counseling
- Serologic tests for syphilis
- Evaluation of sexual partner(s)
- Reevaluation (with laboratory results) in 1 wk

Treat for syphilis and chancroid
- HIV testing and counseling
- Evaluation and treatment of sexual partner(s)
- Abstinence until ulcer heals
- Reevaluation (with laboratory results) in 1 wk

Treat for syphilis
- HIV testing and counseling
- Serologic tests
- Evaluation and treatment of sexual partner(s)
- Abstinence until ulcer heals
- Reevaluation (with laboratory results) in 1 wk

If ulcer not healing, consider
- HIV coinfection
- Syphilis, chancroid
- Acyclovir-resistant or persistent HSV infection

If ulcer not healing, consider
- HIV coinfection
- HSV infection

If ulcer not healing, consider
- HIV coinfection
- Treatment for chancroid

Fig. 3-33 Initial management of genital ulcer disease. *HSV,* Herpes simplex virus; *RPR,* rapid plasma reagin. (From Hoffman IF, Schmitz JL: Genital ulcer disease, management in the HIV era, *Postgrad Med* 98(3):70, 1995.)

GLOMERULAR DISEASE

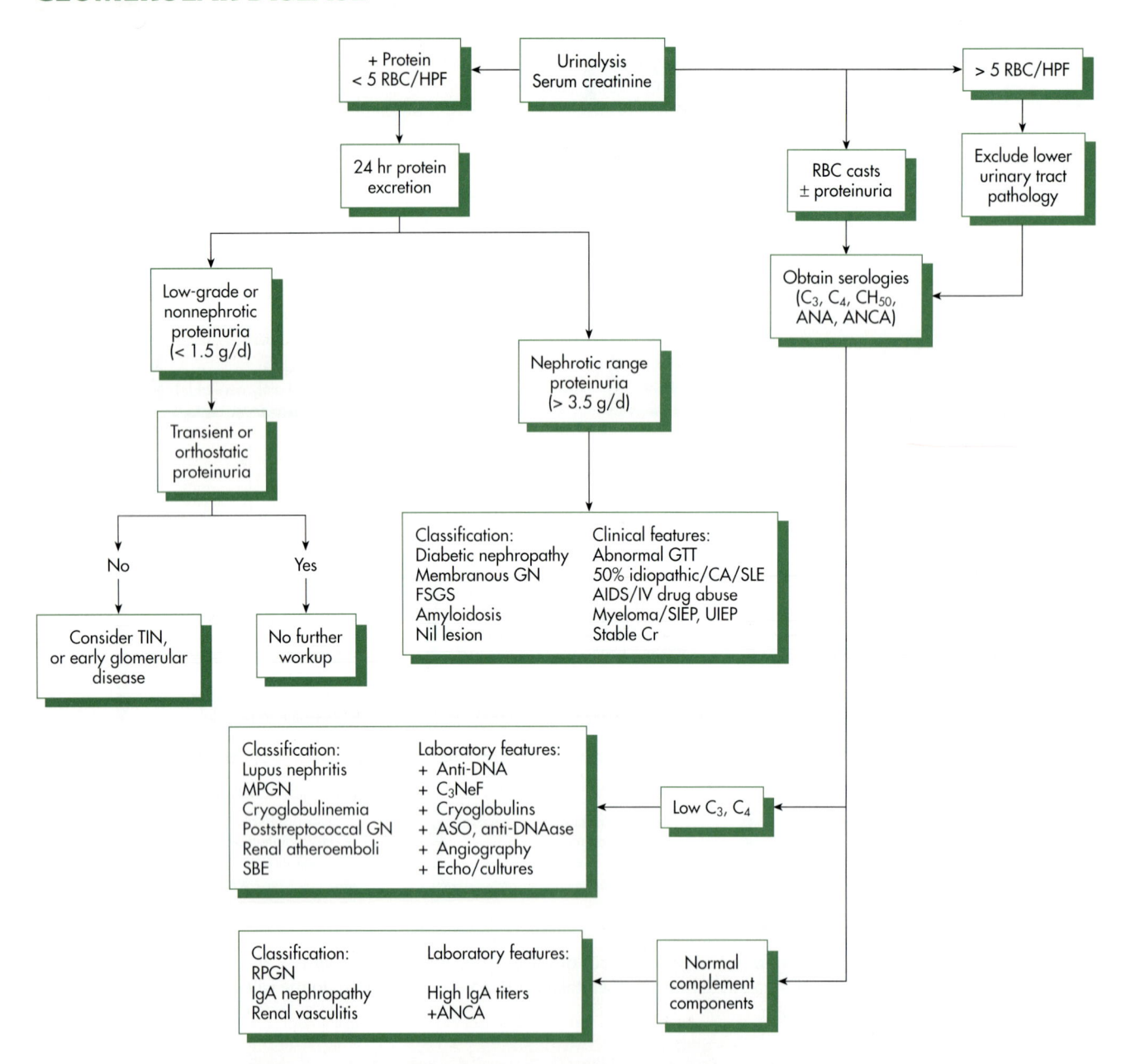

Fig. 3-34 Approach to the differential diagnosis of suspected glomerular disease. *RBC,* Red blood cells; *ANA,* antinuclear antibodies; *ANCA,* antineutrophil cytoplasmic antibodies; *GTT,* glucose tolerance test; *CA,* cancer; *SLE,* systemic lupus erythematosus; *SIEP* and *UIEP,* serum and urine immunoelectrophoresis; *C3NeF,* C3 nephritic factor; *ASO,* antistreptolysin O antibody. A renal biopsy is frequently required to establish the clinical diagnosis. (From Noble J [ed]: *Primary care medicine,* ed 2, St Louis, 1996, Mosby.)

HEAD INJURY

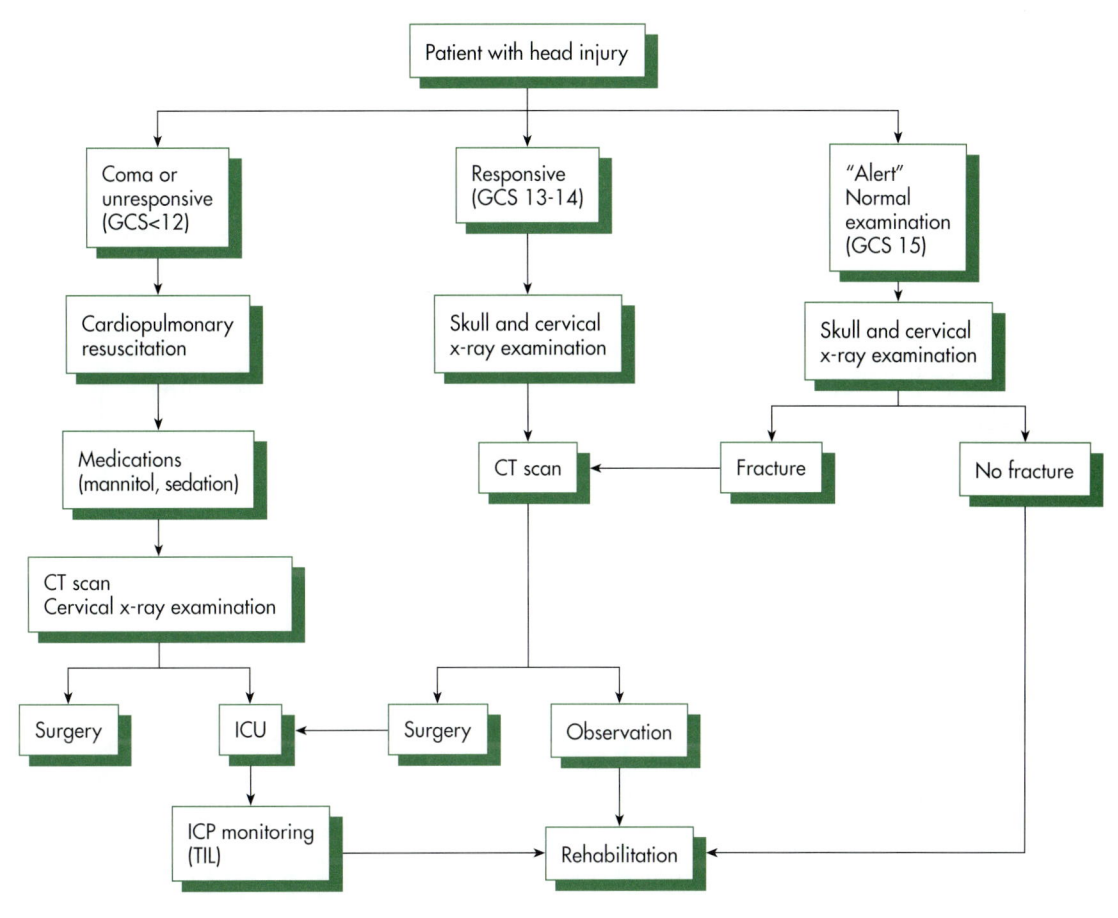

Fig. 3-35 **Management of head injury.** *GCS,* Glasgow coma score; *CT,* computed tomography; *ICU,* intensive care unit; *ICP,* intracranial pressure; *TIL,* therapeutic intensity level. (From Johnson RT, Griffin JW: *Current therapy in neurologic disease,* ed 5, St Louis, 1997, Mosby.)

TABLE 3-5 Glasgow Coma Scale*

EYE OPENING	BEST MOTOR RESPONSE	BEST VERBAL RESPONSE	SCORE
No response	None	None	1
Opens with painful stimulus	Extension (decerebrate rigidity) with painful stimulus	Unintelligible sounds	2
Opens with verbal command	Flexion (decorticate rigidity) with painful stimulus	Use of inappropriate words	3
Opens spontaneously	Withdrawal from noxious stimulus	Confused, disoriented conversation	4
	Localization of pain, pushes away noxious stimulus	Oriented, able to converse	5
	Obeys simple verbal commands	Alert and oriented	6

*Total score is determined by adding the best score from each category (eye opening, best motor response, best verbal response). For example, a patient may:
Open eyes with verbal command   3
Obey simple verbal commands   6
Use inappropriate words   3
TOTAL SCORE   12

716 Hearing loss

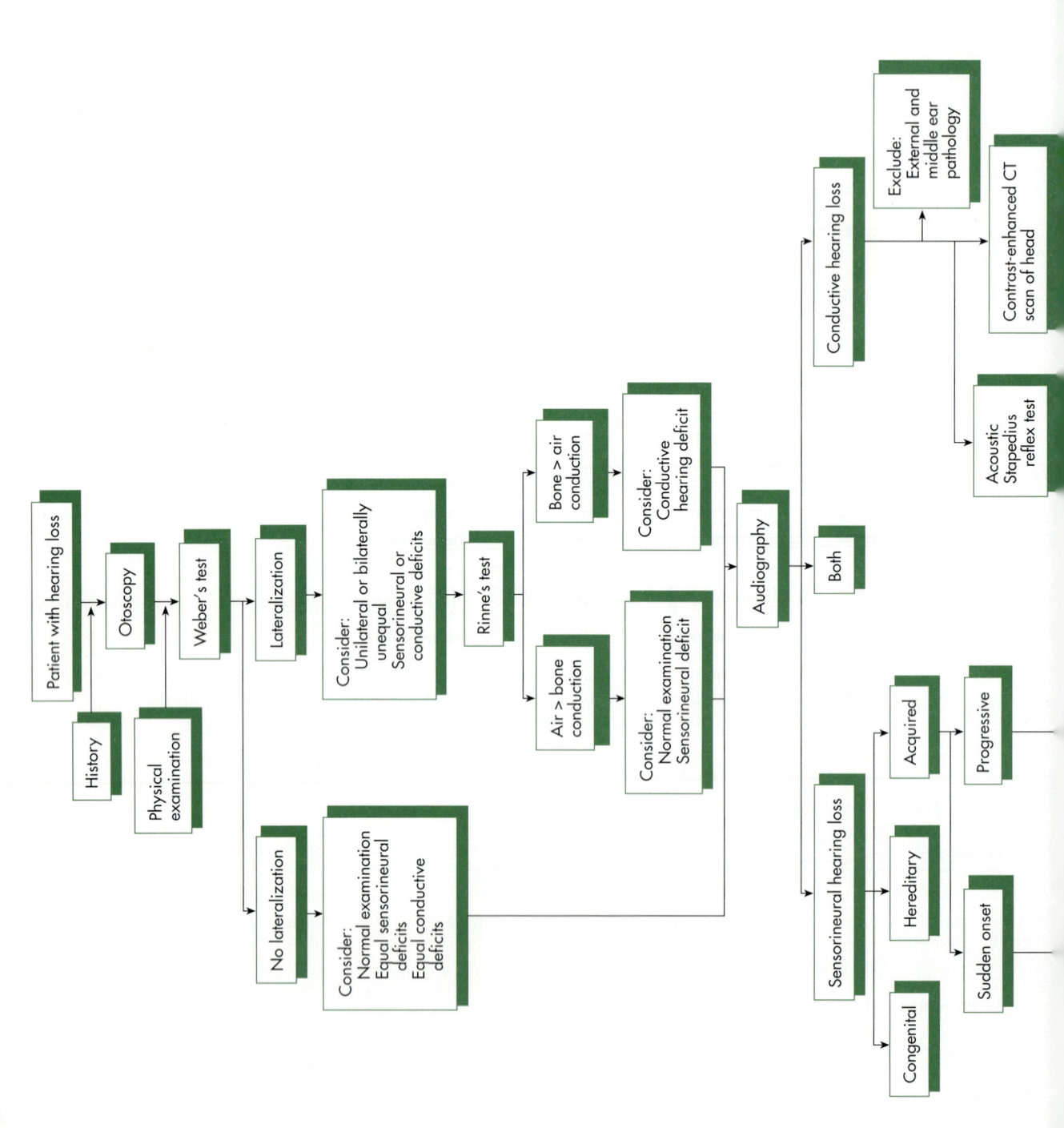

CLINICAL ALGORITHMS

HEARING LOSS

```
Patient with hearing loss
    ↑
  History
  Physical examination
    ↓
  Otoscopy
    ↓
  Weber's test
    ↓
  ┌─ Lateralization ─→ Consider: Unilateral or bilaterally unequal Sensorineural or conductive deficits
  │                         ↓
  │                    Rinne's test
  │                    ┌─ Bone > air conduction ─→ Consider: Conductive hearing deficit
  │                    └─ Air > bone conduction ─→ Consider: Normal examination Sensorineural deficit
  │                                                    ↓
  │                                               Audiography
  │                                               ┌─ Conductive hearing loss ─→ Exclude: External and middle ear pathology ─→ Contrast-enhanced CT scan of head
  │                                               │                                                                       ─→ Acoustic Stapedius reflex test
  │                                               ├─ Both
  │                                               └─ Sensorineural hearing loss
  │                                                       ├─ Acquired ─→ Progressive
  │                                                       │           ─→ Sudden onset
  │                                                       ├─ Hereditary
  │                                                       └─ Congenital
  └─ No lateralization ─→ Consider: Normal examination Equal sensorineural deficits Equal conductive deficits
```

CLINICAL ALGORITHMS

Hearing loss 717

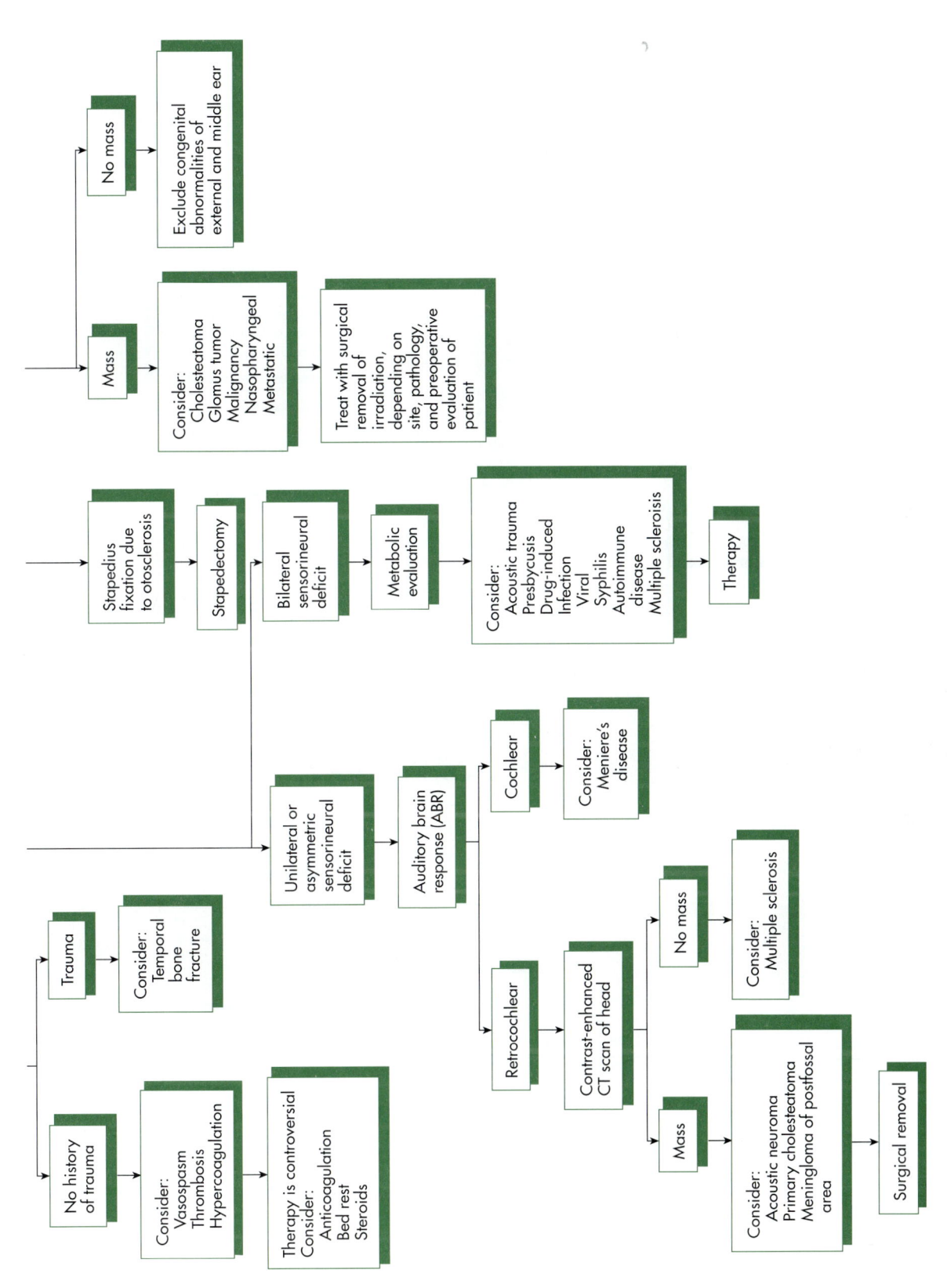

Fig. 3-36 Evaluation of hearing loss. (From Greene HL, Johnson WP, Maricic MJ: *Decision making in medicine*, St Louis, 1993, Mosby.)

HEARTBURN

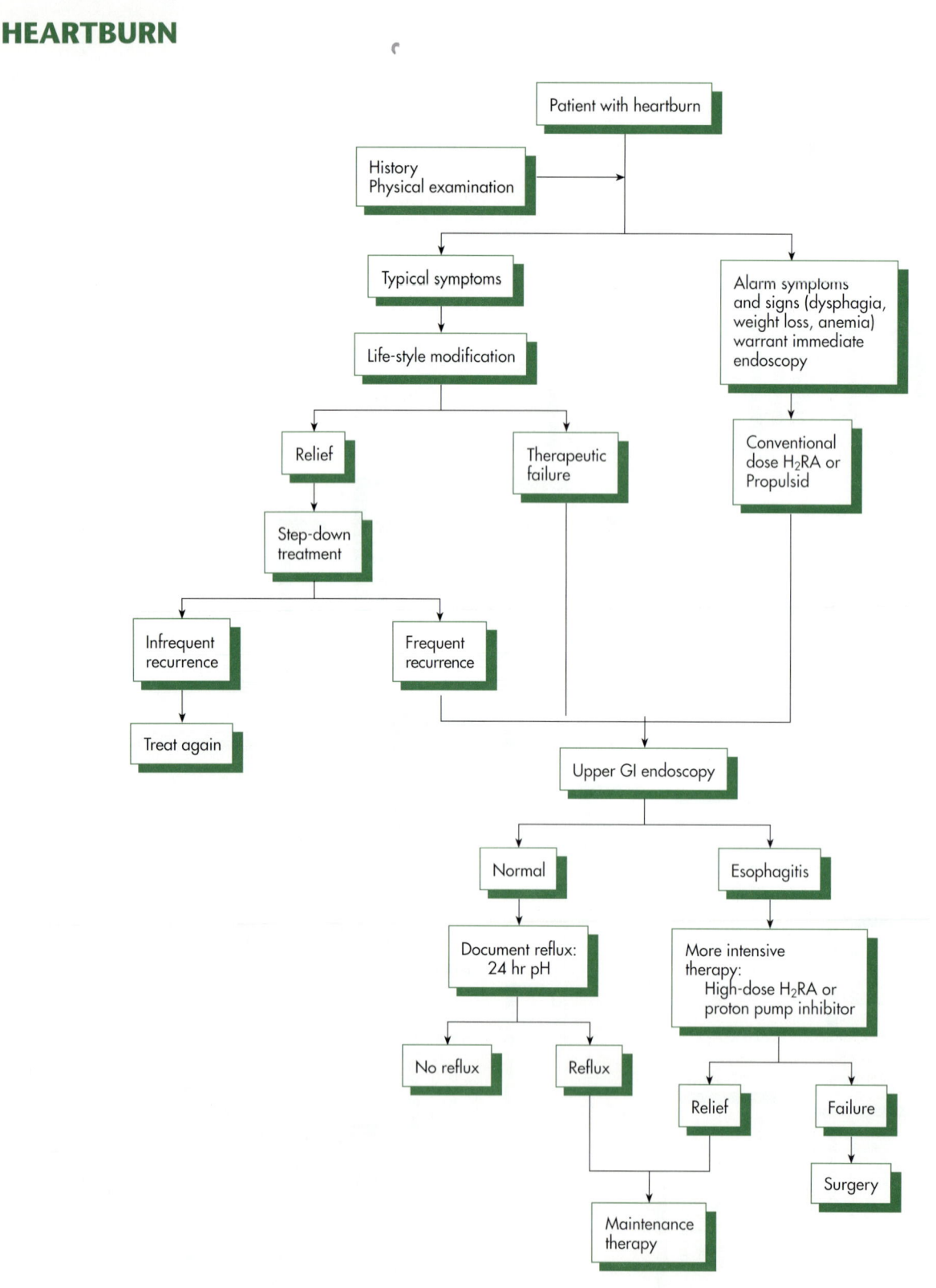

```
Patient with heartburn
    │
    ▼
History
Physical examination
    │
    ├─────────────────────────────────┐
    ▼                                 ▼
Typical symptoms              Alarm symptoms
    │                         and signs (dysphagia,
    ▼                         weight loss, anemia)
Life-style modification       warrant immediate
    │                         endoscopy
    ├──────────┐                      │
    ▼          ▼                      ▼
Relief    Therapeutic            Conventional
    │     failure                dose H₂RA or
    ▼        │                   Propulsid
Step-down    │                      │
treatment    │                      │
    │        │                      │
    ├────────┼──────────┐           │
    ▼        │          ▼           │
Infrequent   │      Frequent        │
recurrence   │      recurrence      │
    │        │          │           │
    ▼        │          │           │
Treat again  │          │           │
             └──────────┴───────────┤
                                    ▼
                            Upper GI endoscopy
                                    │
                         ┌──────────┴──────────┐
                         ▼                     ▼
                      Normal               Esophagitis
                         │                     │
                         ▼                     ▼
                  Document reflux:       More intensive
                     24 hr pH            therapy:
                         │               High-dose H₂RA or
                   ┌─────┴─────┐         proton pump inhibitor
                   ▼           ▼              │
                No reflux   Reflux      ┌─────┴─────┐
                               │        ▼           ▼
                               │      Relief      Failure
                               │        │           │
                               │        │           ▼
                               └────────┤        Surgery
                                        ▼
                                  Maintenance
                                   therapy
```

Fig. 3-37 **Treatment of a patient with heartburn.** (Adapted from Sampliner RE: Heartburn. In Greene HL, Johnson WP, Maricic MJ (eds): *Decision making in medicine*, St Louis, 1993, Mosby.)

HEMATURIA

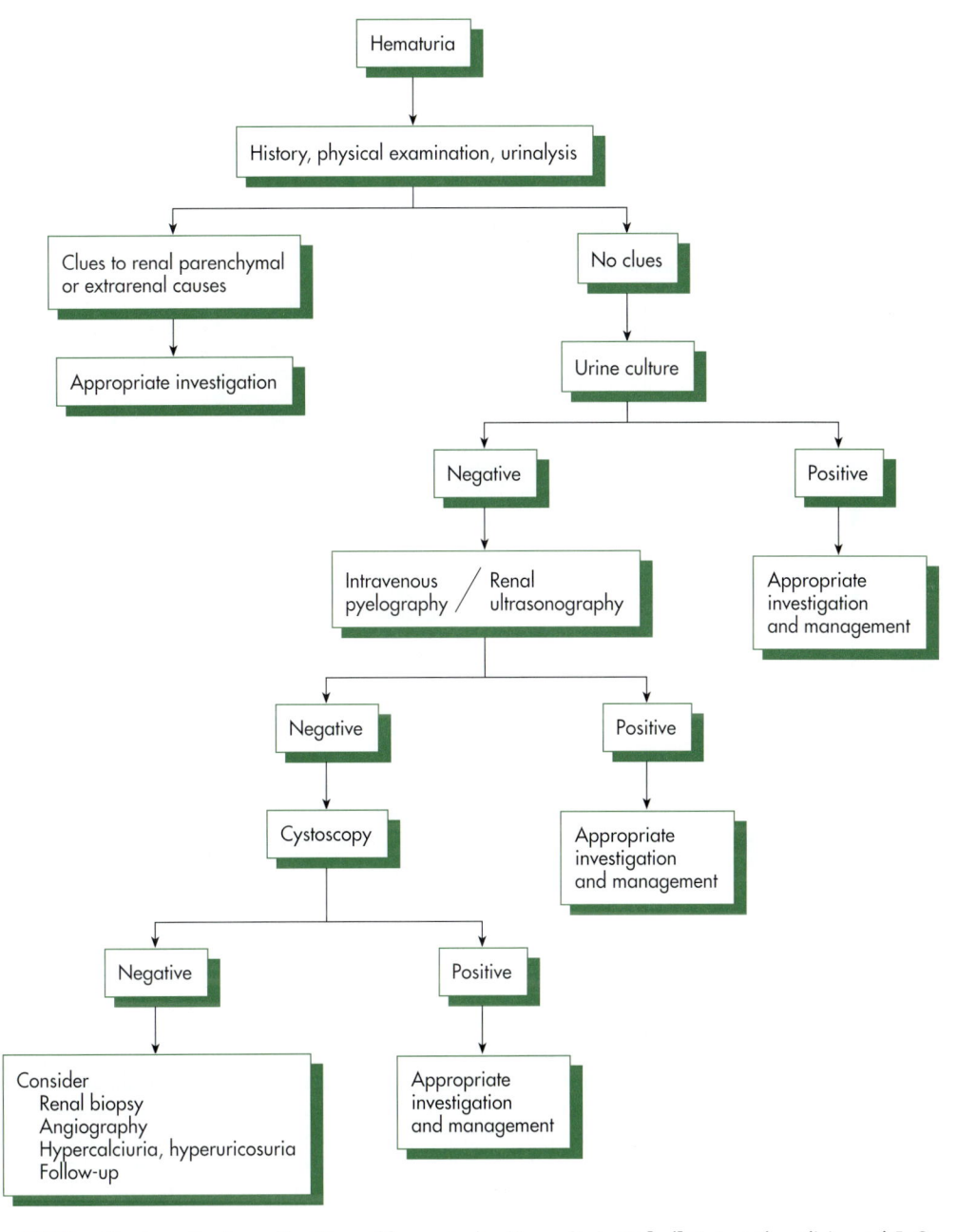

Fig. 3-38 Strategy for investigation of hematuria. (From Stein JH [ed]: *Internal medicine,* ed 5, St Louis, 1998, Mosby.)

HERPETIC AND POSTHERPETIC NEURALGIA

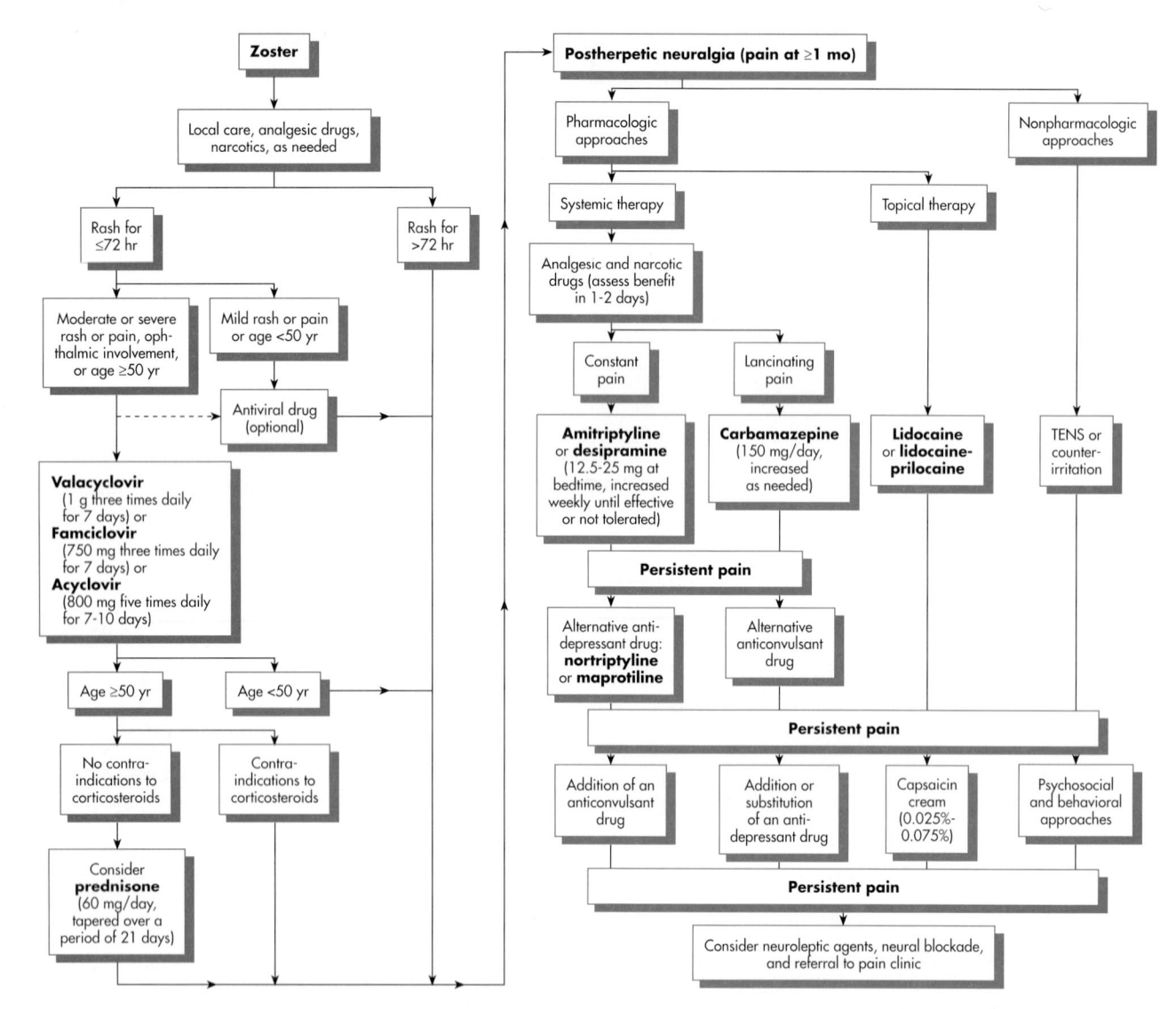

Fig. 3-39 Approaches to the treatment and prevention of acute zoster-associated pain and postherpetic neuralgia. Medications shown in bold have been demonstrated to be effective on the basis of fairly convincing data from controlled trials. The decision to use antiviral drugs in patients with zoster must be individualized, but the prompt use of antiviral therapy in older patients or those with ophthalmic involvement is recommended. Younger patients with mild eruptions and little pain do not require antiviral therapy. Corticosteroids should be considered in older patients if there are no contraindications (e.g., diabetes mellitus, hypertension, or glaucoma). Patients with neuropathic pain within 1 month after the onset of zoster may be treated early, on an empirical basis. The therapeutic approaches for established postherpetic neuralgia are more numerous than those for acute zoster-associated pain, but their value is less well documented. Primary approaches include a topical anesthetic drug and trials of analgesic and narcotic drugs, with the addition of an antidepressant drug if the former prove ineffective, inadequate, or poorly tolerated. *TENS,* Transcutaneous electrical nerve stimulation. (From Kost RG, Straus SE: Postherpetic neuralgia—pathogenesis, treatment, and prevention, *N Engl J Med* 335:32-42, 1996.)

HIRSUTISM

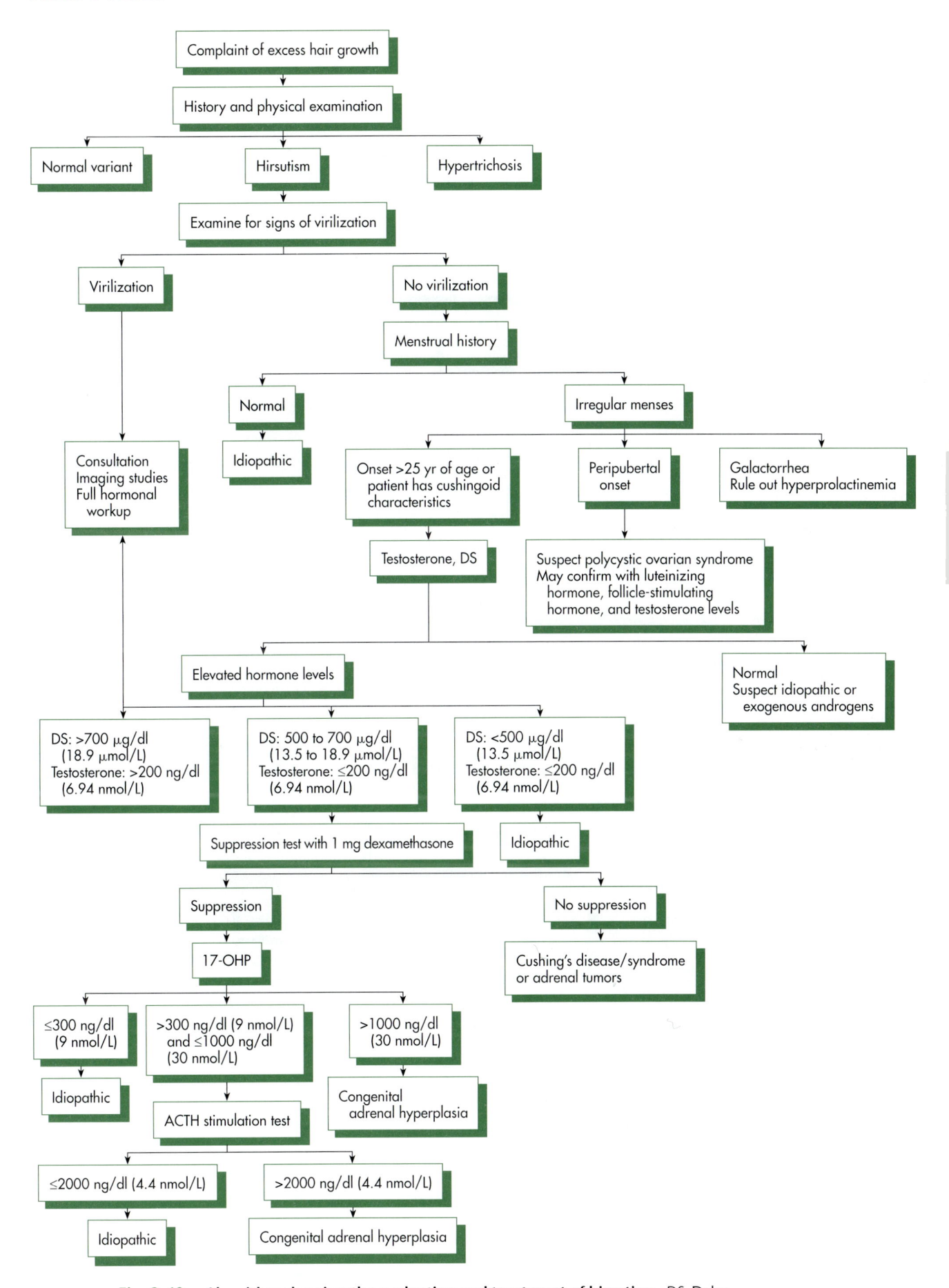

Fig. 3-40 Algorithm showing the evaluation and treatment of hirsutism. *DS*, Dehydroepiandrosterone; *17-OHP*, 17-hydroxyprogesterone; *ACTH*, adrenocorticotropic hormone. (From Gilchrist VJ, Hecht BR: A practical approach to hirsutism, *Am Fam Physician* 52:1837-1846, 1995.)

HYPERCALCEMIA

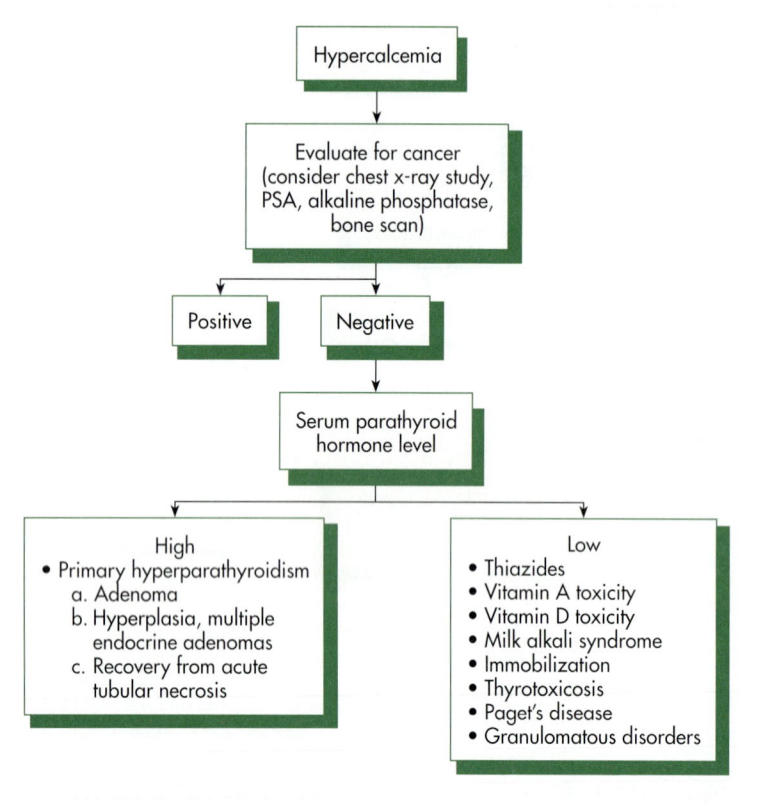

Fig. 3-41 Evaluation of hypercalcemia. (From Wachtel TJ, Stein MD: *Practical guide to the care of the ambulatory patient,* St Louis, 1995, Mosby.)

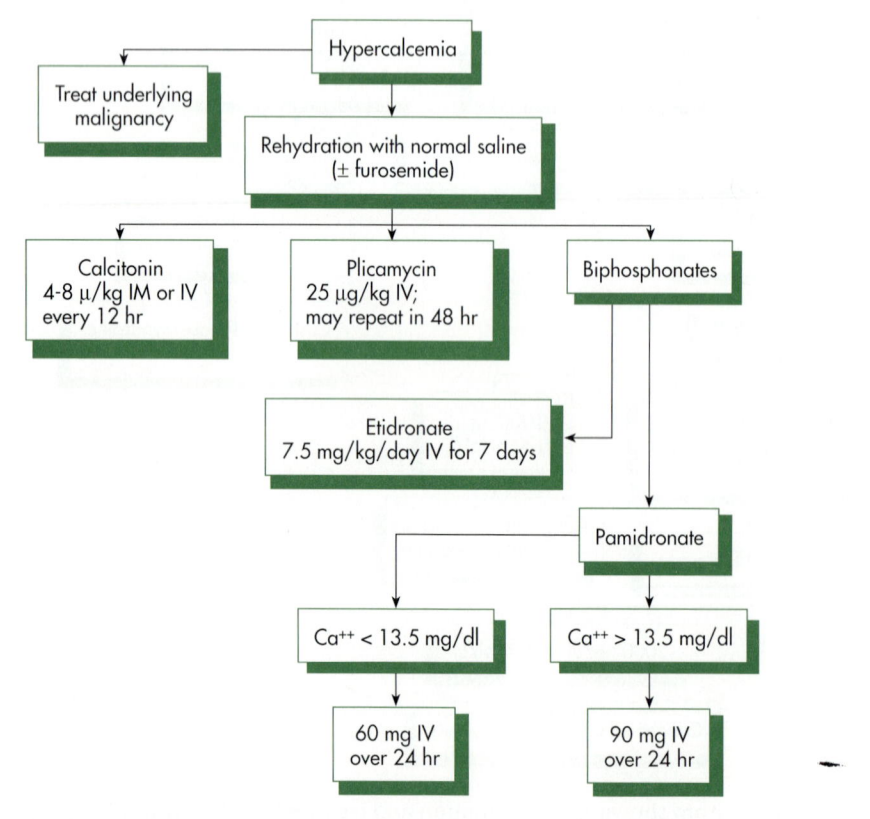

Fig. 3-42 Therapy for hypercalcemia. (From Noble J [ed]: *Primary care medicine,* ed 2, St Louis, 1996, Mosby.)

CLINICAL ALGORITHMS Hypernatremia 723

HYPERNATREMIA

Hypernatremia

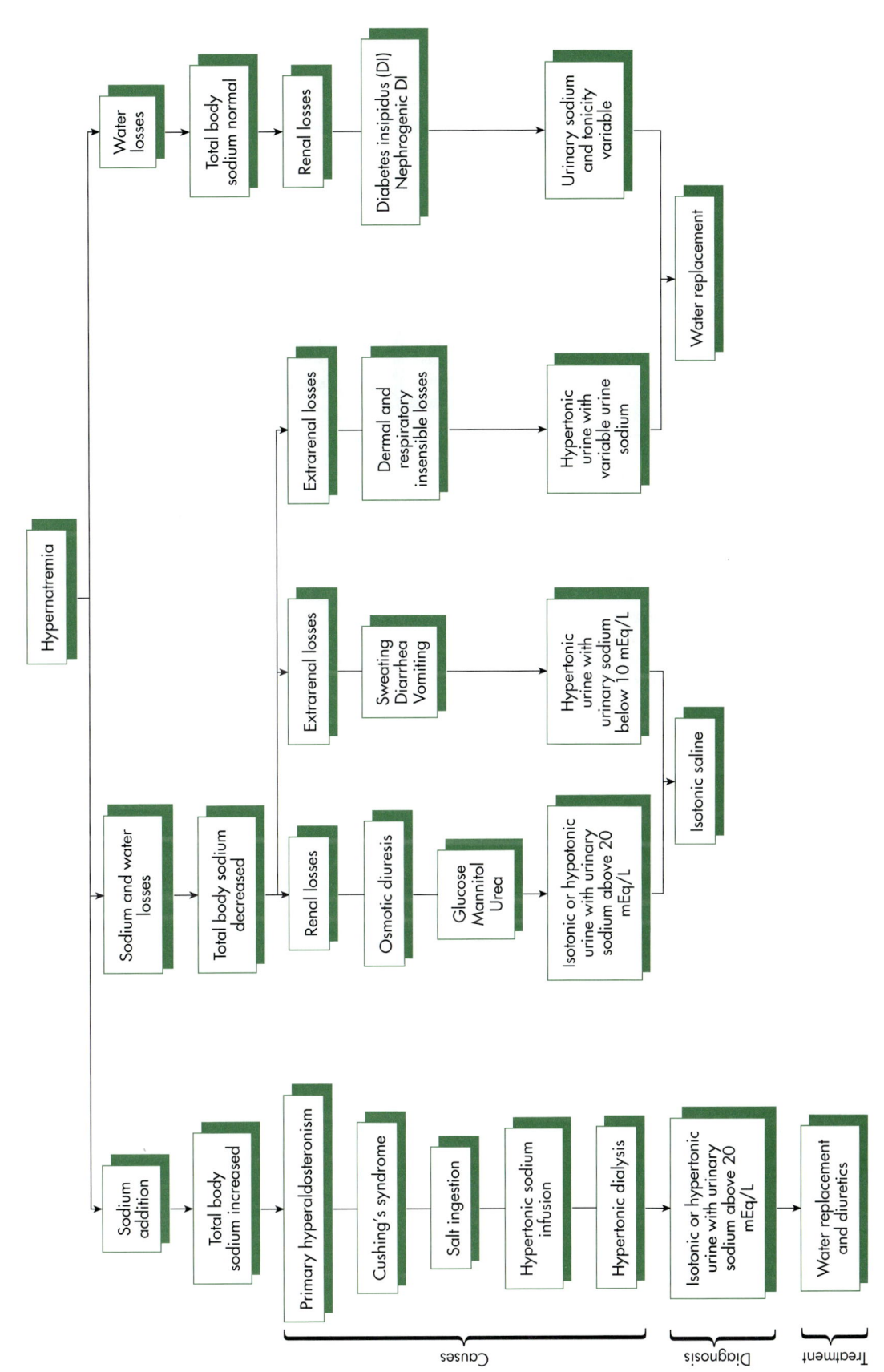

Sodium addition
Total body sodium increased
Causes:
- Primary hyperaldosteronism
- Cushing's syndrome
- Salt ingestion
- Hypertonic sodium infusion
- Hypertonic dialysis

Diagnosis: Isotonic or hypertonic urine with urinary sodium above 20 mEq/L

Treatment: Water replacement and diuretics

Sodium and water losses
Total body sodium decreased

- **Renal losses** → Osmotic diuresis (Glucose, Mannitol, Urea) → Isotonic or hypotonic urine with urinary sodium above 20 mEq/L → Isotonic saline
- **Extrarenal losses** → Sweating, Diarrhea, Vomiting → Hypertonic urine with urinary sodium below 10 mEq/L → Isotonic saline

Water losses
Total body sodium normal

- **Extrarenal losses** → Dermal and respiratory insensible losses → Hypertonic urine with variable urine sodium → Water replacement
- **Renal losses** → Diabetes insipidus (DI), Nephrogenic DI → Urinary sodium and tonicity variable → Water replacement

Fig. 3-43 Evaluation and treatment of hypernatremia. (From Rosen P et al [eds]: Emergency medicine: concepts and clinical practice, St Louis, 1992, Mosby.)

HYPOCALCEMIA

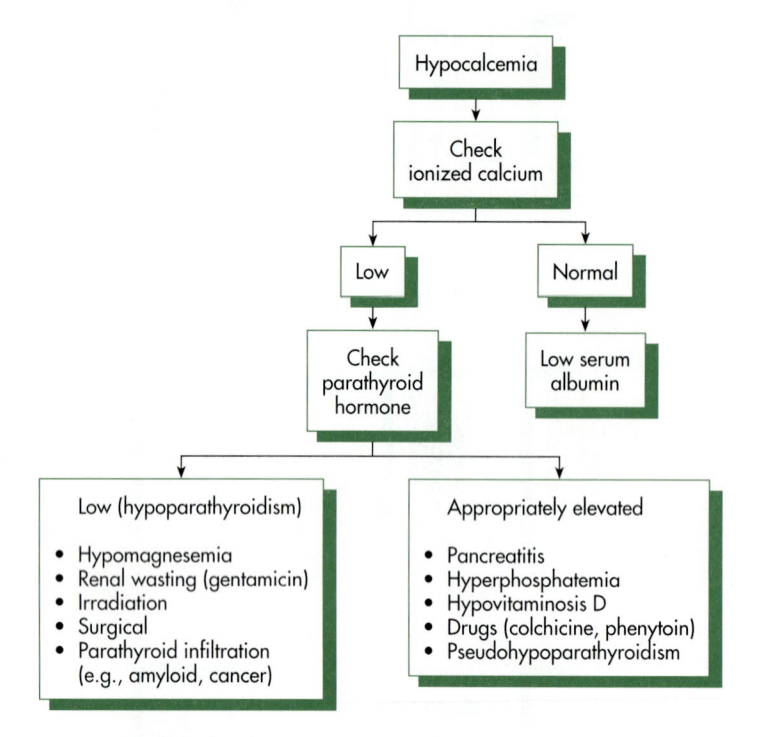

```
                    Hypocalcemia
                         │
                         ▼
                      Check
                  ionized calcium
                    ┌────┴────┐
                    ▼         ▼
                   Low      Normal
                    │         │
                    ▼         ▼
                 Check     Low serum
               parathyroid  albumin
                hormone
              ┌────┴────┐
              ▼         ▼
```

Low (hypoparathyroidism)	Appropriately elevated
• Hypomagnesemia • Renal wasting (gentamicin) • Irradiation • Surgical • Parathyroid infiltration (e.g., amyloid, cancer)	• Pancreatitis • Hyperphosphatemia • Hypovitaminosis D • Drugs (colchicine, phenytoin) • Pseudohypoparathyroidism

Fig. 3-44 **Evaluation of hypocalcemia.** (From Wachtel TJ, Stein MD: *Practical guide to the care of the ambulatory patient,* St Louis, 1995, Mosby.)

HYPOGLYCEMIA, FASTING

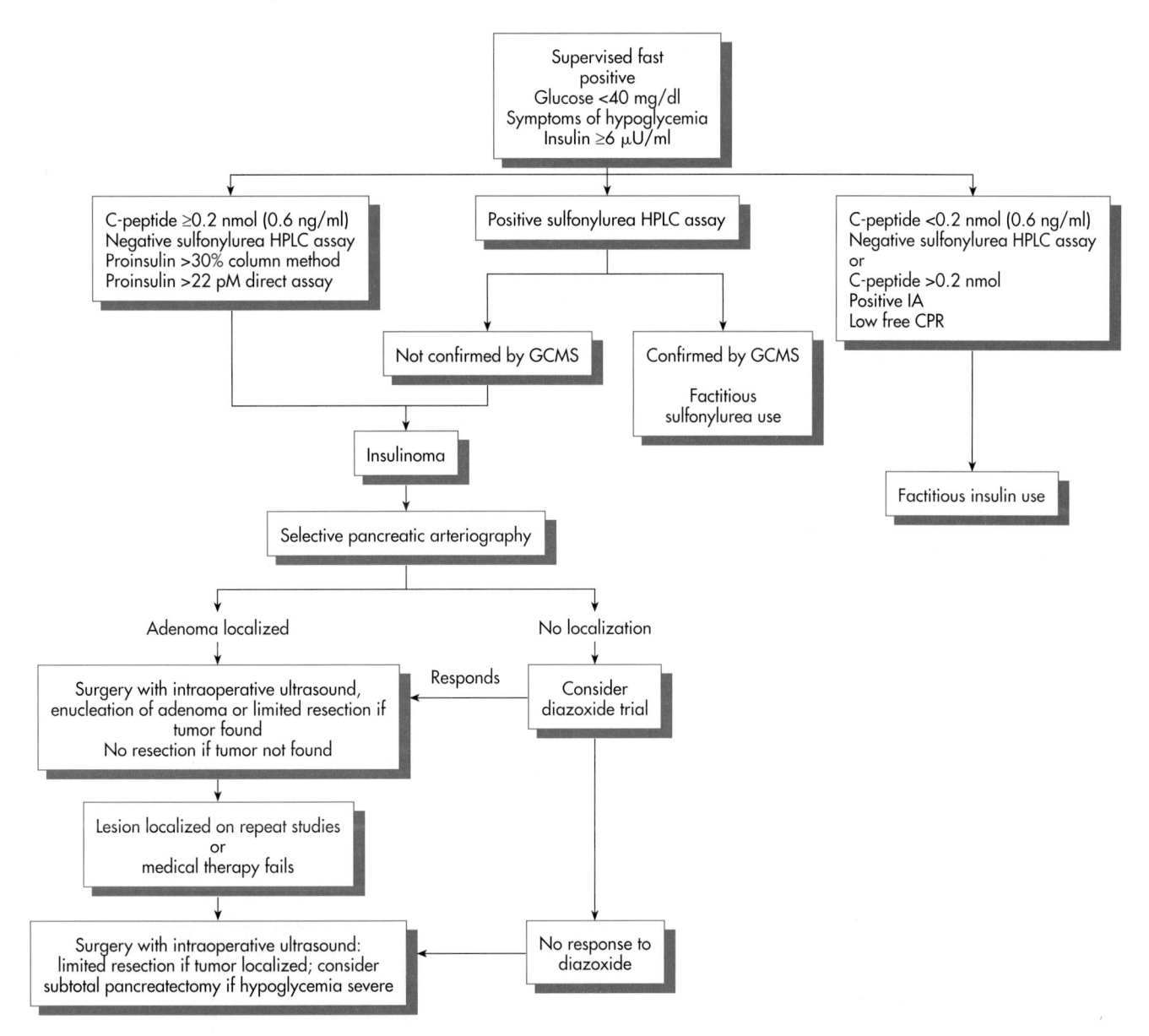

Fig. 3-45 Diagnostic evaluation of patients with documented hypoglycemia and elevated insulin. *CPR*, C-peptide immunoreactivity; *GCMS*, gas chromatography mass spectrometry; *HPLC*, high-pressure liquid chromatography; *IA*, insulin antibodies. (From Moore WT, Eastman RC: *Diagnostic endocrinology*, ed 2, St Louis, 1996, Mosby.)

HYPOKALEMIA

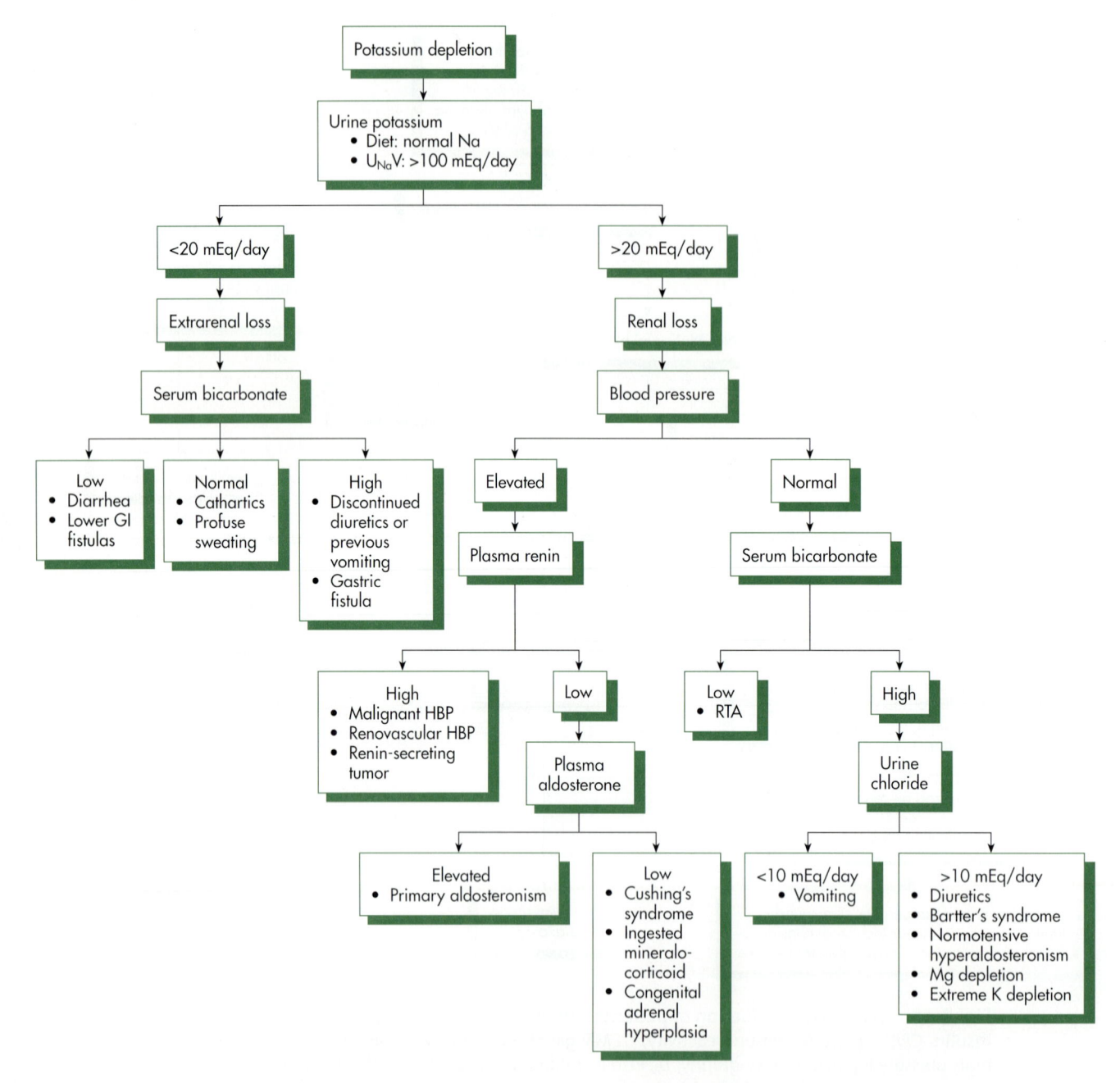

```
                    Potassium depletion
                            │
                    Urine potassium
                    • Diet: normal Na
                    • U_NaV: >100 mEq/day
                    ┌───────┴───────┐
              <20 mEq/day      >20 mEq/day
                    │                │
              Extrarenal loss   Renal loss
                    │                │
              Serum bicarbonate  Blood pressure
          ┌─────┬───┴──┐         ┌──┴──┐
        Low  Normal  High    Elevated  Normal
```

- **<20 mEq/day → Extrarenal loss → Serum bicarbonate**
  - **Low**: Diarrhea; Lower GI fistulas
  - **Normal**: Cathartics; Profuse sweating
  - **High**: Discontinued diuretics or previous vomiting; Gastric fistula

- **>20 mEq/day → Renal loss → Blood pressure**
  - **Elevated → Plasma renin**
    - **High**: Malignant HBP; Renovascular HBP; Renin-secreting tumor
    - **Low → Plasma aldosterone**
      - **Elevated**: Primary aldosteronism
      - **Low**: Cushing's syndrome; Ingested mineralocorticoid; Congenital adrenal hyperplasia
  - **Normal → Serum bicarbonate**
    - **Low**: RTA
    - **High → Urine chloride**
      - **<10 mEq/day**: Vomiting
      - **>10 mEq/day**: Diuretics; Bartter's syndrome; Normotensive hyperaldosteronism; Mg depletion; Extreme K depletion

Fig. 3-46 Diagnostic approach to hypokalemia. Because renal potassium wasting may improve during sodium restriction, diminished potassium excretion is indicative of extrarenal loss only when the diet (and therefore the urine) is rich in sodium. (From Stein JH [ed]: *Internal medicine,* ed 4, St Louis, 1994, Mosby.)

CLINICAL ALGORITHMS　　　　　　　　　　　　　　　　　　　　　　　　　　**Hyponatremia**　727

HYPONATREMIA

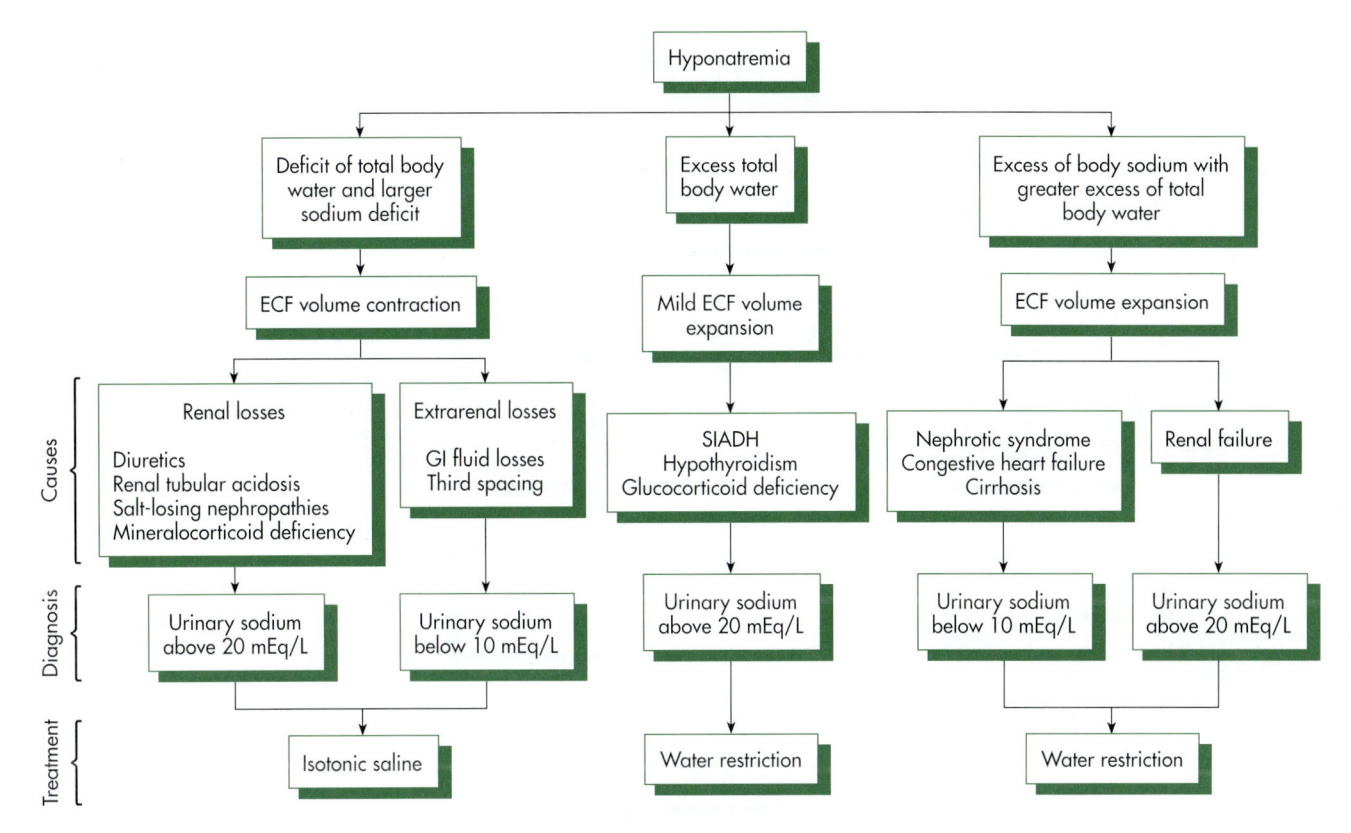

Fig. 3-47 **Evaluation and treatment of asymptomatic, mild hyponatremia.** (From Rosen P et al [eds]: *Emergency medicine: concepts and clinical practice,* St Louis, 1992, Mosby.)

HYPOPHOSPHATEMIA

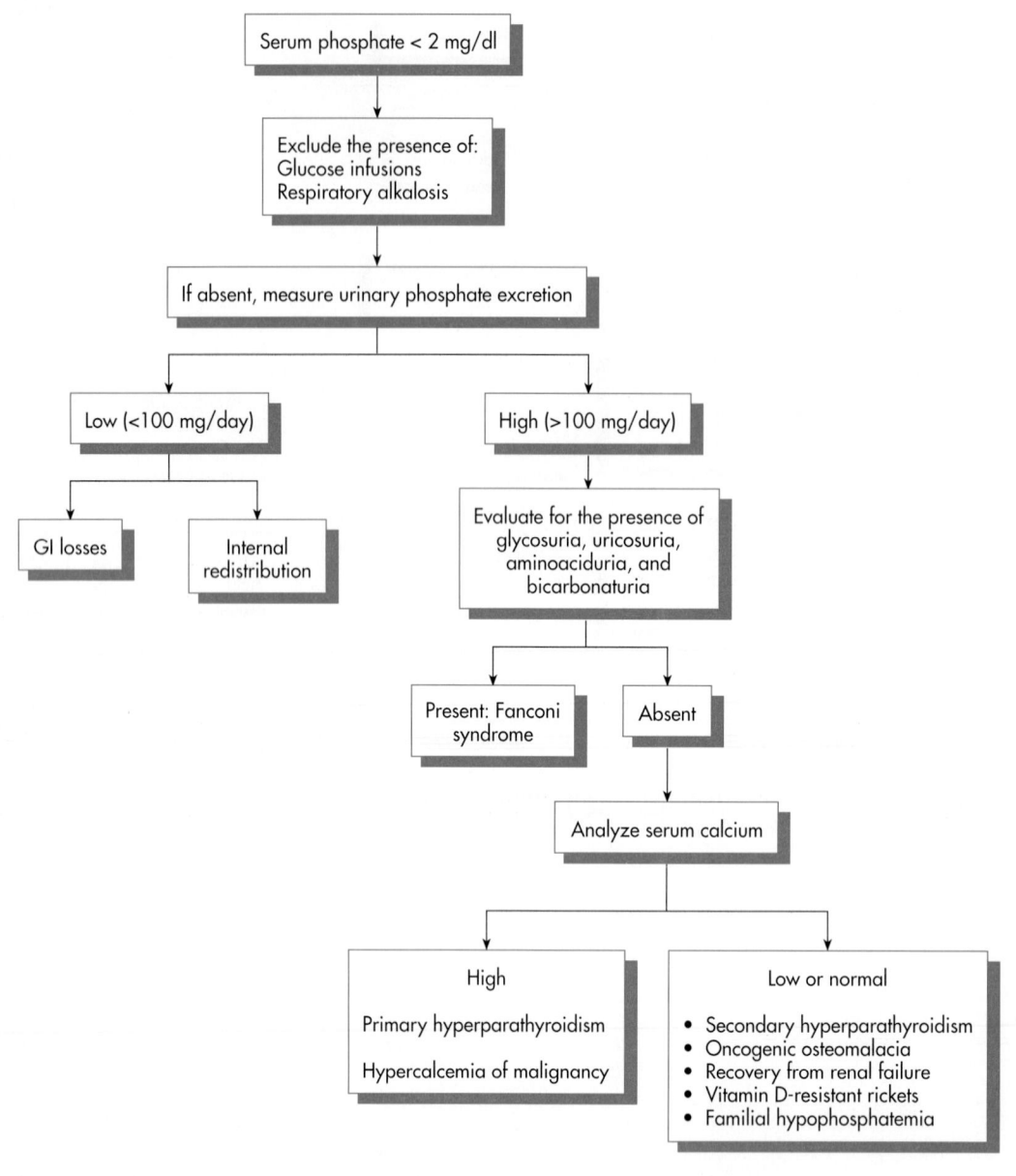

```
                    Serum phosphate < 2 mg/dl
                              │
                              ▼
                    Exclude the presence of:
                       Glucose infusions
                      Respiratory alkalosis
                              │
                              ▼
              If absent, measure urinary phosphate excretion
                    │                        │
                    ▼                        ▼
            Low (<100 mg/day)          High (>100 mg/day)
              │          │                   │
              ▼          ▼                   ▼
          GI losses   Internal        Evaluate for the presence of
                    redistribution     glycosuria, uricosuria,
                                       aminoaciduria, and
                                          bicarbonaturia
                                         │            │
                                         ▼            ▼
                                   Present: Fanconi  Absent
                                     syndrome         │
                                                      ▼
                                               Analyze serum calcium
                                                   │         │
                                                   ▼         ▼
                                                 High    Low or normal
```

High
- Primary hyperparathyroidism
- Hypercalcemia of malignancy

Low or normal
- Secondary hyperparathyroidism
- Oncogenic osteomalacia
- Recovery from renal failure
- Vitamin D-resistant rickets
- Familial hypophosphatemia

Fig. 3-48 **Diagnostic workup of hypophosphatemia.** (From Stein JH [ed]: *Internal medicine,* ed 5, St Louis, 1998, Mosby.)

INFERTILITY

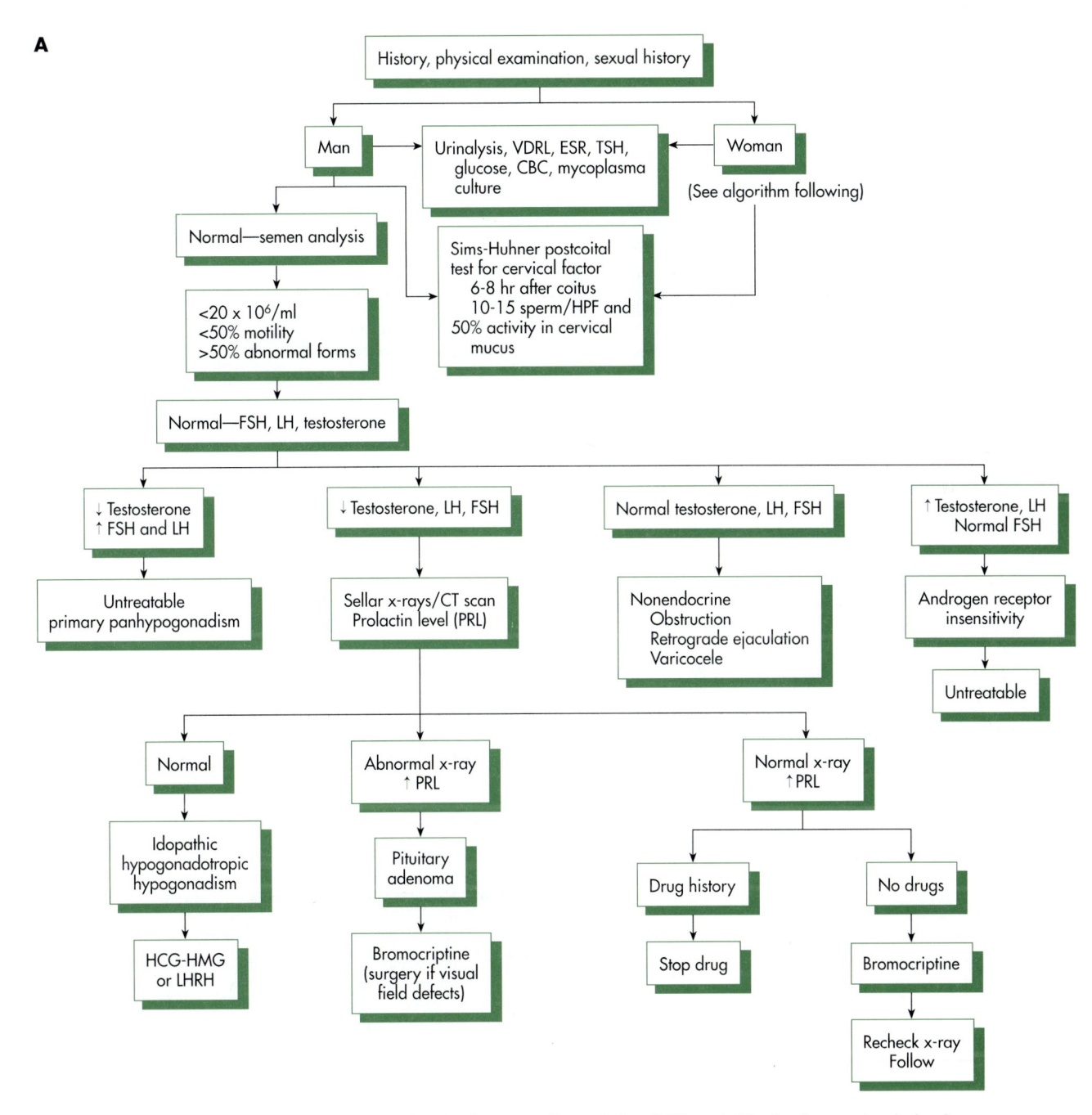

A

```
History, physical examination, sexual history
         │
    ┌────┴────┐
   Man      Woman
    │      (See algorithm following)
    │
Urinalysis, VDRL, ESR, TSH,
glucose, CBC, mycoplasma culture
    │
Normal—semen analysis
    │
<20 × 10⁶/ml
<50% motility
>50% abnormal forms
    │
Sims-Huhner postcoital test for cervical factor
6-8 hr after coitus
10-15 sperm/HPF and 50% activity in cervical mucus
    │
Normal—FSH, LH, testosterone
```

Branches:

- ↓ Testosterone, ↑ FSH and LH → Untreatable primary panhypogonadism
- ↓ Testosterone, LH, FSH → Sellar x-rays/CT scan, Prolactin level (PRL)
  - Normal → Idiopathic hypogonadotropic hypogonadism → HCG-HMG or LHRH
  - Abnormal x-ray, ↑ PRL → Pituitary adenoma → Bromocriptine (surgery if visual field defects)
  - Normal x-ray, ↑ PRL →
    - Drug history → Stop drug
    - No drugs → Bromocriptine → Recheck x-ray Follow
- Normal testosterone, LH, FSH → Nonendocrine / Obstruction / Retrograde ejaculation / Varicocele
- ↑ Testosterone, LH, Normal FSH → Androgen receptor insensitivity → Untreatable

Fig. 3-49 **A, Evaluating infertility in the man.** (From Driscoll CE et al: *The family practice desk reference,* ed 3, St Louis, 1996, Mosby.)

INFERTILITY—cont'd

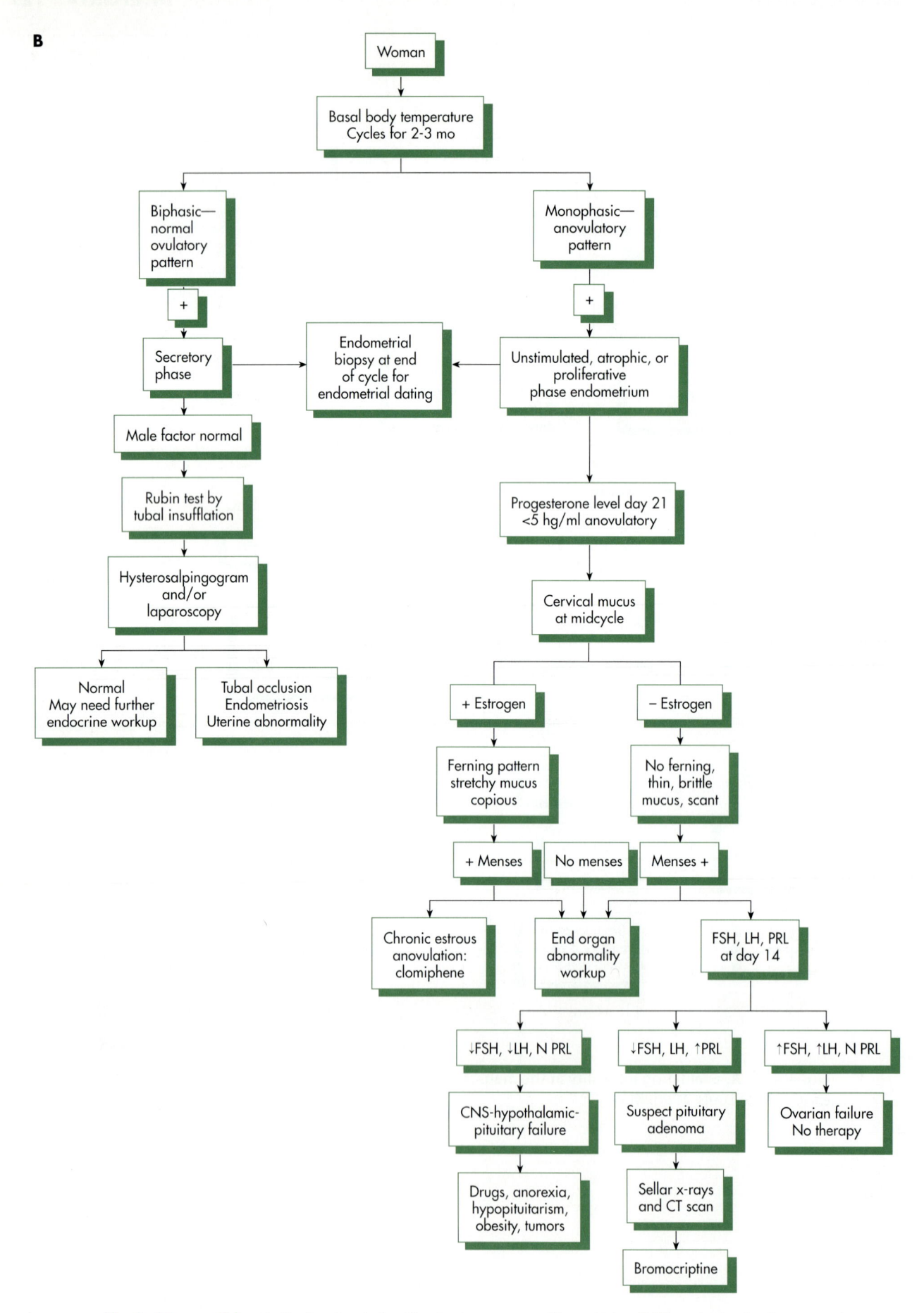

Fig. 3-49—cont'd **B,** Evaluating infertility in the woman. (From Driscoll CE et al: *The family practice desk reference,* ed 3, St Louis, 1996, Mosby.)

CLINICAL ALGORITHMS Jaundice and hepatobiliary disease 731

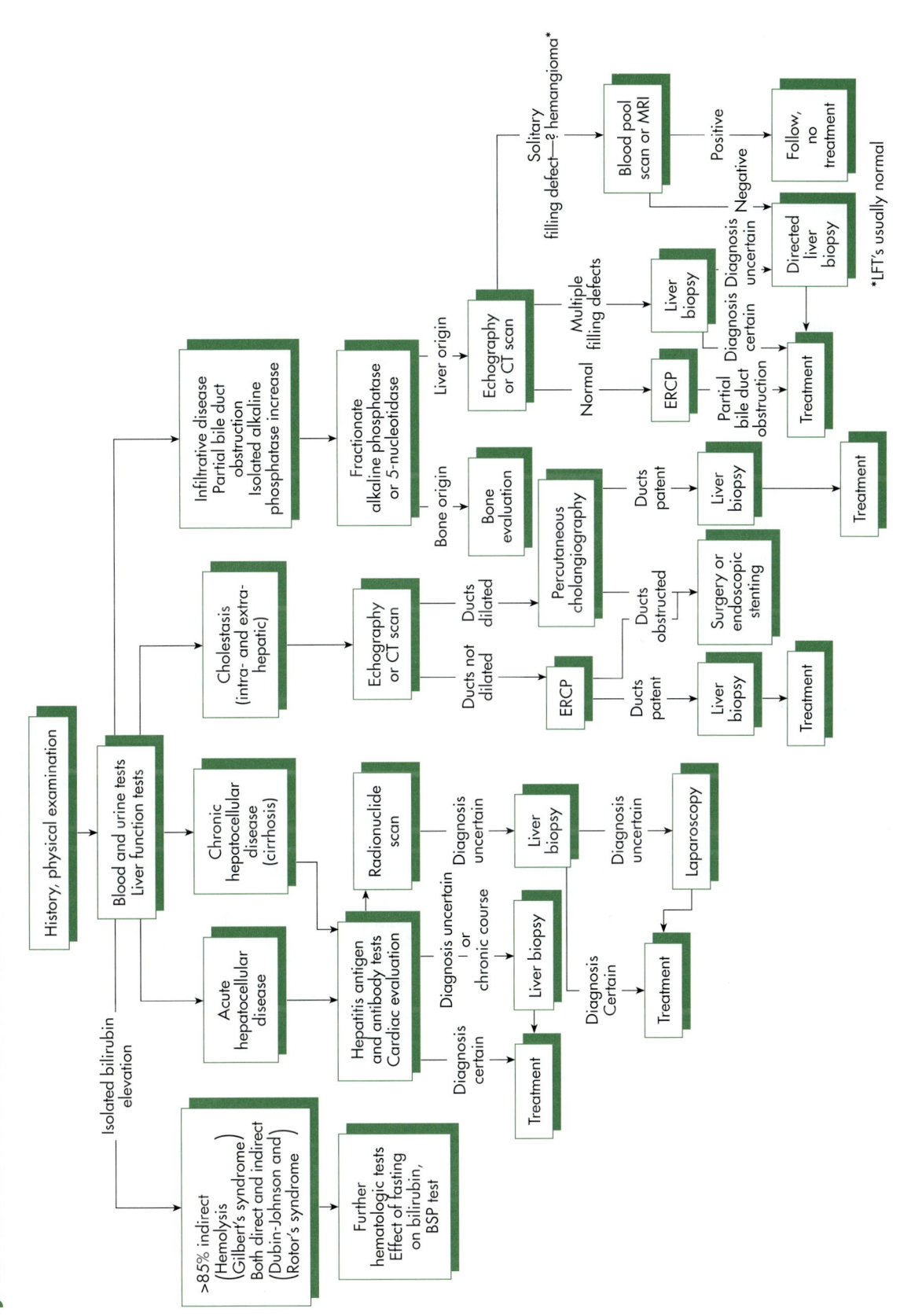

Fig. 3-50 Evaluation of jaundice and hepatobiliary disease. *BSP*, Bromsulphalein; *CT*, computed tomography; *ERCP*, endoscopic retrograde cholangiopancreatography; *LFTs*, liver function tests. (From Stein JH [ed]: *Internal medicine*, ed 4, St Louis, 1994, Mosby.)

LEG ULCER

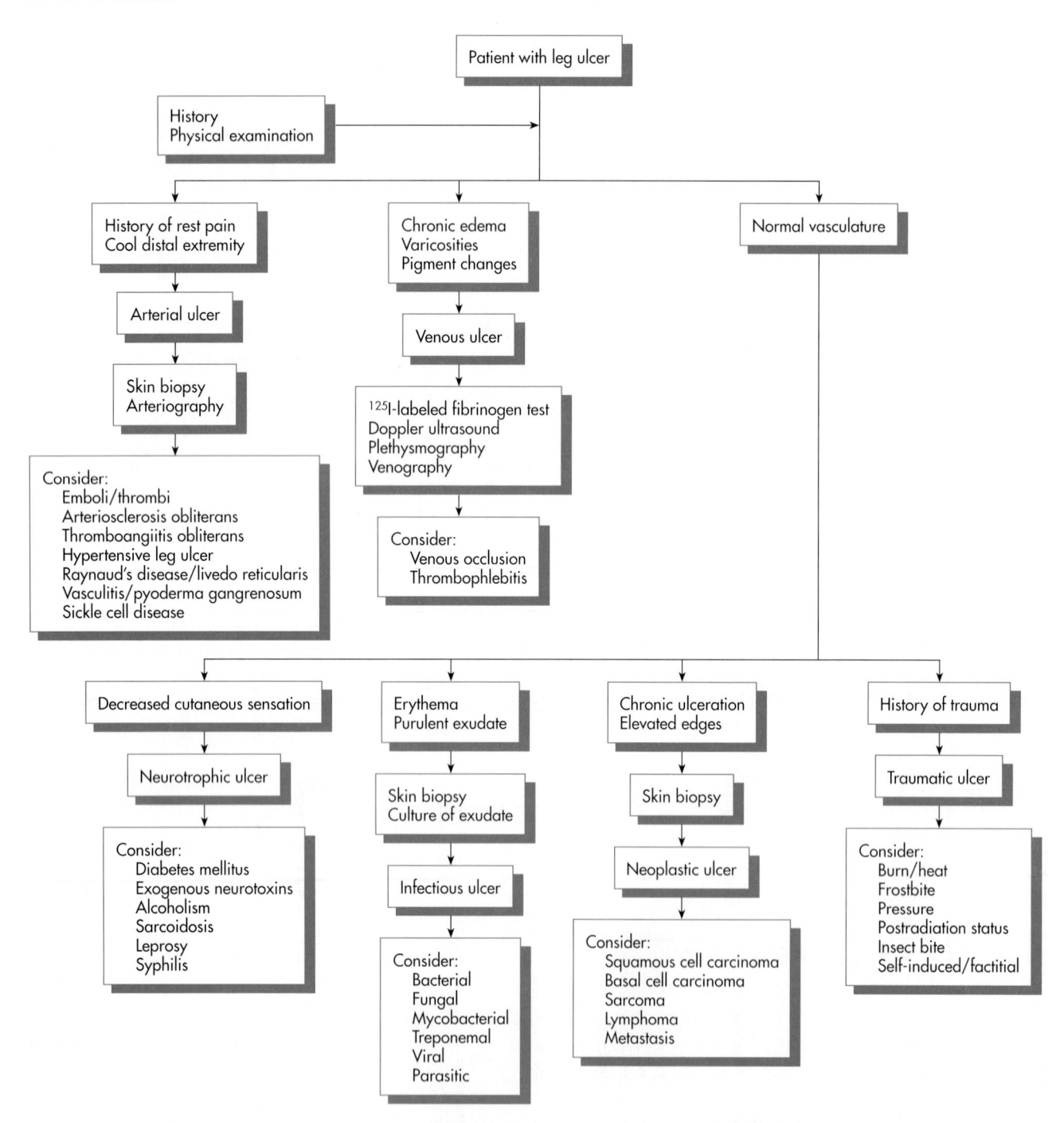

```
                          Patient with leg ulcer
                                   │
      History ─────────────────────┤
      Physical examination         │
                                   │
   ┌───────────────────┬───────────┴───────────┬─────────────────────┐
   │                   │                       │                     │
History of rest pain   Chronic edema      Normal vasculature
Cool distal extremity  Varicosities
   │                   Pigment changes
   │                       │
Arterial ulcer         Venous ulcer
   │                       │
Skin biopsy            ¹²⁵I-labeled fibrinogen test
Arteriography          Doppler ultrasound
   │                   Plethysmography
   │                   Venography
   │                       │
Consider:              Consider:
  Emboli/thrombi         Venous occlusion
  Arteriosclerosis obliterans   Thrombophlebitis
  Thromboangiitis obliterans
  Hypertensive leg ulcer
  Raynaud's disease/livedo reticularis
  Vasculitis/pyoderma gangrenosum
  Sickle cell disease
```

```
   ┌───────────────────┬───────────────────┬─────────────────────┐
   │                   │                   │                     │
Decreased cutaneous    Erythema         Chronic ulceration    History of trauma
sensation              Purulent exudate  Elevated edges
   │                   │                   │                     │
Neurotrophic ulcer     Skin biopsy       Skin biopsy           Traumatic ulcer
   │                   Culture of exudate  │                     │
   │                   │                   │                     │
Consider:              Infectious ulcer   Neoplastic ulcer      Consider:
  Diabetes mellitus    │                   │                      Burn/heat
  Exogenous neurotoxins Consider:         Consider:               Frostbite
  Alcoholism             Bacterial          Squamous cell carcinoma  Pressure
  Sarcoidosis            Fungal             Basal cell carcinoma    Postradiation status
  Leprosy                Mycobacterial      Sarcoma                 Insect bite
  Syphilis               Treponemal         Lymphoma                Self-induced/factitial
                         Viral              Metastasis
                         Parasitic
```

Fig. 3-51 (From Greene HL, Johnson WP, Maricic MJ: *Decision making in medicine*, St Louis, 1993, Mosby.)

LIVER FUNCTION TEST ABNORMALITIES

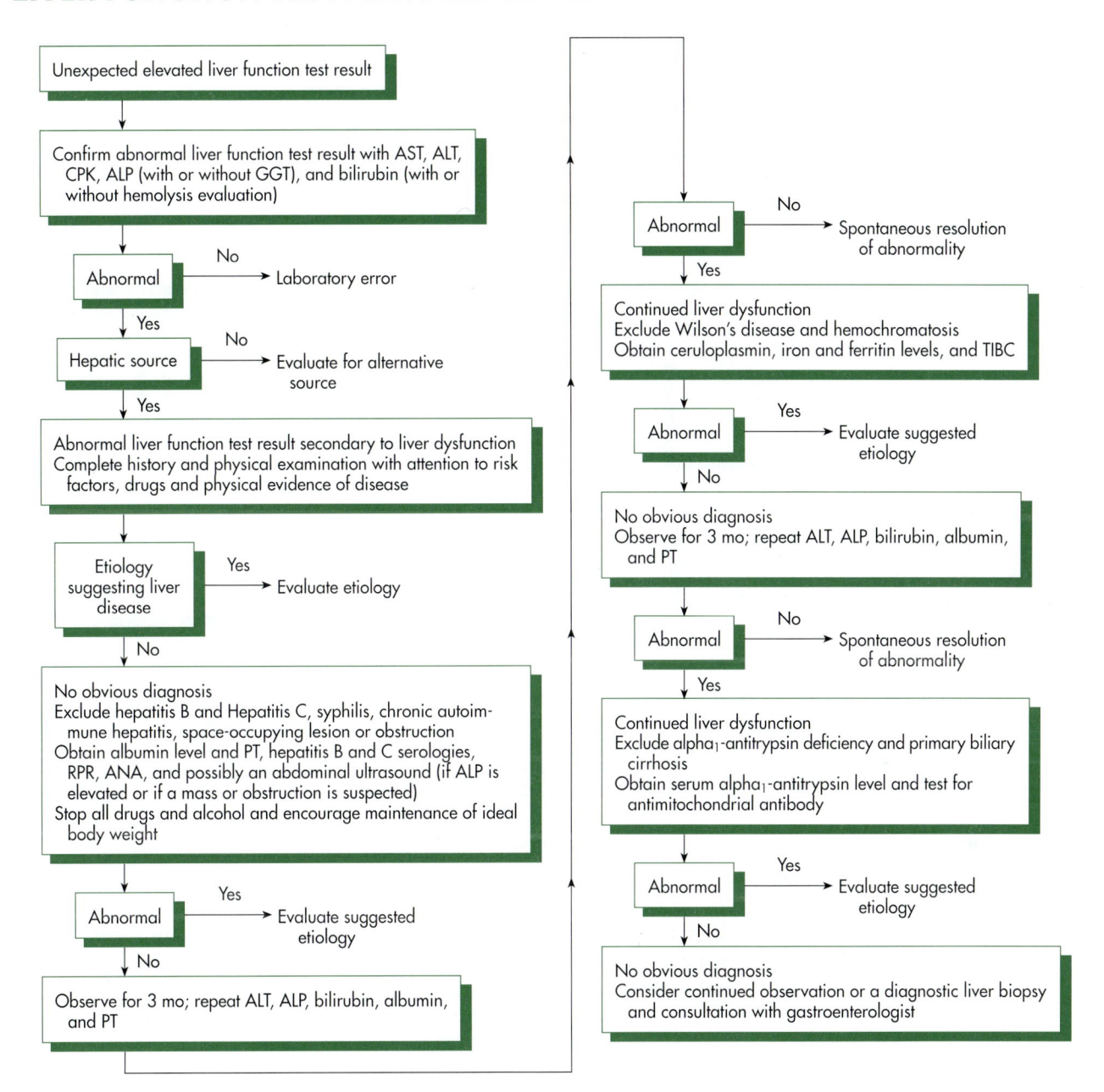

Fig. 3-52 Evaluation of a patient with abnormal results on liver function tests. *AST,* Aspartate transaminase; *ALT,* alanine transaminase, *CPK,* creatine phosphokinase; *ALP,* alkaline phosphatase; *GGT,* gamma glutamyltransferase; *PT,* prothrombin; *RPR,* rapid plasma reagent; *ANA,* antinuclear antibody; *TIBC,* total iron-binding capacity. (From Theal RM, Scott K: Evaluating asymptomatic patients with abnormal liver function test results. *Am Fam Physician* 53:2111-2119, 1996.)

LYMPHADENOPATHY, GENERALIZED

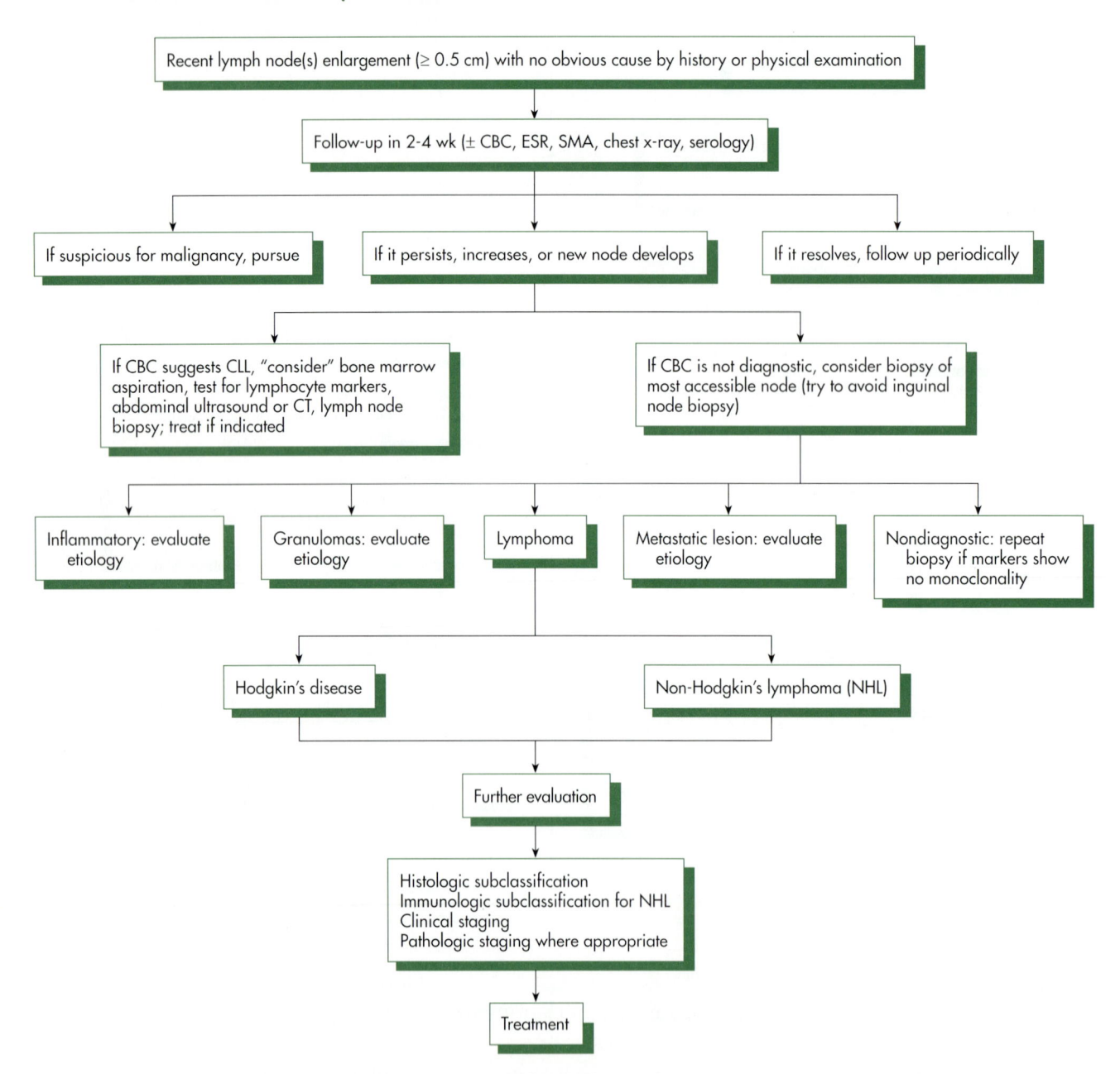

```
Recent lymph node(s) enlargement (≥ 0.5 cm) with no obvious cause by history or physical examination
                                          │
                                          ▼
              Follow-up in 2-4 wk (± CBC, ESR, SMA, chest x-ray, serology)
                    │                     │                     │
                    ▼                     ▼                     ▼
    If suspicious for malignancy,   If it persists, increases,   If it resolves, follow up periodically
    pursue                          or new node develops
                                          │
                    ┌─────────────────────┴─────────────────────┐
                    ▼                                           ▼
    If CBC suggests CLL, "consider" bone marrow         If CBC is not diagnostic, consider biopsy of
    aspiration, test for lymphocyte markers,            most accessible node (try to avoid inguinal
    abdominal ultrasound or CT, lymph node              node biopsy)
    biopsy; treat if indicated
                    │
    ┌───────────┬───┴───────┬──────────────┬──────────────┐
    ▼           ▼           ▼              ▼              ▼
Inflammatory:  Granulomas:  Lymphoma   Metastatic lesion: Nondiagnostic: repeat
evaluate       evaluate                evaluate etiology  biopsy if markers show
etiology       etiology                                   no monoclonality
                            │
                  ┌─────────┴─────────┐
                  ▼                   ▼
          Hodgkin's disease    Non-Hodgkin's lymphoma (NHL)
                        │
                        ▼
                Further evaluation
                        │
                        ▼
        Histologic subclassification
        Immunologic subclassification for NHL
        Clinical staging
        Pathologic staging where appropriate
                        │
                        ▼
                   Treatment
```

Fig. 3-53 Workup of lymphadenopathy. (From Noble J [ed]: *Primary care medicine,* ed 2, St Louis, 1996, Mosby.)

LYMPHADENOPATHY, LOCALIZED

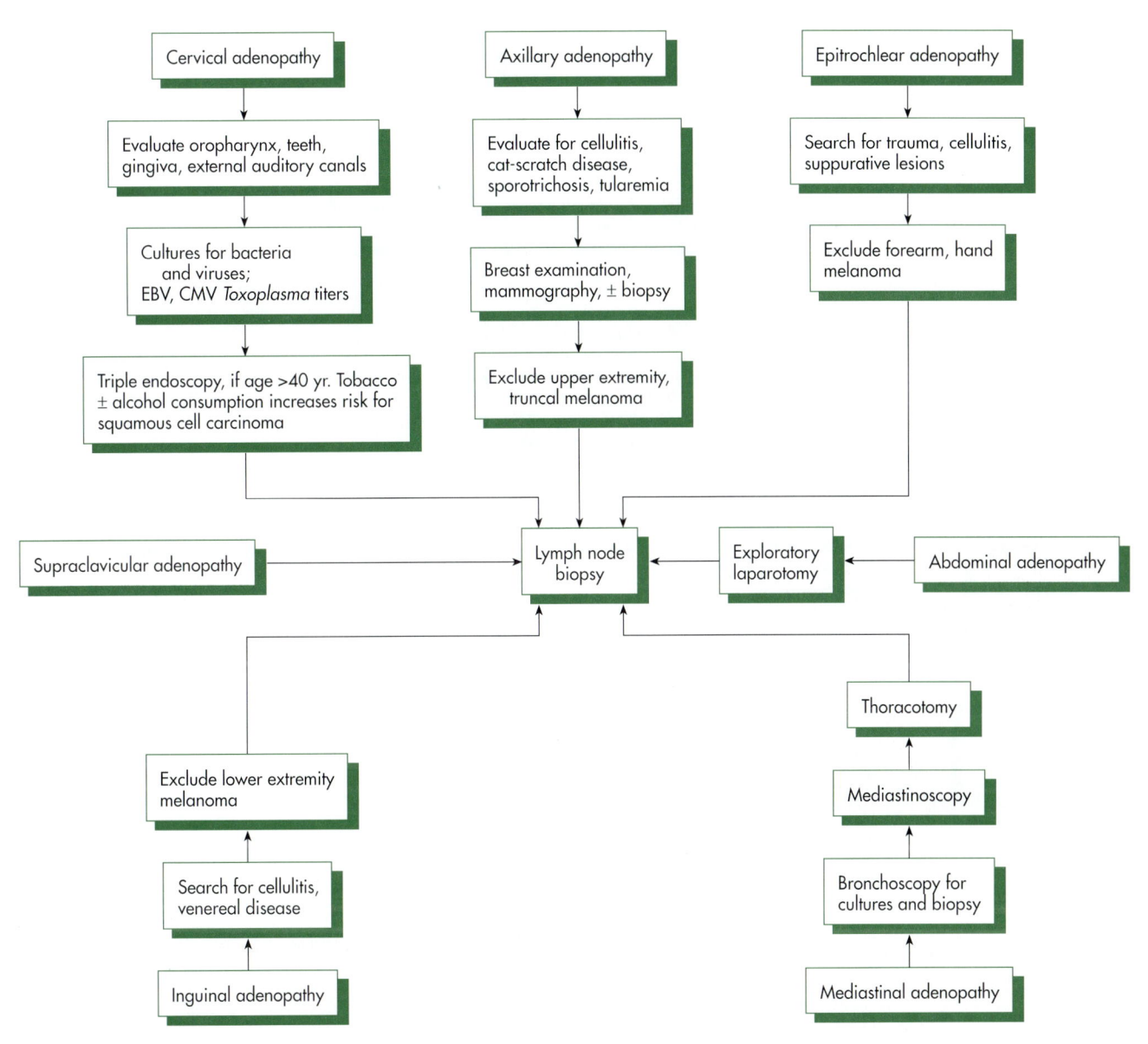

Fig. 3-54 Clinical approach to the patient with localized lymphadenopathy. (From Stein JH [ed]: *Internal medicine,* ed 4, St Louis, 1994, Mosby.)

MACROCYTOSIS

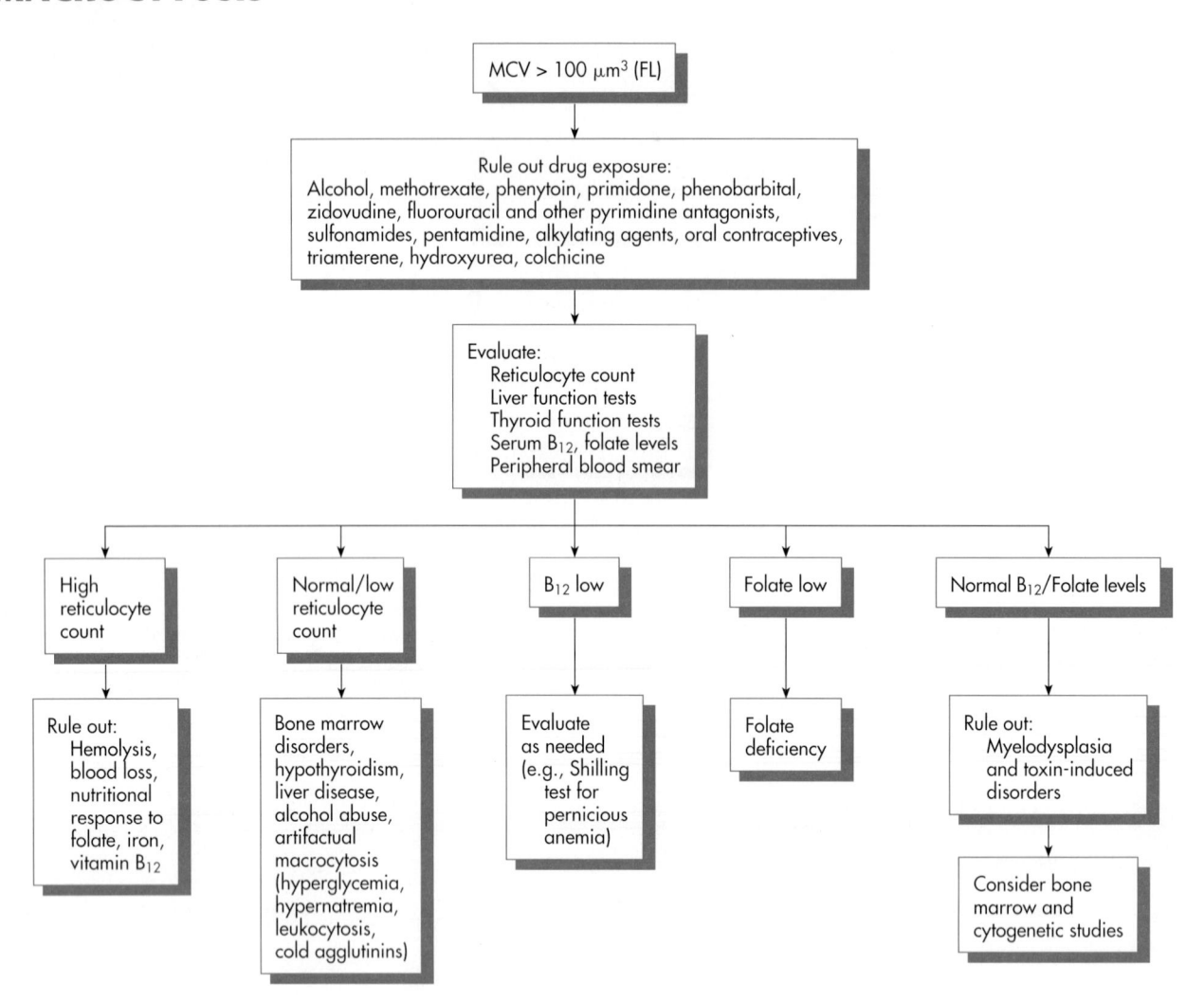

```
                    ┌─────────────────────┐
                    │  MCV > 100 μm³ (FL) │
                    └──────────┬──────────┘
                               ▼
        ┌──────────────────────────────────────────────┐
        │ Rule out drug exposure:                       │
        │ Alcohol, methotrexate, phenytoin, primidone,  │
        │ phenobarbital, zidovudine, fluorouracil and   │
        │ other pyrimidine antagonists, sulfonamides,   │
        │ pentamidine, alkylating agents, oral          │
        │ contraceptives, triamterene, hydroxyurea,     │
        │ colchicine                                    │
        └──────────────────┬───────────────────────────┘
                           ▼
                ┌─────────────────────┐
                │ Evaluate:            │
                │   Reticulocyte count │
                │   Liver function tests│
                │   Thyroid function tests│
                │   Serum B₁₂, folate levels│
                │   Peripheral blood smear│
                └──────────┬──────────┘
```

Branches:

- **High reticulocyte count** → Rule out: Hemolysis, blood loss, nutritional response to folate, iron, vitamin B₁₂

- **Normal/low reticulocyte count** → Bone marrow disorders, hypothyroidism, liver disease, alcohol abuse, artifactual macrocytosis (hyperglycemia, hypernatremia, leukocytosis, cold agglutinins)

- **B₁₂ low** → Evaluate as needed (e.g., Shilling test for pernicious anemia)

- **Folate low** → Folate deficiency

- **Normal B₁₂/Folate levels** → Rule out: Myelodysplasia and toxin-induced disorders → Consider bone marrow and cytogenetic studies

Fig. 3-55 Evaluation of macrocytosis.

MALABSORPTION

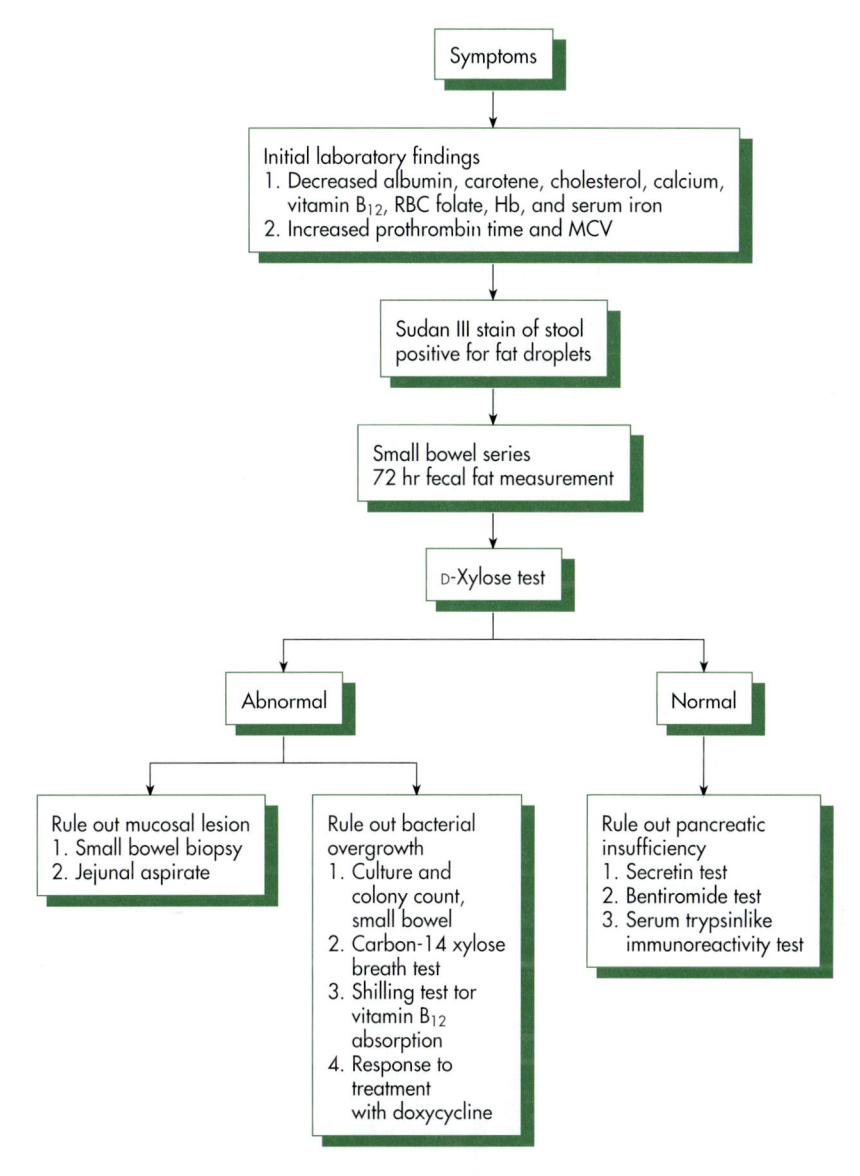

```
                        ┌──────────┐
                        │ Symptoms │
                        └────┬─────┘
                             ▼
   ┌──────────────────────────────────────────────┐
   │ Initial laboratory findings                  │
   │ 1. Decreased albumin, carotene, cholesterol, │
   │    calcium, vitamin B₁₂, RBC folate, Hb,     │
   │    and serum iron                            │
   │ 2. Increased prothrombin time and MCV        │
   └──────────────────────┬───────────────────────┘
                          ▼
              ┌──────────────────────────┐
              │ Sudan III stain of stool │
              │ positive for fat droplets│
              └────────────┬─────────────┘
                           ▼
              ┌──────────────────────────┐
              │ Small bowel series       │
              │ 72 hr fecal fat measurement│
              └────────────┬─────────────┘
                           ▼
                   ┌──────────────┐
                   │ D-Xylose test│
                   └──────┬───────┘
                ┌─────────┴─────────┐
                ▼                   ▼
           ┌──────────┐        ┌────────┐
           │ Abnormal │        │ Normal │
           └────┬─────┘        └───┬────┘
          ┌─────┴──────┐           ▼
          ▼            ▼
```

- Rule out mucosal lesion
  1. Small bowel biopsy
  2. Jejunal aspirate

- Rule out bacterial overgrowth
  1. Culture and colony count, small bowel
  2. Carbon-14 xylose breath test
  3. Shilling test for vitamin B₁₂ absorption
  4. Response to treatment with doxycycline

- Rule out pancreatic insufficiency
  1. Secretin test
  2. Bentiromide test
  3. Serum trypsinlike immunoreactivity test

Fig. 3-56 Diagnostic approach to malabsorption. (From Ferri FF: *Practical guide to the care of the medical patient*, ed 4, St Louis, 1998, Mosby.)

MUSCLE CRAMPS AND ACHES

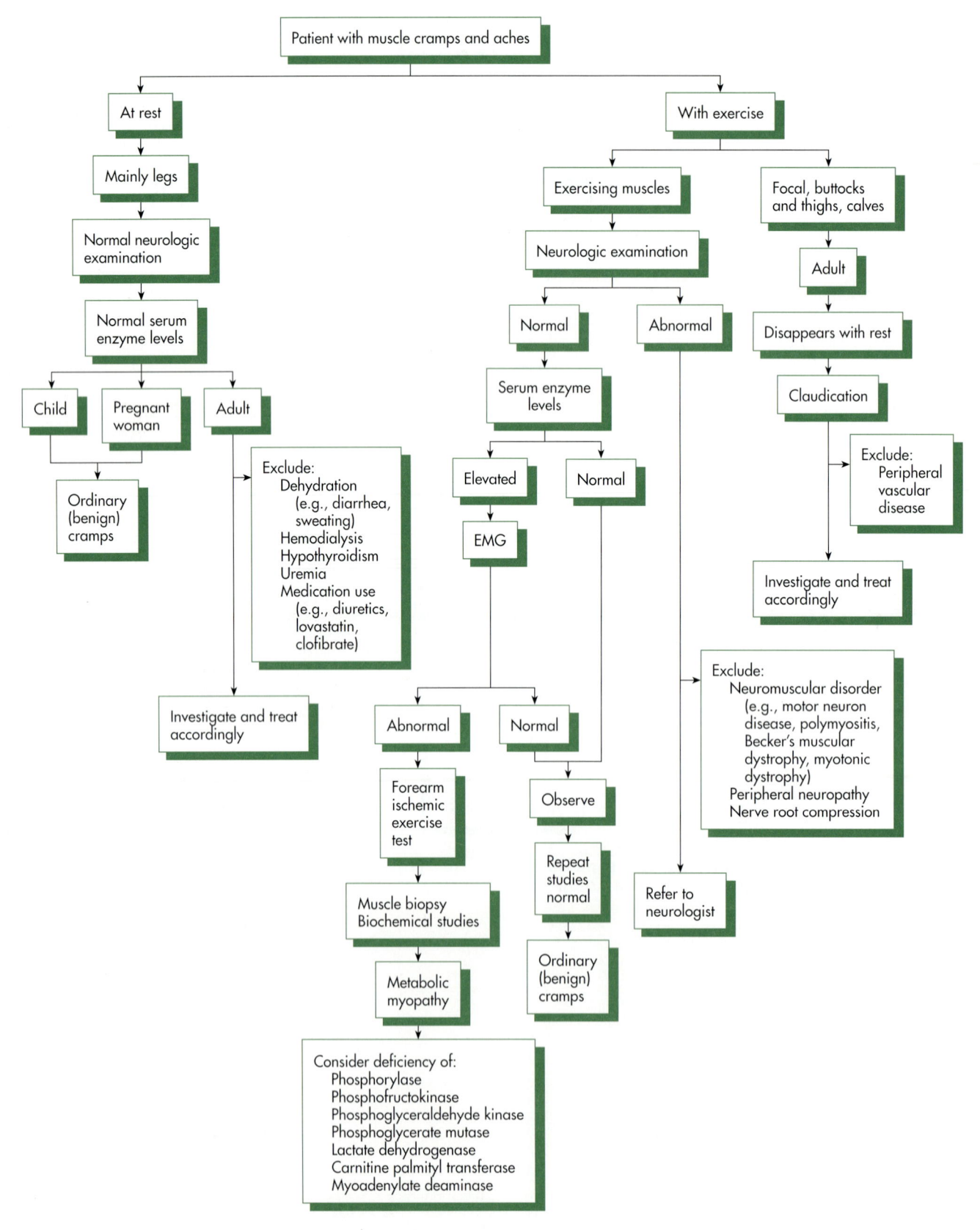

Fig. 3-57 Evaluation of muscle cramps and aches. (From Greene HL, Johnson WP, Maricic MJ: *Decision making in medicine*, St Louis, 1993, Mosby.)

CLINICAL ALGORITHMS **Neck pain** 739

NECK PAIN

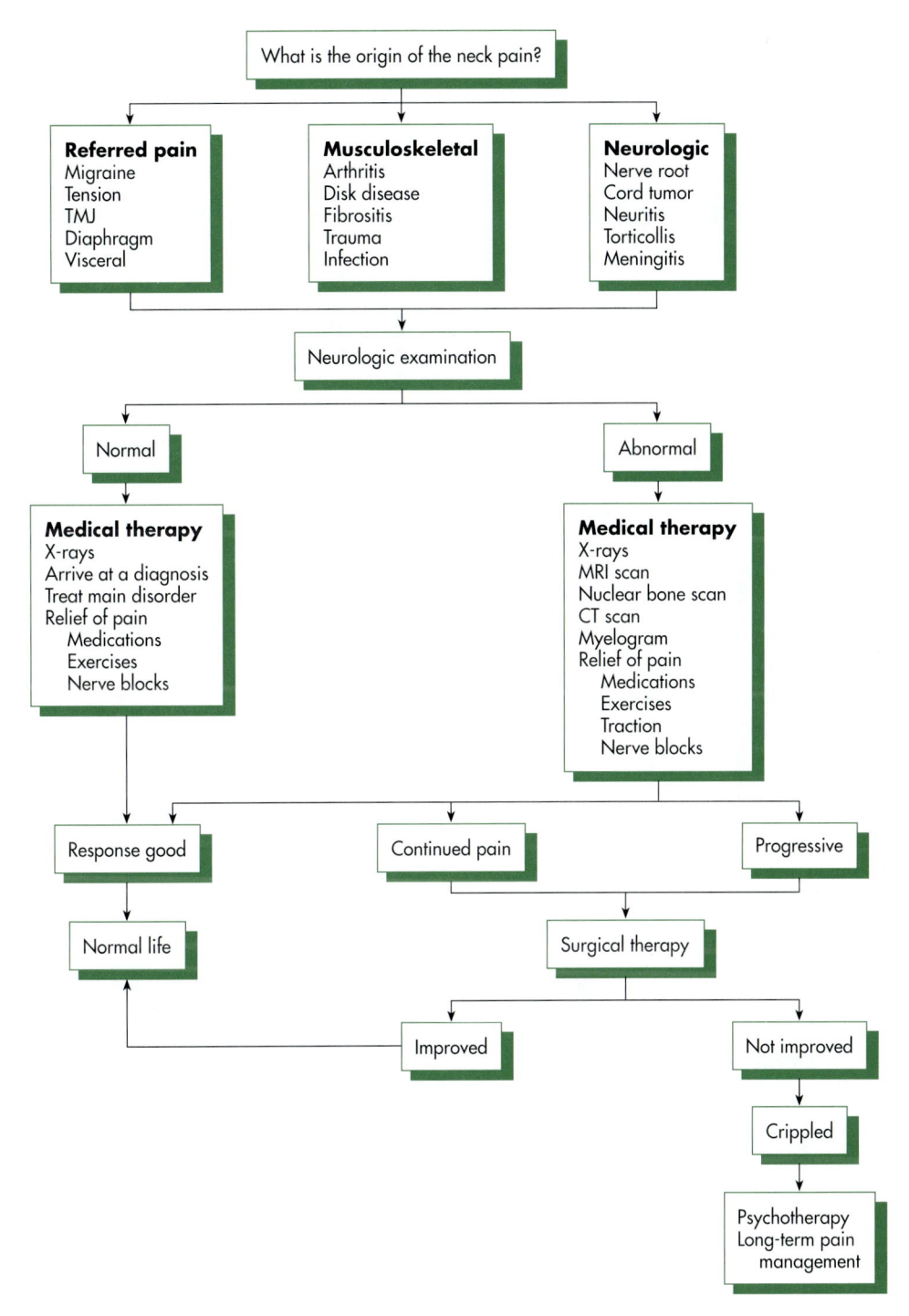

```
                What is the origin of the neck pain?
                                │
         ┌──────────────────────┼──────────────────────┐
         ▼                      ▼                      ▼
   Referred pain          Musculoskeletal           Neurologic
   Migraine               Arthritis                 Nerve root
   Tension                Disk disease              Cord tumor
   TMJ                    Fibrositis                Neuritis
   Diaphragm              Trauma                    Torticollis
   Visceral               Infection                 Meningitis
                                │
                      Neurologic examination
                                │
                  ┌─────────────┴─────────────┐
                  ▼                           ▼
               Normal                      Abnormal
                  │                           │
         Medical therapy             Medical therapy
         X-rays                      X-rays
         Arrive at a diagnosis       MRI scan
         Treat main disorder         Nuclear bone scan
         Relief of pain              CT scan
           Medications               Myelogram
           Exercises                 Relief of pain
           Nerve blocks                Medications
                                       Exercises
                                       Traction
                                       Nerve blocks
                  │              ┌──────────┼──────────┐
                  ▼              ▼                     ▼
           Response good    Continued pain        Progressive
                  │              │                     │
                  ▼              └─────────┬───────────┘
            Normal life                    ▼
                  ▲                  Surgical therapy
                  │                        │
                  │              ┌─────────┴─────────┐
                  │              ▼                   ▼
                  └──────── Improved             Not improved
                                                     │
                                                     ▼
                                                  Crippled
                                                     │
                                                     ▼
                                               Psychotherapy
                                               Long-term pain
                                                 management
```

Fig. 3-58 Diagnosis and therapy for neck pain. (From Stein JH [ed]: *Internal medicine,* ed 4, St Louis, 1994, Mosby.)

740 Nephrolithiasis — CLINICAL ALGORITHMS

NEPHROLITHIASIS

(1) Examination of sediment from urine specimen immediately after voiding
(2) Obtain plain abdominal radiograph, ultrasonogram, and intravenous urogram

Radiolucent stone
(also consider tumor of renal pelvis, blood clot, sloughed renal papilla)

- **Uric acid crystalluria, Urine pH <5.5, Concentrated urine** → **Uric acid stone** (confirm by analysis)
  - Normal serum uric acid → Purine gluttony, Idiopathic uric acid stone, Diarrheal diseases
  - Hyperuricemia → Gout, Malignancy
- **Cystine crystalluria, Acid urine, Positive cyanide nitroprusside test** → **Cystine stone** (confirm by analysis)

Radiodense stone

- **Struvite-apatite crystalluria, Urine pH 7.5, Pyuria and bacilluria** → **Struvite-carbonate apatite stone** (confirm by analysis) → Infection stone due to urease-producing bacilli. Evaluate mechanism for urinary infection. Search for underlying metabolic cause of stone that became secondarily infected

- **Calcium oxalate or apatite crystalluria** → **Calcium oxalate-apatite stone** (confirm by analysis)
  - **Hypercalcemia**
    - High serum PTH, High urine cyclic AMP → Primary hyperparathyroidism
    - Normal or low serum PTH and urine cyclic AMP → Sarcoidosis, other granulomatous diseases, lymphomas [high serum 1,25(OH)$_2$-vitamin D$_3$], Hyperthyroidism (high T$_3$, T$_4$), Myeloma (osteoclast activating factor), Malignant tumor PTH-like peptide in hypercalcemia of malignancy; prostaglandins
  - **Normal serum Ca**
    - **Hypercalciuria** (>300 mg Ca/day or >4 mg Ca/kg/day)
      - Metabolic acidosis (venous blood pH ≤7.34 serum HCO$_3$ ≤22 mEq/L serum Cl ≥108 mEq/L urine pH always ≥6.0 low urine citrate) → Distal renal tubular acidosis
      - No acidosis → Idiopathic hypercalciuria, Renal Ca leak [may include medullary sponge kidney; secondary hyperparathyroidism and activation of 1,25(OH)$_2$-vitamin D$_3$ synthesis]; Renal P leak [activation of 1,25(OH)$_2$-vitamin D$_3$ synthesis; probably indirect]; Absorptive hypercalciuria [mediated via increased 1,25(OH)$_2$-vitamin D$_3$-stimulated intestinal Ca absorption or by augmented gut Ca absorption independent of vitamin D]
    - **Normal urine Ca**
      - Hypocitraturia (<200 mg/day)
      - Hyperoxaluria (urine oxalate >45 mg/day) → Primary hyperoxaluria, Acquired hyperoxaluria, Small bowel disease, Gluttony for oxalate-rich food, Ascorbic acid abuse
      - Hyperuricosuria (urine uric acid >800 mg/day in men; >750 mg/day in women) → Hyperuricosuria and Ca stone syndrome (some also have hypercalciuria)
      - Normal urinary uric acid and oxalate excretion → Idiopathic calcium stone disease. Habitually low fluid intake and thus concentrated urine. ? Deficiency of inhibitor of crystal nucleation or growth. ? Presence of promoter of crystal nucleation or growth

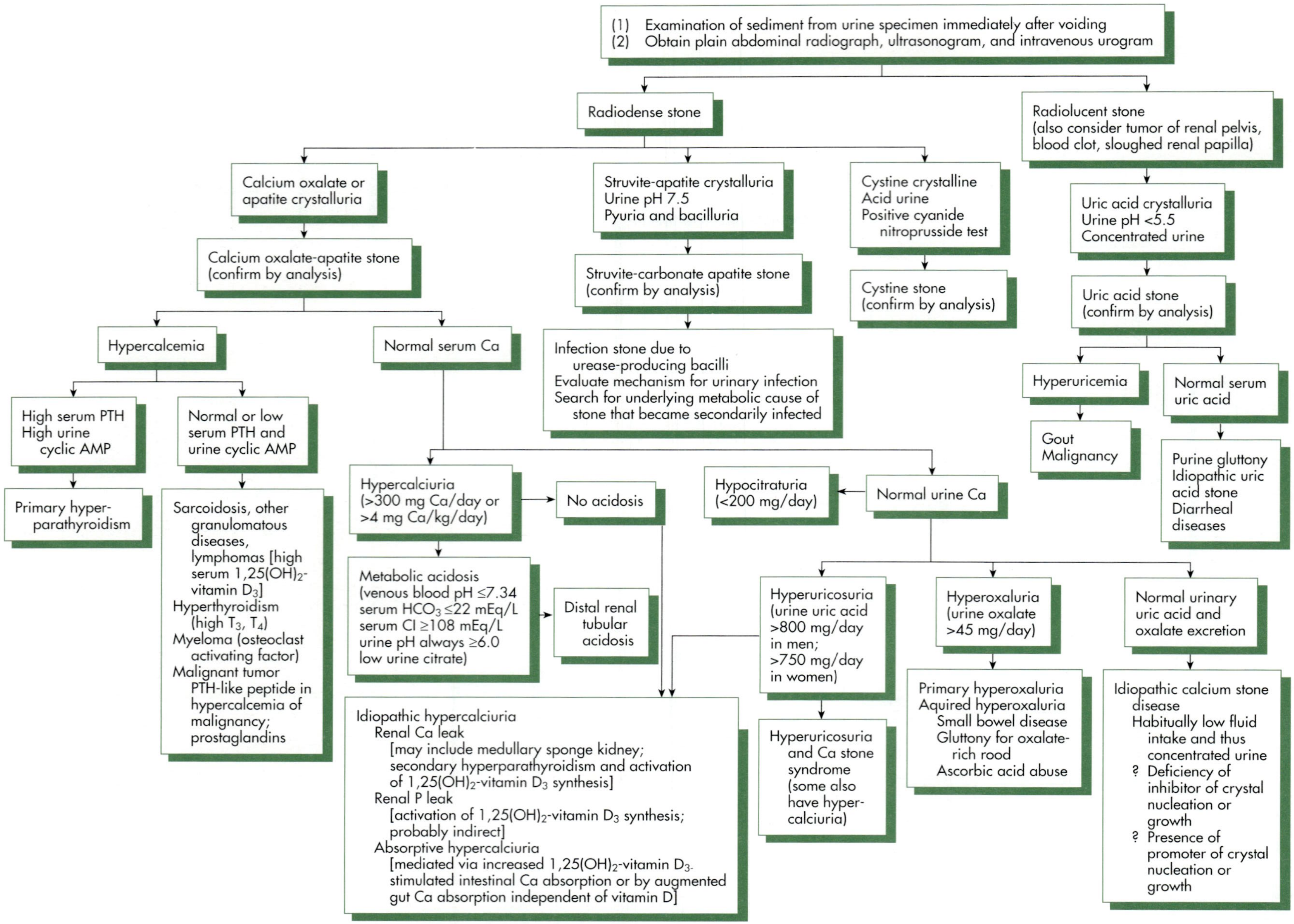

Fig. 3-59 Evaluation of patients with suspected nephrolithiasis (flank pain, ureteral colic, hematuria, fever). (From Stein JH [ed]: *Internal medicine*, ed 4, St Louis, 1994, Mosby.)

CLINICAL ALGORITHMS   Neutropenia   741

NEUTROPENIA

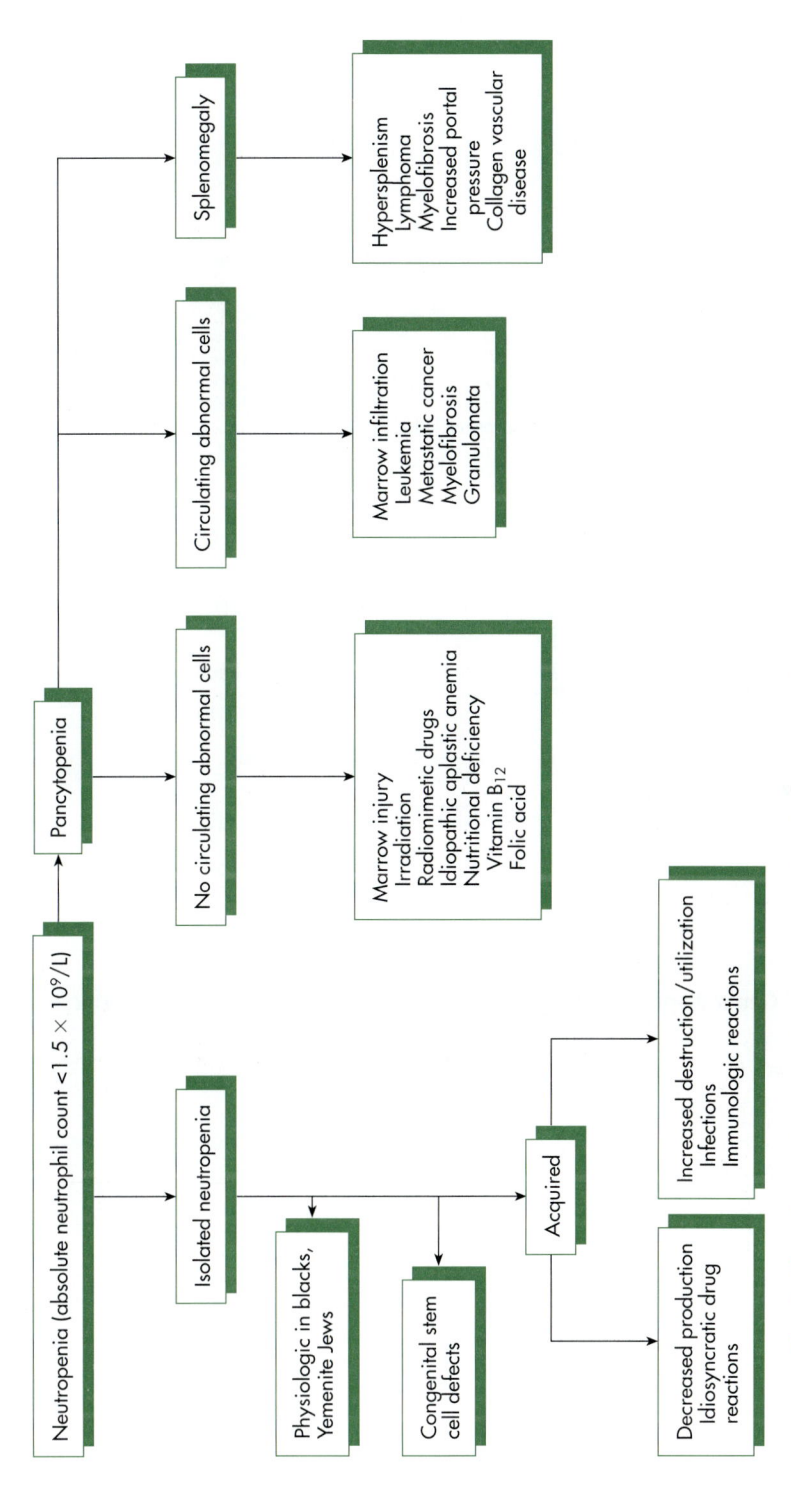

Neutropenia (absolute neutrophil count $<1.5 \times 10^9/L$)

- **Isolated neutropenia**
  - Physiologic in blacks, Yemenite Jews
  - Congenital stem cell defects
  - Acquired
    - Increased destruction/utilization
      - Infections
      - Immunologic reactions
    - Decreased production
      - Idiosyncratic drug reactions

- **Pancytopenia**
  - No circulating abnormal cells
    - Marrow injury
    - Irradiation
    - Radiomimetic drugs
    - Idiopathic aplastic anemia
    - Nutritional deficiency
    - Vitamin B_{12}
    - Folic acid
  - Circulating abnormal cells
    - Marrow infiltration
    - Leukemia
    - Metastatic cancer
    - Myelofibrosis
    - Granulomata
  - Splenomegaly
    - Hypersplenism
    - Lymphoma
    - Myelofibrosis
    - Increased portal pressure
    - Collagen vascular disease

Fig. 3-60 General approach to neutropenia. (From Stein JH [ed]: *Internal medicine*, ed 4, St Louis, 1994, Mosby.)

NEUTROPHILIA

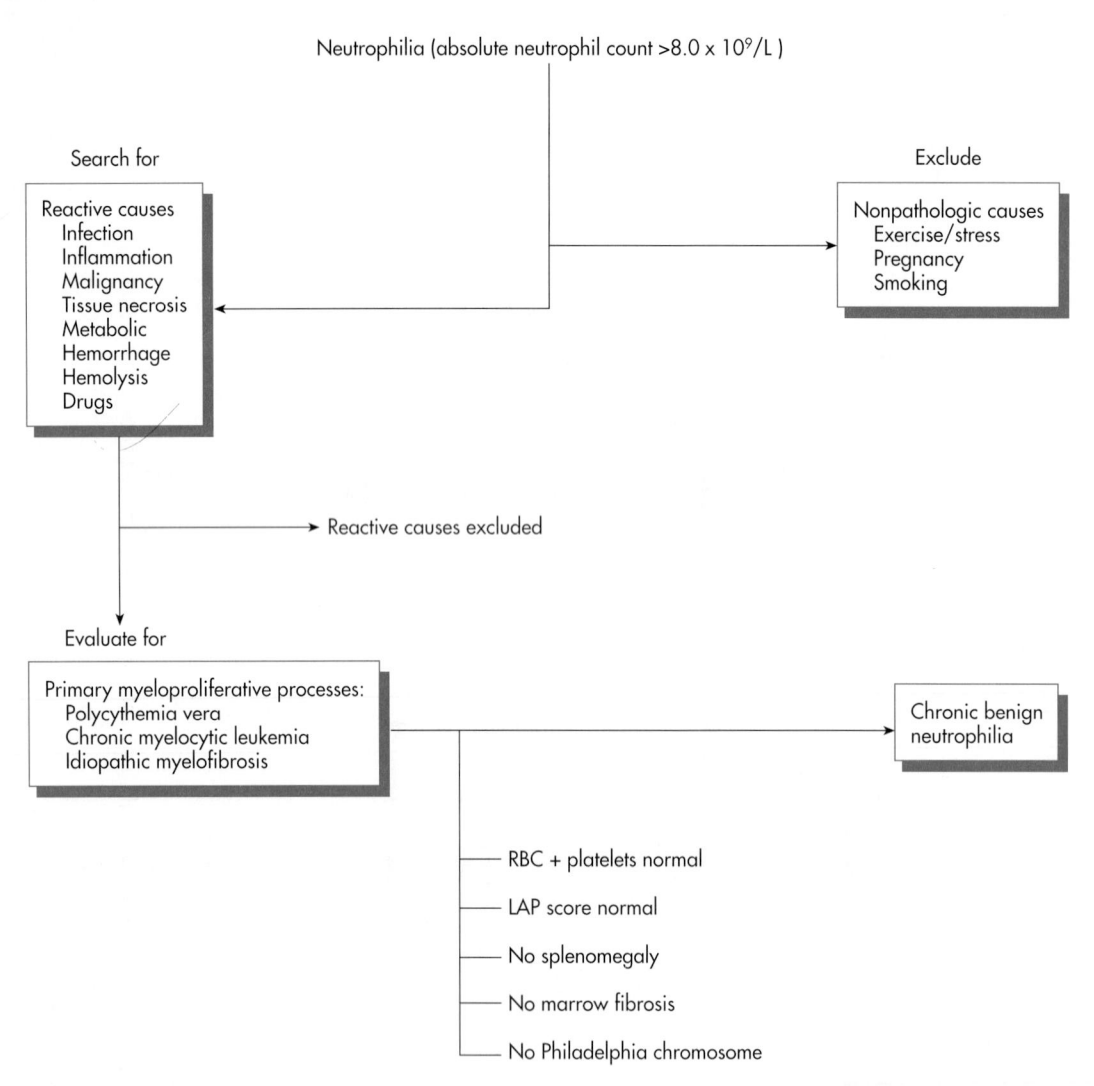

Neutrophilia (absolute neutrophil count >8.0 x 10⁹/L)

Search for
- Reactive causes
  - Infection
  - Inflammation
  - Malignancy
  - Tissue necrosis
  - Metabolic
  - Hemorrhage
  - Hemolysis
  - Drugs

Exclude
- Nonpathologic causes
  - Exercise/stress
  - Pregnancy
  - Smoking

Reactive causes excluded

Evaluate for
- Primary myeloproliferative processes:
  - Polycythemia vera
  - Chronic myelocytic leukemia
  - Idiopathic myelofibrosis

Chronic benign neutrophilia

- RBC + platelets normal
- LAP score normal
- No splenomegaly
- No marrow fibrosis
- No Philadelphia chromosome

Fig. 3-61 **General approach to neutrophilia.** (From Stein JH [ed]: *Internal medicine,* ed 4, St Louis, 1994, Mosby.)

CLINICAL ALGORITHMS

Pain management 743

PAIN MANAGEMENT, CANCER PATIENT

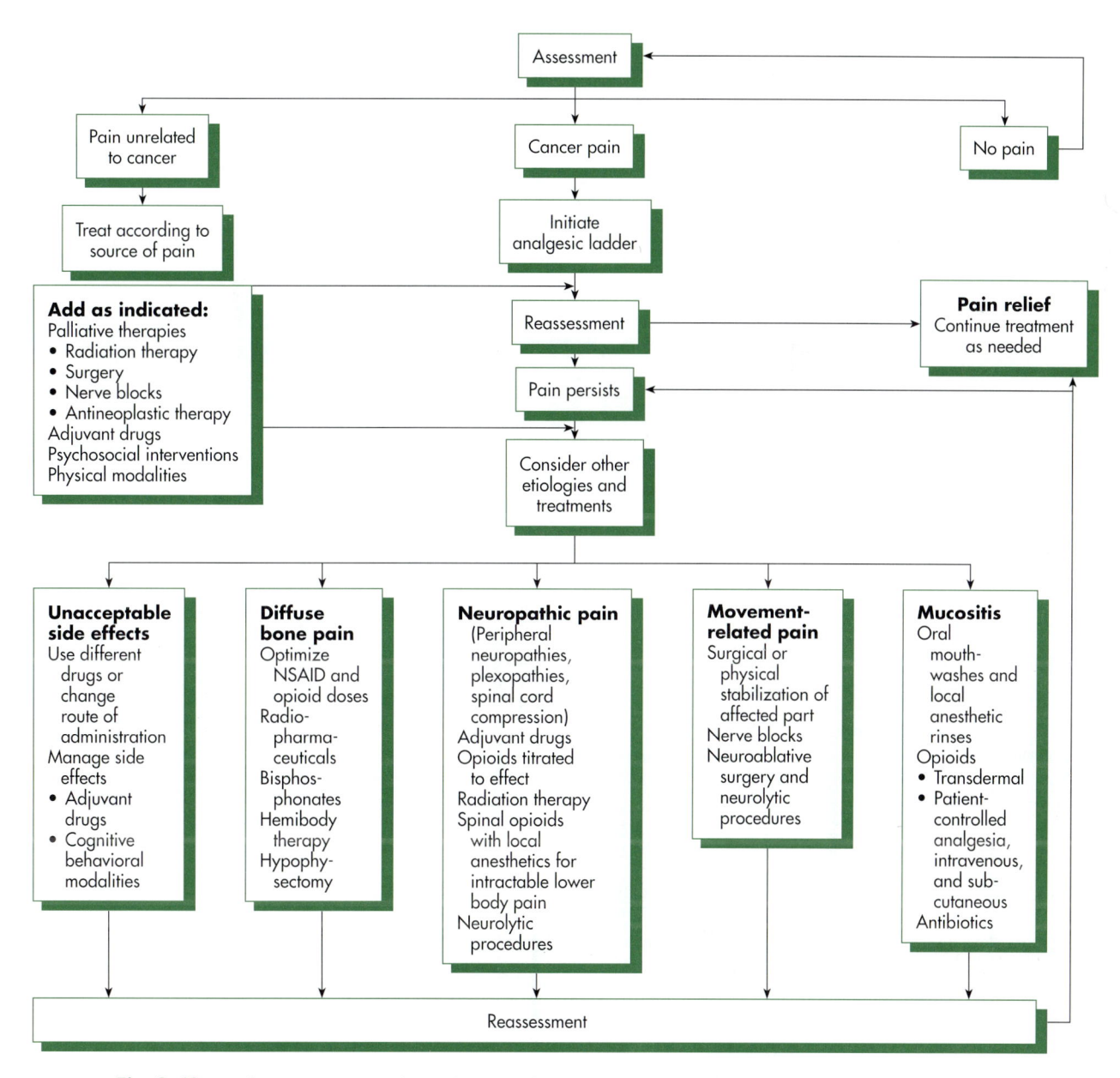

```
                              Assessment
                                  │
        ┌─────────────────────────┼─────────────────────────┐
        ▼                         ▼                         ▼
  Pain unrelated              Cancer pain                 No pain
    to cancer                     │
        │                         ▼
        ▼                     Initiate
  Treat according to         analgesic ladder
   source of pain                 │
                                  ▼                    Pain relief
  Add as indicated:           Reassessment ──────▶   Continue treatment
  Palliative therapies            │                     as needed
  • Radiation therapy             ▼
  • Surgery                   Pain persists ◀─────────────┐
  • Nerve blocks                  │
  • Antineoplastic therapy        ▼
  Adjuvant drugs              Consider other
  Psychosocial interventions  etiologies and
  Physical modalities          treatments
```

Unacceptable side effects	Diffuse bone pain	Neuropathic pain	Movement-related pain	Mucositis
Use different drugs or change route of administration Manage side effects • Adjuvant drugs • Cognitive behavioral modalities	Optimize NSAID and opioid doses Radio-pharma-ceuticals Bisphos-phonates Hemibody therapy Hypophy-sectomy	(Peripheral neuropathies, plexopathies, spinal cord compression) Adjuvant drugs Opioids titrated to effect Radiation therapy Spinal opioids with local anesthetics for intractable lower body pain Neurolytic procedures	Surgical or physical stabilization of affected part Nerve blocks Neuroablative surgery and neurolytic procedures	Oral mouth-washes and local anesthetic rinses Opioids • Transdermal • Patient-controlled analgesia, intravenous, and sub-cutaneous Antibiotics

Reassessment

Fig. 3-62 **Pain management in patients with cancer.** (From Noble J [ed]: *Primary care medicine,* ed 2, St Louis, 1996, Mosby.)

744 Pap smear abnormality

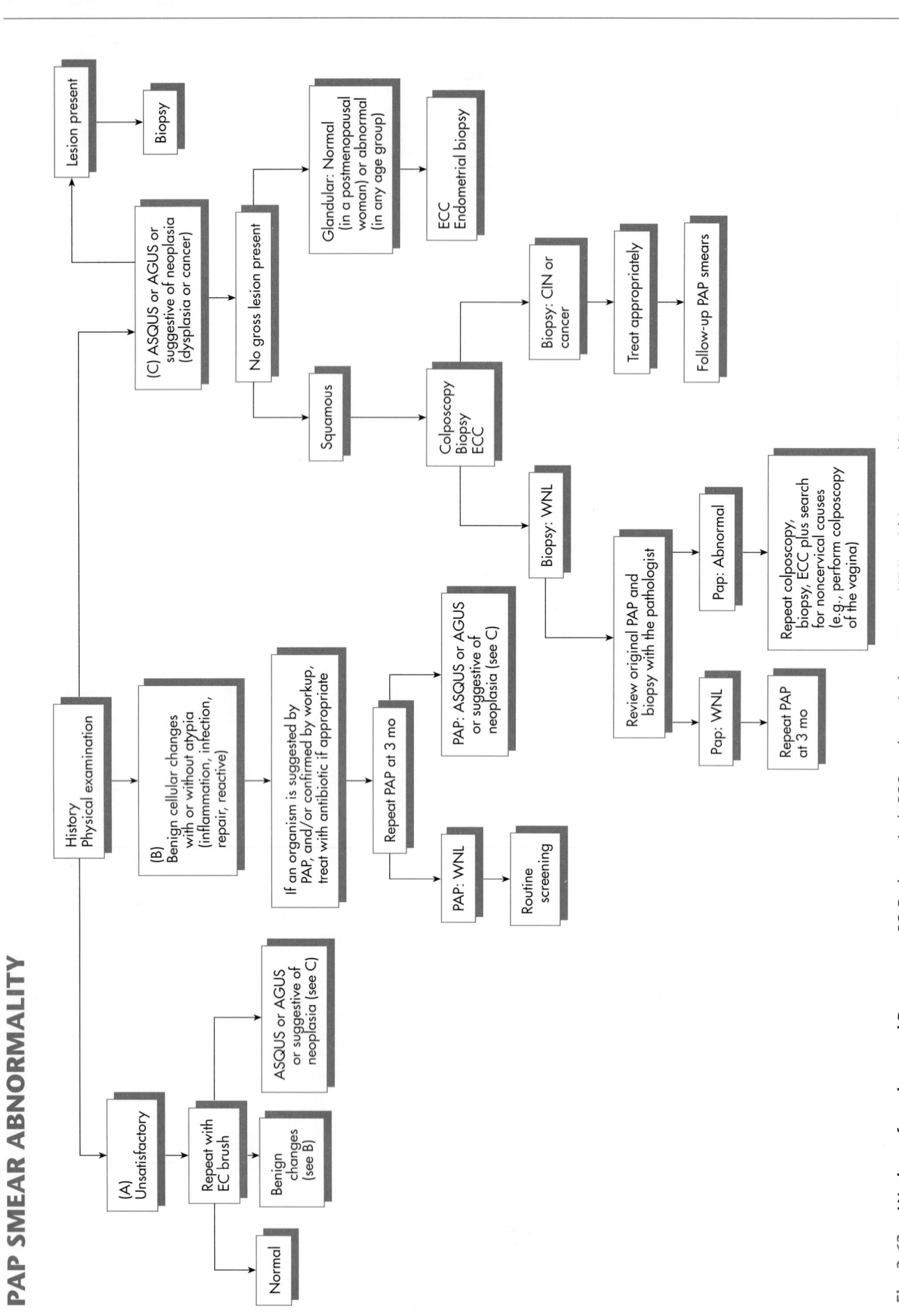

PAP SMEAR ABNORMALITY

Fig. 3-63 **Workup of an abnormal Pap smear.** *EC*, Endocervical; *ECC*, endocervical curettage; *WNL*, within normal limits; *ASQUS* or *AGUS*, atypical squamous cells or atypical glandular cells of undetermined significance. (From Noble J [ed]: *Primary care medicine*, ed 2, St Louis, 1996, Mosby.)

PELVIC MASS

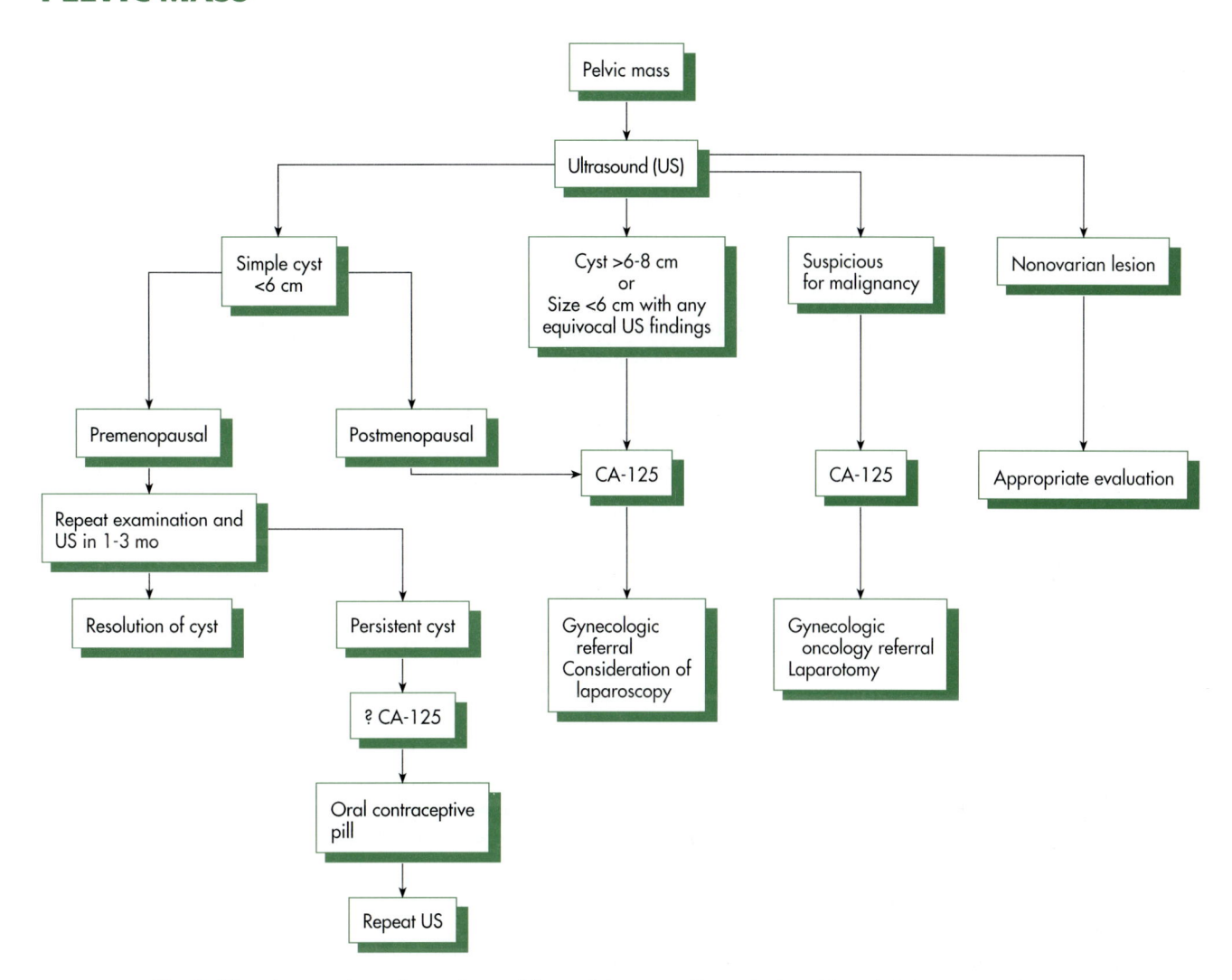

Fig. 3-64 **Approach to the patient with a pelvic mass.** (From Carlson KJ et al: *Primary care of women,* St Louis, 1995, Mosby.)

PELVIC PAIN, REPRODUCTIVE-AGE WOMAN

1. Rapid history and external abdominal examination

- **If surgical abdomen**: consider early ob/gyn/surgery consultation
  - Rupture (ectopic, cyst, abscess)
  - Torsion (adnexal, fibroid)
  - Perforation (uterine)
  - Appendicitis

2. Vital signs

- **If unstable**: Establish venous access and administer fluid bolus
  Spin Hct, type and crossmatch blood as needed
  Consider early ob/gyn/surgery consult without ultrasound
  - Rupture (ectopic, cyst)
  - Septic (abortion, abscess)
  - Placental (previa, abruptio)

3. Complete history, physical examination, and perform pelvic examination

- **If obvious abortion**: consult obstetrician and consider ultrasound
  - Abortion (incomplete, septic)

- **If late pregnancy**: forego pelvic exam
  Check for fetal heart tones
  Consider ultrasound followed by ob/gyn consultation
  - Placenta previa or abruptio
  - Premature labor contractions

4. Laboratory diagnostic workup (pregnancy test, CBC, UA/micro)

- **If pregnant**: consider ultrasound followed by ob/gyn consultation
  - R/I viable intrauterine gestation
  - R/O ectopic pregnancy, abortion, placental problems
  - R/O free intraperitoneal fluid, abscess formation

- **If not pregnant**: consider ultrasound and ob/gyn/surgery consultation
  - R/O gynecologic surgical problems
  - Ovarian cyst rupture, hemorrhage
  - Tubo-ovarian abscess rupture
  - Adnexal or fibroid torsion
  - Uterine perforation

  - Consider nonsurgical gynecologic problems
  - PID, pelvic adhesions, endometriosis, neoplasm, menstrual

  - R/O general surgery problems
  - Appendicitis and complications
  - Other, GI, GU, vascular, orthopedic surgery problems

  - Consider nonsurgical nongynecologic problems
  - Systemic illnesses

Fig. 3-65 Evaluation and management of reproductive-age women with acute pelvic pain.
(From Rosen P et al [eds]: *Emergency medicine: concepts and clinical practice,* ed 4, St Louis, 1998, Mosby.)

POLYCYTHEMIA

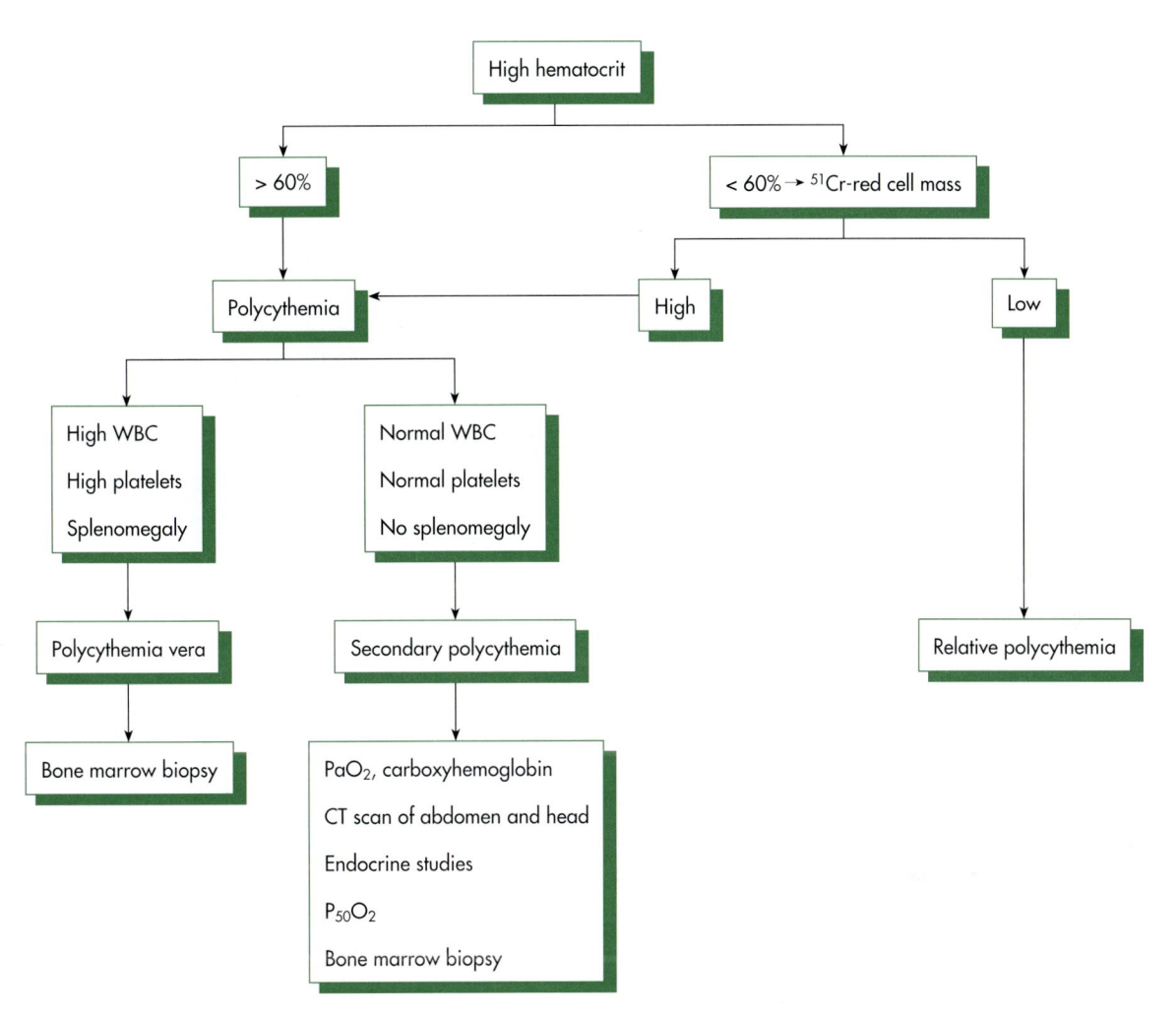

Fig. 3-66 Evaluation of a patient with a high hematocrit. (From Stein JH [ed]: *Internal medicine,* ed 4, St Louis, 1994, Mosby.)

748 Pruritus

CLINICAL ALGORITHMS

PRURITUS, GENERALIZED

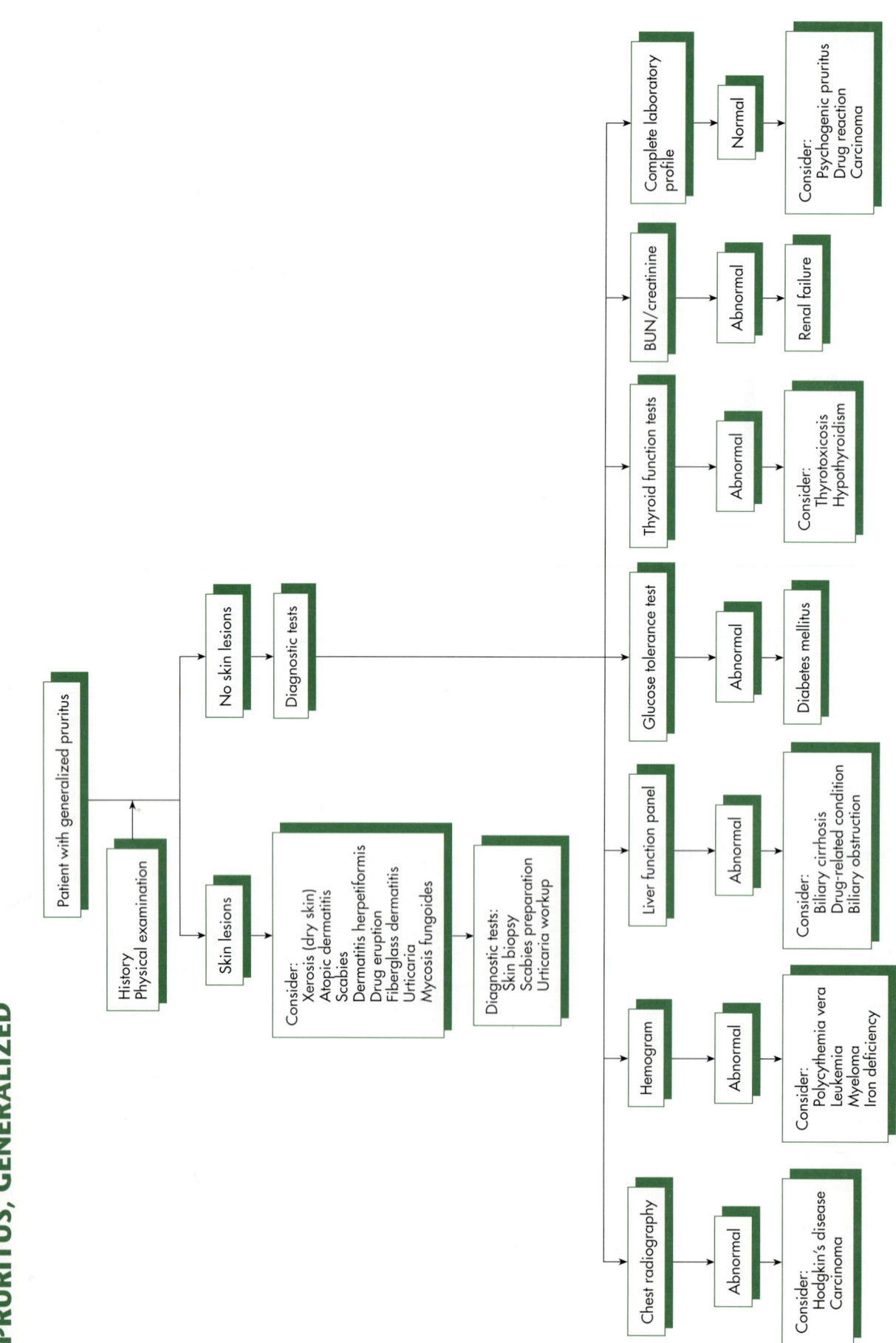

Fig. 3-67 **Evaluation of generalized pruritus.** (From Greene HL, Johnson WP, Maricic MJ: *Decision making in medicine*, St Louis, 1993, Mosby.)

CLINICAL ALGORITHMS

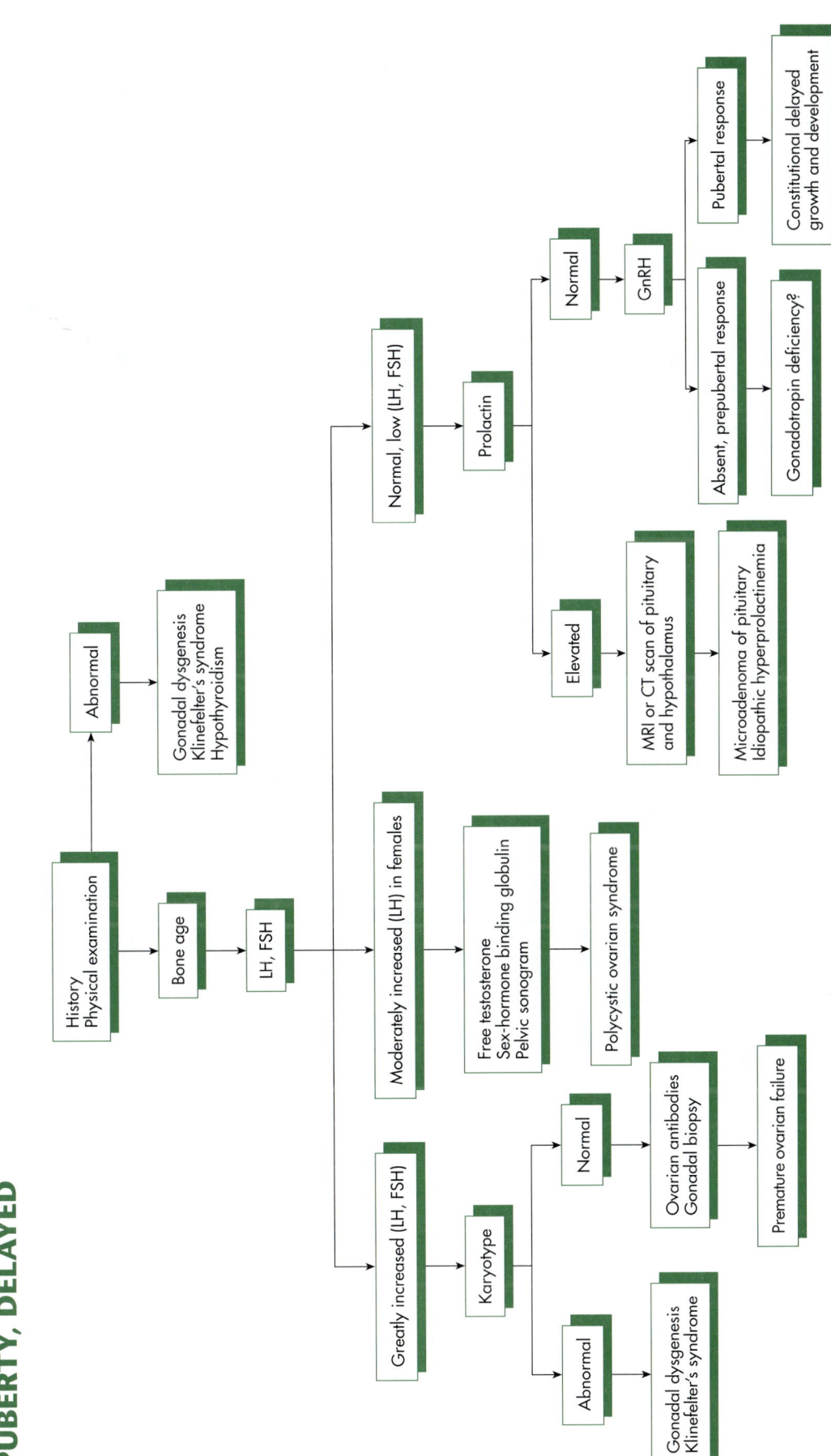

Puberty 749

PUBERTY, DELAYED

Fig. 3-68 Evaluation of patient with delayed puberty. (From Moore WT, Eastman RC: *Diagnostic endocrinology*, ed 2, St Louis, 1996, Mosby.)

PUBERTY, PRECOCIOUS

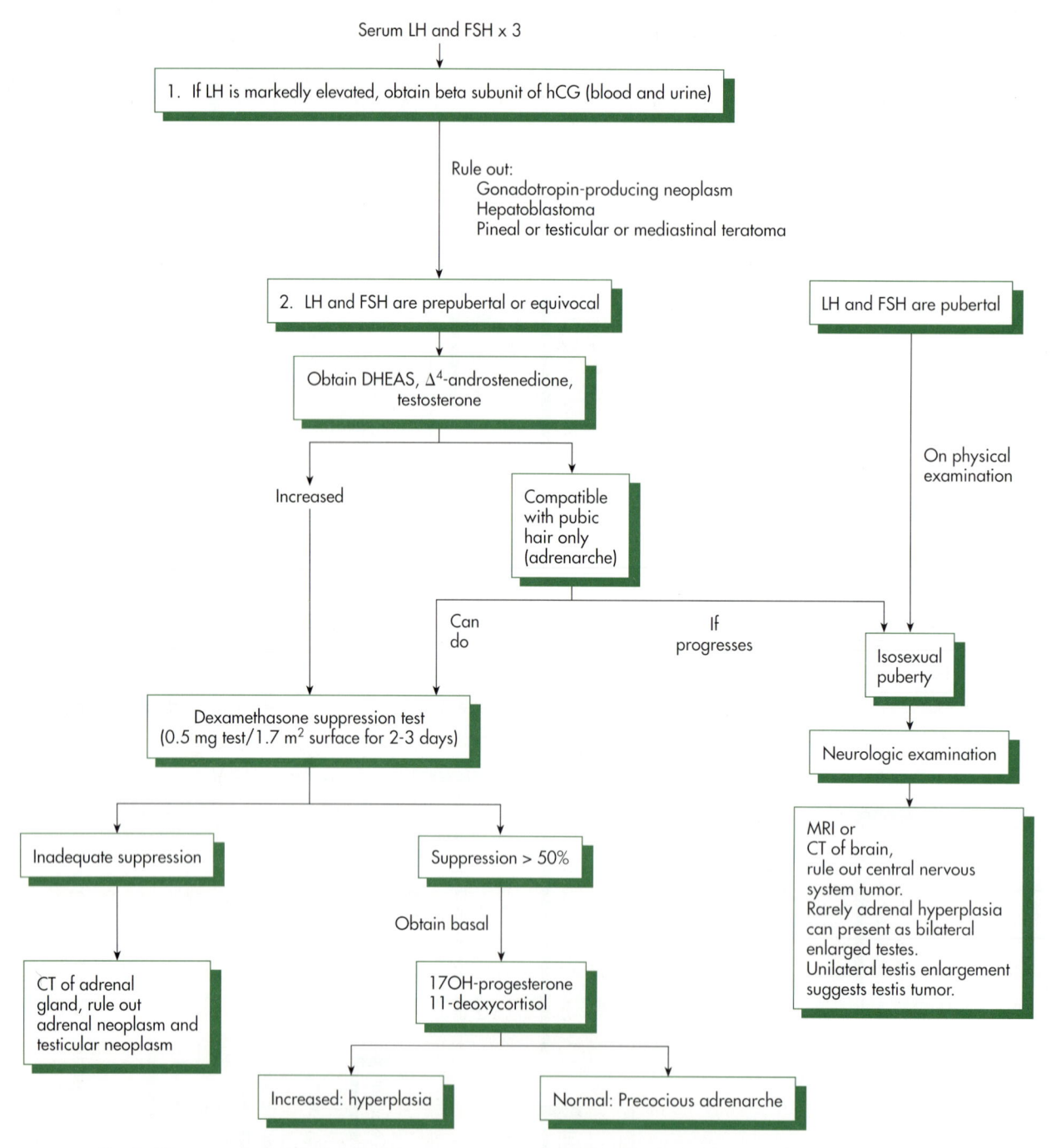

Fig. 3-69 Evaluation of precocious puberty, excluding factitious and iatrogenic causes. (Modified from Odell WD: The physiology of puberty: disorders of the pubertal process. In DeGroot LJ, et al, eds: *Endocrinology*, vol 3, New York, 1979, Grune & Stratton.)

PULMONARY NODULE

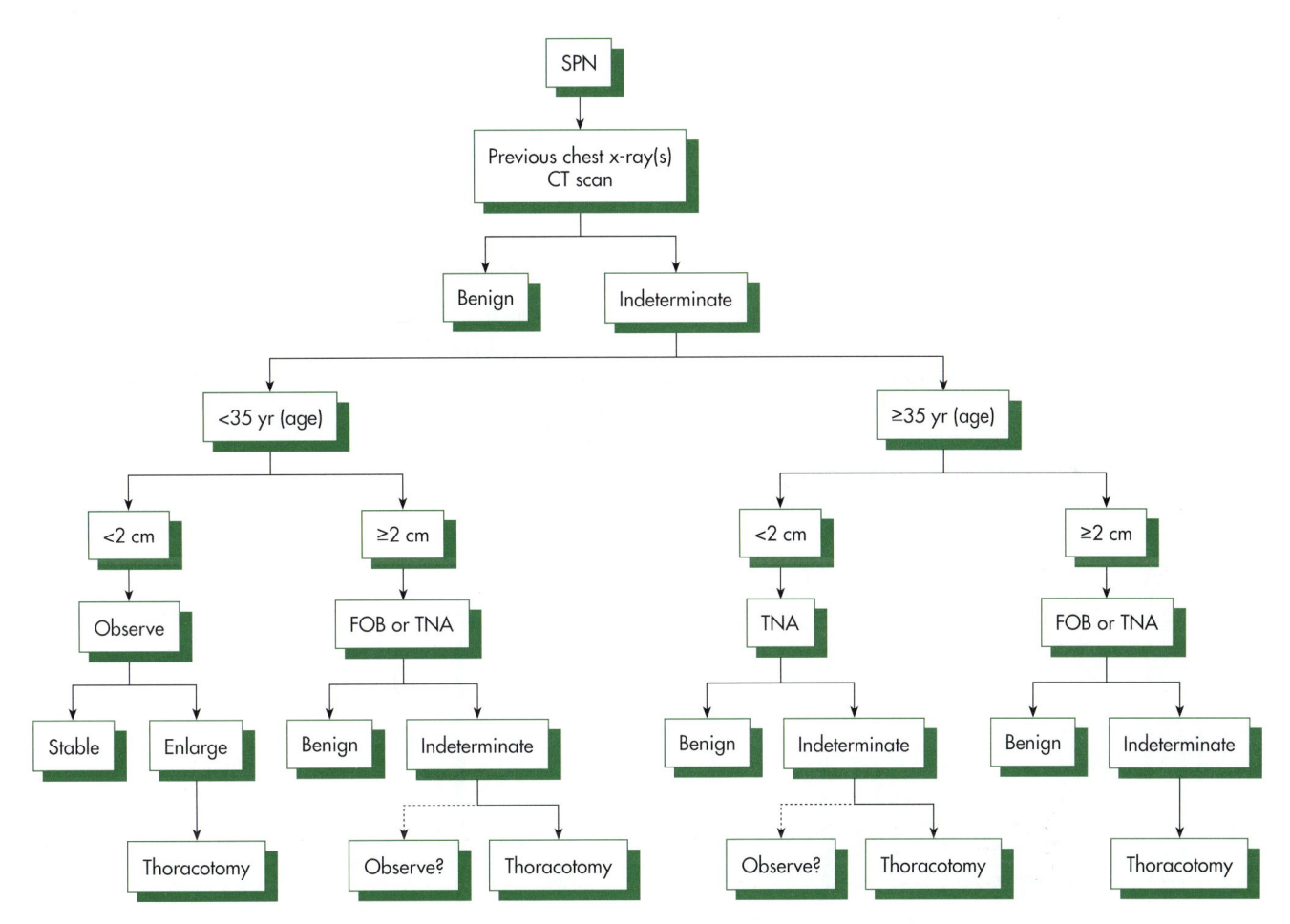

Fig. 3-70 Approach to solitary pulmonary nodule. *FOB,* Fiberoptic bronchoscopy; *SPN,* solitary pulmonary nodule; *TNA,* transthoracic needle aspiration. (From Noble J [ed]: *Primary care medicine,* ed 2, St Louis, 1996, Mosby.)

PULSELESS ELECTRICAL ACTIVITY (PEA)

The term PEA (Pulseless Electrical Activity) has been added to AHA Guidelines in an attempt to *unify* an otherwise complex group of cardiac rhythms. Similarities among the entities included in this group are that they all share a common list of potential etiologies and that they generally respond to the same treatment protocol. It should be noted that this newer term encompasses many rhythms that had previously been designated as EMD (ElectroMechanical Dissociation).

Clinically, the meaning of the term PEA is suggested by its name. Thus, the term is used to describe a group of diverse electrocardiographic rhythms that by definition manifest evidence of Electrical Activity (since they all produce an ECG rhythm) but which are unified by the clinical finding of pulselessness. According to this definition, PEA rhythms must therefore be *nonperfusing*—or at most no more than *minimally* perfusing—(since they are by definition associated with the pulseless state).

Many types of ECG rhythms have been associated with the clinical entity known as PEA. Most of these rhythms can be classified into one of the following groups:

- **EMD Rhythms** - in which there is an organized ECG rhythm (usually with a narrow QRS complex)- but no pulse.
- **Pseudo-EMD Rhythms** - in which the ECG rhythm is associated with at least some meaningful mechanical contraction (as might be evidenced by obtaining a pulse with doppler that is too faint to palpate clinically).
- **Idioventricular** or **Ventricular Escape Rhythms** - in which the QRS complex of the escape rhythm is widened. Atrial activity is absent. There is no pulse. Included in this group are *postdefibrillation* idioventricular rhythms.
- **Bradyasystolic Rhythms** - in which there is profound bradycardia, often with prolonged periods of asystole. There is no pulse.

Key treatment options

Begin/continue CPR
- Early performance of CPR is essential (since by definition PEA is a *non-perfusing* or poorly perfusing rhythm).
- Supportive actions (intubate/establish IV access, etc.).
- Assess blood flow and other clinical parameters (i.e., use of doppler, End-Tidal CO₂, arterial line as possible).

Epinephrine
- Begin with an SDE dose (i.e., 1.0 mg by IV bolus).
- May either repeat SDE (every 3-5 minutes as needed) or increase the dose (i.e., to HDE) if there has been no response.

Search for the cause of PEA
- Consider the most common causes
  a) Inadequate ventilation?
  b) Inadequate circulation?
  c) Metabolic disorder?
- Once detected, try to correct the underlying/precipitating cause.
- Consider empiric volume infusion (since hypovolemia is probably the most common potentially correctable cause of PEA).

Conditions most likely to cause a PEA rhythm

Inadequate ventilation
- Intubation of right mainstem bronchus or other cause of hypoxemia
- Tension pneumothorax (trauma, asthma, patient on ventilator)
- Bilateral pneumothorax (trauma)

Inadequate circulation
- Pericardial effusion with tamponade (trauma, pericarditis, uremia, too vigorous CPR)
- Myocardial rupture or rupture of aortic aneurysm
- Massive pulmonary embolism
- Hypovolemia caused by
  • Acute blood loss (trauma, GI bleeding)
  • Dehydration
  • Septic shock
  • Cardiogenic shock (acute MI, myocardial contusion)
  • Anaphylactic shock
  • Neurogenic shock (cervical spine fracture)

Metabolic disorders
- Electrolyte disturbance (severe hyperkalemia, hypokalemia, hypomagnesemia)
- Persistent severe acidosis (diabetic ketoacidosis, lactic acidosis)
- Overdose of cardiac depressant drugs (tricyclic antidepressants)
- Hypothermia

Consider other options
- Atropine is likely to be helpful only if the PEA rhythm is associated with absolute or relative bradycardia. Give 1 mg IV; may repeat every 3-5 minutes (as needed); up to a total dose of 0.04 mg/kg (= 3mg).
- Pacing is likely to be helpful only if PEA is due to temporarily disturbed conduction (as may occur in some cases of drug overdose).

NOTE: The ECG appearance of a PEA rhythm may provide insight as to the relative likelihood that the condition can be reversed. In general, prognosis tends to be better if the ECG rhythm manifests organized atrial activity (in the form of P waves that conduct), a rate that is not excessively slow, and narrow QRS complexes, provided (of course) that the underlying cause of the PEA rhythm can be identified and corrected.
In contrast, PEA is much more likely to be a preterminal rhythm when organized atrial activity is absent, the QRS complex is wide, and/or bradycardia persists despite medical treatment.

Fig. 3-71 Pulseless electrical activity (PEA). (Adapted from Grauer K, Cavallaro D: *ACLS: Rapid review and case scenarios*, ed 4, St Louis, 1996, Mosby and from American Heart Association ACLS Textbook, 1994.)

PURPURA, PALPABLE

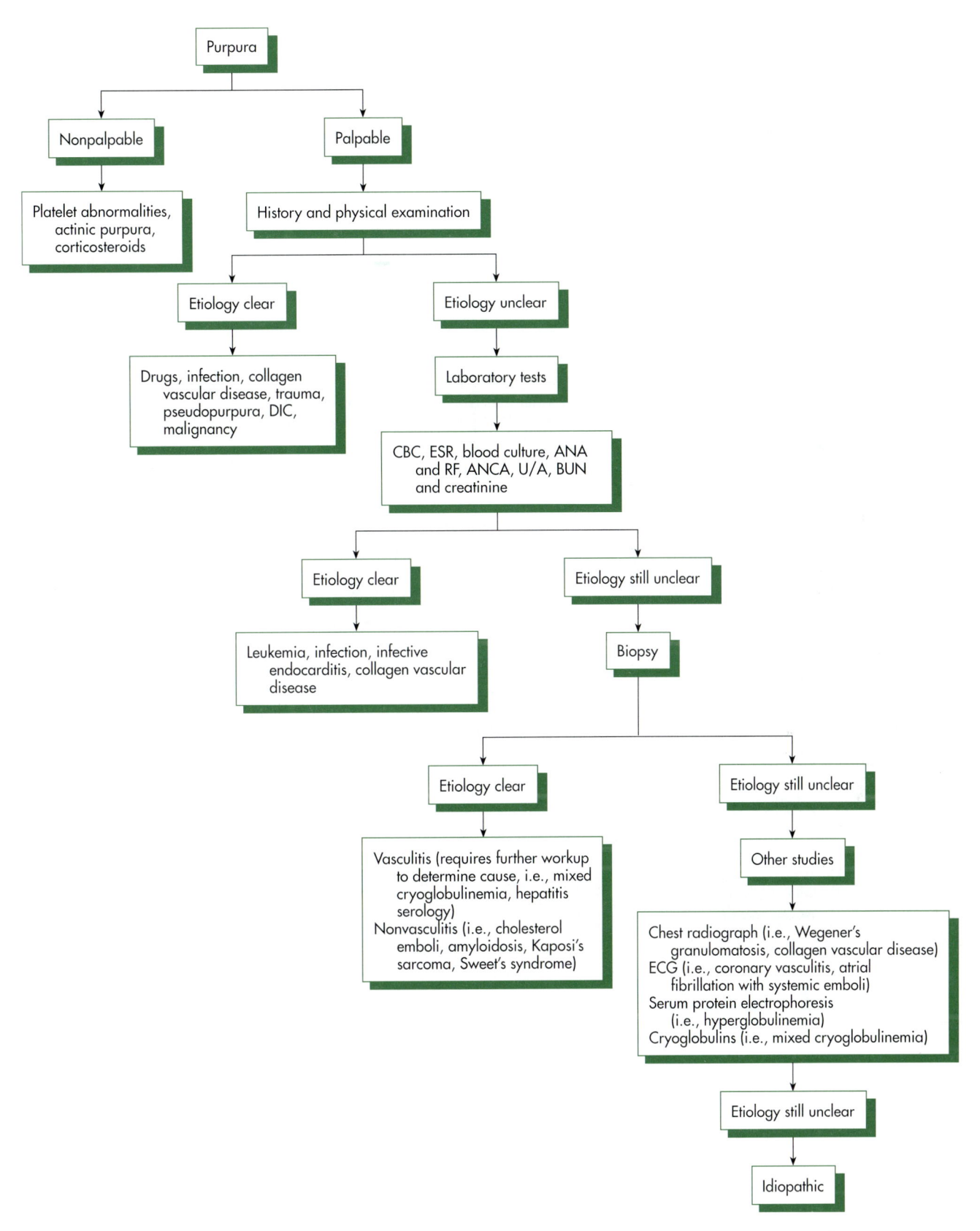

Fig. 3-72 **Diagnostic algorithm for palpable purpura.** *DIC,* Disseminated intravascular coagulation; *CBC,* complete blood cell count; *ESR,* erythrocyte sedimentation rate; *ANA,* antinuclear antibody; *RF,* rheumatoid factor; *ANCA,* antineutrophil cytoplasmic antibody test; *U/A,* urinalysis; *BUN,* blood urea nitrogen; *ECG,* electrocardiogram. (From Stevens GL, Adelman HM, Wallach PM: Palpable purpura: an algorithmic approach, *Am Fam Physician* 52:1355-1362, 1995.)

RHINORRHEA

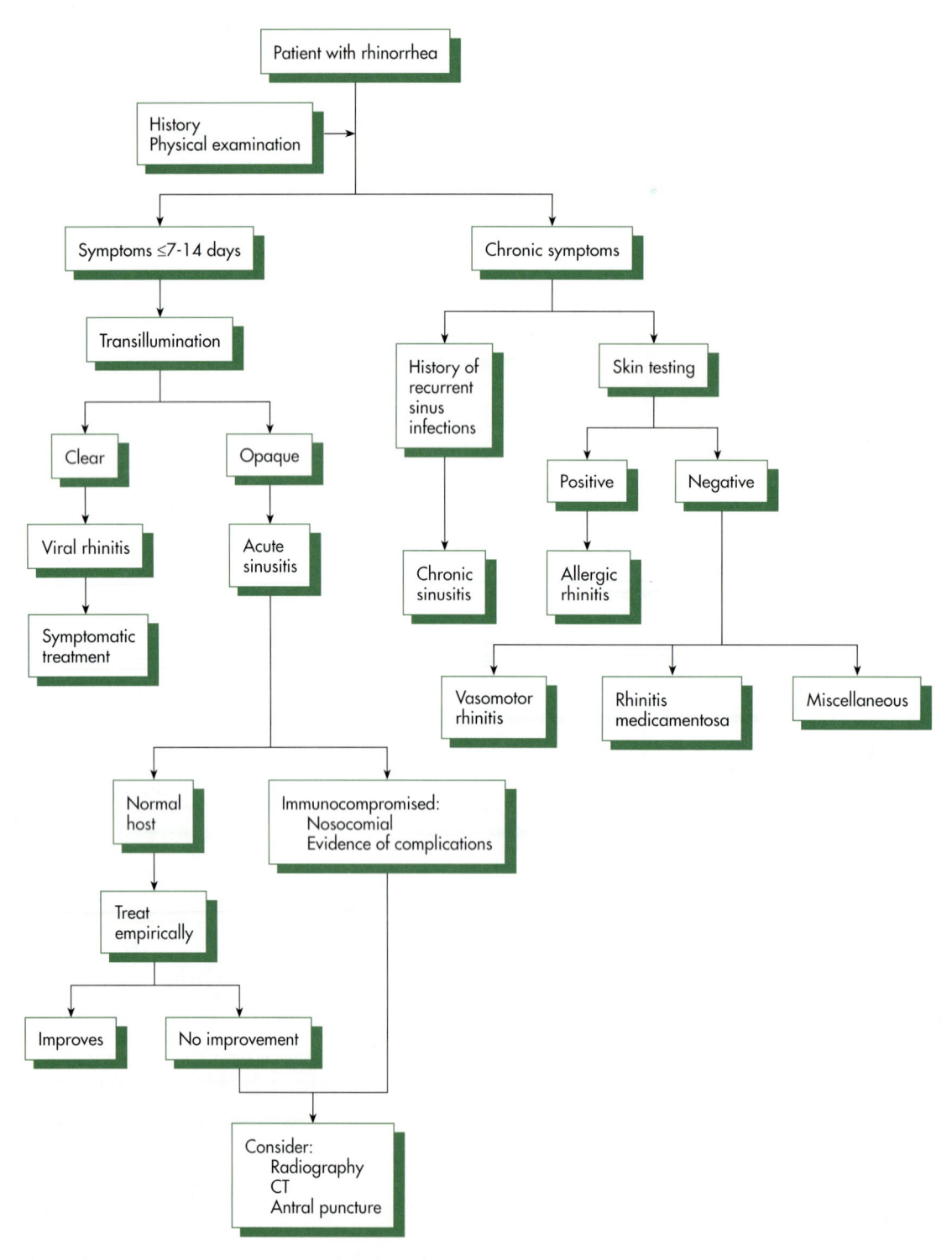

Fig. 3-73 Treatment of a patient with rhinorrhea. (From Noble J [ed]: *Primary care medicine,* ed 2, St Louis, 1996, Mosby.)

CLINICAL ALGORITHMS

SCROTAL MASS

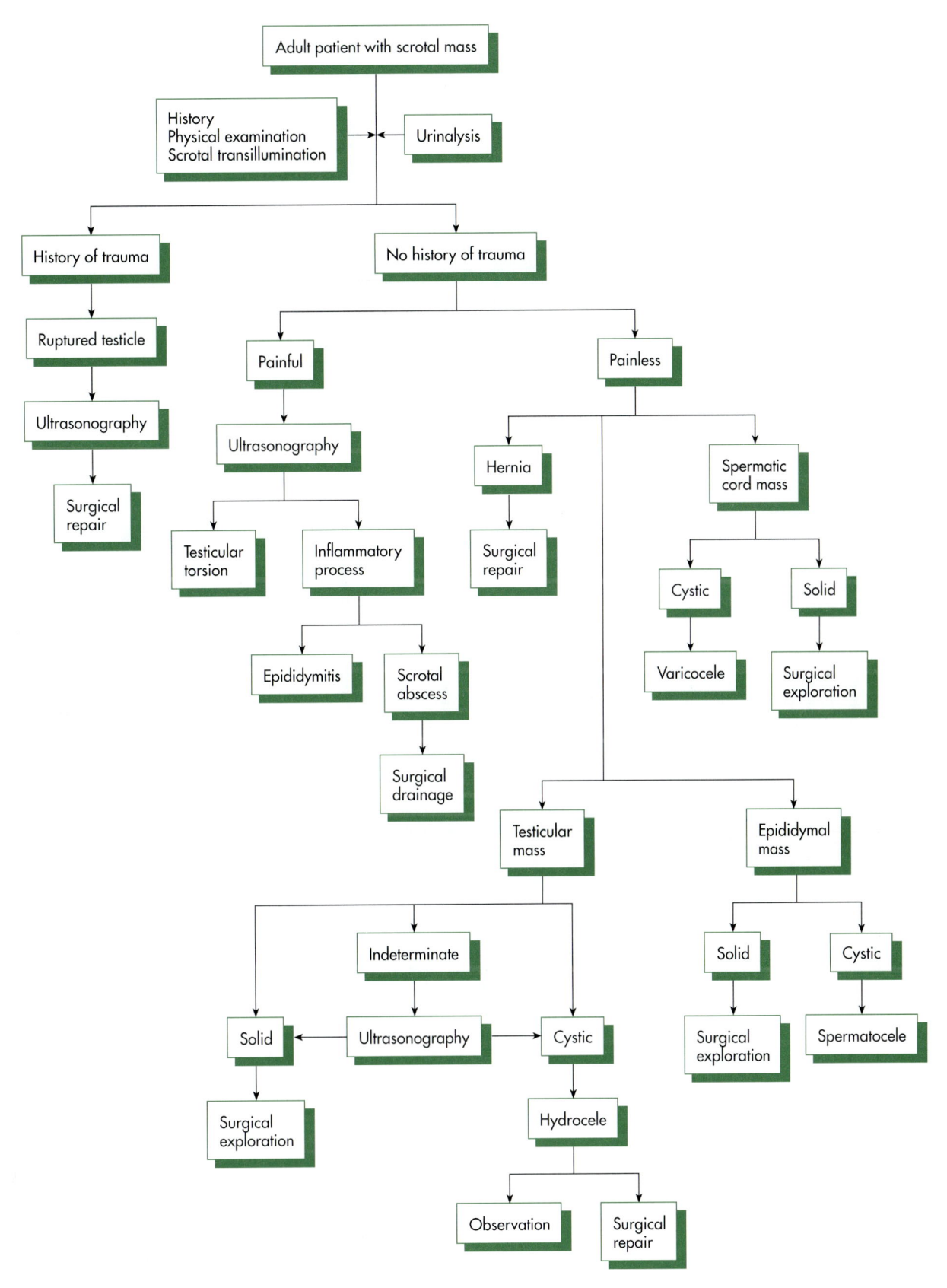

Fig. 3-74 Evaluation of scrotal mass. (From Greene HL, Johnson WP, Maricic MJ: *Decision making in medicine,* St Louis, 1993, Mosby.)

756 Sexual dysfunction

SEXUAL DYSFUNCTION

Fig. 3-75 Evaluation of sexual dysfunction. (From Greene HL, Johnson WP, Maricic MJ: *Decision making in medicine*, St Louis, 1993, Mosby.)

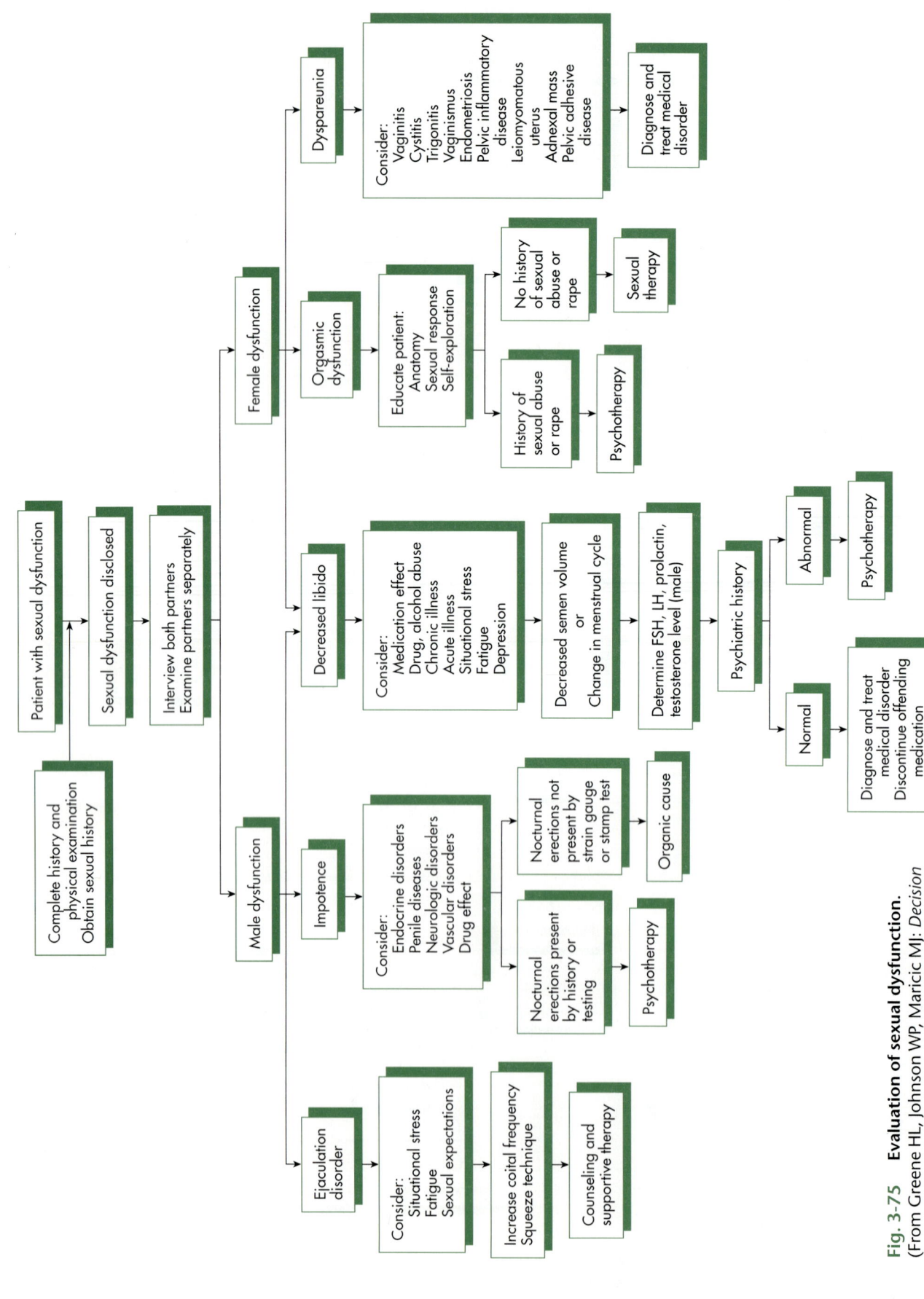

CLINICAL ALGORITHMS

Sleep disorders

SLEEP DISORDERS

A, Patient with sleep disturbance
↓
History
↓
- Insomnia
- Hypersomnia → See Algorithm **B**
- Sleep-associated affective and behavioral disturbance → See Algorithm **C**

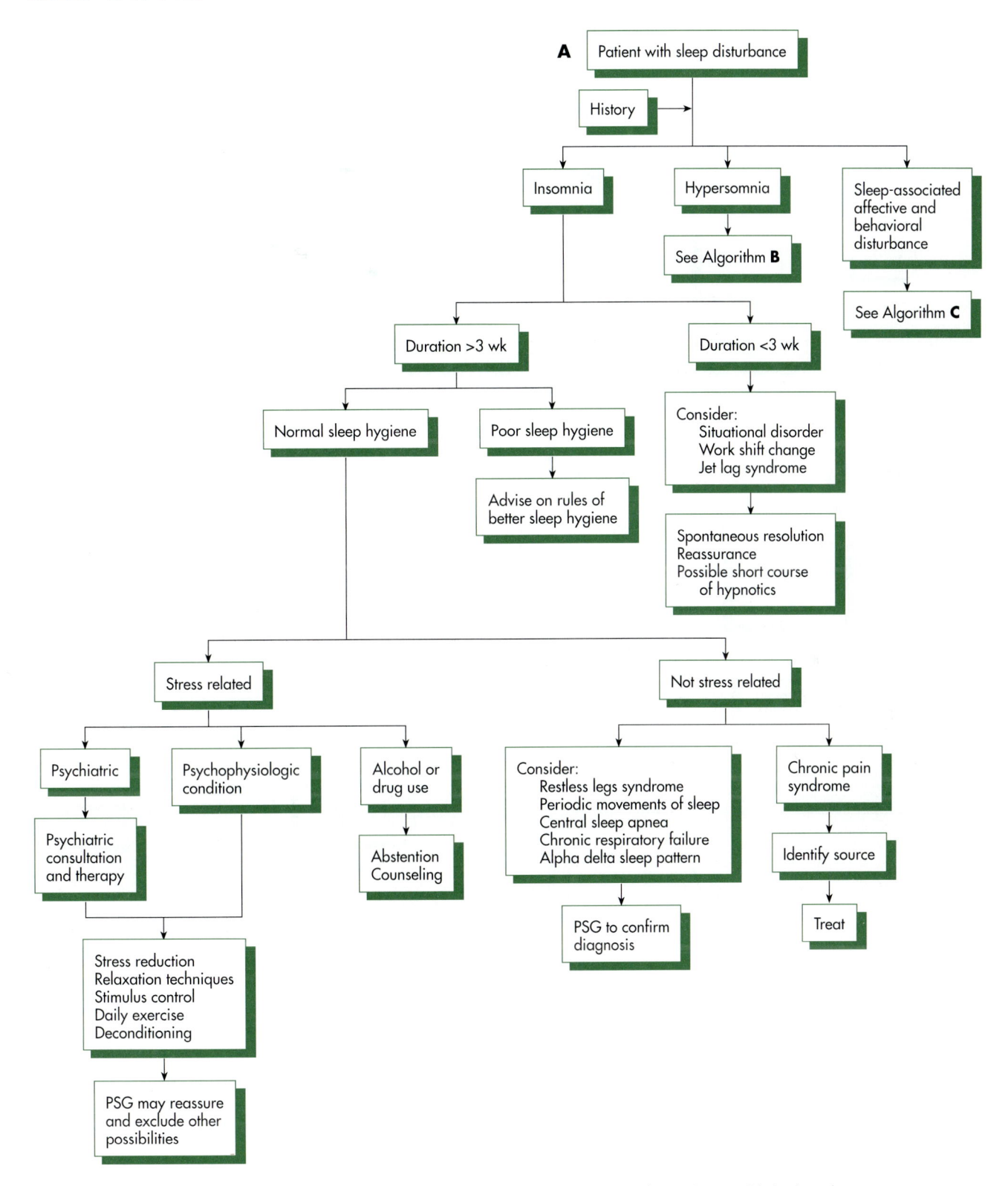

Insomnia:
- Duration >3 wk
  - Normal sleep hygiene
  - Poor sleep hygiene → Advise on rules of better sleep hygiene
- Duration <3 wk
  - Consider:
    - Situational disorder
    - Work shift change
    - Jet lag syndrome
  - Spontaneous resolution
  - Reassurance
  - Possible short course of hypnotics

Normal sleep hygiene:

Stress related:
- Psychiatric → Psychiatric consultation and therapy
- Psychophysiologic condition
- Alcohol or drug use → Abstention Counseling

Stress reduction
Relaxation techniques
Stimulus control
Daily exercise
Deconditioning
↓
PSG may reassure and exclude other possibilities

Not stress related:
- Consider:
  - Restless legs syndrome
  - Periodic movements of sleep
  - Central sleep apnea
  - Chronic respiratory failure
  - Alpha delta sleep pattern
  → PSG to confirm diagnosis
- Chronic pain syndrome → Identify source → Treat

Fig. 3-76 **A, Patient with sleep disturbance.** *PSG*, Polysomnography; *MSLT*, multiple sleep latency tests. (From Greene HL, Johnson WP, Maricic MJ: *Decision making in medicine,* St Louis, 1993, Mosby.)

758 Sleep disorders

SLEEP DISORDERS—cont'd

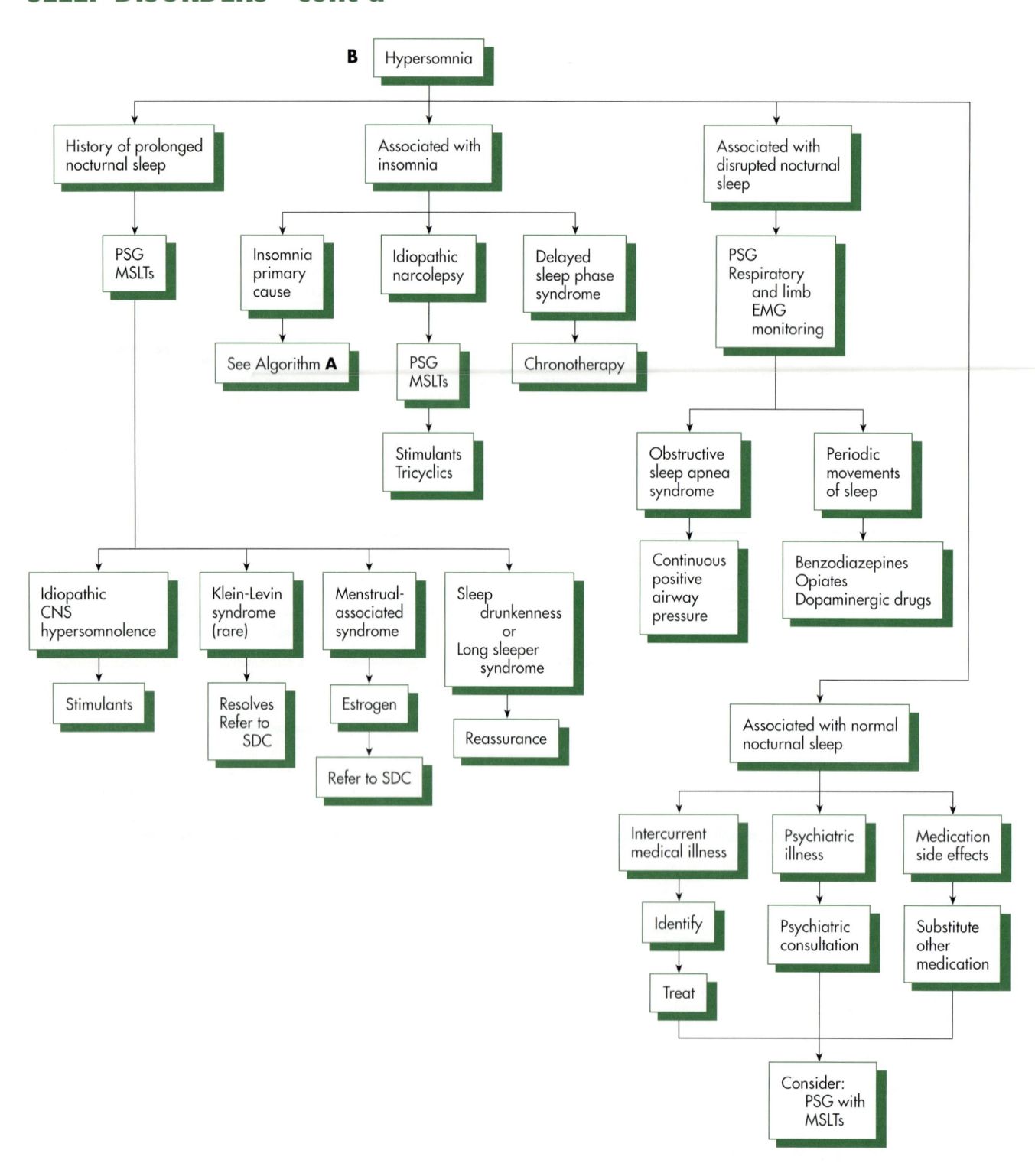

Fig. 3-76—cont'd **B**, Hypersomnia.

SLEEP DISORDERS—cont'd

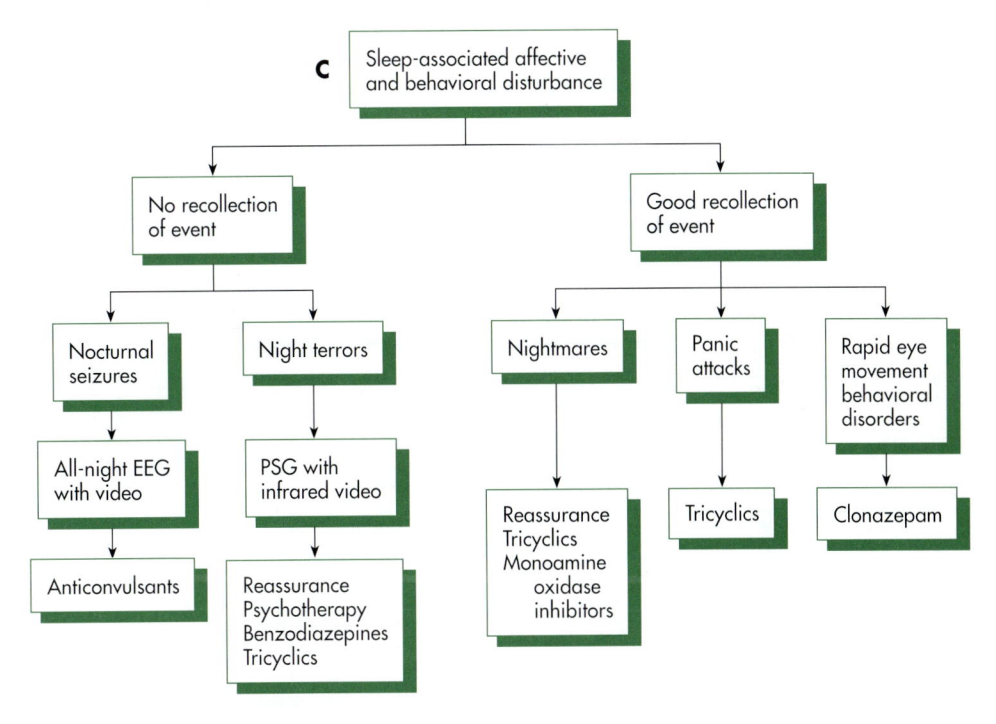

```
                    ┌─────────────────────────┐
                 C  │ Sleep-associated affective│
                    │ and behavioral disturbance│
                    └─────────────────────────┘
                        │                │
            ┌───────────┘                └───────────┐
   ┌────────────────┐                      ┌────────────────┐
   │ No recollection │                      │ Good recollection│
   │    of event     │                      │    of event     │
   └────────────────┘                      └────────────────┘
       │        │                          │        │        │
  ┌─────────┐ ┌──────────┐           ┌──────────┐ ┌────────┐ ┌────────────┐
  │Nocturnal│ │  Night   │           │Nightmares│ │ Panic  │ │ Rapid eye  │
  │seizures │ │ terrors  │           │          │ │attacks │ │ movement   │
  └─────────┘ └──────────┘           └──────────┘ └────────┘ │ behavioral │
       │          │                       │          │      │ disorders  │
       ↓          ↓                       ↓          ↓      └────────────┘
  ┌─────────┐ ┌──────────┐           ┌──────────┐ ┌────────┐       ↓
  │All-night│ │  PSG with│           │Reassurance│ │Tricyclics│ ┌────────────┐
  │EEG with │ │ infrared │           │Tricyclics│ └────────┘  │ Clonazepam │
  │  video  │ │  video   │           │Monoamine │             └────────────┘
  └─────────┘ └──────────┘           │ oxidase  │
       ↓          ↓                  │inhibitors│
  ┌─────────┐ ┌──────────┐           └──────────┘
  │Anticon- │ │Reassurance│
  │vulsants │ │Psychotherapy│
  └─────────┘ │Benzodiazepines│
              │Tricyclics│
              └──────────┘
```

Fig. 3-76—cont'd   **C,** Sleep-associated affective and behavioral disturbance.

SPINAL INJURY, CERVICAL

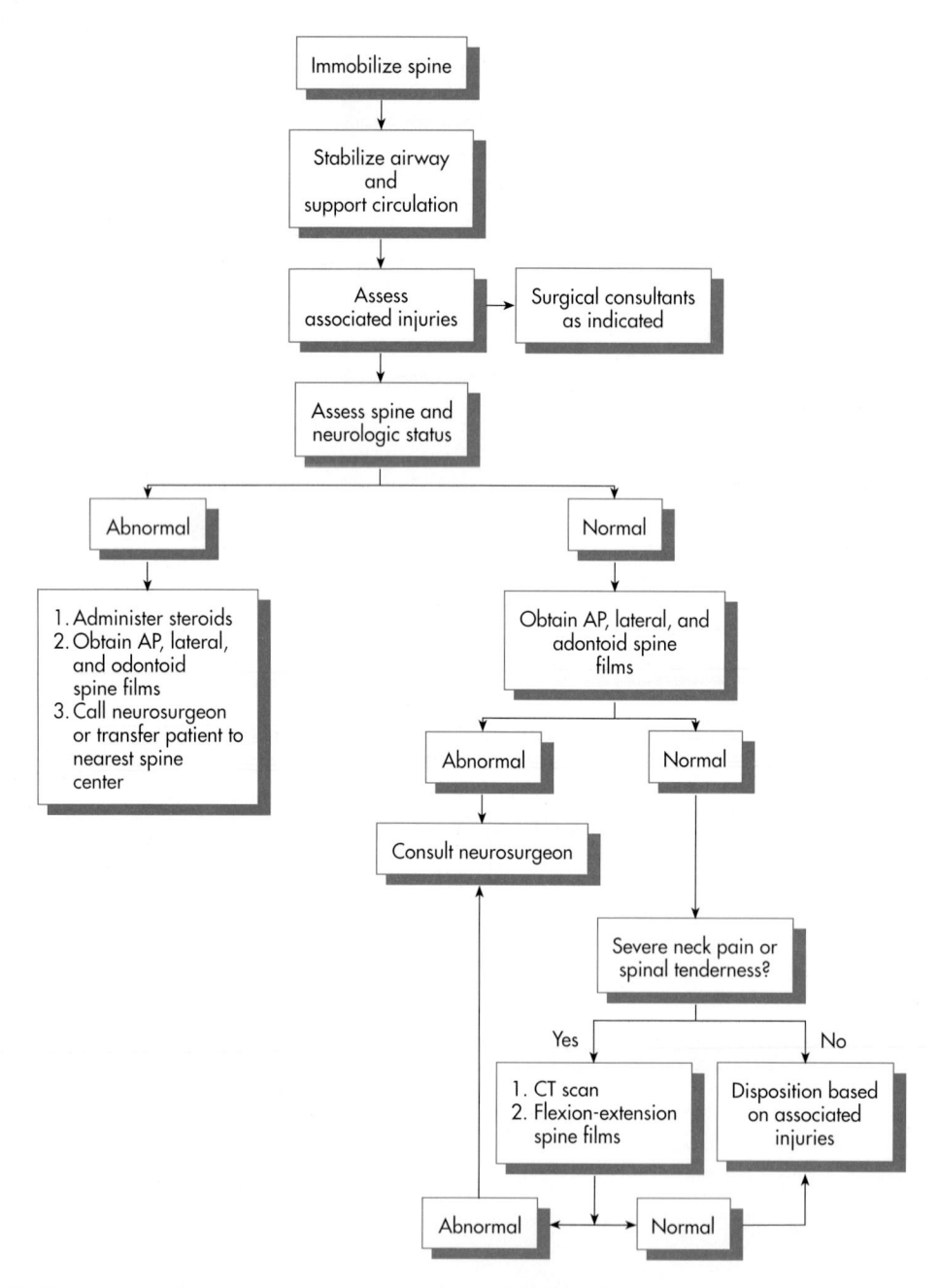

Fig. 3-77 **Approach to patient with suspected cervical spinal injury.** (From Rosen P et al [eds]: *Emergency medicine: concepts and clinical practice,* St Louis, 1997, Mosby.)

SPLENOMEGALY

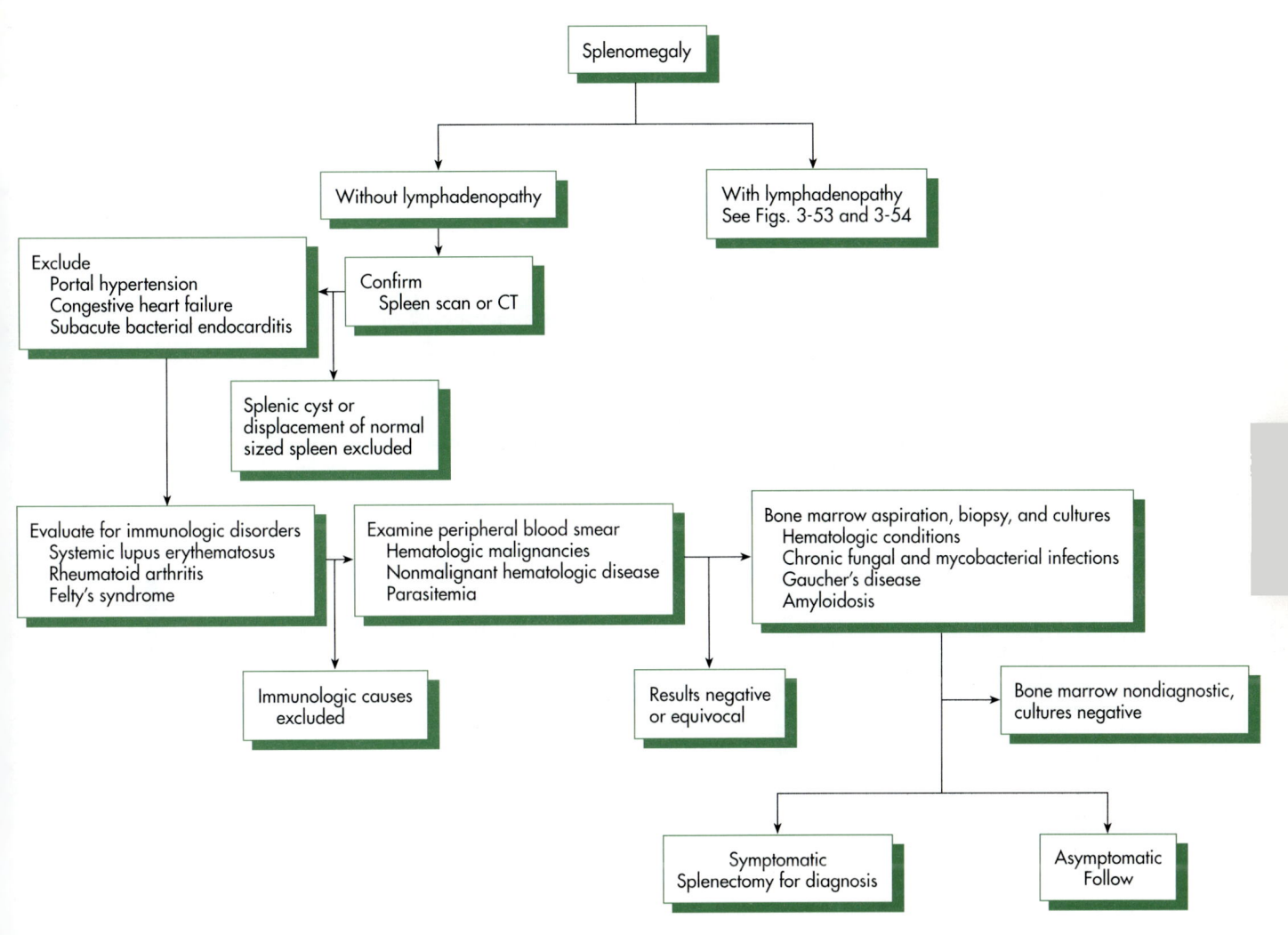

```
                          ┌──────────────┐
                          │ Splenomegaly │
                          └──────┬───────┘
                    ┌────────────┴────────────┐
          ┌─────────▼─────────┐      ┌────────▼─────────────┐
          │ Without            │      │ With lymphadenopathy │
          │ lymphadenopathy    │      │ See Figs. 3-53 and   │
          └─────────┬──────────┘      │ 3-54                 │
                    │                 └──────────────────────┘
         ┌──────────▼──────────┐
         │ Confirm             │
         │ Spleen scan or CT   │
         └──────────┬──────────┘
```

- **Exclude**
  - Portal hypertension
  - Congestive heart failure
  - Subacute bacterial endocarditis

- Splenic cyst or displacement of normal sized spleen excluded

- **Evaluate for immunologic disorders**
  - Systemic lupus erythematosus
  - Rheumatoid arthritis
  - Felty's syndrome

- **Examine peripheral blood smear**
  - Hematologic malignancies
  - Nonmalignant hematologic disease
  - Parasitemia

- **Bone marrow aspiration, biopsy, and cultures**
  - Hematologic conditions
  - Chronic fungal and mycobacterial infections
  - Gaucher's disease
  - Amyloidosis

- Immunologic causes excluded
- Results negative or equivocal
- Bone marrow nondiagnostic, cultures negative

- Symptomatic — Splenectomy for diagnosis
- Asymptomatic — Follow

Fig. 3-78 **Clinical approach to patient with splenomegaly.** (From Stein JH [ed]: *Internal medicine,* ed 5, St Louis, 1998, Mosby.)

TACHYCARDIA, NARROW COMPLEX

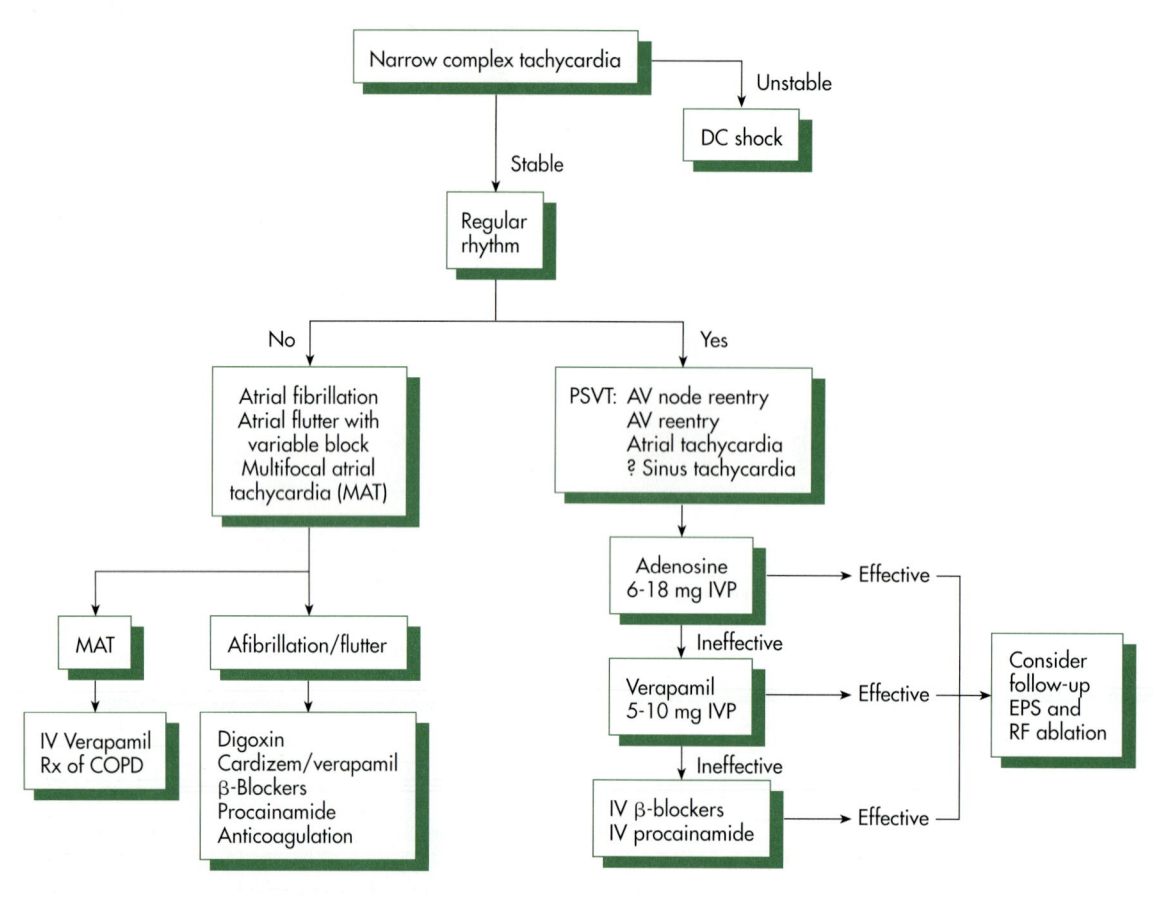

Fig. 3-79 **Evaluation and management of narrow complex tachycardia.** (From Driscoll CE et al: *The family practice desk reference,* ed 3, St Louis, 1996, Mosby.)

CLINICAL ALGORITHMS Tachycardia 763

TACHYCARDIA, WIDE COMPLEX

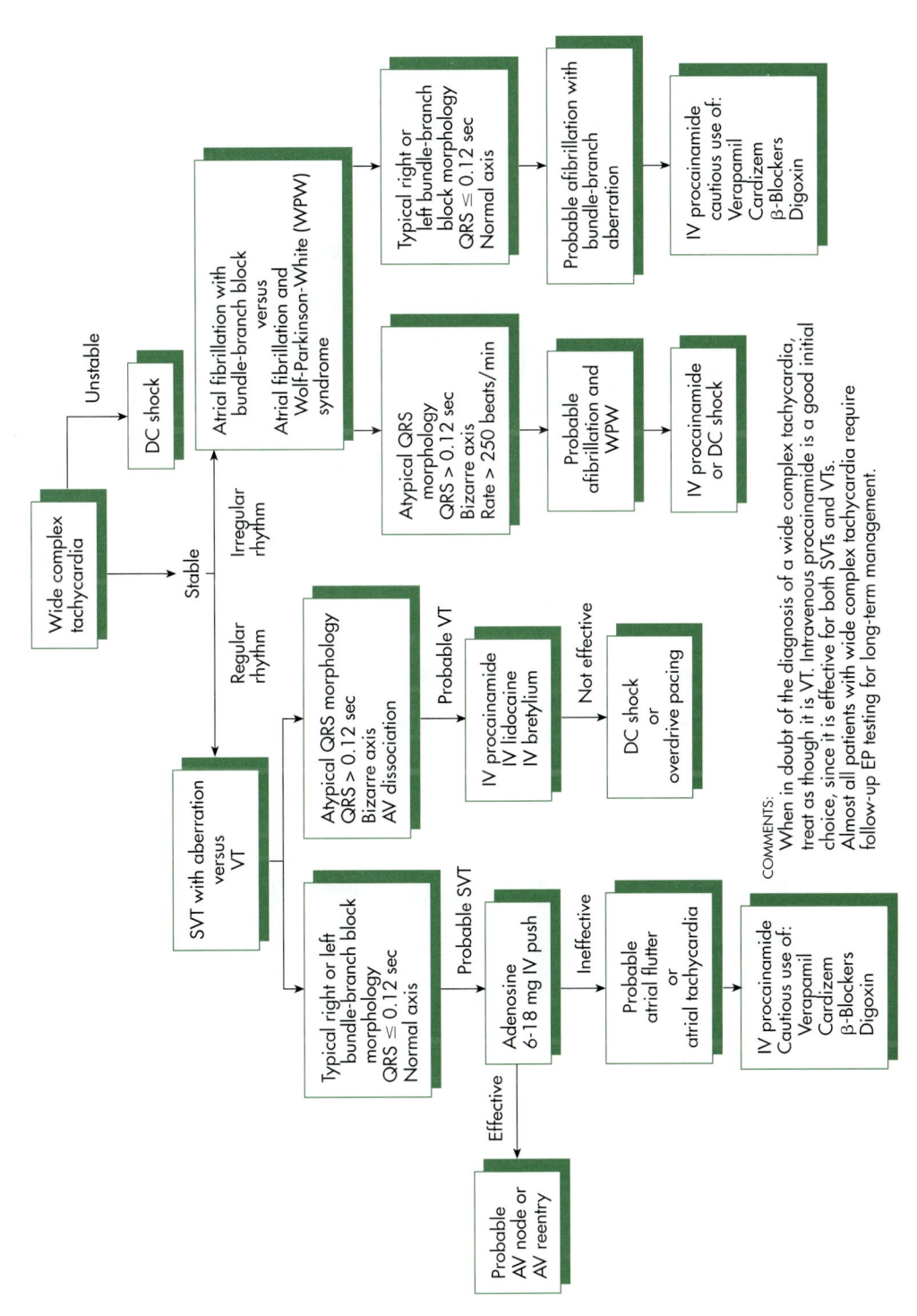

Fig. 3-80 Evaluation and management of wide complex tachycardia. (From Driscoll CE et al: *The family practice desk reference,* ed 3, St Louis, 1996, Mosby.)

Thrombocytopenia

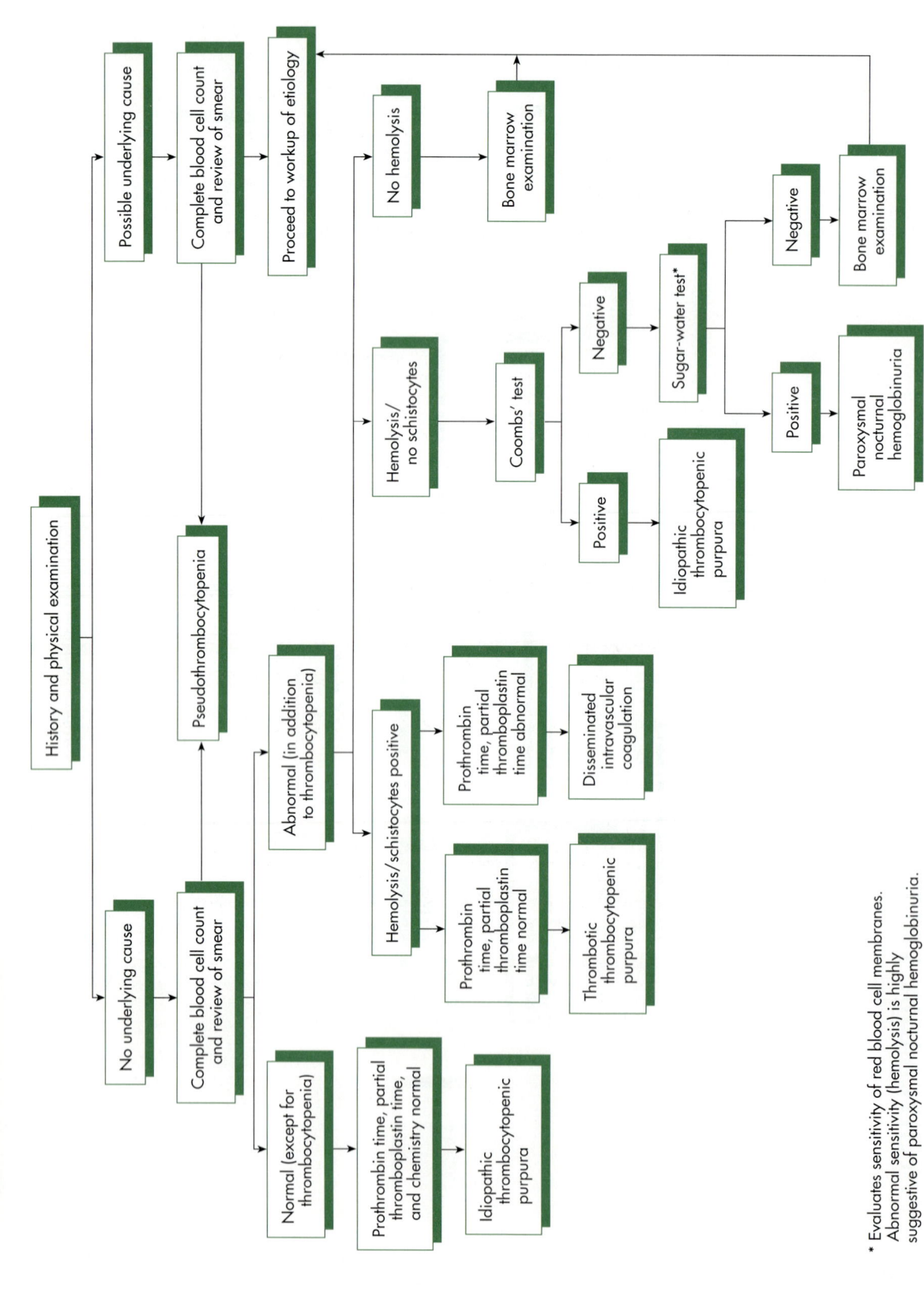

Fig. 3-81 Diagnosis of thrombocytopenia. (From Goldstein KH, Abramson N: Efficient diagnosis of thrombocytopenia, *Am Fam Physician* 53:915-920, 1996.)

*Evaluates sensitivity of red blood cell membranes. Abnormal sensitivity (hemolysis) is highly suggestive of paroxysmal nocturnal hemoglobinuria.

THROMBOLYTIC THERAPY IN ACUTE MI

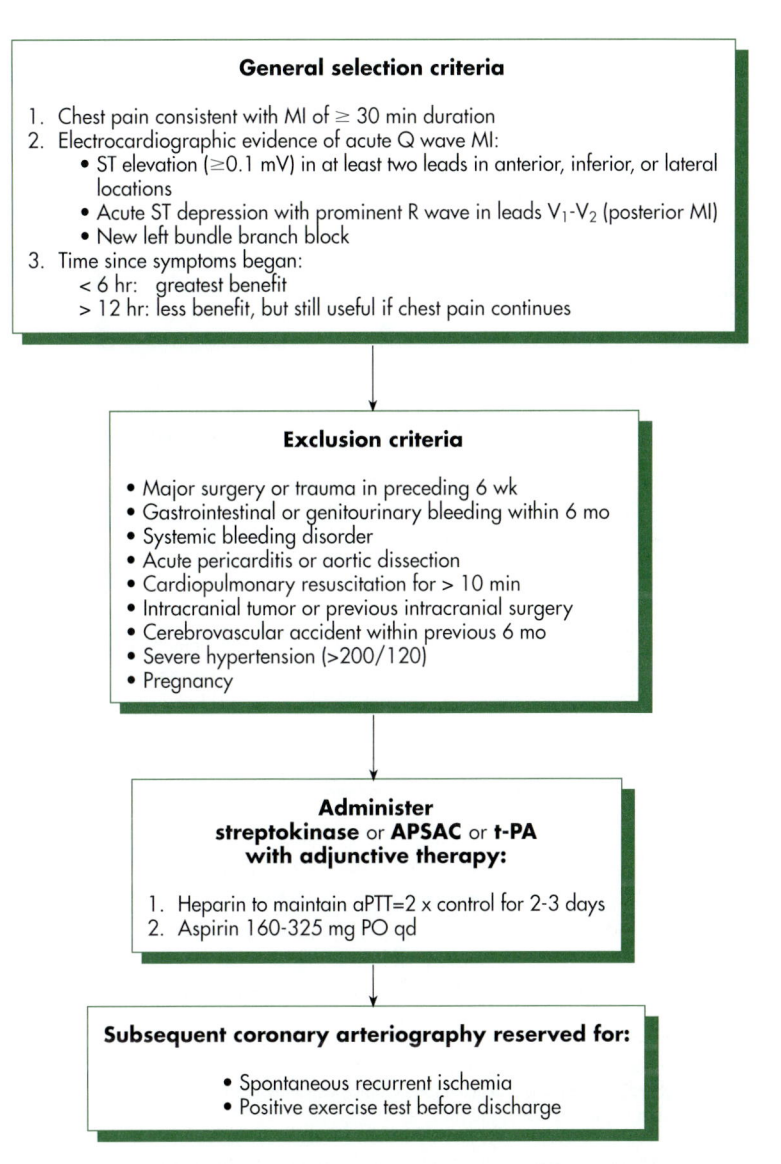

General selection criteria

1. Chest pain consistent with MI of ≥ 30 min duration
2. Electrocardiographic evidence of acute Q wave MI:
   - ST elevation (≥0.1 mV) in at least two leads in anterior, inferior, or lateral locations
   - Acute ST depression with prominent R wave in leads V_1-V_2 (posterior MI)
   - New left bundle branch block
3. Time since symptoms began:
   < 6 hr: greatest benefit
   > 12 hr: less benefit, but still useful if chest pain continues

↓

Exclusion criteria

- Major surgery or trauma in preceding 6 wk
- Gastrointestinal or genitourinary bleeding within 6 mo
- Systemic bleeding disorder
- Acute pericarditis or aortic dissection
- Cardiopulmonary resuscitation for > 10 min
- Intracranial tumor or previous intracranial surgery
- Cerebrovascular accident within previous 6 mo
- Severe hypertension (>200/120)
- Pregnancy

↓

Administer streptokinase or APSAC or t-PA with adjunctive therapy:

1. Heparin to maintain aPTT=2 x control for 2-3 days
2. Aspirin 160-325 mg PO qd

↓

Subsequent coronary arteriography reserved for:

- Spontaneous recurrent ischemia
- Positive exercise test before discharge

Fig. 3-82 Approach to thrombolytic therapy in acute Q wave MI. (From Noble J [ed]: *Primary care medicine,* ed 2, St Louis, 1996, Mosby.)

THYROID DISEASE, NODULAR

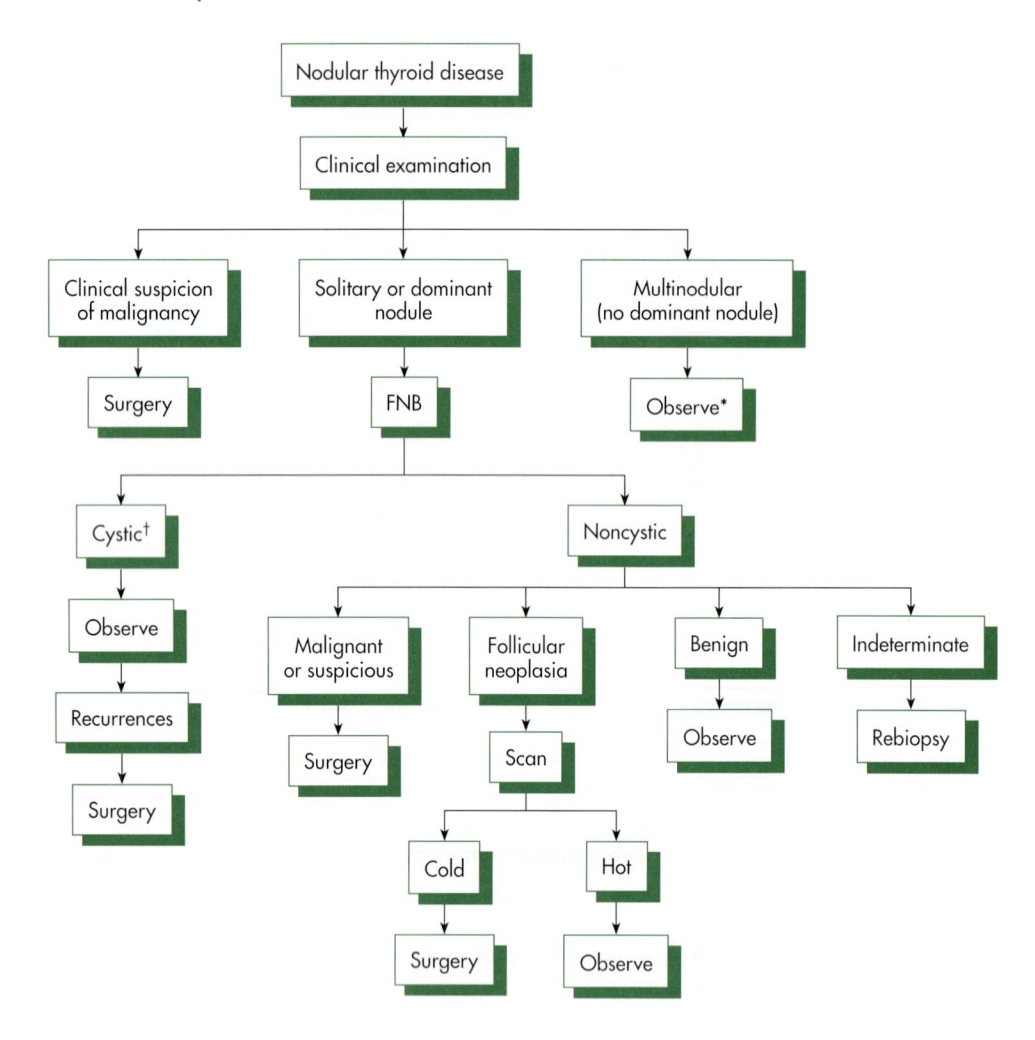

*"Observation" may include attempted suppression with thyroid hormone.
†Disappears completely after aspiration. Aspiration of fluid with only partial reduction in nodule size implies a noncystic nodule.

Fig. 3-83 One cost-effective approach to the management of nodular thyroid disease. (From Moore WT, Eastman RC: *Diagnostic endocrinology,* ed 2, St Louis, 1996, Mosby.)

CLINICAL ALGORITHMS

Thyroid tests 767

THYROID TESTS, DIAGNOSTIC APPROACH

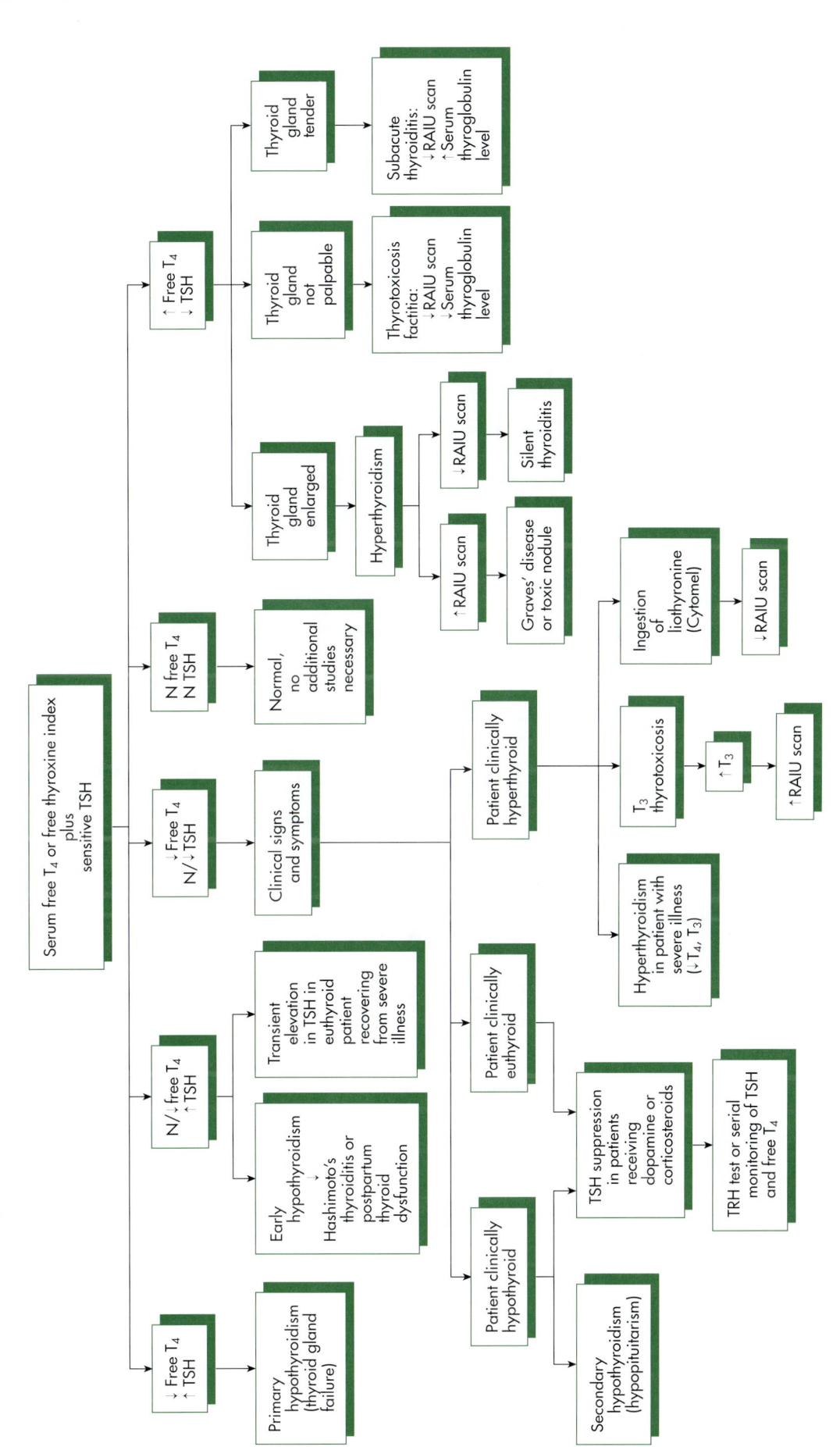

Fig. 3-84 Diagnostic approach to thyroid testing. (From Ferri FF: *Practical guide to the care of the medical patient*, ed 4, St Louis, 1998, Mosby.)

TINNITUS

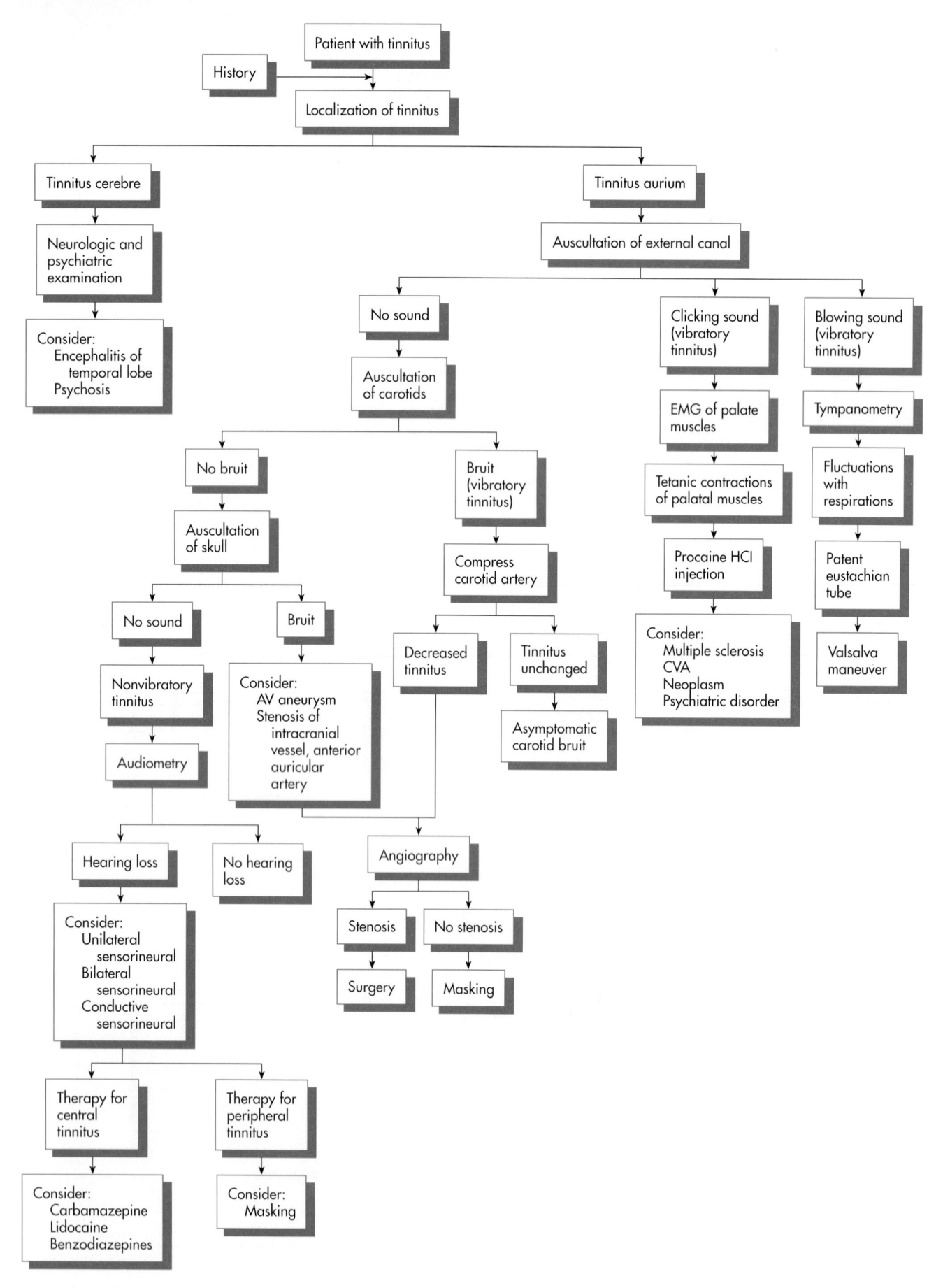

Fig. 3-85 Evaluation of tinnitus. (From Greene HL, Johnson WP, Maricic MJ: *Decision making in medicine,* St Louis, 1993, Mosby.)

CLINICAL ALGORITHMS   Trauma   769

TRAUMA, ABDOMEN

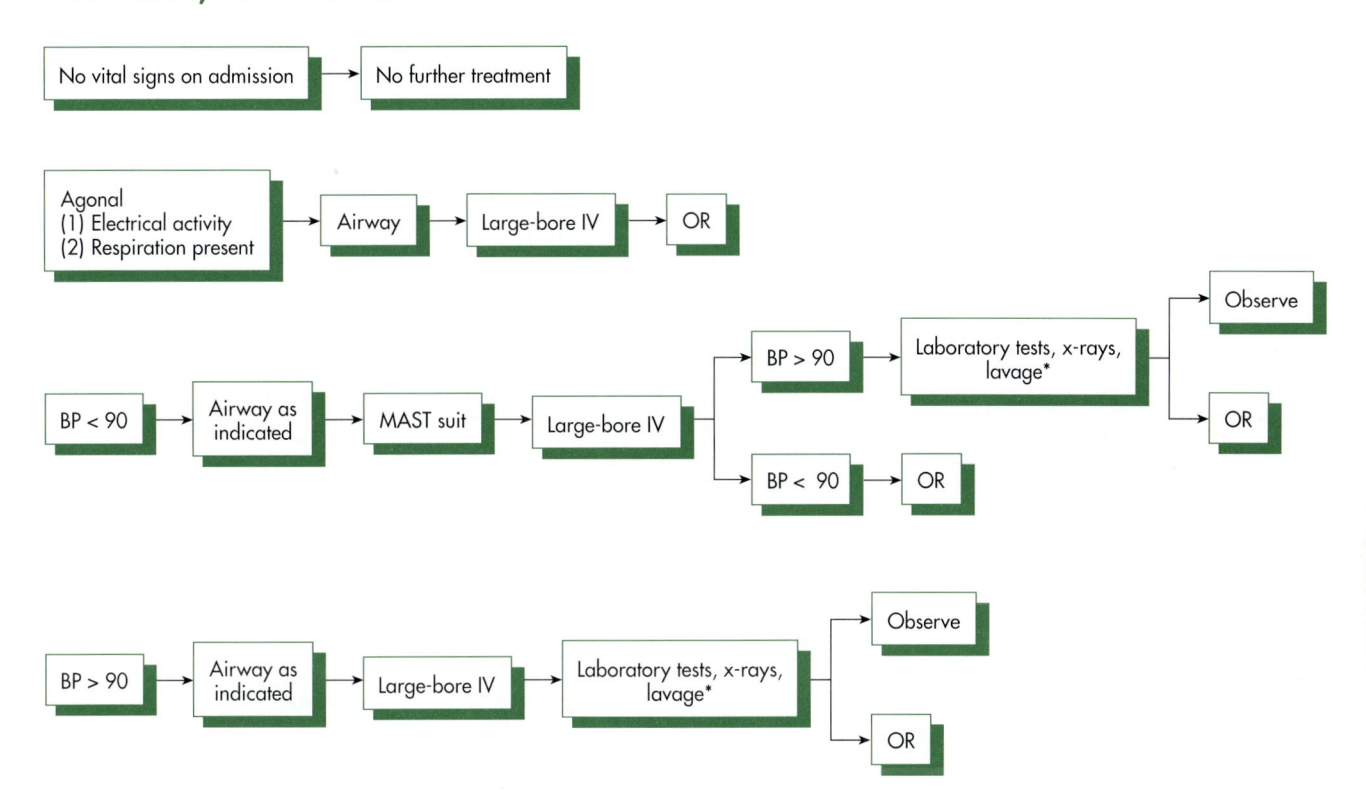

```
No vital signs on admission → No further treatment

Agonal
(1) Electrical activity      → Airway → Large-bore IV → OR
(2) Respiration present

                                                              → BP > 90 → Laboratory tests, x-rays, → Observe
BP < 90 → Airway as → MAST suit → Large-bore IV →                         lavage*                  → OR
          indicated
                                                              → BP < 90 → OR

                                                              → Observe
BP > 90 → Airway as → Large-bore IV → Laboratory tests, x-rays,
          indicated                   lavage*                 → OR
```

*Indications:
(1) ETOH intoxication
(2) Drug intoxication
(3) Head injury
(4) Cord injury
(5) Equivocal examination
(6) Significant trauma on both sides of diaphragm

Fig. 3-86 **Blunt abdominal trauma.** (From Berry SM [ed]: *The Mont Reid surgical handbook,* ed 4, St Louis, 1997, Mosby.)

TRAUMA, CHEST

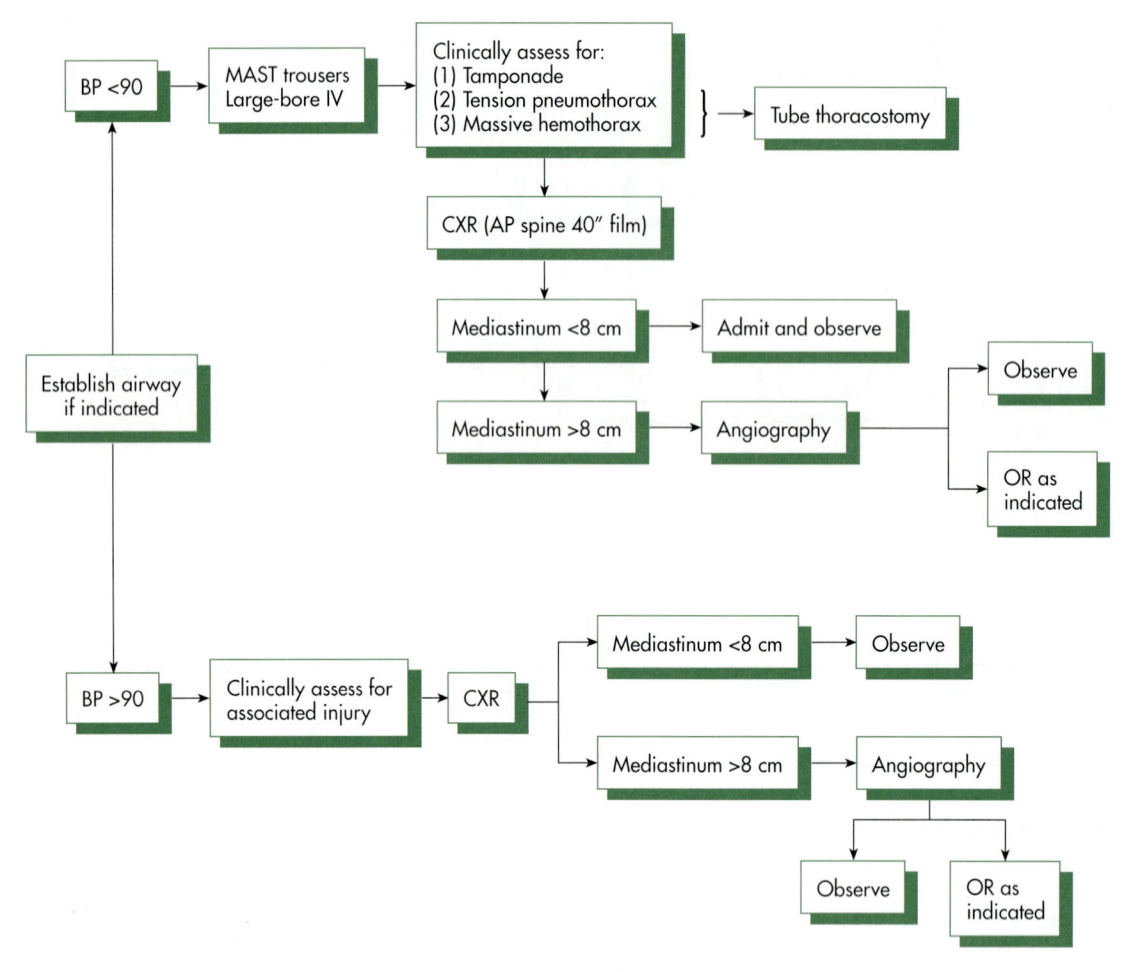

Fig. 3-87 Blunt chest trauma. (From Berry SM [ed]: *The Mont Reid surgical handbook,* ed 4, St Louis, 1997, Mosby.)

CLINICAL ALGORITHMS   Trauma   771

TRAUMA, CHEST—cont'd

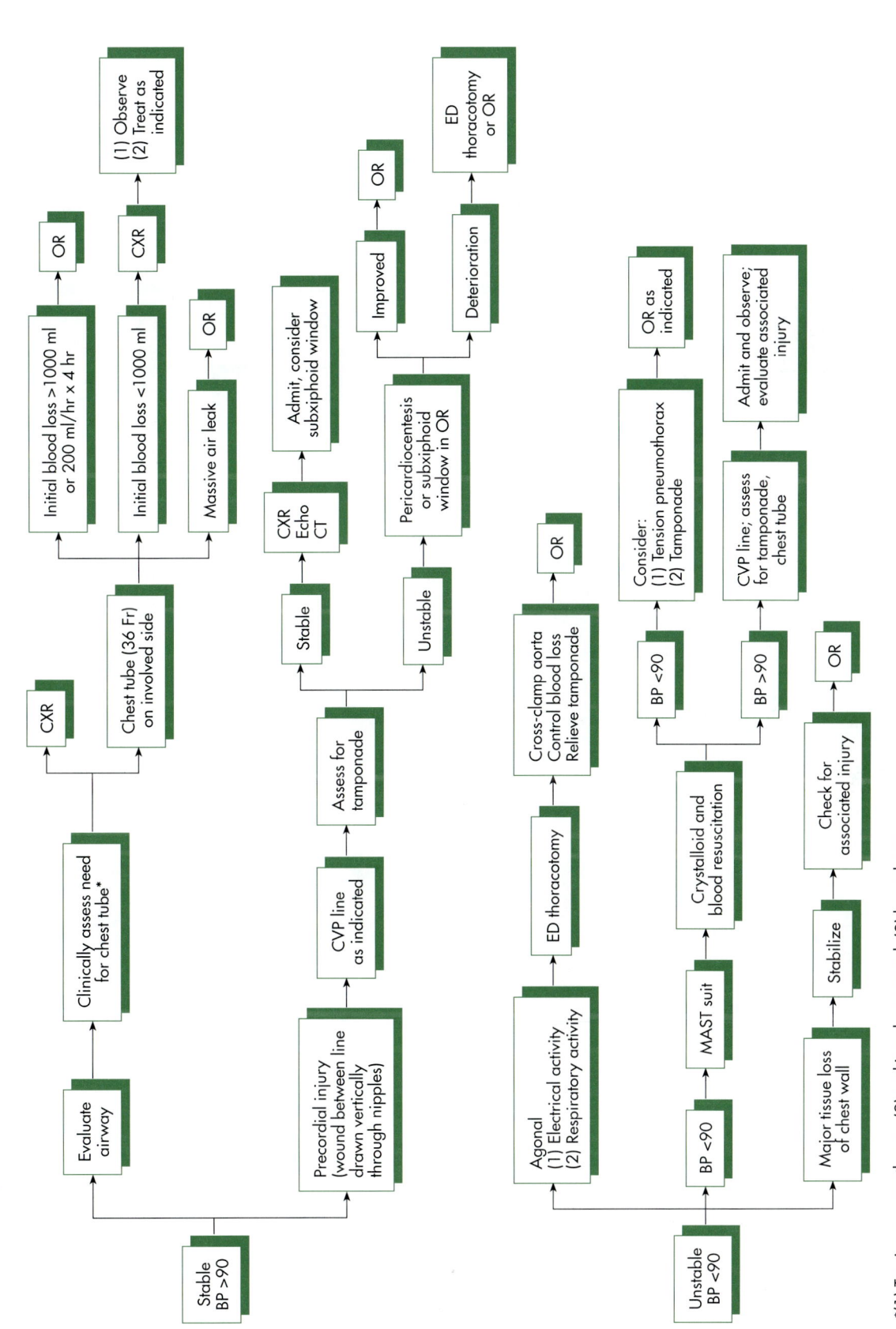

Fig. 3-88 Penetrating chest trauma. (From Berry SM [ed]: *The Mont Reid surgical handbook*, ed 4, St Louis, 1997, Mosby.)

*(1) Tension pneumothorax; (2) sucking chest wound; (3) hemothorax.

772 Trauma

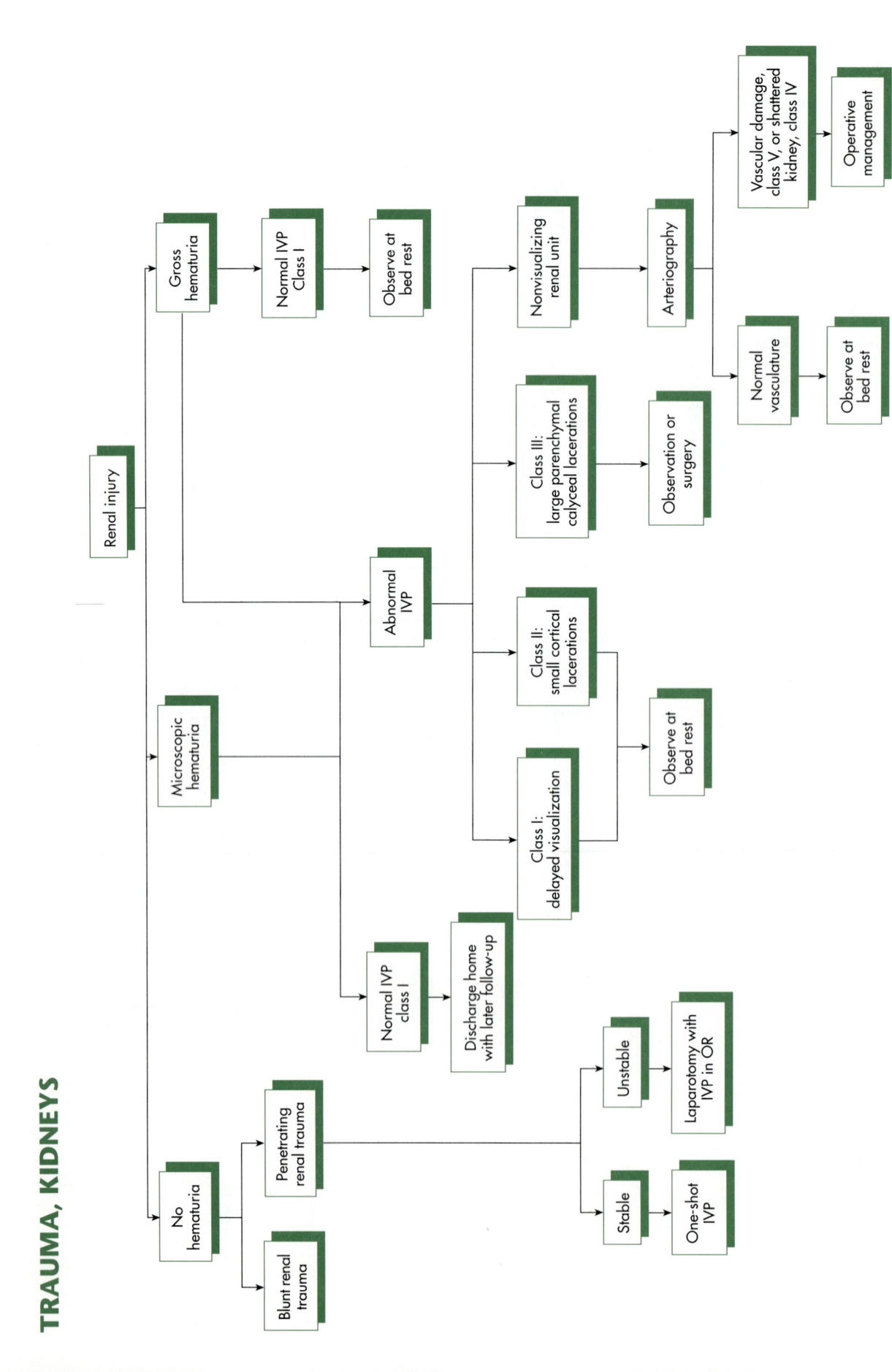

CLINICAL ALGORITHMS

TRAUMA, KIDNEYS

Fig. 3-89 **Treatment of renal trauma.** (From Rosen P et al [eds]: *Emergency medicine: concepts and clinical practice*, St Louis, 1992, Mosby.)

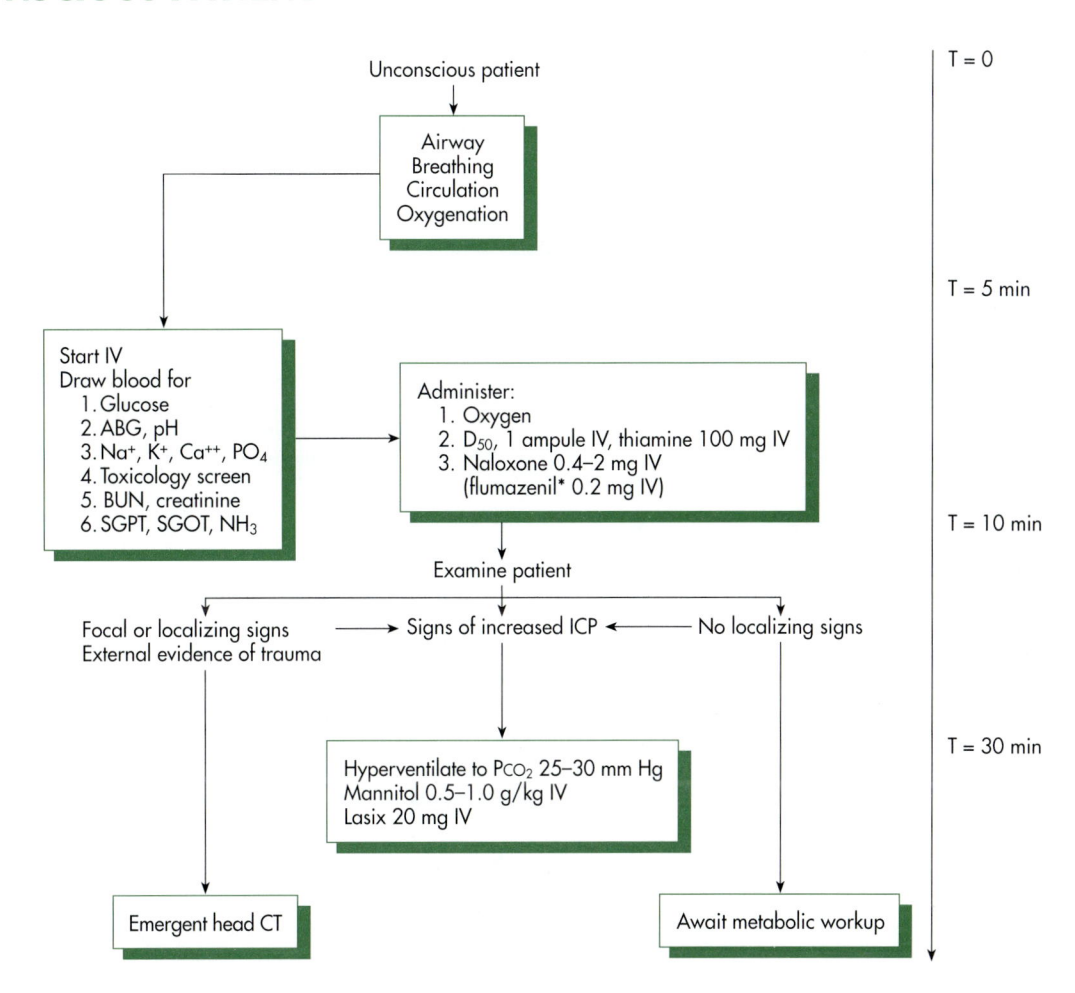

UNCONSCIOUS PATIENT

Fig. 3-90 Approach to the unconscious patient. *ABG,* Arterial blood gas; *BUN,* blood urea nitrogen; *SGPT,* serum glutamic pyruvic transaminase; *SGOT,* serum glutamic oxaloacetic transaminase; *ICP,* intracranial pressure; *CT,* computed tomography. (From Johnson RT, Griffin JW: *Current therapy in neurologic disease,* ed 5, St Louis, 1997, Mosby.)

*Use of flumazenil should not be considered routine because it can precipitate seizures in certain subsets of patients.

URTICARIA, CHRONIC

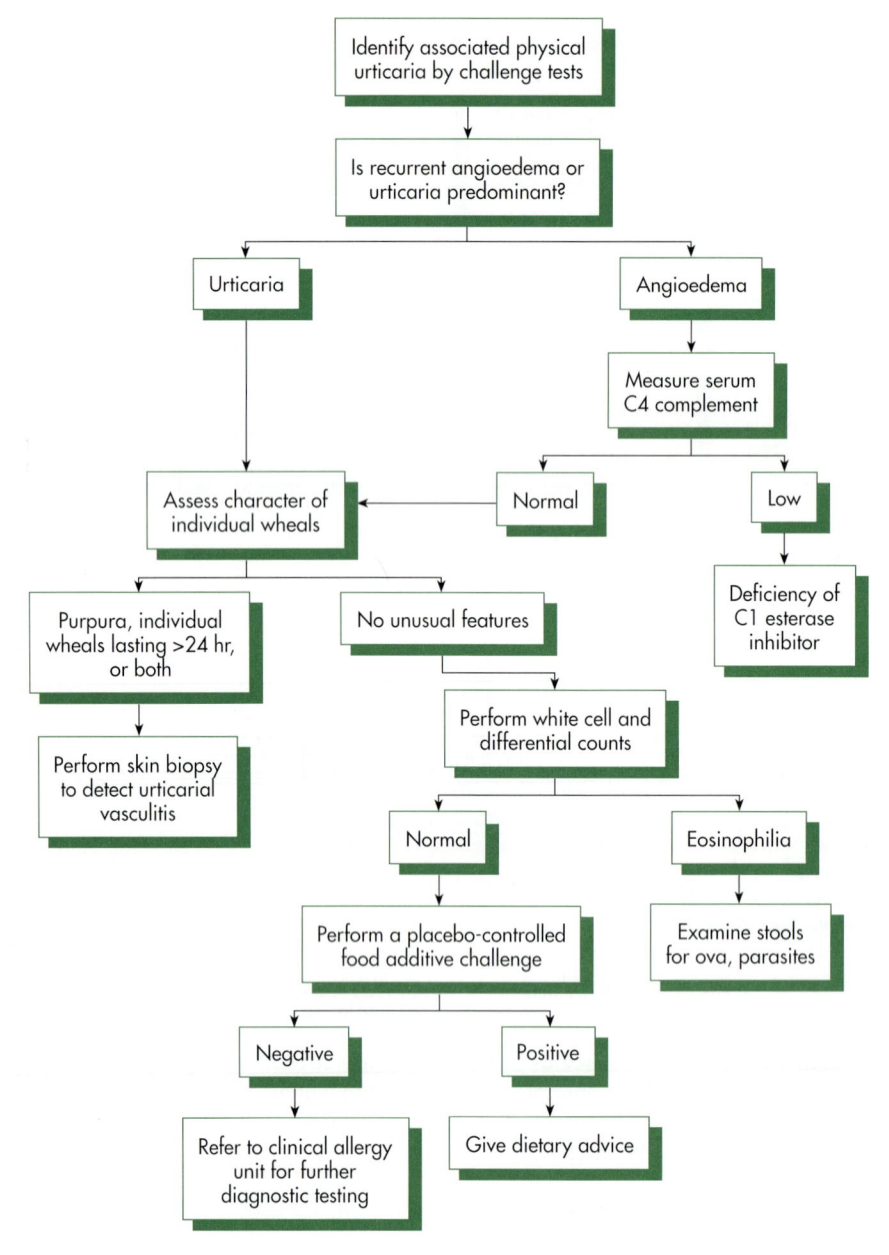

Fig. 3-91 **Investigation and diagnosis of chronic urticaria.** (From Greaves MW: Chronic urticaria, *N Engl J Med* 332:1767-1772, 1995.)

VAGINAL DISCHARGE

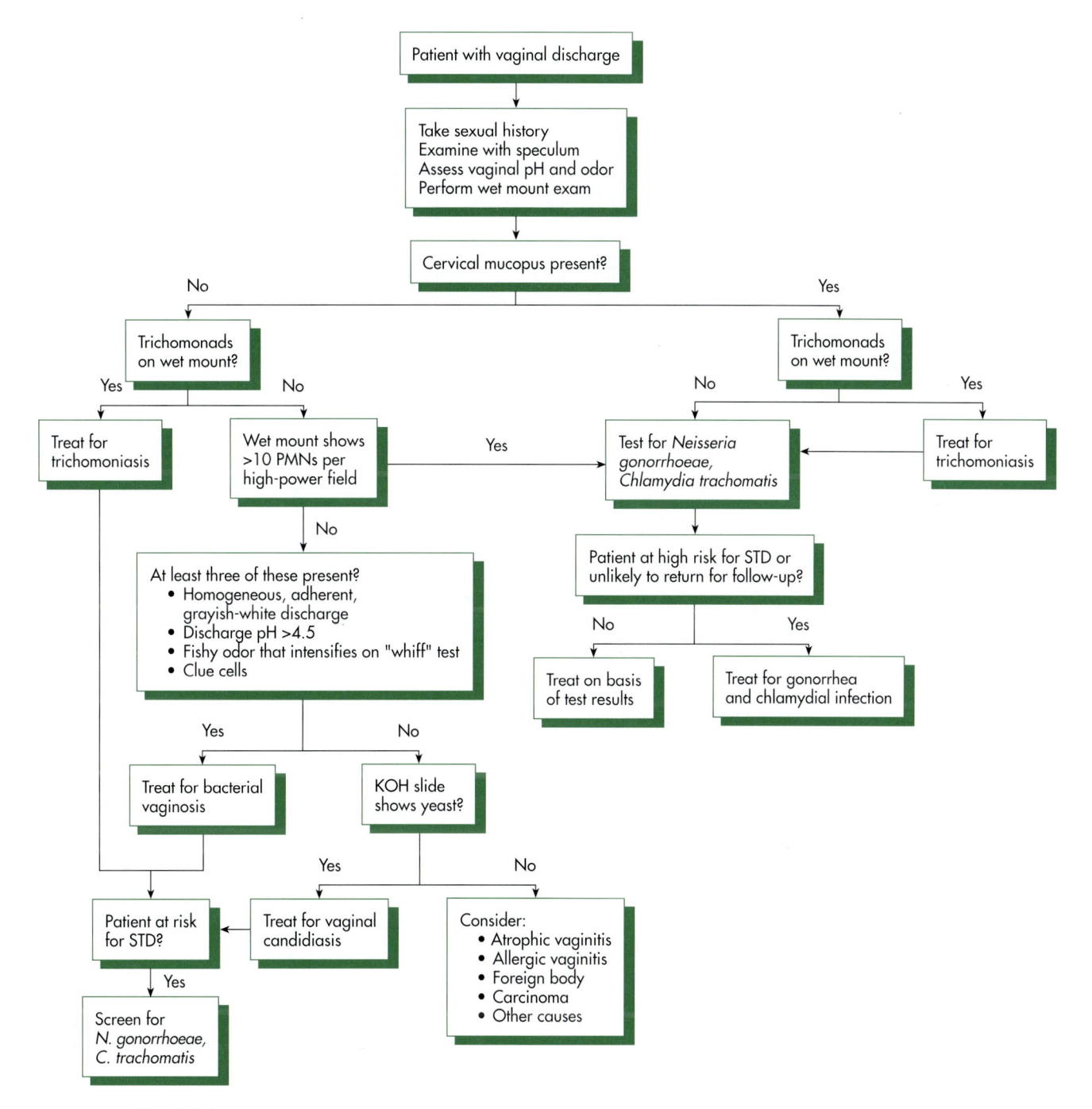

Fig. 3-92 Evaluation of vaginal discharge. *KOH,* Potassium hydroxide; *PMN,* polymorphonuclear leukocyte; *STD,* sexually transmitted disease. (From Fox KK, Behets FMT: Vaginal discharge: how to pinpoint the cause, *Postgrad Med* 98:87-101, 1995.)

VENTRICULAR FIBRILLATION OR PULSELESS VENTRICULAR TACHYCARDIA

Initial actions

- ABCs/perform CPR until defibrillator attached/confirm V Fib.
- Shock (up to 3 times in stacked sequence as needed) for persistent V Fib/ pulseless VT:
    Use energy levels of 200j-200-300j- and then 360 joules.
- NOTE: No pulse check is needed between shocks that are given in stacked sequence.

If V Fib/pulseless VT persists

Continue CPR/Intubate/Establish IV access.
- Epinephrine
    Use an SDE dose (i.e., 1.0 mg by IV bolus) initially.
    May either repeat SDE (every 3-5 minutes as needed) or increase the dose (i.e., to HDE) if there has been no response, choosing between several HDE regimens:
    (1) "Intermediate" dose epinephrine = 2-5 mg IV boluses OR
    (2) Escalating 1-3-5 mg IV boluses OR
    (3) Dosing at 0.1 mg/kg as an IV bolus
- Shock (within 30-60 seconds after first epinephrine dose):
    Use either 360j as a single shock, or may again shock in stacked sequence (with another series of 3 successive shocks at 200-360j).
- NOTE: Use of stacked shocks would be especially appropriate at this time if administration of medication is delayed.

Persistence of V Fib/pulseless VT

- The patient has not responded to:
    Shock (x3); intubation (and ventilation): epinephrine and shock again
- This defines the condition as refractory V Fib. A trial of anti-fibrillatory therapy is now in order.

Consider medications of probable benefit

- Lidocaine
    Give 1.0–1.5 mg/kg (≈50-150 mg) as an initial bolus by IV push. May repeat in 3-5 minutes; although a single dose (at 1.5 mg/kg) IS acceptable in cardiac arrest.
    Resume CPR for 30-60 seconds after giving lidocaine; then shock again.
- AHA Guidelines recommend lidocaine as the antifibrillatory agent of choice for treatment of refractory V Fib. The drug need not be given as a continuous IV infusion until the patient is converted out of V Fib (at which time a prophylactic IV infusion should be started).

Fig. 3-93 **Ventricular fibrillation or pulseless ventricular tachycardia.** (Adapted from Grauer K, Cavallaro D: *ACLS: rapid review and case scenarios,* ed 4, St Louis, Mosby and from American Heart Association ACLS Textbook, 1994.)

VENTRICULAR FIBRILLATION OR PULSELESS VENTRICULAR TACHYCARDIA—cont'd

If lidocaine is ineffective, then consider

- Bretylium
  Give 5 mg/kg (or a single 500 mg IV bolus ≈1 amp), resume CPR for 30-60 seconds, and then shock again.
  A second IV bolus (of 10 mg/kg or ≈1-2 amps) may be given in 5 minutes if V Fib persists (up to a total dose of 30-35 mg/kg).
- May also use magnesium
  Give 1-2 g by IV push, especially for patients with known (or suspected) hypomagnesemia and/or Torsade de Pointes.
- Search for a cause of the arrest (i.e., differential diagnosis)
- Consideration of other measures

Search for a potentially correctable cause of V Fib

Persistence of V Fib at this point in the code should prompt consideration of other factors that could account for the patient's refractory condition. This might include a problem with the ABCs (i.e., a nonpatent airway, asymmetric or absent breath sounds, lack of a pulse with CPR), and/or some other predisposing cause.

- Potentially correctable predisposing causes of refractory V Fib to consider include underlying metabolic disturbance (such as diabetic ketoacidosis or hyperkalemia), hypothermia, hypovolemia, drug overdose (especially of cocaine, tricyclicantidepressants, or narcotics) and/or development of a complication of CPR (such as tension pneumothorax or pericardial tamponade).
- V Fib may also be the end result of (i.e., caused by) many other kinds of processes such as cardiogenic shock (from extensive myocardial infarction), massive pulmonary embolism, ruptured aortic aneurysm, or severe trauma with exsanguinating hemorrhage. Practically speaking, specific diagnosis of these types of conditions is much less important clinically because of the improbability that V Fib resulting from any of these conditions will be amenable to any form of treatment at this point in the code.

Refractory V Fib: other measures to consider

Clinically, it may be helpful to realize that if V Fib persists despite implementation of the actions listed that remaining therapeutic options are relatively limited. There simply is not that much more that can be done. At this point in the process, we suggest consideration of the following measures:

- Continuing epinephrine: Recovery from prolonged cardiopulmonary arrest is unlikely unless coronary perfusion pressure (CPP) is adequate (i.e., ≥15 mm Hg). In the arrested heart, it appears that epinephrine is needed in sufficient amount to achieve such pressures. As a result, the drug should be repeated at least every 3-5 minutes for as long as the patient remains in cardiac arrest. Consideration might also be given to the use of higher doses of drug (i.e., HDE) if the patient fails to respond to SDE doses.
- Considering sodium bicarbonate: Although sodium bicarbonate has been freely used in the past for the treatment of cardiac arrest, recent data strongly question this practice. In fact, a strong case could be made for never administering any sodium bicarbonate at all during cardiopulmonary resuscitation, regardless of what the pH value happens to be. Instead, efforts at correcting acidosis are probably better directed at optimizing ventilation, especially during the early minutes of a code when the major component of acidosis is likely to be respiratory in nature (from hypoventilation). Practically speaking, acceptable indications for use of sodium bicarbonate in the setting of cardiac arrest are limited. They include:
  - Severe metabolic acidosis (usually to a pH value of less than 7.20) that persists beyond the initial phase (i.e., beyond the first 5-15 minutes) of the arrest.
  - Cardiac arrest in a patient known to have a severe preexisting metabolic acidosis prior to the arrest.

NOTE: A number of special resuscitation situations exist in which use of bicarbonate is both appropriate and likely to be helpful. These include hyperkalemia and drug overdose with tricyclic antidepressants or phenobarbital.

Fig. 3-93—cont'd

VENTRICULAR TACHYCARDIA

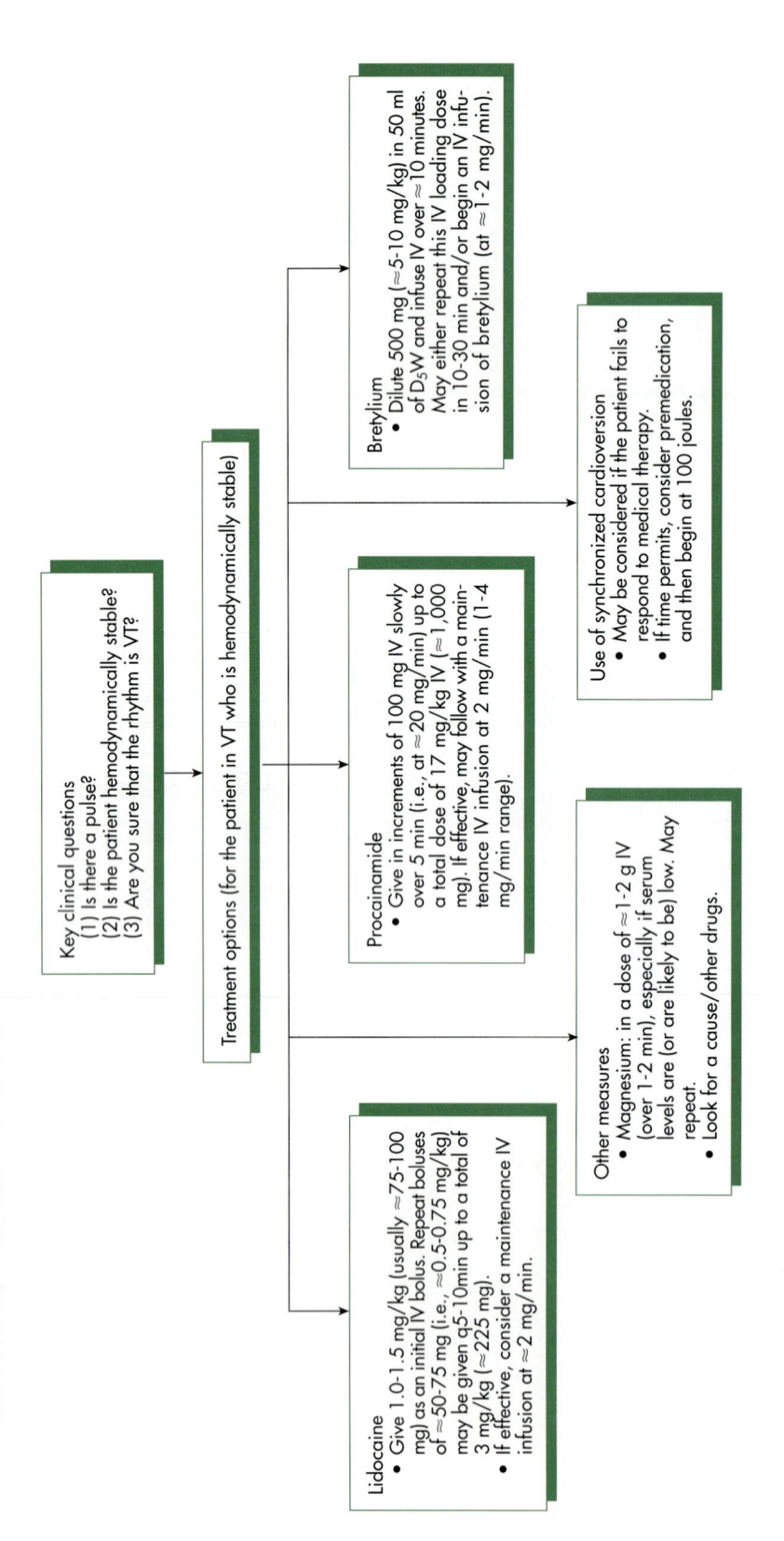

Key clinical questions
(1) Is there a pulse?
(2) Is the patient hemodynamically stable?
(3) Are you sure that the rhythm is VT?

Treatment options (for the patient in VT who is hemodynamically stable)

Lidocaine
- Give 1.0-1.5 mg/kg (usually ≈75-100 mg) as an initial IV bolus. Repeat boluses of ≈50-75 mg (i.e., ≈0.5-0.75 mg/kg) may be given q5-10min up to a total of 3 mg/kg (≈225 mg).
- If effective, consider a maintenance IV infusion at ≈2 mg/min.

Procainamide
- Give in increments of 100 mg IV slowly over 5 min (i.e., at ≈20 mg/min) up to a total dose of 17 mg/kg IV (≈1,000 mg). If effective, may follow with a maintenance IV infusion at 2 mg/min (1-4 mg/min range).

Bretylium
- Dilute 500 mg (≈5-10 mg/kg) in 50 ml of D$_5$W and infuse IV over ≈10 minutes. May either repeat this IV loading dose in 10-30 min and/or begin an IV infusion of bretylium (at ≈1-2 mg/min).

Other measures
- Magnesium: in a dose of ≈1-2 g IV (over 1-2 min), especially if serum levels are (or are likely to be) low. May repeat.
- Look for a cause/other drugs.

Use of synchronized cardioversion
- May be considered if the patient fails to respond to medical therapy.
- If time permits, consider premedication, and then begin at 100 joules.

NOTE: If the patient decompensates at any time during the process of evaluating/treating the tachycardia, STOP and immediately cardiovert.

Fig. 3-94 **Ventricular tachycardia.** (Adapted from Grauer K, Cavallaro D: *ACLS: rapid review and case scenarios,* ed 4, St Louis, 1996, Mosby and from American Heart Association ACLS Textbook, 1994.)

SECTION IV

Laboratory Tests and Interpretation of Results

This section contains over 160 commonly performed laboratory tests. Each test is approached with the following format:
1. Laboratory test
2. Normal range in adult patients
3. Common abnormalities, such as positive test, increased or decreased value
4. Causes of abnormal result

The normal ranges may differ slightly, depending on the laboratory. The reader should be aware of the "normal range" of the particular laboratory performing the test. Every attempt has been made to present current laboratory test data, with emphasis on practical considerations. Normal values are given using the present (traditional) reference interval, followed by the Système Internationale (SI) reference interval, the conversion factor (CF), and the suggested minimum increment (SMI). For example,

TEST	PRESENT REFERENCE INTERVAL	SI REFERENCE INTERVAL	CF	SMI
Fasting glucose	70-110 mg/dl	3.6-6.1 mmol/L	0.05551	0.1 mmol/L

ACETONE (serum or plasma)
Normal:
   Negative
Elevated in:
   DKA, starvation, isopropanol ingestion
ACE LEVEL; see ANGIOTENSIN-CONVERTING ENZYME
ACID-BASE REFERENCE VALUES; see Tables 4-1 and 4-2.

TABLE 4-1 Commonly Used Acid-Base Reference Values for Arterial and Venous Plasma or Serum (Averaged from Various Sources).

	ARTERIAL		VENOUS	
	CONVENTIONAL UNITS	SI UNITS*	CONVENTIONAL UNITS	SI UNITS*
pH	7.40 (7.35-7.45)	7.40 (7.35-7.45)	7.37 (7.32-7.42)	7.37 (7.32-7.42)
P_{CO_2}	40 mm Hg (35-45)	5.33 kPa (4.67-6.10)	45 mm Hg (45-50)	6.10 kPa (5.33-6.67)
P_{O_2}	80-100 mm Hg	10.66 13.33 kPa	40 mm Hg (37-43)	5.33 kPa (4.93-5.73)
HCO_3 (CO_2 combining power)	24 mEq/L (20-28)	24 mmol/L (20-28)	26 mEq/L (22-30)	26 mmol/L (22-30)
CO_2 content	25 mEq/L (22-28)	25 mmol/L (22-28)	27 mEq/L (24-30)	27 mmol/L (24-30)

From Ravel R: *Clinical laboratory medicine,* ed 6, St Louis, 1995, Mosby.
*International system.

TABLE 4-2 Summary of Laboratory Findings in Primary Uncomplicated Respiratory and Metabolic Acid-Base Disorders*

DISORDER	P_{CO_2}	pH	BASE EXCESS
Acute primary respiratory hypoactivity (respiratory acidosis)	Increase	Decrease	Normal/positive
Acute primary respiratory hyperactivity (respiratory alkalosis)	Decrease	Increase	Normal/negative
Uncompensated metabolic acidosis	Normal	Decrease	Negative
Uncompensated metabolic alkalosis	Normal	Increase	Positive
Partially compensated metabolic acidosis	Decrease	Decrease	Negative
Partially compensated metabolic alkalosis	Increase	Increase	Positive
Chronic primary respiratory hypoactivity (compensated respiratory acidosis)	Increase	Normal	Positive
Fully compensated metabolic alkalosis	Increase	Normal	Positive
Chronic primary respiratory hyperactivity (compensated respiratory alkalosis)	Decrease	Normal	Negative
Fully compensated metabolic acidosis	Decrease	Normal	Negative

From Ravel R: *Clinical laboratory medicine,* ed 6, St Louis, 1995, Mosby.
*Base excess results refer to negative (−) values more than −2 and positive (+) values more than +2.

ACID PHOSPHATASE (serum)
Normal range:
0-5.5 U/L (0-90 nkat/L) [CF: 16.67; SMI: 2 nkat/L]
Elevated in:
Carcinoma of prostate, other neoplasms (breast, bone), Paget's disease, osteogenesis imperfecta, malignant invasion of bone, Gaucher's disease, multiple myeloma, myeloproliferative disorders, benign prostatic hypertrophy, prostatic palpation or surgery, hyperparathyroidism, liver disease, chronic renal failure, ITP, bronchitis

ACID SERUM TEST; see HAM TEST

ACTIVATED PARTIAL THROMBOPLASTIN TIME (APTT, aPTT); see PARTIAL THROMBOPLASTIN TIME

ALANINE AMINOTRANSFERASE (ALT, SGPT)
Normal range:
0-35 U/L (0.058 μkat/L) [CF: 0.02 μkat/L]
Elevated in:
Liver disease (hepatitis, cirrhosis, Reye's syndrome), hepatic congestion, infectious mononucleosis, MI, myocarditis, severe muscle trauma, dermatomyositis/polymyositis, muscular dystrophy, drugs (antibiotics, narcotics, antihypertensive agents, heparin, labetalol, lovastatin, NSAIDs, amiodarone, chlorpromazine, phenytoin), malignancy, renal and pulmonary infarction, convulsions, eclampsia, shock liver

ALBUMIN (serum)
Normal range:
4-6 g/dl (40-60 g/L) [CF: 10; SMI: 1 g/L]
Elevated in:
Dehydration (relative increase)
Decreased in:
Liver disease, nephrotic syndrome, poor nutritional status, rapid IV hydration, protein-losing enteropathies (inflammatory bowel disease), severe burns, neoplasia, chronic inflammatory diseases, pregnancy, oral contraceptives, prolonged immobilization, lymphomas, hypervitaminosis A, chronic glomerulonephritis

ALDOLASE (serum)
Normal range:
0-6 U/L (0-100 nkat/L) [CF: 16.67; SMI: 20 nkat/L]
Elevated in:
Muscular dystrophy, rhabdomyolysis, dermatomyositis/polymyositis, trichinosis, acute hepatitis and other liver diseases, MI, prostatic carcinoma, hemorrhagic pancreatitis, gangrene, delirium tremens, burns
Decreased in:
Loss of muscle mass, late stages of muscular dystrophy

ALKALINE PHOSPHATASE (serum)
Normal range:
30-120 U/L (0.5-2 μkat/L) [CF: 0.01667; SMI: 0.1 μkat/L]
Elevated in:
Biliary obstruction, cirrhosis (particularly primary biliary cirrhosis), liver disease (hepatitis, infiltrative liver diseases, fatty metamorphosis), Paget's disease of bone, osteitis deformans, rickets, osteomalacia, hypervitaminosis D, hyperparathyroidism, hyperthyroidism, ulcerative colitis, bowel perforation, bone metastases, healing fractures, bone neoplasms, acromegaly, infectious mononucleosis, CMV infections, sepsis, pulmonary infarction, CHF, hypernephroma, leukemia, myelofibrosis, multiple myeloma, drugs (estrogens, albumin, erythromycin and other antibiotics, cholestasis-producing drugs [phenothiazines]), pregnancy, puberty, others (Boxes 4-1 and 4-2).

> BOX 4-1 Isolated Elevation of Alkaline Phosphatase

ALP Level Increased
AST Level Normal
Total Bilirubin Level Normal
Liver space-occupying lesions
Bone osteoblastic activity increased
Drug-induced (dilantin most common)
Intrahepatic cholestatic process in advanced stage of resolution
Pregnancy (third trimester)
Hyperthyroidism
Hyperparathyroidism

From Ravel R: *Clinical laboratory medicine,* ed 6, St Louis, 1995, Mosby.

> BOX 4-2 Most Common Causes for Alkaline Phosphatase Elevation

Liver and Biliary Tract Origin
Extrahepatic bile duct obstruction
Intrahepatic biliary obstruction
  Liver cell acute injury
  Liver passive congestion
  Drug-induced liver cell dysfunction
Space-occupying lesions
Primary biliary cirrhosis
Sepsis

Bone Origin (Osteoblast Hyperactivity)
Physiologic (rapid) bone growth (childhood and adolescent)
Metastatic tumor with osteoblastic reaction

Fracture healing
Paget's disease of bone

Capillary Endothelial Origin
Granulation tissue formation (active)

Placental Origin
Pregnancy
Some parenteral albumin preparations

Other
Thyrotoxicosis
Benign transient hyperphosphatasemia
Primary hyperparathyroidism

From Ravel R: *Clinical laboratory medicine,* ed 6, St Louis, 1995, Mosby.

Decreased in:
  Hypothyroidism, pernicious anemia, hypophosphatemia, hypervitaminosis D, malnutrition

ALPHA-1-FETOPROTEIN (serum); see α-1 FETOPROTEIN
ALT; see ALANINE AMINOTRANSFERASE
AMMONIA (serum)
Normal range:
  10-80 μg/dl (5-50 μmol/L) [CF: 0.5872; SMI: 5 μmol/L]
Elevated in:
  Hepatic failure, hepatic encephalopathy, Reye's syndrome, portacaval shunt, drugs (diuretics, polymyxin B, methicillin)
Decreased in:
  Drugs (neomycin, lactulose, tetracycline), renal failure
AMYLASE (serum)
Normal range:
  0-130 U/L (0-2.17 μkat/L) [CF: 0.01667; SMI: 0.01 μkat/L]
Elevated in:
  Acute pancreatitis, pancreatic neoplasm, abscess, pseudocyst, ascites, macroamylasemia, perforated peptic ulcer, intestinal obstruction, intestinal infarction, acute cholecystitis, appendicitis, ruptured ectopic pregnancy, salivary gland inflammation, peritonitis, burns, diabetic ketoacidosis, renal insufficiency, drugs (morphine), carcinomatosis (of lung, esophagus, ovary), acute ethanol ingestion, mumps, prostate tumors, post-ERCP, bulimia, anorexia nervosa

Decreased in:
   Advanced chronic pancreatitis, hepatic necrosis, cystic fibrosis

AMYLASE, URINE; *see* **URINE AMYLASE**

ANA; *see* **ANTINUCLEAR ANTIBODY**

ANCA; *see* **ANTINEUTROPHIL CYTOPLASMIC ANTIBODY**

ANGIOTENSIN-CONVERTING ENZYME (ACE level)

Normal range:
   <40 nmol/ml/min (<670 nkat/L) [CF: 16.67; SMI: 10 nkat/L]

Elevated in:
   Sarcoidosis, primary biliary cirrhosis, alcoholic liver disease, hyperthyroidism, hyperparathyroidism, diabetes mellitus, amyloidosis, multiple myeloma, lung disease (asbestosis, silicosis, berylliosis, allergic alveolitis, coccidioidomycosis), Gaucher's disease, leprosy

ANION GAP

Normal range:
   9-14 mEq/L

Elevated in:
   Lactic acidosis, ketoacidosis (DKA, alcoholic starvation), uremia (chronic renal failure), ingestion of toxins (paraldehyde, methanol, salicylates, ethylene glycol), hyperosmolar nonketotic coma, antibiotics (carbenicillin)

Decreased in:
   Hypoalbuminemia, severe hypermagnesemia, IgG myeloma, lithium toxicity, laboratory error (falsely decreased sodium or overestimation of bicarbonate or chloride), hypercalcemia of parathyroid origin, antibiotics (e.g., polymyxin)

ANTICOAGULANT; *see* **CIRCULATING ANTICOAGULANT**

ANTI-DNA

Normal range:
   Absent

Present in:
   SLE, chronic active hepatitis, infectious mononucleosis, biliary cirrhosis

ANTIGLOMERULAR BASEMENT ANTIBODY; *see* **GLOMERULAR BASEMENT MEMBRANE ANTIBODY**

ANTIMITOCHONDRIAL ANTIBODY

Normal range:
   <1:20 titer

Elevated in:
   Primary biliary cirrhosis (85% to 95%), chronic active hepatitis (25% to 30%), cryptogenic cirrhosis (25% to 30%)

ANTINEUTROPHIL CYTOPLASMIC ANTIBODY (ANCA)

Positive test:
   Cytoplasmic pattern (cANCA): positive in Wegener's granulomatosis
   Perinuclear pattern (pANCA): positive in inflammatory bowel disease, primary biliary cirrhosis, primary sclerosing cholangitis, autoimmune chronic active hepatitis, crescenteric glomerulonephritis

ANTINUCLEAR ANTIBODY (ANA)

Normal range:
   <1:20 titer

Positive test:
   SLE (more significant if titer >1:160), drugs (phenytoin, ethosuximide, primidone, methyldopa, hydralazine, carbamazepine, penicillin, procainamide, chlorpromazine, griseofulvin, thiazides), chronic active hepatitis, age over 60 years (particularly age over 80 years), rheumatoid arthritis, scleroderma, mixed connective tissue disease, necrotizing vasculitis, Sjögren's syndrome (SS), tuberculosis, pulmonary interstitial fibrosis. Table 4-3 describes diseases associated with ANA subtypes.

TABLE 4-3 Disease-Associated ANA Subtypes

NUCLEAR LOCATION	DISEASE(S)*
"Native" DNA (dsDNA, or dsDNA/ssDNA complex)	SLE (60%-70%; range, 35%-75%) —also PSS (5%-55%), MCTD (11%-25%), RA (5%-40%), DM (5%-25%), SS (5%)
sNP	SLE (50%) —also other collagen diseases
DNP (DNA-histone complex)	SLE (52%) —also MCTD (8%), RA (3%)
Histones	Drug-induced SLE (95%) —also SLE (30%), RA (15%-24%)
ENA	
Sm	SLE (30%-40%; range, 28%-40%) —also MCTD (0%-8%)
RNP (U1-RNP)	MCTD (in high titer without any other ANA subtype present: 95%-100%) —also SLE (26%-50%), (11%-22%), RA (10%), SS (3%)
SS-A (Ro)†	SS without RA (60%-70%) —also SLE (26%-50%), neonatal SLE (over 95%), PSS (30%), MCTD (50%), SS with RA (9%), PBC (15%-19%)
SS-B (La)	SS without RA (40%-60%) —also SLE (5%-15%), SS with RA (5%)
Scl-70†	PSS (15%-43%)
Centromere†	CREST syndrome (70%-90%; range 57%-96%) —also PSS (4%-20%), PBC (12%)
Nucleolar	PSS (scleroderma) (54%-90%) —also SLE (25%-26%), RA (9%)
RAP (RANA)	SS with RA (60%-76%) —also SS without RA (5%)
Jo-1	Polymyositis (30%)
PM-1	Polymyositis or PMS/PSS overlap syndrome (60%-90%) —also DM (17%)
ssDNA	SLE (60%-70%) —also CAH, infectious mononucleosis, RA, chronic GN, chronic infections, PBC
CYTOPLASMIC LOCATION	**DISEASE(S)**
Mitochondrial	Primary biliary cirrhosis (90%-100%) —also CAH (7%-30%), cryptogenic cirrhosis (30%), acute hepatitis, viral hepatitis (3%), other liver diseases (0%-20%), SLE (5%), SS and PSS (8%)
Microsomal‡	Chronic active hepatitis (60%-80%), Hashimoto's thyroiditis (97%)
Ribosomal	SLE (5%-12%)
Smooth muscle§	Chronic active hepatitis (60%-91%) —also cryptogenic cirrhosis (28%), acute hepatitis, viral hepatitis (5%-87%), infectious mononucleosis (81%), MS (40%-50%), malignancy (67%), PBC (10%-50%)

From Ravel R: *Clinical laboratory medicine*, ed 6, St Louis, 1995, Mosby.
*CAH, Chronic active hepatitis; DM, dermatomyositis; SS, Sjögren's syndrome; PBC, primary biliary cirrhosis; GN, glomerulonephritis; MS, multiple sclerosis.
†Not detected using rat or mouse liver or kidney tissue method.
‡Not detected by cultured cell method.
§Detected by cultured cells but better with rat or mouse tissue.

> BOX 4-3 **Some Etiologies for Aspartate Aminotransferase Values Over 1000 IU/ml**
>
> **Liver Origin**
> Acute hepatitis, viral hepatitis
> Chronic active hepatitis (occasional patients; 16% in one study)
> Reye's syndrome
> Severe liver passive congestion or hypoxia (with or without acute MI, shock, or sepsis)
>
> Drug-induced (e.g., acetaminophen)
> HELLP syndrome of pregnancy (some patients)
>
> **Other**
> First 2-3 days of acute common bile duct obstruction
>
> Acute myocardial infarct (occasional patients)
> Severe rhabdomyolysis

From Ravel R: *Clinical laboratory medicine*, ed 6, St Louis, 1995, Mosby.

ANTI-RNP ANTIBODY; see EXTRACTABLE NUCLEAR ANTIGEN
ANTI-Sm (ANTI-SMITH) ANTIBODY; see EXTRACTABLE NUCLEAR ANTIGEN
ANTI-SMOOTH MUSCLE ANTIBODY; see SMOOTH MUSCLE ANTIBODY
ANTI-STREPTOLYSIN O TITER (STREPTOZYME, ASLO titer)
Normal range for adults:
 <160 Todd units
Elevated in:
 Streptococcal upper airway infection, acute rheumatic fever, acute glomerulonephritis, increased levels of β-lipoprotein
 NOTE: A fourfold increase in titer between acute and convalescent specimens is diagnostic of streptococcal upper airway infection regardless of the initial titer.
ANTITHROMBIN III
Normal range:
 81% to 120% of normal activity; 17-30 mg/dl
Decreased in:
 Hereditary deficiency of antithrombin III, DIC, pulmonary embolism, cirrhosis, thrombolytic therapy, chronic liver failure, postsurgery, third trimester of pregnancy, oral contraceptives, nephrotic syndrome, IV heparin >3 days, sepsis, acute leukemia, carcinoma, thrombophlebitis
Elevated in:
 Warfarin drugs, post-MI
ASLO TITER: see ANTI-STREPTOLYSIN O TITER
ASPARTATE AMINOTRANSFERASE (AST, SGOT)
Normal range:
 0-35 U/L (0-0.58 μkat/L) [CF: 0.01667, SMI: 0.01 μkat/L]
Elevated in:
 Liver disease (hepatitis, cirrhosis, Reye's syndrome), hepatic congestion, infectious mononucleosis, MI, myocarditis, severe muscle trauma, dermatomyositis/polymyositis, muscular dystrophy, drugs (antibiotics, narcotics, antihypertensive agents, heparin, labetalol, lovastatin, NSAIDs, phenytoin, amiodarone, chlorpromazine), malignancy, renal and pulmonary infarction, convulsions, eclampsia, other (Boxes 4-3 and 4-4).
BASOPHIL COUNT
Normal range:
 0.4% to 1% of total WBC; 40-100 mm^3
Elevated in:
 Leukemia, inflammatory processes, polycythemia vera, Hodgkin's lymphoma, hemolytic anemia, after splenectomy, myeloid metaplasia, myxedema
Decreased in:
 Stress, hypersensitivity reaction, steroids, pregnancy, hyperthyroidism, postirradiation

BOX 4-4 Some Etiologies for Aspartate Aminotransferase Elevation

Heart
Acute MI
Pericarditis (active: some cases)

Liver
Hepatitis virus, Epstein-Barr, or cytomegalovirus infection
Active cirrhosis
Liver passive congestion or hypoxia
Alcohol or drug-induced liver dysfunction
Space-occupying lesions (active)
Fatty liver (severe)
Extrahepatic biliary obstruction (early)
Drug-induced

Skeletal Muscle
Acute skeletal muscle injury
Muscle inflammation (infectious or noninfectious)
Muscular dystrophy (active)
Recent surgery
Delirium tremens

Kidney
Acute injury or damage
Renal infarct

Other
Intestinal infarction
Shock
Cholecystitis
Acute pancreatitis
Hypothyroidism
Heparin therapy (60%-80% of cases)

From Ravel R: *Clinical laboratory medicine,* ed 6, St Louis, 1995, Mosby.

BILE, URINE; *see* **URINE BILE**
BILIRUBIN, DIRECT (conjugated bilirubin)
Normal range:
  0-0.2 mg/dl (0-4 μmol/L) [CF: 17.10; SMI: 2 μmol/L]
Elevated in:
  Hepatocellular disease, biliary obstruction, drug-induced cholestasis, hereditary disorders (Dubin-Johnson syndrome, Rotor's syndrome)
BILIRUBIN, INDIRECT (unconjugated bilirubin)
Normal range:
  0-1.0 mg/dl (2-18 μmol/L) [CF: 17.10; SMI: 2 μmol/L]
Elevated in:
  Hemolysis, liver disease (hepatitis, cirrhosis, neoplasm), hepatic congestion secondary to congestive heart failure, hereditary disorders (Gilbert's disease, Crigler-Najjar syndrome), other (Box 4-5)
BILIRUBIN, TOTAL
Normal range:
  0-1.0 mg/dl (2-18 μmol/L) [CF: 17.10, SMI: 2 μmol/L]
Elevated in:
  Liver disease (hepatitis, cirrhosis, cholangitis, neoplasm, biliary obstruction, infectious mononucleosis), hereditary disorders (Gilbert's disease, Dubin-Johnson syndrome), drugs (steroids, diphenylhydantoin, phenothiazines, penicillin, erythromycin, clindamycin, captopril, amphotericin B, sulfonamides, azathioprine, isoniazid, 5-aminosalicylic acid, allopurinol, methyldopa, indomethacin, halothane, oral contraceptives, procainamide, tolbutamide, labetalol), hemolysis, pulmonary embolism or infarct, hepatic congestion secondary to CHF
BILIRUBIN, URINE; *see* **URINE BILE**
BLEEDING TIME (modified Ivy method)
Normal range:
  2 to 9½ min
Elevated in:
  Thrombocytopenia, capillary wall abnormalities, platelet abnormalities (Bernard-Soulier disease, Glanzmann's disease), drugs (aspirin, warfarin, anti-inflammatory medications, streptokinase, urokinase, dextran, β-lactam antibiotics, moxalactam), DIC, cirrhosis, uremia, myeloproliferative disorders, Von Willebrand's disease
BUN; *see* **UREA NITROGEN**
C3; *see* **COMPLEMENT C3**

BOX 4-5 Unconjugated Hyperbilirubinemia

A. **Result of increased bilirubin production** (if normal liver, serum unconjugated bilirubin is usually less than 4 mg/100 ml)
   1. Hemolytic anemia
      a. Acquired
      b. Congenital
   2. Resorption from extravascular sources
      a. Hematomas
      b. Pulmonary infarcts
   3. Excessive ineffective erythropoiesis
      a. Congenital (congenital dyserythropoietic anemias)
      b. Acquired (pernicious anemia, severe lead poisoning; if present, bilirubinemia is usually mild)
B. **Defective hepatic unconjugated bilirubin clearance** (defective uptake or conjugation)
   1. Severe liver disease
   2. Gilbert's syndrome
   3. Crigler-Najjar type I or II
   4. Drug-induced inhibition
   5. Portacaval shunt
   6. Congestive heart failure
   7. Hyperthyroidism (uncommon)

From Ravel R: *Clinical laboratory medicine,* ed 6, St Louis, 1995, Mosby.

BOX 4-6 Selected Etiologies of Hypercalcemia

Relatively Common

Neoplasia (noncutaneous)
  Bone primary
    Myeloma
    Acute leukemia
  Nonbone solid tumors
    Breast
    Lung
    Squamous nonpulmonary
    Kidney
  Neoplasm secretion of parathyroid hormone-related protein (PTHrP, "ectopic PTH")
Primary hyperparathyroidism (PHPT)
Thiazide diuretics
Tertiary (renal) hyperparathyroidism
Idiopathic
Spurious (artifactual) hypercalcemia
  Dehydration
  Serum protein elevation
  Laboratory technical problem

Relatively Uncommon

Neoplasia (less common tumors)
Sarcoidosis
Hyperthyroidism
Immobilization (mostly seen in children and adolescents)
Diuretic phase of acute renal tubular necrosis
Vitamin D intoxication
Milk-alkali syndrome
Addison's disease
Lithium therapy
Idiopathic hypercalcemia of infancy
Acromegaly
Theophylline toxicity

From Ravel R: *Clinical laboratory medicine,* ed 6, St Louis, 1995, Mosby.

C4; *see* **COMPLEMENT C4**

CALCITONIN (serum)

Normal range:
  <100 pg/ml (<100 ng/L) [CF: 1; SMI: 10 ng/L]

Elevated in:
  Medullary carcinoma of the thyroid (particularly if level >1500 pg/ml), carcinoma of the breast, APUDomas, carcinoids, renal failure, thyroiditis

CALCIUM (serum)

Normal range:
  8.8-10.3 mg/dl (2.2-2.58 mmol/L) [CF: 0.2495; SMI: 0.02 mmol/L]
  See Boxes 4-6 and 4-7 for causes of elevated or decreased serum calcium levels. Laboratory findings in conditions affecting serum calcium and phosphorus levels are described in Table 4-4.

BOX 4-7 Selected Etiologies of Hypocalcemia

Artifactual
   Hypoalbuminemia
   Hemodilution
Primary hypoparathyroidism
Pseudohypoparathyroidism
Vitamin D-related
   Vitamin D deficiency
   Malabsorption
Renal failure
Magnesium deficiency
Sepsis
Chronic alcoholism
Tumor lysis syndrome
Rhabdomyolysis
Alkalosis (respiratory or metabolic)
Acute pancreatitis
Drug-induced hypocalcemia
   Large doses of magnesium sulfate
   Anticonvulsants
   Mithramycin
   Gentamicin
   Cimetidine

From Ravel R: *Clinical laboratory medicine,* ed 6, St Louis, 1995, Mosby.

TABLE 4-4 Classic Laboratory Findings in Selected Conditions Affecting Serum Calcium and Phosphorus Levels*

	SERUM CALCIUM	SERUM PHOSPHORUS	ALKALINE PHOSPHATASE	ACIDOSIS	URINE CALCIUM
PHPT	H	N/L†	N/H†		H
Ectopic PTH syndrome	H	L	H		H
Vitamin D excess	H	N/L	N/H		H
Sarcoidosis	N/H	N	H		N/H
Secondary hyperparathyroidism	L/N	H	H	+	H
Tertiary hyperparathyroidism	H	H	H		
Renal acidosis	L/N	N/L	H	+	H
Sprue	L/N	N/L	H		L
Osteomalacia	L/N	L/N	H		L
Paget's disease	N‡	N	H‡		N/H
Metastatic neoplasm to bone§	N/H	N	N/H		N/H
Hypoparathyroidism	L	H	N		L
Osteoporosis	N	N	N		N/H
Hyperthyroidism	N/H	N/H	N/H		N/H

From Ravel R: *Clinical laboratory medicine,* ed 6, St Louis, 1995, Mosby.
*Incidence of these findings varies in individual patients. *H, N,* and *L,* High, normal, and low; second letter, if present, indicates less common finding.
†Alkaline phosphatase level is high and serum phosphate level is low in "textbook cases" of PHPT.
‡PTH normal; ALP normal in 15% of early monostotic stage; Calcium occasionally small increase from immobilization.
§Depends on primary tumor and type of bone lesion produced. Metastatic carcinoma to bone is one of the most common etiologies of hypercalcemia, perhaps the most common.

CALCIUM, URINE; *see* **URINE CALCIUM**

CANCER ANTIGEN 125

Normal range:
   Less than 1.4%
   The cancer antigen 125 (CA 125) test uses an antibody against antigen from tissue culture of an ovarian tumor cell line. Various published evaluations report sensitivity of about 75%-80% in patients with ovarian carcinoma. There is also an appreciable incidence of elevated values in nonovarian malignancies and in certain benign conditions (Box 4-8). Test values may transiently increase during chemotherapy.

CARBON MONOXIDE; *see* **CARBOXYHEMOGLOBIN**

CARBOXYHEMOGLOBIN

Normal range:
   Saturation of hemoglobin <2%; smokers <9% (coma: 50%; death: 80%)

Elevated in:
   Smoking, exposure to smoking, exposure to automobile exhaust fumes, malfunctioning gas-burning appliances

> **BOX 4-8 Elevated CA 125 Levels in Various Conditions**
>
> **Malignant**
> Epithelial ovarian carcinoma, 75%-80% (range 25%-92%, better in serous than mucinous cystadenocarcinoma)
> Endometrial carcinoma, 25%-48% (2%-90%)
> Pancreatic carcinoma, 59%
> Colorectal carcinoma, 20% (15%-56%)
> Endocervical adenocarcinoma, 83%
> Squamous cervical or vaginal carcinoma, 7%-14%
> Lung carcinoma, 32%
> Breast carcinoma, 12%-40%
> Lymphoma, 35%
>
> **Benign**
> Cirrhosis, 40%-80%
> Acute pancreatitis, 38%
> Acute peritonitis, 75%
> Endometriosis, 88%
> Acute pelvic inflammation disease, 33%
> Pregnancy first trimester, 2%-24%
> During menstruation (occasionally)
> Renal failure (?frequency)
> Normal persons, 0.6%-1.4%

From Ravel R: *Clinical laboratory medicine*, ed 6, St Louis, 1995, Mosby.

CARCINOEMBRYONIC ANTIGEN (CEA)
Normal range:
  Nonsmokers: 0-2.5 ng/ml (0-2.5 µg/L) [CF: 1; SMI: 0.1 µg/L]
  Smokers: 0-5 ng/ml (0-5 µg/L) [CF: 1; SMI: 0.1 µg/L]
Elevated in:
  Colorectal carcinomas, pancreatic carcinomas, and metastatic disease usually produce higher elevations (>20 ng/ml)
  Carcinomas of the esophagus, stomach, small intestine, liver, breast, ovary, lung, and thyroid usually produce lesser elevations
  Benign conditions (smoking, inflammatory bowel disease, hypothyroidism, cirrhosis, pancreatitis, infections) usually produce levels <10 ng/ml

CAROTENE (serum)
Normal range:
  50-250 µg/dl (0.9-4.6 µmol/L) [CF: 0.01863; SMI: 0.1 µmol/L]
Elevated in:
  Carotenemia, chronic nephritis, diabetes mellitus, hypothyroidism, nephrotic syndrome, hyperlipidemia
Decreased in:
  Fat malabsorption, steatorrhea, pancreatic insufficiency, lack of carotenoids in diet, high fever, liver disease

CATECHOLAMINES, URINE; see URINE CATECHOLAMINES
CBC; see COMPLETE BLOOD COUNT
CEA; see CARCINOEMBRYONIC ANTIGEN
CEREBROSPINAL FLUID (CSF)
Normal range:
  Appearance: clear
  Glucose: 40-70 mg/dl (2.2-3.9 mmol/L) [CF: 0.055; SMI: 0.1 mmol]
  Protein: 20-45 mg/dl (0.20-0.45 g/L) [CF: 0.01; SMI: 0.1 g/L]
  Chloride: 116-122 mEq/L (116-122 mmol/L) [CF: 1; SMI: 1 mmol/L]
  Pressure: 100-200 mm H_2O
  Cell count (cells/mm^3) and cell type: <6 lymphocytes, no polymorphonucleocytes
  Table 4-5 describes CSF abnormalities in various conditions.

CERULOPLASMIN (serum)
Normal range:
  20-35 mg/dl (200-350 mg/L) [CF: 10; SMI: 10 mg/L]

TABLE 4-5 CSF Abnormalities in Various CNS Conditions

	APPEARANCE	GLUCOSE (MG/DL)	PROTEIN (MG/DL)	CELL COUNT (CELLS/MM³) AND CELL TYPE	PRESSURE (MM HG)
Normal	Clear	50-80	20-45	<6 lymphocytes	100-200
Acute bacterial meningitis	Cloudy	↓↓	↑↑	↑↑ PMN	↑↑
Aseptic (viral) meningitis	Clear/cloudy	N	↑	↑, usually mononuclear cells May be PMN in early stages	N/↑
Hemorrhage	Bloody/xanthochromic	N/↓	↑	↑↑ RBC	↑
Neoplasm	Clear/xanthochromic	N/↓	N/↑	N/↑ lymphocytes	↑↑
Tuberculous meningitis	Cloudy	↓	↑	↑ PMN (early) ↑ lymphocytes (later)	↑
Fungal meningitis	Clear/cloudy	↓	↑	↑ monocytes	↑
Neurosyphilis	Clear/cloudy	N	↑	↑ monocytes	N/↑
Guillain-Barré syndrome	Clear/cloudy	N	↑↑	N/↑ lymphocytes	N

↑, Increased; ↑↑, markedly increased; ↓, decreased; ↓↓, markedly decreased; *N*, normal; *PMN*, polymorphonucleocytes; *RBC*, red blood cells.

Elevated in:
  Pregnancy, estrogens, oral contraceptives, neoplastic diseases (leukemias, Hodgkin's lymphoma, carcinomas), inflammatory states, SLE, primary biliary cirrhosis, rheumatoid arthritis

Decreased in:
  Wilson's disease (values often <10 mg/dl), nephrotic syndrome, advanced liver disease, malabsorption, total parenteral nutrition, Menkes' syndrome

CHLORIDE (serum)

Normal range:
  95-105 mEq/L (95-105 mmol/L) [CF: 1; SMI: 1 mmol/L]

Elevated in:
  Dehydration, excessive infusion of normal saline solution, cystic fibrosis (sweat test), hyperparathyroidism, renal tubular disease, metabolic acidosis, prolonged diarrhea, drugs (ammonium chloride administration, acetazolamide, boric acid, triamterene)

Decreased in:
  CHF, SIADH, Addison's disease, vomiting, gastric suction, salt-losing nephritis, continuous infusion of D_5W, thiazide diuretic administration, diaphoresis, diarrhea, burns, DKA

CHLORIDE, URINE; *see* **URINE CHLORIDE**

CHOLESTEROL, TOTAL

Normal range:
  Varies with age
  Generally <200 mg/dl (<5.20 mmol/L) [CF: 0.02586; SMI: 0.05 mmol/L]

Elevated in:
  Primary hypercholesterolemia, biliary obstruction, diabetes mellitus, nephrotic syndrome, hypothyroidism, primary biliary cirrhosis, high cholesterol diet, pregnancy third trimester, MI, drugs (steroids, phenothiazines, oral contraceptives)

Decreased in:
  Starvation, malabsorption, sideroblastic anemia, thalassemia, abetalipoproteinemia, hyperthyroidism, Cushing's syndrome, hepatic failure, multiple myeloma, polycythemia vera, chronic myelocytic leukemia, myeloid metaplasia, Waldenstrom's macroglobulinemia, myelofibrosis

TABLE 4-6 Some Important Chromosome Abnormalities in Hematopoietic Malignancies

MALIGNANCY	CHROMOSOME ABNORMALITIES	OTHER
CML	t(9;22) (q34;q11)	98% of CML; 25%-33% of adult ALL
CML blast crisis	t(9;22) (q34;q11) with trisomy 8	70% of cases
ANLL (general)	Trisomy 8	Most common ANLL abnormality
ANLL-M2	t(8;21) (q22.1;q27)	10%-18% of patients, often with loss of one sex chromosome
ANLL-M3	t(15;17) (q22;q11)	50%-70% (range 40%-100%) of cases
ANLL-M4	inv(16) (p13;q22)	30% of cases
ANLL-M5	t(9;11) (p22;q23)	35% of cases
ALL-L1	t(1;19) (q23;q13)	Pre-B-cell origin / Pre–Pre-B-cell origin
ALL-L2	t(4;11) (q21;q23) / del (6) (q21;q25)	"Common" B-cell origin
ALL-L3	t(8;14) (q24;q32)	B-cell origin
Myelodysplasia	del (5q)	Most common chromosome abnormality
Burkitt's lymphoma	t(8;14) (q;24;32)	80% of cases, also some cases of small noncleaved non-Burkitt's
Follicular (nodular) lymphoma	t(14;18) (q32;q21)	80%-90% of cases by chromosome analysis, nearly 100% by DNA probe; involves Bcl-2 oncogene on chromosome 18
CLL	Trisomy 12	Most common abnormality
Therapy-related ANLL	del (5q) or del (7q)	90% of cases

From Ravel R: *Clinical laboratory medicine,* ed 6, St Louis, 1995, Mosby.
*Diagnostic abnormality.
CML, Chronic myelogenous leukemia; *ANLL,* acute nonlymphocytic leukemia; *ALL,* acute lymphocytic leukemia; *CLL,* chronic lymphocytic leukemia. M and L followed by a number refers to FAB categories of acute leukemia.

CHOLESTEROL, LOW-DENSITY LIPOPROTEIN; see LOW-DENSITY LIPOPROTEIN CHOLESTEROL
CHOLESTEROL, HIGH-DENSITY LIPOPROTEIN; see HIGH-DENSITY LIPOPROTEIN CHOLESTEROL
CHROMOSOME ABNORMALITIES IN MALIGNANCY; See Table 4-6
CIRCULATING ANTICOAGULANT (lupus anticoagulant)
Normal:
  Negative
Detected in:
  SLE, drug-induced lupus, long-term phenothiazine therapy, multiple myeloma, ulcerative colitis, rheumatoid arthritis, postpartum, hemophilia, neoplasms, chronic inflammatory states, AIDS, nephrotic syndrome
  NOTE: The name is a misnomer because these patients are prone to hypercoagulability and thrombosis.
CK; see CREATINE KINASE
CO; see CARBOXYHEMOGLOBIN
COAGULATION FACTORS; see Table 4-7 for characteristics of coagulation factors

TABLE 4-7 Characteristics of Coagulation Factors

FACTOR	DESCRIPTIVE NAME	SOURCE	APPROXIMATE HALF-LIFE (HR)	FUNCTION
I	Fibrinogen	Liver	120	Substrate for fibrin clot (CP)
II	Prothrombin	Liver (VKD)	60	Serine protease (CP)
V	Proaccelerin, labile factor	Liver	12-36	Cofactor (CP)
VII	Serum prothrombin conversion accelerator, proconvertin	Liver (VKD)	6	(?) Serine protease (EP)
VIII	Antihemophilic factor or globulin	Endothelial cells and (?) elsewhere	12	Cofactor (IP)
IX	Plasma thromboplastin component, Christmas factor	Liver (VKD)	24	Serine protease (IP)
X	Stuart-Prower factor	Liver (VKD)	36	Serine protease (CP)
XI	Plasma thromboplastin antecedent	(?) Liver	40-84	Serine protease (IP)
XII	Hageman factor	(?) Liver	50	Serine protease contact activation (IP)
XIII	Fibrin-stabilizing factor	(?) Liver	96-180	Transglutaminase (CP)
Prekallikrein	Fletcher factor	(?) Liver	?	Serine protease contact activation (IP)
High molecular weight kininogen	Fitzgerald factor, Flaujeac or Williams factor	(?) Liver	?	Cofactor, contact activation (IP)

From Noble J (ed): *Primary care medicine*, ed 2, St Louis, 1996, Mosby.
CP, Common pathway; *VKD,* vitamin K dependent; *EP,* extrinsic pathway; *IP,* intrinsic pathway.

Factor reference ranges:
   V: >10%
   VII: >10%
   VIII: 50% to 170%
   IX: 60% to 136%
   X: >10%
   XI: 50% to 150%
   XII: >30%
   Fig. 4-1 describes the blood coagulation pathways.

COLD AGGLUTININS TITER
Normal range:
   <1:32
Elevated in:
   Primary atypical pneumonia (mycoplasma pneumonia), infectious mononucleosis, CMV infection
   Others: hepatic cirrhosis, acquired hemolytic anemia, frostbite, multiple myeloma, lymphoma, malaria

COMPLEMENT
Normal range:
   C3: 70-160 mg/dl (0.7-1.6 g/L) [CF: 0.01; SMI: 0.1 g/L]
   C4: 20-40 mg/dl (0.2-0.4 g/L) [CF: 0.01; SMI: 0.1 g/L]
Abnormal values:
   See Tables 4-8 and 4-9.

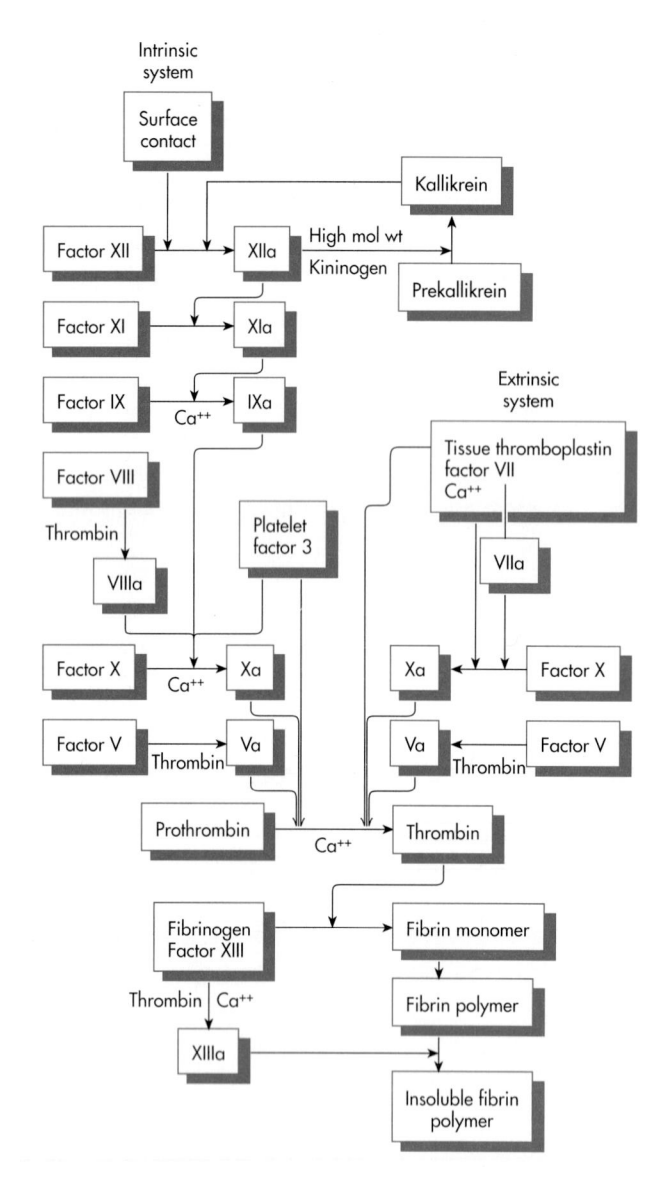

Fig. 4-1 **Blood coagulation pathways.** a, Activated. (From Ravel R: *Clinical laboratory medicine,* ed 6, St Louis, 1995, Mosby.)

TABLE 4-8 **Summary of Complement Deficiencies in Humans and Their Association with Repeated Infection and/or Collagen Disease**

DEFICIENT COMPONENT	PATIENTS	DISEASE/SYMPTOMS
C1r	4	SLE (1), renal disease (1), repeated infections (1)
C1s	2	SLE (2)
C4	3	SLE (3)
C2	23	LE (7), vasculitis (3), MPGN (1), dermatomyositis (1)
C3	4	Repeated infections (3), fever/rash/arthralgias (1)
C5	3	SLE (1), gonococcal disease
C6	5	Relapsing meningococcal meningitis (4), gonococcal disease (1)
C7	5	Raynaud's disease (1), chronic renal disease (1), gonococcal disease (2), SLE (1)
C8	3	SLE (1), gonococcal disease (1)

Adapted with permission from Sonnenwirth AC, Jarrett L (eds): *Gradwohl's clinical laboratory methods and diagnosis,* ed 8, St Louis, 1980, Mosby.
SLE, Systemic lupus erythematosus; *MPGN,* membranoproliferative glomerulonephritis.

TABLE 4-9 General Guide to the Evaluation of C4 and C3 Protein Levels in the Presence of Decreased Hemolytic Complement Activity

NORMAL C4	DECREASED C4
Normal C3	
Alterations in vitro (e.g., improper specimen handling)	Immune complex disease
Coagulation-associated complement consumption	Hypergammaglobulinemic states
Inborn errors (other than C4 or C3)	Cryoglobulinemia
	Hereditary angioedema
	Inborn C4 deficiency
Decreased C3	
Acute glomerulonephritis	Active SLE
Membranoproliferative glomerulonephritis	Serum sickness
Immune complex disease	Chronic active hepatitis
Active SLE	Subacute bacterial endocarditis
Inborn C3 deficiency	Immune complex disease

Adapted with permission from Sonnenwirth AC, Jarrett L (eds): *Gradwohl's clinical laboratory methods and diagnosis*, ed 8, St Louis, 1980, Mosby.

COMPLETE BLOOD COUNT (CBC)
  WBC 3200-9800 mm^3 (3.2-9.8 10^9/L) [CF: 0.001; SMI: 0.1 × 10^9/L]
  RBC
    Male: 4.3-5.9 10^6/mm^3 (4.3-5.9 10^{12}/L) [CF: 1; SMI: 0.1 × 10^{12}/L]
    Female: 3.5-5 10^6/mm^3 (3.5-5 10^{12}/L) [CF: 1; SMI: 0.1 × 10^{12}/L]
  Hemoglobin
    Male: 13.6-17.7 g/dl (136-172 g/L) [CF: 10; SMI: 1 g/L]
    Female: 12-15 g/dl (120-150 g/L) [CF: 10; SMI: 1 g/L]
  Hematocrit
    Male: 39% to 49% (0.39-0.49) [CF: 0.01; SMI: 0.01]
    Female: 33% to 43% (0.33-0.43) [CF: 0.01; SMI: 0.01]
  MCV: 76-100 μm^3 (76-100 fL) [CF: 1; SMI: 1 fL]
  MCH: 27-33 pg (27-33 pg) [CF: 1; SMI: 1 pg]
  MCHC: 33-37 g/dl (330-370 g/L) [CF: 10; SMI: 10 g/L]
  RDW: 11.5% to 14.5%
  Platelet count: 130-400 × 10^3/mm^3 (130-400 × 10^9/L) [CF: 1; SMI: 5 × 10^9/L]
  Differential:
    2-6 stabs (bands, early mature neutrophils)
    60-70 segs (mature neutrophils)
    1-4 eosinophils
    0-1 basophils
    2-8 monocytes
    25-40 lymphocytes
  Table 4-10 describes normal hematologic blood values at various ages.
CONJUGATED BILIRUBIN; *see* BILIRUBIN, DIRECT
COOMBS, DIRECT
Normal:
  Negative
Positive:
  Autoimmune hemolytic anemia, erythroblastosis fetalis, transfusion reactions, drugs (α-methyldopa, penicillins, tetracycline, sulfonamides, levodopa, cephalosporins, quinidine, insulin)

TABLE 4-10 Normal Hematologic Blood Values at Various Ages*

	CORD	DAY 1	DAY 2	DAY 3	DAY 7	DAY 14	DAY 30
Hb (g/100 ml, venous blood)	17.0 (13.5-22)	19.0† (14.5-23)	18.5 (15-23)	18 (14-23)	17.5 (13.5-22)	16.5 (13-21.5)	13.5 (10-17.5)
MCV (Fl)	110 (99-120)	109 (98-119)	115 (101-129)	116 (106-126)	114 (88-140)	106 (86-126)	102 (84-121)
Retics (%)	3-7	1.5-6.5	1.5-6.5	1-5	0-1	0-1	0-1
Nucleated RBCs (% of 100 WBCs)	2-5	1-3	0-1	0	0	0	
Platelets (1000s)	100-290	140-300	150-400		200-470		150-450
WBCs (1000s)	18.1 (9.0-30.0)	18.9 (9.4-34.0)			12.2 (5.0-21.0)	11.4 (5.0-20.0)	10.8 (5.0-19.5)
Neutrophils (% 100 WBCs)	55	60‡			50	40	35
Lymphocytes (% 100 WBCs)	30	30			35	50	55

	MONTH 2	MONTH 3	MONTH 6	MONTH 12	YEAR 5	YEAR 10	ADULT
Hb (g/100 ml, venous blood)	12.0 (10-13.5)	11.3 (9.7-13)	12.0 (10.1-14)	12.0 (10.5-13.5)	12.5 (10.7-14.7)	13.0 (10.8-15.5)	M: 14-18 F: 12-16
MCV (FL)	96 (80-118)		88 (73-100)	79 (71-86)	80 (73-86)	81 (75-87)	90 (80-100)
Retics (%)	0-1						0-1.5
Nucleated RBCs (% of 100 WBCs)	0						0
Platelets (1000s)							150-400
WBCs (1000s)			11.9 (6.0-17.5)	11.4 (6.0-17.5)	8.5 (5.0-14.5)	8.1 (4.5-13.5)	7.5 (4.5-10.5)
Neutrophils (% 100 WBCs)			30	30	50	55	60
Lymphocytes (% 100 WBCs)			60	60	40	40	40

From Ravel R: *Clinical laboratory medicine,* ed 6, St Louis, 1995, Mosby.
*Compiled from various sources. Numbers represent average values; numbers in parentheses indicate reference range.
†Capillary hemoglobin (Hb) is about 2 g higher than venous; the gap then narrows and disappears by day 7. Neonatal Hb is influenced by amount of blood received from the umbilical cord at delivery.
‡Normal neutrophil count is about 25% higher in capillary than venous blood on day 1 and about 10% higher on day 2.

False positive:
 May be seen with cold agglutinins
COOMBS, INDIRECT
Normal:
 Negative
Positive:
 Acquired hemolytic anemia, incompatible cross-matched blood, anti-Rh antibodies, drugs (methyldopa, mefenamic acid, levodopa)
CPK; *see* CREATINE KINASE
COPPER (serum)
Normal range:
 70-140 μg/dl (11-22 μmol/L) [CF: 0.1574, SMI: 0.2 μmol/L]

Decreased in:
  Wilson's disease, Menkes' syndrome, malabsorption, malnutrition, nephrosis, TPN, acute leukemia in remission

Elevated in:
  Aplastic anemia, biliary cirrhosis, SLE, hemochromatosis, hyperthyroidism, hypothyroidism, infection, iron deficiency anemia, leukemia, lymphoma, oral contraceptives, pernicious anemia, rheumatoid arthritis

COPPER, URINE; see URINE COPPER
CORTISOL (plasma)
Normal range:
  Varies with time of collection (circadian variation):
    8 AM: 4-19 µg/dl (110-520 nmol/L) [CF: 27.59; SMI: 10 nmol/L]
    4 PM: 2-15 µg/dl (50-410 nmol/L) [CF: 27.59; SMI: 10 nmol/L]

Elevated in:
  Ectopic ACTH production (i.e., oat cell carcinoma of lung), loss of normal diurnal variation, pregnancy, chronic renal failure
  Iatrogenic, stress, adrenal or pituitary hyperplasia or adenomas

Decreased in:
  Primary adrenocortical insufficiency, anterior pituitary hypofunction, secondary adrenocortical insufficiency, adrenogenital syndromes

C-PEPTIDE
Elevated in:
  Insulinoma, sulfonylurea administration

Decreased in:
  IDDM, factitious insulin administration

CPK; see CREATINE KINASE
C-REACTIVE PROTEIN
Normal range:
  6.8-820 µg/dl (68-8200 µg/L) [CF: 10; SMI: 10 µg/L]

Elevated in:
  Rheumatoid arthritis, rheumatic fever, inflammatory bowel disease, bacterial infections, MI, oral contraceptives, pregnancy third trimester (acute phase reactant), inflammatory and neoplastic diseases

CREATINE KINASE (CK, CPK)
Normal range:
  0-130 U/L (0-2.16 µkat/L) [CF: 0.01667; SMI: 0.01 µkat/L]

Elevated in:
  MI, myocarditis, rhabdomyolysis, myositis, crush injury/trauma, polymyositis, dermatomyositis, vigorous exercise, muscular dystrophy, myxedema, seizures, malignant hyperthermia syndrome, IM injections, CVA, pulmonary embolism and infarction, acute dissection of aorta

Decreased in:
  Steroids, decreased muscle mass, connective tissue disorders, alcoholic liver disease, metastatic neoplasms

CREATINE KINASE ISOENZYMES
CK-MB
  Elevated in: MI, myocarditis, pericarditis, muscular dystrophy, cardiac defibrillation, cardiac surgery, extensive rhabdomyolysis, strenuous exercise (marathon runners), mixed connective tissue disease, cardiomyopathy, hypothermia
  NOTE: CK-MB exists in the blood in two subforms. MB_2 is released from cardiac cells and converted in the blood to MB_1. Rapid assay of CK-MB subforms can

detect MI (CK-MB$_2$ ≥1.0 U/L, with a ratio of CK-MB$_2$/CK-MB$_1$ ≥1.5) within the first 6 hours of onset of symptoms.*

CK-MM
 Elevated in: crush injury, seizures, malignant hyperthermia syndrome, rhabdomyolysis, myositis, polymyositis, dermatomyositis, vigorous exercise, muscular dystrophy, IM injections, acute dissection of aorta

CK-BB
 Elevated in: CVA, subarachnoid hemorrhage, neoplasms (prostate, GI tract, brain, ovary, breast, lung), severe shock, bowel infarction, hypothermia meningitis

CREATININE (serum)
Normal range:
 0.6-1.2 mg/dl (50-110 μmol/L) [CF: 88.4; SMI: 10 μmol/L]
Elevated in:
 Renal insufficiency (acute and chronic), decreased renal perfusion (hypotension, dehydration, CHF), urinary tract infection, rhabdomyolysis, ketonemia
 Drugs (antibiotics [aminoglycosides, cephalosporins], hydantoin, diuretics, methyldopa)
Falsely elevated in:
 DKA, administration of some cephalosporins (e.g., cefoxitin, cephalothin)
Decreased in:
 Decreased muscle mass (including amputees and older persons), pregnancy, prolonged debilitation

CREATININE CLEARANCE
Normal range:
 75-124 ml/min (1.24-2.08 ml/sec) [CF: 0.01667; SMI: 0.02 ml/sec]
Elevated in:
 Pregnancy, exercise
Decreased in:
 Renal insufficiency, drugs (cimetidine, procainamide, antibiotics, quinidine)

CREATININE, URINE; *see* URINE CREATININE
CRYOGLOBULINS (serum)
Normal range:
 Not detectable
Present in:
 Collagen-vascular diseases, CLL, hemolytic anemias, multiple myeloma, Waldenstrom's macroglobulinemia, chronic active hepatitis, Hodgkin's disease

CSF; *see* CEREBROSPINAL FLUID[1]
DRUG MONITORING; *see* Table 4-11
ELECTROLYTES, URINE; *see* URINE ELECTROLYTES
ELECTROPHORESIS, HEMOGLOBIN; *see* HEMOGLOBIN ELECTROPHORESIS
ELECTROPHORESIS, PROTEIN; *see* PROTEIN ELECTROPHORESIS
ENA-COMPLEX; *see* EXTRACTABLE NUCLEAR ANTIGEN
EOSINOPHIL COUNT
Normal range:
 1%-4% eosinophils (0-440/mm^3)
Elevated in:
 Allergy, parasitic infestations (trichinosis, aspergillosis, hydatidosis), angioneurotic edema, drug reactions, warfarin sensitivity, collagen-vascular diseases, acute hypereosinophilic syndrome, eosinophilic nonallergic rhinitis, myelo-

---

*From Puleo PR et al: Use of rapid assay of subforms of creatine kinase MB to diagnose or rule out acute MI, *N Engl J Med* 331:561-566, 1994.

LABORATORY TESTS   Creatinine/Eosinophil count   799

TABLE 4-11 Therapeutic Drug Monitoring Data*

	% PROTEIN BOUND	HALF-LIFE ADULTS	HALF-LIFE CHILDREN	TIME TO PEAK PLASMA LEVEL†	LIVER METABOLISM	TIME TO STEADY STATE ADULTS	TIME TO STEADY STATE CHILDREN	THERAPEUTIC RANGE ADULTS	THERAPEUTIC RANGE CHILDREN	TOXIC LEVELS
Lithium carbonate	0	8-35 hr	—	1-3 hr	No	2-7 days	—	0.8-1.4 mEq/L	—	2.0 mEq/L
Amitriptyline	82-96	17-40 hr	—	4-8 hr	Yes	4-8 days	—	120-250 ng/ml	—	500 ng/ml
Desipramine	73-92	12-54 hr	—	2-8 hr	Yes	2.5-11 days	—	150-250 ng/ml	—	500 ng/ml
Imipramine	80-95	9-24 hr	—	1-2 hr	Yes	2-5 days	—	150-250 ng/ml	—	500 ng/ml
Nortriptyline	93-95	18-93 hr	—	4-8 hr	Yes	4-19 days	—	50-150 ng/ml	—	500 ng/ml
Acetylsalicylic acid	50-90	2-4.5 hr	2-3 hr	1-2 hr	Yes	10-22.5 hr	10-15 hr	Depends on use	Same	300 µg/ml
Acetaminophen	20-30	2-4 hr	2-4 hr	0.5-1.0 hr	Yes	10-20 hr	10-20 hr	Depends on use	Same	250 µg/ml
Theophylline	55-65	3-8 hr	1-8 hr	1-3 hr	Yes	15-20 hr	5-40 hr	10-20 µg/ml	Same	20 µg/ml
Methotrexate	50-70	1.5-15 hr	1.5-15 hr	1-2 hr	No	Varies	Varies	>0.01 µmol	—	10 µmol/24 hr
Carbamazepine	65-85	10-30 hr	8-19 hr	6-18 hr	Yes	2-6 days	2-4 days	8-12 µg/ml	Same	15 µg/ml
Ethosuximide	0	40-60 hr	30-50 hr	1-2 hr	Yes	8-12 days	6-10 days	40-100 µg/ml	Same	150 µg/ml
Phenobarbital	45-50	50-120 hr	40-70 hr	6-18 hr	Yes	11-25 days	8-15 days	15-40 µg/ml	Same	50 µg/ml
Phenytoin	87-93	18-30 hr	12-22 hr	4-8 hr	Yes	4-6 days	2-5 days	10-20 µg/ml	Same	20 µg/ml
Primidone	0-20	4-12 hr	4-6 hr	2-4 hr	Yes	16-60 hr	20-30 hr	5-12 µg/ml	Same	15 µg/ml
Valproic acid	90-95	8-15 hr	6-15 hr	0.5-1.5 hr	Yes	40-75 hr	30-75 hr	50-100 µg/ml	Same	200 µg/ml
Digoxin	10-40	32-51 hr	11-50 hr	1.5-5 hr	20%	7-11 days	2-10 days	0.1-2.0 ng/ml	Same	2.4 ng/ml
Disopyramide	10-80	5-6 hr	—	1-3 hr	Yes	25-30 hr	—	2-5 µg/ml	—	7 µg/ml
Lidocaine	60-70	1-2 hr	—	15-30 min (IM)	Yes	5-10 hr	—	1.5-5.0 µg/ml	—	7 µg/ml
Procainamide (PA)	15	2.2-4 hr	—	1-2 hr	Yes	11-20 hr	—	4-10 µg/ml	—	16 µg/ml
NAPA	10	4-8 hr	—	—	No	22-40 hr	—	9-20 µg/ml	—	—
PA + NAPA	—	—	—	—	—	—	—	10-30 µg/ml	—	30 µg/ml
Propranolol	90-96	2-6 hr	—	1-2 hr	Yes	10-30 hr	—	50-100 ng/ml	—	Variable
Quinidine sulfate	80-90	4-7 hr	—	1.5-2 hr	Yes	20-35 hr	—	2-5 µg/ml§	—	10 µg/ml
Amikacin	0-11	2-3 hr	—	1 hr (IM)	No	10-15 hr	—	15-25 µg/ml	—	35 µg/ml peak 5 µg/ml residual
Gentamicin	0-10	2-3 hr	2-3 hr	1 hr (IM) 0.5 hr (IV)	No	10-15 hr	10-15 hr	5-10 µg/ml	—	12 µg/ml peak 2 µg/ml residual
Tobramycin	0-10	2-3 hr	—	1 hr (IM)	No	10-15 hr	—	5-10 µg/ml	—	Same as gentamicin
Vancomycin	50	4-8 hr	2-3 hr	15 min (IV)	Minor component	—	—	5-10 µg/ml trough 30-40 µg/ml peak	—	80-100 mg/L

From Ravel R: *Clinical laboratory medicine,* ed 6, St Louis, 1995, Mosby.
*Compiled from various sources. *IM,* Intramuscular.
†Oral dose unless otherwise specified.
§More specific methods (HPLC or EMIT).

proliferative disorders, Hodgkin's lymphoma, radiation therapy, NHL, L-tryptophan ingestion, urticaria, pernicious anemia, pemphigus, inflammatory bowel disease, bronchial asthma

EPSTEIN-BARR VIRAL (EBV) INFECTION; *see* Table 4-12, Fig. 4-2, and Box 4-9 for test interpretation

ERYTHROCYTE SEDIMENTATION RATE (ESR; Westergren)

Normal range:
Male: 0-15 mm/hr
Female: 0-20 mm/hr

Elevated in:
Collagen-vascular diseases, infections, MI, neoplasms, inflammatory states (acute phase reactant), hyperthyroidism, hypothyroidism, rouleaux formation

TABLE 4-12   Antibody Tests in EBV Infection

	APPEARANCE*	PEAK	DISAPPEARS
Heterophil Ab	3-5 days after onset of Sx (range, 0-21 days)	During second wk after onset of Sx (1-4 wk)	2-3 mo after onset of Sx (still found at 1 yr in 20% of cases)
VCA-IgM	Beginning of Sx (1 wk before to 1 wk after Sx begin)	During first wk after onset of Sx (0-21 days)	2-3 mo after onset of Sx (1-6 mo)
VCA-IgG	3 days after onset of Sx (0-2 wk)	During second wk after onset of Sx (1-3 wk)	Decline to lower level, then persists for life
EBNA-IgG	3 wk after onset of Sx (1-4 wk)	8 mo after appearance (3-12 mo)	Lifelong
EA-D	5 days after onset of Sx (during first 1-2 wk after onset of Sx)	14-21 days after onset of Sx (1-4 wk)	9 wk after appearance (2-6 mo)
(EBNA-IgM)	(Same as VCA-IgM)	(Same as VCA-IgM)	(Same as VCA-IgM)

From Ravel R: *Clinical laboratory medicine*, ed 6, St Louis, 1995, Mosby.
*Sx, Symptoms.

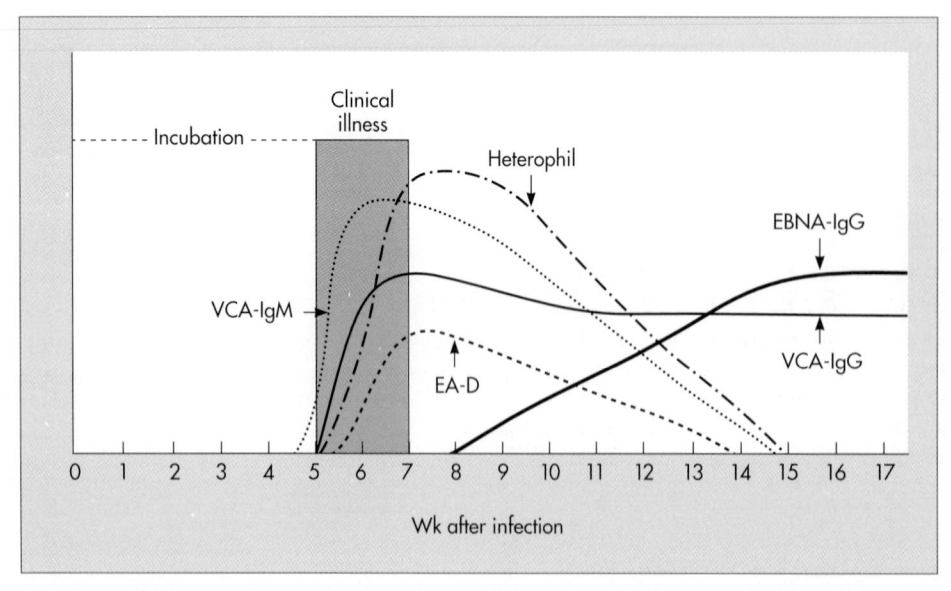

Fig. 4-2   Tests in EBV infection. (From Ravel R: *Clinical laboratory medicine*, ed 6, St Louis, 1995, Mosby.)

> **BOX 4-9 Summary of Epstein-Barr Antibody Test Interpretation**
>
> Never infected (susceptible): VCA-IgM and IgG both negative.
> Presumptive primary infection: clinical symptoms, heterophil positive.
> Primary infection: VCA-IgM positive (EBNA-IgG negative; heterophil positive or negative)
> Reactivated infection: VCA-IgG positive; EBNA-IgG positive; EA-D positive (heterophil negative, VCA-IgM negative)
> Old previous infection: VCA-IgG positive; EBNA-IgG positive; EA-D negative (VCA-IgM negative, heterophil negative)

From Ravel R: *Clinical laboratory medicine,* ed 6, St Louis, 1995, Mosby.

Decreased in:
  Sickle cell disease, polycythemia, corticosteroids, spherocytosis, anisocytosis, hypofibrinogenemia, increased serum viscosity

EXTRACTABLE NUCLEAR ANTIGEN (ENA complex, anti-RNP antibody, anti-Sm, anti-Smith)
Normal:
  Negative
Present in:
  SLE, rheumatoid arthritis, Sjögren's syndrome, mixed connective tissue disease (MCTD)

FDP; *see* **FIBRIN DEGRADATION PRODUCT**

FECAL FAT, QUANTITATIVE (72-hr collection)
Normal range:
  2-6 g/24 hr (7-21 mmol/dl) [CF: 3.515; SMI: 1 mmol/dl]
Elevated in:
  Malabsorption syndrome

FERRITIN (serum)
Normal range:
  18-300 ng/ml (18-300 µg/L) [CF: 1; SMI: 10 µg/L]
Elevated in:
  Hyperthyroidism, inflammatory states, liver disease (ferritin elevated from necrotic hepatocytes), neoplasms (neuroblastomas, lymphomas, leukemia, breast carcinoma), iron replacement therapy, hemochromatosis, hemosiderosis
Decreased in:
  Iron deficiency anemia

α-1 FETOPROTEIN
Normal range:
  0-20 ng/ml (0-20 µg/L) [CF: 1; SMI: 1 µg/L]
Elevated in:
  Hepatocellular carcinoma (usually values >1000 ng/ml), germinal neoplasms (testis, ovary, mediastinum, retroperitoneum), liver disease (alcoholic cirrhosis, acute hepatitis, chronic active hepatitis), fetal anencephaly, spina bifida, basal cell carcinoma, breast carcinoma, pancreatic carcinoma, gastric carcinoma, retinoblastoma, esophageal atresia

FIBRIN DEGRADATION PRODUCT (FDP)
Normal range:
  <10 µg/ml
Elevated in:
  DIC, primary fibrinolysis, pulmonary embolism, severe liver disease
  NOTE: The presence of rheumatoid factor may cause falsely elevated FDP.

FIBRINOGEN
Normal range:
  200-400 mg/dl (2-4 g/L) [CF: 0.01; SMI: 0.1 g/L]

Elevated in:
   Tissue inflammation or damage (acute phase protein reactant), oral contraceptives, pregnancy, acute infection, MI
Decreased in:
   DIC, hereditary afibrinogenemia, liver disease, primary or secondary fibrinolysis, cachexia

FLUORESCENT TREPONEMAL ANTIBODY; see **FTA-ABS**

FOLATE (FOLIC ACID)
Normal range:
   Plasma: 2-10 ng/ml (4-22 nmol/L) [CF: 2.266; SMI: 2 nmol/L]
   RBC: 140-960 ng/ml (550-2200 nmol/L) [CF: 2.266; SMI: 10 nmol/L]
Decreased in:
   Folic acid deficiency (inadequate intake, malabsorption), alcoholism, drugs (methotrexate, trimethoprim, phenytoin, oral contraceptives, azulfadine), vitamin B_{12} deficiency (detective red cell folate absorption), hemolytic anemia
Elevated in:
   Folic acid therapy

FREE T_4; see **T_4, FREE**

FREE THYROXINE INDEX
Normal range:
   1.1-4.3
   See Boxes 4-10 and 4-11 for causes of abnormal results.

GAMMA-GLUTAYL TRANSFERASE (GGT); see **γ-GLUTAMYL TRANSFERASE**

GASTRIN (serum)
Normal range:
   0-180 pg/ml (0-180 ng/L) [CF: 1; SMI: 10 ng/L]
Elevated in:
   Zollinger-Ellison syndrome (gastrinoma), pernicious anemia, hyperparathyroidism, retained gastric antrum, chronic renal failure, gastric ulcer, chronic atrophic gastritis, pyloric obstruction, malignant neoplasms of the stomach, H_2 blockers, omeprazole, calcium therapy, ulcerative colitis, rheumatoid arthritis

---

BOX 4-10 Causes for Increased Thyroxine or Free Thyroxine Values

Laboratory error
Primary hyperthyroidism (T_4/T_3 type)
Severe TBG elevation; some patients with some FT_4 kits
Excess therapy of hypothyroidism
Excessive dose of levothyroxine
Active thyroiditis (subacute, painless, early active Hashimoto's disease); some patients
Familial dysalbuminemic hyperthyroxinemia (some FT_4 kits, especially analog types)
Peripheral resistance to T_4 syndrome
Aminodarone or propranolol; some patients
Postpartem transient toxicosis
Factitious hyperthyroidism
Jod-Basedow (iodine-induced) hyperthyroidism
Severe nonthyroid illness, occasional patients
Acute psychosis (especially paranoid schizophrenia); some patients
T_4 sample drawn 2-4 hr after Synthroid dose
Struma ovarii
Pituitary TSH-secreting tumor; some patients
Certain x-ray contrast media (Telepaque and Oragrafin)
Acute porphyria; some patients
Heparin effect (some T_4 and FT_4 kits)
Amphetamine, heroin, methadone, and PCP abuse; some patients
Perphenazine or 5-fluorouracil; some patients
Antithyroid or anti-IgG heterophil (HAMA*) autoantibodies (some sandwich-method monoclonal antibody kits); occasional patients
"T_4" hyperthyroidism
Hyperemesis gravidarum; about 50% of patients
High altitudes, some patients

From Ravel R: *Clinical laboratory medicine,* ed 6, St Louis, 1995, Mosby.
*Human antimouse antibodies.

> **BOX 4-11** **Causes for Decreased Thyroxine or Free Thyroxine Values**
>
> Laboratory error
> Primary hypothyroidism
> Severe nonthyroid illness;* many patients
> Lithium therapy; some patients
> Severe TBG decrease (congenital, disease, or drug-induced) or severe albumin decrease*
> Dilantin, Depakene, or high-dose salicylate drugs*
> Pituitary insufficiency
> Large doses of inorganic iodide (e.g., SSKI)
> Moderate or severe iodine deficiency
> Cushing's syndrome
> High-dose glucocorticoid drugs; some patients
> Pregnancy, third trimester (low normal or small decrease)
> Addison's disease; some patients (30%)
> Heparin effect (a few FT_4 kits)
> Desipramine or amiodarone drugs; some patients
> Acute psychiatric illness; a few patients

From Ravel R: *Clinical laboratory medicine*, ed 6, St Louis, 1995, Mosby.
*FT_4 less affected than T_4; two-step FT_4 method affected less than analog FT_4 method.

GLOMERULAR BASEMENT MEMBRANE (GBM) ANTIBODY
Normal:
  Negative
Present in:
  Goodpasture's syndrome

GLUCOSE, FASTING
Normal range:
  70-110 mg/dl (3.9-6.1 mmol/L) [CF: 0.05551; SMI: 0.1 mmol/L]
Elevated in:
  Diabetes mellitus, stress, infections, MI, CVA, Cushing's syndrome, acromegaly, acute pancreatitis, glucagonoma, hemochromatosis, drugs (glucocorticoids, diuretics [thiazides, loop diuretics]), glucose intolerance

GLUCOSE, POSTPRANDIAL
Normal range:
  <140 mg/dl (<7.8 mmol/L) [CF: 0.05551; SMI: 0.1 mmol/L]
Elevated in:
  Diabetes mellitus, glucose intolerance
Decreased in:
  Postgastrointestinal resection, reactive hypoglycemia, hereditary fructose intolerance, galactosemia, leucine sensitivity

GLUCOSE TOLERANCE TEST
Normal values above fasting:
  30 min: 30-60 mg/dl (1.65-3.3 mmol/L) [CF: 0.05551; SMI: 0.1 mmol/L]
  60 min: 20-50 mg/dl (1.1-2.75 mmol/L) [CF: 0.05551; SMI: 0.1 mmol/L]
  120 min: 5-15 mg/dl (0.28-0.83 mmol/L) [CF: 0.05551; SMI: 0.1 mmol/L]
  180 min: fasting level or below
Abnormal in:
  Glucose intolerance, diabetes mellitus, Cushing's syndrome, acromegaly, pheochromocytoma, gestational diabetes

GLUCOSE-6-PHOSPHATE DEHYDROGENASE SCREEN (blood)
Normal:
  G_6PD enzyme activity detected
Abnormal:
  If a deficiency is detected, quantitation of G_6PD is necessary; a G_6PD screen may be falsely interpreted as "normal" after an episode of hemolysis because most G_6PD deficient cells have been destroyed.

γ-GLUTAMYL TRANSFERASE (GGT)
Normal range:
  0-30 U/L (0.050 μkat/L) [CF: 0.01667; SMI: 0.01 μkat/L]

Elevated in:
　Chronic alcoholic liver disease, neoplasms (hepatoma, metastatic disease to the liver, carcinoma of the pancreas), SLE, CHF, trauma, nephrotic syndrome, sepsis, cholestasis, drugs (phenytoin, barbiturates), other (Box 4-12 lists additional causes of GGT elevation.)

GLYCATED (GLYCOSYLATED) HEMOGLOBIN (HbA$_{1c}$)

Normal range:
　4.0% to 6.7%

Elevated in:
　Uncontrolled diabetes mellitus (glycated hemoglobin levels reflect the level of glucose control over the preceding 120 days), lead toxicity, alcoholism, iron deficiency anemia, hypertriglyceridemia

Decreased in:
　Hemolytic anemias, decreased RBC survival, pregnancy, acute or chronic blood loss, chronic renal failure, insulinoma, congenital spherocytosis, HbS, HbC, HbD diseases

HAM TEST (acid serum test)

Normal:
　Negative

Positive in:
　Paroxysmal nocturnal hemoglobinuria (PNH)

False positive in:
　Hereditary or acquired spherocytosis, recent transfusion with aged RBCs, aplastic anemia, myeloproliferative syndromes, leukemia, hereditary dyserythropoietic anemia type II (HEMPAS)

HAPTOGLOBIN (serum)

Normal range:
　50-220 mg/dl (0.50-2.2 g/L) [CF: 0.01; SMI: 0.01 g/L]

Elevated in:
　Inflammation (acute phase reactant), collagen-vascular diseases, infections (acute phase reactant), drugs (androgens), obstructive liver disease

Decreased in:
　Hemolysis (intravascular more than extravascular), megaloblastic anemia, severe liver disease, large tissue hematomas, infectious mononucleosis, drugs (oral contraceptives)

HDL; *see* **HIGH-DENSITY LIPOPROTEIN CHOLESTEROL**

BOX 4-12 Some Etiologies for γ-Glutamyltransferase (GGT) Elevation

Liver space-occupying lesions (M-H)* (88%, 45%-100%)†
Alcoholic active liver disease (M, occasionally H) (85%, 63%-100%)
Common bile duct obstruction (M-H) (90%, 62%-100%)
Intrahepatic cholestasis (M-H) (90%, 83%-94%)
Biliary tract acute inflammation (M-H) (95%, 90%-100%)
Acute hepatitis virus hepatitis (M, occasionally H) (95%, 89%-100%)
Infectious mononucleosis (M/S, occasionally H) (90%)
Cytomegalovirus acute infection (S/M) (75%)
Acute pancreatitis (M, occasionally H) (85%, 71%-100%)
Active granulation tissue formation (S-M)
Acetaminophen overdose (S/M)

Dilantin therapy (S, occasionally M) (70%, 58%-90%)
Phenobarbitol (similar to Dilantin)
Severe liver passive congestion (S) (60%)
Reye's syndrome (S) (63%)
Other; all usually S elevations
　Acute MI (5%-30%)
　Tegretol (30%)
　Hyperthyroidism (0%-62%)
　Epilepsy (50%-85%)
　Brain tumor (57%)
　Diabetes mellitus (24%-57%)
　Non-alcohol fatty liver

From Ravel R: *Clinical laboratory medicine,* ed 6, St Louis, 1995, Mosby.
*S, Small (1-3× upper limit); M, moderate (3-5×); H, high (over 5×).
†Percentage of patients, with literature range.

HEMATOCRIT
Normal range:
  Male: 39% to 49% (0.39-0.49) [CF: 0.01; SMI: 0.01]
  Female: 33% to 43% (0.33-0.43) [CF: 0.01; SMI: 0.01]
Elevated in:
  Polycythemia vera, smoking, COPD, high altitudes, dehydration, hypovolemia
Decreased in:
  Blood loss (GI, GU), anemia

HEMOGLOBIN
Normal range:
  Male: 13.6-17.7 g/dl (136-172 g/L) [CF: 10; SMI: 1 g/L]
  Female: 12.0-15.0 g/dl (120-150 g/L) [CF: 10; SMI: 1 g/L]
Elevated in:
  Hemoconcentration, dehydration, polycythemia vera, COPD, high altitudes, false elevations (hyperlipemic plasma, WBC >50,000 mm^3), stress
Decreased in:
  Hemorrhage (GI, GU), anemia
  Fig. 4-3 describes a diagnostic approach to low hemoglobin/hematocrit levels.

HEMOGLOBIN ELECTROPHORESIS
Normal range:
  HbA$_1$: 95%-98%
  HbA$_2$: 1.5%-3.5%
  HbF: <2%
  HbC: absent
  HbS: absent

HEMOGLOBIN, GLYCATED; see GLYCATED HEMOGLOBIN
HEMOGLOBIN, GLYCOSYLATED; see GLYCATED HEMOGLOBIN

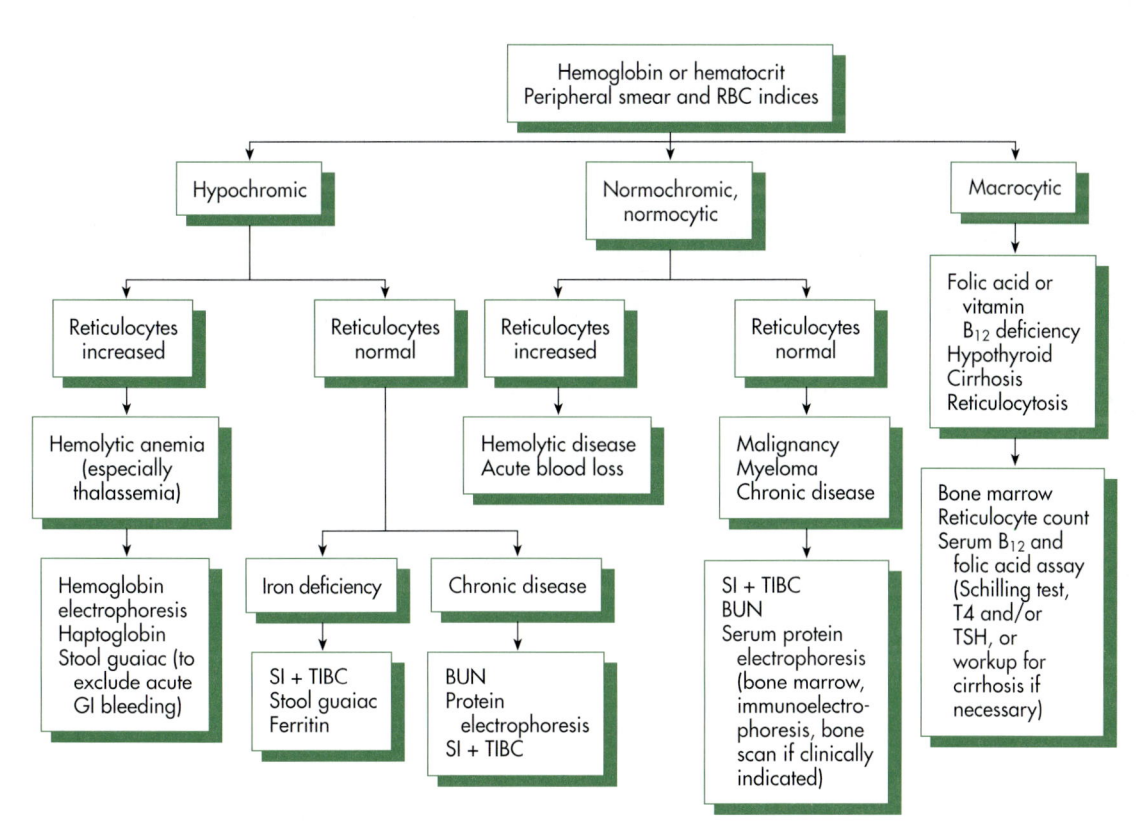

Fig. 4-3 Simplified guide to anemia diagnosis using a minimum of tests aimed at most important disease categories. (From Ravel R: *Clinical laboratory medicine,* ed 6, St Louis, 1995, Mosby.)

HEMOGLOBIN, URINE; see URINE HEMOGLOBIN
HEMOSIDERIN, URINE; see URINE HEMOSIDERIN
HEPATITIS A ANTIBODY
Normal:
    Negative
Present in:
    Viral hepatitis A; can be IgM or IgG (if IgM, acute hepatitis A; if IgG previous infection with hepatitis A); see Boxes 4-13, 4-14, and 4-15 and Fig. 4-4
HEPATITIS A VIRAL INFECTION; see above
HEPATITIS B SURFACE ANTIGEN (HBsAg)
Normal:
    Not detected
Detected in:
    Acute viral hepatitis type B, chronic hepatitis B (Boxes 4-16 through 4-24 and Figs. 4-5 through 4-8)
HEPATITIS B VIRAL INFECTION; see above
HEPATITIS C VIRAL INFECTION; see Boxes 4-25 through 4-27 and Fig. 4-9
HEPATITIS D VIRAL INFECTION; see Boxes 4-28 through 4-30 and Fig. 4-10

BOX 4-13 HAV Antibodies

HAV-IgM Antibody

Appearance

About the same time as clinical symptoms (3-4 wk after exposure, range 14-60 days), or just before beginning of AST/ALT elevation (range 10 days before - 7 days after)

Peak

About 3-4 wk after onset of symptoms (1-6 wk)

Becomes Nondetectable

3-4 mo after onset of symptoms (1-6 mo). In a few cases HAV-IgM antibody can persist as long as 12-14 mo.

HAV-Total Antibody

Appearance

About 3 wk after IgM becomes detectable (therefore about the middle of clinical symptom period to early convalescence)

Peak

About 1-2 mo after onset

Becomes Nondetectable

Remains elevated for life, but can slowly fall somewhat

From Ravel R: *Clinical laboratory medicine*, ed 6, St Louis, 1995, Mosby.

BOX 4-14 Hepatitis A Antigen and Antibodies

HAV-Ag by EM (in stool)
    Shows presence of virus in stool early in infection

HAV-Ab (IgM)
    Current or recent HAV infection
HAV-Ab (total)
    Convalescent or old HAV infection

From Ravel R: *Clinical laboratory medicine*, ed 6, St Louis, 1995, Mosby.

BOX 4-15 Summary: Diagnosis of HAV Infection

Best all-purpose test(s) to diagnose acute HAV infection = HAV-Ab (IgM)

Best all-purpose test(s) to demonstrate past HAV infection/immunity = HAV-Ab (total)

From Ravel R: *Clinical laboratory medicine*, ed 6, St Louis, 1995, Mosby.

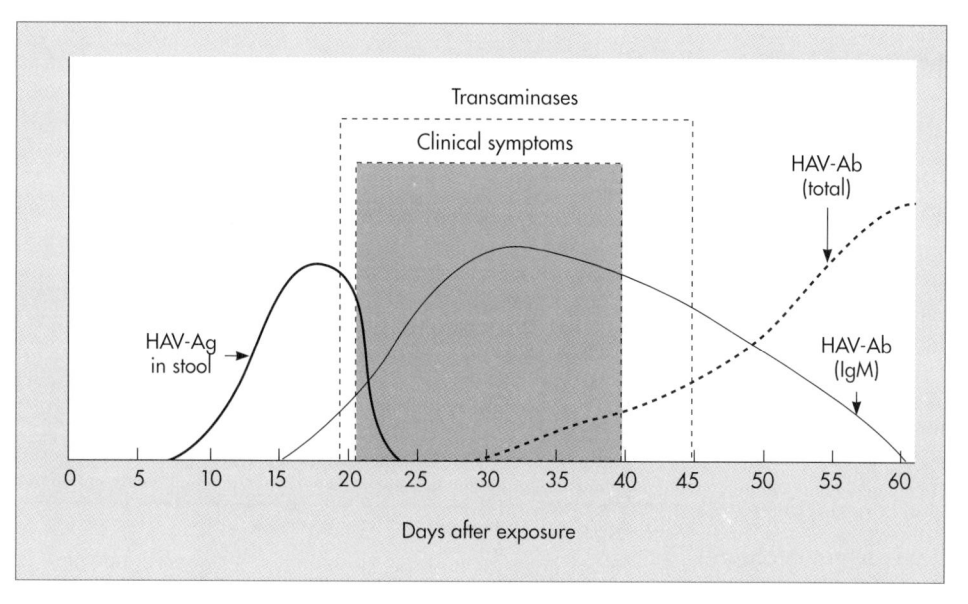

Fig. 4-4 **Serologic tests in HAV infection.** (From Ravel R: *Clinical laboratory medicine,* ed 6, St Louis, 1995, Mosby.)

BOX 4-16 Interpretation of Hepatitis B Serologic Tests

I. HB$_S$Ag positive, HB$_C$Ab negative*
   About 5% (range 0%-17%) of patients with early stage HBV acute infection (HB$_C$Ab rises later)
II. HB$_S$Ag positive, HB$_C$Ab positive, HB$_S$Ab negative
   a. Most of the clinical symptom stage
   b. Chronic HBV carriers without evidence of liver disease ("asymptomatic carriers")
   c. Chronic HBV hepatitis (chronic persistent type or chronic active type)
III. Hb$_S$Ag negative, HB$_C$Ab positive,* HB$_S$Ab negative
   a. Late clinical symptom stage or early convalescence stage (core window)
   b. Chronic HBV infection with HB$_S$Ag below detection levels with current tests
   c. Old previous HBV infection
IV. HB$_S$Ag negative, HB$_C$Ab positive, HB$_S$Ab positive
   a. Late convalescence to complete recovery
   b. Old infection

From Ravel R: *Clinical laboratory medicine,* ed 6, St Louis, 1995, Mosby.
*HB$_C$Ab, Combined IgM + IgG. In some cases (e.g., category III), selective Hb$_C$Ab-IgM assay is useful to differentiate recent and old infection.

BOX 4-17 HB$_S$Ag by Immunoassay

Appearance
2-6 wk after exposure (range 6 days-6 mo). 5%-15% of patients are negative at onset of jaundice

Peak
1-2 wk before to 1-2 wk after onset of symptoms

Becomes Nondetectable
1-3 mo after peak (range 1 wk-5 mo)

From Ravel R: *Clinical laboratory medicine,* ed 6, St Louis, 1995, Mosby.

BOX 4-18 Summary: HBV Surface Antigen and Antibody

HB$_S$Ag by immunoassay
1. Means current active HBV infection.
2. Persistence over 6 mo indicates carrier/chronic HBV infection.

HB$_S$Ag by nucleic acid probe
1. Same significance as detection by immunoassay.
2. Present before and longer than HB$_S$Ag by immunoassay.
3. More reliable marker for increased infectivity than HB$_S$Ag by immunoassay and/or HB$_e$Ag.

From Ravel R: *Clinical laboratory medicine,* ed 6, St Louis, 1995, Mosby.

BOX 4-19 Summary of Hepatitis Test Applications

HB_S

-AG

HB_SAg: shows current active HBV infection.
Persistence over 6 mo indicates carrier/chronic HBV infection.
HBV nucleic acid probe: present before and longer than HB_SAg.
More reliable marker for increased infectivity than HB_SAg and/or HB_eAg.

-Ab

HB_SAb-total: Shows previous healed HBV infection and evidence of immunity.

HB_C

-Ab

HB_CAb-IgM: Shows either acute or very recent infection by HBV.
In convalescent phase of acute HBV, may be elevated when HB_SAg has disappeared (core window).
Negative HB_CAb-IgM with positive HB_SAg suggests either very early acute HBV or carrier/chronic HBV.
HB_CAb-Total: only useful to show past HBV infection if HB_SAg and HB_CAb-IgM are both negative.

HB_e

-Ag

HB_e-AbAg: When present, especially without HB_eAb, suggests increased patient infectivity.
HB_eAb-total: When present, suggests less patient infectivity.

HDV

-Ag

HDV-Ag: shows current infection (acute or chronic) by HDV.
HDV nucleic acid probe: detects antigen before and longer than HDV-Ag by EIA.

-Ab

HDV-Ab (IgM): high elevation in acute HDV; does not persist.
Low or moderate elevation in convalescent HDV; does not persist.
Low to high persistent elevation in chronic HDV (depends on degree of cell injury and sensitivity of the assay).
HDV-Ab (total): High elevation in acute HDV; does not persist.
High persistent elevation in chronic HDV.

HCV

-Ag

HCV nucleic acid probe: shows current infection by HCV (especially using PCR amplification).

-Ab

HCV-Ab (IgG): current, convalescent, or old HCV infection.

HAV

-Ag

HAV-Ag by EM: Shows presence of virus in stool early in infection.

-Ab

HAV-Ab (IgM): current or recent HAV infection.
HAV-Ab (total): convalescent or old HAV infection.

From Ravel R: *Clinical laboratory medicine*, ed 6, St Louis, 1995, Mosby.

BOX 4-20 HB_CAb-IgM

Appearance	Peak	Becomes Nondetectable
About 2 wk (range, 0-6 wk) after HB_SAg appears	About 1 wk after onset of symptoms	3-6 mo after appearance (range 2 wk-2 yr)

From Ravel R: *Clinical laboratory medicine*, ed 6, St Louis, 1995, Mosby.

BOX 4-21 HB_CAb-Total

Appearance	Peak	Becomes Nondetectable
3-4 wk (range 2-10 wk) after HB_SAg appears	3-4 wk after first detection	Elevated throughout life; may have slow decline to lower titers over many years

From Ravel R: *Clinical laboratory medicine*, ed 6, St Louis, 1995, Mosby.

BOX 4-22 HB$_e$Ag

Appearance
About 3-5 days after appearance of HB$_S$Ag

Peak
About the same time as HB$_S$Ag peak

Becomes Nondetectable
About 2-4 wk before HB$_S$Ag disappears in about 70% of cases
About 1-7 days after HB$_S$Ag disappears in about 20% of cases
Accompanies persistent HB$_S$Ag in 30%-50% or more patients who become chronic HBV carriers or have chronic HBV infection; however, may eventually convert to antibody in up to 40% of these patients

From Ravel R: *Clinical laboratory medicine,* ed 6, St Louis, 1995, Mosby.

BOX 4-23 HB$_e$Ab-Total

Appearance
At the same time as or within 1-2 wk (range, 0-4 wk) after e antigen disappears (2-4 wk before HB$_S$Ag loss to 2 wk after HB$_S$Ag loss)

Peak
During HBV core window

Becomes Nondetectable
Persists for several years (4-6 yr)

From Ravel R: *Clinical laboratory medicine,* ed 6, St Louis, 1995, Mosby.

BOX 4-24 Summary: HBV e Antigen and Antibody

HB$_e$Ag
    When present, especially without HB$_e$Ab, suggests increased patient infectivity

HB$_e$Ab-total
    When present, suggests less patient infectivity

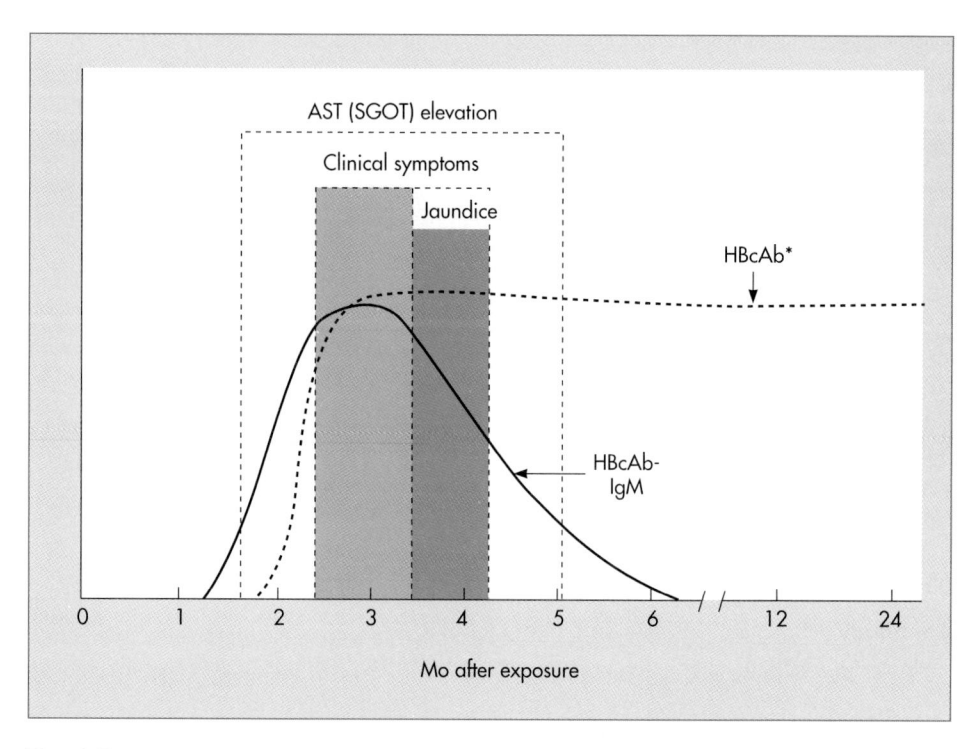

Fig. 4-5 HBV core antibodies. *HB$_C$Ab = HB$_C$Ab-IgM + HB$_C$Ab-IgG (combined). (From Ravel R: *Clinical laboratory medicine,* ed 6, St Louis, 1995, Mosby.)

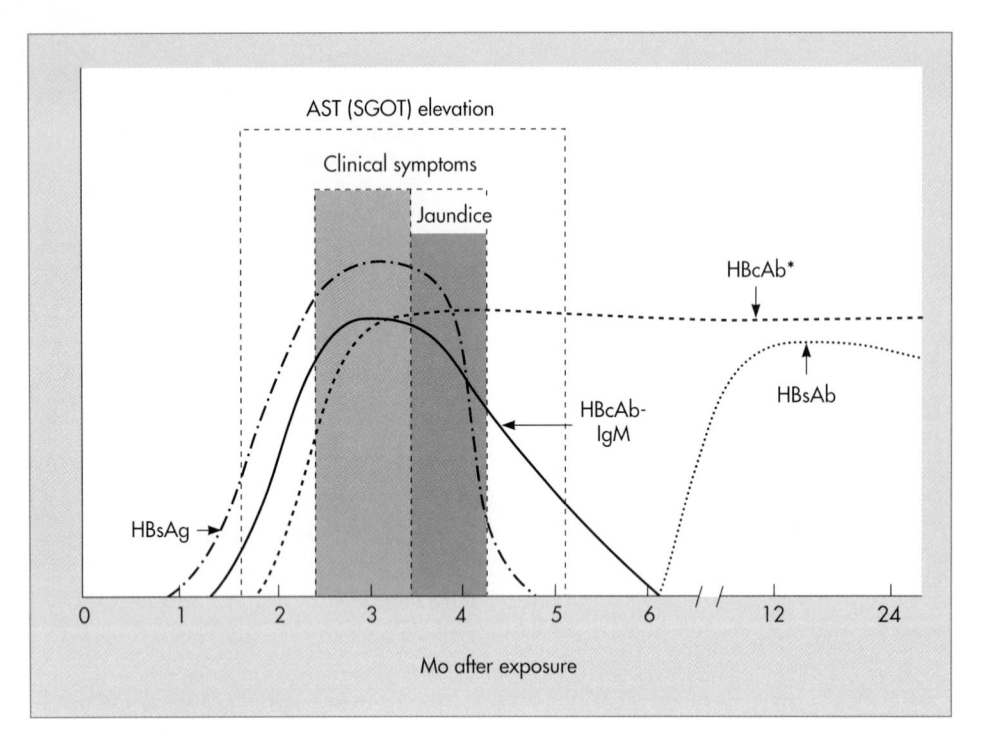

Fig. 4-6 **HBV surface antigen-antibody and core antibodies** (note "core window"). *HB$_C$Ab = HB$_C$Ab-IgM + HB$_C$Ab-IgG (combined). (From Ravel R: *Clinical laboratory medicine,* ed 6, St Louis, 1995, Mosby.)

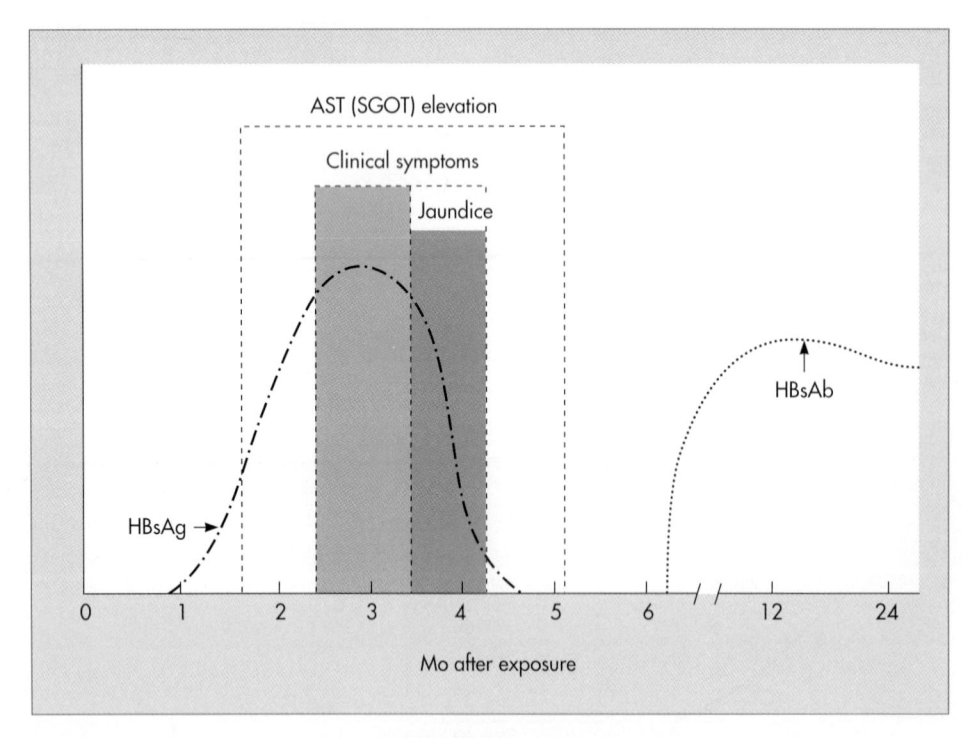

Fig. 4-7 **HBV surface antigen and antibody** (HB$_S$Ag and HB$_S$Ab-total). (From Ravel R: *Clinical laboratory medicine,* ed 6, St Louis, 1995, Mosby.)

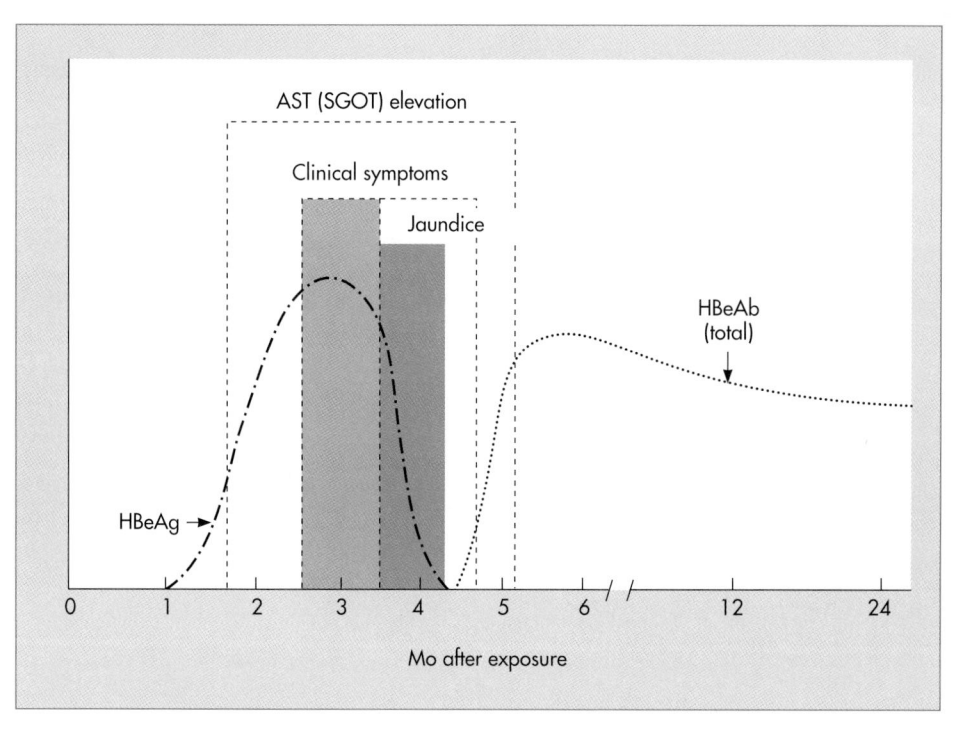

Fig. 4-8 **HBV e antigen and antibody.** (From Ravel R: *Clinical laboratory medicine,* ed 6, St Louis, 1995, Mosby.)

BOX 4-25 **HCV-Ag**

Nucleic Acid Probe (Without PCR)

Appearance: about 3-4 wk after infection (about 1-2 wk later than PCR-enhanced probe)
Becomes nondetectable: near the end of active infection, beginning of convalescence

Nucleic Acid Probe with PCR

Appearance: as early as the second week after infection
Becomes nondetectable: end of active infection, beginning of convalescence

From Ravel R: *Clinical laboratory medicine,* ed 6, St Louis, 1995, Mosby.

BOX 4-26 **HCV-Ab (IgG)**

Second Generation (gen) ELISA

Appearance: About 3-4 mo after infection (about 2-4 wk before first gen tests); 80% by 5-6 wk after symptoms
Becomes nondetectable: 7% lose detectable antibody by 1.5 yr; 7%-66% negative by 4 yr (by first generation tests; more remain elevated and for longer time by second generation tests)

From Ravel R: *Clinical laboratory medicine,* ed 6, St Louis, 1995, Mosby.

BOX 4-27 **Summary: Hepatitis C Antigen and Antibody**

HCV-Ag by nucleic acid probe
 Shows current infection by HCV (especially using PCR amplification)

HCV-Ab (IgG)
 Current, convalescent, or old HCV infection (behaves more like IgM or "total" Ab than usual IgG Ab)

From Ravel R: *Clinical laboratory medicine,* ed 6, St Louis, 1995, Mosby.

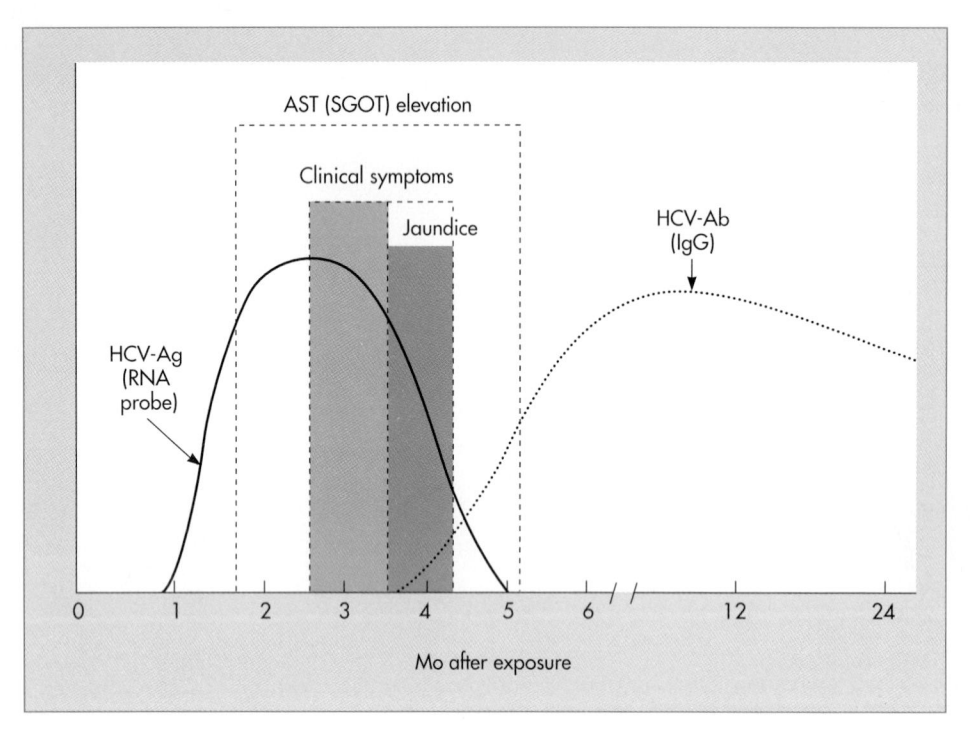

Fig. 4-9 HCV antigen and antibody. (From Ravel R: *Clinical laboratory medicine,* ed 6, St Louis, 1995, Mosby.)

BOX 4-28 Delta Hepatitis Coinfection (Acute HDV + Acute HBV) or Superinfection (Acute HDV + Chronic HBV)

HDV-AG

Detected by DNA probe, less often by immunoassay
Appearance: Prodromal stage (before symptoms); just at or after initial rise in ALT (about a week after appearance of HB_SAg and about the time HB_CAb-IgM level begins to rise)
Peak: 2-3 days after onset
Becomes nondetectable: 1-4 days (may persist until shortly after symptoms appear)

HDV-AB (IgM)

Appearance: about 10 days after symptoms begin (range 1-28 days)

Peak: about 2 wk after first detection
Becomes nondetectable: about 35 days (range 10-80 days) after first detection (most other IgM antibodies take 3-6 mo to become nondetectable)

HDV-AB (Total)

Appearance: about 50 days after symptoms begin (range 14-80 days); about 5 wk after HDV-Ag (range 3-11 wk)
Peak: About 2 wk after first detection
Becomes nondetectable: about 7 mo after first detection (range 4-14 mo)

From Ravel R: *Clinical laboratory medicine,* ed 6, St Louis, 1995, Mosby.

BOX 4-29 Delta Hepatitis Chronic Infection (Chronic HDV + Chronic HBV)

HDV-Ag

Detectable in serum by nucleic acid probe

HDV-Ab (IgM)

Detectable (may need sensitive method; titer depends on degree of virus activity)

HDV-Ab (Total)

Detectable, usually in high titer

From Ravel R: *Clinical laboratory medicine,* ed 6, St Louis, 1995, Mosby.

> **BOX 4-30 Summary: Diagnosis of HDV Infection**
>
> Best current all-purpose screening test = ADV-Ab (total)
>
> Best test to differentiate acute from chronic infection = HDV-Ab (IgM)

From Ravel R: *Clinical laboratory medicine,* ed 6, St Louis, 1995, Mosby.

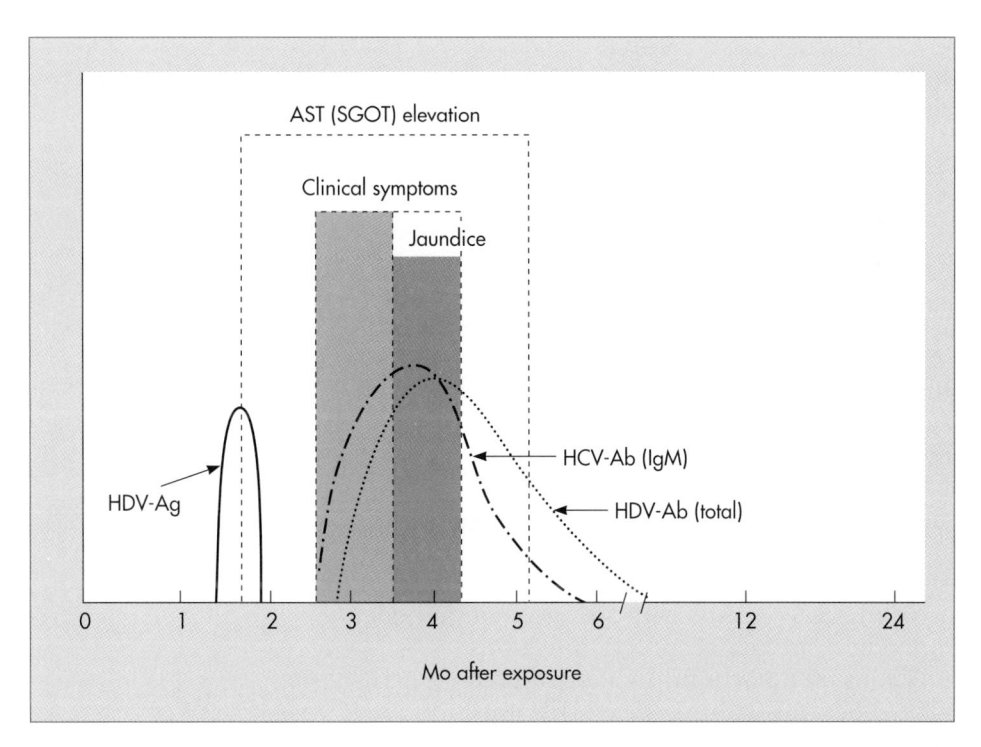

Fig. 4-10 **HDV antigen and antibodies.** (From Ravel R: *Clinical laboratory medicine,* ed 6, St Louis, 1995, Mosby.)

HETEROPHIL ANTIBODY
Normal:
  Negative
Positive in:
  Infectious mononucleosis

HIGH-DENSITY LIPOPROTEIN (HDL) CHOLESTEROL
Normal range:
  Male: 45-70 mg/dl (0.8-1.8 mmol/L) [CF: 0.02586; SMI: 0.05 mmol/L]
  Female: 45-90 mg/dl (0.8-2.35 mmol/L) [CF: 0.02586; SMI: 0.05 mmol/L]
Increased in:
  Use of gemfibrozil, nicotinic acid, estrogens, regular aerobic exercise, small (1 oz) daily alcohol intake
Decreased in:
  Deficiency of apoproteins, liver disease, probucol ingestion, Tangier disease
  NOTE: A cholesterol/HDL ratio ±4.5 is associated with increased risk of coronary artery disease.

HLA ANTIGENS
Associated disorders: see Table 4-13.

HUMAN IMMUNODEFICIENCY VIRUS ANTIBODY, type 1 (HIV-1)
Normal range:
  Not detected
Abnormal result:
  HIV antibodies usually appear in the blood 1-4 mo after infection.

TABLE 4-13 HLA Antigens Associated with Specific Diseases

ANTIGEN	CONDITION	ANTIGEN	CONDITION
HLA-B27	Ankylosing spondylitis	HLA-B8, Dw3	Celiac disease
	Reiter's syndrome	HLA-B8, Dw3	Dermatitis herpetiformis
	Psoriatic arthritis	HLA-B8	Myasthenia gravis
HLA-A10, B18, Dw2	C2 deficiency	HLA-B8	Chronic active hepatitis in children
HLA-A2, B40, Cw3	C4 deficiency	HLA-Drw4	Active chronic hepatitis in adults
HLA-B7, Dw2	Multiple sclerosis	HLA-B13, Bw17	Psoriasis
HLA-A3	Hemochromatosis		

From Cerra FB: *Manual of critical care,* St Louis, 1987, Mosby.

Testing sequence:
1. ELISA is the recommended initial screening test. Sensitivity and specificity are >99%. False positive ELISA may occur with autoimmune disorders, administration of immune globulin manufactured before 1985 within 6 wk of testing, presence of rheumatoid factor, presence of DLA-DR antibodies in multigravida female, administration of influenza vaccine within 3 mo of testing, hemodialysis, positive plasma reagin test, certain medical disorders (hemophilia, hypergammaglobulinemia, alcoholic hepatitis)
2. A positive ELISA is confirmed with Western blot.
False positive Western blot may result from connective tissue disorders, human leukocyte antigen antibodies, polyclonal gammopathies, hyperbilirubinemia, presence of antibody to another human retrovirus, or cross reaction with other nonvirus-derived proteins in healthy persons. Undetermined Western blot may occur in AIDS patients with advanced immunodeficiency (caused by loss of antibodies), and in recent HIV infections.
3. Polymerase chain reaction (PCR) is used to confirm indeterminate Western blot results or negative results in persons with suspected HIV infection.

Fig. 4-11 describes tests in HIV infection.

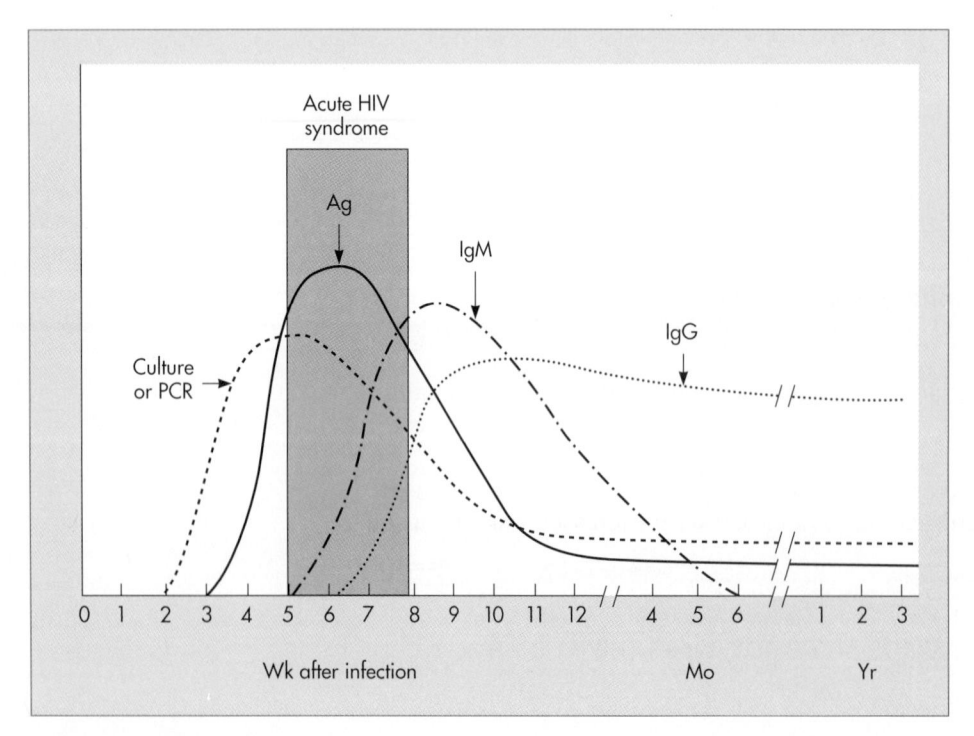

Fig. 4-11 **Tests in HIV-1 infection.** (From Ravel R: *Clinical laboratory medicine,* ed 6, St Louis, 1995, Mosby.)

5-HYDROXYINDOLE-ACETIC ACID, URINE; see URINE 5-HYDROXYINDOLE-ACETIC ACID

IMMUNE COMPLEX ASSAY
Normal:
   Negative
Detected in:
   Collagen-vascular disorders, glomerulonephritis, neoplastic diseases, malaria, primary biliary cirrhosis, chronic acute hepatitis, bacterial endocarditis, vasculitis

IMMUNOGLOBULINS
Normal range:
   IgA: 50-350 mg/dl (0.5-3.5 g/L) [CF: 0.01; SMI: 0.01 g/L]
   IgD: <6 mg/dl (<60 mg/L) [CF: 0.01; SMI: 0.01 g/L]
   IgE: <25 µg/dl (<0.00025 g/L) [CF: 0.01; SMI: 0.01 g/L]
   IgG: 800-1500 mg/dl (8-15 g/L) [CF: 0.01; SMI: 0.01 g/L]
   IgM: 45-150 mg/dl (0.45-1.5 g/L) [CF: 0.01; SMI: 0.01 g/L]
Elevated in:
   IgA: lymphoproliferative disorders, Berger's nephropathy, chronic infections, autoimmune disorders, liver disease
   IgE: allergic disorders, parasitic infections, immunologic disorders, IgE myeloma
   IgG: chronic granulomatous infections, infectious diseases, inflammation, myeloma, liver disease
   IgM: primary biliary cirrhosis, infectious diseases (brucellosis, malaria), Waldenstrom's macroglobulinemia, liver disease
Decreased in:
   IgA: nephrotic syndrome, protein-losing enteropoathy, congenital deficiency, lymphocytic leukemia, ataxia-telangiectasia, chronic sinopulmonary disease
   IgE: hypogammaglobulinemia, neoplasm (breast, bronchial, cervical), ataxia-telangiectasia
   IgG: congenital or acquired deficiency, lymphocytic leukemia, phenytoin, methylprednisolone, nephrotic syndrome, protein-losing enteropathy
   IgM: congenital deficiency, lymphocytic leukemia, nephrotic syndrome

INTERNATIONAL NORMALIZED RATIO (INR)
The INR is a comparative rating of prothrombin time (PT) ratios. The INR represents the observed PT ratio adjusted by the International Reference Thromboplastin. It provides a universal result indicative of what the patient's PT result would have been if measured using the primary World Health Organization International Reference reagent. For proper interpretation of INR values, the patient should be on stable anticoagulant therapy.

Recommended INR ranges:

CONDITION	INR RANGE
Proximal deep vein thrombosis	2-3
Pulmonary embolism	2-3
Transient ischemic attacks	2-3
Atrial fibrillation	2-3
Mechanical prosthetic valves	3-4.5
Recurrent venous thromboembolic disease	3-4.5

IRON-BINDING CAPACITY (TIBC)
Normal range:
   250-460 µg/dl (45-82 µmol/L) [CF: 0.1791; SMI: 1 µmol/L]
Elevated in:
   Iron deficiency anemia, pregnancy, polycythemia, hepatitis, weight loss
Decreased in:
   Anemia of chronic disease, hemochromatosis, chronic liver disease, hemolytic anemias, malnutrition (protein depletion)
   Table 4-14 describes TIBC and serum iron abnormalities.

TABLE 4-14 Serum Iron and Total Iron-Binding Capacity Patterns

SI*↓	TIBC↓	Chronic diseases Uremia
SI↓	TIBC↑	Chronic iron deficiency anemia Pregnancy in third trimester

SI↑	TIBC↓	Hemachromatosis
		Iron therapy overload (TIBC may be normal)
		Hemolytic anemia;
		   thalassemia; lead poisoning;
		   megaloblastic anemia;
		   apalstic, pyridoxine deficiency, or other sideroachrestic anemias

SI↑	TIBC↑	Oral contraceptives Acute hepatitis (some report TIBC is low normal) Chronic hepatitis (some patients)
SI↑	TIBC NL†	B_{12} or folate deficiency
SI↓	TIBC NL	Chronic iron deficiency (some patients) Acute infection, surgery, tissue damage
SI NL	TIBC↑	B_{12}/folate deficiency plus iron deficiency

From Ravel R: *Clinical laboratory medicine,* ed 6, St Louis, 1995, Mosby.
*SI, serum iron.
†NL, normal.

LACTATE DEHYDROGENASE (LDH)
Normal range:
   50-150 U/L (0.82-2.66 μkat/L) [CF: 0.01667; SMI: 0.02 μkat/L]
Elevated in:
   Infarction of myocardium, lung, kidney
   Diseases of cardiopulmonary system, liver, collagen, CNS
   Hemolytic anemias, megaloblastic anemias, transfusions, seizures, muscle trauma, muscular dystrophy, acute pancreatitis, hypotension, shock, infectious mononucleosis, inflammation, neoplasia, intestinal obstruction, hypothyroidism

LACTATE DEHYDROGENASE ISOENZYMES
Normal range:
   LDH_1: 22% to 36% (cardiac, RBC) (0.22-0.36) [CF: 0.01, SMI: 0.01]
   LDH_2: 35% to 46% (cardiac, RBC) (0.35-0.46)
   LDH_3: 13% to 26% (pulmonary) (0.15-0.26)
   LDH_4: 3% to 10% (striated muscle, liver) (0.03-0.1)
   LDH_5: 2% to 9% (striated muscle, liver) (0.02-0.09)
Normal ratios:
   $LDH_1 < LDH_2$
   $LDH_5 < LDH_4$
Abnormal values:
   $LDH_1 > LDH_2$: MI (can also be seen with hemolytic anemias, pernicious anemia, folate deficiency, renal infarct)
   $LDH_5 > LDH_4$: liver disease (cirrhosis, hepatitis, hepatic congestion)

LAP SCORE; *see* LEUKOCYTE ALKALINE PHOSPHATASE
LDH; *see* LACTATE DEHYDROGENASE
LDL; *see* LOW-DENSITY LIPOPROTEIN CHOLESTEROL

LEGIONELLA TITER
Normal:
   Negative
Positive in:
   Legionnaire's disease (presumptive: ≥1:256 titer; definitive: fourfold titer increase to ≥1:128)

LEUKOCYTE ALKALINE PHOSPHATASE
Normal range:
> 13-100 (33-188 U)

Elevated in:
> Leukemoid reactions, neutrophilia secondary to infections (except in sickle cell crisis—no significant increase in LAP score), Hodgkin's disease, polycythemia vera, hairy cell leukemia, aplastic anemia, Down's syndrome, myelofibrosis

Decreased in:
> Acute and chronic granulocytic leukemia, thrombocytopenic purpura, paroxysmal nocturnal hemoglobinuria (PNH), hypophosphatemia, collagen disorders

LEUKOCYTE COUNT; see COMPLETE BLOOD COUNT

LIPASE
Normal range:
> 0-160 U/L (0-2.66 μkat/L) [CF: 0.01667; SMI: 0.02 μkat/L]

Elevated in:
> Acute pancreatitis, perforated peptic ulcer, carcinoma of pancreas (early stage), pancreatic duct obstruction, bowel infarction, intestinal obstruction

LIPOPROTEIN CHOLESTEROL, LOW-DENSITY; see LOW-DENSITY LIPOPROTEIN CHOLESTEROL

LIPOPROTEIN CHOLESTEROL, HIGH-DENSITY; see HIGH-DENSITY LIPOPROTEIN CHOLESTEROL

LOW-DENSITY LIPOPROTEIN (LDL) CHOLESTEROL
Normal range:
> 50-130 mg/dl (1.30-1.68 mmol/L) [CF: 0.02586; SMI: 0.05 mmol/L]

LUPUS ANTICOAGULANT; see CIRCULATING ANTICOAGULANT

LYMPHOCYTES
Normal range:
> 15% to 40%: Total lymphocyte count 800-2600/mm^3
> Total T lymphocyte, 800-2200/mm^3
> CD4 lymphocytes ≥400/mm^3
> CD8 lymphocytes = 200-800/mm^3
> Normal CD4/CD8 ratio is 2.0

Elevated in:
> Chronic infections, infectious mononucleosis and other viral infections, CLL, Hodgkin's disease, ulcerative colitis, hypoadrenalism, ITP

Decreased in:
> AIDS, bone marrow suppression from chemotherapeutic agents or chemotherapy, aplastic anemia, neoplasms, steroids, adrenocortical hyperfunction, neurologic disorders (multiple sclerosis, myasthenia gravis, Guillain-Barré syndrome)

> CD4 lymphocytes are calculated as total WBC × % lymphocytes × % lymphocytes stained with CD4. They are decreased in AIDS and other immune dysfunction.

MAGNESIUM (serum)
Normal range:
> See Box 4-31 for description of magnesium abnormalities. 1.8-3.0 mg/dl (0.80-1.20 mmol/L) [CF: 0.4114; SMI: 0.02 mmol/L]

MEAN CORPUSCULAR VOLUME (MCV)
Normal range:
> 76-100 μm^3 (76-100 fL) [CF: 1; SMI: 1 fL]
> See Tables 4-15 and 4-16 for description of MCV abnormalities.

METANEPHRINES, URINE; see URINE METANEPHRINES

MONOCYTE COUNT
Normal range:
> 2% to 8%

> **BOX 4-31 Magnesium Disorders**
>
> **Magnesium Deficiency**
> Alcoholism
> Malabsorption
> Malnutrition
> IV fluids without magnesium
> Severe diarrhea
> Diabetic ketoacidosis
> Hemodialysis
> Hypercalcemia
> Congestive heart failure
> Artifact (hypoalbuminemia)
>
> Certain medications
>   Loop and thiazide diuretics
>   Cyclosporine
>   Cisplatin
>   Gentamicin
>
> **Magnesium Excess**
> Oliguric renal failure
> Overuse of magnesium-containing compounds
> Artifactual (specimen hemolysis)

From Ravel R: *Clinical laboratory medicine,* ed 6, St Louis, 1995, Mosby.

TABLE 4-15 Some Causes of Increased Mean Corpuscular Volume (Macrocytosis)

CAUSES	% OF ALL MACROCYTOSIS PATIENTS*	% OF MACROCYTOSIS IN EACH DISEASE†
Common		
Folate or B_{12} deficiency	20-30 (5-50)‡	80-90 (4-100)
Chronic liver disease	15-20 (6-28)	25-30 (8-65)
Chronic alcoholism	10-12 (3-15)	60 (26-90)
Cytotoxic chemotherapy	10-15 (2-20)	30-40 (13-82)
Cardiorespiratory abnormality	8 (7-9.5)	?
Reticulocytosis	6-7 (0-15)	Depends on severity
Myelodysplastic syndromes	Frequent over age 40 yr	>60 in RAEB and RARS§
Unexplained	25 (22.5-27)	—
Normal newborn		
Less Common	< 4%	
Noncytotoxic drugs		
Zidovudine		
Phenytoin		30 (14-50)
Azathioprine		
Hypothyroidism		20-30 (8-55)
Chronic leukemia/myelofibrosis		
Radiotherapy for malignancy		
Chronic renal disease (occasional patients)		
Distance-runner macrocytosis (some persons)		
Down syndrome		
Artifactual (e.g., cold agglutinins)		

From Ravel R: *Clinical laboratory medicine,* ed 6, St Louis, 1995, Mosby.
*Percentage of all patients with macrotysis.
†Percentage of patients with each condition listed who have macroytosis.
‡Numbers in parentheses are literature range.
§*RAEB,* Refractory anemia with excessive blasts; *RARS,* refractory anemia with ring sideroblasts (formerly called IASA, or idiopathic acquired sideroblastic anemia).

TABLE 4-16 Some Causes of Decreased Mean Corpuscular Volume (Microcytosis)

COMMON	LESS COMMON
Chronic iron deficiency	Some cases of polycythemia
α- or β-thalassemia (minor)	Some cases of lead poisoning
Anemia of chronic disease	Some cases of congenital spherocytosis
	Some cases of sideroblastic anemia
	Certain abnormal Hbs (Hb E, Hb Lepore)

From Ravel R: *Clinical laboratory medicine,* ed 6, St Louis, 1995, Mosby.

Elevated in:
   Viral diseases, parasites, infections, neoplasms, inflammatory bowel disease, monocytic leukemia, lymphomas, myeloma, sarcoidosis

Decreased in:
   Aplastic anemia, lymphocytic leukemia, glucocorticoid administration

MYOGLOBIN, URINE; *see* **URINE MYOGLOBIN**

NEUTROPHIL COUNT

Normal range:
   50% to 70%
      Subsets
         Stabs (bands, early mature neutrophils): 2% to 6%
         Segs (mature neutrophils): 60% to 70%

Elevated in:
   Acute bacterial infections, acute MI, stress, neoplasms, myelocytic leukemia

Decreased in:
   Viral infections, aplastic anemias, immunosuppressive drugs, radiation therapy to bone marrow, agranulocytosis, drugs (antibiotics, antithyroidals), lymphocytic and monocytic leukemias

5′ NUCLEOTIDASE

Normal range:
   2-16 IU/L (3-27 × 10^{-8} kat/L) [CF: 1.67 × 10^{-8}; SMI: 1 × 10^{-8} kat/L]

Elevated in:
   Biliary obstruction, metastatic neoplasms to liver, primary biliary cirrhosis, renal failure, pancreatic carcinoma, chronic active hepatitis

ONCOGENES

See Table 4-17 for description of common oncogene abnormalities.

OSMOLALITY, SERUM

Normal range:
   280-300 mOsm/kg (280-300 mmol/kg) [CF: 1; SMI: 1 mmol/kg]
   It can also be estimated by the following formula:

$$2([Na] + [K]) + \frac{Glucose}{18} + \frac{BUN}{2.8}$$

Elevated in:
   Dehydration, hypernatremia, diabetes insipidus, uremia, hyperglycemia, mannitol therapy, ingestion of toxins (ethylene glycol, methanol, ethanol), hypercalcemia, diuretics

Decreased in:
   SIADH, hyponatremia, overhydration, Addison's disease, hypothyroidism

OSMOLALITY, URINE; *see* **URINE OSMOLALITY**

PARTIAL THROMBOPLASTIN TIME (PTT), ACTIVATED PARTIAL THROMBOPLASTIN TIME (APTT)

Normal range:
   25-41 sec

TABLE 4-17 Some Currently Important Oncogenes

ONCOGENE	CHROMOSOME LOCATION	OTHER
Neu (HER-2; c-erbB2) (rat neuroblastoma)	17q21	Amplification in 10%-40% of primary cancers; especially breast, ovary, prostate, thyroid, neuroblastoma
bcl-2 (acute B-cell leukemia)	18q21	Involved in translocation t(14;18) (q32q21) in 80%-90% of acute follicular (nodular) non-Hodgkin's lymphoma by chromosome analysis (nearly 100% by DNA probe)
Rb (retinoblastoma)	13q14	Tumor suppressor gene; deletion or mutation results in increased incidence of retinoblastoma, osteosarcoma, breast, endometrial, lung small cell CA*
ras oncogene group (rat sarcoma virus)		
Harvey (c-Ha-ras, H-ras)	11p15	
Kirsten (c-Ki-ras, K-ras)	12p12	
Neuroblastoma (N-ras)	1p22	Mutational activation of ras group member is estimated to occur in 10%-20% of human malignancies; especially lung non-small-cell, kidney, breast, colorectal, prostate; in neuroblastoma, H-ras amplification is paradoxically associated with better prognosis
myc oncogene group (avian myelocytomatosis virus)		
L-myc	1p32	
N-myc	2p	
C-myc	8q24	Amplification in breast CA (37%), neuroblastoma (25%-30%), Burkitt's lymphoma, acute lymphoblastic leukemia of L-3 type
p53	17p13	Tumor suppressor gene; deletion or mutation produces defective gene; increase in colorectal CA (70%-80%), endometrial CA, early-onset breast CA, various others
FAP (familial adenomatous polyposis; also called APC)	5q21	Suppressor gene for familial polyposis and Gardner's syndrome
DCC (deleted in colon cancer)	18q21	Suppressor gene; when deleted, increase in colorectal CA (75%), especially if FAP gene is present
mcc (mutated in colon cancer)	5q21	40% of colon cancer
wt-1 (Wilm's tumor)	11p13	Suppressor gene deletion found in Wilm's tumor; also some cases of breast CA, rhabdomyosarcoma, hepatoblastoma, urinary bladder CA
nf = 1 (neurofibroma)	17q11	Suppressor or gene in von Recklinghausen's disease
RCC (renal cell carcinoma)	3p14	Gene area break in most RCC patients
Meningioma	22q	Partial or full monosomy 22 (specific defect)
Neuroblastoma (83% cases)	del(1p)	Deletion causes loss of suppressor gene
abl (Abelson)	9q	Part of 9, 22 translocation of Philadelphia chromosome

From Ravel R: *Clinical laboratory medicine*, ed 6, St Louis, 1995, Mosby.
*CA, Carcinoma.

Elevated in:
  Heparin therapy, coagulation factor deficiency (I, II, V, VIII, IX, X, XI, XII), liver disease, vitamin K deficiency, DIC, circulating anticoagulant, warfarin therapy, specific factor inhibition (PCN reaction, rheumatoid arthritis), thrombolytic therapy, nephrotic syndrome
  NOTE: Useful to evaluate the intrinsic coagulation system.

pH, URINE; *see* URINE pH
PHOSPHATASE, ACID; *see* ACID PHOSPHATASE
PHOSPHATASE, ALKALINE; *see* ALKALINE PHOSPHATASE

> **BOX 4-32   Selected Disorders Associated with Serum Phosphate Abnormality**
>
> **Phosphate Decrease***
> Parenteral hyperalimentation
> Diabetic acidosis
> Alcohol withdrawal
> Severe metabolic or respiratory alkalosis
> Antacids that bind phosphorus
> Malnutrition with refeeding using low-phosphorus nutrients
> Renal tubule failure to reabsorb phosphate (Fanconi's syndrome; congenital disorder; vitamin D deficiency)
> Glucose administration
> Nasogastric suction
> Malabsorption
> Gram-negative sepsis
> Primary hyperthyroidism
> Chlorothiazide diuretics
> Therapy of acute severe asthma
> Acute respiratory failure with mechanical ventilation
>
> **Phosphate Excess**
> Renal failure
> Severe muscle injury
> Phosphate-containing antacids
> Hypoparathyroidism
> Tumor lysis syndrome

From Ravel R: *Clinical laboratory medicine,* ed 6, St Louis, 1995, Mosby.
*Low phosphate diet can magnify effect of phosphorus-lowering disorders.

PHOSPHATE (serum)
Normal range:
2.5-5 mg/dl (0.8-1.6 mmol/L) [CF: 0.3229; SMI: 0.05 mmol/L]
See Box 4-32 for description of phosphate abnormalities.

PLATELET COUNT
Normal range:
130-400 × 10^3/mm^3 (130-400 × 10^9/L) [CF: 1; SMI: 5 × 10^9/L]

Elevated in:
Neoplasms (GI tract), CML, polycythemia vera, myelofibrosis with myeloid metaplasia, infections, after splenectomy, postpartum, after hemorrhage, hemophilia, iron deficiency, pancreatitis, cirrhosis

Decreased:
A. Increased destruction
   1. Immunologic
      a. Drugs: quinine, quinidine, digitalis, procainamide, thiazide diuretics, sulfonamides, phenytoin, aspirin, penicillin, heparin, gold, meprobamate, sulfa drugs, phenylbutazone, NSAIDs, methyldopa, cimetidine, furosemide, INH, cephalosporins, chlorpropamide, organic arsenicals, chloroquine
      b. ITP
      c. Transfusion reaction: transfusion of platelets with PLA in recipients without PLA-1
      d. Fetal/maternal incompatibility
      e. Vasculitis (e.g., SLE)
      f. Autoimmune hemolytic anemia
      g. Lymphoreticular disorders (e.g., CLL)
   2. Nonimmunologic
      a. Prosthetic heart valves
      b. TTP
      c. Sepsis
      d. DIC
      e. Hemolytic-uremic syndrome
      f. Giant cavernous hemangioma
B. Decreased production
   1. Abnormal marrow
      a. Marrow infiltration (e.g., leukemia, lymphoma, fibrosis)
      b. Marrow suppression (e.g., chemotherapy, alcohol, radiation)

2. Hereditary disorders
   a. Wiskott-Aldrich syndrome: X-linked disorder characterized by thrombocytopenia, eczema, and repeated infections
   b. May-Hegglin anomaly: increased megakaryocytes but ineffective thrombopoiesis
3. Vitamin deficiencies (e.g., vitamin B_{12}, folic acid)

C. Splenic sequestration, hypersplenism
D. Dilutional, secondary to massive transfusion

POTASSIUM (serum)
Normal range:
   3.5-5 mEq/L (3.5-5 mmol/L) [CF: 1; SMI: 0.1 mmol/L]
   See Box 4-33 for causes of potassium abnormalities.

POTASSIUM, URINE; see URINE POTASSIUM

PROLACTIN
Normal range:
   <20 ng/ml (<20 µg/L) [CF: 1; SMI: 1 µg/L]
Elevated in:
   Prolactinomas (level >200 highly suggestive), drugs (phenothiazines, cimetidine, tricyclic antidepressants, metoclopramide, estrogens, antihypertensives [methyldopa], verapamil, haloperidol), postpartum, stress, hypoglycemia, hypothyroidism

PROSTATIC SPECIFIC ANTIGEN (PSA)
Normal range:
   0-4 ng/ml
Elevated in:
   Benign prostatic hypertrophy, carcinoma of prostate, rectal examination, prostate trauma

PROTEIN (serum)
Normal range:
   6-8 g/dl (60-80 g/L) [CF: 10; SMI: 1 g/L]
Elevated in:
   Dehydration, multiple myeloma, Waldenstrom's macroglobulinemia, sarcoidosis, collagen-vascular diseases
Decreased in:
   Malnutrition, low-protein diet, overhydration, malabsorption, pregnancy, severe burns, neoplasms, chronic diseases, cirrhosis, nephrosis

---

BOX 4-33 Clinical Conditions Commonly Associated with Serum Potassium Abnormalities

Hypokalemia
Inadequate intake (cachexia or severe illness of any type)
Intravenous infusion of potassium-free fluids
Renal loss (diuretics; primary aldosteronism)
GI loss (protracted vomiting; severe prolonged diarrhea; GI drainage)
Severe trauma
Treatment of diabetic acidosis without potassium supplements
Treatment with large doses of adrenocorticotropic hormone; Cushing's syndrome
Cirrhosis; some cases of secondary aldosteronism

Hyperkalemia
Renal failure
Dehydration
Excessive parenteral administration of potassium
Artifactual hemolysis of blood specimen
Tumor lysis syndrome
Hyporeninemic hypoaldosteronism
Spironolactone therapy
Addison's disease and salt-losing congenital adrenal hyperplasia
Thrombocythemia

From Ravel R: *Clinical laboratory medicine*, ed 6, St Louis, 1995, Mosby.

PROTEIN ELECTROPHORESIS (serum)
Normal range:
Albumin: 60% to 75% (0.6-0.75) [CF: 0.01; SMI: 0.01]
α-1: 1.7% to 5% (0.02-0.05)
α-2: 6.7% to 12.5% (0.07-0.13)
β: 8.3% to 16.3% (0.08-0.16)
γ: 10.7% to 20% (0.11-0.2)
Albumin: 3.6-5.2 g/dl (36-52 g/L) [CF: 0.01; SMI: 1 g/L]
α-1: 0.1-0.4 g/dl (1-4 g/L)
α-2: 0.4-1 g/dl (4-10 g/L)
β: 0.5-1.2 g/dl (5-12 g/L)
γ: 0.6-1.6 g/dl (6-16 g/L)

Elevated in:
Albumin: dehydration
α-1: neoplastic diseases, inflammation
α-2: neoplasms, inflammation, infection, nephrotic syndrome
β: hypothyroidism, biliary cirrhosis, diabetes mellitus
γ: see IMMUNOGLOBULINS

Decrased in:
Albumin: malnutrition, chronic liver disease, malabsorption, nephrotic syndrome, burns, SLE
α-1: emphysema (α-1 antitrypsin deficiency), nephrosis
α-2: hemolytic anemias (decreased haptoglobin), severe hepatocellular damage
β: hypocholesterolemia, nephrosis
γ: see IMMUNOGLOBULINS
Fig. 4-12 describes serum protein electrophoretic patterns.

PROTHROMBIN TIME (PT)
Normal range:
10-12 sec

Elevated in:
Liver disease, oral anticoagulants (Warfarin), heparin, factor deficiency (I, II, V, VII, X), DIC, vitamin K deficiency, afibrinogenemia, dysfibrinogenemia, drugs (salicylate, chloral hydrate, diphenylhydantoin, estrogens, antacids, phenylbutazone, quinidine, antibiotics, allopurinol, anabolic steroids)

Decreased in:
Vitamin K supplementation, thrombophlebitis, drugs (gluthetimide, estrogens, griseofulvin, diphenhydramine)

PROTOPORPHYRIN (free erythrocyte)
Normal range:
16-36 μg/dl of RBC (0.28-0.64 μmol/L) [CF: 0.0177; SMI: 0.02 μmol/L]

Elevated in:
Iron deficiency, lead poisoning, sideroblastic anemias, anemia of chronic disease, hemolytic anemias, erythropoietic protoporphyria

PSA; *see* PROSTATIC SPECIFIC ANTIGEN
PT; *see* PROTHROMBIN TIME
PTT; *see* PARTIAL THROMBOPLASTIN TIME
RDW; *see* RED BLOOD CELL DISTRIBUTION WIDTH

RED BLOOD CELL (RBC) COUNT
Normal range:
Male: $4.3\text{-}5.9 \times 10^6/mm^3$ ($4.3\text{-}5.9 \times 10^{12}/L$) [CF: 1; SMI: $0.1 \times 10^{12}/L$]
Female: $3.5\text{-}5 \times 10^6/mm^3$ ($3.5\text{-}5 \times 10^{12}/L$) [CF: 1; SMI: $0.1 \times 10^{12}/L$]

Elevated in:
Polycythemia vera, smokers, high altitude, cardiovascular disease, renal cell carcinoma and other erythropoietin-producing neoplasms, stress, hemoconcentration/dehydration

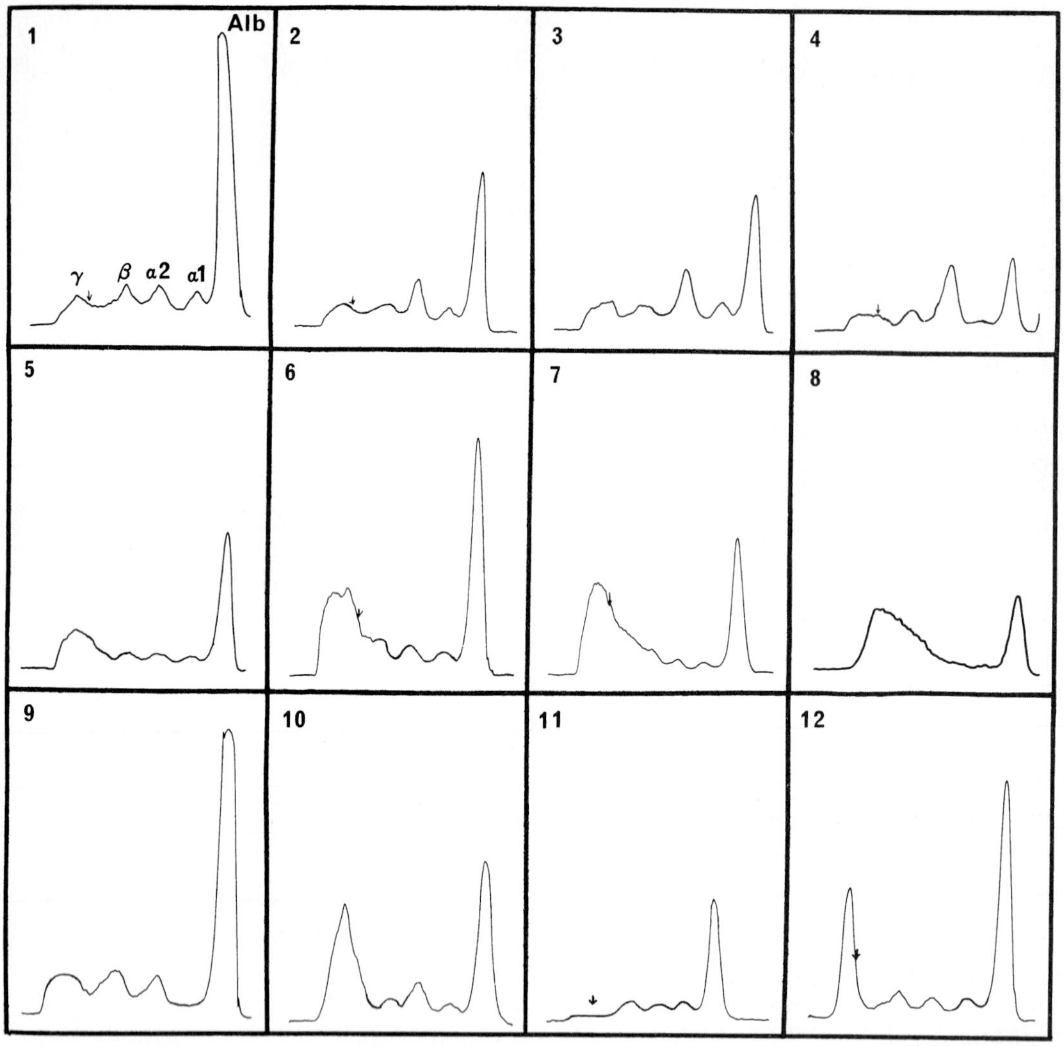

Fig. 4-12 Typical serum protein electrophoretic patterns. *1,* Normal (*arrow* near γ region indicates serum application point). *2,* Acute reaction pattern. *3,* Acute reaction or nephrotic syndrome. *4,* Nephrotic syndrome. *5,* Chronic inflammation, cirrhosis, granulomatous diseases, rheumatoid-collagen group. *6,* Same as 5, but γ elevation is more pronounced. There is also partial (but not complete) β-γ fusion. *7,* Suggestive of cirrhosis but could be found in the granulomatous diseases or the rheumatoid-collagen group. *8,* Characteristic pattern of cirrhosis. *9,* α-1 Antitrypsin deficiency with mild γ elevation suggesting concurrent chronic disease. *10,* Same as 5, but the γ elevation is marked. The configuration of the γ peak superficially mimics that of myeloma, but is more broad-based. There are superimposed acute reaction changes. *11,* Hypogammaglobulinemia or light-chain myeloma. *12,* Myeloma, Waldenstrom's macroglobulinemia, idiopathic or secondary monoclonal gammopathy. (From Ravel R: *Clinical laboratory medicine,* ed 6, St Louis, 1995, Mosby.)

Decreased in:
   Anemias, hemolysis, chronic renal failure, hemorrhage, failure of marrow production

RED BLOOD CELL DISTRIBUTION WIDTH (RDW)
   Measures variability of red cell size (anisocytosis)

Normal range:
   11.5-14.5

Normal RDW and:
   Elevated MCV: aplastic anemia, preleukemia

Normal MCV: normal, anemia of chronic disease, acute blood loss or hemolysis, CLL, CML, nonanemic enzymopathy or hemoglobinopathy
Decreased MCV: anemia of chronic disease, heterozygous thalassemia

Elevated RDW and:
Elevated MCV: vitamin B_{12} deficiency, folate deficiency, immune hemolytic anemia, cold agglutinins, CLL with high count, liver disease
Normal MCV: early iron deficiency, early vitamin B_{12} deficiency, early folate deficiency, anemic globinopathy
Decreased MCV: iron deficiency, RBC fragmentation, HbH disease, thalassemia intermedia

RED BLOOD CELL FOLATE; see FOLATE, RBC

RED BLOOD CELL MASS (VOLUME)
Normal range:
Male: 20-36 ml/kg of BW (1.15-1.21 L/m² BSA)
Female: 19-31 ml/kg of BW (0.95-1.00 L/m² BSA)
Elevated in:
Polycythemia vera, hypoxia (smokers, high altitude, cardiovascular disease), hemoglobinopathies with high oxygen affinity, erythropoietin-producing tumors (renal cell carcinoma)
Decreased in:
Hemorrhage, chronic disease, failure of marrow production, anemias, hemolysis

RED BLOOD CELL MORPHOLOGY; see Fig. 4-13

RENIN (serum)
Elevated in:
Drugs (thiazides, estrogen, minoxidil), chronic renal failure, Bartter's syndrome, pregnancy (normal), pheochromocytoma, renal hypertension, reduced plasma volume, secondary aldosteronism
Decreased in:
Adrenocortical hypertension, increased plasma volume, primary aldosteronism, drugs (propanolol, reserpine, clonidine)
Table 4-18 describes typical renin-aldosterone patterns in various conditions.

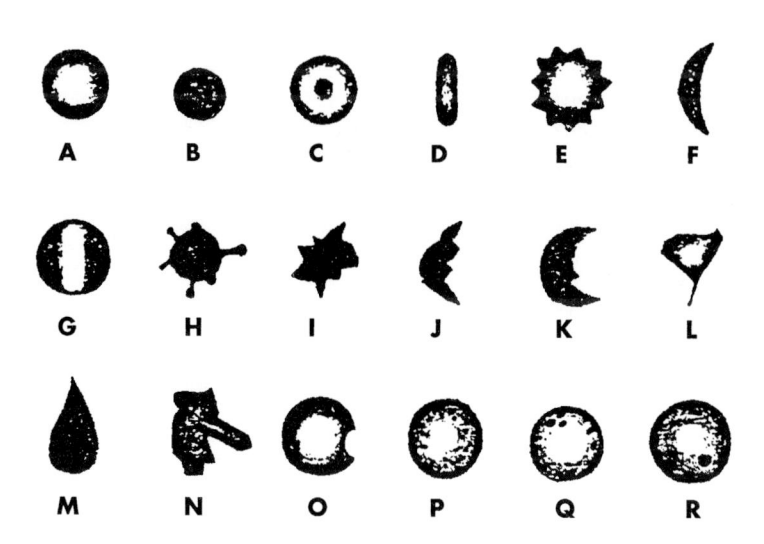

Fig. 4-13 Abnormal RBC.
A, Normal RBC. **B,** Spherocyte. **C,** Target cell. **D,** Elliptocyte. **E,** Echinocyte. **F,** Sickle cell. **G,** Stomatocyte. **H,** Acanthocyte. **I** to **L,** Schistocytes. **M,** Teardrop RBC. **N,** Distorted RBC with Hb C crystal protruding. **O,** Degmacyte. **P,** Basophilic stippling. **Q,** Pappenheimer bodies. **R,** Howell-Jolly body. (From Ravel R: *Clinical laboratory medicine,* ed 6, St Louis, 1995, Mosby.)

TABLE 4-18 Typical Renin-Aldosterone Patterns in Various Conditions

	PLASMA RENIN	ALDOSTERONE
Primary aldosteronism	Low	High
"Low-renin" essential hypertension	Low	Normal
Cushing's syndrome	Low	Low-normal
Licorice ingestion syndrome	Low	Low
High-salt diet	Low	Low
Oral contraceptives	High	Normal
Cirrhosis	High	High
Malignant hypertension	High	High
Unilateral renal disease	High	High
"High-renin" essential hypertension	High	High
Pregnancy	High	High
Diuretic overuse	High	High
Juxtaglomerular tumor (Bartter's syndrome)	High	High
Low-salt diet	High	High
Addison's disease	High	Low
Hypokalemia	High	Low

From Ravel R: *Clinical laboratory medicine*, ed 6, St Louis, 1995, Mosby.

RETICULOCYTE COUNT
Normal range:
  0.5% to 1.5%
Elevated in:
  Hemolytic anemia (sickle cell crisis, thalassemia major, autoimmune hemolysis), hemorrhage, postanemia therapy (folic acid, ferrous sulfate, vitamin B_{12}), chronic renal failure
Decreased in:
  Aplastic anemia, marrow suppression (sepsis, chemotherapeutic agents, radiation), hepatic cirrhosis, blood transfusion, anemias of disordered maturation (iron deficiency anemia, megaloblastic anemia, sideroblastic anemia, anemia of chronic disease)

RHEUMATOID FACTOR
Normal:
  Negative
Present in titer >1:20:
  Rheumatoid arthritis, SLE, chronic inflammatory processes, old age, infections, liver disease, multiple myeloma, sarcoidosis, pulmonary fibrosis, Sjögren's syndrome, other (Box 4-34)

RNP; *see* EXTRACTABLE NUCLEAR ANTIGEN
SCHILLING TEST; *see* Fig. 4-14
SEDIMENTATION RATE; *see* ERYTHROCYTE SEDIMENTATION RATE
SGOT; *see* ASPARTATE AMINOTRANSFERASE
SGPT; *see* ALANINE AMINOTRANSFERASE

SMOOTH MUSCLE ANTIBODY
Normal:
  Negative
Present in:
  Chronic acute hepatitis (≥1:80), primary biliary cirrhosis (≤1:80), infectious mononucleosis

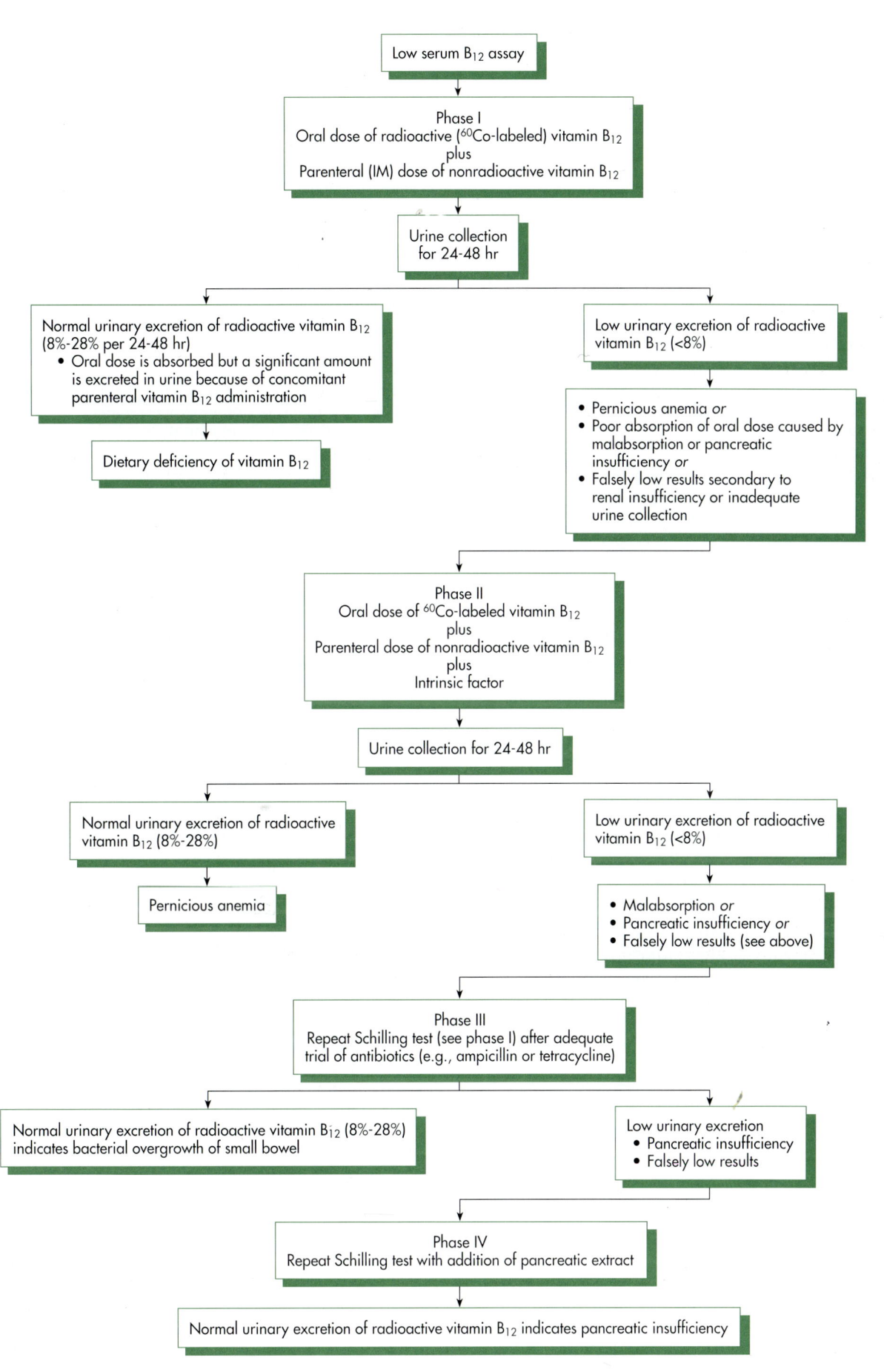

```
                        ┌─────────────────────┐
                        │ Low serum B₁₂ assay │
                        └──────────┬──────────┘
                                   ▼
              ┌────────────────────────────────────────────┐
              │ Phase I                                    │
              │ Oral dose of radioactive (⁶⁰Co-labeled)    │
              │   vitamin B₁₂                              │
              │ plus                                       │
              │ Parenteral (IM) dose of nonradioactive     │
              │   vitamin B₁₂                              │
              └────────────────────┬───────────────────────┘
                                   ▼
                        ┌─────────────────────┐
                        │ Urine collection    │
                        │ for 24-48 hr        │
                        └──────────┬──────────┘
```

Phase I — after urine collection:

- **Normal urinary excretion of radioactive vitamin B₁₂ (8%-28% per 24-48 hr)**
  - Oral dose is absorbed but a significant amount is excreted in urine because of concomitant parenteral vitamin B₁₂ administration
  - → **Dietary deficiency of vitamin B₁₂**

- **Low urinary excretion of radioactive vitamin B₁₂ (<8%)**
  - Pernicious anemia *or*
  - Poor absorption of oral dose caused by malabsorption or pancreatic insufficiency *or*
  - Falsely low results secondary to renal insufficiency or inadequate urine collection

Phase II
Oral dose of ⁶⁰Co-labeled vitamin B₁₂
plus
Parenteral dose of nonradioactive vitamin B₁₂
plus
Intrinsic factor

Urine collection for 24-48 hr

- **Normal urinary excretion of radioactive vitamin B₁₂ (8%-28%)**
  - → **Pernicious anemia**

- **Low urinary excretion of radioactive vitamin B₁₂ (<8%)**
  - Malabsorption *or*
  - Pancreatic insufficiency *or*
  - Falsely low results (see above)

Phase III
Repeat Schilling test (see phase I) after adequate trial of antibiotics (e.g., ampicillin or tetracycline)

- **Normal urinary excretion of radioactive vitamin B₁₂ (8%-28%)** indicates bacterial overgrowth of small bowel

- **Low urinary excretion**
  - Pancreatic insufficiency
  - Falsely low results

Phase IV
Repeat Schilling test with addition of pancreatic extract

- Normal urinary excretion of radioactive vitamin B₁₂ indicates pancreatic insufficiency

Fig. 4-14 Schilling test. (From Ferri FF: *Practical guide to the care of the medical patient,* ed 4, St. Louis, 1998, Mosby.)

BOX 4-34 Diseases in which Rheumatoid Factor is Commonly Present

Rheumatic Diseases
Rheumatoid arthritis
Sjögren's syndrome
Systemic lupus erythematosus
Polymyositis/dermatomyositis
Mixed connective tissue disease
Scleroderma

Infectious Diseases
Subacute bacterial endocarditis
Tuberculosis
Infectious mononucleosis
Hepatitis
Syphilis
Leprosy
Influenza

Malignancies
Lymphoma
Multiple myeloma
Waldenstrom's macroglobulinemia
Postradiation or postchemotherapy

Miscellaneous
Normal adults, especially the elderly
Sarcoidosis
Chronic pulmonary disease (interstitial fibrosis)
Chronic liver disease (chronic active hepatitis, cirrhosis)
Mixed essential cryoglobulinemia
Hypergammaglobulinemic purpura

From Noble J (ed): *Primary care medicine,* ed 2, St Louis, 1996, Mosby.

BOX 4-35 Clinical Situations Frequently Associated with Serum Sodium Abnormalities

I. Hyponatremia
  A. Sodium and water depletion (deficit hyponatremia)
    1. Loss of GI secretions with replacement of fluid but not electrolytes
      a. Vomiting
      b. Diarrhea
      c. Tube drainage
    2. Loss from skin with replacement of fluids but not electrolytes
      a. Excessive sweating
      b. Extensive burns
    3. Loss from kidney
      a. Diuretics
      b. Chronic renal insufficiency (uremia) with acidosis
    4. Metabolic loss
      a. Starvation with acidosis
      b. Diabetic acidosis
    5. Endocrine loss
      a. Addison's disease
      b. Sudden withdrawal of long-term steroid therapy
    6. Iatrogenic loss from serous cavities
      a. Paracentesis or thoracentesis
  B. Excessive water (dilution hyponatremia)
    1. Excessive water administration
    2. CHF
    3. Cirrhosis
    4. Nephrotic syndrome
    5. Hypoalbuminemia (severe)
    6. Acute renal failure with oliguria
  C. Inappropriate antidiuretic hormone (IADH) syndrome
  D. Intracellular loss (reset osmostat syndrome)
  E. False hyponatremia (actually a dilutional effect)
    1. Marked hypertriglyceridemia*
    2. Marked hyperproteinemia*
    3. Severe hyperglycemia

II. Hypernatremia
Dehydration is the most frequent overall clinical finding in hypernatremia.
    1. Deficient water intake (either orally or intravenously)
    2. Excess kidney water output (diabetes insipidus, osmotic diuresis)
    3. Excess skin water output (excess sweating, loss from burns)
    4. Excess GI tract output (severe protracted vomiting or diarrhea without fluid therapy)
    5. Accidental sodium overdose
    6. High-protein tube feedings

From Ravel R: *Clinical laboratory medicine,* ed 6, St Louis, 1995, Mosby.
*Artifact in flame photometry, not in ISE.

SODIUM (serum)
Normal range:
  135-147 mEq/L (135-147 mmol/L) [CF: 1; SMI: 1 mmol/L]
Abnormal:
  see Box 4-35
STREPTOZIME; *see* **ANTI-STREPTOLYSIN O TITER**

SUCROSE HEMOLYSIS TEST (sugar water test)
Normal:
  Absence of hemolysis
Positive in:
  Paroxysmal nocturnal hemoglobinuria (PNH)
  False positive: autoimmune hemolytic anemia, megaloblastic anemias
  False negative: may occur with use of heparin or EDTA

T_3 (TRIIODOTHYRONINE)
Normal range:
  75-220 ng/dl (1.2-3.4 nmol/L) [CF: 0.01536; SMI: 0.1 nmol/L]
Abnormal values:
  see Table 4-19

T_4, FREE (free thyroxine)
Normal range:
  0.8-2.8 ng/dl (10-36 pmol/L) [CF: 12.87; SMI: 1 pmol/L]
Abnormal values:
  see Table 4-19

TESTOSTERONE
Elevated in:
  Adrenogenital syndrome, polycystic ovary disease
Decreased in:
  Klinefelter's syndrome, male hypogonadism

THROMBIN TIME (TT)
Normal range:
  11.3-18.5 sec
Elevated in:
  Thrombolytic and heparin therapy, DIC, hypofibrinogenemia, dysfibrinogenemia

THYROID-STIMULATING HORMONE (TSH)
Normal range:
  2-11 μU/ml (2-11 mU/L) [CF: 1; SMI: 1 mU/L]
Abnormal:
  see Boxes 4-36 and 4-37 and Table 4-19

THYROXINE (T_4)
Normal range:
  4-11 μg/dl (51-142 nmol/L) [CF: 12.87; SMI: 1 nmol/L]
Abnormal values:
  see Table 4-19

TABLE 4-19 **Findings in Thyroid Function Tests in Various Clinical Conditions**

CONDITION	T_4	FT_4I	T_3	FT_3I	TSH	TSI	TRH STIMULATION
Hyperthyroidism							
Graves' disease	↑	↑	↑	↑	↓	+	↓
Toxic nodular goiter	↑	↑	↑	↑	↓	−	↓
Pituitary TSH-secreting tumors	↑	↑	↑	↑	↑	−	↓
T_3 thyrotoxicosis	N	N	↑	↑	↓	+, −	↓
T_4 thyrotoxicosis	↑	↑	N	N	↓	+, −	↓
Hypothyroidism							
Primary	↓	↓	↓	↓	↑	+, −	↑
Secondary	↓	↓	↓	↓	↓, N	−	↓
Tertiary	↓	↓	↓	↓	↓, N	−	N
Peripheral unresponsiveness	↑, N	↑, N	↑, N	↑	↑, N	−	N, ↑

From Tilton RC, Barrows A: *Clinical laboratory medicine*, St Louis, 1992, Mosby.
N, Normal; ↑, increased; ↓, decreased; +, − variable.

> **BOX 4-36** Conditions that Increase Serum Thyroid-Stimulating Hormone Values

Laboratory error
Primary hypothyroidism
Synthroid therapy with insufficient dose; some patients
Lithium or amiodarone; some patients
Hashimoto's thyroiditis in later stage; some patients
Large doses of inorganic iodide (e.g., SSKI)
Severe nonthyroid illness in recovery phase; some patients
Iodine deficiency (moderate or severe)
Addison's disease
TSH specimen drawn in evening (peak of diurnal variation)
Pituitary TSH-secreting tumor
Therapy of hypothyroidism (3-6 wk after beginning therapy [range, 1-8 wk]; sometimes longer when pretherapy TSH is over 100 µU/ml); some patients
Acute psychiatric illness; few patients
Peripheral resistance to T_4 syndrome; some patients
Antibodies (e.g., HAMA) interfering with monoclonal sandwich method of TSH assay
Telepaque (iopanic acid) and Oragrafin (ipodate) x-ray contrast media; some patients
Amphetamines; some patients
High altitudes; some patients

From Ravel R: *Clinical laboratory medicine,* ed 6, St Louis, 1995, Mosby.

> **BOX 4-37** Conditions that Decrease Serum Thyroid-Stimulating Hormone Values*

Laboratory error
T_4/T_3 toxicosis (diffuse or nodular etiology)
Excessive therapy for hypothyroidism
Active thyroiditis (subacute, painless, or early active Hashimoto's disease); some patients
Multinodular goiter containing areas of autonomy; some patients
Severe nonthyroid illness (especially acute trauma, dopamine or glucocorticoid); some patients
T_3 toxicosis
Pituitary insufficiency
Cushing's syndrome (and some patients on high-dose glucocorticoid)
Jod-Basedow (iodine-induced) hyperthyroidism
TSH drawn 2-4 hr after levothyroxine dose; few patients
Postpartem transient toxicosis
Factitious hyperthyroidism
Struma ovarii
Radioimmunoassay, surgery, or antithyroid drug therapy for hyperthyroidism; some patients, 4-6 wk (range 2 wk-2 yr) after the treatment
Interleukin-2 drugs (3%-6% of cases) or α-interferon therapy (1% of cases)
Hyperemesis gravidarum
Amiodarone therapy; some patients

From Ravel R: *Clinical laboratory medicine,* ed 6, St Louis, 1995, Mosby.
*High sensitivity TSH method is assumed.

TIBC; *see* IRON BINDING CAPACITY

TRANSFERRIN
Normal range:
  170-370 mg/dl (1.7-3.7 g/L) [CF: 0.01; SMI: 0.01 g/L]
Elevated in:
  Iron deficiency anemia, oral contraceptive administration, viral hepatitis, late pregnancy
Decreased in:
  Nephrotic syndrome, liver disease, hereditary deficiency, protein malnutrition, neoplasms, chronic inflammatory states, chronic illness, thalassemia, hemochromatosis, hemolytic anemia

TRIGLYCERIDES
Normal range:
  <160 mg/dl (<1.80 mmol/L) [CF: 0.01129; SMI: 0.02 mmol/L]
Elevated in:
  Hyperlipoproteinemias (types I, IIb, III, IV, V), hypothyroidism, pregnancy, estrogens, acute MI, pancreatitis, alcohol intake, nephrotic syndrome, diabetes mellitus, glycogen storage disease
Decreased in:
  Malnutrition, congenital abetalipoproteinemias, drugs (e.g., gemfibrozil, nicotinic acid, clofibrate)

TRIIODOTHYRONINE; see T₃
TSH; see THYROID-STIMULATING HORMONE
TT; see THROMBIN TIME
TUBERCULIN TEST (PPD)
Abnormal results:
see Boxes 4-38 and 4-39 for interpretation
TUMOR MARKERS; see Table 4-20 for description of common tumor markers
UNCONJUGATED BILIRUBIN; see BILIRUBIN, INDIRECT
UREA NITROGEN (BUN)
Normal range:
8-18 mg/dl (3-6.5 mmol/L) [CF: 0.357; SMI: 0.5 mmol/L]
Elevated in:
Drugs (aminoglycosides and other antibiotics, diuretics, lithium, corticosteroids), dehydration, GI bleeding, decreased renal blood flow (shock, CHF, MI), renal disease (glomerulonephritis, pyelonephritis, diabetic nephropathy), urinary tract obstruction (prostatic hypertrophy)
Decreased in:
Liver disease, malnutrition, pregnancy third trimester, overhydration, acromegaly, celiac disease
URIC ACID (serum)
Normal range:
2-7 mg/dl (120-420 μmol/L) [CF: 59.48; SMI: 10 μmol/L]

BOX 4-38 PPD Reaction Size Considered "Positive" (Intracutaneous 5 TU* Mantoux Test at 48 hr)

5 mm or More
HIV infection or risk factors for HIV
Close recent contact with active TB case
Persons with chest x-ray consistent with healed TB

10 mm or More
Foreign-born persons from countries with high TB prevalence in Asia, Africa, and Latin America
IV drug users
Medically underserved low-income population groups (including Native Americans, Hispanics, and African Americans)
Residents of long-term care facilities (nursing homes, mental institutions)
Medical conditions that increase risk for TB (silicosis, gastrectomy, undernourished, diabetes mellitus, high-dose corticosteroids or immunosuppression Rx, leukemia or lymphoma, other malignancies
Employees of long-term care facilities, schools, child-care facilities, health care facilities

15 mm or More
All others not already listed

*TU, Tuberculin units.

BOX 4-39 Factors Associated with False-Negative Tuberculin Tests

Technical Errors
Improper administration
Inaccurate reading
Loss of potency of antigen

Patient-Related Factors (Anergy)
Age (elderly)
Nutritional status
Medications—corticosteroids, immunosuppressive agents
Severe tuberculosis
Coexisting diseases
  HIV infection
  Viral illness or vaccination
  Lymphoreticular malignancies
  Sarcoidosis
  Solid tumors
Lepromatous leprosy
Sjögren's syndrome
Ataxia telangiectasia
Uremia
Primary biliary cirrhosis
Systemic lupus erythematosus
Severe systemic disease of any etiology

From Stein JH (ed): *Internal medicine,* ed 4, St Louis, 1994, Mosby.

TABLE 4-20 Tumor Markers

General Uses:

1. Monitor serial titers before and after therapy. For example, a high preoperative CEA titer that falls to the normal range postoperatively is associated with a better prognosis in breast or colon cancer than is one that remains elevated after local therapy.
2. Serial values are also of use in monitoring (a) the clinical course of disease after local therapy and (b) the response to systemic chemotherapy. A decline in elevated values is usually consistent with tumor regression. Tumor markers are most valuable in monitoring disease not readily assessable by physical examination or simple radiographs.

	CHARACTERISTICS	PRESENCE IN NORMAL SERUM/PLASMA	CONDITIONS IN WHICH ELEVATED SERUM/PLASMA CONCENTRATIONS OCCUR	
			NEOPLASTIC	NONNEOPLASTIC
I. Oncofetal proteins				
1. Carcinoembryonic antigen (CEA)	Glycoprotein (MW 200,000)	<2.5 ng/ml	GI, breast, lung cancers	Inflammatory bowel disease, pancreatitis, gastritis, smoker's chronic bronchitis, alcoholic liver disease, hepatitis
2. Alpha fetoprotein (AFP)	α-Globulin (MW 70,000)	<40 ng/ml	Hepatoma, nonseminomatous testicular cancers	Pregnancy, regenerating liver tissue after viral hepatitis, chemically induced liver necrosis, partial hepatectomy
II. Hormones				
1. Human chorionic gonadotropin, β subunit (β-HCG)	Glycoprotein (MW 45,000); β subunit provides specificity versus LH, FSH, TSH	0	Choriocarcinoma, nonseminomatous testicular cancer, giant cell carcinoma of lung	Pregnancy
2. Ectopic hormones	ACTH, ADH, PTH		Lung, breast, head and neck, cervical cancers	
III. Serum enzymes				
1. Prostatic acid phosphatase (PAP)	Radioimmunoassay detects prostatic isozyme and distinguishes it from acid phosphatases of other organs (e.g., liver, spleen, kidney, small intestine), red and white blood cells, and platelets	0	Prostatic carcinoma	
2. Placental alkaline phosphatase	Biochemically and immunologically similar to that produced by the placenta	0	Seminoma, ovarian cancer	Pregnancy
3. Lactic dehydrogenase (LDH)	Tetramer, two distinct polypeptide chains: H (heart) and M (muscle)		Lymphoma	Hepatitis, MI, muscle injury
IV. Immunoglobulins	Monoclonal elevation (M spike) of complete protein, light or heavy chain, or portions		Multiple myeloma, B cell lymphoma	Monoclonal gammopathy of unknown significance (M-GUS)
V. Tumor-associated antigens				
1. CA-125			Ovarian, lung cancers	Benign gynecologic disease, cirrhosis
2. CA-15.3			Breast, ovarian, lung cancers	
3. Prostate-specific antigen	Glycoprotein (MW 30,000-40,000)		Prostatic carcinoma	Benign prostatic hypertrophy

From Stein JH (ed): *Internal medicine*, ed 4, St Louis, 1994, Mosby.
MW, Molecular weight; *LH,* luteinizing hormone; *FSH,* follicle-stimulating hormone; *TSH,* thyroid-stimulating hormone; *ACTH,* adrenocorticotropic hormone; *ADH,* antidiuretic hormone; *PTH,* parathormone (parathyroid hormone); *GI,* gastrointestinal; *MI,* myocardial infarction.

Elevated in:
Renal failure, gout, excessive cell lysis (chemotherapeutic agents, radiation therapy, leukemia, lymphoma, hemolytic anemia), hereditary enzyme deficiency (hypoxanthine-guanine-phosphoribosyl transferase), acidosis, myeloproliferative disorders, diet high in purines or protein, drugs (diuretics, low doses of ASA, ethambutol, nicotinic acid), lead poisoning, hypothyroidism, Addison's disease, nephrogenic diabetes insipidus, active psoriasis, polycystic kidneys

Decreased in:
Drugs (allopurinol, high doses of ASA, probenecid, warfarin, corticosteroid), deficiency of xanthine oxidase, SIADH, renal tubular deficits (Fanconi's syndrome), alcoholism, liver disease, diet deficient in protein or purines, Wilson's disease, hemochromatosis

URINALYSIS

Normal range:
Color: light straw
Appearance: clear
pH: 4.5-8 (average, 6)
Specific gravity: 1.005-1.030
Microscopic examination:
  RBC: 0-5 (high-power field)
  WBC: 0-5 (high-power field)
  Bacteria (spun specimen): absent
  Casts: 0-4 hyaline (low-power field)
Protein: absent
Ketones: absent
Glucose: absent
Occult blood: absent

URINE AMYLASE

Normal range:
35-260 U Somogyi/hr (6.5-48.1 U/hr) [CF: 0.185; SMI: 1 U/hr]

Elevated in:
Pancreatitis, carcinoma of the pancreas

URINE BILE

Normal:
Absent

Abnormal:
Urine bilirubin: hepatitis (viral, toxic, drug-induced), biliary obstruction
Urine urobilinogen: hepatitis (viral, toxic, drug-induced), hemolytic jaundice, liver cell dysfunction (cirrhosis, infection, metastases)

URINE CALCIUM

Normal range:
<250 mg/24 hr (<6.2 mmol/dl) [CF: 0.02495; SMI: 0.1 mmol/dl]

Elevated in:
Primary hyperparathyroidism, hypervitaminosis D, bone metastases, multiple myeloma, increased calcium intake, steroids, prolonged immobilization, sarcoidosis, Paget's disease, idiopathic hypercalciuria, renal tubular acidosis

Decreased in:
Hypoparathyroidism, pseudohypoparathyroidism, vitamin D deficiency, vitamin D–resistant rickets, diet low in calcium, drugs (thiazide diuretics, oral contraceptives), familial hypocalciuric hypercalcemia, renal osteodystrophy, potassium citrate therapy

URINE cAMP

Elevated in:
Hypercalciuria, familial hypocalciuric hypercalcemia, primary hyperparathyroidism, pseudohypoparathyroidism, rickets

Decreased in:
Vitamin D intoxication, sarcoidosis

URINE CATECHOLAMINES
Normal range:
Norepinephrine: <100 μg/24 hr (<590 nmol/day) [CF: 5.911; SMI: 10 nmol/day]
Epinephrine: <10 μg/24 hr (55 nmol/day) [CF: 5.458; SMI: 5 nmol/day]
Elevated in:
Pheochromocytoma, neuroblastoma, severe stress

URINE CHLORIDE
Normal range:
110-250 mEq/day (110-250 mmol/day) [CF: 1; SMI: 1 mmol/day]
Elevated in:
Corticosteroids, Bartter's syndrome, diuretics, metabolic acidosis, severe hypokalemia
Decreased in:
Chloride depletion (vomiting), colonic villous adenoma, chronic renal failure, renal tubular acidosis

URINE COPPER
Normal range:
<40 μg/24 hr (<0.6 μmol/day) [CF: 0.01574; SMI: 0.2 μmol/day]

URINE CORTISOL, FREE
Normal range:
10-110 μg/24 hr (30-300 nmol/day) [CF: 2.759; SMI: 10 nmol/day]
Elevated:
See CORTISOL (serum)

URINE CREATININE (24 HR)
Normal range:
Male: 0.8-1.8 g/day (7-16 mmol/day) [CF: 8.840; SMI: 0.1 mmol/day]
Female: 0.6-1.6 g/day (5.3-14 mmol/day)
NOTE: Useful test as an indicator of completeness of 24 hr urine collection.

URINE EOSINOPHILS
Normal:
Absent
Present:
Interstitial nephritis, ATN, UTI, kidney transplant rejection, hepatorenal syndrome

URINE GLUCOSE (qualitative)
Normal:
Absent
Present in:
Diabetes mellitus, renal glycosuria (decreased renal threshold for glucose), glucose intolerance

URINE HEMOGLOBIN, FREE
Normal:
Absent
Present in:
Hemolysis (with saturation of serum haptoglobin binding capacity and renal threshold for tubular absorption of hemoglobin)

URINE HEMOSIDERIN
Normal:
Absent
Present in:
Paroxysmal nocturnal hemoglobinuria (PNH), chronic hemolytic anemia, hemochromatosis, blood transfusion, thalassemias

URINE 5-HYDROXYINDOLE-ACETIC ACID (URINE 5-HIAA)
Normal range:
2-8 mg/24 hr (10-40 μmol/day) [CF: 5.23; SMI: 5 μmol/day]

Elevated in:
　Carcinoid tumors, after ingestion of certain foods (bananas, plums, tomatoes, avocados, pineapples, eggplant, walnuts), drugs (MAO inhibitors, phenacetin, methyldopa, glycerol guaiacolate, acetaminophen, salicylates, phenothiazines, imipramine, methocarbamol, reserpine, metamphetamine)

URINE INDICAN
Normal:
　Absent
Present in:
　Malabsorption secondary to intestinal bacterial overgrowth

URINE KETONES (semiquantitative)
Normal:
　Absent
Present in:
　DKA, alcoholic ketoacidosis, starvation, isopropanol ingestion

URINE METANEPHRINES
Normal range:
　0-2.0 mg/24 hr (0-11.0 μmol/day) [CF: 5.458; SMI: 0.5 μmol/day]
Elevated in:
　Pheochromocytoma, neuroblastoma, drugs (caffeine, phenothiazines, MAO inhibitors), stress

URINE MYOGLOBIN
Normal:
　Absent
Present in:
　Severe trauma, hyperthermia, polymyositis/dermatomyositis, carbon monoxide poisoning, drugs (narcotic and amphetamine toxicity), hypothyroidism, muscle ischemia

URINE NITRITE
Normal:
　Absent
Present in:
　Urinary tract infections

URINE OCCULT BLOOD
Normal:
　Negative
Positive in:
　Trauma to urinary tract, renal disease (glomerulonephritis, pyelonephritis), renal or ureteral calculi, bladder lesions (carcinoma, cystitis), prostatitis, prostatic carcinoma, menstrual contamination, hematopoietic disorders (hemophilia, thrombocytopenia), anticoagulants, ASA

URINE OSMOLALITY
Normal range:
　50-1200 mOsm/kg (50-1200 mmol/kg) [CF: 1; SMI: 1 mmol/kg]
Elevated in:
　SIADH, dehydration, glycosuria, adrenal insufficiency, high-protein diet
Decreased in:
　Diabetes insipidus, excessive water intake IV hydration with D_5W, acute renal insufficiency, glomerulonephritis

URINE pH
Normal range:
　4.6-8 (average 6)
Elevated in:
　Bacteriuria, vegetarian diet, renal failure with inability to form ammonia, drugs (antibiotics, sodium bicarbonate, acetazolamide)

Decreased in:
　Acidosis (metabolic, respiratory), drugs (ammonium chloride, methenamine mandelate), diabetes mellitus, starvation, diarrhea

URINE PHOSPHATE
Normal range:
　0.8-2.0 g/24 hr
Elevated in:
　ATN (diuretic phase), chronic renal disease, uncontrolled diabetes mellitus, hyperparathyroidism, hypomagnesemia, metabolic acidosis, metabolic alkalosis, neurofibromatosis, adult-onset vitamin D–resistant hypophosphatemic osteomalacia
Decreased in:
　Acromegaly, acute renal failure, decreased dietary intake, hypoparathyroidism, respiratory acidosis

URINE POTASSIUM
Normal range:
　25-100 mEq/24 hr (25-100 mmol/day) [CF: 1; SMI: 1 mmol/day]
Elevated in:
　Aldosteronism (primary, secondary), glucocorticoids, alkalosis, renal tubular acidosis, excessive dietary potassium intake
Decreased in:
　Acute renal failure, potassium-sparing diuretics, diarrhea, hypokalemia

URINE PROTEIN (quantitative)
Normal range:
　<150 mg/24 hr (<0.15 g/day) [CF: 0.001; SMI: 0.01 g/day]
Elevated in:
　Renal disease (glomerular, tubular, interstitial), CHF, hypertension, neoplasms of renal pelvis and bladder, multiple myeloma, Waldenstrom's macroglobulinemia

URINE SEDIMENT; *see* Fig. 4-15 for evaluation of common abnormalities

URINE SODIUM (quantitative)
Normal range:
　40-220 mEq/day (40-220 mmol/day) [CF: 1; SMI: 1 mmol/day]
Elevated in:
　Diuretic administration, high sodium intake, salt-losing nephritis, acute tubular necrosis, vomiting, Addison's disease, SIADH, hypothyroidism, CHF, hepatic failure, chronic renal failure, Bartter's syndrome, glucocorticoid deficiency, interstitial nephritis caused by analgesic abuse, mannitol, dextran or glycerol therapy, milk-alkali syndrome, decreased renin secretion, postobstructive diuresis
Decreased in:
　Increased aldosterone, glucocorticoid excess, hyponatremia, prerenal azotemia, decreased salt intake

URINE SPECIFIC GRAVITY
Normal range:
　1.005-1.03
Elevated in:
　Dehydration, excessive fluid losses (vomiting, diarrhea, fever), x-ray contrast media, diabetes mellitus, CHF, SIADH, adrenal insufficiency, decreased fluid intake
Decreased in:
　Diabetes insipidus, renal disease (glomerulonephritis, pyelonephritis), excessive fluid intake or IV hydration

URINE VANILLYLMANDELIC ACID (VMA)
Normal range:
　<6.8 mg/24 hr (<35 μmol/day) [CF: 5.046; SMI: 1 μmol/day]

LABORATORY TESTS VDRL/Viscosity 837

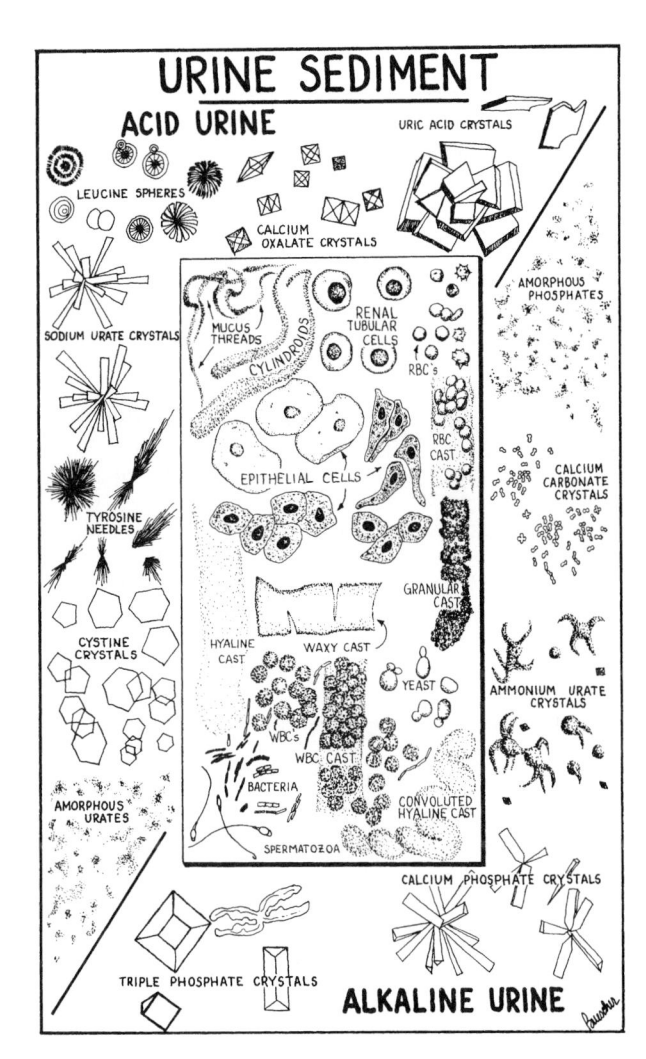

Fig. 4-15 Microscopic examination of urinary sediment. (From Grigorian Greene M: *The Harriet Lane handbook: a manual for pediatric house officers,* ed 12, St Louis, 1991, Mosby. Reproduced with permission from Johns Hopkins Hospital.)

Elevated in:
  Pheochromocytoma, neuroblastoma, ganglioblastoma, drugs (isoproterenol, methocarbamol, levodopa, sulfonamides, chlorpromazine), severe stress, after ingestion of bananas, chocolate, vanilla, tea, coffee

Decreased in:
  Drugs (MAO inhibitors, reserpine, guanethidine, methyldopa)

VDRL

Normal range:
  Negative

Positive test:
  Syphilis, other treponemal diseases (yaws, pina, bejel)
  NOTE: A false-positive test may be seen in patients with SLE and other autoimmune diseases, infectious mononucleosis, HIV, atypical pneumonia, malaria, leprosy, typhus fever, rat-bite fever, relapsing fever.
  NOTE: see Table 4-21 for interpretation of serologic tests for syphilis.

VISCOSITY (serum)

Normal range:
  1.4-1.8 relative to water (1.10-1.22 centipoise)

TABLE 4-21 Interpretation of Serologic Tests for Syphilis*

FINDING		
NONTREPONEMAL TESTS	TREPONEMAL TESTS	INTERPRETATION OF FINDING: IS SYPHILIS PRESENT?*
Nonreactive	Nonreactive	Early primary syphilis is not ruled out by negative serologic tests. Early syphilis is present in 13%-30% of patients who have a negative MHATP test; in about 30% of patients who present with chancre but have a nonreactive reagin test; and in about 10% of patients who have a negative FTA-ABS test. Late syphilis is present in a very small fraction of patients. Adequately treated syphilis in remote past may produce these results, but treponemal tests usually remain reactive.
	Reactive	Observed in about 10% of patients with chancre. The treponemal tests may turn positive shortly before the reagin tests. Reagin tests repeated after several days are generally positive. In adequately treated early syphilis, the reagin test may return to nonreactive within 1-2 yr, whereas the treponemal tests generally do not. Late syphilis is not ruled out by a negative reagin test. The sensitivity of the reagin tests is lower than that of treponemal tests in untreated late syphilis. In secondary syphilis, rarely, a highly reactive serum appears negative when tested undiluted with a reagin test because flocculation is inhibited by relative antibody excess. Not reported to occur with treponemal tests. Quantitative reagin test are positive. False-positive treponemal tests occur in 40% of patients with Lyme disease.
Reactive	Nonreactive Borderline (FTA-ABS)	Finding is not diagnostic of syphilis but constitutes a classic biologic false-positive reaction. Not diagnostic of syphilis: most patients (90%) with this pattern do not develop clinical or serologic evidence of syphilis. Repeat test is indicated. Chronic borderline results are associated with a variety of conditions other than syphilis.
	Beaded (FTA-ABS)	Not diagnostic of syphilis. Seen with collagen vascular disease.
	Reactive	Findings diagnostic of syphilis or other treponemal disease. In adequately treated syphilis, one would expect (1) a sustained fourfold drop in titer of reagin test, although reagin test may remain positive after adequate therapy; (2) treponemal tests remain positive after adequate therapy. Concurrent false-positive results on both nontreponemal and treponemal tests could occur in rare instances. It may be impossible to rule out syphilis in an individual with this test profile.

From Stein JH (ed): *Internal medicine*, ed 4, St Louis, 1994, Mosby.
*Serologic data must always be interpreted in the light of a total clinical evaluation. Diagnosis based on serologic criteria alone is fraught with error. Serologic tests apparently in conflict with clinical diagnosis should be confirmed by repetition or possibly referral to a reference laboratory.

Elevated in:
    Monoclonal gammopathies (Waldenstrom's macroglobulinemia, multiple myeloma), hyperfibrinogenemia, SLE, rheumatoid arthritis, polycythemia, leukemia

VITAMIN B₁₂

Normal:
    190-900 ng/ml
    Vitamin B₁₂ deficiency
        Etiology
            1. pernicious anemia (antibodies against intrinsic factor and gastric parietal cells)
            2. Dietary (strict lacto-ovovegetarians, food faddists)
            3. Malabsorption (achlorhydria, gastrectomy, ileal resection, pancreatic insufficiency, drugs [omeprazole, cholestyramine])
    Falsely low levels occur in patients with severe folate deficiency, in patients using high doses of ascorbic acid, and when cobalamin (Cbl) levels are measured after nuclear medicine studies (radioactivity interferes with cobalamin RIA measurement).

Falsely high or normal levels in patients with cobalamin deficiency can occur in severe liver disease and chronic granulocytic leukemia.

The absence of anemia or macrocytosis does not exclude the diagnosis of cobalamin deficiency.

WBC; see COMPLETE BLOOD COUNT
WESTERGREN; see ERYTHROCYTE SEDIMENTATION RATE
WET-MOUNT MICROSCOPIC PROCEDURES; see Box 4-40
WHITE BLOOD COUNT; see COMPLETE BLOOD COUNT

D-XYLOSE ABSORPTION
Normal range:
21% to 31% excreted in 5 hr (0.21-0.31) [CF: 0.01; SMI: 0.01]
Decreased in:
Malabsorption syndrome

BOX 4-40 **Wet-Mount Microscopic Procedures**

India Ink Preparation

1. Place a drop of specimen on a clean glass slide.
2. Cover with coverslip, preferably a larger size.
3. Place a small drop of India ink on the slide, touching the coverslip; it will be drawn under the coverslip and provide a gradient suspension of the ink particles.
4. Examine using bright-field microscopy; scan the slide to find the point at which suspension is optimal for observing capsules or organisms.

Potassium Hydroxide Preparation

1. Place a small portion of specimen on a clean glass slide.
2. Add a drop of 10% potassium hydroxide solution; if necessary, mix with specimen using an applicator stick.
3. Cover with a coverslip, then heat gently by passing through a flame (do not heat excessively; several minutes or more of setting may be necessary to dissolve material composed of keratin).
4. Examine using bright-field microscopy; adjust substage condenser to optimize contrast.

Methylene Blue Stain for Fecal Leukocytes

1. Place a small portion of liquid stool on a clean glass slide.
2. Add a drop of methylene blue stain and mix with the specimen; place coverslip.
3. Let stand several minutes, then examine with bright-field microscopy.

From Stein JH (ed): *Internal medicine*, ed 5, St Louis, 1998, Mosby.

SECTION V

Clinical Preventive Services

TASK FORCE RATINGS

The Task Force graded the *strength of recommendations* for or against preventive interventions as follows.

STRENGTH OF RECOMMENDATIONS

A There is good evidence to support the recommendation that the condition be specifically considered in a periodic health examination.

B There is fair evidence to support the recommendation that the condition be specifically considered in a periodic health examination.

C There is insufficient evidence to recommend for or against the inclusion of the condition in a periodic health examination, but recommendations may be made on other grounds.

D There is fair evidence to support the recommendation that the condition be excluded from consideration in a periodic health examination.

E There is good evidence to support the recommendation that the condition be excluded from consideration in a periodic health examination.

Data from: US Preventive Services Task Force: *Guide to clinical preventive services: report of the US Preventive Services Task Force,* ed 2, Washington, DC, 1996, US Department of Health and Human Services. Text downloaded from Internet site: http://text.nlm.nih.gov

CONTENTS

A THE PERIODIC HEALTH EXAMINATION
Age-Specific Charts, 843

B SCREENING

Cardiovascular Diseases, 853
1. Screening for Asymptomatic Coronary Artery Disease, 853
2. Screening for High Blood Cholesterol and Other Lipid Abnormalities, 853
3. Screening for Hypertension, 854
4. Screening for Asymptomatic Carotid Artery Stenosis, 855
5. Screening for Peripheral Arterial Disease, 855
6. Screening for Abdominal Aortic Aneurysm, 855

Neoplastic Diseases, 856
7. Screening for Breast Cancer, 856
8. Screening for Colorectal Cancer, 856
9. Screening for Cervical Cancer, 857
10. Screening for Prostate Cancer, 858
11. Screening for Lung Cancer, 858
12. Screening for Skin Cancer—Including Counseling to Prevent Skin Cancer, 858
13. Screening for Testicular Cancer, 859
14. Screening for Ovarian Cancer, 859
15. Screening for Pancreatic Cancer, 859
16. Screening for Oral Cancer, 859
17. Screening for Bladder Cancer, 860
18. Screening for Thyroid Cancer, 860

Metabolic, Nutritional, and Environmental Disorders, 860
19. Screening for Diabetes Mellitus, 860
20. Screening for Thyroid Disease, 860
21. Screening for Obesity, 861
22. Screening for Iron Deficiency Anemia— Including Iron Prophylaxis, 861
23. Screening for Elevated Lead Levels in Childhood and Pregnancy, 862

Infectious Diseases, 863
24. Screening for Hepatitis B Virus Infection, 863
25. Screening for Tuberculous Infection—Including Bacille Calmette-Guérin Immunization, 863
26. Screening for Syphilis, 864
27. Screening for Gonorrhea—Including Ocular Prophylaxis in Newborns, 864
28. Screening for Human Immunodeficiency Virus Infection, 865
29. Screening for Chlamydial Infection—Including Ocular Prophylaxis in Newborns, 866
30. Screening for Genital Herpes Simplex, 867
31. Screening for Asymptomatic Bacteriuria, 868
32. Screening for Rubella—Including Immunization of Adolescents and Adults, 868

Vision and Hearing Disorders, 869
33. Screening for Visual Impairment, 869
34. Screening for Glaucoma, 869
35. Screening for Hearing Impairment, 869

Prenatal Disorders, 870
36. Screening Ultrasonography in Pregnancy, 870
37. Screening for Preeclampsia, 870
38. Screening for D (Rh) Incompatibility, 871
39. Intrapartum Electronic Fetal Monitoring, 871
40. Home Uterine Activity Monitoring, 871

Congenital Disorders, 872
41. Screening for Down Syndrome, 872
42. Screening for Neural Tube Defects—Including Folic Acid/Folate Prophylaxis, 872
43. Screening for Hemoglobinopathies, 873
44. Screening for Phenylketonuria, 874
45. Screening for Congenital Hypothyroidism, 874

Musculoskeletal Disorders, 874
46. Screening for Postmenopausal Osteoporosis, 874
47. Screening for Adolescent Idiopathic Scoliosis, 875

Mental Disorders and Substance Abuse, 875
48. Screening for Dementia, 875
49. Screening for Depression, 875
50. Screening for Suicide Risk, 876
51. Screening for Family Violence, 876
52. Screening for Problem Drinking, 876
53. Screening for Drug Abuse, 878

C COUNSELING
54. Counseling to Prevent Tobacco Use, 880
55. Counseling to Promote Physical Activity, 881
56. Counseling to Promote a Healthy Diet, 881
57. Counseling to Prevent Motor Vehicle Injuries, 883
58. Counseling to Prevent Household and Recreational Injuries, 883
59. Counseling to Prevent Youth Violence, 884
60. Counseling to Prevent Low Back Pain, 885
61. Counseling to Prevent Dental and Periodontal Disease, 885
62. Counseling to Prevent HIV Infection and Other Sexually Transmitted Diseases, 886
63. Counseling to Prevent Unintended Pregnancy, 887
64. Counseling to Prevent Gynecologic Cancers, 887

D IMMUNIZATIONS AND CHEMOPROPHYLAXIS
65. Childhood Immunizations, 889
66. Adult Immunizations—Including Chemoprophylaxis Against Influenza A, 891
67. Postexposure Prophylaxis for Selected Infectious Diseases, 893
68. Postmenopausal Hormone Prophylaxis, 894
69. Aspirin Prophylaxis for the Primary Prevention of Myocardial Infarction, 895
70. Aspirin Prophylaxis in Pregnancy, 895

Part A
THE PERIODIC HEALTH EXAMINATION
Age-Specific Charts

TABLE 5-1   Birth to 10 Years

Interventions considered and recommended for the Periodic Health Examination

Leading causes of death
- Conditions originating in perinatal period
- Congenital anomalies
- Sudden infant death syndrome (SIDS)
- Unintentional injuries (non–motor vehicle)
- Motor vehicle injuries

Interventions for the General Population

Screening

Height and weight *[Ch. 21]*

Blood pressure *[Ch. 3]*

Vision screen (age 3-4 yr) *[Ch. 33]*

Hemoglobinopathy screen (birth)[1] *[Ch. 43]*

Phenylalanine level (birth)[2] *[Ch. 44]*

T_4 and/or TSH (birth)[3] *[Ch. 45]*

Counseling

Injury prevention *[Ch. 57, 58]*
Child safety car seats (age <5 yr)

Lap/shoulder belts (age ≥5 yr)

Bicycle helmet; avoid bicycling near traffic

Smoke detector, flame retardant sleepwear

Hot water heater temperature <120°-130°F

Window/stair guards, pool fence

Safe storage of drugs, toxic substances, firearms and matches

Syrup of ipecac, poison control phone number

CPR training for parents/caretakers

Diet and exercise
Breast-feeding, iron-enriched formula and foods (infants and toddlers) *[Ch. 22, 56]*

Limit fat and cholesterol; maintain caloric balance; emphasize grains, fruits, vegetables (age ≥2 yr) *[Ch. 56]*

Regular physical activity* *[Ch. 55]*

Substance use *[Ch. 54]*
Effects of passive smoking*

Anti-tobacco message*

Dental health *[Ch. 61]*
Regular visits to dental care provider*

Floss, brush with fluoride toothpaste daily*

Advice about baby bottle tooth decay*

Immunizations *[Ch. 65]*
Diphtheria-tetanus-pertussis (DTP)[4]

Oral poliovirus (OPV)[5]

Measles-mumps-rubella (MMR)[6]

H. influenzae type b (Hib) conjugate[7]

Hepatitis B[8]

Varicella[9]

Chemoprophylaxis

Ocular prophylaxis (birth) *[Ch. 27]*

Interventions for High-Risk Populations

Population	Potential Interventions (See detailed high-risk definitions)
Preterm or low birth weight	Hemoglobin/hematocrit (HR1)
Infants of mothers at risk for HIV	HIV testing (HR2)
Low income; immigrants	Hemoglobin/hematocrit (HR1); PPD (HR3)
TB contacts	PPD (HR3)
Native American/Alaska Native	Hemoglobin/hematocrit (HR1); PPD (HR3); hepatitis A vaccine (HR4); pneumococcal vaccine (HR5)
Travelers to developing countries	Hepatitis A vaccine (HR4)
Residents of long-term care facilities	PPD (HR3); hepatitis A vaccine (HR4); influenza vaccine (HR6)
Certain chronic medical conditions	PPD (HR3); pneumococcal vaccine (HR5); influenza vaccine (HR6)
Increased individual or community lead exposure	Blood lead level (HR7)
Inadequate water fluoridation	Daily fluoride supplement (HR8)
Family hx of skin cancer; nevi; far skin, eyes, hair	Avoid excess/midday sun, use protective clothing* (HR9)

[1]Whether screening should be universal or targeted to high-risk groups will depend on the proportion of high-risk individuals in the screening area, and other considerations (See Ch. 43). [2]If done during first 24 hr of life, repeat by age 2 wk. [3]Optimally between day 2 and 6, but in all cases before newborn nursery discharge. [4]2, 4, 6, and 12-18 mo; once between ages 4-6 yr (DTaP may be used at 15 mo and older). [5]2, 4, 6-18 mo; once between ages 4-6 yr. [6]12-15 mo and 4-6 yr. [7]2, 4, 6 and 12-15 mo; no dose needed at 6 mo if PRP-OMP vaccine is used for first 2 doses. [8]Birth, 1 mo, 6 mo; or, 0-2 mo, 1-2 mo later, and 6-18 mo. If not done in infancy: current visit, and 1 and 6 mo later. [9]12-18 mo; or any child without hx of chickenpox or previous immunization. Include information on risk in adulthood, duration of immunity, and potential need for booster doses.
*The ability of clinician counseling to influence this behavior is unproven.

HR1 = Infants age 6-12 mo who are living in poverty, black, Native American or Alaska Native, immigrants from developing countries, preterm and low birth weight infants, infants whose principal dietary intake is unfortified cow's milk (see Ch. 22).

HR2 = Infants born to high-risk mothers whose HIV status is unknown. Women at high risk include past or present injection drug use; persons who exchange sex for money or drugs, and their sex partners; injection drug-using, bisexual, or HIV-positive sex partners currently or in past; persons seeking treatment for STDs; blood transfusion during 1978-1985 (see Ch. 28).

HR3 = Persons infected with HIV, close contacts of persons with known or suspected TB, persons with medical risk factors associated with TB, immigrants from countries with high TB prevalence, medically underserved low-income populations (including homeless), residents of long-term care facilities (see Ch. 25). See Ch. 25 for indications for BCG vaccine.

HR4 = Persons ≥2 yr living in or traveling to areas where the disease is endemic and where periodic outbreaks occur (e.g., countries with high or intermediate endemicity; certain Alaska Native, Pacific Island, Native American, and religious communities). Consider for institutionalized children aged ≥2 yr. Clinicians should also consider local epidemiology (see Ch. 65-67).

HR5 = Immunocompetent persons ≥2 yr with certain medical conditions, including chronic cardiac or pulmonary disease, diabetes mellitus, and anatomic asplenia. Immunocompetent persons ≥2 yr living in high-risk environments or social settings (e.g., certain Native American and Alaska Native populations) (see Ch. 66).

HR6 = Annual vaccination of children ≥6 mo who are residents of chronic care facilities or who have chronic cardiopulmonary disorders, metabolic diseases (including diabetes mellitus), hemoglobinopathies, immunosuppression, or renal dysfunction (see Ch. 66). See Ch. 66 for indications for amantadine/rimantadine prophylaxis.

HR7 = Children about age 12 mo who: (1) live in communities in which the prevalence of lead levels requiring individual intervention, including residential lead hazard control or chelation, is high or undefined; (2) live in or frequently visit a home built before 1950 with dilapidated paint or with recent or ongoing renovation or remodeling; (3) have close contact with a person who has an elevated lead level; (4) live near lead industry or heavy traffic; (5) live with someone whose job or hobby involves lead exposure; (6) use lead-based pottery; or (7) take traditional ethnic remedies that contain lead (see Ch. 23).

HR8 = Children living in areas with inadequate water fluoridation (<0.6 ppm) (see Ch. 61).

HR9 = Persons with a family history of skin cancer, a large number of moles, atypical moles, poor tanning ability, or light skin, hair, and eye color (see Ch. 12).

TABLE 5-2 Ages 11-24 Years

Interventions considered and recommended for the Periodic Health Examination	Leading causes of death Motor vehicle/other unintentional injuries Homicide Suicide Malignant neoplasms Heart diseases

Interventions for the General Population

Screening

Height and weight [Ch. 21]

Blood pressure[1] [Ch. 3]

Papanicolaou (Pap) test[2] (females) [Ch. 9]

Chlamydia screen[3] (females <20 yr) [Ch. 29]

Rubella serology or vaccination hx[4] (females >12 yr) [Ch. 32]

Assess for problem drinking [Ch. 52]

Counseling

Injury prevention [Ch. 57, 58]
Lap/shoulder belts

Bicycle/motorcycle/ATV helmets*

Smoke detector*

Safe storage/removal of firearms* [Ch. 50, 59]

Substance use
Avoid tobacco use [Ch. 54]

Avoid underage drinking and illicit drug use* [Ch. 52, 53]

Avoid alcohol/drug use while driving, swimming, boating, etc.* [Ch. 57, 58]

Sexual behavior [Ch. 62, 63]
STD prevention: abstinence*; avoid high-risk behavior*; condoms/female barrier with spermicide*
Unintended pregnancy: contraception

Diet and exercise

Limit fat and cholesterol; maintain caloric balance; emphasize grains, fruits, vegetables [Ch. 56]

Adequate calcium intake (females) [Ch. 56]

Regular physical activity* [Ch. 55]

Dental health [Ch. 61]
Regular visits to dental care provider*

Floss, brush with fluoride toothpaste daily

Immunizations [Ch. 65, 66]

Tetanus-diphtheria (Td) boosters (11-16 yr)

Hepatitis B[5]

MMR (11-12 yr)[6]

Varicella (11-12 yr)[7]

Rubella[4] (females >12 yr) [Ch. 32]

Chemoprophylaxis

Multivitamin with folic acid (females)

Interventions for High-Risk Populations

Population	Potential Interventions (See detailed high-risk definitions)
High-risk sexual behavior	RPR/VDRL (HR1); screen for gonorrhea (female) (HR2), HIV (HR3), chlamydia (female) (HR4); hepatitis A vaccine (HR5)
Injection or street drug use	RPR/VDRL (HR1); HIV screen (HR3); hepatitis A vaccine (HR5); PPD (HR6); advice to reduce infection risk (HR7)
TB contacts; immigrants; low income	PPD (HR6)
Native Americans/Alaska Natives	Hepatitis A vaccine (HR5); PPD (HR6); pneumococcal vaccine (HR8)
Travelers to developing countries	Hepatitis A vaccine (HR5)
Certain chronic medical conditions	PPD (HR6); pneumococcal vaccine (HR8); influenza vaccine (HR9)
Settings where adolescents and young adults congregate	Second MMR (HR10)
Susceptible to varicella, measles, mumps	Varicella vaccine (HR11); MMR (HR12)
Blood transfusion between 1975-1985	HIV screen (HR3)
Institutionalized persons; health care/lab workers	Hepatitis A vaccine (HR5); PPD (HR6); influenza vaccine (HR9)
Family hx of skin cancer; nevi; fair skin, eyes, hair	Avoid excess/midday sun, use protective clothing* (HR13)
Prior pregnancy with neural tube defect	Folic acid 4.0 mg (HR14)
Inadequate water fluoridation	Daily fluoride supplement (HR15)

[1]Periodic BP for persons aged ≥21 yr. [2]If sexually active at present or in the past: q ≤3 yr. If sexual history is unreliable, begin Pap tests at age 18 yr. [3]If sexually active. [4]Serologic testing, documented vaccination history, and routine vaccination against rubella (preferably with MMR) are equally acceptable alternatives. [5]If not previously immunized: current visit, 1 and 6 mo later. [6]If no previous second dose of MMR. [7]If susceptible to chickenpox.
*The ability of clinician counseling to influence this behavior is unproven.

HR1 = Persons who exchange sex for money or drugs, and their sex partners; persons with other STDs (including HIV); and sexual contacts of persons with active syphilis. Clinicians should also consider local epidemiology (see Ch. 26).

HR2 = Females who have two or more sex partners in the last year; a sex partner with multiple sexual contacts; exchanged sex for money or drugs; or a history of repeated episodes of gonorrhea. Clinicians should also consider local epidemiology (see Ch. 27).

HR3 = Males who had sex with males after 1975; past or present injection drug use; persons who exchange sex for money or drugs, and their sex partners; injection drug-using, bisexual, or HIV-positive sex partner currently or in the past; blood transfusion during 1978-1985; persons seeking treatment for STDs. Clinicians should also consider local epidemiology (see Ch. 28).

HR4 = Sexually active females with multiple risk factors including history of prior STD; new or multiple sex partners; age under 25; nonuse or inconsistent use of barrier contraceptives; cervical ectopy. Clinicians should consider local epidemiology of the disease in identifying other high-risk groups (see Ch. 29).

HR5 = Persons living in, traveling to, or working in areas where the disease is endemic and where periodic outbreaks occur (e.g., countries with high or intermediate endemicity; certain Alaska Native, Pacific Island, Native American, and religious communities); men who have sex with men; injection or street drug users. Vaccine may be considered for institutionalized persons and workers in these institutions, military personnel, and day-care, hospital, and laboratory workers. Clinicians should also consider local epidemiology (see Ch. 66, 67).

HR6 = HIV positive, close contacts of persons with known or suspected TB, health care workers, persons with medical risk factors associated with TB, immigrants from countries with high TB prevalence, medically underserved low-income populations (including homeless), alcoholics, injection drug users, and residents of long-term facilities (see Ch. 25). See Ch. 25 for indications for BCG vaccine.

HR7 = Persons who continue to inject drugs (see Ch. 53).

HR8 = Immunocompetent persons with certain medical conditions, including chronic cardiac or pulmonary disease, diabetes mellitus, and anatomic asplenia. Immunocompetent persons who live in high-risk environments or social settings (e.g., certain Native American and Alaska Native populations) (see Ch. 66).

HR9 = Annual vaccination of residents of chronic care facilities; persons with chronic cardiopulmonary disorders, metabolic diseases (including diabetes mellitus), hemoglobinopathies, immunosuppression, or renal dysfunction; and health care providers for high-risk patients (see Ch. 66). See Ch. 66 for indications for amantadine/rimantadine prophylaxis.

HR10 = Adolescents and young adults in settings where such individuals congregate (e.g., high schools and colleges), if they have not previously received a second dose (see Ch. 65, 66).

HR11 = Healthy persons aged ≥13 yr without a history of chickenpox or previous immunization. Consider serologic testing for presumed susceptible persons aged ≥13 yr (see Ch. 65, 66).

HR12 = Persons born after 1956 who lack evidence of immunity to measles or mumps (e.g., documented receipt of live vaccine on or after the first birthday, laboratory evidence of immunity, or a history of physician-diagnosed measles or mumps) (see Ch. 65, 66).

HR13 = Persons with a family or personal history of skin cancer, a large number of moles, atypical moles, poor tanning ability, or light skin, hair, and eye color (see Ch. 12).

HR14 = Women with prior pregnancy affected by neural tube defect who are planning pregnancy (see Ch. 42).

HR15 = Persons aged <17 yr living in areas with inadequate water fluoridation (<0.6 ppm) (see Ch. 61).

CLINICAL PREVENTIVE SERVICES   The periodic health examination   847

TABLE 5-3 Ages 25-64 Years

Interventions considered and recommended for the Periodic Health Examination	Leading causes of death
	  Malignant neoplasms
	  Heart diseases
	  Motor vehicle and other unintentional injuries
	  Human immunodeficiency virus (HIV) infection
	  Suicide and homicide

Interventions for the General Population

Screening

Blood pressure [Ch. 3]

Height and weight [Ch. 21]

Total blood cholesterol (men age 35-64, women age 45-64) [Ch. 2]

Papanicolaou (Pap) test (women)[1] [Ch. 9]

Fecal occult blood test[2] and/or sigmoidoscopy ($\geq$50 yr) [Ch. 8]

Mammogram $\pm$ clinical breast exam[3] (women 50-69 yr) [Ch. 7]

Assess for problem drinking [Ch. 52]

Rubella serology or vaccination hx[4] (women of childbearing age) [Ch. 32]

Counseling

Substance use
Tobacco cessation [Ch. 54]
Avoid alcohol/drug use while driving, swimming, boating, etc.* [Ch. 57, 58]

Diet and exercise
Limit fat and cholesterol; maintain caloric balance; emphasize grains, fruits, vegetables [Ch. 56]
Adequate calcium intake (women) [Ch. 56]

Regular physical activity* [Ch. 55]

Injury prevention [Ch. 57, 58]
Lap/shoulder belts
Motorcycle/bicycle/ATV helmets*
Smoke detector*
Safe storage/removal of firearms* [Ch. 50, 59]

Sexual behavior [Ch. 62, 63]
STD prevention: avoid high-risk behavior*; condoms/female barrier with spermicide*
Unintended pregnancy: contraception

Dental health [Ch. 61]
Regular visits to dental care provider*
Floss, brush with fluoride toothpaste daily*

Immunizations [Ch. 32, 66]
Tetanus-diphtheria (Td) boosters
Rubella[4] (women of childbearing age)

Chemoprophylaxis
Multivitamin with folic acid (women planning or capable of pregnancy) [Ch. 42]
Discuss hormone prophylaxis (peri- and postmenopausal women) [Ch. 68]

Interventions for High-Risk Populations

Population	Potential Interventions (See detailed high-risk definitions)
High-risk sexual behavior	RPR/VDRL (HR1); screen for gonorrhea (female) (HR2), HIV (HR3), chlamydia (female) (HR4); hepatitis B vaccine (HR5); hepatitis A vaccine (HR6)
Injection or street drug use	RPR/VDRL (HR1); HIV screen (HR3); hepatitis B vaccine (HR5); hepatitis A vaccine (HR6); PPD (HR7); advice to reduce infection risk (HR8)
Low income; TB contacts; immigrants; alcoholics	PPD (HR7)
Native Americans/Alaska Natives	Hepatitis A vaccine (HR6); PPD (HR7); pneumococcal vaccine (HR9)
Travelers to developing countries	Hepatitis B vaccine (HR5); hepatitis A vaccine (HR6)
Certain chronic medical conditions	PPD (HR7); pneumococcal vaccine (HR9); influenza vaccine (HR10)
Blood product recipients	HIV screen (HR3); hepatitis B vaccine (HR5)
Susceptible to measles, mumps, or varicella	MMR (HR11); varicella vaccine (HR12)
Institutionalized persons	Hepatitis A vaccine (HR6); PPD (HR7); pneumococcal vaccine (HR9); influenza vaccine (HR10)
Health care/lab workers	Hepatitis B vaccine (HR5); hepatitis A vaccine (HR6); PPD (HR7); influenza vaccine (HR10)
Family hx of skin cancer; fair skin, eyes, hair	Avoid excess/midday sun, use protective clothing* (HR13)
Previous pregnancy with neural tube defect	Folic acid 4.0 mg (HR14)

[1]Women who are or have been sexually active and who have a cervix: q $\leq$3 yr. [2]Annually. [3]Mammogram q1-2 yr, or mammogram q1-2 yr with annual clinical breast examination. [4]Serologic testing, documented vaccination history, and routine vaccination (preferably with MMR) are equally acceptable.
*The ability of clinician counseling to influence this behavior is unproven.

HR1 = Persons who exchange sex for money or drugs, and their sex partners; persons with other STDs (including HIV); and sexual contacts of persons with active syphilis. Clinicians should also consider local epidemiology (see Ch. 26).

HR2 = Women who exchange sex for money or drugs, or who have had repeated episodes of gonorrhea. Clinicians should also consider local epidemiology (see Ch. 27).

HR3 = Men who had sex with men after 1975; past or present injection drug use; persons who exchange sex for money or drugs, and their sex partners; injection drug-using, bisexual, or HIV-positive sex partner currently or in the past; blood transfusion during 1978-1985; persons seeking treatment for STDs. Clinicians should also consider local epidemiology (see Ch. 28).

HR4 = Sexually active women with multiple risk factors including history of STD; new or multiple sex partners; nonuse or inconsistent use of barrier contraceptives; cervical ectopy. Clinicians should also consider local epidemiology (see Ch. 29).

HR5 = Blood product recipients (including hemodialysis patients), persons with frequent occupational exposure to blood or blood products, men who have sex with men, injection drug users and their sex partners, persons with multiple recent sex partners, persons with other STDs (including HIV), travelers to countries with endemic hepatitis B (see Ch. 66).

HR6 = Persons living in, traveling to, or working in areas where the disease is endemic and where periodic outbreaks occur (e.g., countries with high or intermediate endemicity; certain Alaska Native, Pacific Island, Native American, and religious communities); men who have sex with men; injection or street drug users. Consider for institutionalized persons and workers in these institutions, military personnel, and day-care, hospital, and laboratory workers. Clinicians should also consider local epidemiology (see Ch. 66, 67).

HR7 = HIV positive, close contacts of persons with known or suspected TB, health care workers, persons with medical risk factors associated with TB, immigrants from countries with high TB prevalence, medically underserved low-income populations (including homeless), alcoholics, injection drug users, and residents of long-term care facilities (see Ch. 25). See Ch. 25 for indications for BCG vaccine.

HR8 = Persons who continue to inject drugs (see Ch. 53).

HR9 = Immunocompetent institutionalized persons aged ≥50 yr and immunocompetent persons with certain medical conditions, including chronic cardiac or pulmonary disease, diabetes mellitus, and anatomic asplenia. Immunocompetent persons who live in high-risk environments or social settings (e.g., certain Native American and Alaska Native populations) (see Ch. 66).

HR10 = Annual vaccination of residents of chronic care facilities; persons with chronic cardiopulmonary disorders, metabolic diseases (including diabetes mellitus), hemoglobinopathies, immunosuppression or renal dysfunction; and health care providers for high-risk patients (Ch. 66). See Ch. 66 for indications for amantadine/rimantadine prophylaxis.

HR11 = Persons born after 1956 who lack evidence of immunity to measles or mumps (e.g., documented receipt of live vaccine on or after the first birthday, laboratory evidence of immunity, or a history of physician-diagnosed measles or mumps) (see Ch. 66).

HR12 = Healthy adults without a history of chickenpox or previous immunization. Consider serologic testing for presumed susceptible adults (see Ch. 65, 66).

HR13 = Persons with a family or personal history of skin cancer, a large number of moles, atypical moles, poor tanning ability, or light skin, hair, and eye color (see Ch. 12).

HR14 = Women with previous pregnancy affected by neural tube who are planning pregnancy (see Ch. 42).

CLINICAL PREVENTIVE SERVICES | The periodic health examination 849

TABLE 5-4 Age 65 and Older

Interventions considered and recommended for the Periodic Health Examination	Leading causes of death Heart diseases Malignant neoplasms (lung, colorectal, breast) Cerebrovascular disease Chronic obstructive pulmonary disease Pneumonia and influenza

Interventions for the General Population

Screening

Blood pressure *[Ch. 3]*

Height and weight *[Ch. 21]*

Fecal occult blood test[1] and/or sigmoidoscopy *[Ch. 8]*

Mammogram ± clinical breast exam[2] (women ≤69 yr) *[Ch. 7]*

Papanicolaou (Pap) test (women)[3] *[Ch. 9]*

Vision screening *[Ch. 33]*

Assess for hearing impairment *[Ch. 35]*

Assess for problem drinking *[Ch. 52]*

Counseling

Substance use

Tobacco cessation *[Ch. 54]*

Avoid alcohol/drug use while driving, swimming, boating, etc.* *[Ch. 57, 58]*

Diet and exercise

Limit fat and cholesterol; maintain caloric balance; emphasize grains, fruits, vegetables *[Ch. 56]*

Adequate calcium intake (women) *[Ch. 56]*

Regular physical activity* *[Ch. 55, 58]*

Injury prevention *[Ch. 57, 58]*

Lap/shoulder belts

Motorcycle and bicycle helmets*

Fall prevention*

Safe storage/removal of firearms* *[Ch. 50, 59]*

Smoke detector*

Set hot water heater to <120°-130°F

CPR training for household members

Dental health *[Ch. 61]*

Regular visits to dental care provider*

Floss, brush with fluoride toothpaste daily*

Sexual behavior

STD prevention: avoid high-risk sexual behavior*; use condoms *[Ch. 62]*

Immunizations [Ch. 66]

Pneumococcal vaccine

Influenza[1]

Tetanus-diphtheria (Td) boosters

Chemoprophylaxis

Discuss hormone prophylaxis (peri- and postmenopausal women) *[Ch. 68]*

Interventions for High-Risk Populations

Population	*Potential Interventions (See detailed high-risk definitions)*
Institutionalized persons	PPD (HR1); hepatitis A vaccine (HR2); amantadine/rimantadine (HR4)
Chronic medical conditions; TB contacts; low income; immigrants; alcoholics	PPD (HR1)
Persons ≥75 yr, or ≥70 yr with risk factors for falls	Fall prevention intervention (HR5)
Cardiovascular disease risk factors	Consider cholesterol screening (HR6)
Family hx of skin cancer; nevi; fair skin, eyes, hair	Avoid excess/midday sun, use protective clothing* (HR7)
Native Americans/Alaska Natives	PPD (HR1); hepatitis A vaccine (HR2)
Travelers to developing countries	Hepatitis A vaccine (HR2); hepatitis B vaccine (HR8)
Blood product recipients	HIV screen (HR3); hepatitis B vaccine (HR8)
High-risk sexual behavior	Hepatitis A vaccine (HR2); HIV screen (HR3); hepatitis B vaccine (HR8); RPR/VDRL (HR9)
Injection or street drug use	PPD (HR1); hepatitis A vaccine (HR2); HIV screen (HR3); hepatitis B vaccine (HR8); RPR/VDRL (HR9); advice to reduce infection risk (HR10)
Health care/lab workers	PPD (HR1); hepatitis A vaccine (HR2); amantadine/rimantadine (HR4); hepatitis B vaccine (HR8)
Persons susceptible to varicella	Varicella vaccine (HR11)

[1]Annually. [2]Mammogram q1-2 yr, or mammogram q1-2 yr with annual clinical breast exam. [3]All women who are or have been sexually active and who have a cervix. Consider discontinuation of testing after age 65 yr if previous regular screening with consistently normal results.
*The ability of clinician counseling to influence this behavior is unproven.

HR1 = HIV positive, close contacts of persons with known or suspected TB, health care workers, persons with medical risk factors associated with TB, immigrants from countries with high TB prevalence, medically underserved low-income populations (including homeless), alcoholics, injection drug users, and residents of long-term care facilities (see Ch. 25). See Ch. 25 for indications for BCG vaccine.

HR2 = Persons living in, traveling to, or working in areas where the disease is endemic and where periodic outbreaks occur (e.g., countries with high or intermediate endemicity; certain Alaska Native, Pacific Island, Native American, and religious communities); men who have sex with men; injection or street drug users. Consider for institutionalized persons and workers in these institutions, and day-care, hospital, and laboratory workers. Clinicians should also consider local epidemiology (see Ch. 66, 67).

HR3 = Men who had sex with men after 1975; past or present injection drug use; persons who exchange sex for money or drugs, and their sex partners; injection drug-using, bisexual, or HIV-positive sex partner currently or in the past; blood transfusion during 1978-1985; persons seeking treatment for STDs. Clinicians should also consider local epidemiology (see Ch. 28).

HR4 = Consider for persons who have not received influenza vaccine or are vaccinated late; when the vaccine may be ineffective due to major antigenic changes in the virus; for unvaccinated persons who provide home care for high-risk persons; to supplement protection provided by vaccine in persons who are expected to have a poor antibody response; and for high-risk persons in whom the vaccine is contraindicated (see Ch. 66).

HR5 = Persons aged 75 years and older; or aged 70-74 with one or more additional risk factors including use of certain psychoactive and cardiac medications (e.g., benzodiazepines, antihypertensives); use of ≥4 prescription medications; impaired cognition, strength, balance, or gait. Intensive individualized home-based multifactorial fall prevention intervention is recommended in settings where adequate resources are available to deliver such services (see Ch. 58).

HR6 = Although evidence is insufficient to recommend routine screening in elderly persons, clinicians should consider cholesterol screening on a case-by-case basis for persons ages 65-75 with additional risk factors (e.g., smoking, diabetes, or hypertension) (see Ch. 2).

HR7 = Persons with a family or personal history of skin cancer, a large number of moles, atypical moles, poor tanning ability, or light skin, hair, and eye color (see Ch. 12).

HR8 = Blood product recipients (including hemodialysis patients), persons with frequent occupational exposure to blood or blood products, men who have sex with men, injection drug users and their sex partners, persons with multiple recent sex partners, persons with other STDs (including HIV), travelers to countries with endemic hepatitis B (see Ch. 66).

HR9 = Persons who exchange sex for money or drugs and their sex partners; persons with other STDs (including HIV); and sexual contacts of persons with active syphilis. Clinicians should also consider local epidemiology (see Ch. 26).

HR10 = Persons who continue to inject drugs (see Ch. 53).

HR11 = Healthy adults without a history of chickenpox or previous immunization. Consider serologic testing for presumed susceptible adults (see Ch. 65, 66).

TABLE 5-5 Pregnant Women**

Interventions considered and recommended for the Periodic Health Examination

Interventions for the General Population

Screening

First visit

Blood pressure *[Ch. 3, 37]*

Hemoglobin/hematocrit *[Ch. 22]*

Hepatitis B surface antigen (HBsAg) *[Ch. 24]*

RPR/VDRL *[Ch. 26]*

Chlamydia screen (<25 yr) *[Ch. 29]*

Rubella serology or vaccination history *[Ch. 32]*

D(Rh) typing, antibody screen *[Ch. 38]*

Offer CVS (<13 wk)[1] or amniocentesis (15-18 wk)[1] (age ≥35 yr) *[Ch. 41]*

Offer hemoglobinopathy screening *[Ch. 43]*

Assess for problem or risk drinking *[Ch. 52]*

Offer HIV screening[2] *[Ch. 28]*

Follow-up visits

Blood pressure *[Ch. 3, 37]*

Urine culture (12-16 wk) *[Ch. 31]*

Offer amniocentesis (15-18 wk)[1] (age ≥35 yr) *[Ch. 41]*

Offer multiple marker testing[1] (15-18 wk) *[Ch. 41]*

Offer serum α-fetoprotein[1] (16-18 wk) *[Ch. 42]*

Counseling

Tobacco cessation; effects of passive smoking *[Ch. 54]*

Alcohol/other drug use *[Ch. 52, 53]*

Nutrition, including adequate calcium intake *[Ch. 56]*

Encourage breast-feeding *[Ch. 22, 56]*

Lap/shoulder belts *[Ch. 57]*

Infant safety car seats *[Ch. 57]*

STD prevention: avoid high-risk sexual behavior*; use condoms* *[Ch. 62]*

Chemoprophylaxis

Multivitamin with folic acid[3] *[Ch. 42]*

Interventions for High-Risk Populations

Population	Potential Interventions (See detailed high-risk definitions)
High-risk sexual behavior	Screen for chlamydia (1st visit) (HR1), gonorrhea (1st visit) (HR2), HIV (1st visit) (HR3); HBsAg (3rd trimester) (HR4); RPR/VDRL (3rd trimester) (HR5)
Blood transfusion 1978-1985	HIV screen (1st visit) (HR3)
Injection drug use	HIV screen (HR3); HBsAg (3rd trimester) (HR4); advice to reduce infection risk (HR6)
Unsensitized D-negative women	D(Rh) antibody testing (24-28 wk) (HR7)
Risk factors for Down syndrome	Offer CVS[1] (1st trimester), amniocentesis[1] (15-18 wk) (HR8)
Prior pregnancy with neural tube defect	Offer amniocentesis[1] (15-18 wk), folic acid 4.0 mg[3] (HR9)

[1]Women with access to counseling and follow-up services, reliable standardized laboratories, skilled high-resolution ultrasound, and, for those receiving serum marker testing, amniocentesis capabilities. [2]Universal screening is recommended for areas (states, counties, or cities) with an increased prevalence of HIV infection among pregnant women. In low-prevalence areas, the choice between universal and tangled screening may depend on other considerations (see Ch. 28). [3]Beginning at least 1 mo before conception and continuing through the first trimester.
*The ability of clinician counseling to influence this behavior is unproven.
**See Tables 5-2 and 5-3 for other preventive services recommended for women of this age group.

HR1 = Women with history of STD or new or multiple sex partners. Clinicians should also consider local epidemiology. Chlamydia screen should be repeated in 3rd trimester if at continued risk (see Ch. 29).

HR2 = Women under age 25 with two or more sex partners in the last year, or whose sex partner has multiple sexual contacts; women who exchange sex for money or drugs; and women with a history of repeated episodes of gonorrhea. Clinicians should also consider local epidemiology. Gonorrhea screen should be repeated in the third trimester if at continued risk (see Ch. 27).

HR3 = In areas where universal screening is not performed due to low prevalence of HIV infection, pregnant women with the following individual risk factors should be screened: past or present injection drug use; women who exchange sex for money or drugs; injection drug-using, bisexual, or HIV-positive sex partner currently or in the past; blood transfusion during 1978-1985; persons seeking treatment for STDs (see Ch. 28).

HR4 = Women who are initially HBsAg negative who are at high risk due to injection drug use, suspected exposure to hepatitis B during pregnancy, multiple sex partners (see Ch. 24).

HR5 = Women who exchange sex for money or drugs, women with other STDs (including HIV), and sexual contacts of persons with active syphilis. Clinicians should also consider local epidemiology (see Ch. 26).

HR6 = Women who continue to inject drugs (see Ch. 53).

HR7 = Unsensitized D-negative women (see Ch. 38).

HR8 = Prior pregnancy affected by Down syndrome, advanced maternal age (≥35 yr), known carriage of chromosome rearrangement (see Ch. 41).

HR9 = Women with previous pregnancy affected by neural tube defect (see Ch. 42).

Part B
SCREENING
Cardiovascular Diseases

1. Screening for Asymptomatic Coronary Artery Disease

RECOMMENDATION

There is insufficient evidence to recommend for or against screening middle-aged and older men and women for asymptomatic coronary artery disease, using resting electrocardiography (ECG), ambulatory ECG, or exercise ECG. Recommendations against routine screening can be made on other grounds for individuals who are not at high risk of developing clinical heart disease (see Clinical Intervention). Routine screening is not recommended as part of the periodic health visit or preparticipation sports examination for children, adolescents, or young adults. Clinicians should emphasize proven measures for the primary prevention of coronary disease (see Clinical Intervention).

CLINICAL INTERVENTION

There is insufficient evidence to recommend for or against screening middle-aged and older men and women for asymptomatic coronary artery disease with resting electrocardiography (ECG), ambulatory ECG, or exercise ECG ("C" recommendation). Recommendations against routine screening may be made on other grounds for persons who are not at high risk of developing symptomatic CAD; these grounds include the limited sensitivity and low predictive value of an abnormal resting ECG in asymptomatic persons and the high costs of screening and follow-up. Screening selected high-risk asymptomatic persons (e.g., those with multiple cardiac risk factors) is indicated only where results will influence treatment decisions (e.g., use of aspirin or lipid-lowering drugs in asymptomatic persons). Screening individuals in certain occupations (pilots, truck drivers, etc.) can be recommended on other grounds, including possible benefits to public safety. The choice of specific screening test for asymptomatic CAD is left to clinical discretion: exercise ECG is more accurate than resting ECG but is considerably more expensive.

Routine ECG screening as part of the periodic health visit or preparticipation sports physical is not recommended for asymptomatic children, adolescents, and young adults ("D" recommendation).

Clinicians should emphasize proven measures for the primary prevention of coronary disease in all patients (see Chapter 3, Screening for Hypertension; Chapter 2, Screening for High Blood Cholesterol; Chapter 54, Counseling to Prevent Tobacco Use; Chapter 55, Counseling to Promote Physical Activity; and Chapter 56, Counseling to Promote a Healthy Diet).

2. Screening for High Blood Cholesterol and Other Lipid Abnormalities

RECOMMENDATION

Periodic screening for high blood cholesterol is recommended for all men ages 35-65 and women ages 45-65. There is insufficient evidence to recommend for or against routine screening of asymptomatic persons over age 65, but recommendations to screen healthy men and women ages 65-75 may be made on other grounds (see Clinical Intervention). There is also insufficient evidence to recommend for or against routine screening in children, adolescents, or young adults. Recommendations for screening adolescents and young adults with risk factors for coronary disease, and against routine screening in children, may be made on other grounds (see Clinical Intervention). There is insufficient evidence to recommend for or against routine screening for other lipid abnormalities. All patients should receive periodic screening and counseling regarding other measures to reduce their risk of coronary disease (see Chapter 3, Screening for Hypertension; Chapter 54, Counseling to Prevent Tobacco Use; Chapter 55, Counseling to Promote Physical Activity; and Chapter 56, Counseling to Promote a Healthy Diet).

CLINICAL INTERVENTION

Periodic screening for high blood cholesterol, using specimens obtained from fasting or nonfasting individuals, is recommended for all men ages 35-65 and women ages 45-65 ("B" recommendation). There is insufficient evidence to recommend for or against routine screening in asymptomatic persons after age 65, but screening may be considered on a case-by-case basis ("C" recommendation). Older persons with major CHD risk factors (smoking, hypertension, diabetes) who are otherwise healthy may be more likely to benefit from screening, based on their high risk of CHD and the proven benefits of lowering cholesterol in older persons with symptomatic CHD. Cholesterol levels are not a reliable predictor of risk after age 75, however. There is insufficient evidence to recommend routine screening in children, adolescents, or young adults ("C" recommendation). For adolescents and young adults who have a family history of very high cholesterol, premature CHD in a first-degree relative (before age 50 in men or age 60 in women), or major risk factors for CHD screening may be recommended on other grounds: the greater absolute risk attributable to high cholesterol in such persons and the potential long-term benefits of early life-style interventions in young persons with high cholesterol. Recommendations against routine screening in children may be made on other grounds, including the costs and inconvenience of screening and follow-up, greater potential for adverse effects of treatment, and the uncertain long-term benefits of small reductions in childhood cholesterol levels.

The appropriate interval for periodic screening is not known. Periodic screening is most important when cholesterol levels are increasing (e.g., middle-aged men, perimenopausal women, and persons who have gained weight). An interval of 5 years has been recommended by experts, but longer intervals may be reasonable in low-risk subjects (including those with previously desirable cholesterol levels).

There is insufficient evidence to recommend for or against routine measurement of HDL-C or triglycerides at initial screening ("C" recommendation). For high-risk persons (middle-aged persons with high cholesterol or multiple nonlipid risk factors for CHD), measurement of HDL-C or lipoprotein analysis can be recommended to help identify individuals at highest risk of CHD, in whom individual diet or drug therapy may be indicated.

Decisions about interventions for high cholesterol should be based on at least two measures of cholesterol and assessment of the absolute risk of CHD in each individual. This assessment should take into account the age of the patient (higher risk in men over 45 and women over 55), results of lipoprotein analysis (or ratio of total cholesterol to HDL-C), and the presence and severity of other risk factors for CHD (see above). More specific algorithms for risk assessment have been published. Initial therapy for patients with elevated cholesterol is counseling to reduce consumption of fat (especially saturated fat) and promote weight loss in overweight persons. A two-step dietary program effective in lowering serum cholesterol has been described in detail elsewhere. Benefits of drug therapy are likely to justify costs and potential risks only in persons at high risk of CHD (e.g., middle-aged men and postmenopausal women with very high cholesterol or multiple risk factors). The risks and benefits of drug therapy in asymptomatic persons over 65 have not yet been determined. In postmenopausal women with high cholesterol, estrogen therapy can lower LDL-C and raise HDL-C and is associated with lower risk of CHD in epidemiologic studies (see Chapter 68). Patients should receive information on the potential benefits, costs, and risks of long-term therapy before beginning treatment on cholesterol-lowering drugs.

All adults, adolescents, and children over age 2 years, including those with normal cholesterol levels, should receive periodic counseling regarding dietary intake of fat and saturated fat (see Chapter 56) and other measures to reduce the risk of coronary disease (see Chapters 3, 54, and 55).

3. Screening for Hypertension

RECOMMENDATION

Screening for hypertension is recommended for all children and adults (see Clinical Intervention).

CLINICAL INTERVENTION

Periodic screening for hypertension is recommended for all persons ≥21 years of age ("A" recommendation). The optimal interval for blood pressure screening has not been determined and is left to clinical discretion. Current expert opinion is that adults who are believed to be normotensive should receive blood pressure measurements at least once every 2 years if their last diastolic and systolic blood pressure readings were below 85 and 140 mm Hg, respectively, and annually if the last diastolic blood pressure was 85-89 mm Hg. Sphygmomanometry should be performed in accordance with recommended technique. Hypertension should not be diagnosed on the basis of a single measurement; elevated readings should be confirmed on more than one reading at each of three separate visits. In adults, current blood pressure criteria for the diagnosis of hypertension are an average diastolic pressure of 90 mm Hg or greater and/or an average systolic pressure of 140 mm Hg or greater. Once confirmed, patients should receive appropriate counseling regarding physical activity (Chapter 55), weight reduction and dietary sodium intake (Chapter 56), and alcohol consumption (Chapter 52). Evidence should also be sought for other cardiovascular risk factors, such as elevated serum cholesterol (Chapter 2) and smoking (Chapter 54), and appropriate intervention should be offered when indicated. The decision to begin drug therapy may include consideration of the level of blood pressure elevation, age, and the presence of other cardiovascular disease risk factors (e.g., tobacco use, hypercholesterolemia), concomitant disease (e.g., diabetes, obesity, peripheral vascular disease), or target-organ damage (e.g., left ventricular hypertrophy, elevated creatinine). Antihypertensive drugs should be prescribed in accordance with recent guidelines and with attention to current techniques for improving compliance.

Measurement of blood pressure during office visits is also recommended for children and adolescents ("B" recommendation). This recommendation is based on the proven benefits from the early detection of treatable causes of secondary hypertension;

there is insufficient evidence to recommend for or against routine periodic blood pressure measurement to detect essential (primary) hypertension in this age group. Sphygmomanometry should be performed in accordance with the recommended technique for children, and hypertension should only be diagnosed on the basis of readings at each of three separate visits. In children, criteria defining hypertension vary with age. Age-, sex-, and height-specific blood pressure nomograms for United States children and adolescents have been published.

Routine counseling to promote physical activity (Chapter 55) and a healthy diet (Chapter 56) for the primary prevention of hypertension is recommended for all children and adults.

4. Screening for Asymptomatic Carotid Artery Stenosis

RECOMMENDATION

There is insufficient evidence to recommend for or against screening asymptomatic persons for carotid artery stenosis using the physical examination or carotid ultrasound. For selected high-risk patients, a recommendation to discuss the potential benefits of screening and carotid endarterectomy may be made on other grounds (see Clinical Intervention). All persons should be screened for hypertension (see Chapter 3), and clinicians should provide counseling about smoking cessation (see Chapter 54).

CLINICAL INTERVENTION

There is insufficient evidence to recommend for or against screening asymptomatic persons for carotid artery stenosis, using physical examination or carotid ultrasound ("C" recommendation). A recommendation may be made on other grounds to discuss the potential benefits of screening with high-risk patients (e.g., persons over age 60 at high risk for vascular disease), provided that high-quality vascular surgical care is available (surgical morbidity and mortality less than 3%). These other grounds include the increased prevalence of significant carotid disease, and the possible long-term benefit of endarterectomy in patients with asymptomatic stenosis greater than 60% when performed by qualified surgeons. Patients should be screened and counseled about other risk factors for cerebrovascular disease as discussed in other chapters (see Chapters 3 and 54).

5. Screening for Peripheral Arterial Disease

RECOMMENDATION

Routine screening for peripheral arterial disease in asymptomatic persons is not recommended. Clinicians should be alert to symptoms of peripheral arterial disease in persons at increased risk (see Clinical Intervention) and should evaluate patients who have clinical evidence of vascular disease.

CLINICAL INTERVENTION

Routine screening for peripheral arterial disease in asymptomatic persons is not recommended ("D" recommendation). Clinicians should screen for hypertension (see Chapter 3) and hypercholesterolemia (Chapter 2), and they should provide appropriate counseling regarding the use of tobacco products (Chapter 54), physical activity (Chapter 55), and nutritional risk factors for atherosclerotic disease (Chapter 56). Clinicians should be alert to symptoms of PAD in persons at increased risk (persons over age 50, smokers, diabetics) and evaluate patients who have clinical evidence of vascular disease.

6. Screening for Abdominal Aortic Aneurysm

RECOMMENDATION

There is insufficient evidence to recommend for or against routine screening of asymptomatic adults for abdominal aortic aneurysm with abdominal palpation or ultrasound.

CLINICAL INTERVENTION

There is insufficient evidence to recommend for or against routine screening for abdominal aortic aneurysms with abdominal palpation or ultrasound ("C" recommendation). Recommendations against routine ultrasound screening in the general population may be made on other grounds, such as the low prevalence of clinically significant AAA and the high cost of screening. Although direct evidence that screening for AAA reduces mortality or morbidity is not available in any population, clinicians may decide to screen selected high-risk patients, owing to the significant burden of disease and the availability of effective surgical treatment for large aneurysms. Men over age 60 who have other risk factors (e.g., vascular disease, family history of AAA, hypertension, or smoking) are at highest risk for AAA and death caused by ruptured aneurysms. Screening is not indicated for patients who are not appropriate candidates for major abdominal surgery (e.g., those with severe cardiac or pulmonary disease). If screening is performed, it is not certain whether ultrasound or abdominal palpation is the preferred test. Abdominal palpation is less expensive but also less sensitive than ultrasound. Cost-effectiveness analysis suggests that repeat examination of individuals with a previous normal ultrasound is not indicated.

Neoplastic Diseases

7. Screening for Breast Cancer

RECOMMENDATION

Routine screening for breast cancer every 1-2 years, with mammography alone or mammography and annual clinical breast examination (CBE), is recommended for women aged 50-69. There is insufficient evidence to recommend for or against routine mammography or CBE for women aged 40-49 or aged 70 and older, although recommendations for high-risk women aged 40-49 and healthy women aged ≥70 may be made on other grounds (see Clinical Intervention). There is insufficient evidence to recommend for or against the use of screening CBE alone or the teaching of breast self-examination.

CLINICAL INTERVENTION

Screening for breast cancer every 1-2 years, with mammography alone or mammography and annual clinical breast examination (CBE), is recommended for women aged 50-69 ("A" recommendation). Clinicians should refer patients to mammographers who use low-dose equipment and adhere to high standards of quality control. Such standards have recently been established by the Mammography Quality Standards Act, a federal law mandating that all mammography sites in the United States be accredited through a process approved by the Department of Health and Human Services. There is insufficient evidence to recommend annual CBE alone for women aged 50-69 ("C" recommendation). For women aged 40-49, there is conflicting evidence of fair to good quality regarding clinical benefit from mammography with or without CBE, and insufficient evidence regarding benefit from CBE alone; therefore, recommendations for or against routine mammography or CBE cannot be made based on the current evidence ("C" recommendation). There is no evidence specifically evaluating mammography or CBE in high-risk women under age 50; recommendations for screening such women may be made on other grounds, including patient preference, high burden of suffering, and the higher PPV of screening, which would lead to fewer false positives than are likely to occur from screening women of average risk in this age group. There is limited and conflicting evidence regarding clinical benefit of mammography or CBE for women aged 70-74 and no evidence regarding benefit for women over age 75; however, recommendations for screening women aged 70 and over who have a reasonable life expectancy may be made based on other grounds, such as the high burden of suffering in this age group and the lack of evidence of differences in mammogram test characteristics in older women versus those aged 50-69 ("C" recommendation). There is insufficient evidence to recommend for or against teaching BSE in the periodic health examination ("C" recommendation).

8. Screening for Colorectal Cancer

RECOMMENDATION

Screening for colorectal cancer is recommended for all persons aged 50 and older with annual fecal occult blood testing (FOBT), or sigmoidoscopy (periodicity unspecified), or both (see Clinical Intervention). There is insufficient evidence to determine which of these screening methods is preferable or whether the combination of FOBT and sigmoidoscopy produces greater benefits than does either test alone. There is also insufficient evidence to recommend for or against routine screening with digital rectal examination, barium enema, or colonoscopy, although recommendations against such screening in average-risk persons may be made on other grounds (see Clinical Intervention). Persons with a family history of hereditary syndromes associated with a high risk of colon cancer should be referred for diagnosis and management (see Clinical Intervention).

CLINICAL INTERVENTION

Screening for colorectal cancer is recommended for all persons aged 50 or over ("B" recommendation). Effective methods include FOBT and sigmoidoscopy. There is insufficient evidence to determine which of these screening methods is preferable or whether the combination of FOBT and sigmoidoscopy produces greater benefits than either test alone. Although there is good evidence to support FOBT on an annual basis, there is insufficient evidence to recommend a periodicity for sigmoidoscopy screening. A frequency of every 3-5 years has been recommended by other groups on the basis of expert opinion, and a well-designed case-control study suggests that protection remains unchanged for at least 10 years after rigid sigmoidoscopy. Current evidence suggests that at least some of the benefits of FOBT in reducing colorectal cancer mortality may be achieved through colonoscopic evaluation of abnormal results. Widespread FOBT or sigmoidoscopy screening is therefore likely to generate substantial direct and indirect costs. Appropriate public policy may require consideration of factors other than the scientific evidence of clinical benefit. The appropriate age to discontinue screening has not been determined.

Patients who are offered these tests should receive information about the potential benefits and harms of the procedures, the probability of false-positive results, and the nature of the tests that will be performed if an abnormality is detected. FOBT screening should adhere to current guidelines for dietary restrictions, sample collection, and storage. Although slide rehydration increases the sensitivity of

FOBT, it also decreases specificity, and there is insufficient evidence to determine whether rehydration results in better outcomes than screening with non-rehydrated slides. Sigmoidoscopy should be performed by a trained examiner. The instrument should be selected on the basis of examiner expertise and patient comfort. Longer (e.g., 60-cm instrument) flexible sigmoidoscopes have greater sensitivity and are more comfortable than shorter, rigid sigmoidoscopes.

There is insufficient evidence to recommend for or against routine screening with digital rectal examination, barium enema, or colonoscopy ("C" recommendation). Recommendations against using these tests for screening average-risk persons may be made on other grounds (e.g., availability of alternate tests of proven effectiveness, inaccuracy of digital rectal examination, costs and risks of colonoscopy).

In persons with a single first-degree relative with colon cancer, it is not clear that the modest increase in the absolute risk of cancer justifies routine use of colonoscopy over other screening methods. The increased risk of developing cancer at younger ages may justify beginning screening before age 50 in persons with a positive family history, however, especially when affected relatives developed colorectal cancer at younger ages. Direct evidence of the benefit of screening in younger persons is not available for any group. For persons with a family history of hereditary syndromes associated with a very high risk of colon cancer (i.e., familial polyposis or HNPCC), as well as those previously diagnosed with ulcerative colitis, high-risk adenomatous polyps, or colon cancer, regular endoscopic screening is part of routine diagnosis and management; referral to specialists is appropriate for these high-risk patients.

9. Screening for Cervical Cancer

RECOMMENDATION

Routine screening for cervical cancer with Papanicolaou (Pap) testing is recommended for all women who are or have been sexually active and who have a cervix. Pap smears should begin with the onset of sexual activity and should be repeated at least every 3 years (see Clinical Intervention). There is insufficient evidence to recommend for or against an upper age limit for Pap testing, but recommendations can be made on other grounds to discontinue regular testing after age 65 in women who have had regular previous screenings in which the smears have been consistently normal. There is insufficient evidence to recommend for or against routine screening with cervicography or colposcopy, or for screening for human papilloma virus infection, although recommendations against such screening can be made on other grounds (see Clinical Intervention).

CLINICAL INTERVENTION

Regular Pap tests are recommended for all women who are or have been sexually active and who have a cervix ("A" recommendation). Testing should begin at the age when the woman first engages in sexual intercourse. Adolescents whose sexual history is thought to be unreliable should be presumed to be sexually active at age 18. There is little evidence that annual screening achieves better outcomes than screening every 3 years. Pap tests should be performed at least every 3 years ("B" recommendation). The interval for each patient should be recommended by the physician based on risk factors (e.g., early onset of sexual intercourse, a history of multiple sex partners, low socioeconomic status). (Women infected with human immunodeficiency virus require more frequent screening according to established guidelines.) There is insufficient evidence to recommend for or against an upper age limit for Pap testing, but recommendations can be made on other grounds to discontinue regular testing after age 65 in women who have had regular previous screening in which the smears have been consistently normal ("C" recommendation). Women who have undergone a hysterectomy in which the cervix was removed do not require Pap testing, unless the hysterectomy was performed because of cervical cancer or its precursors. Patients at increased risk because of unprotected sexual activity or multiple sex partners should receive appropriate counseling about sexual practices (see Chapter 62).

The use of an endocervical brush increases the likelihood of obtaining endocervical cells, but there is conflicting evidence that sampling these cells improves sensitivity in detecting cervical neoplasia. Physicians should submit specimens to laboratories that have adequate quality control measures to ensure optimal accuracy in the interpretation and reporting of results. Thorough follow-up of test results should also be ensured, including repeat testing and referral for colposcopy as indicated. Physicians should consider providing patients with a pamphlet or other written information about the meaning of abnormal smears to help ensure follow-up and minimize anxiety over false-positive results.

There is insufficient evidence to recommend for or against routine cervicography or colposcopy screening for cervical cancer in asymptomatic women, nor is there evidence to support routine screening for HPV infection ("C" recommendation). Recommendations against such screening can be made on other grounds, including poor specificity and costs.

10. Screening for Prostate Cancer

RECOMMENDATION

Routine screening for prostate cancer with digital rectal examinations, serum tumor markers (e.g., prostate-specific antigen), or transrectal ultrasound is not recommended.

CLINICAL INTERVENTION

Routine screening for prostate cancer with DRE, serum tumor markers (e.g., PSA), or TRUS is not recommended ("D" recommendation). Patients who request screening should be given objective information about the potential benefits and harms of early detection and treatment. Patient education materials that review this information are available. If screening is to be performed, the best-evaluated approach is to screen with DRE and PSA and to limit screening to men with a life expectancy greater than 10 years. There is currently insufficient evidence to determine the need and optimal interval for repeat screening or whether PSA thresholds must be adjusted for density, velocity, or age.

11. Screening for Lung Cancer

RECOMMENDATION

Routine screening for lung cancer with chest radiography or sputum cytology in asymptomatic persons is not recommended. All patients should be counseled against tobacco use (see Chapter 54).

CLINICAL INTERVENTION

Routine screening of asymptomatic persons for lung cancer with chest radiography or sputum cytology is not recommended ("D" recommendation). All patients should be counseled against tobacco use (see Chapter 54).

12. Screening for Skin Cancer—Including Counseling to Prevent Skin Cancer

RECOMMENDATION

There is insufficient evidence to recommend for or against either routine screening for skin cancer by primary care providers or counseling patients to perform periodic skin self-examinations. A recommendation to consider referring patients at substantially increased risk of malignant melanoma (MM) to skin cancer specialists for evaluation and surveillance may be made on other grounds (see Clinical Intervention). Counseling patients at increased risk of skin cancer to avoid excess sun exposure is recommended, based on the proven efficacy of risk reduction, although the effectiveness of counseling has not been well established. There is insufficient evidence to recommend for or against sunscreen use for the primary prevention of skin cancer.

CLINICAL INTERVENTION

There is insufficient evidence to recommend for or against routine screening for skin cancer by primary care providers using total-body skin examination ("C" recommendation). Clinicians should remain alert for skin lesions with malignant features (i.e., asymmetry, border irregularity, color variability, diameter >6 mm, or rapidly changing lesions) when examining patients for other reasons, particularly patients with established risk factors. Such risk factors include clinical evidence of melanocytic precursor or marker lesions (e.g., atypical moles, certain congenital moles), large numbers of common moles, immunosuppression, a family or personal history of skin cancer, substantial cumulative lifetime sun exposure, intermittent intense sun exposure or severe sunburns in childhood, freckles, poor tanning ability, and light skin, hair, and eye color. Appropriate biopsy specimens should be taken of suspicious lesions.

Persons with melanocytic precursor or marker lesions (e.g., atypical moles [also called dysplastic nevi], certain congenital nevi, familial atypical mole and melanoma syndrome) are at substantially increased risk for MM. A recommendation to consider referring these patients to skin cancer specialists for evaluation and surveillance may be made on the grounds of patient preference or anxiety owing to high burden of suffering, the greater accuracy of TSE when performed by such specialists, and the relatively limited adverse effects from TSE and follow-up skin biopsy, although evidence of benefit from such referral is lacking.

There is also insufficient evidence to recommend for or against counseling patients to perform periodic self-examination of the skin ("C" recommendation). Clinicians may wish to educate patients with established risk factors for skin cancer (see above) concerning signs and symptoms suggesting cutaneous malignancy and the possible benefits of periodic self-examination.

Avoidance of sun exposure, especially between the hours of 10:00 AM and 3:00 PM, and the use of protective clothing such as shirts and hats when outdoors are recommended for adults and children at increased risk of skin cancer (see above) ("B" recommendation). Counseling such patients to avoid excess sun exposure and use protective clothing is recommended, based on the established efficacy of risk reduction from sun avoidance, the potential for large health benefits, low cost, and low risk of adverse effects from such counseling, even though the effectiveness of such counseling is less well established ("C" recommendation).

There is insufficient evidence to recommend for or against counseling patients to use sunscreens to prevent skin cancer ("C" recommendation). The routine use of sunscreens that block both UVA and UVB radiation may be appropriate for persons who have previously had solar keratosis and who cannot avoid sun exposure, in order to prevent additional solar keratoses, which have a small malignant potential.

13. Screening for Testicular Cancer

RECOMMENDATION

There is insufficient evidence to recommend for or against routine screening of asymptomatic men in the general population for testicular cancer by physician examination or patient self-examination. Recommendations to discuss screening options with selected high-risk patients may be made on other grounds (see Clinical Intervention).

CLINICAL INTERVENTION

There is insufficient evidence to recommend for or against routine screening of asymptomatic men for testicular cancer by physician examination or patient self-examination ("C" recommendation). Patients with an increased risk of testicular cancer (those with a history of cryptorchidism or atrophic testes) should be informed of their increased risk of testicular cancer and counseled about the options for screening. Such patients may then elect to be screened or to perform testicular self-examination. Adolescent and young adult males should be advised to seek prompt medical attention if they notice a scrotal abnormality.

14. Screening for Ovarian Cancer

RECOMMENDATION

Routine screening for ovarian cancer by ultrasound, the measurement of serum tumor markers, or pelvic examination is not recommended. There is insufficient evidence to recommend for or against the screening of asymptomatic women at increased risk of developing ovarian cancer.

CLINICAL INTERVENTION

Screening asymptomatic women for ovarian cancer with ultrasound, the measurement of serum tumor markers, or pelvic examination is not recommended ("D" recommendation). There is insufficient evidence to recommend for or against the screening of asymptomatic women at increased risk of ovarian cancer ("C" recommendation).

15. Screening for Pancreatic Cancer

RECOMMENDATION

Routine screening for pancreatic cancer in asymptomatic persons, using abdominal palpation, ultrasonography, or serologic markers, is not recommended.

CLINICAL INTERVENTION

Routine screening for pancreatic cancer in asymptomatic persons, using abdominal palpation, ultrasonography, or serologic markers, is not recommended ("D" recommendation). All patients should be counseled regarding use of tobacco products (see Chapter 54). Counseling to reduce fat and cholesterol intake and to increase intake of fruits and vegetables may be recommended on other grounds (see Chapter 56).

16. Screening for Oral Cancer

RECOMMENDATION

There is insufficient evidence to recommend for or against routine screening of asymptomatic persons for oral cancer by primary care clinicians. All patients should be counseled to discontinue the use of all forms of tobacco (see Chapter 54) and to limit consumption of alcohol (see Chapter 52). Clinicians should remain alert to signs and symptoms of oral cancer and premalignancy in persons who use tobacco or regularly use alcohol.

CLINICAL INTERVENTION

There is insufficient evidence to recommend for or against routine screening of asymptomatic persons for oral cancer by primary care clinicians ("C" recommendation). Although direct evidence of a benefit is lacking, clinicians may wish to include an examination for cancerous and precancerous lesions of the oral cavity in the periodic health examination of persons who chew or smoke tobacco (or did so previously), older persons who drink regularly, and anyone with suspicious symptoms or lesions detected through self-examination. All patients, especially those at increased risk, should be advised to receive a complete dental examination on a regular basis (see Chapter 61). All adolescent and adult patients should be asked to describe their use of tobacco (Chapter 54) and alcohol (Chapter 52). Appropriate counseling should be offered to those persons who smoke cigarettes, pipes, or cigars, those who use chewing tobacco or snuff, and those who have evidence of alcohol abuse. Persons with increased exposure to sunlight should be advised to take protective measures when outdoors to protect their lips and skin from the harmful effects of ultraviolet rays (see Chapter 12).

17. Screening for Bladder Cancer

RECOMMENDATION

Routine screening for bladder cancer with urine dipstick, microscopic urinalysis, or urine cytology is not recommended in asymptomatic persons. All patients who smoke tobacco should be routinely counseled to quit smoking (see Chapter 54).

CLINICAL INTERVENTION

Routine screening for bladder cancer with microscopic urinalysis, urine dipstick, or urine cytology is not recommended in asymptomatic persons ("D" recommendation). Persons working in high-risk professions (e.g., dye or rubber industries) may be eligible for screening at the work site, although the benefit of this has not been determined. Men and women who smoke cigarettes should be advised that smoking significantly increases the risk for bladder cancer, and all smokers should be routinely counseled to quit smoking (see Chapter 54).

18. Screening for Thyroid Cancer

RECOMMENDATION

Routine screening for thyroid cancer using neck palpation or ultrasonography is not recommended for asymptomatic children or adults. There is insufficient evidence to recommend for or against screening persons with a history of external head and neck irradiation in infancy or childhood, but recommendations for such screening may be made on other grounds (see Clinical Intervention).

CLINICAL INTERVENTION

Screening asymptomatic adults or children for thyroid cancer using either neck palpation or ultrasonography is not recommended ("D" recommendation). Although there is insufficient evidence to recommend for or against such screening in asymptomatic persons with a history of external upper body (primarily head and neck) irradiation in infancy or childhood, recommendations for periodic palpation of the thyroid gland in such persons may be made on other grounds, including patient preference or anxiety regarding their increased risk of cancer ("C" recommendation).

Metabolic, Nutritional, and Environmental Disorders

19. Screening for Diabetes Mellitus

RECOMMENDATION

There is insufficient evidence to recommend for or against routine screening for diabetes mellitus in asymptomatic adults. There is also insufficient evidence to recommend for or against universal screening for gestational diabetes mellitus (GDM). Although the benefit of early detection has not been established for any group, clinicians may decide to screen selected persons at high risk of diabetes on other grounds (see Clinical Intervention). Screening with immune markers to identify persons at risk for developing insulin-dependent diabetes is not recommended in the general population.

CLINICAL INTERVENTION

There is insufficient evidence to recommend for or against routine screening for NIDDM in nonpregnant adults ("C" recommendation). Although evidence of a benefit of early detection is not available for any group, clinicians may decide to screen selected persons at high risk of NIDDM on other grounds, including the increased predictive value of a positive test in individuals with risk factors and the potential (although unproven) benefits of reducing asymptomatic hyperglycemia through diet and exercise. Individuals at higher risk of diabetes include obese men and women over 40, patients with a strong family history of diabetes, and members of certain ethnic groups (Native Americans, Hispanics, African Americans). In persons without risk factors, screening for asymptomatic disease is much less likely to be of benefit, owing to the low burden of disease and the poor predictive value of screening tests in low-risk persons. Measurement of fasting plasma glucose is recommended by experts as the screening test of choice; the frequency of screening is left to clinical discretion.

There is also insufficient evidence to recommend for or against routine screening for GDM ("C" recommendation). Although a clear benefit of screening on perinatal morbidity has not been demonstrated for any group, clinicians may decide to screen high-risk pregnant women on other grounds, including the higher burden of disease, and the potential clinical benefits from reducing macrosomia caused by GDM. Risk factors for GDM include obesity, older maternal age, a family history of diabetes, and a history of macrosomia, fetal malformation, or fetal death. The 1-hour 50 g glucose challenge test, with confirmation of abnormal results with a 3-hour 100 g oral glucose tolerance test, is the screening test recommended by expert panels in the United States.

Screening with immune markers to identify asymptomatic individuals at risk for developing IDDM is not recommended in the general population ("D" recommendation).

20. Screening for Thyroid Disease

RECOMMENDATION

Routine screening for thyroid disease with thyroid function tests is not recommended for asymptomatic children or adults. There is insufficient evidence to recommend for or against screening for thyroid disease with thyroid function tests in high-risk patients, but recommendations may be made on other grounds (see Clinical Intervention). Clinicians should remain alert to subtle symptoms and signs of thyroid dysfunction when examining such patients. Screening for congenital hypothyroidism is discussed in Chapter 45.

CLINICAL INTERVENTION

Routine screening for thyroid disease with thyroid function tests is not recommended for asymptomatic children or adults ("D" recommendation). This recommendation does not mean that clinicians should not monitor thyroid function in patients with a previous history of thyroid disease. There is insufficient evidence to recommend for or against screening for thyroid disease with thyroid function tests in high-risk patients, including elderly persons, postpartum women, and persons with Down syndrome, but recommendations may be made on other grounds, such as the higher prevalence of disease and the increased likelihood that symptoms of thyroid disease will be overlooked in these patients ("C" recommendation).

Clinicians should remain alert for subtle or nonspecific symptoms of thyroid dysfunction when examining such patients and maintain a low threshold for diagnostic evaluation of thyroid function. Examples of such symptoms include easy fatigability, weight gain, dry skin or hair, cold intolerance, difficulty concentrating, depression, nervousness, and palpitations. If screening is performed, the preferred test is measurement of thyroid-stimulating hormone (TSH) using a sensitive immunometric or similar assay, because of its superior sensitivity and specificity. Screening for congenital hypothyroidism is discussed in Chapter 45.

21. Screening for Obesity

RECOMMENDATION

Periodic height and weight measurements are recommended for all patients (see Clinical Intervention).

CLINICAL INTERVENTION

Periodic height and weight measurements are recommended for all patients ("B" recommendation). In adults, BMI (body weight in kilograms divided by the square of height in meters) or a table of suggested weights may be used, along with the assessment of other factors such as medical conditions or WHR, as a basis for further evaluation, intervention, or referral to specialists. In adolescents, a BMI exceeding the 85th percentile for age and gender may be used as a basis for further assessment, treatment, or referral. The height (or length if appropriate) and weight of infants and children may be plotted on a growth chart or compared to tables of average weight for height, age, and gender to determine the need for further evaluation, treatment, or referral. The optimal frequency for measuring height and weight in the clinical setting has not been evaluated and is a matter of clinical discretion. There is insufficient evidence to recommend for or against determination of the WHR as a routine screening test for obesity ("C" recommendation).

All patients should receive appropriate counseling to promote physical activity (see Chapter 55) and a healthy diet (see Chapter 56).

22. Screening for Iron Deficiency Anemia—Including Iron Prophylaxis

RECOMMENDATION

Screening for iron deficiency anemia using hemoglobin or hematocrit is recommended for pregnant women and for high-risk infants. There is insufficient evidence to recommend for or against routine screening for iron deficiency anemia in other asymptomatic persons, but recommendations against screening may be made on other grounds (see Clinical Intervention). Encouraging parents to breast-feed their infants and to include iron-enriched foods in the diet of infants and young children is recommended (see also Chapter 56). There is currently insufficient evidence to recommend for or against the routine use of iron supplements for healthy infants or pregnant women.

CLINICAL INTERVENTION

A hemoglobin analysis or hematocrit is recommended for pregnant women at their first prenatal visit ("B" recommendation). There is insufficient evidence to recommend for or against repeated prenatal testing for anemia in asymptomatic pregnant women lacking evidence of medical or obstetric complications ("C" recommendation). Screening for anemia with hemoglobin or hematocrit in high-risk infants, preferably at 6-12 months of age, is also recommended ("B" recommendation). Examples of high-risk infants include infants living in poverty, blacks, Native Americans and Alaska Natives, immigrants from developing countries, preterm and low birth weight infants, and infants whose principal dietary intake is unfortified cow's milk. Although capillary blood specimens are easier to obtain in infants, a venous blood count provides more accurate and reliable data. Serum ferritin testing may be useful as an additional screening test in selected high-risk infants. There is currently insufficient evidence to recommend for or against periodic screening for high-risk infants not found to be anemic at initial screening ("C" recommendation). There is also insufficient evidence to recommend for or against routine testing for anemia in other asymptomatic persons, but recommendations against such screening may be made on the grounds of low prevalence, cost, and potential adverse effects of iron therapy ("C" recommendation).

Guidelines for normal hemoglobin ranges for infants and pregnant women have been published. Appropriate hematologic studies and nutrition counseling should be provided for patients found to have anemia. Compared to other diagnostic tests, serum ferritin has the best sensitivity and specificity for detecting iron deficiency in patients found to be anemic. Screening for hemoglobinopathies is discussed in Chapter 43.

Encouraging mothers to breast-feed their infants and advising parents to include iron-enriched foods in the diet of infants and young children is recommended for the primary prevention of iron deficiency anemia ("B" recommendation). There is also good evidence to recommend breast-feeding based on proven benefits unrelated to iron deficiency (see Chapter 56). Pregnant women should receive specific nutritional guidance to enhance fetal and maternal health (see Chapter 56). There is currently insufficient evidence to recommend for or against the routine use of iron supplements for healthy infants or pregnant women who are not anemic ("C" recommendation).

23. Screening for Elevated Lead Levels in Childhood and Pregnancy

RECOMMENDATION

Screening for elevated lead levels by measuring blood lead at least once at age 12 months is recommended for all children at increased risk of lead exposure. All children with identifiable risk factors should be screened, as should all children living in communities in which the prevalence of blood lead levels requiring individual intervention, including residential lead hazard control or chelation therapy, is high or is undefined (see Clinical Intervention). Evidence is currently insufficient to recommend an exact community prevalence below which targeted screening can be substituted for universal screening. Clinicians can seek guidance from their local or state health department. There is insufficient evidence to recommend for or against routine screening for lead exposure in asymptomatic pregnant women, but recommendations against such screening may be made on other grounds. There is also insufficient evidence to recommend for or against counseling families about the primary prevention of lead exposure, but recommendations may be made on other grounds. Recommendations regarding the primary prevention of lead poisoning by population-wide environmental interventions are beyond the scope of this chapter.

CLINICAL INTERVENTION

Screening for elevated lead levels by measuring blood lead at least once at age 12 months is recommended for all children at increased risk of lead exposure ("B" recommendation). All children with identifiable risk factors should be screened, as should children living in communities in which the prevalence of blood lead levels requiring individual intervention, including chelation therapy or residential lead hazard control, is high or is undefined. If capillary blood is used, elevated lead levels should be confirmed by measurement of venous blood lead. The optimal frequency of screening for lead exposure in children, or for repeated testing of children previously found to have elevated blood lead levels, is unknown and is left to clinical discretion; consideration should be given to the degree of elevation, the interventions provided, and the natural history of lead exposure, including the typical peak in lead levels at 18-24 months of age.

In communities where the prevalence of blood lead levels requiring individual intervention is low, a strategy of targeted screening, possibly using locale-specific questionnaires of known and acceptable sensitivity and specificity, can be used to identify high-risk children who should have blood lead testing. Examples of individual risk factors include: (1) living in or frequently visiting an older home (built before 1950) with dilapidated paint or with recent or ongoing renovation or remodeling, (2) having close contact with a person who has an elevated lead level, (3) living near lead industry or heavy traffic, (4) living with someone whose job or hobby involves lead exposure, (5) using lead-based pottery, or (6) taking traditional ethnic remedies that contain lead. There is currently insufficient evidence to recommend an exact population prevalence below which targeted screening can be substituted for universal screening. The results of cost-benefit analyses, available resources and public health priorities are among the determinants of the prevalence below which targeted screening is recommended for a community. Clinicians can seek guidance from their local or state health department.

There is insufficient evidence to recommend for or against routine screening for lead exposure in asymptomatic pregnant women ("C" recommendation). Recommendations against such screening may be made on the grounds of limited and conflicting evidence regarding the current burden of suffering, high costs, and the potential for adverse effects from intervention.

There is insufficient evidence to recommend for or against trying to prevent lead exposure by counseling families to control lead dust by repeated household cleaning, or to optimize caloric, iron, and calcium intake specifically to reduce lead absorption ("C" recommendation). For high-risk individuals or those living in high-prevalence communities, such recommendations may be made on other grounds, including minimal risk of adverse effects from the cleaning or the dietary advice, and the additional, unrelated benefits from optimizing nutrition (see Chapter 22, Screening for Iron Deficiency Anemia, and Chapter 56, Counseling to Promote a Healthy Diet).

Recommendations regarding community- or population-based interventions for the primary prevention of lead poisoning, assessment of community lead contamination, or the setting of community priorities for lead hazard reduction, are beyond the scope of this document.

Infectious Diseases

24. Screening for Hepatitis B Virus Infection

RECOMMENDATION

Screening with hepatitis B surface antigen (HB$_s$Ag) to detect active (acute or chronic) hepatitis B virus (HBV) infection is recommended for all pregnant women at their first prenatal visit. The test may be repeated in the third trimester in women who are initially HB$_s$Ag-negative and who are at increased risk of HBV infection during pregnancy. Routine screening for HBV infection in the general population is not recommended. Certain persons at high risk may be screened to assess eligibility for vaccination (see Clinical Intervention).

CLINICAL INTERVENTION

Screening with hepatitis B surface antigen (HB$_s$Ag) to detect active (acute or chronic) HBV infection is recommended for all pregnant women at their first prenatal visit ("A" recommendation). The test may be repeated in the third trimester if the woman is initially HB$_s$Ag-negative and engages in high-risk behavior such as injection drug use or if exposure to hepatitis B virus during pregnancy is suspected. Infants born to HB$_s$Ag-positive mothers should receive hepatitis B immune globulin (HBIG) (0.5 ml IM) within 12 hours of birth. Hepatitis B vaccine, at the appropriate dosage, should be administered intramuscularly concurrently with HBIG (at a different injection site). The second and third doses of vaccine should be given 1 and 6 months after the first dose. Depending on the brand of vaccine utilized, the dosage of vaccine given to an infant born to a HB$_s$Ag-positive mother may differ from that given routinely to infants born to HB$_s$Ag-negative mothers. For neonates born to women whose HB$_s$Ag status is unknown at the time of delivery, administering vaccine within 12 hours of birth, using the same dosage as that for infants whose mothers are HB$_s$Ag-positive, is recommended. Maternal testing for HB$_s$Ag should be performed at the same time. If the mother is found to be HB$_s$Ag-positive, HBIG should be administered to her infant as soon as possible and within 7 days of birth. Contacts (sexual or household) of HB$_s$Ag-positive pregnant women should be either vaccinated or tested to determine susceptibility to HBV and vaccinated if susceptible (see also Chapter 67). The decision to do prevaccination testing may be made based on cost-effectiveness analysis.

Routine screening for HBV infection in the general population is not recommended ("D" recommendation). There is insufficient evidence to recommend for or against routinely screening asymptomatic high-risk individuals for HBV infection in order to determine eligibility for vaccination, but recommendations for screening may be made based on cost-effectiveness analyses ("C" recommendation). Such analyses suggest that screening is usually cost-effective in groups with an HBV marker prevalence >20%. See Chapters 65 and 66 for further recommendations on hepatitis B vaccination and Chapter 67 for information about passive and active immunization of persons with possible exposure to HBV-infected individuals or blood products. Counseling on preventive behaviors to reduce the risk of HBV infection and transmission is discussed in Chapter 62.

25. Screening for Tuberculous Infection—Including Bacille Calmette-Guérin Immunization

RECOMMENDATION

Screening for tuberculous infection with tuberculin skin testing is recommended for asymptomatic high-risk persons. Bacille Calmette-Guérin (BCG) vaccination should be considered only for selected high-risk individuals (see Clinical Intervention).

CLINICAL INTERVENTION

Screening for tuberculous infection by tuberculin skin testing is recommended for all persons at increased risk of developing tuberculosis (TB) ("A" recommendation). Asymptomatic persons at increased risk include persons infected with HIV, close contacts of persons with known or suspected TB (including health care workers), persons with medical risk factors associated with TB, immigrants from countries with high TB prevalence (e.g., most countries in Africa, Asia, and Latin America), medically underserved low-income populations (including high-risk racial or ethnic minority populations), alcoholics, injection drug users, and residents of long-term care facilities (e.g., correctional institutions, mental institutions, nursing homes). The Mantoux test involves the intradermal injection of 5 U of tuberculin PPD and the subsequent examination of the injection site 48-72 hours later. Current minimum criteria for a positive skin test, based on observational data and expert opinion, are 15-mm diameter for low-risk individuals, 10-mm diameter for high-risk individuals (e.g., immigrants, medically underserved low-income populations, injection drug users, residents of long-term care facilities, persons with conditions that increase TB risk, infants, and children less than 4 years of age), and 5-mm diameter for persons at very high risk (e.g., persons infected with HIV, persons with abnormal chest radiographs, recent contacts of infected persons). Prior BCG vaccination is not currently considered a valid basis for dismissing positive results. Persons with negative reactions who are at increased risk of anergy (e.g., HIV-infected individuals) can be skin-tested for anergy, but this procedure is now considered optional in current CDC guidelines. Treatment decisions in HIV-infected anergic patients should be made on an individual basis. The frequency of tuberculin skin testing is a matter of clinical discretion.

Persons with a positive PPD test should receive a chest x-ray and clinical evaluation for TB. Those lacking evidence of active infection should receive INH prophylaxis if they meet criteria defined in recent guidelines. Briefly, these criteria recommend INH prophylaxis in persons under 35 years of age who are from high-prevalence countries; medically underserved, low-income, high-prevalence populations; or long-term care facilities. It is also recommended in persons of any age with HIV infection or increased risk of HIV infection, other medical conditions that increase the risk of TB, or close contact with patients with newly diagnosed TB or skin test conversion. Screening for HIV infection may be indicated in recent converters (see Chapter 28). Patients with possible exposure to drug-resistant TB should be treated according to current recommendations for multidrug preventive therapy. Directly observed therapy—observation of the patient by a health care worker as the medication is taken—may be indicated in patients who are unlikely to be compliant.

BCG vaccination against TB should be considered only for tuberculin-negative infants and children who cannot be placed on INH and who have continuous exposure to persons with active disease, those with continuous exposure to patients with organisms resistant to INH or rifampin, and those belonging to groups with a rate of new infections greater than 1% per year and for whom the usual surveillance and treatment programs may not be operationally feasible ("B" recommendation). These groups may also include persons with limited access to or willingness to use health care services.

26. Screening for Syphilis

RECOMMENDATION

Routine serologic screening for syphilis is recommended for all pregnant women and for persons at increased risk of infection (see Clinical Intervention). See Chapter 62 for recommendations on counseling to prevent sexually transmitted diseases.

CLINICAL INTERVENTION

Routine serologic testing for syphilis is recommended for all pregnant women and for persons at increased risk for infection, including commercial sex workers, persons who exchange sex for money or drugs, persons with other STDs (including HIV), and sexual contacts of persons with active syphilis ("A" recommendation). The local incidence of syphilis in the community and the number of sex partners reported by an individual should also be considered in identifying persons at high risk of infection. The optimal frequency for such testing has not been determined and is left to clinical discretion.

All pregnant women should be tested at their first prenatal visit. For women at high risk of acquiring syphilis during pregnancy (e.g., women in the high-risk groups listed above), repeat serologic testing is recommended in the third trimester and at delivery. Follow-up serologic tests should be obtained to document decline in titers after treatment. They should be performed using the same test initially used to document infection (e.g., VDRL or RPR) to ensure comparability.

See Chapter 62 for recommendations on counseling to prevent sexually transmitted diseases.

27. Screening for Gonorrhea—Including Ocular Prophylaxis in Newborns

RECOMMENDATION

Routine screening for *Neisseria gonorrhoeae* is recommended for asymptomatic women at high risk of infection (see Clinical Intervention). All high-risk women should be screened during pregnancy. There is insufficient evidence to recommend for or against screening all pregnant women or screening asymptomatic men. Recommendations to screen selected high-risk young men may be made on other grounds (see Clinical Intervention). Routine screening is not recommended for the general adult population. Ocular antibiotic prophylaxis of all newborn infants is recommended to prevent gonococcal ophthalmia neonatorum.

CLINICAL INTERVENTION

Routine screening for gonorrhea is recommended for asymptomatic women at high risk of infection ("B" recommendation). High-risk groups include commercial sex workers (prostitutes), persons with a history of repeated episodes of gonorrhea, and young women (under age 25) with two or more sex partners in the last year. Actual risk, however, will depend on the local epidemiology of disease. Clinicians may wish to consult local health authorities for guidance in identifying high-risk populations in their community. In communities with high prevalence of gonorrhea, broader screening of sexually active young women may be warranted. Clinicians should remain alert for findings suggestive of cervical infection (e.g., mucopurulent discharge, cervical erythema or friability) during routine pelvic examinations.

Screening is recommended at the first prenatal visit for pregnant women who fall into one of the high-risk categories ("B" recommendation). An additional test in the third trimester is recommended for those at continued risk of acquiring gonorrhea. There is insufficient evidence to recommend for or against universal screening of pregnant women ("C" recommendation). Erythromycin 0.5% ophthalmic ointment, tetracycline 1% ophthalmic ointment, or 1% silver nitrate solution should be applied topically to the eyes of all newborns as soon as possible after birth and no later than 1 hour after birth ("A" recommendation).

There is insufficient evidence to recommend for or against screening high-risk men for gonorrhea ("C" recommendation). In selected clinical settings where asymptomatic infection is highly prevalent in men (e.g., adolescent clinics serving high-risk populations), screening sexually active young men may be recommended on other grounds, including the potential benefits of early treatment for preventing transmission to uninfected sex partners. Screening men with urine leukocyte esterase (LE) dipstick is convenient and inexpensive, but requires confirmation of positive results. Routine screening of men or women is not recommended in the general population of low-risk adults ("D" recommendation). The optimal frequency of screening has not been determined and is left to clinical discretion.

Culture of endocervical specimens is the preferred method for screening asymptomatic women. When EIA or DNA probe tests are used for initial screening, verification of positive results may be necessary, depending on the underlying risk in the patient and potential adverse consequences of a false-positive result. Treatment should employ regimens effective against penicillin- and tetracycline-resistant organisms and should include treatment for coinfection with chlamydia and treatment of sex partners. All sexually active individuals should be counseled about effective means of preventing STDs (see Chapter 62). Clinicians should follow local gonorrhea disease-reporting requirements.

28. Screening for Human Immunodeficiency Virus Infection

RECOMMENDATION

Clinicians should assess risk factors for human immunodeficiency virus (HIV) infection by obtaining a careful sexual history and inquiring about injection drug use in all patients. Periodic screening for infection with HIV is recommended for all persons at increased risk of infection (see Clinical Intervention). Screening is recommended for all pregnant women at risk for HIV infection, including all women who live in states, counties, or cities with an increased prevalence of HIV infection. There is insufficient evidence to recommend for or against universal screening among low-risk pregnant women in low-prevalence areas, but recommendations to counsel and offer screening to all pregnant women may be made on other grounds (see Clinical Intervention). Screening infants born to high-risk mothers is recommended if the mother's antibody status is not known. All patients should be counseled about effective means to avoid HIV infection (see Chapter 62).

CLINICAL INTERVENTION

Clinicians should assess risk factors for HIV infection in all patients by obtaining a careful sexual history and inquiring about drug use. Counseling and testing for HIV should be offered to all persons at increased risk for infection: those seeking treatment for sexually transmitted diseases; men who have had sex with men after 1975; past or present injection drug users; persons who exchange sex for money or drugs, and their sex partners; women and men whose past or present sex partners were HIV-infected, bisexual, or injection drug users; and persons with a history of transfusion between 1978 and 1985 ("A" recommendation).

Pregnant women in these categories, and those from communities (e.g., states, counties, or cities) where the prevalence of seropositive newborns is increased (e.g., $\geq 0.1\%$) should be counseled about the potential benefit to their infant of early intervention for HIV and offered testing as soon as the woman is known to be pregnant ("A" recommendation). Repeat testing may be indicated in the third trimester of pregnancy for women at high risk of recent exposure to HIV. There is insufficient evidence to recommend for or against universal prenatal screening for HIV in low-prevalence communities ("C" recommendation). A policy of offering screening to all pregnant women may be recommended on other grounds, including patient preference, easier implementation, and increased sensitivity compared to screening based on community prevalence and reported risk factors. Careful quality control measures and patient counseling are essential to limit the potential adverse effects from indeterminate and false-positive test results during pregnancy. Testing infants born to high-risk mothers, with permission of mother, is recommended when antibody status of mother is unknown ("B" recommendation).

There is insufficient evidence to recommend for or against routine HIV screening in persons without identified risk factors ("C" recommendation). Recommendations to screen sexually active young women and men in high-risk communities can be made on other grounds, based on the increasing burden of heterosexual transmission and the insensitivity of screening based on self-reported risk factors. Similarly, routine HIV screening may be reasonable in groups such as prisoners, runaway youth, or homeless persons, where the prevalence of high-risk behaviors and HIV is generally high. The definition of high-risk community is imprecise. Clinicians should consult local public health authorities for advice and information on the epidemiology of HIV infection in their communities. More selective screening may be appropriate in low-risk areas. Testing should not be performed in the absence of informed consent and pretest counseling, which should include the purpose of the test, the meaning of reactive and nonreactive results, measures to protect confidentiality, and the need to notify persons at risk. Patients who wish to be tested anonymously should be advised of appropriate testing facilities.

A positive test requires at least two reactive EIAs and confirmation with WB or IFA, performed by experienced laboratories that receive regular external proficiency testing. A separate sample should be submitted for persons found to be seropositive for the first time, to rule out possible error in specimen handling. Patients with indeterminate WB results should be evaluated individually to determine whether findings are likely to represent recent seroconversion. Repeat testing should be performed 3-6 months after indeterminate test results, or sooner if recent seroconversion is suspected. A stable indeterminate WB pattern is not indicative of HIV infection.

Seropositive patients should receive information regarding the meaning of the results, the distinctions between casual nonsexual contact and proven modes of HIV transmission, measures to reduce risk to themselves and others, symptoms requiring medical attention, and available community resources for HIV-infected persons. Clinicians should explore potential barriers to changing high-risk behavior in seropositive and seronegative individuals. Guidelines for HIV counseling have been published by the PHS. Seropositive persons should be evaluated for severity of immune dysfunction and screened for other infectious diseases such as tuberculosis (see Chapter 25). Guidelines for the management of early HIV infection and prevention of opportunistic infections have been published by the Agency for Health Care Policy and Research and the CDC. Arrangements for follow-up medical care are especially important for drug users, who may require assistance in gaining entrance to a drug treatment program (see Chapter 53). All seropositive individuals should be encouraged to notify sex partners, persons with whom injection needles have been shared, and others at risk of exposure. Seropositive cases should be reported confidentially or anonymously to public health officials in accordance with local regulations.

Persons with nonreactive test results should be informed that the risk of acquiring subsequent HIV infection can be prevented by maintaining monogamous sexual relationships with uninfected partners. Other measures to reduce the risk of infection (consistent use of condoms, etc.) should be specifically mentioned (see Chapter 62). The frequency of repeat testing of seronegative individuals is a matter of clinical discretion. Periodic testing is most important in patients who continue high-risk activities. In patients with recent high-risk exposure (e.g., sex with HIV-infected partner), repeat testing at 3 months may be useful to rule out initial false-negative tests.

29. Screening for Chlamydial Infection—Including Ocular Prophylaxis in Newborns

RECOMMENDATION

Routine screening for *Chlamydia trachomatis* infection is recommended for all sexually active female adolescents, high-risk pregnant women, and other asymptomatic women at high risk of infection (see Clinical Intervention). There is insufficient evidence to recommend for or against routine screening in asymptomatic men. Recommendations to screen selected high-risk male adolescents may be made on other grounds (see Clinical Intervention). Routine screening is not recommended for the general adult population. See Chapter 27 for recommendations regarding ocular prophylaxis to prevent ophthalmia neonatorum.

CLINICAL INTERVENTION

Routine screening for asymptomatic infection with *Chlamydia trachomatis* during pelvic examination is recommended for all sexually active female adolescents and for other women at high risk for chlamydial infection ("B" recommendation). Patient characteristics associated with a higher prevalence of infection include: history of prior STD, new or multiple sex partners, age under 25, inconsistent use of barrier contraceptives, cervical ectopy, and being unmarried. Actual risk will depend on number of risk factors and local epidemiology of chlamydial infection. Clinicians may wish to consult local public health authorities for guidance in identifying high-risk populations within their community. Algorithms to identify high-risk women have been published. In clinical settings where the prevalence of infection is known to be high (e.g., some urban family planning clinics), routine screening of all women is appropriate. Clinicians should remain alert for findings suggestive of chlamydial infection (e.g., mucopurulent discharge, cervical erythema, or cervical friability) during pelvic examination of asymptomatic women.

Pregnant women at high risk of infection (including age under 25) should be tested for chlamydia ("B" recommendation). The optimal timing of screening in pregnancy is uncertain. There is insufficient evidence to recommend for or against screening all women during pregnancy ("C" recommendation).

There is insufficient evidence to recommend for or against routine screening in high-risk men ("C" recommendation). In clinical settings where asymptomatic infection is highly prevalent in men (e.g., urban adolescent clinics), screening sexually active young men may be recommended on other grounds, including the potential to prevent transmission to uninfected sex partners. Routine screening for chlamydia is not recommended in the general population of low-risk adults ("D" recommendation).

In women, endocervical specimens should be obtained for cell culture or nonculture assays. Verification of positive nonculture results may be necessary, depending on the underlying risk in the patient and potential adverse consequences of a false-positive result. The choice of screening test for asymptomatic men is left to clinical discretion. Urine LE dipstick is much less expensive than urine assays using EIA, PCR, or LCR, but it is also less sensitive and specific for asymptomatic chlamydial infection. The optimal frequency of testing has not been determined for women or men and is left to clinical discretion.

Routine ocular antibiotic prophylaxis with silver nitrate, erythromycin, or tetracycline is recommended for all newborn infants to prevent ophthalmia neonatorum caused by gonorrhea and is required by law in most states (see Chapter 27). There is insufficient evidence to recommend for or against universal ocular prophylaxis of newborns solely for the prevention of chlamydial conjunctivitis ("C" recommendation).

30. Screening for Genital Herpes Simplex

RECOMMENDATION

Routine screening for genital herpes simplex virus (HSV) infection by viral culture or other tests is not recommended for asymptomatic persons, including asymptomatic pregnant women. There is insufficient evidence to recommend for or against the examination of pregnant women in labor for signs of active genital HSV lesions, although recommendations to do so may be made on other grounds (see Clinical Intervention). See Chapter 62 for recommendations on counseling to prevent sexually transmitted diseases.

CLINICAL INTERVENTION

Routine screening for genital herpes simplex in asymptomatic persons, using culture, serology, or other tests, is not recommended ("D" recommendation). See Chapter 62 for recommendations on counseling to prevent sexually transmitted diseases.

Routine screening for genital herpes simplex infection in asymptomatic pregnant women, by surveillance cultures or serology, is also not recommended ("D" recommendation). Clinicians should take a complete sexual history on all adolescent and adult patients (see Chapter 62).

As part of the sexual history, clinicians should consider asking all pregnant women at the first prenatal visit whether they or their sex partner(s) have had genital herpetic lesions. There is insufficient evidence to recommend for or against routine counseling of women who have no history of genital herpes, but whose partners do have a positive history, to use condoms or abstain from intercourse during pregnancy ("C" recommendation); such counseling may be recommended, however, on other grounds, such as the lack of health risk and potential benefits of such behavior.

There is also insufficient evidence to recommend for or against the examination of all pregnant women for signs of active genital HSV lesions during labor and the performance of cesarean delivery on those with lesions ("C" recommendation); recommendations to do so may be made on other grounds, such as the results of decision analyses and expert opinion. There is not yet sufficient evidence to recommend for or against routine use of systemic acyclovir in pregnant women with recurrent herpes to prevent reactivations near term ("C" recommendation).

31. Screening for Asymptomatic Bacteriuria

RECOMMENDATION

Screening for asymptomatic bacteriuria by urine culture is recommended for all pregnant women (see Clinical Intervention). There is insufficient evidence to recommend for or against routine screening for asymptomatic bacteriuria in diabetic or ambulatory elderly women, but recommendations against such screening may be made on other grounds. Routine screening for asymptomatic bacteriuria in other persons is not recommended.

CLINICAL INTERVENTION

Screening for asymptomatic bacteriuria with urine culture is recommended for pregnant women at 12-16 weeks of gestation ("A" recommendation). The optimal frequency for subsequent periodic urine cultures during pregnancy has not been determined and is left to clinical discretion. The urine specimen should be obtained in a manner that minimizes contamination. Routine screening for asymptomatic bacteriuria with leukocyte esterase or nitrite testing in pregnant women is not recommended because of poor test characteristics compared to urine culture ("D" recommendation).

There is currently insufficient evidence to recommend for or against routine screening for asymptomatic bacteriuria with leukocyte esterase or nitrite testing in ambulatory elderly women or in women with diabetes ("C" recommendation), but recommendations against such screening may be made on other grounds, including a high likelihood of recurrence and the potential adverse effects of antibiotic therapy. Routine screening for bacteriuria with leukocyte esterase or nitrite testing is not recommended for other asymptomatic persons, including school-aged girls ("E" recommendation), institutionalized elderly ("E" recommendation), and other children, adolescents, and adults ("D" recommendation). Screening for asymptomatic bacteriuria with microscopy testing is not recommended ("D" recommendation).

32. Screening for Rubella—Including Immunization of Adolescents and Adults

RECOMMENDATION

Routine screening for rubella susceptibility by history of vaccination or by serology is recommended for all women of childbearing age at their first clinical encounter. Susceptible nonpregnant women should be offered rubella vaccination; susceptible pregnant women should be vaccinated immediately after delivery. An equally acceptable alternative for nonpregnant women of childbearing age is to offer vaccination against rubella without screening (see Clinical Intervention). There is insufficient evidence to recommend for or against screening or routine vaccination of young men in settings where large numbers of susceptible young adults of both sexes congregate, such as military bases and colleges. Routine screening or vaccination of other young men, of older men, and of postmenopausal women is not recommended.

CLINICAL INTERVENTION

All children without contraindications should receive MMR vaccine at age 12-15 months and again at age 4-6 years (see Chapter 65). To reduce further the incidence of congenital rubella syndrome (CRS), screening for rubella susceptibility by history of vaccination or by serology is recommended for all women of childbearing age at their first clinical encounter ("B" recommendation). A documented history of vaccination is more accurate than an undocumented history in determining rubella immunity and is therefore preferred. All susceptible nonpregnant women of childbearing age should be offered vaccination. Susceptible pregnant women should be vaccinated in the immediate postpartum period. An equally acceptable alternative for nonpregnant women of childbearing age is to offer vaccination against rubella without screening ("B" recommendation). The decision of which strategy to use should be tailored to the individual clinician's practice population, depending on the availability of vaccination records, the reliability of the vaccination history, the rate of immunity, the cost of serologic testing, and the cost and likelihood of follow-up vaccination for susceptible persons identified by serologic testing.

There is insufficient evidence to recommend for or against routine screening or vaccination of young men to prevent CRS in settings where large numbers of susceptible young adults of both sexes congregate, such as military bases and colleges ("C" recommendation). Recommendations to give MMR vaccine in these settings may be made on other grounds, however, such as prevention of measles (see Chapter 66). Routine screening or vaccination of other young men, of older men, or of postmenopausal women, is not recommended ("D" recommendation).

Guidelines for the administration of MMR vaccine, and its contraindications, have been published by ACIP. The National Childhood Vaccine Injury Act requires that the date of administration, the manufacturer and lot number, and the name, address, and title of the person administering the vaccine be recorded in the patient's permanent medical record (or in a permanent office log or file).

Vision and Hearing Disorders

33. Screening for Visual Impairment

RECOMMENDATION

Vision screening to detect amblyopia and strabismus is recommended once for all children prior to entering school, preferably between ages 3 and 4. Clinicians should be alert for signs of ocular misalignment when examining infants and children. Screening for diminished visual acuity with the Snellen visual acuity chart is recommended for elderly persons. There is insufficient evidence to recommend for or against screening for diminished visual acuity among other asymptomatic persons, but recommendations against routine screening may be made on other grounds (see Clinical Intervention).

CLINICAL INTERVENTION

Vision screening for amblyopia and strabismus is recommended for all children once before entering school, preferably between ages 3 and 4 years ("B" recommendation). Clinicians should be alert for signs of ocular misalignment when examining all infants and children. Stereoacuity testing may be more effective than visual acuity testing in detecting these conditions.

There is insufficient evidence to recommend for or against routine screening for diminished visual acuity among asymptomatic schoolchildren and nonelderly adults ("C" recommendation). Recommendations against such screening may be made on other grounds, including the inconvenience and cost of routine screening, and the fact that refractive errors can be readily corrected when they produce symptoms.

Routine vision screening with the Snellen acuity test is recommended for elderly persons ("B" recommendation). The optimal frequency for screening is not known and is left to clinical discretion. Selected questions about vision may also be helpful in detecting vision problems in elderly persons, but they do not appear as sensitive or specific as direct assessment of acuity. There is insufficient evidence to recommend for or against routine screening with ophthalmoscopy by the primary care physician in asymptomatic elderly patients ("C" recommendation).

34. Screening for Glaucoma

RECOMMENDATION

There is insufficient evidence to recommend for or against routine screening for intraocular hypertension or glaucoma by primary care clinicians. Recommendations to refer high-risk patients for evaluation by an eye specialist may be made on other grounds (see Clinical Intervention).

CLINICAL INTERVENTION

There is insufficient evidence to recommend for or against routine screening by primary care clinicians for elevated intraocular pressure or early glaucoma ("C" recommendation). Effective screening for glaucoma is best performed by eye specialists who have access to specialized equipment to evaluate the optic disc and measure visual fields. Recommendations may be made on other grounds to refer high-risk patients for evaluation by eye specialists. This recommendation is based on the substantial prevalence of unrecognized glaucoma in these populations, the progressive nature of untreated disease, and expert consensus that reducing intraocular pressure may slow the rate of visual loss in patients with early glaucoma or severe intraocular hypertension. Populations in whom the prevalence of glaucoma is greater than 1% include blacks over age 40 and whites over age 65. Patients with a family history of glaucoma, patients with diabetes, and patients with severe myopia are also at increased risk and may benefit from screening. The optimal frequency for glaucoma screening has not been determined and is left to clinical discretion.

35. Screening for Hearing Impairment

RECOMMENDATION

Screening older adults for hearing impairment by periodically questioning them about their hearing, counseling them about the availability of hearing aid devices, and making referrals for abnormalities when appropriate, is recommended. There is insufficient evidence to recommend for or against routinely screening older adults for hearing impairment using audiometric testing (see Clinical Intervention). There is also insufficient evidence to recommend for or against routinely screening asymptomatic adolescents and working-age adults for hearing impairment. Recommendations against such screening, except for those exposed to excessive occupational noise levels, may be made on other grounds (see Clinical Intervention). Routine hearing screening of asymptomatic children beyond age 3 years is not recommended. There is insufficient evidence to recommend for or against routine screening of asymptomatic neonates for hearing impairment using evoked otoacoustic emission testing or auditory brainstem response. Recommendations to screen high-risk infants may be made on other grounds (see Clinical Intervention). Clinicians examining infants and young children should remain alert for symptoms or signs of hearing impairment.

CLINICAL INTERVENTION

Screening older adults for hearing impairment by periodically questioning them about their hearing, counseling them about the availability of hearing aid devices, and making referrals for abnormalities when appropriate, is recommended ("B" recommendation). The optimal frequency of such screening has not been determined and is left to clinical discretion. An otoscopic examination and audiometric testing should be performed on all persons with evidence of impaired hearing by patient inquiry. Although hand-held devices for audiometry testing (audioscopes) are also sensitive screening tools for hearing deficits, patient inquiry is likely to be a more rapid and less expensive way to screen for hearing loss in older adults. There is therefore insufficient evidence to recommend for or against routinely screening older adults for hearing deficits using audiometry testing ("C" recommendation).

There is insufficient evidence to recommend for or against routinely screening asymptomatic adolescents and working-age adults for hearing impairment ("C" recommendation). Recommendations against such screening, except for those exposed to excessive occupational noise levels, may be made on other grounds, including low prevalence, high cost, and the likelihood that hearing deficits in these individuals will present clinically. Screening of workers for noise-induced hearing loss should be performed in the context of existing work site programs and occupational medicine guidelines.

Routine hearing screening of asymptomatic children beyond age 3 years is not recommended ("D" recommendation). It is recognized, however, that such testing often occurs outside the clinical setting. When this occurs, abnormal test results should be confirmed by repeat testing at appropriate intervals, and all confirmed cases identified through screening referred for ongoing audiologic assessment, selection of hearing aids, family counseling, psychoeducational management, and periodic medical evaluation.

There is insufficient evidence to recommend for or against routine screening of asymptomatic neonates for hearing impairment using evoked otoacoustic emission (EOE) testing or auditory brainstem response (ABR) ("C" recommendation). Recommendations to screen high-risk infants may be made on other grounds, including the relatively high prevalence of hearing impairment, parental anxiety or concern, and the potentially beneficial effect on language development from early treatment of infants with moderate or severe hearing loss. For many high-risk conditions, hearing testing is commonly considered to be part of diagnostic evaluation and management. Risk factors for congenital or perinatally acquired hearing loss include family history of hereditary childhood sensorineural hearing loss; congenital perinatal infection with herpes, syphilis, rubella, cytomegalovirus, or toxoplasmosis; malformations involving the head or neck (e.g., dysmorphic and syndromal abnormalities, cleft palate, abnormal pinna); birth weight below 1500 g; bacterial meningitis; hyperbilirubinemia requiring exchange transfusion; severe perinatal asphyxia (Apgar scores of 0-4 at 1 minute or 0-6 at 5 minutes, absence of spontaneous respirations for 10 minutes, or hypotonia at 2 hours of age); ototoxic medications; and findings associated with a syndrome known to include hearing loss. ABR testing may be useful for all infants who meet at least one of these high-risk criteria or for those who fail EOE testing. High-risk infants should ideally be screened prior to leaving the hospital after birth, but those not tested at birth should be screened before age 3 months with the goal being to initiate rehabilitation by age 6 months as clinically indicated. Clinicians examining any infant or young child should remain alert for symptoms or signs of hearing impairment, including parent/caregiver concern regarding hearing, speech, language, or developmental delay.

Prenatal Disorders

36. Screening Ultrasonography in Pregnancy

RECOMMENDATION

Routine third-trimester ultrasound examination of the fetus is not recommended. There is insufficient evidence to recommend for or against routine ultrasound examination in the second trimester in low-risk pregnant women (see Clinical Intervention).

CLINICAL INTERVENTION

Routine ultrasound examination of the fetus in the third trimester is not recommended, based on multiple trials and metaanalyses showing no benefit for either the pregnant woman or her fetus ("D" recommendation). There is currently insufficient evidence to recommend for or against a single routine midtrimester ultrasound in low-risk pregnant women ("C" recommendation). These recommendations apply to routine screening ultrasonography and not to diagnostic ultrasonography for specific clinical indications (e.g., follow-up evaluation of elevated maternal serum alpha-fetoprotein). Recommendations regarding screening for Down syndrome appear in Chapter 41, and those for neural tube defects appear in Chapter 42.

37. Screening for Preeclampsia

RECOMMENDATION

Screening for preeclampsia with blood pressure measurement is recommended for all pregnant women at the first prenatal visit and periodically throughout the remainder of pregnancy (see Clinical Intervention).

CLINICAL INTERVENTION

Screening for preeclampsia with blood pressure measurement is recommended for all pregnant women at the first prenatal visit and periodically throughout the remainder of pregnancy ("B" recommendation). The optimal frequency for measuring blood pressure in pregnant women has not been determined and is left to clinical discretion; it is most efficient to measure blood pressure on women who are being seen by their clinicians for other reasons. The collection of meaningful blood pressure data requires consistent use of correct technique and a cuff of appropriate size. In addition to the guidelines listed in Chapter 3, the patient should be in the sitting position and the blood pressure should be measured after the patient's arm has rested at heart level for 5 minutes. Further diagnostic evaluation and clinical monitoring, including frequent blood pressure monitoring and urine testing for protein, are indicated if blood pressure does not decrease normally during the middle trimester, if the systolic pressure increases 30 mm Hg above baseline or the diastolic pressure increases 15 mm Hg above baseline, or if the blood pressure exceeds 140/90 mm Hg. Medical interventions should not be prescribed until the diagnosis of preeclampsia is confirmed. See Chapter 70 for recommendations on the use of aspirin prophylaxis in pregnancy.

38. Screening for D (Rh) Incompatibility

RECOMMENDATION

D (formerly Rh) blood typing and antibody screening is recommended for all pregnant women at their first prenatal visit. Repeat antibody screening at 24-28 weeks' gestation is recommended for unsensitized D-negative women (see Clinical Intervention).

CLINICAL INTERVENTION

D blood typing and antibody testing is recommended for all pregnant women at their first prenatal visit, including visits for elective abortion ("A" recommendation). For purposes of blood typing and prophylaxis, D^u- and D-negative blood types should be considered equivalent. Unless the father is known to be D-negative, a repeat D antibody test is recommended for all unsensitized D-negative women at 24-28 weeks' gestation, followed by the administration of a full (300 μg) dose of D immunoglobulin if they are antibody-negative ("B" recommendation). If a D- (or D^u-) positive infant is delivered, the dose should be repeated postpartum, preferably within 72 hours after delivery ("A" recommendation). Unless the father is known to be D-negative, a full dose of D immunoglobulin is recommended for all unsensitized D-negative women after elective abortion (50 μg before 13 weeks) and amniocentesis ("B" recommendation). There is currently insufficient evidence to recommend for or against the routine administration of D immunoglobulin after other obstetric procedures or complications such as chorionic villus sampling, ectopic pregnancy termination, cordocentesis, fetal surgery or manipulation (including external version), antepartum placental hemorrhage, antepartum fetal death, and stillbirth ("C" recommendation).

39. Intrapartum Electronic Fetal Monitoring

RECOMMENDATION

Routine electronic fetal monitoring for low-risk women in labor is not recommended. There is insufficient evidence to recommend for or against intrapartum electronic fetal monitoring for high-risk pregnant women (see Clinical Intervention).

CLINICAL INTERVENTION

Routine electronic fetal monitoring is not recommended for low-risk women in labor when adequate clinical monitoring including intermittent auscultation by trained staff is available ("D" recommendation). There is insufficient evidence to recommend for or against electronic fetal monitoring over intermittent auscultation for high-risk pregnancies ("C" recommendation). For pregnant women with complicated labor (i.e., induced, prolonged, or oxytocin augmented), recommendations for electronic monitoring plus scalp blood sampling may be made on the basis of evidence for a reduced risk of neonatal seizures, although the long-term neurologic benefit to the neonate is unclear and must be weighed against the increased risk to the mother and neonate of operative delivery, general anesthesia, and maternal infection, and a possible increased risk of adverse neurologic outcome in the infant. There is currently no evidence available to evaluate electronic fetal monitoring in comparison to no monitoring.

40. Home Uterine Activity Monitoring

RECOMMENDATION

There is insufficient evidence to recommend for or against home uterine activity monitoring (HUAM) in high-risk pregnancies as a screening test for preterm labor, but recommendations against its use may be made on other grounds (see Clinical Intervention). HUAM is not recommended in normal-risk pregnancies.

CLINICAL INTERVENTION

There is insufficient evidence to recommend for or against HUAM as a screening test for preterm labor in high-risk pregnancies (pregnancies with risk factors for preterm labor), but recommendations against its use may be made on other grounds, including its costs and inconvenience ("C" recommendation). HUAM is not recommended for normal-risk pregnancies (without risk factors for preterm labor) ("D" recommendation).

Congenital Disorders

41. Screening for Down Syndrome

RECOMMENDATION

The offering of amniocentesis or chorionic villus sampling (CVS) for chromosome studies is recommended for pregnant women at high risk for Down syndrome. The offering of screening for Down syndrome by serum multiple-marker testing is recommended for all low-risk pregnant women, and as an alternative to amniocentesis and CVS for high-risk women (see Clinical Intervention). This testing should be offered only to women who are seen for prenatal care in locations that have adequate counseling and follow-up services. There is currently insufficient evidence to recommend for or against screening for Down syndrome by individual serum marker testing or ultrasound examination, but recommendations against such screening may be made on other grounds (see Clinical Intervention).

CLINICAL INTERVENTION

The offering of amniocentesis or CVS for chromosome studies to pregnant women aged 35 years and older and to those at high risk of Down syndrome for other reasons (e.g., previous affected pregnancy, known carriage of a chromosome rearrangement associated with Down syndrome) is recommended ("B" recommendation). In some circumstances, depending on resources, preferences, and other factors, the selection of a different age threshold for offering prenatal diagnosis may be considered. Counseling before the procedure should include a comparison of the risks to the fetus from the procedure and the probability of a chromosome defect given the patient's age or other risk factors, as well as a full discussion of the potential outcomes associated with delivering a child with Down syndrome and of aborting a Down syndrome fetus.

The offering of screening for Down syndrome by maternal serum multiple-marker testing at 15-18 weeks of gestation is recommended for all pregnant women who have access to counseling and follow-up services, skilled high-resolution ultrasound and amniocentesis capabilities, and reliable, standardized laboratories ("B" recommendation). There is currently insufficient evidence to recommend a specific multiple-marker screening protocol. Counseling regarding screening should include information on the procedure itself, the likelihood of follow-up testing with amniocentesis and its associated risks, as well as a full discussion of the potential outcomes associated with delivering a child with Down syndrome and of aborting a Down syndrome fetus. Women with a positive screen should receive detailed information comparing the increased risk of trisomy and the risks of fetal loss from amniocentesis. For women aged 35 years and older, the choice of serum multiple-marker screening versus amniocentesis or CVS for chromosome studies depends on patient preferences and therefore requires a detailed discussion of the potential risks and benefits of each procedure. In particular, the patient should understand the reduced sensitivity of multiple-marker screening for Down syndrome and for other chromosome abnormalities compared to prenatal diagnosis by chromosome studies, and the increased risk of fetal loss or injury with amniocentesis and CVS.

There is currently insufficient evidence to recommend for or against routine ultrasound examination or the use of individual maternal serum markers in pregnant women as screening tests for Down syndrome ("C" recommendation). Recommendations against these tests may be made on other grounds, however, including the availability of other screening tests of proven effectiveness.

42. Screening for Neural Tube Defects— Including Folic Acid/Folate Prophylaxis

RECOMMENDATION

The offering of screening for neural tube defects by maternal serum alpha-fetoprotein (MSAFP) measurement is recommended for all pregnant women who are seen for prenatal care in locations that have adequate counseling and follow-up services available (see Clinical Intervention). Screening with MSAFP may be offered as part of multiple-marker screening (see Chapter 41). There is insufficient evidence to recommend for or against the offering of screening for neural tube defects by midtrimester ultrasound examination to all pregnant women, but recommendations against such screening may be made on other grounds (also see Chapter 36). Daily multivitamins with folic acid to reduce the risk of neural tube defects are recommended for all women who are planning or capable of pregnancy (see Clinical Intervention).

CLINICAL INTERVENTION

The offering of screening for neural tube defects by maternal serum alpha-fetoprotein (MSAFP) measurement at 16-18 weeks' gestation is recommended for all pregnant women who are seen for prenatal care in locations that have adequate counseling and follow-up services, skilled high-resolution ultrasound and amniocentesis capabilities, and reliable, standardized laboratories ("B" recommendation). Women with elevated MSAFP levels should receive a second confirmatory test when time allows (i.e., before 18 weeks of gestation), and high-resolution ultrasound examination by an adequately trained and experienced examiner before amniocentesis is performed. Screening with MSAFP may be offered as part of multiple-marker screening (see Chapter 41). There is currently insufficient evidence to recommend for or against the offering of screening for neural tube defects by routine midtrimester ultrasound examination in pregnant women ("C" recommendation). Recommendations may be made against such screening, except when conducted by expert sonographers at major screening centers, based on its unproven accuracy in other settings, the availability and proven effectiveness of MSAFP screening, and cost. See Chapter 36 for additional recommendations regarding routine ultrasound examination in pregnancy. Pregnant women at high risk of neural tube defects (e.g., those with a previous affected pregnancy) should be referred to specialized centers for appropriate diagnostic evaluation, including high-resolution ultrasound and amniocentesis.

Folic acid supplementation at a dose of 4 mg/day beginning 1-3 months prior to conception and continuing through the first trimester is recommended for women planning pregnancy who have previously had a pregnancy affected by a neural tube defect, to reduce the risk of recurrence ("A" recommendation). It is also recommended that all women planning pregnancy take a daily multivitamin or multivitamin-multimineral supplement containing folic acid at a dose of 0.4-0.8 mg, beginning at least 1 month prior to conception and continuing through the first trimester, to reduce the risk of neural tube defects ("A" recommendation). Taking a daily multivitamin containing 0.4 mg of folic acid is also recommended for all women capable of becoming pregnant, to reduce the risk of neural tube defects in unplanned pregnancies ("B" recommendation). Women taking drugs that interfere with folate metabolism (e.g., methotrexate, pyrimethamine, trimethoprim, phenytoin), women at increased risk of vitamin B_{12} deficiency (e.g., vegans or persons with AIDS), and those with epilepsy whose seizures are controlled by anticonvulsant therapy, should consult with their clinician regarding potential risks and benefits prior to considering folic acid supplementation. There is currently insufficient evidence to recommend for or against counseling women planning or capable of pregnancy to increase their dietary folate consumption to 0.4 mg/day as an alternative to taking multivitamins with folic acid ("C" recommendation). Offering counseling to increase dietary folate intake to women who do not wish to take folic acid supplements may be recommended on other grounds, including low risk, low cost, and likely benefit.

The use of periconceptional multivitamins with folic acid does not necessarily obviate the need to offer screening for neural tube defects during pregnancy, since not all defects will be prevented by prophylaxis.

43. Screening for Hemoglobinopathies

RECOMMENDATION

Neonatal screening for sickle hemoglobinopathies is recommended to identify infants who may benefit from antibiotic prophylaxis to prevent sepsis. Whether screening should be universal or targeted to high-risk groups will depend on the proportion of high-risk individuals in the screening area, the accuracy and efficiency with which infants at risk can be identified, and other characteristics of the screening program. All screening efforts must be accompanied by comprehensive counseling and treatment services. Offering screening for hemoglobinopathies to pregnant women at the first prenatal visit is recommended, especially for those at high risk. There is insufficient evidence to recommend for or against routine screening for hemoglobinopathies in high-risk adolescents and young adults, but recommendations to offer such testing may be made on other grounds (see Clinical Intervention).

CLINICAL INTERVENTION

Screening newborn infants for hemoglobinopathies with hemoglobin electrophoresis or other tests of comparable accuracy on umbilical cord or heel-stick blood specimens is recommended ("A" recommendation). In geographic areas with a very low incidence of hemoglobin disorders, selective screening of newborns may be more efficient than universal screening. Infants with sickle cell disease must receive prompt follow-up, including oral penicillin prophylaxis, diagnostic testing, immunizations, and regular evaluations of growth and nutritional status. Their families should receive genetic counseling regarding testing of family members and risks to future offspring, information about the disease, education about early warning signs of serious complications, and referrals for peer support groups and sources of medical and mental health services.

Offering screening for hemoglobinopathies with hemoglobin electrophoresis or other tests of comparable accuracy to pregnant women at the first prenatal visit is recommended ("B" recommendation), especially for those who are members of racial and ethnic groups with a high incidence of hemoglobinopathies (e.g., individuals of African,

Caribbean, Latin American, Mediterranean, Middle Eastern, or Southeast Asian descent). Carriers identified through testing should be urged to have the father tested and should receive information on the availability of prenatal diagnosis if the father is positive and the fetus is at risk of having a clinically significant hemoglobinopathy.

There is insufficient evidence to recommend for or against screening for hemoglobinopathies in adolescents and young adults from ethnic and racial groups known to be at increased risk for sickle cell disease, thalassemias, and other hemoglobinopathies in order for them to be able to make informed reproductive choices ("C" recommendation). Recommendations to offer such testing may be made on other grounds, including burden of suffering and patient preference. If provided, testing should be accompanied by counseling, which should include a description of the significance of the disease, how it is inherited, the availability of a screening test, and the implications to individuals and their offspring of a positive result.

44. Screening for Phenylketonuria

RECOMMENDATION

Screening for phenylketonuria (PKU) by measurement of phenylalanine level on a dried-blood spot specimen is recommended for all newborns prior to discharge from the nursery. Infants who are tested before 24 hours of age should receive a repeat screening test by 2 weeks of age. There is insufficient evidence to recommend for or against routine prenatal screening for maternal PKU, but recommendations against such screening may be made on other grounds.

CLINICAL INTERVENTION

Screening for phenylketonuria by measurement of phenylalanine level on a dried-blood spot specimen, collected by heel-stick and adsorbed onto filter paper, is recommended for all newborns before discharge from the nursery ("A" recommendation). Infants who are tested in the first 24 hours of age should receive a repeat screening test by 2 weeks of age. Premature infants and those with illnesses optimally should be tested at or near 7 days of age, but in all cases before newborn nursery discharge. All parents should be adequately informed regarding the indications for testing and the interpretation of PKU test results, including the probabilities of false-positive and false-negative findings.

There is insufficient evidence to recommend for or against routine prenatal screening for maternal PKU ("C" recommendation), but recommendations against such screening may be made on other grounds, including the rarity of previously undiagnosed maternal hyperphenylalaninemia, cost, and the potential adverse effects of dietary restriction.

45. Screening for Congenital Hypothyroidism

RECOMMENDATION

Screening for congenital hypothyroidism with thyroid function tests on dried-blood spot specimens is recommended for all newborns in the first week of life (see Clinical Intervention).

CLINICAL INTERVENTION

Screening for congenital hypothyroidism with thyroid function tests performed on dried-blood spot specimens is recommended for all newborns, optimally between days 2 and 6, but in all cases before newborn nursery discharge ("A" recommendation). Blood specimens should be collected by heel-stick, adsorbed onto filter paper, and air dried using standard technique. The choice of which thyroid function test or tests to perform is generally determined by individual state requirements. Testing procedures and follow-up treatment for abnormal results should follow current guidelines. Care should be taken to ensure that those born at home, ill at birth, or transferred between hospitals in the first week of life are appropriately screened before 7 days of age. Normal newborn screening results should not preclude appropriate evaluation of infants presenting with clinical symptoms and signs suggestive of hypothyroidism.

Musculoskeletal Disorders

46. Screening for Postmenopausal Osteoporosis

RECOMMENDATION

There is insufficient evidence to recommend for or against routine screening for osteoporosis with bone densitometry in postmenopausal women. Recommendations against routine screening may be made on other grounds (see Clinical Intervention). All postmenopausal women should be counseled about hormone prophylaxis (see Chapter 68) and be advised of the importance of smoking cessation, regular exercise, and adequate calcium intake (see Chapters 54-56). For those high-risk women who would consider estrogen prophylaxis only to prevent osteoporosis, screening may be appropriate to assist treatment decisions (see Clinical Intervention).

CLINICAL INTERVENTION

There is insufficient evidence to recommend for or against screening for osteoporosis or decreased bone density in asymptomatic, postmenopausal women ("C" recommendation). Recommendations against routine screening may be made on the grounds of the inconvenience and high cost of bone densitometry, and lack of universally accepted criteria for initiating treatment based on bone density measurements. All perimenopausal and postmenopausal women should be counseled about the potential benefits and risks of hormone prophylaxis (see Chapter 68). Although direct evidence of benefit is not available, selective screening may be appropriate for high-risk women who would consider hormone prophylaxis only if they knew they were at high risk for osteoporosis or fracture.

All women should also receive counseling regarding universal preventive measures related to fracture risk, such as dietary calcium and vitamin D intake (Chapter 56), weight-bearing exercise (Chapter 55), and smoking cessation (Chapter 54). Elderly persons should also receive counseling regarding preventive measures to reduce the risk of falls and the severity of fall-related injuries (Chapter 58).

47. Screening for Adolescent Idiopathic Scoliosis

RECOMMENDATION

There is insufficient evidence to recommend for or against routine screening of asymptomatic adolescents for idiopathic scoliosis. Clinicians should remain alert for large spinal curvatures when examining adolescents.

CLINICAL INTERVENTION

There is insufficient evidence to recommend for or against routine screening of asymptomatic adolescents for idiopathic scoliosis ("C" recommendation). The evidence does not support routine visits to clinicians for the specific purpose of scoliosis screening or for performing the examination at specific ages during adolescence. It is prudent for clinicians to include visual inspection of the back of adolescents when it is examined for other reasons. Additional specific inspection maneuvers to screen for scoliosis, such as the forward-bending test, are of unproven benefit.

Mental Disorders and Substance Abuse

48. Screening for Dementia

RECOMMENDATION

There is insufficient evidence to recommend for or against routine screening for dementia with standardized instruments in asymptomatic persons. Clinicians should remain alert for possible signs of declining cognitive function in older patients and evaluate mental status in patients who have problems performing daily activities (see Clinical Intervention).

CLINICAL INTERVENTION

There is insufficient evidence to recommend for or against routine screening for dementia in asymptomatic elderly persons ("C" recommendation). Clinicians should periodically ask patients about their functional status at home and at work, and they should remain alert to changes in performance with age. When possible, information about daily activities should be solicited from family members or other persons. Brief tests such as the MMSE should be used to assess cognitive function in patients in whom the suspicion of dementia is raised by restrictions in daily activities, concerns of family members, or other evidence of worsening function (e.g., trouble with finances, medications, transportation). Possible effects of education and cultural differences should be considered when interpreting results of cognitive tests. The diagnosis of dementia should not be based on results of screening tests alone. Patients suspected of having dementia should be examined for other causes of changing mental status, including depression, delirium, medication effects, and coexisting medical illnesses.

49. Screening for Depression

RECOMMENDATION

There is insufficient evidence to recommend for or against the routine use of standardized questionnaires to screen for depression in asymptomatic primary care patients. Clinicians should maintain an especially high index of suspicion for depressive symptoms in those persons at increased risk for depression (see Clinical Intervention). Physician education in recognizing and treating affective disorders is recommended (see Chapter 50).

CLINICAL INTERVENTION

There is insufficient evidence to recommend for or against the routine use of standardized questionnaires to screen for depression in asymptomatic primary care patients ("C" recommendation). Clinicians should, however, maintain an especially high index of suspicion for depressive symptoms in adolescents and young adults, persons with a family or personal history of depression, those with chronic illnesses, those who perceive or have experienced a recent loss, and those with sleep disorders, chronic pain, or multiple unexplained somatic complaints. Physician education in recognizing and treating affective disorders is recommended (see Chapter 50). Persons with depressive symptoms should be evaluated further and, if diagnosed with major depressive disorder, either treated or referred for treatment.

50. Screening for Suicide Risk

RECOMMENDATION

There is insufficient evidence to recommend for or against routine screening by primary care clinicians to detect suicide risk in asymptomatic persons (see Clinical Intervention). Clinicians should be alert to signs of suicidal ideation in persons with established risk factors. The training of primary care clinicians in recognizing and treating affective disorders is recommended. Clinicians should be alert to signs and symptoms of depression (see Chapter 49) and should routinely ask patients about their use of alcohol and other drugs (Chapters 52 and 53).

CLINICAL INTERVENTION

There is insufficient evidence to recommend for or against routine screening by primary care clinicians to detect suicide risk in asymptomatic persons ("C" recommendation). Clinicians should be alert to evidence of suicidal ideation when the history reveals risk factors for suicide, such as depression, alcohol or other drug abuse, other psychiatric disorder, prior attempted suicide, recent divorce, separation, unemployment, and recent bereavement. Patients with evidence of suicidal ideation should be questioned regarding the extent of preparatory actions (e.g., obtaining a weapon, making a plan, putting affairs in order, giving away prized possessions, preparing a suicide note). It may also be prudent to question the person's family members regarding such actions. Persons with evidence of suicidal intent should be offered mental health counseling and possibly hospitalization.

The training of primary care clinicians in recognizing and treating affective disorders in order to prevent suicide is recommended ("B" recommendation). Clinicians should be alert to signs of depression (see Chapter 49) and other psychiatric illnesses, and they should routinely ask patients about their use of alcohol and other drugs (see Chapters 52 and 53). Patients who are judged to be at risk should receive evaluation for possible psychiatric illness, including substance abuse, and counseling and referral as needed.

Patients who are recognized as having suicidal ideation, or patients who suspect suicidal thoughts in their relatives or friends, should be made aware of available community resources such as local mental health agencies and crisis intervention centers. Parents and homeowners should also be counseled to restrict unauthorized access to potentially lethal prescription drugs and to firearms within the home (also see Chapters 58 and 59).

51. Screening for Family Violence

RECOMMENDATION

There is insufficient evidence to recommend for or against the use of specific screening instruments to detect family violence, but recommendations to include questions about physical abuse when taking a history from adult patients may be made on other grounds (see Clinical Intervention). Clinicians should be alert to the various presentations of child abuse, spouse and partner abuse, and elder abuse.

CLINICAL INTERVENTION

There is insufficient evidence to recommend for or against the use of specific screening instruments for family violence, but including a few direct questions about abuse (physical violence or forced sexual activity) as part of the routine history in adult patients may be recommended on other grounds ("C" recommendation). These other grounds include the substantial prevalence of undetected abuse among adult female patients, the potential value of this information in the care of the patient, and the low cost and low risk of harm from such screening. All clinicians examining children and adults should be alert to physical and behavioral signs and symptoms associated with abuse and neglect. Various guidelines are available to help clinicians in recognizing abuse and neglect in children, spouses/partners, and elders. In all states, suspected cases of child abuse or neglect must be reported to local child protective services agencies. In most states, suspected elder abuse must also be reported. All individuals who present with multiple injuries and an implausible explanation should be evaluated with attention to possible abuse or neglect. Injured pregnant women and elderly patients should receive special consideration for this problem. Suspected cases of abuse should receive proper documentation of the incident and physical findings (e.g., photographs, body maps); treatment of physical injuries; arrangements for counseling by a skilled mental health professional; and the telephone numbers of local crisis centers, shelters, and protective service agencies. The safety of children of victims of abuse should also be ensured.

52. Screening for Problem Drinking

RECOMMENDATION

Screening to detect problem drinking is recommended for all adult and adolescent patients. Screening should involve a careful history of alcohol use and/or the use of standardized screening questionnaires (see Clinical Intervention). Routine measurement of biochemical markers is not recommended in asymptomatic persons. Pregnant women should be advised to limit or cease drinking during pregnancy. Although there is insufficient evidence to prove or disprove harms from light drinking in pregnancy, recommendations that women abstain from alcohol during pregnancy may be made on other grounds (see Clinical Intervention). All persons who use alcohol should be counseled about the dangers of operating a motor vehicle or performing other potentially dangerous activities after drinking alcohol.

CLINICAL INTERVENTION

Screening to detect problem drinking and hazardous drinking is recommended for all adult and adolescent patients ("B" recommendation). Screening should involve a careful history of alcohol use and/or the use of standardized screening questionnaires. Patients should be asked to describe the quantity, frequency, and other characteristics of their use of wine, beer, and liquor, including frequency of intoxication and tolerance to the effects of alcohol. One drink is defined as 12 ounces of beer, a 5-ounce glass of wine, or 1.5 fluid ounces (one jigger) of distilled spirits. Brief questionnaires such as the CAGE or AUDIT may help clinicians assess the likelihood of problem drinking or hazardous drinking (see Table 5-6). Responses suggestive of problem drinking should be confirmed with more extensive discussions with the patient (and family members where indicated) about patterns of use, problems related to drinking, and symptoms of alcohol dependence. Routine measurement of biochemical markers, such as serum GGT, is not recommended for screening purposes. Discussions with adolescents should be approached with discretion to establish a trusting relationship and to respect the patient's concerns about the confidentiality of disclosed information.

All pregnant women should be screened for evidence of problem drinking or risk drinking (2 drinks per day or binge drinking) ("B" recommendation). Including questions about tolerance to alcohol may improve detection of at-risk women. All pregnant women and women contemplating pregnancy should be informed of the harmful effects of alcohol on the fetus and advised to limit or cease drinking. Although there is insufficient evidence to prove or disprove harms from occasional, light drinking during pregnancy, abstinence from alcohol can be recommended on other grounds: possible risk from even low-level exposure to alcohol, lack of harm

TABLE 5-6   **AUDIT Structured Interview***

	SCORE				
QUESTION	0	1	2	3	4
How often do you have a drink containing alcohol?	Never	Monthly or less	2-4 times/mo	2-3 times/wk	4 or more times/wk
How many drinks do you have on a typical day when you are drinking?	None	1 or 2	3 or 4	5 or 6	7-9†
How often do you have 6 or more drinks on one occasion?	Never	Less than monthly	Monthly	Weekly	Daily or almost daily
How often during the last year have you found that you were unable to stop drinking once you had started?	Never	Less than monthly	Monthly	Weekly	Daily or almost daily
How often last year have you failed to do what was normally expected from you because of drinking?	Never	Less than monthly	Monthly	Weekly	Daily or almost daily
How often during the last year have you needed a first drink in the morning to get yourself going after a heavy drinking session?	Never	Less than monthly	Monthly	Weekly	Daily or almost daily
How often during the last year have you had a feeling of guilt or remorse after drinking?	Never	Less than monthly	Monthly	Weekly	Daily or almost daily
How often during the last year have you been unable to remember what happened the night before because you had been drinking?	Never	Less than monthly	Monthly	Weekly	Daily or almost daily
Have you or someone else been injured as a result of your drinking?	Never	Yes, but not in last year (2 points)		Yes, during the last year (4 points)	
Has a relative, doctor, or other health worker been concerned about your drinking or suggested you cut down?	Never	Yes, but not in last year (2 points)		Yes, during the last year (4 points)	

*Score of greater than 8 (out of 41) is suggestive of problem drinking and indicates need for more in-depth assessment. Cut-off of 10 points is recommended by some to provide greater specificity.
†5 points if response is 10 or more drinks on a typical day.

from abstaining, and prevailing expert opinion ("C" recommendation). Women who smoke should be advised that the risk of low birth weight is greatest for mothers who both smoke and drink.

Patients with evidence of alcohol dependence should be referred, where possible, to appropriate clinical specialists or community programs specializing in the treatment of alcohol dependence. Patients with evidence of alcohol abuse or hazardous drinking should be offered brief advice and counseling. Counseling should involve feedback of the evidence of a drinking problem, discussion of the role of alcohol in current medical or psychosocial problems, direct advice to reduce consumption, and plans for regular follow-up. Problems related to alcohol (e.g., physical symptoms, behavioral or mood problems, or difficulties at work and home) should be monitored to determine whether further interventions are needed. There is no single definition of "hazardous" drinking in asymptomatic persons, but successful intervention trials have generally defined 5 drinks per day in men, 3 drinks per day in women, or frequent intoxication to identify persons at risk. Several United States organizations have suggested lower limits for "safe" drinking: 2 drinks per day in men and 1 drink per day in women. All persons who drink should be informed of the dangers of driving or other potentially dangerous activities after drinking (see Chapter 57). The use of alcohol should be discouraged in persons younger than the legal age for drinking ("B" recommendation), although the effectiveness of alcohol abstinence messages in the primary care setting is uncertain.

53. Screening for Drug Abuse

RECOMMENDATION

There is insufficient evidence to recommend for or against routine screening for drug abuse with standardized questionnaires or biologic assays. Including questions about drug use and drug-related problems when taking a history from all adolescent and adult patients may be recommended on other grounds (see Clinical Intervention). All pregnant women should be advised of the potential adverse effects of drug use on the development of the fetus. Clinicians should be alert to signs and symptoms of drug abuse in patients and refer drug abusing patients to specialized treatment facilities where available.

CLINICAL INTERVENTION

There is insufficient evidence to recommend for or against routine screening for drug abuse with standardized questionnaires or biologic assays ("C" recommendation). Including questions about drug use when taking a history from adolescent and adult patients may be recommended on other grounds, including the prevalence of drug use and the serious consequences of drug abuse and dependence. Clinicians should be alert to signs and symptoms of drug abuse and ask about the use of illicit drugs and legal drugs of abuse (e.g., sedatives, stimulants); use of inhalants should be considered in older children, adolescents, and young adults. The quantity, frequency, patterns of consumption, and adverse consequences of drug use (e.g., interference with school or work, evidence of dependence) should be assessed for all patients who report drug use. Clinicians should establish a trusting relationship with patients, approach discussion of drug use in a nonjudgmental manner, and respect the patient's concerns about the confidentiality of disclosed information.

All pregnant women should be advised about the potential risks to the fetus of drug use during pregnancy and the potential to transmit drugs to infants through breast-feeding. Routine drug testing of urine or other body fluids is not recommended as the primary method of detecting drug use in pregnant women or other asymptomatic adults. Selective use of urine testing during pregnancy may be appropriate when the possibility of drug use is suggested by clinical signs and symptoms (e.g., growth retardation, inadequate weight gain, inadequate prenatal care); periodic testing can also help monitor and encourage abstinence in women who have used drugs. Pregnant women who abuse drugs should be advised of the importance of regular prenatal care and be referred for treatment, where available.

Patients should give consent prior to drug testing and be informed of any legal obligations on the part of the clinician to report drug use to child protective agencies or other authorities. Both positive and negative results should be interpreted with understanding of the kinetics of drug metabolism and the limitations of testing methods, and positive screening tests should be confirmed by more reliable methods.

All patients who report potentially harmful use of drugs should be informed of the risks associated with their drug use and advised to cut down or stop. Decisions about treatment should be based on evidence of drug abuse or drug dependence obtained through careful patient interview, including discussion with friends or family members where appropriate. A treatment plan should be developed for the patient and family that is tailored to the drug of abuse and the needs of the patient. Patients with evidence of drug dependence should be referred to appropriate drug-treatment providers and community programs specializing in the treatment of drug dependencies. Persons who continue to inject drugs should be screened periodically for HIV infection and advised of measures that may reduce the risk of infections caused by drug use: use a new sterile syringe with each use, never share or reuse injection equipment, use clean (sterile, if possible) water to prepare drugs, clean the injection site with alcohol prior to injection, and safely dispose of syringes after use (see Chapters 28 and 62). Drug-using patients should be informed of available resources for sterile injection equipment.

Part C
COUNSELING
54. Counseling to Prevent Tobacco Use

RECOMMENDATION

Tobacco cessation counseling on a regular basis is recommended for all persons who use tobacco products. Pregnant women and parents with children living at home also should be counseled on the potentially harmful effects of smoking on fetal and child health. The prescription of nicotine patches or gum is recommended as an adjunct for selected patients. Anti-tobacco messages are recommended for inclusion in health promotion counseling of children, adolescents, and young adults (see Clinical Intervention).

CLINICAL INTERVENTION

A complete history of tobacco use, and an assessment of nicotine dependence among tobacco users, should be obtained from all adolescent and adult patients. Tobacco cessation counseling is recommended on a regular basis for all patients who use tobacco products ("A" recommendation). Pregnant women and parents with children living at home also should be counseled on the potentially harmful effects of smoking on fetal and child health ("A" recommendation). The optimal frequency for performing counseling to prevent tobacco use has not been determined with certainty, but repeated messages over long periods of time are associated with the greatest success in helping patients achieve abstinence. The prescription of nicotine patches or gum is recommended as an adjunct for selected patients ("A" recommendation). There is insufficient evidence to recommend for or against clonidine as an effective adjunct to tobacco cessation counseling ("C" recommendation).

Certain strategies can increase the effectiveness of counseling against tobacco use:

Direct, face-to-face advice and suggestions. The most effective clinician message is a brief, unambiguous, and informative statement on the need to stop using tobacco. If possible, the clinician should also review the short- and long-term health, social, and economic benefits of quitting and foster the tobacco user's belief in his or her ability to stop. The message should address the patient's concerns and any barriers presented by age, social environment, nicotine dependence, and general health. If the patient is not contemplating cessation, then the clinician should try to motivate the patient again at the next visit. If the patient is contemplating stopping, then the clinician should try to get agreement on a specific "quit date" and should prepare the patient for withdrawal symptoms. Patients who have experienced a relapse after previous quit attempts should be reassured that most smokers achieve long-term cessation only after several unsuccessful attempts.

Reinforcement. Schedule "support visits" or follow-up telephone calls, especially during the first 2 weeks when relapse is common.

Office reminders. Use a register system or chart stickers for tobacco users to increase the probability that an anti-tobacco message is delivered at each visit.

Self-help materials. Dispense a variety of effective self-help packages to motivate and aid the majority of tobacco users who quit on their own. These materials are listed in reference works and are available from voluntary organizations in most communities.

Community programs for additional help in quitting. Local hospitals, health departments, community health centers, work sites, commercial services, and voluntary organizations frequently offer smoking cessation programs to which patients can be referred. Clinicians should not, however, refer patients to programs providing treatment of unproven efficacy (e.g., electric shock therapy).

Drug therapy. The prescription of nicotine products as adjuncts to counseling may facilitate cessation by relieving withdrawal symptoms. Persons using the nicotine patch or gum should be advised to stop all tobacco use completely before starting the medication and to carefully store and dispose of products to prevent accidental ingestion by children or pets. The patch should be used on clean, dry, non-hairy skin sites that are alternated daily. A skin site should not be used more frequently than once a week. The patch is generally prescribed for 6-8 weeks over which time the dosage of nicotine is weaned. Those using nicotine gum should be instructed to chew the gum slowly and intermittently to allow proper absorption by the buccal mucosa. While using nicotine gum, patients should not drink or eat acidic substances such as coffee, colas, or citrus juices, which impair nicotine absorption. Nicotine gum is used as needed for up to 3 months, when the risk of relapse is greatest, and then tapered over the next 3 months. In pregnant or nursing patients or patients with a recent myocardial infarction, severe or worsening angina, serious arrhythmias, or vasospastic or endocrine disorders, the potential risks of nicotine adjuncts must be weighed carefully against the known adverse effects of tobacco. Nicotine adjuncts should also be used with caution in persons with peptic ulcer disease, claudication, renal or hepatic insufficiency, or accelerated hypertension. Nicotine gum is contraindicated in patients with active temporomandibular joint disease.

Anti-tobacco messages should be included in health promotion counseling of children, adolescents, and young adults based on the proven efficacy of risk reduction from avoiding tobacco use ("A" recommendation), although the evidence for the effectiveness of clinical counseling to prevent the initiation of tobacco use is less clear ("C" recommendation).

Because school-based programs have been shown to delay initiation of tobacco use, clinicians should support such programs in their communities. Effective school-based programs teach children skills to recognize and resist social pressure to smoke, dip, or chew tobacco as well as to understand the short-term (e.g., bad breath, cost, decreased athletic ability, cough, phlegm production, and shortness of breath) and long-term adverse consequences of tobacco use. Examples of support that clinicians can provide include: becoming aware of programs already in place in local schools and reinforcing their messages with patients and their parents, alerting parents to the existence of such programs, and encouraging parental participation and involvement; serving as a consultant to local schools that implement such programs; developing a list of referrals for tobacco cessation programs for youths; and serving as a community advocate to keep effective programs in place (L.A. Maiman and D. Haynie, National Institutes of Health, personal communication, March 1994).

55. Counseling to Promote Physical Activity

RECOMMENDATION

Counseling patients to incorporate regular physical activity into their daily routines is recommended to prevent coronary heart disease, hypertension, obesity, and diabetes. This recommendation is based on the proven benefits of regular physical activity; the effectiveness of clinician counseling to promote physical activity is not established (see Clinical Intervention).

CLINICAL INTERVENTION

Counseling to promote regular physical activity is recommended for all children and adults. This recommendation is based on the proven efficacy of regular physical activity in reducing the risk for coronary heart disease, hypertension, obesity, and diabetes ("A" recommendation), although there is currently insufficient evidence that counseling asymptomatic primary care patients to incorporate physical activity into their daily routines will have a positive effect on their behavior ("C" recommendation). Clinicians should determine each patient's activity level, ascertain barriers specific to that individual, and provide information on the role of physical activity in disease prevention. The clinician may then assist the patient in selecting appropriate types of physical activity. Factors that should be considered include medical limitations and activity characteristics that both improve health (e.g., increased caloric expenditure, enhanced cardiovascular fitness, low potential adverse effects) and enhance compliance (e.g., low perceived exertion, minimal cost, and convenience).

An emphasis on regular, moderate-intensity physical activity rather than on vigorous exercise is reasonable in sedentary persons. This emphasis encourages a variety of self-directed, moderate-level physical activities (e.g., walking or cycling to work, taking the stairs, raking leaves, mowing the lawn with a power mower, cycling for pleasure, swimming, racket sports) that can be more easily incorporated into an individual's daily routine. An appropriate short-term goal is activity that is a small increase over current levels. Over a period of several months, progression to a level of activity that achieves cardiovascular fitness (e.g., 30 minutes of brisk walking most days of the week) would be ideal. Development and maintenance of muscular strength and joint flexibility is also desirable. Sporadic exercise, especially if extremely vigorous in an otherwise sedentary individual, should be discouraged in favor of moderate-level activities performed consistently.

56. Counseling to Promote a Healthy Diet

RECOMMENDATION

Counseling adults and children over age 2 to limit dietary intake of fat (especially saturated fat) and cholesterol, maintain caloric balance in their diet, and emphasize foods containing fiber (i.e., fruits, vegetables, grain products) is recommended. There is insufficient evidence to recommend for or against counseling the general population to reduce dietary sodium intake or increase dietary intake of iron, beta-carotene, or other antioxidants to improve health outcomes, but recommendations to reduce sodium intake may be made on other grounds. Women should be encouraged to consume recommended quantities of calcium (see Clinical Intervention). Parents should be encouraged to breast-feed their infants. Providing pregnant women with specific nutritional guidelines to enhance fetal and maternal health is recommended. Although there is insufficient evidence to recommend for or against special assessment of the dietary needs and habits of older adults, recommendations to do so can be made on other grounds. There is insufficient evidence that nutritional counseling by physicians has an advantage over counseling by dietitians or community interventions in changing the dietary habits of patients. See Chapter 22 regarding the role of iron during pregnancy and in the diets of newborns and young children, and Chapter 42 regarding the use of folic acid by women of childbearing age. See Chapter 61 regarding intake of refined sugars and adherent carbohydrates that may affect dental health. Counseling regarding alcohol consumption is discussed in Chapter 52.

CLINICAL INTERVENTION

Adults and children over age 2 should limit dietary intake of fat (especially saturated fat) ("A" recommendation) and cholesterol ("B" recommendation), maintain caloric balance in their diet ("B" recommendation), and emphasize fruits, vegetables, and grain products containing fiber ("B" recommendation). Both diet and exercise should be designed to achieve and maintain a desirable weight by keeping caloric intake balanced with energy expenditures. Adolescents and adults, in particular, should reduce total fat intake to less than 30% of total calories and dietary cholesterol to less than 300 mg/day. Saturated fat consumption should be reduced to less than 10% of total calories. To achieve these goals, patients should emphasize consumption of fish, poultry prepared without skin, lean meats, and low-fat dairy products. They should be encouraged to eat a variety of foods, with emphasis on the consumption of whole grain products and cereals, legumes, vegetables, and fruits. Current recommendations from the United States Department of Health and Human Services are for at least five servings of fruits and vegetables and at least six servings of breads, cereals, or legumes each day. Detailed food selection guidelines for healthy eating are published elsewhere.

There is insufficient evidence that, for the general population, reducing dietary sodium intake or increasing dietary intake of iron, beta-carotene, or other antioxidants results in improved health outcomes ("C" recommendation); recommendations to reduce sodium intake may be made on other grounds, including the potential beneficial effects on blood pressure in salt-sensitive persons. See Chapter 61 for information regarding intake of refined sugars and dental health. Women should be encouraged to consume recommended quantities of calcium (adolescents and young adults, 1200-1500 mg/day; adults aged 25-50, 1000 mg/day; postmenopausal women, 1000-1500 mg/day; pregnant and nursing women, 1200-1500 mg/day) ("B" recommendation). Parents should be encouraged to offer breast-feeding to their infants ("A" recommendation). Pregnant women should receive specific nutritional guidelines to enhance fetal and maternal health. See Chapter 22 regarding the role of iron during pregnancy and in the diets of newborns and young children, and see Chapter 42 regarding the use of folic acid by women of childbearing age. There is insufficient evidence to recommend for or against the special assessment of dietary needs and habits of older adults ("C" recommendation), but recommendations to do so can be made on other grounds, such as the increased prevalence of nutrition-related disorders in this age group. Counseling regarding alcohol consumption is discussed in Chapter 52.

There is insufficient evidence that nutritional counseling by physicians, as opposed to counseling by dietitians or community interventions, is effective in changing the dietary habits of patients ("C" recommendation). Clinicians who lack the time or skills to perform a complete dietary history, to address potential barriers to changes in eating habits, and to offer specific guidance on meal planning and food selection and preparation, should either have patients seen by other trained providers in the office or clinic or should refer patients to a registered dietitian or qualified nutritionist for further counseling.

57. Counseling to Prevent Motor Vehicle Injuries

RECOMMENDATION

Counseling all patients, and the parents of young patients, to use occupant restraints (lap/shoulder safety belts and child safety seats), to wear helmets when riding motorcycles, and to refrain from driving while under the influence of alcohol or other drugs is recommended (see Clinical Intervention). There is currently insufficient evidence to recommend for or against counseling patients to prevent pedestrian injuries. See Chapter 58 for recommendations on the prevention of bicycling injuries.

CLINICAL INTERVENTION

Clinicians should regularly urge their patients to use lap/shoulder belts for themselves and their passengers, and for their children who have outgrown safety seats, whenever driving or riding in an automobile, including automobiles equipped with air bags ("A" recommendation for wearing seat belts; "B" recommendation for counseling). Operators of vehicles carrying infants and toddlers should be urged to install and regularly use federally approved child safety seats in accordance with the manufacturer's instructions and the child's size ("A" recommendation for child safety seat use; "B" recommendation for counseling parents). Passengers should not ride in the cargo beds of pickup trucks. Passengers also should not ride in the cargo areas of station wagons or vans except when those areas are fitted with passenger seats and passengers are properly restrained in them with seat belts or child safety seats as appropriate for age. Clinicians may wish to inform their patients of the effectiveness of air bags as a supplement to lap/shoulder belt use in reducing motor vehicle crash-related morbidity and mortality. Rear-facing infant seats should not be placed in the front seat of a car equipped with a passenger-side air bag. Although forward-facing infant seats can be used in this situation, clinicians may wish to inform parents that the safest seating position in the car is the middle of the rear seat. Those who operate or ride on motorcycles should be counseled to wear approved safety helmets; this recommendation is based on the proven efficacy of risk reduction from wearing helmets ("A" recommendation), although the effectiveness of clinician counseling to increase helmet use has not yet been evaluated ("C" recommendation). Recommendations for bicyclists appear in Chapter 58.

All patients should be counseled regarding the dangers of operating a motor vehicle while under the influence of alcohol or other drugs, as well as the risks of riding in a vehicle operated by someone who is under the influence of these substances. This recommendation is based on the proven efficacy of risk reduction ("A" recommendation) and the effectiveness of counseling problem drinkers to reduce alcohol consumption ("B" recommendation) (see Chapter 52); the effectiveness of counseling patients to avoid drinking and driving has not been evaluated ("C" recommendation). Adolescents and young adults in particular should be encouraged to avoid using alcohol or other drugs when driving is anticipated and to discuss with their families transportation alternatives for social activities where alcohol and other drugs are used (also see Chapters 52 and 53). The optimal frequency for counseling patients about motor vehicle injury has not been determined and is left to clinical discretion. Counseling is most important for those at increased risk of motor vehicle injury, such as adolescents and young adults, persons who use alcohol or other drugs, and patients with medical conditions that may impair motor vehicle safety.

There is currently insufficient evidence to recommend for or against counseling patients or their parents in order to reduce pedestrian injuries ("C" recommendation). Recommendations for such counseling for elderly patients and for the parents of school-age and younger children may be made on other grounds, including high burden of suffering, low cost, and lack of adverse effects. One measure that may reduce pedestrian injury risk is wearing brightly colored or reflective clothing to increase visibility to motorists. Educating parents to recognize the developmental limitations on the pedestrian skills of young children and provide appropriate supervision in situations that place children at risk for pedestrian injuries may also be effective in reducing pedestrian injury risk. Although there is insufficient evidence to recommend for or against counseling regarding problem drinking and alcohol use specifically to prevent pedestrian injury ("C" recommendation), such counseling can be recommended on other grounds (see Chapter 52).

58. Counseling to Prevent Household and Recreational Injuries

RECOMMENDATION

Periodic counseling of the parents of children on measures to reduce the risk of unintentional household and recreational injuries is recommended. Counseling to prevent household and recreational injuries is also recommended for adolescents and adults based on the proven efficacy of risk reduction, although the effectiveness of counseling these patients to prevent injuries has not been adequately evaluated. Persons with alcohol or drug problems should be identified, counseled, and monitored (see Chapters 52 and 53). Those who use alcohol or illicit drugs should be warned against engaging in potentially dangerous activities while intoxicated.

Counseling elderly patients on specific measures to prevent falls is recommended based on fair evidence that these measures reduce the risk of falls, although the effectiveness of counseling elders to prevent falls has not been adequately evaluated. More intensive individualized multifactorial intervention is recommended for high-risk elderly patients in settings where adequate resources to deliver such services are available. There is insufficient evidence to recommend for or against the use of external hip protectors to prevent fall injuries. Counseling to prevent motor vehicle and pedestrian injuries is discussed in Chapter 57.

CLINICAL INTERVENTION

Counseling the parents of children on measures to reduce the risk of unintentional injuries from residential fires and hot tap water, drowning, poisoning, bicycling, firearms, and falls is recommended ("B" recommendation). Persons with alcohol or drug problems should be identified, counseled, and monitored, and referred for treatment as appropriate (see Chapters 52 and 53); all adolescents and adults who use alcohol or other drugs should be advised to avoid engaging in potentially dangerous activities (e.g., swimming, boating, handling of firearms, smoking in bed, hunting, bicycling) while intoxicated ("B" recommendation). Counseling regarding other measures to prevent household and recreational injuries is recommended for adolescent and adult (including elderly) patients based on fair evidence for the efficacy of risk reduction ("B" recommendation), although the effectiveness of such counseling has not been adequately evaluated ("C" recommendation). The need to prevent household or recreational injuries should be discussed regularly with patients, although the optimal frequency for such counseling has not been determined and is left to clinical discretion. Clinicians should remain alert to the possibility of abuse or neglect as the etiology of certain household and recreational injuries (see Chapter 51). Illicit drug use, an important risk factor for adolescent and adult poisonings, is discussed in Chapter 53. See also Chapter 50 (Screening for Suicide Risk), Chapter 57 (Counseling to Prevent Motor Vehicle Injuries), and Chapter 59 (Counseling to Prevent Youth Violence).

Specific recommendations to prevent injuries to children include the following measures, many of which are also likely to be effective in preventing injuries to adolescents and adults (including elderly persons). Homeowners should be advised to install smoke detectors in appropriate locations and to test the devices periodically to ensure proper operation. Infants and children should wear flame-resistant nightwear during sleep. Smokers should be advised to cease or reduce smoking (see Chapter 54). Hot water heaters should be set at 120°-130° F. Parents, grandparents, or other patients with children in the home should be advised to keep a 1-ounce bottle of syrup of ipecac, to display the telephone number of the local poison control center, and to place all medications, toxic substances, and matches in child-resistant containers. Bicyclists and parents of children who ride bicycles should be counseled about the importance of wearing approved safety helmets and avoiding riding in motor vehicle traffic. Children and adolescents who ride all-terrain vehicles, and their parents, should be advised to use approved safety helmets and four-wheeled (rather than three-wheeled) machines with smaller engines. Families should be encouraged to install 4-foot four-sided isolation fences with self-latching, self-closing gates around swimming pools, and window guards on windows in buildings that pose high risk for falls. Swimming pool owners and individuals living with or caring for young children or elderly persons should be encouraged to learn cardiopulmonary resuscitation and maneuvers to manage choking incidents. Although there is at present only limited evidence to support removing firearms from the home or keeping them unloaded in a locked compartment for the prevention of unintentional injuries, this intervention can be recommended based on its efficacy for the prevention of violent injuries (see Chapters 50 and 59). Additional interventions likely to be effective but for which there is currently limited evidence of benefit include: avoiding smoking near bedding or upholstery and unsafe handling of smoking materials, installing collapsible gates or other barriers to stairway entrances, observing safe boating practices and wearing personal flotation devices while boating, and wearing orange fluorescent clothing while hunting. Poison-warning stickers intended to deter children from playing with containers of medicine or other poisons (e.g., "Mr. Yuk" stickers) have been found to be ineffective and are not recommended ("D" recommendation).

Counseling elderly patients on measures to reduce the risk of falling, including exercise (particularly training to improve balance), safety-related skills and behaviors, and environmental hazard reduction, along with monitoring and adjusting medications, is recommended based on fair evidence that these measures reduce the likelihood of falling ("B" recommendation), although the effectiveness of routinely counseling elders to prevent falls has not been adequately evaluated ("C" recommendation). Recommendations for regular physical activity in elderly patients without contraindications can also be made based on other proven benefits (see Chapter 55). Intensive individualized home-based multifactorial intervention to reduce the risk of falls is recommended for high-risk elderly patients in settings where adequate resources are available to deliver such services ("B" recommendation). Elderly persons at high risk for falls include those aged 75 years and older; or aged 70-74 with one or more additional risk factors including: use of certain psychoactive and cardiac medications (e.g., benzodiazepines, antihypertensives); use of ≥ 4 prescription medications; impaired cognition, strength, balance, or gait. There is insufficient evidence to recommend for or against the routine use of external hip protectors to prevent fall injuries ("C" recommendation). Once these devices become generally available, recommendations for their use in institutionalized elderly may be made on other grounds, including the large potential benefit and limited adverse effects. There is insufficient evidence to recommend for or against postfall assessment and intervention in institutionalized elderly persons in order to prevent falls ("C" recommendation), but recommendations for such interventions may be made on the basis of other benefits, including reduced hospitalizations and hospital days unrelated to falls. For other recommendations relevant to fall injuries in the elderly, see Chapter 33 (Screening for Visual Impairment), Chapter 46 (Screening for Postmenopausal Osteoporosis), Chapter 48 (Screening for Dementia), Chapter 55 (Counseling to Promote Physical Activity), and Chapter 68 (Postmenopausal Hormone Prophylaxis).

59. Counseling to Prevent Youth Violence

RECOMMENDATION

There is insufficient evidence to recommend for or against clinician counseling of asymptomatic adolescents and adults to prevent morbidity and mortality from youth violence. Adolescent and adult patients should be screened for problem drinking (see Chapter 52). Clinicians should also be alert for symptoms and signs of drug abuse and dependence (see Chapter 53), the various presentations of family violence (see Chapter 51), and suicidal ideation in persons with established risk factors (see Chapter 50).

CLINICAL INTERVENTION

There is currently insufficient evidence to recommend for or against clinician counseling to prevent morbidity and mortality from youth violence ("C" recommendation). Adolescent and adult patients should be screened for problem drinking (see Chapter 52). Clinicians may wish to inform patients (and the parents of child and adolescent patients) of the risk to household members associated with the presence of firearms in the home. Clinicians should also be alert for symptoms and signs of drug abuse and dependence (see Chapter 53), the various presentations of family violence (see Chapter 51), and suicidal ideation in persons with established risk factors (see Chapter 50).

In settings where the prevalence of violence is high, clinicians should ask adolescents and young adults about previous violent behavior or victimization, current alcohol and drug use, and the availability of handguns and other firearms. Clinicians should inform those identified as being at high risk for violence about the risks of violent injury associated with easy access to firearms and with intoxication with alcohol or other drugs.

60. Counseling to Prevent Low Back Pain

RECOMMENDATION

There is insufficient evidence to recommend for or against counseling patients to exercise to prevent low back pain, but recommendations for regular physical activity can be made based on other proven benefits (see Chapter 55). There is also insufficient evidence to recommend for or against the routine use of educational interventions, mechanical supports, or risk factor modification to prevent low back pain (see Clinical Intervention).

CLINICAL INTERVENTION

Although there is some evidence that exercise (flexion, extension, aerobic, or fitness) protects against the development of low back pain, the effect is modest and of unknown duration, and the interventions have not been demonstrated in typical clinical settings. Thus, there is insufficient evidence to recommend for or against counseling patients to exercise specifically to prevent low back pain ("C" recommendation). Recommendations for regular physical activity can be made on other grounds, including its proven efficacy in preventing coronary heart disease, hypertension, obesity, and diabetes (see Chapter 55). There is insufficient evidence to recommend for or against educational interventions or the use of mechanical supports in the prevention of low back pain ("C" recommendation). Given some evidence that mechanical supports may increase the risk of low back pain, recommendations can be made against their use except in the context of comprehensive programs where their use can be carefully monitored to avoid injury. There is insufficient evidence to recommend for or against risk factor modification specifically for the prevention of low back pain ("C" recommendation). Screening for obesity (see Chapter 21) and counseling to prevent tobacco use (see Chapter 54) are recommended based on proven benefits unrelated to low back pain.

Work site screening and job placement practices are beyond the scope of this report.

61. Counseling to Prevent Dental and Periodontal Disease

RECOMMENDATION

Counseling patients to visit a dental care provider on a regular basis, floss daily, brush their teeth daily with a fluoride-containing toothpaste, and appropriately use fluoride for caries prevention and chemotherapeutic mouth rinses for plaque prevention is recommended based on evidence for risk reduction from these interventions. Educating parents to curb the practice of putting infants and children to bed with a bottle is also recommended based on limited evidence of risk reduction. The effectiveness of clinician counseling to change any of these behaviors has not been adequately evaluated. Appropriate dietary fluoride supplements are recommended for children living in communities with inadequate water fluoridation. While examining the oral cavity, clinicians should be alert for obvious signs of oral disease (see Clinical Intervention). Screening for oral cancer is discussed in Chapter 16, and recommendations regarding counseling to promote healthful diets are provided in Chapter 56.

CLINICAL INTERVENTION

Counseling patients to visit a dental care provider on a regular basis is recommended based on evidence for risk reduction from such visits when combined with regular personal oral hygiene ("B" recommendation); the effectiveness of advising patients to visit a dental care provider has not been evaluated ("C" recommendation). There is little evidence regarding the optimal frequency of visits; this recommendation should be made by the patient's dental care provider. Counseling all patients to brush their teeth daily with a fluoride-containing toothpaste and to clean thoroughly between their teeth with dental floss each day is recommended based on the proven efficacy of risk reduction from doing so ("B" recommendation); the effectiveness of clinician counseling to encourage these behaviors has not been adequately evaluated ("C" recommendation). Parents of small children should be encouraged to perform or supervise their children's brushing and to monitor the amount of toothpaste used; wiping the teeth with a piece of gauze or damp cloth is typically recommended for cleaning the teeth of children who are too young to use a toothbrush. Parents of infants and young children should be encouraged to breast-feed (see Chapter 56). Providing advice to parents to put infants and children to bed without a bottle may reduce the risk of baby bottle tooth decay ("B" recommendation). See Chapter 56 for other recommendations regarding counseling to promote a healthy diet.

Clinicians caring for children should ascertain the fluoride concentration of their water supply. For children living in an area with inadequate water fluoridation (<0.6 parts per million [ppm]), the prescription of daily fluoride drops or tablets is recommended ("A" recommendation). According to recently revised guidelines, in communities with a water fluoride concentration of less than 0.3 ppm, the recommended dose is 0.25 mg/day for children 6 months to 3 years of age, 0.50 mg/day for children aged 3-6, and 1.0 mg/day for children aged 6-16. In areas with a water fluoride level of 0.3-0.6 ppm, fluoride supplementation is not recommended for children 6 months to 3 years of age. For older children, the recommended dose is 0.25 mg/day for children aged 3-6 and 0.50 mg/day for children aged 6-16. Some groups have issued more conservative recommendations that limit fluoride supplementation to children age 3 and older living in communities with water fluoride concentrations of less than 0.3 ppm.

When examining the oral cavity, clinicians should be alert for obvious signs of untreated tooth decay or mottling, inflamed or cyanotic gingiva, loose teeth, and severe halitosis, and for signs and symptoms of oral cancer or premalignancy in persons who use tobacco or excessive amounts of alcohol (see Chapter 16). All patients should be counseled to avoid the use of tobacco products (see Chapter 54). When examining children, clinicians should be alert for evidence of early childhood caries (baby bottle tooth decay), mismatching of upper and lower dental arches, crowding or malalignment of the teeth, premature loss of primary posterior teeth (baby molars), and obvious mouth breathing. Patients with these or other suspected abnormalities should be referred to appropriate specialists for further evaluation.

62. Counseling to Prevent HIV Infection and Other Sexually Transmitted Diseases

RECOMMENDATION

All adolescent and adult patients should be advised about risk factors for human immunodeficiency virus (HIV) infection and other sexually transmitted diseases (STDs), and counseled appropriately about effective measures to reduce the risk of infection (see Clinical Intervention). Counseling should be tailored to the individual risk factors, needs, and abilities of each patient. This recommendation is based on the proven efficacy of risk reduction, although the effectiveness of clinician counseling in the primary care setting is uncertain. Individuals at risk for specific STDs should be offered testing in accordance with recommendations on screening for syphilis, gonorrhea, hepatitis B virus infection, HIV infection, and chlamydial infection (see Chapters 24, 26-29). Injection drug users should be advised about measures to reduce their risk and referred to appropriate treatment facilities (see Chapter 53).

CLINICAL INTERVENTION

All adolescent and adult patients should be advised about risk factors for STDs and counseled appropriately about effective measures to reduce risk of infection ("B" recommendation). This recommendation is based on the proven efficacy of risk reduction, although the effectiveness of clinician counseling in the primary care setting has not been evaluated adequately ("C" recommendation). Counseling should be tailored to the individual risk factors, needs, and abilities of each patient. Assessment of risk should be based on a careful sexual and drug use history and consideration of the local epidemiology of STDs. Sexual history should include questions about number and nature of current and past sex partners (including same-sex partners or partners who have injected drugs), any history of past STD infections, the use of condoms or other barrier protection, and particular high-risk sexual practices such as anal intercourse. Patients at risk of STDs should receive information on their risk and be advised about measures to reduce their risk. Effective measures include abstaining from sex, maintaining a mutually faithful monogamous sexual relationship with a partner known to be uninfected, regular use of latex condoms, and avoiding sexual contact with casual partners and high-risk individuals (e.g., injection drug users, commercial sex workers, and persons with numerous sex partners).

Patients who have sex with multiple partners, casual partners, or other persons who may be infected should be advised to use a latex condom at each encounter and to avoid anal intercourse. Condoms need not be recommended to prevent infection in long-standing, mutually monogamous relationships in which neither partner is an injection drug user or is infected with HIV. Patients using condoms should be informed about the importance of using them in accordance with recommended guidelines:

- Handle condoms carefully to avoid damaging with fingernails or sharp objects.
- Use a new condom in good condition for each act of intercourse.
- Place the condom on an erect penis before any intimate contact and unroll completely to the base.
- Leave a space at the tip of the condom and remove air pockets in the space.
- Ensure adequate lubrication during intercourse. Water-based lubricants (e.g., K-Y jelly, spermicidal foam or gel) should be used. Petroleum jelly, mineral oil, hand lotion, baby oil, cold cream, massage oil, and other oil-based lubricants should not be used because they may damage latex condoms.
- Hold condom firmly against base of penis during withdrawal, and withdraw while the penis is still erect so that the condom remains in place.

Women at risk of STDs should be advised of options to reduce their risk in situations when their male partner does not use a condom, including the female condom. Women should be informed that spermicides and female barrier methods (diaphragm or cervical cap) can reduce the risk of gonorrhea and chlamydia but are not likely to be as effective as properly used male condoms, and their effectiveness against HIV and other STDs remains unproven. Pregnant women at risk of STDs should be informed of the potential risks to the fetus of HIV and other sexually transmitted infections (chlamydia, gonorrhea, syphilis, hepatitis B, and herpes) and the importance of being screened for HIV and other STDs during pregnancy.

Advice should be provided as appropriate that using alcohol or drugs can lead to high-risk sexual behavior. Persons who inject drugs should be referred to available drug treatment facilities, warned against sharing drug equipment, and, where possible, referred to sources for uncontaminated injection equipment and condoms. Drug users should be advised of the importance of being tested for HIV, of using condoms regularly with both casual and steady partners, and of following specific steps to reduce the risk of transmitting infection during preparation and injection of drugs (see Chapter 53). All patients at risk for STDs should be offered testing in accordance with recommendations on screening for syphilis, gonorrhea, HIV infection, and chlamydial infection (see Chapters 26-29) and should receive hepatitis B vaccine (see Chapter 66).

63. Counseling to Prevent Unintended Pregnancy

RECOMMENDATION

Periodic counseling about effective contraceptive methods is recommended for all women and men at risk for unintended pregnancy (see Clinical Intervention). Counseling should be based on information from a careful sexual history and should take into account the individual preferences, abilities, and risks of each patient. Sexually active patients should also receive information on measures to prevent sexually transmitted diseases (see Chapter 62).

CLINICAL INTERVENTION

Periodic counseling about effective contraceptive methods is recommended for all women and men at risk for unintended pregnancy ("B" recommendation). Counseling should be based on information from a careful history that includes direct questions about sexual activity, current and past use of contraception, level of concern about pregnancy, and past history of unintended pregnancies. Counseling should take into account the individual preferences, concerns, abilities, and risks of each patient and his or her partner, including risk of STDs (see Chapter 62). Counseling should include a discussion of the risk associated with the patient's current contraceptive practice and, when indicated, available alternatives for more effective contraception. Clinicians should inform adolescent patients that abstinence is the most effective way to prevent unintended pregnancy and STDs, although the effectiveness of abstinence counseling has not been established.

Clear instructions should be provided for the proper use of recommended contraceptive techniques. Hormonal contraceptives, barrier methods used with spermicides, and IUDs should be recommended as the most effective reversible means of preventing pregnancy in sexually active persons. Sexual abstinence, the maintenance of a mutually faithful monogamous sexual relationship, and consistent use of condoms should be emphasized as important measures to reduce the risk of STDs (see Chapter 62). Clinicians should monitor satisfaction and compliance of patients with any chosen form of contraception.

Empathy, confidentiality, and a nonjudgmental, supportive attitude are especially important when discussing issues of sexuality with adolescents. Clinicians should involve young pubertal patients (and their parents, where appropriate) in early, open discussion of sexual development and effective methods to prevent unintended pregnancy and STDs. Clinicians should explore attitudes and expectations of adolescents and other patients who are not currently involved in a sexual relationship to anticipate future need for contraception, and inform them how to obtain information and contraception if they plan to begin engaging in sexual intercourse. Preferably, adolescents should be examined without their parent(s) present. Clinicians providing birth control for minors should take into consideration both the confidentiality of the doctor-patient relationship as well as local legal restrictions when deciding whether to notify parents before prescribing contraception. The optimal frequency of counseling to prevent unintended pregnancy is unknown and is left to clinical discretion.

64. Counseling to Prevent Gynecologic Cancers

RECOMMENDATION

There is insufficient evidence to recommend for or against routine counseling of women about measures for the primary prevention of gynecologic cancers. Clinicians counseling women about contraceptive practices should include information on the potential benefits of oral contraceptives, barrier contraceptives, and tubal sterilization with respect to specific gynecologic cancers (see Chapter 63). Clinicians should also promote other practices (maintaining desirable body weight, smoking cessation, and safe sex practices) that may reduce the incidence of certain gynecologic cancers and have other proven health benefits (see Chapters 21, 54, and 62).

CLINICAL INTERVENTION

There is insufficient evidence to recommend for or against routine counseling of female patients about measures to reduce the risk of cervical, ovarian, and endometrial cancer ("C" recommendation). Clinicians counseling women about contraceptive practices should include information about the potential benefits of specific methods with respect to gynecologic cancers (see Chapter 63). These potential benefits include reduced risks of ovarian and endometrial cancer in women using oral contraceptives, cervical cancer in women who use barrier contraception and spermicides, and ovarian cancer after tubal sterilization. All women should be counseled about effective means to prevent STDs (see Chapter 62) and about the benefits of breast-feeding (see Chapter 56), avoiding obesity (see Chapter 21), and avoiding tobacco use (see Chapter 54).

Part D
IMMUNIZATIONS AND CHEMOPROPHYLAXIS
65. Childhood Immunizations

RECOMMENDATION

All children without established contraindications should receive diphtheria-tetanus-pertussis (DTP), oral poliovirus (OPV), measles-mumps-rubella (MMR), conjugate *Haemophilus influenzae* type b, hepatitis B, and varicella vaccines, in accordance with recommended schedules (see Clinical Intervention). Hepatitis A vaccine is recommended for children and adolescents at high risk for hepatitis A virus (HAV) infection. Pneumococcal vaccine and annual influenza vaccine are recommended for children and adolescents at high risk (see Clinical Intervention and Chapter 66). See Chapter 67 for recommendations on postexposure prophylaxis against selected infectious diseases, and Chapter 25 for recommendations regarding the Bacille Calmette-Guérin (BCG) vaccine.

CLINICAL INTERVENTION

All children without established contraindications should receive diphtheria-tetanus-pertussis (DTP), oral poliovirus (OPV), measles-mumps-rubella (MMR), conjugate *H. influenzae* type b (Hib), hepatitis B, and varicella vaccines ("A" recommendation).

The recommended childhood immunization schedule includes *DTP vaccine* at ages 2 months, 4 months, and 6 months; DTP at 12-18 months or DTaP at 15-18 months; and DTP or DTaP between ages 4 and 6 years, just prior to school entry. A combined tetanus-diphtheria (Td) booster should be administered at age 11-12 years (14-16 years is an acceptable alternative) and periodically in adulthood (see Chapter 66). *OPV vaccine* is recommended at ages 2 months, 4 months, 6-18 months, and 4-6 years.

MMR vaccine should be administered at age 12-15 months and again at 4-6 years of age; 11-12 years is an acceptable alternative for the second dose. Giving the first dose at 15 months may be preferable when compliance with a visit at this age is assured, because efficacy and immunogenicity are slightly higher than at 12 months. Children over 6 years of age who present for care and have not yet received two doses of measles vaccine should be vaccinated with MMR, with the goal that all children will have had two doses of measles or MMR vaccine by 11-12 years of age.

Hib conjugate vaccine should be given at 2, 4, and 6 months (HbOC or PRP-T) or 2 and 4 months (PRP-OMP), with a booster dose at 12-15 months of age using any of the conjugate vaccines. While giving a single conjugate Hib vaccine for the primary series is preferred because of proven clinical efficacy, there is good evidence for the safety and immunogenicity of heterogenous Hib conjugate vaccine series. Therefore, immunization at the recommended intervals (2, 4, 6, and 12-15 months) should not be delayed by efforts to determine the type of vaccine previously received. When this information is unavailable, any of the conjugate vaccines approved for use in infants may be given to complete the series. Licensed combined vaccines (e.g., DTP-HbOC [Tetramune]*) may be substituted for the relevant individual vaccines in cases where both vaccines would normally be given in order to reduce the total number of injections given.

Hepatitis B vaccine is recommended for all infants and for all children and adolescents not previously immunized, particularly those in high-risk populations (see Chapters 24 and 66). For infants, the first dose is recommended at 0-2 months (preferably prior to hospital discharge), the second dose 1-2 months after the first, and the third dose at 6-18 months (preferably at least 4 months after the second dose). Giving hepatitis B vaccine at 0, 1, 2, and 12 months of age is also acceptable. After infancy, the vaccine schedule is at the current visit and 1 and 6 months later. Clinicians may wish to inform parents that booster doses may be required in the future to maintain immunity through adolescence and adulthood.

Varicella vaccine, administered subcutaneously in one 0.5-ml dose, is recommended for routine use in healthy children 12-18 months of age, and in children under age 13 with no reliable history of varicella infection or previous immunization. Clinicians should inform parents that varicella disease in adulthood is associated with increased risk of serious complications, the duration of immunity provided by varicella vaccine has not been established, and booster doses of the vaccine may be required to maintain protection throughout adulthood. Two doses of vaccine delivered 4-8 weeks apart are recommended for healthy adolescents ≥13 years of age with no reliable history of varicella infection or previous vaccination. Given the relatively high prevalence of immunity in adolescents with no history of chickenpox and the results of cost-effectiveness analysis, clinicians may wish to offer serologic testing for varicella susceptibility to history-negative adolescents ≥13 years who are likely to comply with return visits.

Clinicians may wish to conduct an assessment of immunization status for all children at age 11-12, in particular to determine whether the patient needs

---

*Use of trade names is for identification only and does not imply endorsement by the Public Health Service or the US Department of Health and Human Services.

Td, MMR, varicella, or hepatitis B vaccines. Clinicians are referred to published guidelines for details on vaccine contraindications, instructions for immunizing children with medical disorders (including human immunodeficiency virus infection), and modified protocols recommended during community outbreaks or epidemics or for children with delayed immunization.

Hepatitis A vaccine is recommended for all high-risk children aged ≥2 years and all high-risk adolescents ("A" recommendation). High-risk groups include persons living in, traveling to, or working in areas where the disease is endemic and periodic outbreaks occur (e.g., countries with high or intermediate endemicity, Alaska Native, Pacific Islander, and Native American communities, certain religious communities) (see Chapter 66 for additional high-risk groups and recommendations for adult immunization). Hepatitis A vaccination may also be considered for institutionalized persons (e.g., those living in chronic care facilities). Where tracking or identification of high-risk patients is not practical or cost-effective, universal vaccination may be a reasonable policy given the minimal adverse consequences of the vaccine. At this writing, the only licensed hepatitis A vaccine is Havrix (SmithKline Beecham Pharmaceuticals).* Three doses (360 ELISA units/dose), administered intramuscularly, are recommended for persons aged 2-18 years; the second and third doses are given 1 and 6-12 months after the first dose. The need for periodic booster doses has not been established. For persons requiring immediate protection against hepatitis A (e.g., travelers to high-risk areas who have not previously been vaccinated), IG (0.02 ml/kg) should be given simultaneously with the first dose of hepatitis A vaccine, although the clinical efficacy of this approach has not been established. IG can also be recommended as an efficacious intervention for short-term (≤5-6 months) preexposure prophylaxis against hepatitis A (see Chapter 67). While some evidence suggests that the vaccine may be more efficacious than IG, the clinical efficacies of the two regimens have not been directly compared in clinical trials. Other factors to consider in choosing between the two interventions are patient preference, the likely frequency and duration of exposure, the need for immediate protection, and cost.

Annual *influenza vaccine* is recommended for adolescents and children ≥6 months of age who are residents of chronic care facilities or have chronic cardiopulmonary disorders, metabolic diseases (including diabetes mellitus), hemoglobinopathies, immunosuppression, or renal dysfunction ("B" recommendation) (see Chapter 66 for the review of evidence regarding influenza vaccine). Split-virus vaccine is recommended for children ≤12 years; the recommended vaccine dose is 0.25 ml for children 6-35 months of age and 0.5 ml for children ≥3 years of age. Amantadine and rimantadine prophylaxis against influenza A is discussed in Chapter 66.

Pneumococcal vaccine is recommended for immunocompetent adolescents and children (≥2 years of age) with chronic cardiac or pulmonary disease, diabetes mellitus, and anatomic asplenia (excluding sickle cell disease), and those living in special environments or social settings with an identified increased risk of pneumococcal disease (e.g., certain Native American and Alaska Native populations) ("B" recommendation) (see Chapter 66 for the review of evidence regarding pneumococcal vaccine). Routine revaccination is not recommended, but it may be appropriate to consider periodic revaccination in immunocompetent individuals at highest risk for morbidity and mortality from pneumococcal disease (e.g., those with severe chronic disease) who were vaccinated more than 5 years previously. There is insufficient evidence to recommend for or against pneumococcal vaccine as an efficacious vaccine for immunocompromised children ≥2 years of age, but recommendations for vaccinating these persons may be made on other grounds, including high incidence and mortality rates of pneumococcal disease and minimal adverse effects from vaccine ("C" recommendation). Examples of immunocompromised conditions associated with high risk for pneumococcal disease include acquired or congenital immunodeficiency (including HIV infection), sickle cell disease, nephrotic syndrome, chronic renal failure, metastatic or hematologic malignancy, and other conditions associated with immunosuppression, such as organ transplant. It may be appropriate to consider periodic revaccination in these patients, who are likely to have poor initial antibody response and rapid decline of antibodies after vaccination.

See Chapter 25 (Screening for Tuberculous Infection) for recommendations regarding the BCG vaccine. Recommendations on postexposure prophylaxis against selected infectious diseases, including tetanus, hepatitis A, hepatitis B, and Hib, are given in Chapter 67.

---

*Use of trade names is for identification only and does not imply endorsement by the Public Health Service or the US Department of Health and Human Services.

66. Adult Immunizations—Including Chemoprophylaxis Against Influenza A

RECOMMENDATION

Annual influenza vaccine is recommended for all persons aged 65 and older and persons in selected high-risk groups (see Clinical Intervention). Pneumococcal vaccine is recommended for all immunocompetent individuals who are age 65 years and older or otherwise at increased risk for pneumococcal disease (see Clinical Intervention). There is insufficient evidence to recommend for or against pneumococcal vaccine for high-risk immunocompromised individuals, but recommendations for vaccinating these persons may be made on other grounds. The series of combined tetanus-diphtheria toxoids (Td) should be completed for adults who have not received the primary series, and all adults should receive periodic Td boosters. Vaccination against measles and mumps should be provided to all adults born after 1956 who lack evidence of immunity. A second measles vaccination is recommended for adolescents and young adults in settings where such individuals congregate (e.g., high schools and colleges). See Chapter 32 for recommendations for rubella vaccine. Hepatitis B vaccine is recommended for all young adults not previously immunized and for all persons at high risk for infection (see Clinical Intervention). Hepatitis A vaccine is recommended for persons at high risk for hepatitis A virus (HAV) infection (see Clinical Intervention). Varicella vaccine is recommended for susceptible adults (see also Chapter 65). See Chapter 25 for recommendations regarding the Bacille Calmette-Guérin (BCG) vaccine. Recommendations for postexposure prophylaxis against selected infectious diseases are in Chapter 67; see also Chapter 24, Screening for Hepatitis B Virus Infection.

CLINICAL INTERVENTION

Influenza vaccine should be administered annually to all persons ages 65 and older and to persons 6 months of age or older who are residents of chronic care facilities or suffer from chronic cardiopulmonary disorders, metabolic diseases (including diabetes mellitus), hemoglobinopathies, immunosuppression, or renal dysfunction ("B" recommendation). Influenza vaccine is also recommended for health care providers for high-risk patients ("B" recommendation). In persons at high risk for influenza A (e.g., during institutional outbreaks), amantadine or rimantadine prophylaxis (200 mg/day orally) may be started at the time of vaccination and continued for 2 weeks ("B" recommendation). A lower dose (≤100 mg/day) of amantadine is recommended for persons with reduced creatinine clearance and those 65 years of age and older. A reduced dosage (100 mg/day) of rimantadine is indicated for those with reduced renal or hepatic function and for elderly nursing home residents and may also be necessary in healthy persons 65 years and older who experience side effects. Amantadine and rimantadine are most useful as short-term prophylaxis for high-risk persons who have not yet received the vaccine or are vaccinated after influenza A activity in the community has already begun; when the vaccine may be ineffective owing to major antigenic changes in the virus; for unimmunized persons who provide care for high-risk persons; to supplement protection provided by vaccine in persons who are expected to have a poor antibody response; and for high-risk persons in whom the vaccine is contraindicated (i.e., those with anaphylactic hypersensitivity to egg protein). If vaccine is contraindicated, amantadine or rimantadine should be started at the beginning of the influenza season and continued daily for the duration of influenza activity in the community.

Pneumococcal vaccine is recommended for all immunocompetent individuals who are aged 65 years and older or otherwise at increased risk for pneumococcal disease ("B" recommendation). High-risk groups include institutionalized persons ≥50 years of age, persons ≥2 years of age with certain medical conditions, including chronic cardiac or pulmonary disease, diabetes mellitus, and anatomic asplenia (excluding sickle cell disease), and persons ≥2 years of age who live in special environments or social settings with an identified increased risk of pneumococcal disease (e.g., certain Native American and Alaska Native populations). Routine revaccination is not recommended, but it may be appropriate to consider revaccination in immunocompetent individuals at highest risk for morbidity and mortality from pneumococcal disease (e.g., persons ≥75 years of age or with severe chronic disease) who were vaccinated more than 5 years previously. Revaccination with the 23-valent vaccine may be appropriate for high-risk persons who previously received the 14-valent vaccine. There is insufficient evidence to recommend for or against pneumococcal vaccine as an efficacious vaccine for immunocompromised individuals, but recommendations for vaccinating these persons may be made on other grounds, including high incidence and case-fatality rates of pneumococcal disease and minimal adverse effects from the vaccine ("C" recommendation). Immunocompromised conditions associated with high risk for pneumococcal disease include alcoholism, cirrhosis, chronic renal failure, nephrotic syndrome, sickle cell disease, multiple myeloma, metastatic or hematologic malignancy, acquired or congenital immunodeficiency (including HIV infection), and other conditions associated with immunosuppression, such as organ transplant. It may be appropriate to consider periodic revaccination in these high-risk immunocompromised patients, who are likely to have poor initial antibody response and rapid decline of antibodies after vaccination.

The *Td vaccine* series should be completed for patients who have not received the primary series, and all adults should receive periodic Td boosters ("A" recommendation). For persons not previously immunized, the recommended schedule for the primary Td series is 0, 2, and 8-14 months. The optimal interval for booster doses is not established. The standard regimen is to provide a Td booster at least once every 10 years, but in the United States, intervals of 15-30 years between boosters are likely to be adequate in persons who received a complete five-dose series in childhood (see Chapter 65). For international travelers, an interval of 10 years between boosters is recommended.

MMR vaccine should be administered to all persons born after 1956 who lack evidence of immunity to measles (receipt of live vaccine on or after the first birthday, laboratory evidence of immunity, or a history of physician-diagnosed measles) ("A" recommendation). A second measles vaccination is recommended for adolescents and young adults in settings where such individuals congregate (e.g., high schools, technical schools, and colleges), if they have not previously received a second dose (see Chapter 65) ("B" recommendation). The combined MMR vaccine is preferable to monovalent measles vaccine, since many recipients may also be susceptible to mumps or rubella because of inadequate vaccination or primary vaccine failure. Susceptible individuals should be vaccinated against mumps ("B" recommendation). Administration of the MMR or measles vaccine during pregnancy is not recommended. See Chapter 32 for recommendations on rubella screening and vaccination.

Hepatitis B vaccine is recommended for all young adults not previously immunized ("A" recommendation). Hepatitis B vaccine is also recommended for susceptible adults in high-risk groups, including men who have sex with men, injection drug users and their sex partners, persons who have a history of sexual activity with multiple partners in the previous 6 months or have recently acquired another sexually transmitted disease, international travelers to countries where HBV is of high or intermediate endemicity, recipients of certain blood products (including hemodialysis patients), and persons in health-related jobs with frequent exposure to blood or blood products ("A" recommendation). The recommended regimen for the recombinant hepatitis B vaccine is to administer 10 or 20 μg (depending on vaccine product) intramuscularly in the deltoid muscle at the current visit and at 1 and 6 months later. Clinicians should consider testing antibody response to the vaccine in individuals at very high risk from hepatitis B who are likely to have an inadequate antibody response (i.e., chronic renal dialysis patients, injection drug users, HIV-infected patients). Recommendations on screening for HBV infection and prevention of perinatal transmission are in Chapter 24. Recommendations for persons with possible percutaneous or sexual exposure to individuals infected with hepatitis B virus are in Chapter 67.

Hepatitis A vaccine is recommended for all high-risk adults ("B" recommendation). High-risk groups include persons living in, traveling to, or working in areas where the disease is endemic and periodic hepatitis A outbreaks occur (e.g., Alaska Native, Pacific Islander, and Native American communities, certain religious communities, countries with high or intermediate endemicity), men who have sex with men, users of injection or street drugs (depending on local epidemiology), military personnel, and certain hospital and laboratory workers. Hepatitis A vaccine may also be considered for institutionalized persons (e.g., in prisons and institutions for the developmentally disabled) and workers in these institutions and in day care centers. Where tracking or identification of high-risk patients is not practical or cost-effective, universal vaccination may be a reasonable policy given the minimal adverse consequences of the vaccine. At this writing, the only licensed hepatitis A vaccine is Havrix (SmithKline Beecham Pharmaceuticals).* Two doses (1440 ELISA units/dose) at 0 and 6-12 months are recommended for persons over age 18 years. The need for periodic booster doses of the vaccine has not been established. For persons requiring immediate protection against hepatitis A (e.g., travelers to high-risk areas who have not previously been vaccinated), clinicians may wish to consider giving IG simultaneously with the first dose of hepatitis A vaccine, although the clinical efficacy of this approach has not been established. IG can also be recommended as an efficacious intervention for short-term (≤5-6 months) preexposure prophylaxis against hepatitis A (see Chapter 67). While some evidence suggests that the vaccine may be more efficacious than IG, the clinical efficacies of these two interventions have not been directly compared. Other factors to consider in choosing between these two interventions include patient preference, the likely duration of exposure, the need for immediate versus long-term protection, and cost.

Two doses of *varicella vaccine* delivered 4-8 weeks apart are recommended for healthy adults with no history of varicella infection or previous vaccination ("B" recommendation) (see Chapter 65 for the

---

*Use of trademarks is for identification only and does not imply endorsement by the Public Health Service or the US Department of Health and Human Services.

review of evidence regarding varicella vaccine). Vaccination efforts should be targeted to susceptible health care workers and family contacts of immunocompromised individuals, and may also be targeted to susceptible adults who live or work in environments with a high likelihood of varicella transmission (e.g., day care centers, residential institutions, colleges, military bases). Given the high prevalence of immunity in adults with no history of chickenpox and the results of cost-effectiveness analysis (see Chapter 65), clinicians may wish to offer serologic testing for varicella susceptibility to history-negative adults who are likely to comply with return visits.

See Chapter 25 for recommendations regarding the Bacille Calmette-Guérin (BCG) vaccine. Recommendations on postexposure prophylaxis against selected infectious diseases, including tetanus, hepatitis A, and hepatitis B, are given in Chapter 67.

67. Postexposure Prophylaxis for Selected Infectious Diseases

RECOMMENDATION

Postexposure prophylaxis should be provided to selected persons with exposure or possible exposure to *Haemophilus influenzae* type b, hepatitis A, hepatitis B, meningococcal, rabies, or tetanus pathogens (see Clinical Intervention). See Chapter 66 for recommendations on postexposure prophylaxis against influenza A.

CLINICAL INTERVENTION

Postexposure prophylaxis is recommended for selected persons with exposure or possible exposure to *H. influenzae* type b, hepatitis A, hepatitis B, meningococcal, rabies, or tetanus pathogens ("A" recommendation). Details are given below.

H. influenzae Type b Disease. Oral rifampin prophylaxis should be prescribed promptly for patients with Hib disease and for all their household contacts regardless of age, if at least one of the contacts is a child less than 4 years of age who has not been fully vaccinated with a licensed Hib conjugate vaccine. Experts define a household contact as a person residing with the index patient or a nonresident who spent 4 hours or more with the index patient for at least 5 of the 7 days preceding the day of hospital admission of the index patient. The dosage of rifampin for children and adults is 20 mg/kg (maximum 600 mg) as a single daily dose for 4 days. The dose for infants younger than 1 month of age has not been established, but experts recommend reducing the dose to 10 mg/kg/day. Published guidelines also recommend postexposure prophylaxis for all day care attendees and staff, regardless of vaccination status, when 2 or more cases have occurred within 60 days and unvaccinated or incompletely vaccinated children attend. When a single case has occurred in a day care center, rifampin prophylaxis should be given to all attendees and staff only if unvaccinated or incompletely vaccinated children less than 2 years of age are present in the center for at least 25 hours per week. Day care contacts of children with Hib disease should receive rifampin prophylaxis using the same regimen as for household contacts. All children who are less than 5 years of age and who are unvaccinated or incompletely vaccinated should be brought up to date by administration of the recommended doses of a licensed Hib conjugate vaccine (see Chapter 65).

Hepatitis A. Immune globulin should be administered at a dose of 0.02 ml/kg IM as soon as possible within 2 weeks of exposure to sexual and close household contacts of persons with hepatitis A, staff and children at day care centers where a hepatitis A case is recognized, staff and patients at custodial institutions where HAV transmission is documented, and food handlers at food service establishments where a food handler is diagnosed with hepatitis A. Detailed published protocols are available. Hepatitis A vaccine is recommended for persons ≥2 years of age who are at high risk for infection (see Chapters 65 and 66).

Hepatitis B. The use of HBIG and hepatitis B vaccine is recommended to prevent HBV infection in the following circumstances: birth of an infant to a hepatitis B surface antigen (HB$_s$Ag)-positive mother (see Chapter 24), percutaneous or permucosal exposure to HB$_s$Ag-positive blood, sexual exposure to an HB$_s$Ag-positive person, and household exposure of an infant less than 1 year of age to a primary caregiver who has acute HBV infection. For needle sticks and other percutaneous exposures, and for sexual exposures, the precise protocol for postexposure prophylaxis against hepatitis B depends on the nature of the exposure, the availability from the source of exposure of blood for testing, the HB$_s$Ag status of the source, and the hepatitis B vaccination and vaccine-response status of the exposed person. Detailed guidelines are available. See Chapter 24 for detailed recommendations on prenatal screening and perinatal postexposure prophylaxis against HBV infection, and Chapters 65 and 66 for recommendations regarding routine use of hepatitis B vaccine in children and adults.

Meningococcal Infection. Oral rifampin prophylaxis is indicated for household or day care contacts of persons with meningococcal infection, as well as for those with direct exposure to oral secretions (e.g., kissing) of an index patient. The dose is 600 mg for adults, 10 mg/kg for children 1-12 years of age, and 5 mg/kg for infants 3 months to 1 year of age, given twice daily for 2 days (for a total of four doses). Rifampin is contraindicated during pregnancy. There is currently insufficient evidence to recommend for or against the use of ceftriaxone for routine meningococcal prophylaxis ("C" recommendation). Ceftriaxone at a dose of 250 mg IM for adults and 125 mg IM for children is efficacious for eliminating meningococcal carriage of serogroup A strains of meningococcus. In outbreaks caused by serogroup A strains, the use of meningococcal vaccine is recommended in addition to antibiotic prophylaxis for all persons ≥3 months of age. In outbreaks caused by serogroup C, Y, and W-135 strains, vaccination is recommended for persons ≥2 years of age.

Rabies. Postexposure prophylaxis against rabies should be instituted if a possible exposure to rabies has occurred. Criteria for making this assessment, which include the type of animal (e.g., carnivorous wild animals, bats), the circumstances of the attack (e.g., unprovoked attack), and the type of exposure (e.g., bite), are available in published guidelines and from local health departments. HRIG is given at a dose of 20 IU/kg; half of the dose is infiltrated around the wound, and the remainder is given intramuscularly at another site. The upper outer gluteal region of the buttocks is preferred because of the large volume administered. HDCV or RVA is administered in the deltoid muscle in five 1.0 ml injections on days 0, 3, 7, 14, and 28. Persons who were immunized before the incident require only two 1.0 ml doses of vaccine on days 0 and 3, and do not require HRIG. Preexposure prophylaxis with three injections (1.0 ml IM or 0.1 ml intradermally) of vaccine (days 0, 7, and 21 or 28) is recommended for those at high risk of contact with rabies virus, including rabies laboratory workers, veterinarians, animal handlers, and persons planning to spend more than 1 month in countries where rabies is endemic. Persons with frequent exposure should have their antibody level checked every 6 months and receive booster injections if antibody titers are below protective levels. Published guidelines suggest more frequent testing for certain continuously exposed laboratory workers.

Tetanus. All individuals who have not completed a primary vaccination series of at least three doses and who present with wounds should receive 0.5 ml IM adsorbed tetanus toxoid. Diphtheria and tetanus toxoids and whole-cell or acellular pertussis vaccine adsorbed (DTP or DTaP, respectively) or diphtheria and tetanus toxoids adsorbed (DT) (as appropriate) for patients less than 7 years old and tetanus and diphtheria toxoids adsorbed (Td) for patients ≥7 years old, are preferred so that adequate levels of diphtheria and pertussis immunity are maintained (see Chapters 65 and 66). For a wound that is serious and/or contaminated (e.g., with dirt, feces), the incompletely vaccinated patient should receive both vaccine and human TIG (250 units IM at a separate site). Although there is inadequate evidence on which to make a recommendation for or against TIG prophylaxis for clean, minor wounds in inadequately immunized persons, experts recommend against the routine use of human TIG. For individuals presenting with a wound who have completed a primary vaccination series of at least three doses, tetanus toxoid is recommended if more than 10 years have elapsed since the last dose or if only three doses of fluid toxoid (which was used prior to the availability of adsorbed toxoid) were received. There is insufficient evidence to document increased risk after a shorter interval for major or contaminated wounds, but expert opinion supports vaccination when more than 5 years have elapsed. Human TIG is not recommended for persons who have completed a primary vaccination series. All wounds should be properly cleaned and débrided.

Influenza. See Chapter 66 for recommendations regarding the use of amantadine and rimantadine to protect against influenza A.

68. Postmenopausal Hormone Prophylaxis

RECOMMENDATION

Counseling all perimenopausal and postmenopausal women about the potential benefits and risks of hormone prophylaxis is recommended. There is insufficient evidence to recommend for or against hormone therapy for all postmenopausal women. Women should participate fully in the decision-making process, and individual decisions should be based on patient risk factors for disease, clear understanding of the probable benefits and risks of hormone therapy, and patient preferences (see Clinical Intervention).

CLINICAL INTERVENTION

Clinicians should counsel all women around the time of menopause about the possible benefits and risks of postmenopausal hormone therapy and the available treatment options ("B" recommendation). Counseling should include asking about presence and severity of menopausal symptoms (hot flashes, urogenital symptoms), as well as assessing risk factors for heart disease, osteoporosis, and breast cancer. Women should be advised of the probable benefits of hormone therapy on menopausal symptoms, myocardial infarction, and fracture; the increased risks of endometrial cancer with unopposed estrogen; and a possible increased risk of breast cancer. Each woman should consider the relative importance of these benefits and risks, the possible side effects of treatment, and her willingness to take medication for an indefinite period.

Women considering estrogen therapy should be counseled about the available estrogen and progestin preparations and routes of administration. The minimum effective dose of estrogen is 0.625 mg conjugated estrogen or the equivalent once a day. For women who have not had a hysterectomy, progestin therapy or regular endometrial surveillance is recommended to reduce risk of endometrial cancer. The most common progestin regimens include a continuous regimen of daily administration of 2.5 mg medroxyprogesterone acetate (MPA) or equivalent, or a cyclic regimen of 5-10 mg MPA daily for 10-14 days each month. Transdermal estrogen preparations are effective in relieving menopausal symptoms and preventing osteoporosis, but they have less effect on lipids and are of undetermined benefit against heart disease.

All women should receive information about potential alternatives to hormones for treating menopausal symptoms (e.g., vaginal lubricants for dyspareunia, etc.), for preventing osteoporosis (see Chapter 46) and for reducing their risk of heart disease, including screening for high cholesterol (see Chapter 2) and hypertension (see Chapter 3) and counseling to prevent tobacco use and promote physical activity and healthy diet (see Chapters 54-56).

69. Aspirin Prophylaxis for the Primary Prevention of Myocardial Infarction

RECOMMENDATION

There is insufficient evidence to recommend for or against routine aspirin prophylaxis for the primary prevention of myocardial infarction (MI) in asymptomatic persons. Although aspirin reduces the risk of MI in men ages 40-84, its use is associated with important adverse effects, and the balance of benefits and harms is uncertain. If aspirin prophylaxis is considered, clinicians and patients should discuss potential benefits and risks for the individual before beginning its use (see Clinical Intervention).

CLINICAL INTERVENTION

There is insufficient evidence to determine whether the proven benefits of routine aspirin prophylaxis given for the primary prevention of MI in asymptomatic men ages 40 to 84 years outweigh the proven harms, and thus the US Preventive Services Task Force does not recommend for or against its use ("C" recommendation). In men with other risk factors for coronary heart disease who lack contraindications to aspirin use (including allergy to aspirin, history of uncontrolled hypertension, liver or kidney disease, diabetic retinopathy, peptic ulcer or other gastrointestinal disease, bleeding problems, or other risk factors for bleeding or cerebral hemorrhage), the benefits may outweigh the harms. In asymptomatic men without risk factors for coronary heart disease or with relative contraindications to aspirin use, the harms may outweigh the benefits. If aspirin therapy is considered, physicians and patients should understand the potential benefits and risks of aspirin therapy before beginning treatment. At the present time, data are insufficient to support or oppose the use of aspirin prophylaxis for the prevention of MI in women ("C" recommendation). All patients should be encouraged to focus their efforts on modifying primary risk factors for cardiovascular disease such as smoking (Chapter 54), elevated cholesterol (Chapters 2 and 56), and hypertension (Chapter 3).

70. Aspirin Prophylaxis in Pregnancy

RECOMMENDATION

There is insufficient evidence to recommend for or against the routine use of aspirin to prevent preeclampsia or intrauterine growth retardation in pregnant women, including those at high risk (see Clinical Intervention).

CLINICAL INTERVENTION

There is insufficient evidence to recommend for or against routine aspirin prophylaxis in pregnancy for the prevention of either preeclampsia ("C" recommendation) or intrauterine growth retardation ("C" recommendation). Clinicians may wish to inform patients at high risk of preeclampsia that aspirin prophylaxis has been shown to decrease this risk, but such patients should also be informed that aspirin has not been proven to improve overall fetal or maternal outcomes, that one large trial raised the possibility of an increased risk of abruptio placentae, and that aspirin can have additional unpleasant and occasionally serious side effects.

SECTION VI

Review of Medical Literature

The following summaries and editorials are reprinted from the Year Book series published by Mosby–Year Book, Inc., St. Louis, 1997. Materials are grouped by Year Book and organized alphabetically by journal article author.

CONTENTS

YEAR BOOK OF CARDIOLOGY, 901
Edited by: Schlant RC, Collins JJ, Gersh BJ, Graham T, Kaplan NM, Waldo AL

Borghi C et al: Factors Associated with the Development of Stable Hypertension in Young Borderline Hypertensives, 901

Gill JB et al: Prognostic Importance of Myocardial Ischemia Detected by Ambulatory Monitoring Early after Acute Myocardial Infarction, 901

Grossman E et al: Should a Moratorium Be Placed on Sublingual Nifedipine Capsules Given for Hypertensive Emergencies and Pseudoemergencies?, 903

Howard G: Insulin Sensitivity and Atherosclerosis, 903

Williams PT: High-Density Lipoprotein Cholesterol and Other Risk Factors for Coronary Heart Disease in Female Runners, 904

YEAR BOOK OF FAMILY PRACTICE, 905
Edited by: Berg AO, Bowman MA, Davidson RC, Dexter WW, Scherger JE

Abrams SA et al: Absorption by 1-Year-Old Children of an Iron Supplement Given with Cow's Milk or Juice, 905

Ettinger B et al: Reduced Mortality Associated with Long-Term Postmenopausal Estrogen Therapy, 905

Hahn SR et al: The Difficult Patient: Prevalence, Psychopathology, and Functional Impairment, 906

Hemminki E, Meriläinen J: Long-Term Effects of Cesarean Sections: Ectopic Pregnancies and Placental Problems, 907

Hyams JS et al: Abdominal Pain and Irritable Bowel Syndrome in Adolescents: A Community-Based Study, 907

Jamieson DJ, Steege JF: The Prevalence of Dysmenorrhea, Dyspareunia, Pelvic Pain, and Irritable Bowel Syndrome in Primary Care Practices, 908

Joorabchi B, Devries JM: Evaluation of Clinical Competence: The Gap Between Expectation and Performance, 909

Kristiansson P et al: Back Pain During Pregnancy: A Prospective Study, 910

Liberthson RR: Sudden Death from Cardiac Causes in Children and Young Adults, 911

Muller JE: Triggering Myocardial Infarction by Sexual Activity: Low Absolute Risk and Prevention by Regular Physical Exertion, 911

Saigal S et al: Self-Perceived Health Status and Health-Related Quality of Life of Extremely Low-Birth-Weight Infants at Adolescence, 913

Sharpe M et al: Cognitive Behaviour Therapy for the Chronic Fatigue Syndrome: A Randomised Controlled Trial, 913

Werler MM et al: Prepregnant Weight in Relation to Risk of Neural Tube Defects, 914

Ytterstad B: The Harstad Injury Prevention Study: The Epidemiology of Sports Injuries. An 8-Year Study, 915

YEAR BOOK OF GERIATRICS AND GERONTOLOGY, 915
Edited by: Burton JR, Beck JC, Otswald SK, Rabins PV, Reuben DB, Roth J, Shapiro JR, Whitehouse PJ

Bergstrom N et al: Multi-Site Study of Incidence of Pressure Ulcers and the Relationship between Risk Level, Demographic Characteristics, Diagnoses, and Prescription of Preventive Interventions, 915

Graafmans WC et al: Falls in the Elderly: A Prospective Study of Risk Factors and Risk Profiles, 917

Jonker C et al: Memory Complaints and Memory Impairment in Older Individuals, 918

Moore AA, Siu AL: Screening for Common Problems in Ambulatory Elderly: Clinical Confirmation of a Screening Instrument, 919

Nichol KL et al: Immunizations in Long-Term Care Facilities: Policies and Practice, 921

Strawbridge WJ et al: Successful Aging: Predictors and Associated Activities, 922

Tamblyn RM et al: Do Too Many Cooks Spoil the Broth? Multiple Physician Involvement in Medical Management of Elderly Patients and Potentially Inappropriate Drug Combinations, 923

YEAR BOOK OF MEDICINE, 924
Edited by: Klahr S, Cline MJ, Petty TL, Frishman WH, Greenberger NJ, Malawista SE, Mandell GL, O'Rourke RA

Becker U et al: Prediction of Risk of Liver Disease by Alcohol Intake, Sex, and Age: A Prospective Population Study, 924

Bhatia S et al: Malignant Neoplasms Following Bone Marrow Transplantation, 926

Brivet FG et al: Acute Renal Failure in Intensive Care Units—Causes, Outcome, and Prognostic Factors of Hospital Mortality: A Prospective, Multicenter Study, 927

Cavill I: Guidelines for the Prevention and Treatment of Infection in Patients with an Absent or Dysfunctional Spleen, 928

Diabetes Control and Complications Trial Research Group: Effects of Intensive Diabetes Therapy on Neuropsychological Function in Adults in the Diabetes Control and Complications Trial, 929

Fort JM et al: Bowel Habit after Cholecystectomy: Physiological Changes and Clinical Implications, 930

Fries JF et al: Reduction in Long-Term Disability in Patients with Rheumatoid Arthritis by Disease-Modifying Antirheumatic Drug-Based Treatment Strategies, 931

Gabbay FH et al: Triggers of Myocardial Ischemia during Daily Life in Patients with Coronary Artery Disease: Physical and Mental Activities, Anger, and Smoking, 932

Gray-Donald K et al: Nutritional Status and Mortality in Chronic Obstructive Pulmonary Disease, 933

Grodstein F et al: Postmenopausal Estrogen and Progestin Use and the Risk of Cardiovascular Disease, 934

Halm EA: Echocardiography for Assessing Cardiac Risk in Patients Having Noncardiac Surgery, 935

Harding SM et al: Asthma and Gastroesophageal Reflux: Acid Suppressive Therapy Improves Asthma Outcome, 936

Hatala R et al: Once-Daily Aminoglycoside Dosing in Immunocompetent Adults: A Meta-Analysis, 937

Hylek EM et al: An Analysis of the Lowest Effective Intensity of Prophylactic Anticoagulation for Patients with Non-Rheumatic Atrial Fibrillation, 937

Jaakkola MS et al: Effect of Passive Smoking on the Development of Respiratory Symptoms in Young Adults: An 8-Year Longitudinal Study, 938

Jones DC, Hayslett JP: Outcome of Pregnancy in Women with Moderate or Severe Renal Insufficiency, 939

Klag MJ et al: Blood Pressure and End-Stage Renal Disease in Men, 939

Leibowitz G et al: Pre-Clinical Cushing's Syndrome: An Unexpected Frequent Cause of Poor Glycemic Control in Obese Diabetic Patients, 940

Niskanen LK et al: Evolution, Risk Factors, and Prognostic Implications of Albuminuria in NIDDM, 941

Papazian L et al: Effect of Ventilator-Associated Pneumonia on Mortality and Morbidity, 942

Peters RK et al: Long-Term Diabetogenic Effect of Single Pregnancy in Women with Previous Gestational Diabetes Mellitus, 943

Smith JA et al: Pregnancy in Sickle Cell Disease: Experience of the Cooperative Study of Sickle Cell Disease, 944

Stefanski A et al: Early Increase in Blood Pressure and Diastolic Left Ventricular Malfunction in Patients with Glomerulonephritis, 944

Thompson WH et al: Controlled Trial of Oral Prednisone in Outpatients with Acute COPD Exacerbation, 945

Tynell E et al: Acyclovir and Prednisolone Treatment of Acute Infectious Mononucleosis: A Multicenter, Double-Blind, Placebo-Controlled Study, 946

van Boven AJ: Reduction of Transient Myocardial Ischemia with Pravastatin in Addition to the Conventional Treatment in Patients with Angina Pectoris, 947

YEAR BOOK OF NEUROLOGY AND NEUROSURGERY, 947
Edited by: Bradley WG, Wilkins RH

Evans SC et al: MRI of 'Idiopathic' Juvenile Scoliosis: A Prospective Study, 947

Knudsen FU et al: Long-Term Outcome of Prophylaxis for Febrile Convulsions, 948

YEAR BOOK OF OBSTETRICS, GYNECOLOGY, AND WOMEN'S HEALTH, 948
Edited by: Mishell DR, Herbst AL, Kirschbaum TH

Baird DD et al: Vaginal Douching and Reduced Fertility, 948

Bucher HC et al: Effect of Calcium Supplementation on Pregnancy-Induced Hypertension and Preeclampsia: A Meta-Analysis of Randomized Controlled Trials, 949

Creinin MD et al: Methotrexate and Misoprostol for Early Abortion: A Multicenter Trial. I. Safety and Efficacy, 950

Newell M-L et al: Detection of Virus in Vertically Exposed HIV-Antibody-Negative Children, 952

Nygaard IE et al: Efficacy of Pelvic Floor Muscle Exercises in Women with Stress, Urge, and Mixed Urinary Incontinence, 952

Petitti DB et al: Stroke in Users of Low-Dose Oral Contraceptives, 954

Rossing MA et al: Oral Contraceptive Use and Risk of Breast Cancer in Middle-Aged Women, 955

Scott LL et al: Acyclovir Suppression to Prevent Cesarean Delivery after First-Episode Genital Herpes, 956

van der Schouw YT et al: Age at Menopause as a Risk Factor for Cardiovascular Mortality, 956

YEAR BOOK OF PULMONARY DISEASE, 958
Edited by: Petty TL

Bonnefoi H, Smith IE: How Should Cancer Presenting as a Malignant Pleural Effusion Be Managed?, 958

Leatherman JW et al: Muscle Weakness in Mechanically Ventilated Patients with Severe Asthma, 959

Mooe T et al: Sleep-Disordered Breathing in Men with Coronary Artery Disease, 960

Pépin J-L et al: Long-Term Oxygen Therapy at Home: Compliance with Medical Prescription and Effective Use of Therapy, 961

Prandoni P et al: The Long-Term Clinical Course of Acute Deep Venous Thrombosis, 962

Renkema TEJ et al: Effects of Long-Term Treatment with Corticosteroids in COPD, 963

YEAR BOOK OF CARDIOLOGY

FACTORS ASSOCIATED WITH THE DEVELOPMENT OF STABLE HYPERTENSION IN YOUNG BORDERLINE HYPERTENSIVES

Borghi C, Costa FV, Boschi S, et al (Univ of Bologna, Italy)
J Hypertens 14:509-517, 1996

Objective. Although individuals with borderline hypertension frequently progress to stable hypertension, the factors leading to this progression in young individuals, in particular, have not been well studied. Therefore, a prospective analysis of relationships between individual characteristics and development of stable hypertension in a group of young borderline hypertensives was performed.

Methods. Questionnaires regarding family history of hypertension or diabetes mellitus, physical activity, and drinking and smoking habits were administered to 70 non–diet-restricted individuals (average age, 23 years) whose diastolic blood pressure was 10 mm Hg below and 10 mm Hg above 90 mm Hg on at least two occasions. Intracellular sodium level, baseline blood pressure, blood pressure responses to stress, and sensitivity to sodium chloride infusion was determined. Individuals were monitored for an average of 120 months, followed for 10 years, and re-examined to determine the presence of stable hypertension and to establish its prognostic factors.

Results. The percentages of individuals whose diastolic blood pressure increased above 95 mm Hg after 1, 3, 5, 7, and 10 years were 4.3%, 11.4%, 17.1%, 22.8%, and 35.8%, respectively. Borderline hypertensives who progressed to stable hypertension were older (26.9 vs. 21.0 years), had a family history of high blood pressure (92% vs. 64%), were hyperreactors (46% vs. 29%), and were salt sensitive (72% vs. 53%) compared with those who did not develop stable hypertension.

Conclusions. Multivariate analysis showed that in borderline hypertensives, age, salt-sensitivity, hyper-reactivity to stress, a family history of hypertension, and higher intracellular sodium levels are related to the development of stable hypertension. The presence of four or five risk factors identified those at high risk for stable hypertension with a sensitivity of 72%, a specificity of 67%, and an accuracy of 76%.

Commentary

These data are among the few that look prospectively over a reasonably long period (10 years) at the impact of various mechanisms on the progression of hypertension in the absence of interventions. A fundamental, but not fatal, flaw in this study is the manner of selecting the participants with "borderline" hypertension: five sets of blood pressure recordings over 6 months with diastolic blood pressure on at least two occasions below 80 mm Hg and on at least two occasions above 100 mm Hg. These represent considerable variability, but such variability really is not uncommon in patients with "established" hypertension.

Nonetheless, blood pressure tended to elevate significantly in 25 of the 70, and the two groups were compared as to their various features and responses to multiple tests. Beyond the effects of age and family history, sodium sensitivity and intracellular sodium concentration as well as the pressor response to mental stress, were predictive of a rise in blood pressure. Unfortunately, no measures of lipids or insulin/glucose were included; these might have furnished additional predictive power.

The take-home message is that sodium is involved and, unlike response to stress, it can be fairly easily manipulated. Another nail in the coffin of those who say that salt intake is irrelevant.

PROGNOSTIC IMPORTANCE OF MYOCARDIAL ISCHEMIA DETECTED BY AMBULATORY MONITORING EARLY AFTER ACUTE MYOCARDIAL INFARCTION

Gill JB, Cairns JA, Roberts RS, et al
(McMaster Univ, Hamilton, Ont, Canada)
N Engl J Med 334:65-70, 1996

Background. After acute myocardial infarction, survivors are at risk for recurrent infarction, death, and unstable angina for some time. The exercise test is the most common diagnostic test for residual ischemia but cannot be performed in many high risk patients. Detection of myocardial ischemia by ambulatory ECG monitoring could reveal important prognostic information in these patients.

Purpose. The purpose of this study was to determine the incidence of residual myocardial ischemia detected by ambulatory ECG monitoring in survivors of acute myocardial infarction and the prognostic value of this information.

Study Design. The study group consisted of 406 patients from three institutions who had survived acute myocardial infarction for at least 5 days. The average age of these patients was 62 years, and 78% were men. Five to 7 days after infarction, these patients underwent 48 hour ambulatory ECG monitoring, submaximal exercise testing and measurement of left ventricular ejection fraction within 28 days. The study group was followed for 1 year and nonfatal myocardial infarction, hospital admission for unstable angina, and death were study end points.

Findings. The overall 1-year mortality rate was 6%, the rate of death or nonfatal myocardial infarction was 13%, and the rate of death, nonfatal myocardial infarction, or hospital admission for unstable angina was 25%. The incidence of myocardial ischemia detected by ambulatory ECG was 23%. The 1-year mortality rate was 12% among patients with ischemia and 4% among patients without detectable ischemia. The 1-year mortality was 4% among patients with a positive exercise test, 3% among those with a negative exercise test, and 16% among those in whom an exercise test could not be performed. The 1-year mortality was 4% among patients with an ejection fraction greater than 50%, 4% among those with an ejection fraction between 35% and 50%, and 18% among those with an ejection fraction less than 35% (Table 4). With death as the end point, multiple logistic regression revealed that no diagnostic test performed after infarction provided more prognostic information than the standard clinical variables. If nonfatal myocardial infarction and admission to hospital for unstable angina were added, ambulatory ECG monitoring was the only test that contributed additional prognostic information.

Conclusions. In a group of survivors of acute myocardial infarction who underwent ambulatory ECG monitoring, exercise stress testing and measurement of left ventricular ejection fraction, only ambulatory ECG monitoring provided additional prognostic information beyond that provided by standard clinical variables. The detection of residual ischemia by ambulatory ECG was associated with more than double the risk of death, nonfatal myocardial infarction, or hospitalization for unstable angina. These results suggest that ambulatory ECG monitoring should be the screening test of choice after acute myocardial infarction and that exercise testing and measurement of left ventricular ejection fraction should be used only as required.

Commentary

The incidence of ischemia on ambulatory ECG monitoring within 5-7 days among patients with Q wave or non–Q wave infarction (including patients with ST-segment depression) was 23%. Fifty-five percent of the patients received thrombolytic therapy. Although the predictive value of this finding for 1-year cardiac death was low, this improved to 44% when recurrent myocardial infarction and unstable angina were included as outcomes. It would appear, therefore, that a subgroup of patients who are clinically stable are nonetheless at high risk for future events, and that such patients with complex or biologically unstable lesions can be detected by ambulatory electrocardiography. This interesting study also points out the very low predictive accuracy of ST-segment depression on exercise, a finding noted in other studies, particularly among patients who have received thrombolytic or acute reperfusion therapy.

Nonetheless, the role of "routine" ambulatory monitoring in our armamentarium of techniques used for risk stratification after myocardial infarction still needs clarification.[1] In this study, ambulatory monitoring provided incremental information over and above that provided by the exercise ECG, particularly in patients who were unable to exercise.

TABLE 4 Joint Prognostic Value of Ambulatory ECG Monitoring and Measurement of the Left Ventricular Ejection Fraction

ASSESSMENT	DEATH	NONFATAL MI OR DEATH	UNSTABLE ANGINA, NONFATAL MI, OR DEATH
	NUMBER OF PATIENTS/TOTAL NUMBER (%)		
Ejection fraction >50%			
No ischemia	6/178 (3.4)	12/178 (6.7)	31/178 (17.4)
Ischemia	2/46 (4.3)	9/46 (19.6)	16/46 (34.8)
Ejection fraction 35%-50%			
No ischemia	1/91 (1.1)	11/91 (12.1)	18/91 (19.8)
Ischemia	3/24 (12.5)	6/24 (25.0)	12/24 (50.0)
Ejection fraction <35%			
No ischemia	3/20 (15.0)	5/20 (25.0)	6/20 (30.0)
Ischemia	3/13 (23.1)	4/13 (30.8)	8/13 (61.5)
Ejection fraction not measured			
No ischemia	2/22 (9.1)	2/22 (9.1)	4/22 (18.2)
Ischemia	3/12 (25.0)	3/12 (25.0)	6/12 (50.0)
P value			
ECG monitoring, given ejection fraction	0.034	0.002	<0.001
Ejection fraction, given ECG monitoring	0.010	0.083	0.13
Interaction	0.40	0.83	0.59

Courtesy of Gill JB, Cairns JA, Roberts RS, et al: Prognostic importance of myocardial ischemia detected by ambulatory monitoring early after acute myocardial infarction, N Engl J Med 334:65-70, 1996. Reprinted by permission of The New England Journal of Medicine. Copyright 1996, Massachusetts Medical Society.
MI, Myocardial infarction.

What is the relationship of ambulatory ECG monitoring to other tests such as stress echocardiography or stress thallium scintigraphy, and what should be the timing and sequence of these tests? What needs to be emphasized is that the "natural" history of myocardial infarction survivors is changing and improving, and this has a major impact on risk stratification. We cannot necessarily extrapolate from data obtained in the 1970s and 1980s in patients who did not receive acute reperfusion therapy, β-blockers, aspirin, angiotensin-converting enzyme inhibitors, etc. to the current patient population. A new database is needed.

SHOULD A MORATORIUM BE PLACED ON SUBLINGUAL NIFEDIPINE CAPSULES GIVEN FOR HYPERTENSIVE EMERGENCIES AND PSEUDOEMERGENCIES?

Grossman E, Messerli FH, Grodzicki T, et al (Chaim Sheba Med Ctr, Tel Hashomer, Israel; Alton Ochsner Med Found, New Orleans, La; Univ School of Medicine, Kraków, Poland; et al)

JAMA 276:1328-1331, 1996

Objective. Although sublingual nifedipine is commonly used to treat hypertensive emergencies, numerous adverse events have been reported and sublingual absorption of the medication has been shown to be negligible. A literature review of the use of sublingual nifedipine for hypertensive emergencies was conducted.

Antihypertensive Efficacy. Nifedipine is a quick-acting calcium antagonist that lowers arterial blood pressure by peripheral vasodilation. The effect peaks in 30 to 60 minutes and lasts about 6 hours. Monitoring of the drug, equally effective in both sexes and all ages, was not recommended initially because blood pressure lowering was thought to be proportional to initial readings and adverse effects were not thought to be life-threatening.

Administration and Absorption. Sublingual absorption is negligible, but intestinal absorption is faster and results in plasma levels 8 times higher than those achieved with buccal absorption.

Adverse Effects. Adverse effects of buccal or oral nifedipine include an abrupt decrease in arterial pressure, resulting in neurologic deficits, that is exacerbated by hypovolemia and the use of other antihypertensive drugs.

Comment. The FDA has concluded after a review of the literature that dose-response and outcome data on oral nifedipine use are lacking. Nifedipine has not been approved for use in hypertension. The effect of nifedipine is primarily cosmetic. It has been used mainly in pseudoemergencies. In legitimate emergencies, nifedipine use is risky because of its unpredictability. These concerns apply to the short-acting form of the drug, rather than the sustained-release form.

Conclusions. Data show that buccal absorption of nifedipine is poor, its effect on blood pressure lowering is unpredictable, it is not approved by the FDA for the treatment of hypertension, and it is being used mainly in pseudoemergencies.

Commentary

The only good that will likely come from the entire calcium channel blocker (CCB) controversy is the recognition of the potential dangers of short-acting nifedipine, given either sublingually or swallowed (where it is even faster and more potent in lowering blood pressure [BP]). Not that it is that dangerous; the authors were able to uncover only 16 cases of adverse effects in their MEDLINE search from 1966 to 1994, during which time probably 1 million patients received sublingual nifedipine.

But their point is correct: "In true hypertensive emergencies, nifedipine capsules are contraindicated because of the unpredictability of the fall in arterial pressure . . . The routine use of short-acting nifedipine . . . should be abandoned."

So what should the physician do when faced with a hypertensive "emergency?" For the few with a real emergency—those with (rapidly advancing) target organ damage (papilledema, encephalopathy), coronary ischemia, or advancing neurologic damage—admission to an ICU and parenteral antihypertensives are needed. For the large majority—who have very high BP but are in no immediate danger—slower-acting but fast enough oral drugs are available, such as a dose of furosemide, an angiotensin-converting enzyme inhibitor, such as captopril (but not a slow-acting one like lisinopril), or a CCB such as isradipine or felodipine (but not a slow-acting one like amlodipine). Give one or more of these agents, keep the patient around for the few hours it takes for the BP to come down to a safe level (around 170/110 mm Hg), start an effective oral regimen of once-a-day, longer-acting agents, and see the patient in a few days to be sure the drugs are working.

Unfortunately, lots of little ladies in nursing homes and 1 in 30 hospitalized patients[1] are being given sublingual nifedipine whenever their BP is a slightly elevated. The practice should stop. Meanwhile, lots of probably invalid case-control studies incriminate short-acting CCBs for everything bad from angina to zits. None of these putative claims apply to long-acting CCBs, which I believe are safe and should be used when indicated.[2]

REFERENCES
1. Rehman F, Mansoor GA, White WB: Inappropriate physician habits in prescribing oral nifedipine capsules in hospitalized patients, *Am J Hypertens* 9:1035-1039, 1996.
2. Kaplan NM: Do calcium antagonists cause death, gastrointestinal bleeding, and cancer? *Am J Cardiol* 78:932-933, 1996.

INSULIN SENSITIVITY AND ATHEROSCLEROSIS

Howard G, for the IRAS Investigators (Wake Forest Univ, Winston-Salem, NC; Tufts-New England Med Ctr, Boston; Univ of Texas, San Antonio; et al)

Circulation 93:1809-1817, 1996

Introduction. It is thought that reduced insulin sensitivity could be an important risk factor in the development of atherosclerosis. The Insulin Resistance Atherosclerosis Study was conducted to evaluate the relationship between insulin sensitivity and atherosclerosis as defined by the intimal-medial thickness (IMT) of the internal carotid artery (ICA) and the common carotid artery (CCA).

Methods. A triethnic population consisting of 398 black, 457 Hispanic, and 542 non-Hispanic white participants were evaluated at four clinical centers. The B-mode ultrasound was used as a noninvasive measure of intimal thickness of the ICA and CCA. Insulin sensitivity was assessed using an insulin-enhanced frequently sampled IV glucose tolerance test.

Results. In this cohort, non-Hispanic white participants were more insulin sensitive and had lower body fat, compared with their black and Hispanic counterparts. Black participants had higher blood pressure and lipid levels and were more likely to be hypertensive or diabetic, compared with Hispanic and non-Hispanic white participants. A significantly negative relationship between insulin sensitivity and the IMT of the CCA was detected in Hispanic and non-Hispanic white, but not black, participants, even after adjusting for glucose tolerance, measures of body fat, and fasting insulin levels. In all ethnic groups, the relationship between insulin sensitivity and the IMT for the ICA was stronger than for the CCA.

Conclusions. Insulin sensitivity is associated with thinner IMT of the CCA wall in non-Hispanic whites and Hispanics. This association remained after adjustment for traditional cardiovascular risk factors. These findings suggest that insulin resistance may have an independent effect on atherogenesis. It is not certain why a relationship between insulin sensitivity and atherosclerosis is not seen in blacks.

Commentary

These cross-sectional data add to the extensive evidence that reduced insulin sensitivity is associated with (and likely a mechanism for) atherosclerosis. The main attractions of this study are, first, its large size, involving 398 black, 457 Hispanic, and 542 non-Hispanic white subjects and, second, its use of a sensitive indicator of pre-overt atherosclerotic disease, measurement of intimal-medial thickness (IMT) by B-mode ultrasonography of the carotid artery.

The association between insulin resistance and arterial thickness was not totally explained by adjustment for usual risk factors and was strong in Hispanics and non-Hispanic whites but not in blacks. As noted in an editorial by Reaven and Chen,[1] this lack of an association in blacks may be explained by a number of factors, including their baseline characteristics of the greatest degrees of IMT, insulin resistance, obesity, diabetes, and hypertension, all of which could reflect a "plateau effect." They were so affected that relationships between degrees of insulin sensitivity and arterial thickness could no longer be identified. Obviously, longitudinal follow-up, as intended, will clarify the issue.

In keeping with this association, a much higher 5-year mortality rate after coronary angioplasty has been noted in type I or type II diabetics who were being treated with oral hypoglycemic agents (which raise endogenous insulin levels) or with exogenous insulin.[2] Diabetics have greater mortality rates after bypass surgery as well, but their even greater mortality rate after angioplasty suggests that the response of a vessel damaged by angioplasty to high levels of insulin is particularly adverse.

REFERENCES

1. Reaven GM, Chen Y-D I: Insulin resistance, its consequences, and coronary heart disease: must we choose a culprit? *Circulation* 93:1780-1783, 1996.
2. Sobel BE: Potentiation of vasculopathy by insulin: implications from an NHLBI clinical alert, *Circulation* 93:1613-1615, 1996.

HIGH-DENSITY LIPOPROTEIN CHOLESTEROL AND OTHER RISK FACTORS FOR CORONARY HEART DISEASE IN FEMALE RUNNERS

Williams PT   *(Lawrence Berkeley Natl Lab, Berkeley, Calif)*
N Engl J Med 334:1298-1303, 1996

Introduction. Guidelines of the Centers for Disease Control and Prevention state that exercising to the energy equivalent of 8-12 km/wk of running (e.g., 2 miles of brisk walking on most days of the week) will provide most of the health benefits that can be gained from physical activity. Subsequent studies have suggested that additional reductions in coronary risk factors are possible for men with a greater level of physical activity. However, it is unknown whether these findings extend to women. Data from the National Runners' Health Study were used to determine whether exercise beyond the current minimal guidelines provides additional health benefits for women.

Methods. The national cross-sectional survey study included information on kilometers run per week by 1837 female recreational runners. Information on height, weight, cholesterol and triglyceride concentrations, blood pressure, and heart rate were obtained from the women's physicians. The analysis sought a dose-response relationship between distance run per week and the coronary risk factors.

Results. Each additional kilometer run per week by the women in the study was associated with a 0.133 ± 0.020 mg/dl increase in plasma high-density lipoprotein (HDL) concentration. This figure was very close to that previously reported for men in the National Runners' Health Study (0.136 ± 0.006 mg/dl). For women who ran distances of less than 48 km/wk, each 16-km increase in distance led to a significantly higher mean HDL cholesterol level. Mean HDL cholesterol levels were significantly higher for women whose distance exceeded 64 km/wk than for those who ran less than 48 km/wk. In addition, they were more likely to have levels greater than 100, 90, or 80 mg/dl. Premenopausal women who were not using oral contraceptives had significantly higher HDL cholesterol levels as distance per week increased. The same was true for postmenopausal women, with or without estrogen replacement therapy.

Conclusions. Women who exercise above currently recommended minimum levels show significant increases in HDL cholesterol levels, which could lead to additional health benefits. The improvement in HDL cholesterol concentration appears to be independent of menstrual status or estrogen replacement therapy. The difference in mean HDL cholesterol concentration between female runners with the shortest and longest distances per week corresponds to a 29% reduction in the risk of coronary heart disease.

Commentary

Recent data from the National Runners' Health Study suggest that physical activity far in excess of the 2 miles of brisk walking on most days or jogging 8-12 km/wk (recommended by the Centers for Disease Control and Prevention)[1] may provide substantial additional reductions in risk factors.[2] This large study in female runners provides additional evidence that a similar and almost identical dose-response relationship between the level of exercise and HDL-cholesterol concentrations occur in women, irrespective of menstrual status. Moreover, there were beneficial effects on other risk factors such as body mass index and waist-hip circumferences. This study does not prove that running is the cause of the favorable effects, but the association is extremely strong and certainly logical. Such information can be used to justify and indeed support a program of high-level exercise in those women who wish to undertake this form of activity.

REFERENCES

1. Pate RR, Pratt M, Blair SN, et al: Physical activity in public health: a recommendation from the Centers for Disease Control and Prevention and the American College of Sports Medicine, *JAMA* 273:402-407, 1995.
2. Williams PT: Lipoproteins and adiposity show improvement at substantially higher exercise levels than those currently recommended, *Circulation* 90: I-4719, 1994.

YEAR BOOK OF FAMILY PRACTICE

ABSORPTION BY 1-YEAR-OLD CHILDREN OF AN IRON SUPPLEMENT GIVEN WITH COW'S MILK OR JUICE

Abrams SA, O'Brien KO, Wen J, et al (*Baylor College of Medicine, Houston; Texas Children's Hosp, Houston*)
Pediatr Res 39:171-175, 1996

Introduction. There is ongoing concern regarding how to ensure an adequate intake of iron in older infants and toddlers. The problem arises when infants are weaned from formula or breast milk, which usually occurs at about 1 year of age. Few studies have examined the best approaches to iron supplementation for toddlers, but there is some evidence that diluting iron supplement with cow's milk may lead to poor absorption. Iron absorption in 1-year-old children was examined with the use of a 2-tracer stable isotope technique.

Methods. Ten children (mean age, 13 months) who had recently stopped taking formula and started taking cow's milk were included. All received doses of 2 stable isotopically enriched ferrous sulfate, ^{57}Fe and ^{58}Fe, which were given with cow's milk and apple juice, respectively. Two weeks later, the infants returned for measurement of red blood cell iron incorporation of the isotope. The iron absorption calculations assumed that 90% of the absorbed iron was incorporated into the red blood cells.

Results. Iron absorption was 14% for the isotope given with juice vs. 6% for the isotope given with milk, according to paired *t* tests. A significant negative correlation was noted between iron absorption from the dose given with apple juice and the infants' serum level of ferritin. Iron absorption was unrelated to levels of hemoglobin or hematocrit.

Conclusions. Iron supplements for toddlers are better absorbed when given with juice rather than cow's milk. Iron absorption varies among 1-year-old children in relation to their existing iron stores. The way in which cow's milk and ascorbic acid influence iron absorption is unknown.

Commentary

This is as "basic science" an article as you are likely to see in the *Year Book*. I chose this article because it addresses a common problem in a sensible way. I know it is not good form to change practice on the basis of a single article, but this article breaks the rule. If you have an infant or toddler who is receiving iron, give the iron with juice rather than milk. Even then, however, there will be substantial variability in absorption because of variation in existing iron stores.

REDUCED MORTALITY ASSOCIATED WITH LONG-TERM POSTMENOPAUSAL ESTROGEN THERAPY

Ettinger B, Friedman GD, Bush T, et al (*Kaiser Permanente Med Care Program, Oakland, Calif; Univ of Maryland, Baltimore*)
Obstet Gynecol 87:6-12, 1996

Background. There is still considerable controversy regarding the relative risks and benefits of postmenopausal estrogen replacement therapy (ERT). Many of the studies have been limited by having no data on the duration of use or dosage, studying the effects of relatively short-term use, and using relatively young subjects. It was hypothesized that increasing age and use would increase both the risks and benefits of ERT. To examine this hypothesis, the effects of ERT were studied in a cohort of women with well-defined and prolonged postmenopausal estrogen use.

Methods. A group of 232 women were identified who had been born between 1900 and 1915, had begun to use at least 0.3 mg of conjugated estrogens within 3 years of menopause, and had used ERT for at least 5 years. A control group of 222 age-matched women who had not used estrogen or had used it for less than 1 year was identified. Their medical records were reviewed to identify demographic data and health risk factors. In those who died during the study period (1980–1993), the cause of death was determined. Age-specific mortality rates were compared in the 2 cohorts and calculated by duration, recency, and dosage of estrogen use. Mortality rates were also adjusted for mortality risk factors.

Results. The 2 groups had similar demographic profiles. The estrogen users were followed up for a mean of 26.8 years, had a mean age in 1993 of 77.6 years, and had used estrogen for a mean of 17.1 years. The nonusers were followed up for a mean of 17.9 years and had a mean age of 77.4 years. The survival benefit in the estrogen users increased significantly with age (Fig 1). Overall, there was a 46% reduction in age-adjusted mortality risk in the ERT group. The relative risk of mortality was 0.48 with at least 15 years of use and 0.69 with less than 15 years of use. Relative risks were 0.48 for current use, 0.18 for recent use, and 0.55 for remote use. The relative mortality risk was lowest in patients using the lowest dosage; there was no association with mortality risk at the highest dosage. Most of the increased survival was related to the reduced mortality from coronary heart disease and cardiovascular disease. There were no statistically significant differences between the 2 groups in mortality from cancer or other causes, although there was a general trend toward lower mortality in the users group.

Conclusions. Long-term estrogen use in aging women was associated with significantly reduced all-cause mortality, which was primarily due to reduced mortality from coronary heart disease and cardiovascular disease. The survival benefit of estrogen use increased with age and with the duration and recency of use, although the benefit continued for several years after the discontinuation of long-term use. The survival benefits of estrogen use were substantial even after adjustment for health risk factors.

Commentary

Another strongly suggestive, but nonrandomized study. Long-term estrogens continued to be associated with lower mortality, with increasing difference between those taking estrogens and those not taking estrogens as years went by. There was very little use of progesterones. These women were compliers—they continued to take estrogens for many years. The nagging question remains whether it was the ability of physicians to choose healthy women for estrogens or the estrogens themselves that create the lower mortality rates. I suspect estrogens are helpful in lowering mortality, but perhaps not quite as much as this study suggests.

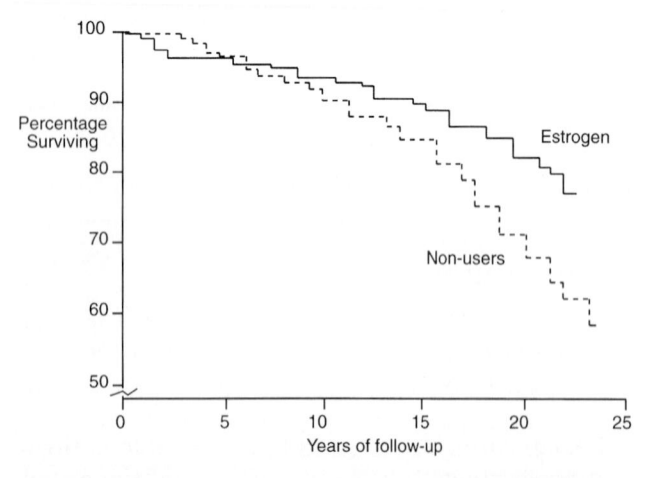

Fig. 1 All-cause mortality in postmenopausal women using estrogen vs. that in matched controls. (Reprinted with permission from *The American College of Obstetricians and Gynecologists.* Ettinger B, Friedman GD, Bush T, et al: Reduced mortality associated with long-term postmenopausal estrogen therapy, *Obstet Gynecol* 87: 6-12, 1996.)

THE DIFFICULT PATIENT: PREVALENCE, PSYCHOPATHOLOGY, AND FUNCTIONAL IMPAIRMENT

Hahn SR, Kroenke K, Spitzer RL, et al (Albert Einstein College of Medicine, Bronx, NY; Uniformed Services Univ, Bethesda, Md; Columbia Univ, NY; et al)
J Gen Intern Med 11:1-8, 1996

Background. The difficult physician-patient relationship has not been adequately studied. The prevalence, psychopathology, and functional impairment of "difficult patients" were documented.

Methods. Six hundred twenty-seven adult patients seen at four primary care clinics were included in the study. Physicians' perceptions of these patients' level of difficulty was assessed using the Difficult Doctor-Patient Relationship Questionnaire. Mental disorders and symptoms among the patients were determined by the Primary Care Evaluation of Mental Disorders (PRIME-MD), and functional status was assessed with the Medical Outcomes Study Short-Form Health Survey (SF-20). Patients also indicated their use of and satisfaction with medical care.

Findings. Ninety-six patients (15%) were rated as difficult by physicians. Sixty-seven percent of these patients had a mental disorder, compared with only 25% of patients considered not difficult. Patient difficulty was especially associated with multisomatoform disorder, panic disorder, dysthymia, generalized anxiety, major depressive disorder, and probable alcohol abuse or dependence. Compared with patients not perceived as difficult, difficult patients were more functionally impaired, used health care services more often, and were less satisfied with care. Demographic characteristics and physical illnesses were unrelated to difficulty. Mental disorders accounted for a great proportion of the excess functional impairment and dissatisfaction in difficult patients.

Conclusions. Patients perceived as difficult by physicians are common in primary care settings. Further research is needed to establish whether improved diagnosis and management of mental disorders in such patients may be of benefit.

Commentary

Most patients with multisomatoform disorder, panic disorder, dysthymic disorder, and generalized anxiety disorder were perceived as difficult by their physicians. Most patients that the physician rated as difficult had one of these disorders, major depression, or alcohol abuse. These difficult patients also had more dysfunction than other patients, even when accounting for their medical problems. These patients were also more likely to be dissatisfied with medical care. I think all of these things are tied together; the patients have mental health symptoms that are not controlled and that affect their interactions with other people, including their physicians. Would that we were terrific at helping them! Perhaps if we more directly recognize the mental health problems contributing to their "problem" status, we could more specifically address the issues, leading to improvement.

LONG-TERM EFFECTS OF CESAREAN SECTIONS: ECTOPIC PREGNANCIES AND PLACENTAL PROBLEMS

Hemminki E, Meriläinen J (Univ of Helsinki)
Am J Obstet Gynecol 174:1569-1574, 1996

Background. Little is known about the long-term effects of cesarean section. There is some evidence that cesarean section decreases fecundity and increases the risk of placenta previa and poor infant outcomes in subsequent pregnancies. The long-term effects of cesarean section on ectopic pregnancy, placenta previa, and abruptio placentae in subsequent pregnancies were evaluated.

Methods and Findings. Finnish registry data were used to identify 16,938 women who had a cesarean section and a group of matched controls. The two groups were compared for the occurrence and outcomes of the subsequent pregnancy from 1987 to 1993. Women with cesarean section were less likely to have a completed pregnancy during follow-up than their matched controls. The risk of ectopic pregnancy was increased in the cesarean section group, with a risk ratio of 1.28. The risk of abruptio placentae was increased as well, both in primiparous women (with risk ratios of 3.22 in a hospital inpatient registry and 2.41 in a birth registry) and nulliparous women (with risk ratios of 4.52 and 3.89, respectively). Primiparous women with cesarean section were also more likely to have placenta previa in their next pregnancy (risk ratios 5.34 and 3.78).

Conclusions. Women who undergo cesarean section are at some increased risk of ectopic pregnancy, and at substantially increased risk of placental problems in their next pregnancy. The consequences of these findings are unclear because there are no previous cohort studies for comparison. The possible negative impact on future pregnancies should be considered in deciding to perform cesarean section.

Commentary

The negative effects of cesarean section are usually stated in terms of intrapartum maternal and fetal risks. This large study from Finland clarifies findings from earlier work that an increased risk occurs for subsequent pregnancies. The modestly increased risk of subsequent ectopic pregnancy and the more substantial risk for abruption of the placenta and placenta previa should be included in the informed consent discussion with women who consider cesarean section. Such increased risk may also be discussed with women who consider procedures that carry an increased risk of cesarean section, such as epidural anesthesia and elective induction of labor. It may not be necessary to explain the risk details fully to women who undergo an urgent cesarean section in labor (not a time for good informed consent), but it could be stated in general that the cesarean section may have some adverse affect on subsequent pregnancies.

ABDOMINAL PAIN AND IRRITABLE BOWEL SYNDROME IN ADOLESCENTS: A COMMUNITY-BASED STUDY

Hyams JS, Burke G, Davis PM, et al (Hartford Hosp, Conn; Connecticut Children's Med Ctr, Hartford; Univ of Connecticut, Hartford)
J Pediatr 129:220-226, 1996

Background. Anecdotal evidence suggests that abdominal pain is common among adolescents, but there are few data on the prevalence of abdominal pain in this population. Previous studies of the clinical and psychological factors associated with recurrent abdominal pain in adolescents have been performed only in those who sought medical care and therefore may not reflect a community-based population. The prevalence of abdominal pain and of a symptom complex consistent with irritable bowel syndrome (IBS) was studied in a community-based population of adolescents, in whom anxiety and depression were also measured.

Methods. Students in the seventh grade and the tenth grade in a midsized suburban town completed three questionnaires that assessed gastrointestinal symptoms, state and trait anxiety, and depression. The symptoms were examined to identify adolescents with IBS, as defined by published criteria. Associations between IBS and anxiety and/or depression were analyzed.

Results. Abdominal pain occurrence in the previous year was reported by 73% of the middle school students and 78% of the high school students and was severe enough to restrict activity in 17% of the middle school students and 24% of the high school students (Table 2). A symptom complex that suggested IBS was present in 8% of the middle school students and 17% of the high school students. Neither abdominal pain nor IBS were significantly related to gender. The anxiety trait scores, but not anxiety state scores, were significantly higher in students with than in those without IBS symptoms in both age groups. Similarly, students of both ages with the symptoms of IBS were more likely to be classified as depressed. Pain severity, frequency, and duration correlated positively with trait anxiety scores, and depressed students had higher ratings for pain severity and frequency than nondepressed students.

Conclusions. Recurrent abdominal pain is common among adolescents, as are the symptoms of IBS. In this population, IBS is significantly associated with trait anxiety and depression, which suggests that interventions that influence anxiety and depression could reduce the prevalence or severity of recurrent abdominal pain and IBS.

Commentary

We've all experienced it as a parent, physician, and perhaps even as an adolescent; evanescent abdominal pain and related symptoms that interrupt school, sports, home, etc. This article caught my attention because IBS is not an entity that I have often ascribed to this age group. I was surprised at how frequently the symptom complex was reported by the study population and how debilitating the symptoms were to those affected (see Table 2). It is interesting that there did not seem to be a gender difference in reported symptoms. The setting of the study (suburban Connecticut) makes me wonder about how much these findings can be generalized. Typically, the focus of my evaluation of adolescent patients with this problem has been to rule out other causes and reassure both patient and parents. The take-home message for me is to not truncate the evaluation with just a "rule out and reassure" stance. These symptoms cause a significant amount of morbidity and should prompt one to look for and address anxiety and depression in this population.

TABLE 2 Abdominal Pain and Other Gastrointestinal Symptoms

	MIDDLE SCHOOL (n = 249)	HIGH SCHOOL (n = 258)
Abdominal pain in last year	73% ± 6%	78% ± 5%
≥6 times	32% ± 6%	37% ± 6%
≥Weekly	13% ± 4%	17% ± 5%
Severe enough to affect activities	24% ± 5%	17% ± 5%
Location*		
Above navel	31% ± 7%	23% ± 6%
Below navel	28% ± 7%	35% ± 6%
Back	41% ± 7%	42% ± 7%
Nocturnal awakening from pain (ever)*	13% ± 5%	15% ± 5%
Duration ≥30 min*	52% ± 7%	51% ± 7%
Nausea†	5% ± 3%	8% ± 3%
Heartburn†	6% ± 3%	5% ± 3%
Acid brash†	8% ± 3%	10% ± 4%

Courtesy of Hyams JS, Burke, G, Davis PM, et al: Abdominal pain and irritable bowel syndrome in adolescents: a community-based study, *J Pediatr* 129:220-226, 1996.
*Percentages refer to subjects reporting abdominal pain at any time during the past year (middle school n = 180, high school n = 120).
†At least once a week or more frequently.

THE PREVALENCE OF DYSMENORRHEA, DYSPAREUNIA, PELVIC PAIN, AND IRRITABLE BOWEL SYNDROME IN PRIMARY CARE PRACTICES

Jamieson DJ, Steege JF (Univ of California, San Francisco; Univ of North Carolina, Chapel Hill)
Obstet Gynecol 87:55-58, 1996

Objective. The frequency of dysmenorrhea, dyspareunia, and lower abdominal pain not associated with menses or intercourse was determined in women of reproductive age.

Methods. A 10-page questionnaire regarding pelvic pain was given to 701 women, aged 18-45 years, who were waiting in gynecologists' or obstetricians' offices; 581 returned usable forms.

Results. Dysmenorrhea was reported by 90% of women; dyspareunia, by 46%; pelvic pain, by 39%; and irritable bowel syndrome, by 12%. Thirty-six percent of 533 menstruating women said they always or frequently had pelvic pain during their periods (Table 2). Lower income women were significantly more likely than higher income women to have dysmenorrhea. Dyspareunia during or after intercourse was reported by 46% of sexually active women and was significantly more common among black women than white women and was

TABLE 2 Prevalence of Pelvic Pain Syndromes

TYPE OF PELVIC PAIN	ALWAYS	OFTEN	SOMETIMES	NEVER
Dysmenorrhea ($n = 533$)	120 (22%)	74 (14%)	288 (54%)	51 (10%)
Dyspareunia, during ($n = 549$)	8 (2%)	22 (4%)	209 (38%)	310 (56%)
Dyspareunia, after ($n = 549$)	2 (0%)	13 (2%)	133 (24%)	401 (73%)
Pelvic pain ($n = 581$)	2 (0%)	40 (7%)	185 (32%)	354 (61%)

Courtesy of Jamieson DJ, Steege JF: The prevalence of dysmenorrhea, dyspareunia, pelvic pain, and irritable bowel syndrome in primary care practices, *Obstet Gynecol* 87:55-58, 1996.
NOTE: Data are presented as *n* (%).

reported significantly more often in the lower income group than in the higher income group. Pelvic pain had the highest prevalence among women aged 26-30 years and was significantly more common among black women than white women.

Conclusions. Pelvic pain is common among women of reproductive age and is not consistently associated with socioeconomic factors. Questions regarding pelvic pain should be a regular part of health care for women.

Commentary

I find the information on the prevalence of symptoms helpful in talking about symptoms with patients. Dysmenorrhea was reported by 90% of these unselected patients. One quarter reported sometimes having dyspareunia after intercourse, and another 38% sometimes had dyspareunia during intercourse. One third reported pelvic pain. I found it surprising that 26% of women had pelvic pain more than 5 days per month, and 10% claimed they missed work at least 1 day per month for noncoital, nonmenstrual pelvic pain. In symptoms so common, most cannot be of major organic significance. We should attempt to prevent "medicalizing" these patients unless the symptoms are particularly severe or frequent. We must be in the position of support, however, and attempt to determine which patients need further workup.

EVALUATION OF CLINICAL COMPETENCE: THE GAP BETWEEN EXPECTATION AND PERFORMANCE

Joorabchi B, Devries JM (*Henry Ford Health System, Detroit; St Joseph Mercy Hosp, Pontiac, Mich*)
Pediatrics 97:179-184, 1996

Objective. The Objective Structured Clinical Examination (OSCE) has been widely used in Europe to evaluate the clinical skills of medical students. The test has seen limited application in the United States. Results of a 3-year experience with the OSCEs in the United States comparing validity, reliability, and faculty expectation vs. performance are reported.

Methods. The 4-hour test was administered in 3 consecutive years to 126 pediatric residents in a

TABLE 6 Resident Performance Based on Minimum Pass Levels: 3-Year Pooled Data

YEAR OF TRAINING	NO. OF RESIDENTS	MPL AS % OF MAXIMUM SCORE	% RESIDENTS BELOW MPL*
1	64	48	41
2	36	57	55
3	26	68	96

Joorabchi B, Devries, JM: Evaluation of clinical competence: the gap between expectation and performance, *Pediatrics* 97:179-184, 1996. (Reproduced by permission of *Pediatrics*, copyright 1996.
*Chi = square, 23.19; P = .000.

community-based program. Monitors graded residents as they interacted with real or simulated patients, interviewing or counseling, examining, performing procedures, handling telephone calls, and interpreting results. The patients evaluated the residents' communication skills and attitudes. Residents were also asked open-ended and multiple-choice questions. Results were compared with other measures of performance.

Results. Content, construct, concurrent validity, and reliability were comparable to those of other measures of performance. In all three tests, there was a significant difference between faculty expectations and resident performance at all levels.

The percentage of residents scoring below the minimum pass level was 41% at 1 year of training, 55% at 2 years, and 96% at 3 years (Table 6). These results compare with other studies of clinical competence. The difference between faculty expectations and resident performance could be the result of poor caliber of the residents, poor quality of the test, unrealistic expectation of faculty, inadequate observations of clinical performance, inaccurate data gathering, or unrealistic standards of faculty.

Conclusions. The difference between faculty expectations and resident performance suggests that a change in educational philosophy toward a more clinically-oriented, learner-directed, problem-based approach is needed.

Commentary

Oh, the difficulties of evaluation, or, how much we expect of our doctors! In this case, residents performed well on rotations and the American Board of Pediatrics examination, yet most (96% of the third-year residents) failed an OSCE examination created by faculty and chief residents. The case examples are provided and seem appropriate, and most examinees felt they had enough time. Almost all studies show that physicians do not perform as well in the examination room as we would like, yet a lot of good medical care happens. Physicians do not ask all the history questions that would be suggested and miss significant physical findings. Certainly, any OSCE test used for licensure or certification will itself need to be evaluated.

BACK PAIN DURING PREGNANCY: A PROSPECTIVE STUDY

Kristiansson P, Svärdsudd K, von Schoultz B *(Uppsala Univ, Sweden; Central Primary Health Care Ctr, Sundsvall, Sweden; Karolinska Hosp, Stockholm)*

Spine 21:702-709, 1996

Objective. The prevalence of back pain during pregnancy ranges from 48% to 90%. The cause is unknown, and few observational studies have been conducted. The natural history of back pain immediately before, during, and immediately after pregnancy was examined in a Swedish prospective cohort study.

Methods. In 1991, 200 pregnant women, 18-42 years of age in two districts completed a questionnaire about back status and were examined in a clinic before, during, and after pregnancy. Pain intensity was measured on two visual analog scales.

Results. Over 76% of women reported back pain at some time during pregnancy. Sixty-one percent reported pain that began during the pregnancy, and another 5.1% reported pain that started during the postpartum period. When pain began during pregnancy, the prevalence of back pain increased from 19% at week 12 to 47% at week 24, increased to 49% at week 36, and decreased to 9.4% after delivery (Fig. 2). Locations of pain included sacral, lumbosacral, lumbar, thoracic, and cervical regions (Fig. 1). Women who had back pain before pregnancy reported pain most commonly in the lumbar and thoracic regions in the first trimester. In the third trimester, the pain patterns were similar to the first group. Those with back pain weighed more than those who had no back pain. Those with back pain that began during pregnancy had significantly more pregnancies than those with no back pain. Pain intensity increased with duration. Younger women reported more pain than older women. Visual analog scores for pain were measured at each

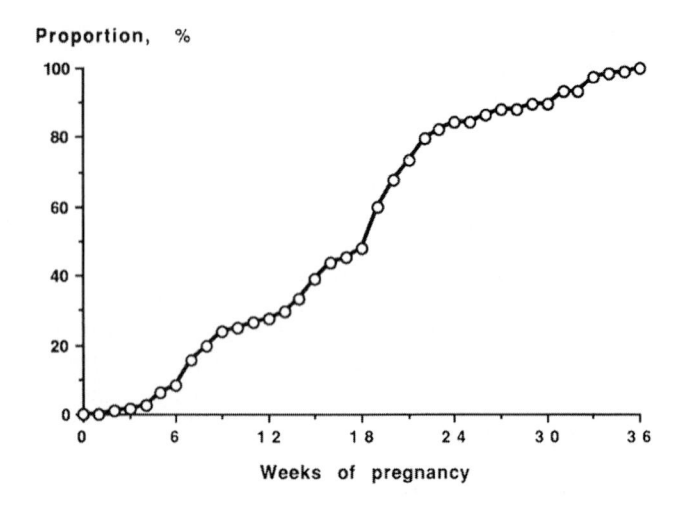

Fig. 2 Cumulative incidence of back pain occurring during pregnancy. (Courtesy of Kristiansson P, Svärdsudd K, von Schoultz B: Back pain during pregnancy: a prospective study, *Spine* 21: 702-709, 1996.)

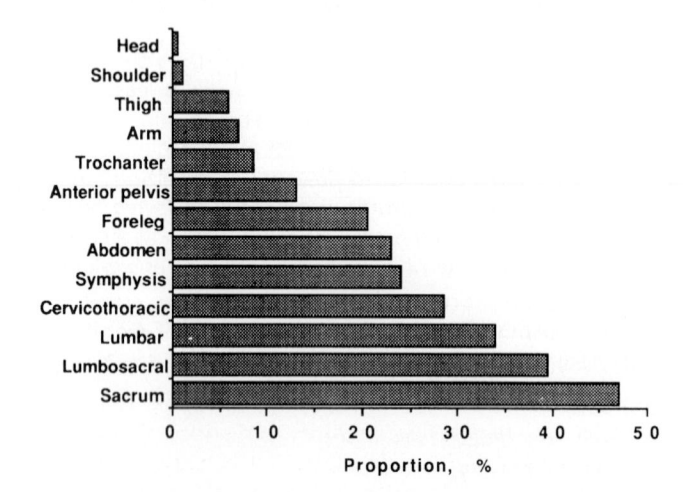

Fig. 1 Distribution and location of reported pain irrespective of time of onset. (Courtesy of Kristiansson P, Svärdsudd K, von Schoultz B: Back pain during pregnancy: a prospective study, *Spine* 21: 702-709, 1996.)

visit. Pain scores were significantly correlated with self-described disability and sick days.

Conclusions. Back pain is common during pregnancy, with approximately 75% of women affected, and its cause is still unknown. The location of pain was different for pain that began during pregnancy and pain that began before pregnancy.

Commentary

This article from Sweden nicely documents when and what type of back pain occurs during pregnancy. Physicians should be on the alert for the development of persistent and severe lumbosacral pain during the middle and end of pregnancy. This often results from subluxation of the sacroiliac joints, which may respond to manipulation.

SUDDEN DEATH FROM CARDIAC CAUSES IN CHILDREN AND YOUNG ADULTS

Liberthson RR (Harvard Med School, Boston; Massachusetts Gen Hosp, Boston)
N Engl J Med 334:1039-1044, 1996

Background. Sudden death in a young person is a rare and shocking event that can have medical and legal ramifications. Although many of these deaths are neither predictable nor preventable, some involve premonitory symptoms, a family history of sudden death at a young age, clinical or ECG abnormalities, or high-risk behavior. Relatively little is known about the demographic characteristics of young people who die suddenly. Current knowledge about sudden cardiac death in children and young adults was reviewed.

Sudden cardiac death in the young. Most sudden cardiac deaths in infants result from complex congenital cardiac lesions. Between the first year and the third decade of life, the most common causes are myocarditis, hypertrophic cardiomyopathy, coronary artery disease, congenital coronary artery anomalies, conduction system abnormalities, mitral valve prolapse, and aortic valve dissection. The incidence of sudden death in patients with congenital heart disease has been declining. Approximately half of patients with sudden death have prodromal symptoms, most commonly chest pain and syncope, and approximately 16% of patients have a family history of sudden death. Young people at risk of sudden death may have various ECG abnormalities, and these should be sought in patients with symptoms, lesions associated with a high risk of sudden death, and a family history of sudden death.

Most sudden deaths in young people result from myocardial or coronary vessel abnormalities, congenital heart lesions, or arrhythmia and conduction disorders, or from high-risk behavior (Table 3). As many as 40% of sudden cardiac deaths result from myocarditis, most frequently caused by infection with the group B coxsackie virus. One study of sudden deaths in young adults found that 23% were caused by coronary artery disease, almost always in young men with no history of angina pectoris or myocardial infarction. An ectopic origin of the left or right coronary artery in the left or right aortic sinus of Valsalva is the most common congenital coronary artery anomaly causing sudden death. Congenital heart lesions responsible for sudden death include pulmonary vascular obstruction, tetralogy of Fallot, and transposition of the great arteries after atrial switch operation. Arrhythmia and conduction abnormalities include congenital long QT syndrome and Wolff-Parkinson-White syndrome. High-risk behaviors that can lead to sudden death in young people include physical exertion by patients with structural heart disease, cocaine use, and eating disorders.

Summary. The rare problem of sudden cardiac death in young people is usually caused by one of a small list of disorders. Associated lesions, prodromal symptoms, family history of sudden death, and high-risk behaviors may provide important clues that a patient is at risk of sudden death.

Commentary

The recent sudden death of prominent athletes has caused concern regarding the health and safety of children and young adults performing maximal physical exercise during athletics. It would be nice if there were a single diagnosis and a single method for detecting the potentially lethal condition. As this review article so clearly states, the causes of sudden death in young athletes are multiple and require a more comprehensive approach. A careful history, physical examination, ECG, and echocardiogram may become a routine part of screening for athletes in high-risk sports. This evaluation can be done inexpensively in a well-organized delivery system.

TRIGGERING MYOCARDIAL INFARCTION BY SEXUAL ACTIVITY: LOW ABSOLUTE RISK AND PREVENTION BY REGULAR PHYSICAL EXERTION

Muller JE, for the Determinants of Myocardial Infarction Onset Study Investigators (Harvard Med School, Boston; Harvard School of Public Health, Boston)
JAMA 275:1405-1409, 1996

Background. Although there are anecdotal reports that sexual activity has triggered myocardial infarction (MI), there are minimal data about this association. Therefore, this association was analyzed with data from the Myocardial Infarction Onset Study, a large study investigating the relative risk of several potential triggers.

TABLE 3 Common Cardiac Causes of Sudden Death in Young Persons and Clinical Correlates*

CAUSE	FAMILY HISTORY OF SUDDEN DEATH	PRODROMAL SYNCOPE	PRODROMAL CHEST PAIN	ELECTROCARDIOGRAPHIC ABNORMALITY
Myocardial abnormality				
Hypertophic cardiomyopathy	+	+	−	+
Myocarditis	−	+	+	+
Dilated cardiomyopathy	+	+	−	+
Right ventricular cardiomyopathy	+	+	−	+
Congenital coronary-artery anomaly				
Coronary artery disease	+	−	+	+
Kawasaki's disease	−	−	+	+
Origin of left or right coronary artery in right or left sinus of Valsalva	−	+	+	−
Anomalous origin of left coronary artery in pulmonary artery	−	+	+	+
Congenital heart disease				
Pulmonary vascular obstruction	−	+	−	+
Tetralogy of Fallot	−	+	−	+
Transposed great arteries with atrial-switch operation	−	+	−	+
Aortic stenosis	−	+	+	+
Mitral-valve prolapse	+	+	+	+
Marfan's syndrome	+	−	+	
Arrhythmia or conduction-system abnormality				
Long-QT syndrome	+	+	−	+
Ventricular preexcitation	−	+	−	+
Ventricular tachycardia	−	+	−	+
Sinus-node dysfunction	−	+	−	+
Heart block	−	+	−	+
High-risk behavior				
Use of cocaine or tricyclic agents	−	+	+	−
Bulimia or anorexia nervosa	−	+	−	+

Courtesy of Liberthson RR: Sudden death from cardiac causes in children and young adults, *N Engl J Med* 334:1039-1044, 1996. Reprinted by permission of *The New England Journal of Medicine*. Copyright 1996, Massachusetts Medical Society.
*Plus sign denotes the presence of a clinical correlate.

Methods. The Onset Study collected data from 22 community hospitals and 23 tertiary care centers regarding 1774 patients within 1 week of their MIs. The interviewers identified the time of onset of symptoms of MI and the timing and intensity of exposure to potential triggers. Information was gathered about sexual activity within the 26 hours preceding the onset of symptoms and about the usual frequency of sexual activity and of strenuous exercise. The change in risk of MI associated with sexual activity was analyzed to determine relative risk and the induction time for this risk factor.

Results. Data were available on 858 sexually active patients, of whom 79 (9%) had sexual activity within the 24 hours preceding MI and 27 (3%) had sexual activity within the 2 hours preceding MI. The relative risk of MI was increased only during the 2 hours immediately after sexual activity; during this period the relative risk was 2.5. However, the relative risk of MI within that 2-hour period was reduced to 1.9 in patients who engaged in strenuous physical exertion twice per week and to 1.2 in patients who exercised 3 times per week. The relative risk was similar among patients with or without a prior MI and among patients with or without a history of angina.

Conclusions. Sexual activity can act as a trigger for MI within 2 hours, when the relative risk of MI is slightly and transiently increased. However, regular exercise can significantly reduce the risk of MI associated with sexual activity.

Commentary

As the commercial tabloids know all too well, any article with sex in the title grabs our attention. When this article came out in *JAMA*, it made the local television news with the lead, "It's okay for heart patients to have sex." The true importance of this study, however, is to those patients with known coronary artery disease or a history of MI whose anxiety about the dangers of sexual intercourse are very real. This large study of 1700 patients in 45 hospitals looked at the time relationship of sexual activity to recent onset myocardial infarction. The study did show an increased risk during the period immediately after sexual intercourse. This risk was no greater, however, than the risk from other exercises. The more important news is that the relative risk is low and the absolute risk is extremely low (1 chance in a million).

Perhaps the most important finding in this study was the protective effect of a regular exercise program to reduce the risk of myocardial infarction after sexual intercourse. Perhaps we can learn from our Madison Avenue colleagues and use sex as the incentive for our post-MI patients to engage in a supervised exercise program.

SELF-PERCEIVED HEALTH STATUS AND HEALTH-RELATED QUALITY OF LIFE OF EXTREMELY LOW-BIRTH-WEIGHT INFANTS AT ADOLESCENCE

Saigal S, Feeny D, Rosenbaum P, et al
(McMaster Univ, Hamilton, Ont, Canada)
JAMA 276:453-459, 1996

Introduction. Extremely low-birth-weight (ELBW) infants born in the first years of improved survival are now teenagers. Reports on how these children are doing usually are based on the opinions of parents and teachers and on the results of psychometric tests given to the children. The patient's perspective is an increasingly important component of assessment in all areas of medicine. The health status and health-related quality of life (HRQL) of a cohort of ELBW children was determined from their own perspectives as teenagers using direct interview.

Methods. One hundred and forty-one teenagers from a cohort of 169 ELBW survivors born between 1977 and 1982 and 124 of 145 well-matched normal control subjects were interviewed regarding their self-reported, subjectively defined personal health status and HRQL.

Results. Forty-one of 150 ELBW survivors had neurosensory impairments: 19 with cerebral palsy, 6 with hydrocephalus, 14 with cognitive impairments, 5 with autism, 5 with unilateral blindness, 9 with bilateral blindness, and 2 with deafness. One adolescent was in a group home and four were in a foster home. Most adolescents (94%) were attending a regular school where children with disabilities were integrated with all other children. Proxy responses were needed from parents for nine children who were severely impaired and unable to give self-reports. Compared with control subjects, adolescents who were ELBW infants described a significantly greater number of attributes affected and more severe and complex limitations in cognition, sensation, self-care, and pain. Most adolescents who were ELBW infants (excluding the nine who were unable to give self-reports) and most control subjects rated their HRQL as satisfactory (71% vs. 73%).

Conclusions. Overall, teenagers who were ELBW infants were positive about their HRQL, despite the fact that many experienced neurosensory impairments. These are the first reported findings on health status and quality of life from the perspective of those who were born prematurely.

Commentary

This article joins quite a literature on the follow-up of ELBW infants. Its particular strengths are the geographically defined population base, the extraordinary attention to tracking down patients years later, and the meticulous attention to valid quality measures. I am most impressed by the similarities, rather than the differences, in quality of life between ELBW and normal-birth-weight teenagers. I have three overall comments. First, the results, positive though they are, provide weak and indirect evidence that administering intensive care to all ELBW infants is a good idea. Editorialists writing in the same issue urge that such treatment still be considered investigational.[1] Second, the self-report nature of the study leaves open the question of whether ELBW teenagers may be denying their true feelings by inflating their quality of life scores. Third, keep in mind that these patients were mostly white, middle-class Canadians; who knows whether the findings might generalize to some of the more heterogeneous or disadvantaged populations in the United States? Thus, I consider the findings to be reassuring, but incomplete. We are making progress in understanding the outcomes of these infants, but have a long way to go. More long-term, population-based research needs to be conducted using both subjective and objective measures.

REFERENCE
1. Tyson JE, Broyles RS: Progress in assessing the long-term outcome of extremely low-birth-weight infants, *JAMA* 276: 492-493, 1996.

COGNITIVE BEHAVIOUR THERAPY FOR THE CHRONIC FATIGUE SYNDROME: A RANDOMISED CONTROLLED TRIAL

Sharpe M, Hawton K, Simkin S, et al   *(Warneford Hosp, Oxford, England; John Radcliffe Hosp, Oxford, England; Univ of Oxford, England)*
BMJ 312:22-26, 1996

Background. The cause of chronic fatigue syndrome continues to be a subject of controversy. However, cognitive behavior therapy may be useful in its treatment. Such therapy is based on the hypothesis that inaccurate beliefs, ineffective coping behavior, negative mood states, social problems, and pathophysiologic processes interact to perpetuate the syndrome. The goal of cognitive behavior therapy is to help patients reassess their understanding of the illness and adopt more effective coping behaviors. The efficacy and acceptability of adding cognitive behavior therapy to the medical care of patients with this syndrome were investigated.

Methods. Sixty patients referred consecutively and meeting criteria for chronic fatigue syndrome were included in the randomized, controlled trial. Medical treatment consisted of evaluation, advice, and follow-up in general practice. Patients randomly assigned to cognitive behavior therapy were offered 16 individual weekly sessions in addition to the standard care. All but two randomly assigned patients accepted the treatment. Final assessments were performed at 12 months. Outcome measures included the attainment of normal daily functioning and clinically significant functional improvement.

Findings. Intention to treat analysis indicated that 73% of the recipients of cognitive behavior therapy attained a satisfactory outcome, compared to 27% of patients receiving only medical care. Improvements in patients' conditions persisted after cognitive behavior therapy was completed. Patients receiving cognitive behavior therapy evidenced more change in illness beliefs and coping behavior previously associated with poor outcomes than patients receiving medical care alone.

Conclusions. The addition of cognitive behavior therapy to the medical management of chronic fatigue syndrome is acceptable to patients. Such treatment appears to result in a sustained reduction in functional impairment.

Commentary

Not much has been shown to be effective for chronic fatigue syndrome, so a positive report deserves careful scrutiny. This is a nicely designed randomized trial showing that cognitive behavioral therapy works and by a wide margin. Nearly three quarters of the patients improved with therapy compared to about one quarter receiving usual care—a threefold difference that is both statistically and clinically significant. The treatment protocol, however, was daunting: 16 1-hour sessions over 4 months. Few family physicians are qualified to provide the treatment, and even fewer would have the time. Still, given what we know about the frequent use of medical services by patients with this condition under usual care, the extraordinary investment in time for treatment is probably worth it. I think that this article provides compelling arguments for your consulting mental health providers to set up a similar program for these uncommon but high-need patients.

Also, be aware that the definition of the syndrome is still under development. A recent study by Komaroff's group in Boston has suggested further refinements in the case definition used by the Centers for Disease Control and Prevention, i.e., eliminating need for muscle weakness, arthralgias, and sleep disturbance and adding anorexia and nausea.

REFERENCE

1. Komaroff AL et al: An examination of the working case definition of chronic fatigue syndrome, *Am J Med* 100:56-64, 1996.

PREPREGNANT WEIGHT IN RELATION TO RISK OF NEURAL TUBE DEFECTS

Werler MM, Louik C, Shapiro S, et al (*Boston Univ School of Public Health, Brookline, Mass*)
JAMA 275:1089-1092, 1996

Objective. It has been suggested that obesity may increase the risk of having a pregnancy affected by a neural tube defect (NTD). This is an important public health question because obesity is common and NTDs are among the most frequent and severe congenital malformations. The role played by folate intake is important to determine as well. The effect of maternal obesity on risk of NTDs was evaluated in 2 case-control studies: one conducted as part of a birth defect surveillance program and the other as part of a population-based study.

Surveillance study. A total of 604 fetuses or infants with an NTD diagnosed within 6 months of delivery, 1658 control fetuses or infants with other major malformations, and 93 controls without major malformations were studied. Women with body weights of 50-59 kg were used as the reference group. The relative risk of NTDs for women weighing 80-89 kg was 1.9 (95% confidence interval, 1.2-2.9). For women weighing 110 kg or more, the relative risk was 4.0 (95% confidence interval, 1.6-9.9). The risk of NTDs related to body weight applied to women who did and did not receive the recommended level of 400 µg of folate daily. For women with body weights of less than 70 kg who took 400 µg of folate or more, the risk of NTDs decreased by 40%. For women weighing more than 70 kg, taking the recommended folate level did not reduce the risk of NTDs.

Population-based study. A total of 538 fetuses and infants with NTDs and 539 controls without malformations were studied. The mothers were interviewed within an average of 5 months after their term delivery date. The risk of NTD was approximately doubled for obese women, compared with those with a body mass index of 29 kg/m^2 or less. The odds ratio was 1.9, with a 95% confidence interval of 1.3-2.9. The obesity-associated increase in risk was unrelated to vitamins containing folic acid, diabetes, use of diet pills, dietary folic acid intake, or a previous NTD pregnancy. The odds ratio was unaffected by adjustment for maternal age, education, gravity, vitamin use, and alcohol use. The link between maternal obesity and NTD was greater for spina bifida and other less common NTDs than for anencephaly.

Conclusions. Mothers with heavier prepregnancy body weights are at increased risk of NTDs; the risk appears to be doubled for obese women, independent of the effects of folate intake. This modest effect probably makes a significant contribution to the number of NTDs in the population, because about 10% of women are obese when they become pregnant.

Commentary

The discovery of the association between folic acid intake and NTDs was a major contribution to our knowledge in maternity care in the last few years These important studies indicate that prepregnant obesity may be as great a risk factor as a low folic acid intake, and its presence may override the benefit of folic acid ingestion. These findings underscore the importance of preconception care, in particular the treatment of obesity before pregnancy. With many successful family planning methods to choose from, the alert family physician should work with women of childbearing age to achieve an optimal health status before pregnancy. This now includes avoiding obesity and ingesting folic acid.

THE HARSTAD INJURY PREVENTION STUDY: THE EPIDEMIOLOGY OF SPORTS INJURIES, AN 8-YEAR STUDY

Ytterstad B   (Univ of Tromsø, Norway)

Br J Sports Med 30:64-68, 1996

Background. Sports-related injuries are the second leading cause of injuries in Norway. The World Health Organization has stressed the importance of injury control, and the goal for Europe is to reduce morbidity and mortality from accidents by 25% or more. Reliable epidemiologic data are needed for injury prevention programs. National data are of limited value for local prevention programs because different populations have different epidemiologic characteristics. The epidemiology of sports injuries during an 8-year period was described, and the effectiveness of a downhill skiing safety program was evaluated.

Methods. A community with a population of approximately 22,500 was studied. During a period of 8 years, sports injuries treated in a hospital were prospectively reported. Demographic and injury data were recorded, including type of activity, place of injury, and equipment used. A prevention program aimed at downhill skiers was evaluated.

Results. There were 2234 sports injuries reported of 12,977 unintentional injuries. Of all individuals with sports injuries, more than 63% were males. Approximately 75% of sports injuries involved falls and trauma resulting from contact with objects or other individuals. Almost 50% were sprains or dislocations, more than 23% were open wounds, excoriations, or contusions, almost 18.5% were fractures, and approximately 2.5% were concussions or more serious brain injury. Two thirds of injuries occurred in team sports, and soccer accounted for almost 45% of all sports injuries. Downhill skiing injuries had a higher mean score on the injury scale than all other sports combined. After adjusting for exposure, injury rates for downhill skiing decreased by 15% after the downhill skiing safety program was implemented.

Conclusions. Hospital recording of injuries is feasible and provides valuable information for evaluating the effectiveness of sports injury prevention programs. Local epidemiologic data on injuries can improve community programs aimed at preventing sports injuries. Further research is needed to fully evaluate the effectiveness of the downhill skiing safety program.

Commentary

Sports and athletic activities are an integral and important part of our daily lives. I am never sure whether I am wearing my sports medicine or family practice hat when treating the strain or sprain of one of my long-term patients. I am sure, though, that more can be accomplished with prevention (a familiar refrain) in this area. There are many sports injury surveillance initiatives out there. Most of the effective ones, however, are collecting data on organized, usually competitive, athletes, for example, the National Collegiate Athletic Association.

This study intrigued me for several reasons. It is a long-term though modest-scale surveillance of recreational sports injuries with interventions aimed at decreasing injuries based on the surveillance data. The common weakness of sports injury surveillance studies are in the definitions of injury and denominator. What qualifies as a reportable event—any injury, or only a time loss injury? What qualifies as a contact—one ski run, or a whole day? In this study only emergency department data were recorded, and no denominator was ever identified. These are significant confounders. Nevertheless, the population studied was easily captured (250 km north of the Arctic Circle!), and the design seemed successful in identifying and modifying risk factors (in skiing) to reduce apparent injury rates. This is a good example of adapting a study to local conditions and using surveillance techniques to make an impact on the health of our recreational athletes in the community—preventive sports medicine.

YEAR BOOK OF GERIATRICS AND GERONTOLOGY

MULTI-SITE STUDY OF INCIDENCE OF PRESSURE ULCERS AND THE RELATIONSHIP BETWEEN RISK LEVEL, DEMOGRAPHIC CHARACTERISTICS, DIAGNOSES, AND PRESCRIPTION OF PREVENTIVE INTERVENTIONS

Bergstrom N, Braden B, Kemp M, et al   (*Univ of Nebraska, Omaha; Creighton Univ, Omaha, Neb; Rush Univ, Chicago; et al*)

J Am Geriatr Soc 44:22-30, 1996

Background. Differences in past studies have made it difficult to compile consistent data on the incidence and etiology of pressure ulcers. The inci-

TABLE 1 Demographic Characteristics of Randomly Selected Subjects According to Pressure Ulcer Outcome (0, 1, 2) and Clinical Setting

PRESSURE ULCER OUTCOME	TERTIARY CARE (n = 306) 0*	1†	2‡	VAMC (n = 282) 0*	1†	2‡	NURSING HOME (n = 255) 0*	1†	2‡	TOTAL (n = 843) 0*	1†	2‡
Age												
n	280	9	17	261	8	13	194	18	43	735	35	73
X	53.8	61.7	61.2	62.4	65.6	65.9	73.0	73.6	79.7	61.9	68.7	72.9
SD	17.9	20.8	15.5	11.5	6.9	15.6	12.0	8.6	9.3	16.2	13.3	14.6
Range	19-99	28-84	36-86	25-91	54-73	42-102	29-92	56-91	55-95	19-99	38-91	36-102
F, df, P	(2.17, [2,303], P = NS)			(0.85, [2,279], P = NS)			(6.29, [2,252], P = .002)			(18.1, [2,840], P = .0001)		
Braden Scale Source												
n	280	9	17	261	8	13	194	18	43	735	35	73
X	19.4	19.8	17.4	20.5	17.9	15.4	19.3	17.4	16.1	19.8	18.1	16.3
SD	2.7	5.1	4.0	2.4	4.1	3.5	2.4	2.5	2.6	2.5	3.7	3.2
Range	11-23	8-23	9-23	11-23	12-23	9-22	9-23	12-21	10-22	8-23	8-23	9-23
F, df, P	(0.01, [2,303], P = NS)			(9.24, [2,279], P = .0001)			(13.19, [2,252], P = .0001)			(59.92, [2,840], P = .0001)		
Sex												
% Male	90	3	7	92	3	5	9	8	13	89	4	7
% Female	93	3	4	100	0	0	74	6	20	84	4	12
	(NS)			(NS)			(NS)			(χ^2 = 6.175, [2], P = .05)		
Race												
% White	89	4	7	92	4	4	74	8	18	85	5	10
% Black	100	0	0	93	0	7	91	3	6	95	<1	4
% Other	100	0	0	100	0	0	100	0	0	100	0	0
	(NS)			(NS)			(NS)			(P = <.003)		

Courtesy of Bergstrom N, Braden B, Kemp M, et al: Multi-site study of incidence of pressure ulcers and the relationship between risk level, demographic characteristics, diagnoses, and prescription of preventive interventions, *J Am Geriatr Soc* 44(1):22-30, 1996.
*0 = No pressure ulcer.
†1 = Stage I pressure ulcer present on 2 consecutive observations.
‡2 = Stage II pressure ulcer present on at least 1 observation.

dence of pressure ulcers in varied populations, demographic characteristics, and the impact of primary diagnosis on the development of pressure ulcers were determined in a cohort study.

Methods. A total of 843 patients were randomly selected from two skilled nursing homes, two university tertiary care hospitals, and two Veterans' Administration Medical Centers (VAMCs). The patients had no pressure ulcers on admission. Sixty-three percent of the patients were male, and 79% were white. The mean age was 63 years (Table 1).

Findings. Pressure ulcers developed in 12.8% of the patients. The incidence was 8.5% in tertiary care centers, 7.4% in VAMCs, and 23.9% in nursing homes. In a logistic regression analysis, factors that predicted pressure ulcers were lower Braden Scale scores, older age, and white race. When the Braden Scale score was included in the regression, primary diagnosis did not significantly predict the development of pressure ulcers. Braden Scale scores and white race predicted use of turning, whereas Braden Scale scores, white race, and female sex predicted use of pressure reduction (Tables 3, 4, and 6).

TABLE 3 Logistic Regression Predicting Pressure Ulcer Development Using Demographic Characteristics, Braden Scale Score, and Preventive Measures

	OR	95% CI	χ^2	P
Variables in Model				
Turning Prescription	.68	0.37-1.22	1.68	.195
Pressure Reduction	.80	0.49-1.30	0.81	.368
Braden Scale	1.30	1.19-1.41	36.05	<.001
Age	.97	0.95-0.98	15.56	<.001
Race	2.73	1.25-5.98	6.29	.012
Sex	0.93		0.08	.773
Intercept			1.60	.206
Model χ^2			121.80	<.001
Degrees of Freedom			6	

Courtesy of Bergstrom N, Braden B, Kemp M, et al: Multi-site study of incidence of pressure ulcers and the relationship between risk level, demographic characteristics, diagnoses, and prescription of preventive interventions, *J Am Geriatr Soc* 44(1):22-30, 1996.

TABLE 4 Logistic Regression Models Predicting Pressure Ulcer Development Using the Braden Score or Mobility and Activity Subscale Scores and Selected Primary Diagnoses

	BRADEN SCALE NOT IN MODEL				BRADEN SCALE IN MODEL			
	OR	95% CI	χ^2	P	OR	95% CI	χ^2	P
Variables in Model								
Braden Scale					1.37	1.28, 1.48	75.76	<.001
Mobility	1.72	1.27-2.33	12.21	<.001				
Activity	1.46	1.13-1.88	8.20	.004				
Cardiovascular Diagnosis	2.49	1.14-5.48	5.18	.023				
Intercept			5.5	.018			36.31	<.001
Model χ^2			48.04	<.001			85.36	<.001
Degrees of Freedom			2				1	

Courtesy of Bergstrom N, Braden B, Kemp M, et al: Multi-site study of incidence of pressure ulcers and the relationship between risk level, demographic characteristics, diagnoses, and prescription of preventive interventions, *J Am Geriatr Soc* 44(1):22-30, 1996.

TABLE 6 Logistic Regression Predicting Prescriptive Practices in Pressure Ulcer Prevention Based on Level of Risk (Braden Scale Score), Age, Race, and Sex

	TURNING				PRESSURE REDUCTION			
	OR	95% CI	χ^2	P	OR	95% CI	χ^2	P
Variables in models								
Braden Scale	1.6	1.45-1.73	103.83	<.001	1.29	1.22-1.37	73.80	<.001
Age	.99	0.98-1.01	.02	.893	1.00	0.99-1.01	0.21	.645
Race	2.66	1.21-5.81	6.02	.014	1.90	1.26-2.86	9.39	.002
Sex	.94	0.58-1.53	.06	.806	.32	0.23-0.43	50.64	<.001
Intercept			38.61	<.001			22.75	<.001
Model χ^2			161.66	<.001			168.57	<.001
Degrees of Freedom			4				4	

Courtesy of Bergstrom N, Braden B, Kemp M, et al: Multi-site study of incidence of pressure ulcers and the relationship between risk level, demographic characteristics, diagnoses, and prescription of preventive interventions, *J Am Geriatr Soc* 44(1):22-30, 1996.

Conclusions. The basis of prescriptive decisions for the prevention of pressure ulcers should be risk assessment rather than primary diagnosis or demographic factors. Risk assessment should enable health care providers to make better use of turning and support surfaces.

Commentary

Pressure ulcers are a persistent and costly threat to institutionalized frail elderly, and the annual cost of pressure ulcer treatment in the United States is as high as $7 million. The 1992 publication of the Agency for Health Care Policy and Research Clinical Practice Guidelines: *Pressure Ulcers in Adults: Prediction and Prevention,* established the standard for assessment and prevention in all settings.[1] The nurse researchers in this article found an average incidence rate of 12.8% in a sample of 843 residents followed up for up to 4 weeks in six long-term care settings in three geographical regions. These findings, together with those of Olson, Langemo, Burd, et al., who found an incidence rate of 13.4% over 2 weeks for patients admitted to an acute care setting,[2] emphasize the importance of implementing a formal system of need assessment and aggressive prevention protocols for all institutionalized elderly on admission to the facility.

REFERENCES

1. Panel for the Prediction and Prevention of Pressure Ulcers in Adults: *Pressure ulcers in adults: prediction and prevention,* Clinical Practice Guideline, No 3, Rockville, Md, Agency for Health Care Policy and Research, 1992 Public Health Service, US Department of Health and Human Services, AHCPR publication 92-0047.
2. Olson B, Langemo D, Burd C, et al: Pressure ulcer incidence in an acute care setting, *J Wound Ostomy Continence Nurs* 23:15-22, 1996.

FALLS IN THE ELDERLY: A PROSPECTIVE STUDY OF RISK FACTORS AND RISK PROFILES

Graafmans WC, Ooms ME, Hofstee HMA, et al
(Vrije Universiteit, Amsterdam; Academisch Ziekenhuis Vrije Universiteit, Amsterdam)
Am J Epidemiol 143:1129-1136, 1996

Background. Falls among the elderly can result in injury, social isolation, and psychological difficulty. Important risk factors for falls include impairment in mobility and cognition and the use of medication. Risk factors and risk profiles were prospectively studied.

Methods. Falls among 354 individuals aged 70 years and older were registered during a 28-week period in 1992. All individuals were living in homes or apartments for the elderly in the Amsterdam area.

Findings. One hundred twenty-six individuals (36%) had a total of 251 falls. Fifty-seven of them had two or more falls. Mobility impairment was associated with falls, with an odds ratio (OR) of 2.1, and was especially associated with recurrent falls (OR, 5.0). Dizziness on standing also was associated with falls and recurrent falls, with ORs of 2.1 for each. Several risk factors were associated with recurrent falls only, including history of stroke (OR, 3.4), poor mental state (OR, 2.4), and postural hypotension (OR, 2.0). When all of the aforementioned risk factors were present, an elderly individual had an 84% probability of recurrent falls in a 28-week period, compared with 3% when none of these risk factors were present. The probability of recurrent falls ranged from 11% to 29% when predicted by number of falls occurring the previous year. Neither falls nor recurrent falls were strongly associated with physical activity, the use of high-risk medication, or the use of vitamin D_3, which was allocated randomly to the participants.

Conclusions. The risk profiles established in this study predicted a large range of probabilities of falls, especially recurrent falls. Impairment of mobility was the major risk factor. Improving mobility may help prevent recurrent falls.

Commentary

Falls remain a major problem in the elderly; they cause injuries, primarily fractures; a fear of falling; and social isolation. Previous studies have shown that mobility impairment, cognitive impairment, and use of medication are important risk factors for falls.

This study, a prospective one carried out in Amsterdam, carefully identified falls and examined the role of potential risk factors in both single falls and recurrent falls. The authors subsequently combined these factors to form risk profiles. The study analyzed two different outcome measures in an institutionalized population that appears to be comparable to that of a residential care facility in this country. The two outcome measures were at least one fall vs. none and recurrent falls vs. one fall or less. The study shows that a history of stroke, postural hypotension, disabilities of the lower extremities, and impaired cognitive function increases the risk of recurrent falls; it also shows that the mobility items were more strongly related to recurrent falls than to single falls.

It is interesting that the use of medication in this study did not reveal a strong relationship with falls or recurrent falls, in striking contrast to many other studies.[1-4] It is difficult to determine the reason for this difference, although this group of authors used medications at baseline, whereas most other studies have identified medication use at the time of the fall.

The most important message of this and other studies[5,6] is that recurrent falls may be especially amenable to preventive strategies. Mobility impairment is the strongest risk factor and perhaps the easiest to change in a prevention program that includes exercise, and recent studies have showed its effectiveness in terms of averting falls, but none have showed its effectiveness in the prevention of fractures.

REFERENCES

1. Grisso JA, Kelsey JL, Strom BL, et al: Risk factors for falls as a cause of hip fracture in women: The Northeast Hip Fracture Study Group, *N Engl J Med* 324:1326-1331, 1991.
2. Tinetti ME, Speechley M, Ginter SF: Risk factors for falls among elderly persons living in the community, *N Engl J Med* 319:1701-1707, 1988.
3. Prudham D, Evans JG: Factors associated with falls in the elderly: a community study, *Age Ageing* 10:141-146, 1981.
4. Granek E, Baker SP, Abbey H, et al: Medications and diagnoses in relation to falls in a long-term care facility, *J Am Geriatr Soc* 35:503-511, 1987.
5. Tinetti ME, Baker DI, McAvay G, et al: A multifactorial intervention to reduce the risk of falling among elderly people living in the community, *N Engl J Med* 331:821-827, 1994.
6. MacRae PG, Feltner ME, Reinsch S: A 1-year exercise program for older women: effects on falls, injuries, and physical performance, *J Aging Phys Activity* 2:127-142, 1994.

MEMORY COMPLAINTS AND MEMORY IMPAIRMENT IN OLDER INDIVIDUALS

Jonker C, Launer LJ, Hooijer C, et al
(Free Univ, Amsterdam, The Netherlands; Erasmus Univ, Rotterdam, The Netherlands)
J Am Geriatr Soc 44:44-49, 1996

Background. Interpretation of an older patient's complaint of memory loss may be complex. Individuals with dementia are more likely to complain about their memory than are those without dementia, but evidence also exists that individuals may complain about their memory for other reasons, such as depression. Nondemented, nondepressed individuals living in the community are proportionately the largest group at risk for memory impairment. The relationship between complaints about memory and cognitive test performance was evaluated in such a population.

Methods. Of the 4051 participants in the Amsterdam Study on the Elderly (65-85 years of age), 2537 respondents who were neither demented nor depressed were included in the analysis. Answers to questions about the presence or absence of memory complaints and memory-related problems were classified into four categories of subjective memory complaints. Cognitive function was assessed by deriving subscales based on questions from the CAMCOG and several other mental status tests.

Results. Memory complaints and problems were noted for 22.1% of nondemented, nondepressed individuals, compared with 36.7% of depressed individuals and 46.4% of demented individuals. Cognitive subscales correlated negatively with age and positively with premorbid verbal intelligence. Scores were higher for men than for women on most cognitive tests. After adjustment for these associations, individuals with self-reported memory complaints and memory problems, compared with those without memory complaints or problems, showed increased risk of poor performance in recall, factual memory, time and place orientation, and concentration, but there was no increased risk of poor performance at language, verbal abstraction, or copying design.

Discussion. Individuals living in the community who are neither depressed nor demented and who have complaints about memory perform less well on cognitive tests than do those without memory complaints. Individuals reporting both memory complaints and memory-related problems perform even less well on cognitive tests. Asking questions about memory complaints as well as memory-related problems may identify a wider group at risk. This distinction may be important because older individuals sometimes perceive their memory to be generally impaired, yet specific questioning about activities reveals substantially less impairment. Subjective memory complaints should be considered a potential indicator of memory impairment signaling a need for follow-up.

Commentary

The Amsterdam Study on the Elderly has been a useful community-based study of elderly individuals. In this portion of the study, the researchers address an important topic for clinicians: the prognostic value of subjective memory complaints. When do such complaints portend that a neurologically significant memory problem will occur in the future? Some of us have been touting the clinical pearl that if the family complains about the patient's memory, the problem is likely to be early dementia, whereas if the patient complains about his or her own memory, the problem is more likely to be depression.

In this study, individuals with depression were not studied and the CAMCOG was used to assess cognition. Although the authors include a number of caveats about their finding, they present the concern that subjective memory complaints can warn of subsequent dementia. For nondepressed individuals, the clinician would do well to consider referral to a neuropsychologist or at least a follow-up visit in 6 months.

SCREENING FOR COMMON PROBLEMS IN AMBULATORY ELDERLY: CLINICAL CONFIRMATION OF A SCREENING INSTRUMENT

Moore AA, Siu AL *(Univ of California, Los Angeles; Mount Sinai School of Medicine, New York)*
Am J Med 100:438-443, 1996

Introduction. Functional deficits are better able to predict patient outcomes after hospitalization than admitting diagnoses. Existing instruments for measuring health status and function in elderly patients have not been useful for physicians in clinical practice. An instrument was developed and tested to determine if nonphysician office staff could effectively evaluate the functional ability of ambulatory elderly patients seen in physicians' offices.

Methods. A literature review was conducted to identify problems that typically contribute to functional disability. Easy-to-administer screening measures were developed for eight problems often missed during traditional physical examination: malnutrition/weight loss, visual impairment, hearing loss, cognitive impairment, urinary incontinence, depression, physical disability, and reduced leg mobility. A research assistant administered the screening to patients before they were seen by a geriatrician. These physicians were blinded to results of the screening performed by the research assistant. Results of the screening were compared with the geriatrician's evaluation. This was considered the gold standard. Geriatricians were then allowed to see the screening results and were given the opportunity to revise the original assessment. The sensitivity, specificity, and predictive value of the blinded and unblinded geriatric assessments were compared.

Results. The mean age of the 109 patients in the study population was 79 years. The screening package (Table 1) took 8-12 minutes to administer. The interrater agreement per item ranged from 77% to 100%. Sensitivities were 0.65-0.93 (blinded) and 0.70-0.95 (unblinded). Specificities were 0.50-0.95 (blinded) and 0.64-0.95 (unblinded). The prevalence rate for the functional deficits measured ranged from 21% to 72%. The positive predictive values for items in the screening tool ranged from 0.60 and 0.91. The negative predictive values for same ranged between 0.77 and 0.96. Depending on the educational and skill level of the employee doing these screenings, it was estimated that the direct cost per patient screened in a clinical practice would be $1 to $7.

Conclusions. The screening instrument developed to assess functional status in elderly patients in a clinical practice was inexpensive, short, and easy to use. Its validity and reliability were good. In a clinical setting, this tool could help physicians focus on the problems that commonly compromise the health and functioning of elderly patients.

Commentary

As pressure mounts for physicians to increase their productivity, concerns have been raised about the ability to provide comprehensive care within a shorter amount of time. Several recent efforts have been made to reduce the burden of work for the physicians by delegating some of their traditional

TABLE 1 Screening Package Characteristics

PROBLEM	SCREENING MEASURE	POSITIVE SCREEN	SUPPORTING DATA
Vision	2 Parts: Ask: "Do you have difficulty driving, or watching television, or reading, or doing any of your daily activities because of your eyesight?" If yes, then: Test each eye with Snellen chart while patient wears corrective lenses (if applicable)	Yes to question and inability to read greater than 20/40 on Snellen chart.	Question: derived from some of the most reliable items on the Boston Activities of Daily Vision Scale; test-retest reliability is 0.8; Snellen chart: "gold" standard.
Hearing	Use audioscope set at 40 dB. Test hearing using 1,000 and 2,000 Hz	Inability to hear 1,000 or 2,000 Hz in both ears or either of these frequencies in one ear.	In physicians' offices: sensitivity = 0.94; specificity = 0.72.
Leg mobility	Time the patient after asking: "Rise from the chair. Walk 20 feet briskly, turn, walk back to the chair and sit down."	Unable to complete task in 15 seconds.	Modified version of the "Up & Go"; inter-rater and test-retest reliability = 0.99; good correlations with other measures of gait and balance (-0.6 to -0.8).
Urinary incontinence	2 Parts: Ask: "In the last year, have you ever lost your urine and gotten wet?" If yes, then ask: "Have you lost urine on at least 6 separate days?"	Yes to both questions.	83% agreement between patient response and urologic assessment.
Nutrition/weight loss	2 Parts: Ask: "Have you lost 10 lbs. over the past 6 months without trying to do so?" Weigh the patient.	Yes to the question or weight <100 lb.	Question: relative risk of death = 2.0* (NHEFS); weight: PPV of malnutrition = 0.99.
Memory	Three-item recall	Unable to remember all three items after 1 minute.	Likelihood ratios: recalls all 3 = 0.06; recalls 2 = 0.5; recalls <2 = 3.1.
Depression	Ask: "Do you often feel sad or depressed?"	Yes to the question.	Sensitivity = 0.78; specificity = 0.87.
Physical disability	Six questions: "Are you able to: "Do strenuous activities like fast walking or bicycling?" "Do heavy work around the house like washing windows, walls, or floors?" "Go shopping for groceries or clothes?" "Get to places out of walking distance?" "Bathe, either a sponge bath, tub bath, or shower?" "Dress, like putting on a shirt, buttoning and zipping, or putting on shoes?"	Yes to any of the questions.	Coefficient of scalability 0.86; coefficient of reproducibility 0.96; test-retest reliability 0.88; good correlation with other measures of physical function 0.63-0.89.

Reprinted by permission of the publisher from Moore AA, Siu AL: Screening for common problems in ambulatory elderly: clinical confirmation of a screening instrument, *Am J Med* 100:438-443, Copyright 1996 by Excerpta Medica, Inc.
*Personal communication from Tamara B. Harris, M.D.
NHEFS, National Health Epidemiologic Follow-up Study; PPV, positive predictive value.

tasks to office staff. Two years ago, Miller et al. reported a screening procedure that used individual instruments that had, by and large, been validated in other studies.[1] That battery required 21 minutes of an office assistant's time. Moore and Siu here report an even briefer screen that requires 10 minutes to administer and covers many of the common syndromes affecting older persons. These instruments, and others that will undoubtedly be developed, may prove extremely useful in ensuring that geriatric problems are not overlooked. However, their value depends on proper implementation and appropriate action based on the results of the screen. Practitioners or health care systems must be willing to invest the costs to release office staff to perform the screens, or hire additional staff to administer them. Moreover, clinicians must know how to respond when screening indicates a potential problem, including the appropriate subsequent diagnostic and therapeutic steps.

REFERENCE
1. Miller DK, Brunworth D, Brunworth DS, et al: Efficiency of geriatric case-finding in a private practitioner's office, J Am Geriatr Soc 43:533-537, 1995.

IMMUNIZATIONS IN LONG-TERM CARE FACILITIES: POLICIES AND PRACTICE

Nichol KL, Grimm MB, Peterson DC   (VA Med Center, Minneapolis; Minnesota Dept of Health, Minneapolis, Minn)

J Am Geriatr Soc 44:349-355, 1996

Introduction. The residents of long-term care facilities may be vulnerable to vaccine-preventable diseases, especially influenza, pneumococcal pneumonia, and tetanus. Recognition of the importance of immunization in this population prompted an investigation of the policies and practices regarding resident and employee vaccinations in long-term care institutions.

Methods. A questionnaire was mailed to all 445 long-term care facilities for adults in Minnesota. Information was requested on immunization policies and programs for the residents and the employees, attitudes toward immunizations, and 12-month vaccination rates for influenza, pneumococcal pneumonia, and tetanus/diphtheria among residents and for influenza, tetanus, and hepatitis B among employees.

Results. The questionnaire was returned by 90% of the facilities. Among residents, the mean 12-month immunization rates were 84% for influenza vaccination, 11.9% for pneumococcal vaccination, and 2.9% for tetanus/diphtheria vaccination (Table 1). The vaccination rates improved significantly in institutions with formal, written vaccination policies or facility-wide standing orders and in facilities not requiring written consent for immunization. Influenza vaccination was considered very important and cost-effective by most of the facilities, whereas the tetanus/diphtheria vaccination was typically considered much less important and cost-effective. Although 86.1% of the facilities had an influenza vaccination program for employees, there was only a 33% 12-month vaccination rate among employees. The other 12-month vaccination rates among employees were 23.2% for hepatitis B and 1.7% for tetanus/diphtheria. Employee vaccination rates were improved in facilities offering on-site vaccination and free vaccination and in facilities providing in-service education regarding immunization.

TABLE 1 Long-Term Care Facilities' Immunization Activities for Residents

	PERCENT OF FACILITIES ($n = 399$)
Written policies for vaccination	
Influenza	69.3
Pneumococcal	33
Tetanus/diphtheria	16.3
Routine assessment of immunization status	
Influenza	
All residents	94.3
New residents admitted during immunization season	65
Pneumococcal	
Residents ≥65 years	38.9
Residents with chronic cardiopulmonary disease	14.8
Tetanus/diphtheria—primary series	
New residents	6
Tetanus/diphtheria—boosters	
Residents with chronic skin ulceration	2.3
Residents with acute skin trauma	21.4
12-month vaccination rates (spring 1992-spring 1993)	
Influenza	84
Pneumococcal	11.9
Tetanus/diphtheria	2.9
Assessment of vaccination rates included as part of quality assurance/ quality improvement activities	
Influenza	40.4
Pneumococcal	7.9
Tetanus/diphtheria	2.6

Courtesy of Nichol KL, Grimm MB, Peterson DC: Immunizations in long-term care facilities: policies and practice, J Am Geriatr Soc 44(4):349-355, 1996.

Conclusions. Because infectious diseases contribute significantly to the morbidity and mortality of residents of long-term care facilities, the vaccination policies and practices are of vital importance in protecting the health of this vulnerable population. Therefore, long-term care institutions should implement programs to increase immunization rates among both residents and employees.

Commentary

Residents in nursing homes represent an important target population for vaccinations. Traditionally, such facilities have not had a great rate of immunizing their residents. However, with increased attention to the importance of immunization, vaccination rates have improved considerably in recent years. This study adds to our knowledge of what strategies result in the highest vaccination rates. It is important because it represents a statewide survey that included 399 nursing homes. The greatest immunization rates of patients occurred in those nursing homes when there were written immunization policies, standing orders for vaccine administration, and no requirement for written consent for the administration of a vaccine.

The record on immunization of nursing home staff is not as good as it is for patients. It should be. Health care providers should serve as role models for excellent preventive care, and furthermore, we owe it to our patients to protect them by taking immunization ourselves. In the current study, several strategies improved the vaccination rate among employees. Those strategies were the following: offering the vaccine on site, not charging for administration of the agent, and providing an educational program on the importance and safety of vaccination.

This is an important article to get into the hands of all medical and nursing directors.

SUCCESSFUL AGING: PREDICTORS AND ASSOCIATED ACTIVITIES

Strawbridge WJ, Cohen RD, Shema SJ, et al (*California Public Health Found, Berkeley; California Dept of Health Services, Berkeley*)
Am J Epidemiol 144:135-141, 1996

Introduction. A growing interest in preventing disease and promoting health in older individuals has led to an examination of "successful" aging. Although there is no agreed-upon standard for what constitutes successful aging, the definition adopted for this study assumes the ability to perform without difficulty all the basic physical activities expected of an adult. A group of men and women aged 65-95 years was followed up for 6 years to determine predictors of successful aging.

Methods. Study participants were members of the Alameda County Study, a longitudinal investigation of factors related to health and mortality. In 1984, 508 cohort members aged 65 years or older completed questionnaires covering matters of health, sociodemographic variables, and behavioral and psychosocial factors. At 6-year follow-up, 356 of the 381 surviving members of the 1984 cohort responded to a second questionnaire. Those who were aging successfully could execute 13 basic activities without difficulty or assistance and five physical performance activities with no more than a little difficulty.

Results. The group of survivors had a mean age of 71.9 years and included 209 women (59%) and 147 men (41%); 88% were white and 12% were black. Whereas nearly 60% were scored as aging successfully in 1984, that proportion decreased to 35% in 1990. Eighteen individuals showed improvement, moving from not aging successfully in 1984 to aging successfully in 1990. There was a strong relationship between baseline successful aging and follow-up successful aging. After adjusting for baseline status, sex, and age, positive predictors of successful aging in 1990 were income above the lowest quintile, 12 or more years of education, and white ethnicity. After adjusting for all variables, behavioral and psychosocial predictors were the absence of depression, having close personal contacts, and walking often for exercise (Table 2). The likelihood of successful aging was reduced by the presence of certain chronic medical conditions.

Conclusions. Individuals who age successfully and are able to function independently have a good quality of life. Many do paid or volunteer work and participate regularly in activities they enjoy. Their physical health status is generally high, they are not too tired to do things they enjoy, and they report feeling pleasure and excitement more than depression.

TABLE 2 Baseline Predictors of 1990 Successful Aging for 356 Alameda Study Cohort Members Aged 65-95 Years at Baseline Interviewed in 1984 and 1990

1984 BASELINE PREDICTOR	OR*	95% CI*
Baseline Successful Aging and Sociodemographic Predictors		
Baseline successful aging	7.21	4.06-12.78
White ethnicity	2.12	0.93-4.86
Income above lowest quintile	2.01	0.99-4.11
Aged 65-74 years compared with older	1.82	1.02-3.27
≥12 years of education	1.67	0.98-2.84
Male sex	1.30	0.79-2.11
Married	0.82	0.45-1.51
Chronic Conditions		
Diabetes	0.10	0.01-0.79
Asthma	0.27	0.05-1.36
Stroke	0.34	0.07-1.61
Chronic obstructive pulmonary disease	0.41	0.17-0.97
Arthritis	0.43	0.26-0.71
Hearing problems	0.48	0.25-0.89
Cancer	0.73	0.36-1.49
Behavioral and Psychosocial Predictors		
Not often depressed	1.82	1.05-3.16
Has five or more close personal contacts	1.76	1.02-3.02
Often walks for exercise	1.70	0.98-2.96
Moderate alcohol use	1.48	0.83-2.62
Does not currently smoke cigarettes	1.22	0.60-2.47

Courtesy of Strawbridge WJ, Cohen RD, Shema SJ, et al: Successful aging: Predictors and associated activities, *Am J Epidemiol* 144:135-141, 1996.
OR, odds ratio; CI, confidence interval.
Based upon logistic regression models. All models include age, sex, and baseline successful aging. Behavioral and psychosocial predictors also include adjustments for ethnicity, income, education, and number of chronic conditions.

Commentary

Why do some persons age successfully whereas others do not? The authors of this study used prospective Alameda County Study data to identify predictors of successful aging, as defined by functional status and physical performance measures, during the subsequent 6 years. The strongest predictor was successful aging at the baseline interview. Other predictors included white ethnicity, younger age (65-74 years compared with 75 years or older), the absence of specific chronic conditions (diabetes, arthritis, chronic obstructive pulmonary disease, or hearing problems), and specific behavioral or psychosocial factors ("not often depressed," five or more close personal contacts, and walking often for exercise). As expected, those who had aged successfully were more engaged in work and leisure activities, had fewer sick days and saw doctors less frequently, and had better mental health. Although some of these predictors are immutable, others (e.g., walking for exercise, increasing personal contacts) may be changed. Perhaps the more important question is whether better management of the chronic diseases associated with unsuccessful aging can make a difference.

DO TOO MANY COOKS SPOIL THE BROTH? MULTIPLE PHYSICIAN INVOLVEMENT IN MEDICAL MANAGEMENT OF ELDERLY PATIENTS AND POTENTIALLY INAPPROPRIATE DRUG COMBINATIONS

Tamblyn RM, McLeod PJ, Abrahamowicz M, et al
(McGill Univ, Montreal)
Can Med Assoc J 154:1177-1184, 1996

Introduction. Problems can occur in prescribing medication for older patients who have a number of medical problems and are receiving care from several physicians. Without monitoring by a single pharmacy or primary care physician, a patient may be prescribed potentially inappropriate drug combinations (PIDCs) or two drugs from the same group. Factors that increase or decrease the risk of a PIDC were retrospectively examined in a cross-sectional study.

Methods. Study participants were drawn from elderly Medicare registrants in 12 geographically defined health care regions in Quebec. Those eligible had visited at least one physician in 1990, were not living in a health care institution for the entire year, and had received at least one prescription for a cardiovascular drug, a psychotropic drug, or a nonsteroidal antiinflammatory drug (NSAID). Data were obtained by reviewing physician and prescription claims. A PIDC was defined as a drug combination with established or probable evidence of a risk of adverse interaction and which could not normally be justified to achieve safe and effective treatment in an elderly patient.

Results. A total of 51,587 patients, 82% of the sample of eligible participants, had been prescribed drugs from one or more of the three drug groups studied. These patients had a mean age of 74.7 years and received a median of seven different drugs each. Most had a single primary care physician and had prescriptions filled at a single pharmacy, but two thirds had two or more prescribing physicians during the study period. Overall, 17.4% of patients had at least one PIDC during the year. Those receiving a psychotropic drug were most likely to have a PIDC, and the most common PIDC was concurrent prescription of two benzodiazepines. In all three drug groups (Fig. 1), the number of prescribing physicians was the most important risk factor for a PIDC. Use of a single dispensing pharmacy lowered the risk of a PIDC in all drug groups, whereas the presence of a single primary care physician lowered the risk for cardiovascular and psychotropic PIDCs (Table 3).

Conclusions. For elderly patients, the risk of a PIDC increases with the number of physicians involved in their care. Use of a single dispensing pharmacy and having a primary care physician can lower this risk.

TABLE 3 Proportion of Patients With a Single Primary Care Physician or a Single Dispensing Pharmacy Who Had a PIDC, by Type of Drug Combination

VARIABLE	CARDIOVASCULAR	PSYCHOTROPIC	NSAID
Single primary care physician			
Yes	5.1	18.3	3.8
No	7.1	22.1	4.0
Odds ratio	0.70*	0.79*	0.94
Single dispensing pharmacy			
Yes	5.0	18.7	3.5
No	7.2	22.4	4.6
Odds ratio	0.68*	0.79*	0.75*

TYPE OF DRUG COMBINATION: % OF PATIENTS WITH A PIDC

Courtesy of Tamblyn RM, McLeod PJ, Abrahamowicz M, et al: Do too many cooks spoil the broth? multiple physician involvement in medical management of elderly patients and potentially inappropriate drug combinations, Can Med Assoc J 154:1177-1184, 1996.
*$P < 0.001$.

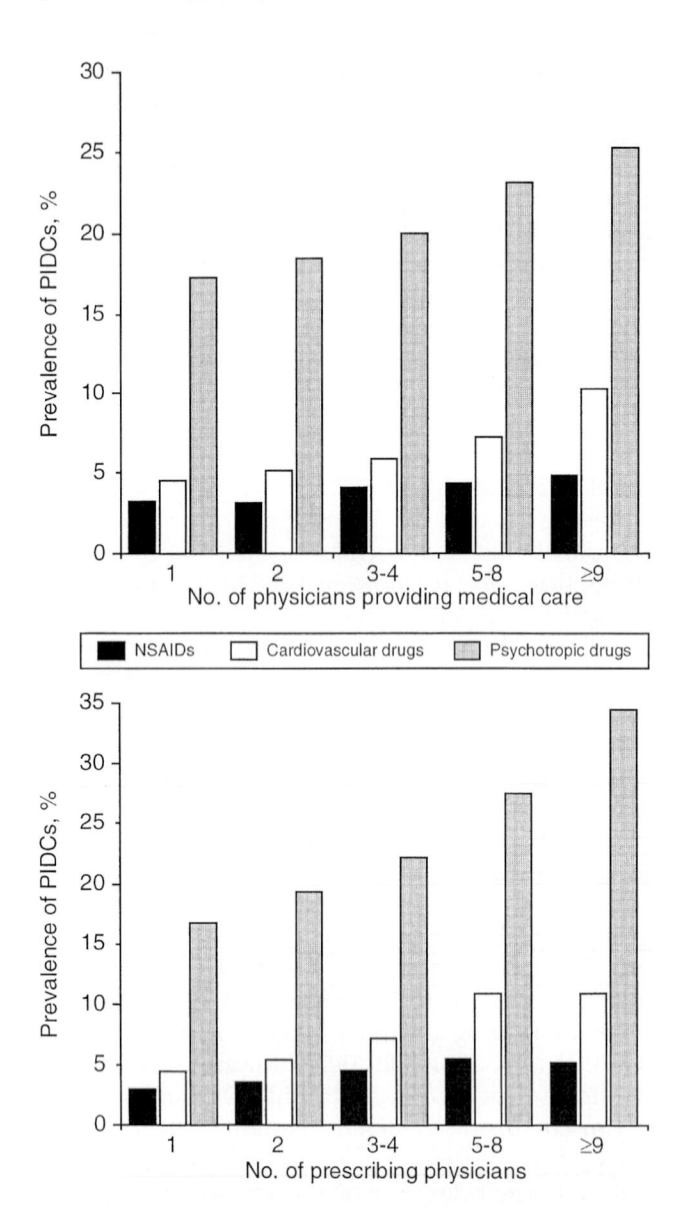

Fig. 1 Prevalence of potentially inappropriate drug combinations (PIDCs) by number of physicians providing medical care *(top)* and number of prescribing physicians *(bottom)*, by type of drug combination. *NSAIDs,* nonsteroidal antiinflammatory drugs. (Courtesy of Tamblyn RM, McLeod PJ, Abrahamowicz M, et al: Do too many cooks spoil the broth? multiple physician involvement in medical management of elderly patients and potentially inappropriate drug combinations, *Can Med Assoc J* 154:1177-1184, 1996.)

Commentary

Among the arguments for identification of a primary care physician is the fragmentation of care provided when many physicians are involved. One particularly risky consequence of receiving care from many physicians is drug prescribing without adequate consideration of the medications that the patient is already receiving from another physician. Communication between providers may be inadequate. Moreover, patients may not accurately relate what medications they are taking and may use multiple pharmacies to fill their prescriptions.

In this study, researchers in Canada examined PIDCs as determined by expert reviewers and then examined the impact of having a single primary care physician to coordinate the care, as well as the impact of having a single pharmacy to monitor dispensing. Most of the PIDCs involved using multiple drugs of the same class or having the same physiologic effect (e.g., potassium-sparing diuretic with potassium supplement). Their results indicate that the greater the number of physicians providing medical care or prescribing medications, the higher the risk of PIDCs for cardiovascular drugs, psychotropic drugs, or NSAIDs. Having a single primary care physician reduced the odds of a cardiovascular or a psychotropic PIDC by 30% and 21%, respectively. Having a single dispensing pharmacy reduced the odds of a cardiovascular, a psychotropic, or an NSAID drug PIDC by 32%, 21%, and 25%, respectively. These findings indicate the need for better coordination of medical care and a network system among pharmacies to ensure that duplication and potential adverse drug interactions are brought to the attention of patients' physicians.

YEAR BOOK OF MEDICINE

PREDICTION OF RISK OF LIVER DISEASE BY ALCOHOL INTAKE, SEX, AND AGE: A PROSPECTIVE POPULATION STUDY

Becker U, Deis A, Sørensen TIA, et al *(Univ of Copenhagen; Danish Committee for the Assessment of Sub-Standard Lives, Copenhagen; Copenhagen Health Services)*
Hepatology 23:1025-1029, 1996

Background.—The risk of alcohol-induced liver damage is known to increase with the amount of alcohol consumed, but the dose-effect relationship has not been determined. A large population-based cohort underwent 12-year follow-up to assess the association between self-reported current alcohol intake and the risk of future liver disease.

Patients and Methods.—The study population was drawn from the Copenhagen City Heart Study. Complete information was available for 13,285 individuals between 30 and 79 years of age who completed the alcohol intake questionnaire. Participants were asked to respond to multiple-choice questions concerning the frequency and type (beer, wine, or spirits) of alcohol consumption. After 12 years, register-based information was obtained on death or hospital discharge with a liver-related diagnosis suggestive of alcohol-induced liver disease. The risk function between alcohol intake and liver diseases was analyzed by using multiplicative Poisson regression models.

Results.—There were 261 cases of alcohol-induced liver disease (184 men and 77 women), resulting in

Alcoholic cirrhosis

Alcoholic liver disease

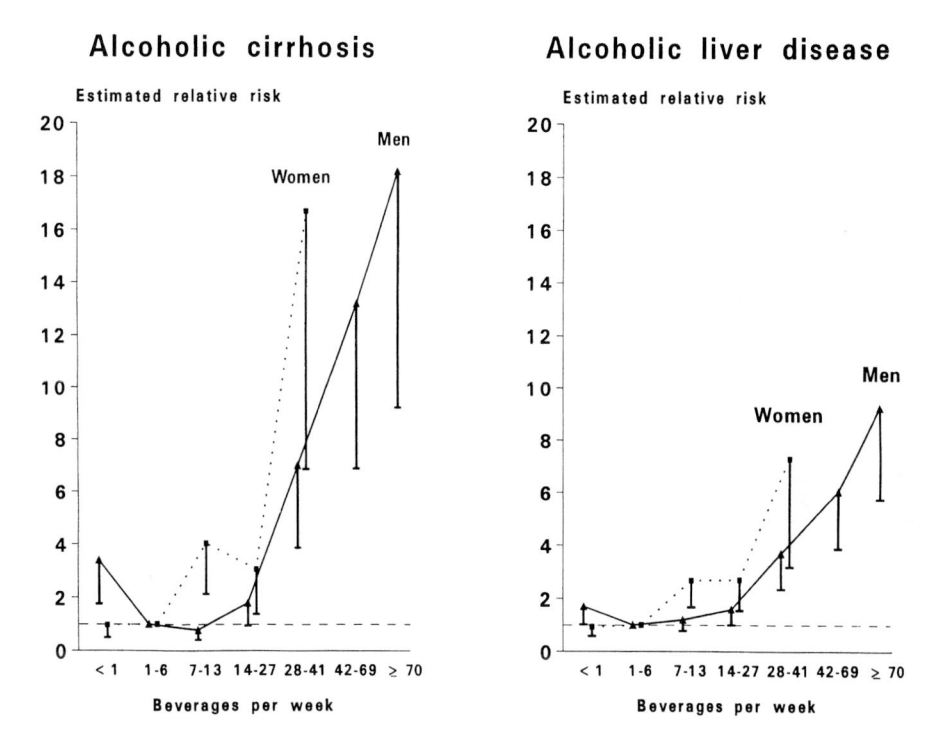

Fig. 1 Relative risk estimates for development of alcohol-induced cirrhosis and alcohol-induced liver disease as a function of the individual alcohol intake classified as <1 beverage (<12 g); 1 to 6 beverages (12-72 g); 7 to 13 beverages (84-156 g); 14 to 27 beverages (168-24 g); 28 to 41 beverages (336-492 g); 42 to 69 beverages (504-828 g); ≥70 beverages (≥840 g). The group with an alcohol intake of 1 to 6 beverages per week is the reference group (relative risk, >1). The vertical lines are estimated lower than 95% confidence limits. (Courtesy of Becker U, Deis A, Sørensen TIA, et al: Prediction of risk of liver disease by alcohol intake, sex, and age: a prospective population study, *Hepatology* 23:1025-1029, 1996.)

TABLE 1 Alcohol Intake by Sex, Number of Incident Cases of Alcohol-Induced Liver Disease, and Cirrhosis

ALCOHOL INTAKE	MEN (n)	WOMEN (n)	ALCOHOL-INDUCED LIVER DISEASE MEN (n)	ALCOHOL-INDUCED LIVER DISEASE WOMEN (n)	ALCOHOL-INDUCED CIRRHOSIS MEN (n)	ALCOHOL-INDUCED CIRRHOSIS WOMEN (n)
Beverages per week (g alcohol per week)						
<1 (<12)	625	2,472	15	17	10	5
1-6 (12-72)	1,183	3,079	18	23	6	7
7-13 (84-156)	1,825	1,019	32	20	7	9
14-27 (168-324)	1,234	543	29	11	11	4
28-41 (336-492)	585	72	31	4	20	3
42-69 (504-828)	388	29	34	1	25	0
≥70 (≥840)	211	20	25	1	17	0
TOTAL	6,051	7,234	184	77	96	28

Courtesy of Becker U, Deis A, Sørensen TIA, et al: Prediction of risk of liver disease by alcohol intake, sex, and age: a prospective population study, *Hepatology* 23:1025-1029, 1996.

98 deaths during the observation period. Alcohol-induced cirrhosis occurred in 96 men and 28 women, yielding incidence rates of 0.2% per year in men and 0.03% per year in women (Table 1). Risk for the development of cirrhosis and liver disease was lowest among those whose alcohol intake ranged from 1 to 6 beverages per week. Above this level, a steep dose-dependent increase in relative risk was observed (Fig. 1). With an intake of 7-13 beverages per week for women and 14-27 beverages per week for men, the relative risk was higher than 1. For any given level of alcohol intake, the relative

risk of alcohol-related liver disease and alcohol-induced cirrhosis was significantly higher for women than for men.

Conclusions. Both men and women had a dose-dependent increase in the relative risk of alcohol-induced liver disease. Previous studies have indicated that women are more vulnerable to alcohol, and in this cohort the risk increased more steeply for women than for men with increasing alcohol intake.

Commentary

This carefully done study provides additional support for the concept that the likelihood of the development of alcoholic liver disease is directly related to dose and duration of alcohol use. I think it is important for physicians to quantify a patient's alcohol intake in a manner similar to the quantifying of cigarette consumption. A simple and easy to use reference system is as follows: 1 oz of whiskey, gin, or vodka contains up to 10-11 g of alcohol, one 12-oz can of beer has 10-11 g of alcohol, and 4 oz of wine has 10-11 g of alcohol. Thus, a patient drinking 6 bottles of beer per day is ingesting approximately 60-66 g of alcohol per day. One dose of alcohol in each of the above quantities is equivalent to 1 unit. More potent ales and beers may have as many as 12 g per bottle, so this number could rise to 72 g per day.

There is evidence to support the concept that more than 30 g of alcohol per day is capable of causing liver injury in women, and more than 60 g of alcohol per day is capable of effecting liver injury in men. Most authorities have suggested that alcohol consumption in quantities greater than 3 units per day or 21 units per week constitutes excessive consumption of alcohol.

That factors other than alcohol consumption are important in the development of alcoholic liver disease is clearly evident. One such factor is hepatitis C, which potentiates the likelihood of the development of alcoholic liver disease. It would have been interesting if Becker et al. had carried out additional studies to determine the proportion of their patients with alcohol-induced liver disease who actually were hepatitis C-positive. Similar prospective studies should surely take this factor, as well as other factors, into consideration.

MALIGNANT NEOPLASMS FOLLOWING BONE MARROW TRANSPLANTATION

Bhatia S, Ramsay NKC, Steinbuch M, et al
(Univ of Minnesota, Minneapolis)
Blood 87:3633-3639, 1996

Background. As survival after bone marrow transplantation (BMT) improves, problems are arising with post-BMT neoplasms. A low but significant risk of second neoplasms has been reported among patients who have undergone BMT for leukemias and aplastic anemias. A large BMT cohort was studied to assess the incidence of post-BMT neoplasms and to identify any associated host or treatment factors.

Methods. A total of 2150 recipients of BMT during a 20-year period were studied, including 1063 patients who received allogeneic marrow from related donors, 227 who received unrelated donor grafts, and 750 who received autologous marrow. Conditioning regimens varied. Any post-BMT malignancies were recorded, and the risk of and factors associated with these neoplasms were analyzed. Forty percent of the cohort were alive at a median follow-up of 3 years, with a total of 5025 person-years of follow-up after BMT.

Findings. A total of 53 post-BMT neoplasms developed in 51 patients in the cohort, compared with 4.3 expected in the general population, for a standardized incidence ratio of 11.6. There were 22 cases of B-cell lymphoproliferative disorder, 17 solid nonhematopoietic tumors, 10 cases of myelodysplastic syndrome, two cases of non-Hodgkin's lymphoma, and 1 case each of acute myelogenous leukemia and Hodgkin's disease. The 13-year actuarial incidence of post-BMT malignancy was estimated at 10% ± 2% (Fig. 1).

At 4 years, the cumulative probability of B-cell lymphoproliferative disorder leveled off at 1.6%. This risk was independently associated with in vitro T-cell bone marrow depletion (relative risk [RR] 11.9); HLA mismatch (RR 8.9); use of antithymocyte globulin to prevent graft-vs.-host disease (RR 5.9), and the preparative regimen (RR 2.5). The 13-year cumulative probability of solid malignancies was about 6% ± 2%. The most common solid tumor was malignant melanoma, (standardized incidence ratio 10.3). By 9 years, the actuarial incidence of myelodysplastic syndrome/acute myelogenous

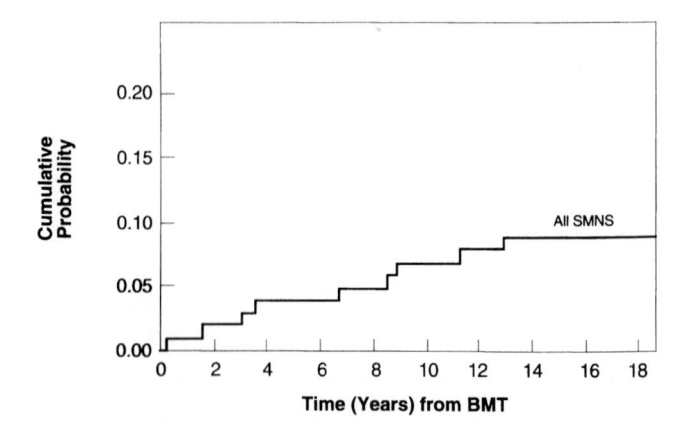

Fig. 1 Cumulative probability of second malignant neoplasms *(SMNs)* in 2150 patients undergoing bone marrow transplantation. (Courtesy of Bhatia S, Ramsay NKC, Steinbuch M, et al: Malignant neoplasms following bone marrow transplantation, *Blood* 87:3633-3639, 1996.)

leukemia leveled off at about 2%, occurring most frequently in older patients with Hodgkin's disease or non-Hodgkin's lymphoma who received autologous peripheral-blood stem cells.

Conclusions. Survivors of BMT are at risk of later malignancies. Post-BMT malignant neoplasms may contribute significantly to the overall morbidity and mortality of BMT. Future research should focus on screening techniques and ways of identifying patients at increased risk. The increased risk of leukemia and lymphoma is unlikely to persist beyond the first decade after BMT, but the risk of radiation-associated solid tumors may continue to increase.

Commentary

In this analysis of more than 2100 recipients of BMT, 51 subsequently had malignant disease. This is more than tenfold the expected incidence of 4.3 cases. Almost half of the neoplasms were B-cell disorders, and about one third were solid tumors. The actuarial probability of a second neoplasm developing by 13 years was nearly 10%, with the probability of a solid tumor being between 5% and 6%.

Of the 51 malignant disorders, 10 were myelodysplastic syndromes. These were seen mostly in recipients of autologous blood stem cell transplantation for Hodgkin's disease or non-Hodgkin's lymphomas.

These are important observations and indicate that there is an additional long-term complication of BMT—a complication that was anticipated but not well documented.

ACUTE RENAL FAILURE IN INTENSIVE CARE UNITS—CAUSES, OUTCOME, AND PROGNOSTIC FACTORS OF HOSPITAL MORTALITY: A PROSPECTIVE, MULTICENTER STUDY

Brivet FG, and The French Study on Acute Renal Failure
(A Béclère Univ Hosp, Clamart, France; et al)
Crit Care Med 24:192-198, 1996

Background. Acute renal failure continues to have a high, perhaps even rising, mortality. Previous reports of acute renal failure have differed in their descriptions of the patient population, definitions of acute renal failure, definitions of outcome variables, and coexisting diseases.

Methods. The causes, prognostic factors, and outcomes of severe acute renal failure were prospectively studied. The study included all patients with severe acute renal failure from 20 French ICUs during a 6-month period. To be enrolled in the study, patients without preexisting renal disease had to have a serum creatinine concentration of 3.5 mg/dl or more and/or a blood urea nitrogen concentration of 100 mg/dl or more. Patients with previous chronic renal insufficiency (i.e., a serum creatinine concentration of greater than 1.8 mg/dl) had to have a blood urea nitrogen or serum creatinine concentration increasing to 100% above the baseline value. Patients whose basal serum creatinine concentration exceeded 3.4 mg/dl were excluded. Data collected included the patients' previous health status and any preexisting organ dysfunction, along with the type and cause of acute renal failure. The Simplified Acute Physiology Score, Acute Physiology and Chronic Health Evaluation Score, and number of organ system failures were assessed, and prognostic factors were identified by univariate and stepwise logistic regression analysis.

Results. Of 360 patients with acute renal failure identified, 217 were enrolled in the study at the time of ICU admission and 143 were enrolled afterward. About 60% of patients had a history of health problems in the 3 months preceding admission. Seventy-eight percent were admitted for medical reasons. The type of acute renal failure was renal in 78% of patients, prerenal in 17%, and postrenal in 5%. Forty-eight percent of patients received renal replacement therapy, and 58% died in the hospital. Factors predicting death on stepwise logistic regression were advanced age, altered previous health status, hospitalization before ICU admission, delayed acute renal failure, sepsis, oliguria, and severity of illness, as measured by the previously mentioned scoring systems (Table 3).

TABLE 3. Multivariate Predictors of Acute Renal Failure (ARF) Hospital Mortality

VARIABLE	β	ODDS RATIO	95% CI
Constant	−3.742	—	—
Age (45 vs. 65 yrs)	0.021	1.55	1.32-1.81
Previous altered health status	0.856	2.35	1.37-4.07
Hospitalization before ICU admission	0.795	2.22	1.32-3.72
ARF occurring during ICU stay	1.089	2.97	1.72-5.13
Septic cause	0.842	2.32	1.37-3.93
SAPS at inclusion (15 vs. 20)	0.084	1.54	1.36-1.75
Oliguria	0.791	2.22	1.28-3.84

Courtesy of Brivet FG, and The French Study on Acute Renal Failure: acute renal failure in intensive care units—causes, outcome, and prognostic factors of hospital mortality: a prospective, multicenter study, *Crit Care Med* 24:192-198, 1996.
CI, confidence interval; *SAPS*, Simplified Acute Physiology Score.

Conclusions. Patients with acute renal failure severe enough to require ICU admission continue to have a high hospital mortality rate. Prognostic factors in this group of patients are identified and should be included in future trials of acute renal failure. Important factors to assess include patient age; previous health status; disease characteristics, i.e., initial or delayed acute renal failure, oliguria, or sepsis; and the severity of illness at baseline, as reflected by physiologic scoring systems.

Commentary

Acute renal failure is a clinical syndrome characterized by a marked decrease in renal function during a period of hours or days. Despite considerable advances in renal replacement therapy and in the management of critically ill patients, the mortality rate associated with acute renal failure remains high and may have even increased in the last two decades. The syndrome of acute renal failure can develop before or during hospitalization; it is found in about 5% of patients admitted to medical and surgical services. Hospital-acquired acute renal failure may be recognized by a sudden rise in blood urea nitrogen or serum creatinine or a sudden reduction in urine volume. When urine volume is less than 400 ml/day or 20 ml/hr, it is termed oliguric renal failure.

This multicenter study from France examined the prognostic factors that may determine the outcome of patients with acute renal failure admitted to hospitals during the 1990s. The results indicate that the mortality rate of acute renal failure remains high, about 58%. This figure is not dissimilar from that of other recent reports.[1,2] In certain populations of patients with acute renal failure, however, lower mortality rates have been reported. Reasons for the high mortality rate in some series include: the older age of referred patients, sepsis, and an increasing incidence of multi-organ failure. In this study, the number of survivors exceeded that of nonsurvivors when the patients were younger than 30 years of age. In patients between the ages of 30 and 45 years, the number of survivors and nonsurvivors was equal. Among patients older than 45 years, more died than survived. The mean age of survivors in this study was 54.1 years as compared with 64.5 years for the 210 patients who did not survive.

In this controlled prospective study, the authors emphasize seven predictive factors associated with severe acute renal failure requiring transfer of patients to an ICU. These factors include age, previous health status, hospitalization before transfer to the ICU the late occurrence of acute renal failure, sepsis, oliguria, and severity of illness at the time of inclusion in the study. Hypotension and the need for mechanical ventilation were found to be predictors of a worse prognosis in a multivariate analysis when severity of the illness was not assessed by physiologic scales or when the scales were unpredictive at admission.

One note of caution should be interjected here. The causes of acute renal failure in elderly individuals may be somewhat different from those in younger individuals; for example, atheroembolic disease may be a more common cause of renal failure in the elderly, and other complications related to age may influence the outcome in these patients as compared with younger individuals. Regardless, the mortality of acute renal failure remains high. Preventive measures and acute awareness of the settings in which this entity occurs may be important in improving survival in this population of patients.

REFERENCES

1. Rasmussen HH, Pitt EA, Ibels LS, et al: Prediction of outcome in acute renal failure by discriminant analysis of clinical variables, *Arch Intern Med* 145:2015-2018, 1985.
2. Liano F, Gallego A, Pascual J, et al: Prognosis of acute tubular necrosis: an extended prospectively contrasted study, *Nephron* 63: 21-31, 1993.

GUIDELINES FOR THE PREVENTION AND TREATMENT OF INFECTION IN PATIENTS WITH AN ABSENT OR DYSFUNCTIONAL SPLEEN

Cavill I, for the Working Party of the British Committee for Standards in Haematology Clinical Haematology Task Force *(British Committee for Standards in Haematology, London)*
BMJ 312:430-434, 1996

Introduction. Patients who have undergone splenectomy have a lifelong risk of major, life-threatening infections. Most serious infections are caused by *Streptococcus pneumoniae, Haemophilus influenzae,* or *Neisseria meningitidis*. The British Committee for Standards in Haematology has recommended ways to prevent and treat infections in patients with absent or dysfunctional spleens.

Methods. The MEDLINE and Excerpta Medica databases were searched to locate published data about infections in patients with absent or dysfunctional spleens. The guideline development group was convened by the British Committee for Standards in Haematology and was comprised of representatives from a range of medical specialties chosen for their expertise. Recommendations from the group and findings from published evidence were used to formulate the guidelines.

Findings. The guidelines stress preventive measures to avoid the development of postsplenectomy infections. Routine immunizations, especially against pneumonococcal, *Haemophilus influenzae,* and influenza, are not contraindicated and are recommended in children younger than 16 years and in patients with impaired immune function. Antibiotic prophylaxis is also recommended, particularly during the first 2 years after splenectomy. Patients should be instructed to begin antibiotic therapy, such as amoxicillin or penicillin, when signs and symptoms of infection begin. Precautions against infection are also needed during travel; patients with absent or dysfunctional spleens are at high risk for falciparum malaria, and use of appropriate antimalarial prophylaxis is especially important. Other potential sources of infection, such as animal or tick bites, must also be recognized and appropriate measures taken. Serious infections require immediate medical care. Parenteral penicillin is recommended for patients with suspected pneumococcal, meningococcal, or other serious infections. If resistance or allergy is suspected, or if the patient has been receiving prophylactic antibiotics, a cephalosporin (cefotaxime or ceftriaxone) should be used.

Commentary

This expert group in Britain has put together a set of guidelines based on evaluation of the current literature and the opinions of representative experts. I have one major disagreement with their recommendations for the treatment for suspected infection. In this era when it is relatively common (in many areas approximately 20%) for pneumococcal strains to be at least moderately resistant to penicillin, I believe that patients with no spleens who have suspected serious infection should be treated with a parenteral third-generation cephalosporin (either cefotaxime or ceftriaxone) to cover the pneumococcus, *Hemophilus influenzae*, and the meningococcus.

EFFECTS OF INTENSIVE DIABETES THERAPY ON NEUROPSYCHOLOGICAL FUNCTION IN ADULTS IN THE DIABETES CONTROL AND COMPLICATIONS TRIAL

The Diabetes Control and Complications Trial Research Group (Bethesda, Md)
Ann Intern Med 124:379-388, 1996

Objective. Intensive therapy for insulin-dependent diabetes mellitus (IDDM) delays the onset of diabetic retinopathy, nephropathy, and neuropathy but increases the risk for severe hypoglycemia. Previous studies have shown that severe hypoglycemia is associated with a transient reduction in cognitive function. However, the long-term effects of intensive therapy for IDDM on cognitive function have not been well studied. Using data from the multicenter Diabetes Control and Complications Trial, the long-term effects of intensive therapy for IDDM on neuropsychological performance were examined.

Patients. The study population consisted of 1441 adolescents and young adults with IDDM, ages 13-39 years, of whom 711 were randomly assigned to receive intensive therapy and 730 to receive conventional therapy. Only patients who had had IDDM for 1-15 years, with no or minimal retinopathy or nephropathy at baseline, were entered into the trial. Intensive treatment consisted of three or more insulin injections per day or continuous subcutaneous insulin infusion, and four or more blood glucose tests per day. Conventional therapy consisted of 1 or 2 daily insulin injections. Patients with a history of substance abuse, psychological disturbances, or recurrent hypoglycemia with coma or seizure were excluded. All episodes of severe hypoglycemia had to be reported as soon as possible. Patients underwent an extensive series of neuropsychological tests, with known sensitivity for neurocognitive deficits associated with hypoglycemia, at baseline; at years 2, 5, and 7; and at the end of the study. Eight cognitive domain scores were derived from the test results. Regression analysis was used to examine the association between the number of hypoglycemic episodes and neuropsychological performance. Follow-up ranged from 3.5 to 9 years; the mean was 6.5 years.

Results. Intensive diabetes therapy was not associated with the development of clinically important cognitive impairment or with an increased risk of worsening of neuropsychological function. There was no difference in performance on neuropsychological testing between the intensively treated patients and the conventionally treated patients. Patients who had frequent hypoglycemic episodes did not perform differently than those who did not have repeated episodes of hypoglycemia.

Conclusions. Intensive diabetes therapy with its attendant risk of severe hypoglycemia is not associated with clinically important cognitive impairment.

Commentary

We know that repeated episodes of hypoglycemia can cause hypoglycemia unawareness, so that blood glucose concentrations fall more before the common autonomic symptoms—palpitations, tremor, sweating, and anxiety—occur. The patient is therefore more likely to have neuroglycopenic symptoms—fatigue, dizziness, confusion, difficulty speaking and concentrating; and, ultimately, convulsions and coma. This study from the Diabetes Control and Complications Trial examined the possibility that repeated episodes of hypoglycemia can cause permanent brain injury, as has been suggested to occur, especially in children.[1,2]

The goals of therapy in the intensive therapy group were fasting and postprandial blood glucose concentrations less that 120 mg/dl (6.7 mmol/L) and 180 mg/dl (10 mmol/L), respectively, normal glycosylated hemoglobin values, and no severe hypoglycemia. In the conventional therapy group, the goals were no symptoms of hyperglycemia and no severe hypoglycemia. The neuropsychological testing done on these patients was exhaustive, taking up to 5 hours, and included tests of learning ability, memory, attention, motor speed, verbal fluency, and problem solving. From these results, global ratings of change were made by neuropsychologists unaware of treatment group assignment.

Most patients in either treatment group had no change in neuropsychological rating, but a few had a lower rating and a very few had a higher rating. The lack of overall change is reassuring. More important, there were no differences in ratings among the patients who had severe hypoglycemia and those who did not. Severe hypoglycemia was defined as an episode in which the patient required the assistance of another person and also had either a blood glucose concentration less than 50 mg/dl (2.8 mmol/L) or symptoms reversed by glucose administration (about one third of these episodes involved a seizure, suspected seizure, or coma). Episodes with less severe symptoms were not counted because the correlation with blood glucose values is very poor.[3] Severe hypoglycemia occurred about 3 times more often in the intensive therapy group (61 vs. 19 episodes per 100 patient-years).

These results mean that the occurrence of neuropsychological dysfunction in young adults with diabetes should not be attributed to hypoglycemia, and other causes should be sought. The results may not apply to children or older adults, or even to these patients if they continue to have episodes of severe hypoglycemia. In addition, there are many other reasons to avoid severe hypoglycemia, ranging from its autonomic and neuroglycopenic symptoms to the risk of injury or medical catastrophe to the induction of hypoglycemia unawareness, which only increases the risk of severe hypoglycemia.

REFERENCES
1. Langan SJ, Deary IJ, Hepburn DA, et al: Cumulative cognitive impairment following recurrent severe hypoglycemia in adult patients with insulin-treated diabetes, *Diabetologia* 34:337-344, 1991.
2. Rovet JF, Erhlich RM, Hoppe M: Specific intellectual defects in children with early onset diabetes mellitus, *Child Dev* 59:226-234, 1988.
3. Pramming S, Thorsteinsson B, Bendtson I, et al: The relationship between symptomatic and biochemical hypoglycaemia in insulin-dependent diabetic patients, *J Intern Med* 228:641-646, 1990.

BOWEL HABIT AFTER CHOLECYSTECTOMY: PHYSIOLOGICAL CHANGES AND CLINICAL IMPLICATIONS

Fort JM, Azpiroz F, Casellas F, et al
(Autonomous Univ, Barcelona)
Gastroenterology 111:617-622, 1996

Background. A 2-year prospective study estimated that persistent diarrhea develops in approximately 8% of patients undergoing elective cholecystectomy; the true incidence could be higher because milder cases may not be reported. To elucidate the pathophysiology of postcholecystectomy diarrhea, the effects of cholecystectomy on both transit time and bowel habits were examined.

Methods. Five experimental groups of patients were included in the study: 29 patients before and 1 month after uncomplicated cholecystectomy; 22 patients 4 years after cholecystectomy; 14 patients with postcholecystectomy diarrhea; and two control groups consisting of five patients with acute infectious diarrhea and 13 patients before and 1 month after other elective surgery. A modified radiopaque pellet method was used to measure colonic transit, and the standard lactulose breath H_2O test was used to measure orocecal transit.

Results. Colonic transit was substantially accelerated (51 hours before vs. 38 hours after) and orocecal transit was slightly delayed (80 minutes before vs. 103 minutes after) 1 month after cholecystectomy as opposed to before (Fig. 1). Four years after cholecystectomy, similar colonic and orocecal transit times were measured. Patients with postcholecystectomy diarrhea and patients with acute infectious diarrhea had similar acceleration in colonic transit time (Fig. 3). Gut transit was not affected by

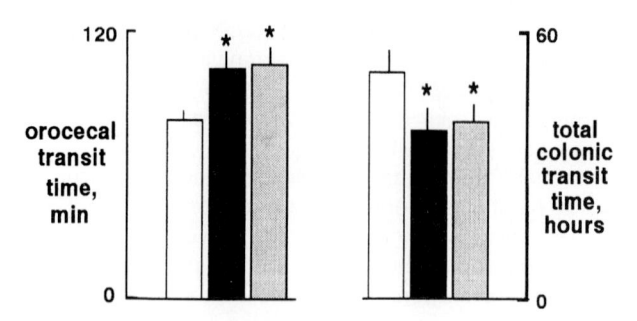

Fig. 1 Effect of cholecystectomy on orocecal and total colonic transit time. One month after cholecystectomy *(solid column),* patients had slower orocecal and faster colonic transit than before cholecystectomy *(open column).* Transit times in patients 4 years after cholecystectomy *(shaded column)* were similar to transit times after 1 month. Values are expressed as mean ± standard error. *$P \leq 0.05$ vs. before cholecystectomy. (Courtesy of Fort JM, Azpiroz F, Casellas F, et al: Bowel habit after cholecystectomy: physiological changes and clinical implications, *Gastroenterology* 111:617-622, 1996.)

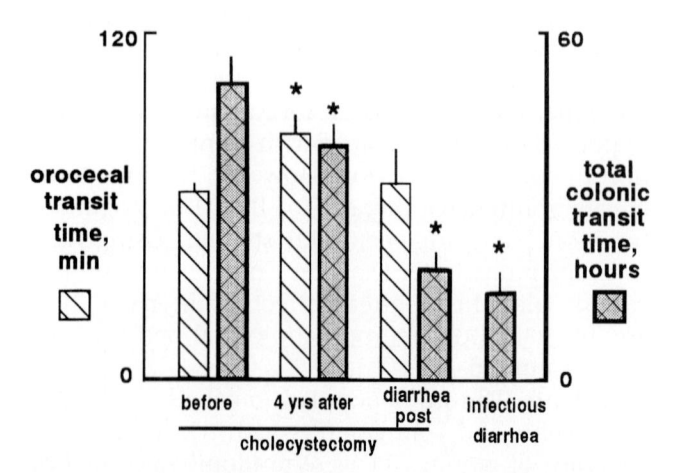

Fig. 3 Orocecal transit time and total colonic transit time in patients with postcholecystectomy diarrhea. Colonic transit was in the range of patients with infectious diarrhea, markedly faster than in patients before cholecystectomy and 4 years after cholecystectomy. In contrast to the latter, orocecal transit was not prolonged in patients with postcholecystectomy diarrhea. Values are expressed as mean ± standard error. *$P \leq 0.05$ vs. before cholecystectomy. (Courtesy of Fort JM, Azpiroz F, Casellas F, et al: Bowel habit after cholecystectomy: physiological changes and clinical implications, *Gastroenterology* 111:617-622, 1996.)

surgery per se. Postcholecystectomy diarrhea occurred in 12% of this study population.

Conclusions. These data suggest that cholecystectomy shortens gut transit time by accelerating passage of the fecal bolus through the colon, with marked acceleration in the right colon. Cholecystectomy may cause an increase in colonic bile output and a shift in bile acid composition toward the more diarrheogenic secondary bile acids. A substantial fraction of patients having cholecystectomy were aware of a change in bowel function after surgery, although all did not consider the change to have a significant effect on their lives (a few patients who had previously experienced constipation considered the effect positive).

Commentary

This study clearly demonstrates that cholecystectomy induces persistent changes in gut transit and that these changes effect a noticeable modification of bowel habits. The major change is accelerated transit in the right colon. This colonic effect is apparently caused by an increase in colonic bile acid input, in turn related to an increased enterohepatic cycling of bile acid cycles after removal of the gallbladder.

The authors also conducted a phone survey of 148 patients who had undergone cholecystectomy 4 years previously, and this survey showed that 47 patients (32%) had noted a change in bowel habits, i.e., either an increase in defecation frequency or decreased stool consistency. Further, in 18 patients (12%), the diarrhea was severe enough, i.e., three or more watery movements per day, to be classified as postcholecystectomy diarrhea. This finding is in accord with previous surveys,[1] which have reported that in approximately 8% of patients undergoing elective cholecystectomy, persistent diarrhea develops. In this setting, treatment with a bile acid sequestering agent, such as cholestyramine, is often effective in ameliorating troublesome diarrhea.

REFERENCE
1. Ros E, Zambon D: Postcholecystectomy symptoms: a prospective study of gallstone patients before and two years after surgery, *Gut* 28:1500-1504, 1987.

REDUCTION IN LONG-TERM DISABILITY IN PATIENTS WITH RHEUMATOID ARTHRITIS BY DISEASE-MODIFYING ANTIRHEUMATIC DRUG-BASED TREATMENT STRATEGIES

Fries JF, Williams CA, Morfeld D, et al *(Stanford Univ, Calif; Univ of Saskatchewan, Saskatoon, Sask, Canada)*

Arthritis Rheum 39:616-622, 1996

Background. Recently, there has been a trend in the management of rheumatoid arthritis toward using disease-modifying antirheumatic drugs (DMARDs) initially rather than using them only after initial management with traditional nonsteroidal antiinflammatory drugs (NSAIDs). However, there is little research evidence comparing the efficacy of the new and old strategies. The effectiveness of consistent DMARD treatment was evaluated with prospectively collected data from a large patient population followed up longitudinally.

Methods. Data were collected at eight centers on 2888 patients, who were followed up for as long as 20 years (average follow-up, 9 years). All the patients completed at least two Health Assessment Questionnaires at least 6 months apart. The patients were divided into groups defined by the type and length of treatment with DMARDs, NSAIDs, or prednisone. Associations between the last Disability Index value and the treatment groups were analyzed with bivariate and multivariate stepwise linear regressions.

Results. Although baseline disability values were highest in the DMARD and prednisone groups, DMARD treatment was most strongly associated with lower final disability values (Fig. 1). Among the patients treated with DMARD, those receiving only consistent DMARD therapy had a final disability level 30% lower than those treated with DMARDs on only one visit. These associations were not affected by the duration of disease at the first visit, suggesting that DMARD therapy is effective even when therapy is delayed. Patients treated consistently with NSAIDs had slightly increasing dis-

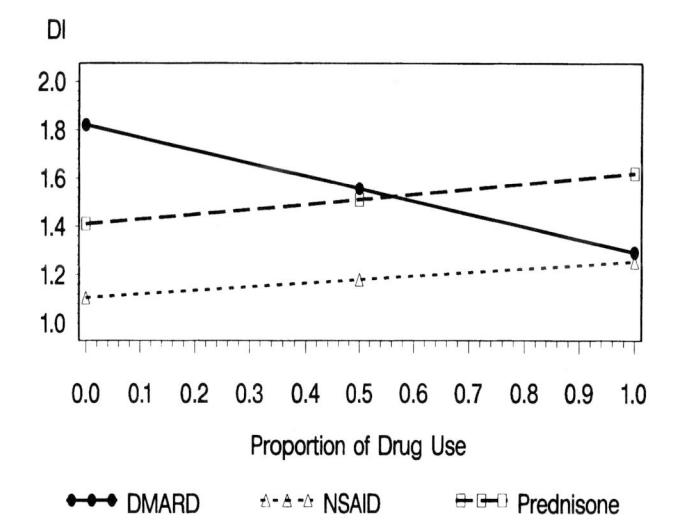

Fig. 1 Regression lines from bivariate analyses, showing the association of the proportion of encounters under different medication regimens with final Disability Index (DI) levels. Proportion of visits during disease-modifying antirheumatic drug (DMARD) use is associated with improved long-term disability values ($P < 0.0001$), proportion of visits during use of four arbitrarily selected nonsteroidal antiinflammatory drugs (NSAIDs) shows little association ($P = 0.36$), and proportion of visits under a regimen of prednisone is associated with poorer long-term disability levels ($P = 0.0005$). (Courtesy of Fries JF, Williams CA, Morfeld D, et al: Reduction in long-term disability in patients with rheumatoid arthritis by disease-modifying antirheumatic drug-based treatment strategies, *Arthritis Rheum* 39:616-622, 1996.)

ability values, whereas prednisone treatment was strongly associated with poor disability outcome. In stepwise linear regression analysis, DMARD therapy was the most powerful predictor of outcome after initial disability, age, and disease duration.

Conclusions.—Consistent DMARD use is strongly associated with improved long-term disability outcomes in patients with rheumatoid arthritis. Therefore, this strategy should be encouraged as first-line therapy in this patient population.

Commentary

The traditional NSAID-based "therapeutic pyramid" was based on the premise that rheumatoid arthritis is a benign, nonfatal, slowly evolving, often spontaneously remitting illness that is often responsive to simple therapy. Hence, patients were initially given an extended trial of NSAIDs; when these agents failed to control disease activity they were followed by sequential trials of agents such as chloroquine derivatives, oral and IM gold, D-penicillamine, and sulfasalazine, and only then by immunosuppressive or cytotoxic agents such as corticosteroids, azathioprine, or methotrexate. This therapeutic march from NSAIDs through the tiers of so-called DMARDs might take 5 years or more. However, rheumatoid arthritis is no longer viewed as globally benign and indolent; it is often rapidly debilitating, may result in irreversible anatomic abnormalities in as little as 2 years, and in its more severe forms has a markedly increased mortality, approximating that of 3-vessel coronary artery disease. Moreover, long-term NSAIDs have proven to be more toxic, and the later agents less so, than initially believed. This is the basis for changes in strategy toward the use of DMARDs early and in combination.

How does one evaluate whether the newer strategies are better than the older one when the outcomes of greatest interest—functional disability and premature mortality—are so delayed? The authors point out that a proper randomized controlled trial would entail 8-10 years, large numbers of patients, and great expense; would miss new therapeutic opportunities developed during its course; and would be ethically questionable. Their alternative was to use existing longitudinal observational data sets, identifying and adjusting for their selection and other biases. In this thoughtfully considered analysis, viewed by the authors as preliminary, consistent use of DMARDs was associated with better long-term disability outcomes, whereas consistent prednisone use (prednisone, like DMARDs, is perhaps likely to be received more frequently by more seriously affected patients) was associated with worse outcomes (see Fig. 1).

TRIGGERS OF MYOCARDIAL ISCHEMIA DURING DAILY LIFE IN PATIENTS WITH CORONARY ARTERY DISEASE: PHYSICAL AND MENTAL ACTIVITIES, ANGER AND SMOKING

Gabbay FH, Krantz DS, Kop WJ, et al (Uniformed Services Univ, Bethesda, Md; Cedars-Sinai Med Ctr, Los Angeles; Georgetown Univ, Washington, DC; et al)
J Am Coll Cardiol 27:585–592, 1996

Background.—Transient myocardial ischemia occurs in patients with coronary artery disease during many activities, not just strenuous exercise. Studies have shown that cold, mental stress, anger, and cigarette smoking can trigger myocardial ischemia. Few studies have investigated the effect of emotional states or mental stress on ischemia during daily life. In two ambulatory monitoring studies, the potency of specific physical activities and emotions as triggers of myocardial ischemia could not be determined because of the study design. There is little information on the effect of cigarette smoking on ischemia. The potency of physical activity, mental activity, emotional states, and cigarette smoking as triggers of ischemia was investigated.

Methods.—The study included 63 patients between 43 and 77 years of age with coronary artery disease. Patients kept a validated structured diary of physical and mental activities and moods. All patients underwent ECG monitoring. Physical and mental activities were evaluated and classified according to five levels of intensity.

Results.—Ischemia occurred most often during activities that were moderately intense. Most of the patients' time was spent in physical and mental activities of low intensity, but the risk of ischemia was the highest during intense physical activities and stressful mental activities. The amount of time in ischemia was higher for activities of high intensity. The amount of time in ischemia was 5% for high-intensity activities and 0.2% for low-intensity activities. Strenuous physical activity and intense anger were strong ischemia triggers. At the onset of ischemia, heart rates increased with the intensity of the activity or mental state. Among patients who smoked, the risk of ischemia was more than 5 times as high when the patients were actually smoking (Fig. 5). Coffee and alcohol consumption were also associated with ischemia, but after controlling for concurrent cigarette smoking, this relationship disappeared.

Conclusions.—During daily life, ischemia can be triggered in patients with coronary artery disease by activities of high and low intensity. Anger and smoking are strong triggers of ischemia. Mental activities are as important as physical activities in triggering ischemia. Coffee and alcohol consumption are associated with ischemia only when associated with smoking. The diary system used in this investigation was previously validated in a series of studies. However, this method still relies on patient self-report.

Commentary

Myocardial infarction and sudden death often occur without a precipitating cause; with careful probing, however, it does appear that specific "triggers" may precipitate a myocardial infarction in a large minority of cases; these include time of day (early awakening hours), physical and mental

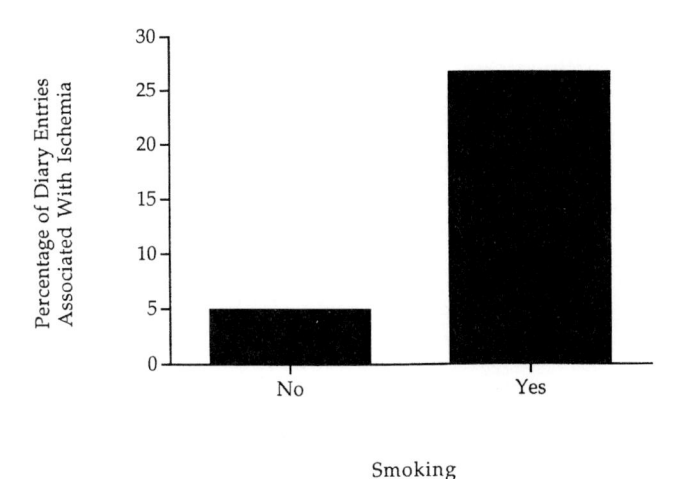

Fig. 5.— The percentage of diary entries associated with ischemic episodes by reports of smoking for six smokers in the sample. The percentage of diary entries associated with ischemia was more than 5 times as high when patients reported smoking as when they did not ($P < 0.0001$). (Reprinted with permission from the American College of Cardiology, courtesy of Gabbay FH, Krantz DS, Kop WJ, et al: Triggers of myocardial ischemia during daily life in patients with coronary artery disease: physical and mental activities, anger and smoking, J Am Coll Cardiol 27:585-592, 1996.)

stress, sexual intercourse, cold, and smoking (including "crack"). It was recently reported that the Northridge, California earthquake was a significant trigger of sudden cardiac death.[1]

This article by Gabbay et al. reports on an increased incidence of myocardial ischemia during daily life activities, including strenuous exercise, anger, and smoking (see Fig. 5). Cessation of smoking, behavioral modification, and regular exercise may protect against the triggers of myocardial infarction.[2]

REFERENCES
1. Leor J, Poole K, Kloner RA: Sudden cardiac death triggered by an earthquake, N Engl J Med 334:413-419, 1996.
2. Mittleman MA, Maclure M, Tofler GH, et al: Triggering of acute myocardial infarction onset by episodes of anger, Circulation 92:1729-1755, 1995.

NUTRITIONAL STATUS AND MORTALITY IN CHRONIC OBSTRUCTIVE PULMONARY DISEASE

Gray-Donald K, Gibbons L, Shapiro SH, et al
(McGill Univ, Montreal; Montreal Chest Inst)
Am J Respir Crit Care Med 153:961-966, 1996

Objective.—Many patients with chronic obstructive pulmonary disease (COPD) have low body weight and other signs of malnutrition. Survival rates are reduced in patients with low body weight, but it is unknown whether this association is independent of other factors related to survival. Nutritional status was studied as a prognostic factor in patients with severe COPD.

Methods.—The research subjects were drawn from a study of 348 patients with severe COPD who underwent measurement of lung function and body weight as part of a study of negative pressure ventilation. One hundred eighty-four patients were admitted to the hospital, where baseline diffusing capacity, maximal inspiratory and expiratory mouth pressures, and blood gases were measured. Cox regression analysis was done to assess body weight and other variables as predictors of survival.

Results.—One hundred sixty-two patients died during follow-up. For the total cohort, survival was independently related to body mass index (BMI) (with a hazard ratio of 0.73 for a 5-kg/m^2 increase in body weight) and home oxygen therapy (with a hazard ratio of 0.39 for patients not receiving oxygen) (Fig. 1). The more extensive data available on the hospitalized patients found that increased Paco$_2$ and low BMI, maximal inspiratory mouth pressure, and diffusing capacity were significant predictors of respiratory mortality. Factors not related to survival included Pao$_2$, measured while the patient was receiving oxygen; forced expiratory volume in 1 second (FEV$_1$); maximal expiratory mouth pressure; age; smoking; and sex. Body mass index was not a significant predictor of total mortality, but all the other predictors remained the same.

Conclusions.—In patients with severe COPD, low body weight is associated with an increased risk of respiratory mortality. Hypercapnia, decreased inspiratory muscle strength, and reduced diffusing capacity are significant factors as well. Only controlled trials of long-term nutritional support can determine whether poor nutrition has a causal effect or is only an indicator of disease severity.

Commentary

Low body weight associated with advanced COPD has been shown to be an adverse prognostic factor. This was first reported more than 30 years ago[1] and confirmed 20 years later in the intermittent positive pressure breathing trial.[2] In recent years, the nutrition status of patients with advanced COPD has been studied extensively.[3-6] In general, poor nutrition is more common in emphysema and chronic bronchitis.[5] Thus far, evidence of improved rates of survival with calorie repletion has not been shown.[6] Short-term nutrition intervention in advanced COPD has been shown to restore the immune response in selected patients with advanced COPD.[7]

This study emphasizes that total body weight was also associated with increased mortality rates. Total body weight may be improved by dietary augmentation. However, whether mortality can be changed by any dietary or pharmacologic alterations remains to be determined. Recently, the use of anabolic steroids given in conjunction with dietary supplementation seems to augment nonfat body weight

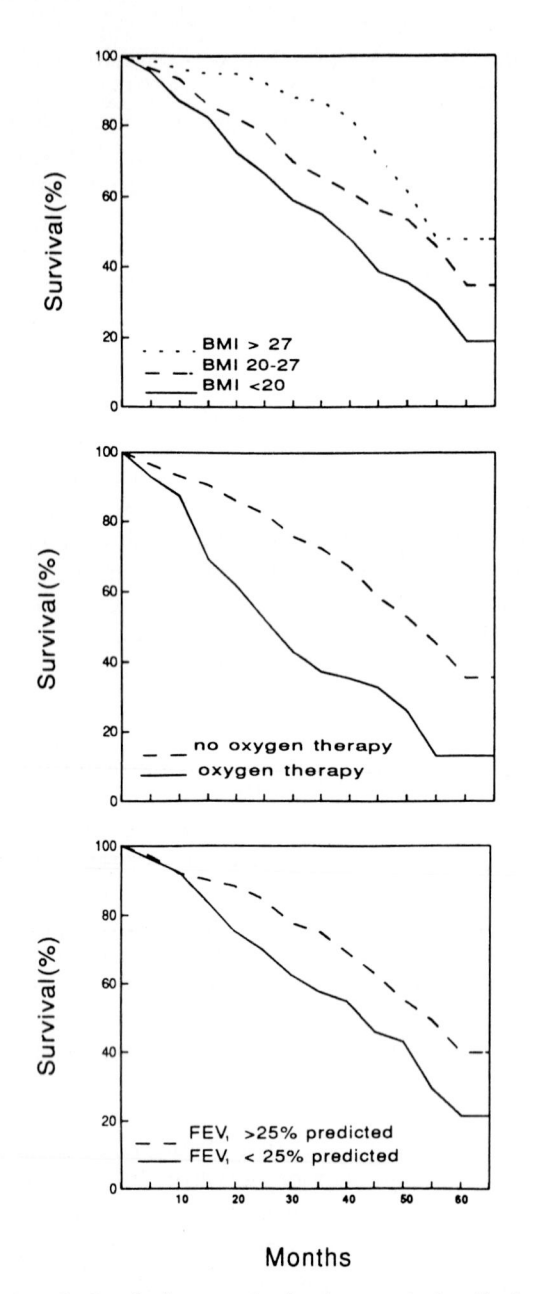

Fig. 1 **A,** Survival curves for body mass index (kg/m²); **B,** use of supplemental oxygen; and **C,** forced expiratory volume in 1 second (FEV₁) percent predicted. *BMI*, body mass index. (Courtesy of Gray-Donald K, Gibbons L, Shapiro SH, et al: Nutritional status and mortality in chronic obstructive pulmonary disease, *Am J Respir Crit Care Med* 153:961-966, 1996.)

compared with nutrition support alone.[8] Thus, there may be a reawakening of interest in improving not only the nutrition status, but also the body mass, of patients with severe weight loss from COPD. Further studies on the global value of nutrition supplementation and steroids, such as in exacerbations of disease, hospitalization, and survival will be needed to help establish the value of this approach to advanced COPD.

REFERENCES

1. Renzetti AD, McClement JH, Lilt BD: Mortality in relation to respiratory function in chronic obstructive lung disease, *Am J Med* 41:115-129, 1966.
2. Wilson D, Rogers RM, Wright EC, et al: Body weight in chronic obstructive pulmonary disease, *Am Rev Respir Dis* 139:1435-1438, 1989.
3. Hunter AM, Cary M, Larsh HW: The nutritional status of patients with chronic obstructive pulmonary disease, *Am Rev Respir Dis* 124:376-381, 1981.
4. Schols AMWJ, Soeters PB, Dingemans AMC, et al: Prevalence and characteristics of nutritional depletion in patients with stable COPD eligible for pulmonary rehabilitation, *Am Rev Respir Dis* 147:1151-1156, 1993.
5. Openbrier DR, Irwin MM, Rogers RM, et al: Nutritional status and lung function in patients with emphysema and chronic bronchitis, *Chest* 83:17-22, 1983.
6. Braun SR, Dixon RM, Kiem NL, et al: Predictive clinical value of nutritional assessment factors in COPD, *Chest* 85:353-357, 1984.
7. Fuenzalida CE, Petty TL, Jones ML: The immune response to short-term nutritional intervention in advanced chronic obstructive disease, *Am Rev Respir Dis* 142:49-56, 1990.
8. Schols AM, Soeters PB, Mostert R, et al: Physiologic effects of nutritional support and anabolic steroids in patients with chronic obstructive pulmonary disease: a placebo-controlled randomized trial, *Am J Respir Crit Care Med* 152:1268-1274, 1995.

POSTMENOPAUSAL ESTROGEN AND PROGESTIN USE AND THE RISK OF CARDIOVASCULAR DISEASE

Grodstein F, Stampfer MJ, Manson JE, et al (Harvard Med School, Boston; Harvard School of Public Health, Boston)
N Engl J Med 335:453-461, 1996

Background.—Research has shown a correlation between estrogen therapy in postmenopausal women and a reduced risk of heart disease. The effect of combined estrogen and progestin on the risk of cardiovascular disease, however, has not been studied thoroughly.

Methods.—A total of 59,337 participants in the Nurses' Health Study were assessed to determine the relation between cardiovascular disease and postmenopausal hormone treatment. The women, aged 30-55 years at baseline, were followed up for 16 years. Between 1976 and 1992, 770 women had myocardial infarction or died of coronary disease, and 572 had strokes.

Findings.—According to a proportional-hazards model, women taking estrogen with progestin had a marked reduction in the risk of major coronary heart disease compared with women not using hormones or using estrogen alone. The multivariate adjusted relative risks were 0.39 and 0.60, respectively. However, the use of combined hormones or estrogen alone was not associated with stroke (Fig. 1).

Conclusions.—In relatively young postmenopausal women, the addition of progestin to estrogen apparently does not attenuate the cardioprotec-

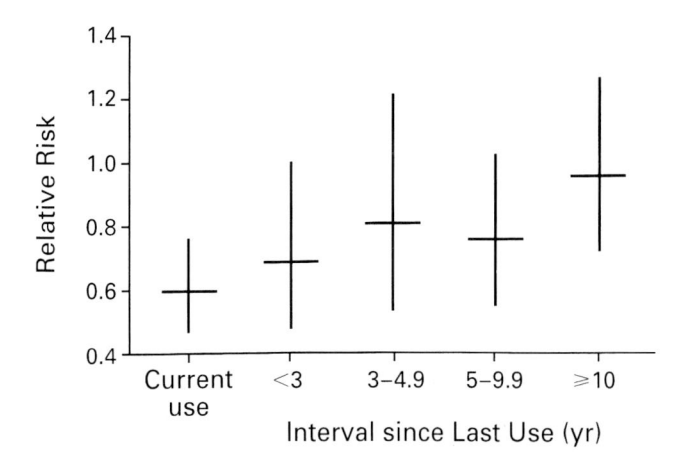

Fig. 1.—Relative risk of major coronary heart disease among current hormone users and among past users, according to the interval since last use. Data are for 1976 to 1992. *Horizontal bars* indicate relative risks, and *vertical bars* indicate 95% confidence intervals. (Reprinted by permission of *The New England Journal of Medicine*, from Grodstein F, Stampfer MJ, Manson JE, et al: Postmenopausal estrogen and progestin use and the risk of cardiovascular disease, *N Engl J Med* 335: 453-461, copyright 1996, Massachusetts Medical Society.)

tive effects of hormone treatment. However, the cardiovascular benefits of postmenopausal hormone therapy must be weighed against the possible risks (such as breast cancer), especially in long-term and older users.

Commentary

Hormone replacement (estrogen with or without progestin) is being evaluated as a means for reducing the risk of cardiovascular disease in postmenopausal women. Multiple epidemiologic studies have demonstrated that postmenopausal women who take estrogen have a lower risk of cardiovascular disease than women who do not use estrogen. A controversy exists as to whether the addition of progestins adds to or detracts from the cardioprotective effects of estrogen alone. Progestin can counteract the endometrial bleeding problems seen with estrogen use.

This report from the Nurses' Health Study demonstrates that the addition of progestin does not attenuate the cardiovascular benefits of estrogen, although the combination or estrogen alone did not appear to attenuate the risk of stroke.

Whether estrogen replacement, with and without progestin, alters the risk of cardiovascular disease is being addressed definitively in the prospective Women's Health Initiative, which is nearing its final recruitment numbers and is scheduled to be completed in 2005. This study will also be evaluating the effects of hormone replacement on memory loss, stroke incidence, cancer incidence, and fracture risk.

ECHOCARDIOGRAPHY FOR ASSESSING CARDIAC RISK IN PATIENTS HAVING NONCARDIAC SURGERY

Halm EA, for the Study of Perioperative Ischemia Research Group (*Massachusetts Gen Hosp, Boston; et al*)
Ann Intern Med 125:433-441, 1996

Introduction.—Patients undergoing noncardiac operations sometimes experience serious and potentially fatal cardiac complications. Several diagnostic tests have been proposed to assess cardiac risk before noncardiac surgery, including transthoracic echocardiography. However, the role of this preoperative test is still unclear. The prognostic value of echocardiography to assess cardiac risk in patients undergoing noncardiac surgery was evaluated.

Methods.—The prospective cohort study included 339 consecutive men at a VA medical center who were scheduled for major noncardiac surgery. All had known or suspected coronary artery disease. History, physical examination, ECG, and laboratory data were available on each patient. The echocardiograms were analyzed to determine the left ventricular systolic ejection fraction, any regional wall motion abnormalities, and left ventricular hypertrophy. After surgery, the patients were followed up for the occurrence of ischemic events, including cardiac death, nonfatal myocardial infarction, and unstable angina; congestive heart failure; and ventricular tachycardia. The prognostic value and operating characteristics of preoperative echocardiography were assessed.

Results.—Ischemic events occurred in 3% of patients, congestive heart failure in 8%, and ventricular tachycardia in 8%. None of the echocardiographic variables were significantly associated with ischemic events. Univariate analysis suggested that an ejection fraction of less than 40% increased the risk of all cardiac outcomes, of congestive heart failure, and of ventricular tachycardia. After multivariate analyses to adjust for clinical risk factors, ejection fraction still predicted all cardiac outcomes—odds ratio 2.5—but was not significantly associated with congestive heart failure or ventricular tachycardia. Wall motion score was also a risk factor for all cardiac events combined, odds ratio 1.3. An ejection fraction of less than 40% was 28% to 31% sensitive and 87% to 89% specific in predicting all types of adverse outcomes. However, its operating characteristics were poor. Echocardiography did not provide any clinically useful predictive information in addition to that supplied by clinical risk factors.

Conclusions.—Echocardiography is not useful in assessing the risk of cardiac complications in patients undergoing noncardiac surgery. It adds no predictive information to that provided by clinical risk models, and it performs poorly as a diagnostic test. Echocardiography should not be included in the cost-effective approach to cardiac risk assessment.

Commentary

This study shows that in patients with coronary artery disease undergoing noncardiac surgery, a preoperative echocardiogram provides no additional information. Simple predictive models of congestive heart failure and known clinical risk factors could predict outcome.[1]

In an era of cost containment, a routine echocardiogram is not part of a preoperative assessment in patients with known or suspected coronary disease. Other noninvasive tests such as dipyridamole-thallium scintigraphy and ambulatory monitoring for myocardial ischemia have been suggested to be useful in preoperative assessment but, similar to echocardiography, they may not provide any more useful information.

REFERENCE

1. Mangano DT, Goldman L: Preoperative assessment of the patient with known coronary disease, *N Engl J Med* 333:1750-1756, 1996.

ASTHMA AND GASTROESOPHAGEAL REFLUX: ACID SUPPRESSIVE THERAPY IMPROVES ASTHMA OUTCOME

Harding SM, Richter JE, Guzzo MR, et al
(Univ of Alabama, Birmingham)
Am J Med 100:395-405, 1996

Background. Gastroesophageal reflux disease (GERD) is a common, and often overlooked, exacerbating factor in asthma. Antireflux therapy has the potential to improve the symptoms of asthmatic patients. A prospective cohort study was performed in asthmatic patients with reflux symptoms to determine the optimal acid suppressive therapy dosage, the amount and time course of improvement in asthma symptoms, and the predictive factors of improvement.

Methods. Thirty asthmatic patients with GERD were recruited from the outpatient pulmonary clinic at the University of Alabama Hospital. The study group patients underwent baseline esophageal manometry, dual-probe 24-hour esophageal pH testing, barium esophogram, and pulmonary spirometry, and completed a demographic questionnaire. During the 4 weeks before treatment, patients recorded their reflux and asthma symptom scores and their peak expiratory flow rates (PEFs) when they awakened, 1 hour after dinner, and at bedtime. After this initial 4-week period, patients began with 20 mg of omeprazole, a proton pump inhibitor, daily, and the dose was titrated until acid suppression could be detected by a 24-hour pH test. Patients remained at this dosage for 3 months. Patients were considered to respond if asthma symptoms were reduced at least 20% and/or PEF was increased by at least 20%.

Results. During the course of this study, 73% of the patients responded to the acid suppressive therapy with either a reduction in asthma symptoms or an increase in PEF. The average acid suppressive dose of omeprazole was 27 mg/day, with 27% of the patients requiring more than 20 mg/day. Two patients required 60 mg/day. The presence of regurgitation or excessive proximal esophageal reflux predicted an asthma response to acid suppressive therapy with 100% sensitivity, 100% negative predictive value, 44% specificity, and a positive predictive value of 79%.

Conclusions. Patients with asthma should be screened for gastroesophageal reflux, because the majority of these patients may have improvement in asthma symptoms with acid suppressive therapy. If reflux is detected, patients should receive acid suppressive therapy with omeprazole, up to 60 mg/day, for at least 3 months. Gastroesophageal reflux appears to be a common exacerbating influence on asthma, and acid suppressive therapy can improve asthma symptoms and pulmonary function in the majority of these patients. Further research is needed to understand the link between asthma and gastroesophageal reflux.

Commentary

Both asthma and gastroesophageal reflux are common diseases. With the advent of ambulatory pH monitoring, it is now evident that gastroesophageal reflux is not only common in patients with asthma but may be a triggering factor.[1-4] The ability to suppress acid production by proton pump inhibitors offers a rational and practical approach to therapy. The present article strongly indicates that most asthmatic patients with demonstrable reflux can be improved by acid production suppression, often with higher than the usual doses used in peptic ulcer disease. Thus, patients who are not responding well to use of inhaled steroids or inflammatory mediator blockers such as cromolyn sodium or nedocromil sodium should be studied for esophageal reflux, particularly if they have symptoms of heartburn. However, it must be emphasized that many asthmatic patients with clinically significant gastroesophageal reflux do not have symptoms of heartburn; thus, the suspicion that GERD is present should be based on lack of expected responses to anti-asthma maintenance medications.

REFERENCES

1. Mays EE: Intrinsic asthma in adults: association with gastroesophageal reflux, *JAMA* 236:2626-2628, 1976.
2. Sontag SJ, O'Connell S, Khandelwal S, et al: Most asthmatics have gastroesophageal reflux with or without bronchodilator therapy, *Gastroenterology* 99:613-620, 1990.
3. Harding SM, Richter JE: Gastroesophageal reflux disease and asthma, *Sem Gastrointest Dis* 3:139-150, 1992.
4. Sontag SJ, Schnell TG, Miller TQ, et al: Prevalence of esophagitis in asthmatics, *Gut* 33:872-876, 1992.

ONCE-DAILY AMINOGLYCOSIDE DOSING IN IMMUNOCOMPETENT ADULTS: A META-ANALYSIS

Hatala R, Dinh T, Cook DJ
(McMaster Univ, Hamilton, Ont, Canada)
Ann Intern Med 124:717-725, 1996

Background. Aminoglycoside antibiotics are an essential component in the treatment of severe bacterial infections. Dosing strategies must balance the achievement of adequate serum levels to inhibit bacterial growth with a minimal trough serum concentration to prevent ototoxicity and nephrotoxicity. Studies comparing the efficacy and toxicity of once-daily with conventional aminoglycoside dosing strategies have reported conflicting results. Because many of these studies were too small to have sufficient power, the data of randomized, clinical trials were synthesized in a meta-analysis.

Methods. MEDLINE searches identified 17 randomized, controlled trials comparing efficacy and safety outcome measures of an IV once-daily regimen with a standard regimen of aminoglycoside treatment of infected, immunocompetent adults. The articles were scored by two reviewers for methodologic quality. Pooled risk ratios were calculated for each outcome with homogeneity in the individual study risk ratios. The heterogeneity of risk ratios for outcome assessments was evaluated for the influence of differing methodologic quality, different aminoglycosides used, different coadministered antibiotic classes, and different primary sources of infection.

Results. There was a pooled risk ratio of 1.02 for bacteriologic cure. There were heterogeneous individual trial results for clinical cure, which could not be explained by the influences of methodologic quality, the aminoglycoside used, the coadministered antibiotic, or the infection site. Therefore, a common risk ratio for clinical cure was not calculated. The pooled mortality risk ratio was 0.91, favoring once-daily dosing. The pooled risk ratios for nephrotoxicity and for ototoxicity were 0.87 and 0.67, respectively, both favoring once-daily aminoglycoside dosing.

Conclusions. Once-daily and standard aminoglycoside dosing regimens have equivalent efficacy, but once-daily dosing may reduce mortality and toxicity. However, the wide and overlapping confidence intervals indicate a need for more studies to more precisely estimate these risks.

Commentary

This is another meta-analysis agreeing that aminoglycosides given once daily appear to be equivalent in efficacy and may be less toxic than standard (usually 3 times a day) dosing. It should be emphasized that studies using animal models of endocarditis have not indicated equivalent efficacy of once-daily dosing with multiple dosing. Thus, once-daily dosing of aminoglycosides is not presently recommended for therapy of endocarditis.

AN ANALYSIS OF THE LOWEST EFFECTIVE INTENSITY OF PROPHYLACTIC ANTICOAGULATION FOR PATIENTS WITH NONRHEUMATIC ATRIAL FIBRILLATION

Hylek EM, Skates SJ, Sheehan MA, et al
(Massachusetts Gen Hosp, Boston; Harvard Med School, Boston)
N Engl J Med 335:540-546, 1996

Background. Because the risk of hemorrhage in patients with atrial fibrillation increases with the intensity of anticoagulation, determining the lowest intensity of anticoagulation for preventing ischemic stroke would be useful. Because the risk of ischemic stroke is low in patients taking anticoagulant medications, prospective studies are difficult to perform. Therefore, the relationship between the intensity of anticoagulation, as reflected by the international normalized ratio (INR) and the risk of stroke, was analyzed in a case-control study.

Methods. Seventy-four patients discharged with both atrial fibrillation and ischemic stroke diagnoses between 1989 and 1994 were each matched with three control patients receiving anticoagulation therapy for nonrheumatic atrial fibrillation who did not have stroke. Their records were reviewed to collect information on the INR, duration of warfarin therapy, and demographic and clinical characteristics. The relationships between various INRs and stroke were analyzed in univariate and multivariate models.

Results. The risk of stroke increased sharply as the INR values decreased below 2.0, with a nearly doubled risk with INRs of 1.7, a nearly three fold risk with INRs of 1.5, and a seven fold risk with INRs of 1.3, compared with INRs of 2.0 (Table 4). In multiple logistic regression analysis with other correlates of stroke, the significance of the INR in predicting stroke changed little. Other independent predictors of stroke risk included previous stroke, diabetes mellitus, hypertension, and current smoking.

Conclusions. Anticoagulant prophylaxis at INRs of 2.0 or greater is effective in preventing stroke, whereas the risk of stroke increases significantly with less intense anticoagulation. Previous studies have found rapidly increasing risk of hemorrhage associated with INRs exceeding 4.0-5.0. Therefore, maintaining the INR between 2.0 and 3.0 is recommended as the optimal anticoagulation strategy to provide adequate prevention of both ischemic stroke and major hemorrhage.

TABLE 4   Adjusted Odds Ratios for Ischemic Stroke According to the INR

INR	ODDS RATIO (95% CI)*
1.0	17.6 (7.9-39.3)
1.1	11.9 (6.0-23.8)
1.2	8.3 (4.6-15.0)
1.3	6.0 (3.6-9.8)
1.4	4.4 (2.9-6.6)
1.5	3.3 (2.4-4.6)
1.6	2.5 (1.9-3.3)
1.7	2.0 (1.6-2.4)
1.8	1.5 (1.4-1.7)
1.9	1.2 (1.2-1.3)

From Hylek EM, Skates SJ, Sheehan MA, et al: An analysis of the lowest effective intensity of prophylactic anticoagulation for patients with nonrheumatic atrial fibrillation, N Engl J Med 335:540-546. Reprinted by permission of The New England Journal of Medicine, copyright 1996, Massachusetts Medical Society.
INR, International normalized ratio; CI, confidence interval.
Odds ratios are the odds of ischemic stroke among patients with the INR in question as compared with the patients with an INR of 2.0.

Commentary

This study provides data for supporting the target INR of between 2.0 and 3.0 as an optimal level of prophylactic anticoagulation with warfarin for patients with nonrheumatic atrial fibrillation. There is no question that anticoagulation can reduce the risk of emboli, and there is probably an underutilization of this treatment, especially in older subjects who are at the highest risk for stroke.[1]

REFERENCE
1. Golzari H, Cebul RD, Bahler RC: Atrial fibrillation: restoration and maintenance of sinus rhythm and indications for anticoagulation therapy, Ann Intern Med 125:311-327, 1996.

EFFECT OF PASSIVE SMOKING ON THE DEVELOPMENT OF RESPIRATORY SYMPTOMS IN YOUNG ADULTS: AN 8-YEAR LONGITUDINAL STUDY

Jaakkola MS, Jaakkola JJK, Becklake MR, et al
(Finnish Inst of Occupational Health, Helsinki; Univ of Helsinki; McGill Univ, Montreal)
J Clin Epidemiol 49:581-586, 1996

Purpose. The evidence that exposure to environmental tobacco smoke (ETS) causes respiratory symptoms is relatively strong in children. However, studies of the effects of passive smoking in adults have yielded conflicting results. There have been no longitudinal studies to determine whether passive smoking during adolescence or adulthood is related to respiratory symptoms. Such a study was performed, with an emphasis on the potential dose-response relationship.

Methods. One hundred seventeen younger adults who had never smoked completed a questionnaire on respiratory health. The subjects' ages at baseline ranged from 15 to 40 years. Eight years later, the subjects were reevaluated; respiratory symptoms were noted, including wheezing, dyspnea, cough, and phlegm production. Information on exposure to ETS at home and at work was gathered as well. Multivariate logistic regression analyses, with controls for age, sex, atopy, and other respiratory symptoms, were performed to seek associations between ETS exposure and respiratory symptoms.

Results. Sixty-two percent of subjects were exposed to ETS at home or at work. These subjects had a significantly greater cumulative incidence of respiratory symptoms, except for phlegm production. One third of initially asymptomatic subjects had one or more respiratory symptoms during follow-up. The risk of dyspnea increased with increasing ETS exposure—the odds ratio was 2.37 for subjects exposed to an average of 10 cigarettes per day. The other symptoms also became more frequent at higher levels of ETS exposure, but these associations were not significant.

Conclusions. Passive smoking at home or work appears to increase the rate of respiratory symptoms in young adults. At least for dyspnea, the harmful effects of ETS may occur in dose-dependent fashion. Efforts to prevent exposure to ETS must continue into young adulthood.

Commentary

Passive smoking has conclusively been shown to cause respiratory disease in children.[1-8] This study offers evidence of the harmful effect of passive smoking in young adults. We must come to the reasonable conclusion that passive smoking is a true health hazard for patients with asthma, cystic fibrosis, chronic obstructive pulmonary disease, or lung cancer.

REFERENCES
1. Samet JM, Marbury MC, Spengler JD: Health effects and sources of indoor air pollution. Part I, Am Rev Respir Dis 136:1486-1508, 1987.
2. Spitzer WO, Lawrence V, Dales R, et al: Links between passive smoking and disease: a best-evidence synthesis, a report of the Working Group on Passive Smoking, Clin Invest Med 13:17-42, 1990.
3. Respiratory Health Effects of Passive Smoking: Lung Cancer and Other Disorders. Washington, DC, EPA/600/6-90/006F, US Environmental Protection Agency, Office of Health and Environmental Assessment, Office of Research and Development, 1992.
4. Weiss ST, Tager IB, Speizer FE, et al: Persistent wheeze: its relationship to respiratory illness, cigarette smoking and level of pulmonary function in a population sample of children, Am Rev Respir Dis 122:697-707, 1980.
5. Dodge R: The effects of indoor pollution on Arizona children, Arch Environ Health 37:151-155, 1982.
6. Ware JH, Dockery DW, Spiro A III, et al: Passive smoking, gas cooking, and respiratory health of children living in six cities, Am Rev Respir Dis 129:366-374, 1984.
7. Charlton A: Children's coughs related to parental smoking, BMJ 288:1647-1649, 1984.

8. Burchfiel CM, Higgins MW, Keller JB, et al: Passive smoking in childhood: respiratory conditions and pulmonary function in Tecumseh, Michigan, *Am Rev Respir Dis* 133:966-973, 1986.

OUTCOME OF PREGNANCY IN WOMEN WITH MODERATE OR SEVERE RENAL INSUFFICIENCY

Jones DC, Hayslett JP (Yale Univ, New Haven, Conn)
N Engl J Med 335:226-232, 1996

Background. The presence of moderate to severe renal disease in a pregnant woman reportedly both accelerates the underlying disease and markedly reduces fetal survival. Six medical centers collaborated to establish the types of complications occurring during pregnancy in such patients.

Methods. Maternal and obstetric complications and pregnancy outcomes were examined for 67 women with primary renal disease (82 pregnancies). All participants had experienced gestation lasting beyond the first trimester and showed initial serum creatinine concentrations of at least 1.4 mg/dl.

Results. Mean serum creatinine concentrations among these women increased from 1.9 mg/dl in early pregnancy to 2.5 mg/dl in the third trimester. Between baseline and the third trimester of pregnancy, the frequency of high-grade proteinuria increased from 23% to 41% and frequency of hypertension from 28% to 48%. Pregnancy-related loss of maternal renal function occurred in 43% of the 57 women (70 pregnancies) for whom data were available during pregnancy and immediately postpartum. Rapid acceleration of maternal renal insufficiency occurred in eight of these pregnancies. In the overall group, risk of accelerated progression to end-stage renal failure was highest for women with a baseline pregnancy serum creatinine concentration above 2 mg/dl. Infant survival rate was 93%, with a 59% incidence of preterm delivery and a 37% incidence of growth retardation.

Conclusions. Increased risk of complications as a result of deteriorating renal function, hypertension, and obstetric complications is present for pregnant women with moderate or severe renal insufficiency. Despite increased incidences of preterm delivery and growth retardation, however, infant survival is high.

Commentary

Normal pregnancy is rare in women whose serum creatinine and urea are greater than 3 mg/dl and 36 mg/dl, respectively. Women with mild reductions in renal function (serum creatinine levels of 1.4 mg/dl or less) usually have a successful obstetric outcome, and pregnancy usually does not substantially alter the natural history of their renal disease.[1] On the other hand, this report indicates that women with renal disease and serum creatinine values that exceed 1.4 mg/dl frequently have hypertension and increased proteinuria, and about half of the women included in this study sustained a more rapid decline in glomerular filtration rate as assessed by a fall in creatinine clearance of greater than 25%. Of note is the finding that in 75% of the women the decline in renal function did not reverse after delivery and in many instances progressed further. There was a high rate of preterm delivery and of fetal growth retardation. As pointed out in an accompanying editorial,[2] "the good news in this report is that with advances in the care of newborn babies, fetal survival has improved remarkably." This, of course, is the result of substantial advances in neonatal care in the past decade.

REFERENCES

1. Katz AI, Davison JM, Hayslett JP, et al: Pregnancy in women with kidney disease, *Kidney Int* 18:192-206, 1980.
2. Epstein FH: Pregnancy and renal disease, *N Engl J Med* 38:277-278, 1996.

BLOOD PRESSURE AND END-STAGE RENAL DISEASE IN MEN

Klag MJ, Whelton PK, Randall BL, et al (Johns Hopkins Univ, Baltimore, Md; Univ of Minnesota, Minneapolis; Univ of Texas, Houston; et al)
N Engl J Med 334:13-18, 1996

Introduction. For the estimated 190,000 Americans who, in 1991, were dialyzed or underwent renal transplantation for end-stage kidney disease, hypertension was second only to diabetes as an underlying cause. These conditions accounted for 29% and 36% of cases, respectively.

Objective. The risk of end-stage renal failure was related to blood pressure levels in a prospective series of 332,544 men aged 35-57 years who were screened in the mid-1970s for entry into the Multiple Risk Factor Intervention Trial, a randomized primary prevention study intended to show how controlling high blood pressure affects the risk of coronary heart disease.

Methods. At the time of screening, three blood pressure readings were taken using a standard mercury device, and the average of the last two readings was used for analysis. Data on patients treated for end-stage renal disease were taken from the national registry of the Health Care Financing Administration, and data on deaths resulting from renal failure were derived from the National Death Index and the Social Security Administration.

Findings. A total of 814 men were treated for, or died of, end-stage renal disease during an average follow-up of 16 years. There was a strong association with higher blood pressure, which persisted after controlling for age and other baseline factors. The steep risk gradient associated with systolic blood pressure far exceeded the apparent influence of diastolic pressure. Those having a systolic pressure of 210 mm Hg or higher or a diastolic pressure of 120 mm Hg or above had a relative risk of end-stage renal disease of 22. The increased risk could not be ascribed to disease developing shortly after screening. In men entering the study, the association was not altered by adjusting for the baseline serum creatinine and urinary protein excretion.

Conclusions. Elevated blood pressure—particularly systolic pressure—is a strong independent risk factor for end-stage renal disease in middle-aged men.

Commentary

It is now well appreciated that hypertension accelerates the progression of chronic renal disease. This study extends somewhat our knowledge of the link between blood pressure and renal disease. A higher blood pressure, as measured carefully on a single occasion, was a strong independent risk factor for end-stage renal disease. There was a correlation between the degree of risk and the level of blood pressure readings.

Although there is a long history in medicine indicating that malignant hypertension is linked to an increased risk of renal failure, several recent trials indicate that relatively mild increases in blood pressure may substantially affect the progression of renal disease and lead to end-stage renal failure. This is particularly true in patients with proteinuria. In this paper, Klag et al. also found that older age, lower income, higher serum cholesterol concentrations, cigarette smoking, diabetes mellitus, and black race were, likewise, associated with an increased risk of end-stage renal disease.

There is no question that adequate control of hypertension is important in markedly decreasing the risk for cardiovascular disease; this paper points out that primary prevention of mild to slightly severe hypertension may also forestall or delay the onset of end-stage renal disease. Consequently, early identification, early treatment, and continuous monitoring of blood pressure in patients with hypertension is important in an effort to decrease or markedly delay the incidence of cardiovascular events, strokes, and end-stage renal failure.

PRE-CLINICAL CUSHING'S SYNDROME: AN UNEXPECTED FREQUENT CAUSE OF POOR GLYCAEMIC CONTROL IN OBESE DIABETIC PATIENTS

Leibowitz G, Tsur A, Chayen SD, et al
(Hebrew Univ, Jerusalem)
Clin Endocrinol (Oxf) 44:717-722, 1996

Introduction. Although Cushing's syndrome is thought to be a rare cause of uncontrolled diabetes mellitus, its prevalence in obese patients with uncontrolled diabetes has not been studied. To examine this issue, a retrospective analysis of patients with endogenous Cushing's syndrome and a cross-sectional study of obese patients with poorly controlled diabetes were conducted.

Methods. The clinical and biochemical data of all 63 patients with Cushing's syndrome who were treated at the study institution during the past 15 years were reviewed for the presence of diabetes and the symptoms leading to the diagnosis of Cushing's syndrome. In the cross-sectional study, 90 obese patients with uncontrolled diabetes were evaluated for the presence of Cushing's syndrome. All underwent an overnight 1-mg dexamethasone suppression test; 2- and 8-mg dexamethasone suppression tests and imaging studies were performed in those with nonsuppressible serum cortisol concentrations (>140 nmol/L [5 µg/dl]).

Results. Eleven of the patients with Cushing's syndrome (17.5%) had diabetes mellitus, including seven with pituitary tumors (Cushing's disease), two with ectopic corticotropin production, and one with adrenal adenoma; the etiology in the remaining patient was unclear. Two patients had long-standing diabetes without the classic physical characteristics of Cushing's syndrome. All these patients had a marked improvement in glycemic control when their Cushing's syndrome was cured.

In 85 of the 90 obese patients with diabetes, serum cortisol suppression after 1 mg of dexamethasone was normal. Among the remaining five patients, Cushing's syndrome was confirmed in three. Surgical treatment of Cushing's syndrome in these three patients led to improved glycemic control.

Conclusions. Preclinical Cushing's syndrome in obese patients with poorly controlled diabetes may be more common than previously believed. When common causes of poor glycemic control are ruled out in such patients, an overnight dexamethasone suppression test may be useful.

Commentary

This study addressed two questions: What is the frequency of diabetes mellitus in patients with Cushing's syndrome, and what is the frequency of Cushing's syndrome in patients with diabetes? The answer to the former—17.5%—is similar to what has been found in other studies.[1] The answer to the latter—3.3%—is hardly high, but given the very large number of patients with (mostly) non-insulin-dependent diabetes mellitus (NIDDM) in most populations, Cushing's syndrome could be a good deal more common than is generally believed.

The 90 diabetic patients who underwent the overnight dexamethasone suppression test, a well-accepted screening test for Cushing's syndrome, were not randomly selected. They had been referred to a specialty clinic, were obese, and had high glycosylated hemoglobin values despite treatment with insulin (37 patients), an oral hypoglycemic drug (46 patients), or diet (four patients) for unstated periods of time (three were newly diagnosed). Of the three patients found to have Cushing's syndrome, two had Cushing's disease and one had an adrenal adenoma. None were suspected to have Cushing's syndrome, although several had facial plethora or hypertension, hardly specific signs of cortisol excess. (The frequency of these findings in those who did not have Cushing's syndrome is not stated.)

There are many obese patients with NIDDM who are poorly controlled, and many reasons why they are poorly controlled, of which improper diet, inability to lose weight, and inadequate drug or insulin therapy are surely the most common. Should they all be screened for Cushing's syndrome? Although the overnight screening test is simple and reliable, its sensitivity and specificity are not 100%, nor are those of the other accepted screening test, 24-hour urinary cortisol excretion.[2] Thus, widespread screening for a low-frequency illness is sure to result in many false positive test results. Rather than routine screening of patients with NIDDM, therefore, it would seem more prudent to be alert to its presence and screen only those patients who have more than just hard-to-control hyperglycemia, at least until these results are confirmed and the minimal cortisol excess in these patients is known to do something more than just make hyperglycemia harder to control.

REFERENCES

1. Ross EJ, Linch DC: Cushing's syndrome—killing disease: discriminatory value of signs and symptoms aiding early diagnosis, *Lancet* 2:646-649, 1982.
2. Kaye TB, Crapo L: Cushing's syndrome: an update on diagnostic tests, *Ann Intern Med* 112:434-444, 1990.

EVOLUTION, RISK FACTORS, AND PROGNOSTIC IMPLICATIONS OF ALBUMINURIA IN NIDDM

Niskanen LK, Parviainen M, Penttilä I, et al
(Univ of Kuopio, Finland)
Diabetes Care 19:486-493, 1996

Background. Good metabolic and blood pressure control can prevent or arrest the progression of albuminuria in patients with insulin-dependent diabetes mellitus (IDDM). However, the evolution and determinants of albuminuria in patients with non-insulin-dependent diabetes mellitus (NIDDM) have not been defined clearly. To characterize better the course and impact of albuminuria in patients with NIDDM, the incidence, determinants, and impact on cardiovascular mortality were evaluated in a 10-year study of patients with newly diagnosed NIDDM and nondiabetic subjects.

Methods. A total of 133 patients with newly diagnosed NIDDM and 144 nondiabetic subjects were examined at baseline and 5 and 10 years later. The examinations included a history of cardiovascular diseases, information about drugs, and measurements of body mass index, plasma glucose and insulin concentrations and urinary albumin excretion.

Results. At the time of diagnosis, the patients with NIDDM had a higher urinary albumin excretion than did the nondiabetic subjects. Albuminuria was present in 21% of the diabetic patients and 1.4% of the nondiabetic subjects at baseline, in 21% of the patients and 7% of the nondiabetic subjects at 5 years, and in 33% of the patients and 12% of the nondiabetic subjects at 10 years. In the diabetic patients, the incidence of microalbuminuria and macroalbuminuria increased significantly between 5 and 10 years of follow-up (Fig. 1). The 10-year urinary albumin excretion value was significantly and independently associated with fasting plasma glucose and fasting plasma insulin concentrations in diabetic patients, whereas fasting plasma insulin concentrations and systolic blood pressure were the most important predictors of urinary albumin excretion in the nondiabetic subjects. There were 28 cardiovascular deaths in the diabetic group and four in the nondiabetic group. Albuminuria at baseline and at 5 years was significantly associated with cardiovascular mortality in the patients, even after adjusting for other risk factors.

Conclusions. Poor glycemic control is the strongest predictor of the development of microalbuminuria in patients with NIDDM, whereas hypertension is the strongest predictor of microalbuminuria in nondiabetic subjects. Microalbuminuria is

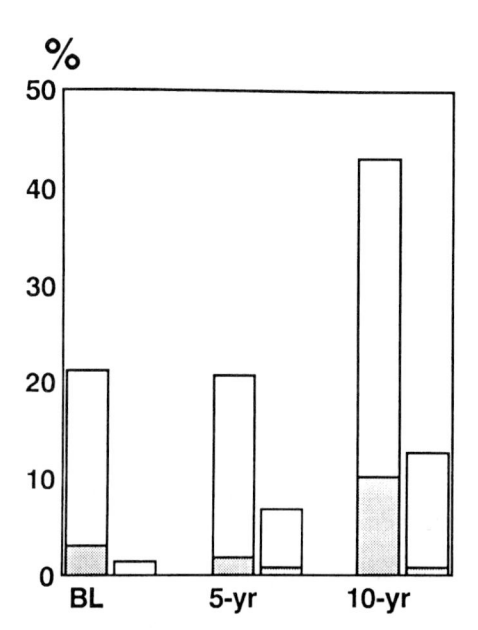

Fig. 1 Cumulative incidence of microalbuminuria and macroalbuminuria in diabetic *(left bars)* and nondiabetic *(right bars)* subjects during follow-up. *Open bars,* urinary albumin excretion (UAE) 30-300 mg/24 hours or 20-200 µg/min; *speckled bars,* UAE greater than 300 mg/24 hr or greater than 200 µg/min. *BL,* baseline. (Courtesy of Niskanen LK, Parviainen M, Penttilä I, et al: Evolution, risk factors, and prognostic implications of albuminuria in NIDDM, *Diabetes Care* 19:486-493, 1996.)

an important risk factor for cardiovascular death in patients with NIDDM.

Commentary

The approximately 30% of patients with IDDM destined to have end-stage renal disease usually have microalbuminuria after having diabetes for about 10 years, macroalbuminuria after 15-20 years, and end-stage renal disease after about 25 years. In contrast, some patients with NIDDM have microalbuminuria at the time of diagnosis. Because the onset of NIDDM is usually insidious, many if not all the patients have had diabetes for years before the diagnosis is made. Also, progression of microalbuminuria to end-stage renal disease is much less predictable in patients with NIDDM.

The results of this study confirm and extend some of these comments. The study is unique in that the patients were followed up for 10 years from the time of diagnosis of NIDDM and there was a matched group of normal subjects. Only a few of the latter had microalbuminuria at any time. Although the fraction of diabetic patients with microalbuminuria or macroalbuminuria changed little in 5 years, it increased substantially from 5 to 10 years (see Fig. 1). At 10 years, only 5% of the patients had an elevated serum creatinine concentration, and only 1% had died of nephropathy, although the overall death rate was 27% (as compared with 6% in the control group), mostly from cardiovascular disease. The degree of hyperglycemia (measured as the fasting plasma glucose concentration at baseline and 5 years and glycosylated hemoglobin at 5 years) was the only predictor of microalbuminuria and macroalbuminuria at 10 years (in a 10-year U.S. study, not begun at the time of diagnosis, the predictors were hyperglycemia, hypertension, and smoking[1]). The only explanation for the lack of increase in microalbuminuria or macroalbuminuria (measured as both their frequency and mean urinary albumin excretion) in the first 5 years of the study that I can think of is antidiabetic treatment, which for most patients was an oral hypoglycemic drug; however, the mean fasting plasma glucose concentration increased 18 mg/dl (1 mmol/L) during this interval.

Albuminuria may not be as strong a predictor of end-stage renal disease in NIDDM patients as it is in patients with IDDM, but there is likely to be a relationship, and end-stage renal disease in patients with NIDDM is the single most common indication for chronic hemodialysis or renal transplantation in the United States. Therefore, microalbuminuria should be tested for regularly in patients with NIDDM and, when detected, intervention undertaken. The interventions should include more vigorous efforts at control of hyperglycemia and treatment with an angiotensin-converting enzyme inhibitor in both normotensive and hypertensive patients.[2]

REFERENCES

1. Klein R, Klein BEK, Moss SE, et al: Ten-year incidence of gross proteinuria in people with diabetes, *Diabetes* 44:916-923, 1995.
2. Ravid M, et al: Long-term stabilizing effect of angiotensin-converting enzyme inhibition on plasma creatinine and on proteinuria in normotensive type II diabetic patients, *Ann Intern Med* 118:577-581, 1993.

EFFECT OF VENTILATOR-ASSOCIATED PNEUMONIA ON MORTALITY AND MORBIDITY

Papazian L, Bregeon F, Thirion X, et al
(Hôpital Sainte-Marguerite, Marseille, France)
Am J Respir Crit Care Med 154:91-97, 1996.

Background. Mechanical ventilation is a substantial risk factor for acquiring pneumonia. However, the effects of ventilator-associated pneumonia (VAP) on mortality and morbidity are controversial, with studies hampered by methodologic difficulties. The mortality and excess hospital stay attributable to VAP were examined in a matched case-control study.

Methods. Data were collected prospectively on patients admitted to the ICU between 1989 and 1993. During the study, 97 immunocompetent patients who had been mechanically ventilated for more than 48 hours received a diagnosis of VAP based on clinical, biologic, and radiologic evidence plus the isolation of a causative microorganism. Of these 97 patients, 85 were matched with a control patient without VAP. Cases and controls were matched for diagnosis, indication for mechanical ventilation, age (within 5 years), sex, Acute Physiology and Chronic Health Evaluation (APACHE) II score on admission (within 5 points), duration of ventilation, and date of admission (within 1 year). Mortality and hospital and ICU length of stay were compared.

Results. Death occurred in the ICU in 40% of the case patients and 38.8% of the control patients, and in the hospital in 41% of each group. Of the 37 pairs with a discordant outcome, the case patient died in 19 pairs. Mortality rates increased with increased APACHE II scores, but mortality rates were similar among cases and controls at each level of the APACHE II score. Similarly, there were no significant differences in mortality rates between cases and controls when analyzed by early or late onset of pneumonia, by medical or surgical diagnosis, or by the responsible organisms. However, compared with control patients, case patients had longer durations of mechanical ventilation and ICU stays.

Conclusions. Ventilator-associated pneumonia does not increase mortality, which is determined by other host factors, but does increase the cost of care because of its association with longer mechanical ventilation and ICU stays.

Commentary

Although VAP is a common complication of critically ill patients who require mechanical ventilatory support and is believed to increase length of hospital stay and mortality, this

LONG-TERM DIABETOGENIC EFFECT OF SINGLE PREGNANCY IN WOMEN WITH PREVIOUS GESTATIONAL DIABETES MELLITUS

Peters RK, Kjos SL, Xiang A, et al
(Univ of Southern California, Los Angeles)
Lancet 347:227-230, 1996

Background. The progressive metabolic changes occurring during pregnancy lead to marked insulin resistance. Women in whom gestational diabetes develops have insufficient pancreatic β-cell reserve to increase insulin secretion in the presence of pregnancy-related insulin resistance. The effects of subsequent pregnancies on the risk of non-insulin-dependent diabetes mellitus (NIDDM) in women with a history of gestational diabetes (and thus with a high prevalence of pancreatic β-cell dysfunction) were evaluated.

Methods. The study subjects were 666 Hispanic women with gestational diabetes who received care at a high-risk family planning clinic at the Los Angeles County Hospital. Each woman was followed up from the time of her last postpartum visit until her last clinic visit or until she developed diabetes, as defined by the National Diabetes Data Group criteria. During follow-up, the women underwent annual examination, which included weighing and oral glucose tolerance testing. Additional pregnancies and other risk factors for diabetes were evaluated for their long-term diabetogenic effects. The other risk factors included antepartum oral glucose tolerance, highest fasting plasma glucose, and gestational age at diagnosis during the index pregnancy; postpartum body mass index; and glucose tolerance, weight change, breast-feeding, and oral contraceptive use during follow-up.

Results. The mean duration of follow-up was 7.5 years, during which time 87 of the women completed another pregnancy. Seven of these women developed NIDDM immediately after the additional pregnancy. The women with an additional pregnancy had a subsequent annual NIDDM incidence rate of 31%, as compared with 12% for the cohort overall. Additional pregnancy increased the rate ratio of NIDDM to 3.3, according to proportional hazards regression analysis, as compared with women without an additional pregnancy and after adjustment for other diabetes risk factors. The rate ratio for NIDDM also increased by 2.0 for each 10 lb gained during follow-up, after adjustment for the additional pregnancy and other risk factors.

Conclusions. For women with a history of gestational diabetes, a subsequent pregnancy more than triples the risk of developing NIDDM. This increase occurs independent of the well-recognized effects of weight gain and other risk factors. The findings suggest that episodes of insulin resistance may play a role in the decreasing β-cell function in patients at high risk for NIDDM.

Commentary

Pregnancy is a state of reversible insulin resistance, caused largely by placental hormones (human placental lactogen, estrogen, progesterone) and prolactin. In most pregnant women, insulin secretion increases sufficiently so that plasma glucose concentrations remain normal. In approximately 3% of pregnant women, however, gestational diabetes develops because their insulin secretory capacity is limited and they therefore cannot secrete enough insulin to maintain euglycemia. Almost all women who have gestational diabetes become euglycemic after delivery, but their glucose tolerance is not entirely normal,[1] and permanent diabetes (usually non-insulin-dependent diabetes) ultimately develops in approximately 35% to 50%.

The results of this study indicate that in women who have gestational diabetes during a pregnancy, a subsequent pregnancy substantially increases the risk of permanent diabetes. Although the study was done in Hispanic women, in whom the incidence of diabetes is high, I see no reason to doubt that the results are also applicable to other women. One factor contributing to this increase in risk was the greater nongestational weight gain in the women who had a subsequent pregnancy. But that is not the whole story. As the authors point out, their results also indicate that in women with limited insulin secretory capacity, a several-month period of insulin resistance further impairs β-cell function. The likely mechanism is glucose toxicity. (Among women in general, increasing parity is not associated with an increased risk of diabetes.[2])

Minimizing insulin resistance and hyperglycemia during pregnancy may therefore not only reduce morbidity and mortality in the fetus, but also help to preserve β-cell function in the mother. This argues not only for more aggressive treatment of gestational diabetes, but also more vigorous efforts to reduce insulin resistance in a woman who has had gestational diabetes when she is not pregnant and to make contraception available, should the woman wish it.

REFERENCES

1. Kjos SL, Peters RK, Xiang A, et al: Predicting future diabetes in Latino women with gestational diabetes, *Diabetes* 44:586-591, 1995.
2. Manson JE, Rimm EB, Colditz GA, et al: Parity and incidence of non-insulin-dependent diabetes mellitus, *Am J Med* 93:13-18, 1992.

PREGNANCY IN SICKLE CELL DISEASE: EXPERIENCE OF THE COOPERATIVE STUDY OF SICKLE CELL DISEASE

Smith JA, Espeland M, Bellevue R, et al (Harlem Hosp Ctr-Columbia Univ, New York; Bowman Gray School of Medicine, Winston-Salem, NC; State Univ of New York Health Science Ctr, Brooklyn; et al)

Obstet Gynecol 87:199-204, 1996

Background. Previous reports vary as to the maternal and fetal mortality and complications associated with sickle cell disease in pregnant women. The maternal and fetal outcomes of 445 pregnancies from the Cooperative Study of Sickle Cell Disease were studied.

Methods. Pregnant women from 19 centers were recruited for the prospective study. Information on the patients' steady state and on sickle- and non-sickle-related events was collected by a structured study protocol. Antepartum and intrapartum complications were assessed for pregnancies carried to delivery. The fetal outcomes of gestational age, birth weight, and Apgar score were assessed, along with the effects of genotype on event rates.

Outcome. Sixty-four percent of pregnancies progressed to delivery; about 29% ended in elective abortion, 7% in miscarriage, and 1% in stillbirth. The rates of non-sickle-related complications in the study group, both antepartum and intrapartum, were similar to those of a group of black women without sickle cell disease. Two of the pregnant women died, one as a direct result of her sickle cell disease. Sickle-related maternal morbidity was the same during pregnancy as before. Of pregnancies carried to term, 99% resulted in the birth of a live neonate. Mothers with the SS genotype had small-for-gestational-age (SGA) infants in 21% of cases. Genotype had no significant effect on 5-minute Apgar score. The risk factors for having an SGA neonate were preeclampsia and acute anemic events.

Conclusions. Women with all major genotypes of sickle cell disease tolerate pregnancy well. The offspring appear to be healthy, although those whose mothers have the SS genotype are at increased risk of being SGA. Thus, the previous recommendation that women with sickle cell disease should avoid pregnancy or have an abortion seems unwarranted. However, further study is needed to define the possible interactions of risk factors for SGA status and the long-term outcomes of infants at risk.

Commentary

This is a useful article for those who deal with sickle cell disease, because previous studies of this subject have been limited by small sample size and analysis restricted to regional experiences. This study brings together the results from 19 different centers treating sickle cell disease. Interestingly, this analysis of 445 pregnancies found that the antepartum and intrapartum complications were the same in women with sickle cell disease and appropriately matched controls. Moreover, the frequency of complications related to sickle cell disease was the same during pregnancy as it was during the nonpregnant condition.

A total of 64% of the pregnancies went to term and delivery and 99% of these resulted in a live birth. Overall, the results were surprisingly good, although about 1 in 5 of the neonates had a low birth weight for their gestational age. Attention to prevention of preeclampsia and severe anemia may result in even better statistics for outcome of pregnancy in sickle cell disease.

EARLY INCREASE IN BLOOD PRESSURE AND DIASTOLIC LEFT VENTRICULAR MALFUNCTION IN PATIENTS WITH GLOMERULONEPHRITIS

Stefanski A, Schmidt KG, Waldherr R, et al
(Ruperto Carola Univ, Heidelberg, Germany)
Kidney Int 50:1321-1326, 1996

Background. In patients with diabetic nephropathy, blood pressure progressively increases before normal blood pressure (140/90 mm Hg) is transgressed. Information on such blood pressure characteristics is not available for patients with glomerulonephritis.

Methods. Twenty untreated patients with biopsy-proven primary chronic glomerulonephritis (GN) were examined. All had a casual blood pressure of less than 140/90 mm Hg and normal glomerular filtration rate by inulin clearance. A group of normotensive, healthy individuals matched for body mass index, sex, and age comprised a control group.

Findings. Patients with GN had significantly greater median 24-hour, daytime, and nocturnal sleeping time mean arterial pressure values than the controls. However, the increased blood pressure did not exceed the upper limit of normal. On echocardiography, posterior wall thickness and ventricular septal thickness were significantly greater in the patients. The patients had a significantly lower early diastolic-to-late diastolic ratio of mitral valve peak inflow velocity.

Conclusions. The increased ambulatory blood pressure documented in patients with primary chronic GN is associated with evidence of target organ damage in the heart. In patients with GN, blood pressure appears to increase initially within the normotensive range. These findings argue for early antihypertensive intervention, but controlled trials of the safety and efficacy of such an approach are needed.

Commentary

This study provides evidence for an increase in blood pressure, although not beyond normal limits set by the World Health Organization, in individuals with biopsy-proven IgA glomerulonephritis who have normal values of glomerular filtration rate. The postulate that the blood pressure levels found in patients with incipient glomerulonephritis are inappropriately high is supported by the presence of damage in target organs. Measurements of the thickness of the wall of the left ventricle revealed significantly higher values in the patients with glomerulonephritis. This study did not address the mechanisms underlying the increase in blood pressure. Inappropriate activity of pressor systems (angiotensin II, endothelin intrarenally) or sodium retention as a consequence of the renal pathologic condition should be considered. The need for antihypertensive therapy early in the course of IgA glomerulonephritis may be justified. However, as pointed out by the authors, controlled trials to test the efficacy and safety of lowering blood pressure in such patients are needed.

CONTROLLED TRIAL OF ORAL PREDNISONE IN OUTPATIENTS WITH ACUTE COPD EXACERBATION

Thompson WH, Nielson CP, Carvalho P, et al
(Univ of Washington, Seattle; Veterans Affairs Med Ctr, Boise, Idaho)
Am J Respir Crit Care Med 154:407-412, 1996

Background.—Corticosteroids are an accepted treatment for acute exacerbations of chronic obstructive pulmonary disease (COPD), but the benefits of this treatment have not been proven. Corticosteroids were tested for their efficacy in the outpatient treatment of COPD exacerbations.

Methods.—The randomized, double-blind, placebo-controlled trial included 27 patients with acute exacerbations of COPD. All continued to take their regular medications and increased their use of β-agonists. The patients were assigned to receive 9 days of treatment with either oral prednisone, in a tapering course from 60 to 20 mg, or placebo. The results were assessed by spirometry, arterial blood gas tensions, a chemistry panel, a complete blood count, and dyspnea scores. Patients who required hospitalization for deteriorating respiratory status or lack of subjective improvement in dyspnea were considered treatment failures.

Results.—Patients in the prednisone group had a faster rate of improvement in partial pressure of oxygen in arterial blood (PaO_2) (Fig. 1), alveolar-arterial oxygen gradient, forced expiratory volume in 1 second (Fig. 2), and peak expiratory flow. The treatment failure rate was 57% with placebo vs. 0% with prednisone. The steroid-treated patients had more rapid improvement in dyspnea as well (Fig. 3). In the non-steroid-treated patients, the eosinophil count before the start of treatment was associated with a poor response to treatment.

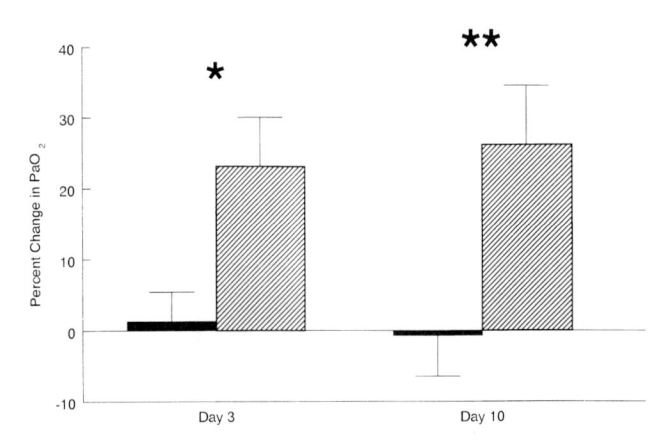

Fig. 1—Percent change from day 1 ($\pm$ SE) in partial pressure of oxygen in arterial blood (PaO_2) on days 3 and 10 for placebo *(black bar)* and prednisone *(hatched bar)* groups. The difference between the two groups was significant on both days 3 and 10 (*$P = 0.02$, **$P = 0.002$). (Courtesy of Thompson WH, Nielson CP, Carvalho P, et al: Controlled trial of oral prednisone in outpatients with acute COPD exacerbation, *Am J Respir Crit Care Med* 154:407-412, 1996.)

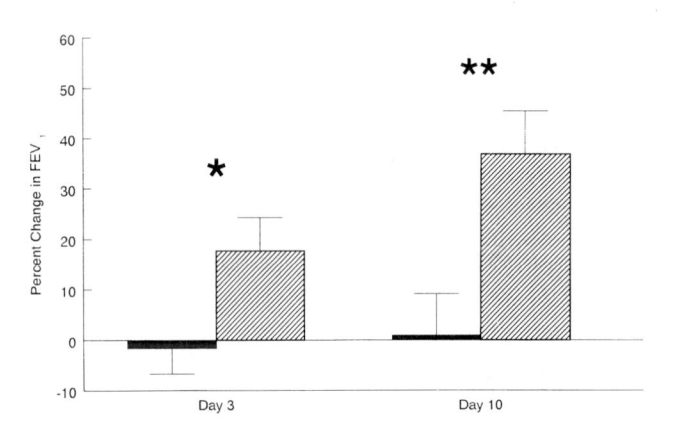

Fig. 2—Percent change from day 1 ($\pm$ SE) in forced expiratory volume in 1 second (FEV_1) on days 3 and 10 for placebo *(black bar)* and prednisone *(hatched bar)* groups. The difference between the two groups was not quite statistically significant on day 3 (*$P = 0.05$) but was significant on day 10 (**$P = 0.01$). (Courtesy of Thompson WH, Nielson CP, Carvalho P, et al: Controlled trial of oral prednisone in outpatients with acute COPD exacerbation, *Am J Respir Crit Care Med* 154:407-412, 1996.)

Conclusions.—Outpatient oral prednisone therapy accelerates recovery from acute exacerbations of COPD. Steroid treatment results in quicker improvement of respiratory measurements, a lower treatment failure rate, and improvements in subjec-

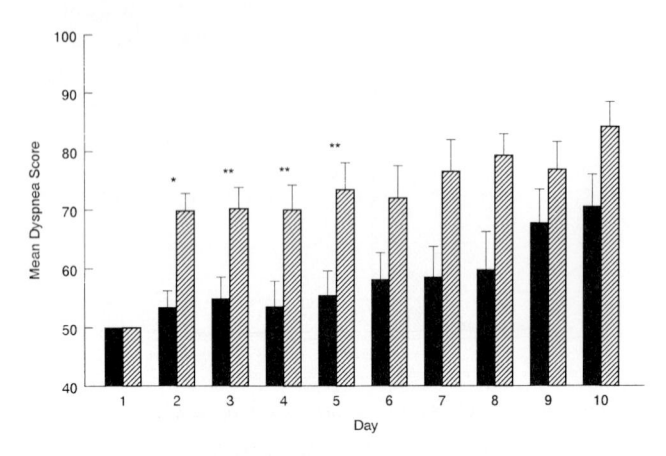

Fig. 3 Mean (± SE) dyspnea scale scores on days 1 through 10 for the placebo *(black bar)* and prednisone *(hatched bar)* groups. The difference between the two groups was significant only on day 2 after Bonferroni's correction for multiple comparisons (*P = 0.01, **P = 0.05-0.10). (Courtesy of Thompson WH, Nielson CP, Carvalho P, et al: Controlled trial of oral prednisone in outpatients with acute COPD exacerbation, *Am J Respir Crit Care Med* 154:407-412, 1996.)

tive dyspnea. The mechanisms of prednisone's benefits in this situation are unknown.

Commentary

This is a carefully designed, randomized, controlled clinical trial of corticosteroids used in outpatients with acute exacerbations of COPD. The rationale for the use of corticosteroids in COPD has been well described.[1] This study draws conclusions quite different from those of Murata et al.,[2] who showed that the randomized use of IV corticosteroids did not prevent the need for hospitalization in exacerbations of chronic bronchitis. However, the study is confirmatory of the often-quoted trial by Albert, who used methylprednisolone in hospitalized patients, showing small but statistically and clinically significant improvements in outcome.[3] Thus, this paper adds further credence to the common use of short courses of corticosteroids in exacerbations of chronic bronchitis.

Elsewhere in the world, particularly in Europe, exacerbations of chronic bronchitis would be treated empirically with antibiotics. Whether this practice is rational has been debated, but in another controlled clinical trial,[4] antibiotics were shown to be effective in some but not all cases of patients with exacerbations of COPD. It would be of interest to design a study comparing antibiotics with corticosteroids alone and in combination to better define the type of patient most likely to respond to the nonspecific antiinflammatory effects of corticosteroids or the antimicrobial and possibly associated antiinflammatory effects of antibiotic therapy.

REFERENCES

1. Hudson LD, Monti CM: Rationale and use of corticosteroids in chronic obstructive pulmonary disease, *Med Clin North Am* 74:661-690, 1990.
2. Murata GH, Gorby MS, Chick TW, et al: Intravenous and oral corticosteroids for the prevention of relapse after treatment of decompensated COPD: effect on patients with a history of multiple relapses, *Chest* 98:845-849, 1990.
3. Albert RK, Martin TR, Lewis SW: Controlled clinical trial of methylprednisolone in patients with chronic bronchitis and acute respiratory insufficiency, *Ann Intern Med* 92:753-758, 1980.
4. Anthonisen NR, Manfreda J, Warren CPW: Antibiotic therapy in exacerbations of chronic obstructive pulmonary disease, *Ann Intern Med* 106:196-204, 1987.

ACYCLOVIR AND PREDNISOLONE TREATMENT OF ACUTE INFECTIOUS MONONUCLEOSIS: A MULTICENTER, DOUBLE-BLIND, PLACEBO-CONTROLLED STUDY

Tynell E, Aurelius E, Brandell A, et al *(Karolinska Institutet, Danderyd, Sweden; Huddinge Univ, Sweden; Univ of Stockholm; et al)*
J Infect Dis 174:324-331, 1996

Background.—Infectious mononucleosis can produce mild symptoms or even be fatal in immunodeficient patients. The safety and efficacy of treatment with acyclovir and prednisolone in patients with IM were investigated in a double-blind study.

Methods.—Ninety-four patients, 14-30 years of age, with clinical features of infectious mononucleosis and symptoms of 7 days or less in duration were enrolled. By random assignment, patients received placebo or oral acyclovir, 800 mg 5 times a day, plus prednisolone, 0.7 mg/kg for the first 4 days and reduced by 0.1 mg/kg on consecutive days for another 6 days.

Findings.—Shedding of oropharyngeal Epstein-Barr virus (EBV) was significantly inhibited during active treatment. However, combination treatment had no effect on duration of general illness, sore throat, weight loss, or absence from school or work. Treatment also had no effect on the frequency of latent EBV-infected B lymphocytes in peripheral blood or the histocompatibility leukocyte antigen-restricted EBV-specific cellular immunity, determined 6 months after disease onset.

Conclusions.—Acyclovir and prednisolone therapy appears to be of limited value in patients with mild to moderate symptoms of infectious mononucleosis. Further studies of this treatment in patients with infectious mononucleosis and complications requiring intensive care are warranted.

Commentary

Mononucleosis is a common infection that is usually self-limited and relatively benign. Some patients, however, are debilitated and ill for a long time, and rare serious complications may occur. Previous studies have suggested that corticosteroids can reduce the duration of fever and increase the rate of resolution of constitutional symptoms. Corticosteroids result in high levels of viral excretion, and there are reports that cases of myocarditis and encephalitis have occurred in steroid-treated patients, so infectious diseases physicians have been reluctant to advocate corticosteroid treatment. The investigators reasoned that, if acyclovir was added to prednisolone, they could demonstrate the effect of corticosteroids and blunt the viral replication. Combination therapy did decrease viral replication, but combination therapy did not benefit the patients. Corticosteroid therapy should be reserved for those patients with mononucleosis who have impending airway obstruction, severe thrombocytopenia, or hemolytic anemia.

REDUCTION OF TRANSIENT MYOCARDIAL ISCHEMIA WITH PRAVASTATIN IN ADDITION TO THE CONVENTIONAL TREATMENT IN PATIENTS WITH ANGINA PECTORIS

van Boven AJ, on behalf of the REGRESS Study Group
(Univ Hospital Groningen, The Netherlands; et al)
Circulation 94:1503-1505, 1996

Background. Treatment to reduce cholesterol levels can reduce morbidity and mortality in patients who have or are at high risk of coronary heart disease. However, the potential antiischemic effects of lipid-lowering therapy are unknown. The effects of cholesterol-lowering therapy on transient myocardial ischemia were studied.

Methods. The prospective, randomized, placebo-controlled trial included 768 men (mean age, 56 years) with coronary artery disease and stable angina pectoris. All had serum cholesterol levels of 155-310 mg/dl. All patients received standard antianginal therapy, including medication, percutaneous transluminal angioplasty, and/or coronary artery bypass grafting. In addition, they were randomly assigned to receive 2 years of treatment with pravastatin, 40 mg once daily, or placebo. The effects of treatment on transient myocardial ischemia were analyzed by 48-hour ambulatory ECG monitoring.

Results. From baseline to 2 years, the prevalence of transient myocardial ischemia decreased from 28% to 19% in the pravastatin group and increased from 20% to 23% in the placebo group. The odds ratio for recurrent ischemia was 0.62, with a 95% confidence interval of 0.41-0.93. The mean number of ischemic episodes decreased by 1.23 in the pravastatin group and 0.53 in the placebo group; the average duration of ischemia decreased from 80 to 42 minutes with pravastatin and from 60 to 42 minutes with placebo. Total ischemic burden fell from 41 to 22 mm/min with pravastatin and from 34 to 26 mm/min with placebo. Pravastatin significantly reduced the risk of ischemia—odds ratio 0.45, 95% confidence interval 0.22-0.91—after adjustment for independent risk factors.

Conclusions. Lipid-lowering therapy with pravastatin reduces transient ischemia in men with coronary artery disease, this randomized study finds. Pravastatin significantly reduces the number of ischemic episodes, the duration of ischemia, and the total ischemic burden even in patients who have received optimal antianginal therapy. The mechanism of these effects is unknown but could involve normalization of coronary endothelial function.

Commentary

This study shows that lipid-lowering therapy with pravastatin reduces transient myocardial ischemia detected by ambulatory ECG monitoring. The possible mechanisms for this action include regression of atherosclerotic plaques and attenuation of coronary endothelial dysfunction with lipid-lowering therapy. Multiple studies are now in progress evaluating lipid-lowering therapy, specifically the statins, as a treatment in patients with both symptomatic and asymptomatic ischemia. The postinfarction trials using statins have clearly shown their beneficial actions in preventing coronary thrombotic events. A vascular plaque stabilizing action appears to be an important effect of statin benefit, which may go well beyond just lipid lowering.

YEAR BOOK OF NEUROLOGY AND NEUROSURGERY

MRI OF 'IDIOPATHIC' JUVENILE SCOLIOSIS: A PROSPECTIVE STUDY

Evans SC, Edgar MA, Hall-Craggs MA, et al
(Middlesex Hosp, London)
J Bone Joint Surg (Br) 78B:314-317, 1996

Objective. Juvenile idiopathic scoliosis is relatively uncommon. With the availability of MRI, studies have found a preponderance of syringomyelia, often associated with Chiari I malformation, in the juvenile age group. Recent reviews have identified a possible association between syringomyelia and some cases of idiopathic scoliosis. Patients with juvenile scoliosis were prospectively studied by MRI.

Methods. The study included 31 consecutive patients with idiopathic scoliosis detected between the ages of 4 and 12 years. Twenty-four were girls (mean age 9 years), and seven were boys (mean age 7 years). All underwent MRI scanning of the hind brain and spinal cord to seek evidence of syrinx formation, spinal dysraphism, and cord neoplasms.

Results. Twenty-six percent of patients had a significant neuroanatomic abnormality detected on MRI. Six of these eight patients had Chiari I malformation associated with a syrinx, one had isolated Chiari I malformation, and one had astrocytoma of the cervical spinal cord. Four of these patients had a left-sided thoracic curve compared with only 3 of 23 patients with normal neuroanatomical findings. None of the clinical features examined could distinguish between patients with and without MRI abnormalities. Unilateral absence of abdominal reflexes was found in 12% of patients with neuroanatomic abnormalities and 9% of those without.

Conclusions. Magnetic resonance imaging of the hind brain and spinal cord detects Chiari I malformation and other neuroanatomic abnormalities in many patients with apparent "idiopathic" juvenile scoliosis. It is potentially dangerous to undertake surgical treatment of scoliosis in a patient with undecompressed syringomyelia, and significant improvement may follow decompression of the foramen magnum. Thus, MRI scanning should be mandatory for all patients with juvenile-onset scoliosis.

Commentary

Evans et al. reminded us that juvenile scoliosis is not always idiopathic and that preoperative assessment by MRI may reveal the cause and lead to safer surgical treatment.

LONG-TERM OUTCOME OF PROPHYLAXIS FOR FEBRILE CONVULSIONS

Knudsen FU, Paerregaard A, Anderson R, et al
(Glostrup Univ, Denmark)
Arch Dis Child 74:13-18, 1996

Background. Major cohort studies have shown that long-term outcomes are normal for most children with febrile convulsions. As a result, long-term prophylaxis with antiepileptic agents has been abandoned for the most part. However, febrile convulsions may be associated with more subtle adverse outcomes in motor, neurologic, intellectual, or cognitive functions. In addition, it is unknown whether medical intervention in early childhood affects long-term prognosis, including the occurrence of subsequent epilepsy. These questions were investigated in a randomized, controlled, long-term follow-up study.

Methods and findings. Follow-up data were collected from 289 children 12 years after randomization to intermittent prophylaxis (group 1) or no prophylaxis (group 2). All had had febrile convulsions in early childhood. At follow-up mean age in group 1 was 14 years and in group 2 was 14.1 years. Body weight, height, and head circumference were also comparable between groups. The groups also had very similar findings on neurologic assessment, the Stott motor test of fine and gross motor development, the Wechsler Intelligence Scale for children (including verbal intelligence quotient [IQ], performance IQ, and full-scale IQ), a neuropsychologic test battery (including short- and long-term, auditory, and visual memory), and visuomotor tempo, computer reaction time, and reading tests. Scholastic achievement was also comparable between groups. The incidence of epilepsy in 0.7% in group 1 and 0.8% in group 2.

Conclusions. Type of treatment of febrile convulsions in early childhood did not affect the occurrence of subsequent epilepsy or long-term neurologic, motor, intellectual, cognitive, and scholastic abilities. Thus, in the long term, preventing new febrile convulsions appears to be no better than abbreviating them.

Commentary

Epileptologists, who see adults with refractory seizures, often elicit a history of febrile seizures during infancy and believe that a causal relationship exists. Child neurologists, who see children with febrile seizures, know that they are rarely a precursor of epilepsy. This is one of the few prospective long-term (12 years) follow-up studies of febrile convulsions. It confirmed that febrile seizures have a benign outcome whether they are simple or complex (prolonged, multiple, partial) or whether or not they are prevented with diazepam. Febrile seizures do not beget afebrile seizures unless both are caused by an underlying brain disorder.

YEAR BOOK OF OBSTETRICS, GYNECOLOGY, AND WOMEN'S HEALTH

VAGINAL DOUCHING AND REDUCED FERTILITY

Baird DD, Weinberg CR, Voigt LF, et al *(Natl Inst of Environmental Health Sciences, Research Triangle Park, NC; Univ of Washington, Seattle)*
Am J Public Health 86:844-850, 1996

Background. In one national survey, 37% of American women of childbearing age reported douching. Eighteen percent douched at least once a week. However, this common practice may have adverse effects. It has been associated with an increased risk of chlamydia infection, pelvic inflammatory disease, and ectopic pregnancy. The relationship between vaginal douching and fertility was investigated.

Methods. To avoid problems inherent in studying patients who are infertile, the fertility of douchers and nondouchers was compared by collecting data on the number of months parous women required to become pregnant. This method was expected to underestimate the effect of douching on fertility because women who were sterile were excluded. Eight hundred forty women participated.

Findings. Compared with nondouchers, douchers were 30% less likely to become pregnant each month they tried to conceive. This association persisted after adjustment for covariates and was not

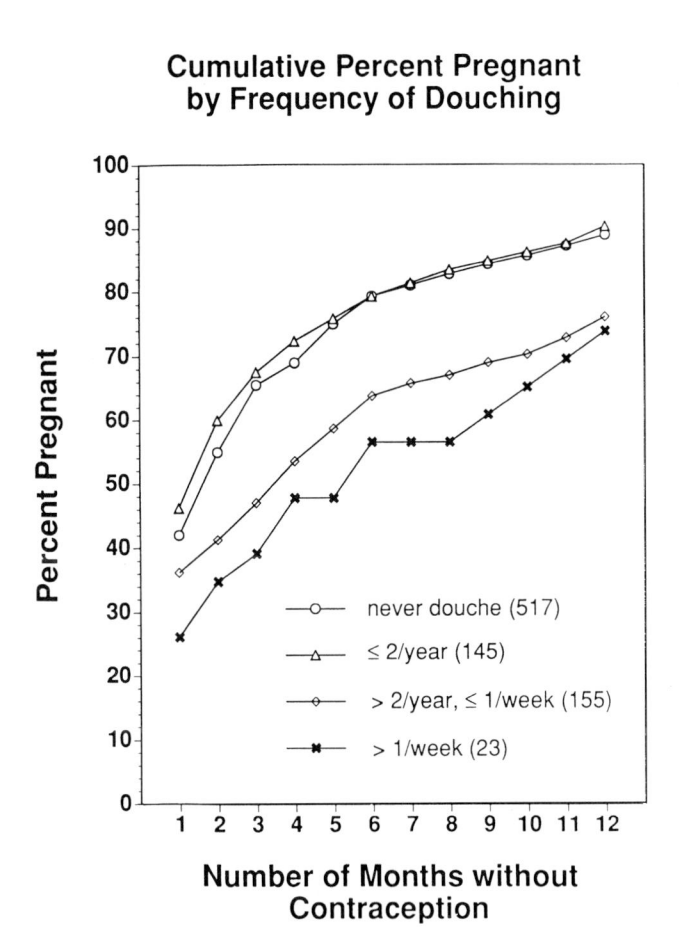

Fig. 1 Unadjusted cumulative percentage pregnant each month for women in four groups determined by their frequency of douching. (Courtesy of Baird DD, Weinberg CR, Voigt LF, et al: Vaginal douching and reduced fertility, *Am J Public Health* 86:844-850, copyright 1996, American Public Health Association.)

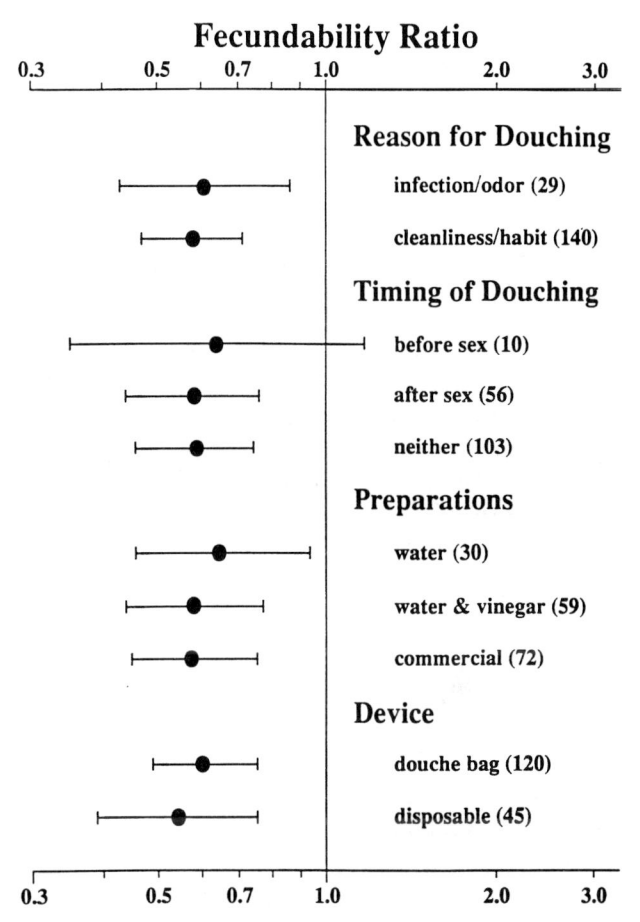

Fig. 2 Adjusted fecundability ratios (with 95% confidence intervals) for groups of women with different douching habits. (Courtesy of Baird DD, Weinberg CR, Voigt LF, et al: Vaginal douching and reduced fertility, *Am J Public Health* 86:844-850, copyright 1996, American Public Health Association.)

explained by douching for medical reasons. The reduction in fertility was unassociated with the type of douching preparation used. Monthly fertility was reduced by 50% among women 18-24 years of age, 29% among those 25-29 years of age, and 6% among those 30-39 years of age. These age differences were significant (Figs. 1 and 2).

Conclusions. In this series, douching was associated with decreased fertility. Additional research is needed to determine whether this relationship is causal and, if so, the degree to which pelvic infection mediates it.

Commentary

In prior epidemiologic studies, the environmental factors of cigarette smoking and caffeine ingestion have each been shown to independently decrease female fecundability. The data in this study indicate that vaginal douching with any liquid material also reduces fecundability, especially in women of young reproductive age. Thus, the woman in an infertile couple should be advised to stop smoking, stop drinking caffeinated beverages, and avoid vaginal douching.

EFFECT OF CALCIUM SUPPLEMENTATION ON PREGNANCY-INDUCED HYPERTENSION AND PREECLAMPSIA: A META-ANALYSIS OF RANDOMIZED CONTROLLED TRIALS

Bucher HC, Guyatt GH, Cook RJ, et al (McMaster Univ, Hamilton, Ont, Canada; Univ of Waterloo, Kitchener, Ont, Canada)
JAMA 275:1113-1117, 1996

Background. A recent meta-analysis concluded that calcium supplementation reduced the proportion of women with new-onset hypertension and preeclampsia in pregnancy. However, that analysis was limited in its assessment of the studies' validity, and in its exploration of the reasons the findings varied. Because new randomized trials of calcium supplementation in pregnancy have been reported since that meta-analysis was published, a new systemic overview was conducted.

Data Sources. Publications were identified through a MEDLINE and EMBASE search of studies published between 1966 and 1994. The authors of eligible trials were contacted to ensure data accuracy and completeness. Fourteen randomized studies were included in the analysis, with a total of 2459 women enrolled in these studies. Unpublished trials were also identified with the help of the eligible trial authors.

Data Synthesis. Differences in blood pressure changes between patients receiving calcium and those in control groups were weighted by the inverse of the variance. The pooled analysis demonstrated a −5.4 mm Hg decrease in systolic blood pressure and a −3.44 mm Hg decline in diastolic pressure. Compared with women given placebo, women given calcium supplementation had a 0.38 odds ratio for the development of preeclampsia.

Conclusions. Systolic and diastolic blood pressures, as well as preeclampsia, are reduced by calcium supplementation during pregnancy. Calcium supplementation should be considered for pregnant women at risk of preeclampsia. However, more studies are needed to establish the effect of calcium on maternal and fetal morbidity.

Commentary

This meta-analysis by a group of McMaster University scientists follows the application of that technique to a series of studies of the effect of 1-2 g per day of calcium supplement on nonpregnant individuals. There they found significant reduction in systolic blood pressure in the randomized patients receiving calcium supplementation, an average of −1.27 mm Hg. No significant change in diastolic blood pressure appeared to result and the authors concluded the effects were too small to support recommending calcium supplementation to patients with mild hypertension. Here, they find the results sufficiently compelling to recommend 1.5-2 g of calcium supplement per day in pregnancy in an effort to prevent preeclampsia. The inevitable problems of meta-analysis in aggregating heterogeneous studies, as though there were no differences among them, appear somewhat larger here than in the earlier publication. Strong evidence for data heterogeneity was found for both systolic and diastolic blood pressure and a number of covariants were found, especially in the diastolic blood pressure data.

As before, unpublished data that had not been peer reviewed were included for analysis by the investigators. Most important, observer blinding to test vs. placebo status was not required for entry. This increased the likelihood that observer bias played a role in the conclusions. Two preliminary reports were included, in addition to three studies where blood pressure measurements were deemed inadequate but ". . . reported data about adverse outcomes that we did include" was entered. What this means is unclear. Criteria for the diagnosis of preeclampsia, not a trivial matter, are not described. A pooled estimate of reduced risk of preeclampsia of 0.3 seems large for the relatively small reductions in mean blood pressure identified here. These data have been used to justify a prospective randomized trial of calcium supplement designed to evaluate morbidity outcome variables. Perhaps that will bolster the recommendations made here with what seems to be arguable evidence.

METHOTREXATE AND MISOPROSTOL FOR EARLY ABORTION: A MULTICENTER TRIAL. I. SAFETY AND EFFICACY

Creinin MD, Vittinghoff E, Keder L, et al
(Univ of Pittsburgh, Pa; Univ of California, San Francisco; Women's Health Care Services, Wichita, Kansas)
Contraception 53:321-327, 1996

Background. Several studies have shown that IM injection of methotrexate 50 mg/m^2 followed by misoprostol insertion induces abortion in the first 56 days of gestation. However, the safety and efficacy of this procedure have yet to be assessed at multiple sites using a single protocol.

Methods. The current multicenter study included 300 pregnant women seeking elective abortion. Seven days after the IM injection of methotrexate, 50 mg/m^2, the patients returned for vaginally administered misoprostol, 800 μg. Four 200-g tablets were placed into the vagina through a speculum. As the speculum was removed, the tablets were pushed into the posterior fornix with a large cotton swab. Patients were permitted to get up immediately after misoprostol was administered. A vaginal ultrasound examination was performed 1 and 5 days later. A surgical abortion was done when cardiac activity was still present after the second ultrasonography. Patients returned 4 weeks later for a follow-up assessment.

Findings. Overall, abortion occurred with no need for surgery in 87.7% of the women. The complete abortion rate was 90.6% in women with gestations of less than 49 days and 81.6% in women with gestations of 50-56 days. In 65% of women, abortion occurred within 24 hours of the initial or repeat misoprostol dose. In the remaining 22.7% of women who aborted, abortion was delayed by a mean of 23.6 days. The success rate after the first misoprostol dose was greater between days 43 and 56 compared to before day 43 (Table 3). In almost all the women, bleeding and/or cramping began within 3.3 hours after the first misoprostol dose.

Patients in whom the procedure was immediately successful had vaginal bleeding lasting a mean of 10 days and spotting for a mean of 4 days. In women with delayed abortion, vaginal bleeding lasted a mean of 7 days and spotting a mean of 4 days. None of the women needed a transfusion. In a univariate analysis, gravidity of less than 3, lower gestational age, and lower serum β-human chorionic gonadotropin on the day of methotrexate injection significantly predicted treatment success (Fig. 1).

Conclusions. Methotrexate followed by misoprostol is an effective and safe alternative to surgical abortion and the use of antiprogestins and prostaglandin for medical abortion. The adverse effects of methotrexate and misoprostol administration were minimal.

Commentary

This large multicenter study confirms the fact that the sequential use of a single IM injection of methotrexate followed by vaginally administered misoprostol is an effective method of electively terminating a pregnancy of less than 7 weeks gestational age from onset of the last menses, with a success rate of about 90%. Problems with this medical therapy are the fact that only two thirds of the women aborted within 24 hours of the last misoprostol dose. Most of the remaining one third of women who do abort do not do so until 2-3 weeks later. In addition, the women who do abort bleed an average of about 2 weeks and in some instances for as long as 6-8 weeks. Finally, about one third of the women experience nausea, vomiting, or diarrhea. Koppersmith et al.[1] reported that about two thirds of women in early pregnancy treated with vaginal misoprostol alone, without methotrexate, had a successful abortion within 48 hours without the gastrointestinal side effects of methotrexate. These investigators did not extend their study beyond that time period but performed vaginal evacuation of the uterine cavity if abortion had failed to occur within 12 hours after receiving the last study medication. Until an antiprogestin is available for use in the United States, if a woman wishes to terminate her pregnancy medically, perhaps vaginal misoprostol alone without methotrexate should still be given. For the one third of women who fail to abort, uterine evacuation can be performed to avoid the prolonged duration of uterine bleeding and need for careful evaluation, as well as avoiding the side effects of methotrexate.

TABLE 3 Cumulative Abortion Rate (N = 300)

	ABORTION RATE	INCOMPLETE ABORTION*
Before misoprostol	2 (0.7%)	
After first dose of misoprostol†	158 (52.7%)	4 (2.5%)
After second dose of misoprostol†	203 (67.7%)	8 (3.9%)
By follow-up on day 14	209 (69.7%)	8 (3.8%)
By day 21	232 (77.3%)	11 (4.7%)
By day 28	263 (87.7%)	13 (4.9%)
By day 35	275 (91.7%)	13 (4.7%)
By day 80	277 (92.3%)	14 (5.1%)

Reprinted by permission of the publisher from Creinin MD, Vittinghoff E, Keder L, et al: Methotrexate and misoprostol for early abortion: a multicenter trial. I. Safety and efficacy, *Contraception* 53:321-327, 1996. Copyright 1996 by Elsevier Science Inc.
*Includes 1 patient with a surgical aspiration for hemorrhage (day 9).
†Within 24 hours of misoprostol administration.

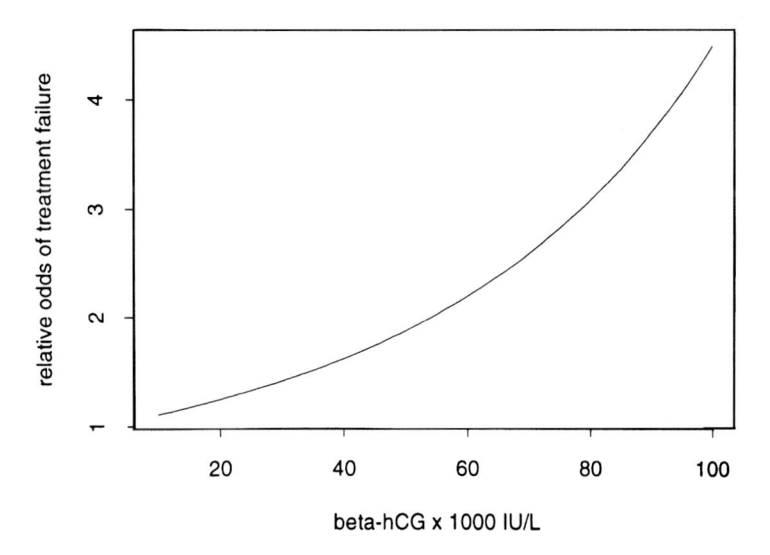

Fig. 1 Odds of treatment failure based on serum β-human chorionic gonadotropin (β-hCG) on the day of methotrexate injection. (Reprinted by permission from Creinin MD, Vittinghoff E, Keder L, et al: Methotrexate and misoprostol for early abortion: a multicenter trial. I. Safety and efficacy, *Contraception* 53:321-327, 1996. Copyright 1996 by Elsevier Science Inc.)

DETECTION OF VIRUS IN VERTICALLY EXPOSED HIV-ANTIBODY-NEGATIVE CHILDREN

Newell M-L, Dunn D, De Maria A, et al (Inst of Child Health, London; Univ of Genoa, Italy; Univ of Padua, Italy; et al)
Lancet 347:213-215, 1996

Introduction. Fetuses can acquire HIV infection from their HIV-infected mothers in utero or during delivery. However, cases of neonates acquiring HIV by vertical transmission with subsequently cleared infection have been reported. To investigate the frequency of HIV virus clearance, the progress of infants born to HIV-infected mothers was followed from birth.

Methods. At four centers participating in the European Collaborative Study, 299 infants with HIV-infected mothers, born over a 9-year period, were classified as HIV-antibody-negative. Of these, 264 were tested with virus culture or polymerase chain reaction at least once before the age of 3 months.

Results. Of the 264 infants tested, nine had at least one virus culture or polymerase chain reaction sample revealing HIV positivity, and demonstrated subsequent seroreversion (Table 3). Six infants demonstrated a pattern consistent with viral clearance, with positive virus tests early in life and later seroreversion. The other three infants demonstrated no clear pattern, with virus detected intermittently and later in life. All nine infants were fed exclusively by bottle, had no HIV-related symptoms, and had received no antiviral treatment, and all but one were delivered vaginally.

Conclusions. There was a 2.7% incidence of infants of HIV mothers who clear HIV or tolerate virus. In current pediatric practice, the parents of these infants are informed that their infant is HIV-negative. Further study of these infants may provide insight into the mechanisms of virus clearance and have implications for vaccine development.

Commentary

Although individual cases of apparently vertically infected HIV-1-positive infants spontaneously becoming HIV-negative have appeared, this is the first systematic study sufficiently large to allow rate estimates of that phenomenon. If the rate of spontaneous clearance of virus is high, estimates of vertical transmission based on viral culture and polymerase chain reaction analysis of newborn blood in the first month or two of life are higher than the actual rates. If newborn viral clearance takes place, as it most commonly does before 18 months of life, it indicates a possible role for passively transferred maternal antibody in the prevention of fetal infection given the presence of fetal virus. If that is not what is involved, there is an entirely new, currently unrecognized set of operations at work in the neonate that may have important implications for infected adults.

The data were derived from four European centers participating in the European Collaborative Study of HIV-positive pregnancy.[1] During the period from 1985 to 1994, 264 infants were tested every 3 months for 18 months or until HIV-negative, and 219 of these had at least two viral cultures. The crude rate for conversion of neonates initially HIV-positive both by viral culture and polymerase chain reaction was 3.4%. When corrections were made, excluding those with only one positive culture and estimating the likelihood of error based on the two positive tests occurring by random chance, the clearance rate was 2.7%. An additional finding reported gratuitously here is that of 857 infants followed for 1700 child-years, an average of about 2 years each, none who were antibody-negative—whether or not they were originally antibody-positive—ever reverted to be antibody-positive. This suggests a low rate of horizontal transmission among those mother-infant pairs. An important study, this work will spawn a great deal of mechanistic investigation.

EFFICACY OF PELVIC FLOOR MUSCLE EXERCISES IN WOMEN WITH STRESS, URGE, AND MIXED URINARY INCONTINENCE

Nygaard IE, Kreder KJ, Lepic MM, et al (Univ of Iowa, Iowa City)
Am J Obstet Gynecol 174:120-125, 1996

Background. The Agency for Health Care Policy and Research recommends that nonsurgical treatment be attempted in patients with urinary incontinence before resorting to surgical intervention. Pelvic muscle exercises have been found to be effective for the treatment of stress incontinence in previous studies, with reported success rates ranging from 31% to 97%. To evaluate, on the basis of intent to treat, the efficacy of a 3-month pelvic floor muscle exercise program as first-line intervention among women with stress, urge, or mixed urinary incontinence, a prospective, randomized study was performed. The ability of a specially designed audiotape to improve compliance and exercise effect also was assessed.

Patients and Methods. Seventy-one patients evaluated in two tertiary care center referral clinics for urinary incontinence were enrolled in the study. Genital prolapse past the vaginal introitus was not observed in any patient. Patients were randomly assigned to pelvic floor exercise with or without the use of a 270-minute audiotape that featured technique tips, reminders, and exercise (contraction/relaxation) cues. The number of incontinent episodes, evaluated by means of a 3-day voiding diary, served as the main outcome measure.

Results. Fifty-five women completed the entire 3-month exercise program. For all 71 participants, the mean number of incontinent episodes decreased from 3.1 to 2.3 per day. Among the 55 patients who completed the entire 3-month program, the mean number of incontinent episodes decreased from 2.6

TABLE 3   Laboratory Data on 9 Seronegative Children Who Tested Positive by Virus Culture or Polymerase Chain Reaction on at Least 1 Sample

CHILD	AGE (MONTHS) AT LOSS OF ANTIBODY	NUMBER OF SAMPLES IN WHICH VIRUS DETECTED	TEST RESULTS BY VIRUS-CULTURE/PCR (AGE IN MONTHS)				
A	8-10	2	+/ND (1)	ND/+ (2)	ND/− (10)	−/− (13)	−/− (29)	−/ND (55)	−/ND (64)
B	3-16	2	+/+ (3)	+/+ (6)	−/− (16)	−/− (18)	−/− (24)		
C	9-11	2	+/ND (0)	−/ND (3)	−/+ (5)	−/− (9)	−/ND (11)	−/ND (15)	−/− (20)	−/− (25)
D	12-15	1	−/− (0)	+/+ (1)	−/− (4)	−/ND (6)	−/− (9)	−/ND (12)	−/ND (15)	−/ND (23)
E	11-16	1	−/ND (B)	+/ND (3)	−/ND (26)	ND/− (50)			
F	7-18	1	+/ND (4)					
G	15-17	3	+/ND (3)	+/− (6)	+/+ (12)	−/− (24)	−/− (30)	−/− (45)	ND/− (47)	−/− (68)	−/− (72)
H	8-11	4	+/ND (0)	−/ND (3)	−/ND (8)	+/ND (14)	+/ND (17)	−/ND (25)	ND/+ (47)	−/ND (23)
I	5-8	2	−/ND (B)	+/ND (1)	−/ND (5)	−/ND (8)	−/ND (11)	−/ND (14)	−/ND (17)	−/ND (56)
							−/ND (32)	+/ND (39)		

Courtesy of Newell M-L, Dunn D, De Maria A, et al.: Detection of virus in vertically exposed HIV-antibody-negative children, *Lancet*, 347:213-215, copyright by The Lancet 1996.
B, birch; *ND*, not done; *PCR*, polymerase chain reaction.

to 1.3 per day. Six months after program completion, 10 women with stress incontinence had undergone surgical treatment. Among the 27 patients with genuine stress incontinence who were not treated surgically, 12 indicated that their improvement was good and declined further therapy. No differences in outcome or compliance were noted among women who had and had not exercised with the aid of the audiotape.

Conclusions. Six months after completing a 3-month course of pelvic floor muscle exercises, one third of the program participants expressed satisfaction with their outcome. Use of the specially designed audiotape did not enhance the success rate or decrease the dropout rate. The exercises performed were similarly effective for all patients, regardless of urodynamic diagnosis. Additional studies are needed to determine inexpensive methods that could be used to improve the success rate of this risk-free, economical, and easy-to-provide therapy.

Commentary

When evaluating published results of anti-incontinence treatments, the reader should pay attention to the reported results. Although many published reports on operative procedures for stress urinary incontinence report cure and failure, or cure improvement and failure (cure is being completely dry), most reports on Kegel exercises report an improvement, or put together improvement and cure in one group.

This study reports improvement in more than 50% of patients. However, improvement included reduction of the number of leaking episodes from 2.6 to 1.7 for stress urinary incontinence, from 3.5 to 2.3 for detrusor instability, and from 3.9 to 3.2 for mixed incontinence. These women were not dry. They were less wet than before. In the absence of a control group (which, as Fantl et al.[1] showed, helped 25% of patients), improvement occurred in approximately 33% of patients who felt that pelvic floor training helped them to the point that they wanted to continue and wished no other treatment. For the practicing physician, this is a very important message. One in three women was satisfied with the results of the training program and wished not to have surgery. These numbers should be discussed with patients after a diagnosis is established and treatment plans are made.

REFERENCE

1. Fantl JA, Wyman JF, McClish DK, et al: Efficacy of bladder training in older women with urinary incontinence, *JAMA* 265:609-613, 1991.

STROKE IN USERS OF LOW-DOSE ORAL CONTRACEPTIVES

Petitti DB, Sidney S, Bernstein A, et al (Kaiser Permanente Med Care Program, Southern California, Pasadena; Kaiser Permanente Med Care Program, Northern California, Oakland)
N Engl J Med 335:8-15, 1996

Background. In previous research, the use of oral contraceptives (OCs) has been associated with an increased risk of stroke. However, that research studied only OCs containing more estrogen than is now generally used. The relationship between stroke and OC use was examined in a large HMO in which high-estrogen OCs were rarely used.

Methods. The population-based, case-control study included female patients (age range, 15-44 years) who had and had not experienced strokes, fatal and nonfatal. Data on the use of OCs were gathered in interviews.

Findings. Four hundred eight strokes occurred among 1.1 million women during 3.6 million woman-years, for an incidence of 11.3 strokes per 100,000 woman-years. Two hundred ninety-five women with stroke and their matched control subjects were interviewed. Compared with former users and women who had never used OCs, current OC users had an odds ratio of 1.18 for ischemic stroke, after adjustment for other risk factors for stroke. The adjusted odds ratio was 1.14 for hemorrhagic stroke. Current OC use and smoking interacted positively to affect hemorrhagic stroke risk (Table 4).

Conclusions. Overall, current low-estrogen OC use does not seem to increase the risk of hemorrhagic stroke. This study confirms that the incidence of stroke among young women is low.

Commentary

In the 1960s, soon after their introduction, high estrogen dose oral contraceptive formulations were found to be causally linked to venous thromboembolism. In the 1970s, reports were published showing that women ingesting these high steroid dose formulations also were at an increased relative risk of having stroke and myocardial infarction develop. Subsequent studies showed that the increased risk of myocardial infarction was only significantly increased among women older than 35 years who also smoked and ingested high-dose formulations. It was also shown that the cause of the myocardial infarction in oral contraceptive users was due to arterial thrombosis, not accelerated atherosclerosis, brought about by the thrombophilic effect of the estrogenic component. The magnitude of the thrombophilic effect, as well as the extent of risk of venous thrombophlebitis, were both found to be directly correlated to the amount of estrogen in the formulation. Data regarding the risk of stroke with oral contraceptive use are less clear. Some studies show an increased risk of only thrombotic stroke, whereas others found an increased risk of only hemorrhagic stroke. The effect of age, smoking, and existing hypertension on the risk of stroke with oral contraceptive use is also not well defined, perhaps because these factors affect the risk of hemorrhagic and thrombotic stroke differently. The results of this large case-control study, which indicate no significant increase in risk of either thrombotic or hemorrhagic stroke among women using low estrogen dose oral contraceptives and a low overall incidence of these events among women of reproductive age, are very reassuring.

TABLE 4 Adjusted Odds Ratios for Ischemic Infarction and Hemorrhagic Stroke, According to Oral Contraceptive Use*

VARIABLE	ISCHEMIC INFARCTION† NO. OF WOMEN WITH STROKE	NO. OF MATCHED CONTROLS	OR (95% CI)	HEMORRHAGIC STROKE‡ NO. OF WOMEN WITH STROKE	NO. OF MATCHED CONTROLS	OR (95% CI)
Current use vs. non-current use						
Current use	17	43	1.18 (0.54-2.59)	21	50	1.14 (0.60-2.16)
Noncurrent use§	125	335	1.00	127	346	1.00
Current use vs. past use and no use¶						
Current use	14	43	0.65 (0.25-1.70)	14	50	1.02 (0.37-2.82)
Past use	82	271	0.49 (0.25-0.98)	81	272	0.89 (0.41-1.91)
No use§	28	64	1.00	14	74	1.00
Any use vs. no use¶						
Any use	96	314	0.52 (0.27-1.00)	95	322	0.91 (0.43-1.93)
No use§	28	64	1.00	14	74	1.00

From Petitti DB, Sidney S, Bernstein A, et al: Stroke in uses of low-dose oral contraceptives, N Engl J Med 335:8-15. Reprinted by permission of *The New England Journal of Medicine*. Copyright 1996, Massachusetts Medical Society.
OR, odds ratio; CI, confidence interval.
*Women with missing values not included. Current use denotes use in the month before the index date. Noncurrent use includes past use and no use.
†Odds ratios have been adjusted for the presence or absence of treated hypertension, the presence or absence of treated diabetes, smoking status, race or ethnic group, and body mass index.
‡Odds ratios have been adjusted for the presence or absence of treated hypertension, the presence or absence of treated diabetes, smoking status, race or ethnic group.
§Reference category.
¶Women for whom proxy respondents were interviewed have been excluded.

ORAL CONTRACEPTIVE USE AND RISK OF BREAST CANCER IN MIDDLE-AGED WOMEN

Rossing MA, Stanford JL, Weiss NS, et al (Fred Hutchinson Cancer Research Ctr, Seattle; Univ of Washington, Seattle)
Am J Epidemiol 144:161-164, 1996

Introduction.—The women who first used oral contraceptives when they became available in the 1960s are now middle aged, the time of life when breast cancer is most frequent. However, little is known about the effects of oral contraception on breast cancer risk. The potential link between contraceptive use and breast cancer risk in middle age was evaluated in a case-control study.

Methods.—The population-based study included women in Washington State who were 50 to 64 years old in 1988-1990. There were 537 breast cancer cases and 492 disease-free control subjects. The women were interviewed in detail about their use of oral contraceptives, among other variables.

Results.—The two groups were similar in the proportion of women who had ever used oral contraceptives, the total duration of oral contraceptive use, the time since last use, or the age at first or last use. Women whose first use of oral contraceptives was within 20 years of their interview had a slightly increased risk of breast cancer; otherwise, risk did not increase with decreasing time since last use. Oral contraceptive use did not affect breast cancer risk among women in different 5-year age strata, and there was no significant effect when various subgroups of women were compared (i.e., those with vs. without a family history of breast cancer, parous vs. nulliparous women, and users vs. nonusers of hormone replacement therapy).

Conclusions.—Among women who were of reproductive age when oral contraceptives first became available, the use of birth control pills does not seem to increase the risk of breast cancer during middle age. This is true even for women who use oral contraceptives relatively later during their reproductive years (i.e., after age 40).

Commentary

The information from the massive collaborative reanalysis of data from 54 epidemiologic studies, approximately 90% of all the epidemiologic information published on the topic, as well as the data from the case-control study in Washington State are reassuring about the risk of breast cancer associated with use of oral contraceptives (OC). As observed in the large Cancer and Steroid Hormone Study done in the United States several years ago, OC use, like early first term pregnancy, may slightly increase the risk of breast cancer when a woman is young and the incidence of the disease is low. Early first term pregnancy has also been shown to have a protective effect against the development of breast cancer in women of older age when the disease is most prevalent and thus reduces the lifetime risk of developing this cancer. Data are not yet available that analyze the effect of OC use on lifetime risk of breast cancer or the risk in women older than age 60. However, the data on breast cancer risk and OC use in middle-aged women, when the disease is more common than in younger women, indicate that there is no effect of OC use on risk of this disease.

It is hoped that OCs, like first term pregnancy at an early age, will prove to reduce the lifetime risk of breast cancer. In the meantime, women should be reassured by the results of these studies that use of oral contraceptives does not affect the risk of breast cancer developing 10 years after stopping use as well as after age 50 when the disease becomes more common. It is also reassuring that, like previous studies, neither of these analyses showed that OC use affected the risk of breast cancer among women with a family history of breast cancer.

ACYCLOVIR SUPPRESSION TO PREVENT CESAREAN DELIVERY AFTER FIRST-EPISODE GENITAL HERPES

Scott LL, Sanchez PJ, Jackson GL, et al
(Univ of Texas, Dallas)
Obstet Gynecol 87:69-73, 1996

Background. It is currently recommended that pregnant women with visible genital herpes lesions or prodromal symptoms at the time of labor have their offspring delivered by cesarean section to prevent possible transmission of the herpes virus (HSV) to the neonate. Gravida patients without visible lesions or prodromal symptoms are allowed to continue in labor because they have a low incidence of neonatal HSV transmission.

Objective. The study objective was to determine whether suppressive acyclovir therapy given to gravidas at term who had their first episode of genital HSV infection during pregnancy would decrease the need for cesarean section for that indication.

Methods. In 46 pregnant women who were experiencing their first episode of genital herpes during pregnancy, the diagnosis was confirmed by positive cultures for HSV. The patients were randomly assigned in double-blind fashion to regimens of acyclovir 400 mg or placebo 3 times a day. Twenty-one patients assigned to receive acyclovir and 25 assigned to receive placebo completed the study and yielded assessable results. Study medication was initiated at 36 weeks' gestation and continued until delivery. Vaginal delivery was performed if there was no clinical recurrence of herpes and if no other contraindications were present; otherwise, a cesarean section was performed. Cultures for HSV were obtained from the neonate's conjunctiva, oropharynx, and rectum 24 to 72 hours after delivery. Neonates were also examined for evidence of acyclovir toxicity. The neonate's medical status was reviewed 1 month after delivery.

Results. None of the 21 patients treated with acyclovir had clinical evidence of recurrent genital herpes at the time of delivery, and all had vaginal deliveries. On the other hand, 9 of the 25 (36%) of those treated with placebo had clinical evidence of recurrent genital herpes at delivery and underwent cesarean section. The difference favoring the acyclovir group was highly statistically significant. No neonate had evidence of herpes infection or acyclovir toxicity either shortly after delivery or 1 month postpartum.

Conclusions. In comparison with treatment with placebo, suppressive acyclovir therapy initiated at 36 weeks' gestation and continued until delivery significantly reduced the need for cesarean section for recurrent genital herpes. None of the neonates in the study manifested evidence of herpes infection, and none of those treated with acyclovir had evidence of acyclovir toxicity.

Commentary

It is clear that nonpregnant individuals with recurrent genital herpes have decreased frequency of recurrence when they take prophylactic acyclovir. So, it is not surprising that there is suggestion of value in its prophylactic use in pregnancy. The only questions are issues of fetal safety associated with the use of 1.2 g of acyclovir every day for an average of 3.6 weeks during the third trimester. Certainly, the drug appears safe for pregnant women, and the lack of evident fetal effect in the 21 women treated here is encouraging.

It is important that the study was blinded to patients and physicians, but the need for cesarean section in women in labor without lesions but with "prodromal symptoms" of recurrent herpes is arguable. Because no patients without lesions had positive cultures at the time of delivery, some needless cesarean sections were probably done. Although it is impossible to tell how many women without lesions but with prodromal symptoms were in the placebo group, it appears they were disproportionately distributed there and may well have biased the conclusion. At any rate, more data, with patient management based on visible cultured lesions at the time of delivery, would be vital. Note that only 1 of 9 patients with visible lesions at the time of abdominal delivery proved in fact to have a positive culture. The principal value of the study is the evidence of safety to mother and fetus.

AGE AT MENOPAUSE AS A RISK FACTOR FOR CARDIOVASCULAR MORTALITY

van der Schouw YT, van der Graaf Y, Steyerberg EW, et al
(Utrecht Univ, The Netherlands; Erasmus Univ, Rotterdam, The Netherlands; Academic Hosp, Utrecht, The Netherlands)
Lancet 347:714-718, 1996

Background. Estrogen deficiency after menopause may lead to an increased risk of cardiovascular disease. However, previous studies have been inconclusive, largely because of short postmenopausal follow-up periods. The link between age at menopause and cardiovascular mortality was investigated in a study with a median follow-up of 16 years.

Methods. The research subjects came from a cohort of 12,115 postmenopausal women living in one Dutch city between 1974 and 1977. The analysis included 1199 women who went through menopause during follow-up, which lasted from 1 to 20 years. The women were followed up through regular screening visits, at which information on menopausal status, age at menopause, medication use, cardiovascular risk factors, and indicators of ovarian function was obtained. The link between age at menopause and total cardiovascular mortality was analyzed, with information on deaths obtained from the research subjects' family physicians.

Results. The women in the various strata of age at menopause (which ranged from 39 years and younger to 55 years and older) were similar in the baseline characteristics. Risk of cardiovascular mortality was significantly increased for women with early menopause (Fig. 1). Women with menopause at age 40-44 had a 5.7% annual hazard of cardiovascular death at age 70, compared with 4.3% for those with menopause at age 55 or older. Each 1-year delay in menopause carried a 2% decrease in the annual hazard of cardiovascular death. Age at menopause had a reasonably linear effect on cardiovascular mortality—the effects of a 1-year delay were approximately the same at age 50 as at age 40. Age at menopause clearly affected cardiovascular mortality at age 65; however, by age 80 this effect had disappeared.

Conclusions. Early menopause is associated with an increased risk of cardiovascular mortality. Early menopause is an independent risk factor for cardiovascular mortality, and seems to play a more important role at younger biologic ages. Age at menopause has no effect on cardiovascular mortality for women who have undergone hysterectomy and an increased effect for those who have had oophorectomy. The impact of smoking on cardiovascular mortality is strong enough to eliminate the effects of early menopause.

Commentary

There have been no prospective randomized clinical trials demonstrating that exogenous estrogen replacement therapy (ERT) given to postmenopausal women reduces the risk of cardiovascular disease. However, a meta-analysis of 31 observational studies has shown that postmenopausal women taking ERT have only half the risk of having a myocardial infarction that women not taking ERT have. In addition to providing a favorable lipid profile, there are several other mechanisms whereby exogenous estrogen prevents acceleration of coronary artery atherosclerosis. The results of this study indicate that endogenous estrogen is also protective against cardiovascular disease because women with early menopause have a significantly greater risk of cardiovascular death

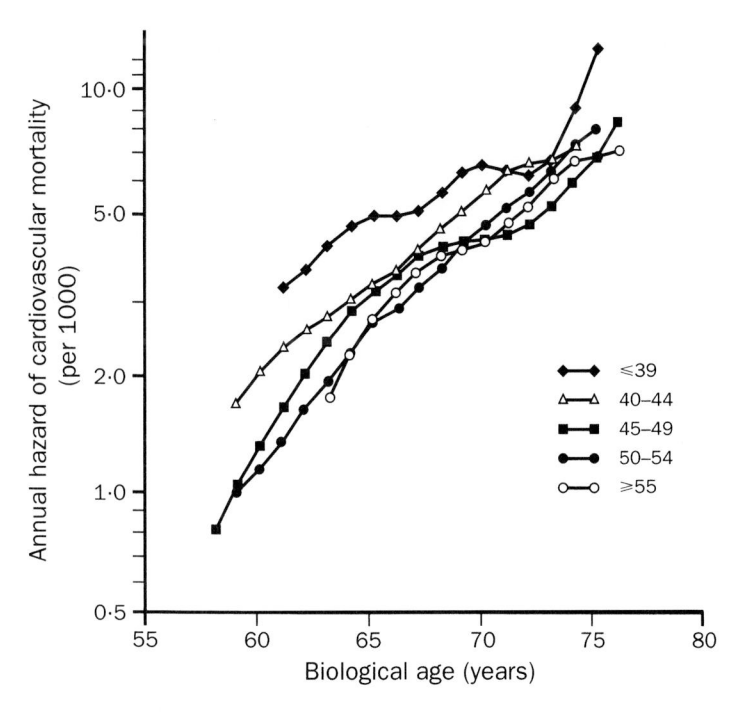

Fig. 1 Annual hazard of cardiovascular mortality (logarithmic scale) in relation to age at menopause. For proportional hazards, the lines should be parallel. (Courtesy of van der Schouw YT, van der Graaf Y, Steyerberg EW, et al: Age at menopause as a risk factor for cardiovascular mortality, *Lancet* 347:714-718, copyright by The Lancet 1996.)

between the ages of 60 and 75 years than women who become menopausal after age 50. Thus, women who became menopausal younger than age 45 should be particularly encouraged to ingest ERT.

YEAR BOOK OF PULMONARY DISEASE

HOW SHOULD CANCER PRESENTING AS A MALIGNANT PLEURAL EFFUSION BE MANAGED?

Bonnefoi H, Smith IE
(Royal Marsden NHS Trust, Surrey, England)
Br J Cancer 74:832-835, 1996

Background. Malignant pleural effusion from an unknown primary is a common finding in patients with cancer. The value of extensive investigations to identify the primary is unclear, and there is no established treatment policy. Therefore, the management of these patients, the natural history of disease, and the response to palliative chemotherapy were investigated in a retrospective study.

Methods. The records of 42 consecutive patients referred with a malignant pleural effusion and no evidence of a primary between 1985 and 1994 were reviewed. Investigations to identify a primary included CT scan of the thorax in 32 patients, fiber optic bronchoscopy in 23, abdominal CT scan or ultrasound in 37, mammography in 10, and pelvic ultrasound in 10 patients. Thirty-seven patients received chemotherapy. Symptoms were assessed after each course of treatment by the patients. Objective response was defined as the absence of reaccumulated pleural fluid on chest radiographs.

Results. The primary was identified in only 15 patients and was lung cancer in all cases. The lung cancer was detected by 11 of 32 CT thoracic scans and 3 of 23 fiberoptic bronchoscopies. No primaries were detected by abdominal CT or ultrasound scans, mammography, or pelvic ultrasound. A symptomatic response was noted by 78% of the 37 patients who received chemotherapy, including 22% with complete response. An objective response occurred in 86% of the patients. The median duration of both symptom and objective response was 6 months. The median overall survival was 12 months for the entire group (Fig. 1), 7.5 months in patients with lung cancer, and 16 months in patients with no detected primary (Fig. 2).

Conclusions. A malignant pleural effusion with no identifiable primary site is associated with a poor prognosis. Although a CT scan of the thorax appears to be the most effective investigation technique for identifying a lung primary, a more extensive investigation is likely to be unrewarding. Palliative chemotherapy provides useful short-term relief of symptoms in most patients.

Commentary

This study gives the outcome of a large number of patients who were seen with a malignant pleural effusion. An encouraging feature of this study is the overall survival rate (see

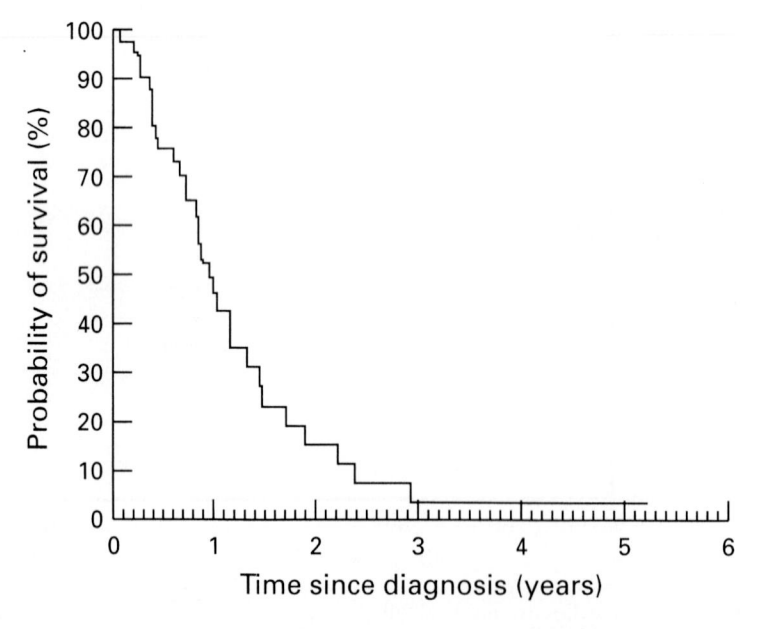

Fig. 1 Overall survival since diagnosis. All patients, *n* = 42. (Courtesy of Bonnefoi H, Smith IE: How should cancer presenting as a malignant pleural effusion be managed? *Br J Cancer* 74:832-835, 1996.)

Fig. 1), which was better than one might have expected. The overall survival rate was much worse when a primary carcinoma was found than when it was not found (see Fig. 2). It was impressive that palliation could be achieved in the majority of patients.

MUSCLE WEAKNESS IN MECHANICALLY VENTILATED PATIENTS WITH SEVERE ASTHMA

Leatherman JW, Fluegel WL, David WS, et al
(Hennepin County Med Ctr, Minneapolis)
Am J Respir Crit Care Med 153:1686-1690, 1996

Background. Diffuse muscle weakness may develop in patients undergoing mechanical ventilation for severe asthma because of acute myopathy. Authorities debate whether corticosteroid treatment or neuromuscular paralysis causes myopathy. Also, it is not clear whether the chemical structure of the drug used to induce paralysis affects the risk of myopathy. The incidence of clinically significant weakness in patients given corticosteroids alone vs. corticosteroids plus a neuromuscular blocking agent (NMBA), the effects of paralysis duration on the incidence of muscle weakness, and the relative risk of muscle weakness in patients paralyzed with atracurium vs. an aminosteroid NMBA were determined.

Methods and Findings. One hundred seven consecutive episodes of mechanical ventilation for severe asthma were assessed in this retrospective cohort study. Corticosteroid plus NMBA treatment was associated with a much greater incidence of muscle weakness when compared with corticosteroid treatment alone. The 20 patients with weakness were paralyzed significantly longer than the 49 patients given an NMBA with no subsequent weakness (Fig. 2). Paralysis lasted for more than 24 hours in 18 of these 20 patients. The use of atracurium to achieve paralysis did not reduce the incidence of weakness when compared with the use of an aminosteroid NMBA.

Conclusions. Corticosteroid-treated patients with severe asthma subjected to prolonged neuromuscular paralysis are at significant risk of muscle weakness. The use of atracurium does not decrease the risk of weakness.

Commentary

This study shows an astonishing incidence of acute myopathy in patients mechanically ventilated for status asthmaticus and who received both large doses of corticosteroids and neuromuscular blockade. Muscle weakness appears to be a myopathy and not the neuropathy of long-standing critical illness with sepsis and multiorgan system failure.[1] I continue to wonder why neuromuscular blockade is so popular in the management of acute respiratory failure, particularly in severe asthma and the acute respiratory distress syndrome, because my own experience over many years has indicated that neuromuscular blockade is not often needed to provide patient comfort. What is needed is a proper interface of the ventilator to meet the needs of the patient and the judicious use of analgesic agents, most notably morphine in sufficient dosage to reduce the pain and discomfort associated with intubation and mechanical ventilation.

It appears to me that the widespread use of neuromuscular blockade is more for the convenience of the medical staff

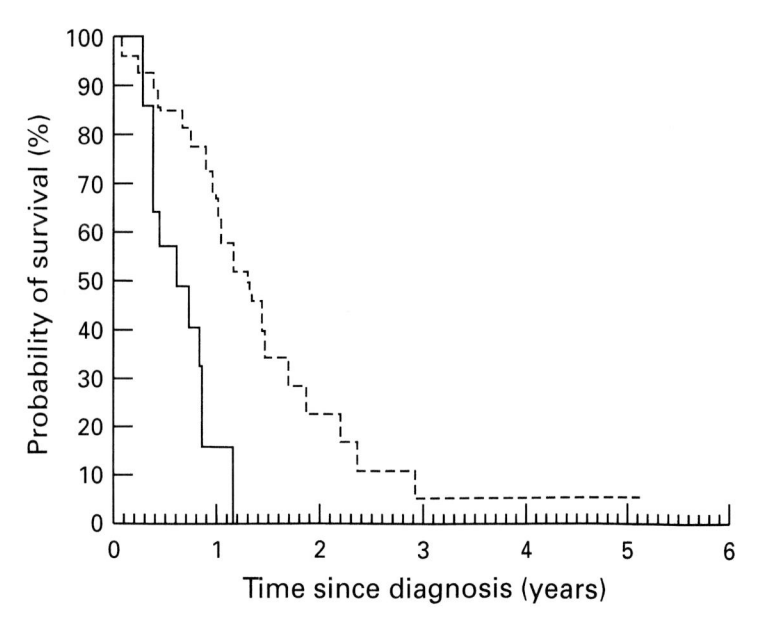

Fig. 2 Overall survival since diagnosis. *Solid line* indicates primary found, $n = 15$; *dashed line*, primary not found, $n = 27$. (Courtesy of Bonnefoi H, Smith IE: How should cancer presenting as a malignant pleural effusion be managed? *Br J Cancer* 74:832-835, 1996.)

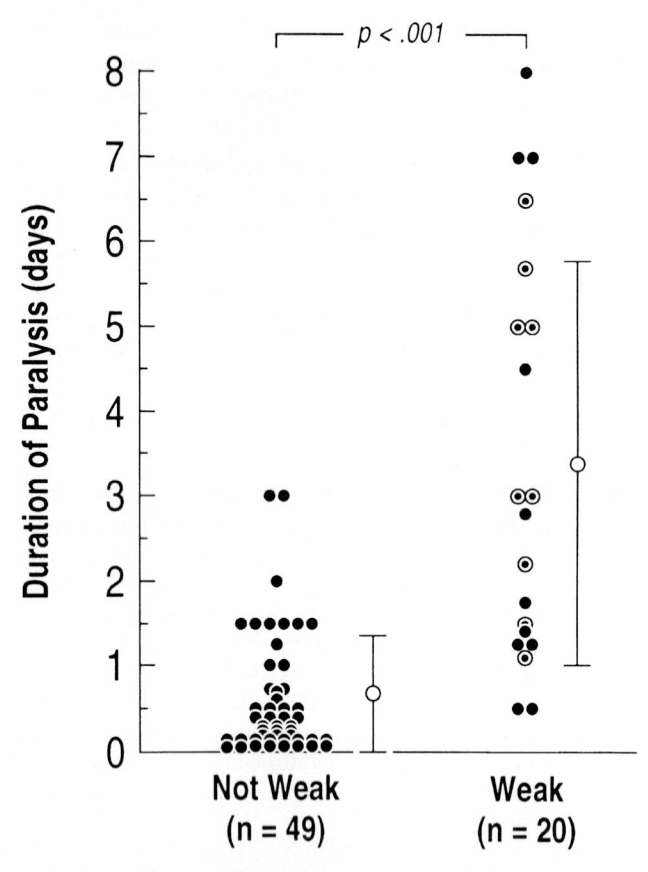

Fig. 2.—Duration of paralysis in weak and nonweak patients who had received a neuromuscular blocking agent, with length of paralysis shown for individual patients and mean ± SD for both groups. Weak patients had a significantly longer duration of paralysis than did nonweak patients ($P < 0.001$). Patients in whom severe weakness developed are *circled*. (Courtesy of Leatherman JW, Fluegel WL, David WS, et al: Muscle weakness in mechanically ventilated patients with severe asthma, *Am J Respir Crit Care Med* 153:1686-1690, 1996.)

or perhaps a cover-up for inexperience rather than a medical necessity. The morbidity associated with neuromuscular blockade is underscored by this article, which also indicates that newer, nonsteroidal NMBAs such as atracurium are as likely to be associated with myopathy as older agents. I continue to believe that the dynamic hyperinflation that occurs in asthma and chronic obstructive pulmonary disease can be overcome by skilled ventilator adjustments, with or without the strategy of permissive hypercapnia, which is a reasonable ventilator strategy.[2]

REFERENCES

1. Zochodne DW, Bolton CF, Well GA, et al: Critical illness polyneuropathy: a complication of sepsis and multiple organ failure, *Brain* 110:819-842, 1987.
2. Tuxen DV: Permissive hypercapnic ventilation, *Am J Respir Crit Care Med* 150:870-874, 1994.

SLEEP-DISORDERED BREATHING IN MEN WITH CORONARY ARTERY DISEASE

Mooe T, Rabben T, Wiklund U, et al
(Norrland Univ Hosp, Umeå, Sweden)
Chest 109:659-663, 1996

Purpose.—Previous studies have suggested that sleep apnea may increase cardiovascular morbidity and mortality. Various hemodynamic changes accompany episodes of apnea, and sympathetic nervous system activation may occur as well. There is little information on how sleep apnea affects patients with coronary artery disease (CAD), who may be adversely affected by these changes. Sleep apnea and nocturnal hypoxemia were evaluated in men with symptomatic CAD, including an examination of the link between disordered breathing and CAD.

Methods.—The case-control study included a random sample of 142 men (mean age, 58 years) who were undergoing coronary angiography for angina pectoris. All had angiographically verified CAD. Fifty age-matched controls without evidence of heart disease were studied as well. Sleep studies were performed in both groups, with desaturations and apneas assessed by pulse oximetry, oronasal thermistors, a body position indicator, and body and respiratory movement recorders. The CAD patients and controls were compared for the number of arterial oxygen desaturations of 4% or more per hour of sleep, as well as the oxygen desaturation index (ODI) and the number of episodes of apnea or hypopnea per hour of sleep, or apnea-hypopnea index (AHI).

Results.—An ODI of 5 or greater was present in 39% of the men with CAD, compared with 22% of the controls. The mean ODI value was 6.4 in patients vs. 2.7 in controls. An AHI of 10 or greater was recorded in 37% of patients and 20% of controls. Disordered breathing was significantly more severe in obese individuals. Factors significantly predicting CAD on multiple logistic regression analysis were ODI, AHI, body mass index, and hypertension. Patients in the highest quartiles of ODI and AHI were about 4 times more likely to have symptomatic CAD than were those in the lowest quartile.

Conclusions.—Sleep-disordered breathing is common among men with CAD. Sleep apnea is significantly associated with nocturnal hypoxemia and CAD, even after adjustment for other factors. The adverse effects of sleep-disordered breathing in patients with CAD—in terms of ischemia, arrhythmias, and prognosis—remain to be determined.

Commentary

The adverse effects of sleep-disordered breathing in patients with CAD have been previously reported.[1-3] Occult sleep-disordered breathing is commonly found in patients with stable congestive heart failure.[4] The cardiopulmonary consequences of obstructive sleep apnea include both breathing dysrhythmias and increased ventricular ectopic activity and the risk of sudden death.[5] Thus, this study adds to a body of previously published observations that suggest that both obstructive sleep apnea and significant hypoxemia are common in CAD. This can set up a vicious cycle when obstructive sleep apnea is associated with hypertension and arrhythmia production. Thus, a high index of suspicion should be directed toward any patient with CAD with a history of snoring, morning headaches, unexplained erythrocytosis, daytime somnolence, and impotence, which are all hallmarks of sleep apnea. A variety of treatments are available to correct the phenomenon of sleep apnea. Continuous positive airway pressure at either one or two levels is popular with or without supplemental oxygen. Even new oral prosthetic devices hold promise.

In spite of the associations described in this report, it should be kept in mind that sleep apnea, hypoxia, and oxygen desaturation are also fairly common in normal individuals, mostly men.[6]

REFERENCES

1. He J, Kryger MH, Zorick FJ, et al: Mortality and apnea index in obstructive sleep apnea: experience in 385 male patients, Chest 94:9-14, 1988.
2. Partimen M, Jamieson A, Guillenminault C: Long-term outcome for obstructive sleep apnea syndrome patients: mortality, Chest 94:1200-1204, 1988.
3. Hung J, Whitford EG, Parsons RW, et al: Association of sleep apnea with myocardial infarction in men, Lancet 336:261-264, 1990.
4. Shahrokh J, Parker TJ, Wexler L, et al: Occult sleep-disordered breathing in stable congestive heart failure, Ann Intern Med 122:487-492, 1995.
5. Shepard JW: Cardiopulmonary consequences of obstructive sleep apnea, Mayo Clin Proc 65:1250-1259, 1990.
6. Block AJ, Boysen PG, Wynne JW, et al: Sleep apnea, hypopnea and oxygen desaturation in normal subjects: a strong male predominance, N Engl J Med 300:513-517, 1979.

LONG-TERM OXYGEN THERAPY AT HOME: COMPLIANCE WITH MEDICAL PRESCRIPTION AND EFFECTIVE USE OF THERAPY

Pépin J-L, Barjhoux CE, Deschaux C, et al
(CHU de Grenoble, France)
Chest 109:1144-1150, 1996

Objective.—Although long-term oxygen therapy (LTOT) improves survival and quality of life for patients with respiratory failure and chronic obstructive pulmonary disease (COPD), it is expensive and requires substantial patient cooperation. Because compliance is so important, patient characteristics and medical orders affecting compliance were prospectively evaluated.

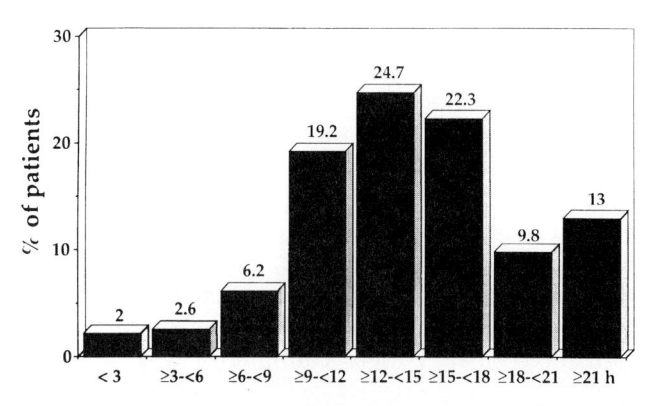

Data of effective duration of daily oxygen therapy achieved by the patients

Fig. 1 Data of effective duration of daily oxygen therapy achieved by the patients. The mean duration is 14.5 ± 5 hours. Only 45% of patients had long-term oxygen therapy for more than 15 hours. (Courtesy of Pépin J-L, Barjhoux CE, Deschaux C, et al: Long-term oxygen therapy at home: compliance with medical prescription and effective use of therapy, Chest 109:1144-1150, 1996).

Methods.—Prescribing physicians received questionnaires about their criteria, and 930 patients with COPD (167 female) aged 40-80 years received visits from respiratory technicians to determine oxygen use during inside and outside activities during a 3-month period. Patients using LTOT less than 15 hr/day were termed "ineffective users." Arterial blood gases and airflow obstruction were determined.

Results.—Patients used oxygen for 36 months on average for hypoxemia, hypercapnia, and severe airflow obstruction (Fig. 1). Physicians prescribed oxygen therapy based on blood gas measurements in 72% of patients and based on severe disability in 23% of patients. Oxygen therapy was prescribed for 16 hours on average and for more than 12 hours for 98% of patients. Only 36% of patients were instructed to use oxygen during toileting, 24% at meals, and 37% for leisure activities. Mean oxygen use was 91% of prescribed oxygen use. More than half of patients changed the duration of their oxygen use: 297 who reduced the time because they believed the therapy was ineffective had a significantly higher mean partial pressure of oxygen in arterial blood (Pa_{O_2}) (56.9 mm Hg) than the others; 175 who increased their intake time had a significantly lower Pa_{O_2} (53.3 mm Hg); 210 could not tolerate treatment either because of headache or noise. Effective users were significantly more hypoxic (Pa_{O_2} = 54.5 vs. 56.9 mm Hg), more hypercapnic (Pa_{CO_2} = 47.9 vs. 46.4 mm Hg), and more obstructed (forced expiratory volume in 1 second/vital capacity = 39.5% vs. 44.8%) than ineffective users. Effective users had more severe disease and more severe obstruction than ineffective users. Effectiveness of therapy also depended on a prescribed use of at least 15 hr/day, follow-up education, smoking cessation, oxygen use during all domestic activities, length of treatment, and tolerance for therapy.

Conclusions. More explicit directions plus follow-up education and reinforcement are important in ensuring patient compliance with LTOT at home.

Commentary

This study documents that LTOT is not used more than 15 hours per day in the majority of patients. The problems with poor adherence to the prescribed duration of oxygen therapy are attributed to poor patient instruction and equally negligent patient compliance. This is disappointing because of the well-established fact that oxygen improves survival in COPD. The longer daily use, i.e., more than 17 hours per day, provided the best survival in comparisons between two controlled clinical trials, i.e., the British Medical Research Council and Nocturnal Oxygen Therapy Trial.[1,2] The present study does document that the more severely impaired patients tended to use oxygen more faithfully, probably because they noticed greater clinical benefit from more continuous oxygen usage with truly portable devices. The use of transtracheal oxygen in selected patients may also lead to better acceptance of oxygen as an effective therapeutic agent that should be used continuously in patients with past serious manifestations of chronic stable hypoxemia including poor exercise tolerance, cor pulmonale, erythrocytosis, and morning headaches, or with any obvious degree of intellectual deterioration, which may respond to continuous long-term oxygen therapy.

REFERENCES

1. Report of the Medical Research Council Working Party: Long term domiciliary oxygen therapy in chronic cor pulmonale complicating chronic bronchitis and emphysema, *Lancet* 1:681-685, 1981.
2. Nocturnal Oxygen Therapy Trial Group: Continuous or nocturnal oxygen therapy in hypoxemic chronic obstructive lung disease, *Ann Intern Med* 93:391-398, 1980.

THE LONG-TERM CLINICAL COURSE OF ACUTE DEEP VENOUS THROMBOSIS

Prandoni P, Lensing AWA, Cogo A, et al
(Univ Hosp of Padua, Italy; Academic Med Ctr, Amsterdam)
Ann Intern Med 125:1-7, 1996

Background. The long-term risk for recurrent venous thromboembolism and the incidence and severity of postthrombotic sequelae in patients with symptomatic deep venous thrombosis (DVT) have not been thoroughly studied. The clinical course of a first episode of symptomatic DVT in a large series of patients with long-term follow-up was described.

Methods and Findings. Three hundred fifty-five consecutive patients were followed up prospectively for 8 years. At 2, 5, and 8 years, the cumulative incidence of recurrent venous thromboembolism was 17.5%, 24.6%, and 30.3%, respectively. Cancer and impaired coagulation inhibition increased the risk for recurrent venous thromboembolism, the corresponding hazard ratios being 1.72 and 1.44. Surgery and recent trauma or fracture were correlated with a reduced risk. The cumulative incidence of postthrombotic syndrome was 22.8% at 2 years, 28% at 5 years, and 29.1% at 8 years. The risk for the postthrombotic syndrome was also strongly corre-

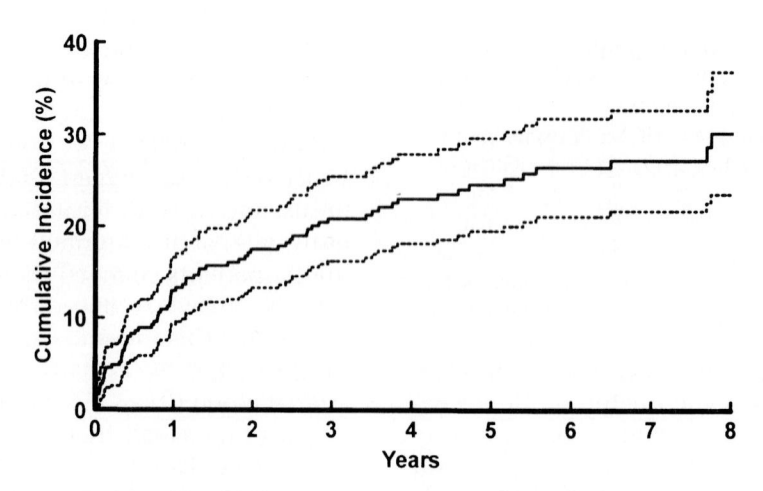

Fig. 1 The cumulative incidence of recurrent venous thromboembolism in patients with a first episode of symptomatic deep venous thrombosis. The *dashed lines* represent the 95% confidence intervals. (Courtesy of Prandoni P, Lensing AWA, Cogo A, et al: The long-term clinical course of acute deep venous thrombosis, *Ann Intern Med* 125:1-7, 1996.)

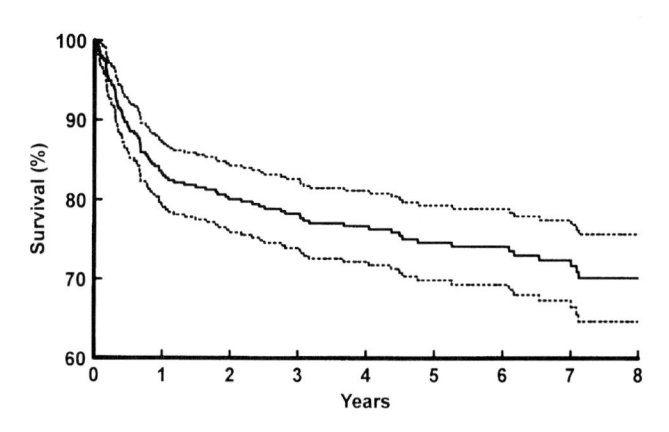

Fig. 3 Survival in patients with a first episode of symptomatic deep venous thrombosis. The *dashed lines* represent the 95% confidence intervals. (Courtesy of Prandoni P, Lensing AWA, Cogo A, et al: The long-term clinical course of acute deep venous thrombosis, Ann Intern Med 125:1-7, 1996.)

lated with the development of ipsilateral recurrent DVT. Eight-year survival was 70.2%. Cancer raised the risk of death, with a hazard ratio of 8.1 (Figs. 1 and 3).

Conclusions. The risk for recurrent venous thromboembolism in patients with symptomatic DVT is high and persists for many years. This is especially true for patients with no transient risk factors for DVT. Almost one third of patients have postthrombotic syndrome, which is strongly associated with ipsilateral recurrent DVT. The use of short-course anticoagulation treatment in patients with symptomatic DVT should be reconsidered.

Commentary

This study demonstrates considerable postthromboembolic morbidity and mortality. It is unique in its size and duration of follow-up. Because venous thrombosis and pulmonary embolism are the same disease, this study appropriately questions the modern popularity of short-term anticoagulation after an episode of thromboembolism, even if risk factors are transient.[1] This study differs from the conclusions of an earlier evaluation of long-term follow-up, which suggested that death occurred in only a small minority of patients but with the caveat "when properly diagnosed and treated."[2] This study suggests long-term, controlled clinical trials of low-dose anticoagulation to evaluate long-term morbidity and mortality.

REFERENCES
1. Moser KL, Fedullo PF, LitteJohn JK, et al: Frequent asymptomatic pulmonary embolism in patients with deep venous thrombosis, JAMA 271:223-225, 1994.
2. Carson JL, Kelley MA, Duff A, et al: The clinical course of pulmonary embolism, N Engl J Med 326:1240-1245, 1992.

EFFECTS OF LONG-TERM TREATMENT WITH CORTICOSTEROIDS IN COPD
Renkema TEJ, Schouten JP, Koëter GH, et al
(Univ of Groningen, The Netherlands)
Chest 109:1156-1162, 1996

Background. The effectiveness of corticosteroid therapy in patients with nonallergic chronic obstructive pulmonary disease (COPD) remains controversial. This randomized, blinded, controlled clinical trial assessed the effectiveness of corticosteroid therapy in patients with COPD.

Study Group. Male patients with COPD were recruited from a pulmonary medicine outpatient clinic. Patients were excluded if they were older than 70 years of age, were receiving continuous corticosteroid therapy, or had another condition that would confound interpretation of the results of the study. All patients were smokers or ex-smokers.

Study Design. After a 3-month period without any corticosteroids, baseline measurements were performed and then patients were allocated blindly by computer randomization to a 2-year regimen of inhaled budesonide, inhaled budesonide plus oral prednisolone, or placebo. Patients were assessed every 2 months by physical examination, spirometry, and a history that included a standardized questionnaire. Patients were maintained on their standard medications.

Results. Of the initial 58 participants in this study, 11 dropped out. There were significantly more withdrawals because of pulmonary problems in the placebo group than in the treatment groups. The median decline in forced expiratory volume in 1 second (FEV_1) was 60 ml/yr in the placebo group, 40 ml/yr in the budesonide plus prednisolone group, and 30 ml/yr in the budesonide group. Treatment with corticosteroids significantly reduced pulmonary symptoms. Morning plasma cortisol levels remained within the normal range in all groups.

Conclusions. This controlled, clinical trial demonstrated some benefit of long-term daily treatment with inhaled corticosteroids in nonallergic patients with COPD. Lung function decline was less in the group receiving corticosteroid treatment than in the placebo group. These results suggest that further studies on the effectiveness of corticosteroid treatment should be carried out with larger groups of patients with COPD.

Commentary

Some time ago, the senior author of this study offered the suggestion that corticosteroids could retard the rate of decline of ventilatory function in advanced COPD and, possibly, in less severe degrees of the disease.[1,2] That corticosteroids are occasionally effective in patients believed to have COPD and not bronchial asthma has been previously reported,[3,4] but only a minority of patients with clinically diagnosed COPD are truly steroid responsive[5] as judged by objective improvements in airflow FEV_1.

This study is important because it is a randomized, controlled clinical trial, unlike the previous reports on steroid efficacy. In this study, both ex-smokers and continuing smokers had a reduced decline in FEV_1 with budesonide, compared with placebo. The addition of 5 mg of prednisolone to budesonide not only produced no additional benefit but, in fact, appeared to be less effective than budesonide alone for reasons that are not explained. In any case, this report should be taken as *preliminary* evidence that inhaled corticosteroids can be valuable in retarding the rate of decline in FEV_1 in moderate COPD, as judged by the selection criteria for this investigation. A much broader study is needed to confirm these preliminary results, and two such studies are currently under way in Europe (EUROSCOP)[6] and in the United States (Lung Health II).

REFERENCES

1. Postma DS, Steenhuis EJ, van der Weele LTH, et al: Severe chronic airflow obstruction: can corticosteroids slow down progression? *Eur J Respir Dis* 67:56-64, 1985.
2. Postma DS, Peters I, Steenhuis EJ, et al: Moderately severe chronic airflow obstruction: can corticosteroids slow down progression? *Eur Respir J* 1:22-26, 1988.
3. Mendella LA, Manfreda J, Warren CPW, et al: Steroid response in stable chronic obstructive pulmonary disease, *Ann Intern Med* 96:17-21, 1982.
4. Petty TL, Brink GA, Miller MW, et al: Objective functional improvement in chronic airway obstruction, *Chest* 57:216-223, 1970.
5. Sahn SA: Corticosteroids in chronic bronchitis and pulmonary emphysema, *Chest* 73:389-396, 1978.
6. Pauwels RA, Lofdahl CG, Pride NB, et al: European Respiratory Society Study on Chronic Obstructive Pulmonary Disease (EUROSCOP): hypothesis and design, *Eur Respir J* 5:1254-1261, 1992.

SECTION VII

Medications: Comparison Tables

BIBLIOGRAPHY

Drug facts and comparisons, St Louis, 1996, Facts and Comparisons.
Ellsworth AJ et al: *Mosby's medical drug reference,* St Louis, 1997, Mosby.
McEvoy GK, American Hospital Formulary Service: *Drug information,* Bethesda, Md, 1995, American Society of Hospital Pharmacists.
Physicians GenRx, St Louis, 1997, Mosby.
United States Pharmacopeial Convention: USP dispensing information, Vol I, *Drug information for the health care professional,* ed 16, Easton, Pa, 1996, Mack Publishing.

ACE INHIBITORS

TABLE 7-1 ACE Inhibitors

AGENT	PREPARATIONS	INITIAL DOSAGE (PO)	ONSET OF ACTION (MIN)	TIME OF PEAK EFFECT ON BP LEVELS (HR)	EFFECTIVE HALF-LIFE (HR)	COST*
Benazepril (Lotensin)	tab: 5, 10, 20, 40 mg	HTN: 10 mg qd	60	1-2	10-11	$$
Captopril (Capoten)	tab: 12.5, 25, 50, 100 mg	HTN: 25 mg bid CHF; 12.5 mg tid	15-30	1-2	2	$$$$ $$ (generic)
Enalapril (Vasotec)	tab: 2.5, 5, 10, 20 mg; inj: 125 mg/ml	HTN: 5 qd CHF; 2.5 mg bid	60-120	4-8	11	$$$
Fosinopril (Monopril)	tab: 10, 20 mg	HTN: 10 mg	60	2-4	12	$
Lisinopril (Prinivil, Zestril)	tab: 5, 10, 20, 40 mg	HTN: 10 mg qd CHF; 5 mg qd	60	2-7	12	$$
Moexipril (Univasc)	tab: 7.5, 15 mg	HTN: 7.5 mg qd	60-120	1-2	2-9	$
Quinapril (Accupril)	tab: 5, 10, 20, 40 mg	HTN: 10 mg qd CHF; 5 mg bid	60	1-2	3	$
Ramipril (Altace)	cap: 1.25, 2.5, 5, 10	HTN: 2.5 mg qd	60-120	2-4	13-17	$
Trandolapril (Mavik)	tab: 1, 2, 4 mg	HTN: 1-2 mg qd	60-120	4-10	6-10	$

HTN, Hypertension; *CHF*, congestive heart failure.
*Cost of low-dose therapy per month; *$*, <$30; *$$*, $31-40; *$$$*, $41-50; *$$$$*, >$50.

ACID SECRETION INHIBITORS

TABLE 7-2 Acid Secretion Inhibitors

AGENT	PREPARATIONS	DOSAGE	COST
H2 Blockers			
Cimetidine (Tagamet)	tab: 200, 300, 400, 800 mg liq: 300 mg/5 ml inj: 300 mg/2 ml tab: Tagamet HB 200 mg (OTC)	Active peptic ulcer disease: 800 mg qhs Maintenance: 400 mg qhs IV: 300 mg q6-8h or total dose administered as continuous infusion over 24 hr	$ (Generic)
Famotidine (Pepcid)	tab: 20, 40 mg oral susp: 40 mg/5 ml inj: 10 mg/ml tab: Pepcid AC 10 mg (OTC)	Active peptic ulcer disease: 40 mg qhs Maintenance: 20 mg qhs IV: 20 mg q12h or total dose administered as continuous infusion over 24 hr	$$
Nizatidine (Axid)	Pulvules: 150, 300 mg tab: Axid XR 75 mg (OTC)	Active peptic ulcer: 300 mg qhs Maintenance: 150 mg qhs	$$
Ranitidine (Zantac)	tab: 150, 300 mg susp: 15 mg/ml inj: 25 mg/ml effervescent tab: 150 mg granules: 150 mg tab: Zantac 75 mg (OTC)	Active peptic ulcer: 300 mg qhs Maintenance: 150 mg qhs IV: 50 mg q6-8h or total dose administered as continuous infusion over 24 hr	$$
Proton Pump Inhibitors			
Lansoprazole (Prevacid)	cap: 15, 30 mg	Duodenal ulcer: 15 mg qd Erosive esophagitis: 30 mg qd Zollinger-Ellison: 60 mg qd	$$$
Omeprazole (Prilosec)	cap: 10, 20 mg	Duodenal ulcer: 20 mg qd Gastric ulcer: 40 mg qd GERD: 20 mg qd Zollinger-Ellison: 60 mg qd *H. pylori* eradication: 40 mg qd (with clarithromycin) for 2 wk, then 20 mg qd for 2 wk	$$$

From Ferri F: *Practical guide to the care of the medical patient*, ed 4, St Louis, 1998, Mosby.
$, Least expensive; $$$, most expensive.

ADRENERGIC ANTAGONISTS

TABLE 7-3 Adrenergic Antagonists*

AGENT	PREPARATIONS	INITIAL DOSAGE	COMMENTS	COST†
Clonidine (Catapres)	tab: 0.1, 0.2, 0.3 mg transdermal therapeutic system (TTS): 1 (2.5 mg), 2 (5 mg), 3 (7.5 mg)	PO: 0.1 mg bid patch: TTS-1, apply one every 7 days	Centrally acting α-blocker	$ $$$$ (patch)
Doxazosin (Cardura)	tab: 1, 2, 4, 8 mg	1 mg qd	Selective α-1-adrenergic blocker	$$$
Guanabenz (Wytensin)	tab: 4, 8 mg	4 mg bid	Centrally acting α-blocker	$$
Guanadrel (Hylorel)	tab: 10, 25 mg	5-10 mg bid	Peripherally acting α-blocker	$$$$
Guanethidine (Ismelin)	tab: 10, 25 mg	10-25 mg qd	Peripherally acting α-blocker	$
Guanfacine (Tenex)	tab: 1, 2 mg	1 mg qd at hs	Centrally acting α-blocker	$$
Labetalol (Normodyne, Trandate)	tab: 100, 200, 300 mg inj: 5 mg/ml	PO: 100 mg bid IV: 200 mg by slow injection over 2 min	Combined α- and β-adrenergic blocker	$$ $$$$
Methyldopa (Aldomet)	tab: 125, 250, 500 mg inj: 250 mg/5 ml	PO: 250 mg bid-tid IM/IV: 125-250 mg q6h	Centrally acting α-blocker	$
Prazosin (Minipress)	cap: 1, 2, 5 mg	1 mg hs (first dose), then 1 mg bid-tid	α-1-adrenergic blocker	$
Reserpine (Serpasil)	tab: 0.1, 0.25 mg	0.5 mg daily for 1-2 wk, then reduce dosage to 0.1 0.25 mg qd	Peripherally acting α-blocker	$
Terazosin (Hytrin)	cap: 1, 2, 5, 10 mg	1 mg hs (first dose), then increase to 2 mg qd after 3 days	α-1-adrenergic blocker	$$$

*Refer to Table 7-15 for description of β-adrenergic antagonists.
†Cost to pharmacist for 1 mo of low-dose therapy: $, <$20; $$, $21-$31; $$$, $32-$41; $$$$, >$41.

ANTIARRHYTHMIC AGENTS

TABLE 7-4 Antiarrhythmic Agents, Electrophysiologic Effects

DRUG	PR	QRS	QT	SINUS RATE	CLASS	DRUG	PR	QRS	QT	SINUS RATE	CLASS
Amiodarone	↑	↑	↑	↓	III	Procainamide	N/↑	↑	↑	N	Ia
Bretylium	N	N	N	N	III	Propafenone	↑	↑	N/↑	N	Ic
Digitalis	N/↑	N	N/↓	N/↓	—	Propranolol	N/↑	N	N/↓	↓	II
Disopyramide	N/↑	↑	↑	N/↑	Ia	Quinidine	N/↑	↑	↑	N/↓	Ia
Flecainide	↑	↑	N/↑	N	Ic	Sotalol	↑	N	↑	↓	III
Lidocaine	N	N	N	N	Ib	Tocainide	N	N	N/↓	N	Ib
Mexiletine	N	N	N	—	Ib	Verapamil	↑	N	N	↓	IV
Moricizine	↑	↑	N	N/↑	I						

From Ferri F: *Practical guide to the care of the medical patient*, ed 4, St Louis, 1998, Mosby.
↑, Increase; ↓, decrease; N, no change.

ANTIBIOTIC DOSAGE

TABLE 7-5 Dosage of Antimicrobial Agents

DRUG	NORMAL UNIT DOSE (ROUTE)	NORMAL DOSE INTERVAL (HR)	ADJUSTED MAXIMUM DOSE IN RENAL FAILURE GFR >50 ML/MIN	GFR 10-50 ML/MIN	GFR <10 ML/MIN	REMOVAL BY DIALYSIS
Aminoglycosides						
Gentamicin tobramycin[a]	1.0-1.7 mg/kg (IM/IV)	8	1.0-1.7 mg/kg q(8 × creatinine)h or (1.0-1.7 mg/kg ÷ creatinine) q8h[b]			Yes (H, P)[c]
Netilmicin[a]	1.3-2.2 mg/kg (IM, IV)	8	1.3-2.2 mg/kg q(8 × creatinine)h or (1.3-2.2 mg/kg ÷ creatinine) q8h[b]			Yes (H, P)[d]
Kanamycin, amikacin[a]	5 mg/kg (IM, IV)	8	5 mg/kg q(8 × creatinine)h or (5 mg/kg ÷ creatinine) q 8h[b]			Yes (H, P)[e]
Azithromycin	250-500 mg (PO)	24	Unknown	Unknown	Unknown	Unknown
Carbapenems, carbacephems						
Imipenem	0.5-1 (IV)	6	0.5 q6h[f]	0.5 q8-12h	0.25-0.5 q12h[g]	Yes (H)
Loracarbef	0.2-0.4g (PO)	12	NC	0.2g q12-24h	0.2g q72-120h	Yes (H)
Cephalosporins						
Cefaclor	0.25-0.5 g (PO)	8	NC	NC	NC	Yes (H)
Cefadroxil	0.5-1.0 g (PO)	12	NC	0.5 g q12-24h	0.5 g q36h	Yes (H)
Cefamandole	1-2 g (IM, IV)	4	1-2 g q6h	1-2 g q6-8h	0.5-1.0 g q8-12h	Yes (H), no (P)
Cefazolin	0.5-1.5 g (IM, IV)	8	0.5-1.0 g q8h	0.5-1.0 g q12h	0.5-1.0 g q24-48h	Yes (H), no (P)
Cefixime	400 mg (PO)	24	NC[i]	300 mg q24h[j]	200 mg q24h[k]	No (H, P)
Cefmetazole	2 g (IV)	6-12	1-2 g q12h	1-2 g q16-24h	1-2 g q48h	Yes (H)
Cefonicid	1-2 g (IM, IV)	24	NC	1 g q24-48h	0.25-1.0 g q72-120h	No (H)
Cefoperazone	1-3 g (IM, IV)	8	NC	NC	NC	Yes (H)
Ceforanide	0.5-1.0 g (IM, IV)	12	NC	1 g q24-48h	1 g q48-72h	Yes (H)
Cefotaxime	1-2 g (IM, IV)	6	NC	1-2 g q6-12h	1-2 g q12-24h	Yes (H), no (P)
Cefotetan	2 g (IV, IM)	12	NC	1-2 g q12-24h	1-2 g q48h	Yes (H)
Cefoxitin	1-2 g (IM, IV)	4	1-2 g q6h	1-2 g q8-24h	0.5-1.0 g q12-48h	Yes (H), no (P)
Cefpodoxime	0.1-0.4g (PO)	12	NC	n	n	Yes (H)
Cefprozil	250-500 mg (PO)	12-24	NC	125-250 mg q12-24h[h]	125-250 mg q12-24h	Yes (H)
Ceftazidime	0.5-2.0 g (IM, IV)	8	0.5-2.0 g q8h	0.5-2.0 g q12-24h	0.5-2.0 g q36-48h	Yes (H, P)
Ceftizoxime	1-2 g (IM, IV)	6	1-2 g q8h	1 g q12h	0.5 g q12-24h	Yes (H), no (P)
Ceftriaxone	1-2 g (IM, IV)	12-24	NC	NC	NC	No (H)
Cefuroxime	0.75-1.5 g (IM, IV)	6	NC	0.75-1.5 g q8-12h	0.75 g q24h	Yes (H, P)
Cephalexin	0.25-0.5 g (PO)	6	NC	NC	NC	Yes (H, P)
Cephalothin	1-2 g (IV)	4	1-2 g q6h	1-2 g q6h	1 g q8-12h	Yes (H, P)
Cephapirin	1-2 g (IV)	4	1-2 g q6h	1-2 g q6h	1 g q8-12h	Yes (H, P)
Cephradine	1-2 g (IV)	4	1-2 g q6h	1 g q6h	1 g q12h	Yes (H, P)
	0.25-0.5 g (PO)	6	NC	NC	NC	
Chloramphenicol	0.25-1.0 g (PO, IV)	6	NC	NC	NC	Yes (H), no (P)
Clarithromycin	250-500 mg (PO)	12	Unknown	Unknown	Unknown	Unknown
Clindamycin	0.6 g (IM, IV)	6-8	NC	NC	NC	No (H, P)
	0.15-0.3 g (PO)	6	NC	NC	NC	
Erythromycin	0.5-1.0 g (IV)	6	NC	NC	NC	No (H, P)
	0.25-0.5 g (PO)	6	NC	NC	NC	
Metronidazole	15 mg/kg load (IV), then 7.5 mg/kg (IV)	6	NC	NC	NC	Yes (H), no (P)
Monobactams						
Aztreonam	1-2 g (IV)	8	NC	1 g q8h	0.5 g q6-12h	Yes (H, P)
Nitrofurantoin	50-100 mg (PO)	6	NC	Avoid[o]	Avoid[o]	Yes (H)

TABLE 7-5 Dosage of Antimicrobial Agents—cont'd

DRUG	NORMAL UNIT DOSE (ROUTE)	NORMAL DOSE INTERVAL (HR)	ADJUSTED MAXIMUM DOSE IN RENAL FAILURE GFR >50 ML/MIN	GFR 10-50 ML/MIN	GFR <10 ML/MIN	REMOVAL BY DIALYSIS
Penicillins						
Amoxicillin	0.25-0.5 g (PO)	8	NC	0.25-0.5 g q12h	0.25 g q12h	Yes (H), No (P)
Ampicillin	0.5-2.0 g (IM, IV)	4	NC	0.5-2.0 g q8h	0.5-2.0 g q12h	Yes (H), no (P)
	0.25-0.5 g (PO)	6	NC	0.25-0.5 g q8h	0.25-0.5 g q12h	
Azlocillin	2-3 g (IM, IV)	4	NC	3 g q6h	3 g q12h	Yes (H), no (P)
Carbenicillin	2-5 g (IM, IV)	4	NC	2-5 g q6h	2 g q8-12h	Yes (H, P)
Indanyl-carbenicillin	0.5-1.0 g (PO)	6	NC	NC	Avoid	
Cloxacillin	0.5-1.0 g (PO)	6	NC	NC	NC	No (H, P)
Dicloxacillin	0.25-0.5 g (PO)	6	NC	NC	NC	No (H, P)
Methicillin	1-2 g (IM, IV)	4	NC	NC	1-2 g q8-12h	No (H, P)
Mezlocillin	2-3 g (IM, IV)	4	NC	3 g q6-8h	2 g q6-8h	Yes (H), No (P)
Nafcillin	1-2 g (IM, IV)	4	NC	NC	NC	No (H, P)
Oxacillin	1-2 g (IM, IV)	4	NC	NC	NC	No (H, P)
	0.5-1.0 g (PO)	6	NC	NC	NC	
Penicillin G	0.4-4.0 million units (IM, IV)	4	NC	NC	2 million U q4h	Yes (H), No (P)
Penicillin V	0.25-0.5 g (PO)	6	NC	NC	NC	Yes (H), No (P)
Piperacillin	2-3 g (IM, IV)	4	NC	3 g q6h	3 g q8h	Yes (H)
Ticarcillin	2-3 g (IM, IV)	4	NC	2-3 g q6h	2 g q12h	Yes (H, P)
Polymyxins						
Polymyxin B	1.5-2.5 mg/kg/day (IV)	Continuous infusion	Avoid	Avoid	Avoid	No (H), Yes (P)
Colistin	0.8-1.7 mg/kg IM	8	Avoid	Avoid	Avoid	No (H), Yes (P)
Quinolones						
Nalidixic acid	0.5-1.0 g (PO)	6	NC	NC	Avoid	Unknown
Ciprofloxacin	250-750 mg (PO)	12	NC	250-500 mg q12h[l]	250-500 mg q18h[m]	
	200-400 mg (IV)	12	NC	200-400 mg q18-24h[m]	200-400 mg q18-24h[m]	No (<14%) (H, P)
Lomefloxacin	400 mg (PO)	24	NC	200 q24h	Unknown	No (<14%) (H, P)
Norfloxacin	400 mg (PO)	12	NC	400 q24h	400 q24h	No (<14%) (H, P)
Ofloxacin	200-400 mg (PO, IV)	12	NC	200-400 mg q24h	100-200 mg q24h	No (<14%) (H, P)
Sulfisoxazole	1 g (PO)	6	NC	1 g q8-12h	1 g q12-24h	Yes (H, P)
Tetracyclines						
Tetracycline	0.25-0.5 g (PO, IV)	6	0.25-0.5 g q8-12h	Avoid	Avoid	No (H, P)
Doxycycline	100 mg (PO, IV)	12-24	NC	NC	NC	No (H, P)
Trimethoprim-sulfamethoxazole	2-3 mg TMP/kg (IV)	6	NC	2-3 mg TMP/kg q12h	Avoid	Yes (H), No (P)
	160/800 mg (PO)	12	NC	160/800 mg q24h	Avoid	
Trimethoprim	100 mg (PO)	12	NC	100 mg q24h	Avoid	Yes (H), No (P)
Vancomycin[a]	1 g (IV)	12	1 g q24-72h[a]	1 g q72-240h[a]	1 g q240h[a]	No (H, P)

From Stein JH et al: *Internal medicine*, ed 5, St Louis, 1998, Mosby.
[a]Serum level monitoring is recommended for therapy of the patient with renal impairment.
[b]When using the latter formula, a normal unit dose is necessary initially. Both formulas are valid estimates only if serum creatinine reflects GFR accurately.
[c]After an initial loading dose, therapeutic levels can be maintained by administering a dose of 1 mg/kg after each hemodialysis or by adding 5 μg/ml to the peritoneal dialysis fluid.
[d]After an initial loading dose, therapeutic levels can be maintained by administering a dose of 1.5 mg/kg after each hemodialysis or by adding 7.5 μg/ml to the peritoneal dialysis fluid.
[e]After an initial loading dose, therapeutic levels can be maintained by administering a dose of 3.5 mg/kg after each hemodialysis or by adding 20 μg/ml to the peritoneal dialysis fluid.
[f]Dose adjustment generally required for Ccr < 70 ml/min/1.73 m^2.
[g]This range applies to Ccr 6-20 ml/min/1.73 m^2, the upper range may be associated with increased risk of seizures. The drug should not be used when Ccr <5 ml/min/1.73 m^2 unless the patient is receiving hemodialysis.
[h]50% standard dose recommended for GFR ≤ 30 ml/min.
[i]If Ccr ≥ 60 ml/min.
[j]If Ccr 21-60 ml/min.
[k]If Ccr < 20 ml/min.
[l]If Ccr 30-50 ml/min.
[m]If Ccr 5-29 ml/min.
[n] Administer dose q24h for Ccr < 30 ml/min; for patients receiving hemodialysis, give three times weekly after dialysis.
[o] Avoid if Ccr < 60 ml/min.
GFR, Glomerular filtration rate; *H*, hemodialysis; *P*, peritoneal dialysis; *NC*, no change; *TMP*, trimethoprim.

ANTICONVULSANTS

TABLE 7-6 Anticonvulsants

AGENT	PREPARATIONS	DOSAGE (PO)	PRINCIPAL USE	HALF-LIFE	THERAPEUTIC LEVEL (µG/ML)	TOXIC LEVEL (µG/ML)
Carbamazepine (Tegretol)	tab: 200 mg; chew tab: 100 mg; susp: 100 mg/5 ml	Initial: 200 mg bid; Maintenance: 800-1200 mg/day	Partial complex and seizures grand mal	20 hr ± 5 hr	2-10	>12
Clonazepam (Klonopin)	tab: 0.5, 1, 2, mg	Initial: 0.5 mg tid; Maintenance: 1.5-2.0 mg/day	Absence, myoclonic, atonic seizures	30 hr ± 10 hr	15-60	>100
Ethosuximide (Zarontin)	cap: 250 mg; syrup: 250 mg/5 ml	Initial: 500 mg/day; Maintenance: 1-1.5 g/day	Absence seizures	48 hr ± 12 hr	40-100	>150
Fosphenytoin (Cerebyx)	inj: 50 mg phenytoin equivalent (PE) units/ml (fosphenytoin sodium 75 mg/ml, equivalent to phenytoin sodium 50 mg/ml for IV infusion or IM inj)	Loading: 10-20 mg PE/kg IV (max 150 mg PE/min) or IM; Maintenance: 1-6 mg PE/kg/day	Control of status epilepticus seizures during surgery	8 min IV, 33 min IM	NA	NA
Gabapentin (Neurontin)	cap: 100, 300	Initial: 300 mg hs on day 1, 300 mg bid on day 2, 300 mg tid on day 3, then adjust as needed; Maintenance: 900-1800 mg/day divided into three doses	Adjunct in partial seizures with or without secondary generalization	4 hr-12 hr	2-3	>3
Lamotrigine (Lamictal)	tab: 25, 100, 150, 200 mg	Initial: 50 mg qd when used with enzyme-inducing drugs (AEDS) but not in combination with valproate; 25 mg qod when used with AEDS plus valproate	Refractory partial seizures in adults	24 hr	2-4	>4
Phenobarbital	tab: 8, 16, 32, 65, 100 mg; cap: 16 mg; elixir: 15 mg/5 ml	50-100 mg bid-tid	Tonic-clonic and partial seizures	96 hr ± 12 hr	15-35	>60
Phenytoin (Dilantin)	Kapseals: 30, 100 mg; susp: 125 mg/5 ml; chew tab: 50 mg; pediatr susp: 30 mg/5 ml	Loading dose: 1 g divided in 3 doses (400, 300, 300) administered at 2 hr intervals; Maintenance: 100 mg tid	Generalized tonic-clonic (grand mal), simple partial, and complex partial seizures	24 hr ± 12 hr	10-20	>30
Primidone (Mysoline)	tab: 50, 250 mg; susp: 250 mg/5 ml	Initial: 100-125 mg at hs, increase to bid on day 4, tid on day 7, then 250 mg tid on day 10; Maintenance: 250 mg tid	Partial complex and tonic-clonic seizures	10 hr ± 5 hr	5-10	>12
Valproic acid	cap: 250 mg, 500; syrup: 250 mg/5 ml	Initial: 15 mg/kg/day; Maintenance: 10-60 mg/kg	Tonic clonic and absence seizures	8 hr ± 2 hr	50-100	>200

ANTIDEPRESSANTS

TABLE 7-7 Antidepressants

AGENT	PREPARATIONS	INITIAL DOSAGE	CLASS	SEDATING EFFECT	ANTI-CHOLINERGIC EFFECT	ORTHOSTATIC EFFECT	EFFECT ON CARDIAC FUNCTION	AVERAGE ELIMINATION HALF-LIFE (HR)
Amitriptyline (Elavil)	tab: 10, 25, 50, 75, 100, 150 mg inj: 10 mg/ml	10-75 mg qhs	Tricyclic	++++	++++	++++	++++	24
Amoxapine (Asendin)	tab: 25, 50, 100, 150 mg	25-50 mg bid-tid	Heterocyclic	++	+	+++	++	10
Bupropion (Wellbutrin)	tab: 75, 100 mg	100 mg bid	Aminoketone	+	+	+	+	14
Desipramine (Norpramin)	tab: 10, 25, 50, 75, 100, 150 mg	10-50 mg qd	Tricyclic	+	+	++	+	18
Doxepin (Adapin, Sinequan)	cap: 10, 25, 50, 75, 100, 150 mg	10-25 mg tid	Tricyclic	++++	+++	+++	+++	17
Fluoxetine (Prozac)	Cap: 10, 20 mg Oral sol: 20 mg/5 ml	20 mg qd	Serotonin reuptake inhibitor (SSRI)	0	+	0	0	96
Imipramine (Tofranil)	tab: 10, 25, 50 mg cap: Tofranil-PM 75, 100, 125, 150 mg inj: 25 mg/2 ml	75 mg qd	Tricyclic	+++	+++	+++	++++	22
Maprotiline (Ludiomil)	tab: 25, 50, 75 mg	50-75 mg qd	Heterocyclic	++	++	+++	++	43
Mirtazapine (Remeron)	tab: 15, 30 mg	15 mg qhs	Tetracyclic	++++	++	+	+++	NA
Nefazodone (Serzone)	tab: 100, 150, 200, 250 mg	100 mg bid	Phenylpiperazine	++	+	+	+	3
Nortriptyline (Pamelor)	cap: 10, 25, 50, 75 mg liq: 10 mg/5 ml	10 mg qd	Tricyclic	+++	++	+	++	26
Paroxetine (Paxil)	tab: 10, 20, 30, 40 mg	10-20 mg qd	SSRI	0	+	0	0	24
Protriptyline (Vivactil)	tab: 5, 10 mg	5 mg tid	Tricyclic	+	+++	++	++	76
Sertraline (Zoloft)	tab: 50, 100 mg	50 mg qd	SSRI	+	0	0	0	24
Trazodone (Desyrel)	tab: 50, 100, 150, 300 mg	50 mg tid	Heterocyclic	+++	+	++	+	8
Venlafaxine (Effexor)	tab: 25, 37.5, 50, 75, 100 mg	25 mg tid or 37.5 mg bid	Phenylethylamine	++	++	0	0	5

0, None; +, weak; ++, mild; +++, moderate; ++++, strong.

ANTIDIABETIC AGENTS

TABLE 7-8 Antidiabetic Agents, Oral

DRUG	PREPARATIONS (MG)	STARTING DOSE (MG/DAY)	MAXIMUM DAILY DOSE	DURATION OF ACTION (HR)	HALF-LIFE ($T_{1/2}$)	EXCRETION	COST*	THERAPEUTIC CLASS
Acarbose (Precose)	tab: 50, 100	25	300 mg	6-12	2	Urine, feces	$$$$	Alpha-glucosidase inhibitor†
Chlorpropamide (Diabinese)	tab: 100, 250	100	750 mg	≥36	35	Urine	$ (generic)	Sulfonylurea‡ (first generation)
Glimepiride (Amaryl)	tab: 1, 2, 4	1	8 mg	24	9	Urine, feces	$$$$	Sulfonylurea‡ (second generation)
Glipizide (Glucotrol)	tab: 5, 10	5	40 mg	12-24	3-7	Urine (88%)	$$$	Sulfonylurea‡ (second generation)
Glyburide (Diabeta, Micronase)	tab: 1.25, 2.5, 5	2.5	20 mg	Up to 24	4-10	Urine feces	$$	Sulfonylurea‡ (second generation)
Glyburide, micronized (Glynase Prestab)	tab: 1.5, 3, 6	1.5-3	12 mg	Up to 24	4-10	Urine, feces	$$$$	Sulfonylurea‡ (second generation)
Metformin (Glucophage)	tab: 500, 850	500	2250 mg	12-24	6	Urine (90%)	$$$$	Biguanide§
Tolazamide (Tolinase)	tab: 100, 250, 500	100	1000 mg	12-14	7	Urine	$ (generic)	Sulfonylurea‡ (first generation)
Tolbutamide (Orinase)	tab: 250, 500	500	3000 mg	12-14	6	Urine	$ (generic)	Sulfonylurea‡ (first generation)
Troglitazone (Rezulin)	tab: 200, 400	200	600 mg	6-12	16-34	Feces (85%)	$$$$	Thiazolidinedione‖ (Glitazone)

*Cost to pharmacist for 1 mo of therapy (low dose): $, <$20; $$, $20-$30; $$$, $31-$40, $$$$, >41.
†α-Glucosidase inhibitor: major mechanism of action is delay of GI absorption of glucose.
‡Sulfonylurea: major mechanism of action is stimulation of pancreatic insulin production and increased tissue sensitivity to insulin.
§Biguanide: major mechanism of action is decreased hepatic glucose production and increased glucose uptake.
‖Thiazolidinedione: major mechanism of action is decreased insulin resistance.

ANTIEMETICS

TABLE 7-9 Antiemetics

AGENT	PREPARATIONS	USUAL ADULT DOSAGE	CLASS
Chlorpromazine (Thorazine)	tab: 10, 25, 50, 100, 200 mg spansule: 30, 75, 150, 200, 300 mg syrup: 10 mg/5 ml supp: 25, 100 mg inj: 25 mg/ml	PO: 10 mg q4h IM: 25 mg q4h until vomiting stops PR: 25 mg q6h	Phenothiazine
Granisetron (Kytril)	inj: 1 mg/ml tab: 1 mg	IV: 10 µg/kg over 5 min, starting within 30 min of beginning chemotherapy PO: 1 mg up to 1 hr before chemotherapy, then 1 mg 12 hr after	Selective 5-HT3 receptor antagonist
Hydroxyzine (Vistaril)	cap: 25, 50, 100 mg syrup: 25 mg/5 ml	PO: 25-50 mg q6-8h IM: 50 mg q6-8h	Antihistamine
Meclizine (Antivert, Bonine)	tab: 12.5, 25, 32, 50 mg tab, chew: 25 mg cap: 30 mg	PO: 12.5-25 mg q4-6hr	Antihistamine, anticholinergic
Metoclopramide (Reglan)	tab: 5, 10 mg syrup: 5 mg/5 ml inj: 5 mg/5 ml	PO: 10 mg q8h IM/IV: 10 mg q6-8h	Benzamide antidopaminergic
Ondansetron (Zofran)	inj: 40 mg/vial tab: 4, 8 mg syrup: 5 mg/5 ml	IV: 0.15 mg/kg, infused over 15 min, given 3 times 4 hr apart beginning 30 min before cancer chemotherapy PO: 8 mg q4h for 3 doses beginning 30 min before chemotherapy, then 8 mg q8h for 24-48 hr after chemotherapy is completed	Selective 5-HT3 receptor antagonist
Prochlorperazine (Compazine)	tab: 5, 10, 25 mg spansule: 10, 15, 30 mg syrup: 5 mg/5 ml supp: 2.5, 5, 25 mg inj: 10 mg/2 ml	PO: 5-10 mg q6-8h PR: 25 mg bid IM: 5-10 mg q3-4h (do not exceed 40 mg/day) IV: 2.5-10 mg by slow IV injection (5 mg/min; do not exceed 40 mg/day)	Phenothiazine
Promethazine (Phenergan)	tab: 12.5, 25, 50 mg supp: 12.5, 25, 50 mg syrup: 6.25 mg/5 ml	PO: 25 mg 30-60 min before travel Maintenance: 25 mg bid	Phenothiazine
Thiethylperazine (Torecan)	tabs: 10 mg supp: 10 mg inj: 10 mg/2 ml	PO/PR: 10 mg q8h IM: 10 mg q8h	Phenothiazine
Trimethobenzamide (Tigan)	cap: 100, 250 mg supp: 200 mg inj: 100 mg/ml	PO: 250 mg q6-8h PR: 200 mg q6-8h IM: 200 mg q6-8h	Trimethobenzamide

From Ferri F: *Practical guide to the care of the medical patient,* ed 4, St Louis, 1998, Mosby.

ANTIHISTAMINES

TABLE 7-10 Antihistamines for Allergic Rhinitis

AGENT	PREPARATIONS	DOSAGE	SEDATION	ANTICHOLINERGIC EFFECT	CLASS	COST
Brompheniramine (Dimetane)	tab: 4 mg elixir: 2 mg/5 ml Extentab: 8, 12 mg	4 mg q4-6h Extentab: 8-12 mg q12h	+	++	Alkylamine	$ (Generic)
Chlorpheniramine (Chlor-Trimeton)	tab: 4 mg syrup: 2.5 mg/5 ml 12 mg	4 mg q4-6h Repetab: 8-12 mg q12h	+	++	Alkylamine	$ (Generic)
Dexchlorpheniramine (Polaramine)	tab: 2 mg syrup: 2 mg/5 ml Repetab: 4, 6 mg	2 mg q4-6h Repetab: 4-6 mg q8h	+	++	Alkylamine	$ (Generic)
Clemastine (Tavist-1)	tab: 1, 2 mg syrup: 0.5 mg/5 ml	1-2 mg bid	++	+++	Ethanolamine	$$$
Diphenhydramine (Benadryl)	tab: 25 mg cap: 50 mg elixir: 12.5 mg/5 ml	25-50 mg q6-8h	+++	+++	Ethanolamine	$ (Generic)
Astemizole (Hismanal)	tab: 10 mg	10 mg qd	0	0	Benzimidazole	$$$$
Cetirizine (Zyrtec)	tab: 5, 10 mg syrup: 1 mg/ml	5-10 mg qd	0	0	Metabolite of hydroxyzine	$$$$
Fexofenadine (Allegra)	cap: 60 mg	60 mg bid	0	0	Metabolite of terfenadine	$$$$
Loratadine (Claritin)	tab: 10 mg syrup: 1 mg/ml	10 mg qd	0	0	Selective H_1-receptor antagonist	$$$$

From Ferri F: *Practical guide to the care of the medical patient,* ed 4, St Louis, 1998, Mosby.
+, Low; ++, moderate; +++, high; $, least expensive; $$$$, most expensive.

ANTIPSYCHOTICS

TABLE 7-11 Antipsychotics

AGENT	PREPARATIONS	DOSAGE	CLASS/FREQUENT ADVERSE EFFECTS
Chlorpromazine (Thorazine)	tab: 10, 25, 50, 100, 200 mg cap: 30, 75, 150, 200, 300 mg syrup: 10 mg/5 ml inj: 25 mg/ml supp: 25, 100 mg	Initial: 10-25 mg PO tid Acute agitation: 25 mg IM; repeat in 1 hr if necessary	Phenothiazine, aliphatic Drowsiness, anticholinergic effects, postural hypotension
Clozapine (Clozaril)	tab: 25, 100 mg	Initial: 25 mg qd-bid	Tricyclic dibenzodiazepine Agranulocytosis
Fluphenazine (Prolixin)	tab: 1, 2.5, 5, 10 mg conc: 5 mg/ml inj: 2.5 mg/ml	Initial: 0.5-1 mg tid IM: 1.25 mg	Phenothiazine, piperazine Extrapyramidal effects, akathisia, dystonia
Haloperidol (Haldol)	tab: 0.5, 1, 2, 5, 10, 20 mg conc: 2 mg/ml inj: 5 mg/ml	Initial: 0.5 mg bid-tid Acute agitation: 2-5 mg IM	Butyrophenone Extrapyramidal effects, dystonia, akathisia
Lithium	cap: 150, 300, 600 mg tab: 150, 300 mg	300 mg tid	Thirst, fine tremor, GI irritation, mild diarrhea, leukocytosis, polyuria
Mesoridazine (Serentil)	tab: 10, 25, 50, 100 mg conc: 25 mg/ml inj: 25 mg/ml	PO: psychosis, 50 mg tid initially; psychoneurosis, 10 mg tid initially IM: 25 mg, may repeat in 30-60 min	Piperidine phenothiazine Tardive dyskinesia, anticholinergic and extrapyramidal effects
Olanzapine (Zyprexa)	tab: 5, 7.5, 10 mg	Initial: 5-10 mg PO	Thienobenzodiazepine Somnolence, dizziness, constipation, hypotension
Perphenazine (Trilafon)	tab: 2, 4, 8, 16 mg conc: 16 mg/5 ml inj: 5 mg/ml	Initial 4-8 mg tid	Phenothiazine, piperazine Extrapyramidal effects, akathisia, dystonia
Risperidone (Risperdal)	tab: 2, 3, 4 mg	Initial: 1 mg bid on day 1, then 2 mg bid on day 2, then 3 mg bid; usual range is 4-6 mg/day, max 16 mg/day	Benzisoxazole derivative Anxiety, somnolence, extrapyramidal and anticholinergic effects, orthostatic hypotension
Thioridazine (Mellaril)	tab: 10, 15, 25, 50, 100, 150, 200 mg conc: 30, 100 mg/ml susp: 25 mg/5 ml	10-100 mg tid	Phenothiazine, piperidine Drowsiness, anticholinergic effects, postural hypotension
Thiothixene (Navane)	cap: 1, 2, 5, 10, 20 mg conc: 5 mg/ml inj: 2, 5 mg/ml	Initial: 2 mg tid Acute agitation: 4 mg IM	Thioxanthene Extrapyramidal effects, akathisia, dystonia, anticholinergic effects
Trifluoperazine (Stelazine)	tab: 1, 2, 5, 10 mg conc: 10 mg/ml	Initial: 2-5 mg bid Acute agitation: 1-2 mg IM	Phenothiazine, piperazine Extrapyramidal effects, akathisia, dystonia

From Ferri F: *Practical guide to the care of the medical patient*, ed 4, St Louis, 1998, Mosby.

ANTIRETROVIRAL AGENTS

TABLE 7-12 Antiretroviral Agents for HIV Infection

MEDICATION	THERAPEUTIC CLASS	PREPARATIONS	INITIAL DOSE	MAJOR TOXICITIES	COST TO THE PHARMACIST PER MO OF THERAPY
Didanosine (ddI, Videx)	Nucleoside analog	chew tab: 25, 50, 100, 150 mg	Weight ≥ 60 kg, tab: 200 mg bid; powder: 250 mg bid Weight < 60 kg, tab: 125 mg bid; powder: 167 mg bid	Peripheral neuropathy, pancreatitis, liver failure, retinal depigmentation and vision change in children, diarrhea	$150-$200
Lamivudine (3TC, Epivir)	Nucleoside analog	tab: 150 mg	Weight ≥ 50 kg: 150 mg bid with AZT Weight < 50 kg: 2 mg/kg bid with AZT	Headache, nausea, insomnia, fatigue, neuropathy, myalgias	$200-$250
Stavudine (d4T, Zerit)	Nucleoside analog	cap: 15, 20, 30, 40 mg	Weight ≥ 60 kg: 40 mg bid Weight < 60 kg: 30 mg bid	Peripheral neuropathy, aminotransferase elevation	$200-$250
Zalcitabine (ddC, Hivid)	Nucleoside analog	tab: 0.375, 0.75 mg	0.75 mg tid	Esophageal ulcers, peripheral neuropathy, pancreatitis, exacerbation of hepatic dysfunction	$200-$250
Zidovudine (AZT, Retrovir)	Nucleoside analog	cap, gel: 100 mg syr: 50 mg/5 ml IV infusion: 10 mg/ml	100 mg q4h or 200 mg tid; give IV infusion over 1 hr, 1 mg/kg q4h for symptomatic infection	Bone marrow suppression, myopathy, myositis, cholestatic hepatitis	$250-$300 (for oral therapy)
Indinavir (Crixivan)	Protease inhibitor	cap: 200, 400 mg	800 mg tid	Bilirubin elevation (10% of patients), kidney stones (3% of patients)	$400-$500
Nelfinavir (Viracept)	Protease inhibitor	tab: 250 mg oral powder: 50 mg/kg	750 mg tid	Diarrhea, nausea, abdominal pain, flatulence, rash	>$400
Ritonavir (Norvir)	Protease inhibitor	cap: 100 mg	600 mg bid	Nausea, vomiting, diarrhea, paresthesias, elevation of lipids and transaminases, altered taste	$650-$700
Saquinavir (Invirase)	Protease inhibitor	cap: 200 mg	600 mg bid	Diarrhea, nausea, abdominal pain	$550-$600

TABLE 7-12 Antiretroviral Agents for HIV Infection—cont'd

MEDICATION	THERAPEUTIC CLASS	PREPARATIONS	INITIAL DOSE	MAJOR TOXICITIES	COST TO THE PHARMACIST PER MO OF THERAPY
Delarvidine (Rescriptor)	Non-nucleoside reverse transcriptase inhibitor	tab: 100 mg	400 mg tid	Rash, GI upset	>$400
Nevirapine (Viramune)	Non-nucleoside reverse transcriptase inhibitor	tab: 200 mg	200 mg qd	Rash, fever, nausea, headaches	$150-$250

ANTISEPTIC SOLUTIONS

TABLE 7-13 Antiseptic Solutions

AGENTS	ANTIMICROBIAL ACTIVITY	MECHANICS OF ACTION	TISSUE TOXICITY	INDICATIONS AND CONTRAINDICATIONS
Povidone-iodine solution (iodine complexes) (Betadine)	Available as a 10% solution with polyvinylpyrolidine (povidone) containing 1% free iodine with broad rapid-onset antimicrobial activity	Potent germicide in low concentrations	Will decrease PMN migration and life span at concentration >1% May cause systemic toxicity at higher concentrations; questionable toxicity at 1% concentration	Probably a safe and effective wound cleanser at a 1% concentration 10% solution is effective to prepare the skin about the wound
Povidone-iodine surgical scrub	Same as the solution	Same	Toxic to open wounds	Best as a hand cleaner; never use in open wounds
Nonionic detergents Pluronic F-68 Shur Clens	Ethyleneoxide is 80% of its molecular weight It has no antimicrobial activity	Wound cleanser	No toxicity to open wounds, eyes, or intravenous solutions	It appears to be an effective, safe wound cleanser
Hydrogen peroxide	3% solution in water has brief germicidal activity	Oxidizing agent that denatures protein	Toxic to open wound	Should not be used on wounds after the initial cleaning, may be used to clean intact skin
Hexachlorophene (pHiso Hex) (polychlorinated bis-phenol)	Bacteriostatic (2% to 5%) Greater activity against gram-positive organisms	Interruption of bacterial electron transport and disruption of membrane-bound enzymes	Little skin toxicity; the scrub form is damaging to open wound	Never use scrub solution in open wounds Very good preoperative hand preparation
Alcohols	Low-potency antimicrobial most effective as a 70% ethyl and 70% isopropyl alcohol solution	Denatures protein	Will kill irreversibly and function as a fixative	No role in routine care
Phenols	Bacteriostatic >0.2% Bactericidal >1% Fungicidal 1.3%	Denatures protein	Extensive tissue necrosis and systemic toxicity	Never use >2% aqueous phenol or >4% phenol plus glycerol

From Rosen P et al: *Emergency medicine*, ed 3, St Louis, 1997, Mosby.

BENZODIAZEPINES

TABLE 7-14 Benzodiazepines

AGENT	PREPARATIONS	EQUIVALENT DOSE	DOSAGE	HALF-LIFE (HR)	MAIN INDICATION	COST
Alprazolam (Xanax)	tab: 0.25, 0.5, 1, 2 mg	0.5	0.25-0.5 mg tid	14	Anxiety	$$$$ $$ (generic)
Chlordiazepoxide (Librium)	cap: 5, 10, 25 mg amp: 100 mg/5 ml	10	5-25 mg qid	48-96	Anxiety	$ (generic)
Clonazepam (Klonopin)	tab: 0.5, 1, 2 mg	0.5	0.5-1 mg tid	18-50	Anxiety	$$$$ $$ (generic)
Clorazepate (Tranxene)	tab: 3.75, 7.5, 15 mg; long-acting (Tranxene SD): 11.25, 22.5 mg	7.5	tab: 3.75-15 mg tid Tranxene SD: 11.25-22.5 mg qd	48-96	Anxiety	$ (generic)
Diazepam (Valium)	tab: 2, 5, 10 mg amp: 5 mg/ml	5	2-10 mg bid-qid	48-96	Anxiety	$ (generic)
Estazolam (ProSom)	tab: 1, 2 mg	1	0.5-2 mg qhs	10-24	Insomnia	$$$$
Flurazepam (Dalmane)	cap: 15, 30 mg	15	15-30 mg hs	48-72	Insomnia	$$ (generic)
Lorazepam (Ativan)	tab: 0.5, 1, 2, mg inj: 2, 4 mg/ml	1	1 mg bid-tid	10-20	Anxiety	$ (generic)
Oxazepam (Serax)	tab: 15 mg cap: 10, 15, 30 mg	15	10-15 mg tid-qid	8-12	Anxiety	$$ (generic)
Prazepam (Centrax)	tab: 10 mg cap: 5, 10, 20 mg	10	10 mg bid-tid	30-60	Anxiety	$$$$
Quazepam (Doral)	tab: 7.5, 15 mg	7.5	7.5-1.5 mg hs	15-35	Insomnia	$$$$
Temazepam (Restoril)	cap: 7.5, 15, 30 mg	15	7.5-15 mg hs	10-20	Insomnia	$$ (generic)
Triazolam (Halcion)	tab: 0.125, 0.25 mg	0.25	0.125-0.25 mg hs	2-5	Insomnia	$$$$

From Ferri F: *Practical guide to the care of the medical patient,* ed 4, St Louis, 1998, Mosby.
$, Least expensive; $$$$, most expensive.

β-ADRENERGIC BLOCKING AGENTS

TABLE 7-15 β-Adrenergic Blocking Agents

DRUG	ORAL PREPARATIONS	INITIAL DOSAGE	MAINTENANCE DOSAGE	CARDIO-SELECTIVITY	ISA	LIPID SOLUBILITY	ELIMINATION HALF-LIFE (HR)	PRIMARY EXCRETION ROUTE	COST*
Acebutolol (Sectral)	cap: 200, 400 mg qd	400 mg qd	200-800 mg	Yes	Yes	+	6-12	Renal	$$$
Atenolol (Tenormin)	tab: 50, 100 mg	50 mg qd	50-100 mg qd	Yes	No	+	6-9	Renal	$$
Betaxolol (Kerlone)	tab: 10, 20 mg	10 mg qd	20 mg qd	Yes	No	++	16	Hepatic	$
Bisoprolol (Zebeta)	tab: 5, 10 mg	2.5 mg qd	5 mg qd	Yes	No	+	9-12	Renal	$$$
Carteolol (Cartrol)	tab: 2.5, 5 mg	2.5 mg qd	2.5-5 mg qd	No	Yes	+	6-12	Renal	$$$$$
Carvedilol (Coreg)	tab: 3.125, 6.25, 12.5, 25 mg	3.125 mg bid	12.5 mg bid	No	No	+	6-8	Feces	$$$$$
Labetalol (Normodyne, Trandate)	tab: 100, 200, 300 mg	100 mg bid	200-400 mg bid	No	No	++	3-4	Hepatic	$$
Metoprolol (Lopressor, Toprol XL)	tab: 50, 100, 200 mg	100 mg qd	50-200 mg/day	Yes	No	++	3-4	Hepatic	$$
Nadolol (Corgard)	tab: 20, 40, 80 mg	40 mg qd	40-80 mg qd	No	No	+	14-24	Renal	$$$$
Penbutolol (Levatol)	tab: 20 mg	20 mg qd	20 mg qd	No	Yes	++	5	Renal	$$$$$
Pindolol (Visken)	tab: 5, 10 mg	5 mg bid	5-10 mg bid	No	Yes	++	3-4	hepatic/renal	$$$$$
Propranolol (Inderal)	tab: 10, 20, 60, 80, 90 mg	10-20 mg bid	40-320 mg bid	No	No	+++	3-4	Hepatic	$
Sotalol (Betapace)	tab: 80, 160, 240 mg	80 mg bid	160-320 mg/day	—	No	+	12	Renal	$$$$$
Timolol (Blocadren)	tab: 5, 10	10 mg	10-20 mg bid	No	No	+	4-5	Hepatic	$$

From Ferri F: *Practical guide to the care of the medical patient,* ed 4, St Louis, 1998, Mosby.
+, Low; ++, medium; +++, high; *ISA,* intrinsic sympathomimetic activity.
*Cost to pharmacist per month of low-dose therapy: $, <$20; $$, $2-$30; $$$, $31-$40; $$$$, $41-$50; $$$$$, >$50.

CALCIUM CHANNEL BLOCKERS

TABLE 7-16 Calcium Channel Blockers

AGENT	ORAL PREPARATIONS	INITIAL DOSAGE	MYOCARDIAL CONTRACTILITY	CHEMICAL CLASS	AV NODAL CONDUCTION	CARDIAC OUTPUT	PERIPHERAL VASODILATION	SAFE FOR CONCOMITANT USE WITH β-BLOCKER	COST*	HALF-LIFE (HR)
Amlodipine (Norvasc)	tab: 2.5, 5, 10 mg	HTN: 5 mg qd Angina: 5-10 mg qd	↑	Dihydropyridine	N	↑	++	++	$$$$	30-50
Diltiazem (Cardizem, Dilacor, Tiazac)	tab: 30, 60, 90, 120 mg cap, SR: 120, 180, 240, 300, 360	Angina: 30 mg qid HTN: 120-300 mg/day	→	Benzothiazepine	→	N/↑	+	+	$$ (Generic) $$$$	3.5-7
Felodipine (Plendil)	tab: 5, 10 mg	HTN: 2.5, 5 mg qd	↑	Dihydropyridine	N	↑	++	++	$$$	11-16
Isradipine (DynaCirc)	cap: 2.5, 5 mg SR cap: 5, 10 mg	HTN: 2.5 mg bid	N	Dihydropyridine	N	↑	++	++	$$$	8-9
Nicardipine (Cardene)	cap: 20, 30 mg cap, SR: 30, 45 mg (bid)	Angina: 20 mg tid HTN: 40-120 mg/day	N	Dihydropyridine	N/↑	↑	++	++	$$$	2-4
Nifedipine (Procardia, Adalat)	cap: 10, 20 mg tab, XR: 30, 60, 90	Angina: 10 mg tid HTN: 30-90 mg/day	→	Dihydropyridine	N	↑	++	++	$$ (Generic)	1.9-5
Nisoldipine (Sular)	tab: 10, 20, 30, 40 mg	HTN: 20 mg qd	N	Dihydropyridine	N	N	+++	++	$$	7-12
Verapamil (Calan, Isoptin, Verelan, Covera-HS)	tab: 40, 80, 120 mg caplet, SR: 120 mg cap: 120, 180, 240, 360 mg	Angina: 40 mg tid HTN: 120-360 mg/day	↓↓	Diphenylalkylamine	↓↓	↓↑	+	0	$ (Generic) $$$	3-7

From Ferri F: *Practical guide to the care of the medical patient*, ed 4, St Louis, 1998, Mosby.
SR, XR, Extended release preparation; ↑, increase; ↓, decrease; *N*, no significant effect; *0*, least; *+++*, most; *HTN*, hypertension.
*Cost to pharmacist per month of low-dose therapy: $, <$30; $$, $31-$40; $$$, $41-$50; $$$$, >$50.

CEPHALOSPORINS

TABLE 7-17 Cephalosporins

AGENT	PREPARATIONS	USUAL DOSAGE RANGE (NORMAL RENAL FUNCTION)*	GENERATION	HALF-LIFE (HR)
Cefadroxil (Ultracef, Duricef)	cap: 500 mg tab: 1 g oral susp: 125, 250, 500 mg/5 ml	PO: 1 g qd-bid	First	1.3
Cefazolin (Ancef, Kefzol)	inj: 250, 500 mg, 1 g	IV: 500 mg-1.5 g q6-8h	First	2.0
Cefepime (Maxipime)	inj: 500 mg, 1 g, 2 g	IV: 500 mg-2 g q12h	Fourth	2.0
Ceftibuten (Cedax)	cap: 400 mg susp: 90, 180 mg/5 ml	PO: 400 mg q24h	Third	2.0
Cephalexin (Keflex)	Pulvules: 250, 500 mg susp: 125, 250 mg/5 ml tab: 250 mg, 500 mg, 1 g	PO: 250 mg-1 g q6h	First	1.0
Cephalothin (Keflin)	inj: 1, 2 g	IV: 500 mg-2 g q4-6h	First	0.6
Cephapirin (Cefadyl)	inj: 500 mg, 1 g, 2 g	IV: 500 mg-2 g q4-6h	First	0.5
Cephradine (Velosef, Anspor)	cap: 250, 500 mg susp: 125, 250 mg/5 ml inj: 250, 500 mg, 1 g	PO: 250-500 mg q6h KV: 500 mg-2 g q4-6h	First	1.0
Cefaclor (Ceclor)	Pulvules: 250, 500 mg susp: 125, 250 mg/5 ml	PO: 250-500 mg q8h	Second	1.0
Cefamandole (Mandol)	inj: 500 mg, 1 g, 2 g	IV: 500 mg-1 g q4-6h	Second	0.8
Cefmetazole (Zefazone)	inj: 1, 2 g	IV: 2 g q6-12h	Second	1.5
Cefonicid (Monocid)	inj: 500 mg, 1 g	IV: 1-2 g q24h	Second	4.0
Ceforanide (Precef)	inj: 500 mg, 1 g	IV: 0.5-1 g q12h	Second	2.9
Cefotetan (Cefotan)	inj: 1, 2 g	IV: 1-3 g q12h	Second	4.0
Cefoxitin (Mefoxin)	inj: 1, 2 g	IV: 1-2 g q6-8h	Second	0.8
Cefpodoxime (Vantin)	tab: 100, 200 mg susp: 50 mg, 100 mg/5 ml	PO: 100-200 mg q12h	Second	2-3
Cefprozil (Cefzil)	tab: 250, 500 mg	PO: 250-500 mg q12h	Second	1.3
Cefuroxime (Zinacef, Ceftin)	inj: 750 mg tab: 125, 250, 500 mg	IV: 750 mg-1.5 g q8h PO: 250-500 mg bid	Second	1.5
Loracarbef (Lorabid)	cap: 200 mg	PO: 200-400 mg q12h	Second	1.0
Cefixime (Suprax)	tab: 100, 400 mg susp: 100 mg/5 ml	400 mg qd	Third	3-4
Cefoperazone (Cefobid)	inj: 1, 2 g	IV: 1-4 g bid	Third	2.0
Cefotaxime (Claforan)	inj: 1, 2 g	IV; 1 g q12h-2g q4h	Third	1.0
Ceftazidime (Fortaz)	inj: 500 mg, 1, 2 g	IV: 1-2 g q8h	Third	1.8
Ceftizoxime (Cefizox)	inj: 1, 2 g	IV; 1-4 g q8h	Third	1.7
Ceftriaxone (Rocephin)	inj: 250 mg, 500 mg, 1 g, 2 g	IV: 1-2 g qd	Third	8.0

Modified from Stein JH (ed): *Internal medicine*, ed 4, St Louis, 1994, Mosby.

CHEMOTHERAPEUTIC AGENTS

TABLE 7-18 Chemotherapeutic Agents, Toxicity

DRUG	BONE MARROW TOXICITY	SKIN* NECROSIS	SKIN* RASHES	SKIN* HAIR	GI TRACT† MUCOSITIS	GI TRACT† NAUSEA AND VOMITING	HEPATIC
Actinomycin D	3	3	3	3	3	3	0
Amsacrine (AMSA)	2	3	0	3	1	1	1
Ara-C (cytarabine)	3	0	0	0	2	2	3
L-Asparaginase	0	0	0	0	0	2	3
Azathioprine	—						3
Bleomycin	0	0	3	2	3	1	0
Busulfan	—	0	2	0	0	1	1
Carboplatin	3	0	1	1	0	1	0
Carmustine (BCNU)	3	2	2	1	0	3	3
Chlorambucil	2	0	1	0	0	1	1
Cisplatin	1	0**	0	0	0	3	0
Cyclophosphamide	3	0	1	3	1	2	1
Dacarbazine (DTIC)	1	2	0	0	0	3	2
Deoxycoformycin	1	0	1	0	0	1	2
Daunomycin/doxorubicin	3	3	3	3	3	3	0
Etoposide/teniposide	2	2	0	1	1	1	2
Fludarabine	2	0	2	0	1	2	1
Fluorouracil	1-2	1	2	2	3	1	2
Hexamethylmelamine	1	0	0	0	0	1	0
Hydroxyurea	3	0	1	1	0	1	0
Ifosfamide	2	0	0	3	1	2	1
Lomustine (CCNU)	3	0	0	0	0	3	3
Melphalan	3	0	0	0	0	1	1
Mercaptopurine	2	0	1	0	2	1	3
Methotrexate	1-2	0	1	1	3	1	3
Mithramycin	1	2	2	0	2	3	3
Mitomycin C	1	3	1	0	0	1	0
Mitotane	—	0	1	0	0	2	0
Mitoxantrone	2	3	0	1	2	2	1
Nitrogen mustard	3	3	2	1	1	3	0
Procarbazine	2	0	1	0	0	2	0
Streptozocin	1	2	0	0	0	3	3
Taxol (paclitaxel)	3		1	3	2	2	2
Thioguanine (6-TG)	2	0	1	0	2	1	2
Thiotepa		0	0	1	0	0	0
Vincristine	1	3	0	2	1	1	2
Vinblastine	3	3	0	2	2	1	0
Vindesine	2	3	0	2	1	1	0

From Noble J (ed): *Primary care medicine,* ed 2, St Louis, 1996, Mosby.
0, Very mild or very rare; 1, occasional, usually not severe; 2, moderately severe; 3, frequent or severe; *SIADH,* syndrome of inappropriate antidiuretic hormone; *MAO,* monoamine oxidase; *RTA,* renal tubular acidosis; *XRT,* radiation therapy.
*Necrosis if extravasated, or phlebitis; rashes, pruritus, changes in pigmentation; alopecia.
†Stomatitis.
‡Arrhythmias or congestive heart failure.
§Hypersensitivity reactions.
‖CNS toxicity.
¶Peripheral neuropathy.
#Toxicity unique to agent.
**High drug concentration infusion.

Chemotherapeutic agents

				NEUROLOGIC		
CARDIAC‡	ALLERGIC§	PULMONARY FIBROSIS	NEPHROTIC	CENTRAL‖	PERIPHERAL¶	OTHER#
1	0	0	0	0	0	Fever, radiation recall
3	0	0	0	1	0	Cardiac arrhythmias
0	1	2	0	2	2	Fever, conjunctivitis
0	2	0	0	2	0	Fever, coagulopathy, pancreatitis
2		1	0	0	0	—
1	1	3	0	1	0	Pericarditis, fever
0	0	2	0	0	0	Addisonian syndrome, cataracts
0	2	0	0	1	1	Cumulative myelosuppression
0	0	2	2	2	0	Prolonged nausea and vomiting
0	1	1	0	1	0	
1	3	0	3	2	3	Vascular toxicity, prolonged nausea and vomiting
0	1	2	0	0	0	Fever, SIADH, cystitis
0	0	0	0	1	0	Flulike syndrome
0	1	—	2	1	0	
3	1	0	0	0	0	Radiation recall
0	2	0	0	1	2	
0	1	1	1	3	1	
1	1	0	0	2	1	Conjunctivitis
0	0	0	0	2	2	
0	1	0	0	1	0	
1	1	0	2	2	1	Prolonged nausea and vomiting, cystitis, fever
0	0	1	2	0	0	Prolonged nausea and vomiting
0	1	1	0	0	0	
0	0	0	0	0	0	
0	1	2	2	2	0	Fever, conjunctivitis
0	0	0	3	0	0	Coagulopathy, fever
1	0	2	2	0	0	Hemolytic-uremic syndrome
0	1	0	0	2	0	Adrenal insufficiency
1	0	0	0	0	0	
0	0	0	0	1	0	
0	2	2	0	2	2	MAO inhibitor
0	0	0	3	0	0	Prolonged nausea and vomiting; proximal RTA
3	3	0	—	0	0	Cardiac arrhythmias, fever
0	0	0	0	0	0	
0	0	0	0	0	0	
1	0	0	0	2	3	Hepatotoxic with XRT, SIADH
0	0	1	0	0	1	
0	0	1	0	2	3	

CONTRACEPTIVES, ORAL

TABLE 7-19 Contraceptives, Oral

BRAND NAME AND REGIMEN	ESTROGEN	AMOUNT (μG)	PROGESTIN	AMOUNT (MG)
Monophasic*				
Loestrin 1/20, 21, 28Fe	EE	20	NETA	1.0
Loestrin 1.5/30, 21, 28Fe	EE	30	NETA	1.5
Nordette-21, -28	EE	30	LNG	0.15
Lo/Ovral, 21, 28	EE	30	NG	0.3
Levlen, 21, 28	EE	30	LNG	0.15
Levora, 21, 28	EE	30	LNG	0.15
Desogen, 28	EE	30	DSG	0.15
Ortho-Cept, 21, 28	EE	30	DSG	0.15
Genora 1/35, 21, 28	EE	35	NET	1.0
Genora 0.5/35, 21, 28	EE	35	NET	0.5
N.E.E. 1/35, 21, 28	EE	35	NET	1.0
Nelova 1/35E, 21, 28	EE	35	NET	1.0
Nelova 0.5/35E, 21, 28	EE	35	NET	0.5
Norethin 1/35E, 21, 28	EE	35	NET	1.0
Norinyl 1+35, 21, 28	EE	35	NET	1.0
Ortho-Novum 1/35, 21, 28	EE	35	NET	1.0
Brevicon, 21, 28	EE	35	NET	0.5
Modicon, 21, 28	EE	35	NET	0.5
Ovcon-35, 21, 28	EE	35	NET	0.4
Demulen 1/35, 21, 28	EE	35	EDDA	1.0
Ortho-Cyclen, 21, 28	EE	35	NGS	0.25
Genora 1/50, 21, 28	ME	50	NET	1.0
Nelova 1/50M, 21, 28	ME	50	NET	1.0
Norethin 1/50M, 21, 28	ME	50	NET	1.0
Norinyl 1+50, 21, 28	ME	50	NET	1.0
Ortho-Novum 1/50, 21, 28	ME	50	NET	1.0
Ovcon-50, 21, 28	EE	50	NET	1.0
Demulen 1/50, 21, 28	EE	50	EDDA	1.0
Ovral, 21, 28	EE	50	NG	0.5
Biphasic†				
Jenest-28	7-EE	35	7-NET	0.5
	14-EE	35	14-NET	1.0
Nelova 10/11, 21, 28	10-EE	35	10-NET	0.5
	11-EE	35	11-NET	1.0
Ortho-Novum 10/11, 21, 28	10-EE	35	10-NET	0.5
	11-EE	35	11-NET	1.0

Continued

TABLE 7-19 Contraceptives, Oral—cont'd

BRAND NAME AND REGIMEN	ESTROGEN	AMOUNT (MG)	PROGESTIN	AMOUNT (MG)
Triphasic‡				
Tri-Norinyl, 21, 28	7-EE	35	7-NET	0.5
	9-EE	35	9-NET	1.0
	5-EE	35	5-NET	0.5
Ortho-Novum 7/7/7, 21, 28	7-EE	35	7-NET	0.5
	7-EE	35	7-NET	0.75
	7-EE	35	7-NET	1.0
Tri-Levlen, 21, 28	6-EE	30	6-LNG	0.05
	5-EE	40	5-LNG	0.075
	10-EE	30	10-LNG	0.125
Triphasil, 21, 28	6-EE	30	6-LNG	0.05
	5-EE	40	5-LNG	0.075
	10-EE	30	10-LNG	0.125
Ortho Tri-Cyclen	7-EE	35	7-NGS	0.180
	7-EE	35	7-NGS	0.215
	7-EE	35	7-NGS	0.250
Progestin Only (Minipill)				
Micronor			NET	0.35
Nor-Q.D.			NET	0.35
Ovrette			NG	0.075

From Danakas GT: *Practical guide to the care of the gynecologic/obstetric patient,* St Louis, 1997, Mosby.
*Monophasic: provides a fixed dosage of estrogen to progestin throughout the cycle.
†Biphasic: Estrogen amount remains the same throughout the cycle. In first half of cycle, decreased progestin/estrogen ratio allows endometrial proliferation. In second half of cycle, increased ratio provides adequate secretory development.
‡Triphasic estrogen amount remains the same or varies and progestin amount varies throughout cycle.
EE, Ethinyl estradiol; *ME,* mestranol; *NET,* norethindrone; *NETA,* norethindrone acetate; *EDDA,* ethynodiol diacetate; *NG,* norgestrel; *LNG,* levonorgestrel; *DSG,* desogestrel; *NGS,* norgestimate.

CORTICOSTEROIDS

TABLE 7-20 Corticosteroid Comparison Chart

DRUG	EQUIVALENT ANTIINFLAMMATORY DOSAGES (MG)	GLUCO-CORTICOID POTENCY	MINERALO-CORTICOID POTENCY	ROUTE OF ADMINISTRATION
Prednisone	10.0	4.0	0.8	PO
Hydrocortisone (Solu-Cortef)	40.0	1.0	1.0	PO, IM, IV
Methylprednisolone (Solu-Medrol)	8.0	5.0	0.5	PO, IM, IV
Dexamethasone (Decadron)	1.5	30.0	0.0	PO, IV
Cortisone	50.0	0.8	0.8	PO, IM

From Ferri F: *Practical guide to the care of the medical patient,* ed 4, St Louis, 1998, Mosby.

DIURETICS

TABLE 7-21 Diuretics

CLASS	AGENT	PREPARATIONS	DOSAGE (MG/DAY)	SITE OF ACTION	COST*
Thiazide	Chlorothiazide (Diuril)	tab: 250, 500 mg susp: 250 mg/5 ml	125-500	Distal tubule	$
	Hydrochlorothiazide (Esidrix)	tab: 25, 50, 100	12.5-50	Distal tubule	$
	Hydrochlorothiazide (Microzide)	tab: 12.5 mg	12.5 mg qd	Distal tubule	$$
	Methyclothiazide (Enduron)	tab: 2.5, 5 mg	2.5-5	Distal tubule	$$
Phthalimidine derivative	Chlorthalidone (Hygroton)	tab: 25, 50, 100 mg	12.5-50	Distal tubule	$$$
Quinazoline	Metolazone (Diulo, Zaroxolyn, Mykrox)	tab: 2.5, 5, 10 mg tab: 0.5 mg (Mykrox)	2.5-10 0.5 (Mykrox)	Cortical diluting site and proximal convoluted tubule	$$
Indoline	Indapamide (Lozol)	tab: 1.25, 2.5 mg	2.5-5	Distal tubule	$$$
Loop	Bumetanide (Bumex)	tab: 0.5, 1, 2 mg inj: 0.25 mg/ml	0.5-5 PO/IV/IM	Ascending limb of loop of Henle	$$ $$$
	Ethacrynic acid (Edecrin)	tab: 25, 50 mg	25-100	Ascending limb of loop of Henle	$$
	Furosemide (Lasix)	tab: 20, 40, 80 mg oral sol: 10 mg/ml inj: 10 mg/ml	20-160 PO/IV/IM	Ascending limb of loop of Henle	$ $$$ $$$
	Torsemide (Demadex)	tab: 5, 10, 20, 100 mg inj: amp 20, 50 mg	10-20 mg PO/IV	Ascending limb of loop of Henle	$$$
Carbonic anhydrase inhibitors	Acetazolamide (Diamox)	tab: 125, 250 mg	250 mg-1 g	Carbonic anhydrase inhibitor	$$
	Methazolamide (Neptazane)	tab: 25, 50 mg	100-300 mg	Carbonic anhydrase inhibitor	$$$
Potassium-sparing	Amiloride (Midamor)	tab: 5 mg	5-10	Distal tubule	$$
	Spironolactone (Aldactone)	tab: 25, 50, 100	25-100	Distal tubule	$$
	Triamterene (Dyrenium)	cap: 50, 100	50-150	Distal tubule	$$

From Ferri F: *Practical guide to the care of the medical patient*, ed 4, St Louis, 1998, Mosby.
*Cost to pharmacist per month of therapy: $, <$20; $$, $21-$30; $$$, >$30.

FLUOROQUINOLONES

TABLE 7-22 Fluoroquinolones

AGENT	PREPARATION	DOSAGE	HALF-LIFE (HR)	EXCRETION	COST FOR 10 DAYS (PO) $
Cinoxacin (Cinobac)	cap: 250, 500 mg	UTI: 250 mg q6h or 500 mg q12h	1.5	Urine	40-90
Ciprofloxacin (Cipro)	tab: 100, 250, 500, 750 mg inj: 200, 400 mg sol, ophth: 0.3%, 2.5 ml	UTI: 250-500 mg q12h Bone, joint, skin, respiratory tract: 500-750 mg q12h Infectious diarrhea: 500 mg q12h Simple cystitis: 100 mg q12h for 3 days Ocular: 1 gtt 5-6 times/day	4	Urine, feces	70-190
Enoxacin (Penetrex)	tab: 200, 400 mg	UTI: 200-400 mg q12h	3-6	Urine	60-90
Levofloxacin (Levaquin)	tab: 250, 500 mg inj: 25 mg/ml	Bronchitis: 500 mg PO qd for 7 days Pneumonia: 500 mg PO qd for 7-14 days Sinusitis: 500 mg PO qd for 7-14 days Skin and skin structure 500 mg PO qd for 7-10 days	6	Urine	60-90
Lomefloxacin (Maxaquin)	tab: 400 mg	Cystitis, complicated UTI: 400 mg qd Acute bacterial exacerbation of chronic bronchitis: 400 mg qd	6-8	Urine	60-90
Norfloxacin (Noroxin)	tab: 400 mg sol, ophth: 0.3%, 5 ml	UTI: 400 mg q12h Uncomplicated gonorrhea: 800 mg, single dose Ocular: 1 gtt qid	4	Urine, feces	60-90
Ofloxacin (Floxin)	tab: 200, 300, 400 mg inj: 200, 400 mg sol, ophth: 0.3%, 5 ml	UTI: 200 mg q12h Prostatitis: 300 mg q12h Acute uncomplicated gonorrhea: 400 mg single dose Cervicitis/urethritis: 300 mg q12h Pneumonia, exacerbation of chronic bronchitis: 400 mg q12h	5-10	Urine	70-180
Sparfloxacin (Zagam)	tab: 200 mg	Community-acquired pneumonia, bacterial exacerbations of chronic bronchitis: 400 mg on day 1, then 200 mg qd	6-9	Urine (50%)	60-90

INSULIN PREPARATIONS

TABLE 7-23　Insulin Preparations

PREPARATION	ONSET OF ACTION*	DURATION OF ACTION*	PEAK EFFECT*
Rapid-acting			
Human insulin analog (Humalog)	<15 min	3.5-4.5 hr	1 hr
Regular (crystalline zinc)	30-60 min	5-7 hr	2-4 hr
Semilente	30 min-3 hr	12-16 hr	4-8 hr
Intermediate-acting			
NPH	2 hr	18-28 hr	6-12 hr
Lente	2-4 hr	24-28 hr	6-12 hr
Long-acting			
Ultralente	4-6 hr	36 + hr	12-16 hr
Mixture of NPH and regular (50/50 mixture, 70/30 mixture)	30 min	24 hr	2-12 hr (70/30) 3-5 hr (50/50)

From Ferri F: *Practical guide to the care of the medical patient*, ed 4, St Louis, 1998, Mosby.
*After subcutaneous injection. The onset, duration of action, and peak effect vary with each patient and are influenced by the site and depth of injection and the concentration and volume.

MEDICATIONS: COMPARISON TABLES

LAXATIVES

TABLE 7-24 Preparations Used in the Symptomatic Treatment of Constipation or Fecal Impaction

TYPE	ACTION	GENERIC AGENT	BRAND	DAILY DOSE	PRECAUTIONS
Bulk agents	Increase in stool water, bulk, and rate of bowel transit	Bran/fiber		10 g/day × 7 days, then 20 g/day PO	Bulk agents require adequate fluid intake, 1.5-2.0 L/day, to prevent worsening of the constipation or development of obstruction or impaction
		Psyllium	Metamucil Hydrocil Fiberall	Up to 30 g/day in divided doses PO	
		Methylcellulose	Citrucel Collogel Hydrolose	Up to 6 g/day in divided doses PO	
Lubricants	Inhibit colonic water absorption and coats stool for easier passage	Mineral oil	Zymenol Kondremul	15-30 ml/once or twice per day PO	Contraindicated in debilitated patients or those with swallowing problems; aspiration causes lipoid pneumonia; may impair absorption of fat-soluble vitamins
Stool softeners	Soften stool and some gut secretory and stimulant effect	Docusete sodium Docusete calcium Docusete potassium	Colace Surfak Dialose	50-360 mg PO	Little evidence in literature supporting effectiveness; may be directly hepatotoxic or potentiate hepatotoxicity of other drugs
Irritants	Stimulate motility and increase gut mucosal secretion of sodium and water	Senna extract Phenolphthalein	Senekot Ex-lax Feen-a-mint Correctol	1-2 tab or tsp PO 130-275 mg PO	Chronic use may cause myenteric plexus neuronal damage and major motility dysfunction, "cathartic colon"
		Bisacodyl	Dulcolax Carter's Pills	5-15 mg PO	
		Danthron Castor oil	Dorbane Neoloid	75-150 mg PO 50-60 ml PO	

Continued

TABLE 7-24 Preparations Used in the Symptomatic Treatment of Constipation or Fecal Impaction—cont'd

TYPE	ACTION	GENERIC AGENT	BRAND	DAILY DOSE	PRECAUTIONS
Osmotic agents	Osmotically draw fluid into the bowel lumen, increasing intraluminal pressure and stimulating peristalsis	Magnesium salts Citrate Hydroxide Sulfate	Citrate of magnesia Milk of magnesia Epsom salts	200 ml PO 15-30 ml PO 240-300 ml PO	Magnesium toxicity in patients with renal insufficiency All osmotic agents require good fluid intake for maximal effect
		Nonabsorbable sugars Lactulose	Cephulac Chronulac	15-30 ml PO bid	Monitor glucose level
		Sorbitol (70% sol) Polyethylene Glycol-saline solution	Golytely Colyte	15-30 ml PO bid 2-6 L PO	
Suppositories	Local irritant or osmotic effect	Glycerine Bisacodyl	Dulcolax	3 g PR 10 mg PR	May cause rectal irritation
Enemas	Local irritant, osmotic, or lubricating effect	Tap water or saline enemas Sodium salts Phosphate Sulfate Mineral oil	Fleets Enema Phospho-soda	100-200 mg PR 120 ml PR 60-120 ml PR	Hot water, soap, or hydrogen peroxide enemas should never be used because they irritate the rectal mucosa and may cause bleeding; sodium salts may cause fluid overload in patients with CHR; phosphates may affect the serum phosphorous and calcium levels; phosphate enemas should not be used in patients with renal insufficiency

From Rosen P et al: *Emergency medicine*, ed 3, St Louis, 1997, Mosby.

LIPID-LOWERING AGENTS

TABLE 7-25   Lipid-Lowering Agents

AGENT	PREPARATIONS	INITIAL DOSAGE	MECHANISM OF ACTION	EFFECT	COST*
Atorvastatin (Lipitor)	tab: 10, 20, 40 mg	10 mg qd	HMG-CoA reductase inhibitor (Statin)	↓↓ LDL ↑ HDL ↓ Triglycerides	$$$$
Cholestyramine	Questran powder; 378 g cans or packets containing 4 g of cholestyramine in 9 g of powder Questran Light: 210 g can or packets containing 4 g of cholestyramine in 5 g of powder	Powder: one packet or scoopful (4 g) qd mixed with water or other fluids	Bile acid sequestrant	↓ LDL N/↑ triglycerides	$$$ $$$$ (Packets)
Colestipol (Colestid)	granules: 500 mg bottles or packets containing 5 g of granules tab: 1 g	15 g bid 2 g qd-bid	Bile acid sequestrant	↓ LDL N/↑ triglycerides	$$$
Fluvastatin (Lescol)	cap: 20, 40 mg	20 mg qd in evening	HMG-CoA reductase inhibitor (Statin)	↓↓ LDL ↑ HDL	$$$
Gemfibrozil (Lopid)	tab: 600 mg cap: 300 mg	600 mg bid	↑ Intravascular breakdown of VLDL	↓↓ Triglycerides ↓ LDL ↑ HDL	$$ (Generic)
Lovastatin† (Mevacor)	tab: 10, 20, 40 mg	20 mg qd in evening	HMG-CoA reductase inhibitor (Statin)	↓↓ LDL ↑ HDL	$$$$
Nicotinic acid (Niacin)	tab: 100, 250, 500 mg cap: 250, 300, 400, 500 mg	100 mg tid with or following meals; if tolerated, gradually increase dose to 1 g tid	Decreases synthesis of VLDL and clearance of HDL	↓ LDL ↓ Triglycerides ↑ HDL	$ (Generic)
Pravastatin† (Pravachol)	tab: 10, 20, 40 mg	10 mg qd in evening	HMG-CoA reductase inhibitor (Statin)	↓↓ LDL ↑ HDL	$$$$
Probucol (Lorelco)	tab: 250, 500 mg	250-500 bid	Enhances LDL metabolism	↓ LDL ↓ HDL	$$$
Simvastatin† (Zocor)	tab: 5, 10, 20, 40 mg	5 mg qd in evening	HMG-CoA reductase inhibitor (Statin)	↓↓ LDL ↑ HDL	$$$$

From Ferri F: *Practical guide to the care of the medical patient,* ed 4, St Louis, 1998, Mosby.
*Cost to pharmacist per month of low-dose therapy: $, <$20; $$, $21-$40; $$$, $41-$50; $$$$, >$51.
$According to the World Health Organization—defined daily doses of HMGs, Lovastatin, 30 mg = Pravastatin, 20 mg = Simvastatin, 15 mg. *N,* No change.

MACROLIDE ANTIBIOTICS

TABLE 7-26 Macrolide Antibiotics

MACROLIDE	ORAL PREPARATIONS	DOSAGE	PRIMARY ROUTE OF EXCRETION	HALF-LIFE (HR)	COST* ($)
Azithromycin (Zithromax)	cap: 250 mg susp: 100, 200 mg/5 ml	500 mg on day 1, then 250 mg qd for 4 days	Biliary	65-70	40-50
Clarithromycin (Biaxin)	tab: 250, 500 mg susp: 125, 250 mg/5 ml	250-500 mg q12h 500 mg tid for *H. pylori* therapy	Renal	3-8	70-100
Dirithromycin (Dynabac)	cap: 250 mg	500 mg qd	Fecal, renal	30-44	40-60
Erythromycin	tab, cap: 200, 250, 333, 500 mg susp: 200, 400 mg/5 ml	1-2 g/day in 3 to 4 divided doses	Biliary	1-2	<20 (generic)

*Cost to pharmacist for 10-day dose.

NARCOTIC ANALGESICS

TABLE 7-27 Narcotic Analgesic Comparison Chart

DRUG	EQUIVALENT PO DOSE (MG)	DURATION OF ANALGESIA (HR)	PREPARATIONS	DOSAGE
PO Analgesics				
Codeine	200	4-6	tab: 15, 30, 60 mg	15-60 mg q6h
Hydromorphone (Dilaudid)	7.5	4-6	tab: 2, 4, 8 mg	2-4 mg q6h
Levorphanol (Levo-Dromoran)	4	4-7	tab: 2 mg	4 mg q6-8h
Meperidine (Demerol)	300	4-6	tab: 50, 100 mg; syrup: 50 mg/5 ml	50-150 mg q3-4h
Methadone (Dolophine)	20	3-5	tab: 5, 10 mg; tab: 10, 15, 30	10-30 mg q4h; 10-30 mg q4h
Morphine	60	4-7	Sust Rel tab (MS contin): 30, 60, 100, 200 mg	MS contin: 30-100 mg q12h
Pentazocine (Talwin Nx)	180	4-7	tab: 50 mg	50 mg q3-4h
Propoxyphene (Darvon)	240	4-6	cap: 65 mg	65 mg q4h
IM Analgesics (Conversion from PO to IM: Codeine, 200 mg PO = 130 mg IM)				
Codeine	130	4-6	inj: 30, 60 mg	15-60 mg IM/IV/SC
Buprenorphine (Buprenex)	0.3	3-6	inj: 0.3 mg/ml	0.3 mg IM q6h
Butorphanol (Stadol)	2.0	3-6	inj: 1, 2 mg/ml	2 mg IM q3-4h
Dezocine (Dalgan)	10	3-6	inj: 5, 10, 15 mg/ml	5-20 mg IM q3-6h
Hydromorphone (Dilaudid)	1.5	4-5	inj: 1, 2, 4 mg/ml	1-2 mg IM q4-6h
Levorphanol (Levo-Dromoran)	2	4-6	inj: 2 mg/ml	2 mg q6-8h
Meperidine (Demerol)	75	4-6	inj: 25, 50, 75, 100 mg/ml	50-100 mg IM/SC q3-4h
Methadone (Dolophine)	10	3-5	inj: 10 mg/ml	2.5-10 mg IM/SC q3-4h
Morphine	10	4-6	inj: 0.5, 1, 2, 3, 4, 5, 8, 10, 15 mg	10 mg q4h
Oxymorphone (Numorphan)	1.1	3-5	inj: 1, 1.5 mg/ml	1-1.5 mg IM/SC q4-6h
Pentazocine (Talwin Nx)	60	4-6	inj: 30 mg/ml	30 mg IM/SC/IV q3-4h

Combination analgesics

DRUG	CONTENT (MG)
Tylenol with Codeine no. 2	Acetaminophen 300, Codeine 15
Tylenol with Codeine no. 3	Acetaminophen 300, Codeine 30
Tylenol with Codeine no. 4	Acetaminophen 300, Codeine 60
Percocet	Acetaminophen 325, oxycodone HCl 5
Percodan	Aspirin 325, oxycodone HCl 5
Tylox	Acetaminophen 500, oxycodone HCl 5
Darvocet N-100	Acetaminophen 650, propoxyphene napsylate 100
Talwin Compound	Aspirin 325, pentazocine HCl 12.5
Vicodin	Acetaminophen 500 mg, hydrocodone bitartrate 5 mg
Lortab liquid	Acetaminophen 120 mg, hydrocodone bitartrate 2.5 mg
Talacen	Pentazocine 25mg, acetaminophen 650 mg
Talwin Compound	Pentazocine 12.5 mg, aspirin 325 mg
Transdermal (Duragesic)	Fentanyl 25, 50, 75, 100 µg/hr; Dosage: initially 25 µg/hr; may be worn for 72 hr

From Ferri F: *Practical guide to the care of the medical patient*, ed 4, 1998, Mosby.

NITRATES

TABLE 7-28 Nitrates for Angina

DRUG	DOSAGE AND PREPARATIONS	ONSET OF ACTION (MIN)	DURATION OF ACTION
Nitroglycerin			
Sublingual (Nitrostat)	0.15-0.6 mg q5min prn (0.15, 0.3, 0.4, 0.6 mg)	1-3	½-1 hr
Isordil sublingual	2.5-5 mg prn q2-3h (tab: 2.5, 5, 10 mg)	2-5	1-3 hr
Lingual aerosol (Nitrolingual spray)	0.4 mg/metered dose prn (200 metered doses/inhal)	1-3	½-1 hr
2% ointment (Nitro-bid)	2.5-12.5 cm q4-6h (20, 60 g tubes)	30	3-10 hr
Transdermal (Transderm Nitro, Nitro-dur, Nitrodisc, Minitran, Deponit)	Infusion system 0.1 mg/hr (2.5 mg/24 hr) 0.2 mg/hr (5 mg/24 hr) 0.3 mg/hr (7.5 mg/24 hr) 0.4 mg/hr (10 mg/24 hr) 0.6 mg/hr (15 mg/24 hr)	30-60	Up to 24 hr
Isosorbide dinitrate (Isordil)	10-40 mg q6h (tab: 5, 10, 20, 30, 40 mg)	30	3-6 hr
Isosorbide mononitrate (Monoket, Ismo, Imdur)	10-20 mg bid with doses 7 hr apart (Monoket tabs 10, 20 mg) 20 mg bid with doses 7 hr apart (Ismo tab 20 mg) 60 mg qd (Imdur tab 60 mg)	30-60	12-14 hr
Intravenous (Tridil, Nitrostat)	50 mg/500 ml; initiate infusion at 5 µg/min	1-2	3-5 min

From Ferri F: *Practical guide to the care of the medical patient*, ed 4, 1998, Mosby.

MEDICATIONS: COMPARISON TABLES
Nonsteroidal antiinflammatory drugs (NSAIDS)

NONSTEROIDAL ANTIINFLAMMATORY DRUGS (NSAIDS)

TABLE 7-29 Nonsteroidal Antiinflammatory Drugs (NSAIDs)

AGENTS	PREPARATIONS	DOSAGE	PLASMA HALF-LIFE (HR) OF REGULAR PREPARATION	CHEMICAL CLASS	COST*	METABOLISM
Aspirin	tab: 325, 500, 650, 800, 975 mg supp: 325, 650	325-650 mg q4h	9-16	Salicylate	$	Liver
Diclofenac (Voltaren, Cataflam)	tab: 25, 50, 75 mg Ext. Rel tab (Voltaren XR): 100 mg	50-75 mg bid	2	Phenylacetic	$$$$	Bile 35%, kidney 65%
Diflunisal (Dolobid)	tab: 250, 500 mg	250-500 mg q8-12h	8-12	Salicylate	$$$	Liver
Etodolac (Lodine)	cap: 200, 300, 400, 500 mg Ext Rel tab (Lodine XL): 400, 600 mg	200-400 mg q6-8h 800-1200 mg qd (Lodine XL)	7.3	Indoleacetic acid	$$$$$	Kidney, bile
Fenopren (Nalfon)	tab: 600 mg	200-600 mg tid-qid	3	Propionic acid	$$$$	Liver
Flurbiprofen (Ansaid)	tab: 50, 100 mg	100 mg bid-tid	5	Propionic acid	$$$$	Liver, kidney
Ibuprofen (Motrin)	tab: 200, 300, 400, 600, 800 mg susp: 100 mg/5 ml	200-800 mg tid-qid	2	Propionic acid	$ (generic)	Liver, kidney
Indomethacin (Indocin)	cap: 25, 50, 75 mg (SR) supp: 50 mg susp: 25 mg/5 ml	PO: 25-50 mg tid (SR qd-bid) PR: 50 mg qd	5-6	Indoleacetic acid	$ (generic)	Liver
Ketoprofen (Orudis, Oruvail)	cap: 25, 50, 75 mg Controlled release cap (Oruvail) 100, 150, 200 mg tab (Actron): 12.5 mg	50-75 mg tid 200 mg qd	2 1-4	Propionic acid	$$$$$	Kidney

Continued

TABLE 7-29 Nonsteroidal Antiinflammatory Drugs (NSAIDs)—cont'd

AGENTS	PREPARATIONS	DOSAGE	PLASMA HALF LIFE (HR) OF REGULAR PREPARATION	CHEMICAL CLASS	COST*	METABOLISM
Ketorolac (Toradol)	Prefilled syringe: 15, 30, 60 mg tab: 10 mg	30-60 mg IM initially followed by 15-30 mg IM q6h PO: 10 mg q6h	4-6	Propionic acid	$$$$$	Kidney
Meclofenamate (Meclomen)	cap: 50, 100 mg	50 mg q4-6h	4	Fenamic acid	$$$$	Liver
Nabumetone (Relafen)	tab: 500, 750 mg	1000 mg as single dose qd	20-30	Naphthylkanone	$$$$$	Liver
Naproxen (Naprosyn, Anaprox, Aleve, Naprelan)	tab: 250, 375, 500 mg susp: 125 mg/5 ml Naprelan (controlled release): 375, 500 mg Anaprox tabs: 275, 550 mg	250-500 mg bid 275-550 mg bid 750-1000 mg qd (Naprelan)	12-15	Propionic acid	$$$ $ (Generic)	Kidney
Oxaprozin (Daypro)	tab: 600 mg	1200 mg as single dose qd	42-50	Propionic acid	$$$$$	Liver
Piroxicam (Feldene)	10, 20 mg	20 mg qd	40	Oxicam	$ (Generic)	Liver
Salsalate (Disalcid)	tab: 500, 750 mg cap: 500 mg	1500 mg bid	3-16	Salicylate	$ (Generic)	Liver
Sulindac (Clinoril)	tab: 150, 200 mg	150-200 mg bid	16	Indoleacetic acid	$ (Generic)	Enterohepatic
Tolmetin (Tolectin)	tab: 200, 400, 600 mg	200-600 mg tid	2	Indoleacetic acid	$$$$$	Liver

From Ferri F: *Practical guide to the care of the medical patient,* ed 4, St Louis, 1998, Mosby.
*Cost to pharmacist for a 30-day supply: $, <$30; $$, $31-$40; $$$, $41-$50; $$$$, $51-$60; $$$$$, >$61.

TOPICAL STEROID PREPARATIONS

TABLE 7-30 Topical Steroid Preparations

AGENT	COMMON BRAND NAMES	POTENCY
Betamethasone		
Betamethasone valerate 0.01%	Valisone cream, lotion 0.01%	Low
Betamethasone valerate 0.1%	Valisone cream, ointment 0.1%	Intermediate
Betamethasone benzoate 0.025%	Benisone gel, Uticort gel (0.1%)	Intermediate
Betamethasone dipropionate 0.05% to 0.1%	Diprosone cream (0.05%) Diprosone aerosol (0.1%)	High
Betamethasone dipropionate augmented 0.05%	Diprolene ointment, gel 0.05%	Ultra-high
Desoximetasone		
Desoximetasone 0.05%	Topicort LP cream, gel 0.05%	Intermediate
Desoximetasone 0.25%	Topicort cream, ointment	High
Fluocinolone		
Fluocinolone acetonide 0.01%	Synalar cream, solution 0.01%	Low
Fluocinolone acetonide 0.025%	Synalar ointment 0.025%	Intermediate
Fluocinolone acetonide 0.2%	Synalar HP cream 0.2%	High
Fluocinonide 0.05%	Lidex cream, gel 0.05%	High
Hydrocortisone		
Hydrocortisone base or acetate 0.5%	Corticaine cream 0.5%	Low
Hydrocortisone base or acetate 1, 2.5%	Hytone cream 1%, 2.5%	Low
Hydrocortisone valerate 0.2%	Westcort cream, ointment 0.2%	Intermediate
Triamcinolone		
Triamcinolone acetonide 0.025%	Aristocort, Kenalog cream, ointment 0.025%	Low
Triamcinolone acetonide 0.1%	Aristocort, Kenalog cream, ointment 0.1%	Intermediate
Triamcinolone acetonide 0.5%	Aristocort, Kenalog cream, ointment 0.5%	High

From Ferri F: *Practical guide to the care of the medical patient,* ed 4, St Louis, 1998, Mosby.
NOTE: Most of these preparations are available in 15 g tubes.

VENTRICULAR ARRHYTHMIA THERAPEUTIC AGENTS

TABLE 7-31 Ventricular Arrhythmia Agents (Oral)

AGENT	ORAL DOSAGE	ELIMINATION HALF-LIFE	GROUP	ECG MANIFESTATIONS	TOXIC SERUM LEVELS (μG/ML)
Amiodarone (Cordarone)	Loading: 800-1600 mg/day for 1-3 wk, then 600-800 mg/day for 4 wk Maintenance: 100-400 mg/day	26-107 days	III	Prolonged QRS, QT, and PR: sinus bradycardia	—
Disopyramide (Norpace)	100-200 mg q6h	7-10 hr; 7-15 hr for sustained relase form	IA	Prolonged QRS, QT, and PR (+/−)	>9
Encainide (Enkaid)	Initially: 25 mg q8h Maintenance: 25-50 mg q8h	1-2 hr	IC	Prolonged QRS, PR	—
Flecainide (Tambocor)	Initially: 100 mg q12h Maintenance: 100-200 mg q12h	12-26 hr	IC	Prolonged QRS, PR	>1
Mexiletine (Mexitil)	Initially: 100-200 mg q8h Maintenance: 100-300 mg q6-12h	10-12 hr	IB	No significant change	>2
Moricizine (Ethmozine)	200-300 mg q8h	1.5-3.5 hr	I	Prolonged QRS, PR	—
Procainamide (Pronestyl)	50 mg/kg/day in divided doses q3-4h (q6h for slow-release form)	3-4 hr; 6 hr for sustained-release form	IA	Prolonged QRS, QT, and PR (+/−)	>16
Propafenone (Rythmol)	Initially: 150 mg q8h; dosage may be increased at a minimum of 3-4 day intervals to 225 mg q8h	2-10 hr	IC	Prolonged QRS, PR	—
Quinidine sulfate	200-400 mg q4-6h	6-11 hr	IA	Prolonged QRS, QT, and PR (+/−)	>8
Sotalol (Betapace)	Initially: 80 mg bid Maximum: 320 mg/day	12 hr	II, III	Prolonged PR, QT	—
Tocainide (Tonocard)	Initially 200-400 mg q8h Maintenance: 200-600 mg q8h	12 hr	IB	No significant change	>10

From Ferri F: *Practical guide to the care of the medical patient,* ed 4, St Louis, 1998, Mosby.

TABLE 7-32 IV Agents Used in Treating Ventricular Arrhythmias

DRUG	INDICATIONS	DOSAGE	ONSET OF ACTION	THERAPEUTIC PLASMA LEVEL (μG/ML)
Lidocaine (Xylocaine)	Ventricular tachyarrhythmias	Loading: 1 mg/kg bolus followed by infusion at 1-4 mg/min	Immediate	2-5
Bretylium (Bretylol)	Life-threatening refractory ventricular fibrillation or tachycardia	5 mg/kg slow bolus followed by infusion at 2 mg/min	5 minutes for significant antifibrillatory effect; may be delayed up to 2 hr for prevention of ventricular arrhythmias	1.33
Procainamide (Pronestyl)	Ventricular tachyarrhythmias	100 mg slow IV bolus followed by infusion at 1-4 mg/min	Immediate	3-10
Phenytoin (Dilantin)	Digitalis-induced ventricular arrhythmias	125-250 mg slow bolus q15min prn to maximum of 750 mg/hr	Immediate	5-20

From Ferri F: *Practical guide to the care of the medical patient,* ed 4, St Louis, 1998, Mosby.

APPENDIX

Essential Facts and Formulas

APPENDIX

DISEASE PREVENTION
Childhood Immunization Schedule

TABLE A-1 Recommended Childhood Immunization Schedule United States, January-December 1998*

AGE ▶ VACCINE ▼	BIRTH	1 MO	2 MO	4 MO	6 MO	12 MO	15 MO	18 MO	4-6 YR	11-12 YR	14-16 YR
Hepatitis B[2,3]	Hep B-1										
		Hep B-2		Hep B-3						Hep B[3]	
Diphtheria, Tetanus, Pertussis[4]			DTaP or DTP	DTaP or DTP	DTaP or DTP	DTaP or DTP[4]			DTaP or DTP	Td	
H. influenzae type b[5]			Hib	Hib	Hib[5]	Hib[5]					
Polio[6]			Polio	Polio		Polio[6]			Polio		
Measles, Mumps, Rubella[7]						MMR			MMR[7]	MMR[7]	
Varicella[8]						Var				Var[8]	

From Advisory Committee on Immunization Practices (ACIP), the American Academy of Pediatricians (AAP), and the American Academy of Family Physicians (AAFP): Recommended childhood immunization schedule, *Pediatrics* 47:10, Jan 1998.

*Approved by the Advisory Committee on Immunization Practices (ACIP), the American Academy of Pediatrics (AAP), and the American Academy of Family Physicians (AAFP). Vaccines[1] are listed under the routinely recommended ages. Bars indicate range of acceptable ages for vaccination. Shaded bars indicate vaccines to be assessed and administered if necessary.

[1]This schedule indicates the recommended age for routine administration of currently licensed childhood vaccines; vaccines are listed under the ages for which they are routinely recommended. Catch-up immunization should be done during any visit when feasible. Some combination vaccines are available and may be used whenever administration of all components of the vaccine is indicated. Providers should consult the manufacturers' package inserts for detailed recommendations.

[2]**Infants born to HBsAg-negative mothers** should receive 2.5 μg of Merck vaccine (Recombivax HB) or 10 μg of SmithKline Beecham (SB) vaccine (Engerix-B). The 2nd dose should be administered ≥ 1 mo after the 1st dose.
Infants born to HBsAg-positive mothers should receive 0.5 mL hepatitis B immune globulin (HBIG) within 12 hrs of birth, and either 5 μg of Merck vaccine (Recombivax HB) or 10 μg of SB vaccine (Engerix-B) at a separate site. The 2nd dose is recommended at 1-2 mos of age and the 3rd dose at 6 mos of age.
Infants born to mothers whose HBsAg status is unknown should receive either 5 μg of Merck vaccine (Recombivax HB) or 10 μg of SB vaccine (Engerix-B) within 12 hrs of birth. The 2nd dose of vaccine is recommended at 1 mo of age and the 3rd dose at 6 mos of age. Blood should be drawn at the time of delivery to determine the mother's HBsAg status; if it is positive, the infant should receive HBIG as soon as possible (no later than 1 wk of age). The dosage and timing of subsequent vaccine doses should be based upon the mother's HBsAg status.

[3]Children and adolescents who have not been vaccinated against hepatitis B in infancy may begin the series during any childhood visit. Those who have not previously received 3 doses of hepatitis B vaccine should initiate or complete the series during the 11-12 year-old visit. The 2nd dose should be administered at least 1 mo after the 1st dose, and the 3rd dose should be administered at least 4 mos after the 1st dose and at least 2 mos after the 2nd dose.

[4]DTaP (diphtheria and tetanus toxoids and acellular pertussis vaccine) is the preferred vaccine for all doses in the vaccination series, including completion of the series in children who have received ≥1 dose of whole-cell DTP vaccine. Whole-cell DTP is an acceptable alternative to DTaP. The 4th dose of DTaP may be administered as early as 12 mo of age, provided 6 months have elapsed since the 3rd dose, and if the child is considered unlikely to return at 15-18 mos of age. Td (tetanus and diphtheria toxoids, absorbed, for adult use) is recommended at 11-12 years of age if at least 5 years have elapsed since the last dose of DTP, DTaP, or DT. Subsequent routine Td boosters are recommended every 10 years.

[5]Three *H. influenzae* type b (Hib) conjugate vaccines are licensed for infant use. If PRP-OMP (PedvaxHIB [Merck]) is administered at 2 and 4 mos of age, a dose at 6 mos is not required.

[6]Two poliovirus vaccines are currently licensed in the US: inactivated poliovirus vaccine (IPV) and oral poliovirus vaccine (OPV). The following schedules are all acceptable by the ACIP, the AAP, and the AAFP, and parents and providers may choose among them:
  1. IPV at 2 and 4 mos; OPV at 12-18 mos and 4-6 yr
  2. IPV at 2, 4, 12-18 mos, and 4-6 yr
  3. OPV at 2, 4, 6-18 mos, and 4-6 yr

The ACIP routinely recommends schedule 1. IPV is the only poliovirus vaccine recommended for immunocompromised persons and their household contacts.

[7]The 2nd dose of MMR is routinely recommended at 4-6 yrs of age or at 11-12 yrs of age, but may be administered during any visit, provided at least 1 month has elapsed since receipt of the 1st dose and that both doses are administered at or after 12 mo of age. Those who have not previously received the second dose should complete the schedule no later than the routine visit to a health care provider at age 11 to 12 yr.

[8]Susceptible children may receive Varicella vaccine (Var) at any visit after the first birthday, and those who lack a reliable history of chickenpox should be immunized during the 11-12 year-old visit. Susceptible children ≥ 13 years of age should receive 2 doses, at least 1 mo apart.

Immunizations for Adults

TABLE A-2 Immunizations for Adults in the United States ≥18 Years of Age

NAME	PRIMARY SCHEDULE AND BOOSTER(S)	INDICATIONS	SIDE EFFECTS
Tetanus/diphtheria adsorbed toxoid (Td)	Two 0.5 ml IM doses 1 mo apart and third dose 6-12 mo after the second; booster every 10 yr.	All adults; check for receipt of primary series in refugees, immigrants, foreign born.	Local erythema and pain; rarely anaphylaxis, neuropathy, encephalopathy.
Measles (as MMR) live virus	One 0.5 ml SC dose; second dose at least 1 mo later (or immunity by antibody titers or physician-diagnosed measles).	Adults born after 1956 need one dose; an additional dose is given on entering school, a long-term correctional facility, health care work, during outbreaks, and for foreign travel; adults born before 1957 are considered immune, but giving one dose to health care workers at risk of exposure may be prudent.	Local erythema and pain, low-grade fever, rash, arthralgias from 1 to 21 days postvaccination; rarely, high fever from 5 to 21 days postvaccination.
Mumps (as MMR) live virus	One 0.5 ml SC dose (or immunity by antibody titers or physician-diagnosed mumps).	All adults born after 1956; adults born before 1957 are considered immune.	As for measles.
Rubella (as MMR) live virus	One 0.5 ml SC dose (or immunity by antibody titers).	All adults.	As for measles.
Polio (OPV), live virus, oral; (IPV), inactivated virus	IPV preferred for primary vaccination. Two 0.5 ml SC doses 1 to 2 mo apart and third dose 6-12 mo after the second; one booster dose for travelers.	Adults generally considered immune; indicated for health care workers exposed to the virus, unimmunized persons whose children receive OPV, travelers to high-risk countries.	Rarely, poliomyelitis (OPV); local pain and erythema, rarely fever (IPV).
Hepatitis B, recombinant DNA–derived surface antigen particles	Two IM doses 1 mo apart and third dose 5 mo after the second; higher dose and more frequent schedule for persons with chronic renal failure approaching dialysis; check postvaccination antibody titers in health care workers, immunocompromised, HIV-infected, and persons with chronic renal failure; yearly titers with boosters as needed for persons on dialysis.	Persons with multiple sex partners or sexually transmitted diseases, male homosexuals, injection drug users, persons whose sex partner is in a high-risk group, frequent recipients of blood products, persons on hemodialysis, Native Alaskans, health care or public safety workers with frequent blood or body fluid exposures, institutionalized developmentally disabled and their staff, household and sexual contacts of chronically infected carriers (for contacts of acutely infected persons see Table 3-4); consider for persons from an endemic area residing in a similar cultural community in the US; certain travelers to high-risk areas.	Local erythema and pain; rarely fever.

Modified from *MMWR* 40 (RR-12):60, 82, 1991 and MMWR 42 (RR-4):16, 1993; and from Noble J (ed): *Primary care medicine,* ed 2, St Louis, 1996, Mosby.
IM, Intramuscular; *SC,* subcutaneous; *ID,* intradermal.
*If able, it is prudent to wait to vaccinate until after the first trimester to minimize any concern about teratogenicity. "Pregnancy" as a contraindication also includes the time 3 months before conception.
†Includes persons with congenital immunodeficiency, leukemia, lymphoma, generalized malignancy receiving chemotherapy or radiation, persons on high-dose steroids or receiving immunosuppressive therapy for any reason; does not include persons with functional or anatomic asplenia or complement component deficiency.

CONTRAINDICATIONS	PREGNANCY*	HIV INFECTION	SEVERE IMMUNOCOMPROMISE†
Neurologic or anaphylactic reaction to a previous dose (can be given TIG for postexposure prophylaxis).	Recommended; no confirmed risk to fetus.	Recommended.	Recommended.
Anaphylaxis to chicken eggs or neomycin (contact dermatitis to neomycin is not a contraindication); severe reaction to a previous dose.	Contraindicated; no confirmed risk to fetus; vaccination of susceptible women should be part of postpartum care.	Recommended/considered.	Contraindicated.
As for measles.	As for measles.	As for measles.	As for measles.
As for measles; rubella vaccine from human diploid cells can be given to persons with anaphylaxis to chicken eggs.	As for measles.	As for measles.	As for measles.
Anaphylactic reaction to a previous dose, to neomycin or streptomycin (and for IPV, polymyxin B) (contact dermatitis to these antibiotics is not a contraindication); household contacts and close nursing personnel of immunocompromised persons should be given IPV, not OPV.	Use IPV; if immediate protection in less than 4 wk is needed, then use OPV; no confirmed risk to fetus.	Use IPV; OPV contraindicated.	Use IPV; OPV contraindicated.
Anaphylactic reaction to common baker's yeast.	Use if indicated; no reported risk to fetus.	Use if indicated (check postvaccination antibody titer).	Use if indicated (check postvaccination antibody (titer).

Continued

TABLE A-2 Immunizations for Adults in the United States ≥18 Years of Age—cont'd

NAME	PRIMARY SCHEDULE AND BOOSTER(S)	INDICATIONS	SIDE EFFECTS
Pneumococcal bacterial polysaccharide	One 0.5 ml IM or SC dose; consider revaccination after 6 yr for persons at highest risk of fatal disease (splenic dysfunction or anatomic asplenia) or declining antibody levels (nephrotic, chronic renal failure, transplant recipients).	Adults over 65 yr; persons with chronic pulmonary disease, cardiovascular disease, diabetes, alcoholism, cirrhosis, chronic renal failure, nephrotic syndrome, organ transplantation, functional or anatomic asplenia, or immunocompromise for any reason; homeless persons and Native Alaskans.	Local erythema and pain; low-grade fever.
Influenza inactivated virus	One 0.5 ml IM dose, seasonally.	As for pneumococcal vaccine with the exception of some Native Alaskans; caregivers and household contacts of persons for whom the vaccine is indicated, health care workers and visiting nurses, travelers to the tropics or southern hemisphere who are at risk of poor outcome if infected.	Local erythema and pain, malaise, low-grade fever, headache.
Hemophilus influenza type b (HbCV) bacterial polysaccharide, conjugated	Dose for adults has not been determined; generally one 0.5 ml IM dose is used.	Adults at highest theoretic risk; functional or anatomic asplenia, severe non-HIV immunocompromise; consider in HIV-infected persons.	Local erythema and pain, malaise, fever.
Meningococcal bacterial polysaccharide (serogroups A, C, W135, and Y)	One 0.5 ml SC dose; duration of immunity unknown.	Adults with functional or anatomic asplenia or with terminal complement component deficiency; prophylaxis during outbreaks if serogroup represented in the vaccine; travelers to endemic areas.	
Rabies human diploid cell vaccine (HDCV), rabies vaccine adsorbed (RVA)	Preexposure prophylaxis: 1.0 ml IM doses (HDCV or RVA) on days 0, 7, and 28; or 0.1 ml ID doses (HDCV) on days 0, 7, and 21 or 28; one booster dose or check antibody titers every 2 yr; chloroquine can interfere with immunity. Postexposure prophylaxis: wound care first, then: if received appropriate preexposure prophylaxis or previous postexposure prophylaxis—two 1.0 ml IM doses (HDCV or RVA) on days 0 and 3. All other persons—HRIG (20 IU/kg) half dose to infiltrate the wound and half the dose IM, with five 0.1 ml IM doses (HDCV or RVA) on days 0, 3, 7, 14, and 28.	Veterinarians, animal handlers, certain laboratory workers, travelers for greater than 1 mo to countries where rabies is endemic in domesticated animals. Any significant exposure.	Local erythema and pain (in 75%), malaise, fever, headache, abdominal pain, myalgias, dizziness (in 5%-40%), anaphylaxis (in 0.1%); mild immune complex hypersensitivity reaction in persons given a booster (in 6%).

CONTRAINDICATIONS	PREGNANCY*	HIV INFECTION	SEVERE IMMUNOCOMPROMISE†
More severe local reactions in persons revaccinated in less than 14 mo.	Use if indicated; unknown risk to fetus.	Recommended.	Recommended.
Severe reaction to a previous dose; anaphylaxis to chicken eggs.	Use if indicated; do not delay if influenza season imminent; no confirmed risk to fetus.	Recommended.	Recommended.
Hypersensitivity reaction to the conjugated protein carriers.	Use if high risk of infection; unknown risk to fetus.	Consider.	Recommended.
None to date.	Use if high risk of infection; unknown risk to fetus.	Use if indicated.	Use if indicated.
Severe reaction to a previous dose; consult public health department if postexposure prophylaxis is needed.	Use if indicated; unknown risk to fetus.	Use if indicated (check postvaccination antibody titer).	Use if indicated (check postvaccination antibody titer).

Continued

TABLE A-2 Immunizations for Adults in the United States ≥18 Years of Age—cont'd

NAME	PRIMARY SCHEDULE AND BOOSTER(S)	INDICATIONS	SIDE EFFECTS
Hepatitis A inactivated virus	1.0 ml dose; booster in 6 mo.	Certain travelers to high-risk areas, certain occupations at risk.	Local erythema and pain.
Yellow fever live virus	One 0.5 ml SC dose 10 days to 10 yr before travel; booster dose every 10 yr; avoid mosquitoes; space 3 wk from cholera vaccine.	Certain travelers to areas where yellow fever is endemic.	Low-grade fever, headache, myalgias (in 2%-5%), encephalitis (extremely rare).
Japanese encephalitis inactivated virus	Three 0.5 ml SC doses on days 0, 7, and 30; last dose to precede travel by 10 days; need for boosters unknown; avoid mosquitoes.	Certain travelers to areas where Japanese encephalitis is endemic.	Local erythema and pain, fever, malaise, nausea, abdominal discomfort; anaphylaxis precautions.
Cholera inactivated bacteria	Two 0.5 ml IM or SC doses; or two 0.2 ml ID doses given 1 to 4 wk apart; booster dose every 6 mo; careful food and water selection; space 3 wk from yellow fever vaccine.	Travelers to areas that require vaccination or certain travelers at high risk.	Local erythema and pain, fever, malaise.
Typhoid live bacteria, oral; inactivated bacteria, parenteral	Four oral doses on days 0, 2, 4, and 6 with the series repeated every 5 yr; or two 0.5 ml SC doses 4 wk apart or three SC doses at weekly intervals with a 0.5 ml SC or 0.1 ml ID booster every 3 yr; careful food and water selection.	Certain travelers to high risk areas, certain laboratory workers, household contacts of a chronic carrier.	Live—nausea, abdominal discomfort, rash; inactivated—local pain and erythema, rare fever, malaise, headache.
Plague infected bacteria	One 1.0 ml IM dose followed by a 0.2 ml dose at 1 mo and another 3 to 6 mo after the second; if the exposure is ongoing 6 mo later, give two 0.2 ml doses 6 mo apart, then a dose every 1 to 2 yr.	Certain laboratory workers, certain travelers to high-risk areas.	Local erythema and pain, fever, malaise, headache (in 10%).
Anthrax inactivated bacteria	Six SC doses, three given at 2 wk intervals and three given at 6 mo intervals; yearly booster.	Persons working with imported animal hides.	Local erythema and pain.

CONTRAINDICATIONS	PREGNANCY*	HIV INFECTION	SEVERE IMMUNOCOMPROMISE†
Severe reaction to a previous dose.	No data; unknown risk to fetus.	Use if indicated; pooled IG may be preferred.	Use if indicated; pooled IG may be preferred.
Severe reaction to a previous dose; anaphylaxis to chicken eggs.	Postponement of travel is preferable; vaccinate if at high risk; attempt waiver if at low risk; unknown risk to fetus.	Contraindicated if HIV is symptomatic; weigh risk vs benefit if HIV is asymptomatic.	Contraindicated.
Severe reaction to a previous dose; persons with atopy are at risk of severe reactions.	Weigh risk vs benefit; unknown risk to fetus.	Weigh risk vs benefit.	Weigh risk vs benefit.
Severe reaction to a previous dose.	Use if high risk of infection; unknown risk to fetus.	Use if indicated.	Use if indicated.
None to date.	Use if high risk of infection; no confirmed risk to fetus.	Use parenteral if at high risk; oral is contraindicated.	Use parenteral if at high risk; oral is contraindicated.
Hypersensitivity to casein, beef protein, soya, phenol, or formaldehyde.	Use if high risk of infection; no reported risk to fetus.	Use if indicated.	Use if indicated.
Severe reaction to a previous dose.	No data; unknown risk to fetus.	Use if indicated.	Use if indicated.

Immunizations during Pregnancy

TABLE A-3 Immunization during Pregnancy

IMMUNOBIOLOGIC AGENT	RISK FROM DISEASE TO PREGNANT WOMAN	RISK FROM DISEASE TO FETUS OR NEONATE	TYPE OF IMMUNIZING AGENT	RISK FROM IMMUNIZING AGENT TO FETUS	INDICATIONS FOR IMMUNIZATION DURING PREGNANCY	DOSE SCHEDULE	COMMENTS
Live Virus Vaccines							
Measles	Significant morbidity, low mortality; not altered by pregnancy	Significant increase in abortion rate; may cause malformations	Live attenuated virus vaccine	None confirmed	Contraindicated (see immune globulins)	Single dose SC, preferably as measles-mumps-rubella*	Vaccination of susceptible women should be part of post-partum care
Mumps	Low morbidity and mortality; not altered by pregnancy	Probable increased rate of abortion in first trimester	Live attenuated virus vaccine	None confirmed	Contraindicated	Single dose SC, preferably as measles-mumps-rubella	Vaccination of susceptible women should be part of post-partum care
Poliomyelitis	No increased incidence in pregnancy, but may be more severe if it does occur	Anoxic fetal damage reported; 50% mortality in neonatal disease	Live attenuated virus (oral polio vaccine [OPV]) and enhanced potency inactivated virus (e-IPV) vaccine†	None confirmed	Not routinely recommended for women in US, except persons at increased risk of exposure	*Primary:* Two doses of e-IPV SC at 4-8 wk intervals and a third dose 6-12 mo after the second dose. *Immediate protection:* One dose OPV orally (in outbreak setting)	Vaccine indicated for susceptible pregnant women traveling in endemic areas or in other high-risk situations
Rubella	Low morbidity and mortality; not altered by pregnancy	High rate of abortion and congenital rubella syndrome	Live attenuated virus vaccine	None confirmed	Contraindicated	Single dose SC, preferably as measles-mumps-rubella	Teratogenicity of vaccine is theoretic, not confirmed to date; vaccination of susceptible women should be part of post-partum care
Yellow fever	Significant morbidity and mortality; not altered by pregnancy	Unknown	Live attenuated virus vaccine	Unknown	Contraindicated except if exposure is unavoidable	Single dose SC	Postponement of travel preferable to vaccination, if possible

Immunizations during pregnancy

Inactivated Virus Vaccines

Influenza	Possible increase in morbidity and mortality during epidemic of new antigenic strain	Possible increased abortion rate; no malformations confirmed	Inactivated virus vaccine	None confirmed	Women with serious underlying diseases; public health authorities to be consulted for current recommendation	One dose IM every year
Rabies	Near 100% fatality; not altered by pregnancy	Determined by maternal disease	Killed virus vaccine	Unknown	Indications for prophylaxis not altered by pregnancy; each case considered individually	Public health authorities to be consulted for indications, dosage, and route of administration
Hepatitis B	Possible increased severity during third trimester	Possible increase in abortion rate and prematurity; neonatal hepatitis can occur; high risk of newborn carrier state	Recombinant vaccine	None reported	Pre- and post-exposure for women at risk of infection	Three- or four-dose series IM	Used with hepatitis B immune globulin for some exposures; exposed newborn needs vaccination as soon as possible

Inactivated Bacterial Vaccines

Cholera	Significant morbidity and mortality; more severe during third trimester	Increased risk of fetal death during third-trimester maternal illness	Killed bacterial vaccine	None confirmed	Indications not altered by pregnancy; vaccination recommended only in unusual outbreak situations	Single dose SC or IM, depending on manufacturer's recommendations when indicated
Plague	Significant morbidity and mortality; not altered by pregnancy	Determined by maternal disease	Killed bacterial vaccine	None reported	Selective vaccination of exposed persons	Public health authorities to be consulted for indications, dosage, and route of administration

Continued

From *ACOG Technical Bulletin*, no. 160, Oct 1991.
*Two doses necessary for adequate vaccination of students entering institutions of higher education, newly hired medical personnel, and international travelers.
†Inactivated polio vaccine recommended for nonimmunized adults at increased risk.
SC, Subcutaneously; *PO*, orally; *IM*, intramuscularly; *ID*, intradermally.

TABLE A-3 Immunization during Pregnancy—cont'd

IMMUNOBIOLOGIC AGENT	RISK FROM DISEASE TO PREGNANT WOMAN	RISK FROM DISEASE TO FETUS OR NEONATE	TYPE OF IMMUNIZING AGENT	RISK FROM IMMUNIZING AGENT TO FETUS	INDICATIONS FOR IMMUNIZATION DURING PREGNANCY	DOSE SCHEDULE	COMMENTS
Inactivated Bacterial Vaccines—cont'd							
Pneumococcus	No increased risk during pregnancy; no increase in severity of disease	Unknown	Polyvalent polysaccharide vaccine	No data available on use during pregnancy	Indications not altered by pregnancy; vaccine used only for high-risk individuals	In adults, one SC or IM dose only; consider repeat dose in 6 yr for high-risk individuals	
Typhoid	Significant morbidity and mortality; not altered by pregnancy	Unknown	Killed or live attenuated oral bacterial vaccine	None confirmed	Not recommended routinely except for close, continued exposure or travel to endemic areas	*Killed;* *Primary:* Two injections SC at least 4 wk apart *Booster:* Single dose SC or ID (depending on type of product used) every 3 yr *Oral;* *Primary:* Four doses on alternate days *Booster:* Schedule not yet determined	
Toxoids							
Tetanus, diphtheria	Severe morbidity; tetanus mortality 30%, diphtheria mortality 10%; unaltered by pregnancy	Neonatal tetanus mortality 60%	Combined tetanus-diphtheria toxoids preferred: adult tetanus-diphtheria formulation	None confirmed	Lack of primary series, or no booster within past 10 yr	*Primary:* Two doses IM at 1-2 mo interval with a third dose 6-12 mo after the second *Booster:* Single dose IM every 10 yr, after completion of primary series	Updating of immune status should be part of antepartum care

Specific Immune Globulins

Hepatitis B	Possible increased severity during third trimester	Possible increase in abortion rate and prematurity; neonatal hepatitis can occur; high risk of carriage in newborn	Hepatitis B immune globulin	None reported	Postexposure prophylaxis	Depends on exposure; consult Immunization Practices Advisory Committee recommendations (IM)	Usually given with HBV vaccine; exposed newborn needs immediate postexposure prophylaxis
Rabies	Near 100% fatality; not altered by pregnancy	Determined by maternal disease	Rabies immune globulin	None reported	Postexposure prophylaxis	Half dose at injury site, half dose in deltoid	Used in conjunction with rabies killed virus vaccine
Tetanus	Severe morbidity; mortality 21%	Neonatal tetanus mortality 60%	Tetanus immune globulin	None reported	Postexposure prophylaxis	One dose IM	Used in conjunction with tetanus toxoid
Varicella	Possible increase in severe varicella pneumonia	Can cause congenital varicella with increased mortality in neonatal period; very rarely causes congenital defects	Varicella-zoster immune globulin (obtained from the American Red Cross)	None reported	Can be considered for healthy pregnant women exposed to varicella to protect against maternal, not congenital, infection	One dose IM within 96 hr of exposure	Indicated also for newborns of mothers who developed varicella within 4 days before delivery or 2 days after delivery; approximately 90%-95% of adults are immune to varicella; not indicated for prevention of congenital varicella

Continued

TABLE A-3 Immunization during Pregnancy—cont'd

Standard Immune Globulins

IMMUNOBIOLOGIC AGENT	RISK FROM DISEASE TO PREGNANT WOMAN	RISK FROM DISEASE TO FETUS OR NEONATE	TYPE OF IMMUNIZING AGENT	RISK FROM IMMUNIZING AGENT TO FETUS	INDICATIONS FOR IMMUNIZATION DURING PREGNANCY	DOSE SCHEDULE	COMMENTS
Hepatitis A	Possible increased severity during third trimester	Probable increase in abortion rate and prematurity; possible transmission to neonate at delivery if mother is incubating the virus or is acutely ill at that time	Standard immune globulin	None reported	Postexposure prophylaxis	0.02 ml/kg IM in one dose of immune globulin	Immune globulin should be given as soon as possible and within 2 wk of exposure; infants born to mothers who are incubating the virus or are acutely ill at delivery should receive one dose of 0.5 ml as soon as possible after birth
Measles	Significant morbidity, low mortality; not altered by pregnancy	Significant increase in abortion rate; may cause malformations	Standard immune globulin	None reported	Postexposure prophylaxis	0.25 ml/kg IM in one dose of immune globulin, up to 15 ml	Unclear if it prevents abortion; must be given within 6 days of exposure

Administration of Vaccines and Immune Globulins

TABLE A-4 Administration of Multiple Vaccines and Immune Globulins

VACCINE COMBINATION	RECOMMENDED MINIMUM INTERVAL BETWEEN DOSES
≥2 killed vaccines	None. May be administered simultaneously or at any interval between doses. (If possible, cholera, parenteral typhoid, and plague vaccines should be given on separate occasions to avoid accentuating their side effects.)
Killed and live vaccines	None. May be administered simultaneously or at any interval between doses. (Cholera vaccine with yellow fever vaccine is the exception. These vaccines should be given separately at least 3 wk apart; otherwise the antibody response to each may be suboptimal.)
≥2 live vaccines	May be administered simultaneously. If given separately, there must be an interval at least 4 wk between them. However, OPV can be administered at any time before, with, or after an MMR or oral typhoid, if indicated.
Live vaccine and PPD	May be administered simultaneously. If given separately, the PPD should be given 4 to 6 wk after the live vaccine.
Immune globulin and killed vaccine	None. May be administered simultaneously or at any interval between doses.
Immune globulin and live vaccine	Should not be given together. The live vaccine should be given a minimum of 2 wk before the immune globulin. If the live vaccine is to be given after the immune globulin, the minimum time that should elapse between administration is dose dependent and is outlined in Table 8-5. Of note, OPV, oral typhoid, and yellow fever are exceptions to these recommendations and can be given any time before, during, or after an immune globulin-containing product.

Modified from *MMWR* 43(RR-1):15-16, 1994.

Administration of vaccines and immune globulins

TABLE A-5 Suggested Intervals between Administration of Immune Globulin Preparations for Various Indications and Vaccines Containing Live Measles Virus*

INDICATION	DOSE (INCLUDING MG IgG/KG)	TIME INTERVAL (MO) BEFORE MEASLES VACCINATION
Tetanus (TIG) prophylaxis	250 units (10 mg IgG/kg) IM	3
Hepatitis A (IG) prophylaxis		
Contact prophylaxis	0.02 ml/kg (3.3 mg IgG/kg) IM	3
International travel	0.06 ml/kg (10 mg IgG/kg) IM	3
Hepatitis B prophylaxis (HBIG)	0.06 ml/kg (10 mg IgG/kg) IM	3
Rabies immune globulin (HRIG)	20 IU/kg (22 mg IgG/kg) IM	4
Varicella prophylaxis (VZIG)	125 units/10 kg (20-40 mg IgG/kg) IM (maximum 625 units)	5
Measles prophylaxis (IG)		
Standard (i.e., nonimmunocompromised contact)	0.25 ml/kg (40mg IgG/kg) IM	5
Immunocompromised contact	0.50 ml/kg (80 mg IgG/kg) IM	6
Blood transfusion:		
Red blood cells (RBCs), washed	10 ml/kg (negligible IgG/kg) IV	0
RBCs, adenine-saline added	10 ml/kg (10 mg IgG/kg) IV	3
Packed RBCs (Hct 65%)†	10 ml/kg (60 mg IgG/kg) IV	6
Whole blood cells (Hct 35%-50%)†	10 ml/kg (80-100 mg IgG/kg) IV	6
Plasma/platelet products	10 ml/kg (160 mg IgG/kg) IV	7
Replacement therapy for immune deficiencies	300-400 mg/kg IV‡ (as IGIV)	8
Treatment of:		
Immune thrombocytopenic purpura§	400 mg/kg IV (as IGIV)	8
Immune thrombocytopenic purpura§	1000 mg/kg IV (as IGIV)	10
Kawasaki disease	2 g/kg IV (as IGIV)	11

From *MMWR* 45(RR-12),1996.
*This table is not intended for determining the correct indications and dosage for the use of immune globulin preparations. Unvaccinated persons may not be fully protected against measles during the entire suggested time interval, and additional doses of immune globulin and/or measles vaccine may be indicated after measles exposure. The concentration of measles antibody in a particular immune globulin preparation can vary by lot. The rate of antibody clearance after receipt of an immune globulin preparation also can vary. The recommended time intervals are extrapolated from an estimated half-life of 30 days for passively acquired antibody and an observed interference with the immune response to measles vaccine for 5 mo after a dose of 80 mg IgG/kg.
†Assumes a serum IgG concentration of 16 mg/ml.
‡Measles vaccination is recommended for most HIV-infected children who do not have evidence of severe immunosuppression, but it is contraindicated for patients who have congenital disorders of the immune system.
§Formerly referred to as idiopathic thrombocytopenic purpura.

Vaccinations for International Travel

TABLE A-6 Vaccinations for International Travel

DISEASE*	AREAS AFFECTED†	PROPHYLAXIS RECOMMENDED‡
Tetanus	All	All travelers: vaccine series/booster.
Measles	All	Born after 1956: ensure immunity by antibody titer, diagnosed measles, or two doses of vaccine.
Rubella	All	All travelers: ensure immunity by antibody titer or vaccine.
Mumps	All	Born after 1956: ensure immunity by antibody titer, diagnosed mumps, or one dose of vaccine.
Poliomyelitis	Developing countries not in the western hemisphere but including Peru and Colombia; tropics at risk all year; temperate zones have increased cases in summer and fall	All travelers: vaccine series/booster.
Hepatitis B	5%-20% of population are carriers—Africa, Middle East except Israel, all Southeast Asia, Amazon basin, Haiti, Dominican Republic; 1%-5% of population are carriers—South Central and Southwest Asia, Israel, Japan, the Americas, Russia, eastern and southern Europe	Travelers for more than 6 mo and having close contact with the population or staying less time but having higher risk activities (sex, close household contact, seeking dental or medical care): vaccine series.
Hepatitis A	Developing countries	Travelers to rural areas, eating and drinking in settings of poor sanitation: hepatitis A vaccine or pooled IG prophylaxis.
Influenza	Tropics throughout the year; southern hemisphere April to September	Travelers for whom vaccine is otherwise indicated: give the current vaccine and revaccinate in fall as usual.
Meningococcus*	Tanzania, Kenya, sub-Saharan Africa from Mali to Ethiopia; required for pilgrims to Mecca, Saudi Arabia, during the hajj	All travelers: vaccine.
Rabies	Endemic dog rabies exist in parts of Mexico, El Salvador, Guatemala, Peru, Colombia, Ecuador, India, Nepal, Philippines, Sri Lanka, Thailand, Viet Nam	Travelers staying for more than 30 days or at high risk of exposure: vaccine series/booster.
Yellow fever*	North and central South America, forest-savannah zones of Africa, some countries in Africa, Asia and Middle East require travelers from endemic areas to be vaccinated	All travelers: vaccine/booster at approved Yellow Fever Vaccination Center.
Japanese encephalitis	Seasonally in most areas of Asia; in temperate zones the incidence is increased in summer and early fall; in the tropics occurs all year	Travelers to high-risk rural areas, staying outdoors or during the transmission season: vaccine series.
Cholera*	Certain undeveloped countries	If required by local authorities, one dose usually suffices. Primary series only for those living in high-risk areas under poor sanitary conditions or those with compromised gastric defense mechanisms (achlorhydria, antacid therapy or previous ulcer surgery): booster every 6 mo.
Typhoid fever	Many countries of Asia, Africa, Central and South America	Travelers with prolonged stay in rural areas with poor sanitation: vaccine series/booster.
Plague	Africa, Asia, Americas in rural mountainous or upland areas	Travelers with research or field activities that bring them in contact with rodents: vaccine series/booster. Consider taking tetracycline (500 mg qid) for chemoprophylaxis (inferred from clinical experience in treating plague).

From Noble J (ed): *Primary care medicine*, ed 2, St Louis, 1996, Mosby.

*Only yellow fever vaccine is required for entry by any country, cholera vaccine may be required by some local authorities, and meningococcus vaccine is only required for pilgrims to Mecca, Saudi Arabia, during the hajj. However, it is important to follow the recommendations for other vaccines for disease prevention. If a required vaccine is contraindicated or withheld for any reason, attempts should be made to obtain a waiver from the country's consulate or embassy.

†Because areas affected can change, and for more specific details, consult the CDC's traveler's hotline or the most recent edition of *Health Information for the International Traveler*.

‡For detailed information concerning the administration of individual vaccines, consult the text under each vaccine.

Hepatitis B Prophylaxis

TABLE A-7 Recommendations for Hepatitis B Prophylaxis after Percutaneous or Permucosal Exposure to Blood

EXPOSED PERSON	TREATMENT OF EXPOSED PERSON BASED ON STATUS OF SOURCE		
	HBsAG-POSITIVE SOURCE	HBsAG-NEGATIVE SOURCE	SOURCE NOT TESTED OR SOURCE UNKNOWN
Unvaccinated	One dose of HBIG*; initiate hepatitis B vaccine†	Initiate hepatitis B vaccine†	Initiate hepatitis B vaccine†
Previously vaccinated			
Known responder	Test exposed person for anti-HBsAg‡ 1. If adequate, no treatment 2. If inadequate, hepatitis B vaccine booster dose	No treatment	No treatment
Known nonresponder	Two doses of HBIG or one dose of HBIG plus one dose of hepatitis B vaccine	No treatment	If known high-risk source, may treat as if source were HBsAg positive
Response unknown	Test exposed person for anti-HBsAg† 1. If adequate, no treatment 2. If inadequate, one dose of HBIG plus hepatitis B vaccine booster dose	No treatment	Test exposed person for anti-HBsAg‡ 1. If adequate, no treatment 2. If inadequate, hepatitis B vaccine booster dose

Adapted from Recommendations of the Immunization Practices Advisory Committee (ACIP): *MMWR* 40(RR-13):22, 1991.
*HBIG dose, 0.006 ml/kg intramuscularly.
†See Table 8-8 for hepatitis B vaccine dose.
‡Adequate anti-HBsAg level is ≥10 mIU.
HBsAg, Hepatitis B surface antigen; *anti-HBsAg*, antibody to hepatitis B surface antigen; *HBIG*, hepatitis B immune globulin.

TABLE A-8 Recommended Doses of Currently Licensed Hepatitis B Vaccines

POPULATION GROUP	RECOMBIVAX HB* DOSE IN µG (DOSE IN ML)	ENGERIX-B* DOSE IN µG (DOSE IN ML)
Infants of HBsAg-negative mothers and children <11 yr	2.5 (0.25)	10 (0.5)
Infants of HBsAg-positive mothers; prevention of perinatal infection	5 (0.5)	10 (0.5)
Children and adolescents 11-19 yr	5 (0.5)	20 (1.0)
Adults ≥20 yr	10 (1.0)	20 (1.0)
Dialysis patients and other immunocompromised persons	40†	40‡

Adapted from Recommendations of the Immunization Practices Advisory Committee (ACIP): *MMWR* 40(RR-13):7, 1991.
*Both vaccines are routinely administered in a three-dose series of 0, 1, and 6 mo. Engerix-B is also licensed for a four-dose series administered at 0, 1, 2, and 12 mo.
†Special formulation.
‡Two 1.0 ml doses administered at one site in a four-dose schedule at 0, 1, 2, and 6 mo.

TABLE A-9 Recommended Schedule of Hepatitis B Immunoprophylaxis to Prevent Perinatal Transmission

POPULATION GROUP	VACCINE DOSE	AGE OF INFANT
Infants born to HBsAg-positive mothers	First dose	Birth (within 12 hr)
	HBIG†	Birth (within 12 hr)
	Second dose	1 mo
	Third dose	6 mo‡
Infants born to mothers not screened for HBsAg§	First dose	Birth (within 12 hr)
	HBIG‡	If mother is HBsAg positive, administer HBIG to infant as soon as possible, not later than 1 wk after birth
	Second dose	1-2 mo‖
	Third dose	6 mo‡

Adapted from Recommendations of the Immunization Practices Advisory Committee (ACIP): *MMWR* 40(RR-13):12, 1991.
*See Table 8-8 for appropriate vaccine dose.
†HBIG is given in a dose of 0.5 ml, administered intramuscularly at a site different from that used for vaccine.
‡If four-dose schedule (Engerix-B) is used, the third dose is administered at 2 mo of age and the fourth dose at 12-18 mo.
§First vaccine dose is the same as the dose for an HBsAg-positive mother (see Table 8-8). If mother is HBsAg positive, continue that dose; if mother is HBsAg negative, use appropriate dose from Table 8-8.
‖Infants of women who are HBsAg negative can be vaccinated at 2 mo of age.
HbsAg, Hepatitis B surface antigen; *HBIG,* hepatitis B immune globulin.

HIV Chemoprophylaxis after Occupational Exposure

TABLE A-10 HIV Chemoprophylaxis after Occupational Exposure

TYPE OF EXPOSURE	SOURCE	ANTIRETROVIRAL PROPHYLAXIS	REGIMEN
Percutaneous	Blood		
	Highest risk*	Recommend	AZT† plus 3TC plus IDV
	Increased risk	Recommend	AZT plus 3TC ± IDV‡
	No increased risk	Offer	AZT plus 3TC
	Fluid containing visible blood, other potentially infectious fluid, or tissue	Offer	AZT plus 3TC
	Other body fluid (e.g., urine)	Do not offer	
Mucous membrane	Blood	Offer	AZT plus 3TC ± IDV‡
	Fluid containing visible blood, other potentially infectious fluid, or tissue	Offer	AZT ± 3TC
	Other body fluid (e.g., urine)	Do not offer	
Skin, increased risk§	Blood	Offer	AZT plus 3TC ± IDV‡
	Fluid containing visible blood, other potentially infectious fluid, or tissue	Offer	AZT ± 3TC
	Other body fluid (e.g., urine)	Do not offer	

From Update: Provisional Public Health Service recommendations for chemoprophylaxis after occupational exposure to HIV, *MMWR* 45:468-472, 1996.
*Highest risk, both large volume of blood and blood containing high HIV titer; increased risk, exposure to either large volume of blood or high HIV titer; no increased risk, neither large blood volume nor high HIV titer.
†Regimens include AZT, 200 mg tid; 3TC, 150 mg bid; IDV, 800 mg tid (or saquinavir mesylate [Invirase], 600 mg tid if IDV is not available.) Treatment should continue for 4 wk.
‡Possible toxicity of additional drug may not be warranted.
§Prolonged contact, extensive area of contact, skin integrity compromised, or high titer of HIV in blood or other fluids.
AZT, Zidovudine (Retrovir); *3TC,* lamivudine (Epivir); *IDV,* indinavir sulfate (Crixivan).

Endocarditis Prophylaxis

> **BOX A-1 Cardiac Conditions Associated With Endocarditis**
>
> **Endocarditis Prophylaxis Recommended**
> *High-Risk Category*
>
> Prosthetic cardiac valves, including bioprosthetic and homograft valves
> Previous bacterial endocarditis
> Complex cyanotic congenital heart disease (e.g., single ventricle states, transposition of the great arteries, tetralogy of Fallot)
> Surgically constructed systemic pulmonary shunts or conduits
>
> *Moderate-Risk Category*
>
> Most other congenital cardiac malformations (other than above and below)
> Acquired valvar dysfunction (e.g., rheumatic heart disease)
> Hypertrophic cardiomyopathy
> Mitral valve prolapse with valvar regurgitation and/or thickened leaflets
>
> **Endocarditis Prophylaxis Not Recommended**
> *Negligible-Risk Category (No Greater Risk Than the General Population)*
>
> Isolated secundum atrial septal defect
> Surgical repair of atrial septal defect, ventricular defect, or patent ductus arteriosus (without residua beyond 6 mo)
> Previous coronary artery bypass graft surgery
> Mitral valve prolapse without valvar regurgitation
> Physiologic, functional, or innocent heart murmurs
> Previous Kawasaki disease without valvar dysfunction
> Previous rheumatic fever without valvar dysfunction
> Cardiac pacemakers (intravascular and epicardial) and implanted defibrillators

From Dajani AS et al: Prevention of bacterial endocarditis, recommendations by the American Heart Association, *JAMA* 277:1794-1801, 1997.

> **BOX A-2 Dental Procedures and Endocarditis Prophylaxis**
>
> **Endocarditis Prophylaxis Recommended***
>
> Dental extractions
> Periodontal procedures including surgery, scaling and root planing, probing, and recall maintenance
> Dental implant placement and reimplantation of avulsed teeth
> Endodontic (root canal) instrumentation of surgery only beyond the apex
> Subgingival placement of antibiotic fibers or strips
> Initial placement of orthodontic bands—but not brackets
> Intraligamentary local anesthetic injections
> Prophylactic cleaning of teeth or implants where bleeding is anticipated
>
> **Endocarditis Prophylaxis Not Recommended**
>
> Restorative dentistry† (operative and prosthodontic) with or without retraction cord‡
> Local anesthetic injections (nonintraligamentary)
> Intracanal endodontic treatment; post–placement and buildup
> Placement of rubber dams
> Postoperative suture removal
> Placement of removable prosthodontic or orthodontic appliances
> Taking of oral impressions
> Fluoride treatments
> Taking of oral radiographs
> Orthodontic appliance adjustment
> Shedding of primary teeth

From Dajani AS et al: Prevention of bacterial endocarditis, recommendations by the American Heart Association, *JAMA* 277:1794-1801, 1997.
*Prophylaxis is recommended for patients with high- and moderate-risk cardiac conditions.
†This includes restoration of decayed teeth (filling cavities) and replacement of missing teeth.
‡Clinical judgment may indicate antibiotic use in selected circumstances that may create significant bleeding.

BOX A-3 Other Procedures and Endocarditis Prophylaxis

Endocarditis Prophylaxis Recommended

Respiratory tract

Tonsillectomy and/or adenoidectomy
Surgical operations that involve respiratory mucosa
Bronchoscopy with a rigid bronchoscope

Gastrointestinal Tract*

Sclerotherapy for esophageal varices
Esophageal stricture dilation
Endoscopic retrograde cholangiography* with biliary obstruction
Biliary tract surgery
Surgical operations that involve intestinal mucosa

Genitourinary Tract

Prostatic surgery
Cystoscopy
Urethral dilation

Endocarditis Prophylaxis Not Recommended

Respiratory Tract

Endotracheal intubation
Bronchoscopy with a flexible bronchoscope, with or without biopsy†
Tympanostomy tube insertion

Gastrointestinal Tract

Transesophageal echocardiography†
Endoscopy with or without gastrointestinal biopsy†

Genitourinary Tract

Vaginal hysterectomy†
Vaginal delivery†
Cesarean section
In uninfected tissue:
  Urethral catheterization
  Uterine dilatation and curettage
  Therapeutic abortion
  Sterilization procedures
  Insertion or removal of intrauterine devices

Other

Cardiac catheterization, including balloon angioplasty
Implanted cardiac pacemakers, implanted defibrillators, and coronary stents
Incision or biopsy of surgically scrubbed skin
Circumcision

From Dajani AS et al: Prevention of bacterial endocarditis, recommendations by the American Heart Association, *JAMA* 277:1794-1801, 1997.
*Prophylaxis is recommended for high-risk patients; optional for medium-risk patients.
†Prophylaxis is optional for high-risk patients.

TABLE A-11 Prophylactic Regimens for Dental, Oral, Respiratory Tract, or Esophageal Procedures

SITUATION	AGENT	REGIMEN*
Standard general prophylaxis	Amoxicillin	Adults: 2.0 g; children: 50 mg/kg orally 1 h before procedure
Unable to take oral medications	Ampicillin	Adults: 2.0 g intramuscularly (IM) or intravenously (IV); children: 50 mg/kg IM or IV within 30 min before procedure
Allergic to penicillin	Clindamycin or	Adults: 600 mg; children: 20 mg/kg orally 1 h before procedure
	Cephalexin† or cefadroxil† or	Adults: 2.0 g; children: 50 mg/kg orally 1 h before procedure
	Azithromycin or clarithromycin	Adults: 500 mg; children: 15 mg/kg orally 1 h before procedure
Allergic to penicillin and unable to take oral medications	Clindamycin or	Adults: 600 mg; children: 20 mg/kg IV within 30 min before procedure
	Cefazolin†	Adults 1.0 g; children: 25 mg/kg IM or IV within 30 min before procedure

From Dajani AS et al: Prevention of bacterial endocarditis, recommendations by the American Heart Association, *JAMA* 277:1794-1801, 1997.
*Total children's dose should not exceed adult dose.
†Cephalosporins should not be used in individuals with immediate-type hypersensitivity reaction (urticaria, angioedema, or anaphylaxis) to penicillins.

TABLE A-12 Prophylactic Regimens or Genitourinary Gastrointestinal (Excluding Esophageal) Procedures

SITUATION	AGENTS*	REGIMEN†
High-risk patients	Ampicillin plus gentamicin	Adults: ampicillin 2.0 g intramuscularly (IM) or intravenously (IV) plus gentamicin 1.5 mg/kg (not to exceed 120 mg) within 30 min of starting the procedure; 6 h later, ampicillin 1 g IM/IV or amoxicillin 1 g orally
		Children: ampicillin 50 mg/kg IM or IV (not to exceed 2.0 g) plus gentamicin 1.5 mg/kg within 30 min of starting the procedure; 6 h later, ampicillin 25 mg/kg IM/IV or amoxicillin 25 mg/kg orally
High-risk patients allergic	Vancomycin plus gentamicin	Adults: vancomycin 1.0 g IV over 1-2 h plus gentamicin 1.5 mg/kg IV/IM (not to exceed 120 mg); complete injection/infusion within 30 min of starting the procedure
		Children: vancomycin 20 mg/kg IV over 1-2 h plus gentamicin 1.5 mg/kg IV/IM; complete injection/infusion within 30 min of starting the procedure
Moderate-risk patients	Amoxicillin or ampicillin	Adults: amoxicillin 2.0 g orally 1 h before procedure, or ampicillin 2.0 g IV/IV within 30 min of starting the procedure
		Children: amoxicillin 50 mg/kg orally 1 h before procedure, or ampicillin 50 mg/kg IM/IV within 30 min of starting the procedure
Moderate-risk patients allergic to ampicillin/amoxicillin	Vancomycin	Adults: vancomycin 1.0 g IV over 1-2 h; complete infusion within 30 min of starting the procedure
		Children: vancomycin 20 mg/kg IV over 1-2 h; complete infusion within 30 min of starting the procedure

From Dajani AS et al: Prevention of bacterial endocarditis, recommendations by the American Heart Association, *JAMA* 277:1794-1801, 1997.
*Total children's dose should not exceed adult dose.
†No second dose of vacomycin or gentamicin is recommended.

PATIENT EVALUATION
Mini-Mental State Examination

Mini–Mental State Examination

I. Orientation (maximum score: 10)
Ask "What is today's date?" Then ask specifically for parts omitted, such as "Can you also tell me what season it is?"

Ask "Can you tell me the name of this hospital?"
"What floor are we on?"
"What town (or city) are we in?"
"What county are we in?"
"What state are we in?"

II. Registration (maximum score: 3)
Ask the patient if you may test his memory. Then say "ball," "flag," "tree" clearly and slowly, allowing about 1 sec for each. After you have said all three words, ask the patient to repeat them. This first repetition determines the score (0–3), but continue to say them (up to six trials) until the patient can repeat all three words. If he does not eventually learn all three, recall cannot be meaningfully tested.

III. Attention and calculation (maximum score: 5)
Ask the patient to begin at 100 and count backward by 7. Stop after five subtractions (93, 86, 79, 72, 65). Score one point for each correct number.

If the subject cannot or will not perform this task, ask him to spell the word "world" backward (D, L, R, O, W). Score one point for each correctly placed letter, e.g. DLROW = 5, DLORW = 3.
Record how the patient spelled "world" backward: _____
   D L R O W

IV. Recall (maximum score: 3)
Ask the patient to recall the three words you previously asked him to remember (learned in Registration).

V. Language (maximum score: 9)
Naming: Show the patient a wristwatch and ask "What is this?" Repeat for a pencil. Score one point for each item named correctly.

Repetition: Ask the patient to repeat "No if's, and's or but's. "Score one point for correct repetition.

Three–stage command: Give the patient a piece of blank paper and say "Take the paper in your right hand, fold it in half and put it on the floor." Score one point for each action performed correctly.

Reading: On a blank piece of paper, print the sentence "Close your eyes" in letters large enough for the patient to see clearly. Ask the patient to read it and do what it says. Score correct only if he actually closes his eyes.

Writing: Give the patient a blank piece of paper and ask him to write a sentence. It is to be written spontaneously. It must contain a subject and verb and make sense. Correct grammar and punctuation are not necessary.

Copying: On a clean piece of paper, draw intersecting pentagons as illustrated, each side measuring about 1 inch, and ask the patient to copy it exactly as it is. All 10 angles must be present and two must intersect to score 1 point. Tremor and rotation are ignored.

Date (e.g., January 21)........ 1 ____
Year .... 2 ____
Month .... 3 ____
Day (e.g., Monday) .... 4 ____
Season .... 5 ____
Hospital .... 6 ____
Floor .... 7 ____
Town/city .... 8 ____
County .... 9 ____
State.................................. 10 ____

"ball" .... 11 ____
"flag" .... 12 ____
"tree" .... 13 ____

Number of trials: _____

"93" .... 14 ____
"86" .... 15 ____
"79" .... 16 ____
"72" .... 17 ____
"65" .... 18 ____
       or
Number of correctly
placed letters.................... 19 ____

"ball" .... 20 ____
"flag" .... 21 ____
"tree" .... 22 ____

Watch .... 23 ____
Pencil................................ 24 ____

Repetition .... 25 ____

Takes in right hand........... 26 ____
Folds in half...................... 27 ____
Puts on the floor............... 28 ____

Closes eyes .... 29 ____

Writes sentence................ 30 ____

Draws pentagons .... 31 ____

Score: Add number of correct responses. In Section III, include items 14 through 18 or item 19, not both. (maximum total score: 30).

Total score: _____

Level of consciousness: ____coma ____stupor ____drowsy ____alert

Interpretation: Traditionally, using a cutoff score of 23 out of 30, the sensitivity and specificity of the MMSE has been reported to be 87% and 82%, respectively, for detecting delirium or dementia in hospitalized patients. However, cognitive performance as measured by the MMSE varies within the population by age and education. To adjust for these variables it has been proposed that a cutoff score of 19 is appropriate for those with 0-4 yr of schooling and will identify those individuals performing below the level of 75% of their peers; the cutoff score should be 23 for those with 5-8 yr of education, 27 for those with 9-12 yr of schooling. A score below 29 would be abnormal in 75% of those with a college education.

Fig. A-1 Mini-mental state examination. (From Folstein MF, Folstein SE, McHugh PR: Mini-mental state: a practical method for grading the cognitive state of patients for the clinician, *J Psychiatr Res* 12:189-198, 1975.)

Orthopedic Maneuvers

> **BOX A-4** **Orthopedic Maneuvers**
>
> **Knee Valgus Stress Test** — To test medial collateral ligament
> - Patient: Supine, leg extended and supported by examiner
> - Examiner: Beside extremity tested, with one hand on distal lateral femur and other on medial tibia below the joint line
> - Technique: Apply medial pressure on femur while distracting tibia laterally. Note amount of opening of medial knee. It should be minimal. Compare with other leg.
>
> **Knee Varus Stress Test** — To test lateral collateral ligament
> - Patient: Supine, leg extended and supported by examiner
> - Examiner: Beside extremity tested, with one hand on distal medial femur and other on the lateral tibia below the joint line
> - Technique: Apply lateral pressure on the femur while distracting the tibia medially. Note amount of opening of lateral knee. It should be minimal. Compare to other leg.
>
> **Straight Leg Raise** — To test for protrusion of disk causing radicular pain
> - Patient: Supine
> - Examiner: Gently hold leg at knee and ankle
> - Technique: Slowly raise the leg through 60 degrees of motion. Pain will be felt if positive between 30 and 60 degrees in back, hip, and leg.
>
> **Spurling Test** — To test for cervical or foramen restriction
> - Patient: Seated on stool
> - Examiner: Standing with hands on patient's head
> - Technique: Apply downward pressure with neck straight, left, left posterior, right, right posterior. Elicited pain or neurologic symptom is positive test.
>
> **McMurray Sign** — To test for tears in medial and lateral menisci
> - Patient: Supine and relaxed with knee completely bent
> - Examiner: Standing at the side of the injured limb
> - Technique: Grasp the heel and rotate the foot externally while abducting the leg and extending the knee. A click or pain is significant for lateral tear. Opposite maneuver can be positive for medial tear and is done by rotating the foot internally and abducting the leg while extending the knee.
>
> **Apprehension Test** — To test for patella subluxation
> - Patient: Seated
> - Examiner: Hand on affected patella
> - Technique: Gently push the patella laterally. A start of apprehension is positive. If negative, examiner can extend the knee and then passively flex the knee while gently pushing the patella laterally.
>
> **Anterior Drawer Sign** — To test the anterior cruciate
> - Patient: Supine, hip flexed 45 degrees, knee flexed 90 degrees
> - Examiner: Sitting on patient's ipsilateral foot
> - Technique: Place hands around the tibia just below the joint line. Apply anterior force and note the amount of anterior motion. Always compare with other knee.
>
> **Lachman Test** — When the knee cannot be flexed
> - Patient: Supine, hip, and knee extended
> - Examiner: Standing beside patient
> - Technique: Grasp the femur with one hand and the tibia below the joint line. Apply a distracting force to the tibia and note the excursion.
>
> **Posterior Drawer Sign** — To test the posterior cruciate
> - Patient: Supine, hip flexed 45 degrees, knee flexed 90 degrees
> - Examiner: Sitting on patient's ipsilateral foot
> - Technique: Same as anterior drawer sign, except apply posterior force on tibia.

From Driscoll CE et al: *The family practice desk reference*, ed 3, St Louis, 1996, Mosby.

Office Hearing Tests

TABLE A-13 Office Hearing Tests

TEST	METHOD	INTERPRETATION
Weber's test	512 Hz tuning fork placed on top of the head; patient is asked which ear tone is heard	*Normal:* sound heard in midline *Conductive loss:* sound heard on affected side *Neurosensory loss:* sound heard on unaffected side
Rinne's test	512 Hz tuning fork held against mastoid; when sound is no longer heard, duration of bone conduction is noted; fork transferred to ½ inch from ear; air conduction should be twice as long as bone and louder	*Air > bone:* normal (+) test *Bone > air:* conductive hearing loss (−) test
Whispered voice	Occlude opposite ear; whisper softly, from 2 feet away; do not use a question that is answered by "yes" or "no"	Usually indicates 20 dB hearing loss if not perceived
Watch tick	Hold watch 2 inches from ear	Indicates high-frequency loss if not perceived; if heard, 98% chance of hearing all lower frequencies normally
Schwabach's test	512 Hz tuning fork is pressed alternately to examiner's mastoid, then to patient's mastoid	When hearing is normal, both patient and examiner cease to hear the tuning fork at the same time; if patient hears the tuning fork longer than an examiner with normal hearing, this indicates middle ear (conductive) loss; if examiner with normal hearing hears the tuning fork longer, the patient has sensorineural loss

From Driscoll CE et al: *The family practice desk reference,* ed 3, St Louis, 1996, Mosby.

Screening of Geriatric Patients for Hearing Handicaps

BOX A-5 **Hearing Handicap Inventory for the Elderly-Screening Version (HHIE-S)***

	YES (4)	SOMETIMES (2)	NO (0)
1. Does a hearing problem cause you to feel embarrassed when meeting new people?	___	___	___
2. Does a hearing problem cause you to feel frustrated when talking to members of your family?	___	___	___
3. Do you have difficulty hearing when someone speaks in a whisper?	___	___	___
4. Do you feel handicapped by a hearing problem?	___	___	___
5. Does a hearing problem cause you difficulty when visiting friends, relatives, or neighbors?	___	___	___
6. Does a hearing problem cause you to attend religious services less often than you would like?	___	___	___
7. Does a hearing problem cause you to have arguments with family members?	___	___	___
8. Does a hearing problem cause you difficulty when listening to TV or radio?	___	___	___
9. Do you feel that any difficulty with your hearing limits or hampers your personal or social life?	___	___	___
10. Does a hearing problem cause you difficulty when in a restaurant with relatives or friends?	___	___	___

From Ventry IM, Weinstein BE: Identification of elderly people with hearing problems, *Am Speech-Language-Hearing Assoc* 25:37, 1983.
*Range of total points, 0-40; 0-8, no self-perceived handicap; 10-22, mild to moderate handicap; 24-40, significant handicap.

International Prostate Symptom Score (I-PSS)

Patient name:	Not at all	Less than 1 time in 5	Less than half the time	About half the time	More than half the time	Almost always	Your score
1. Incomplete emptying Over the past month, how often have you had a sensation of not emptying your bladder completely after you finished urinating?	0	1	2	3	4	5	
2. Frequency Over the past month, how often have you had to urinate again less than 2 hr after you finished urinating?	0	1	2	3	4	5	
3. Intermittency Over the past month, how often have you found you stopped and started again several times when you urinated?	0	1	2	3	4	5	
4. Urgency Over the past month, how often have you found it difficult to postpone urination?	0	1	2	3	4	5	
5. Weak stream Over the past month, how often have you had a weak urinary stream?	0	1	2	3	4	5	
6. Straining Over the past month, how often have you had to push or strain to begin urination?	0	1	2	3	4	5	

	None	1 time	2 times	3 times	4 times	5 or more times	
7. Nocturia Over the past month, how many times did you most typically get up to urinate from the time you went to bed at night until the time you got up in the morning?	0	1	2	3	4	5	
Total I-PSS score =							

Quality of life due to urinary symptoms	Delighted	Pleased	Mostly satisfied	Mixed—about equally satisfied and dissatisfied	Mostly dissatisfied	Unhappy	Terrible
If you were to spend the rest of your life with your urinary condition just the way it is now, how would you feel about that?	0	1	2	3	4	5	6

The I-PSS is based on the answers to seven questions concerning urinary symptoms.
Each question allows the patient to choose one out of five answers indicating increasing severity of the particular symptom. The answers are assigned points from 0 to 5. The total score can therefore range from 0 to 35 (asymptomatic to very symptomatic).
Furthermore, the International Consensus Committee (ICC) recommends the use of only a single question to assess the quality of life. The answers to this question range from "delighted" to "terrible" or 0 to 6. Although this single question may or may not capture the global impact of BPH symptoms or quality of life, it may serve as a valuable starting point for a doctor-patient conversation.
The ICC strongly recommends that all physicians who counsel patients suffering from symptoms of prostatism use these measures not only during the intitial interview but also during and after treatment to monitor treatment response.

Fig. A-2 **International prostate symptom score (I-PSS).** (From Noble J (ed): *Textbook of primary care medicine,* ed 2, St Louis, 1996, Mosby.)

Katz Index of Activities of Daily Living

> **BOX A-6 Katz Index of Activities of Daily Living***
>
> 1. **Bathing (sponge bath, tub bath, or shower)**
>   a. Receives no assistance (gets in and out of tub by self if tub is usual means of bathing)
>   b. Receives assistance in bathing only one part of body such as the back or a leg
>   c. Receives assistance in bathing more than one part of body or is not bathed
> 2. **Continence**
>   a. Controls urination and bowel movement completely by self
>   b. Has occasional "accidents"
>   c. Needs supervision to keep urine or bowel control, uses catheter, or is incontinent
> 3. **Dressing (gets clothes from closets and drawers, including underclothes, outer garments; uses fasteners, including braces, if worn)**
>   a. Gets clothes and gets completely dressed without assistance
>   b. Gets clothes and gets dressed without assistance except in tying shoes
>   c. Receives assistance in getting clothes or getting dressed or stays partly or completely undressed
> 4. **Eating**
>   a. Feeds self without assistance
>   b. Feeds self except for assistance in cutting meat or buttering bread
>   c. Receives assistance in feeding or is fed partly or completely by using tubes or intravenous fluids
> 5. **Toileting (going to the "toilet room" for bowel and urine elimination; cleaning self after elimination and arranging clothes)**
>   a. Goes to "toilet room," cleans self, and arranges clothes without assistance (may use object for support such as cane, walker, or wheelchair and may manage night bedpan or commode and emptying same in morning)
>   b. Receives assistance in going to "toilet room," cleaning self, or arranging clothes after elimination or receives assistance in using night bedpan or commode
>   c. Does not go to room termed "toilet" for the elimination process
> 6. **Transferring**
>   a. Moves in and out of bed or chair without assistance (may use object for support such as cane or walker)
>   b. Moves in and out of bed or chair with assistance
>   c. Does not get out of bed

*Response *a*, 3 points; *b*, 2 points; *c*, 1 point; maximum score, 18 points.

Evaluation for Alcohol Abuse

BOX A-7 Short Michigan Alcoholism Screening Test (SMAST)

	YES	NO
1. Do you feel you are a normal drinker? (By normal we mean do you drink less than or as much as most other people.)	(0 point)	(1 point)
2. Do others who are important to you ever worry or complain about your drinking?	(1 point)	(0 point)
3. Do you ever feel bad about your drinking?	(1 point)	(0 point)
4. Do friends or relatives think you are a normal drinker?	(0 point)	(1 point)
5. Are you always able to stop drinking when you want to?	(0 point)	(1 point)
6. Have you ever attended a meeting of Alcoholics Anonymous (AA) for yourself?	(3 points)	(0 point)
7. Has your drinking ever created problems between you and others who are important to you?	(1 point)	(0 point)
8. Have you ever gotten into trouble at work because of your drinking?	(1 point)	(0 point)
9. Have you ever neglected your obligations, your family, or your work for 2 or more days in a row because you were drinking?	(1 point)	(0 point)
10. Have you ever gone to anyone for help about your drinking?	(3 points)	(0 point)
11. Have you ever been in a hospital because of your drinking?	(3 points)	(0 point)
12. Have you ever been arrested for drunken driving, driving while intoxicated, or driving while under the influence of alcoholic beverages?	(1 point)	(0 point)
13. Have you ever been arrested, even for a few hours, because of other drunken behavior?	(1 point)	(0 point)

SCORING SYSTEM

0-1 POINT—NORMAL
2 POINTS—POSSIBLY ALCOHOLIC
3 OR MORE POINTS—PROBABLY ALCOHOLIC

Modified from Selzer ML: The Michigan alcoholism screening test: the quest for a new diagnostic instrument; *Am J Psychiatry* 127:1653-1658;1971.

BOX A-8 CAGE Survey

Are You . . .

C utting down or feel the need to?
A nnoyed when people criticize your drinking?
G uilty about your drinking?
E ye-opening with a drink in the morning?

If you answered yes to any question, there is high probability of alcoholism.

From Ewing JA: Detecting alcoholism: the CAGE questionnaire, *JAMA* 252:1905-1907, 1984.

BOX A-9 Scale for Assessing Severity of Alcohol Withdrawal Syndrome

Patient name _____
Date _____ Time (24 hr clock, midnight = 00:00) _____
Pulse or heart rate, taken for 1 min: _____
Blood pressure _____

Total CIWA-Ar Score _____
Rater's initials _____
Maximum possible score: 67

Nausea and vomiting—Ask "Do you feel sick to your stomach? Have you vomited?" Observation.
0 no nausea and no vomiting
1 mild nausea with no vomiting
2
3
4 intermittent nausea with dry heaves
5
6
7 constant nausea, frequent dry heaves and vomiting

Tremor—Arms extended and fingers spread apart. Observation.
0 no tremor
1 not visible, but can be felt fingertip-to-fingertip
2
3
4 moderate, with patient's arms extended
5
6
7 severe, even with arms not extended

Paroxysmal sweats—Observation.
0 no sweat visible
1 barely perceptible sweating, palms moist
2
3
4 beads of sweat obvious on forehead
5
6
7 drenching sweats

Anxiety—Ask "Do you feel nervous?" Observation.
0 no anxiety, at ease
1 mildly anxious
2
3
4 moderately anxious or guarded, so anxiety is inferred
5
6
7 equivalent to acute panic states, as seen in severe delirium or acute schizophrenic reactions

Agitation—Observation.
0 normal activity
1 somewhat more than normal activity
2
3
4 moderately fidgety and restless
5
6
7 paces back and forth during most of the interview or constantly thrashes about

Tactile disturbances—Ask "Have you any itching, pins-and-needles sensations, burning, numbness, or a feeling of bugs crawling on or under your skin?" Observation.
0 none
1 very mild itching, pins and needles, burning, or numbness
2 mild itching, pins and needles, burning, or numbness
3 moderate itching, pins and needles, burning, or numbness
4 moderately severe hallucinations
5 severe hallucinations
6 extremely severe hallucinations
7 continuous hallucinations

Auditory disturbances—Ask "Are you more aware of sounds around you? Are they harsh? Do they frighten you? Are you hearing anything that is disturbing to you? Are you hearing things you know are not there?" Observation.
0 not present
1 very mild harshness or ability to frighten
2 mild harshness or ability to frighten
3 moderate harshness or ability to frighten
4 moderately severe hallucinations
5 severe hallucinations
6 extremely severe hallucinations
7 continuous hallucinations

Visual disturbances—Ask "Does the light appear to be too bright? Is its color different? Does it hurt your eyes? Are you seeing anything that is disturbing to you? Are you seeing things you know are not there?" Observation.
0 not present
1 very mild sensitivity
2 mild sensitivity
3 moderate sensitivity
4 moderately severe hallucinations
5 severe hallucinations
6 extremely severe hallucinations
7 continuous hallucinations

Headache, fullness in head—Ask "Does your head feel different? Does it feel like there is a band around your head?" Do not rate for dizziness or lightheadedness. Otherwise, rate severity.
0 not present
1 very mild
2 mild
3 moderate
4 moderately severe
5 severe
6 very severe
7 extremely severe

Orientation and clouding of sensorium—Ask "What day is this? Where are you? Who am I?"
0 oriented and can do serial additions
1 cannot do serial additions or is uncertain about date
2 disoriented for date by no more than 2 calendar days
3 disoriented for date by more than 2 calendar days
4 disoriented for place and/or person

Adapted from Sullivan JT et al: *Assessment of alcohol withdrawal: the revised clinical institute withdrawal assessment for alcohol scale (CIWA-Ar)*. Br J Addiction 84:1353, 1989.

Hamilton Anxiety Scale

BOX A-10 Hamilton Anxiety Rating Scale

Instructions: This checklist is to assist the physician or psychiatrist in evaluating each patient as to his or her degree of anxiety and pathologic condition. Please fill in the appropriate rating:
None, 0; mild, 1; moderate, 2; severe, 3; severe, grossly disabling, 4.

The Hamilton Anxiety Rating Scale can help physicians quantify their patient's anxiety symptoms. A score of 18 or greater reflects a significant level of anxiety.

ITEM		RATING	ITEM		RATING
Anxious	Worries, anticipation of the worst, fearful anticipation, irritability	_____	Cardiovascular symptoms	Tachycardia, palpitations, pain in chest, throbbing of vessels, fainting feelings, missing beat	_____
Tension	Feelings of tension, fatigability, startle response, moved to tears easily, trembling, feelings of restlessness, inability to relax	_____	Respiratory symptoms	Pressure or constriction in chest, choking feelings, sighing, dyspnea	_____
Fears	Of dark, of strangers, of being left alone, of animals, of traffic, of crowds	_____	Gastrointestinal symptoms	Difficulty in swallowing, wind, abdominal pain, burning sensations, abdominal fullness, nausea, vomiting, borborygmi, looseness of bowels, loss of weight, constipation	_____
Insomnia	Difficulty in falling asleep, broken sleep, unsatisfying sleep and fatigue on waking, dreams, nightmares, night terrors	_____	Genitourinary symptoms	Frequency of micturition, urgency of micturition, amenorrhea, menorrhagia, development of frigidity, premature ejaculation, loss of libido, impotence	_____
Intellectual (cognitive)	Difficulty in concentration, poor memory	_____			
Depressed mood	Loss of interest, lack of pleasure in hobbies, depression, early waking, diurnal swing	_____	Autonomic symptoms	Dry mouth, flushing, pallor, tendency to sweat, giddiness, tension headache, raising of hair	_____
Somatic (muscular)	Pains and aches, twitching, stiffness, myoclonic jerks, grinding of teeth, unsteady voice, increased muscular tone	_____	Behavior at interview	Fidgeting, restlessness or pacing, tremor of hands, furrowed brow, strained face, sighing or rapid respiration, facial pallor, swallowing, belching, brisk tendon jerks, dilated pupils, exophthalmos	_____
Somatic (sensory)	Tinnitus, blurring of vision, hot and cold flushes, feelings of weakness, picking sensation	_____			

Additional comments:

Investigator's signature: _____

From Hamilton M: The assessment of anxiety states by rating, *Br J Med Psychol* 32:50, 1959.

Zung Depression Scale

Instructions: Read each sentence carefully. For each statement, check the bubble in the column that best corresponds to how often you have felt that way during the past 2 wk.

For statements 5 and 7, if you are on a diet, answer as if you were not.

Please check a response for each of the 20 items.

Patient name _____

Age _____

Sex _____

Date _____

#	Statement	None or a little of the time	Some of the time	Good part of the time	Most or all of the time
1	I feel downhearted, blue, and sad	○ 1	○ 2	○ 3	○ 4
2	Morning is when I feel the best	○ 4	○ 3	○ 2	○ 1
3	I have crying spells or feel like it	○ 1	○ 2	○ 3	○ 4
4	I have trouble sleeping through the night	○ 1	○ 2	○ 3	○ 4
5	I eat as much as I used to	○ 4	○ 3	○ 2	○ 1
6	I enjoy looking at, talking to, and being with attractive women/men	○ 4	○ 3	○ 2	○ 1
7	I notice that I am losing weight	○ 1	○ 2	○ 3	○ 4
8	I have trouble with constipation	○ 1	○ 2	○ 3	○ 4
9	My heart beats faster than usual	○ 1	○ 2	○ 3	○ 4
10	I get tired for no reason	○ 1	○ 2	○ 3	○ 4
11	My mind is as clear as it used to be	○ 4	○ 3	○ 2	○ 1
12	I find it easy to do the things I used to do	○ 4	○ 3	○ 2	○ 1
13	I am restless and can't keep still	○ 1	○ 2	○ 3	○ 4
14	I feel hopeful about the future	○ 4	○ 3	○ 2	○ 1
15	I am more irritable than usual	○ 1	○ 2	○ 3	○ 4
16	I find it easy to make decisions	○ 4	○ 3	○ 2	○ 1
17	I feel that I am useful and needed	○ 4	○ 3	○ 2	○ 1
18	My life is pretty full	○ 4	○ 3	○ 2	○ 1
19	I feel that others would be better off if I were dead	○ 1	○ 2	○ 3	○ 4
20	I still enjoy the things I used to do	○ 4	○ 3	○ 2	○ 1

Raw score

SDS index

SDS Index	Equivalent Clinical Global Impressions
Below-50	Within normal range, no psychopathology
50-59	Presence of minimal to mild depression
60-69	Presence of moderate to marked depression
70 and over	Presence of severe to extreme depression

Conversion of Raw Scores to the SDS Index

Raw Score	SDS Index	Raw Score	SDS Index	Raw Score	SDS Index	Raw Score	SDS Index	Raw Score	SDS Index
20	25	32	40	44	55	56	70	68	85
21	26	33	41	45	56	57	71	69	86
22	28	34	43	46	58	58	73	70	88
23	29	35	44	47	59	59	74	71	89
24	30	36	45	48	60	60	75	72	90
25	31	37	46	49	61	61	76	73	91
26	33	38	48	50	63	62	78	74	92
27	34	39	49	51	64	63	79	75	94
28	35	40	50	52	65	64	80	76	95
29	36	41	51	53	66	65	81	77	96
30	38	42	53	54	68	66	83	78	98
31	39	43	54	55	69	67	84	79	99
								80	100

Fig. A-3 Zung self-rating depression scale. (From Zung WWR: A self-rating depression scale, *Arch Gen Psychiatry* 12:63-70, 1965.)

Geriatric Depression Scale

BOX A-11 The Geriatric Depression Scale (GDS)—Short Form

Choose the best answer for how you felt over the past week.

PLEASE CIRCLE ONE

1. Are you basically satisfied with your life?	Yes	No
2. Have you dropped many of your activities and interests?	Yes	No
3. Do you feel that your life is empty?	Yes	No
4. Do you often get bored?	Yes	No
5. Are you in good spirits most of the time?	Yes	No
6. Are you afraid that something bad is going to happen to you?	Yes	No
7. Do you feel happy most of the time?	Yes	No
8. Do you often feel helpless?	Yes	No
9. Do you prefer staying at home to going out and doing new things?	Yes	No
10. Do you feel you have more problems with memory than most people?	Yes	No
11. Do you think it is wonderful to be alive now?	Yes	No
12. Do you feel pretty worthless the way you are now?	Yes	No
13. Do you feel full of energy?	Yes	No
14. Do you feel that your situation is hopeless?	Yes	No
15. Do you think that most people are better off than you are?	Yes	No

Scoring: A score of 0-5 is normal; a score above 5 suggests depression.
One point for each of the following answers:

1. No	4. Yes	7. No	10. Yes	13. No
2. Yes	5. No	8. Yes	11. No	14. Yes
3. Yes	6. Yes	9. Yes	12. Yes	15. Yes

From Yesavage JA, et al: *J Psychiatr Res* 17:37-49, 1982-1983.

Evaluation for Sports Participation

BOX A-12 Classification of Sports by Contact

CONTACT/COLLISION		LIMITED CONTACT		NONCONTACT	
Basketball	Lacrosse	Baseball	Racquetball	Archery	Orienteering
Boxing*	Martial arts	Bicycling	Skating	Badminton	Power lifting
Driving	Rodeo	Cheerleading	Ice	Body building	Race walking
Field hockey	Rugby	Canoeing/kayaking	Inline	Bowling	Riflery
Football	Ski jumping	(white water)	Roller	Canoeing/kayaking	Rope jumping
Flag	Soccer	Fencing	Skiing	(flat water)	Running
Tackle	Team handball	Field	Cross-country	Crew/rowing	Sailing
Ice hockey	Water polo	High jump	Downhill	Curling	Scuba diving
	Wrestling	Pole vault	Water	Dancing	Strength training
		Floor hockey	Softball	Field	Swimming
		Gymnastics	Squash	Discus	Table Tennis
		Handball	Ultimate Frisbee	Javelin	Tennis
		Horseback riding	Volleyball	Shot put	Track
			Windsurfing/surfing	Golf	Weight lifting

From American Academy of Pediatrics, Committee on Sports Medicine and Fitness: Medical conditions affecting sports participation; *Pediatrics* 94(5): 757-760, 1994.
*Participation not recommended.

APPENDIX Evaluation for sports participation

TABLE A-14 Medical Conditions and Sports Participation

This table is designed to be understood by medical and nonmedical personnel. In the *Explanation* section below, "needs evaluation" means that a physician with appropriate knowledge and experience should assess the safety of a given sport for an athlete with the listed medical condition. Unless otherwise noted, this is because of the variability of the severity of the disease or of the risk of injury among the specific sports in Box 8-12, or both.

CONDITION	MAY PARTICIPATE?
Atlantoaxial instability (instability of the joint between cervical vertebrae 1 and 2) *Explanation:* Athlete needs evaluation to assess risk of spinal cord injury during sports participation.	Qualified yes
Bleeding disorder *Explanation:* Athlete needs evaluation.	Qualified yes
Cardiovascular diseases	
Carditis (inflammation of the heart) *Explanation:* Carditis may result in sudden death with exertion.	No
Hypertension (high blood pressure) *Explanation:* Those with significant essential (unexplained) hypertension should avoid weight and power lifting, body building, and strength training. Those with secondary hypertension (hypertension caused by a previously identified disease) or severe essential hypertension need evaluation.	Qualified yes
Congenital heart disease (structural heart defects present at birth) *Explanation:* Those with mild forms may participate fully; those with moderate or severe forms, or who have undergone surgery, need evaluation.	Qualified yes
Dysrhythmia (irregular heart rhythm) *Explanation:* Athlete needs evaluation because some types require therapy or make certain sports dangerous, or both.	Qualified yes
Mitral valve prolapse (abnormal heart valve) *Explanation:* Those with symptoms (chest pain, symptoms of possible dysrhythmia) or evidence of mitral regurgitation (leaking) on physical examination need evaluation. All others may participate fully.	Qualified yes
Heart murmur *Explanation:* If the murmur is innocent (does not indicate heart disease), full participation is permitted. Otherwise, the athlete needs evaluation (see congenital heart disease and mitral valve prolapse above).	Qualified yes
Cerebral palsy *Explanation:* Athlete needs evaluation.	Qualified yes
Diabetes mellitus *Explanation:* All sports can be played with proper attention to diet, hydration, and insulin therapy. Particular attention is needed for activities that last 30 min or more.	Yes
Diarrhea *Explanation:* Unless disease is mild, no participation is permitted, because diarrhea may increase the risk of dehydration and heat illness. See "Fever" below.	Qualified no
Eating disorders Anorexia nervosa Bulimia nervosa *Explanation:* These patients need both medical and psychiatric assessment before participation.	Qualified yes
Eyes Functionally one-eyed athlete Loss of an eye Detached retina Previous eye surgery or serious eye injury *Explanation:* A functionally one-eyed athlete has a best corrected visual acuity of <20/40 in the worse eye. These athletes would suffer significant disability if the better eye was seriously injured as would those with loss of an eye. Some athletes who have previously undergone eye surgery or had a serious eye injury may have an increased risk of injury because of weakened eye tissue. Availability of eye guards approved by the American Society for Testing Materials (ASTM) and other protective equipment may allow participation in most sports, but this must be judged on an individual basis.	Qualified yes

Continued

TABLE A-14 Medical Conditions and Sports Participation—cont'd

CONDITION	MAY PARTICIPATE?
Fever	No
Explanation: Fever can increase cardiopulmonary effort, reduce maximum exercise capacity, make heat illness more likely, and increase orthostatic hypotension during exercise. Fever may rarely accompany myocarditis or other infections that may make exercise dangerous.	
Heat Illness, hx of	Qualified yes
Explanation: Because of the increased likelihood of recurrence, the athlete needs individual assessment to determine the presence of predisposing conditions and to arrange a prevention strategy.	
HIV infection	Yes
Explanation: Because of the apparent minimal risk to others, all sports may be played that the state of health allows. In all athletes, skin lesions should be properly covered, and athletic personnel should use universal precautions when handling blood or body fluids with visible blood.	
Kidney: absence of one	Qualified yes
Explanation: Athlete needs individual assessment for contact/collision and limited contact sports.	
Liver: enlarged	Qualified yes
Explanation: If the liver is acutely enlarged, participation should be avoided because of risk of rupture. If the liver is chronically enlarged, individual assessment is needed before collision/contact or limited contact sports are played.	
Malignancy	Qualified yes
Explanation: Athlete needs individual assessment.	
Musculoskeletal disorders	Qualified yes
Explanation: Athlete needs individual assessment.	
Neurologic	
History of serious head or spine trauma, severe or repeated concussions, or craniotomy.	Qualified yes
Explanation: Athlete needs individual assessment for collision/contact or limited contact sports, and also for noncontact sports if there are deficits in judgment or cognition. Recent research supports a conservative approach to management of concussion.	
Convulsive disorder, well controlled	Yes
Explanation: Risk of convulsion during participation is minimal.	
Convulsive disorder, poorly controlled	Qualified yes
Explanation: Athlete needs individual assessment for collision/contact or limited contact sports. Avoid the following noncontact sports: archery, riflery, swimming, weight or power lifting, strength training, or sports involving heights. In these sports, occurrences of a convulsion may be a risk to self or others.	
Obesity	Qualified yes
Explanation: Because of the risk of heat illness, obese persons need careful acclimatization and hydration.	
Organ transplant recipient	Qualified yes
Explanation: Athlete needs individual assessment.	
Ovary: absence of one	Yes
Explanation: Risk of severe injury to the remaining ovary is minimal.	
Respiratory	
Pulmonary compromise including cystic fibrosis	Qualified yes
Explanation: Athlete needs individual assessment, but generally all sports may be played if oxygenation remains satisfactory during a graded exercise test. Patients with cystic fibrosis need acclimatization and good hydration to reduce the risk of illness.	
Asthma	Yes
Explanation: With proper medication and education, only athletes with the most severe asthma will have to modify their participation.	
Acute upper respiratory infection	Qualified yes
Explanation: Upper respiratory obstruction may affect pulmonary function. Athlete needs individual assessment for all but mild disease. See "Fever" above.	
Sickle cell disease	Qualified yes
Explanation: Athlete needs individual assessment. In general, if status of the illness permits, all but high exertion, collision/contact sports may be played. Overheating, dehydration, and chilling must be avoided.	

TABLE A-14 Medical Conditions and Sports Participation—cont'd

CONDITION	MAY PARTICIPATE?
Sickle cell trait *Explanation:* It is unlikely that individuals with sickle cell trait (AS) have an increased risk of sudden death or other medical problems during athletic participation except under the most extreme conditions of heat, humidity, and possibly increased altitude. These individuals, like all athletes, should be carefully conditioned, acclimatized, and hydrated to reduce any possible risk.	Yes
Skin: boils, herpes simplex, impetigo, scabies, molluscum contagiosum *Explanation:* While the patient is contagious, participation in gymnastics with mats, martial arts, wrestling, or other collision/contact or limited contact sports is not allowed. Herpes simplex virus probably is not transmitted via mats.	Qualified yes
Spleen, enlarged *Explanation:* Patients with acutely enlarged spleens should avoid all sports because of risk of rupture. Those with chronically enlarged spleens need individual assessment before playing collision/contact or limited contact sports.	Qualified yes
Testicle: absent or undescended *Explanation:* Certain sports may require a protective cup.	Yes

From American Academy of Pediatrics, Committe on Sports Medicine and Fitness: Medical Conditions affecting sports participation, *Pediatrics* 94(5): 757-760, 1994.

GROWTH AND DEVELOPMENT
Developmental Milestones

TABLE A-15 Developmental Assessment and Guidance

AGE	GROSS MOTOR	VISUAL MOTOR	LANGUAGE	SOCIAL	GUIDANCE
1 mo	Raises head slightly from prone, makes crawling movements, lifts chin up	Has tight grasp, follows to midline	Alert to sound (e.g., by blinking, moving, startling)	Regards face, spontaneous smile	Car seats, fever control, thermometers, talking to baby, sleeping, stimulating mobiles
2 mo	Holds chin in midline, lifts chest off table, head up 45 degrees	No longer clenches fist tightly, follows object past midline	Smiles after being stroked or talked to	Acts increasingly alert, recognizes parent, may smile spontaneously	
3 mo	Supports self on forearms in prone, holds head up steadily	Holds hand open at rest, pulls at clothing, follows in circular fashion, puts hands together	Coos (produces long vowel sounds in musical fashion), squeals, laughs	Reaches for familiar people or objects; anticipates feeding, regards own hand	Car seats, diet, stimulating safe toys, babysitters
4-5 mo	Rolls front to back, back to front, sits well when propped, supports on wrists, shifts weight, can bear weight on legs	Move arms in unison to grasp, touches cube placed on table, follows 180 degrees	4 mo: orients to voice 5 mo: orients to bell, says "ah goo," razzes	Enjoys looking around environment	
6 mo	Sits well, puts feet in mouth in supine position	Reaches with either hand, transfers, uses raking grasp	Babbles (imitates speech sounds) 8 mo: says "mama/dada" indiscriminately	Works for toy, feeds self, recognizes strangers	Car seats, stair gates, electric cord and outlet covers, crawling, stranger anxiety, peek-a-boo, banging toys
9 mo	Creeps, crawls, cruises, pulls to feet, likes to stand, pivots when sitting	Uses overhand pincer grasp, probes with forefinger, holds bottle, finger-feeds	Imitates sounds 10 mo: waves bye-bye	Starts to explore environment	Car seats, water bath safety, finger-foods, cup weaning, teeth care, first book, appropriate discipline, ipecac
11 mo	Stands for 2 sec		Follows one-step command with gesture, says "mama/dada" discriminately		
12 mo	Walks alone or with hand held, pivots when sitting, cooperates with dressing	Uses mature pincer grasp, throws objects, lets go of toys, hand release	One word	Imitates actions, comes when called, cooperates with dressing, indicates wants, plays ball with examiner	Car seats, books, water safety, burns, scalds, diet, decreases appetite, riding toys, pull toys, temper tantrums, nightmares, toilet training
13 mo	Stands alone		Two words		
14 mo	Stoops and recovers, walks well				
15 mo	Walks well, creeps upstairs, walks backwards	Scribbles in imitation of examiner	Follows one-step command without gesture, uses two words	Drinks from cup	

TABLE A-15 Developmental Assessment and Guidance—cont'd

AGE	GROSS MOTOR	VISUAL MOTOR	LANGUAGE	SOCIAL	GUIDANCE
18 mo	Runs, throws toy from standing without falling	Turns 2-3 pages at a time, fills spoon and feeds self	Uses three words, points to one body part when named, uses mature jargoning, includes intelligible words	Copies parent in tasks (e.g., sweeping, dusting), plays in company of other children, uses spoon, fork	
21 mo	Squats in play, goes up steps, kicks ball forward	Builds tower of two blocks, drinks well from cup	Points to three body parts, uses two-word combination	Asks to have food and to go to toilet	
24 mo	Walks up and down steps without help, throws ball overhand	Turns pages one at a time, removes shoes, pants, etc., build tower of six cubes	Uses 50 words, two-word sentences, three pronouns; names objects in pictures		Car seats, books, playground safety, babysitter, giving up blanket, etc., appropriate discipline, learning to play with others
30 mo	Jumps with both feet off floor, throws ball overhand	Unbuttons, holds pencil in adult fashion, differentiates horizontal and vertical lines	Appropriate use of pronouns, understands concept of "1," repeats two digits	Tells first and last names when asked, gets drink without help	
3 yr	Pedal tricycle, can alternate feet when going up steps	Dresses and undresses partially, dries hands if reminded, draws a circle	Tells story about experiences, knows his or her sex	Shares toys, takes turns, plays well with others	
4 yr	Hops, skips, alternates feet going down stairs	Buttons clothing fully, catches ball	Knows all colors, says song or poem from memory	Tells "tall tales"; plays cooperatively with a group of children	Consideration should be given to discussing "private" areas and setting limits for those areas
5 yr	Skips, alternating feet; jumps over low obstacles	Ties shoes, spreads with knife	Prints first name, asks meaning of words, prepares cereal	Plays competitive games, abides by rules, likes to help in household tasks	

Modified from *The Harriet Lane handbook*, ed 14, Chicago, 1996, Mosby.

1040 Physical growth curves

APPENDIX

Physical Growth Curves

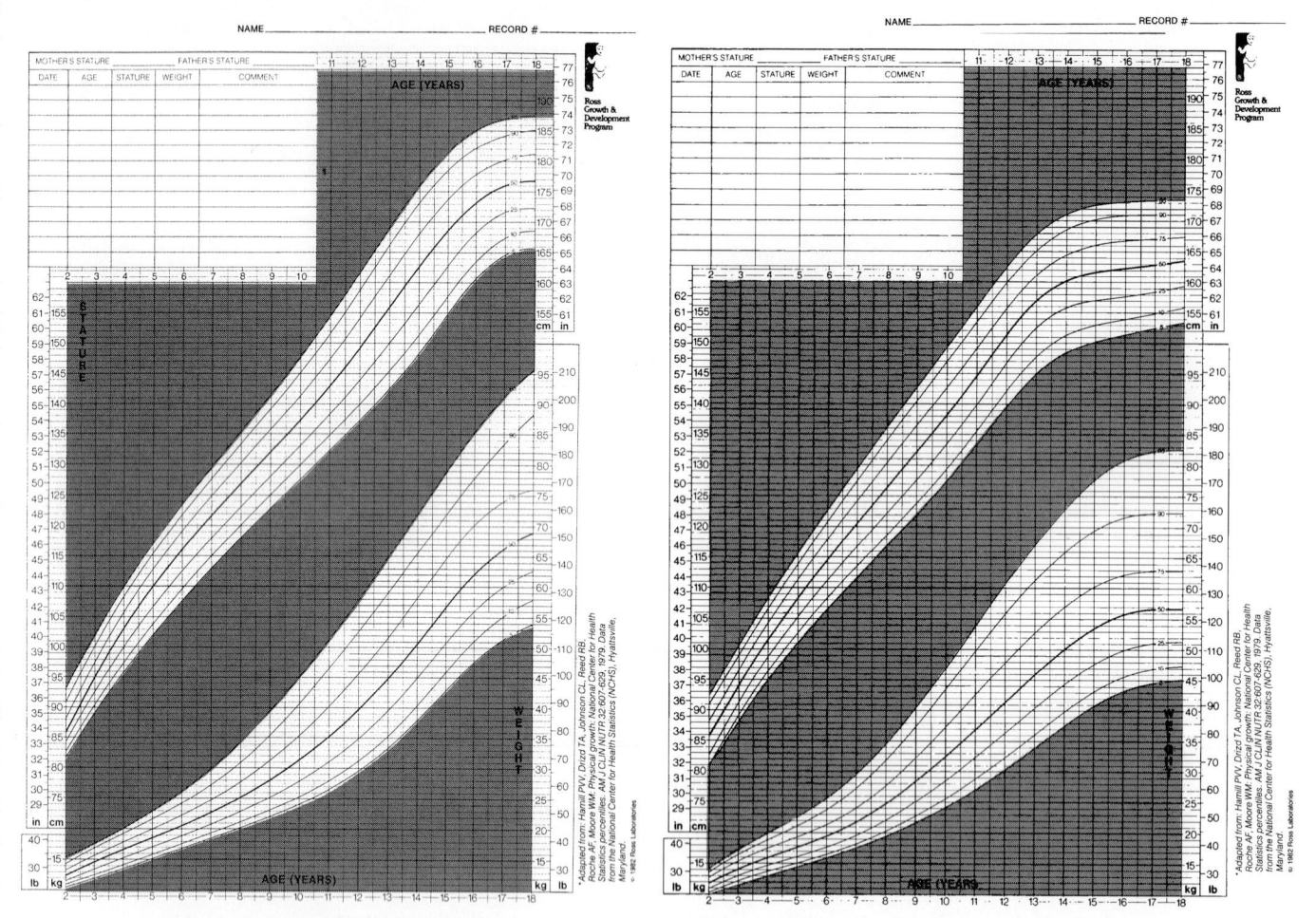

Fig. A-4 Physical growth curves and NCHS percentiles for children, age 2 through 18 years, for height and weight. **A**, Boys. **B**, Girls.

APPENDIX Sexual maturation stages 1041

Sexual Maturation Stages

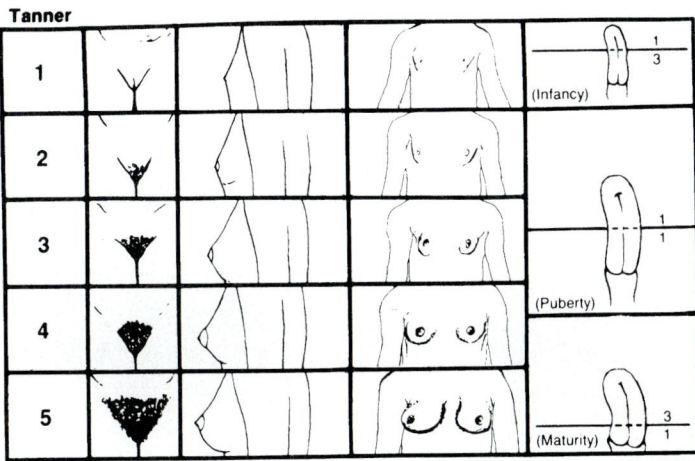

Tanner	Pubic Hair	Breast
1	Infantile pattern. No true pubic hair present, although there may be a fine downy hair distribution.	Infantile or childhood pattern.
2	Sparse growth of lightly pigmented hair, longer than the fine down of the previous stage, appearing on the mons or the labia.	Early pubertal breast development, sometimes referred to as a "breast bud." A small mound of breast tissue causes a visible elevation.
3	The pubic hair becomes darker, coarser, and curlier. Distribution is still minimal.	The areola and the breast undergo more definite pronouncement in size, with a continuous rounded contour.
4	The pubic hair is adult in character, but not yet as widely distributed as in most adults.	The areola and nipple enlarge further and form a secondary mound projecting above the contour of the remainder of the breast.
5	The pubic hair is distributed in the typical adult female pattern, forming an inverse triangle.	The adult breast stage. The secondary mound visible in the preceding stage has now blended into a smooth contour of the breast.

Fig. A-5 Sexual maturation of girl. This may be assessed using the normal appearance of the external genitalia as described by Tanner and the usual expected sequence and tempo. (From Driscoll CE et al: *The family practice desk reference,* ed 3, St Louis, 1996, Mosby.)

BOX A-13 Genital Development (Male)

Stage I Preadolescent; testes, scrotum, and penis about same size and proportion as in early childhood.
Stage II Enlargement of scrotum and testes; skin of scrotum reddens and changes in texture; little or no enlargement of penis (11.64 + 1.07).
Stage III Enlargement of penis, first mainly in length; further growth of testes and scrotum (12.85 + 1.04).
Stage IV Increased size of penis with growth in breadth and development of glans; further enlargement of testes and scrotum and increased darkening of scrotal skin (13.77 + 1.02).
Stage V Genitalia adult in size and shape (14.92 + 1.10).

From *Harriet Lane handbook,* ed 14, St Louis, 1996, Mosby.

MEDICAL TABLES, GRAPHS, AND FORMULAS
Commonly Used Formulas

> **BOX A-14 Commonly Used Formulas**
>
> 1. Calculation of creatinine clearance (CCr)
>
> $$\text{CCr (male)} = \frac{(140 - \text{Age}) \times \text{Wt (in kg)}}{\text{Serum creatinine} \times 72}$$
>
> $$\text{CCr (female)} = 0.85 \times \text{CCr (male)}$$
>
> 2. Alveolar-arterial oxygen gradient (Aa gradient)
>
> $$\text{Aa gradient} = \left[(713)(\text{FIo}_2) - \left(\frac{\text{Paco}_2}{0.8}\right)\right] - \text{Pao}_2$$
>
> Normal Aa gradient = 5-15 mm
> FIo_2 = Fraction of inspired oxygen (normal = 0.21-1.0)
> Paco_2 = Arterial carbon dioxide tension (normal = 35-45 mm Hg)
> Pao_2 = Arterial partial pressure oxygen (normal = 70-100 mm Hg)
> Differential diagnosis of Aa gradient:
>
> | ABNORMALITY | 15% O$_2$ | 100% O$_2$ |
> |---|---|---|
> | Diffusion defect | Increased gradient | Correction of gradient |
> | Ventilation/perfusion mismatch | Increased gradient | Partial or complete correction of gradient |
> | Right-to-left shunt (intracardiac or pulmonary) | Increased gradient | Increased gradient (no correction) |
>
> 3. Anion gap (AG)
>
> $$\text{AG} = \text{Na}^+ - (\text{Cl}^- + \text{HCO}_3^-)$$
>
> 4. Fractional excretion of sodium
>
> $$\text{FE}_{\text{Na}} = \frac{U_{\text{Na}}/P_{\text{Na}}}{U_{\text{Cr}}/P_{\text{Cr}}} \times 100$$
>
> 5. Serum osmolality
>
> $$\text{Osm} = 2\,(\text{Na}^+ + \text{K}^+) + \frac{\text{Glucose}}{18} + \frac{\text{BUN}}{2.8}$$
>
> 6. Corrected sodium in hyperglycemic patients
>
> $$\text{Corrected Na}^+ = \text{Measured Na}^+ + 1.6 \times \frac{\text{Glucose} - 140}{100}$$
>
> 7. Water deficit in hypernatremic patients
>
> $$\text{Water deficit (in liters)} = 0.6 \times \text{Body weight (kg)} \times \left(\frac{\text{Measured serum sodium}}{\text{Normal serum sodium}} - 1\right)$$

APPENDIX   Acid-base map/Nomogram for calculation of body surface area   1043

Acid-Base Map

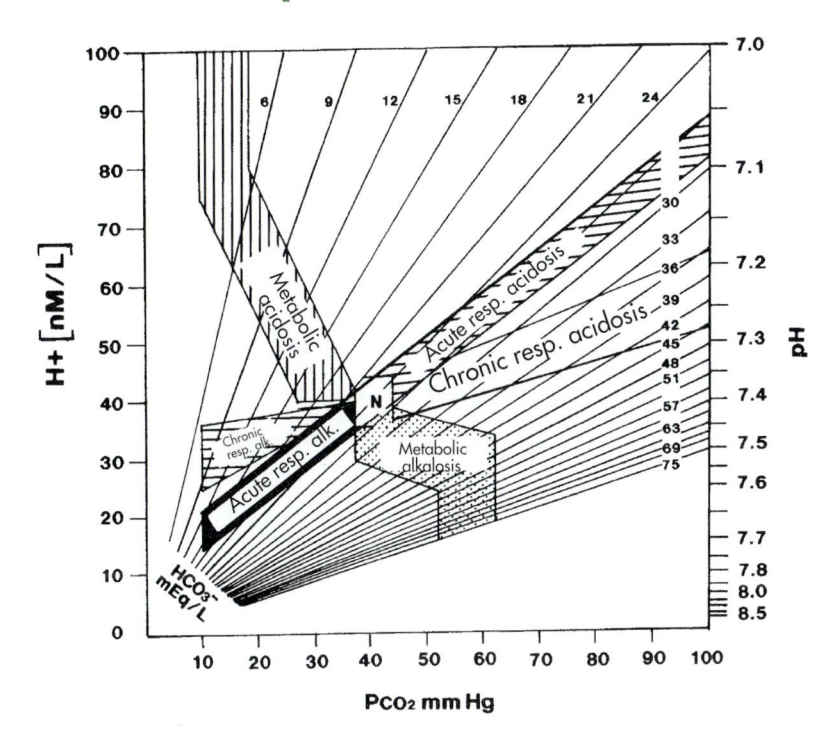

Fig. A-6   **Acid-base map.** *N*, Normal values. (From Koutlas TC (ed): *The Mont Reid surgical handbook,* ed 3, St Louis, 1994, Mosby.)

Nomogram for Calculation of Body Surface Area

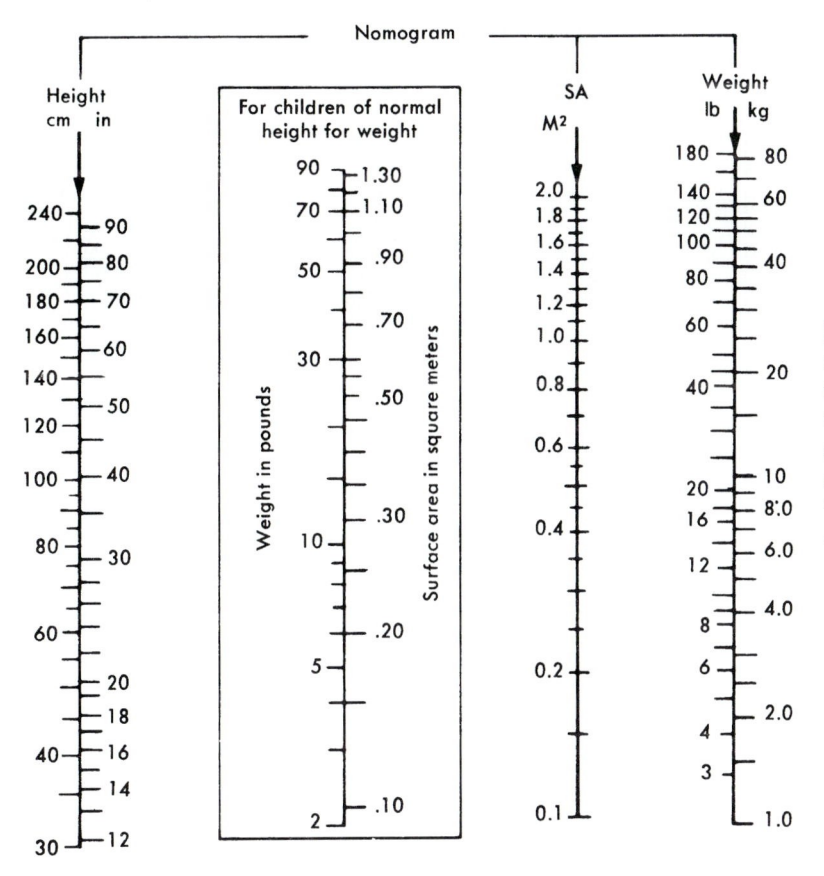

Fig. A-7   **Nomogram for evaluation of body surface area (BSA).** Place a straight edge from the patient's height in the left column to his weight in the right column. The point of intersection on the body surface area column indicates the BSA. (Reproduced from Behrman RE, Vaughn VC (eds): *Nelson's textbook of pediatrics,* ed 15, Philadelphia, 1996, Saunders.)

Events of the Cardiac Cycle

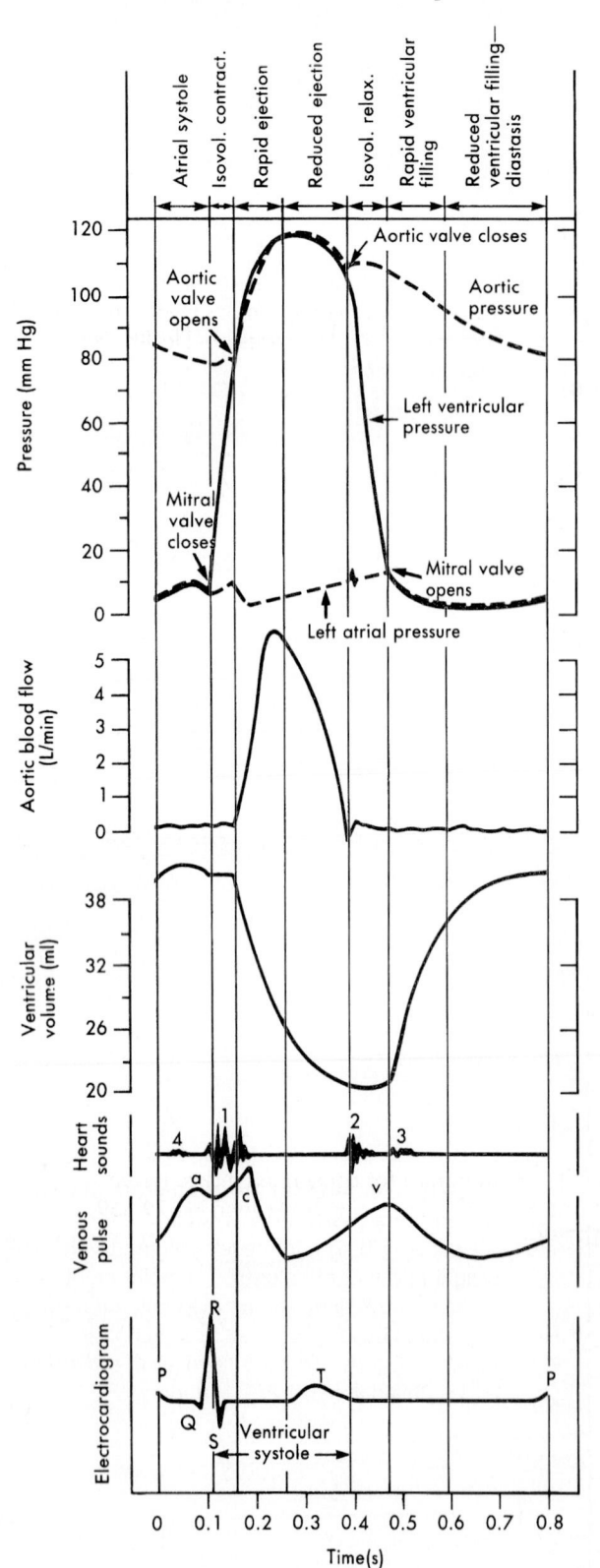

Fig. A-8 Events of the cardiac cycle. Left atrial, aortic, and left ventricular pressure pulses are correlated in time with aortic flow, ventricular volume, heart sounds, venous pulse, and electrocardiogram to provide a complete cardiac cycle in the dog. (From Berne RM, Levy MN: *Cardiovascular physiology,* ed 6, St Louis, 1992, Mosby.)

Spinal Dermatomes

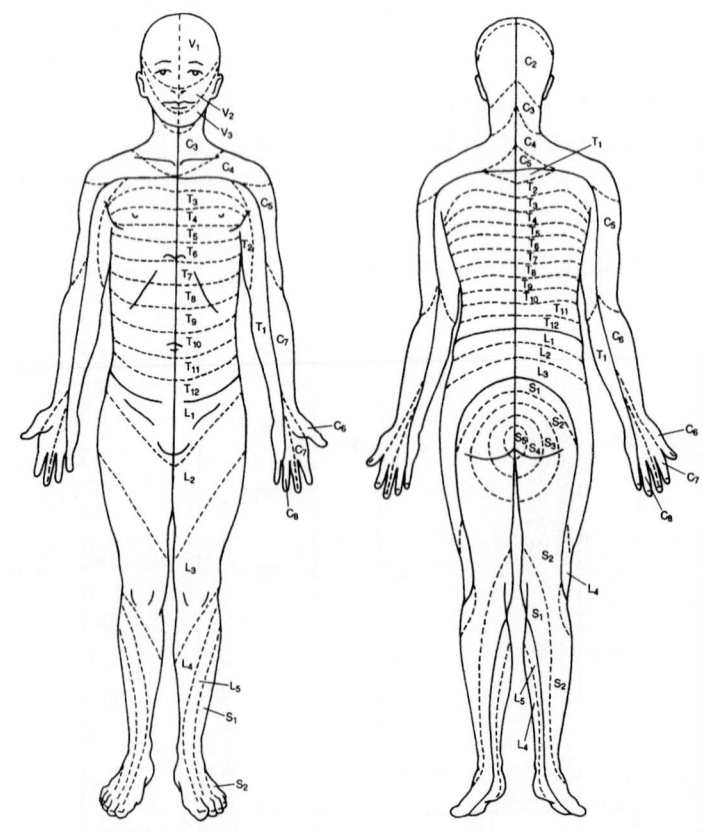

Fig. A-9 Spinal dermatomes. (From *Harriet Lane handbook,* ed 12, St Louis, 1991, Mosby.)

NUTRITION
Food Guide Pyramid

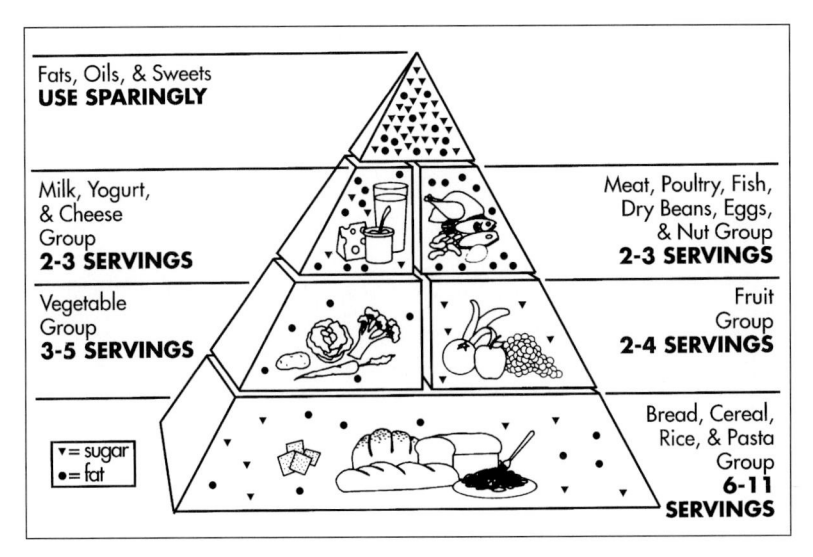

Fig. A-10 **Food Guide Pyramid: guide to daily food choices.** (From US Department of Agriculture, US Department of Health and Human Services.)

Nomogram for Body Mass Index

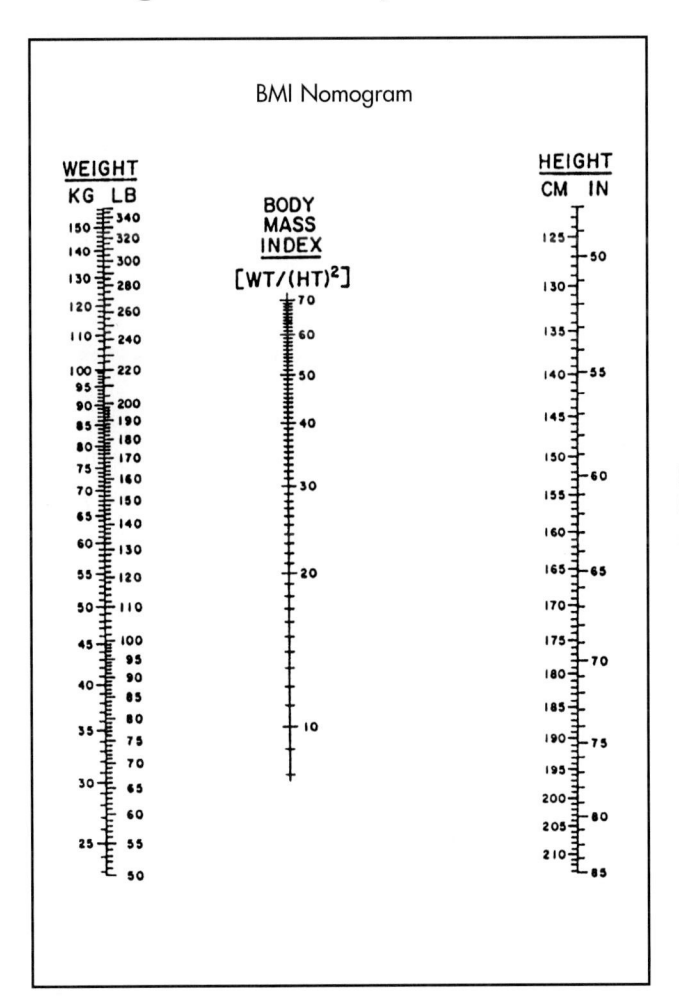

Fig. A-11 **Nomogram for body mass index.** (From Bray GA: *Obesity in America,* NIH Publication No 79-359, Nov 1979.)

Nutritional Assessment

TABLE A-16 Nutritional Assessment

MEASUREMENT	ASSESSMENT
A. Anthropometric measurements	
1. Weight (kg)	Body weight status
2. Height (cm)	Desirable weight of adults
3. Weight/height ratio	Body weight status
4. %Ideal body weight = $\dfrac{\text{Actual weight}}{\text{Ideal body weight}} \times 100$	
5. %Usual body weight = $\dfrac{\text{Actual weight}}{\text{Usual weight}} \times 100$	
6. %Weight change = $\dfrac{\text{Usual weight} - \text{Actual weight}}{\text{Usual weight}} \times 100$	
7. Arm circumference (cm)	
8. %Standard arm circumference = $\dfrac{\text{Actual arm circumference}}{\text{Standard arm circumference}} \times 100$	Body weight status
9. Triceps skinfold (mm)	Body fatness Men: 8-23 mm Women: 10-30 mm
10. %Standard triceps skinfold = $\dfrac{\text{Actual triceps skinfold}}{\text{Standard triceps skinfold}} \times 100$	
11. Arm muscle circumference (mm) = Arm circumference (mm) $- 0.314 \times$ Triceps skinfold (mm)	Lean muscle mass Midarm muscle circumference (120-140 mm)
12. %Standard arm muscle circumference = $\dfrac{\text{Actual arm muscle circumference}}{\text{Standard arm muscle circumference}} \times 100$	
B. Laboratory measurements	
1. Total iron-binding capacity (TIBC) (µg/dl)	Labile or visceral protein status Protein-calorie malnutrition
2. Serum transferrin = $(0.8 \times \text{TIBC}) - 43$ (mg/dl)	Visceral protein status Protein-calorie malnutrition
3. Serum albumin (g/dl)	Visceral protein status Protein-calorie malnutrition
4. White blood cell count (WBC/mm^3)	
5. Total lymphocyte count = $\dfrac{\text{\%Lymphocytes} \times \text{WBC}}{100}$	Immune function
6. 24 hr urinary creatinine (mg)	Ideal urinary creatinine values
7. Creatinine height index = $\dfrac{\text{Actual urinary creatinine}}{\text{Ideal urinary creatinine}} \times 100$	Muscle or lean body mass
8. 24 hr urinary nitrogen (g)	Body protein status
9. Nitrogen balance = $\dfrac{\text{Protein intake}}{6.25} - (\text{Urinary urea nitrogen} + 4)$	Body protein status
10. Basal energy expenditure	Used to derive total caloric needs
11. Complete blood count (CBC)	Anemia: Normocytic Microcytic Macrocytic
12. Skin tests Purified protein derivative (PPD) *Candida* Spp. Dinitrochlorobenzene (DNCB)	Immune function

From Stein JH (ed): *Internal medicine*, ed 5, St Louis, 1998, Mosby.

Recommended Daily Dietary Allowances

TABLE A-17 Recommended Daily Dietary Allowances of the Food and Nutrition Board, National Academy of Sciences–National Research Council,* *Designed for the maintenance of good nutrition of practically all healthy people in the United States*

	AGE (YR)	ENERGY (KCAL)†	PROTEIN (G)	A ACTIVITY (RE)‡	A ACTIVITY (IU)	D ACTIVITY (IU)	E ACTIVITY‖ (IU)	C (MG)	FOLA-CIN¶ (μG)	NIA-CIN# (MG)	RIBO-FLAVIN (MG)	THIA-MINE (MG)
Infants	0-0.5	kg × 115	kg × 2.2	420§	1400	400	3	35	30	6	0.4	0.3
	0.5-1	kg × 105	kg × 2	400	2000	400	4	35	45	8	0.6	0.5
Children	1-3	1300	23	400	2000	400	5	45	100	9	0.8	0.7
	4-6	1700	30	500	2500	400	6	45	200	11	1	0.9
	7-10	2400	34	700	3300	400	7	45	300	16	1.4	1.2
Males	11-14	2700	45	1000	5000	400	8	50	400	18	1.6	1.4
	15-18	2800	56	1000	5000	400	10	60	400	18	1.7	1.4
	19-22	2900	56	1000	5000	300	10	60	400	19	1.7	1.5
	23-50	2700	56	1000	5000		10	60	400	18	1.6	1.4
	51+	2400	56	1000	5000		10	60	400	16	1.4	1.2
Females	11-14	2200	46	800	4000	400	8	50	400	15	1.3	1.1
	15-18	2100	46	800	4000	400	8	60	400	14	1.3	1.1
	19-22	2100	44	800	4000	300	8	60	400	14	1.3	1.1
	23-50	2000	44	800	4000		8	60	400	13	1.2	1
	51+	1800	44	800	4000		8	60	400	13	1.2	1
Pregnant		+300	+30	1000	5000	600	10	80	800	+2	+0.3	+0.4
Lactating		+500	+20	1200	7000	600	10	100	500	+5	+0.5	+0.5

WATER-SOLUBLE VITAMINS				MINERALS**							
B_6 (MG)	B_{12} (MG)	BIOTIN (μG)	PANTOTHENIC ACID (MG)	Ca (MG)	P (MG)	I (μG)	Fe (MG)	Mg (MG)	Zn (MG)	Cu (MG)	Mn (MG)
0.3	0.5	35	3	360	240	40	10	50	3	0.6	0.6
0.6	1.5	50	3	540	360	50	15	70	5	0.6	0.6
0.9	2	65	5	800	800	70	15	150	10	1	1
1.3	2.5	85	10	800	800	90	10	200	10	1.5	1.5
1.6	3	120	10	800	800	120	10	250	10	1.5	1.5
1.8	3	200	10	1200	1200	150	18	350	15	2	4
2	3	200	10	1200	1200	150	18	400	15	2	4
2.2	3	200	10	800	800	150	10	350	15	2	4
2.2	3	200	10	800	800	150	10	350	15	2	4
2.2	3	200	10	800	800	150	10	350	15	2	4
1.8	3	200	10	1200	1200	150	18	300	15	2	4
2	3	200	10	1200	1200	150	18	300	15	2	4
2	3	200	10	800	800	150	18	300	15	2	4
2	3	200	10	800	800	150	18	300	15	2	4
2	3	200	10	800	800	150	10	300	15	2	4
2.6	4	200	10	1200	1200	175	18+††	450	20	2	4
2.5	4	200	10	1200	1200	200	18	450	25	2	4

*The allowances are intended to provide for individual variations among most normal persons as they live in the United States under usual environmental stresses. Diets should be based on a variety of common foods to provide other nutrients for which human requirements have been less well defined.
†Kilojoules (kJ) = 4.2 × kcal.
‡Retinol equivalents.
§Assumed to be all as retinol in milk during the first 6 mo of life. All subsequent intakes are assumed to be one half as retinol and one half as β-carotene when calculated from international units. As retinol equivalents, three fourths are as retinol and one fourth as β-carotene.
‖Total vitamin E activity, estimated to be 80% as α-tocopherol and 20% other tocopherols.
¶The folacin allowances refer to dietary sources as determined by *Lactobacillus casei* assay. Pure forms of folacin may be effective in doses less than one fourth of the recommended dietary allowance.
#Although allowances are expressed as niacin, it is recognized that on the average 1 mg of niacin is derived from each 60 mg of dietary tryptophan.
**Recommended daily allowances are now available for fluoride, selenium, molybdenum, and chromium.
††This increased requirement cannot be met by ordinary diets; therefore the use of supplemental iron is recommended.

Height-Weight Correlations for Adults

TABLE A-18　Height-Weight Correlations for Adults

MEN 25-59 YR

HEIGHT (FT/IN)	SMALL FRAME (LB)*	MEDIUM FRAME (LB)*	LARGE FRAME (LB)*
5'2"	128-134	131-141	138-150
5'3"	130-136	133-143	140-153
5'4"	132-138	135-145	142-156
5'5"	134-140	137-148	144-160
5'6"	136-142	139-151	146-164
5'7"	138-145	142-154	149-168
5'8"	140-148	145-157	152-172
5'9"	142-151	148-160	155-176
5'10"	144-154	151-163	158-180
5'11"	146-157	154-166	161-184
6'0"	149-160	157-170	164-188
6'1"	152-164	160-174	168-192
6'2"	155-168	164-178	172-197
6'3"	158-172	167-182	176-202
6'4"	162-176	171-187	181-207

*In indoor clothing weighing 5 lb, shoes with 1" heels.

WOMEN 25-59 YR

HEIGHT (FT/IN)	SMALL FRAME (LB)*	MEDIUM FRAME (LB)*	LARGE FRAME (LB)*
4'10"	102-111	109-121	118-131
4'11"	103-113	111-123	120-134
5'0"	104-115	113-126	122-137
5'1"	106-118	115-129	125-140
5'2"	108-121	118-132	128-143
5'3"	111-124	121-135	131-147
5'4"	114-127	124-138	134-151
5'5"	117-130	127-141	137-155
5'6"	120-133	130-144	140-159
5'7"	123-136	133-147	143-163
5'8"	126-139	136-150	146-167
5'9"	129-142	139-153	149-170
5'10"	132-145	142-156	152-173
5'11"	135-148	145-159	155-176
6'0"	138-151	148-162	158-179

From Driscoll CE et al: *The family practice desk reference*, ed 3, St Louis, 1996, Mosby.
*In indoor clothing weighing 3 lb, shoes with 1" heels.

Commercial Formulas for Nutritional Support

TABLE A-19 Examples of Commercial Formulas for Nutritional Support

FORMULA	PROTEIN	FAT	CARBOHYDRATE	LACTOSE
Complete Defined-Formula Diets				
Milk Base: Moderate Residue, Intact Protein				
Carnation Instant Breakfast (Carnation)	55.2	27.6	124.1	84.0
Compleat (Sandoz)	40.2	40.2	119.6	24.4
Enfamil (Mead Johnson)	22.2	54.6	103.3	103.3
Meritene (Sandoz)	60.4	33.3	114.6	80.0
Sustacal (powder) (Mead Johnson)	57.0	25.9	133.3	93.0
Lactose-Free, Low-Residue, Intact Protein, Protein Isolates				
Compleat-Modified (Sandoz)	40.1	32.0	130.8	0
Enrich (Ross)	36.1	34.8	147.3	0
Ensure (Ross)	35.1	35.1	136.8	0
Ensure HN (Ross)	41.9	33.4	133.2	0
Ensure Plus (Ross)	36.6	35.5	133.3	0
Ensure Plus HN (Ross)	41.7	33.3	133.3	0
Isocal (Mead Johnson)	32.1	41.1	126.2	0
Isocal HN (Mead Johnson)	41.5	42.4	116.0	0
Isomil (Ross)	26.4	54.4	101.5	0
Jevity (Ross)	41.9	34.7	143.1	0
Magnacal (Sherwood Medical)	35.0	40.0	125.0	0
Osmolite (Ross)	35.0	36.2	136.8	0
Osmolite HN (Ross)	41.9	34.7	133.2	0
Portagen (Mead Johnson)	34.6	47.5	114.8	0
Resource (Sandoz)	34.9	34.9	136.7	0
Prosobee (Mead Johnson)	30.0	53.0	100.0	0
Similac (Ross)	23.8	53.6	108.8	0
Sustacal (Mead Johnson)	60.3	22.8	138.6	0
Traumacal (Mead Johnson)	55.3	45.3	94.6	0
Ultracal (Mead Johnson)	41.5	42.4	116.0	0
Lactose-Free, Low-Residue, Hydrolyzed Protein, Amino Acids				
Critical HN (Mead Johnson)	35.8	5.0	207.5	0
Nutramigen (Mead Johnson)	28.0	39.0	134.0	0
Pregestimil (Mead Johnson)	28.5	41.0	134.0	0
Reabilan (O'Brien/KMI)	31.0	39.0	131.0	0
Vital HN (Ross)	41.7	10.8	185.0	0
Vivonex T.E.N. (Sandoz)	38.2	2.8	206.0	0
Formula for Special Metabolic Indications				
Amin-Aid (Kendall McGaw)	9.9	23.6	187.0	0
Hepatic-Aid II (Kendall McGaw)	37.5	30.8	143.3	0
Lofenalac (Mead Johnson)	32.5	39.8	129.2	0
Phenyl-Free (Mead Johnson)	50.0	16.8	162.5	0
Pulmocare (Ross)	42.0	61.3	70.7	0
Replena (Ross)	14.8	47.2	126.2	0
Travasorb Renal (Clintec)	17.1	13.3	202.7	0
Travasorb Hepatic (Clintec)	26.4	13.2	193.2	0
Supplementary Feedings				
Casec (Mead Johnson)	237.6	5.4	0.0	0
Citrotein (Doyle)	60.5	2.6	184.2	0
Controlyte (Doyle)	0.0	48.0	143.0	0
MCT Oil (Mead Johnson)	0.0	120.5	0.0	0
Microlipid (Sherwood Medical)	0.0	111.0	0.0	0
Pedialyte (Ross)	0.0	0.0	250.0	0
Polycose (Ross)	0.0	0.0	250.0	0
Propac (Sherwood Medical)	189.9	20.5	0.0	0
Sumacal (Sherwood Medical)	0.0	0.0	250.0	0

Grams per 100 kcal.

From Stein JH (ed): *Internal medicine*, ed 4, St Louis, 1994, Mosby.

ONCOLOGY
Breast Self-Examination

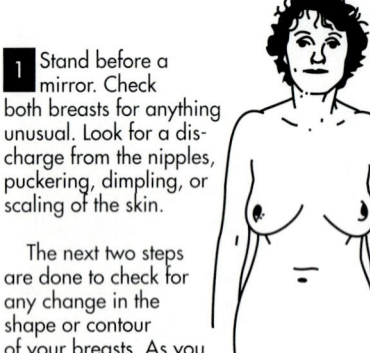

1 Stand before a mirror. Check both breasts for anything unusual. Look for a discharge from the nipples, puckering, dimpling, or scaling of the skin.

The next two steps are done to check for any change in the shape or contour of your breasts. As you do them, you should be able to feel your chest muscles tighten.

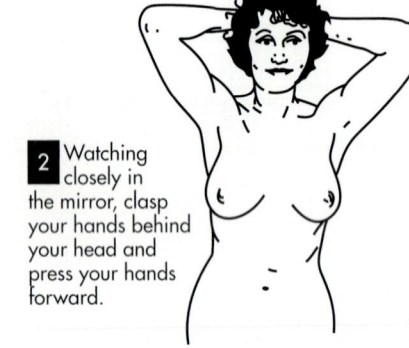

2 Watching closely in the mirror, clasp your hands behind your head and press your hands forward.

3 Next, press your hands firmly on your hips and bow slightly toward the mirror as you pull your shoulders and elbows forward.

Some women do the next part of the exam in the shower. Your fingers will glide easily over soapy skin, so you can concentrate on feeling for changes inside the breast.

4 Raise your left arm. Use three or four fingers of your right hand to feel your left breast firmly, carefully, and thoroughly. Beginning at the outer edge, press the flat part of your fingers in small circles, moving the circles slowly around the breast. Gradually work toward the nipple. Be sure to cover the whole breast. Pay special attention to the area between the breast and the underarm, including the underarm area itself. Feel for any unusual lump or mass under the skin.

5 Gently squeeze the nipple and look for a discharge. (If you have any discharge during the month—whether or not it is during BSE—see your doctor.) Repeat the exam on your right breast.

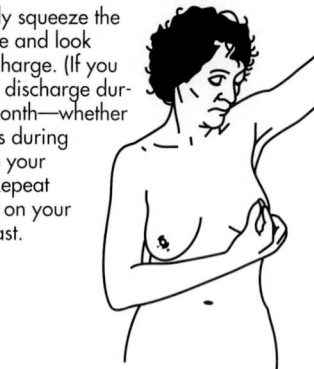

6 Steps 4 and 5 should be repeated lying down. Lie flat on your back, with your left arm over your head and a pillow or folded towel under your left shoulder. This position flattens the breast and makes it easier to check it. Use the same circular motion described above. Repeat on your right breast.

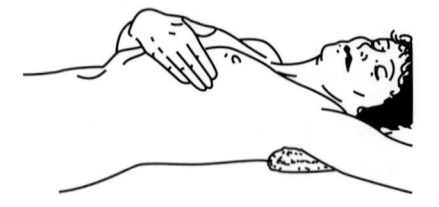

Fig. A-12   **Breast self-examination (BSE).** (Redrawn from NIH Publication No. 91-1556, Oct 1990.)

Cancer Risk Factor Screening for Women

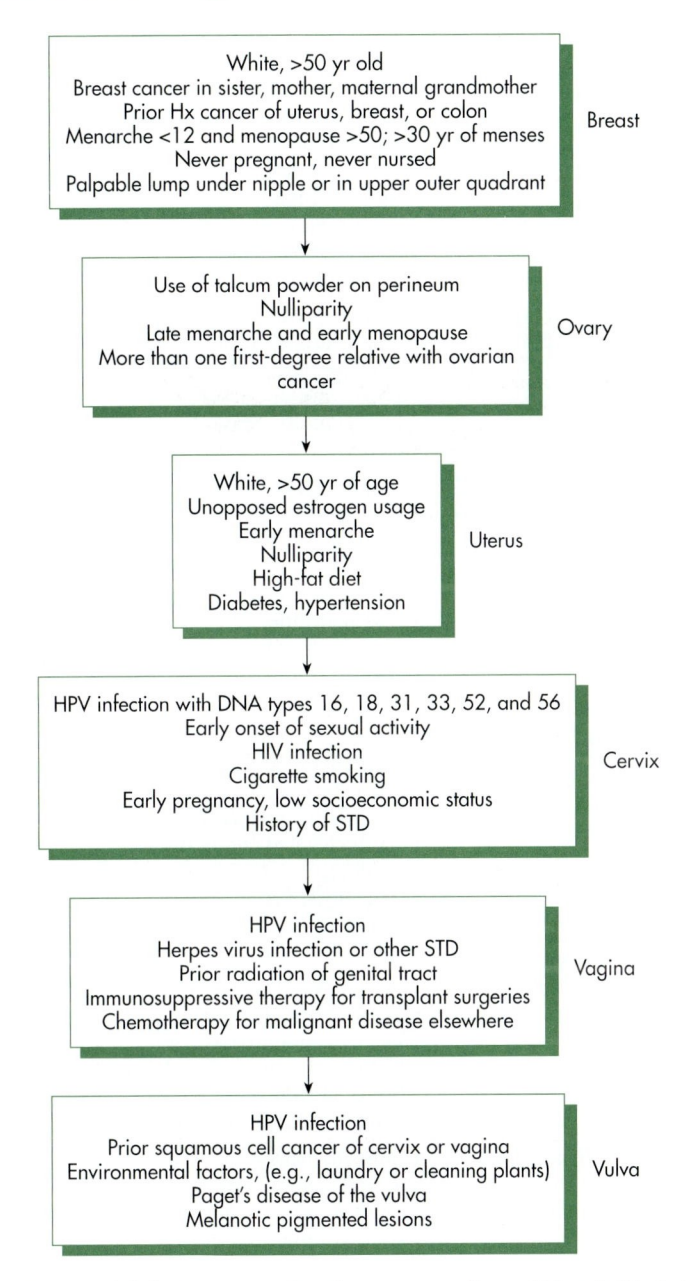

Breast
- White, >50 yr old
- Breast cancer in sister, mother, maternal grandmother
- Prior Hx cancer of uterus, breast, or colon
- Menarche <12 and menopause >50; >30 yr of menses
- Never pregnant, never nursed
- Palpable lump under nipple or in upper outer quadrant

Ovary
- Use of talcum powder on perineum
- Nulliparity
- Late menarche and early menopause
- More than one first-degree relative with ovarian cancer

Uterus
- White, >50 yr of age
- Unopposed estrogen usage
- Early menarche
- Nulliparity
- High-fat diet
- Diabetes, hypertension

Cervix
- HPV infection with DNA types 16, 18, 31, 33, 52, and 56
- Early onset of sexual activity
- HIV infection
- Cigarette smoking
- Early pregnancy, low socioeconomic status
- History of STD

Vagina
- HPV infection
- Herpes virus infection or other STD
- Prior radiation of genital tract
- Immunosuppressive therapy for transplant surgeries
- Chemotherapy for malignant disease elsewhere

Vulva
- HPV infection
- Prior squamous cell cancer of cervix or vagina
- Environmental factors, (e.g., laundry or cleaning plants)
- Paget's disease of the vulva
- Melanotic pigmented lesions

Fig. A-13 Cancer risk factor screening for women. (From Driscoll CE et al: *The family practice desk reference,* ed 3, St Louis, 1996, Mosby.)

Possible Strategies for Follow-up of Selected Cancers

TABLE A-20 Possible Strategies for Follow-up of Selected Cancers

CANCER SITE	FOLLOW-UP FREQUENCY	REGIMEN FOR EACH FOLLOW-UP VISIT	ADDITIONAL FOLLOW-UP
Prostate	Every 3-4 mo × 3 yr; then every 6 mo × 2 yr; then annually	Complete history Physical examination Complete blood count Hepatic transaminases Alkaline phosphatase PSA	
Breast	Every 3 mo × 3 yr; then every 6 mo × 2 yr; then annually	Complete history Physical examination Complete blood count Hepatic transaminases Alkaline phosphatase Calcium	Mammography every 12 mo; CXR every 6-12 mo
Lung	Every 3 mo × 3 yr; then every 6 mo × 3 yr; then annually	Complete history Physical examination Complete blood count Hepatic transaminases Alkaline phosphatase BUN/creatinine Calcium phosphate CXR	Chest CT with cuts through the liver and adrenals every 6-12 mo
Colorectal	Every 3 mo × 2 yr; then every 6 mo × 3 yr; then annually	Complete history Physical examination Complete blood count Hepatic transaminases Alkaline phosphatase CEA (if elevated before surgery) Sigmoidoscopy (if S/P anterior resection of rectal lesion)	CXR annually Colonoscopy (every 3-6 mo after surgery in patients with obstructing lesion) or Colonoscopy (at 1 yr after surgery; if negative then every 2-3 yr in patients without an obstructing lesion)
Bladder	Every 3 mo × 2 yr; then every 6 mo × 3 yr; then annually	Complete history Physical examination Complete blood count Hepatic transaminases Alkaline phosphatase BUN/creatinine Urinalysis, urine cytology	Cystoscopy and urethral washings with each visit (when organ has been preserved)
Uterine cervix	Every 3 mo × 1 yr; then every 4 mo × 1 yr; then every 6 mo × 3 yr; then annually	Complete history Physical examination Complete blood count Hepatic transaminases Alkaline phosphatase BUN/creatinine Urinalysis CXR Colposcopy	Abdominal/pelvic CT every 6-12 mo × 3-5 yr
Testicular	Every 1 mo × 1 yr; then every 2 mo × 1 yr; then every 3-6 mo thereafter	Complete history Physical examination Complete blood count Hepatic transaminases Alkaline phosphatase CXR Serum tumor markers (α-fetoprotein, β-subunit of human chorionic gonadotropin)	Abdominal/pelvic CT every 2-3 mo × 1 yr; then every 6 mo

TABLE A-20 Possible Strategies for Follow-up of Selected Cancers—cont'd

CANCER SITE	FOLLOW-UP FREQUENCY	REGIMEN FOR EACH FOLLOW-UP VISIT	ADDITIONAL FOLLOW-UP
Oropharyngeal	Every 1 mo × 1 yr; then every 2-3 mo × 2 yr; then every 6 mo × 2 yr; then annually	Complete history Physical examination	CXR Indirect laryngoscopy Sputum cytology
Skin (melanoma)	Every 3 mo × 2 yr; then every 6 mo × 4 yr; then annually	Complete history Physical examination Complete blood count Hepatic transaminases Alkaline phosphatase	

From Noble J (ed): *Primary care medicine*, ed 2, St Louis, 1996, Mosby.
BUN, Blood urea nitrogen; *CXR,* chest x-ray; *CT,* computed tomography; *CEA,* carcinoembryonic antigen.

EMERGENCY MEDICINE
Toxicology Treatment Protocols

TABLE A-21 Prevention of Absorption

MODALITIES	AGENTS/METHODS	DOSAGE	COMMENTS
Gastric emptying	Ipecac	*Peds:* <15 mo: 10 ml PO >15 mo: 15 ml PO *Adults:* 30-60 ml PO	Contraindicated in comatose or seizing patients, in caustic ingestions, or children <9 mo old
	Lavage Ewald tubes *Peds:* 24-28 FR	*Peds:* 2-3 ml/kg aliquots of warmed saline	Protect airway
	Adults: 36-40 FR	*Adults:* 2-3 ml/kg aliquots	
Binding of toxin	Activated charcoal	*Peds:* 30-50 g PO *Adults:* 50-100 g PO 1 g/kg	1. Contraindicated in caustic ingestions 2. May bind acetylcysteine 3. Ineffective in methanol/iron ingestions 4. Pulse doses q2-4h. Effective for drugs with significant enterohepatic recirculation
Neutralizers [used in place of activated charcoal]	Sodium formaldehyde sulfoxylate	20 g ampule PO	Mercury poisoning
	Sodium bicarbonate lavage	300 ml 10% solution left in stomach after lavage	Iron poisoning
	Potassium permanganate	100 mg/1000 ml of saline or water for lavage	Poisoning from nicotine, cyanide, quinine, physiostigmine, strychnine
	Starch solution	75 mg/1000 ml of saline or water for lavage	Iodine poisoning
Cathartics	Magnesium sulfate Magnesium citrate	*Peds:* 250 mg/kg *Adults:* 30 g (300 ml of 10% solution)	Contraindicated in renal failure, gastrointestinal bleeding, or ileus
	Sorbitol	*Adults:* 40 ml of 70% W/W solution *Peds (up to 6 yr old):* 20 ml of 70% W/W solution	

Modified from Rosen P et al (eds): *Emergency medicine: concepts and clinical practice*, ed 3, St Louis, 1997, Mosby.

TABLE A-22 Forced Diuresis (Understand Limited Benefits). Poisonings that Require Immediate Dialysis: Methyl Alcohol, Ethylene Glycol, *Amanita phalloides* Ingestion

	NEUTRAL DIURESIS (NS OR LR IV TO MAINTAIN URINE OUTPUT OF 3-6 ML/KG/HR)	ACID DIURESIS (MAINTAIN URINE pH 5.5-6.5)	ALKALINE DIURESIS
Agents	Furosemide IV *Peds:* 1 mg/kg *Adults:* 40 mg Mannitol IV *Peds:* 750 mg/kg *Adults:* 20-50 g	Ascorbic acid *Adults:* 0.5-2.0 g PO or IV q6h Ammonium chloride IV *Peds:* 75 mg/kg per dose (max 1.5 g) q6h (max dose: 6-8 g/24 hr) *Adults:* 20 mg/kg per dose (max 4 g) q2-6h HCl via CVP *Adults:* 0.2 mEq/kg	Bicarbonate 1-2 mEq/kg IV
	Give furosemide and IV fluids when urine reaches desired pH		
Indicated in poisonings from:	Bromides Isoniazid	Phencyclidine (PCP) Strychnine Amphetamines Quinine Quinidine	Salicylates Phenobarbital Lithium
Precautions	Avoid volume depletion	Avoid volume depletion Contraindicated in rhabdomyolysis or myoglobinuria	Avoid volume depletion Monitor and replace urinary K^+ losses

Modified from Rosen P et al (eds): *Emergency medicine: concepts and clinical practice,* ed 3, St Louis, 1997, Mosby.

TABLE A-23 Antidotes

POISON	ANTIDOTE	DOSAGE	INDICATIONS	COMMENTS
Acetaminophen	Acetylcysteine	*Load:* 140 mg/kg PO *Maint:* 70 mg/kg PO q4h × 17 doses	1. Toxic APAP levels 2. Estimated ingestion >140 mg/kg (10 g in adults)	1. Most effective within 12 hr of ingestion.
Anticholinergics (atropine)	Physostigmine	*Adult:* 1-2 mg IV over 2 min. Repeat q10 min (max dose: 4 mg/30 min) *Peds:* 0.5 mg IV over 2 min. May repeat dose q10min to max dose of 2 mg	1. Cardiac dysrhythmia refractory to lidocaine 2. Unstable SVT 3. Refractory seizures 4. Prolonged CNS effects	1. May induce convulsions and bradycardia (cholinergic crisis). Use with caution.
Arsenic/mercury/gold	BAL (dimercaprol)	3-5 mg/kg IM q4h × 2 days		1. Treatment may induce nausea, vomiting, headache, dysesthesia, and hypertension.
Benzodiazepines	Flumazenil	*Adult:* 1 mg IV	1. Benzodiazepine overdose	1. Patient should rapidly awake if benzodiazepines are responsible for obtunded state.
β-blocker	Glucagon	*Load:* 3-10 mg IV over 2 min *Infuse:* 2-5 mg over 1 hr, taper over 12 hr	1. Bradycardia or heart block 2. Refractory hypotension	1. Antiemetic or NG tube for glycogen-induced vomiting (30%-50% incidence).
Carbon monoxide	Oxygen	100% O_2 by tight mask Hyperbaric O_2 at 3 atmospheres	1. COHb > 25% 2. COHb > 15% + history of cardiac diseases 3. Acute ECG changes 4. CNS symptoms 5. Metabolic acidosis + exposure 6. Abnormal thermoregulation 7. P_{O_2} >60 mm Hg 8. Pregnancy with symptoms or COHb > 10% 9. CO + cyanide or other metabolic toxin	1. Indications for admission are same as for hyperbaric treatment.
Cholinergic	Atropine	*Adult:* 2 mg IV q10-30 min until stable *Peds:* 0.05 mg/kg IV q10-30 min	1. SLUDGE syndrome 2. Muscarinic effects	1. Blocks acetylcholine. 2. Expect results in 10 min. 3. Physiologic antidote.
	Pralidoxime (2-PAM)	*Adult:* 1 g/100 cc NS IV over 30 min *Peds:* 25-50 mg/kg IV over 30 min	1. Organophosphates 2. Nicotine effects of twitching, respiratory paralysis, and areflexia	1. Not for carbamate poisoning. 2. Nicotinic and muscarnic effects. 3. Specific antidote. 4. Give atropine before 2-PAM.

Modified from Rosen P et al (eds): *Emergency medicine: concepts and clinical practice,* ed 3, St Louis, 1997, Mosby.

Treatment Guidelines for STDs Following Sexual Assault

TABLE A-24 Management of Sexual Assault: Treatment Guidelines for Sexually Transmitted Diseases

DISEASE	PROPHYLACTIC ANTIBIOTICS RECOMMENDED TREATMENT	ALTERNATIVES
Gonorrhea	Ceftriaxone 250 mg IM once	Cefixime 400 mg PO once
Pharyngeal, rectal		
Urogenital		Spectinomycin 2 g IM once*
Pregnancy	Same	Same
Chlamydia		
Urethral, cervical, rectal	Doxycycline 100 mg PO bid × 7 days	Azithromycin 1 g PO once†
		Erythromycin 500 mg PO qid × 7 days
Pregnancy	Erythromycin 500 mg PO qid × 7 days	Erythromycin ethylsuccinate 800 mg PO qid × 7 days‡
		Amoxicillin 500 mg PO tid × 7 days
Trichomonas	Metronidazole (Flagyl) 2 g PO once	Flagyl 500 mg PO bid × 7 days
Pregnancy		
First trimester	Wait until after first trimester, then treat	
Second and third trimesters	Oral Flagyl	
Bacterial Vaginosis	Flagyl 500 mg PO bid × 7 days	Clindamycin cream 2%, one vaginal application qhs × 7 days
		Clindamycin 300 mg PO bid × 7 days
		Flagyl 2 g PO once
Pregnancy		
First trimester	Clindamycin cream	
Second and third trimesters	Oral or vaginal Flagyl	
Hepatitis B		
Immune globulin§	0.06 ml/kg single IM dose within 14 days of exposure	
Vaccination§	Three doses, each 1 ml IM in the deltoid muscle at 0, 1, 6 mo	

Modified from Centers for Disease Control and Prevention: *MMWR* 42 (No RR-14):3184, 1993.
*Not effective against pharyngeal gonorrhea nor against incubating syphilis.
†Safety during pregnancy not been established.
‡Can switch to 250 mg PO qid for 14 days if not tolerated; erythromycin estolate is contraindicated during pregnancy.
§Both safe in pregnancy.

Bite Wounds Guidelines

> **BOX A-15 Bite Wounds Guidelines**
>
> ### Treatment
>
> #### Preexposure Prophylaxis
>
> Preexposure prophylaxis is important for spelunkers, veterinarians, and virologists. Human diploid vaccine should be given. The neutralizing antibody titer should be followed to ensure immunity in high-risk or exposed individuals.
>
> #### Postexposure Prophylaxis
>
> After exposure the following questions must be asked:
> 1. What is the status of animal rabies in the locale where the exposure took place? (This may require a call to your public health department.)
> 2. Was the attack provoked or unprovoked?
> 3. Of what species was the animal?
> 4. What was the state of health of the animal?
>
> Most animals transmit rabies virus in saliva only a few days before becoming ill themselves (dog and skunk, 5 days; fox, 3 days; cat, 1 day); bats, however, may harbor the virus for many months.
>
> #### Bites by household pets
>
> If the dog or cat is healthy and available for observation for 10 days, do not treat the patient unless the animal develops rabies. An exception to this rule is bites to the head, where an incubation period of 4 days has been reported and prophylaxis should begin immediately. At the first sign of rabies in the animal, treat the patient with rabies immune globulin (RIG) and human diploid cell vaccine (HDCV). The symptomatic animal should be killed and tested as soon as possible.
>
> If the pet is rabid or suspected to be rabid, or a pet from outside the United States (especially Latin America, Africa, and most of Asia), treat with RIG and HDCV.
>
> #### Bites by wild animals
>
> All skunks, bats, foxes, coyotes, raccoons, bobcats, and other carnivores should be regarded as rabid unless laboratory tests prove negative. Treat the patient with RIG and HDCV.
>
> #### Bites by other animals
>
> Consider other animals (e.g., livestock, rodents, lagomorphs) individually. Local and state public health officials should be consulted on the need for prophylaxis. Bites by the following almost never call for antirabies prophylaxis: squirrels, hamsters, guinea pigs, gerbils, chipmunks, rats, mice and other rodents, rabbits, and hares.
>
> ### Specifics of Treatment
>
> 1. The most important step is to cleanse the wound immediately and with a brush and soap to remove as much virus as possible. Rinse well, then perform a second scrub with soap or alcohol, *which is rabicidal*. This reduces the risk of rabies by as much as 90%.
> 2. If vaccine treatment is indicated, both RIG and HDCV should be given as soon as possible, regardless of interval after exposure.
>
> The administration of RIG is the more urgent procedure. If HDCV is not immediately available, start RIG and give HDCV as soon as it is obtained. RIG is given at a total dose of 20 IU/kg, with half infiltrated at the wound site and half IM in the arm or thigh. This passive immunization results in the early appearance of antibody but also inhibits the development of the active antibody from the human diploid vaccine, thus the reason for prolonged dosage of the vaccines.
>
> Active immunization is accomplished with the HDCV. It is given intramuscularly for a total of five doses, on days 0, 3, 7, 14, and 28. Serum for rabies antibody testing should be collected 2 weeks after the fifth dose. If there is no antibody response, give an additional booster.

From Noble J (ed): *Primary care medicine,* ed 2, St Louis, 1996, Mosby.

Thrombolytic Therapy in AMI

BOX A-16 Qualifying Criteria for the Use of Thrombolytic Therapy in AMI

Age <75 Yr Old*

Risk of developing a major hemorrhagic complication progressively increases with increasing age

Symptom Onset Within 6 Hr

History of new-onset (ischemic-sounding) chest pain of at least 30 min duration that is not relieved by sublingual nitroglycerin

Symptom onset should be less than 6 hr before the time of presentation (and ideally less than 3-4 hr).

Patients with either intermittent chest pain (i.e., "stuttering" infarction) and/or persistent chest pain of *greater than* 6 hr duration may still be candidates for thrombolytic therapy if the clinical picture suggests that AMI is still in the process of evolving.

Definitive Evidence of AMI in Progress

Definitive ECG changes (i.e., ≥ 1 mm of ST segment elevation in ≥ two contiguous leads)

- Identifies patients who are most likely to benefit from thrombolytic therapy
- Minimizes chance of misdiagnosing conditions such as acute pericarditis or dissecting aneurysm, and inappropriately treating with thrombolytic therapy

Strongly consider repeating the ECG if the history is highly suggestive of AMI and the initial tracing fails to show definitive changes

Strongly consider repeating the ECG if chest pain completely resolves following nitroglycerin to verify that ST segment elevation is still present (i.e., to rule out coronary spasm)

If readily available, echocardiography may occasionally help diagnose AMI in patients who do not demonstrate definitive ECG changes (although these patients are less likely to benefit from thrombolytic therapy)

No Absolute Contraindications to Thrombolytic Therapy

From Grauer K, Cavallaro D (eds): *ACLS certification preparation*, St Louis, 1993, Mosby.
*The cutoff for age should not be absolute, however, since the incidence and mortality of AMI *also* increase with age. The decision of whether to treat a patient over 75 may therefore need to be individualized.

BOX A-17 Contraindications to the Use of Thrombolytic Therapy in AMI (Adapted from the ACC/AHA Task Force Report, 1990)

Absolute Contraindications

Active bleeding disorder
Recent trauma or surgery (i.e., within the previous 2 wk)
Suspected aortic aneurysm/acute pericarditis
Prolonged or traumatic CPR
Recent head trauma or known intracranial neoplasm
Previous allergic reaction to the thrombolytic agent being considered (i.e., streptokinase or APSAC)
Excessive hypertension (i.e., BP *remains* >180/110 mm Hg)
History of recent CVA/TIA (i.e., within the previous 6 mo) or of a cerebrovascular accident known to be hemorrhagic
Diabetic hemorrhagic retinopathy or other hemorrhagic ophthalmologic condition
Pregnancy

Relative Contraindications

Relatively recent trauma or surgery (i.e., performed *more than* 2 wk before the time of presentation)
Long-term history of severe hypertension
Active peptic ulcer disease (but *without* known GI bleeding)
History of remote CVA/TIA (i.e., more than 6 mo ago)
Known bleeding diathesis or current use of anticoagulants
Cardiopulmonary resuscitation of relatively short duration (<10 min)
Significant liver dysfunction
Prior exposure to streptokinase or APSAC (especially within the preceding 6 to 9 mo)*

From Grauer K, Cavallaro D (eds): *ACLS certification preparation*, St Louis, 1993, Mosby.
*Non-streptokinase-containing agents (i.e., rt-PA, urokinase; etc.) may be used again without concern for developing an allergic reaction.

Burn Area Estimation

TABLE A-25 Rule of Nines

AREA	%*	AREA	%*
Head and neck	9	Posterior chest and abdomen	18
Right upper extremity	9	Genitals	1
Left upper extremity	9	Right lower extremity	18
Anterior chest and abdomen	18	Left lower extremity	18
		TOTAL	100

*The percentages are added to determine the extent of burn injury in the patient.

TABLE A-26 Lund-Browder Chart for Burn Estimate (Percentage of Body Surface Area)

AREA	0-1	1-4	5-9	10-15	ADULT
Head	19	17	13	10	7
Neck	2	2	2	2	2
Anterior trunk	13	17	13	13	13
Posterior trunk	13	13	13	13	13
Right buttock	2½	2½	2½	2½	2½
Left buttock	2½	2½	2½	2½	2½
Genitalia	1	1	1	1	1
Right upper arm	4	4	4	4	4
Left upper arm	4	4	4	4	4
Right lower arm	3	3	3	3	3
Left lower arm	3	3	3	3	3
Right hand	2½	2½	2½	2½	2½
Left hand	2½	2½	2½	2½	2½
Right thigh	5½	6½	8½	8½	9½
Left thigh	5½	6½	8½	8½	9½
Right leg	5	5	5½	6	7
Left leg	5	5	5½	6	7
Right foot	3½	3½	3½	3½	3½
Left foot	3½	3½	3½	3½	3½

From Noble J (ed): *Primary care medicine,* ed 2, St Louis, 1996, Mosby.

COMMUNITY RESOURCES

> **BOX A-18** **Community Resources Used by Family Physician's Patients**
>
> **Physical Health Care**
>
> Child development clinics—diagnoses of various handicaps
> County health department—TB and STD case follow-up
> Community dental services
> National Black Women's Health Project (1-800-275-2947)
> Public health nurses—immunization program
> Planned Parenthood and family planning clinics—contraception and venereal disease treatment (1-800-230-7526)
> Veterinarian—zoonoses control
> Women-infants-children (WIC) programs providing food supplements
>
> **Home Care**
>
> Hospice—terminal illness care
> Homemakers, Inc.—housekeeping assistance
> Home Intravenous Therapy Team
> La Leche League—breastfeeding (1-800-525-3243)
> Medical equipment and supply companies—home oxygen and sick care items
> Manpower Health Care Services
> Occupational therapist
> Visiting Nurses Association—home nursing assistance
> Others listed in Yellow Pages under "nurses" or "health"
>
> **Social Services**
>
> Aid to Dependent Children (ADC)
> Child Welfare Services—foster care, child abuse intervention
> Department of Public Assistance
> Eldercare Locator (1-800-677-1116)
> Food Stamp Program—food assistance
> General Assistance to Unemployed (GAU)
> Health Foundation National Clearinghouse on Postsecondary Education for People with Disabilities (1-800-544-3284)
> Hill-Burton Funds—free or reduced hospital services provided by some hospitals
> Lutheran Social Services—social and psychologic services
> Medicaid—financial aid for medical services
> Medicare Hotline (1-800-638-6833)
> National Council for Adoption
> National Information Center for Children/Youth with Disabilities
> National Information Clearinghouse for Infants with Disabilities and Life-Threatening Conditions (1-800-922-9234)
> National Rehabilitation Information Center (1-800-346-2742)
> United Cerebral Palsy Association (1-800-872-5827)
>
> **Psychologic Services**
>
> Al-Anon (1-800-443-4525)
> Al-Anon Family Groups (1-800-356-9996)
> Alcohol and Drug Information Referral Line (1-800-252-6465)
> Association for Retarded Citizens
> Cocaine Hotline (1-800-262-2463)
> Community mental health services
> Crisis center—all types of emotional problems
> Marriage and family service
> National Clearinghouse on Family Support/Children's Mental Health (1-800-628-1696)
> National Council on Alcoholism and Drug Dependence Hopeline (1-800-622-2255)
> National Down Syndrome Congress (1-800-232-6372)
> National Down Syndrome Society (1-800-221-4602)
> National Institute on Drug Abuse Hotline (1-800-662-4357)
> National Runaway Switchboard (1-800-621-4000)
> Parents Anonymous, Inc.
> Pastoral care through local churches
> Phoenix Society for Burn Survivors (1-800-888-2876)
> Rape crisis center—sexual assault
>
> **Disease-Related Associations and General Information Services**
>
> Alzheimer's Association (1-800-272-3900)
> American Cancer Society (1-800-227-2345)
> American Diabetes Association (1-800-232-3472)
> American Heart Association (1-800-242-8721)
> American Liver Foundation (1-800-223-0179)
> American Lung Association (1-800-362-1643-Iowa only)
> American Parkinson Disease Association (1-800-223-2732)
> American Society for Deaf Children (1-800-942-2732)
> Birthright (1-800-848-5683)
> Cancer Information and Counseling Line (1-800-525-3777)
> Cancer Information Service of the National Cancer Institute (1-800-422-6237)
> Candlelighters Childhood Cancer Foundation (1-800-366-2223)
> CDC National AIDS Clearinghouse (1-800-458-5231)
> CDC National AIDS Hotline (1-800-342-2437)
>   Deaf Consumers (1-800-243-7889)
>   Spanish-Speaking Consumers (1-800-344-7432)
> CDC National Sexually Transmitted Diseases Hotline (1-800-227-8922)
> Cystic Fibrosis Foundation (1-800-344-4823)
> Easter Seals
> Epilepsy Foundation of America (1-800-332-1000)
> Hearing AID Help Line (1-800-521-5247)
> International Shriners Hospital (1-800-237-5055)
> Leukemia Society of America (1-800-955-4572)
> Lupus Foundation of America, Inc. (1-800-558-0121)
> Multiple Sclerosis Association (1-800-798-6677, Iowa only)
> Muscular Dystrophy Association
> National Abortion Federation Hotline (1-800-772-9100)
> National Center for the Blind (1-800-638-7518)
> National Marrow Donor Program for Cancer Patients (1-800-654-1247)
> National Organization for Rare Disorders (1-800-999-6673)
> National Parkinson Foundation (1-800-327-4545)
> National Spinal Cord Injury Hotline (1-800-962-9629)
> Senior Citizens Center

From Driscoll CE et al: *The family practice desk reference,* ed 3, St Louis, 1996, Mosby.

APPENDIX Community resources/Treatment of bacterial endocarditis 1061

BOX A-18 Community Resources Used by Family Physician's Patients—cont'd

Disease-Related Associations and General Information Services—cont'd

Simon Foundation for Continence/Help for Incontinent People (1-800-237-4666)
Social Security Office
Spina Bifida Association of America (1-800-621-3141)
United Ostomy Association (1-800-826-0826)
United Way (1-703-836-7100)
University of Iowa Cancer Information Service (1-800-237-1225)

Volunteer Groups
Y-ME for Breast Cancer (1-800-221-2141)

Short-Term Emergency Assistance
American Red Cross (1-202-737-8300)
Community churches
Community food pantry
REACT and Civil Defense
Salvation Army (1-703-684-5500)

TREATMENT OF BACTERIAL ENDOCARDITIS

TABLE A-27 Current Recommendations for Treatment of Bacterial Endocarditis

ANTIBIOTICS	DOSAGE*	ADMINISTRATION	DURATION	COMMENTS
Penicillin-Susceptible Viridans Streptococci and *Streptococcus bovis* (MIC ≤0.1 μg/ml)				
1. Penicillin G	2 million U q4h	IV	4 wk	Preferred in patients >65 yr old and those with renal or eight cranial nerve impairment, heart failure, or CNS complications; effective for other penicillin-susceptible non-viridans streptococci
2. Penicillin G and gentamicin†	2 million U q4h 1 mg/kg (not to exceed 80 mg) q8h	IV IV	2 wk 2 wk	Uncomplicated patient: age <65 yr; no renal or eighth cranial nerve impairment; no CNS complication; no severe heart failure; not nutritionally deficient variant; viridans streptococci and *S. bovis* only
3. Penicillin G and gentamicin†	2 million U q4h 1 mg/kg (not to exceed 80 mg) q8h	IV IV	4 wk 2 wk	Nutritionally deficient variants; relapse complications such as shock or extracardiac focus of infection; 6 wk of penicillin for prosthetic valve infection
4. Vancomycin‡	15 mg/kg (not to exceed 1 g) q12h	IV	4 wk	Penicillin allergy
5. Cefazolin§	1-2 g q8h	IV	4 wk	Penicillin allergy
6. Ceftriaxone§	2 g once daily	IV or IM	4 wk	Uncomplicated patient with viridans streptococci; candidate for outpatient therapy; penicillin allergy
Strains of Viridans Streptococci and *S. bovis* Relatively Resistant to Penicillin G (0.1 μg/ml <MIC <0.5 μg/ml)				
1. Penicillin G and gentamicin†	2 million U q4h 1 mg/kg (not to exceed 80 mg) q8h	IV IV	4 wk 2 wk	For MIC >0.5 μg/ml, treat same as enterococcus; for prosthetic valve infection, give 6 wk of penicillin and 6 wk of gentamicin

From Stein JH (ed): *Internal medicine*, ed 4, St Louis, 1994, Mosby.
*Dosages are for patients with normal renal function.
†Streptomycin, 500 mg q12h IM, may be used instead of gentamicin. Gentamicin doses should be adjusted to achieve a peak serum concentration of 3 μg/ml and streptomycin a peak serum concentration of 20 μg/ml.
‡Vancomycin peak serum concentrations 1 hr after infusion should be in the range of 30-45 μg/ml.
§Cephalosporins should be avoided in patients with an immediate-type hypersensitivity reaction to penicillin.
‖This use of rifampin is not listed in the manufacturer's official directive.
¶*Haemophilus* sp, *Actinobacillus actinomycelemcomitans*, *Cardiobacterium hominis*, *Eikenella corrodens*, *Kingella kingii*.
MIC, Minimum inhibitory concentration.

Continued

TABLE A-27 Current Recommendations for Treatment of Bacterial Endocarditis—cont'd

ANTIBIOTICS	DOSAGE*	ADMINISTRATION	DURATION	COMMENTS
Strains of Viridans Streptococci and *S. bovis* Relatively Resistant to Penicillin G (0.1 μg/ml <MIC <0.5 μg/ml)—cont'd				
2. Vancomycin‡	15 mg/kg (not to exceed 1 g) q12h	IV	4 wk	Penicillin allergy; avoidance of gentamicin
3. Cefazolin§	1-2 g q8h	IV	4 wk	Penicillin allergy; avoidance of gentamicin
Enterococcal *(E. faecalis)* (or Viridans Streptococci with MI ≤0.5 μg/ml)				
1. Penicillin G	4 million U q4h	IV	4-6 wk	Increase to 6-8 wk for symptoms longer than 3 mo, complicated course, or prosthetic valve infection; some would use ampicillin, but no evidence of superiority available
and gentamicin†	1 mg/kg (not to exceed 80 mg) q8h	IV	4-6 wk	
2. Vancomycin‡	15 mg/kg (not to exceed 1 g) q12h	IV	4-6 wk	Penicillin allergy
and gentamicin†	1 mg/kg (not to exceed 80 mg) q8h	IV	4-6 wk	
Staphylococcus aureus				
1. Nafcillin	1.5 g q4h	IV	4 wk	Methicillin-susceptible strain; increase duration to 6 wk for complicated infection; omit gentamicin for significant renal impairment; some recommend gentamicin for 5-7 days
and gentamicin†	1 mg/kg (not to exceed 80 mg) q8h	IV	3-5 days	
2. Vancomycin‡	15 mg/kg (not to exceed 1 g) q12h	IV	4-6 wk	Penicillin allergy or methicillin-resistant strain; increase duration to 6 wk or longer for complicated infection
3. Cefazolin§	2 g q8h	IV	4-6 wk	Penicillin allergy; increase duration to 6 wk for complicated infection
4. Nafcillin	1.5 g q4h	IV	2 wk	Methicillin-susceptible strain; IV drug user, tricuspid valve infection only, no extrapulmonary infection, no renal impairment
and gentamicin†	1 mg/kg (not to exceed 80 mg) q8h	IV	3-5 days	
5. Nafcillin	1.5 g q4h	IV	6-8 wk	Prosthetic valve infected with methicillin-susceptible strain; for methicillin-resistant strain, substitute vancomycin for nafcillin
and rifampin*	300 mg q12h	PO or IV	6 wk	
and gentamicin†	1 mg/kg (not to exceed 80 mg) q8h	IV	2 wk	
Coagulase-Negative Staphylococci or Prosthetic Valve Infection				
1. Nafcillin	1.5 g q4h	IV	6-8 wk	Methicillin-susceptible strain; vancomycin recommended in case of uncertain methicillin susceptibility
and rifampin	300 mg q12h	PO or IV	6-8 wk	
gentamicin†	1 mg/kg (not to exceed 80 mg) q8h	IV	2 wk	
2. Vancomycin‡	15 mg/kg (not to exceed 1 g) q12h	IV	6-8 wk	Methicillin-resistant strain; penicillin allergy
and rifampin‖	300 mg q12h	PO or IV	6-8 wk	
and gentamicin‡	1 mg/kg (not to exceed 80 mg) q8h	IV	2 wk	
HACEK Group¶				
1. Ampicillin	2 g q4h	IV	4 wk	Definitive regimen determined by in vitro susceptibilities
and gentamicin†	1 mg/kg not to exceed 80 mg) q8h	PO or IV	4 wk	
2. Ceftriaxone§	2 g once daily	IV or IM	6 wk	Penicillin allergy

MEDICAL RECORD ABBREVIATIONS

a	arterial
A₂	aortic second sound
Aa	alveolar/arterial
āā	of each
AAA	abdominal aortic aneurysm
AB	apical beat
ABC	airway, breathing, circulation
abd	abdomen
ABG	arterial blood gas
ABI	ankle-brachial reflex
abn	abnormal
ABVD	doxorubicin (Adriamycin), bleomycin, vinblastine, dacarbazine (DTIC)
ac	before meals
AC	abdominal circumference
A/C	assist control
ACE	angiotension-converting enzyme, adrenocortical extract
acet	acetone
aCL	anticardiolipin (antibody)
ACOG	American College of Obstetricians and Gynecologists
ACLS	advanced cardiovascular life support
ACT	activated clotting time
ACTH	adrenocorticotropic hormone
ACV	Assist Control Ventilation
ADA	American Dental Association, American Diabetic Association, American Dietetic Association
ADH	antidiruetic hormone
ADL	activities of daily living
ad lib	as desired, freely
adm	admission
ADPKD	autosomal dominant polycystic kidney disease
AF	atrial fibrillation
AFB	acid-fast bacilli
AFP	alpha-fetoprotein
A/G	albumin/globulin ratio
AG	anion gap
AICP	autoimplantable cardioverter/defibrillator
AIDP	acute inflammatory demyelinating polyneuropathy
AIDS	acquired immune deficiency syndrome
AJ	ankle jerk
AKA	above-knee amputation
AL	arterial line
alb	albumin
alk phos	alkaline phosphatase
ALL	acute lymphoblastic leukemia
ALS	amotrophic lateral sclerosis
ALT	alanine aminotransferase
AM	morning
AMA	against medical advice, American Medical Association, Anti-Mitochondrial Antibody
AMI	acute myocardial infarction
AML	acute myelogenous leukemia
amp	ampule
AMP	adenosine monophosphate
amt	amount
amy	amylase
ANA	antinuclear antibody
ANCA	antineutrophil cytoplasmic antibody
ANLL	acute nonlymphocytic leukemia
Anti-SMA	Anti-smooth muscle antibody
AODM	adult-onset diabetes mellitus
AOP	aortic pressure
A&P	auscultation and percussion
AP	anteroposterior
APA	aldosterone-producing adenoma
APAG	antipseudomonal aminoglycosidic penicillin
appt	appointment
APRV	airway pressure release ventilation
APSAC	anisoylated plasminogen/streptokinase activator complex
APS	Anti-phospholipid syndrome
APTT	activated partial thromboplastin time
APUD	amine precursor uptake decarboxylase
aq	water
AR	aortic regurgitation
ARC	AIDS-related complex
ARDS	acute respiratory distress syndrome
ARF	acute renal failure
ARM	artificial rupture of membranes
ARPKD	autosomal recessive polycystic kidney disease
ART	assessment, review, and treatment
AS	Atriosystolic, aortic stenosis
asa	aspirin
ASA	American Society of Anesthesiologists
ASCUS	atypical squamous cells of undetermined significance
ASH	asymmetric septal hypertrophy
ASHD	arteriosclerotic heart disease
ASO (also ASLO)	antistreptolysin O
AST	aspartate aminotransferase
at fib	atrial fibrillation
ATC	around the clock
ATD	antithyroid drugs
ATG	antithymocyte globulin
ATN	acute tubular necrosis
AV	arteriovenous, atrioventricular
AVM	arteriovenous malformation
AVP	arginine vasopressin
AZT	zidovudine
B	black
ba	barium
BA	bone age
BACOD	bleomycin, doxorubicin (Adriamycin), cyclophosphamide, vincristine (Oncovin), dexamethasone
BACOP	bleomycin, doxorubicin (Adriamycin), cyclophosphamide, vincristine (Oncovin), prednisone
BAER	brain stem auditory evoked response

BAL	British anti-Lewisite (dimercaprol)	CEA	carcinoembryonic antigen, carotid end arterectomy
BAO	basic acid output	CF	complement fixation, conversion factor
BBB	bundle branch block	CFS	chronic fatigue syndrome
BC	blood culture	CGL	chronic granulocytic (myelogenous) leukemia
BCG	bacillus Calmette-Guérin	CHD	congenital heart disease, coronary heart disease
BCNU	carmustine	CHF	congestive heart failure
BCP	birth control pill	cho	carbohydrate
BE	barium enema	CHOP	cyclophosphamide, doxorubicin, vincristine (Oncovin), prednisone
BEE	basal energy expenditure	CI	cardiac index
bid	two times a day	CIDP	chronic idiopathic demyelinating radiculonecropathy
bilat	bilateral	CIE	counterimmunoelectrophoresis
bili	bilirubin	CIN	cervical intraepithelial neoplasia
BKA	below-knee amputation	CK	creatine kinase
Bl s	blood sugar	CK-MB	creatine kinase, myocardial band
BM	bowel movement	cl	clear
BMI	body mass index	Cl^-	chloride
BMR	basal metabolic rate	CLL	chronic lymphocytic leukemia
BP	blood pressure, bullous pemphigoid	cm	centimeter
BPH	benign prostatic hypertrophy	CM	costal margin
bpm	beats per minute	CMF	cyclophosphamide, methotrexate, 5-fluorouracil
BR	bed rest	CML	chronic myelogenous leukemia
BRP	bathroom privileges	CMV	cytomegalovirus, controlled mechanical ventilation
BS or bs	breath sounds	CNS	central nervous system
BSA	body surface area	CO	cardiac output, carbon monoxide
BSO	bilateral salpingo-oophorectomy	c/o	complains of
BTB	break-through bleeding	CO_2	carbon dioxide
BTL	bilateral tubal ligation	CoA	coenzyme A
BUN	blood urea nitrogen	COMLA	cyclophosphamide, vincristine (Oncovin), methotrexate, leucovorin, cytosine arabinoside
BW	body weight	conc	concentrate
Bx	biopsy	COPD	chronic obstructive pulmonary disease
$\bar{c}$	with	CPAP	continuous positive airway pressure
C	centigrade	CPK	creatine phosphokinase
C3 to C9	protein components of complement system	CPR	cardiopulmonary resuscitation
Ca	cancer	Cr	creatinine
CA	chronologic age	CR	cardiorespiratory
Ca^{+2}	calcium	CRH	corticotropin releasing hormone
C/A	Clinitest and acetone	C&S	culture and sensitivity
CAB	coronary artery bypass	CSD	cat-scratch disease
CABG	coronary artery bypass graft	CSF	cerebrospinal fluid
CAD	coronary artery disease	CSM	carotid sinus massage
CAF	cyclophosphamide, doxorubicin (Adriamycin), 5-fluorouracil	C/sec	cesarean section
cal	calorie	CT	computed tomography
cAMP	cyclic adenosine monophosphate	CTS	Carpal tunnel syndrome
cap	capsule	Cu	copper
CAT	computerized axial tomography	CV	cardiovascular
cath	catheterization	cva	costovertebral angle
CAV	cyclophosphamide, doxorubicin (Adriamycin), vincristine	CVA	cerebrovascular accident
CBC	complete blood cell count	CVP	central venous pressure
CBD	common bile duct	CXR	chest x-ray
CBE	clinical breast examination	cysto	cystoscopy
Cbl	cobalamin	D&C	dilation and curettage
cc	cubic centimeter	D/C	discontinue
CC	chief complaint		
CCr	creatine clearance		
CCU	coronary care unit		
CD4	helper-inducer T cells		
CD8	suppressor-cytotoxic T cells		
CDC	Centers for Disease Control		

Medical record abbreviations

D&S	dilation and suction	EF	ejection fraction
DAT	diet as tolerated	EIA	electroimmunoassay
DBIL	direct bilirubin	EKG	electrocardiogram
DCF	2′ deoxycoformycin	elect	electrolyte
DDAVP	desmopressin	ELISA	enzyme-linked immunoassay
ddI	dideoxyinosine	elix	elixir
DEC	diethylcarbamazine	EMD	electromechanical dissociation
DES	diethylstilbestrol	EMG	electromyogram
DFA	direct fluorescent antibody	EMS	emergency medical services
DGI	disseminated gonococcal infection	ENT	ear, nose, and throat
DH	dermatitis herpetiformis	EOE	evoked otoacoustic emission
DHPG	ganciclovir	EOM	extraocular movements
DI	diabetes insipidus	EP	ectopic pregnancy
Dial	dialysis	EPO	erythropoietin
DIC	disseminated intravascular coagulation	EPS	extrapyramidal symptoms
DIF	direct immunofluorescence	ER	emergency room, estrogen receptor
dil	dilute	ERCP	endoscopic retrograde cholangiopancreatography
DIP	distal interphalangeal, desquamative interstitial pneumonitis	ERS	evacuation retained secundines
DKA	diabetic ketoacidosis	ESR	erythrocyte sedimentation rate
DL_{CO}	diffusing capacity of lung for carbon monoxide	ESRD	end-stage renal disease
dl	deciliter	EST, ECT	electroshock therapy
DLE	drug-related lupus erythematosus	EUA	examination under anesthesia
DM	diabetes mellitus	et al	and others
DNA	deoxyribonucleic acid	ext	extract, extremities
DNR	do not resuscitate	F	fahrenheit
DNCB	dinitrochlorobenzene	FBS	fasting blood sugar
DOA	dead on arrival	FDP	fibrin degradation product
DOT	directly observed therapy	Fe	iron
DP	dorsalis pedis	FE	fractional excretion
DPT	diphtheria, pertussis, tetanus	FEV	forced expiratory volume
DR	delivery room	FF	force fluids
DRE	digital rectal examination	FFP	fresh frozen plasma
ds	double strand	FH	family history
DSD	dry sterile dressing	FHC	family health center
DT	diphtheria tetanus; delirium tremens	FHH	familial hypercalciuric hypercalcemia
DTIC	dacarbazine	FHM	fetal heart monitor
DTR	deep tendon reflex	FHR	fetal heart rate
DTs	delirium tremens	FIGO	International Federation of Gynecologists and Obstetricians
DU	duodenal ulcer		
DUB	dysfunctional uterine bleeding	FIo_2	fraction of inspired oxygen
DVT	deep vein thrombosis	fl	fluid, femtoliter
D_5NS	dextrose in 5% normal saline	fL	femtoliter
D_5W	dextrose (5%) in water	FMF	familial Mediterranean fever
Dx	diagnosis	FNA	fine needle aspiration
EACA	epsilon aminocaproic acid	FOBT	fecal occult blood testing
EBA	epidermolysis bullosa acquisita	FS	frozen section
EBL	estimated blood loss	FSH	follicle-stimulating hormone
EBV	Epstein-Barr virus	FTA-ABS	fluorescent treponemal antibody absorbed
ECF	extended care facility, extracellular fluid	FTI	free thyroxine index
ECG	electrocardiogram	5-FU	5-fluorouracil
ECHO	etoposide, cyclophosphamide, hydroxydavnomycin (doxorubicin), and Oncovin (vincristine); echocardiogram	FUO	fever of undetermined origin
		FVC	forced vital capacity
		FWB	full weight bearing
ECM	erythema chronicum migrans	fx	fracture
ED	emergency department	g	gram
EDC	estimated date of confinement	Ga	gallium
EDTA	ethylene diamine tetraacetate	GA	general anesthesia
EEG	electroencephalogram	GB	gallbladder
EENT	eyes, ears, nose, and throat	GBM	glomerular basement membrane

GBS	Guillain-Barré syndrome		H&P	history and physical exam
Gc	gonococcus		HPI	history of present illness
GERD	gastroesophageal reflux disease		HPV	human papilloma virus
GFR	glomerular filtration rate		HR	heart rate
GGT	γ-glutamyltransferase		HRS	hepatorenal syndrome
GGTP	γ-glutamyltranspeptidase		hs	hour of sleep (at bedtime)
GH	growth hormone		HSV	herpes simplex virus
GI	gastrointestinal		ht	height
GIP	gastric inhibitory polypeptide		HTN	hypertension
GITS	gastrointestinal therapeutic system		hx	history
glu	glucose		I&D	incision and drainage
GN	graduate nurse, glomerulonephritis		IABP	intraaortic balloon pump
GNR	gram-negative rods		IBC	iron-binding capacity
Gn-RH	gonadotropin-releasing hormone		IBD	inflammatory bowel disease
G_6PD	glucose-6-phosphate dehydrogenase		IBS	irritable bowel syndrome
GPA	guided percutaneous aspiration		ICP	intracranial pressure
gr	grain		ICU	intensive care unit
GSW	gunshot wound		ID	intradermal
gtt	drop		IDDM	insulin-dependent diabetes mellitus
GTT	glucose tolerance test		IF	idiopathic flushing
GU	genitourinary		IFA	immunofluorescent assay
GVHD	graft versus host disease		Ig	immunoglobulin
G/W enema	glycerine and water enema		IgA	immunoglobulin A
Gyn	gynecology		IGF	insulinlike growth factor
H_2	histamine$_2$		IHA	idiopathic hyperaldosteronism
H_2RA	histamine-2 receptor agonists		IHSS	idiopathic hypertrophic subaortic stenosis
H/A	headache		IIM	idiopathic inflammatory myopathy
HA	hyperalimentation, height age		ILD	interstitial lung disease
HAV	hepatitis A virus		IM	intramuscular
Hb	hemoglobin		Imp	impression
HB_cAg	hepatitis B core antigen		IMV	intermittent mandatory ventilation
HB_sAg	hepatitis B surface antigen		inf	infusion
HBIG	hepatitis B immune globulin		inh	inhalation
HBP	high blood pressure		INH	isonicotinoylhydrazine (isoniazid)
HBV	hepatitis B virus		inj	injection
HC	head circumference		INR	International Normalized ratio
hCG	human chorionic gonadotropin		I&O	intake and output
HCO_3^-	bicarbonate		IOP	intraocular pressure
hct	hematocrit		IPC	intermittent pneumatic compression
HCV	hepatitis C virus		IPG	impedance plethysmography
HD	hospital discharge		iPLP	parathyroid hormone–like protein by radioimmunoassay
HDL	high-density lipoprotein			
HDV	hepatitis D virus		IPPB	intermittent positive pressure breathing
HEENT	head, eyes, ears, nose, and throat		iPTH	parathyroid hormone by radioimmunoassay
HEMPAS	hereditary erythroblastic multinuclearity associated with positive acidified serum		IQ	intelligence quotient
			IRV	inverse ratio ventilation
Hg	hemoglobin		ISG	immune serum globulin
H/H	hemoglobin/hematocrit		ITP	idiopathic thrombocytopenic purpura
5-HIAA	5-hydroxyindoleacetic acid		IUD	intrauterine device
HIDA	hepatoiminodiacetic acid		IUGR	Intrauterine growth restriction
HIV	human immunodeficiency virus		IUP	intrauterine pregnancy
H&L	heart and lungs		IV	intravenous
HLA	human leukocyte antigen		IVC	inferior vena cava
HMG-CoA	3-hydroxy-3-methylglutaryl coenzyme A		IVP	intravenous pyelogram
HNP	herniated nucleus pulposus		J	joule
HNPCC	hereditary nonpolyposis colorectal cancer syndrome		JG	juxtaglomerular
			JRA	juvenile rheumatoid arthritis
H_2O	water		JVD	jugular venous distention
H_2O_2	hydrogen peroxide		JVP	jugular vein pulse
HOCM	hypertrophic obstructive cardiomyopathy		kat	katal (mole/sec)
HORF	high-output renal failure		K^+	potassium

kg	kilogram
KJ	knee jerk
KOH	potassium hydroxide
17-KS	17-ketosteroid
KUB	kidney, ureter, and bladder
l	left
L	liter
LA	left atrium
lab	laboratory
lac	laceration
LAD	left axis deviation
LAHB	left anterior hemiblock
lap	laparotomy
LAP	leukocyte alkaline phosphatase
LAV	lymphadenopathy-associated virus (same as HIV)
lb	pound
LBP	low back pain
LBBB	left bundle branch block
LDH	lactate dehydrogenase
LDL	low-density lipoprotein
LE	leukocyte esterase
LEEP	Loop electrosurgical excision procedure
LES	lower esophageal sphincter
LFT	liver function test
LGI	lower gastrointestinal
LGV	lymphogranuloma venereum
LH	luteinizing hormone
LHRH	luteinizing hormone–releasing hormone
Li	lithium
Lip	lipid
liq	liquid
LLL	left lower lobe
LLQ	left lower quadrant
LMD	local medical doctor
LMP	last menstrual period
LNMP	last normal menstrual period
LOC	level of consciousness
LP	lumbar puncture
LPHB	left posterior hemiblock
LPN	licensed practical nurse
LSB	left sternal border
LUL	left upper lobe
LUQ	left upper quadrant
LVEDP	left ventricular end diastolic pressure
LVH	left ventricular hypertrophy
m	murmur
M	midnight, monoclonal
M1 to M7	categories of ANLL
MAC	*Mycobacterium avium* complex
MACE	methotrexate, doxorubicin (Adriamycin), cyclophosphamide, epipodophyllotoxin
MAO	monoamine oxidase
MAP	mean arterial pressure
MAT	multifocal atrial tachycardia
max	maximum
MB	izoenzyme of cardiac origin
MBC	minimum bactericidal concentration
MCA	middle cerebral artery
MCL	midclavicular line
MCP	metacarpophalangeal
MCTD	mixed connective tissue disease
MCV	mean corpuscular volume
med	medication
MED	medical, minimum erythema dose
MEN	multiple endocrine neoplasia
mEq	milliequivalent
MERSA	methicillin-resistant *Staphylococcus aureus*
mets	metastases
MF	maturation factor
mg	milligram
MG	myasthenia gravis
Mg^{2+}	magnesium
MH	malignant hyperthermia
MHTAP	microhemagglutination assay for antibody to *Treponema pallidum*
MI	myocardial infarction
MIBG	meta-iodobenzyl guanidine
MIC	minimum inhibitory concentration
MIDCAB	minimally invasive direct coronary artery bypass
min	minute
mixt	mixture
μkat	microkatal (micromole/sec)
ml	milliliter
ML	malignant lymphoma
μmol	micromole
mm	millimeter
mM, mmol	millimole
MMSE	Mini-Mental State Examination
MN	mononeuropathy
MNMP	mononeuropathy multiplex
mod	moderate
MODS	multiple organ dysfunction syndrome
MOM	milk of magnesia
MOPP	mechlorethamine, vincristine (Oncovin), procarbazine, prednisone
mOsm	milliosmol
MP	metacarpophalangeal
MPGN	membrane proliferative glomerulonephritis
MPTP	analog of meperidine (used by drug addicts)
MR	mitral regurgitation
MRA	magnetic resonance angiography
MRI	magnetic resonance imaging
MRSA	methicillin-resistant *Staphylococcus aureus*
MS	multiple sclerosis, mitral stenosis, mental status
MSU	monosodium urate
MTBE	methy *tert*-butyl ether
MTC	medullary thyroid carcinoma
MTP	metatarsophalangeal
MUGA	multiple gated (image) acquisition (analysis)
MVA	motor vehicle accident
MVP	mitral valve prolapse; mitomycin, vinblastine, cisplatin (Platinol)
MVV	maximum voluntary ventilation
N	normal
NA	not applicable
Na^+	sodium

NaHCO$_3$	sodium bicarbonate	p̄	pulse
NAPA	N-acetyl-procainamide, N-acetyl-paraaminophenol	P wave	part of the electrocardiographic cycle representing atrial depolarization (stimulation)
NAS	no added sodium	P$_2$	pulmonic second sound
NB	newborn	Pa$_{CO_2}$	partial pressure of CO$_2$ in arterial blood
NCP	nursing care plan	Pa$_{O_2}$	partial pressure of O$_2$ in arterial blood
NCS	nerve conduction study	P&A	percussion and auscultation
NCV	nerve conduction velocity	PA	pernicious anemia, posteroanterior, pulmonary artery
NEC	necrotizing enterocolitis		
neg	negative	PAD	peripheral arterial disease
NETT	nasal endotracheal tube	PADP	pulmonary artery diastolic pressure
Neuro	neurology	PAM	pulse amplitude modulation
ng	nanogram	pap	Papanicolaou
NG	nasogastric	PAP	pulmonary artery pressure
NGU	nongonococcal urethritis	para	number of pregnancies
NH$_3$	ammonia	PAS	paraaminosalicylic acid
NHL	non-Hodgkin's lymphoma	PASP	pulmonary artery systolic pressure
NIDDM	non–insulin-dependent diabetes mellitus	PAT	paroxysmal atrial tachycardia
		PAWP	pulmonary artery wedge pressure
NIH	National Institutes of Health	PBC	primary biliary cirrhosis
NKA	no known allergy	pc	after meals
nkat	nanokatal (nanomole/sec)	P$_{CO_2}$	carbon dioxide tension
NKDA	no known drug allergy	PCP	*Pneumocystis carinii* pneumonia, phencyclidine
NM	neuromuscular		
NME	necrolytic migratory erythema	PCR	polymerase chain reaction
no	number	PCT	porphyria cutanea tarda
NO	nitrous oxide	PCWP	pulmonary capillary wedge pressure
noc	night	PE	physical exam, pulmonary embolism
NPH	normal pressure hydrocephalus, neutral protamine Hagedorn (insulin)	PEARL	pupils equal and reactive to light
		ped	pediatric
NPO	nothing by mouth	PEEP	positive end-expiratory pressure
NS	normal saline	PEFR	peak expiratory flow rate
NSAID	nonsteroidal antiinflammatory drug	PEG	percutaneous endoscopic gastrostomy
NSILA	nonsuppressable insulinlike activity	per	by
NSR	normal sinus rhythm	PERRLA	pupils equal, round, reactive to light and accommodation
NTG	nitroglycerin		
NYHA	New York Heart Association	PFT	pulmonary function test
OA	oral airway	pg	picogram
OAF	osteoclast activating factor	PGE	prostaglandin E
OB	obstetrics	PH	past history
OD	overdose, right eye	phos	phosphorus
OETT	oral endotracheal tube	PHP	pseudohypoparathyroidism
17-OHCD	17-hydroxycorticosteroid	PHR	peak heart rate
25-OHD	1,25-dihydroxyvitamin D	PI	present illness
oint	ointment	PID	pelvic inflammatory disease
OOB	out of bed	PIP	proximal interphalangeal
OOP	out on pass	PKU	phenylketonuria
OPD	outpatient department	PLA	plasminogen activator
opt	optimum	PLP	parathyroid hormone–like protein
ophth	ophthalmology	PM	afternoon
OR	operating room	PMI	point of maximum impulse
Oral	oral surgery	PML	polymorphous light eruption
ORIF	open reduction with internal fixation	PMN	polymorphonuclear leukocyte
Orth or ortho	orthopedics	PMP	previous menstrual period
OS	left eye, opening snap	PM & R	physical medicine and rehabilitation
osm	osmolality	PMR	polymyalgia rheumatica
OT	occupational therapy	PND	paroxysmal nocturnal dyspnea
OTC	over-the-counter	PNH	paroxysmal nocturnal hemoglobinuria
OU	each eye	PO	by mouth
oz	ounce	postop	postoperative
p	after	P$_{O_2}$	oxygen tension

Medical record abbreviations

PP	postpartum	RAN	resident's admission note
PPD	purified protein derivative	RAP	right atrial pressure
PPNG	penicillinase-producing *Neisseria gonorrhoeae*	RBBB	right bundle branch block
		RBC	red blood cells
PR	per rectum, pulmonic regurgitation, progesterone receptor	RDS	respiratory distress syndrome
		RDW	red cell distribution width
PR interval	part of electrocardiographic cycle from onset of atrial depolarization to onset of ventricular depolarization	R&E	round and equal
		readm	readmission
		REM	rapid eye movement
PRA	plasma renin activity	RF	rheumatoid factor
preop	preoperative	Rh	Rhesus blood factor
prep	preparation	RIA	radio immunoassay
PROM	premature rupture of membranes	RL	Ringer's lactate
prn	as needed	RIND	reversible ischemic neurologic deficit
PRSP	penicillinase-resistant synthetic penicillin	RLL	right lower lobe
		RLQ	right lower quadrant
PS	pulmonic stenosis	RML	right middle lobe
PSA	prostatic specific antigen	RN	registered nurse
PSC	primary sclerosing cholangitis	RNA	ribonucleic acid
PSGN	poststreptococcal glomerulonephritis	R/O	rule out
psi	pounds per square inch	ROM	range of motion
PSV	pressure support ventilation	ROS	review of systems
PSVT	paroxysmal supraventricular tachycardia	RPGN	rapidly progressive glomerulonephritis
		RPI	reticulocyte production index
Psych or psych	psychiatry	RPR	rapid plasma reagin
pt	patient	rpt	repeat
PT	prothrombin time, physical therapy, posterior tibia	RPT	registered physical therapist
		RR	recovery room
PTA	prior to admission	RSR	regular sinus rhythm
PTC	percutaneous transhepatic cholangiography	RSV	respiratory syncytial virus
		rt-PA	recombinant tissue plasminogen activator
PTCA	percutaneous transluminal coronary angioplasty	R/T	related to
		rT_3	reverse triiodothyronine
Pth	pathology	RTA	renal tubular acidosis
PTH	parathormone	RTC	return to clinic
PTRA	percutaneous transluminal renal angioplasty	RUL	right upper lobe
		RUQ	right upper quadrant
PTT	partial thromboplastin time	RV	right ventricle, residual volume
PTU	propylthiouracil	RVH	renovascular hypertension, right ventricular hypertrophy
PUD	peptic ulcer disease		
PVNS	pigmented villonodular synovitis	Rx	therapy, treatment, prescription
PWP	pulmonary wedge pressure	S_1	first heart sound
PVC	premature ventricular contraction	S_2	second heart sound
PVR	pulmonary vascular resistance	S_3	third heart sound
PX	physical	S_4	fourth heart sound
q	every	s̄	without
qd	every day	S/A	sugar and acetone
qh	every hour	SA	sinoatrial
qhs	every bed time	SACE	serum angiotensin-converting enzyme
qid	four times a day	SAH	subarachnoid hemorrhage
qns	quantity not sufficient	sat	saturated
qod	every other day	SB	stillbirth
qs	quantity sufficient	SBE	subacute bacterial (infective) endocarditis
QRS	part of electrocardiographic wave representing ventricular depolarization (stimulation)	SBP	spontaneous bacterial peritonitis
		SBT	serum bactericidal titer
		SC	subcutaneous
r	right	SCP	standard care plan
R	respiratory rate (per min)	SFEMG	single fiber electromyography
RA	rheumatoid arthritis, right atrium	SGA	small for gestational age
RAI	radioactive iodine	SGOT	serum glutamic oxaloacetic transaminase (aspartate aminotransferase, AST)
RAIU	radioactive iodine uptake		

SI	Système Internationale
SIADH	syndrome of inappropriate secretion of antidiuretic hormone
SIMV	synchronized intermittent mandatory ventilation
SIRS	systemic inflammatory response syndrome
SGPT	serum glutamic pyruvate transaminase (alanine aminotransferase, ALT)
SL	sublingual
SLA	soluble liver antigens
SLE	systemic lupus erythematosus
SLR	straight leg raising
SMA	superior mesenteric artery
SMAST	short Michigan alcholism screening test
SMI	suggested minimum increment
SMS	somatostatin
SNF	skilled nursing facility
SO_2	oxygen saturation
SOB	short of breath
SOC	state of consciousness
sol	solution
S/P	status post
SPECT	single photon emission computed tomography
SQ	subcutaneous
SR	slow release
SRM	spontaneous rupture membranes
s̄s̄	half
S/S	signs and symptoms
SS	Sjögren's syndrome
SSE	soap suds enema
SSKI	saturated solution potassium iodide
SSRI	selective serotonin reuptake inhibitors
SSS	sick sinus syndrome
ST segment	part of electrocardiographic cycle representing the beginning of ventricular repolarization (recovery)
stat	immediately
STD	sexually transmitted disease
STS	serologic test for syphilis
subcu	subcutaneous
supp	suppository
Surg	surgery
SURT	sarcoidosis of upper respiratory tract
susp	suspension
SVC	superior vena cava
SVR	systemic vascular resistance
SVT	supraventricular tachycardia
Sx	symptoms
syr	syrup
T wave	part of the ECG cycle, representing a portion of ventricular repolarization (recovery)
T_3	triiodothyronine
T_4	thyroxine
T&A	tonsillectomy and adenoidectomy
tab	tablet
TAH	total abdominal hysterectomy
TB	tuberculosis
TBG	thyroxine-binding globulin, total blood gases
TBIL	total bilirubin
TBNa	total body sodium
Tbsp	tablespoon
TBW	total body water
T/C	throat culture
temp	temperature
TENS	transcutaneous electrical nerve stimulation
TFT	thyroid function test
Tg	thyroglobulin
THBR	thyroid hormone-binding ratio
TIA	transient ischemic attack
TIBC	total iron-binding capacity
tid	three times daily
tinc	tincture
TIPS	transjugular intrahepatic portosystemic shunt
TLC	total lung capacity
TM	tympanic membrane
TMJ	temporomandibular joint
TmP	renal threshold for phosphorus
TMP-SMX	trimethoprim/sulfamethoxazole
TNG	toxic multinodular goiter
TNM	tumor-nodes-metastases
TO	telephone order
TOA	Tuboovarian abscess
top	topical
tPA	tissue plasminogen activator
TP	total protein
TPE	therapeutic plasma exchange, tropical pulmonary eosinophilia
TPI	*Treponema pallidum* immobilization
TPN	total parenteral nutrition
TPR	temperature, pulse, and respiration
TR	tricuspid regurgitation
TRAP	tartrate-resistant acid phosphatase
TRF	thyrotropin releasing factor
T_3RIA	triiodothyronine level by radioimmunoassay
T_3RU	T_3 resin uptake
TRH	thyrotropin-releasing hormone
TRIG	triglycerides
TRUS	transrectal ultrasound
TS	tricuspid stenosis
TSAb	thyroid-stimulating antibodies
TSE	testicular self-examination
TSH	thyroid-stimulating hormone
tsp	teaspoon
TT	thrombin time
TTP	thrombotic thrombocytopenic purpura, ribothymidine 5'triphosphate
TTS	transdermal therapeutic system
TUR	transurethral resection
TURBT	transurethral resection of bladder tumor
TURP	transurethral resection prostate
TU	tuberculin unit
TV	tidal volume
TWAR	*Chlamydia psittaci*
Tx	therapy
U	unit
UA	umbilical artery
U/A	urinalysis

UFH	unfractionated heparin	WBC	white blood (cell) count
UGI	upper gastrointestinal	w/c	wheel chair
UICC	international union against cancer	WD	well developed
ung	ointment	WF	white female
U/P	urine/plasma ratio (concentration)	WHO	World Health Organization
URAC	uric acid	WN	well nourished
URI	upper respiratory tract infection	WNL	within normal limits
USP	United States Pharmacopeia	WPW	Wolff Parkinson White
UTI	urinary tract infection	wt	weight
UV	ultraviolet	y/o	years old
v	mixed venous	×	times
V	volume	ZDV	zidovudine
vag hyst	vaginal hysterectomy	Z-E	Zollinger-Ellison (syndrome)
VAIN	vaginal intraepithelial neoplasia		
VAMP	vincristine, doxorubicin (Adriamycin), methylprednisolone		
VAT	ventricular activation time		
VD	venereal disease		
VDRL	Venereal Disease Research Laboratories (test for syphilis)		
VC	vital capacity		
VER	visual evoked response		
VF	ventricular fibrillation		
VIN	vulvar intraepithelial neoplasia		
VIP	vasoactive intestinal polypeptide		
VLDL	very low density lipoprotein		
VMA	vanillylmandelic acid		
VPC	ventricular premature contraction		
VO	verbal order		
VP-16	epipodophyllotoxin		
vs	visit		
VS	vital signs		
VSD	ventricular septal defect		
VT/VF	ventricular tachycardia/fibrillation		
VVC	vulvovaginal candidiasis		
W	white		

Symbols

@	at
++	moderate amount
+++	large amount
0	zero, none
°	degree
♀	female
♂	male
#	number
↑	increased
↓	decreased
>	greater than
<	less than
μ or μm	micron (micrometer)
+	positive, presence
"	second
'	minute
ø	absence of
✔	check
−	negative, absence
△	changes

NOTICE: The science of medicine is constantly evolving. Every attempt has been made by the author and consultants to ensure that this manual includes the latest recommendations from the medical literature. Doses of drugs and treatment recommendations have been carefully reviewed. **However, it is strongly recommended that the reader become completely familiar with the manufacturer's product information when prescribing any of the drugs described in this manual.** This recommendation is especially important with new or infrequently used drugs. As new information becomes available, changes in treatment modalities invariably follow; therefore when choosing a particular treatment, the reader should consider not only the information provided in this manual but also any recently published medical literature on the subject.

Index

A

AAA; *see* Abdominal aortic aneurysm
Abbreviations, list of, 1063-1071
Abdomen, acute; *see* Peritonitis, secondary
Abdominal aortic aneurysm
  basic information about, 36
  diagnosis of, 36, 855
  screening for, 855
  treatment of, 36
Abdominal distention
  from mechanical obstruction, 537
  from nonmechanical obstruction, 537
Abdominal pain
  in adolescents, 539, 907-908, 908*t*
  in children, 539
  diffuse, 537
  from drugs and toxins, 538
  epigastric, 537
  evaluation of, *671*
  extraabdominal, 538
  functional, 538
  hematologic, 538
  in infants, 539
  infectious, 538
  intraabdominal, 538
  left lower quadrant, 538
  left upper quadrant, 537
  localized, 537-538
  metabolic, 538
  periumbilical, 537-538
  poorly localized, 538
  in pregnancy, 539
  referred, 538
  right lower quadrant, 538
  right upper quadrant, 537
  suprapubic, 537
Abdominal trauma, blunt, evaluation of, *769*
A beta lipoproteinemia in differential diagnosis of Friederich's ataxia, 190
Abortion; *see also* Miscarriage, spontaneous
  early, methotrexate and misoprostol for, 950-951, *951*
  recurrent, potential causes of, 540
  threatened, in differential diagnosis of ectopic pregnancy, 164
Abortive insanity; *see* Obsessive-compulsive disorder
Abruptio placentae, 3
  basic information about, 3
  diagnosis of, 3
  treatment of, 3

Page numbers in italics indicate illustrations; *t* indicates tables.

Abscess
  breast; *see* Breast abscess
  in differential diagnosis of brain neoplasm, 76
  in differential diagnosis of colorectal cancer, 127
  in differential diagnosis of echinococcosis, 162
  in differential diagnosis of hemorrhoids, 217
  in differential diagnosis of spontaneous bacterial peritonitis, 360
  hepatic, in differential diagnosis of babesiosis, 64
  liver, in differential diagnosis of cholangitis, 115
  parapharyngeal, in differential diagnosis of nonneoplastic neck mass, 626*t*
  pelvic, 4-5
    basic information about, 4
    diagnosis of, 4
    treatment of, 4
  perinephric, in differential diagnosis of pyelonephritis, 401
  peritonsillar, in differential diagnosis of epiglottitis, 176
  retropharyngeal, in differential diagnosis of nonneoplastic neck mass, 626*t*
Abuse
  child; *see* Child abuse
  drug; *see* Drug abuse
  geriatric; *see* Geriatric abuse
Acanthosis nigricans, history, manifestations, and malignancy associated with, 564*t*
Acarbose, preparations, dosage, duration of action, half-life, excretion, cost, class, 975*t*
Accidents; *see also* Injuries
  counseling to prevent
    household and recreational, 883-884
    motor vehicle, 882-883
Accupril; *see* Quinapril
ACE inhibitors, dosage, onset of action, peak effect, half-life, cost, 967*t*
Acebutolol, preparations, dosage, cardioselectivity, lipid solubility, half-life, excretion, cost, 981*t*
Acetaminophen, drug monitoring data for, 799*t*
Acetaminophen poisoning
  antidotes for, dosage and indications, 1055*t*
  basic information about, 10
  diagnosis of, 10
  treatment of, 10
Acetylsalicylic acid, drug monitoring data for, 799*t*

Achalasia in differential diagnosis of Chagas' disease, 109
Achilles tendinitis in differential diagnosis of deep vein thrombosis, 473
Achilles tendon rupture
  basic information about, 11
  diagnosis of, 11
  treatment of, 11
Acid phosphatase, laboratory findings for, 782-783
Acid secretion inhibitors, preparations, dosage, cost, 968*t*
Acid-base disorders
  metabolic, laboratory findings in, 781*t*
  respiratory, laboratory findings in, 781*t*
Acid-base map, *1043*
Acid-base reference values for arterial and venous plasma or serum, 781*t*
Acidosis
  anion gap, 540
  lactic, 541
  metabolic, 541
  metabolic/respiratory, laboratory findings in, 781*t*
  renal tubular; *see* Renal tubular acidosis
  respiratory, 542
  uremic, in differential diagnosis of diabetic ketoacidosis, 151
Acne rosacea; *see also* Rosacea
  in differential diagnosis of acne vulgaris, 12
Acne vulgaris
  basic information about, 12
  diagnosis of, 12
  in differential diagnosis of folliculitis, 187
  in differential diagnosis of rosacea, 422
  treatment of, 12
Acneiform eruptions, drug-induced, 565
Acoustic neuroma
  in differential diagnosis of Meniere's disease, 292
  in differential diagnosis of Ramsay Hunt syndrome, 403
Acquired immunodeficiency syndrome; *see also* Human immunodeficiency virus
  basic information about, 13
  diagnosis of, 13
  diarrhea in patients with, 569
  in differential diagnosis of nonneoplastic neck mass, 627*t*
  infectious diseases in patients with, 604*t*-605*t*
  neuropathies associated with, 631*t*
  treatment of, 13
Acrochordon in differential diagnosis of warts, 529
Acrodermatitis chronica atrophicans; *see* Lyme disease

1073

Index

Acromegaly
  basic information about, 14
  diagnosis of, 14
  differential diagnosis of, 366
  neuropathies associated with, 631t
  treatment of, 14, 367
Actinic keratosis in differential diagnosis of squamous cell carcinoma, 450
Actinomyces in differential diagnosis of nonneoplastic neck mass, 627t
Actinomycin D, toxicity of, 984t-985t
Activated partial thromboplastin time, laboratory values, 819-820
Activities of daily living, Katz Index of, 1029
Acute abdomen; see also Peritonitis, secondary
  in differential diagnosis of Addison's disease, 15
Acute fatty metamorphosis; see Pregnancy, fatty liver of
Acute lymphoblastic leukemia; see Leukemia, acute lymphoblastic
Acute myocardial infarction; see also Myocardial infarction
  in differential diagnosis of myocarditis, 316
  pain from, in differential diagnosis of herpes zoster, 228
  prognostic importance of myocardial ischemia following, 901-903
  thrombolytic therapy in, 765, 1058
Acute necrotizing encephalitis; see Encephalitis, acute viral
Acute renal failure; see Renal failure, acute
Acute respiratory distress syndrome, 410-411
  basic information about, 410
  diagnosis of, 410
  in differential diagnosis of congestive heart failure, 130
  in differential diagnosis of viral pneumonia, 376
  treatment of, 411
Acute tubular necrosis in differential diagnosis of hepatorenal syndrome, 223
Acute yellow atrophy; see Pregnancy, fatty liver of
Acyclovir for acute infectious mononucleosis, 946-947
Adalat; see Nifedipine
Adapin; see Doxepin
Addiction; see Drug abuse
Addison's disease
  basic information about, 15
  diagnosis of, 15
  renin-aldosterone patterns in, 826t
  treatment of, 15
Adenitis, mesenteric, in differential diagnosis of Crohn's disease, 140
Adenocarcinoma
  in situ, in differential diagnosis of cervical dysplasia, 104
  of lung, 277
  of vagina; see Vaginal malignancy
  of vulva; see Vulvar cancer
Adenoma, pituitary; see Pituitary adenoma
Adenomyosis
  in differential diagnosis of dysfunctional uterine bleeding, 159
  in differential diagnosis of dysmenorrhea, 161
  in differential diagnosis of endometriosis, 170
Adenopathy in differential diagnosis of nonneoplastic neck mass, 626t
Adenosarcoma; see Uterine malignancy

Adenovirus
  ages affected, prodrome, morphology, distribution, diagnosis, 574t
  in differential diagnosis of influenza, 257
  in differential diagnosis of tularemia, 501
Adenovirus pneumonia in differential diagnosis of human granulocytic ehrlichiosis, 237
Adhesions
  in differential diagnosis of colorectal cancer, 127
  in differential diagnosis of dysmenorrhea, 161
Adhesive capsulitis; see Frozen shoulder
Adnexal torsion in differential diagnosis of pelvic inflammatory disease, 352
Adnexitis; see Pelvic inflammatory disease
Adolescents
  abdominal pain and irritable bowel syndrome in, 907-908, 908t
  assessing for drug abuse, 878
  counseling about contraception, 887
  extremely low-birth-weight infants as, self-perceived health status of, 913
  idiopathic scoliosis in, screening recommendations for, 875
  sudden death from cardiac causes in, 911
  violence of, counseling to prevent, 884-885
Adrenal abnormalities in differential diagnosis of menopause, 297
Adrenal mass, 542
  evaluation of, 672
Adrenarche, premature, in differential diagnosis of precocious puberty, 383
Adrenergic antagonists, preparations, dosage, cost, 969t
Adrenocortical insufficiency, primary, in differential diagnosis of Addison's disease, 15
Adrenogenital syndrome in differential diagnosis of Cushing's syndrome, 142
Adult respiratory distress syndrome; see Acute respiratory distress syndrome
AF; see Atrial fibrillation
Affective disorders, sleep-associated, 759
A-fib; see Atrial fibrillation
African trypanosomiasis in differential diagnosis of Chagas' disease, 109
Aging
  and development of stable hypertension, 901
  successful, predictors and associated activities, 922t, 922-923
Agoraphobia/panic, 16-17
  basic information about, 16
  diagnosis of, 16
  treatment of, 16-17
Alanine aminotransferase, laboratory findings in, 782
Albumin
  laboratory findings in, 782
  serum, assessment of, 1046t
Albuminuria in NIDDM, evolution, risk factors, and prognostic implications, 941, 941-942
Alcohol abuse; see also Alcoholism; Problem drinking
  in cirrhosis of liver, 121
  evaluation of, 1030
  high-risk sexual behavior and, 887
  injuries due to, counseling to prevent, 883-884
  suicide risk and, 876
Alcohol use
  motor vehicle operation and, 882-883
  oral cancer and, 859

Alcohol use—cont'd
  predicting liver disease by, 924-926, 925, 925t
Alcohol withdrawal syndrome; see also Delirium tremens
  in differential diagnosis of hepatic encephalopathy, 218
  in differential diagnosis of thyrotoxic storm, 478
  scale for assessing severity of, 1031
Alcoholic delirium; see Delirium tremens
Alcoholic hepatitis, liver function tests in, 618t
Alcoholic ketoacidosis in differential diagnosis of diabetic ketoacidosis, 151
Alcoholic polyneuritic psychosis; see Korsakoff's psychosis
Alcoholic pseudo-Cushing's syndrome in differential diagnosis of Cushing's syndrome, 142
Alcoholism
  basic information about, 18
  diagnosis of, 18
  in differential diagnosis of pernicious anemia, 33
  treatment of, 18
Alcohols, antimicrobial activity, mechanics of action, toxicity, indications and contraindications, 979t
Aldolase, laboratory findings in, 782
Aldomet; see Methyldopa
Aldosteronism
  primary
    basic information about, 19
    diagnosis of, 19
    treatment of, 19
    renin-aldosterone patterns in, 826t
Aleve; see Naproxen
Alkaline phosphatase
  elevation of
    causes of, 783
    isolated, 783
  laboratory findings for, 782-783
Alkalosis
  metabolic, 542, 781t
  respiratory, 543, 781t
Alkaptonuria of axial skeleton, characteristics of, 549t
Allegra; see Fexofenadine
Allen-Masters syndrome in differential diagnosis of dysmenorrhea, 161
Allergic alveolitis in differential diagnosis of diffuse interstitial lung disease, 153
Allergic blepharitis in differential diagnosis of blepharitis, 73
Allergic contact dermatitis; see Dermatitis, contact
Allergic rhinitis, drug therapy for; see Antihistamines
Allergies
  antibiotic, management of, 1023t, 1024t
  in differential diagnosis of hordeolum, 236
  in differential diagnosis of pruritus ani, 392
  eosinophilia due to, 573
Alopecia
  androgenetic, differential diagnosis of, 544t
  drug-induced, 565
  nonscarring, 543t-544t
  scarring, 543t
Alopecia areata, differential diagnosis of, 544t
Alpha$_2$ antiplasmin, disorders of, inheritance, incidence, bleeding symptoms, test results, treatment, 562t

Index

5-Alpha-reductase deficiency, phenotypes, karyotypes, inheritance, hormone levels, pathogenesis, 546t
Alprazolam, preparations, dosage, half-life, indication, cost, 980t
ALS; see Amyotrophic lateral sclerosis
Altace; see Ramipril
Alveolar-arterial oxygen gradient, formula for, 1042
Alveolitis
　allergic, in differential diagnosis of diffuse interstitial lung disease, 153
　extrinsic allergic, granulomatous disorders due to, 584
Alzheimer's disease
　basic information about, 20
　diagnosis of, 20
　in differential diagnosis of Creutzfeldt-Jakob disease, 139
　in differential diagnosis of Parkinson's disease, 347
　encephalopathy in, in differential diagnosis of HIV, 232
　treatment of, 20
Amaryl; see Glimepiride
Amaurosis fugax
　basic information about, 21
　diagnosis of, 21
　treatment of, 21
Amblyopia
　basic information about, 22
　diagnosis of, 22
　screening recommendations for, 869
　treatment of, 22
Amebiasis
　basic information about, 23
　clinical features, diagnosis, and treatment, 582t
　diagnosis of, 23
　in differential diagnosis of babesiosis, 64
　in differential diagnosis of granuloma inguinale, 206
　treatment of, 23
Amebic dysentery; see Amebiasis
Amebic liver abscess in differential diagnosis of typhoid fever, 504
Amenorrhea
　differential diagnosis of, 544t-545t
　evaluation of, 673
American trypanosomiasis; see Chagas' disease
Amikacin
　dosage for, and dialysis removal, 971t
　drug monitoring data for, 799t
Aminoglycosides
　dosage for, and dialysis removal, 971t
　in immunocompromised host, 937
Amiodarone
　dosage, half-life, ECG manifestations, toxicity, 1000t
　electrophysiologic effects of, 969t
Amitriptyline
　drug monitoring data for, 799t
　preparations, dosage, class, effects, half-life, 974t
AML; see Leukemia, acute myelogenous
Amlodipine, preparations, dosage, effects, class, cost, half-life, 982t
Ammonia, laboratory findings in, 783
Amnesia, causes of, 545
Amniocentesis
　for Down syndrome screening, 872
　for neural tube defects, 872-873
Amniotic fluid embolism in differential diagnosis of eclampsia, 163
Amoxapine, preparations, dosage, class, effects, half-life, 974t
Amoxicillin, dosage for, and dialysis removal, 972t

Amphetamine abuse in differential diagnosis of pheochromocytoma, 363
Ampicillin, dosage for, and dialysis removal, 972t
Amsacrine, toxicity of, 984t-985t
Amsterdam Study on the Elderly, 918-919
Amylase
　laboratory findings for, 783-784
　urine, 833
Amyloidosis
　basic information about, 24
　diagnosis of, 24
　in differential diagnosis of acute glomerulonephritis, 200
　in differential diagnosis of hypothyroidism, 251
　in differential diagnosis of Sheehan's syndrome, 437
　primary, in differential diagnosis of temporal arteritis, 465
　treatment of, 24
Amyotrophic lateral sclerosis
　basic information about, 25
　diagnosis of, 25
　in differential diagnosis of syringomyelia, 459
　treatment of, 25
Anaerobic infection(s), 26-27
　basic information about, 26
　diagnosis of, 26
　treatment of, 26-27
Anagen arrest in differential diagnosis of alopecia, 544t
Anal fissure
　basic information about, 28
　diagnosis of, 28
　treatment of, 28
Anal fistula
　in differential diagnosis of hemorrhoids, 217
　in differential diagnosis of pilonidal disease, 365
Anal papillae, hypertrophied, in differential diagnosis of hemorrhoids, 217
Anal ulcer; see Anal fissure
Analgesics, narcotic, equivalent dose, duration, preparations, dosage, 995t
Anaphylactoid reaction; see Anaphylaxis
Anaphylaxis
　basic information about, 29
　diagnosis of, 29
　treatment of, 29
Anaplastic carcinoma of thyroid; see Thyroid carcinoma
Anaprox; see Naproxen
Anarthritic rheumatoid syndrome; see Polymyalgia rheumatica
Ancef; see Cefazolin
Androgen insensitivity, micropenis due to, 622
Androgen resistance syndromes, 546t
Anemia
　aplastic
　　basic information about, 30
　　diagnosis of, 30
　　treatment of, 30
　autoimmune hemolytic, basic information about, 31
　diagnosis of, 805
　evaluation of, 674
　hemolytic, in differential diagnosis of Gilbert's disease, 196
　hereditary, in differential diagnosis of hemochromatosis, 215
　iron deficiency
　　basic information about, 32
　　clinical and laboratory features, 547t
　　diagnosis of, 32

Anemia—cont'd
　iron deficiency—cont'd
　　in differential diagnosis of lead poisoning, 267
　　in differential diagnosis of sickle cell anemia, 34
　　screening recommendations for, 861-862
　　treatment of, 32
　megaloblastic, causes of, 547-548
　pernicious
　　basic information about, 33
　　diagnosis of, 33
　　in differential diagnosis of myasthenia gravis, 312
　　treatment of, 33
　sickle cell, 34-35; see also Sickle cell disease
　　basic information about, 34
　　diagnosis of, 34
　　treatment of, 34-35
Anergy, cutaneous, causes of, 548
Aneurysm
　abdominal aortic; see also Abdominal aortic aneurysm
　carotid artery, in differential diagnosis of cavernous sinus thrombosis, 97
　in differential diagnosis of migraine, 210
　dissecting
　　in differential diagnosis of peptic ulcer disease, 354
　　in differential diagnosis of pericarditis, 356
　ventricular, in differential diagnosis of mitral valve prolapse, 302
Anger, myocardial ischemia triggered by, 932-933
Angiitis, hypersensitivity, neuropathies associated with, 631t
Angina pectoris, 37-38
　basic information about, 37
　classification of, 37
　diagnosis of, 37
　in differential diagnosis of peptic ulcer disease, 354
　in differential diagnosis of pericarditis, 356
　nitrates for, dosage, preparations, onset of action, duration of action, 996t
　during noncardiac surgery, 935
　reducing transient myocardial ischemia in, with pravastatin, 947
　treatment of, 37-38
　unstable, in differential diagnosis of GERD, 194
Angioedema in differential diagnosis of epiglottitis, 176
Angiofibroma in differential diagnosis of acne vulgaris, 12
Angiostrongylus cantonensis in tissue infections, epidemiology, transmission, manifestations, diagnosis, treatment, 629t
Angiostrongylus costaricensis in tissue infections, epidemiology, transmission, manifestations, diagnosis, treatment, 629t
Angiotensin-converting enzyme, laboratory findings in, 784
Anion gap
　formula for, 1042
　laboratory findings for, 784
Anion gap acidosis, 540
Anisakis in tissue infections, epidemiology, transmission, manifestations, diagnosis, treatment, 629t
Anisocoria, causes of, 549

1076 Index

Ankle
  fracture of
    basic information about, 39
    diagnosis of, 39
    treatment of, 39
  sprain of
    basic information about, 40
    diagnosis of, 40
    treatment of, 40
Ankylosing spondylitis
  basic information about, 41
  characteristics of, 549t, 656t
  course and distribution, 551t
  diagnosis of, 41
  in differential diagnosis of low back pain, 554t
  in differential diagnosis of psoriatic arthritis, 52
  in differential diagnosis of Reiter's syndrome, 406
  treatment of, 41
Anogenital warts; see Condyloma acuminatum
Anorectal fissure; see Anal fissure
Anorectal fistula
  basic information about, 42
  diagnosis of, 42
  treatment of, 42
Anorectal gonorrhea, clinical features, diagnosis, and treatment, 582t
Anorectal lesions in differential diagnosis of encopresis, 167
Anorectal syphilis, clinical features, diagnosis, and treatment, 582t
Anorexia nervosa, 43-44
  basic information about, 43
  diagnosis of, 43
  in differential diagnosis of Addison's disease, 15
  evaluation of, 675
  treatment of, 43-44
Ansaid; see Flurbiprofen
Anserine bursitis, knee pain due to, findings, diagnosis, and management, 612t
Anspor; see Cephradine
Anterior cord syndrome, 445
Anterior drawer sign, 1026
Anthrax in differential diagnosis of tularemia, 501
Anthrax vaccine, schedule, indications, side effects, contraindications, during pregnancy, with HIV infection, in immunocompromised patient, 1010t-1011t
Antiarrhythmic agents, electrophysiologic effects of, 969t
Antibiotics
  dosage for, and dialysis removal, 971t-972t
  macrolide, preparations, dosage, excretion, half-life, cost, 994t
Anticholinergic poisoning, antidotes for, dosage and indications, 1055t
Anticoagulant, circulating, laboratory findings, 792
Anticonvulsants, preparations, dosage, use, half-life, therapeutic level, toxic level, 973t
Antidepressants, preparations, dosage, class, effects, half-life, 974t
Antidiabetic agents, preparations, dosage, duration of action, half-life, excretion, cost, class, 975t
Antidiuretic hormone, inappropriate secretion of
  basic information about, 254
  diagnosis of, 254
  treatment of, 254

Anti-DNA, laboratory findings for, 784
Antidotes, dosage and indications for, 1055t
Antiemetics, preparations, dosage, class, 976t
Antihistamines, preparations, dosage, effects, class, cost, 977t
Antineutrophil cytoplasmic antibody, laboratory findings for, 784
Antinuclear antibodies
  abnormalities of, 676
  disease-associated subtypes of, 785t
  laboratory findings for, 784
Antipsychotics, preparations, dosage, class, adverse effects, 978t
Antiretroviral agents, therapeutic class, preparations, dosage, toxicities, cost, 970t
Antirheumatic drugs, disease-modifying; see Disease-modifying antirheumatic drugs
Antiseptic solutions, antimicrobial activity, mechanics of action, toxicity, indications and contraindications, 979t
Anti-streptolysin O titer, laboratory findings, 786
Antithrombin III, laboratory findings, 786
Antivert; see Meclizine
Anxiety
  abdominal pain and irritable bowel syndrome associated with, 907-908
  basic information about, 45
  diagnosis of, 45
  in differential diagnosis of chronic fatigue syndrome, 119
  in differential diagnosis of premenstrual syndrome, 386
  in differential diagnosis of pruritus ani, 392
  in differential diagnosis of Sjögren's syndrome, 442
  Hamilton Scale for assessing, 1032
  treatment of, 45
Anxiety attacks; see Agoraphobia; Panic
Anxiety disorders
  in differential diagnosis of asthma, 56
  in differential diagnosis of drug abuse, 7
  in differential diagnosis of Graves' disease, 207
  in differential diagnosis of hyperthyroidism, 247
  in differential diagnosis of lead poisoning, 267
  in differential diagnosis of obsessive-compulsive disorder, 325
  in differential diagnosis of pheochromocytoma, 363
  in differential diagnosis of phobias, 364
  in differential diagnosis of pulmonary embolism, 399
  and difficult physician-patient relationship, 907
Aorta, abdominal, aneurysm of; see Abdominal aortic aneurysm
Aortic aneurysm, ruptured or dissecting, in differential diagnosis of acute pancreatitis, 344
Aortic dissection, acute, in differential diagnosis of angina pectoris, 37
Aortic insufficiency; see Aortic regurgitation
Aortic regurgitation
  basic information about, 46
  diagnosis of, 46
  treatment of, 46
Aortic sclerosis in differential diagnosis of aortic stenosis, 47
Aortic stenosis
  basic information about, 47
  diagnosis of, 47
  treatment of, 47

Aortic valvular stenosis; see Aortic stenosis
Apathetic hyperthyroidism in differential diagnosis of Addison's disease, 15
Aphthous stomatitis
  in differential diagnosis of herpangina, 224
  in differential diagnosis of herpes simplex infection, 225
Aplasia cutis in differential diagnosis of alopecia, 543t
Apnea, sleep; see Sleep apnea
Appendicitis
  acute
    basic information about, 48
    diagnosis of, 48
    treatment of, 48
  in differential diagnosis of acute pancreatitis, 344
  in differential diagnosis of benign ovarian tumor, 341
  in differential diagnosis of ectopic pregnancy, 164
  in differential diagnosis of endometriosis, 170
  in differential diagnosis of pelvic abscess, 4
  in differential diagnosis of pelvic inflammatory disease, 352
  in differential diagnosis of preeclampsia, 384
  in differential diagnosis of pyelonephritis, 401
  in differential diagnosis of secondary peritonitis, 359
  in differential diagnosis of spontaneous bacterial peritonitis, 360
  in differential diagnosis of urolithiasis, 510
Apprehension test, 1026
Ara-C, toxicity of, 984t-985t
Arboviral encephalitis; see also Encephalitis, acute viral
  basic information about, 166
  diagnosis of, 166
  treatment of, 166
ARDS; see Acute respiratory distress syndrome
ARF; see Renal failure, acute
Argentaffinoma syndrome; see Carcinoid syndrome
Aristocort; see Triamcinolone
Arm(s), swelling of, differential diagnosis of, 657t
Arm circumference, calculation of, 1046t
Arrhythmias
  in differential diagnosis of agoraphobia/panic, 16
  drug therapy for; see Antiarrhythmic agents
  sports participation and, 1035t
  sudden cardiac death due to, 911, 912t
Arsenic poisoning, antidotes for, dosage and indications, 1055t
Artefaktkrankheit; see Munchausen's syndrome
Arterial insufficiency in differential diagnosis of deep vein thrombosis, 473
Arteriosclerosis obliterans in differential diagnosis of leg pain, 615t
Arteriosclerotic peripheral vascular disease in differential diagnosis of thromboangiitis obliterans, 471
Arteriovenous malformations
  in differential diagnosis of colorectal cancer, 127
  in differential diagnosis of migraine, 210
Arteritis
  cranial, neuropathies associated with, 631t

Arteritis—cont'd
  in differential diagnosis of cluster headache, 209
  necrotizing; see Polyarteritis nodosa
  temporal
    basic information about, 465
    diagnosis of, 465
    treatment of, 465
Arthralgia, diagnosis of, 677
Arthritis; see also Osteoarthritis; Rheumatoid arthritis
  of axial skeleton, characteristics of, 549t
  crystal-induced, characteristics of, 550t
  in differential diagnosis of rotator cuff syndrome, 423
  in differential diagnosis of spondyloarthropathies, 655
  with GI disease, characteristics of, 656t
  granulomatous
    basic information about, 49
    diagnosis of, 49
    treatment of, 49
  of hip, in differential diagnosis of lumbar disc syndromes, 276
  infectious
    basic information about, 50
    diagnosis of, 50
    in differential diagnosis of bursitis, 85
    in differential diagnosis of Charcot's joint, 111
    in differential diagnosis of gout, 205
    treatment of, 50
  juvenile rheumatoid
    basic information about, 51
    characteristics of, 549t
    diagnosis of, 51
    in differential diagnosis of Legg-Calvé-Perthes disease, 268
    in differential diagnosis of rheumatic fever, 419
    treatment of, 51
  monoarticular, differential diagnosis of, 550
  oligoarticular, differential diagnosis of, 550
  polyarticular, causes of, 551t
  psoriatic
    of axial skeleton, 549t
    basic information about, 52
    characteristics of, 656t
    course and distribution, 551t
    diagnosis of, 52
    in differential diagnosis of Reiter's syndrome, 406
    treatment of, 52
  reactive; see Reiter's syndrome
  rheumatoid; see Rheumatoid arthritis
  septic; see also Arthritis, infectious
    in differential diagnosis of Legg-Calvé-Perthes disease, 268
Arthritis-tenosynovitis, gonococcal, in differential diagnosis of Reiter's syndrome, 406
Arthropathy, neuropathic; see Charcot's joint
Arthrosis; see Arthritis; Osteoarthritis
Artifactual illness; see Munchausen's syndrome
Artificial insemination; see Insemination, therapeutic
Asbestosis
  basic information about, 54
  diagnosis of, 54
  treatment of, 54
Ascariasis
  basic information about, 55
  diagnosis of, 55
  in differential diagnosis of hookworm, 235
  treatment of, 55

Ascending cholangitis; see Cholangitis
Ascites
  algorithm for, 678
  causes of, 552
ASD; see Atrial septal defect
Asendin; see Amoxapine
Aseptic meningitis; see Meningitis, viral
ASH; see Cardiomyopathy, hypertrophic
Asherman's syndrome
  in differential diagnosis of amenorrhea, 544t
  in differential diagnosis of menopause, 297
L-Asparaginase, toxicity of, 984t-985t
Aspartate aminotransferase
  elevated, causes for, 786t, 787
  laboratory findings, 786
Asperger's syndrome in differential diagnosis of autistic disorder, 63
Aspergillosis infection in differential diagnosis of tracheitis, 488
Aspiration in differential diagnosis of acute bronchitis, 82
Aspirin
  for angina pectoris, 38
  dosage and indications, 44t
  preparations, dosage, half-life, class, cost, metabolism, 997t
  for preventing myocardial infarction, 895
  for preventing preeclampsia or intrauterine growth retardation, 895
Astemizole, preparations, dosage, effects, class, cost, 977t
Asthma, 56-57
  basic information about, 56
  diagnosis of, 56
  in differential diagnosis of acute bronchitis, 82
  in differential diagnosis of bronchiectasis, 81
  in differential diagnosis of chronic obstructive pulmonary disease, 120
  in differential diagnosis of congestive heart failure, 130
  in differential diagnosis of cystic fibrosis, 143
  in differential diagnosis of pulmonary edema, 398
  gastroesophageal reflux as factor in, 936
  granulomatosis associated with, 585t-586t
  muscle weakness in mechanically ventilated patients with, 959-960, 960
  pharmacologic management of, 56-57
  treatment of, 56-57
Asystole, evaluation of, 679
Ataxia
  causes of, 552
  Friedreich's; see Friedreich's ataxia
  locomotor; see Tabes dorsalis
Atelectasis
  basic information about, 58
  diagnosis of, 58
  in differential diagnosis of asbestosis, 54
  treatment of, 58
Atenolol, preparations, dosage, cardioselectivity, lipid solubility, half-life, excretion, cost, 981t
Atherosclerosis
  coronary
    in differential diagnosis of dilated cardiomyopathy, 89
    in differential diagnosis of hypertrophic cardiomyopathy, 90
    in differential diagnosis of restrictive cardiomyopathy, 91
  insulin sensitivity and, 903-904
Ativan; see Lorazepam

Atlantoaxial instability, sports participation and, 1035t
Atopic dermatitis; see Dermatitis, atopic
Atopic eczema; see Dermatitis, atopic
Atopic neurodermatitis; see Dermatitis, atopic
Atorvastatin, preparations, dosage, mechanism of action, effect, cost, 993t
Atrial fibrillation
  basic information about, 59
  diagnosis of, 59
  in differential diagnosis of atrial flutter, 60
  nonrheumatic, prophylactic anticoagulation for, 937-938, 938t
  treatment of, 59
Atrial flutter
  basic information about, 60
  diagnosis of, 60
  in differential diagnosis of atrial fibrillation, 59
  treatment of, 60
Atrial premature beats in differential diagnosis of atrial fibrillation, 59
Atrial septal defect
  basic information about, 61
  diagnosis of, 61
  in differential diagnosis of mitral stenosis, 301
  treatment of, 61
Atrioventricular block, third-degree; see Heart block, complete
Attention deficit disorder; see Attention deficit hyperactivity disorder
Attention deficit hyperactivity disorder
  basic information about, 62
  diagnosis of, 62
  in differential diagnosis of lead poisoning, 267
  treatment of, 62
AUDIT structured interview for assessing problem drinking, 877t
Auditory brainstem response, 870
Autism; see Autistic disorder
Autistic disorder
  basic information about, 63
  diagnosis of, 63
  treatment of, 63
Autoimmune disease in differential diagnosis of myelodysplastic syndromes, 313
Autoimmune disorders, eosinophilia due to, 573
Autoimmune inner ear syndrome in differential diagnosis of Meniere's disease, 292
Autoimmune thrombocytopenic purpura; see Idiopathic thrombocytopenic purpura
Autoimmune thyroiditis; see Thyroiditis
Avascular necrosis
  in differential diagnosis of rotator cuff syndrome, 423
  knee pain due to, findings, diagnosis, and management, 612t
Axid; see Nizatidine
Azathioprine, toxicity of, 984t-985t
Azithromycin
  dosage for, and dialysis removal, 971t
  preparations, dosage, excretion, half-life, cost, 994t
Azlocillin, dosage for, and dialysis removal, 972t
Azotemia, prerenal, in differential diagnosis of hepatorenal syndrome, 223
AZT; see Zidovudine
Aztreonam, dosage for, and dialysis removal, 971t

B

Babesiosis, 64-65
  basic information about, 64
  diagnosis of, 64-65
  in differential diagnosis of human granulocytic ehrlichiosis, 237
  in differential diagnosis of Lyme disease, 279
  prevention of, 65
  treatment of, 65
Bacillary dysentery; see Shigellosis
Bacille Calmette-Guérin immunization, recommendations for, 863-864
Bacillus cereus pneumonia in differential diagnosis of pulmonary tuberculosis, 498
Back pain
  counseling to prevent, 885
  further management of, *686*
  initial evaluation of, *680*
  low, differential diagnosis of, 553t-554t
  during pregnancy, *910*, 910-911
  slow-to-recover, *684*
  surgical considerations with persistent sciatica, *685*
  symptom control methods, 683t
  symptoms of potentially serious conditions, *681*
  treatment and follow-up, *682*
Bacteremia
  in differential diagnosis of bacterial meningitis, 294
  in differential diagnosis of infective endocarditis, 168
  nosocomial, 323
Bacteria; see also specific genera and species
  granulomatous disorders due to, 584
Bacterial endocarditis; see Endocarditis, infective
Bacterial epididymitis, nonspecific; see Epididymitis
Bacterial infection
  anaerobic; see Anaerobic infection(s)
  in differential diagnosis of ulcerative colitis, 505
Bacterial keratitis; see Corneal ulceration
Bacterial meningitis in differential diagnosis of leptospirosis, 169
Bacterial tracheobronchitis; see Tracheitis
Bacterial vaginosis; see Vaginosis, bacterial
Bacteriuria
  asymptomatic, 509
  screening recommendations for, 868
Bacteroides, infections due to, 26
Baker's cyst; see also Bursitis
  ruptured, in differential diagnosis of deep vein thrombosis, 473
Balanitis
  basic information about, 66
  diagnosis of, 66
  treatment of, 66
Balanitis xerotica obliterans in differential diagnosis of balanitis, 66
Balding; see Alopecia
Balloon valvuloplasty for aortic stenosis, 47
Bang's disease; see Brucellosis
Bannworth's syndrome; see Lyme disease
Bartholin gland carcinoma; see Vulvar cancer
Bartholinitis, gonococcal; see Gonorrhea
Bartholin's gland abscess in differential diagnosis of anorectal fistula, 42
Bartter's syndrome, renin-aldosterone patterns in, 826t
Basal cell carcinoma
  basic information about, 67
  diagnosis of, 67
  in differential diagnosis of acne vulgaris, 12

Basal cell carcinoma—cont'd
  in differential diagnosis of melanoma, 291
  treatment of, 67
  of vulva; see Vulvar cancer
Basal cell nevus syndrome in differential diagnosis of basal cell carcinoma, 67
Basal energy expenditure, assessment of, 1046t
Basophil count, laboratory findings, 786
Battered elder syndrome; see Geriatric abuse
"Battered-child syndrome"; see Child abuse
Bazex's syndrome, history, manifestations, and malignancy associated with, 564t
BCC; see Basal cell carcinoma
Bedsores; see Pressure ulcers
Bed-wetting; see Enuresis
Behavioral disorders, sleep-associated, *759*
Behçet's disease
  course and distribution, 551t
  in differential diagnosis of acute viral encephalitis, 166
  in differential diagnosis of glossitis, 202
  in differential diagnosis of herpes simplex infection, 225
Bell's palsy
  basic information about, 68
  diagnosis of, 68
  in differential diagnosis of Ramsay Hunt syndrome, 403
  treatment of, 68
Benadryl; see Diphenhydramine
Benazepril, dosage, onset of action, peak effect, half-life, cost, 967t
Benign chest wall pain syndrome; see Costochondritis
Benign prostatic hypertrophy in differential diagnosis of prostate cancer, 389
Benisone; see Betamethasone
Benzodiazepine poisoning, antidotes for, dosage and indications, 1055t
Benzodiazepines, preparations, dosage, half-life, indication, cost, 980t
Beta-adrenergic blocking agents
  mechanism of action of, 38
  preparations, dosage, cardioselectivity, lipid solubility, half-life, excretion, cost, 981t
Beta-blocker poisoning, antidotes for, dosage and indications, 1055t
Betamethasone, brand names and potency, 999t
Betapace; see Sotalol
Betaxolol, preparations, dosage, cardioselectivity, lipid solubility, half-life, excretion, cost, 981t
Biaxin; see Clarithromycin
Bicycling, injuries due to, counseling to prevent, 884
Biliary colic
  in differential diagnosis of acute pancreatitis, 344
  in differential diagnosis of cholangitis, 115
Biliary liver disease in differential diagnosis of irritable bowel syndrome, 259
Biliary neoplasm in differential diagnosis of cholecystitis, 116
Biliary sepsis; see Cholangitis
Biliary tract disease in pregnancy, characteristics of, 617t
Bilirubin
  direct, laboratory values, 787
  indirect, laboratory values, 787
  total, laboratory values, 787
  urine; see Urine bile
Bipolar disorder
  basic information about, 69
  diagnosis of, 69

Bipolar disorder—cont'd
  in differential diagnosis of attention deficit hyperactivity disorder, 62
  treatment of, 69
Birth, breech, 80
Birth control; see Contraception
Bisoprolol, preparations, dosage, cardioselectivity, lipid solubility, half-life, excretion, cost, 981t
Bite wounds
  basic information about, 70
  diagnosis of, 70
  treatment of, 70, 1057
Bladder, distended, in differential diagnosis of benign ovarian tumor, 341
Bladder cancer, 71-72
  basic information about, 71
  diagnosis of, 71-72
  follow-up strategies for, 1052t
  screening recommendations for, 860
  treatment of, 72
Blastomyces dermatitidis in differential diagnosis of coccidioidomycoses, 125
Bleeding; see also Hemorrhage
  in early pregnancy, *687*
  gastrointestinal, *688*
    causes by location, 555
    diagnostic considerations by age, 556t
  uterine; see Dysfunctional uterine bleeding
  vaginal; see Vaginal bleeding
Bleeding disorders; see also Clotting factor disorders; Coagulopathies
  congenital, *692*
  diagnosis based on routine screening tests, 555t
Bleeding time, laboratory values, 787
Bleomycin, toxicity of, 984t-985t
Blepharitis
  allergic, in differential diagnosis of cavernous sinus thrombosis, 97
  basic information about, 73
  diagnosis of, 73
  treatment of, 73
Blindness; see Visual loss
Blocadren; see Timolol
Blood, peripheral, lymphocyte abnormalities in, 620t
Blood pressure; see also Hypertension
  end-stage renal disease and, 939-940
  measurement of, 854-855
  in pregnant women, 871
Blood transfusion
  administration of, 1018t
  repeated, in differential diagnosis of hemochromatosis, 215
Blood values, normal, by age group, 796t
Blue nevus in differential diagnosis of melanoma, 291
Body mass index, nomogram for, *1045*
Body surface area, nomogram for calculating, *1043*
Body weight; see Weight
Boeck's sarcoid; see Sarcoidosis
Bone, neoplastic metastasis to, laboratory findings for calcium and phosphorus, 789t
Bone disease
  metastatic, in differential diagnosis of primary malignant bone tumor, 74
  Paget's; see Paget's disease of bone
Bone infarction in differential diagnosis of osteomyelitis, 332
Bone infection; see Osteomyelitis
Bone marrow, infiltrative diseases of, in differential diagnosis of acute myelogenous leukemia, 271
Bone marrow transplantation, malignant neoplasms following, *926*, 926-927

Bone tumors
   in differential diagnosis of multiple myeloma, 306
   primary malignant
      basic information about, 74
      diagnosis of, 74
      treatment of, 74
Bonine; see Meclizine
Bonnevie-Ullrich-Turner syndrome; see Turner's syndrome
Botulism
   basic information about, 75
   diagnosis of, 75
   in differential diagnosis of Guillain-Barré syndrome, 208
   treatment of, 75
Bowel obstruction in differential diagnosis of secondary peritonitis, 359
BPH; see Prostatic hyperplasia, benign
Brachial neuritis
   in differential diagnosis of cervical disc syndromes, 103
   in differential diagnosis of frozen shoulder, 191
   in differential diagnosis of thoracic outlet syndrome, 470
Brain, metastasis to, in differential diagnosis of hepatic encephalopathy, 218
Brain abscess
   in differential diagnosis of bacterial meningitis, 294
   in differential diagnosis of infective endocarditis, 168
Brain neoplasms
   basic information about, 76
   diagnosis of, 76
   in differential diagnosis of bulimia nervosa, 84
   in differential diagnosis of cavernous sinus thrombosis, 97
   in differential diagnosis of eclampsia, 163
   in differential diagnosis of Korsakoff's psychosis, 262
   in differential diagnosis of listeriosis, 275
   treatment of, 76
Brain stem encephalitis; see Encephalitis, acute viral
Branchial cleft cysts in differential diagnosis of thyroid nodule, 476
Breast
   discharge from nipples, 693
   Paget's disease of; see Paget's disease of breast
   routine screen or palpable mass evaluation, 697-698
Breast abscess
   basic information about, 77
   diagnosis of, 77
   treatment of, 77
Breast cancer, 78-79
   basic information about, 78
   diagnosis of, 78
   follow-up strategies for, 1052t
   hormone therapy and, 894-895
   oral contraceptive use and, 955-956
   during pregnancy and lactation, 79
   radiologic screening and evaluation, 695-696
   screening and evaluation, 693, 694, 856
   treatment of, 78-79
Breast disease, fibrocystic; see Fibrocystic breast disease
Breast feeding
   dental health and, 885
   iron supplements after weaning from, 905
   promoting, 881
   recommendations for, 861-862
Breast mass, differential diagnosis of, 556
Breast self-examination, 1050

Breathing, sleep-disordered, in men with coronary artery disease, 960-961
Breech birth
   basic information about, 80
   diagnosis of, 80
   treatment of, 80
Bretylium
   electrophysiologic effects of, 969t
   for ventricular arrhythmias, indications, dosage, onset of action, therapeutic plasma levels, 1001t
Bretylol; see Bretylium
Brevicon, estrogen and progestin content of, 986t
Briquet's syndrome; see Somatization disorder
Brodie's abscess in differential diagnosis of osteomyelitis, 332
Brompheniramine, preparations, dosage, effects, class, cost, 977t
Bronchial asthma; see Asthma
Bronchiectasis
   basic information about, 81
   diagnosis of, 81
   in differential diagnosis of chronic obstructive pulmonary disease, 120
   treatment of, 81
Bronchiolitis
   in differential diagnosis of acute bronchitis, 82
   in differential diagnosis of bacterial pneumonia, 370
Bronchitis
   acute
      basic information about, 82
      diagnosis of, 82
      treatment of, 82
   chronic; see also Chronic obstructive pulmonary disease
      in differential diagnosis of bacterial pneumonia, 370
      in differential diagnosis of bronchiectasis, 81
Bronchoalveolar cancer of lung, 277
Bronchospasm; see Asthma
Bronze diabetes; see Hemochromatosis
Brown-Sequard syndrome, 445
Brucellosis
   basic information about, 83
   diagnosis of, 83
   in differential diagnosis of acute viral encephalitis, 166
   in differential diagnosis of human granulocytic ehrlichiosis, 237
   in differential diagnosis of miliary tuberculosis, 496
   in differential diagnosis of nonneoplastic neck mass, 627t
   in differential diagnosis of salmonellosis, 424
   in differential diagnosis of tularemia, 501
   in differential diagnosis of typhoid fever, 504
   treatment of, 83
Brugia malayi in tissue infections, epidemiology, transmission, manifestations, diagnosis, treatment, 629t
Budd-Chiari syndrome in differential diagnosis of fatty liver of pregnancy, 181
Buerger's disease; see Thromboangiitis obliterans
Bulimia nervosa
   basic information about, 84
   diagnosis of, 84
   treatment of, 84
Bullae, differential diagnosis of, 649
Bullous diseases, differential diagnosis of, 557t

Bullous myringitis in differential diagnosis of otitis externa, 335
Bullous pemphigoid
   in differential diagnosis of impetigo, 253
   in differential diagnosis of urticaria, 512
BUN; see Urea nitrogen
Buprenex; see Buprenorphine
Buprenorphine, equivalent dose, duration, preparations, dosage, 995t
Bupropion, preparations, dosage, class, effects, half-life, 974t
Burkitt's lymphoma, chromosomal abnormalities in, 792t
Burns, estimation of area, 1059t
Bursitis
   basic information about, 85
   diagnosis of, 85
   in differential diagnosis of osteoarthritis, 330
   knee pain due to, findings, diagnosis, and management, 612t
   subacromial, in differential diagnosis of shoulder pain, 648t
   treatment of, 85
Busulfan, toxicity of, 984t-985t
Butorphanol, equivalent dose, duration, preparations, dosage, 995t

C
Cachexia in differential diagnosis of Lambert-Eaton syndrome, 265
CAGE survey, 1030
Calan; see Verapamil
Calcitonin, laboratory values, 788
Calcium
   conditions affecting levels of, laboratory findings in, 789t
   dietary intake of, 881
   laboratory values, 788
Calcium channel blocking agents
   mechanism of action of, 38
   preparations, dosage, effects, class, cost, half-life, 982t
Calcium oxalate-induced arthritis, characteristics of, 550t
Calcium pyrophosphate deposition disease; see also Pseudogout
   characteristics of, 550t
Calcium supplements and pregnancy-induced hypertension and preeclampsia, 949-950
Campylobacter jejuni, food poisoning due to, 188
Cancer; see also Carcinoma; Malignancy; Neoplastic disease; specific cancers
   bladder; see Bladder cancer
   chemotherapy for; see Chemotherapeutic agents
   in differential diagnosis of dysfunctional uterine bleeding, 159
   in differential diagnosis of pulmonary tuberculosis, 498
   follow-up strategies for, 1052t
   internal, cutaneous signs of, 564t
   metastatic, in differential diagnosis of granulomatous arthritis, 49
   pain management in, 743
Cancer antigen 125
   laboratory findings, 789
   levels in various conditions, 790
Cancer risk factor assessment for women, 1051
Candida intertrigo in differential diagnosis of cellulitis, 99
Candida septicemia, history, rash characteristics and distribution, clinical findings, diagnostic aids, 578t
Candida vaginitis in differential diagnosis of vaginitis, 663t

Candidiasis
  basic information about, 86
  cutaneous, in differential diagnosis of folliculitis, 187
  diagnosis of, 86
  in differential diagnosis of atopic dermatitis, 146
  in differential diagnosis of psoriasis, 397
  in differential diagnosis of tinea cruris, 480
  treatment of, 86
  vulvovaginal, in differential diagnosis of trichomoniasis, 492
Candidosis; see Candidiasis
Capillary hemangioma in differential diagnosis of Kaposi's sarcoma, 260
Capital femoral osteochondrosis; see Legg-Calvé-Perthes disease
Capoten; see Captopril
Capsulitis, adhesive; see also Frozen shoulder
  in differential diagnosis of shoulder pain, 648t
Captopril, dosage, onset of action, peak effect, half-life, cost, 967t
Carbamazepine
  drug monitoring data for, 799t
  preparations, dosage, use, half-life, therapeutic level, toxic level, 973t
Carbapenems, dosage for, and dialysis removal, 971t
Carbenicillin, dosage for, and dialysis removal, 972t
Carbon monoxide poisoning, antidotes for, dosage and indications, 1055t
Carbonic anhydrase inhibitors, class, preparations, dosage, site of action, cost, 978t
Carboplatin, toxicity of, 984t-985t
Carboxyhemoglobin, laboratory findings, 789
Carbuncle in differential diagnosis of pilonidal disease, 365
Carcinoembryonic antigen, laboratory findings, 790
Carcinoid flush in differential diagnosis of rosacea, 422
Carcinoid syndrome
  basic information about, 87
  diagnosis of, 87
  in differential diagnosis of pheochromocytoma, 363
  treatment of, 87
Carcinoid tumor
  in differential diagnosis of Crohn's disease, 140
  in differential diagnosis of lung neoplasm, 277
Carcinoma; see also Cancer; Malignancy; Neoplastic disease; specific types
  basal cell; see Basal cell carcinoma
  breast; see Breast cancer
  in differential diagnosis of anorexia nervosa, 43
  in differential diagnosis of granuloma inguinale, 206
  in differential diagnosis of nephrotic syndrome, 319
  inflammatory, in differential diagnosis of breast abscess, 77
  intraductal, 79
  metastatic
    in differential diagnosis of hyperosmolar coma, 243
    in differential diagnosis of multiple myeloma, 306
    in differential diagnosis of non-Hodgkin's lymphoma, 284
    in differential diagnosis of ovarian cancer, 340

Carcinoma—cont'd
  microinvasive, in differential diagnosis of cervical dysplasia, 104
Cardene; see Nicardipine
Cardiac arrest, code status determination preceding, 699
Cardiac cycle, events of, 1044
Cardiac failure; see Congestive heart failure
Cardiac murmurs
  causes of, 558
  response to physiologic interventions, 558t
  sports participation and, 1035t
Cardiac tamponade
  basic information about, 88
  diagnosis of, 88
  treatment of, 88
Cardiogenic pulmonary edema; see Pulmonary edema
Cardiogenic shock in differential diagnosis of septicemia, 436
Cardiology, year book of, 899, 901-905
Cardiomyopathy
  in differential diagnosis of cardiac tamponade, 88
  in differential diagnosis of Chagas' disease, 109
  in differential diagnosis of myocarditis, 316
  dilated
    basic information about, 89
    diagnosis of, 89
    treatment of, 89
  hypertrophic
    basic information about, 90
    diagnosis of, 90
    in differential diagnosis of aortic stenosis, 47
    in differential diagnosis of mitral regurgitation, 300
    treatment of, 90
  restrictive
    basic information about, 91
    diagnosis of, 91
    treatment of, 91
Cardiovascular disease
  in differential diagnosis of anxiety, 45
  in differential diagnosis of costochondritis, 138
  mortality from
    and age and menopause, 956-958, 957
    estrogen replacement therapy and, 906
  risk of, estrogen replacement therapy and, 934-935, 935
  sports participation and, 1035t
Cardioversion for atrial fibrillation, 59
Cardizem; see Diltiazem
Cardura; see Doxazosin
Caries, dental, counseling to prevent, 885-886
Carmustine, toxicity of, 984t-985t
Carotene, laboratory findings, 790
Carotid artery aneurysm in differential diagnosis of cavernous sinus thrombosis, 97
Carotid artery stenosis, asymptomatic, screening for, 855
Carotid sinus syncope; see Carotid sinus syndrome
Carotid sinus syndrome
  basic information about, 92
  diagnosis of, 92
  treatment of, 92
Carpal tunnel syndrome
  basic information about, 93
  with cervical radiculopathy, 103
  diagnosis of, 93
  in differential diagnosis of amyloidosis, 24

Carpal tunnel syndrome—cont'd
  in differential diagnosis of cervical disc syndromes, 103
  in differential diagnosis of thoracic outlet syndrome, 470
  treatment of, 93
Carteolol, preparations, dosage, cardioselectivity, lipid solubility, half-life, excretion, cost, 981t
Cartrol; see Carteolol
Carvedilol, preparations, dosage, cardioselectivity, lipid solubility, half-life, excretion, cost, 981t
Cataflam; see Diclofenac
Catapres; see Clonidine
Cataract
  basic information about, 94
  diagnosis of, 94
  treatment of, 94
Catatonia in differential diagnosis of neuroleptic malignant syndrome, 321
Catecholamines, urine, 834
Cat-scratch disease, 95-96
  basic information about, 95
  diagnosis of, 95-96
  in differential diagnosis of acute viral encephalitis, 166
  in differential diagnosis of nonneoplastic neck mass, 627t
  in differential diagnosis of tularemia, 500
  treatment of, 96
Cauda equina syndrome, 445
  back pain due to, 681t
Cavernous sinus thrombosis
  basic information about, 97
  diagnosis of, 97
  treatment of, 97
CBC; see Complete blood count
Ceclor; see Cefaclor
Cecum, perforated, in differential diagnosis of acute appendicitis, 48
Cedax; see Ceftibuten
Cefaclor
  dosage for, and dialysis removal, 971t
  preparations, dosage, generation, half-life, 983t
Cefadroxil
  dosage for, and dialysis removal, 971t
  preparations, dosage, generation, half-life, 983t
Cefadyl; see Cephapirin
Cefamandole
  dosage for, and dialysis removal, 971t
  preparations, dosage, generation, half-life, 983t
Ceftazidime, dosage for, and dialysis removal, 971t
Cefazolin
  dosage for, and dialysis removal, 971t
  preparations, dosage, generation, half-life, 983t
Cefepime, preparations, dosage, generation, half-life, 983t
Cefixime
  dosage for, and dialysis removal, 971t
  preparations, dosage, generation, half-life, 983t
Cefizox; see Ceftizoxime
Cefmetazole
  dosage for, and dialysis removal, 971t
  preparations, dosage, generation, half-life, 983t
Cefobid; see Cefoperazone
Cefonicid
  dosage for, and dialysis removal, 971t
  preparations, dosage, generation, half-life, 983t

Index

Cefoperazone
  dosage for, and dialysis removal, 971t
  preparations, dosage, generation, half-life, 983t
Ceforanide
  dosage for, and dialysis removal, 971t
  preparations, dosage, generation, half-life, 983t
Cefotan; see Cefotetan
Cefotaxime
  dosage for, and dialysis removal, 971t
  preparations, dosage, generation, half-life, 983t
Cefotetan
  dosage for, and dialysis removal, 971t
  preparations, dosage, generation, half-life, 983t
Cefoxitin
  dosage for, and dialysis removal, 971t
  preparations, dosage, generation, half-life, 983t
Cefpodoxime, preparations, dosage, generation, half-life, 983t
Cefprozil
  dosage for, and dialysis removal, 971t
  preparations, dosage, generation, half-life, 983t
Ceftazidime, preparations, dosage, generation, half-life, 983t
Ceftibuten, preparations, dosage, generation, half-life, 983t
Ceftin; see Cefuroxime
Ceftizoxime
  dosage for, and dialysis removal, 971t
  preparations, dosage, generation, half-life, 983t
Ceftriaxone, preparations, dosage, generation, half-life, 983t
Cefuroxime
  dosage for, and dialysis removal, 971t
  preparations, dosage, generation, half-life, 983t
Cefzil; see Cefprozil
Celiac sprue
  basic information about, 98
  diagnosis of, 98
  in differential diagnosis of Crohn's disease, 140
  in differential diagnosis of cystic fibrosis, 143
  in differential diagnosis of tropical sprue, 494
  treatment of, 98
Cellulitis
  basic information about, 99
  diagnosis of, 99
  in differential diagnosis of bursitis, 85
  in differential diagnosis of deep vein thrombosis, 473
  in differential diagnosis of gout, 205
  in differential diagnosis of thrombophlebitis, 472
  of eyelid, in differential diagnosis of hordeolum, 236
  orbital, in differential diagnosis of cavernous sinus thrombosis, 97
  treatment of, 99
Central cord syndrome, 445
Central nervous system
  fungal infections in, host factors, neurologic presentation, 581t
  lesions of, dementia associated with, laboratory diagnosis of, 567t
  primary tumors of; see Brain neoplasm
Central nervous system disease in differential diagnosis of amblyopia, 22
Cephalexin
  dosage for, and dialysis removal, 971t

Cephalexin—cont'd
  preparations, dosage, generation, half-life, 983t
Cephalgia, histaminic; see Headache, cluster
Cephalosporins
  dosage for, and dialysis removal, 971t
  preparations, dosage, generation, half-life, 983t
Cephalothin
  dosage for, and dialysis removal, 971t
  preparations, dosage, generation, half-life, 983t
Cephapirin
  dosage for, and dialysis removal, 971t
  preparations, dosage, generation, half-life, 983t
Cephradine
  dosage for, and dialysis removal, 971t
  preparations, dosage, generation, half-life, 983t
Cerebellar ataxia in differential diagnosis of Friedrich's ataxia, 190
Cerebral anoxia
  in differential diagnosis of hepatic encephalopathy, 218
  in differential diagnosis of Korsakoff's psychosis, 262
Cerebral degeneration; see Alzheimer's disease
Cerebral lesions in differential diagnosis of toxoplasmosis, 486
Cerebral palsy
  basic information about, 100
  diagnosis of, 100
  in differential diagnosis of encopresis, 167
  sports participation and, 1035t
  treatment of, 100
Cerebral toxoplasmosis in differential diagnosis of listeriosis, 275
Cerebrospinal fluid
  abnormalities of, differential diagnosis of, 559t
  laboratory findings, 790, 791t
Cerebrovascular accident; see also Stroke
  basic information about, 101
  diagnosis of, 101
  in differential diagnosis of botulism, 75
  in differential diagnosis of hepatic encephalopathy, 218
  in differential diagnosis of hyperosmolar coma, 243
  in differential diagnosis of hypothermia, 250
  in differential diagnosis of malaria, 287
  in differential diagnosis of myxedema coma, 317
  in differential diagnosis of poliomyelitis, 378
  treatment of, 101
Cerebyx; see Fosphenytoin
Cervical cancer
  basic information about, 102
  counseling to prevent, 887-888
  diagnosis of, 102
  in differential diagnosis of abruptio placentae, 3
  in differential diagnosis of cervical polyps, 106
  in differential diagnosis of dysfunctional uterine bleeding, 159
  in differential diagnosis of estrogen deficient vulvovaginitis, 525
  follow-up strategies for, 1052t
  screening for, 857
  treatment of, 102
Cervical disc syndromes
  basic information about, 103
  diagnosis of, 103

Cervical disc syndromes—cont'd
  in differential diagnosis of frozen shoulder, 191
  treatment of, 103
Cervical dysplasia, 104
  basic information about, 104
  diagnosis of, 104-105
  treatment of, 105
Cervical intraepithelial neoplasia; see Cervical cancer; Cervical dysplasia
Cervical polyps
  basic information about, 106
  diagnosis of, 106
  in differential diagnosis of cervical cancer, 102
  in differential diagnosis of dysfunctional uterine bleeding, 159
  in differential diagnosis of dysmenorrhea, 161
  in differential diagnosis of endometrial cancer, 169
  treatment of, 106
Cervical radiculopathy
  in differential diagnosis of carpal tunnel syndrome, 93
  in differential diagnosis of epicondylitis, 174
  in differential diagnosis of rotator cuff syndrome, 423
  in differential diagnosis of thoracic outlet syndrome, 470
Cervical spine disorders
  in differential diagnosis of tension-type headache, 211
  evaluation of, 760
Cervical spondylotic myelopathy in differential diagnosis of amyotrophic lateral sclerosis, 25
Cervical stenosis in differential diagnosis of dysmenorrhea, 161
Cervical trauma in differential diagnosis of abruptio placentae, 3
Cervicitis
  basic information about, 107
  diagnosis of, 107
  in differential diagnosis of bacterial vulvovaginitis, 524
  in differential diagnosis of trichomonas vulvovaginitis, 528
  gonococcal; see Gonorrhea
  mucopurulent, in differential diagnosis of trichomoniasis, 492
  nongonococcal mucopurulent, in differential diagnosis of gonorrhea, 203
  treatment of, 107
Cervicography, recommendations for, 857
Cervix, elongated, in differential diagnosis of uterine prolapse, 515
Cesarean section
  criteria for, 80
  ectopic pregnancies following, 907
  preventing, after first-episode genital herpes, 956
Cestode infection
  epidemiology, transmission, clinical presentation, diagnosis, and treatment, 559t
  transmission, clinical findings, diagnosis, treatment, 607t
Cetirizine, preparations, dosage, effects, class, cost, 977t
CFS; see Chronic fatigue syndrome
Chagas' disease, 108-109
  basic information about, 108
  diagnosis of, 109
  treatment of, 109
Chalazion in differential diagnosis of hordeolum, 236

Chancre, soft; see Chancroid
Chancroid
  basic information about, 110
  diagnosis of, 110
  in differential diagnosis of tularemia, 500
  treatment of, 110
Change of life; see Menopause
Charcot-Marie-Tooth disease
  basic information about, 112
  diagnosis of, 112
  treatment of, 112
Charcot's joint
  basic information about, 111
  diagnosis of, 111
  in differential diagnosis of osteomyelitis, 332
  treatment of, 111
Check-rein shoulder; see Frozen shoulder
Chemicals
  in differential diagnosis of glossitis, 202
  granulomatous disorders due to, 584
Chemoprophylaxis
  ages 11-24 years, 845t-846t
  ages 25-64 years, 847t-848t
  age 65 and older, 849t-850t
  for infectious diseases, 893-894
Chemotherapeutic agents, toxicity of, 984t-985t
Cherry-red epiglottitis; see Epiglottitis
Chest pain
  in children, cardiac and noncardiac causes of, 560
  in differential diagnosis of pulmonary embolism, 399
  nonpleuritic, cardiac and noncardiac causes of, 560
  pleuritic, cardiac and noncardiac causes of, 560
Chest trauma, evaluation of, 770-771
Chest wall pain syndrome, benign; see Costochondritis
CHF; see Congestive heart failure
Chickenpox; see also Varicella
  ages affected, prodrome, morphology, distribution, diagnosis, 574t
  basic information about, 113
  diagnosis of, 113
  in differential diagnosis of impetigo, 253
  treatment of, 113
Child(ren)
  blood pressure measurement in, 854-855
  CHD screening in, 853
  cholesterol screening in, 853-854
  counseling to prevent tobacco use by, 880-881
  elevated lead levels in, screening for, 862-863
  HIV-antibody-negative, detection of virus in, 952, 953t
  immunizations for, 889-890
  iron supplements in, 905
  sudden death from cardiac causes in, 911
Child abuse
  basic information about, 5
  diagnosis of, 5
  screening for, 876
  treatment of, 6
Child maltreatment syndrome, 5; see also Child abuse; Pedophilia
Child molestation; see Pedophilia
Childhood autism; see Autistic disorder
Childhood disintegration disorder in differential diagnosis of autistic disorder, 63
Chlamydia genital infection
  basic information about, 114
  diagnosis of, 114
  reducing risk of, 887
  screening recommendations for, 866-867

Chlamydia genital infection—cont'd
  treatment of, 114
  after sexual assault, 1056t
Chlamydia pneumonia
  in differential diagnosis of coccidioidomycoses, 125
  in differential diagnosis of *Mycoplasma* pneumonia, 372
  in differential diagnosis of psittacosis, 396
Chlamydia trachomatis in differential diagnosis of gonorrhea, 203
Chlorambucil, toxicity of, 984t-985t
Chloramphenicol
  adverse effects of, 27
  dosage for, and dialysis removal, 971t
Chlordiazepoxide, preparations, dosage, half-life, indication, cost, 980t
Chloride
  laboratory findings, 791
  urine, 834
Chlorpheniramine, preparations, dosage, effects, class, cost, 977t
Chlorpromazine
  antiemetic use of, preparations, dosage, class, 976t
  antipsychotic use of, preparations, dosage, class, adverse effects, 978t
Chlorpropamide, preparations, dosage, duration of action, half-life, excretion, cost, class, 975t
Chlor-Trimeton; see Chlorpheniramine
Cholangitis
  basic information about, 115
  diagnosis of, 115
  in differential diagnosis of acute pancreatitis, 344
  in differential diagnosis of spontaneous bacterial peritonitis, 360
  treatment of, 115
Cholecystectomy, bowel habit after, 930, 930-931
Cholecystitis
  acute, in differential diagnosis of cholangitis, 115
  basic information about, 116
  diagnosis of, 116
  in differential diagnosis of hyperemesis gravidarum, 241
  in differential diagnosis of pericarditis, 356
  in differential diagnosis of secondary peritonitis, 359
  in differential diagnosis of spontaneous bacterial peritonitis, 360
  treatment of, 116
Cholelithiasis
  basic information about, 117
  diagnosis of, 117
  in differential diagnosis of chronic pancreatitis, 346
  in differential diagnosis of peptic ulcer disease, 354
  treatment of, 117
Cholera
  basic information about, 118
  diagnosis of, 118
  treatment of, 118
Cholera vaccine
  for international travel, 1019t
  during pregnancy, 1013t
  schedule, indications, side effects, contraindications, during pregnancy, with HIV infection, in immunocompromised patient, 1010t-1011t
Cholestasis
  intrahepatic
    liver function tests in, 618t
    in pregnancy, characteristics of, 617t

Cholestasis—cont'd
  of pregnancy, in differential diagnosis of fatty liver of pregnancy, 181
Cholesteatoma in differential diagnosis of labyrinthitis, 263
Cholesterol; see also Lipoprotein
  high levels of, interventions for, 854
  high-density lipoprotein, in female runners, 904-905
  as predictor of CHD risk, 853
  screening for, 853-854
    in children, 853-854
  total, laboratory findings, 791
Cholestyramine, preparations, dosage, mechanism of action, effect, cost, 993t
Cholinergic poisoning, antidotes for, dosage and indications, 1055t
Chondrocalcinosis; see Pseudogout
Chondromalacia, knee pain due to, findings, diagnosis, and management, 612t
Chondromatosis, synovial, knee pain due to, findings, diagnosis, and management, 613t
Chondrosarcoma, 74
Chorea
  drug-induced, in differential diagnosis of Huntington's chorea, 238
  Huntington's; see Huntington's chorea
  manifestations, differential diagnosis, tests, treatment, 596t
Choreoathetosis, manifestations, differential diagnosis, tests, treatment, 596t
Chorionic villus sampling, recommendations for, 872
Chorioretinitis in differential diagnosis of toxoplasmosis, 486
Choroid, inflammatory lesions of; see Retinal detachment
Christmas disease; see Hemophilia
Chromosomal disorders
  in differential diagnosis of Turner's syndrome, 502
  in hematopoietic malignancies, 792t
Chromosome studies for Down syndrome, 872
Chronic fatigue syndrome; see also Epstein-Barr virus infection
  basic information about, 119
  cognitive behavior therapy for, 913-914
  diagnosis of, 119
  in differential diagnosis of Lyme disease, 279
  in differential diagnosis of myasthenia gravis, 312
  treatment of, 119
Chronic obstructive pulmonary disease
  basic information about, 120
  diagnosis of, 120
  in differential diagnosis of asthma, 56
  in differential diagnosis of cardiac tamponade, 88
  in differential diagnosis of congestive heart failure, 130
  in differential diagnosis of pulmonary edema, 398
  in differential diagnosis of sleep apnea, 443
  long-term corticosteroid treatment of, 963-964
  mortality from, nutritional status and, 933-934, 934
  prednisone for, 945, 945-946, 946
  treatment of, 120
Chronic renal failure; see Renal failure, chronic
Churg-Strauss syndrome
  differential diagnosis of, 585t-586t
  neuropathies associated with, 631t

Cicatricial pemphigoid, differential diagnosis of, 557t
Cigarette smoking; see Smoking
Cimetidine, preparations, dosage, cost, 968t
Cinobac; see Cinoxacin
Cinoxacin, preparation, dosage, half-life, excretion, cost, 989t
Cipro; see Ciprofloxacin
Ciprofloxacin
  dosage for, and dialysis removal, 972t
  preparation, dosage, half-life, excretion, cost, 989t
Circulating anticoagulant, laboratory findings, 792
Cirrhosis, 121-122
  basic information about, 121
  diagnosis of, 121-122
  in differential diagnosis of acute glomerulonephritis, 200
  in differential diagnosis of congestive heart failure, 130
  in differential diagnosis of hemochromatosis, 215
  predicting, by alcohol intake, 924-925, 925, 925t
  treatment of, 122
Cisplatin, toxicity of, 984t-985t
Claforan; see Cefotaxime
Clap; see Gonorrhea
Clarithromycin
  dosage for, and dialysis removal, 971t
  preparations, dosage, excretion, half-life, cost, 994t
Claritin; see Loratadine
Claudication
  basic information about, 123
  diagnosis of, 123
  in differential diagnosis of leg pain, 615t
  treatment of, 123
Clemastine, preparations, dosage, effects, class, cost, 977t
Climacteric ovarian failure; see Menopause
Clindamycin, dosage for, and dialysis removal, 971t
Clinical breast examination; see also Breast cancer
  recommendations for, 856
Clinical competence, evaluation of, 909t, 909-910
Clinical preventive services, 841-895; see also Congenital disorders; Counseling; Environmental disorders; Immunizations; Infectious disease; Mental disorders; Metabolic disorders; Musculoskeletal disorders; Neoplastic disease; Nutritional disorders; Prenatal disorders
  Task Force ratings of, 841
Clinoril; see Sulindac
CLL; see Leukemia, chronic lymphocytic
Clonazepam, preparations, dosage
  half-life, indication, cost, 980t
  use, half-life, therapeutic level, toxic level, 973t
Clonidine, preparations, dosage, cost, 969t
Clonorchis sinensis, epidemiology, transmission, manifestations, diagnosis, treatment, 660t
Clorazepate, preparations, dosage, half-life, indication, cost, 980t
Clostridium botulinum
  food poisoning due to, 188
  infections due to, 26
Clostridium difficile, infections due to, 26
Clostridium perfringens, infections due to, 26
Clostridium septicum, infections due to, 26
Clostridium tertium, infections due to, 26
Clostridium tetani, infections due to, 26

Clotting factor disorders; see also Coagulopathies
  in differential diagnosis of hemophilia, 216
  in differential diagnosis of von Willebrand's disease, 522
Clotting factor VIII deficiency hemophilia; see Hemophilia
Clotting factor IX hemophilia; see Hemophilia
Clotting factor XIII deficiency, diagnosis of, 555t
Clotting factors
  characteristics of, 793t
  reference ranges, 793
Cloxacillin, dosage for, and dialysis removal, 972t
Clozapine, preparations, dosage, class, adverse effects, 978t
Clozaril; see Clozapine
Clubbing, causes of, 561
Cluster headache; see Headache, cluster
CML; see Leukemia, chronic myelogenous
CO_2, average values for arterial and venous plasma or serum, 781t
CO_2 narcosis in differential diagnosis of myxedema coma, 317
Coagulation, pathways for, 794
Coagulation factors; see Clotting factors
Coagulopathies; see also Bleeding disorders; Clotting factor disorders
  congenital, inheritance, incidence, symptoms, test results, treatment, 561t-562t
  consumptive; see Disseminated intravascular coagulation
  in differential diagnosis of dysfunctional uterine bleeding, 159
Coat's disease; see Retinal hemorrhage
Cobalamin deficiency, etiopathophysiologic classification of, 547
Cocaine abuse in differential diagnosis of pheochromocytoma, 363
Cocaine intoxication in differential diagnosis of heat exhaustion/heat stroke, 214
Coccidioidomas in differential diagnosis of coccidioidomycoses, 125
Coccidioidomycoses, 124-126
  basic information about, 124-125
  diagnosis of, 125
  in differential diagnosis of pulmonary tuberculosis, 498
  treatment of, 126-127
Coccygeal sinus in differential diagnosis of pilonidal disease, 365
Code status, determination before cardiac arrest, 699
Codeine, equivalent dose, duration, preparations, dosage, 995t
Cognitive behavior therapy for chronic fatigue syndrome, 913-914
Cognitive function, effect of intensive diabetes therapy on, 929-930
Cold, myocardial ischemia triggered by, 932-933
Cold agglutinins titer, laboratory findings, 793
Colestid; see Colestipol
Colestipol, preparations, dosage, mechanism of action, effect, cost, 993t
Colic, biliary
  in differential diagnosis of acute pancreatitis, 344
  in differential diagnosis of cholangitis, 115
Colistin, dosage for, and dialysis removal, 972t

Colitis
  antibiotic-induced; see Pseudomembranous colitis
  in differential diagnosis of secondary peritonitis, 359
  ischemic, in differential diagnosis of diverticular disease, 156
  pseudomembranous; see Pseudomembranous colitis
  ulcerative; see Ulcerative colitis
Collagen disorders in differential diagnosis of sarcoidosis, 426
Collagenous colitis in differential diagnosis of Crohn's disease, 140
Collagen-vascular disease
  in differential diagnosis of miliary tuberculosis, 496
  in differential diagnosis of septicemia, 436
Collagen-vascular disease cataract; see Cataract
Colon
  diverticula of; see Diverticulitis
  irritable; see Irritable bowel syndrome
Colon cancer; see Colorectal cancer
Colonoscopy, recommendations for, 857
Colorado tick fever in differential diagnosis of human granulocytic ehrlichiosis, 237
Colorectal cancer, 127-128
  in differential diagnosis of Crohn's disease, 140
  in differential diagnosis of diverticular disease, 156
  in differential diagnosis of irritable bowel syndrome, 259
  follow-up strategies for, 1052t
  in high-risk population, 857
  screening for, 856-857
Colposcopy, recommendations for, 857
Coma
  differential diagnosis of, 562
  in differential diagnosis of status epilepticus, 451
  hepatic; see Hepatic encephalopathy
  hyperosmolar; see Hyperosmolar coma
Comedone, defined, 653t
Community resources, 1060-1061
Compartment syndrome in differential diagnosis of claudication, 123
Compazine; see Prochlorperazine
Complement
  deficiencies of, infection and/or collagen disease associated with, 794t
  laboratory findings, 793
Complement C3, levels in decreased hemolytic complement activity, 795t
Complement C4, levels in decreased hemolytic complement activity, 795t
Complete blood count
  assessment of, 1046t
  normal values in, 795
Concentration camp syndrome; see Posttraumatic stress disorder
Condoms, counseling about use of, 824
Conduction system abnormalities, sudden cardiac death due to, 912t
Condyloma acuminatum; see also Warts
  basic information about, 129
  diagnosis of, 129
  in differential diagnosis of cervical dysplasia, 104
  treatment of, 129
Condyloma lata
  in differential diagnosis of granuloma inguinale, 206
  in differential diagnosis of warts, 529
Congenital anomalies presenting as neck masses, differential diagnosis of, 628t

Congenital cataract; see Cataract
Congenital disorders, screening recommendations for, 872-874
Congenital heart disease
  sports participation and, 1035t
  sudden cardiac death due to, 911, 912t
Congenital polycystic disease in differential diagnosis of echinococcosis, 162
Congenital rubella syndrome, prevention of, 868
Congestive cardiomyopathy; see Cardiomyopathy, dilated
Congestive heart failure, 130-131
  basic information about, 130
  diagnosis of, 130
  in differential diagnosis of asthma, 56
  in differential diagnosis of chronic obstructive pulmonary disease, 120
  in differential diagnosis of diffuse interstitial lung disease, 153
  in differential diagnosis of hypothyroidism, 251
  in differential diagnosis of pulmonary embolism, 399
  in differential diagnosis of sleep apnea, 443
  during noncardiac surgery, 935
  secondary to mitral stenosis, 131
  treatment of, 130-131
Conjunctivitis
  basic information about, 132
  diagnosis of, 132
  in differential diagnosis of episcleritis, 177
  in differential diagnosis of primary closed-angle glaucoma, 199
  in differential diagnosis of red eye, 640t
  in differential diagnosis of uveitis, 516
  treatment of, 132
Connective tissue disease
  course and distribution, 551t
  in differential diagnosis of fibromyalgia, 184
  mixed
    basic information about, 303
    diagnosis of, 303
    treatment of, 303
Conn's syndrome; see Aldosteronism, primary
Consciousness, loss of; see Syncope
Constipation
  agents used in treatment of; see Laxatives
  causes of, 563
Consumptive coagulopathy; see Disseminated intravascular coagulation
Contact dermatitis; see Dermatitis, contact
Contraception, 133-134
  basic information about, 133
  counseling about, 887
  diagnosis for, 133
  gynecologic cancers and, 887-888
  treatment options, 133-134
Contraceptive devices
  intrauterine
    in differential diagnosis of dysfunctional uterine bleeding, 159
    in differential diagnosis of dysmenorrhea, 161
  oral; see Oral contraceptives
Contractures, Dupuytren's; see Dupuytren's contracture
Contusion, corneal; see Corneal abrasion
Conus medullaris syndrome, 445
Conversion disorder
  basic information about, 135
  diagnosis of, 135
  in differential diagnosis of anorexia nervosa, 43

Conversion disorder—cont'd
  in differential diagnosis of somatization disorder, 444
  treatment of, 135
Convulsions, febrile, prophylaxis for, 948
Coombs, direct, laboratory values, 795-796
COPD; see Chronic obstructive pulmonary disease
Copper
  laboratory values, 796-797
  urine, 834
Cordarone; see Amiodarone
Coreg; see Carvedilol
Corgard; see Nadolol
Corneal abrasion
  basic information about, 136
  diagnosis of, 136
  in differential diagnosis of ocular foreign body, 326
  treatment of, 136
Corneal contusion; see Corneal abrasion
Corneal disease
  in differential diagnosis of amblyopia, 22
  in differential diagnosis of primary closed-angle glaucoma, 199
Corneal erosion; see Corneal abrasion
Corneal lesions
  in differential diagnosis of cataract, 94
  in differential diagnosis of conjunctivitis, 132
Corneal ulceration
  basic information about, 137
  diagnosis of, 137
  in differential diagnosis of corneal abrasion, 136
  in differential diagnosis of ocular foreign body, 326
  in differential diagnosis of red eye, 640t
  treatment of, 137
Coronary artery anomalies, sudden cardiac death due to, 912t
Coronary artery bypass surgery, indications for, 38
Coronary artery disease
  asymptomatic, screening for, 853
  mortality from, estrogen replacement therapy and, 906
  prevention of, 853
  risk factors for, 853
  sleep-disordered breathing in, 960-961
Coronary occlusion; see Myocardial infarction
Coronary stents, benefits and risks of, 38
Coronary thrombosis; see Myocardial infarction
Corpus luteum cysts in differential diagnosis of ectopic pregnancy, 164
Corticaine; see Hydrocortisone
Corticosteroid therapy for COPD, 963-964
Corticosteroids, comparison chart for, 987t
Corticotropin-secreting pituitary adenoma, 366
Cortisol, laboratory values, 797
Cortisone, comparison chart for, 987t
Corynebacterium vaginalis vaginitis; see Vaginosis, bacterial
Corynebacterium vaginosis; see Vulvovaginitis, bacterial
Costochondritis
  basic information about, 138
  diagnosis of, 138
  treatment of, 138
Costosternal chondrodynia; see Costochondritis
Costosternal syndrome; see Costochondritis
Cough
  causes of, 563
  chronic, assessment and management, 702
  whooping; see Pertussis

Counseling
  to prevent dental and periodontal disease, 885-886
  to prevent gynecologic cancers, 887-888
  to prevent HIV infection and other sexually transmitted diseases, 886-887
  to prevent household and recreational injuries, 883-884
  to prevent low back pain, 885
  to prevent motor vehicle injuries, 882-883
  to prevent tobacco use, 880-881
  to prevent unintended pregnancies, 887
  to prevent youth violence, 884-885
  for problem drinking, 878
  to promote healthy diet, 881-882
  to promote physical activity, 881
Covera-HS; see Verapamil
Coxa plana; see Legg-Calvé-Perthes disease
Coxiella burnetti pneumonia in differential diagnosis of Mycoplasma pneumonia, 372
Coxsackie virus infection
  ages affected, prodrome, morphology, distribution, diagnosis, 574t
  in differential diagnosis of herpes simplex infection, 225
C-peptide, laboratory values, 797
Crack, myocardial ischemia triggered by, 932-933
Cramps
  leg, nocturnal, 614
  menstrual; see Dysmenorrhea
  muscle, evaluation of, 738
Cranial arteritis; see also Arteritis, temporal
  neuropathies associated with, 631t
Cranial nerve lesions in differential diagnosis of myasthenia gravis, 312
C-reactive protein, laboratory values, 797
Creatine kinase, elevated, evaluation of, 703
Creatine kinase isoenzymes, laboratory values, 797-798
Creatinine
  laboratory values, 798
  urinary, assessment of, 1046t
Creatinine clearance
  formula for, 1042
  laboratory values, 798
  urine, 834
Creatinine height index, assessment of, 1046t
Creutzfeldt-Jakob disease
  basic information about, 139
  diagnosis of, 139
  treatment of, 139
CRF; see Renal failure, chronic
Crigler-Najjar syndrome in differential diagnosis of Gilbert's disease, 196
Crimean-Congo fever in differential diagnosis of yellow fever, 533
Crixivan; see Indinavir
Crohn's disease
  basic information about, 140
  diagnosis of, 140
  in differential diagnosis of ulcerative colitis, 505
  treatment of, 140
Croup
  in differential diagnosis of epiglottitis, 176
  in differential diagnosis of pertussis, 361
  in differential diagnosis of tracheitis, 488
  pseudomembranous; see Tracheitis
Crusts
  differential diagnosis of, 651
  genital, differential diagnosis of, 583t
Cryoglobulinemia
  in differential diagnosis of polyarteritis nodosa, 379
  neuropathies associated with, 631t

Cryoglobulins, laboratory values, 798
Cryptococcosis
    basic information about, 141
    diagnosis of, 141
    in differential diagnosis of *Pneumocystis carinii* pneumonia, 374
    treatment of, 141
Cryptococcus in differential diagnosis of acute viral encephalitis, 166
Cryptosporidiosis with HIV infection, 709t
Crystal deposition diseases, course and distribution, 551t
C-section; *see* Cesarean section
CSS; *see* Carotid sinus syndrome
Cushing's disease/syndrome
    basic information about, 142
    diagnosis of, 142
    differential diagnosis of, 366
    preclinical, and glycemic control in obese diabetic patients, 940-941
    renin-aldosterone patterns in, 826t
    treatment of, 142
Cutaneous anergy, causes of, 548
CVA; *see* Cerebrovascular accident; Stroke
Cyanosis, causes of, 566
Cycloid psychosis; *see* Bipolar disorder
Cyclophosphamide, toxicity of, 984t-985t
Cystectomy, indications for, 72
Cysticercosis; *see* Tapeworm
Cystic changes; *see* Fibrocystic breast disease
Cystic diseases, renal, characteristics of, 642t
Cystic fibrosis
    basic information about, 143
    diagnosis of, 143
    in differential diagnosis of acute bronchitis, 82
    in differential diagnosis of bronchiectasis, 81
    in differential diagnosis of celiac disease, 98
    in differential diagnosis of chronic obstructive pulmonary disease, 120
    in differential diagnosis of lactose intolerance, 264
    treatment of, 143
Cystic hygroma in differential diagnosis of congenital anomalies presenting as neck masses, 628t
Cystic neoplasms in differential diagnosis of echinococcosis, 162
Cysticercosis, epidemiology, transmission, clinical presentation, diagnosis, and treatment, 559t
Cystitis, interstitial
    in differential diagnosis of bladder cancer, 71
    in differential diagnosis of endometriosis, 170
    in differential diagnosis of urinary tract infection, 509
Cysts
    adventitial, in differential diagnosis of leg pain, 615t
    Baker's; *see* Bursitis
    corpus luteum, in differential diagnosis of ectopic pregnancy, 164
    defined, 653t
    dermoid, in differential diagnosis of congenital anomalies presenting as neck masses, 628t
    in differential diagnosis of colorectal cancer, 127
    in differential diagnosis of thyroid nodule, 476
    epididymal, in differential diagnosis of epididymitis, 175
    hemorrhagic, in differential diagnosis of endometriosis, 170
    mucous, in differential diagnosis of nail disorders, 625t

Cysts—cont'd
    ovarian, in differential diagnosis of dysmenorrhea, 161
    perianal sebaceous, in differential diagnosis of anorectal fistula, 42
    sebaceous; *see* Sebaceous cyst
    thyroglossal duct, in differential diagnosis of congenital anomalies presenting as neck masses, 628t
Cytomegalovirus infection
    in differential diagnosis of nonneoplastic neck mass, 627t
    in differential diagnosis of tracheitis, 488
    with HIV infection, 709t
Cytomegalovirus mononucleosis in differential diagnosis of Epstein-Barr virus infections, 178

D

D incompatibility; *see also* Rh incompatibility
    screening recommendations for, 871
Dacarbazine, toxicity of, 984t-985t
Dacryocystitis in differential diagnosis of hordeolum, 236
Dalgan; *see* Dezocine
Dalmane; *see* Flurazepam
Darvocet N-100, contents of, 995t
Darvon; *see* Propoxyphene
Daunomycin/doxorubicin, toxicity of, 984t-985t
Daydreaming in differential diagnosis of absence seizure disorder, 432
Daypro; *see* Oxaprozin
ddC; *see* Zalcitabine
ddI; *see* Didanosine
De Quervain's thyroiditis; *see* Thyroiditis
Death, sudden, from cardiac causes, in children and adolescents, 911
Decadron; *see* Dexamethasone
Deep vein thrombosis
    basic information about, 473
    diagnosis of, 473
    in differential diagnosis of cellulitis, 99
    long-term clinical course of, 962, 962-963, 963
    treatment of, 473
Deer-fly fever; *see* Tularemia
Deficiency states in differential diagnosis of Guillain-Barré syndrome, 208
Degenerative joint disease; *see* Arthritis; Joint disease, degenerative; Osteoarthritis
Dehydration in hypernatremic patients, formula for, 1042
Delirium
    alcoholic; *see* Delirium tremens
    differential diagnosis of, 566
    in differential diagnosis of hepatic encephalopathy, 218
Delirium tremens
    basic information about, 144
    diagnosis of, 144
    in differential diagnosis of rabies, 402
    treatment of, 144
Delta hepatitis
    chronic infection, 812
    coinfection or superinfection, 812
Delusional disorder in differential diagnosis of schizophrenia, 428
Delusions in differential diagnosis of obsessive-compulsive disorder, 325
Dementia
    causes of, laboratory diagnosis of, 567t
    diagnostic tests, 705t
    in differential diagnosis of AIDS, 13
    in differential diagnosis of Alzheimer's disease, 20
    in differential diagnosis of Creutzfeldt-Jakob disease, 139

Dementia—cont'd
    in differential diagnosis of hypothyroidism, 251
    in differential diagnosis of Korsakoff's psychosis, 262
    in differential diagnosis of major depression, 145
    encephalopathy in, in differential diagnosis of HIV, 232
    management algorithm, *704*
    memory loss and, 918-919
    multiinfarct, in differential diagnosis of amyloidosis, 24
    screening recommendations for, 875
Dementia praecox; *see* Schizophrenia
Demerol; *see* Meperidine
Demodex folliculorum in differential diagnosis of blepharitis, 73
Demulen, estrogen and progestin content of, 986t
Demyelination in differential diagnosis of AIDS, 13
Dengue fever
    in differential diagnosis of malaria, 287
    in differential diagnosis of yellow fever, 533
Dental disorders
    counseling to prevent, 885-886
    in differential diagnosis of trigeminal neuralgia, 493
Dental health
    ages 11-24 years, 845t
    interventions for, 843t
        ages 25-64 years, 847t-848t
        ages 65 and older, 849t-850t
Dental procedures
    endocarditis prophylaxis and, 1022
    prophylactic regimens for, 1023t
Deoxycoformycin, toxicity of, 984t-985t
Deoxycorticosterone-producing tumor in differential diagnosis of primary aldosteronism, 19
Depression
    abdominal pain and irritable bowel syndrome associated with, 907-908
    assessment of
        in elderly, 920t, 1034
        recommendations for, 875
    in differential diagnosis of Addison's disease, 15
    in differential diagnosis of AIDS, 13
    in differential diagnosis of Alzheimer's disease, 20
    in differential diagnosis of anorexia nervosa, 43
    in differential diagnosis of chronic fatigue syndrome, 119
    in differential diagnosis of drug abuse, 7
    in differential diagnosis of hypothyroidism, 251
    in differential diagnosis of myxedema coma, 317
    in differential diagnosis of obsessive-compulsive disorder, 325
    in differential diagnosis of premenstrual syndrome, 386
    in differential diagnosis of sleep apnea, 443
    drug therapy for; *see* Antidepressants
    major
        basic information about, 145
        diagnosis of, 145
        treatment of, 145
    memory loss and, 918-919
    persons at risk for, 875
    suicide risk and, 876
    Zung Scale for assessing, *1033*
Depressive episode; *see* Depression, major
Deprivation amblyopia; *see* Amblyopia

1086 Index

Dermatitis
  atopic
    basic information about, 146
    diagnosis of, 146
    in differential diagnosis of contact dermatitis, 147
    treatment of, 146
  chronic, in differential diagnosis of Paget's disease of breast, 343
  contact
    basic information about, 147
    diagnosis of, 147
    differential diagnosis of, 568t
    in differential diagnosis of atopic dermatitis, 146
    in differential diagnosis of erythema multiforme, 180
    in differential diagnosis of hordeolum, 236
    in differential diagnosis of impetigo, 253
    in differential diagnosis of psoriasis, 397
    in differential diagnosis of rosacea, 422
    in differential diagnosis of scabies, 427
    treatment of, 147
  differential diagnosis of, 568t
  in differential diagnosis of psoriasis, 397
  in differential diagnosis of scabies, 427
  exfoliative, drug-induced, 565
  seborrheic; see Seborrheic dermatitis
  stasis, in differential diagnosis of Kaposi's sarcoma, 260
Dermatitis artefacta; see Munchausen's syndrome
Dermatitis herpetiformis
  differential diagnosis of, 557t
  in differential diagnosis of atopic dermatitis, 146
  in differential diagnosis of chickenpox, 113
  in differential diagnosis of scabies, 427
Dermatofibroma in differential diagnosis of Kaposi's sarcoma, 260
Dermatomyositis
  complement deficiencies associated with, 794t
  in differential diagnosis of trichinosis, 491
  history, manifestations, and malignancy associated with, 564t
Dermatophyte fungal infections in differential diagnosis of folliculitis, 187
Dermatosis, acute febrile neutrophilic, history, manifestations, and malignancy associated with, 564t
Dermoid cysts in differential diagnosis of congenital anomalies presenting as neck masses, 628t
Desipramine
  drug monitoring data for, 799t
  preparations, dosage, class, effects, half-life, 974t
Desogen, estrogen and progestin content of, 986t
Desoximetasone, brand names and potency, 999t
Desyrel; see Trazodone
Detergents, nonionic, antimicrobial activity, mechanics of action, toxicity, indications and contraindications, 979t
Developmental delay, workup for, 706
Dexamethasone, comparison chart for, 987t
Dexchlorpheniramine, preparations, dosage, effects, class, cost, 977t
Dezocine, equivalent dose, duration, preparations, dosage, 995t
d4T; see Stavudine

Diabeta; see Glyburide
Diabetes
  bronze; see Hemochromatosis
  neuropathies associated with, 631t
Diabetes insipidus
  basic information about, 148
  diagnosis of, 148
  in differential diagnosis of diabetes mellitus, 149
  treatment of, 148
Diabetes mellitus, 149-150
  bacteriuria screening and, 868
  basic information about, 149
  diagnosis of, 149-150
  in differential diagnosis of acute glomerulonephritis, 200
  in differential diagnosis of diabetes insipidus, 148
  in differential diagnosis of Graves' disease, 207
  in differential diagnosis of hyperthyroidism, 247
  in differential diagnosis of pruritus ani, 392
  in differential diagnosis of retinitis pigmentosa, 414
  drug therapy for; see Antidiabetic agents
  gestational
    long-term effect of, 943
    screening for, 860
  insulin-dependent
    intensive therapy for, effect on neuropsychological function, 929-930
    screening recommendations for, 860
  intensive therapy for, effect on neuropsychological function, 929-930
  non-insulin-dependent
    albuminuria in, evolution, risk factors, and prognostic implications of, 941, 941-942
    screening recommendations for, 860
  in obese patients, Cushing's syndrome and, 142, 940-941
  screening recommendations for, 860
  sports participation and, 1035t
  treatment of, 150
Diabetic ketoacidosis, 151-152
  basic information about, 151
  diagnosis of, 151
  in differential diagnosis of acute pancreatitis, 344
  in differential diagnosis of hyperosmolar coma, 243
  in differential diagnosis of preeclampsia, 384
  treatment of, 151-152
Diabetic retinopathy
  basic information about, 416
  diagnosis of, 416
  in differential diagnosis of macular degeneration, 285
  treatment of, 416
Diabinese; see Chlorpropamide
Diarrhea
  acute, diagnosis of, 707
  bloody, in differential diagnosis of shigellosis, 438
  chronic
    diagnosis of, 708
    with HIV infection, 709
  Clostridium difficile in, 26
  in differential diagnosis of cholera, 118
  in differential diagnosis of giardia, 195
  in differential diagnosis of renal tubular acidosis, 409
  drug-induced, 568
  in patients with AIDS, 569

Diarrhea—cont'd
  postcholecystectomy, pathophysiology of, 930, 930-931
  sports participation and, 1035t
Diazepam, preparations, dosage, half-life, indication, cost, 980t
DIC; see Disseminated intravascular coagulation
Diclofenac, preparations, dosage, half-life, class, cost, metabolism, 997t
Dicloxacillin, dosage for, and dialysis removal, 972t
Didanosine, therapeutic class, preparations, dosage, toxicities, cost, 970t
Diet
  age 11-24 years, 845t
  healthy, counseling to promote, 881-882
  interventions for, 843t
    age 25-64 years, 847t-848t
    age 65 and older, 849t-850t
  recommended allowances for, 1047t
Difficult Doctor-Patient Relationship Questionnaire, 906
Diffuse interstitial lung disease; see Lung disease, diffuse interstitial
Diflunisal, preparations, dosage, half-life, class, cost, metabolism, 997t
Digital rectal examination
  for colorectal cancer, 856-857
  for prostate cancer, 858
Digitalis, electrophysiologic effects of, 969t
Digoxin, drug monitoring data for, 799t
Dilacor; see Diltiazem
Dilantin; see Phenytoin
Dilaudid; see Hydromorphone
Diltiazem, preparations, dosage, effects, class, cost, half-life, 982t
Dimetane; see Brompheniramine
Diphenhydramine, preparations, dosage, effects, class, cost, 977t
Diphtheria
  basic information about, 154
  diagnosis of, 154
  in differential diagnosis of epiglottitis, 176
  in differential diagnosis of Guillain-Barré syndrome, 208
  in differential diagnosis of tracheitis, 488
  in differential diagnosis of tularemia, 501
  treatment of, 154
Diphtheria vaccine during pregnancy, 1014t
Diphtheria-tetanus-pertussis vaccine, recommendations for, for children, 889
Diprolene; see Betamethasone
Diprosone; see Betamethasone
Dirithromycin, preparations, dosage, excretion, half-life, cost, 994t
Disability, deliberate; see Munchausen's syndrome
Disalcid; see Salsalate
Discharge, vaginal, evaluation of, 775
Discoid lupus erythematosus in differential diagnosis of alopecia, 543t
Disease-modifying antirheumatic drugs and reduced disability in rheumatoid arthritis, 931, 931-932
Disopyramide
  dosage, half-life, ECG manifestations, toxicity, 1000t
  drug monitoring data for, 799t
  electrophysiologic effects of, 969t
Disorders of initiating and maintaining sleep; see Insomnia
Disseminated intravascular coagulation
  basic information about, 155
  diagnosis based on routine screening tests, 555t

Disseminated intravascular coagulation—cont'd
  diagnosis of, 155
  in differential diagnosis of thrombotic thrombocytopenic purpura, 474
  treatment of, 155
Diuresis, forced, 1054t
Diuretic overuse, renin-aldosterone patterns in, 826t
Diuretics
  class, preparations, dosage, site of action, cost, 978t
  in differential diagnosis of primary aldosteronism, 19
Diverticulitis, 156
  basic information about, 156
  diagnosis of, 156
  in differential diagnosis of acute appendicitis, 48
  in differential diagnosis of benign ovarian tumor, 341
  in differential diagnosis of colorectal cancer, 127
  in differential diagnosis of Crohn's disease, 140
  in differential diagnosis of irritable bowel syndrome, 259
  in differential diagnosis of pelvic abscess, 4
  in differential diagnosis of secondary peritonitis, 359
  in differential diagnosis of ulcerative colitis, 505
  in differential diagnosis of urolithiasis, 510
  treatment of, 156
Diverticulosis, 156
Dizziness, differential diagnosis of, 569
DKA; see Diabetic ketoacidosis
Dolobid; see Etodolac
Dolophine; see Methadone
Domestic violence; see also Child abuse; Geriatric abuse
  screening for, 876
Donovanosis; see Granuloma inguinale
Doral; see Quazepam
Double-crush syndrome, 103
Douching, vaginal, reduced fertility and, 948-949, 949
Down syndrome
  basic information about, 157
  diagnosis of, 157
  screening recommendations for, 872
  treatment of, 157
Doxazosin, preparations, dosage, cost, 969t
Doxepin, preparations, dosage, class, effects, half-life, 974t
Doxycycline, dosage for, and dialysis removal, 972t
DPT vaccine, schedule for children, 1005t
Dracunculiasis medinensis in tissue infections, epidemiology, transmission, manifestations, diagnosis, treatment, 629t
Dribble, postvoid, 256
Drinking, problem; see Alcohol abuse; Alcoholism; Problem drinking
Drug(s); see also specific drugs
  anaphylaxis due to; see Anaphylaxis
  diarrhea associated with, 568
  flushing due to, 580
  gynecomastia associated with, 587
  pleural effusions due to, 635
  polyneuropathy due to, 635
  potentially inappropriate, with multiple physician management of elderly, 923t, 923-924, 924
Drug abuse, 7-8
  by adolescents, 878, 884-885
  basic information about, 7

Drug abuse—cont'd
  in cirrhosis of liver, 121
  diagnosis of, 7
  in differential diagnosis of anxiety, 45
  high-risk sexual behavior and, 887
  injuries due to, counseling to prevent, 883-884
  during pregnancy, 878
  screening recommendations for, 878-879
  suicide risk and, 876
  treatment of, 7-8, 878-879
Drug eruptions
  in differential diagnosis of erythema multiforme, 180
  in differential diagnosis of pityriasis rosea, 368
  in differential diagnosis of psoriasis, 397
  in differential diagnosis of rosacea, 422
  in differential diagnosis of urticaria, 512
Drug hypersensitivity
  arthritis due to, course and distribution, 551t
  in differential diagnosis of ascariasis, 55
Drug intoxication
  in differential diagnosis of hypothermia, 250
  in differential diagnosis of myxedema coma, 317
  in differential diagnosis of Tourette's syndrome, 483
Drug monitoring, data for, 799t
Drug rash in differential diagnosis of chickenpox, 113
Drug reaction
  in differential diagnosis of Hodgkin's disease, 233
  in differential diagnosis of juvenile rheumatoid arthritis, 51
Drug use, motor vehicle operation and, 882-883
Drug withdrawal in differential diagnosis of thyrotoxic storm, 478
Drug-induced cataract; see Cataract
Dry eye syndrome in differential diagnosis of blepharitis, 73
DTP vaccine
  for preventing tetanus, 894
  recommendations for children, 889
DTs; see Delirium tremens
DUB; see Dysfunctional uterine bleeding
Duchenne's muscular dystrophy; see Muscular dystrophy
Duct carcinoma in situ, 79
Duodenal ulcer; see Peptic ulcer disease
Dupuytren's contracture
  basic information about, 158
  diagnosis of, 158
  treatment of, 158
DVT; see Deep vein thrombosis
Dynabac; see Dirithromycin
DynaCirc; see Isradipine
Dysentery, bacillary; see Shigellosis
Dysfibrinogenemia
  characteristics and causes, 594
  in differential diagnosis of disseminated intravascular coagulation, 155
Dysfunctional uterine bleeding, 159-160
  basic information about, 159
  diagnosis of, 159-160
  in differential diagnosis of ectopic pregnancy, 164
  in differential diagnosis of spontaneous miscarriage, 446
  treatment of, 160
Dyshidrosis, differential diagnosis of, 568t
Dysmenorrhea
  basic information about, 161
  diagnosis of, 161

Dysmenorrhea—cont'd
  prevalence of, in primary care practices, 908-909, 909t
  treatment of, 161
Dysmyelopoietic syndrome; see Myelodysplastic syndromes
Dyspareunia, prevalence of, in primary care practices, 908-909, 909t
Dyspepsia
  in differential diagnosis of peptic ulcer disease, 354
  nonulcer
    in differential diagnosis of cholelithiasis, 117
    in differential diagnosis of gastritis, 193
Dysphagia, causes of, 570
Dysplasias, hereditary, in differential diagnosis of myelodysplastic syndromes, 313
Dysplastic nevi
  in differential diagnosis of melanoma, 291
  and risk of skin cancer, 858
Dyspnea
  causes of, 570
  passive smoking and, 938
  psychogenic
    in differential diagnosis of dilated cardiomyopathy, 89
    in differential diagnosis of hypertrophic cardiomyopathy, 90
    in differential diagnosis of restrictive cardiomyopathy, 91
Dysrhythmias; see Arrhythmias
Dysthymic disorders
  in differential diagnosis of chronic fatigue syndrome, 119
  and difficult physician-patient relationship, 907
Dystonia
  focal, manifestations, differential diagnosis, tests, treatment, 596t-597t
  paroxysmal, manifestations, differential diagnosis, tests, treatment, 597t
  segment/generalized, manifestations, differential diagnosis, tests, treatment, 597t
Dystonic reaction in differential diagnosis of tetanus, 466
Dysuria, differential diagnosis of, 571

E

Early infantile autism; see Autistic disorder
Eating disorders; see also Anorexia nervosa; Bulimia nervosa; Obesity
  sports participation and, 1035t
Eaton-Lambert syndrome; see Lambert-Eaton myasthenic syndrome
ECG monitoring of myocardial ischemia after acute myocardial infarction, 901-903, 902t
Echinococcosis
  basic information about, 162
  diagnosis of, 162
  treatment of, 162
Echinococcus granulosus infection, epidemiology, transmission, clinical presentation, diagnosis, and treatment, 559t
Echinococcus multilocularis infection, epidemiology, transmission, clinical presentation, diagnosis, and treatment, 559t
ECHO virus infection, ages affected, prodrome, morphology, distribution, diagnosis, 574t
Echocardiography for assessing cardiac risk during noncardiac surgery, 935-936

Index

Eclampsia
  basic information about, 163
  diagnosis of, 163
  in differential diagnosis of fatty liver of pregnancy, 181
  in differential diagnosis of thrombotic thrombocytopenic purpura, 474
  in pregnancy, characteristics of, 617t
  treatment of, 163
Ecthyma in differential diagnosis of impetigo, 253
Ectocervicitis; see Cervicitis
Ectopic pregnancy; see Pregnancy, ectopic
Ectopic thyroid in differential diagnosis of thyroid carcinoma, 475
Eczema; see also Dermatitis, atopic
  in differential diagnosis of impetigo, 253
  in differential diagnosis of Paget's disease of breast, 343
  in differential diagnosis of pediculosis, 350
  in differential diagnosis of scabies, 427
  in differential diagnosis of tinea corporis, 479
  nummular
    in differential diagnosis of contact dermatitis, 147
    in differential diagnosis of pityriasis rosea, 368
Eczematous eruptions, drug-induced, 565
Eczematous otitis externa; see Otitis externa
Edema
  in differential diagnosis of lymphedema, 281
  in differential diagnosis of nephrotic syndrome, 319
  generalized
    causes of, 571
    evaluation of, 710
  of lower extremities, causes of, 571
  pulmonary; see Pulmonary edema
  regional, evaluation of, 711
Effexor; see Venlafaxine
Effort syndrome; see Posttraumatic stress disorder
Ehrlichiosis
  in differential diagnosis of babesiosis, 64
  in differential diagnosis of Lyme disease, 279
  human granulocytic; see Human granulocytic ehrlichiosis
  human monocytic, in differential diagnosis of human granulocytic ehrlichiosis, 237
Eikenella corrodens pneumonia in differential diagnosis of pulmonary tuberculosis, 498
Ejaculation, premature
  basic information about, 165
  diagnosis of, 165
  treatment of, 165
Elavil; see Amitriptyline
Elder abuse; see also Geriatric abuse
  screening for, 876
Elderly
  ambulatory, screening for common problems in, 919-921, 920t
  assessing
    for dementia, 875
    for depression, 1034
    with hearing handicaps, 1027
  counseling, to prevent household/recreational injuries, 884
  falls by, risk factors and risk profiles for, 917-918
  insomnia in, causes of, 606t
  memory complaints and memory impairment in, 918-919

Elderly—cont'd
  multiple physician involvement in management of, 923t, 923-924, 924
Elephantiasis; see also Lymphedema
  in differential diagnosis of filariasis, 185
EM; see Erythema multiforme
Embolism
  amniotic fluid, in differential diagnosis of eclampsia, 163
  in differential diagnosis of amaurosis fugax, 21
  pulmonary; see Pulmonary embolism
Emergency medicine
  antidotes in, 1055t
  forced diuresis, 1054t
  toxicology treatment protocols, 1053t
Emphysema; see Chronic obstructive pulmonary disease
Empyema, subdural, in differential diagnosis of bacterial meningitis, 294
Enalapril, dosage, onset of action, peak effect, half-life, cost, 967t
Encainide, dosage, half-life, ECG manifestations, toxicity, 1000t
Encephalitis
  acute necrotizing; see Encephalitis, acute viral
  acute viral
    basic information about, 166
    diagnosis of, 166
    treatment of, 166
  in differential diagnosis of febrile seizures, 435
  in differential diagnosis of hepatic encephalopathy, 218
  in differential diagnosis of myxedema coma, 317
  postinfectious, in differential diagnosis of Tourette's syndrome, 483
Encephalitis lethargica; see Encephalitis, acute viral
Encephalopathic states in differential diagnosis of narcolepsy, 318
Encephalopathy
  congenital static; see Cerebral palsy
  in differential diagnosis of status epilepticus, 451
  hepatic, 218
  subacute spongiform, 139
  toxic, dementia associated with, laboratory diagnosis of, 567t
  viral, in differential diagnosis of rabies, 402
  Wernicke's, 532
Encopresis
  basic information about, 167
  diagnosis of, 167
  treatment of, 167
Endocarditis
  arthritis due to, course and distribution, 551t
  bacterial
    in differential diagnosis of rheumatic fever, 419
    treatment of, 1061t-1062t
  cardiac conditions associated with, 1022
  in differential diagnosis of bacterial meningitis, 294
  in differential diagnosis of tularemia, 501
  infective
    basic information about, 168
    diagnosis of, 168
    history, rash characteristics and distribution, clinical findings, diagnostic aids, 578t
    treatment of, 168
  prophylaxis of
    contraindications to, 1022, 1023
    dental procedures and, 1022

Endocarditis—cont'd
  prophylaxis of—cont'd
    miscellaneous medical procedures and, 1023
  subacute bacterial, in differential diagnosis of chronic fatigue syndrome, 119
Endocervicitis; see Cervicitis
Endocrine disorders
  in differential diagnosis of anorexia nervosa, 43
  in differential diagnosis of dysfunctional uterine bleeding, 159
Endolymphatic hydrops; see Meniere's disease
Endometrial cancer
  basic information about, 169
  counseling to prevent, 887-888
  diagnosis of, 169
  in differential diagnosis of estrogen deficient vulvovaginitis, 525
  hormone therapy and, 894-895
  treatment of, 169
Endometrial hyperplasia in differential diagnosis of dysfunctional uterine bleeding, 159
Endometrial polyps in differential diagnosis of cervical polyps, 106
Endometrial stromal sarcoma; see Uterine malignancy
Endometriosis, 170-171
  basic information about, 170
  diagnosis of, 170
  in differential diagnosis of bladder cancer, 71
  in differential diagnosis of diverticular disease, 156
  in differential diagnosis of dysmenorrhea, 161
  in differential diagnosis of ectopic pregnancy, 164
  in differential diagnosis of irritable bowel syndrome, 259
  in differential diagnosis of ovarian cancer, 340
  in differential diagnosis of pelvic inflammatory disease, 352
  in differential diagnosis of ulcerative colitis, 505
  treatment of, 170-171
Endometritis
  basic information about, 172
  diagnosis of, 172
  in differential diagnosis of pyelonephritis, 401
  treatment of, 172
Endomyocardial fibrosis in differential diagnosis of amyloidosis, 24
Endomyometritis; see Endometritis
Endoperimetritis; see Endometritis
Endophthalmitis in differential diagnosis of retinoblastoma, 415
Enkaid; see Encainide
Enoxacin, preparation, dosage, half-life, excretion, cost, 989t
Enteric fever; see Salmonellosis; Typhoid fever
Enteritis
  in differential diagnosis of acute appendicitis, 48
  radiation
    in differential diagnosis of Crohn's disease, 140
    in differential diagnosis of ulcerative colitis, 505
  regional; see Crohn's disease
Enterocolitis in differential diagnosis of amebiasis, 23

Index

Enteropathic arthropathy, course and distribution, 551*t*
Enteroviral infection
 ages affected, prodrome, morphology, distribution, diagnosis, 574*t*
 in differential diagnosis of human granulocytic ehrlichiosis, 237
 in differential diagnosis of poliomyelitis, 378
 in differential diagnosis of Ramsay Hunt syndrome, 403
Entrapment neuropathies in differential diagnosis of carpal tunnel syndrome, 93
Enuresis
 basic information about, 173
 diagnosis of, 173
 nocturnal, 256
 treatment of, 173
Environmental disorders, screening for, 860-863
Environmental tobacco smoke, effect on respiratory symptoms in young adults, 938
Eosinophil count, laboratory values, 798, 800
Eosinophilia
 causes of, 573
 in differential diagnosis of ascariasis, 55
Eosinophilic gastroenteritis in differential diagnosis of celiac disease, 98
Epicondylitis
 basic information about, 174
 diagnosis of, 174
 treatment of, 174
Epidermal necrolysis, drug-induced, 565
Epidermoid cyst in differential diagnosis of thyroid nodule, 476
Epidermolysis bullosa acquisita, differential diagnosis of, 557*t*
Epididymal cysts in differential diagnosis of epididymitis, 175
Epididymitis
 basic information about, 175
 diagnosis of, 175
 treatment of, 175
Epidural abscess in differential diagnosis of low back pain, 554*t*
Epiglottitis
 basic information about, 176
 diagnosis of, 176
 in differential diagnosis of pertussis, 361
 in differential diagnosis of tracheitis, 488
 treatment of, 176
Epilepsy
 differential diagnosis of, 572*t*
 in differential diagnosis of febrile seizures, 435
 in differential diagnosis of heat exhaustion/heat stroke, 214
Episcleritis
 basic information about, 177
 diagnosis of, 177
 in differential diagnosis of conjunctivitis, 132
 in differential diagnosis of uveitis, 516
 treatment of, 177
Epistaxis, causes of, 573
Epivir; *see* Lamivudine
Epstein-Barr virus infection; *see also* Chronic fatigue syndrome
 ages affected, prodrome, morphology, distribution, diagnosis, 575*t*
 basic information about, 178
 diagnosis of, 178
 in differential diagnosis of acute myelogenous leukemia, 271
 in differential diagnosis of viral meningitis, 295

Epstein-Barr virus infection—cont'd
 tests in, *800-801*
 treatment of, 178
Erb's muscular dystrophy, 311
Erectile dysfunction
 basic information about, 179
 diagnosis of, 179
 treatment of, 179
Erosion, differential diagnosis of, 651
Erosive gastritis; *see* Gastritis
Erysipelas; *see* Cellulitis
Erythema
 in differential diagnosis of urticaria, 512
 genital, differential diagnosis of, 583*t*
Erythema gyratum repens, history, manifestations, and malignancy associated with, 564*t*
Erythema infectiosum, ages affected, prodrome, morphology, distribution, diagnosis, 574*t*
Erythema multiforme
 basic information about, 180
 diagnosis of, 180
 differential diagnosis of, 557*t*
 in differential diagnosis of glossitis, 202
 in differential diagnosis of tinea corporis, 479
 in differential diagnosis of toxic shock syndrome, 484
 drug-induced, 565
 treatment of, 180
Erythema nodosum
 arthritis due to, course and distribution, 551*t*
 in differential diagnosis of thrombophlebitis, 472
 drug-induced, 565
Erythrasma in differential diagnosis of tinea cruris, 480
Erythrocyte sedimentation rate, laboratory values, 800-801
Erythrocytes, distribution width, *824*
Erythrocytosis, differential diagnosis of, 635*t*
Erythroderma, history, manifestations, and malignancy associated with, 564*t*
Erythromycin
 dosage for, and dialysis removal, 971*t*
 preparations, dosage, excretion, half-life, cost, 994*t*
Erythroplasia of Queyrat in differential diagnosis of balanitis, 66
Erythropoietin-producing states in differential diagnosis of polycythemia vera, 380
Escherichia coli, food poisoning due to, 188
Esophageal cancer in differential diagnosis of GERD, 194
Esophageal procedures, prophylactic regimens for, 1023*t*
Esophageal spasm in differential diagnosis of GERD, 194
Esophagitis
 in differential diagnosis of GERD, 194
 peptic; *see* Gastroesophageal reflux disorder
 reflux, in differential diagnosis of gastric cancer, 192
Esotropia; *see* Strabismus
Essential headache; *see* Headache, tension-type
Essential hypertension; *see* Hypertension
Estazolam, preparations, dosage, half-life, indication, cost, 980*t*
Estrogen, increased production of, gynecomastia associated with, 587
Estrogen replacement therapy, 297-298
 alternatives to, 895
 benefits and risks of, 894-895

Estrogen replacement therapy—cont'd
 long-term postmenopausal, reduced mortality associated with, 10, 905-906
 postmenopausal, and risk of cardiovascular disease, 934-935, *935*
Ethmozine; *see* Moricizine
Ethosuximide
 drug monitoring data for, 799*t*
 preparations, dosage, use, half-life, therapeutic level, toxic level, 973*t*
Etodolac, preparations, dosage, half-life, class, cost, metabolism, 997*t*
Etoposide/teniposide, toxicity of, 984*t*-985*t*
Evoked otoacoustic emission testing, 870
Ewing's sarcoma, 74
Exanthematous eruptions, drug-induced, 565
Exanthems, differential diagnosis of, 574*t*-575*t*
Excoriation, defined, 653*t*
Exercise
 ages 11-24 years, 845*t*
 counseling to promote, 881
 and high-density lipoprotein levels, 904-905
 interventions for, 843*t*
  ages 25-64 years, 847*t*-848*t*
  ages 65 and older, 849*t*-850*t*
 pelvic floor muscle, for urinary incontinence, 952, 954
 and risk of myocardial infarction associated with sexual activity, 912-913
Exfoliative dermatitis, drug-induced, 565
Exophthalmus, thyroid, in differential diagnosis of cavernous sinus thrombosis, 97
Exotropia; *see* Strabismus
Extractable nuclear antigen, laboratory values, 801
Extrinsic pathway defect, diagnosis based on routine screening tests, 555*t*
Eye disorders, sports participation and, 1035*t*
Eye pain, causes of, 576*t*
Eyelid abscess in differential diagnosis of hordeolum, 236
Eyelid malignancy in differential diagnosis of blepharitis, 73
Eyeworm infections, epidemiology, transmission, manifestations, diagnosis, treatment, 629*t*

F

Facial flushing in differential diagnosis of rosacea, 422
Facial pain
 causes of, 576*t*
 classification of, 589
Facial paralysis
 causes of, 576
 idiopathic; *see* Bell's palsy
Factitious disorder; *see also* Munchausen's syndrome
 in differential diagnosis of conversion disorder, 135
Factitious hyponatremia in differential diagnosis of inappropriate secretion of antidiuretic hormone, 254
Factors, clotting; *see* Clotting factors
Fallopian tube disorders in differential diagnosis of Meigs' syndrome, 290
Falls
 by elderly, risk factors and risk profiles for, 917-918
 injuries due to, counseling to prevent, 883-884
Familial Mediterranean fever, arthritis due to, course and distribution, 551*t*

Family planning; see Contraception
Family practice, year book of, 905-915
Family violence; see also Child abuse;
   Geriatric abuse
   screening for, 876
Famotidine, preparations, dosage, cost, 968t
Fasciitis, necrotizing, in differential
   diagnosis of cellulitis, 99
Fasciola hepatica, epidemiology,
   transmission, manifestations,
   diagnosis, treatment, 660t
Fascioscapulohumeral disease; see Muscular
   dystrophy
Fat, limiting intake of, 881
Fatigue in differential diagnosis of absence
   seizure disorder, 432
Fatty liver of pregnancy; see Pregnancy, fatty
   liver of
Febrile convulsions, prophylaxis for, 948
Febrile mucocutaneous syndrome; see
   Stevens-Johnson syndrome
Febrile seizure, benign; see Seizures, febrile
Fecal fat, quantitative, laboratory values,
   801
Fecal impaction, agents used in treatment
   of; see Laxatives
Fecal incontinence; see Encopresis
Fecal occult blood testing, 712
   recommendations for, 856
Feldene; see Piroxicam
Felodipine, preparations, dosage, effects,
   class, cost, half-life, 982t
Femoral neck fracture
   basic information about, 182
   diagnosis of, 182
   treatment of, 182
Fenopren, preparations, dosage, half-life,
   class, cost, metabolism, 997t
Ferritin, laboratory values, 801
Fertility, reduced, vaginal douching and,
   948-949, 949
Fetal death, causes of, 80
Fetal hydantoin syndrome in differential
   diagnosis of Turner's syndrome, 502
α-1-Fetoprotein, laboratory values, 801
Fetus; see also Pregnancy; Prenatal disorders
   abruptio placentae and, 3
   HIV-antibody-negative, detection of virus
      in, 952, 953t
   intrapartum electronic monitoring of,
      871
   ultrasound evaluation of, 870
Fever
   cat-scratch; see Cat-scratch disease
   in differential diagnosis of juvenile
      rheumatoid arthritis, 51
   drug-induced, 580
   hemorrhagic, in differential diagnosis of
      babesiosis, 64
   life-threatening diseases associated with,
      differential diagnosis of, 577t-579t
   rheumatic; see Rheumatic fever
   San Joaquin Valley; see
      Coccidioidomycoses
   sports participation and, 1036t
   of unknown origin
      causes of, 580
      in differential diagnosis of infective
         endocarditis, 168
      in differential diagnosis of psittacosis,
         396
      without localizing manifestations, in
         differential diagnosis of brucellosis,
         83
Fexofenadine, preparations, dosage, effects,
   class, cost, 977t
Fibrin degradation product, laboratory
   values, 801

Fibrinogen
   deficiency of, diagnosis of, 555t
   disorders of, inheritance, incidence,
      bleeding symptoms, test results,
      treatment, 561t
   laboratory values, 801-802
Fibroadenoma in differential diagnosis of
   breast cancer, 78
Fibrocystic breast disease
   basic information about, 183
   diagnosis of, 183
   in differential diagnosis of breast cancer,
      78
   treatment of, 183
Fibroids, uterine; see Uterine fibroids;
   Uterine myomas
Fibroma, infantile digital, in differential
   diagnosis of warts, 529
Fibromyalgia
   basic information about, 184
   diagnosis of, 184
   in differential diagnosis of Lyme disease,
      279
   treatment of, 184
Fibrosarcoma, 74
Fibrositis; see also Fibromyalgia
   in differential diagnosis of shoulder pain,
      648t
Fibrous dysplasia in differential diagnosis of
   Paget's disease of bone, 342
Fibrous thyroiditis; see Thyroiditis
Filariasis, 185-186
   basic information about, 185
   diagnosis of, 185-186
   in differential diagnosis of lymphangitis,
      2880
   treatment of, 186
Fire, injuries due to, counseling to prevent,
   883-884
Firearms, injuries from, counseling to
   prevent, 884-885
Fissures
   differential diagnosis of, 651
   in differential diagnosis of hemorrhoids,
      217
Fistula-in-ano, 42
Fistulas
   anorectal, 42
   classification of, 42
   in differential diagnosis of urinary tract
      infection, 509
Flea bites in differential diagnosis of scabies,
   427
Flecainide
   dosage, half-life, ECG manifestations,
      toxicity, 1000t
   electrophysiologic effects of, 969t
Floxin; see Ofloxacin
Flu; see Influenza
Fludarabine, toxicity of, 984t-985t
Fluocinolone, brand names and potency,
   999t
Fluocinonide, brand names and potency,
   999t
Fluoridation, water, counseling about,
   885-886
Fluoroquinolones, preparation, dosage, half-
   life, excretion, cost, 989t
Fluorouracil, toxicity of, 984t-985t
Fluoxetine, preparations, dosage, class,
   effects, half-life, 974t
Fluphenazine, preparations, dosage, class,
   adverse effects, 978t
Flurazepam, preparations, dosage, half-life,
   indication, cost, 980t
Flurbiprofen, preparations, dosage, half-life,
   class, cost, metabolism, 997t
Flush syndrome; see Carcinoid syndrome

Flushing
   differential diagnosis of, 580
   facial, in differential diagnosis of rosacea,
      422
   history, manifestations, and malignancy
      associated with, 564t
   idiopathic, in differential diagnosis of
      carcinoid syndrome, 87
Fluvastatin, preparations, dosage,
   mechanism of action, effect, cost,
   993t
FOBT; see Fecal occult blood testing
Folate
   laboratory values, 802
   neural tube defects and, 914-915
   supplementary, for preventing neural
      tube defects, 872-873
Folate deficiency, etiopathophysiologic
   classification of, 547-548
Folic acid
   neural tube defects and, 914-915
   supplementary, for preventing neural
      tube defects, 872-873
Folic acid deficiency in differential diagnosis
   of pernicious anemia, 33
Follicular carcinoma of thyroid; see Thyroid
   carcinoma
Follicular conjunctivitis; see Conjunctivitis
Folliculitis
   bacterial, in differential diagnosis of
      alopecia, 543t
   basic information about, 187
   diagnosis of, 187
   in differential diagnosis of acne vulgaris,
      12
   in differential diagnosis of impetigo, 253
   treatment of, 187
Folliculitis decalvans in differential
   diagnosis of alopecia, 543t
Food, anaphylaxis due to; see Anaphylaxis
Food guide pyramid, 1045
Food poisoning
   bacterial, 188-189
      basic information about, 188-189
      diagnosis of, 189
      treatment of, 189
   staphylococcal, in differential diagnosis of
      toxic shock syndrome, 484
Foreign body
   in differential diagnosis of corneal
      abrasion, 136
   in differential diagnosis of otitis externa,
      335
   in differential diagnosis of prepubescent
      vulvovaginitis, 527
   ocular
      basic information about, 326
      diagnosis of, 326
      treatment of, 326
Foreign body aspiration
   in differential diagnosis of asthma, 56
   in differential diagnosis of bronchiectasis,
      81
   in differential diagnosis of epiglottitis,
      176
   in differential diagnosis of laryngitis,
      266
   in differential diagnosis of pertussis, 361
Formulas, commonly used, 1042
Fortax; see Ceftazidime
Fosinopril, dosage, onset of action, peak
   effect, half-life, cost, 967t
Fosphenytoin, preparations, dosage, use,
   half-life, therapeutic level, toxic level,
   973t
Fracture(s)
   acute, in differential diagnosis of
      osteochondritis dissecans, 331

Fracture(s)—cont'd
  ankle
    basic information about, 39
    diagnosis of, 39
    treatment of, 39
  in differential diagnosis of osteomyelitis, 332
  femoral neck; see Femoral neck fracture
  knee pain due to, findings, diagnosis, and management, 611t
Free thyroxine index
  increased, causes of, 802
  laboratory values, 802
Frequency-urgency syndrome
  in differential diagnosis of bladder cancer, 71
  in differential diagnosis of urinary tract infection, 509
Friedreich's ataxia
  basic information about, 190
  diagnosis of, 190
  treatment of, 190
Frozen shoulder
  basic information about, 191
  diagnosis of, 191
  treatment of, 191
Functional illness; see Conversion disorder
Functional incontinence of stool, 255; see also Encopresis
Fungal arthritis in differential diagnosis of granulomatous arthritis, 49
Fungal infection
  of central nervous system, host factors, neurologic presentation, 581t
  in differential diagnosis of AIDS, 13
  in differential diagnosis of coccidioidomycoses, 125
  in differential diagnosis of Crohn's disease, 140
  in differential diagnosis of lung neoplasm, 277
Fungal keratitis; see Corneal ulceration
Fungal meningitis, CSF abnormalities in, 559t
Fungal vaginitis in differential diagnosis of bacterial vulvovaginitis, 524
Fungus(i), granulomatous disorders due to, 584
Furuncle in differential diagnosis of pilonidal disease, 365
Fusobacterium, infections due to, 26

G

Gabapentin, preparations, dosage, use, half-life, therapeutic level, toxic level, 973t
Gais-Böck's syndrome in differential diagnosis of polycythemia vera, 380
Galactorrhea, causes of, 582t
Gallbladder disease; see also Cholecystitis
  in differential diagnosis of fatty liver of pregnancy, 181
  in differential diagnosis of preeclampsia, 384
Gallstones; see Cholelithiasis
Gangrene, presenile; see Thromboangiitis obliterans
Gardnerella vaginalis vaginitis; see Vaginosis, bacterial
Gardnerella vaginosis; see Vulvovaginitis, bacterial
Gastric cancer
  basic information about, 192
  diagnosis of, 192
  treatment of, 192
Gastric ulcer; see Peptic ulcer disease
Gastrin, laboratory values, 802

Gastritis
  basic information about, 193
  diagnosis of, 193
  in differential diagnosis of peptic ulcer disease, 354
  in differential diagnosis of pernicious anemia, 33
  hypertrophic, in differential diagnosis of gastric cancer, 192
  treatment of, 193
Gastrocnemius muscle rupture in differential diagnosis of Achilles tendon rupture, 11
Gastroenteritis
  in differential diagnosis of cholera, 118
  in differential diagnosis of ectopic pregnancy, 164
  in differential diagnosis of fatty liver of pregnancy, 181
  in differential diagnosis of malaria, 287
  in differential diagnosis of motion sickness, 305
  in differential diagnosis of preeclampsia, 384
  in differential diagnosis of salmonellosis, 425
  in differential diagnosis of trichinosis, 491
  E. coli, in differential diagnosis of thrombotic thrombocytopenic purpura, 474
  eosinophilic, in differential diagnosis of celiac disease, 98
  viral, in differential diagnosis of bacterial food poisoning, 189
Gastroesophageal reflux disorder
  basic information about, 194
  diagnosis of, 194
  in differential diagnosis of cholelithiasis, 117
  in differential diagnosis of gastric cancer, 192
  in differential diagnosis of gastritis, 193
  in differential diagnosis of peptic ulcer disease, 354
  in differential diagnosis of sleep apnea, 443
  as factor in asthma, 936
  treatment of, 194
Gastrointestinal bleeding, 688
  causes by location, 555
  diagnostic considerations by age, 556t
Gastrointestinal disorders
  in differential diagnosis of angina pectoris, 37
  in differential diagnosis of anorexia nervosa, 43
  in differential diagnosis of bulimia nervosa, 84
  in differential diagnosis of costochondritis, 138
  in differential diagnosis of dysfunctional uterine bleeding, 159
  in differential diagnosis of pericarditis, 356
  in differential diagnosis of pseudomembranous gout, 395
  in differential diagnosis of pulmonary embolism, 399
Gastrointestinal procedures
  endocarditis prophylaxis and, 1023
  prophylactic regimens for, 1024t
Gastroparesis in differential diagnosis of gastritis, 193
Gaucher's disease in differential diagnosis of osteomyelitis, 332
Gay bowel syndrome
  clinical features, diagnosis, and treatment, 582t

Gay bowel syndrome—cont'd
  in differential diagnosis of Crohn's disease, 140
  in differential diagnosis of ulcerative colitis, 505
GBS; see Guillain-Barré syndrome
GC; see Gonorrhea
Gemfibrozil, preparations, dosage, mechanism of action, effect, cost, 993t
Generalized anxiety disorder; see Anxiety; Anxiety disorders
Geniculate herpes; see Ramsay Hunt syndrome
Genital herpes; see Herpes simplex infection
Genital herpes simplex infection; see Herpes simplex infection
Genital infections; see *Chlamydia* genital infection; other specific STDs
Genital lesions, differential diagnosis of, 583t
Genital prolapse; see Uterine prolapse
Genital tract, malignancy of, in differential diagnosis of endometrial cancer, 169
Genital ulcers, management of, 713
Genital warts; see Condyloma acuminatum
Genitourinary procedures
  endocarditis prophylaxis and, 1023
  prophylactic regimens for, 1024t
Genora, estrogen and progestin content of, 986t
Gentamicin
  dosage for, and dialysis removal, 971t
  drug monitoring data for, 799t
GERD; see Gastroesophageal reflux disorder
Geriatric abuse
  basic information about, 9
  diagnosis of, 9
  treatment of, 9
Geriatric Depression Scale, 1034
Geriatrics, year book of, 915-924
Germ cell tumor; see Ovarian cancer
Gerontology, year book of, 915-924
Gerstmann-Sträussler syndrome; see Creutzfeldt-Jakob disease
Gestational diabetes mellitus
  long-term effect of, 943
  screening recommendations for, 860
Giant cell arteritis, 465
Giardiasis
  basic information about, 195
  diagnosis of, 195
  treatment of, 195
Gilbert's disease
  basic information about, 196
  diagnosis of, 196
  liver function tests in, 618t
  treatment of, 196
Gilles de la Tourette syndrome; see Tourette's syndrome
Gingival hyperplasia in differential diagnosis of gingivitis, 197
Gingivitis
  basic information about, 197
  diagnosis of, 197
  treatment of, 197
Glands, epithelial abnormalities of, in differential diagnosis of cervical dysplasia, 104
Glasgow Coma Scale, 715t
Glaucoma
  acute angle, in differential diagnosis of corneal abrasion, 136
  chronic open-angle
    basic information about, 198
    diagnosis of, 198
    treatment of, 198

Index

Glaucoma—cont'd
  in differential diagnosis of amaurosis fugax, 21
  in differential diagnosis of conjunctivitis, 132
  in differential diagnosis of episcleritis, 177
  in differential diagnosis of ocular foreign body, 326
  in differential diagnosis of red eye, 640t
  in differential diagnosis of retinoblastoma, 415
  in differential diagnosis of uveitis, 516
  open-angle, in differential diagnosis of primary closed-angle glaucoma, 199
  persons at risk for, 869
  primary closed-angle
    basic information about, 199
    diagnosis of, 199
    treatment of, 199
  screening recommendations for, 869
  secondary, in differential diagnosis of chronic open-angle glaucoma, 198
Glimepiride
  preparations, dosage, duration of action, excretion, cost, 977t
Glipizide, preparations, dosage, duration of action, half-life, excretion, cost, class, 975t
Glomerular basement membrane antibody, laboratory values, 803
Glomerular disease, differential diagnosis of, 714
Glomerulonephritis
  acute
    basic information about, 200
    diagnosis of, 200-201
    treatment of, 201
  blood pressure and diastolic left ventricular malfunction in, 944-945
  in differential diagnosis of infective endocarditis, 168
  in differential diagnosis of preeclampsia, 384
  in differential diagnosis of pyelonephritis, 401
  in differential diagnosis of trichinosis, 491
  idiopathic rapidly progressive, in differential diagnosis of Goodpasture's syndrome, 204
Glossitis
  basic information about, 202
  diagnosis of, 202
  treatment of, 202
Glucophage; see Metformin
Glucose
  fasting, laboratory values, 803
  postprandial, laboratory values, 803
Glucose tolerance test, laboratory values, 803
Glucose-6-phosphate dehydrogenase screen, laboratory values, 803
Glucotrol; see Glipizide
γ-Glutamyl transferase
  elevated, etiologies for, 804
  laboratory values, 803-804
Gluten enteropathy; see Celiac sprue
Glyburide, preparations, dosage, duration of action, half-life, excretion, cost, class, 975t
Glycated (glycosylated) hemoglobin, laboratory values, 804
Glycemic control
  and development of microalbuminuria in NIDDM, 941-942
  in obese diabetic patients with preclinical Cushing's syndrome, 940-941
Glycemic index, 150
Glynase Prestab; see Glyburide

Gnathostoma spinigerum in tissue infections, epidemiology, transmission, manifestations, diagnosis, treatment, 629t
Goiter
  causes of, 584
  multinodular
    in differential diagnosis of thyroid carcinoma, 475
    in differential diagnosis of thyroid nodule, 476
Gold poisoning, antidotes for, dosage and indications, 1055t
Golfer's elbow; see Epicondylitis
Gonadal failure, gynecomastia associated with, 587
Gonococcal infection
  complement deficiencies associated with, 794t
  disseminated, history, rash characteristics and distribution, clinical findings, diagnostic aids, 577t
  knee pain due to, findings, diagnosis, and management, 611t
Gonococcal ophthalmia neonatorum, prevention of, 864
Gonorrhea
  anorectal, clinical features, diagnosis, and treatment, 582t
  basic information about, 203
  diagnosis of, 203
  in differential diagnosis of chlamydia genital infections, 114
  in differential diagnosis of prepubescent vulvovaginitis, 527
  reducing risk of, 887
  screening recommendations for, 864-865
  treatment of, 203
    after sexual assault, 1056t
Goodpasture's syndrome
  basic information about, 204
  diagnosis of, 204
  in differential diagnosis of Wegener's granulomatosis, 531
  treatment of, 204
Gout
  basic information about, 205
  diagnosis of, 205
  in differential diagnosis of cellulitis, 99
  in differential diagnosis of osteomyelitis, 332
  knee pain due to, findings, diagnosis, and management, 610t
  treatment of, 205
Gouty arthritis
  characteristics of, 550t
  in differential diagnosis of pseudogout, 394
  in differential diagnosis of psoriatic arthritis, 52
Gowers' disease; see Muscular dystrophy
Grand mal seizure; see Seizure disorder, generalized tonic-clonic
Granisetron, preparations, dosage, class, 976t
Granulation tissue in differential diagnosis of Kaposi's sarcoma, 260
Granulocytopenia in differential diagnosis of pharyngitis/tonsillitis, 362
Granuloma, midline, in differential diagnosis of Wegener's granulomatosis, 531
Granuloma annulare
  in differential diagnosis of erythema multiforme, 180
  in differential diagnosis of tinea corporis, 479

Granuloma inguinale
  basic information about, 206
  diagnosis of, 206
  in differential diagnosis of chancroid, 110
  treatment of, 206
Granulomas
  in differential diagnosis of cat-scratch disease, 95
  pulmonary nodules due to, 639t
Granulomatosis, Wegener's, in differential diagnosis of asthma, 56
Granulomatous arthritis, 49
Granulomatous disorders
  classification of, 584
  in differential diagnosis of coccidioidomycoses, 125
  in differential diagnosis of hyperparathyroidism, 244
  in differential diagnosis of lung neoplasm, 277
Granulomatous lung disease
  differential diagnosis of, 585t-586t
  in differential diagnosis of Wegener's granulomatosis, 531
Granulomatous thyroiditis; see Thyroiditis
Granulomatous uveitis; see Uveitis
Graves' disease
  basic information about, 207
  diagnosis of, 207
  in differential diagnosis of thyroiditis, 477
  treatment of, 207
Groin pain, differential diagnosis of, 587
Gross stress reaction; see Posttraumatic stress disorder
Growth and development, developmental milestones in, 1038t-1039t
Growth hormone-releasing hormone, ectopic production of, in differential diagnosis of acromegaly, 14
Growth hormone-secreting pituitary adenoma, 366
Guanabenz, preparations, dosage, cost, 969t
Guanadrel, preparations, dosage, cost, 969t
Guanethidine, preparations, dosage, cost, 969t
Guanfacine, preparations, dosage, cost, 969t
Guillain-Barré syndrome
  basic information about, 208
  CSF abnormalities in, 559t, 791t
  diagnosis of, 208
  in differential diagnosis of Bell's palsy, 68
  in differential diagnosis of botulism, 75
  in differential diagnosis of poliomyelitis, 378
  in differential diagnosis of rabies, 402
  treatment of, 208
Guinea worm in tissue infections, epidemiology, transmission, manifestations, diagnosis, treatment, 629t
Gynecologic cancer; see also specific types
  counseling about, 887-888
Gynecology, year book of, 900
Gynecomastia, differential diagnosis of, 587

H

H_2 blockers, preparations, dosage, cost, 968t
Haemophilus influenzae type b disease, chemoprophylaxis of, 893
Haemophilus influenzae type b vaccine
  for children, recommendations for, 889, 1005t
  schedule, indications, side effects, contraindications, during pregnancy, with HIV infection, in immunocompromised patient, 1008t-1009t

Index 1093

Haemophilus influenzae vaccine for patients with absent or dysfunctional spleen, 928
Haemophilus vaginalis vaginitis; *see* Vaginosis, bacterial
Haemophilus vaginosis; *see* Vulvovaginitis, bacterial
Hair loss; *see* Alopecia
Hairy cell leukemia
 basic information about, 274
 diagnosis of, 274
 in differential diagnosis of aplastic anemia, 30
 in differential diagnosis of chronic lymphocytic leukemia, 272
 lymphocyte abnormalities in, 620t
 treatment of, 274
Halcion; *see* Triazolam
Haldol; *see* Haloperidol
Halitosis, causes of, 588
Haloperidol, preparations, dosage, class, adverse effects, 978t
HAM test, laboratory values, 804
Hamartoma in differential diagnosis of breast cancer, 78
Hamilton Anxiety Scale, 1032
Hand-foot-mouth disease in differential diagnosis of herpangina, 224
Haptoglobin, laboratory values, 804
Harstad Injury Prevention Study, 915
Hashimoto's thyroiditis; *see* Thyroiditis
Hay fever; *see* Rhinitis, allergic
HCO₃, average values for arterial and venous plasma or serum, 781t
HDV infection, diagnosis of, 813
Head injury, management of, 715
Head trauma
 in differential diagnosis of Bell's palsy, 68
 in differential diagnosis of eclampsia, 163
 in differential diagnosis of heat exhaustion/heat stroke, 214
 in differential diagnosis of Tourette's syndrome, 483
Headache
 classification of, 589
 cluster
  basic information about, 209
  diagnosis of, 209
  treatment of, 209
 differential diagnosis of, 588t
 migraine; *see* Migraine
 tension-type
  basic information about, 211
  diagnosis of, 211
  treatment of, 211
Health examination; *see* Periodic health examination
Hearing, screening in ambulatory elderly, 920t
Hearing disorders, 869-870
Hearing impairment
 risk factors for, 870
 screening recommendations for, 869-870
Hearing loss
 causes of, 590
 in differential diagnosis of otosclerosis, 339
 evaluation of, 716-717
 screening geriatric patients with, 1027
Hearing test, in-office, 1027t
Heart attack; *see* Myocardial infarction
Heart block
 complete
  diagnosis of, 212
  information about, 212
  treatment of, 212

Heart block—cont'd
 second-degree
  basic information about, 213
  diagnosis of, 213
  treatment of, 213
Heart failure; *see* Congestive heart failure
Heart murmurs; *see* Cardiac murmurs
Heartburn, treatment of, 718
Heat exhaustion/heat stroke
 basic information about, 214
 diagnosis of, 214
 in differential diagnosis of neuroleptic malignant syndrome, 321
 sports participation and, 1036t
 treatment of, 214
Heat illness; *see* Heat exhaustion/heat stroke
Heavy metal neuropathy in differential diagnosis of Guillain-Barré syndrome, 208
Height-weight correlations, 1048t
Helicobacter pylori gastritis; *see* Gastritis
Helicobacter pylori infection in differential diagnosis of pernicious anemia, 33
HELLP syndrome
 in differential diagnosis of fatty liver of pregnancy, 181
 in pregnancy, characteristics of, 617t
Helminths
 eosinophilia due to, 573
 intestinal, transmission, clinical findings, diagnosis, treatment, 607t-608t
Hemachromatosis in differential diagnosis of Sheehan's syndrome, 437
Hemangioma
 capillary, in differential diagnosis of Kaposi's sarcoma, 260
 in differential diagnosis of congenital anomalies presenting as neck masses, 628t
 vertebral, in differential diagnosis of Paget's disease of bone, 342
Hematocrit
 high, evaluation of, 747
 laboratory values, 805
 low, evaluation of patient with, 674
 during pregnancy, 861
Hematologic values, normal, by age group, 796t
Hematoma
 in differential diagnosis of deep vein thrombosis, 473
 in differential diagnosis of Kaposi's sarcoma, 260
 in differential diagnosis of pelvic abscess, 4
 subdural, in differential diagnosis of hepatic encephalopathy, 218
Hematopoietic malignancy, chromosome abnormalities in, 792t
Hematuria
 causes of, 590
 evaluation of, 719
 TICS in diagnosis of, 590
Hemiballismus, manifestations, differential diagnosis, tests, treatment, 596t
Hemidiaphragm, elevated, causes of, 572
Hemiparesis, causes of, 590
Hemiplegia, causes of, 590
Hemochromatosis
 basic information about, 215
 diagnosis of, 215
 in differential diagnosis of Addison's disease, 15
 treatment of, 215
Hemoglobin
 analysis in pregnant women, 861
 laboratory values, 805

Hemoglobin electrophoresis, laboratory values, 805
Hemoglobin S disease; *see* Anemia, sickle cell
Hemoglobinopathies
 in differential diagnosis of hemolytic transfusion reaction, 489
 in differential diagnosis of polycythemia vera, 380
 screening newborn for, 873-874
Hemoglobinuria, paroxysmal nocturnal, in differential diagnosis of myelodysplastic syndromes, 313
Hemolysis, liver function tests in, 618t
Hemolytic anemia in differential diagnosis of Gilbert's disease, 196
Hemolytic leukemia, autoimmune, in differential diagnosis of aplastic anemia, 31
Hemolytic-uremic syndrome
 in differential diagnosis of acute glomerulonephritis, 200
 in differential diagnosis of disseminated intravascular coagulation, 155
 in differential diagnosis of fatty liver of pregnancy, 181
 in differential diagnosis of idiopathic thrombocytopenic purpura, 252
 in differential diagnosis of preeclampsia, 384
 in differential diagnosis of thrombotic thrombocytopenic purpura, 474
 in differential diagnosis of toxic shock syndrome, 484
Hemophilia
 basic information about, 216
 diagnosis of, 216
 inheritance, incidence, bleeding symptoms, test results, treatment, 561t-562t
 treatment of, 216
Hemoptysis, causes of, 591
Hemorrhage; *see also* Bleeding
 cerebral, CSF abnormalities in, 791t
 CSF abnormalities in, 559t
 in differential diagnosis of retinal detachment, 412
 intraparenchymal, in differential diagnosis of subarachnoid hemorrhage, 454
 during pregnancy; *see* Pregnancy, vaginal bleeding during
 retinal, 413
 subarachnoid
  basic information about, 454
  diagnosis of, 454
  treatment of, 454
 subconjunctival, in differential diagnosis of episcleritis, 177
 subarachnoid, in differential diagnosis of migraine, 210
Hemorrhagic fever
 in differential diagnosis of Stevens-Johnson syndrome, 452
 in differential diagnosis of yellow fever, 533
Hemorrhagic gastritis; *see* Gastritis
Hemorrhoids
 basic information about, 217
 diagnosis of, 217
 treatment of, 217
Hemosiderosis in differential diagnosis of sarcoidosis, 426
Henoch-Schönlein purpura, arthritis due to, course and distribution, 551t
Heparin for unstable angina, 38
Hepatic abscess in differential diagnosis of cholecystitis, 116

Hepatic coma; see Hepatic encephalopathy
Hepatic encephalopathy
  basic information about, 218
  diagnosis of, 218
  treatment of, 218
Hepatic failure in differential diagnosis of septicemia, 436
Hepatic necrosis in differential diagnosis of disseminated intravascular coagulation, 155
Hepatic nephropathy; see Hepatorenal syndrome
Hepatitis
  alcoholic, liver function tests in, 618t
  delta, 812
  in differential diagnosis of acetaminophen poisoning, 10
  in differential diagnosis of cholangitis, 115
  in differential diagnosis of cholecystitis, 116
  in differential diagnosis of chronic fatigue syndrome, 119
  in differential diagnosis of fatty liver of pregnancy, 181
  in differential diagnosis of hyperemesis gravidarum, 241
  in differential diagnosis of malaria, 287
  in differential diagnosis of pericarditis, 356
  in differential diagnosis of psittacosis, 396
  nonviral
    in differential diagnosis of hepatitis B, 220
    in differential diagnosis of hepatitis C, 222
  in pregnancy, characteristics of, 617t
  summary of test applications, 808
  viral
    in differential diagnosis of babesiosis, 64
    in differential diagnosis of human granulocytic ehrlichiosis, 237
    in differential diagnosis of leptospirosis, 169
    in differential diagnosis of yellow fever, 533
Hepatitis A
  basic information about, 219
  chemoprophylaxis of, 893
  diagnosis of, 219
  treatment of, 219
Hepatitis A antibody, laboratory values, 806
Hepatitis A inactivated virus, schedule, indications, side effects, contraindications, during pregnancy, with HIV infection, in immunocompromised patient, 1010t-1011t
Hepatitis A vaccine
  administration of, 1018t
  for international travel, 1019t
  during pregnancy, 1016t
  recommendations for
    for adults, 892
    for children, 890
Hepatitis A virus
  antibodies to, laboratory evaluation, 806
  antigen, laboratory evaluation, 806
  diagnosis of, 806
  serologic tests for, 807
Hepatitis B
  arthritis due to, course and distribution, 551t
  basic information about, 220
  chemoprophylaxis of, 893
  diagnosis of, 220-221
  screening recommendations for, 863
  serologic tests, 807

Hepatitis B—cont'd
  surface antigen and antibody, 807
  treatment of, 221
  after sexual assault, 1056t
Hepatitis B surface antigen
  by immunoassay, 807
  laboratory values, 806
Hepatitis B vaccine
  administration of, 1018t
  for adults, schedule, indications, side effects, contraindications, during pregnancy, with HIV infection, in immunocompromised patient, 1006t
  after exposure to blood, 1020t
  for international travel, 1019t
  during pregnancy, 1013t, 1015t
  for preventing perinatal transmission, 1021t
  recommendations for
    for adults, 892
    for children, 889
  recommended dosages, 1020t
  schedule for children, 1005t
Hepatitis B virus
  antibodies, 809
  surface antigen-antibody and core antibodies, 810
Hepatitis B$_c$Ab, total, laboratory findings, 808
Hepatitis B$_c$Ab-IgM, laboratory findings, 808
Hepatitis B$_e$
  antigen and antibody, 811
  antigen and antibody summary, 809
Hepatitis B$_e$Ab
  laboratory findings, 809
  total, laboratory findings, 809
Hepatitis C
  alcohol-induced liver disease and, 926
  basic information about, 222
  diagnosis of, 222
  treatment of, 222
Hepatitis C virus, antigen and antibody, 811, 812
Hepatitis C virus-Ab, second generation ELISA detection, 811
Hepatitis C virus-Ag, nucleic acid probe detection, 811
Hepatitis E in differential diagnosis of hepatitis A, 219
Hepatitis viruses
  in differential diagnosis of hepatitis A, 219
  in differential diagnosis of hepatitis C, 222
Hepatobiliary disease, evaluation of, 731
Hepatocellular necrosis, liver function tests in, 618t
Hepatomegaly, causes of, 591
Hepatorenal syndrome
  basic information about, 223
  diagnosis of, 223
  treatment of, 223
Hereditary cataract, 94
Hereditary motor and sensory neuropathy, 112
Hernia
  in differential diagnosis of acute appendicitis, 48
  in differential diagnosis of endometriosis, 170
  groin pain related to, 587
Herniated disk, differential diagnosis of, 553t
Heroin overdose in differential diagnosis of congestive heart failure, 130
Herpangina
  basic information about, 224
  diagnosis of, 224

Herpangina—cont'd
  in differential diagnosis of herpes simplex infection, 225
Herpes digitalis; see Herpes simplex infection
Herpes gestationis
  differential diagnosis of, 557t
  in differential diagnosis of urticaria, 512
Herpes gladiatorum; see Herpes simplex infection
Herpes iris; see Stevens-Johnson syndrome
Herpes labialis; see Herpes simplex infection
Herpes simplex blepharitis in differential diagnosis of blepharitis, 73
Herpes simplex infection, 225-226
  basic information about, 225
  clinical features, diagnosis, and treatment, 582t
  diagnosis of, 225-226
  in differential diagnosis of chancroid, 110
  in differential diagnosis of corneal ulceration, 137
  in differential diagnosis of gonococcal urethritis, 506
  in differential diagnosis of herpangina, 224
  in differential diagnosis of herpes zoster, 228
  in differential diagnosis of hordeolum, 236
  in differential diagnosis of impetigo, 253
  in differential diagnosis of nongonococcal urethritis, 507
  in differential diagnosis of Ramsay Hunt syndrome, 403
  in elderly, in differential diagnosis of tracheitis, 488
  genital
    basic information about, 227
    diagnosis of, 227
    management of, 713
    preventing cesarean delivery and, 956
    screening recommendations for, 867
    treatment of, 227
  treatment of, 226
Herpes ulcers
  in differential diagnosis of corneal abrasion, 136
  in differential diagnosis of ocular foreign body, 326
Herpes zoster infection
  basic information about, 228
  diagnosis of, 228
  in differential diagnosis of angina pectoris, 37
  in differential diagnosis of herpes simplex infection, 225
  history, manifestations, and malignancy associated with, 564t
  treatment of, 228
Herpes zoster oticus, 403
Herpetic geniculate ganglionitis, 403
Herpetic neuralgia, treatment of, 720
Heterophil antibody, laboratory findings, 813
Hexachlorophene, antimicrobial activity, mechanics of action, toxicity, indications and contraindications, 979t
Hexamethylmelamine, toxicity of, 984t-985t
Hexosaminidase deficiency in differential diagnosis of amyotrophic lateral sclerosis, 25
Hib conjugate vaccine, recommendations for, for children, 889
Hidradenitis suppurativa
  in differential diagnosis of anorectal fistula, 42

Hidradenitis suppurativa—cont'd
 in differential diagnosis of pilonidal
  disease, 365
High altitude retinopathy; see Retinal
  hemorrhage
High blood pressure; see Hypertension
High-density lipoprotein(s), laboratory
  findings, 813
High-risk populations, 843t-844t
 ages 25-64 years, interventions for,
  847t-848t
 gonorrhea screening in, 865
 periodic health examination of, for
  pregnant women, 851t-852t
 potential interventions for, ages 11-24
  years, 845t
 sudden cardiac death in, 912t
 syphilis screening for, 864
Hip, arthritis of, in differential diagnosis of
  lumbar disc syndromes, 276
Hip pain
 causes of, 592
 referred, in differential diagnosis of
  Osgood-Schlatter disease, 329
Hirschsprung's disease in differential
  diagnosis of encopresis, 167
Hirsutism
 differential diagnosis of, 592
 evaluation and treatment of, 721
Hismanal; see Astemizole
Histaminic cephalgia; see Headache, cluster
Histoplasma capsulatum in differential
  diagnosis of coccidioidomycoses, 125
Histoplasmosis, 229-231
 acute pulmonary, in differential diagnosis
  of histoplasmosis, 230
 basic information about, 229-230
 diagnosis of, 230-231
 in differential diagnosis of macular
  degeneration, 285
 in differential diagnosis of *Pneumocystis
  carinii* pneumonia, 374
 in differential diagnosis of pulmonary
  tuberculosis, 498
 in differential diagnosis of tularemia, 501
 treatment of, 231
Hives; see Urticaria
Hivid; see Zalcitabine
HLA antigens
 diseases associated with, 814t
 testing sequence, 814
Hoarseness, causes of, 593
Hodgkin's disease, 233-234
 basic information about, 233
 diagnosis of, 233-234
 in differential diagnosis of non-Hodgkin's
  lymphoma, 284
 in differential diagnosis of sarcoidosis,
  426
 treatment of, 234
Home care, community resources for,
  1060-1061
Home uterine activity monitoring,
  screening recommendations for,
  871-872
Hookworm
 basic information about, 235
 diagnosis of, 235
 treatment of, 235
Hordeolum
 basic information about, 236
 diagnosis of, 236
 treatment of, 236
Hormone therapy; see also Estrogen
  replacement therapy
 alternatives to, 895
 postmenopausal, 894-895
Horton's headache, 209

Hospital addiction syndrome; see
  Munchausen's syndrome
Hospital-acquired infections; see
  Nosocomial infections
Housemaid's knee; see Bursitis
HRS; see Hepatorenal syndrome
HUAM; see Home uterine activity
  monitoring
Human granulocytic ehrlichiosis
 basic information about, 237
 diagnosis of, 237
 treatment of, 237
Human immunodeficiency virus
 acute retroviral syndrome of, in
  differential diagnosis of
  mononucleosis, 304
 antibody to, laboratory findings, 813
 chemoprophylaxis of, after occupational
  exposure, 1021t
Human immunodeficiency virus 1, tests of,
  814
Human immunodeficiency virus infection
 ages 11-24 years, 845t-846t
 basic information about, 232
 chronic diarrhea in patients with, 709
 counseling to prevent, 886
 diagnosis of, 232
 in differential diagnosis of chronic fatigue
  syndrome, 119
 in differential diagnosis of Epstein-Barr
  virus infections, 178
 in differential diagnosis of Sheehan's
  syndrome, 437
 pathogens associated with, 709t
 screening recommendations for, 865-866
 sports participation and, 1036t
 tetanus/diphtheria vaccine and, 1007t
 treatment of, 232
 vertically infected fetuses showing HIV-
  antibody-negative, 952, 953t
Human monocytic ehrlichiosis in
  differential diagnosis of human
  granulocytic ehrlichiosis, 237
Human papilloma virus infection, screening
  for, 857
Huntington's chorea
 basic information about, 238
 diagnosis of, 238
 treatment of, 238
Huntington's disease; see Huntington's
  chorea
Hydatid disease; see also Echinococcosis
 epidemiology, transmission, clinical
  presentation, diagnosis, and
  treatment, 559t
Hydatidiform molar gestation in differential
  diagnosis of spontaneous miscarriage,
  446
Hydradenitis in differential diagnosis of
  breast abscess, 77
Hydrocephalus
 dementia associated with, laboratory
  diagnosis of, 567t
 normal pressure
  basic information about, 239
  diagnosis of, 239
  treatment of, 239
Hydrocortisone
 brand names and potency, 999t
 comparison chart for, 987t
Hydrogen peroxide, antimicrobial activity,
  mechanics of action, toxicity,
  indications and contraindications,
  979t
Hydromorphone, equivalent dose, duration,
  preparations, dosage, 995t
Hydronephrosis in differential diagnosis of
  pyelonephritis, 401

Hydrophobia; see Rabies
Hydroxyapatite arthropathy, characteristics
  of, 550t
5-Hydroxyindole-acetic acid, urine; see
  Urine 5-hydroxyindole-acetic acid
Hydroxyurea, toxicity of, 984t-985t
Hydroxyzine, preparations, dosage, class,
  976t
Hylorel; see Guanadrel
Hymen, imperforate, in differential
  diagnosis of dysmenorrhea, 161
Hyperactivity; see Attention deficit
  hyperactivity disorder
Hyperaldosteronism; see also Aldosteronism,
  primary
 basic information about, 249
 diagnosis of, 249
 treatment of, 249
Hyperbilirubinemia, unconjugated,
  conditions associated with, 788
Hypercalcemia
 causes of, 244
 in differential diagnosis of hepatic
  encephalopathy, 218
 etiologies of, 788
 evaluation of, 722
 laboratory differential diagnosis of,
  593t
 treatment of, 722
Hypercapnia, persistent, causes of, 594
Hypercholesteremia; see
  Hypercholesterolemia
Hypercholesterinemia; see
  Hypercholesterolemia
Hypercholesterolemia
 basic information about, 240
 diagnosis of, 240
 treatment of, 240
Hypercoagulable states, causes of, 594
Hyperemesis gravidarum
 basic information about, 241
 diagnosis of, 241
 in pregnancy, characteristics of, 617t
 treatment of, 241
Hyperglycemia
 corrected sodium in patients with,
  formula for, 1042
 stress, in differential diagnosis of diabetes
  mellitus, 149
Hyperinsulinism, differential diagnosis of,
  595t
Hyperkalemia, causes of, 822, 1146
Hyperkeratosis in differential diagnosis of
  cervical dysplasia, 104
Hyperkeratosis paraneoplastica, history,
  manifestations, and malignancy
  associated with, 564t
Hyperkinetic movement disorders,
  manifestations, differential diagnosis,
  tests, treatment, 596t-597t
Hyperlipidemia; see Hyperlipoproteinemia
Hyperlipoproteinemia
 primary
  basic information about, 242
  diagnosis of, 242
  treatment of, 242
 type II familial; see Hypercholesterolemia
Hypermagnesemia, causes of, 598
Hypernatremia
 causes of, 828
 evaluation and treatment of, 723
 water deficit in patients with, formula for,
  1042
Hyperosmolar coma
 basic information about, 243
 diagnosis of, 243
 treatment of, 243

Hyperosmolar nonketotic state; see also
     Hyperosmolar coma
  in differential diagnosis of diabetic
     ketoacidosis, 151
Hyperparathyroidism
  basic information about, 244
  diagnosis of, 244
  in differential diagnosis of
     agoraphobia/panic, 16
  in differential diagnosis of osteoporosis,
     333
  in differential diagnosis of Paget's disease
     of bone, 342
  in differential diagnosis of rickets, 421
  laboratory findings for calcium and
     phosphorus, 789t
  treatment of, 244
Hyperpigmentation, postinflammatory, in
     differential diagnosis of Kaposi's
     sarcoma, 260
Hyperplasia, atypical, in differential
     diagnosis of endometrial cancer, 169
Hypersensitivity angiitis, neuropathies
     associated with, 631t
Hypersensitivity pneumonitis
  in differential diagnosis of asthma, 56
  in differential diagnosis of bacterial
     pneumonia, 370
Hypersomnia, evaluation of, 758
Hypersplenism
  in differential diagnosis of aplastic
     anemia, 30
  in differential diagnosis of idiopathic
     thrombocytopenic purpura, 252
Hypertension, 245-246
  basic information about, 245
  diagnosis of, 245, 854
  in differential diagnosis of acute
     glomerulonephritis, 200
  in differential diagnosis of macular
     degeneration, 285
  in differential diagnosis of
     pheochromocytoma, 363
  end-stage renal disease and, 939-940
  in glomerulonephritis, 944-945
  "high-renin" essential, renin-aldosterone
     patterns in, 826t
  idiopathic intracranial, in differential
     diagnosis of tension-type headache,
     211
  intervention for, 854
  "low-renin" essential, renin-aldosterone
     patterns in, 826t
  malignant
     in differential diagnosis of nephrotic
       syndrome, 319
     in differential diagnosis of thrombotic
       thrombocytopenic purpura, 474
     renin-aldosterone patterns in, 826t
  pregnancy-induced; see also Preeclampsia
     calcium supplementation and, 949-950
  pulmonary, in differential diagnosis of
     atrial septal defect, 61
  renovascular, in differential diagnosis of
     primary aldosteronism, 19
  screening for, 854-855
  sports participation and, 1035t
  stable, factors associated with
     development of, in young borderline
     hypertensives, 901
  treatment of, 245-246
Hypertensive emergencies
  recommended treatment of, 903
  sublingual nifedipine for, 903
Hyperthermia; see also Heat exhaustion/heat
     stroke
  malignant; see also Neuroleptic malignant
     syndrome

Hyperthermia—cont'd
  malignant—cont'd
     in differential diagnosis of heat
       exhaustion/heat stroke, 214
Hyperthyroidism, 247-248
  apathetic, in differential diagnosis of
     Addison's disease, 15
  basic information about, 247
  diagnosis of, 247
  in differential diagnosis of
     agoraphobia/panic, 16
  in differential diagnosis of Graves'
     disease, 207
  in differential diagnosis of rickets, 421
  factitious, in differential diagnosis of
     thyroiditis, 477
  laboratory findings for calcium and
     phosphorus, 789t
  thyroid function test results in, 829t
  treatment of, 247-248
Hypertrichosis, differential diagnosis of, 592
Hypertrichosis lanuginosa, history,
     manifestations, and malignancy
     associated with, 564t
Hypertrophic cardiomyopathy
  in differential diagnosis of aortic stenosis,
     47
  in differential diagnosis of mitral
     regurgitation, 300
Hypertrophic gastritis in differential
     diagnosis of gastric cancer, 192
Hypertrophic obstructive cardiomyopathy;
     see Cardiomyopathy, hypertrophic
Hypertrophic pulmonary osteoarthropathy,
     course and distribution, 551t
Hyperventilation, persistent, causes of, 598
Hypocalcemia
  in differential diagnosis of tetanus, 466
  etiologies of, 789
  evaluation of, 724
  laboratory differential diagnosis of, 599t
Hypochondriasis
  in differential diagnosis of Munchausen's
     syndrome, 210
  in differential diagnosis of obsessive-
     compulsive disorder, 325
Hypoglycemia
  in differential diagnosis of epilepsy, 572t
  in differential diagnosis of hepatic
     encephalopathy, 218
  in differential diagnosis of hypothermia,
     250
  in differential diagnosis of myxedema
     coma, 317
  in differential diagnosis of transient
     ischemic attack, 490
  fasting, diagnosis of, 725
Hypoglycemia syndromes, test results for,
     600t
Hypogonadism
  causes of, 601
  hypergonadotropic, micropenis due to,
     622
Hypokalemia
  causes of, 602, 822
  diagnosis of, 726
  in differential diagnosis of primary
     aldosteronism, 19
  renin-aldosterone patterns in, 826t
Hyponatremia
  causes of, 828
  evaluation and treatment of, 727
  factitious, in differential diagnosis of
     inappropriate secretion of
     antidiuretic hormone, 254
  with hypervolemia, in differential
     diagnosis of inappropriate secretion
     of antidiuretic hormone, 254

Hypoparathyroidism
  in differential diagnosis of hypocalcemia,
     599t
  laboratory findings for calcium and
     phosphorus, 789t
Hypophosphatemia, diagnosis of, 728
Hypoplastic anemia; see Anemia, aplastic
Hypoplastic myelodysplastic syndrome in
     differential diagnosis of aplastic
     anemia, 30
Hypothalamic amenorrhea in differential
     diagnosis of amenorrhea, 545t
Hypothalamic dysfunction in differential
     diagnosis of menopause, 297
Hypothermia
  basic information about, 250
  diagnosis of, 250
  in differential diagnosis of septicemia,
     436
  treatment of, 250
Hypothyroidism
  basic information about, 251
  congenital, screening recommendations
     for, 874
  diagnosis of, 251
  in differential diagnosis of allergic
     rhinitis, 420
  in differential diagnosis of chronic
     obstructive pulmonary disease, 120
  in differential diagnosis of encopresis, 167
  in differential diagnosis of idiopathic
     thrombocytopenic purpura, 252
  in differential diagnosis of major
     depression, 145
  in differential diagnosis of menopause,
     297
  in differential diagnosis of narcolepsy, 318
  neuropathies associated with, 631t
  thyroid function test results in, 829t
  treatment of, 251
Hypovolemia in differential diagnosis of
     inappropriate secretion of
     antidiuretic hormone, 254
Hypovolemic shock in differential diagnosis
     of Addison's disease, 15
Hypoxemia in differential diagnosis of
     polycythemia vera, 380
Hysteria; see also Conversion disorder
  in differential diagnosis of rabies, 402
  in differential diagnosis of tetanus, 466
Hysterical conversion; see Conversion
     disorder
Hysterical paralysis in differential diagnosis
     of Guillain-Barré syndrome, 208
Hytone; see Hydrocortisone
Hytrin; see Terazosin

I

IBD; see Inflammatory bowel disease
IBS; see Irritable bowel syndrome
Ibuprofen, preparations, dosage, half-life,
     class, cost, metabolism, 997t
IDDM; see Diabetes mellitus
Idiopathic facial paralysis; see Bell's palsy
Idiopathic flushing in differential diagnosis
     of carcinoid syndrome, 87
Idiopathic hypertension; see Hypertension
Idiopathic hypertrophic subaortic stenosis;
     see Cardiomyopathy, hypertrophic
Idiopathic rapidly progressive
     glomerulonephritis in differential
     diagnosis of Goodpasture's
     syndrome, 204
Idiopathic thrombocytopenic purpura
  basic information about, 252
  diagnosis of, 252
  treatment of, 252
Ifosfamide, toxicity of, 984t-985t

Index 1097

IgE-mediated rhinitis; *see* Rhinitis, allergic
Imbalance in differential diagnosis of dizziness, 569
Imipenem
 adverse effects of, 27
 dosage for, and dialysis removal, 971*t*
Imipramine
 drug monitoring data for, 799*t*
 preparations, dosage, class, effects, half-life, 974*t*
Immune complex assay, laboratory findings, 815
Immune deficiencies, replacement therapy for, administration of, 1018*t*
Immune globulin preparations, administration of, 1017*t*, 1018*t*
Immune thrombocytopenic purpura, 252
 treatment of, 1018*t*
Immunizations, 889-893; *see also* specific vaccines
 administration of, 1017*t*, 1018*t*
 for adults, 891-893
 in immunocompromised patient, 1006*t*
 schedule, indications, side effects, contraindications, during pregnancy, with HIV infection, 1006*t*
 age 11-24 years, 845*t*
 age 25-64 years, 847*t*-848*t*
 age 65 and older, 849*t*-850*t*
 anaphylaxis due to; *see* Anaphylaxis
 Bacille Calmette-Guérin, 863-864
 for children, 889-890
 for hepatitis B, 863
 for high-risk populations, 845*t*-846*t*
  age 65 and older, 849*t*-850*t*
 for international travel, 1019*t*
 interventions for, 843*t*
 in long-term care facilities, 921*t*, 921-922
 during pregnancy, 1012*t*-1016*t*
 rubella, 868-869
 schedule for children, 1005*t*
Immunocompromised host, 845*t*-846*t*; *see also* Acquired immunodeficiency syndrome; Human immunodeficiency virus infection
 aminoglycoside dosing in, 937
 infectious diseases in, 604*t*-605*t*
 tetanus/diphtheria vaccine and, 1007*t*
Immunodeficiency states
 in differential diagnosis of cystic fibrosis, 143
 eosinophilia due to, 573
Immunoglobulin G antiphospholipid antibodies, characteristics and causes, 594
Immunoglobulins, laboratory findings, 815
Immunologic disorders, granulomatous disorders due to, 584
Impetigo
 basic information about, 253
 diagnosis of, 253
 differential diagnosis of, 557*t*
 in differential diagnosis of chickenpox, 113
 in differential diagnosis of contact dermatitis, 147
 in differential diagnosis of herpes simplex infection, 225
 in differential diagnosis of Ramsay Hunt syndrome, 403
 treatment of, 253
Impetigo vulgaris; *see* Impetigo
Impingement syndrome, 423; *see also* Rotator cuff syndrome
Impotence; *see also* Erectile dysfunction
 causes of, 603
Incest in differential diagnosis of pedophilia, 351

Incontinence, 255-256
 basic information about, 255-256
 diagnosis of, 256
 fecal; *see* Encopresis
 treatment of, 256
 urinary; *see also* Enuresis
  pelvic floor muscle exercises and, 952, 954
  screening in ambulatory elderly, 920*t*
Indanyl-carbenicillin, dosage for, and dialysis removal, 972*t*
Inderal; *see* Propranolol
Indinavir, therapeutic class, preparations, dosage, toxicities, cost, 970*t*
Indocin; *see* Indomethacin
Indoline, class, preparations, dosage, site of action, cost, 978*t*
Indomethacin, preparations, dosage, half-life, class, cost, metabolism, 997*t*
Infant(s)
 extremely low-birth-weight, self-perceived health status of during adolescence, 913
 high-risk, screening for iron deficiency anemia, 861
Infantile paralysis; *see* Poliomyelitis
Infection(s)
 from bite wounds, 70
 cestode, epidemiology, transmission, clinical presentation, diagnosis, and treatment, 559*t*
 chronic, in differential diagnosis of Addison's disease, 15
 congenital, in differential diagnosis of toxoplasmosis, 486
 dementia associated with, laboratory diagnosis of, 567*t*
 in differential diagnosis of acute viral encephalitis, 166
 in differential diagnosis of anorexia nervosa, 43
 in differential diagnosis of Bell's palsy, 68
 in differential diagnosis of diverticular disease, 156
 in differential diagnosis of heat exhaustion/heat stroke, 214
 in differential diagnosis of ocular foreign body, 326
 in differential diagnosis of polyarteritis nodosa, 379
 eosinophilia due to, 573
 hospital-acquired; *see* Nosocomial infections
 intestinal, in differential diagnosis of amebiasis, 23
 knee pain due to, findings, diagnosis, and management, 611*t*
 prevention and treatment of, in patients with absent or dysfunctional spleen, 928-929
 primary, in differential diagnosis of temporal arteritis, 465
 trematode, epidemiology, transmission, manifestations, diagnosis, treatment, 660*t*
Infectious arthritis
 in differential diagnosis of gout, 205
 in differential diagnosis of osteoarthritis, 330
Infectious diseases; *see also* specific diseases
 immunizations against; *see also* Immunizations; specific vaccines
  in long-term care facilities, 921*t*, 921-922
 in immunocompromised hosts, 604*t*-605*t*
 postexposure prophylaxis for, 893-894
 screening recommendations for, 863-868
 in travelers, 605*t*

Infectious hepatitis; *see* Hepatitis A
Infectious keratitis; *see* Corneal ulceration
Infectious mononucleosis; *see* Epstein-Barr virus infection; Mononucleosis
Infertile male syndrome, phenotypes, karyotypes, inheritance, hormone levels, pathogenesis, 546*t*
Infertility; *see also* Insemination, therapeutic
 diagnosis of, 468
 endometriosis-associated, 171
 female, evaluation of, *730*
 male, evaluation of, *729*
Inflammatory bowel disease; *see also* Crohn's disease; Ulcerative colitis
 in differential diagnosis of celiac disease, 98
 in differential diagnosis of cholelithiasis, 117
 in differential diagnosis of colorectal cancer, 127
 in differential diagnosis of diverticular disease, 156
 in differential diagnosis of lactose intolerance, 264
 in differential diagnosis of pseudomembranous gout, 395
 in differential diagnosis of secondary peritonitis, 359
 in differential diagnosis of tropical sprue, 494
Influenza
 basic information about, 257
 chemoprophylaxis of, 894
 diagnosis of, 257
 in differential diagnosis of acute bronchitis, 82
 in differential diagnosis of human granulocytic ehrlichiosis, 237
 in differential diagnosis of leptospirosis, 169
 in differential diagnosis of malaria, 287
 treatment of, 257
Influenza inactivated virus, schedule, indications, side effects, contraindications, during pregnancy, with HIV infection, in immunocompromised patient, 1008*t*-1009*t*
Influenza vaccine
 for international travel, 1019*t*
 for patients with absent or dysfunctional spleen, 928
 during pregnancy, 1013*t*
 recommendations for
  for adults, 891
  for children, 890
 for residents of long-term care facilities, 921*t*
Inguinal adenitis in differential diagnosis of lymphogranuloma venereum, 283
Injuries
 household and recreational, counseling to prevent, 883-884
 motor vehicle, counseling to prevent, 882-883
 sports, Harstad study of epidemiology of, 915
Injury prevention, interventions for, 843*t*
 age 11-24 years, 845*t*
 age 25-64 years, 847*t*-848*t*
 age 65 and older, 849*t*-850*t*
Insanity, abortive; *see* Obsessive-compulsive disorder
Insect bites
 in differential diagnosis of impetigo, 253
 in differential diagnosis of lymphangitis, 280
 in differential diagnosis of urticaria, 512

Insemination
  therapeutic (frozen donor semen)
    basic information about, 467
    diagnosis of, 467
    treatment of, 467
  therapeutic (husband/partner)
    basic information about, 468
    diagnosis of, 468
    treatment of, 468-469
Insomnia; see also Sleep apnea; Sleep disorders
  basic information about, 258
  diagnosis of, 258
  in elderly, causes of, 606t
  treatment of, 258
Insulin, elevated, diagnosis of, 725
Insulin preparations, onset of action, duration, peak effect, 990t
Insulin sensitivity, atherosclerosis and, 903-904
Insulin therapy, effect on cognitive function, 929-930
Insulin-dependent diabetes mellitus; see Diabetes mellitus, insulin-dependent
Intensive care units, acute renal failure in, 927t, 927-928
Intermittent claudication; see Claudication
International prostate symptom score, 1028
Interstitial cystitis in differential diagnosis of bladder cancer, 71
Interstitial fibrosis in differential diagnosis of bronchiectasis, 81
Interstitial lung disease
  in differential diagnosis of amyloidosis, 24
  diffuse; see Lung disease, diffuse interstitial
Interstitial nephritis, acute, in differential diagnosis of acute glomerulonephritis, 200
Intertrigo in differential diagnosis of tinea cruris, 480
Intervertebral disks, herniated, differential diagnosis of, 553t
Intestinal infection in differential diagnosis of amebiasis, 23
Intestinal obstruction
  in differential diagnosis of acute appendicitis, 48
  in differential diagnosis of acute pancreatitis, 344
  in differential diagnosis of cholangitis, 115
Intestines
  helminth infestations of, 607t-608t
  pseudo-obstruction of, 608
Intracapsular fracture; see Femoral neck fracture
Intracranial mass
  in differential diagnosis of cluster headache, 209
  in differential diagnosis of febrile seizures, 435
  in differential diagnosis of tension-type headache, 211
Intracranial mass lesion in differential diagnosis of cryptococcosis, 141
Intracranial pressure, increased, headache associated with, 589
Intracranial tumor in differential diagnosis of bacterial meningitis, 294
Intracranial venous sinus thrombosis; see Cavernous sinus thrombosis
Intrahepatic cholestasis
  liver function tests in, 618t
  in pregnancy, characteristics of, 617t

Intrauterine contraceptive devices
  in differential diagnosis of dysfunctional uterine bleeding, 159
  in differential diagnosis of dysmenorrhea, 161
Intrauterine growth retardation, aspirin for preventing, 895
Intrinsic pathway defect, diagnosis based on routine screening tests, 555t
Invirase; see Saquinavir
Iritis
  in differential diagnosis of conjunctivitis, 132
  in differential diagnosis of red eye, 640t
Iron deficiency anemia; see Anemia, iron deficiency
Iron supplements
  absorption in 1-year-old children, 905
  recommendations for, 861-862
Iron-binding capacity, laboratory findings, 815, 816t
Irradiation in differential diagnosis of myelodysplastic syndromes, 313
Irritable bowel syndrome
  in adolescents, 907-908, 908t
  basic information about, 259
  diagnosis of, 259
  in differential diagnosis of celiac disease, 98
  in differential diagnosis of diverticular disease, 156
  in differential diagnosis of endometriosis, 170
  in differential diagnosis of lactose intolerance, 264
  in differential diagnosis of pseudomembranous gout, 395
  in differential diagnosis of ulcerative colitis, 505
  prevalence of, in primary care practices, 908-909, 909t
  treatment of, 259
Irritable heart; see Posttraumatic stress disorder
Irritant contact dermatitis; see Dermatitis, contact
Ischemia, myocardial; see Myocardial ischemia
Ischemic bowel disease
  in differential diagnosis of amebiasis, 23
  in differential diagnosis of ulcerative colitis, 505
Ischemic colitis
  in differential diagnosis of Crohn's disease, 140
  in differential diagnosis of diverticular disease, 156
Ismelin; see Guanethidine
Isoenzymes, creatine kinase, laboratory values, 797-798
Isoptin; see Verapamil
Isordil sublingual, dosage, preparations, onset of action, duration of action, 996t
Isosorbide dinitrate, dosage, preparations, onset of action, duration of action, 996t
Isosorbide mononitrate, dosage, preparations, onset of action, duration of action, 996t
Isradipine, preparations, dosage, effects, class, cost, half-life, 982t
ITP; see Idiopathic thrombocytopenic purpura

J

Jacksonian seizures, 434
Japanese encephalitis vaccine
  for international travel, 1019t
  schedule, indications, side effects, contraindications, during pregnancy, with HIV infection, in immunocompromised patient, 1010t-1011t
Jaundice
  causes of, 591, 609
  evaluation of, 731
  obstructive, liver function tests in, 618t
Jeep disease; see Pilonidal disease
Jenest-28, estrogen and progestin content of, 986t
Jock itch; see Tinea cruris
Joint disease, degenerative; see also Charcot's joint
  in differential diagnosis of bursitis, 85
  in differential diagnosis of claudication, 123
Jugular vein
  distention of, causes of, 609
  thrombus of, in differential diagnosis of nonneoplastic neck mass, 626t
Juvenile chronic arthritis; see Arthritis, juvenile rheumatoid
Juvenile idiopathic scoliosis, 947-948
Juvenile polyarthritis; see Arthritis, juvenile rheumatoid
Juvenile rheumatoid arthritis; see Arthritis, juvenile rheumatoid

K

Kanamycin, dosage for, and dialysis removal, 971t
Kanner's autism, 63
Kaposi's sarcoma
  basic information about, 260
  diagnosis of, 260
  in differential diagnosis of thrombophlebitis, 472
  treatment of, 260
Katz Index of Activities of Daily Living, 1029
Kawasaki's syndrome
  ages affected, prodrome, morphology, distribution, diagnosis, 575t
  in differential diagnosis of toxic shock syndrome, 484
  treatment of, 1018t
Keflex; see Cephalexin
Keflin; see Cephalothin
Kefzol; see Cefazolin
Kenalog; see Triamcinolone
Keratitis
  in differential diagnosis of uveitis, 516
  infectious; see Corneal ulceration
Keratoacanthoma
  in differential diagnosis of basal cell carcinoma, 67
  in differential diagnosis of squamous cell carcinoma, 450
Keratosis
  actinic, in differential diagnosis of squamous cell carcinoma, 450
  hypertrophic actinic, in differential diagnosis of warts, 529
  multiple seborrheic, history, manifestations, and malignancy associated with, 564t
  seborrheic, in differential diagnosis of melanoma, 291
Keratosis biliaris in differential diagnosis of folliculitis, 187
Kerlone; see Betaxolol

Ketoacidosis, diabetic; *see* Diabetic ketoacidosis
Ketones, urine, laboratory findings, 835
Ketoprofen, preparations, dosage, half-life, class, cost, metabolism, 997t
Ketorolac, preparations, dosage, half-life, class, cost, metabolism, 998t
Kidney(s); *see also* renal entries
　cystic disease of, 642t
　pelvic
　　in differential diagnosis of benign ovarian tumor, 341
　　in differential diagnosis of ovarian cancer, 340
　trauma to, evaluation of, *772*
Kidney disease, sports participation and, 1036t
Kidney stone in differential diagnosis of cholangitis, 115
Klinefelter's syndrome
　basic information about, 261
　diagnosis of, 261
　treatment of, 261
Klonopin; *see* Clonazepam
Knee pain, causes of, 610t-613t
Knee valgus stress test, 1026
Knee varus stress test, 1026
Korsakoff's psychosis, 262
KS; *see* Kaposi's sarcoma
Kytril; *see* Granisetron

L
Labetalol
　preparations, dosage, cardioselectivity, lipid solubility, half-life, excretion, cost, 969t, 981t
Laboratory tests, 779-839
　for acetone, 781
　acid phosphatase, 782-783
　for acid-base values in arterial and venous plasma or serum, 781t
　alkaline phosphatase, 782-783
　for primary uncomplicated respiratory and metabolic acid-base disorders, 781t
Labyrinthine disease in differential diagnosis of transient ischemic attack, 490
Labyrinthine fistula in differential diagnosis of labyrinthitis, 263
Labyrinthitis
　basic information about, 263
　diagnosis of, 263
　in differential diagnosis of mastoiditis, 289
　in differential diagnosis of motion sickness, 305
　treatment of, 263
　viral, in differential diagnosis of Meniere's disease, 292
Lachman test, 1026
Lactase deficiency; *see* Lactose intolerance
Lactate dehydrogenase, laboratory findings, 816
Lactation, breast cancer during, 79
Lactational/puerperal abscess, 77
Lactic acidosis, 540
Lactose intolerance
　basic information about, 264
　diagnosis of, 264
　in differential diagnosis of diverticular disease, 156
　treatment of, 264
Lambert-Eaton myasthenic syndrome
　basic information about, 265
　diagnosis of, 265
　treatment of, 265

Lamictal; *see* Lamotrigine
Lamivudine, therapeutic class, preparations, dosage, toxicities, cost, 970t
Lamotrigine, preparations, dosage, use, half-life, therapeutic level, toxic level, 973t
Landouzy-Dejerine disease; *see* Muscular dystrophy
Lansoprazole, preparations, dosage, cost, 968t
Large cell carcinoma of lung, 277
Larva migrans in tissue infections, epidemiology, transmission, manifestations, diagnosis, treatment, 629t
Laryngitis
　basic information about, 266
　diagnosis of, 266
　treatment of, 266
Laryngocele
　in differential diagnosis of congenital anomalies presenting as neck masses, 628t
　in differential diagnosis of thyroid nodule, 476
Laryngotracheitis; *see* Laryngitis
Laryngotracheobronchitis
　in differential diagnosis of laryngitis, 266
　membranous; *see* Tracheitis
Laxative abuse in differential diagnosis of celiac disease, 98
Laxatives, action, generic agent, brands, daily dose, precautions, 991t-992t
Lead axonal neuropathy in differential diagnosis of amyotrophic lateral sclerosis, 25
Lead poisoning
　basic information about, 267
　diagnosis of, 267
　screening recommendations for, 862-863
　treatment of, 267
Left ventricular ejection fraction, prognostic value of, 902t
Leg(s), swelling of, differential diagnosis of, 657t
Leg cramps, nocturnal, 614
Leg mobility, screening in ambulatory elderly, 920t
Leg pain, with exercise, 615t
Leg ulcers
　differential diagnosis of, 616
　evaluation of, *732*
Legg-Calvé-Perthes disease
　basic information about, 268
　diagnosis of, 268
　treatment of, 268
Legionella in differential diagnosis of psittacosis, 396
Legionella pneumonia in differential diagnosis of *Mycoplasma* pneumonia, 372
Legionella titer, laboratory findings, 816
Legionnaire's disease
　in differential diagnosis of human granulocytic ehrlichiosis, 237
　in differential diagnosis of leptospirosis, 169
　in differential diagnosis of toxic shock syndrome, 484
Leiomyoma; *see also* Uterine myomas
　in differential diagnosis of dysfunctional uterine bleeding, 159
　in differential diagnosis of dysmenorrhea, 161
　in differential diagnosis of pelvic abscess, 4
　in differential diagnosis of uterine malignancy, 513

Leiomyosarcoma; *see also* Uterine malignancy
　in differential diagnosis of uterine myomas, 514
Leishmaniasis
　in differential diagnosis of Chagas' disease, 109
　in differential diagnosis of malaria, 287
Leprosy
　in differential diagnosis of Bell's palsy, 68
　neuropathies associated with, 631t
Leptospirosis
　basic information about, 269
　diagnosis of, 269
　in differential diagnosis of babesiosis, 64
　in differential diagnosis of human granulocytic ehrlichiosis, 237
　in differential diagnosis of nonneoplastic neck mass, 627t
　in differential diagnosis of toxic shock syndrome, 484
　in differential diagnosis of yellow fever, 533
　treatment of, 269
Lermoyez's syndrome; *see* Meniere's disease
Lescol; *see* Fluvastatin
Leser-Trélat sign, history, manifestations, and malignancy associated with, 564t
Leukemia
　acute lymphoblastic
　　basic information about, 270
　　diagnosis of, 270
　acute lymphocytic, in differential diagnosis of acute myelogenous leukemia, 271
　acute myelogenous
　　basic information about, 271
　　diagnosis of, 271
　　in differential diagnosis of acute lymphoblastic leukemia, 170
　　treatment of, 271
　acute myeloid; *see* Leukemia, acute myelogenous
　acute nonlymphoblastic; *see* Leukemia, acute myelogenous
　acute nonlymphocytic; *see* Leukemia, acute myelogenous
　chromosomal abnormalities in, 792t
　chronic granulocytic; *see* Leukemia, chronic myelogenous
　chronic lymphocytic
　　basic information about, 272
　　diagnosis of, 272
　　in differential diagnosis of chronic myelogenous leukemia, 273
　　treatment of, 272
　chronic myelogenous
　　basic information about, 273
　　diagnosis of, 273
　　treatment of, 273
　in differential diagnosis of osteoporosis, 333
　in differential diagnosis of sickle cell anemia, 34
　hairy cell; *see* Hairy cell leukemia
　hypoplastic acute lymphoblastic, in differential diagnosis of aplastic anemia, 30
　hypoplastic acute myeloid, in differential diagnosis of aplastic anemia, 30
　lymphocyte abnormalities in, 620t
　prolymphocytic, in differential diagnosis of chronic lymphocytic leukemia, 272
Leukemic reticuloendotheliosis; *see* Hairy cell leukemia
Leukemoid reaction in differential diagnosis of acute myelogenous leukemia, 271

Leukocyte alkaline phosphatase, laboratory findings, 817
Leukocyte count; see Complete blood count
Leukocyte oxidase defect, granulomatous disorders due to, 584
Leukocytoclastic vasculitis, drug-induced, 565
Leukoplakia in differential diagnosis of balanitis, 66
Leukorrhea, physiologic, in differential diagnosis of prepubescent vulvovaginitis, 527
Levaquin; see Levofloxacin
Levatol; see Penbutolol
Levlen, estrogen and progestin content of, 986t
Levo-Dromoran; see Levorphanol
Levofloxacin, preparation, dosage, half-life, excretion, cost, 989t
Levora, estrogen and progestin content of, 986t
Levorphanol, equivalent dose, duration, preparations, dosage, 995t
LGV; see Lymphogranuloma venereum
Librium; see Chlordiazepoxide
Lice; see Pediculosis
Lichen planopilaris in differential diagnosis of alopecia, 543t
Lichen planus
  in differential diagnosis of balanitis, 66
  in differential diagnosis of erythema multiforme, 180
  in differential diagnosis of nail disorders, 625t
  in differential diagnosis of pityriasis rosea, 368
  erosive, differential diagnosis of, 557t
Lichen planus-like eruptions, drug-induced, 565
Lichen sclerosis
  in differential diagnosis of estrogen deficient vulvovaginitis, 525
  in differential diagnosis of pruritus vulvae, 393
Lichen simplex chronicus
  in differential diagnosis of atopic dermatitis, 146
  in differential diagnosis of contact dermatitis, 147
Lichenification, defined, 653t
Lichenoid eruptions, drug-induced, 565
Licorice ingestion syndrome, renin-aldosterone patterns in, 826t
Lidex; see Fluocinonide
Lidocaine
  drug monitoring data for, 799t
  electrophysiologic effects of, 969t
  for ventricular arrhythmias, indications, dosage, onset of action, therapeutic plasma levels, 1001t
Ligamentous injury, knee pain due to, findings, diagnosis, and management, 611t
Lightheadedness in differential diagnosis of dizziness, 569
Limb-girdle muscular dystrophy; see Muscular dystrophy
Linear IgA bullous dermatosis, differential diagnosis of, 557t
Linitis plastica; see Gastric cancer
Lipase, laboratory findings, 817
Lipid abnormalities, screening for, 853-854
Lipid-lowering agents, preparations, dosage, mechanism of action, effect, cost, 993t
Lipitor; see Atorvastatin

Lipoprotein
  high-density
    exercise and, 904-905
    laboratory findings, 813
  low-density, laboratory findings, 817
Liposarcoma, 74
Lisinopril, dosage, onset of action, peak effect, half-life, cost, 967t
Listeriosis
  basic information about, 275
  diagnosis of, 275
  treatment of, 275
Lithium, preparations, dosage, class, adverse effects, 978t
Lithium carbonate, drug monitoring data for, 799t
Little's disease; see Cerebral palsy
Liver
  cirrhosis of; see Cirrhosis
  fatty, of pregnancy, 181
Liver abscess
  amebic
    in differential diagnosis of salmonellosis, 424
    in differential diagnosis of typhoid fever, 504
    in differential diagnosis of cholangitis, 115
Liver disease
  in differential diagnosis of acetaminophen poisoning, 10
  in differential diagnosis of Gilbert's disease, 196
  in differential diagnosis of pruritus ani, 392
  liver function tests in, 618t
  predicting risk of, 924-926, 925, 925t
  in pregnancy, characteristics of, 617t
  sports participation and, 1036t
Liver failure in differential diagnosis of myxedema coma, 317
Liver function tests, abnormalities of, 733
Loa loa in tissue infections, epidemiology, transmission, manifestations, diagnosis, treatment, 629t
Lobar nephronia; see Pyelonephritis
Locomotor ataxia; see Tabes dorsalismain
Loestrin, estrogen and progestin content of, 986t
Löffler's syndrome in differential diagnosis of ascariasis, 55
Lomefloxacin
  dosage for, and dialysis removal, 972t
  preparation, dosage, half-life, excretion, cost, 989t
Lomustine, toxicity of, 984t-985t
Long-term care facilities, immunizations in, 921t, 921-922
Loop diuretics, class, preparations, dosage, site of action, cost, 978t
Lo/Ovral, estrogen and progestin content of, 986t
Lopid; see Gemfibrozil
Lopressor; see Metoprolol
Lorabid; see Loracarbef
Loracarbef
  preparations, dosage, half-life, 983t
Loracarbet, preparations, dosage, generation, half-life, 983t
Loratadine, preparations, dosage, effects, class, cost, 977t
Lorazepam, preparations, dosage, half-life, indication, cost, 980t
Lorelco; see Probucol
Lortab liquid, contents of, 995t
Lotensin; see Benazepril
Lou Gehrig's disease; see Amyotrophic lateral sclerosis

Lovastatin, preparations, dosage, mechanism of action, effect, cost, 993t
Low back pain; see also Lumbar disc syndromes
  counseling to prevent, 885
  differential diagnosis of, 553t-554t
Low-density lipoprotein, laboratory findings, 817
Ludiomil; see Maprotiline
Lues; see Syphilis
Lumbar disc syndromes; see also Low back pain
  basic information about, 276
  diagnosis of, 276
  treatment of, 276
Lung(s); see also pulmonary entries
  lesions of, 639
  solitary nodules of, causes of, 639t
Lung abscess
  in differential diagnosis of bronchiectasis, 81
  in differential diagnosis of lung neoplasm, 277
Lung cancer
  in differential diagnosis of asbestosis, 54
  in differential diagnosis of bronchiectasis, 81
  screening for, 858
Lung disease
  chronic, in differential diagnosis of restrictive cardiomyopathy, 91
  diffuse interstitial
    basic information about, 153
    diagnosis of, 153
    in differential diagnosis of asthma, 56
    treatment of, 153
  granulomatous, differential diagnosis of, 585t-586t
  interstitial, in differential diagnosis of amyloidosis, 24
Lung neoplasm, 277-278
  in differential diagnosis of bacterial pneumonia, 370
  metastatic, in differential diagnosis of lung neoplasm, 277
  primary, 277-278
    basic information about, 277
    diagnosis of, 277-278
    treatment of, 278
Lung-Browder chart for burn estimate, 1059t
Lupus anticoagulant; see Circulating anticoagulant
Lupus encephalitis in differential diagnosis of acute viral encephalitis, 166
Lupus erythematosus, discoid, in differential diagnosis of alopecia, 543t
Lyme arthritis in differential diagnosis of juvenile rheumatoid arthritis, 51
Lyme disease
  arthritis due to, course and distribution, 551t
  basic information about, 279
  diagnosis of, 279
  in differential diagnosis of acute viral encephalitis, 166
  in differential diagnosis of bacterial meningitis, 294
  in differential diagnosis of chronic fatigue syndrome, 119
  in differential diagnosis of human granulocytic ehrlichiosis, 237
  in differential diagnosis of listeriosis, 275
  history, rash characteristics and distribution, clinical findings, diagnostic aids, 578t

Lyme disease—cont'd
  knee pain due to, findings, diagnosis, and management, 611t
  neuropathies associated with, 631t
  treatment of, 279
Lymphadenitis, nonbacterial regional; see Cat-scratch disease
Lymphadenopathy
  in differential diagnosis of toxoplasmosis, 486
  generalized, 619, 734
  localized, 619, 735
Lymphangitic carcinomatosis
  in differential diagnosis of acute respiratory distress syndrome, 410
  in differential diagnosis of diffuse interstitial lung disease, 153
Lymphangitis
  basic information about, 280
  diagnosis of, 280
  in differential diagnosis of deep vein thrombosis, 473
  in differential diagnosis of thrombophlebitis, 472
  treatment of, 280
Lymphatic filariasis; see also Filariasis
  epidemiology, transmission, manifestations, diagnosis, treatment, 629t
Lymphedema
  basic information about, 281
  congenital, in differential diagnosis of Turner's syndrome, 502
  diagnosis of, 281
  in differential diagnosis of deep vein thrombosis, 473
  in differential diagnosis of swollen limbs, 657t
  treatment of, 282
Lymphoblastic leukemia, hypoplastic acute, in differential diagnosis of aplastic anemia, 30
Lymphocytes
  abnormalities of, in peripheral blood, 620t
  assessment of, 1046t
  laboratory findings, 817
Lymphocytic hypophysitis in differential diagnosis of Sheehan's syndrome, 437
Lymphocytic thyroiditis; see Thyroiditis
Lymphogranuloma inguinale in differential diagnosis of vulvar cancer, 523
Lymphogranuloma venereum
  basic information about, 283
  clinical features, diagnosis, and treatment, 582t
  diagnosis of, 283
  in differential diagnosis of tularemia, 500
  treatment of, 283
Lymphoma
  adult T cell, in differential diagnosis of chronic lymphocytic leukemia, 272
  chromosomal abnormalities in, 792t
  cutaneous, in differential diagnosis of Kaposi's sarcoma, 260
  in differential diagnosis of celiac disease, 98
  in differential diagnosis of Crohn's disease, 140
  in differential diagnosis of Epstein-Barr virus infections, 178
  in differential diagnosis of hairy cell leukemia, 274
  in differential diagnosis of malaria, 287
  in differential diagnosis of miliary tuberculosis, 496
  in differential diagnosis of mononucleosis, 304

Lymphoma—cont'd
  in differential diagnosis of multiple myeloma, 306
  in differential diagnosis of osteoporosis, 333
  in differential diagnosis of polyarteritis nodosa, 379
  in differential diagnosis of sarcoidosis, 426
  gastric, 192
    in differential diagnosis of gastritis, 193
  lymphocyte abnormalities in, 620t
  non-Hodgkin's; see Non-Hodgkin's lymphoma
  splenic, in differential diagnosis of chronic myelogenous leukemia, 273
  tonsillar hypertrophy in, in differential diagnosis of pharyngitis/tonsillitis, 362
Lymphomatoid granulomatosis, differential diagnosis of, 585t-586t
Lymphoproliferative disorders in differential diagnosis of idiopathic thrombocytopenic purpura, 252
Lymphoreticulosis, benign inoculation; see Cat-scratch disease

M

Macrocytosis
  causes of, 818t
  evaluation of, 736
Macroglobulinemia, Waldenström's
  in differential diagnosis of chronic lymphocytic leukemia, 272
  lymphocyte abnormalities in, 620t
Macrolide antibiotics, preparations, dosage, excretion, half-life, cost, 994t
Macular degeneration
  basic information about, 285
  diagnosis of, 285
  treatment of, 285
Macules, differential diagnosis of, 649
Magnesium
  diseases involving deficiency or excess of, 818
  laboratory findings, 817
Magnesium deficiency, causes of, 603
Malabsorption syndromes
  classification of, 621
  diagnosis of, 737
  in differential diagnosis of AIDS, 13
  in differential diagnosis of lead poisoning, 267
  in differential diagnosis of pernicious anemia, 33
Malaria, 286-288
  basic information about, 286
  diagnosis of, 287
  in differential diagnosis of babesiosis, 64
  in differential diagnosis of salmonellosis, 424
  in differential diagnosis of tularemia, 501
  in differential diagnosis of typhoid fever, 504
  in differential diagnosis of yellow fever, 533
  treatment of, 287-288
Male erectile disorder; see Erectile dysfunction
Malignancy; see also Cancer; Carcinoma; Neoplastic disease; specific types
  in differential diagnosis of hyperparathyroidism, 244
  hematopoietic, chromosome abnormalities in, 792t
  internal, cutaneous signs of, 564t
  knee pain due to, findings, diagnosis, and management, 613t
  sports participation and, 1036t

Malignant hypertension
  in differential diagnosis of nephrotic syndrome, 319
  in differential diagnosis of thrombotic thrombocytopenic purpura, 474
  renin-aldosterone patterns in, 826t
Malignant hyperthermia; see also Neuroleptic malignant syndrome
  in differential diagnosis of heat exhaustion/heat stroke, 214
Malignant melanoma; see also Melanoma
  in differential diagnosis of retinal hemorrhage, 413
  in high-risk population, 858
Malingering
  in differential diagnosis of conversion disorder, 135
  in differential diagnosis of Munchausen's syndrome, 210
Malta fever; see Brucellosis
Mammary dysplasia; see Fibrocystic breast disease
Mammogram
  abnormal, evaluating, 696
  in evaluation of breast discharge, 694
Mammography, recommendations for, 856
Mammography Quality Standards Act, 856
Mandol; see Cefamandole
Mania
  in differential diagnosis of bipolar disorder, 69
  in differential diagnosis of drug abuse, 7
Manic-depression; see Bipolar disorder
Mantoux test, positive, 831
Maprotiline, preparations, dosage, class, effects, half-life, 974t
Marie's disease; see Acromegaly
Marie-Strumpell disease; see Ankylosing spondylitis
Market men's disease; see Tularemia
Mass lesions
  in differential diagnosis of cerebrovascular accident, 101
  in differential diagnosis of transient ischemic attack, 490
Mastitis, chronic cystic; see Fibrocystic breast disease
Mastocytosis, primary nasal, 643t-644t
Mastoiditis
  basic information about, 289
  diagnosis of, 289
  in differential diagnosis of otitis externa, 335
  treatment of, 289
Maternal serum alpha-fetoprotein, measurement of, 872-873
Mavik; see Trandolapril
Maxaquin; see Lomefloxacin
Maxipime; see Cefepime
Maze procedure, 59
McArdle syndrome in differential diagnosis of leg pain, 615t
McMurray sign, 1026
MDS; see Myelodysplastic syndromes
Mean corpuscular volume
  decreased, causes of, 819t
  increased, causes of, 818t
  laboratory findings, 817
Measles
  ages affected, prodrome, morphology, distribution, diagnosis, 574t
  in differential diagnosis of trichinosis, 491
Measles vaccine
  administration of, 1018t
  for international travel, 1019t
  during pregnancy, 1012t, 1016t

Measles-mumps-rubella vaccine,
    for adults
        in immunocompromised patient, 1006t
        recommendations for, 892
            schedule, indications, side effects, contraindications, during pregnancy, with HIV infection, 1006t
    for children, recommendations for, 889, 1005t
    recommendations for, 868-869
Mechanical ventilation, pneumonia associated with, 942-943
Meckel's diverticulitis in differential diagnosis of acute appendicitis, 48
Meclizine, preparations, dosage, class, 976t
Meclofenamate, preparations, dosage, half-life, class, cost, metabolism, 998t
Meclomen; see Meclofenamate
Medial collateral ligament instability in differential diagnosis of epicondylitis, 174
Mediastinal masses/widening, causes of, 622
Medical literature, review of, 897-964; see also Year books
Medical records, abbreviations used in, 1063-1071
Medications
    in differential diagnosis of bacterial meningitis, 294
    in differential diagnosis of viral meningitis, 295
Medicine, year book of, 924-947
Mediterranean fever, familial, arthritis due to, course and distribution, 551t
Medullary carcinoma of thyroid; see Thyroid carcinoma
Mefoxin; see Cefoxitin
Megacolon in differential diagnosis of Chagas' disease, 109
Megaloblastic anemia; see also Anemia, pernicious
    causes of, 547-548
Meigs' syndrome
    basic information about, 290
    diagnosis of, 290
    treatment of, 290
Melanocytic precursor, skin cancer risk and, 858
Melanoma
    basic information about, 291
    diagnosis of, 291
    in differential diagnosis of basal cell carcinoma, 67
    in differential diagnosis of Kaposi's sarcoma, 260
    in differential diagnosis of nail disorders, 625t
    follow-up strategies for, 1053t
    treatment of, 291
    of vagina; see Vaginal malignancy
    of vulva; see Vulvar cancer
Melioidosis in differential diagnosis of pulmonary tuberculosis, 498
Melkersson-Rosenthal syndrome in differential diagnosis of Bell's palsy, 68
Mellaril; see Thioridazine
Melphalan, toxicity of, 984t-985t
Membrane(s), ruptured, in differential diagnosis of abruptio placentae, 3
Membranous laryngotracheobronchitis; see Tracheitis
Memory
    impairment of, in elderly, 918-919
    screening in ambulatory elderly, 920t
Meniere's disease
    basic information about, 292
    diagnosis of, 292

Meniere's disease—cont'd
    in differential diagnosis of labyrinthitis, 263
    treatment of, 292
Meningioma
    basic information about, 293
    diagnosis of, 293
    treatment of, 293
Meningitis
    bacterial
        basic information about, 294
        diagnosis of, 294
        in differential diagnosis of leptospirosis, 169
        in differential diagnosis of viral meningitis, 295
        treatment of, 294
    complement deficiencies associated with, 794t
    CSF abnormalities in, 559t, 791t
    in differential diagnosis of acute viral encephalitis, 166
    in differential diagnosis of Bell's palsy, 68
    in differential diagnosis of cavernous sinus thrombosis, 97
    in differential diagnosis of cryptococcosis, 141
    in differential diagnosis of febrile seizures, 435
    in differential diagnosis of hepatic encephalopathy, 218
    in differential diagnosis of infective endocarditis, 168
    in differential diagnosis of listeriosis, 275
    in differential diagnosis of malaria, 287
    in differential diagnosis of migraine, 210
    in differential diagnosis of psittacosis, 396
    in differential diagnosis of sporotrichosis, 448
    in differential diagnosis of subarachnoid hemorrhage, 454
    viral
        basic information about, 295
        diagnosis of, 295
        treatment of, 295
Meningocele; see Meningomyelocele
Meningococcal bacterial polysaccharide, schedule, indications, side effects, contraindications, during pregnancy, with HIV infection, in immunocompromised patient, 1008t-1009t
Meningococcal infection, chemoprophylaxis of, 893-894
Meningococcemia
    ages affected, prodrome, morphology, distribution, diagnosis, 575t
    in differential diagnosis of human granulocytic ehrlichiosis, 237
    in differential diagnosis of toxic shock syndrome, 484
    history, rash characteristics and distribution, clinical findings, diagnostic aids, 577t
Meningococcus vaccine for international travel, 1019t
Meningomyelocele
    basic information about, 296
    diagnosis of, 296
    treatment of, 296
Meniscal tear, knee pain due to, findings, diagnosis, and management, 612t
Menopause
    age at, and risk of mortality from cardiovascular disease, 956-958, 957
    basic information about, 297
    diagnosis of, 297

Menopause—cont'd
    estrogen replacement therapy following reduced mortality and, 10, 905-906
        and risk of cardiovascular disease, 934-935, 935
    hormone therapy following, 894-895
    osteoporosis following, screening recommendations for, 874-875
    treatment of, 297-298
Menstrual cramps; see Dysmenorrhea
Mental disorders; see also specific disorders
    and difficult physician-patient relationship, 907
    screening recommendations for, 875-879
Mental status, changes in, in differential diagnosis of amyloidosis, 24
Meperidine, equivalent dose, duration, preparations, dosage, 995t
Mercaptopurine, toxicity of, 984t-985t
Mercury poisoning, antidotes for, dosage and indications, 1055t
Mesenteric adenitis in differential diagnosis of Crohn's disease, 140
Mesoridazine, preparations, dosage, class, adverse effects, 978t
Metabolic abnormalities in differential diagnosis of eclampsia, 163
Metabolic acidosis, 540
    in differential diagnosis of diabetic ketoacidosis, 151
    in differential diagnosis of renal tubular acidosis, 409
    laboratory findings in, 781t
Metabolic alkalosis, 542
    laboratory findings in, 781t
Metabolic cataract; see Cataract
Metabolic disorders
    dementia associated with, laboratory diagnosis of, 567t
    in differential diagnosis of motion sickness, 305
    screening for, 860-863
Metaplasia in differential diagnosis of cervical dysplasia, 104
Metatarsalgia
    basic information about, 299
    diagnosis of, 299
    treatment of, 299
Metazoa, granulomatous disorders due to, 584
Metformin, preparations, dosage, duration of action, half-life, excretion, cost, class, 975t
Methadone, equivalent dose, duration, preparations, dosage, 995t
Methicillin, dosage for, and dialysis removal, 972t
Methotrexate
    drug monitoring data for, 799t
    for early abortion, 950-951, 951
    toxicity of, 984t-985t
Methyldopa, preparations, dosage, cost, 969t
Methylprednisolone, comparison chart for, 987t
Metoclopramide, preparations, dosage, class, 976t
Metoprolol, preparations, dosage, cardioselectivity, lipid solubility, half-life, excretion, cost, 981t
Metritis; see Endometritis
Metronidazole, dosage for, and dialysis removal, 971t
Mevacor; see Lovastatin
Mexiletine
    dosage, half-life, ECG manifestations, toxicity, 1000t
    electrophysiologic effects of, 969t

Mexitil; *see* Mexiletine
Mezlocillin, dosage for, and dialysis removal, 972*t*
MI; *see* Myocardial infarction
Michigan Alcoholism Screening Test, 1030
Microcytosis, causes of, 819*t*
Micronase; *see* Glyburide
Micronor, progestin content of, 987*t*
Micropenis, causes of, 622
Microsporidiosis with HIV infection, 709*t*
Migraine
  basic information about, 210
  diagnosis of, 210
  differential diagnosis of, 588*t*
  in differential diagnosis of cavernous sinus thrombosis, 97
  in differential diagnosis of cerebrovascular accident, 101
  in differential diagnosis of cluster headache, 209
  in differential diagnosis of epilepsy, 572*t*
  in differential diagnosis of partial seizure disorder, 434
  in differential diagnosis of tension-type headache, 211
  in differential diagnosis of transient ischemic attack, 490
  in differential diagnosis of viral meningitis, 295
  treatment of, 210
Migrainous vertigo in differential diagnosis of Meniere's disease, 292
Milia, defined, 653*t*
Miliaris in differential diagnosis of folliculitis, 187
Miliary tuberculosis in differential diagnosis of malaria, 287
Milk intolerance; *see* Lactose intolerance
Milk-alkali syndrome in differential diagnosis of hyperparathyroidism, 244
Minerals, recommended daily allowances for, 1047*t*
Mini-Mental State Examination, *1025*
Minipress; *see* Prazosin
Miosis, causes of, 623
Mirtazapine, preparations, dosage, class, effects, half-life, 974*t*
Miscarriage, spontaneous; *see also* Abortion
  basic information about, 446
  diagnosis of, 446-447
  treatment of, 447
Misoprostol for early abortion, 950-951, *951*
Mithramycin, toxicity of, 984*t*-985*t*
Mitomycin C, toxicity of, 984*t*-985*t*
Mitotane, toxicity of, 984*t*-985*t*
Mitoxantrone, toxicity of, 984*t*-985*t*
Mitral click murmur syndrome; *see* Mitral valve prolapse
Mitral insufficiency; *see* Mitral regurgitation
Mitral regurgitation
  basic information about, 300
  diagnosis of, 300
  in differential diagnosis of aortic stenosis, 47
  treatment of, 300
Mitral stenosis
  basic information about, 301
  congestive heart failure secondary to, 131
  diagnosis of, 301
  treatment of, 301
Mitral valve prolapse
  basic information about, 302
  diagnosis of, 302
  sports participation and, 1035*t*
  treatment of, 302
Müllerian anomalies in differential diagnosis of amenorrhea, 544*t*

MMR vaccine; *see* Measles-mumps-rubella vaccine
Mnemonics, TICS, 590
Mobitz type II block; *see* Heart block, second-degree
Modicon, estrogen and progestin content of, 986*t*
Moexipril, dosage, onset of action, peak effect, half-life, cost, 967*t*
Moles, atypical, and risk of skin cancer, 858
Mollaret's meningitis in differential diagnosis of acute viral encephalitis, 166
Molluscum contagiosum
  in differential diagnosis of basal cell carcinoma, 67
  in differential diagnosis of blepharitis, 73
  in differential diagnosis of warts, 529
Monilethrix in differential diagnosis of pediculosis, 350
Monilial vulvovaginitis; *see* Vulvovaginitis, fungal
Moniliasis; *see* Candidiasis
Monobactams, dosage for, and dialysis removal, 971*t*
Monocid; *see* Cefonicid
Monoclonal gammopathy of undetermined significance in differential diagnosis of multiple myeloma, 306
Monocyte count, laboratory findings, 817
Mononucleosis; *see also* Epstein-Barr virus infection
  acyclovir and prednisolone for treating, 946-947
  basic information about, 304
  diagnosis of, 304
  in differential diagnosis of bacterial meningitis, 294
  in differential diagnosis of chronic fatigue syndrome, 119
  in differential diagnosis of diphtheria, 154
  in differential diagnosis of HIV, 232
  in differential diagnosis of nonneoplastic neck mass, 626*t*-627*t*
  in differential diagnosis of psittacosis, 396
  in differential diagnosis of sarcoidosis, 426
  in differential diagnosis of tularemia, 501
  in differential diagnosis of viral meningitis, 295
  infectious
    ages affected, prodrome, morphology, distribution, diagnosis, 575*t*
    lymphocyte abnormalities in, 620*t*
  treatment of, 304
Monopril; *see* Fosinopril
Moraxella infection in differential diagnosis of corneal ulceration, 137
Moricizine
  dosage, half-life, ECG manifestations, toxicity, 1000*t*
  electrophysiologic effects of, 969*t*
Morphine, equivalent dose, duration, preparations, dosage, 995*t*
Morton's neuroma in differential diagnosis of tarsal tunnel syndrome, 464
Mosaic warts; *see* Warts
Motion sickness
  basic information about, 305
  diagnosis of, 305
  treatment of, 305
Motor vehicle injuries, counseling to prevent, 882-883
Motor-verbal tic disorder; *see* Tourette's syndrome
Motrin; *see* Ibuprofen
Mouth, cancer of; *see* Oral cancer

Movement disorders, hyperkinetic, manifestations, differential diagnosis, tests, treatment, 596*t*-597*t*
MR; *see* Mitral regurgitation
MS; *see* Mitral stenosis; Multiple sclerosis
Mucopurulent cervicitis; *see* Cervicitis
Mucormycosis in differential diagnosis of cavernous sinus thrombosis, 97
Mucous cysts in differential diagnosis of nail disorders, 625*t*
Mullerian system, congenital malformation of, in differential diagnosis of dysmenorrhea, 161
Mullerian tumors, malignant mixed; *see* Uterine malignancy
Multiple myeloma, 74
  basic information about, 306
  diagnosis of, 306
  in differential diagnosis of low back pain, 553*t*
  in differential diagnosis of osteoporosis, 333
  in differential diagnosis of temporal arteritis, 465
  treatment of, 306
Multiple sclerosis
  basic information about, 307
  diagnosis of, 307
  in differential diagnosis of acute viral encephalitis, 166
  in differential diagnosis of Bell's palsy, 68
  in differential diagnosis of chronic fatigue syndrome, 119
  in differential diagnosis of Meniere's disease, 292
  in differential diagnosis of myasthenia gravis, 312
  in differential diagnosis of syringomyelia, 459
  treatment of, 307
Multisomatoform disorder and difficult physician-patient relationship, 907
Mumps, 308-309
  basic information about, 308
  diagnosis of, 308-309
  treatment of, 309
Mumps vaccine; *see also* Measles-mumps-rubella vaccine
  for international travel, 1019*t*
  during pregnancy, 1012*t*
Munchausen by proxy; *see* Munchausen's syndrome
Munchausen's syndrome
  basic information about, 310
  diagnosis of, 310
  in differential diagnosis of somatization disorder, 444
  treatment of, 310
Muscle contraction headache; *see* Headache, tension-type
Muscle cramps/aches
  in differential diagnosis of claudication, 123
  evaluation of, *738*
  headache associated with, 589
Muscle weakness
  causes of, 623
  in mechanically ventilated patients with asthma, 959-960, *960*
Muscular atrophy, peroneal, 112
Muscular dystrophy
  basic information about, 311
  diagnosis of, 311
  treatment of, 311
Musculoskeletal disorders
  in differential diagnosis of angina pectoris, 37

1104 Index

Musculoskeletal disorders—cont'd
  screening recommendations for, 874-875
  sports participation and, 1036t
MVP; *see* Mitral valve prolapse
Myasthenia gravis
  basic information about, 312
  diagnosis of, 312
  in differential diagnosis of anxiety, 45
  in differential diagnosis of botulism, 75
  in differential diagnosis of chronic fatigue syndrome, 119
  in differential diagnosis of Lambert-Eaton syndrome, 265
  treatment of, 312
Mycobacteria
  atypical, in differential diagnosis of nonneoplastic neck mass, 627t
  granulomatous disorders due to, 584
Mycobacterium avium complex with HIV infection, 709t
Mycobacterium disease in differential diagnosis of lung neoplasm, 277
Mycobacterium tuberculosis in differential diagnosis of coccidioidomycoses, 125
Mycoplasma in differential diagnosis of psittacosis, 396
Mycoplasma pneumonia
  basic information about, 372
  diagnosis of, 372-373
  in differential diagnosis of coccidioidomycoses, 125
  treatment of, 373
Mydriasis, causes of, 624
Myelitis
  causes of, 624
  syphilitic, in differential diagnosis of amyotrophic lateral sclerosis, 25
Myelodysplasia
  chromosomal abnormalities in, 792t
  in differential diagnosis of pernicious anemia, 33
Myelodysplastic syndromes
  basic information about, 313
  diagnosis of, 313
  in differential diagnosis of acute myelogenous leukemia, 271
  in differential diagnosis of chronic myelogenous leukemia, 273
  in differential diagnosis of idiopathic thrombocytopenic purpura, 252
  treatment of, 313
Myelomeningocele in differential diagnosis of encopresis, 167
Myelopathy, causes of, 624
Myocardial abnormalities, sudden cardiac death due to, 912t
Myocardial infarction, 314-315
  acute; *see* Acute myocardial infarction
  aspirin for preventing, 895
  basic information about, 314
  diagnosis of, 314
  in differential diagnosis of acute pancreatitis, 344
  in differential diagnosis of peptic ulcer disease, 354
  in differential diagnosis of pulmonary embolism, 399
  during noncardiac surgery, 935
  sexual activity associated with, 911-913
  treatment of, 314-315
Myocardial ischemia
  activities triggering, 932-933, *933*
  prognostic importance of, after acute myocardial infarction, 901-903
  ST segment elevation in, 657t
  transient, pravastatin for reducing, 947
Myocarditis
  basic information about, 316
  diagnosis of, 316

Myocarditis—cont'd
  in differential diagnosis of amyloidosis, 24
  in differential diagnosis of toxoplasmosis, 486
  treatment of, 316
Myofascial pain syndrome; *see* Fibromyalgia
Myoma, prolapsed, in differential diagnosis of cervical polyps, 106
Myopathy
  in differential diagnosis of Addison's disease, 15
  in differential diagnosis of myasthenia gravis, 312
Myositis ossificans in differential diagnosis of swollen limbs, 657t
Myotonic muscular dystrophy; *see* Muscular dystrophy
Mysoline; *see* Primidone
Myxedema; *see* Hypothyroidism
Myxedema coma
  basic information about, 317
  diagnosis of, 317
  in differential diagnosis of hyperosmolar coma, 243
  in differential diagnosis of hypothermia, 250
  treatment of, 317
Myxoma, left atrial, in differential diagnosis of mitral stenosis, 301

N

Nabumetone, preparations, dosage, half-life, class, cost, metabolism, 998t
Nadolol, preparations, dosage, cardioselectivity, lipid solubility, half-life, excretion, cost, 981t
Nafcillin, dosage for, and dialysis removal, 972t
Nail disorders, differential diagnosis of, 625t
Nalfon; *see* Fenopren
Nalidixic acid, dosage for, and dialysis removal, 972t
Naprelan; *see* Naproxen
Naprosyn; *see* Naproxen
Naproxen, preparations, dosage, half-life, class, cost, metabolism, 998t
Narcolepsy
  basic information about, 318
  diagnosis of, 318
  in differential diagnosis of epilepsy, 572t
  in differential diagnosis of sleep apnea, 443
  treatment of, 318
Narcotic analgesics, equivalent dose, duration, preparations, dosage, 995t
Nasal polyps in differential diagnosis of chronic rhinitis, 644
Nausea, causes of, 625
Navane; *see* Thiothixene
Neck masses
  congenital anomalies presenting as, differential diagnosis of, 628t
  nonneoplastic, differential diagnosis of, 626t-627t
Neck pain, evaluation and treatment of, *739*
Necrolytic migratory erythema, history, manifestations, and malignancy associated with, 564t
Necrotizing fasciitis in differential diagnosis of cellulitis, 99
Necrotizing sarcoid granulomatosis, differential diagnosis of, 585t-586t
N.E.E., estrogen and progestin content of, 986t
Nefazodone, preparations, dosage, class, effects, half-life, 974t
Neglect, child; *see* Child abuse

Neisseria gonorrhoeae; *see also* Gonorrhea
  screening recommendations for, 864-865
Neisseria infection, arthritis due to, course and distribution, 551t
Nelova, estrogen and progestin content of, 986t
Nematodes
  in differential diagnosis of filariasis, 185
  intestinal, transmission, clinical findings, diagnosis, treatment, 607t-608t
  tissue infections due to, 629t
Neonate; *see* Newborn
Neoplastic disease; *see also* Cancer; Carcinoma; Malignancy; specific types
  after bone marrow transplantation, *926*, 926-927
  bone metastasis of, laboratory findings for calcium and phosphorus, 789t
  cerebral, CSF abnormalities in, 791t
  cervical intraepithelial; *see* Cervical cancer
  CSF abnormalities in, 559t
  in differential diagnosis of acute bronchitis, 82
  in differential diagnosis of AIDS, 13
  in differential diagnosis of alopecia, 543t
  in differential diagnosis of atelectasis, 58
  in differential diagnosis of Bell's palsy, 68
  in differential diagnosis of cholelithiasis, 117
  in differential diagnosis of chronic obstructive pulmonary disease, 120
  in differential diagnosis of glossitis, 202
  in differential diagnosis of hemorrhoids, 217
  in differential diagnosis of osteochondritis dissecans, 331
  in differential diagnosis of otitis externa, 335
  in differential diagnosis of peptic ulcer disease, 354
  in differential diagnosis of ulcerative colitis, 505
  in differential diagnosis of Wegener's granulomatosis, 531
  endocrine, in differential diagnosis of primary aldosteronism, 19
  eosinophilia due to, 573
  flushing due to, 580
  granulomatous disorders due to, 584
  mediastinal, 622
  metastatic, 622
    in differential diagnosis of hyperthyroidism, 247
  pulmonary nodules due to, 639t
  screening for, 856-860
Nephritis
  acute bacterial; *see* Pyelonephritis
  acute interstitial, in differential diagnosis of acute glomerulonephritis, 200
  salt-losing, in differential diagnosis of Addison's disease, 15
Nephrolithiasis; *see also* Urolithiasis
  in differential diagnosis of preeclampsia, 384
  in differential diagnosis of pyelonephritis, 401
  evaluation of, *740*
Nephronia, lobar; *see* Pyelonephritis
Nephropathy, hepatic, 223
Nephrotic syndrome
  basic information about, 319
  diagnosis of, 319
  in differential diagnosis of congestive heart failure, 130
  in differential diagnosis of hypothyroidism, 251
  treatment of, 319

Nerve entrapment syndrome, 93
    in differential diagnosis of endometriosis, 170
Netilmicin, dosage for, and dialysis removal, 971t
Neural tube defects
    prevention of, 872-873
    risk of, prepregnant weight and, 914-915
    screening recommendations for, 872-873
Neuralgia
    cranial, headache associated with, 589
    herpetic and postherpetic, treatment of, 720
    postherpetic, in differential diagnosis of cluster headache, 209
    sphenopalatine; see Headache, cluster
Neurasthenia in differential diagnosis of myasthenia gravis, 312
Neuritis, brachial
    in differential diagnosis of cervical disc syndromes, 103
    in differential diagnosis of frozen shoulder, 191
Neuroacanthocytosis in differential diagnosis of Huntington's chorea, 238
Neuroblastoma
    basic information about, 320
    diagnosis of, 320
    treatment of, 320
Neurodermatitis, atopic; see Dermatitis, atopic
Neurogenic bladder in differential diagnosis of bladder cancer, 71
Neurolabyrinthitis, viral; see Labyrinthitis
Neuroleptic malignant syndrome
    basic information about, 321
    diagnosis of, 321
    in differential diagnosis of bacterial meningitis, 294
    treatment of, 321
Neurologic deficit
    focal, causes of, 630
    multifocal, causes of, 630
Neurologic disorders
    dementia in, laboratory diagnosis of, 567t
    in differential diagnosis of bulimia nervosa, 84
    sports participation and, 1036t
Neurology, year book of, 900, 947-948
Neuroma, acoustic
    in differential diagnosis of Meniere's disease, 292
    in differential diagnosis of Ramsay Hunt syndrome, 403
Neuronopathy, acute vestibular; see Labyrinthitis
Neurontin; see Gabapentin
Neuropathic arthropathy; see also Charcot's joint
    in differential diagnosis of pseudogout, 394
Neuropathy
    in differential diagnosis of Charcot-Marie-Tooth disease, 112
    diseases associated with, 631t
    entrapment, in differential diagnosis of carpal tunnel syndrome, 93
    heavy metal, in differential diagnosis of Guillain-Barré syndrome, 208
    hereditary motor and sensory; see also Charcot-Marie-Tooth disease
        in differential diagnosis of Friedrich's ataxia, 190
    lead axonal, in differential diagnosis of amyotrophic lateral sclerosis, 25
    multifocal motor, in differential diagnosis of amyotrophic lateral sclerosis, 25

Neuropathy—cont'd
    optic; see also Optic neuritis
        in differential diagnosis of chronic open-angle glaucoma, 198
    peripheral, in differential diagnosis of amyloidosis, 24
    ulnar, in differential diagnosis of epicondylitis, 174
Neurosis, anxiety; see Anxiety; Anxiety disorders
Neurosurgery, year book of, 900, 947-948
Neurosyphilis
    CSF abnormalities in, 559t, 791t
    in differential diagnosis of major depression, 145
    tabetic; see Tabes dorsalis
Neutropenia, evaluation of, 741
Neutrophil count, laboratory values, 819
Neutrophilia, evaluation of, 742
Nevirapine, therapeutic class, preparations, dosage, toxicities, cost, 970t
Newborn; see also Congenital disorders
    hepatitis B immunizations for, 863
    ocular prophylaxis in, 866-867
    screening for hemoglobinopathies, 873-874
    screening for hypothyroidism, 874
    screening for phenylketonuria, 874
Newborn conjunctivitis; see Conjunctivitis
NGU; see Urethritis, nongonococcal
NHL; see Non-Hodgkin's lymphoma
Niacin; see Nicotinic acid
Nicardipine, preparations, dosage, effects, class, cost, half-life, 982t
Nicotine dependence, assessing, 880
Nicotinic acid, preparations, dosage, mechanism of action, effect, cost, 993t
NIDDM; see Diabetes mellitus
Nifedipine
    adverse effects of, 903
    gingival hyperplasia due to, 197
    preparations, dosage, effects, class, cost, half-life, 982t
    sublingual, for hypertensive emergencies and pseudoemergencies, 903
Nipple, florid papillomatosis of, in differential diagnosis of Paget's disease of breast, 343
Nisoldipine, preparations, dosage, effects, class, cost, half-life, 982t
Nitrates
    for angina, dosage, preparations, onset of action, duration of action, 996t
    mechanism of action of, 38
Nitrofurantoin, dosage for, and dialysis removal, 971t
Nitrogen, urinary, assessment of, 1046t
Nitrogen balance, assessment of, 1046t
Nitrogen mustard, toxicity of, 984t-985t
Nitroglycerin, dosage, preparations, onset of action, duration of action, 996t
Nizatidine, preparations, dosage, cost, 968t
Nocturnal enuresis, 256
Nodular lymphangitis; see Lymphangitis
Nodules, differential diagnosis of, 650
Nomogram for calculating body surface area, 1043
Non-A, B hepatitis, transfusion-related; see Hepatitis C
Non-Hodgkin's lymphoma
    basic information about, 284
    diagnosis of, 284
    in differential diagnosis of Hodgkin's disease, 233
    treatment of, 284
Non-insulin-dependent diabetes mellitus; see Diabetes mellitus, non-insulin-dependent

Nonionic detergents, antimicrobial activity, mechanics of action, toxicity, indications and contraindications, 979t
Nonketotic hyperosmolar coma; see Hyperosmolar coma
Nonproliferative diabetic retinopathy; see Diabetic retinopathy
Nonsteroidal antiinflammatory drugs
    preparations, dosage, half-life, class, cost, metabolism, 997t-998t
    and reduced disability in rheumatoid arthritis, 931, 931-932
Noonan syndrome in differential diagnosis of Turner's syndrome, 502
Nordette-21, estrogen and progestin content of, 986t
Norethin, estrogen and progestin content of, 986t
Norfloxacin
    dosage for, and dialysis removal, 972t
    preparation, dosage, half-life, excretion, cost, 989t
Norinyl, estrogen and progestin content of, 986t
Normodyne; see Labetalol
Noroxin; see Norfloxacin
Norpace; see Disopyramide
Norpramin; see Desipramine
Nor-Q.D., progestin content of, 987t
Nortriptyline
    drug monitoring data for, 799t
    preparations, dosage, class, effects, half-life, 974t
Norvasc; see Amlodipine
Norvir; see Ritonavir
Nosocomial infections, 322-324
    basic information about, 322
    diagnosis of, 322-324
    treatment of, 324
NSAIDs; see Nonsteroidal antiinflammatory drugs
Nuclear antigen, extractable, laboratory values, 801
5'Nucleotidase, laboratory values, 819
Nucleus pulposus, degenerative disease of, characteristics of, 549t
Nummular dermatitis, differential diagnosis of, 568t
Nummular eczema in differential diagnosis of contact dermatitis, 147
Numorphan; see Oxymorphone
Nutcracker esophagus in differential diagnosis of GERD, 194
Nutritional assessment
    in ambulatory elderly, 920t
    anthropometric and laboratory measurements in, 1046t
Nutritional counseling, 881-882
Nutritional disorders, screening for, 860-863
Nutritional status and mortality from COPD, 933-934, 934
Nutritional support, commercial formulas for, 1049t
Nystagmus, causes of, 631

O

Oat cell carcinoma of lung, 277
Obesity
    causes of, 666
    in diabetic patients
        Cushing's syndrome and, 142, 940-941
    and risk of neural tube defects in fetus, 914-915
    screening recommendations for, 861
    sports participation and, 1036t

1106 Index

Obsessive-compulsive disorder
  basic information about, 325
  diagnosis of, 325
  treatment of, 325
Obstetrics, year book of, 900
Obstructive jaundice, liver function tests in, 618t
Occlusion amblyopia; see Amblyopia
Occult blood
  fecal, evaluation of, 712
  urine, laboratory findings, 835
Ocular muscular dystrophy; see Muscular dystrophy
Oculopharyngeal muscular dystrophy; see Muscular dystrophy
Ofloxacin
  dosage for, and dialysis removal, 972t
  preparation, dosage, half-life, excretion, cost, 989t
Ohara's disease; see Tularemia
Oliguric renal failure; see Hepatorenal syndrome
Olivopontocerebellar atrophy in differential diagnosis of Huntington's chorea, 238
Omeprazole, preparations, dosage, cost, 968t
Onchocerca volvulus in tissue infections, epidemiology, transmission, manifestations, diagnosis, treatment, 629t
Oncogenes, chromosome location and comments on, 820t
Oncology; see Cancer; Carcinoma; Malignancy; Neoplastic disease; specific cancers
Ondansetron, preparations, dosage, class, 976t
Onychomycosis in differential diagnosis of nail disorders, 625t
Ophthalmia neonatorum, gonococcal, prevention of, 864
Opisthorchis, epidemiology, transmission, manifestations, diagnosis, treatment, 660t
Optic atrophy
  basic information about, 327
  diagnosis of, 327
  treatment of, 327
Optic neuritis
  basic information about, 328
  diagnosis of, 328
  treatment of, 328
Optic neuropathy
  in differential diagnosis of amblyopia, 22
  in differential diagnosis of chronic open-angle glaucoma, 198
OPV vaccine, recommendations for children, 889
Oral cancer, screening recommendations for, 859
Oral contraceptives
  breast cancer and, 955-956
  estrogen and progestin content of, 986t-987t
  low-dose, stroke in users of, 954, 955t
  renin-aldosterone patterns in, 826t
  use of, 700-701
Oral hygiene, counseling about, 885-886
Oral poliovirus vaccine; see Poliomyelitis vaccine
Oral procedures, prophylactic regimens for, 1023t
Orbital cellulitis in differential diagnosis of cavernous sinus thrombosis, 97
Orbital tumors in differential diagnosis of strabismus, 453
Orchitis in differential diagnosis of epididymitis, 175

Organ transplant, sports participation and, 1036t
Organic amblyopia; see Amblyopia
Orinase; see Tolbutamide
Ornithosis; see Psittacosis
Oropharyngeal cancer, follow-up strategies for, 1053t
Ortho Tri-Cyclen, estrogen and progestin content of, 987t
Ortho-Cept, estrogen and progestin content of, 986t
Ortho-Cyclen, estrogen and progestin content of, 986t
Ortho-Novum, estrogen and progestin content of, 986t, 987t
Orthopedic maneuvers, 1026
Orudis; see Ketoprofen
Oruvail; see Ketoprofen
Osgood-Schlatter disease
  basic information about, 329
  diagnosis of, 329
  knee pain due to, findings, diagnosis, and management, 612t
Osmolality
  serum, laboratory values, 819
  urine, 835
Osmotic diuresis in differential diagnosis of diabetes insipidus, 148
Osteitis deformans; see Paget's disease of bone
Osteoarthritis; see also Arthritis
  basic information about, 330
  diagnosis of, 330
  in differential diagnosis of carpal tunnel syndrome, 93
  in differential diagnosis of Charcot's joint, 111
  in differential diagnosis of costochondritis, 138
  in differential diagnosis of fibromyalgia, 184
  in differential diagnosis of gout, 205
  in differential diagnosis of pseudogout, 394
  in differential diagnosis of shoulder pain, 648t
  erosive, in differential diagnosis of psoriatic arthritis, 52
  knee pain due to, findings, diagnosis, and management, 613t
  treatment of, 330
Osteoarthrosis; see Arthritis; Osteoarthritis
Osteochondritis dissecans
  basic information about, 331
  diagnosis of, 331
  treatment of, 331
Osteochondrosis; see Osteochondritis dissecans
  capital femoral; see Legg-Calvé-Perthes disease
Osteogenesis imperfecta in differential diagnosis of osteoporosis, 333
Osteoma cutis in differential diagnosis of acne vulgaris, 12
Osteomalacia
  in differential diagnosis of osteoporosis, 333
  laboratory findings for calcium and phosphorus, 789t
Osteomyelitis
  basic information about, 332
  diagnosis of, 332
  in differential diagnosis of cellulitis, 99
  in differential diagnosis of Charcot's joint, 111
  in differential diagnosis of infective endocarditis, 168
  in differential diagnosis of low back pain, 554t

Osteomyelitis—cont'd
  in differential diagnosis of Paget's disease of bone, 342
  in differential diagnosis of pilonidal disease, 365
  in differential diagnosis of primary malignant bone tumor, 74
  treatment of, 332
Osteonecrosis, knee pain due to, findings, diagnosis, and management, 612t
Osteoporosis, 333-334
  basic information about, 333
  diagnosis of, 333
  in differential diagnosis of rickets, 421
  hormonal therapy and, 894-895
  laboratory findings for calcium and phosphorus, 789t
  postmenopausal, screening recommendations for, 874-875
  prevention of, 875, 895
  treatment of, 333-334
Osteosarcoma, 74
Ostium primum, 61
Ostium secundum, 61
Otitis externa, 335-336
  basic information about, 335
  diagnosis of, 335-336
  in differential diagnosis of mastoiditis, 289
  in differential diagnosis of otitis media, 338
  treatment of, 336
Otitis in differential diagnosis of Ramsay Hunt syndrome, 403
Otitis media, 337-338
  basic information about, 337
  diagnosis of, 338
  in differential diagnosis of mastoiditis, 289
  in differential diagnosis of Meniere's disease, 292
  treatment of, 338
Otomycosis; see Otitis externa
Otosclerosis
  basic information about, 339
  diagnosis of, 339
  treatment of, 339
Otospongiosis; see Otosclerosis
Ovarian abnormalities in differential diagnosis of menopause, 297
Ovarian cancer
  basic information about, 340
  counseling to prevent, 887-888
  diagnosis of, 340
  in differential diagnosis of Meigs' syndrome, 290
  screening for, 859
  treatment of, 340
Ovarian cyst
  in differential diagnosis of dysmenorrhea, 161
  in differential diagnosis of ovarian cancer, 340
  in differential diagnosis of pyelonephritis, 401
  ruptured
    in differential diagnosis of ectopic pregnancy, 164
    in differential diagnosis of pelvic inflammatory disease, 352
Ovarian disorders in differential diagnosis of Meigs' syndrome, 290
Ovarian failure, premature, in differential diagnosis of amenorrhea, 544t
Ovarian neoplasm
  in differential diagnosis of menopause, 297
  in differential diagnosis of uterine myomas, 514

Ovarian torsion in differential diagnosis of benign ovarian tumor, 341
Ovarian tumor
　benign
　　basic information about, 341
　　diagnosis of, 341
　　treatment of, 341
　in differential diagnosis of pelvic abscess, 4
Ovaries, absence of, sports participation and, 1036t
Ovcon, estrogen and progestin content of, 986t
Overflow incontinence, 255
Overweight; see also Obesity
　causes of, 666
Ovral, estrogen and progestin content of, 986t
Ovrette, progestin content of, 987t
Oxacillin, dosage for, and dialysis removal, 972t
Oxaprozin, preparations, dosage, half-life, class, cost, metabolism, 998t
Oxazepam, preparations, dosage, half-life, indication, cost, 980t
Oxygen therapy, long-term, at home, 961, 961-962
Oxymorphone, equivalent dose, duration, preparations, dosage, 995t

P

Paget's disease
　of bone
　　basic information about, 342
　　diagnosis of, 342
　　treatment of, 342
　of breast
　　basic information about, 343
　　diagnosis of, 343
　　in differential diagnosis of cellulitis, 99
　　treatment of, 343
　in differential diagnosis of hyperparathyroidism, 244
　in differential diagnosis of osteoporosis, 333
　in differential diagnosis of vulvar cancer, 523
　laboratory findings for calcium and phosphorus, 789t
Pain
　abdominal
　　in differential diagnosis of abdominal aorta aneurysm, 36
　　evaluation of, 671
　back; see Back pain
　eye, causes of, 576t
　facial
　　causes of, 576t
　　classification of, 589
　groin, differential diagnosis of, 587
　hip, causes of, 592
　knee, causes of, 610t-613t
　leg, with exercise, 615t
　low back
　　counseling to prevent, 885
　　differential diagnosis of, 553t-554t
　neck, evaluation and treatment of, 739
　pelvic
　　causes of, 633
　　evaluation of, 746
　rectal, causes of, 640
　referred, in differential diagnosis of otitis media, 338
　shoulder, diagnosis, evaluation, treatment, 648t
Pain disorder in differential diagnosis of somatization disorder, 444
Pain management in cancer patient, 743

Painful arc syndrome; see Rotator cuff syndrome
Painful periods; see Dysmenorrhea
Palindromic rheumatism, course and distribution, 551t
Palsy; see Bell's palsy
Pamelor; see Nortriptyline
PAN; see Polyarteritis nodosa
Pancreatic cancer
　in differential diagnosis of chronic pancreatitis, 346
　screening recommendations for, 859
Pancreatic insufficiency in differential diagnosis of lactose intolerance, 264
Pancreatitis
　acute, 344-345
　　basic information about, 344
　　diagnosis of, 344-345
　　treatment of, 345
　chronic
　　basic information about, 346
　　diagnosis of, 346
　　treatment of, 346
　in differential diagnosis of cholangitis, 115
　in differential diagnosis of cholelithiasis, 117
　in differential diagnosis of gastritis, 193
　in differential diagnosis of hyperemesis gravidarum, 241
　in differential diagnosis of irritable bowel syndrome, 259
　in differential diagnosis of peptic ulcer disease, 354
　in differential diagnosis of secondary peritonitis, 359
　in differential diagnosis of septicemia, 436
Pancytopenia, causes of, 632
Panic; see Agoraphobia/panic
Panic attack
　defined, 16
　in differential diagnosis of phobias, 364
Panic disorder
　defined, 16
　and difficult physician-patient relationship, 907
Panniculitis in differential diagnosis of thrombophlebitis, 472
Pap smear
　abnormal; see also Cervical dysplasia
　　cervical polyps and, 106
　　workup of, 744
　recommendations for, 857
Papillae, hypertrophied anal, in differential diagnosis of hemorrhoids, 217
Papillary carcinoma of thyroid; see Thyroid carcinoma
Papillary conjunctivitis; see Conjunctivitis
Papillary necrosis in differential diagnosis of urinary tract infection, 509
Papilledema, causes of, 632
Papillitis, optic, 328
Papilloma, squamous, in differential diagnosis of cervical polyps, 106
Papillomatosis, florid, of nipple, in differential diagnosis of Paget's disease of breast, 343
Papules
　differential diagnosis of, 650
　genital, differential diagnosis of, 583t
Paracetamol poisoning; see Acetaminophen poisoning
Paraganglioma; see Pheochromocytoma
Paragonimiasis in differential diagnosis of pulmonary tuberculosis, 498
Paragonimus westermani, epidemiology, transmission, manifestations, diagnosis, treatment, 660t

Parainfluenza virus infection in differential diagnosis of influenza, 257
Paralysis
　ascending; see Guillain-Barré syndrome
　congenital spastic; see Cerebral palsy
　facial, causes of, 576
　hysterical, in differential diagnosis of Guillain-Barré syndrome, 208
　idiopathic facial; see Bell's palsy
　infantile; see Poliomyelitis
　tick, in differential diagnosis of botulism, 75
Paralysis agitans; see Parkinson's disease
Paraneoplastic pemphigus, differential diagnosis of, 557t
Paraphilia
　in differential diagnosis of obsessive-compulsive disorder, 325
　in differential diagnosis of pedophilia, 351
Paraplegia, causes of, 632
Parasitic infection
　in differential diagnosis of celiac disease, 98
　in differential diagnosis of chronic fatigue syndrome, 119
　in differential diagnosis of Crohn's disease, 140
　in differential diagnosis of pruritus ani, 392
　in differential diagnosis of pseudomembranous gout, 395
　in differential diagnosis of tropical sprue, 494
　in differential diagnosis of ulcerative colitis, 505
Parasomnia in differential diagnosis of sleep apnea, 443
Parathesias, causes of, 633
Paratyphoid fever in differential diagnosis of human granulocytic ehrlichiosis, 237
Parkinsonism, secondary, in differential diagnosis of Parkinson's disease, 347
Parkinson's disease
　basic information about, 347
　diagnosis of, 347
　in differential diagnosis of anxiety, 45
　treatment of, 347-348
Paronychia in differential diagnosis of nail disorders, 625t
Parotitis; see Mumps
Paroxetine, preparations, dosage, class, effects, half-life, 974t
Paroxysmal atrial tachycardia
　basic information about, 349
　diagnosis of, 349
　treatment of, 349
Paroxysmal nocturnal hemoglobinuria in differential diagnosis of myelodysplastic syndromes, 313
Paroxysmal vertigo in differential diagnosis of epilepsy, 572t
Partial thromboplastin time, laboratory values, 819-820
Partner abuse, screening for, 876
Passovoy, disorders of, inheritance, incidence, bleeding symptoms, test results, treatment, 562t
PAT; see Paroxysmal atrial tachycardia
Patellar tendinitis in differential diagnosis of Osgood-Schlatter disease, 329
Patent ductus arteriosus in differential diagnosis of aortic regurgitation, 46
Patient(s), difficult
　Difficult Doctor-Patient Relationship Questionnaire for assessing, 906
　prevalence, psychopathology, and functional impairment, 906-907
Paxil; see Paroxetine

1108 Index

PCO$_2$, average values for arterial and venous plasma or serum, 781t
PCP; see *Pneumocystis carinii* pneumonia
Pediculosis
 basic information about, 350
 diagnosis of, 350
 in differential diagnosis of scabies, 427
 treatment of, 350
Pedophilia
 basic information about, 351
 diagnosis of, 351
 treatment of, 351
Pelvic abscess, 4-5
 basic information about, 4
 diagnosis of, 4
 treatment of, 4
Pelvic adhesions in differential diagnosis of endometriosis, 170
Pelvic congestion syndrome in differential diagnosis of dysmenorrhea, 161
Pelvic inflammatory disease
 basic information about, 352
 diagnosis of, 352-353
 in differential diagnosis of dysmenorrhea, 161
 in differential diagnosis of ectopic pregnancy, 164
 in differential diagnosis of endometriosis, 170
 in differential diagnosis of pyelonephritis, 401
 in differential diagnosis of secondary peritonitis, 359
 in differential diagnosis of urolithiasis, 510
 treatment of, 353
Pelvic masses
 differential diagnosis of, 633
 in differential diagnosis of Meigs' syndrome, 290
 evaluation of, 745
Pelvic organ prolapse; see Uterine prolapse
Pelvic pain
 causes of, 633
 evaluation of, 746
 prevalence of, in primary care practices, 908-909, 909t
Pemphigoid
 bullous, differential diagnosis of, 557t
 cicatricial, differential diagnosis of, 557t
 in differential diagnosis of Stevens-Johnson syndrome, 452
Pemphigus in differential diagnosis of Stevens-Johnson syndrome, 452
Pemphigus foliaceus, differential diagnosis of, 557t
Pemphigus vulgaris
 differential diagnosis of, 557t
 in differential diagnosis of erythema multiforme, 180
 in differential diagnosis of impetigo, 253
Penbutolol, preparations, dosage, cardioselectivity, lipid solubility, half-life, excretion, cost, 981t
Penetrex; see Enoxacin
Penicillin(s)
 alternatives to, 1023t
 dosage for, and dialysis removal, 972t
Penicillin G, dosage for, and dialysis removal, 972t
Penicillin V, dosage for, and dialysis removal, 972t
Penis, carcinoma of, in differential diagnosis of balanitis, 66
Pentazocine, equivalent dose, duration, preparations, dosage, 995t
Pepcid; see Famotidine
Peptic esophagitis; see Gastroesophageal reflux disorder

Peptic ulcer disease
 basic information about, 354
 diagnosis of, 354-355
 in differential diagnosis of acute pancreatitis, 344
 in differential diagnosis of cholelithiasis, 117
 in differential diagnosis of chronic pancreatitis, 346
 in differential diagnosis of gastric cancer, 192
 in differential diagnosis of gastritis, 193
 in differential diagnosis of GERD, 194
 in differential diagnosis of irritable bowel syndrome, 259
 in differential diagnosis of preeclampsia, 384
 perforated, in differential diagnosis of spontaneous bacterial peritonitis, 360
 treatment of, 345, 355
Peptostreptococcus, infections due to, 26
Percocet, contents of, 995t
Percodan, contents of, 995t
Percutaneous transluminal coronary angioplasty, indications for, 38
Perianal abscess in differential diagnosis of pilonidal disease, 365
Periarteritis nodosa; see also Polyarteritis nodosa
 neuropathies associated with, 631t
Periarthritis; see Frozen shoulder
Pericapsulitis; see Frozen shoulder
Pericardial abnormalities
 in differential diagnosis of cardiac tamponade, 88
 in differential diagnosis of dilated cardiomyopathy, 89
 in differential diagnosis of hypertrophic cardiomyopathy, 90
 in differential diagnosis of restrictive cardiomyopathy, 91
Pericardial tamponade in differential diagnosis of pulmonary embolism, 399
Pericarditis
 basic information about, 356
 constrictive, in differential diagnosis of mitral valve prolapse, 302
 diagnosis of, 356
 in differential diagnosis of infective endocarditis, 168
 in differential diagnosis of peptic ulcer disease, 354
 in differential diagnosis of pulmonary embolism, 399
 pain from, in differential diagnosis of herpes zoster, 228
 ST segment elevation in, 657t
 treatment of, 356-357
Perinephric abscess in differential diagnosis of pyelonephritis, 401
Periodic health examination
 age 11-24 years, 845t
 age 25-64 years, 847t-848t
 age 65 and older, 849t-850t
 age-specific charts for, 843t-850t
 contents of, 842
 for general population, 843t
 for high-risk populations, 843t
 for pregnant women, 851t-852t
Periodontal disease, counseling to prevent, 885-886
Peripheral arterial disease, asymptomatic, screening for, 855
Peripheral conversion, increased, gynecomastia associated with, 587
Peripheral neuropathy
 basic information about, 358
 diagnosis of, 358

Peripheral neuropathy—cont'd
 in differential diagnosis of amyloidosis, 24
 in differential diagnosis of tarsal tunnel syndrome, 464
 treatment of, 358
Peripheral vascular disease
 arteriosclerotic, in differential diagnosis of thromboangiitis obliterans, 471
 in differential diagnosis of tarsal tunnel syndrome, 464
Peripheral vascular insufficiency in differential diagnosis of cellulitis, 99
Peritoneal cancer in differential diagnosis of ovarian cancer, 340
Peritonitis
 secondary
  basic information about, 359
  diagnosis of, 359
  in differential diagnosis of spontaneous bacterial peritonitis, 360
  treatment of, 359
 spontaneous bacterial
  basic information about, 360
  diagnosis of, 360
  treatment of, 360
Peritonsillar abscess in differential diagnosis of epiglottitis, 176
Pernicious anemia; see Anemia, pernicious
Peroneal muscular atrophy, 112
Perphenazine, preparations, dosage, class, adverse effects, 978t
Pertussis
 basic information about, 361
 diagnosis of, 361
 treatment of, 361
Petechia, differential diagnosis of, 653t
Petit mal seizures; see Seizure disorder, absence
Petrositis in differential diagnosis of mastoiditis, 289
pH, average values for arterial and venous plasma or serum, 781t
Pharyngitis
 bacterial, in differential diagnosis of herpangina, 224
 basic information about, 362
 diagnosis of, 362
 in differential diagnosis of acute bronchitis, 82
 in differential diagnosis of Epstein-Barr virus infections, 178
 in differential diagnosis of mononucleosis, 304
 in differential diagnosis of tularemia, 501
 streptococcus, in differential diagnosis of diphtheria, 154
 treatment of, 362
 viral, in differential diagnosis of diphtheria, 154
Phenergan; see Promethazine
Phenobarbital
 drug monitoring data for, 799t
 preparations, dosage, use, half-life, therapeutic level, toxic level, 973t
Phenols, antimicrobial activity, mechanics of action, toxicity, indications and contraindications, 979t
Phenylketonuria, screening recommendations for, 874
Phenytoin
 drug monitoring data for, 799t
 gingival hyperplasia due to, 197
 preparations, dosage, use, half-life, therapeutic level, toxic level, 973t
 for ventricular arrhythmias, indications, dosage, onset of action, therapeutic plasma levels, 1001t

Index

Pheochromocytoma
　basic information about, 363
　diagnosis of, 363
　in differential diagnosis of
　　agoraphobia/panic, 16
　in differential diagnosis of Graves'
　　disease, 207
　in differential diagnosis of
　　hyperthyroidism, 247
　in differential diagnosis of primary
　　aldosteronism, 19
　in differential diagnosis of thyrotoxic
　　storm, 478
　treatment of, 363
Phlebitis; *see* Thrombophlebitis, superficial
Phobias
　basic information about, 364
　diagnosis of, 364
　treatment of, 364
Phosphatase; *see* Acid phosphatase; Alkaline
　phosphatase
Phosphate
　laboratory findings, 821
　serum abnormalities of, disorders
　　associated with, 821
Phosphorus, conditions affecting levels of,
　laboratory findings in, 789*t*
Photosensitivity
　differential diagnosis of, 634*t*
　in differential diagnosis of atopic
　　dermatitis, 146
Photosensitivity eruptions, drug-induced,
　565
PHPT, laboratory findings for calcium and
　phosphorus, 789*t*
Phthalimidine derivative, class,
　preparations, dosage, site of action,
　cost, 978*t*
Phthiriasis palpebrarum in differential
　diagnosis of blepharitis, 73
Phthirus pubis in differential diagnosis of
　blepharitis, 73
Physical activity, counseling to promote,
　881
Physical disability, screening in ambulatory
　elderly, 920*t*
Physical growth curves, *1040*
Physician-patient relationship, difficult,
　factors affecting, 906-907
Pilar casts in differential diagnosis of
　pediculosis, 350
Piles; *see* Hemorrhoids
Pilonidal disease
　basic information about, 365
　diagnosis of, 365
　treatment of, 365
Pilonidal sinus in differential diagnosis of
　anorectal fistula, 42
Pinodolol, preparations, dosage,
　cardioselectivity, lipid solubility, half-
　life, excretion, cost, 981*t*
Pinworms
　in differential diagnosis of prepubescent
　　vulvovaginitis, 527
　in differential diagnosis of pruritus
　　vulvae, 393
Piperacillin, dosage for, and dialysis
　removal, 972*t*
Piroxicam, preparations, dosage, half-life,
　class, cost, metabolism, 998*t*
Pituitary adenoma
　basic information about, 366
　diagnosis of, 366-367
　treatment of, 367
Pituitary infarction in differential diagnosis
　of amenorrhea, 545*t*
Pituitary tumor
　in differential diagnosis of amenorrhea,
　　545*t*

Pituitary tumor—cont'd
　in differential diagnosis of menopause,
　　297
Pityriasis alba in differential diagnosis of
　tinea versicolor, 481
Pityriasis rosea
　basic information about, 368
　diagnosis of, 368
　in differential diagnosis of erythema
　　multiforme, 180
　in differential diagnosis of tinea corporis,
　　479
　in differential diagnosis of tinea
　　versicolor, 481
　treatment of, 368
Pityriasis versicolor; *see* Tinea versicolor
Placenta, separation of, 3
Placenta previa in differential diagnosis of
　abruptio placentae, 3
Placental disorders after cesarean section,
　907
Plague in differential diagnosis of tularemia,
　501
Plague vaccine
　for international travel, 1019*t*
　during pregnancy, 1013*t*
　schedule, indications, side effects,
　　contraindications, during pregnancy,
　　with HIV infection, in
　　immunocompromised patient,
　　1010*t*-1011*t*
Plantar corns in differential diagnosis of
　warts, 529
Plantar fasciitis in differential diagnosis of
　tarsal tunnel syndrome, 464
Plantaris tendon rupture in differential
　diagnosis of Achilles tendon rupture,
　11
Plaque, differential diagnosis of, 650
Plasma cell myeloma; *see* Bone tumor,
　primary malignant; Multiple
　myeloma
Plasmacytoma; *see* Bone tumor, primary
　malignant
Plasminogen activator inhibitor, disorders
　of, inheritance, incidence, bleeding
　symptoms, test results, treatment,
　562*t*
Platelet count
　falsely low, in differential diagnosis of
　　idiopathic thrombocytopenic
　　purpura, 252
　laboratory findings, 821-822
Platelet function disorders
　diagnosis based on routine screening
　　tests, 555*t*
　in differential diagnosis of hemophilia,
　　216
　in differential diagnosis of von
　　Willebrand's disease, 522
Plendil; *see* Felodipine
Pleural effusions
　drug-induced, 635
　encapsulated, in differential diagnosis of
　　atelectasis, 58
　exudative/transudative, 634
　malignant, management of, *958*, 958-959,
　　959
Pleuritis
　in differential diagnosis of pulmonary
　　embolism, 399
　pain from
　　in differential diagnosis of herpes
　　　zoster, 228
　　in differential diagnosis of *Mycoplasma*
　　　pneumonia, 372
Plumbism; *see* Lead poisoning
PMS; *see* Premenstrual syndrome

Pneumococcal bacterial polysaccharide,
　schedule, indications, side effects,
　contraindications, during pregnancy,
　with HIV infection, in
　immunocompromised patient,
　1008*t*-1009*t*
Pneumococcus infection in differential
　diagnosis of corneal ulceration, 137
Pneumococcus pneumonia in differential
　diagnosis of *Mycoplasma* pneumonia,
　372
Pneumococcus vaccine
　for patients with absent or dysfunctional
　　spleen, 928
　during pregnancy, 1014*t*
　recommendations
　　for adults, 891
　　for children, 890
　　for residents of long-term care facilities,
　　　921*t*
Pneumoconioses
　in differential diagnosis of asbestosis, 54
　in differential diagnosis of sarcoidosis,
　　426
Pneumocystis carinii pneumonia
　basic information about, 374
　diagnosis of, 374
　in differential diagnosis of cryptococcosis,
　　141
　treatment of, 374
Pneumonia
　adenovirus, in differential diagnosis of
　　human granulocytic ehrlichiosis,
　　237
　aspiration
　　basic information about, 369
　　diagnosis of, 369
　　treatment of, 369
　atypical; *see* Pneumonia, viral
　bacterial
　　basic information about, 370
　　diagnosis of, 370-371
　　in differential diagnosis of psittacosis,
　　　396
　　in differential diagnosis of viral
　　　pneumonia, 376
　　treatment of, 371
　community-acquired, in differential
　　diagnosis of coccidioidomycoses,
　　125
　in differential diagnosis of acute
　　bronchitis, 82
　in differential diagnosis of acute
　　pancreatitis, 344
　in differential diagnosis of asthma, 56
　in differential diagnosis of atelectasis, 58
　in differential diagnosis of congestive
　　heart failure, 130
　in differential diagnosis of cystic fibrosis,
　　143
　in differential diagnosis of influenza, 257
　in differential diagnosis of lung
　　neoplasm, 277
　in differential diagnosis of malaria, 287
　in differential diagnosis of pertussis, 361
　in differential diagnosis of pulmonary
　　embolism, 399
　Mycoplasma; *see Mycoplasma* pneumonia
　necrotizing, in differential diagnosis of
　　pulmonary tuberculosis, 498
　nonbacterial; *see* Pneumonia, viral
　nosocomial, 323
　with pleurisy, in differential diagnosis of
　　pericarditis, 356
　Pneumocystis carinii; *see Pneumocystis carinii*
　　pneumonia
　ventilator-associated, effect on mortality
　　and morbidity, 942-943

1110 Index

Pneumonia—cont'd
  viral
    basic information about, 375-376
    diagnosis of, 376
    treatment of, 377
Pneumonitis
  in differential diagnosis of toxoplasmosis, 486
  hypersensitivity
    in differential diagnosis of asthma, 56
    in differential diagnosis of bacterial pneumonia, 370
  viral, in differential diagnosis of acute respiratory distress syndrome, 410
Pneumothorax
  in differential diagnosis of pericarditis, 356
  in differential diagnosis of pulmonary embolism, 399
PO_2, average values for arterial and venous plasma or serum, 781*t*
Poisoning
  acetaminophen; *see* Acetaminophen poisoning
  injuries due to, counseling to prevent, 883-884
  lead; *see* Lead poisoning
  treatment protocols for, 1053*t*
Polaramine; *see* Dexchlorpheniramine
Poliomyelitis
  basic information about, 378
  diagnosis of, 378
  in differential diagnosis of Guillain-Barré syndrome, 208
  in differential diagnosis of rabies, 402
  treatment of, 378
Poliomyelitis vaccine
  for adults, schedule, indications, side effects, contraindications, during pregnancy, with HIV infection, in immunocompromised patient, 1006*t*
  for children
    recommendations for, 889
    schedule for, 1005*t*
  for international travel, 1019*t*
  during pregnancy, 1012*t*
Polyarteritis nodosa
  basic information about, 379
  diagnosis of, 379
  treatment of, 379
Polyarthritis, juvenile; *see* Arthritis, juvenile rheumatoid
Polychondritis, relapsing, arthritis due to, course and distribution, 551*t*
Polycystic disease, congenital, in differential diagnosis of echinococcosis, 162
Polycystic ovarian syndrome
  in differential diagnosis of amenorrhea, 545*t*
  in differential diagnosis of menopause, 297
Polycythemia(s)
  differential diagnosis of, 635*t*, *747*
  primary; *see* Polycythemia vera
Polycythemia vera
  basic information about, 380
  diagnosis of, 380, *747*
  differential diagnosis of, 635*t*
  treatment of, 380
Polydipsia, primary, in differential diagnosis of diabetes insipidus, 148
Polyglucosan body disease in differential diagnosis of amyotrophic lateral sclerosis, 25
Polymorphous light eruption in differential diagnosis of photosensitivity, 634*t*
Polymyalgia rheumatica
  basic information about, 381
  diagnosis of, 381

Polymyalgia rheumatica—cont'd
  in differential diagnosis of fibromyalgia, 184
  in differential diagnosis of rheumatoid arthritis, 53
  treatment of, 381
Polymyositis
  in differential diagnosis of Lambert-Eaton syndrome, 265
  in differential diagnosis of myasthenia gravis, 312
  in differential diagnosis of polymyalgia rheumatica, 381
Polymyxin B, dosage for, and dialysis removal, 972*t*
Polyneuropathy
  acute; *see* Guillain-Barré syndrome
  in differential diagnosis of lead poisoning, 267
  drug-induced, 635
  hereditary, in differential diagnosis of Guillain-Barré syndrome, 208
  idiopathic dominantly inherited hypertrophic; *see* Charcot-Marie-Tooth disease
  symmetric, 636
Polyps
  cervical; *see* Cervical polyps
  nasal, in differential diagnosis of chronic rhinitis, 644
  rectal, in differential diagnosis of hemorrhoids, 217
Polyradiculopathy in differential diagnosis of peripheral nerve dysfunction, 358
Polyuria
  causes of, 636
  in differential diagnosis of enuresis, 173
Popliteal artery entrapment syndrome in differential diagnosis of leg pain, 615*t*
Popliteal swelling, causes of, 636
Popliteal synovial membrane, ruptured, in differential diagnosis of swollen limbs, 657*t*
Poradenitis inguinalis; *see* Lymphogranuloma venereum
Porphyria cutanea tarda in differential diagnosis of photosensitivity, 634*t*
Porphyromonas, infections due to, 26
Posterior drawer sign, 1026
Posterior fossa, masses of, in differential diagnosis of trigeminal neuralgia, 493
Postherpetic neuralgia
  in differential diagnosis of cluster headache, 209
  treatment of, *720*
Postphlebitic syndrome
  in differential diagnosis of deep vein thrombosis, 473
  in differential diagnosis of swollen limbs, 657*t*
Posttraumatic stress disorder
  basic information about, 382
  diagnosis of, 382
  treatment of, 382
Potassium
  laboratory findings, 822
  serum abnormalities of, disorders associated with, 822
  urine, 836
Potassium-sparing diuretics, class, preparations, dosage, site of action, cost, 978*t*
Pott's disease; *see* Arthritis, granulomatous
Povidone-iodine solution, antimicrobial activity, mechanics of action, toxicity, indications and contraindications, 979*t*

Povidone-iodine surgical scrub, antimicrobial activity, mechanics of action, toxicity, indications and contraindications, 979*t*
PPD; *see* Purified protein derivative
Pravachol; *see* Pravastatin
Pravastatin
  preparations, dosage, mechanism of action, effect, cost, 993*t*
  for reducing transient myocardial ischemia in angina pectoris, 957
Prazepam, preparations, dosage, half-life, indication, cost, 980*t*
Prazosin, preparations, dosage, cost, 969*t*
Precef; *see* Ceforanide
Precocious puberty
  basic information about, 383
  causes of, 638
  diagnosis of, 383
  evaluation of, *750*
  treatment of, 383
Precose; *see* Acarbose
Prednisolone for acute infectious mononucleosis, 946-947
Prednisone
  for acute COPD exacerbation, *945*, 945-946, *946*
  comparison chart for, 987*t*
  and reduced disability in rheumatoid arthritis, *931*, 931-932
Preeclampsia, 384-385
  aspirin for preventing, 895
  basic information about, 384
  calcium supplementation and, 949-950
  diagnosis of, 384-385
  in differential diagnosis of acute glomerulonephritis, 200
  in differential diagnosis of fatty liver of pregnancy, 181
  in differential diagnosis of thrombotic thrombocytopenic purpura, 474
  in pregnancy, characteristics of, 617*t*
  screening recommendations for, 870-871
  treatment of, 385
Pregnancy
  aspirin prophylaxis in, 895
  assessing alcohol use during, 877-878
  back pain during, *910*, 910-911
  blood pressure measurement in, 871
  breast cancer during, 79
  cholestasis of, in differential diagnosis of fatty liver of pregnancy, 181
  D incompatibility testing in, 871
  in differential diagnosis of idiopathic thrombocytopenic purpura, 252
  in differential diagnosis of uterine myomas, 514
  drug abuse during, 878
  early, bleeding in, *687*
  ectopic
    after cesarean sections, 907
    basic information about, 164
    diagnosis of, 164
    in differential diagnosis of benign ovarian tumor, 341
    in differential diagnosis of dysmenorrhea, 161
    in differential diagnosis of endometriosis, 170
    in differential diagnosis of pelvic inflammatory disease, 352
    in differential diagnosis of spontaneous miscarriage, 446
    in differential diagnosis of urolithiasis, 510
    ruptured, in differential diagnosis of secondary peritonitis, 359
    treatment of, 164
  electronic fetal monitoring during, 871

Pregnancy—cont'd
  elevated lead levels during, screening for, 862-863
  fatty liver of
    basic information about, 181
    diagnosis of, 181
    in differential diagnosis of preeclampsia, 384
    treatment of, 181
  gestational diabetes mellitus in, long-term effect of, 943
  gonorrhea screening during, 865
  hematocrit during, 861
  hemoglobin analysis during, 861
  hepatitis B screening during, 863
  HIV screening during, 865-866
  home uterine activity monitoring in, 871-872
  hypertension and preeclampsia in, calcium supplementation and, 949-950
  immunizations during, 1012t-1016t
  liver disease in, characteristics of, 617t
  maternal weight prior to, and risk of neural tube defects, 914-915
  periodic health examination during, 851t-852t
    for high-risk populations, 851t-852t
  renin-aldosterone patterns in, 826t
  screening during
    for bacteriuria, 868
    for chlamydial infection, 867
    for Down syndrome, 872
    for genital herpes simplex infection, 867
    for neural tube defects, 872-873
  screening for iron deficiency anemia during, 861
  seizures of; see Eclampsia
  sickle cell disease in, 944
  syphilis screening during, 864
  tetanus/diphtheria vaccine during, 1007t
  toxemia of; see also Preeclampsia
    in differential diagnosis of nephrotic syndrome, 319
  ultrasonography during, 870
  unintended, counseling to prevent, 887
  vaginal bleeding during, 662
    basic information about, 517
    diagnosis of, 517
    treatment of, 517
  in women with moderate/severe renal insufficiency, 939
Pregnancy-induced hypertension; see Preeclampsia
Preleukemia; see Myelodysplastic syndromes
Premenopausal state
  in differential diagnosis of Graves' disease, 207
  in differential diagnosis of hyperthyroidism, 247
Premenstrual syndrome
  basic information about, 386
  diagnosis of, 386
  treatment of, 386-387
Prenatal disorders, 870-872
Pressure ulcers
  demographic characteristics of subjects, according to outcome and clinical setting, 916t
  incidence of, factors influencing, 915-917
  predicting development of, 916t, 917t
  predicting prescriptive practices in prevention of, 917t
Presyncope
  in differential diagnosis of dizziness, 569
  in differential diagnosis of partial seizure disorder, 434
Prevacid; see Lansoprazole

Prevotella, infections due to, 26
Prilosec; see Omeprazole
Primary adrenocortical insufficiency in differential diagnosis of Addison's disease, 15
Primidone
  drug monitoring data for, 799t
  preparations, dosage, use, half-life, therapeutic level, toxic level, 973t
Prinivil; see Lisinopril
Prinzmetal's variant, 37
Problem drinking; see also Alcohol abuse; Alcoholism
  AUDIT structured interview for assessing, 877t
  during pregnancy, 877-878
  referring patients with, 878
  screening for, 876-878
Probucol, preparations, dosage, mechanism of action, effect, cost, 993t
Procainamide
  dosage, half-life, ECG manifestations, toxicity, 1000t
  drug monitoring data for, 799t
  electrophysiologic effects of, 969t
  for ventricular arrhythmias, indications, dosage, onset of action, therapeutic plasma levels, 1001t
Procarbazine, toxicity of, 984t-985t
Procardia; see Nifedipine
Prochlorperazine, preparations, dosage, class, 976t
Proctitis in differential diagnosis of lymphogranuloma venereum, 283
Proctocolitis, idiopathic; see also Ulcerative colitis
  in differential diagnosis of pelvic inflammatory disease, 352
Progestin and beneficial effects of estrogen replacement therapy, 934-935
Prolactin
  increased, gynecomastia associated with, 587
  laboratory findings, 822
Prolactinoma, 366
  basic information about, 388
  diagnosis of, 388
  differential diagnosis of, 366
  in differential diagnosis of amenorrhea, 545t
  treatment of, 367, 388
Proliferative diabetic retinopathy; see Diabetic retinopathy
Prolixin; see Fluphenazine
Promethazine, preparations, dosage, class, 976t
Pronestyl; see Procainamide
Propafenone
  dosage, half-life, ECG manifestations, toxicity, 1000t
  electrophysiologic effects of, 969t
Propoxyphene, equivalent dose, duration, preparations, dosage, 995t
Propranolol
  drug monitoring data for, 799t
  electrophysiologic effects of, 969t
  preparations, dosage, cardioselectivity, lipid solubility, half-life, excretion, cost, 981t
ProSom; see Estazolam
Prostate cancer
  basic information about, 389
  diagnosis of, 389
  in differential diagnosis of benign prostatic hyperplasia, 390
  follow-up strategies for, 1052t
  screening for, 858
  treatment of, 389

Prostate stones in differential diagnosis of prostate cancer, 389
Prostate symptom score, international, *1028*
Prostatic hyperplasia, benign
  basic information about, 390
  diagnosis of, 390-391
  treatment of, 391
Prostatic hypertrophy; see Prostatic hyperplasia, benign
Prostatic specific antigen, laboratory findings, 822
Prostatitis
  in differential diagnosis of benign prostatic hyperplasia, 390
  in differential diagnosis of prostate cancer, 389
Prosthetic valves, endocarditis due to, 168
Protein
  C-reactive, 797
  serum
    electrophoretic patterns, *824*
    laboratory findings, 822
Protein C deficiency, characteristics and causes, 594
Protein electrophoresis, laboratory values, 823
Protein S deficiency, characteristics and causes, 594
Proteinuria, causes of, 637
Prothrombin, disorders of, inheritance, incidence, bleeding symptoms, test results, treatment, 561t
Prothrombin time, laboratory values, 823
Proton pump inhibitors, preparations, dosage, cost, 968t
Protoporphyrin, laboratory values, 823
Protozoa, granulomatous disorders due to, 584
Protozoal infection
  in differential diagnosis of acute viral encephalitis, 166
  in differential diagnosis of ulcerative colitis, 505
Protriptyline, preparations, dosage, class, effects, half-life, 974t
Prozac; see Fluoxetine
Pruigo nodularis in differential diagnosis of Kaposi's sarcoma, 260
Pruritus
  causes of, 637
  evaluation of, *748*
  history, manifestations, and malignancy associated with, 564t
Pruritus ani
  basic information about, 392
  diagnosis of, 392
  treatment of, 392
Pruritus vulvae
  basic information about, 393
  diagnosis of, 393
  treatment of, 393
Pseudo-Cushing's syndrome, alcoholic, in differential diagnosis of Cushing's syndrome, 142
Pseudofolliculitis barbae in differential diagnosis of folliculitis, 187
Pseudogout
  basic information about, 394
  characteristics of, 550t
  diagnosis of, 394
  in differential diagnosis of cellulitis, 99
  in differential diagnosis of gout, 205
  knee pain due to, findings, diagnosis, and management, 610t
  treatment of, 394
Pseudohemophilia; see von Willebrand's disease
Pseudohypoaldosteronism in differential diagnosis of hypoaldosteronism, 249

Index

Pseudohypoparathyroidism in differential diagnosis of hypocalcemia, 599t
Pseudomembranous colitis
  basic information about, 395
  diagnosis of, 395
  in differential diagnosis of Crohn's disease, 140
  treatment of, 395
Pseudomembranous conjunctivitis; *see* Conjunctivitis
Pseudomembranous croup; *see* Tracheitis
Pseudomonas infection in differential diagnosis of corneal ulceration, 137
Pseudomonas septicemia, history, rash characteristics and distribution, clinical findings, diagnostic aids, 577t-578t
Pseudoneurologic illness; *see* Conversion disorder
Pseudoobstruction in differential diagnosis of encopresis, 167
Pseudoseizure in differential diagnosis of eclampsia, 163
Pseudoxanthomylastica; *see* Retinal hemorrhage
Psittacosis
  basic information about, 396
  diagnosis of, 396
  in differential diagnosis of tularemia, 501
  treatment of, 396
Psoriasis
  basic information about, 397
  diagnosis of, 397
  in differential diagnosis of atopic dermatitis, 146
  in differential diagnosis of balanitis, 66
  in differential diagnosis of basal cell carcinoma, 67
  in differential diagnosis of cellulitis, 99
  in differential diagnosis of contact dermatitis, 147
  in differential diagnosis of nail disorders, 625t
  in differential diagnosis of pityriasis rosea, 368
  in differential diagnosis of tinea corporis, 479
  in differential diagnosis of tinea cruris, 480
  treatment of, 397
Psoriatic arthritis; *see* Arthritis, psoriatic
Psychiatric disorders; *see also* specific disorders
  in differential diagnosis of drug abuse, 7
  in differential diagnosis of rabies, 402
  in differential diagnosis of thyrotoxic storm, 478
Psychogenic headache; *see* Headache, tension-type
Psychogenic rheumatism; *see* Fibromyalgia
Psychogenic spells in differential diagnosis of epilepsy, 572t
Psychologic disorders in differential diagnosis of endometriosis, 170
Psychomotor seizures, 434
Psychomyogenic headache; *see* Headache, tension-type
Psychosis
  cycloid; *see* Bipolar disorder
  in differential diagnosis of bipolar disorder, 69
  in differential diagnosis of obsessive-compulsive disorder, 325
  in differential diagnosis of pedophilia, 351
  Korsakoff's, 262
Psychosomatic illness; *see* Conversion disorder

PTH syndrome, ectopic, laboratory findings for calcium and phosphorus, 789t
Pubertas praecox; *see* Precocious puberty
Puberty
  delayed
    causes of, 638
    evaluation of, 749
  precocious; *see* Precocious puberty
PUD; *see* Peptic ulcer disease
Pulmonary disease
  chronic, in differential diagnosis of hypertrophic cardiomyopathy, 90
  in differential diagnosis of angina pectoris, 37
  in differential diagnosis of costochondritis, 138
  frank, in differential diagnosis of dilated cardiomyopathy, 89
  year book of, 900, 958-964
Pulmonary edema
  basic information about, 398
  cardiogenic, in differential diagnosis of acute respiratory distress syndrome, 410
  diagnosis of, 398
  in differential diagnosis of bacterial pneumonia, 370
  treatment of, 398
Pulmonary embolism
  basic information about, 399
  diagnosis of, 399-400
  in differential diagnosis of asthma, 56
  in differential diagnosis of bacterial pneumonia, 370
  in differential diagnosis of cardiac tamponade, 88
  in differential diagnosis of chronic obstructive pulmonary disease, 120
  in differential diagnosis of congestive heart failure, 130
  in differential diagnosis of *Mycoplasma* pneumonia, 372
  in differential diagnosis of pulmonary edema, 398
  in differential diagnosis of septicemia, 436
  pain from, in differential diagnosis of herpes zoster, 228
  treatment of, 400
Pulmonary fibrosis in differential diagnosis of pulmonary edema, 398
Pulmonary function abnormalities, laboratory findings in, 639t
Pulmonary hypertension in differential diagnosis of atrial septal defect, 61
Pulmonary infarction in differential diagnosis of pericarditis, 356
Pulmonary nodule, evaluation of, 751
Pulmonary regurgitation in differential diagnosis of mitral regurgitation, 300
Pulmonary stenosis in differential diagnosis of atrial septal defect, 61
Pulseless electrical activity, evaluation of, 752
Pupillary block glaucoma; *see* Glaucoma, primary closed-angle
Purified protein derivative
  assessment of, 1046t
  vaccine
    administration of, 1017t
Purpura
  causes of, 640
  differential diagnosis of, 653t
  immune thrombocytopenic; *see* Idiopathic thrombocytopenic purpura
  palpable, diagnosis of, 753

Purpura—cont'd
  thrombotic thrombocytopenic; *see* Thrombotic thrombocytopenic purpura
Purulent otitis media; *see* Otitis media
Pustules, differential diagnosis of, 649
Pyelonephritis
  basic information about, 401
  diagnosis of, 401
  in differential diagnosis of cholangitis, 115
  in differential diagnosis of hyperemesis gravidarum, 241
  in differential diagnosis of preeclampsia, 384
  in differential diagnosis of urolithiasis, 510
  recurrent, 509
  treatment of, 401
Pyoderma; *see also* Impetigo
  staphylococcal, in differential diagnosis of acne vulgaris, 12
Pyoderma gangrenosum, history, manifestations, and malignancy associated with, 564t
Pyogenic arthritis; *see* Arthritis, infectious
Pyogenic granuloma in differential diagnosis of Kaposi's sarcoma, 260
Pyelonephrosis; *see* Pyelonephritis
Pyosalpinx; *see* Pelvic inflammatory disease
Pyrophosphate arthropathy; *see* Pseudogout

Q

Q fever
  in differential diagnosis of human granulocytic ehrlichiosis, 237
  in differential diagnosis of *Mycoplasma* pneumonia, 372
  in differential diagnosis of tularemia, 501
Quazepam, preparations, dosage, half-life, indication, cost, 980t
Quinapril, dosage, onset of action, peak effect, half-life, cost, 967t
Quinazoline, class, preparations, dosage, site of action, cost, 978t
Quinidine, electrophysiologic effects of, 969t
Quinidine sulfate
  dosage, half-life, ECG manifestations, toxicity, 1000t
  drug monitoring data for, 799t
Quinolones, dosage for, and dialysis removal, 972t

R

Rabbit fever; *see* Tularemia
Rabies
  basic information about, 402
  chemoprophylaxis of, 894
  diagnosis of, 402
  treatment of, 402
Rabies human diploid cell vaccine, schedule, indications, side effects, contraindications, during pregnancy, with HIV infection, in immunocompromised patient, 1008t-1009t
Rabies immune globulin, administration of, 1018t
Rabies vaccine
  for international travel, 1019t
  during pregnancy, 1013t, 1015t
Radial nerve compression in differential diagnosis of epicondylitis, 174
Radiation enteritis
  in differential diagnosis of Crohn's disease, 140

Radiation enteritis—cont'd
  in differential diagnosis of ulcerative colitis, 505
Radiculopathy
  cervical
    in differential diagnosis of carpal tunnel syndrome, 93
    in differential diagnosis of epicondylitis, 174
    in differential diagnosis of thoracic outlet syndrome, 470
  proximal, in differential diagnosis of tarsal tunnel syndrome, 464
Ramipril, dosage, onset of action, peak effect, half-life, cost, 967t
Ramsay Hunt syndrome
  basic information about, 403
  diagnosis of, 403
  treatment of, 403
Ranitidine, preparations, dosage, cost, 968t
Ranula in differential diagnosis of congenital anomalies presenting as neck masses, 628t
Rash, life-threatening diseases associated with, differential diagnosis of, 577t-579t
Rasmussen encephalitis; see Encephalitis, acute viral
Rat-bite fever in differential diagnosis of tularemia, 500
Raynaud's disease, complement deficiencies associated with, 794t
Raynaud's phenomenon
  basic information about, 404
  diagnosis of, 404-405
  treatment of, 405
Reactive airway disease; see Asthma
Rebound headache in differential diagnosis of tension-type headache, 211
Recommended daily dietary allowances, 1047t
Rectal cancer; see Colorectal cancer
Rectal pain, causes of, 640
Rectal polyp in differential diagnosis of hemorrhoids, 217
Rectal prolapse
  in differential diagnosis of encopresis, 167
  in differential diagnosis of hemorrhoids, 217
Red blood cell distribution width, laboratory values, 824-825
Red blood cells
  mass, laboratory values, 825
  morphology, laboratory values, 825
Red eye; see also Conjunctivitis
  differential diagnosis of, 640t
Reflex sympathetic dystrophy
  in differential diagnosis of carpal tunnel syndrome, 93
  in differential diagnosis of thoracic outlet syndrome, 470
Reflux esophagitis; see Gastroesophageal reflux disorder
Refractive amblyopia; see Amblyopia
Refractory anemia; see Anemia, aplastic
Reglan; see Metoclopramide
Reifenstein syndrome, phenotypes, karyotypes, inheritance, hormone levels, pathogenesis, 546t
Reiter's syndrome
  of axial skeleton, characteristics of, 549t
  basic information about, 406
  characteristics of, 656t
  course and distribution, 551t
  diagnosis of, 406
  in differential diagnosis of balanitis, 66
  knee pain due to, findings, diagnosis, and management, 610t
  treatment of, 406

Relafen; see Nabumetone
Relapsing fever in differential diagnosis of human granulocytic ehrlichiosis, 237
Remeron; see Mirtazapine
Renal acidosis, laboratory findings for calcium and phosphorus, 789t
Renal calculus in differential diagnosis of pelvic inflammatory disease, 352
Renal carbuncle; see Pyelonephritis
Renal colic; see also Urolithiasis
  in differential diagnosis of acute pancreatitis, 344
  pain from, in differential diagnosis of herpes zoster, 228
Renal disease
  complement deficiencies associated with, 794t
  in differential diagnosis of dysfunctional uterine bleeding, 159
  in differential diagnosis of nephrotic syndrome, 319
  end-stage, blood pressure and, 939-940
  renin-aldosterone patterns in, 826t
Renal failure
  acute
    basic information about, 407
    diagnosis of, 407
    in intensive care units, 927t, 927-928
    mortality from, 928
    treatment of, 407
  chronic
    basic information about, 408
    diagnosis of, 408
    in differential diagnosis of diffuse interstitial lung disease, 153
    treatment of, 408
  in differential diagnosis of disseminated intravascular coagulation, 155
  in differential diagnosis of myelodysplastic syndromes, 313
  in differential diagnosis of myxedema coma, 317
  oliguric; see Hepatorenal syndrome
  serum and radiographic abnormalities in, 641t
  urinary abnormalities in, 642t
Renal insufficiency in pregnant women, 939
Renal pulmonary disease, drug-induced, in differential diagnosis of Goodpasture's syndrome, 204
Renal tubular acidosis
  basic information about, 409
  diagnosis of, 409
  treatment of, 409
Renin-aldosterone patterns in various conditions, 826t
Renin-secreting tumor in differential diagnosis of primary aldosteronism, 19
Repolarization, early, ST segment elevation in, 657t
Reserpine, preparations, dosage, cost, 969t
Resistant ovary syndrome in differential diagnosis of amenorrhea, 545t
Respiratory acidosis, 542
  in differential diagnosis of renal tubular acidosis, 409
  laboratory findings in, 781t
Respiratory alkalosis, 543
  laboratory findings in, 781t
Respiratory disease in differential diagnosis of agoraphobia/panic, 16
Respiratory disorders, sports participation and, 1036t
Respiratory distress syndrome, acute; see Acute respiratory distress syndrome
Respiratory failure, hypoventilatory, causes of, 642

Respiratory infections
  in differential diagnosis of chronic obstructive pulmonary disease, 120
  passive smoking and, 938
Respiratory procedures
  endocarditis prophylaxis and, 1023
  prophylactic regimens for, 1023t
Respiratory syncytial virus in differential diagnosis of influenza, 257
Restoril; see Temazepam
Reticulocyte count, laboratory values, 826
Reticuloendotheliosis, leukemic; see Hairy cell leukemia
Retinal detachment
  basic information about, 412
  diagnosis of, 412
  in differential diagnosis of retinoblastoma, 415
  in differential diagnosis of uveitis, 516
  treatment of, 412
Retinal hemorrhage
  basic information about, 413
  diagnosis of, 413
  treatment of, 413
Retinal lesions in differential diagnosis of cataract, 94
Retinal trauma; see Retinal hemorrhage
Retinal vein/artery, occlusion of, in differential diagnosis of amaurosis fugax, 21
Retinitis pigmentosa
  basic information about, 414
  diagnosis of, 414
  treatment of, 414
Retinoblastoma
  basic information about, 415
  diagnosis of, 415
  treatment of, 415
Retinopathy
  diabetic; see Diabetic retinopathy
  in differential diagnosis of uveitis, 516
  high altitude, 413
  toxic, in differential diagnosis of retinitis pigmentosa, 414
Retrobulbar neuritis; see Optic neuritis
Retroperitoneal adenitis in differential diagnosis of lymphogranuloma venereum, 283
Retroperitoneal cyst/neoplasm in differential diagnosis of benign ovarian tumor, 341
Retrovir; see Zidovudine
Retroviral infections, drug therapy for; see Antiretroviral agents
Rett's syndrome in differential diagnosis of autistic disorder, 63
Reye's syndrome in differential diagnosis of fatty liver of pregnancy, 181
Rezulin; see Troglitazone
Rh incompatibility; see also D incompatibility
  basic information about, 417
  diagnosis of, 417
  treatment of, 417
Rhabdomyolysis
  basic information about, 418
  diagnosis of, 418
  treatment of, 418
Rheumatic carditis; see Rheumatic fever
Rheumatic fever
  acute, in differential diagnosis of toxic shock syndrome, 484
  arthritis due to, course and distribution, 551t
  basic information about, 419
  diagnosis of, 419
  in differential diagnosis of infective endocarditis, 168

Rheumatic fever—cont'd
  in differential diagnosis of juvenile rheumatoid arthritis, 51
  in differential diagnosis of Reiter's syndrome, 406
  treatment of, 419
Rheumatic heart disease in differential diagnosis of atrial septal defect, 61
Rheumatism
  nonarticular; see Fibromyalgia
  psychogenic; see Fibromyalgia
Rheumatoid arthritis
  of axial skeleton, characteristics of, 549t
  basic information about, 53
  course and distribution, 551t
  diagnosis of, 53
  in differential diagnosis of Charcot's joint, 111
  in differential diagnosis of chronic fatigue syndrome, 119
  in differential diagnosis of fibromyalgia, 184
  in differential diagnosis of gout, 205
  in differential diagnosis of polymyalgia rheumatica, 381
  in differential diagnosis of pseudogout, 394
  in differential diagnosis of psoriatic arthritis, 52
  in differential diagnosis of Reiter's syndrome, 406
  in differential diagnosis of rheumatic fever, 419
  juvenile; see Arthritis, juvenile rheumatoid
  knee pain due to, findings, diagnosis, and management, 610t
  neuropathies associated with, 631t
  reduced disability in, with drug-based treatment, 931, 931-932
  treatment of, 53
Rheumatoid disease in differential diagnosis of Sheehan's syndrome, 437
Rheumatoid factor
  diseases associated with, 828
  laboratory values, 826
Rheumatoid syndrome, anarthritic; see Polymyalgia rheumatica
Rhinitis
  allergic
    basic information about, 420
    diagnosis of, 420
    drug therapy for, 977t
    treatment of, 420
  atrophic, in differential diagnosis of chronic rhinitis, 645t
  chronic, classification and therapy of, 643t-646t
  in differential diagnosis of asthma, 56
  eosinophilic allergic, findings, diagnosis, therapy, 643t
  eosinophilic nonallergic, findings, diagnosis, therapy, 643t
  structurally related, in differential diagnosis of chronic rhinitis, 645t
Rhinitis medicamentosa
  in differential diagnosis of allergic rhinitis, 420
  in differential diagnosis of chronic rhinitis, 645t
Rhinorrhea, treatment of, 754
Rhodococcus equi pneumonia in differential diagnosis of pulmonary tuberculosis, 498
Rickets
  basic information about, 421
  diagnosis of, 421

Rickets—cont'd
  in differential diagnosis of hypocalcemia, 599t
  treatment of, 421
Riedel's thyroiditis; see Thyroiditis
Rift Valley fever in differential diagnosis of yellow fever, 533
Right ventricular infarction in differential diagnosis of cardiac tamponade, 88
Ringworm; see Tinea corporis; Tinea cruris
Rinne's test, method and interpretation, 1027t
Risperdal; see Risperidone
Risperidone, preparations, dosage, class, adverse effects, 978t
Ritonavir, therapeutic class, preparations, dosage, toxicities, cost, 970t
River blindness, epidemiology, transmission, manifestations, diagnosis, treatment, 629t
Rocephin; see Ceftriaxone
Rocky Mountain spotted fever
  ages affected, prodrome, morphology, distribution, diagnosis, 575t
  in differential diagnosis of bacterial meningitis, 294
  in differential diagnosis of human granulocytic ehrlichiosis, 237
  in differential diagnosis of toxic shock syndrome, 484
  in differential diagnosis of viral meningitis, 295
  history, rash characteristics and distribution, clinical findings, diagnostic aids, 577t
Rosacea
  basic information about, 422
  diagnosis of, 422
  treatment of, 422
Roseola exanthem, ages affected, prodrome, morphology, distribution, diagnosis, 574t
Rotator cuff syndrome
  basic information about, 423
  diagnosis of, 423
  in differential diagnosis of cervical disc syndromes, 103
  in differential diagnosis of frozen shoulder, 191
  in differential diagnosis of shoulder pain, 648t
  treatment of, 423
RTA; see Renal tubular acidosis
Rubella
  ages affected, prodrome, morphology, distribution, diagnosis, 574t
  arthritis due to, course and distribution, 551t
  screening recommendations for, 868
Rubella vaccine; see also Measles-mumps-rubella vaccine
  for international travel, 1019t
  during pregnancy, 1012t
Rule of Nines, 1059t
Rythmol; see Propafenone

S

Salicylate poisoning in differential diagnosis of diabetic ketoacidosis, 151
Salivary gland infection in differential diagnosis of nonneoplastic neck mass, 626t
Salivary gland neoplasm in differential diagnosis of sialadenitis, 439
Salmonella
  in differential diagnosis of infective endocarditis, 168
  food poisoning due to, 188

Salmonellosis
  basic information about, 424
  diagnosis of, 424-425
  in differential diagnosis of babesiosis, 64
  treatment of, 425
Salpingitis; see Pelvic inflammatory disease
Salsalate, preparations, dosage, half-life, class, cost, metabolism, 998t
Salt deficiency, renin-aldosterone patterns in, 826t
Salt excess, renin-aldosterone patterns in, 826t
Salt-losing nephritis in differential diagnosis of Addison's disease, 15
San Joaquin Valley fever; see Coccidioidomycoses
Saquinavir, therapeutic class, preparations, dosage, toxicities, cost, 970t
Sarcoid granulomatosis, necrotizing, differential diagnosis of, 585t-586t
Sarcoidosis
  arthritis due to, course and distribution, 551t
  basic information about, 426
  CNS, in differential diagnosis of listeriosis, 275
  diagnosis of, 426
  in differential diagnosis of bacterial pneumonia, 370
  in differential diagnosis of Bell's palsy, 68
  in differential diagnosis of coccidioidomycoses, 125
  in differential diagnosis of diffuse interstitial lung disease, 153
  in differential diagnosis of granulomatous arthritis, 49
  in differential diagnosis of Hodgkin's disease, 233
  in differential diagnosis of listeriosis, 275
  in differential diagnosis of lung neoplasm, 277
  in differential diagnosis of pulmonary edema, 398
  in differential diagnosis of pulmonary tuberculosis, 498
  in differential diagnosis of Sheehan's syndrome, 437
  granulomatosis associated with, 585t-586t
  laboratory findings for calcium and phosphorus, 789t
  neuropathies associated with, 631t
  treatment of, 426
Sarcoma
  in differential diagnosis of cervical polyps, 106
  Kaposi's; see Kaposi's sarcoma
  of vagina; see Vaginal malignancy
  vulvar; see Vulvar cancer
Scabies
  basic information about, 427
  diagnosis of, 427
  in differential diagnosis of atopic dermatitis, 146
  in differential diagnosis of chickenpox, 113
  in differential diagnosis of contact dermatitis, 147
  in differential diagnosis of impetigo, 253
  in differential diagnosis of pediculosis, 350
  treatment of, 427
Scalded-skin syndrome
  in differential diagnosis of Stevens-Johnson syndrome, 452
  in differential diagnosis of toxic shock syndrome, 484
Scales, differential diagnosis of, 651

Scarlet fever
  ages affected, prodrome, morphology, distribution, diagnosis, 575t
  in differential diagnosis of toxic shock syndrome, 484
Scars, differential diagnosis of, 652
SCC; see Squamous cell carcinoma
Schilling test, 827
Schistosomes, epidemiology, transmission, manifestations, diagnosis, treatment, 660t
Schistosomiasis in differential diagnosis of lymphogranuloma venereum, 283
Schizophrenia, 428-429
  basic information about, 428
  childhood-onset, in differential diagnosis of autistic disorder, 63
  diagnosis of, 428-429
  in differential diagnosis of anorexia nervosa, 43
  in differential diagnosis of bulimia nervosa, 84
  treatment of, 429
Schwabach's test, method and interpretation, 1027t
Scleritis
  basic information about, 430
  diagnosis of, 430
  in differential diagnosis of conjunctivitis, 132
  in differential diagnosis of episcleritis, 177
  in differential diagnosis of uveitis, 516
  treatment of, 430
Sclerodermal renal crisis in differential diagnosis of acute glomerulonephritis, 200
Scleromalacia perforans; see Scleritis
Sclerosis, disseminated; see Multiple sclerosis
Scoliosis
  adolescent idiopathic, screening recommendations for, 875
  basic information about, 431
  diagnosis of, 431
  in differential diagnosis of endometriosis, 170
  juvenile idiopathic, 947-948
  treatment of, 431
Scrotal mass, treatment of, 755
Sebaceous cyst
  in differential diagnosis of breast abscess, 77
  perianal, in differential diagnosis of anorectal fistula, 42
Sebaceous hyperplasia
  in differential diagnosis of acne vulgaris, 12
  in differential diagnosis of basal cell carcinoma, 67
Seborrheic dermatitis
  in differential diagnosis of atopic dermatitis, 146
  in differential diagnosis of contact dermatitis, 147
  in differential diagnosis of pediculosis, 350
  in differential diagnosis of rosacea, 422
  in differential diagnosis of scabies, 427
  in differential diagnosis of tinea cruris, 480
  in differential diagnosis of tinea versicolor, 481
Seborrheic keratoses
  in differential diagnosis of melanoma, 291
  in differential diagnosis of warts, 529
  multiple, history, manifestations, and malignancy associated with, 564t

Sectral; see Acebutolol
Sedatives in differential diagnosis of narcolepsy, 318
Seizure disorders
  absence
    basic information about, 432
    diagnosis of, 432
    treatment of, 432
  in differential diagnosis of agoraphobia/panic, 16
  in differential diagnosis of sleep apnea, 443
  generalized tonic-clonic
    basic information about, 433
    diagnosis of, 433
    treatment of, 433
  partial
    basic information about, 434
    diagnosis of, 434
    treatment of, 434
Seizures
  in differential diagnosis of bacterial meningitis, 294
  in differential diagnosis of cerebrovascular accident, 101
  in differential diagnosis of narcolepsy, 318
  in differential diagnosis of transient ischemic attack, 490
  in differential diagnosis of viral meningitis, 295
  drug therapy for; see Anticonvulsants
  febrile
    basic information about, 435
    diagnosis of, 435
    treatment of, 435
  of pregnancy; see Eclampsia
Self-injurious behavior in differential diagnosis of Munchausen's syndrome, 210
Self-murder; see Suicide
Self-wetting; see Enuresis
Semen, frozen donor; see Insemination, therapeutic (frozen donor semen)
Senile cataract; see Cataract
Senile chorea in differential diagnosis of Huntington's chorea, 238
Sepsis; see also Septicemia
  biliary; see Cholangitis
  in differential diagnosis of Addison's disease, 15
  in differential diagnosis of hyperosmolar coma, 243
  in differential diagnosis of secondary peritonitis, 359
Septal obstruction in differential diagnosis of allergic rhinitis, 420
Septic arthritis; see also Arthritis, infectious
  in differential diagnosis of Legg-Calvé-Perthes disease, 268
Septic diskitis in differential diagnosis of low back pain, 554t
Septic shock; see also Septicemia
  in differential diagnosis of toxic shock syndrome, 484
Septicemia
  basic information about, 436
  Candida, history, rash characteristics and distribution, clinical findings, diagnostic aids, 578t
  diagnosis of, 436
  Pseudomonas, history, rash characteristics and distribution, clinical findings, diagnostic aids, 577t
  staphylococcal, history, rash characteristics and distribution, clinical findings, diagnostic aids, 577t
  treatment of, 436

Serax; see Oxazepam
Serentil; see Mesoridazine
Serpasil; see Reserpine
Sertraline, preparations, dosage, class, effects, half-life, 974t
Serum albumin, assessment of, 1046t
Serum hepatitis; see Hepatitis B
Serum osmolality, formula for, 1042
Serum sickness
  in differential diagnosis of erythema multiforme, 180
  in differential diagnosis of juvenile rheumatoid arthritis, 51
  in differential diagnosis of nephrotic syndrome, 319
  in differential diagnosis of rheumatic fever, 419
  in differential diagnosis of Stevens-Johnson syndrome, 452
Serum transferrin, assessment of, 1046t
Serum tumor markers
  for ovarian cancer, 859
  for prostate cancer, 858
Serzone; see Nefazodone
Sex cord stromal tumor; see Ovarian cancer
Sexual abuse; see also Child abuse; Pedophilia
  in differential diagnosis of prepubescent vulvovaginitis, 527
Sexual assault, STD treatment following, 1056t
Sexual behavior
  ages 11-24 years, 845t
  counseling about, 886-887
  high-risk
    ages 11-24 years, 845t-846t
    ages 25-64 years, 847t-848t
  interventions for, ages 25-64 years, 847t-848t
  Papanicolaou testing and, 857
Sexual dysfunction; see also Erectile dysfunction
  evaluation of, 756
Sexual intercourse, myocardial infarction associated with, 911-912
Sexual maturation stages
  female, 1041
  male, 1041
Sexually transmitted diseases; see also Chlamydia genital infection; Condyloma acuminatum; other STDs
  counseling to prevent, 886
  in differential diagnosis of dysfunctional uterine bleeding, 159
  treatment of, after sexual assault, 1056t
Sexually transmitted epididymitis; see Epididymitis
"Shaken baby syndrome"; see Child abuse
Sheehan's syndrome
  basic information about, 437
  diagnosis of, 437
  treatment of, 437
Shell shock; see Posttraumatic stress disorder
Shigella, food poisoning due to, 188
Shigellosis
  basic information about, 438
  diagnosis of, 438
  treatment of, 438
Shin splints in differential diagnosis of leg pain, 615t
Shingles; see Herpes zoster infection
Shock
  anaphylactic; see Anaphylaxis
  septic; see Septicemia
Short bowel syndrome in differential diagnosis of celiac disease, 98

Short stature, differential diagnosis of, 647t
Shoulder
 frozen, 191
 instability of, in differential diagnosis of rotator cuff syndrome, 423
Shoulder pain, diagnosis, evaluation, treatment, 648t
SIADH; see Antidiuretic hormone, inappropriate secretion of
Sialadenitis
 basic information about, 439
 diagnosis of, 439
 treatment of, 439
Sialolithiasis in differential diagnosis of sialadenitis, 439
Sicca syndrome; see Sjögren's syndrome
Sickle cell crisis in differential diagnosis of disseminated intravascular coagulation, 155
Sickle cell disease; see also Anemia, sickle cell
 pregnancy in, 944
 screening newborn for, 873-874
 sports participation and, 1036t
Sickle cell trait, sports participation and, 1037t
Sideroblastic anemia in differential diagnosis of iron deficiency anemia, 32
Siderosis in differential diagnosis of asbestosis, 54
Sigmoidoscopy, recommendations for, 856-857
Silicosis
 in differential diagnosis of asbestosis, 54
 in differential diagnosis of pulmonary tuberculosis, 498
Simvastatin, preparations, dosage, mechanism of action, effect, cost, 993t
Sinequan; see Doxepin
Sinus venous defect, 61
Sinusitis
 basic information about, 440
 diagnosis of, 440-441
 differential diagnosis of, 588t
 in differential diagnosis of acute bronchitis, 82
 in differential diagnosis of allergic rhinitis, 420
 in differential diagnosis of chronic rhinitis, 644-645t
 in differential diagnosis of Wegener's granulomatosis, 531
 treatment of, 441
Sjögren's syndrome
 basic information about, 442
 diagnosis of, 442
 in differential diagnosis of acute viral encephalitis, 166
 neuropathies associated with, 631t
 treatment of, 442
SJS; see Stevens-Johnson syndrome
Skin; see also cutaneous entries
 drug-induced eruptions of, 565
Skin cancer; see also Basal cell carcinoma; Squamous cell carcinoma
 ages 11-24 years, 845t-846t
 follow-up strategies for, 1053t
 screening and prevention, 858-859
Skin disorders
 in differential diagnosis of glossitis, 202
 sports participation and, 1037t
Skin lesions, differential diagnosis of
 primary, 649
 secondary, 651
 special, 653t
SLE; see Systemic lupus erythematosus

Sleep apnea
 basic information about, 443
 diagnosis of, 443
 in differential diagnosis of chronic obstructive pulmonary disease, 120
 in differential diagnosis of narcolepsy, 318
 treatment of, 443
Sleep disorders; see also Insomnia
 in elderly, 606t
 evaluation of, 757-759
 in men with coronary artery disease, 960-961
Small cell carcinoma of lung, 277
Smoking; see also Tobacco use
 counseling to prevent, 880-881
 in differential diagnosis of polycythemia vera, 380
 myocardial ischemia triggered by, 932-933, 933
 passive, effect on respiratory symptoms in young adults, 938
Snake bite in differential diagnosis of lymphangitis, 2880
Social phobia in differential diagnosis of drug abuse, 7
Social services, community resources for, 1060-1061
Sodium
 corrected, in hyperglycemia patients, formula for, 1042
 in development of stable hypertension, 901
 dietary intake of, 881-882
 fractional excretion of, formula for, 1042
 serum, laboratory findings, 828
 serum abnormalities of, conditions associated with, 828
 urine, laboratory findings, 836
Soft tissue tumor in differential diagnosis of Dupuytren's contracture, 158
Soft-tissue infection, nosocomial, 323-324
Solar lentigo in differential diagnosis of melanoma, 291
Soldier's heart; see Posttraumatic stress disorder
Solu-Cortef; see Hydrocortisone
Solu-Medrol; see Methylprednisolone
Somatization disorder
 basic information about, 444
 diagnosis of, 444
 in differential diagnosis of conversion disorder, 135
 persistent; see Conversion disorder
 treatment of, 444
Somatoform disorders in differential diagnosis of Munchausen's syndrome, 210
Sore throat; see Pharyngitis
Sotalol
 electrophysiologic effects of, 969t
 preparations, dosage, cardioselectivity, lipid solubility, half-life, excretion, cost, 981t
 for ventricular arrhythmias, dosage, half-life, ECG manifestations, toxicity, 1000t
Sparfloxacin, preparation, dosage, half-life, excretion, cost, 989t
Spastic colon; see Irritable bowel syndrome
Specific gravity, urine, laboratory findings, 836
Sphenopalatine neuralgia; see Headache, cluster
Spherocytosis, causes of, 654
Sphincteric incontinence, 255-256
Spinal cord compression
 basic information about, 445
 diagnosis of, 445

Spinal cord compression—cont'd
 in differential diagnosis of poliomyelitis, 378
 treatment of, 445
Spinal cord disorders
 in differential diagnosis of amyotrophic lateral sclerosis, 25
 in differential diagnosis of cerebral palsy, 100
Spinal cord tumor
 in differential diagnosis of syringomyelia, 459
 in differential diagnosis of tabes dorsalis, 462
Spinal dermatomes, 1044
Spinal injury, cervical, evaluation of, 760
Spinal muscular atrophy in differential diagnosis of syringomyelia, 459
Spinal pain
 radicular, in differential diagnosis of osteoarthritis, 330
 referred, in differential diagnosis of fibromyalgia, 184
Spinal sclerosis; see Tabes dorsalis
Spinal stenosis
 in differential diagnosis of amyotrophic lateral sclerosis, 25
 in differential diagnosis of claudication, 123
 in differential diagnosis of low back pain, 554t
Spirochetes, granulomatous disorders due to, 584
Spleen
 absent or dysfunctional, infection management in patients with, 928-929
 enlarged, sports participation and, 1037t
Splenic lymphoma in differential diagnosis of chronic myelogenous leukemia, 273
Splenomegaly
 causes of, 654
 evaluation of, 761
Spondyloarthropathy
 characteristics of, 656t
 differential diagnosis for, 655
 knee pain due to, findings, diagnosis, and management, 610t
 reactive, in differential diagnosis of low back pain, 554t
 seronegative; see also Ankylosing spondylitis; Reiter's syndrome
 comparison of, 656t
 in differential diagnosis of rheumatoid arthritis, 53
Spondylosis deformans of axial skeleton, characteristics of, 549t
Spongiform encephalopathy, subacute; see Creutzfeldt-Jakob disease
Sporotrichoid lymphangitis; see Lymphangitis
Sporotrichosis
 basic information about, 448
 diagnosis of, 448-449
 in differential diagnosis of tularemia, 500
 treatment of, 449
Sports
 injuries due to, counseling to prevent, 883-884
 participation in
  assessing, 1034
  medical conditions and, 1035t-1037t
Sports injuries, Harstad study of epidemiology of, 915
Spouse abuse, screening for, 876

Sprain
  ankle
    basic information about, 40
    diagnosis of, 40
    treatment of, 40
  soft-tissue, in differential diagnosis of lumbar disc syndromes, 276
Sprue
  celiac; see Celiac sprue
  in differential diagnosis of lactose intolerance, 264
  in differential diagnosis of pseudomembranous gout, 395
  in differential diagnosis of ulcerative colitis, 505
  laboratory findings for calcium and phosphorus, 789t
  tropical
    basic information about, 494
    diagnosis of, 494
    treatment of, 494
Spurling test, 1026
Squamous cell carcinoma
  basic information about, 450
  diagnosis of, 450
  in differential diagnosis of nail disorders, 625t
  in differential diagnosis of warts, 529
  of lung, 277
  treatment of, 450
  of vagina; see Vaginal malignancy
  of vulva; see Vulvar cancer
Squamous cell hyperplasia
  in differential diagnosis of estrogen deficient vulvovaginitis, 525
  in differential diagnosis of pruritus vulvae, 393
Squamous intraepithelial lesion; see Cervical dysplasia
Squamous papilloma in differential diagnosis of cervical polyps, 106
SS; see Sjögren's syndrome
ST segment, elevation of, differential diagnosis of, 657t
Stadol; see Butorphanol
Staphylococcal pyoderma in differential diagnosis of acne vulgaris, 12
Staphylococcal scalded skin syndrome, ages affected, prodrome, morphology, distribution, diagnosis, 575t
Staphylococcal septicemia, history, rash characteristics and distribution, clinical findings, diagnostic aids, 577t
Staphylococcus infection in differential diagnosis of corneal ulceration, 137
Stasis dermatitis
  differential diagnosis of, 568t
  in differential diagnosis of Kaposi's sarcoma, 260
Stasis skin changes; see Varicose veins
Stature
  short, causes of, 647t
  tall, causes of, 658t
Status asthmaticus; see also Asthma
  defined, 56
Status epilepticus
  basic information about, 451
  diagnosis of, 451
  treatment of, 451
Stavudine, therapeutic class, preparations, dosage, toxicities, cost, 970t
Stelazine; see Trifluoperazine
Steroid acne in differential diagnosis of acne vulgaris, 12
Steroids, topical, brand names and potency, 999t
Stevens-Johnson syndrome
  basic information about, 452
  diagnosis of, 452

Stevens-Johnson syndrome—cont'd
  differential diagnosis of, 557t
  in differential diagnosis of herpes simplex infection, 225
  in differential diagnosis of toxic shock syndrome, 484
  treatment of, 452
Still's disease; see also Arthritis, juvenile rheumatoid
  in differential diagnosis of rheumatic fever, 419
Stings, anaphylaxis due to; see Anaphylaxis
Stomach cancer; see Gastric cancer
Stomatitis, aphthous
  in differential diagnosis of herpangina, 224
  in differential diagnosis of herpes simplex infection, 225
Stone disease in differential diagnosis of bladder cancer, 71
Stool, functional incontinence of; see Encopresis
Strabismus
  basic information about, 453
  diagnosis of, 453
  in differential diagnosis of retinoblastoma, 415
  screening recommendations for, 869
  treatment of, 453
Strabismus amblyopia; see Amblyopia
Straight leg raise, 1026
Streptococcus, infections due to, 26
Streptococcus pharyngitis in differential diagnosis of diphtheria, 154
Streptozime; see Anti-streptolysin O titer
Streptozocin, toxicity of, 984t-985t
Stress
  in development of stable hypertension, 901
  myocardial ischemia triggered by, 932-933
Stress fracture in differential diagnosis of deep vein thrombosis, 473
Stress headache; see Headache, tension-type
Stress hyperglycemia in differential diagnosis of diabetes mellitus, 149
Stress incontinence, 255
Stress polycythemia in differential diagnosis of polycythemia vera, 380
Strictures in differential diagnosis of colorectal cancer, 127
Stroke; see also Cerebrovascular accident
  in differential diagnosis of Bell's palsy, 68
  in differential diagnosis of brain neoplasm, 76
  heat; see Heat exhaustion/heat stroke
  ischemic, lowest effective prophylactic anticoagulation therapy for, 937-938, 938t
  in users of low-dose oral contraceptives, 954, 955t
Strongyloidiasis
  in differential diagnosis of hookworm, 235
  in tissue infections, epidemiology, transmission, manifestations, diagnosis, treatment, 629t
Strychnine poisoning in differential diagnosis of tetanus, 466
Stye; see Hordeolum
Subacromial joint, internal derangement of; see Rotator cuff syndrome
Subacute bacterial endocarditis in differential diagnosis of chronic fatigue syndrome, 119
Subacute spongiform encephalopathy; see Creutzfeldt-Jakob disease
Subarachnoid hemorrhage in differential diagnosis of migraine, 210
Subareolar abscess; see Breast abscess

Subdural hematoma in differential diagnosis of hepatic encephalopathy, 218
Substance abuse; see also Alcoholism; Drug abuse
  in differential diagnosis of eclampsia, 163
  screening recommendations for, 875-879
Substance dependence in differential diagnosis of drug abuse, 7
Substance use
  ages 11-24 years, 845t
  in high-risk populations, ages 25-64 years, 847t-848t
  interventions for
    ages 25-64 years, 847t-848t
    ages 65 and older, 849t-850t
Sucrose hemolysis test, laboratory findings, 829
Sudden cardiac death
  in children and adolescents, 911
  in young persons, common causes of, 912t
Sudden death, events triggering, 932-933
Suicide
  basic information about, 455
  diagnosis of, 455
  treatment of, 455
Suicide risk, screening recommendations for, 876
Sular; see Nisoldipine
Sulcus tumor
  in differential diagnosis of frozen shoulder, 191
  in differential diagnosis of thoracic outlet syndrome, 470
Sulfisoxazole, dosage for, and dialysis removal, 972t
Sulindac, preparations, dosage, half-life, class, cost, metabolism, 998t
Sunscreens, skin cancer prevention and, 859
Suppurative adenitis in differential diagnosis of lymphogranuloma venereum, 283
Suppurative cholangitis; see Cholangitis
Supraglottitis; see also Epiglottitis
  in differential diagnosis of laryngitis, 266
Suprascapular nerve entrapment in differential diagnosis of rotator cuff syndrome, 423
Supraspinatus syndrome; see Rotator cuff syndrome
Supraventricular tachycardia; see Paroxysmal atrial tachycardia
Suprax; see Cefixime
Surgery, noncardiac, cardiac risk in, 935-936
Surgical abdomen; see Peritonitis, secondary
Surreptitious illness; see Munchausen's syndrome
Survivor syndrome; see Posttraumatic stress disorder
Sweet's syndrome, history, manifestations, and malignancy associated with, 564t
Swelling of limbs, differential diagnosis of, 657t
Swimmer's ear; see Otitis externa
Swimming, injuries due to, counseling to prevent, 883-884
Sycosis barbae; see Folliculitis
Sydenham's chorea
  in differential diagnosis of Huntington's chorea, 238
  in differential diagnosis of Tourette's syndrome, 483
Synalar; see Fluocinolone
Syncope
  basic information about, 456
  carotid sinus; see Carotid sinus syndrome
  diagnosis of, 456-457
  in differential diagnosis of epilepsy, 572t

1118 Index

Syncope—cont'd
　in differential diagnosis of generalized tonic-clonic seizure disorder, 433
　treatment of, 457
Syndrome X, 37
Synovial chondromatosis, knee pain due to, findings, diagnosis, and management, 613t
Synovial fluid, abnormalities of, laboratory diagnosis of, 658t
Synovitis
　pigmented villonodular, knee pain due to, findings, diagnosis, and management, 613t
　toxic, in differential diagnosis of Legg-Calvé-Perthes disease, 268
Syphilis
　anorectal, clinical features, diagnosis, and treatment, 582t
　basic information about, 458
　diagnosis of, 458
　in differential diagnosis of acute viral encephalitis, 166
　in differential diagnosis of chancroid, 110
　in differential diagnosis of erythema multiforme, 180
　in differential diagnosis of herpes simplex infection, 225
　in differential diagnosis of nonneoplastic neck mass, 627t
　in differential diagnosis of psoriasis, 397
　in differential diagnosis of retinitis pigmentosa, 414
　in differential diagnosis of scabies, 427
　in differential diagnosis of tinea corporis, 479
　in differential diagnosis of tularemia, 500
　screening recommendations for, 864
　secondary
　　in differential diagnosis of granuloma inguinale, 206
　　in differential diagnosis of pityriasis rosea, 368
　　in differential diagnosis of tinea versicolor, 481
　serologic tests for
　　interpretation of, 838t
　　laboratory findings, 837
　treatment of, 458
Syphilitic myelitis in differential diagnosis of amyotrophic lateral sclerosis, 25
Syringomyelia
　basic information about, 459
　diagnosis of, 459
　in differential diagnosis of amyotrophic lateral sclerosis, 25
　treatment of, 459
Systemic inflammatory response syndrome; see Septicemia
Systemic lupus erythematosus
　basic information about, 460
　complement deficiencies associated with, 794t
　course and distribution, 551t
　diagnosis of, 460-461
　in differential diagnosis of acute glomerulonephritis, 200
　in differential diagnosis of bacterial meningitis, 294
　in differential diagnosis of chronic fatigue syndrome, 119
　in differential diagnosis of disseminated intravascular coagulation, 155
　in differential diagnosis of fatty liver of pregnancy, 181
　in differential diagnosis of Goodpasture's syndrome, 204
　in differential diagnosis of idiopathic thrombocytopenic purpura, 252

Systemic lupus erythematosus—cont'd
　in differential diagnosis of juvenile rheumatoid arthritis, 51
　in differential diagnosis of photosensitivity, 634t
　in differential diagnosis of polyarteritis nodosa, 379
　in differential diagnosis of preeclampsia, 384
　in differential diagnosis of psoriasis, 397
　in differential diagnosis of rheumatic fever, 419
　in differential diagnosis of rheumatoid arthritis, 53
　in differential diagnosis of rosacea, 422
　in differential diagnosis of tinea corporis, 479
　in differential diagnosis of viral meningitis, 295
　neuropathies associated with, 631t
　treatment of, 461
Systemic necrotizing vasculitis in differential diagnosis of Goodpasture's syndrome, 204

T

T_3, laboratory findings, 829
T_4, laboratory findings, 829
T cell lymphoma in differential diagnosis of chronic lymphocytic leukemia, 272
Tabes dorsalis
　basic information about, 462
　diagnosis of, 462
　in differential diagnosis of syringomyelia, 459
　treatment of, 462
Tachycardia
　multifocal atrial, in differential diagnosis of atrial fibrillation, 59
　narrow complex, evaluation and management, 762
　during noncardiac surgery, 935
　paroxysmal atrial, in differential diagnosis of atrial flutter, 60
　pulseless ventricular, evaluation of, 776-777
　supraventricular; see Paroxysmal atrial tachycardia
　ventricular, evaluation of, 778
　wide complex, evaluation and management, 763
Taenia solium infection, epidemiology, transmission, clinical presentation, diagnosis, and treatment, 559t
Tagamet; see Cimetidine
Talacen, contents of, 995t
Talar dome fracture; see Osteochondritis dissecans
Tall stature, causes of, 658
Talwin Compound, contents of, 995t
Talwin Nx; see Pentazocine
Tambocor; see Flecainide
Tapeworm
　basic information about, 463
　diagnosis of, 463
　treatment of, 463
Tardive dyskinesia, manifestations, differential diagnosis, tests, treatment, 596t
Tarsal tunnel syndrome
　basic information about, 464
　diagnosis of, 464
　treatment of, 464
Tavist-1; see Clemastine
Taxol, toxicity of, 984t-985t
TB; see Tuberculosis
3TC; see Lamivudine
Teenagers; see Adolescents
Tegretol; see Carbamazepine

Telangiectasia, differential diagnosis of, 653t
Telogen effluvium in differential diagnosis of alopecia, 544t
Temazepam, preparations, dosage, half-life, indication, cost, 980t
Temporal arteritis; see Arteritis, temporal
Tendinitis
　Achilles, in differential diagnosis of deep vein thrombosis, 473
　bicipital, in differential diagnosis of shoulder pain, 648t
　in differential diagnosis of bursitis, 85
　in differential diagnosis of carpal tunnel syndrome, 93
　in differential diagnosis of fibromyalgia, 184
　in differential diagnosis of osteoarthritis, 330
　in differential diagnosis of tarsal tunnel syndrome, 464
　patellar, in differential diagnosis of Osgood-Schlatter disease, 329
　rotator cuff, in differential diagnosis of cervical disc syndromes, 103
Tenex; see Guanfacine
Tennis elbow; see Epicondylitis
Tenormin; see Atenolol
Tension-type headache; see Headache, tension-type
Teratoma
　in differential diagnosis of congenital anomalies presenting as neck masses, 628t
　in differential diagnosis of meningomyelocele, 296
Terazosin, preparations, dosage, cost, 969t
Testicles
　absent or undescended, sports participation and, 1037t
　size variations in, causes of, 659
Testicular cancer
　follow-up strategies for, 1052t
　screening for, 859
Testicular feminization, phenotypes, karyotypes, inheritance, hormone levels, pathogenesis, 546t
Testicular torsion in differential diagnosis of epididymitis, 175
Testosterone, laboratory values, 829
Tetanus
　basic information about, 466
　chemoprophylaxis of, 894
　diagnosis of, 466
　in differential diagnosis of rabies, 402
　treatment of, 466
Tetanus vaccine
　administration of, 1018t
　for international travel, 1019t
　during pregnancy, 1014t, 1015t
Tetanus/diphtheria vaccine
　for adults
　　in immunocompromised patients, 1006t-1007t
　　recommendations, 892
　　schedule, indications, side effects, contraindications, during pregnancy, with HIV infection, 1006t-1007t
　for residents of long-term care facilities, 921t
Tetracyclines, dosage for, and dialysis removal, 972t
Thalassemia in differential diagnosis of sickle cell anemia, 34
Thalassemia trait
　clinical and laboratory features, 547t
　in differential diagnosis of iron deficiency anemia, 32
Thelarche, premature, in differential diagnosis of precocious puberty, 383

Index

Theophylline, drug monitoring data for, 799t
Thiazide diuretics
  class, preparations, dosage, site of action, cost, 978t
  in differential diagnosis of hyperparathyroidism, 244
Thiethylperazine, preparations, dosage, class, 976t
Thioguanine, toxicity of, 984t-985t
Thioridazine, preparations, dosage, class, adverse effects, 978t
Thiotepa, toxicity of, 984t-985t
Thiothixene, preparations, dosage, class, adverse effects, 978t
Thoracic outlet syndrome
  basic information about, 470
  diagnosis of, 470
  in differential diagnosis of cervical disc syndromes, 103
  in differential diagnosis of shoulder pain, 648t
  treatment of, 470
Thorazine; see Chlorpromazine
Thrombin time, laboratory values, 829
Thromboangiitis obliterans
  basic information about, 471
  diagnosis of, 471
  in differential diagnosis of leg pain, 615t
  treatment of, 471
Thrombocytopenia
  causes of, 659
  diagnosis of, 555t, 764
Thrombocytopenic purpura in differential diagnosis of disseminated intravascular coagulation, 155
Thromboembolism, pulmonary; see Pulmonary embolism
Thrombolytic therapy for acute myocardial infarction, 765, 1058
  contraindications to, 1058
Thrombophlebitis; see also Cavernous sinus thrombosis
  deep venous; see Deep vein thrombosis
  in differential diagnosis of cellulitis, 99
  in differential diagnosis of swollen limbs, 657t
  migratory, history, manifestations, and malignancy associated with, 564t
  superficial
    basic information about, 472
    diagnosis of, 472
    in differential diagnosis of deep vein thrombosis, 473
    treatment of, 472
Thrombosis
  cavernous sinus; see Cavernous sinus thrombosis
  coronary; see Myocardial infarction
  deep vein; see Deep vein thrombosis
  intracerebral, in differential diagnosis of eclampsia, 163
Thrombotic thrombocytopenic purpura
  basic information about, 474
  diagnosis of, 474
  in differential diagnosis of idiopathic thrombocytopenic purpura, 252
  treatment of, 474
Thrush; see Candidiasis
Thyroglossal duct cyst
  in differential diagnosis of congenital anomalies presenting as neck masses, 628t
  in differential diagnosis of thyroid nodule, 476
Thyroid, cold nodules of, differential diagnosis of, 659

Thyroid carcinoma
  basic information about, 475
  diagnosis of, 475
  in differential diagnosis of thyroid nodule, 476
  in differential diagnosis of thyroiditis, 477
  screening recommendations for, 860
  treatment of, 475
Thyroid disease
  in differential diagnosis of fibromyalgia, 184
  nodular, management of, 766
  screening recommendations for, 860-861
  symptoms of, 861
  tests in diagnosis of, 767
Thyroid exophthalmus in differential diagnosis of cavernous sinus thrombosis, 97
Thyroid function tests, findings in various conditions, 829t
Thyroid nodule
  basic information about, 476
  diagnosis of, 476
  treatment of, 476
Thyroid storm in differential diagnosis of heat exhaustion/heat stroke, 214
Thyroiditis
  basic information about, 477
  diagnosis of, 477
  in differential diagnosis of chronic fatigue syndrome, 119
  in differential diagnosis of Graves' disease, 207
  in differential diagnosis of thyroid carcinoma, 475
  lymphocytic, in differential diagnosis of thyroid carcinoma, 475
  treatment of, 477
Thyroid-stimulating hormone
  decreased, conditions associated with, 830
  increased, conditions associated with, 830
  laboratory values, 829
Thyrotoxic ophthalmopathy in differential diagnosis of myasthenia gravis, 312
Thyrotoxic storm
  basic information about, 478
  diagnosis of, 478
  treatment of, 478
Thyrotoxicosis; see also Graves' disease; Hyperthyroidism
  in differential diagnosis of pheochromocytoma, 363
Thyrotropin-secreting pituitary adenoma, 366
Thyroxine, laboratory values, 829
Thyroxine index
  decreased, causes of, 803
  free; see Free thyroxine index
TIA; see Transient ischemic attack
Tic disorders
  in differential diagnosis of obsessive-compulsive disorder, 325
  in differential diagnosis of Tourette's syndrome, 483
Tic douloureux; see Trigeminal neuralgia
Ticarcillin, dosage for, and dialysis removal, 972t
Tick paralysis in differential diagnosis of botulism, 75
TICS mnemonic, 590
Tietze's syndrome in differential diagnosis of costochondritis, 138
Tigan; see Trimethobenzamide
Timolol, preparations, dosage, cardioselectivity, lipid solubility, half-life, excretion, cost, 981t
Tinea capitis in differential diagnosis of alopecia, 543t

Tinea circinata; see Tinea corporis
Tinea corporis
  basic information about, 479
  diagnosis of, 479
  in differential diagnosis of impetigo, 253
  in differential diagnosis of pityriasis rosea, 368
  treatment of, 479
Tinea cruris
  basic information about, 480
  diagnosis of, 480
  treatment of, 480
Tinea in differential diagnosis of psoriasis, 397
Tinea versicolor
  basic information about, 481
  diagnosis of, 481
  in differential diagnosis of pityriasis rosea, 368
  in differential diagnosis of tinea cruris, 480
  treatment of, 481
Tinnitus, evaluation of, 768
Tobacco use; see also Smoking
  bladder cancer and, 860
  counseling to prevent, 880-881
  oral cancer and, 859
Tobramycin
  dosage for, and dialysis removal, 971t
  drug monitoring data for, 799t
Tocainide
  dosage, half-life, ECG manifestations, toxicity, 1000t
  electrophysiologic effects of, 969t
Tofranil; see Imipramine
Tolazamide, preparations, dosage, duration of action, half-life, excretion, cost, class, 975t
Tolbutamide, preparations, dosage, duration of action, half-life, excretion, cost, class, 975t
Tolectin; see Tolmetin
Tolinase; see Tolazamide
Tolmetin, preparations, dosage, half-life, class, cost, metabolism, 998t
Tonocard; see Tocainide
Tonsillitis
  basic information about, 362
  diagnosis of, 362
  in differential diagnosis of herpangina, 224
  lingual, in differential diagnosis of epiglottitis, 176
  treatment of, 362
Topicort; see Desoximetasone
Toprol XL; see Metoprolol
Toradol; see Ketorolac
Torecan; see Thiethylperazine
Torticollis
  basic information about, 482
  diagnosis of, 482
  treatment of, 482
Total iron-binding capacity, assessment of, 1046t
Total lymphocyte count, assessment of, 1046t
Tourette's syndrome
  basic information about, 483
  diagnosis of, 483
  treatment of, 483
Toxemia; see also Eclampsia
  of pregnancy; see also Preeclampsia
  in differential diagnosis of nephrotic syndrome, 319
Toxic amblyopia; see Amblyopia
Toxic cataract; see Cataract

Toxic epidermal necrolysis in differential
  diagnosis of toxic shock syndrome,
  484
Toxic erythema in differential diagnosis of
  Stevens-Johnson syndrome, 452
Toxic retinopathy in differential diagnosis
  of retinitis pigmentosa, 414
Toxic shock syndrome
  basic information about, 484
  diagnosis of, 484-485
  history, rash characteristics and
    distribution, clinical findings,
    diagnostic aids, 578t
  treatment of, 485
Toxic synovitis in differential diagnosis of
  Legg-Calvé-Perthes disease, 268
Toxicity in differential diagnosis of
  myelodysplastic syndromes, 313
Toxicology treatment protocols, 1053t
Toxoplasmosis
  basic information about, 486
  cerebral, in differential diagnosis of
    listeriosis, 275
  diagnosis of, 486-487
  in differential diagnosis of acute viral
    encephalitis, 166
  in differential diagnosis of Epstein-Barr
    virus infections, 178
  in differential diagnosis of
    mononucleosis, 304
  in differential diagnosis of nonneoplastic
    neck mass, 627t
  in differential diagnosis of tularemia, 500
  treatment of, 487
Tracheitis
  bacterial, in differential diagnosis of
    laryngitis, 266
  basic information about, 488
  diagnosis of, 488
  treatment of, 488
Tracheobronchitis, bacterial; see Tracheitis
Trachomatis, chlamydia, in differential
  diagnosis of gonorrhea, 203
Trandate; see Labetalol
Trandolapril, dosage, onset of action, peak
  effect, half-life, cost, 967t
Transdermal, contents of, 995t
Transferrin
  laboratory values, 830
  serum, assessment of, 1046t
Transfusion reaction, hemolytic
  basic information about, 489
  diagnosis of, 489
  treatment of, 489
Transfusion-related non-A, B hepatitis; see
  Hepatitis C
Transient ischemic attack
  basic information about, 490
  diagnosis of, 490
  in differential diagnosis of cerebrovascular
    accident, 101
  in differential diagnosis of epilepsy, 572t
  in differential diagnosis of partial seizure
    disorder, 434
  treatment of, 490
Transplantation, bone marrow, malignant
  neoplasms following, 926, 926-927
Transverse vaginal septum in differential
  diagnosis of dysmenorrhea, 161
Tranxene; see Clorazepate
Trauma
  blunt abdominal, evaluation of, 769
  chest, evaluation of, 770-771
  in differential diagnosis of alopecia, 543t
  in differential diagnosis of amenorrhea,
    545t
  in differential diagnosis of cavernous
    sinus thrombosis, 97

Trauma—cont'd
  in differential diagnosis of diabetic
    retinopathy, 416
  in differential diagnosis of macular
    degeneration, 285
  to kidneys, evaluation of, 772
Traumatic cataract; see Cataract
Traumatic neurosis; see Posttraumatic stress
  disorder
Travelers, infectious diseases in, 605t
Trazodone, preparations, dosage, class,
  effects, half-life, 974t
Trematodes
  in tissue infections, epidemiology,
    transmission, manifestations,
    diagnosis, treatment, 660t
  transmission, clinical findings, diagnosis,
    treatment, 607t
Tremor
  causes of, 660
  essential, in differential diagnosis of
    Parkinson's disease, 347
Triamcinolone, brand names and potency,
  999t
Triazolam, preparations, dosage, half-life,
  indication, cost, 980t
Triceps skinfold, measurement of, 1046t
Trichinella spiralis in tissue infections,
  epidemiology, transmission,
  manifestations, diagnosis, treatment,
  629t
Trichinosis
  basic information about, 491
  diagnosis of, 491
  treatment of, 491
Trichomonas vaginitis; *see also* Vulvovaginitis,
  trichomonas
  in differential diagnosis of bacterial
    vulvovaginitis, 524
  in differential diagnosis of fungal
    vulvovaginitis, 526
  in differential diagnosis of vaginitis, 663t
Trichomonas vulvovaginitis in differential
  diagnosis of prepubescent
  vulvovaginitis, 527
Trichomoniasis
  basic information about, 492
  diagnosis of, 492
  in differential diagnosis of candidiasis, 86
  in differential diagnosis of nongonococcal
    urethritis, 507
  treatment of, 492
  after sexual assault, 1056t
Trichonodosis in differential diagnosis of
  pediculosis, 350
Trichotillomania in differential diagnosis of
  alopecia, 543t
Trick; *see* Trichomoniasis
Tricuspid regurgitation in differential
  diagnosis of mitral regurgitation, 300
Trifluoperazine, preparations, dosage, class,
  adverse effects, 978t
Trigeminal neuralgia
  basic information about, 493
  diagnosis of, 493
  in differential diagnosis of cluster
    headache, 209
  treatment of, 493
Triglycerides, laboratory values, 830
Triiodothyronine, laboratory findings, 829
Trilafon; *see* Perphenazine
Tri-Levlen, estrogen and progestin content
  of, 987t
Trimethobenzamide, preparations, dosage,
  class, 976t
Trimethoprim, dosage for, and dialysis
  removal, 972t
Trimethoprim-sulfamethoxazole, dosage for,
  and dialysis removal, 972t

Tri-Norinyl, estrogen and progestin content
  of, 987t
Triphasil, estrogen and progestin content of,
  987t
Trisomy 21; *see* Down syndrome
Troglitazone, preparations, dosage, duration
  of action, half-life, excretion, cost,
  class, 975t
Tropical bubo; *see* Lymphogranuloma
  venereum
Tropical enteropathy; *see* Sprue, tropical
Trypanosomiasis, American; *see* Chagas'
  disease
TTP; *see* Thrombotic thrombocytopenic
  purpura
Tubal sterilization, gynecologic cancers and,
  887-888
Tuberculin test
  false-negative, factors associated with, 831
  positive, 831
Tuberculosis
  in differential diagnosis of AIDS, 13
  in differential diagnosis of asthma, 56
  in differential diagnosis of bronchiectasis,
    81
  in differential diagnosis of chronic fatigue
    syndrome, 119
  in differential diagnosis of infective
    endocarditis, 168
  in differential diagnosis of lung
    neoplasm, 277
  in differential diagnosis of menopause,
    297
  in differential diagnosis of nonneoplastic
    neck mass, 627t
  in differential diagnosis of *Pneumocystis
    carinii* pneumonia, 374
  in differential diagnosis of salmonellosis,
    424
  in differential diagnosis of sarcoidosis,
    426
  in differential diagnosis of tularemia, 500,
    501
  in differential diagnosis of typhoid fever,
    504
  in differential diagnosis of vulvar cancer,
    523
  miliary
    basic information about, 495
    diagnosis of, 496
    in differential diagnosis of malaria,
      287
    treatment of, 496
  pulmonary
    basic information about, 497-498
    diagnosis of, 498-499
    treatment of, 499
  screening recommendations for, 863-864
Tuberculous abscess in differential diagnosis
  of breast abscess, 77
Tuberculous arthritis; *see* Arthritis,
  granulomatous
Tuberculous meningitis, CSF abnormalities
  in, 559t, 791t
Tubo-ovarian abscess, 4; *see also* Pelvic
  inflammatory disease
  in differential diagnosis of benign ovarian
    tumor, 341
Tubular necrosis, acute, in differential
  diagnosis of hepatorenal syndrome,
  223
Tularemia
  basic information about, 500
  diagnosis of, 500-501
  in differential diagnosis of human
    granulocytic ehrlichiosis, 237
  in differential diagnosis of nonneoplastic
    neck mass, 627t
  treatment of, 501

Index

Tumor markers
  laboratory findings, 832t, 833
  uses of, 832
Tumors
  back pain due to, 681t
  brain; see Brain neoplasms
  in differential diagnosis of diabetic retinopathy, 416
  in differential diagnosis of lumbar disc syndromes, 276
  in differential diagnosis of migraine, 210
  in differential diagnosis of miliary tuberculosis, 496
  in differential diagnosis of retinal detachment, 412
  in differential diagnosis of retinoblastoma, 415
  mediastinal, causes of, 622
  metastatic, in differential diagnosis of brain neoplasm, 76
  nonneoplastic, of neck, differential diagnosis of, 626t-627t
  soft tissue, in differential diagnosis of Dupuytren's contracture, 158
Turner's syndrome, 502-503
  basic information about, 502
  diagnosis of, 502-503
  in differential diagnosis of amenorrhea, 544t
  treatment of, 593
Twisted neck; see Torticollis
Tylenol, with codeine, contents of, 995t
Tylox, contents of, 995t
Typhoid fever; see also Salmonellosis
  basic information about, 504
  diagnosis of, 504
  in differential diagnosis of babesiosis, 64
  in differential diagnosis of human granulocytic ehrlichiosis, 237
  in differential diagnosis of malaria, 287
  in differential diagnosis of miliary tuberculosis, 496
  in differential diagnosis of psittacosis, 396
  in differential diagnosis of tularemia, 501
  in differential diagnosis of yellow fever, 533
  treatment of, 504
Typhoid vaccine
  for international travel, 1019t
  during pregnancy, 1014t
  schedule, indications, side effects, contraindications, during pregnancy, with HIV infection, in immunocompromised patient, 1010t-1011t
Typhus in differential diagnosis of human granulocytic ehrlichiosis, 237

U

Ulcerative colitis
  basic information about, 505
  diagnosis of, 505
  in differential diagnosis of Crohn's disease, 140
  treatment of, 505
Ulcers
  anal; see Anal fissure
  corneal
    in differential diagnosis of corneal abrasion, 136
    in differential diagnosis of ocular foreign body, 326
    in differential diagnosis of red eye, 640t
  differential diagnosis of, 651
  genital
    differential diagnosis of, 583t
    management of, 713

Ulcers—cont'd
  leg
    differential diagnosis of, 616
    evaluation of, 732
  necrotic, in differential diagnosis of granuloma inguinale, 206
  peptic; see Peptic ulcer disease
  perforated, in differential diagnosis of acute appendicitis, 48
  pressure; see Pressure ulcers
Ulcus molle; see Chancroid
Ullrich-Turner syndrome; see Turner's syndrome
Ulnar nerve compression in differential diagnosis of thoracic outlet syndrome, 470
Ulnar neuropathy in differential diagnosis of epicondylitis, 174
Ultrasonography in pregnancy, screening recommendations for, 870
Unconscious patient, evaluation and management, 773
Unipolar depression; see Depression, major
Univasc; see Moexipril
Urea nitrogen, laboratory values, 831
Uremia in differential diagnosis of hepatic encephalopathy, 218
Uremic acidosis in differential diagnosis of diabetic ketoacidosis, 151
Urethral strictures in differential diagnosis of benign prostatic hyperplasia, 390
Urethritis
  in differential diagnosis of urinary tract infection, 509
  gonococcal; see also Gonorrhea
    basic information about, 506
    diagnosis of, 506
    treatment of, 506
  male-chlamydial, in differential diagnosis of trichomoniasis, 492
  nongonococcal
    basic information about, 507
    diagnosis of, 507
    in differential diagnosis of chlamydia genital infections, 114
    in differential diagnosis of gonorrhea, 203
    treatment of, 507
Urge incontinence, 255
Uric acid, serum, laboratory values, 831
Urinary creatinine, assessment of, 1046t
Urinary incontinence; see also Enuresis
  pelvic floor muscle exercises and, 952, 954
  screening in ambulatory elderly, 920t
Urinary nitrogen, assessment of, 1046t
Urinary tract infection, 508-509
  basic information about, 508-509
  diagnosis of, 509
  in differential diagnosis of bladder cancer, 71
  in differential diagnosis of pelvic inflammatory disease, 352
  in differential diagnosis of urolithiasis, 510
  treatment of, 509
Urinary tract infections, nosocomial, 323
Urine amylase, laboratory findings, 833
Urine bile, laboratory findings, 833
Urine calcium, laboratory findings, 833
Urine cAMP, laboratory findings, 833
Urine catecholamines, laboratory findings, 834
Urine chloride, laboratory findings, 834
Urine copper, laboratory findings, 834
Urine cortisol, free, laboratory findings, 834
Urine creatinine, laboratory findings, 834
Urine eosinophils, laboratory findings, 834

Urine glucose, laboratory findings, 834
Urine hemoglobin, free, laboratory findings, 834
Urine hemosiderin, laboratory findings, 834
Urine 5-hydroxyindole-acetic acid, laboratory findings, 834-835
Urine indican, laboratory findings, 835
Urine ketones, laboratory findings, 835
Urine metanephrines, laboratory findings, 835
Urine myoglobin, laboratory findings, 835
Urine nitrite, laboratory findings, 835
Urine occult blood, laboratory findings, 835
Urine osmolality, laboratory findings, 835
Urine pH, laboratory findings, 835-836
Urine phosphate, laboratory findings, 836
Urine potassium, laboratory findings, 836
Urine sediment, laboratory findings, 837
Urine sodium, laboratory findings, 836
Urine specific gravity, laboratory findings, 836
Urine vanillylmandelic acid, laboratory findings, 836-837
Urolithiasis; see also Nephrolithiasis
  basic information about, 510
  diagnosis of, 510-511
  treatment of, 511
Uropathy, obstructive, causes of, 661
Urticaria
  basic information about, 512
  chronic, evaluation and management, 774
  diagnosis of, 512
  in differential diagnosis of chickenpox, 113
  in differential diagnosis of erythema multiforme, 180
  in differential diagnosis of Stevens-Johnson syndrome, 452
  drug-induced, 565
  etiologic classification of, 661
  history, manifestations, and malignancy associated with, 564t
  treatment of, 512
Uterine activity monitoring, home, screening recommendations for, 871-872
Uterine bleeding, dysfunctional; see Dysfunctional uterine bleeding
Uterine cancer; see Endometrial cancer; Uterine malignancy
Uterine descensus; see Uterine prolapse
Uterine disorders in differential diagnosis of Meigs' syndrome, 290
Uterine fibroids; see also Uterine myomas
  in differential diagnosis of benign ovarian tumor, 341
  in differential diagnosis of ectopic pregnancy, 164
  in differential diagnosis of ovarian cancer, 340
  prolapsed
    in differential diagnosis of cervical cancer, 102
Uterine malignancy
  basic information about, 513
  diagnosis of, 513
  treatment of, 513
Uterine myomas
  basic information about, 514
  diagnosis of, 514
  treatment of, 514
Uterine prolapse
  basic information about, 515
  diagnosis of, 515
  treatment of, 515

Uterine synechiae in differential diagnosis of amenorrhea, 544t
UTI; see Urinary tract infection
Uticort; see Betamethasone
Uveitis; see also Retinal detachment
  basic information about, 516
  diagnosis of, 516
  in differential diagnosis of retinoblastoma, 415
  treatment of, 516

V

Vaccinations; see Immunizations; specific vaccines
Vaginal bleeding
  abnormal
    differential diagnosis of, 662t
    during pregnancy, 662
  anovulatory, 691
  intermenstrual, 689-690
  ovulatory, 689
Vaginal cuff abscess, 4
Vaginal discharge, evaluation of, 775
Vaginal douching, reduced fertility and, 948-949, 949
Vaginal malignancy
  basic information about, 518
  diagnosis of, 518
  treatment of, 518
Vaginal neoplasia in differential diagnosis of dysfunctional uterine bleeding, 159
Vaginal trauma in differential diagnosis of abruptio placentae, 3
Vaginismus
  basic information about, 519
  diagnosis of, 519
  treatment of, 519
Vaginitis
  atrophic; see also Vulvovaginitis, estrogen deficient
    in differential diagnosis of endometrial cancer, 169
    in differential diagnosis of fungal vulvovaginitis, 526
  differential diagnosis of, 663t
  in differential diagnosis of pruritus vulvae, 393
  in differential diagnosis of urinary tract infection, 509
  in differential diagnosis of vaginal malignancy, 518
Vaginosis
  bacterial; see also Vulvovaginitis, bacterial
    basic information about, 520
    diagnosis of, 520
    in differential diagnosis of candidiasis, 86
    in differential diagnosis of fungal vulvovaginitis, 526
    in differential diagnosis of prepubescent vulvovaginitis, 527
    in differential diagnosis of trichomonas vulvovaginitis, 528
    in differential diagnosis of trichomoniasis, 492
    in differential diagnosis of vaginitis, 663t
    treatment of, 520
  treatment of, after sexual assault, 1056t
Valisone; see Betamethasone
Valium; see Diazepam
Valproic acid
  drug monitoring data for, 799t
  preparations, dosage, use, half-life, therapeutic level, toxic level, 973t
Valvular disorders
  in differential diagnosis of aortic regurgitation, 46

Valvular disorders—cont'd
  in differential diagnosis of dilated cardiomyopathy, 89
  in differential diagnosis of hypertrophic cardiomyopathy, 90
  in differential diagnosis of mitral stenosis, 301
  in differential diagnosis of myocarditis, 316
  in differential diagnosis of restrictive cardiomyopathy, 91
Valvuloplasty, balloon, for aortic stenosis, 47
Vancomycin
  dosage for, and dialysis removal, 972t
  drug monitoring data for, 799t
Vantin; see Cefpodoxime
Vaquez disease; see Polycythemia vera
Varicella; see also Chickenpox
  ages affected, prodrome, morphology, distribution, diagnosis, 574t
  in differential diagnosis of herpes simplex infection, 225
Varicella vaccine
  administration of, 1018t
  during pregnancy, 1015t
  recommendations
    for adults, 892-893
    for children, 889
  schedule for children, 1005t
Varicella zoster virus in differential diagnosis of warts, 529
Varicose veins
  basic information about, 521
  diagnosis of, 521
  in differential diagnosis of deep vein thrombosis, 473
  treatment of, 521
Vascular disease
  dementia in, laboratory diagnosis of, 567t
  in differential diagnosis of diabetic retinopathy, 416
Vascular insufficiency in differential diagnosis of labyrinthitis, 263
Vascular lesions; see also Retinal detachment
  in differential diagnosis of melanoma, 291
Vascular malformations in differential diagnosis of trigeminal neuralgia, 493
Vascular occlusion
  in differential diagnosis of carpal tunnel syndrome, 93
  mesenteric, in differential diagnosis of acute pancreatitis, 344
Vasculitis
  classification of, 663t
  complement deficiencies associated with, 794t
  in differential diagnosis of thrombotic thrombocytopenic purpura, 474
  leukocytoclastic, drug-induced, 565
  systemic, in differential diagnosis of septicemia, 436
  systemic necrotizing, in differential diagnosis of Goodpasture's syndrome, 204
  urticarial, in differential diagnosis of urticaria, 512
Vasotec; see Enalapril
VDRL, laboratory findings, 837
Veins, varicose; see Varicose veins
Velosef; see Cephradine
Venereal warts; see Condyloma acuminatum
Venlafaxine, preparations, dosage, class, effects, half-life, 974t
Venous claudication in differential diagnosis of leg pain, 615t

Venous insufficiency, chronic; see Varicose veins
Venous occlusive disease in differential diagnosis of congestive heart failure, 130
Ventilation, mechanical, pneumonia associated with, 942-943
Ventricular arrhythmias
  drug therapy for, dosage, half-life, ECG manifestations, toxicity, 1000t
  IV agents for, indications, dosage, onset of action, therapeutic plasma levels, 1001t
Ventricular failure, causes of, 664
Ventricular fibrillation, evaluation of, 776-777
Ventricular infarction, right, in differential diagnosis of cardiac tamponade, 88
Ventricular septal defect
  in differential diagnosis of aortic stenosis, 47
  in differential diagnosis of mitral regurgitation, 300
Ventricular tachycardia, evaluation of, 778
Verapamil
  electrophysiologic effects of, 969t
  preparations, dosage, effects, class, cost, half-life, 982t
Verelan; see Verapamil
Verruca plana; see Warts
Verruca plantaris; see Warts
Verruca vulgaris; see Warts
Verrucous carcinoma of vulva; see Vulvar cancer
Vertebrobasilar disease in differential diagnosis of Meniere's disease, 292
Vertigo; see also Meniere's disease
  benign positional, in differential diagnosis of labyrinthitis, 263
  causes of, 664
  in differential diagnosis of dizziness, 569
  paroxysmal, in differential diagnosis of epilepsy, 572t
  physiologic; see Motion sickness
Vesicles
  differential diagnosis of, 649
  genital, differential diagnosis of, 583t
Vesicoureteral reflux in differential diagnosis of urinary tract infection, 509
Vestibular neuronopathy, acute; see Labyrinthitis
Vibrio cholerae, food poisoning due to, 188
Vibrio parahaemolyticus, food poisoning due to, 188
Vicodin, contents of, 995t
Videx; see Didanosine
Vidian neuralgis; see Headache, cluster
Villonodular synovitis, pigmented, knee pain due to, findings, diagnosis, and management, 613t
Vinblastine, toxicity of, 984t-985t
Vincristine, toxicity of, 984t-985t
Vindesine, toxicity of, 984t-985t
Violence; see also specific types of abuse
  family, screening for, 876
  youth, counseling to prevent, 884-885
Viral arthritis in differential diagnosis of juvenile rheumatoid arthritis, 51
Viral diseases
  in differential diagnosis of hepatitis B, 220
  in differential diagnosis of hepatitis C, 222
Viral exanthem in differential diagnosis of pityriasis rosea, 368
Viral hepatitis
  in differential diagnosis of fatty liver of pregnancy, 181

Viral hepatitis—cont'd
  in differential diagnosis of leptospirosis, 169
  in differential diagnosis of yellow fever, 533
Viral infection
  in differential diagnosis of acute myelogenous leukemia, 271
  in differential diagnosis of chronic lymphocytic leukemia, 272
  in differential diagnosis of Hodgkin's disease, 233
  in differential diagnosis of idiopathic thrombocytopenic purpura, 252
  in differential diagnosis of Lyme disease, 279
  in differential diagnosis of non-Hodgkin's lymphoma, 284
  in differential diagnosis of rheumatic fever, 419
  in differential diagnosis of Wegener's granulomatosis, 531
Viral keratitis; see Corneal ulceration
Viral labyrinthitis in differential diagnosis of Meniere's disease, 292
Viral neurolabyrinthitis; see Labyrinthitis
Viral pharyngitis in differential diagnosis of diphtheria, 154
Viral pneumonitis in differential diagnosis of lung neoplasm, 277
Viral respiratory infections in differential diagnosis of psittacosis, 396
Viral syndrome
  in differential diagnosis of hairy cell leukemia, 274
  in differential diagnosis of motion sickness, 305
Viramune; see Nevirapine
Viscosity, serum, laboratory findings, 837-838
Vision, screening in ambulatory elderly, 920t
Vision disorders, 869-870
Visken; see Pindolol
Vistaril; see Hydroxyzine
Visual field defects, causes of, 665
Visual impairment, screening recommendations for, 869
Visual loss, causes of, 666
Vitamin B$_{12}$, laboratory findings, 838-839
Vitamin B$_{12}$ deficiency
  in differential diagnosis of pernicious anemia, 33
  in differential diagnosis of tabes dorsalis, 462
Vitamin B$_{12}$/folate deficiency in differential diagnosis of myelodysplastic syndromes, 313
Vitamin D deficiency in differential diagnosis of hypocalcemia, 599t
Vitamin D intoxication in differential diagnosis of hyperparathyroidism, 244
Vitamin K deficiency in differential diagnosis of disseminated intravascular coagulation, 155
Vitamin K deficiency in differential diagnosis of hemophilia, 216
Vitamins, recommended daily allowances for, 1047t
Vitiligo in differential diagnosis of tinea versicolor, 481
Vivactil; see Protriptyline
Vogt-Koyangai-Harada syndrome in differential diagnosis of acute viral encephalitis, 166
Voltaren; see Diclofenac

Vomiting
  causes of, 625, 666
  drug therapy for; see Antiemetics
  psychogenic, in differential diagnosis of bulimia nervosa, 84
von Willebrand's disease
  basic information about, 522
  diagnosis of, 522, 555t
  treatment of, 522
von Willebrand's factor, disorders of, inheritance, incidence, bleeding symptoms, test results, treatment, 561t
Vulvar atrophy in differential diagnosis of vulvar cancer, 523
Vulvar cancer
  basic information about, 523
  diagnosis of, 523
  in differential diagnosis of estrogen deficient vulvovaginitis, 525
  in differential diagnosis of pruritus vulvae, 393
  treatment of, 523
Vulvar disorders in differential diagnosis of dysfunctional uterine bleeding, 159
Vulvar dystrophies in differential diagnosis of vulvar cancer, 523
Vulvitis in differential diagnosis of pruritus vulvae, 393
Vulvodynia; see Pruritus vulvae
Vulvovaginitis
  bacterial
    basic information about, 524
    diagnosis of, 524
    treatment of, 524
  estrogen deficient
    basic information about, 525
    diagnosis of, 525
    treatment of, 525
  fungal
    basic information about, 526
    diagnosis of, 526
    treatment of, 526
  gonococcal; see Gonorrhea
  prepubescent
    basic information about, 527
    diagnosis of, 527
    treatment of, 527
  trichomonas
    basic information about, 528
    diagnosis of, 528
    treatment of, 528

W

Waldenström's macroglobulinemia
  in differential diagnosis of chronic lymphocytic leukemia, 272
  lymphocyte abnormalities in, 620t
Warts; see also Condyloma acuminatum
  basic information about, 529
  diagnosis of, 529
  in differential diagnosis of hemorrhoids, 217
  dysplastic, in differential diagnosis of condyloma acuminatum, 129
  treatment of, 529-530
Watch tick test, method and interpretation, 1027t
Water deficit in hypernatremic patients, formula for, 1042
Water-rat trapper's disease; see Tularemia
Weaver's bottom; see Bursitis
Weber's test, method and interpretation, 1027t
Wegener's granulomatosis
  basic information about, 531
  diagnosis of, 531

Wegener's granulomatosis—cont'd
  differential diagnosis of, 585t-586t
  in differential diagnosis of allergic rhinitis, 420
  in differential diagnosis of asthma, 56
  in differential diagnosis of Goodpasture's syndrome, 204
  neuropathies associated with, 631t
  treatment of, 531
Weight
  ideal, calculation of, 1046t
  and mortality from COPD, 934
  recommendations for, 861
Weight gain, causes of, 666
Weight loss
  causes of, 667
  screening in ambulatory elderly, 920t
Wellbutrin; see Bupropion
Well's disease; see Leptospirosis
Wenckebach block; see Heart block, second-degree
Wernicke-Korsakoff syndrome; see Korsakoff's psychosis; Wernicke's encephalopathy
Wernicke's encephalopathy
  basic information about, 532
  diagnosis of, 532
  treatment of, 532
Westcort; see Hydrocortisone
Wet-mount microscopic procedures, 839
Wheals; see also Urticaria
  differential diagnosis of, 649
Wheezing, causes of, 667
Whipple's disease
  arthritis due to, course and distribution, 551t
  in differential diagnosis of celiac disease, 98
  in differential diagnosis of tropical sprue, 494
White blood cell count; see also Complete blood count
  assessment of, 1046t
Whooping cough; see Pertussis
Wild hare disease; see Tularemia
Wilms' tumor in differential diagnosis of neuroblastoma, 320
Wilson's disease in differential diagnosis of Huntington's chorea, 238
Women's health, year book of, 900
Wounds, bite; see Bite wounds
Wry neck; see Torticollis
Wuchereria bancrofti in tissue infections, epidemiology, transmission, manifestations, diagnosis, treatment, 629t
Wytensin; see Guanabenz

X

Xanax; see Alprazolam
Xeroderma pigmentosa in differential diagnosis of basal cell carcinoma, 67
Xerotic dermatitis, differential diagnosis of, 568t
Xylocaine; see Lidocaine
D-Xylose absorption, laboratory findings, 839

Y

Year books; see also specific areas of practice
  of cardiology, 899, 901-905
  of family practice, 899, 905-915
  of geriatrics and gerontology, 899, 915-924
  of medicine, 899-900, 924-947
  of neurology and neurosurgery, 900, 947-948

Year books—cont'd
　of obstetrics, gynecology, and women's health, 900, 948-958
　of pulmonary disease, 900, 958-964
Yellow fever
　basic information about, 533
　diagnosis of, 533
　treatment of, 533
Yellow fever live virus, schedule, indications, side effects, contraindications, during pregnancy, with HIV infection, in immunocompromised patient, 1010t-1011t
Yellow fever vaccine
　for international travel, 1019t
　during pregnancy, 1012t

Yersinia enterocolitica, food poisoning due to, 188
Youth violence, counseling to prevent, 884-885
Yuppie flu; *see* Chronic fatigue syndrome

Z

Zagam; *see* Sparfloxacin
Zalcitabine, therapeutic class, preparations, dosage, toxicities, cost, 970t
Zantac; *see* Ranitidine
Zarontin; *see* Ethosuximide
Zebeta; *see* Bisoprolol
Zefazone; *see* Cefmetazole
Zerit; *see* Stavudine
Zestril; *see* Lisinopril

Zidovudine
　after HIV occupational exposure, 1021t
　therapeutic class, preparations, dosage, toxicities, cost, 970t
Zinacef; *see* Cefuroxime
Zithromax; *see* Azithromycin
Zocor; *see* Simvastatin
Zofran; *see* Ondansetron
Zollinger-Ellison syndrome in differential diagnosis of celiac disease, 98
Zoloft; *see* Sertraline
Zung Depression Scale, *1033*
Zyrtec; *see* Cetirizine